FAMILY HOME CARE BOXES

GUIDELINES BOXES

NURSING CARE PLANS

CONGRATULATIONS

You now have access to Mosby's "Get Smart" Bonus Package!

Here's what's included to help you "Get Smart"

sign on at:

www.mosby.com/MERLIN/Wong/essentials/

A Website just for you as you learn pediatric nursing with the 5th edition of Whaley & Wong's *Essentials of Pediatric Nursing*

what you will receive:

Whether you're a student, an instructor, or a clinician, you'll find information just for you. Things like:
- Content Updates ➡ Links to Related Products
- Author Information . . . and more

plus:

 **WebLinks**

An exciting new program that allows you to directly access hundreds of active websites keyed specifically to the content of this book. The WebLinks are continually updated, with new ones added as they develop **Simply peel off the sticker on this page and register with the listed passcode.**

If tab is removed, you cannot return this book to Mosby, Inc.

Free CD-ROM Companion

with every copy of Whaley & Wong's *Essentials of Pediatric Nursing*, 5th Edition

If passcode sticker is removed, this textbook cannot be returned to Mosby, Inc.

With a Strong Emphasis on Clinical and Functional Relevance, this Valuable CD-ROM Features:

Critical Thinking Exercises
Case Studies
Nursing Care Plans to Build and Individualize
Anatomy Reviews
Procedures and Guidelines to Print and Carry

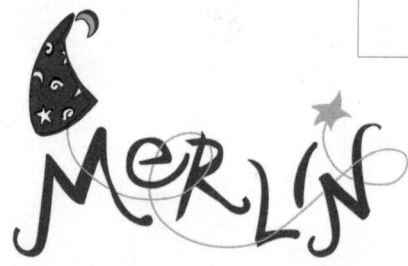

MERLIN

Mosby's **E**lectronic **R**esource **L**inks & **I**nformation **N**etwork

Mosby

WHALEY & WONG'S
ESSENTIALS OF
Pediatric Nursing

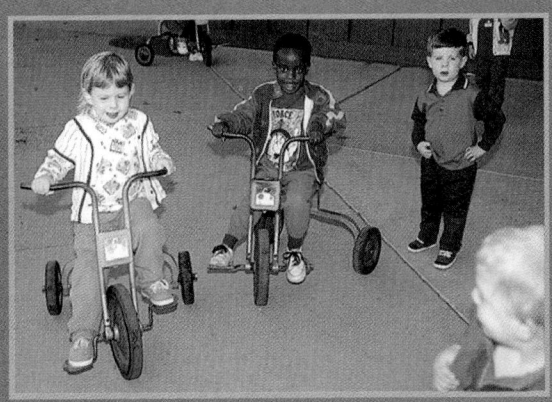

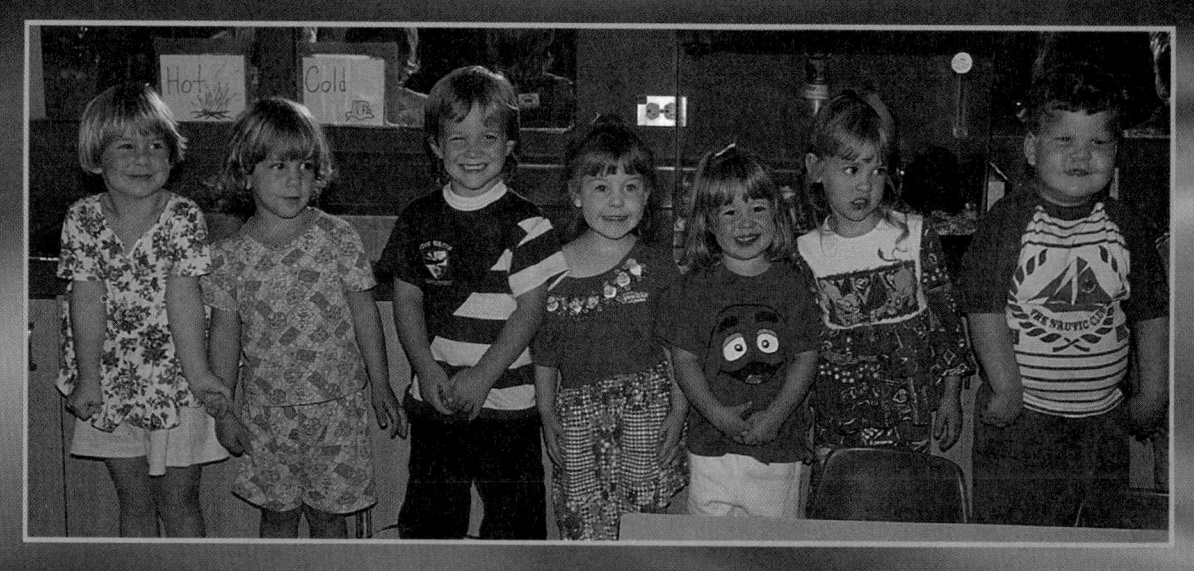

WHALEY & WONG'S
ESSENTIALS OF
Pediatric Nursing

DONNA L. WONG, PhD, RN, PNP, CPN, FAAN

Nursing Consultant
The Children's Hospital at Saint Francis;
Adjunct Associate Professor
Department of Pediatrics
University of Oklahoma College of Medicine—Tulsa;
Clinical Associate Professor
University of Oklahoma College of Nursing;
Adjunct Associate Professor and Consultant
Oral Roberts University Anna Vaughn School of Nursing
Tulsa, Oklahoma

FIFTH EDITION
illustrated in full color

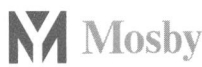 Mosby

St. Louis Baltimore Boston Carlsbad Chicago Naples New York Philadelphia Portland
London Madrid Mexico City Singapore Sydney Tokyo Toronto Wiesbaden

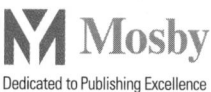
Dedicated to Publishing Excellence

A NOTE TO THE READER:

The author and publisher have made every attempt to check dosages and nursing content for accuracy. Because the science of pharmacology is continually advancing, our knowledge base continues to expand. Therefore we recommend that the reader always check product information for changes in dosage or administration before administering any medication. This is particularly important with new or rarely used drugs.

FIFTH EDITION

Printed in the United States of America

Mosby-Year Book, Inc.
11830 Westline Industrial Drive
St. Louis, Missouri 63146

ISBN 0-323-01058-X

99 00 01 02 / 9 8 7 6 5 4 3 2

To

*my husband, **Ting**,*
for the unconditional love, intellectual enlightenment,
and support that make it all possible

*my daughter, **Nina**,*
for being the kind of daughter parents dream about

*my mother, **Madeline**,*
for making the first typed manuscript a reality
and encouraging me to be a steel magnolia

*my beloved father, **Rudy**,*
for being a parent, partner, and friend—I miss you

*my beloved grandmother, **Ida**,*
who at 95 years of age made finger puppets
so we can give atraumatic care

D.L.W.

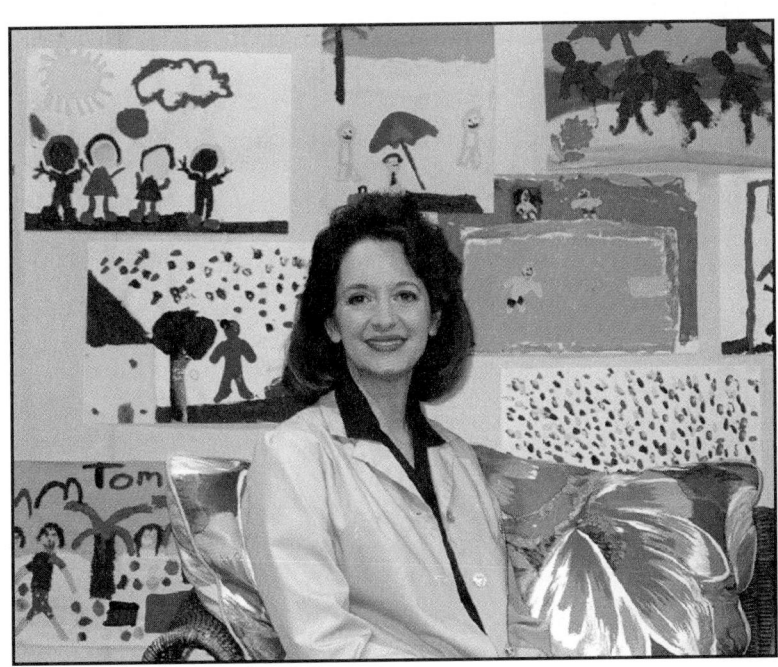

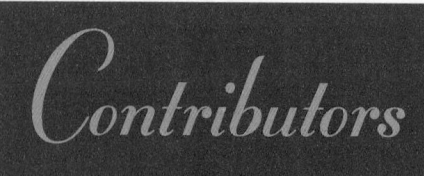
Contributors

Elizabeth Ahmann, ScD, RN
Senior Lecturer
Columbia University
School of Nursing
New York, New York;
Consultant, Child and Family Health
Washington, D.C.;
Section Editor, *Pediatric Nursing*
Pitman, New Jersey

Natalie Cloutman Arnold, MSN, RN, PNP
Instructor, Nursing Division
Tulsa Community College
Tulsa, Oklahoma

Annette C. Bollig, MSN, RN
Director, Critical Care Nursing
Children's Hospital of Wisconsin
Milwaukee, Wisconsin

Lynn B. Clutter, MSN, RN,C, CNS
Family-Child Health Consultant
Independent Practice;
Adjunct Faculty
Oral Roberts University
Anna Vaughn School of Nursing
Tulsa, Oklahoma

Lydia DeSantis, PhD, RN
Associate Professor
University of Miami
School of Nursing
Miami, Florida

Pamela A. DiVito-Thomas, MS, RN
Instructor
Oral Roberts University
Anna Vaughn School of Nursing
Tulsa, Oklahoma

Laurie E. Doerner, MSN, RN
Instructor
Oral Roberts University
Anna Vaughn School of Nursing;
Consultant, Private Practice
Pediatrics, Home Care, Infusion Therapy, and Quality
  Improvement
Tulsa, Oklahoma

Jeanne O'Connor Egan, MSN, RN
Pediatric Clinical Specialist
Children's National Medical Center
Washington, D.C.

Teresa L. Hall, MS, RN
Nursing Supervisor
Hathaway Children's Services
Sylmar, California

Renee Covey Harrison, MS, RN
Assistant Professor, Nursing Division
Tulsa Community College
Tulsa, Oklahoma

Caryn Stoermer Hess, MS, RN
Nursing Consultant
Englewood, Colorado

Marilyn Hockenberry-Eaton, PhD, RN, PNP, FAAN
Director, Pediatric Nurse Practitioner Services
Texas Children's Hospital
Houston, Texas

Ellen F. Johnsen, BA, RNC
Instructor, Tulsa Training Center
Oklahoma State University
Tulsa, Oklahoma

Christina Algiere Kasprisin, MS, RN
College of Nursing
University of Vermont
Burlington, Vermont

Nancy E. Kline, MS, RN, CPNP
Oncology Nurse Practitioner
Texas Children's Hospital;
Instructor of Pediatrics
Baylor College of Medicine
Houston, Texas

Laura L. Kuensting, MSN(R), RN
Pediatric Clinical Nurse Specialist
Emergency Services
Christian Hospitals;
Staff Nurse
Emergency Services
Cardinal Glennon Children's Hospital
St. Louis, Missouri

Shona Swenson Lenss, BSN, RN
Attention Deficit/Hyperactivity Disorder Nurse
  Coordinator
Cheyenne Children's Clinic
Cheyenne, Wyoming

Lynn E. Mattis, MSN, RN
Clinical Nurse Specialist
Division of Pediatric Gastroenterology/Nutrition
Department of Pediatrics
The Johns Hopkins Hospital
Baltimore, Maryland

Patricia O'Brien, MSN, RNC, PNP
Cardiovascular Clinical Nurse Specialist
Cardiovascular Program
Children's Hospital
Boston, Massachusetts

Kathryn A. Perry, MSN, APRN, RN,C, CNS
Clinical Nurse Specialist for Child
  Neurology
Children's Medical Center
Tulsa, Oklahoma

Judy Holt Rollins, MS, RN
Consultant, Rollins & Associates, Inc.;
Coordinator, Studio G
Georgetown University Medical Center;
Adjunct Instructor
Georgetown University School of Medicine
Washington, D.C.;
Associate Editor, *Pediatric Nursing*
Pitman, New Jersey

Cynthia Hylton Rushton, PhD, RN,C, FAAN
Clinical Nurse Specialist in Ethics
The Johns Hopkins Children's Center
Baltimore, Maryland

Mercedes Sandaval, PhD
Chairperson, Arts and Sciences Department
Inter-American Center
Miami-Dade Community College
Miami, Florida

Donna P. Smith, MS, RN
Genetic Counselor
H.A. Chapman Institute of Medical Genetics
Tulsa, Oklahoma

Judith A. Vessey, PhD, RN,C, DPNP
Professor, Program Director
Advanced Practice Nursing Program
The Johns Hopkins University
School of Nursing
Baltimore, Maryland

Krena Hunter White, MS, MA, RN
Assistant Professor, Nursing Division
Tulsa Community College
Tulsa, Oklahoma

David Wilson, MS, RN,C
Instructor
Oral Roberts University
Anna Vaughn School of Nursing
Tulsa, Oklahoma

Marilyn L. Winkelstein, PhD, RN
Associate Professor
University of Maryland
School of Nursing
Baltimore, Maryland

Susan B. Zekauskas, MSN, RN, PNP
Pediatric Nurse Consultant;
Assistant Professor, Nursing Division
Tulsa Community College
Tulsa, Oklahoma

Preface

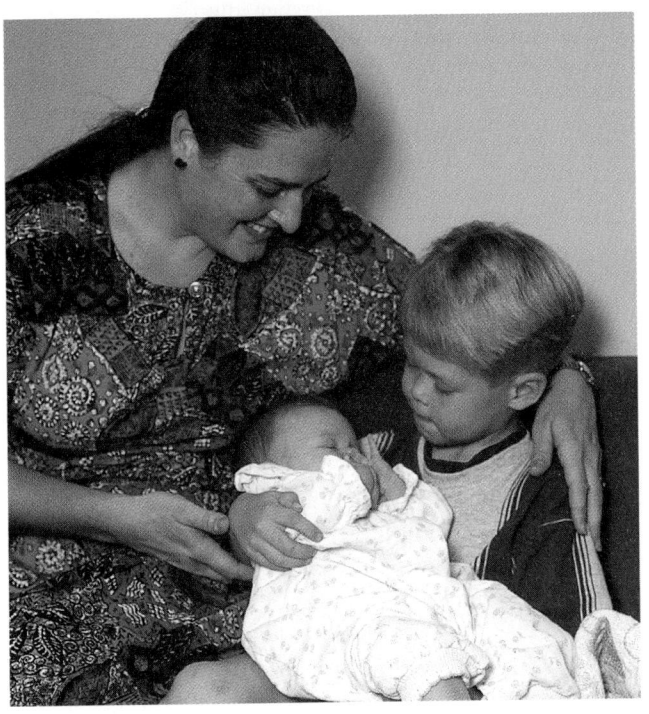

In offering this fifth edition of *Essentials of Pediatric Nursing*, we are grateful for the support given to the book over the years. While carefully preserving aspects of the book that have met with such universal acceptance—its state-of-the-art, research-based information; its strong, integrated focus on the family; its logical and user-friendly organization; and its easy reading style—we have continued the approach toward revision that began in the fourth edition. We have enlisted the assistance of 27 expert nurse specialists to revise, rewrite, or write portions of the text on areas undergoing rapid and complex change, such as case management, genetics, community and home care, high-risk newborn care, and adolescent issues. At the same time, we have not compromised the strengths of a text that has been used with great satisfaction by thousands of students and nurses. We carefully supervised each of the revisions and in many cases reorganized and revised the material ourselves to maintain the consistent organization and writing style that, over the years, have proved so effective in the teaching of pediatric nursing. We remain acutely aware that, in the end, the purpose of the book is to teach.

To that end, we have tried to meet the increasing demands of faculty and students to teach and to learn in an environment characterized by rapid change, enormous amounts of information, fewer clinical facilities, more need for community

SPECIAL FEATURES

Much effort has been directed toward making this book easy to teach from and, more important, easy to learn from. In this edition the following new features have been added to benefit educators, students, and practitioners.

- A functional and attractive FULL-COLOR DESIGN visually enhances the organization of each chapter, as well as the special features.
- Many of the COLOR PHOTOGRAPHS are new, and anatomic drawings are easy to follow, with color appropriately used to illustrate important aspects, such as saturated and desaturated blood. As an example, the full-color heart illustrations in Chapter 25 clearly depict congenital cardiac defects and associated hemodynamic changes.
- FAMILY HOME CARE boxes help nurses and students teach parents about the special needs of their infants and children.
- THINKING CRITICALLY ABOUT . . . boxes replace the Challenging Tradition boxes in the fourth edition. They continue to present key research information that refutes or questions traditional pediatric nursing practices, and the reader is challenged to think critically and improve practice by questioning traditional nursing procedures that are without scientific basis. Such information is valuable to the beginning student, who learns and begins to question before traditional practices become ingrained, and to the practicing nurse, who can refine care based on presented information.
- CRITICAL THINKING EXERCISES describe brief scenarios of child-family-nurse interactions that depict real-life clinical situations. From the synthesis of the topical content and a critical analysis of possible options, the reader chooses the best intervention and learns to make clinical judgments. Immediately following the scenario is the rationale for the correct answer and explanations for the incorrect options.
- CULTURAL AWARENESS boxes integrate concepts of culturally sensitive care throughout the text. The emphasis is on the clinical application of the information, whether it focuses on toilet training or on male or female circumcision.
- ATRAUMATIC CARE boxes emphasize the importance of providing competent care without creating undue physical and psychologic distress. Although many of the boxes provide suggestions for managing pain, atraumatic care also considers approaches to promoting self-esteem and preventing embarrassment.

- NURSING CARE PLANS include RATIONALES for nursing interventions that are not immediately evident to the student. This has strengthened the connection between the text and the interventions in the care plans. All care plans have been revised by one contributor, Caryn Hess, to maintain consistency throughout the book and include patient and family goals and the most recent NANDA nursing diagnoses.

Numerous pedagogic devices that enhance student learning have been retained from the previous edition:

- CHAPTER OUTLINES with page numbers begin each chapter, which allows readers to quickly locate topics of interest.
- RELATED TOPICS allow readers to turn to any chapter where a given topic is discussed. At the beginning of the chapter, readers will see the topic listed in the RELATED TOPICS section, indicating the chapter or chapters where the appropriate discussion(s) can be found. On turning to the cross-referenced chapter(s), readers will find the topic listed in the chapter outline with a page number.
- LEARNING OBJECTIVES in each chapter provide the reader with a basic guideline for the major points presented in and learned from the chapter.
- NURSING ALERTS call the reader's attention to considerations that if ignored could lead to a deteriorating or emergency situation. Key assessment data, risk factors, and danger signs are among the kinds of information included.
- NURSING TIPS present handy information of a nonemergency nature that makes patients more comfortable and the nurse's job a little easier.
- GUIDELINES boxes summarize important nursing interventions for a variety of situations and conditions.
- EMERGENCY TREATMENT boxes are flagged by colored thumb tabs and are listed on the inside front cover, enabling the reader to quickly locate interventions for crisis situations.
- FAMILY FOCUS boxes present issues of special significance to families who have a child with a particular disorder. This feature is another method of highlighting the needs or concerns of families that should be addressed when family-centered care is provided.
- FYI (For Your Information) segments present information of interest that may help one understand a concept or increase an interest in reading about a condition. Unlike the Nursing Alerts, which present essential information, the FYIs present information that is optional for the reader and again help prioritize what information is most essential for the reader to assimilate.
- KEY TERMS are highlighted throughout each chapter to reinforce student learning.
- Hundreds of TABLES and BOXES highlight key concepts and nursing interventions.
- KEY POINTS, located at the end of each chapter, help the reader summarize major points, make connections, and synthesize information.
- A highly detailed, cross-referenced INDEX allows readers to quickly access discussions.

- PRINTED ENDPAPERS on the inside front and back covers provide information nurses refer to often, such as vital signs and blood pressure, as well as listings of some of the text's features and their page numbers.

experiences, and less time. To help students to quickly locate essential information, we retained most of the features used in the last edition, and many new ones have been added. Most importantly, this text encourages students to *think critically.*

The new features, Thinking Critically About . . . boxes and Critical Thinking Exercises, focus on research issues and judgment decisions. The process of critical thinking is explained in Chapter 2.

ORGANIZATION AND REVISIONS

In general, this fifth edition incorporates the basic organization and presentation of content from previous editions. The early chapters of the book emphasize normal growth and maturation and some common health and developmental problems encountered at various age levels. Following these early chapters is a new chapter (20) on home care. Later chapters focus on serious health problems of infants and children that frequently require hospitalization and/or home care. The role of the nurse and the role of the family in all aspects of the child's health care and in all health care settings are emphasized throughout. The units and their respective chapters reflect the organization of wellness to illness.

UNIT ONE provides a longitudinal view of the child as an individual on a continuum of developmental changes from birth through adolescence and as a member of a family unit maturing within a culture and a community. Chapter 1 includes a discussion of morbidity and mortality in infancy and childhood, including Canadian child mortality, and child health care from a historical perspective. Because of the importance of injuries as the leading cause of death in children, an overview of this topic is included. This book is about families with children, and to set this tone early, the philosophy of family-centered care is emphasized. This book is also about providing atraumatic care—care that minimizes the psychologic and physical stress that health promotion and illness treatment can inflict. Features such as Family Focus and Atraumatic Care boxes bring these philosophies to life throughout the text. Finally, we address the philosophy of delivering nursing care. We believe strongly that children and families need consistent caregivers. To extend this concept of primary care nursing beyond traditional settings, especially into the home, the model of case management is introduced.

In Chapter 2 the presentation of the nursing process prepares the reader for its continued application to nursing care of children throughout the remainder of the book. A unique feature of this chapter is its focus on the application of critical thinking to the nursing process. In addition, the revised definition of nursing is included.

Chapter 3 expands the discussion of social, cultural, and religious influences on child development and health promo-

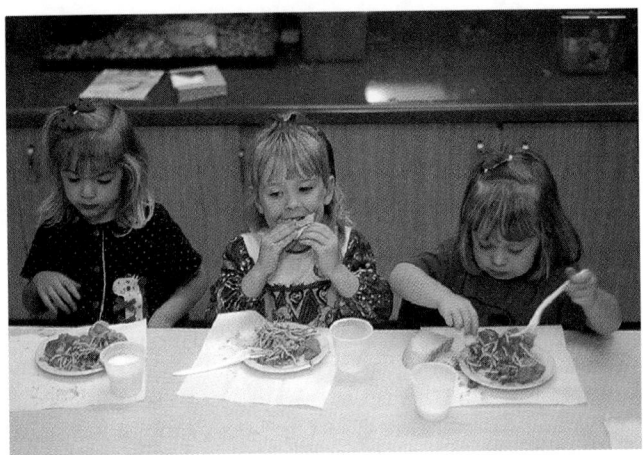

tion, including socioeconomic factors, customs and folkways, and health beliefs and practices. Additional information on culturally sensitive communication is presented, as well as several Cultural Awareness boxes and Critical Thinking Exercises, to make the material relevant for the reader. Chapter 4, devoted to the family, further emphasizes the importance of this social group on the health and welfare of children. Family theories establish the tone of the chapter, which has been expanded to include more on family stress theory and the Typology Model of Adjustment and Adaptation.

The basic overview of child development in Chapter 5 maintains the same general organization and expands on the theoretic approach to personality development and learning. Biologic systems development is deemphasized in this chapter and discussed more fully in relation to major systems dysfunction later in the book. Important revisions include discussions of stress, coping, environmental hazards, and the influence of mass media on children.

UNIT TWO is concerned with the principles and skills of nursing assessment, including communication and interviewing, observation, physical and behavioral assessment, and health guidance. Chapter 6 contains guidelines for communicating with both children and their families and a detailed description of a health assessment, including an extensive discussion of family assessment and nutritional assessment. Chapter 7 continues to provide a comprehensive approach to physical examination and developmental assessment, with new material added on measurement of temperature and the Denver II, which now replaces the Denver Developmental Screening Test.

UNIT THREE stresses the importance of the neonatal period, a time of greatest risk to survival, and includes the addition of several health concerns encountered in the vulnerable first month of life. Chapter 8 contains several updated areas, reflecting current issues and developments, such as early postpartum discharge and car restraint safety such as air bags. The strong emphasis on the family remains, with additional attention given to the latest research on bonding.

Chapter 9 stresses the nurse's role in care of the high-risk newborn and the importance of acute observations to the survival of this vulnerable group of infants. Rapid advances in the field of neonatal care have mandated extensive revision with a greater sensitivity to the diverse needs of infants, from those with extremely low birth weight to those of normal ges-

tational age. A discussion of infant stress, including pain and developmental care, is provided. Updates in this chapter more clearly describe dermatologic problems, new thinking regarding hyperbilirubinemia and inborn errors of metabolism, and advances in the understanding of genetic diseases. A table on prenatal testing procedures has been added.

UNITS FOUR through **SIX** present the major developmental stages outlined in Unit One, which are expanded to provide a broader concept of these stages and the health problems most often associated with them. Special emphasis is placed on the preventive aspects of care. The chapters on health promotion follow a standard approach that is used consistently for each age-group. New areas and those receiving expanded coverage are injury prevention, nutrition, cognitive development, alternate child care arrangements, and dental health. As the book goes to press, major changes in the immunization schedule are current through September 1996.

The chapters on health problems in these units reflect primarily more typical and age-related concerns. We rewrote the information on many disorders to reflect recent changes. Examples include sudden infant death syndrome, lead poisoning, wound healing, Lyme disease, attention deficit-hyperactivity disorder, contraception, teenage pregnancy, drug abuse, and suicide.

UNIT SEVEN deals with children who have the same developmental needs as growing children but who, because of congenital or acquired physical, cognitive, or sensory impairment, require alternative interventions to facilitate development. Chapter 18 reflects current trends in the care of families and children with chronic illness or disability, such as home care, normalizing children's lives, focusing on developmental needs, enabling and empowering families, and providing early intervention. It also focuses on the impact of life-threatening illness and death on the child and family. The sections on hospice and home care, the child's right to die, and the impact of the death on siblings have been expanded.

The content in Chapter 19 on cognitive and sensory impairments includes a revised discussion on fragile X syndrome. Chapter 20 is now devoted to home care. It presents an overview of home care with specific interventions for the nurse to function successfully in this increasingly important environment. The focus is on building family-nurse partnerships.

UNIT EIGHT is concerned with the impact of hospitalization on the child and the family and continues to present a comprehensive overview of the stressors imposed by hospitalization and nursing interventions to prevent or eliminate them. Chapter 21 has expanded discussions of pain assessment and management that include adjuvant medications or coanalgesics, EMLA, conscious sedation, assessment of pain by parents, and patient-controlled analgesia. The section on discharge planning and home care provides the basic concepts for implementing home care for children with complex health needs and complements Chapter 20. Chapter 22 continues to present information on the safe implementation of procedures with children. We have tried to include as much available research as possible to base the nursing interventions on scientific findings, not traditional practice. Major additions to this important chapter are sections on maintaining healthy skin; venous access devices, including peripherally inserted central catheters (PICC lines); pulse oximetry; and the Cen-

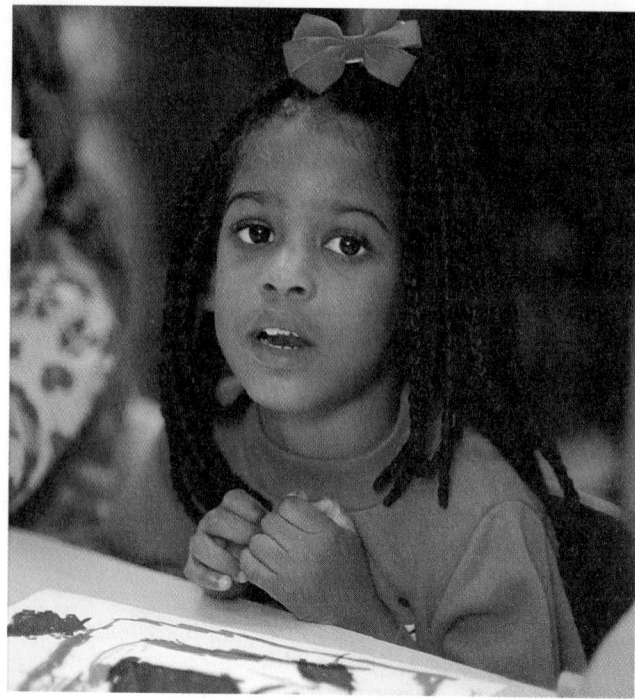

ters for Disease Control and Prevention's 1996 guidelines for infection control.

UNITS NINE through TWELVE consider serious health problems of infants and children primarily from the biologic systems orientation, which has the practical organizational value of permitting health problems and nursing considerations to relate to specific pathophysiologic disturbances. Important additions and revisions include discussions of respiratory syncytial virus (RSV); tuberculosis; asthma; cystic fibrosis; oral rehydration therapy; short bowel syndrome; seizures; acquired immunodeficiency syndrome (AIDS); diabetes mellitus; growth disorders; burns; scoliosis; latex allergy; and use of folic acid to prevent neural tube defects.

Extensive appendixes are also included and contain information on family assessment, patterns of inheritance, developmental assessment, growth measurements, common laboratory values, recommended daily dietary allowances (RDAs), NANDA-approved diagnoses, and, a new addition, several foreign-language translations of the FACES Pain Rating Scale. All of the appendix material reflects the most current versions of forms, charts, and values.

UNIFYING PRINCIPLES

Several unifying principles have guided the organizational structure of this book since its inception. These principles have been strengthened in the revision to produce a text that is consistent in approach throughout each chapter.

The Family as the Unit of Care
The child is an integral member of the family unit. Nursing care is most effective when it is rendered with the belief that the family is the unit of care. This belief permeates the book. When a child is healthy, the child's health is enhanced when the family is a fully functioning, health-promoting system. The family unit can be manifested in a myriad of structures; each has the potential to provide a caring, supportive environment in which the child can grow, mature, and maximize his or her human potential.

In addition to family-centered care being integrated into every chapter, an entire chapter is devoted to understanding the family as the basic unit in children's lives. Another chapter discusses the social, cultural, and religious influences that have an impact on family beliefs. Separate sections in another chapter deal in depth with family communication and family assessment. The impact of illness, hospitalization, home care, and the death of a child are covered extensively in three additional chapters. The needs of the family are emphasized throughout the text under Nursing Considerations in a separate section on family support. Numerous Family Home Care boxes are included to assist nurses in providing helpful information to families. Family Focus boxes present unique aspects of a condition as viewed by the family or the nurse.

An Integrated Approach to Development
Children are whole people. No book on pediatric nursing is complete without extensive coverage of communication, nutrition, play, safety, dental care, sexuality, sleep, self-esteem, and, of course, parenting. Nurses promote the healthy expression of all these dimensions of personhood and need to understand how these functions are expressed by different children at different developmental ages and stages. Effective parenting depends on the parent's knowledge of development, and it is often the nurse's responsibility to provide parents with a developmental awareness of their children's needs. For these reasons, coverage of the many dimensions of childhood are integrated within the growth and development chapters, rather than being presented in separate chapters. Safety concerns, for instance, are much different for a toddler than for an adolescent. Sleep needs change with age, as do nutritional needs. As a result, the units on each age of childhood contain complete information on all these functions as they relate to the specific age. Using the integrated approach, students gain an appreciation for the unique characteristics and needs of children at every age and stage.

Focus on Wellness and Illness
In a pediatric nursing text, a focus on illness is expected. Children become ill, and nurses typically are involved in helping children get well. However, it is not sufficient to prepare students to care primarily for sick children. First, health is more than the absence of disease. Being healthy is being whole in mind, body, and spirit. Therefore the majority of the first half of the book is devoted to discussions that promote physical, psychosocial, mental, and spiritual wellness. Much emphasis is placed on anticipatory guidance of parents to prevent injury or illness in the child.

Second, health care is more than ever focused on prevention. The objectives set forth in the "Healthy People 2000" report clearly establish a health care agenda in which solutions to medical/social problems lie in preventive strategies, not in more or better treatment.

Third, health care is moving from acute care settings to the community, the home, ambulatory centers, and clinics. Nurses must be prepared to function in all areas. To be suc-

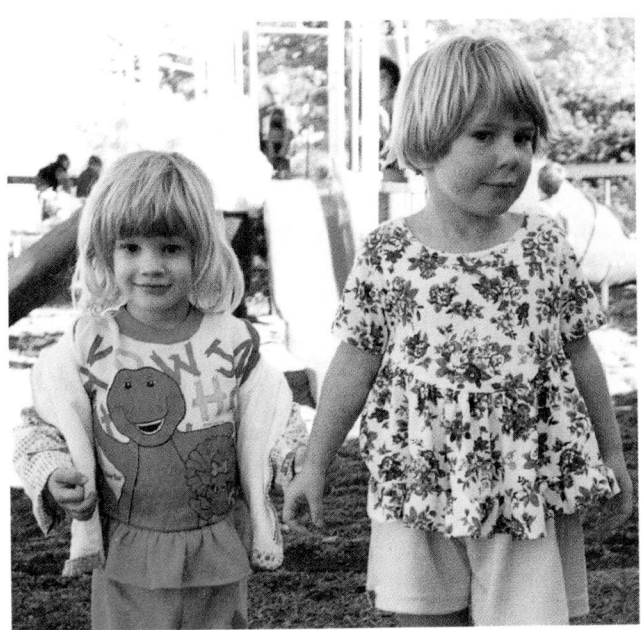

cessful, they must understand the pathophysiology, diagnosis, and treatment of health conditions. Competent nursing care flows from this knowledge and is enhanced by an awareness of childhood development, family dynamics, and communication skills.

Nursing Care

Although the information in this text incorporates information from numerous disciplines (medicine, pathophysiology, pharmacology, nutrition, psychology, sociology), its primary purpose is to provide information on the nursing care of children and families. Discussions of all disorders conclude with a section on Nursing Considerations. In addition, 23 care plans have been included in this fifth edition. Taken together, these features provide coverage of the nursing care for most diseases, disorders, conditions, and crises of childhood. In a sense, by emphasizing specific health problems through the vehicle of care plans, students gain an intuitive sense of the major health problems of childhood.

The purpose of the care plans, like every other feature of the book, is to teach, to convey information. They include all the current nursing diagnoses approved by NANDA through its Twelfth Conference that have a potential bearing on the health problem. For every diagnosis, appropriate patient goals, extensive possible interventions with rationales, and sample evaluation outcomes are presented. Thus a complete range of nursing care is presented within the context of a care plan and the nursing process.

For almost every health problem for which a Nursing Care Plan is included, the surrounding narrative text is presented according to the nursing process. In these instances specific headings for assessment, nursing diagnoses, planning, implementation, and evaluation, with identifying logos for each step, present appropriate information that is then amplified in the Nursing Care Plan, presented in a standard nursing practice context. Because adequate discussion of each step of the nursing process requires considerable space and repeti-

tion, less common conditions or disorders involving more medical than nursing care are not organized according to the nursing process but are presented in the same structure as used in previous editions. This decision also helps maintain a manageable book size despite the addition of numerous new features and expanded discussions of material that were necessary for this revision. The care plans provide excellent prototypes for standards of nursing practice.

The Critical Role of Research

This revision is the product of an exhaustive review of the literature published since the book was last revised. So that information is accurate and current, the majority of citations are less than 5 years old, and many chapters have entries within 1 year of publication. Examples of current "cutting edge" information are recommendations from the American Academy of Pediatrics on immunizations, folic acid supplementation, perinatal human immunodeficiency virus (HIV) testing, asthma, tuberculosis, and sleep position. The section on pain reflects guidelines from the Agency for Health Care Policy and Research (AHCPR) and the American Pain Society. The new discussions on skin care reflect the AHCPR's guidelines on pressure ulcers. Infection control has been completely rewritten to reflect the latest Centers for Disease Control and Prevention guidelines. Cardiopulmonary resuscitation and first aid for choking are based on the 1994 recommendations of the American Heart Association.

The efforts toward updating content have also been extended toward updating the address of every resource listed in the text. Despite this meticulous checking, it is inevitable that some information will change during this edition's publication. Therefore, telephone numbers for each organization are included to facilitate the reader's access to an organization.

CANADIAN CONTENT

The fifth edition of this text includes Canadian statistics regarding infant and child health in Chapter 1 and the latest Canadian immunization schedules in Chapter 10. Throughout the text numerous Canadian resource organizations are also provided. These efforts have been made in an attempt to make the text as valuable as possible to Canadian readers.

TEACHING/LEARNING PACKAGE

For the fifth edition of this text, an extensive number of ancillary products for instructors and students to use in class and clinical settings is offered:

Mosby/Wong Web Site. In keeping in step with the "superhighway" of information, we have developed through Mosby's web site a special service that provides updates, bibliographies, abstracts, announcements, additional resources, and links to other sources of relevant Internet information. Through the Internet you simply use the location address of Mosby's home page (www.mosby.com) to access up-to-date, state-of-the-art information pertaining to pediatric nursing. With the touch of a few keys, this text is continually updated and enhanced through the world of cyberspace.

Instructor's Resource Kit. This innovative resource kit for the instructor holds the following components:

- *Instructor's Manual,* with learning objectives, chapter outlines and accompanying teaching strategies, and learning activities.
- *Test Bank,* with more than 1000 multiple-choice stand-alone test items. An answer key with page-number references to the textbook is included.
- *Pediatric Updates,* which describe the very latest research findings, guidelines, or approaches to caring for children and their families. Instructors will receive a new set of *Pediatric Updates* twice a year. Each update is keyed to the chapter in the text where the topic is found.
- *Critical Thinking Exercises,* which are in addition to the Critical Thinking Exercises found in the text. Situations and four choices for interventions are described, with the correct answer and rationale provided on the back side of the page.
- *Case Studies,* with the case and related questions on the front side of the page and answers on the back.
- *Pediatric Video* content summaries for the *Whaley & Wong's Pediatric Nursing Video Series* and content summary of the **Pediatric Assessment Interactive Video Disc.**

Overhead Transparencies. Full-color transparency acetates focus on key material in the text, helping instructors to increase student understanding.

Computerized Test Bank. Available in IBM and Macintosh, ESA Test is the computerized version of the *Test Bank* from the *Instructor's Resource Kit.* Complete with a user's guide, ESA Test allows instructors to edit, add, delete, or select questions on the computer.

Available for purchase:

Study Guide. This comprehensive and challenging study aid presents multiple-choice and matching questions to review content along with Critical Thinking Case Studies. The *Study Guide* also includes questions related to *Whaley and Wong's Pediatric Nursing Video Series* to help students test their knowledge after viewing. Answers are located at the back for the students' reference. All pages are perforated and can be removed as needed.

Whaley and Wong's Pediatric Nursing Video Series. This set of six individual videotapes, each approximately 20 minutes in length, provides students with an opportunity to see nurses, children, and families in actual clinical settings. The series is narrated by Donna Wong, and topics include Communication with Children and Families, Growth and Development, Family-Centered Care, Medications and Injections, Pain Assessment and Management, and Pediatric Assessment.

Pediatric Assessment Interactive Videodiscs. These videodiscs were developed and produced by The Fuld Institute for Technology in Nursing Education. Three case studies help students master the transition from the classroom to the actual practice setting.

Pediatric Quick Reference. This handy pocket-size reference provides quick access to information needed in the clinical setting.

Wong & Whaley's Clinical Manual of Pediatric Nursing, ed. 4. This Manual contains a wealth of information for use as a reference for students and in the clinical setting, including over 80 Nursing Care Plans, home care instructions that can be copied and given to families, detailed descriptions of nursing skills and procedures, a copy of the Wong-Baker FACES Pain Rating Scale, and much, much more!

● ● ●

Just as children and their families bring with them a vast and unique background that affects their role within the health care system, so it is that each nurse brings to each child and family an individual set of characteristics and values that will affect their relationship. Although I have attempted to present a total picture of the child in each age-group both in wellness and in illness, no one child, family, or nurse will be found in this book. I hope that each page, chapter, and unit builds a foundation on which the nurse can begin to construct the ideal of comprehensive, atraumatic, and individualized nursing care for infants, children, adolescents, and their families.

Donna L. Wong

Acknowledgments

With each edition of *Essentials of Pediatric Nursing*, more and more of my colleagues have become involved in the revision of the book. I am grateful to the many nursing faculty members, practitioners, and students who have offered their comments, recommendations, and suggestions. Many of the staff nurses and clinical specialists I meet are the "silent heroes" who teach me so much about the preventive, bedside, and home care that children and families need to recover. I am especially indebted to the contributors who revised selected chapters of this edition and to the reviewers for their constructive criticism and suggestions.

I especially thank Peggy Cook, librarian at Hillcrest Medical Center, Tulsa, Oklahoma, for the scores of computer searches and hundreds of articles she provided, as well as the many citations she checked for accuracy, which made it possible to update the content through 1996. I also thank Gail Russell, librarian, and Dwight Vance, drug information pharmacist at Saint Francis Hospital, for their efforts in searching the literature.

Not only have numerous individuals helped make the book current and accurate, several people have contributed to making the book attractive with the addition of color photographs. Thanks go to Pat Watson, Linda Goodwin, Tim Yancy, and Ting Wong for the beautiful color photography; to Lynn Clutter, Debi Lammert, and Linda Goodwin for coordinating the photography sessions at the Children's Hospital at Saint Francis, Ave Maria House, and several other facilities in Tulsa, Oklahoma; and to the health professionals, children, and parents who generously allowed us to take photographs.

No book is ever a reality without the dedication and perseverance of the editorial staff, and although it is impossible to list every individual at Mosby who has made exceptional efforts to produce this text, I am especially grateful to Sally Schrefer, Shelly Hayden, Jenny Doll, Mark Spann, Judi Lang, and Linda Ierardi for their support and commitment to excellence. A very special nurse colleague, Pamela DiVito-Thomas, has joined me during the revision of this book. Among her many talents as my associate, she brought her knowledge of nursing and critical thinking to this edition. In addition, I thank my typists, Lynne Murtha and Nina Wong, for the superb job they did and for their efforts in meeting deadlines.

Finally, I thank my family—Ting and Nina—for the unselfish love, endless patience, and quiet understanding that allow me to devote such a large part of my life to my career. Truly, without their willingness to assume many of the tasks necessary to produce a textbook and their sacrifices that allowed me the time needed to revise it, this book would never have been completed.

Donna L. Wong

Brief Contents

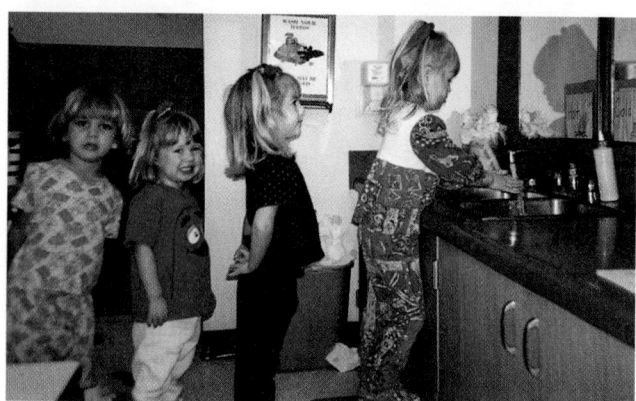

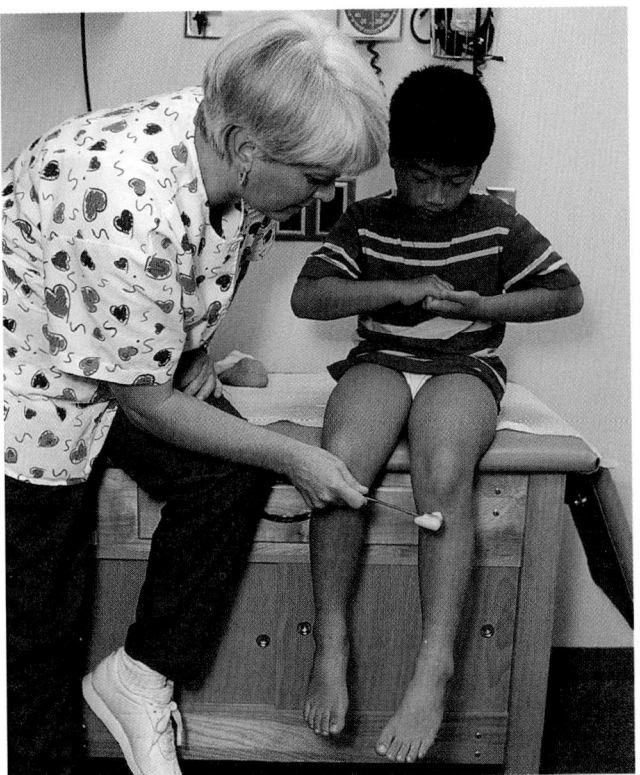

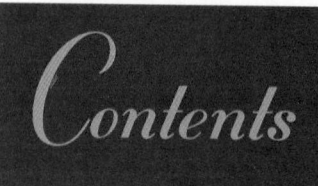

Contents

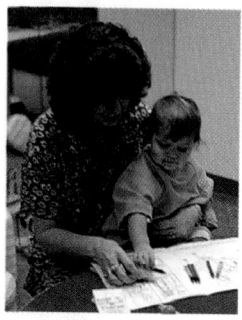

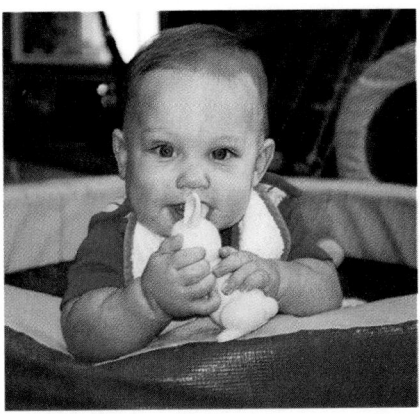

UNIT TWO
ASSESSMENT OF THE CHILD AND FAMILY

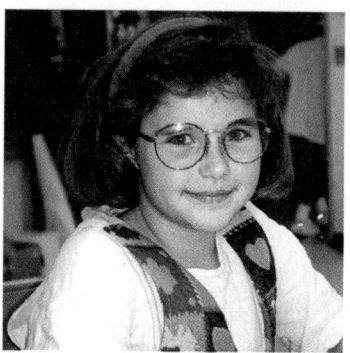

UNIT THREE
THE NEWBORN

UNIT FOUR
INFANCY

CHAPTER 10
Health Promotion of the Infant and Family 287

CHAPTER 11
Health Problems of Infants 335

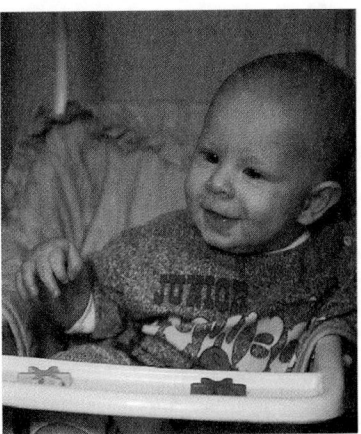

UNIT FIVE
EARLY CHILDHOOD

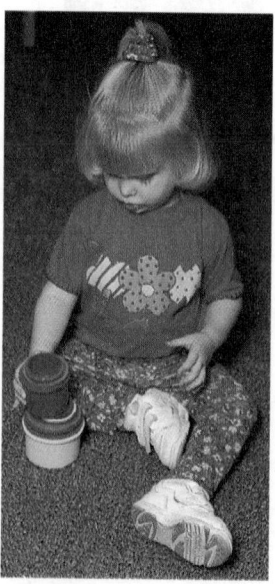

UNIT SIX
MIDDLE CHILDHOOD AND ADOLESCENCE

UNIT SEVEN
THE CHILD AND FAMILY WITH SPECIAL NEEDS

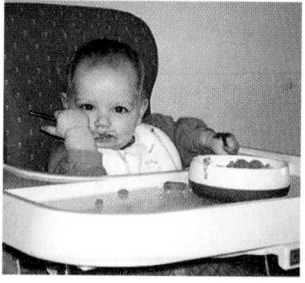

UNIT EIGHT
IMPACT OF HOSPITALIZATION ON THE CHILD AND FAMILY

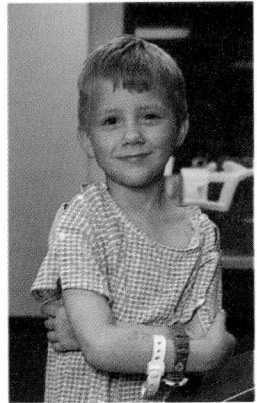

CHAPTER 22
Pediatric Variations of
Nursing Interventions 672

UNIT NINE
THE CHILD WITH PROBLEMS RELATED TO THE TRANSFER OF OXYGEN AND NUTRIENTS

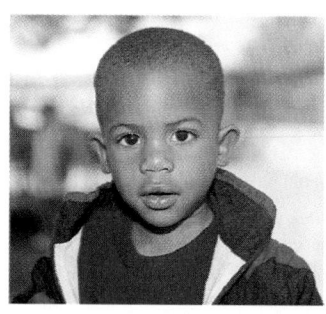

UNIT TEN
THE CHILD WITH PROBLEMS RELATED TO THE PRODUCTION AND CIRCULATION OF BLOOD

CHAPTER 26
The Child with Hematologic or Immunologic Dysfunction 903

UNIT ELEVEN
THE CHILD WITH A DISTURBANCE OF REGULATORY MECHANISMS

CHAPTER 27
The Child with Genitourinary Dysfunction 951

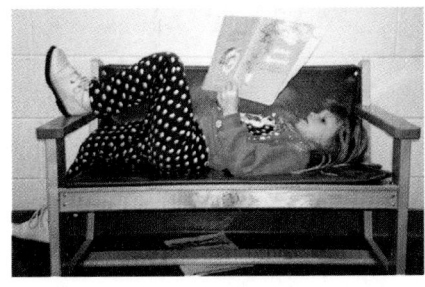

CHAPTER 28
The Child with Cerebral Dysfunction 982

CHAPTER 29
The Child With Endocrine Dysfunction 1034

CHAPTER 30
The Child with Integumentary Dysfunction 1066

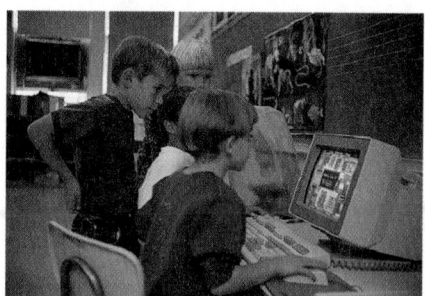

UNIT TWELVE
THE CHILD WITH A PROBLEM THAT INTERFERES WITH PHYSICAL MOBILITY

APPENDIXES

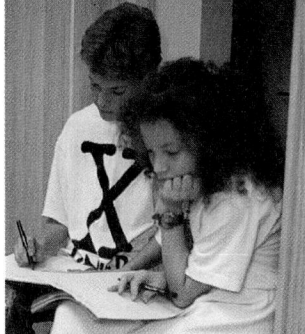

WHALEY & WONG'S

ESSENTIALS OF

Pediatric Nursing

Chapter 1

PERSPECTIVES OF PEDIATRIC NURSING

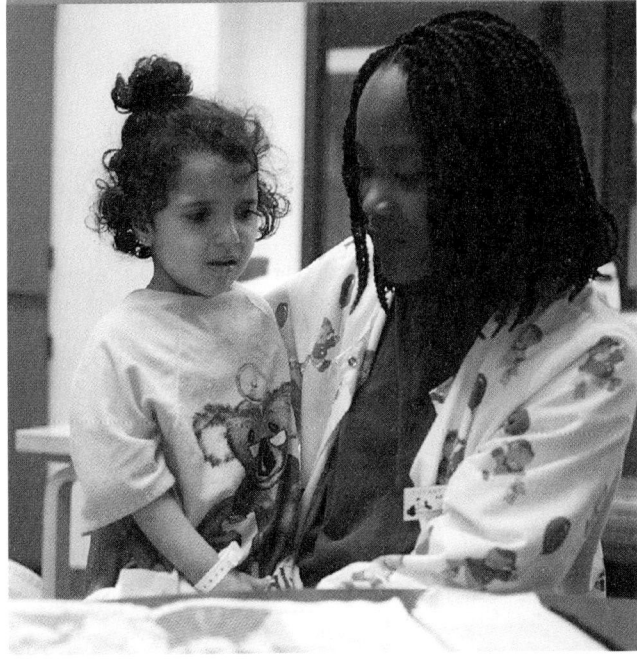

RELATED TOPICS

LEARNING OBJECTIVES
On completion of this chapter the reader will be able to:

- Define the terms *mortality* and *morbidity*
- Identify two ways that knowledge of mortality and morbidity can improve child health

- List three major causes of death during infancy, early childhood, later childhood, and adolescence
- List two major causes of illness during childhood

- Outline four events that were significant in the evolution of child health care in the U.S.
- Describe five broad functions of the pediatric nurse in promoting the health of children

1

HEALTH DURING CHILDHOOD

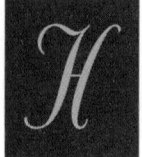 ealth is a complex phenomenon. As defined by the *World Health Organization (WHO)*, it is "a state of complete physical, mental, and social well-being and not merely the absence of disease." Despite this broad definition, however, health is traditionally assessed by observing *mortality* (death) and *morbidity* (illness) over a period of time. Therefore the *presence* of disease becomes a prime indicator of health.

Information concerning mortality and morbidity is of importance to nurses. Such data yield significant information about (1) the causes of death and illness, (2) high-risk age-groups for certain disorders or hazards, (3) advances in treatment and prevention, and (4) specific areas of health counseling. Nurses who are aware of such information can better guide their planning and delivery of care.

"HEALTHY PEOPLE 2000"

Although the health of people, including children, in the United States has improved dramatically during the twentieth century, there remains cause for concern. There is a growing awareness that many of the serious domestic problems, such as acquired immunodeficiency syndrome (AIDS), drug abuse, violence, and unwanted pregnancies, have a direct effect on the health of the nation. Most importantly, the solutions to these problems do not lie in better or more innovative medical treatment, but in *prevention*.

In 1990 "Healthy People 2000" (1991) was issued. It sets the following three broad goals for public health over the 1990s: (1) increase the span of healthy life for Americans, (2) reduce health disparities among Americans, and (3) achieve access to preventive services for all Americans.

Three broad approaches—health promotion, health protection, and preventive services—are employed to achieve the 22 priority areas, which contain approximately 300 measurable objectives. Selected objectives pertaining to pediatrics include improving nutritional and infant health, reducing unintentional injuries, improving oral health, reducing and controlling human immunodeficiency virus (HIV) infection, preventing sexually transmitted diseases, increasing immunization against and preventing infectious diseases, and improving clinical preventive services by reducing barriers to health care (Mason and McGinnis, 1990). All health professionals, especially nurses, in any practice setting should be aware of the priority areas and work toward improving the health of U.S. children. Since the main intervention is prevention, many of the strategies nurses use, such as counseling, education, and screening, can be implemented *independently* to help achieve these goals.

MORTALITY

Figures describing rates of occurrence for events such as death in children are often referred to as *vital statistics. Mortality statistics* describe the incidence or number of individuals who have died over a specific period of time. They are usually presented as rates per 100,000 because of their lower frequency

---

Pamela DiVito-Thomas, MS, RN, assisted in the revision of this chapter.

of occurrence. Such rates are calculated from a sample of death certificates.

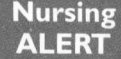 **Nursing ALERT**   Because of the complexity of compiling such data, statistics may vary in different reports and should be interpreted cautiously. For example, figures may be *estimated* (from previously collected data), *provisional* (from temporary current data), or *final* (from complete provisional data). Final statistics are often published 2 or more years after data collection.

Infant Mortality

The *infant mortality rate* is the number of deaths per 1000 live births during the first year of life. It may be further divided into *neonatal mortality* (<28 days of life) and *postneonatal mortality* (28 days to 11 months). In the United States there has been a dramatic decrease in infant mortality. At the beginning of the twentieth century the rate was about 200 infant deaths per 1000 live births. In 1994 the number dropped to 7.9 deaths per 1000 live births, the lowest rate ever recorded in the United States. This decrease has resulted primarily from improvements in perinatal care, such as treatment of respiratory distress syndrome, and fewer deaths from sudden infant death syndrome (SIDS).

From a worldwide perspective the United States lags significantly behind other developed countries. In 1992 it ranked last among the 22 countries with the lowest infant death rates, with Japan having the lowest rate (Table 1-1).

TABLE 1-1. Infant mortality for 22 countries with populations over 2.5 million, 1992 (rate per 1000 live births)

COUNTRY	RATE
Japan	4.5
Singapore	5.0*
Sweden	5.4*
Finland	5.6 (1990)
Norway	5.9
Canada	6.1
Germany	6.2
Netherlands	6.3
Hong Kong	6.4
Switzerland	6.4
France	6.5
Denmark	6.5*
United Kingdom	6.6
Ireland	6.6
Australia	7.0
New Zealand	7.3*
Spain	7.4 (1991)
Austria	7.5
Belgium	7.5*
Italy	8.3*
Greece	8.4*
United States of America	8.5

From Wegman ME: Annual summary of vital statistics—1993, *Pediatrics* 94(6):802, 1994.
*Provisional data.

This is far behind neighboring countries, such as Canada, which ranked sixth. Over several years the rank of the U.S. has fallen. Although the reason is unknown, a major difference between the United States and the other 21 countries is that they all have a national health program (Wegman, 1994).

Birth weight is considered the major determinant of neonatal death in technologically developed countries and is closely related to gestational age (Wilcox and Skjaerven, 1992). The relationship between birth weight (and gestational age) and mortality shows that the lower the birth weight, the higher the mortality. The relatively high incidence of low birth weight (LBW) (<2500 g) in the United States is considered a key factor in its higher neonatal mortality rates when compared with other countries. Access to and use of high-quality prenatal care is the single most promising preventive strategy to decrease early delivery and infant mortality (Naeye, 1993). Other factors that increase the risk of infant mortality include black race, male gender, short or long gestation, birth order (all but second), maternal age (younger or older), and lower level of maternal education (Schoendorf and others, 1992).

Although there has been a steady and significant decline in infant mortality, the number of deaths occurring in the first year of life is still proportionately high when compared with death rates at other ages (Table 1-2). This is also true of other countries, such as Canada (Table 1-3). In the United States and Canada the death rate for infants under 1 year of age is greater than the rates for individuals ages 1 through 54 years. It is not until age 55 and over that the death rate begins to exceed the rate for infants.

During the first half of the 1900s neonatal mortality rates had not shown the remarkable reduction observed in postneonatal infant mortality. In the early 1960s attention was focused on perinatal health care in an effort to decrease the number of neonatal deaths. As a result neonatal mortality declined from 20 per 1000 live births in 1950 to 5 per 1000 live births in 1994 (Guyer and others, 1995). As Table 1-4 demonstrates, most of the 10 leading causes of death during infancy continue to occur during the perinatal period. The first four causes—congenital anomalies, sudden infant death syndrome, disorders related to short gestation and unspecified low birth weight, and respiratory distress syndrome—accounted for about half of all deaths of infants under 1 year of age in 1992.

Although a number of perinatal problems have benefited from improved treatment, congenital anomalies continue to be a leading cause of infant mortality, accounting for more than 20% of those deaths. The incidence of the majority of birth defects has remained substantially the same. Some, such as heart defects, have been rising, but the increase is the result of improved methods of detection, not increased births of affected infants (Khoury and Erickson, 1992). The defects anencephaly and spina bifida are expected to decrease as much as 50% with the current recommendation of folic acid supplementation for all women of childbearing age (see Spina Bifida [Myelomeningocele] Chapter 32). Most birth defects are associated significantly with low birth weight; therefore, prevention of congenital anomalies depends to a large extent on reducing the number of LBW infants (Mili and others, 1991).

TABLE 1-2. Death rates by age, United States, 1994 (estimated rates per 100,000)

AGE (YEARS)	RATE	AGE (YEARS)	RATE
Under 1	811.1	45-54	452.3
1-4	44.5	55-64	1,139.0
5-14	22.7	65-74	2,590.9
15-24	99.6	75-84	5,909.7
25-34	141.0	85 and over	15,312.6
35-44	239.5		

From Singh GK and others: Annual summary of births, marriages, divorces, and deaths: United States, 1994. *Monthly vital statistics report* 43(13):6, Hyattsville, MD, 1995, National Center for Health Statistics.

TABLE 1-3. Death rates for children, Canada, 1988 (rates per 100,000)

AGE (YEARS)	RATE		
	TOTAL	MALE	FEMALE
Under 1	717.9	801.6	630.0
1-4	41.4	45.9	36.2
5-9	21.7	26.8	16.4
10-14	24.6	31.0	17.8
15-19	70.8	103.4	36.3
20-24	90.5	138.8	41.1

Data from Canadian Center for Health Information, Statistics Canada, 1988.

TABLE 1-4. Leading causes of death in infants under 1 year of age, United States, 1992 (rate per 100,000 live births)

RANK	CAUSES OF DEATH	RATE
1	Congenital anomalies	183.2
2	Sudden infant death syndrome	120.3
3	Disorders relating to short gestation and unspecified low birth weight	99.3
4	Respiratory distress syndrome	50.8
5	Newborn affected by maternal complications of pregnancy	35.9
6	Newborn affected by complications of placenta, cord, and membranes	24.4
7	Infections specific to the perinatal period	22.2
8	Accidents and adverse effects	20.1
9	Intrauterine hypoxia and birth asphyxia	15.1
10	Pneumonia and influenza	14.8

From Kochanek KD, Hudson BL: Advance report of final mortality statistics, 1992. *Monthly vital statistics report* 43(6):65, Hyattsville, MD, 1995, National Center for Health Statistics.

TABLE 1-5. Leading causes of death in children at selected age intervals, United States, 1992 (rates per 100,000)

RANK	AGES 1-4	RATE	AGES 5-14	RATE	AGES 15-24	RATE
	All causes	43.6	All causes	22.5	All causes	95.6
1	Injuries	15.9	Injuries	9.3	Injuries	37.8
2	Congenital anomalies	5.5	Cancer	3	Homicide	22.2
3	Cancer	3.1	Homicide	1.6	Suicide	13
4	Homicide	2.8	Congenital anomalies	1.2	Cancer	5
5	Heart disease	1.8	Heart disease	0.8	Heart disease	2.7
	HIV infection (7)*	1			HIV infection (6)*	1.6

From Kochanek KD, Hudson BL: Advance report of final mortality statistics, 1992. *Monthly vital statistics report,* 43(6):23, Hyattsville, MD, 1995, National Center for Health Statistics.
*HIV (Human immunodeficiency virus); rank in parentheses.

When infant death rates are categorized according to race, a disturbing difference is seen. The infant mortality for whites is considerably lower than for all other races in the United States, with blacks having twice the rate for whites. Although the infant mortality of both groups has declined, the gap has remained fairly constant. Unfortunately, data on minority groups are less readily available. For example, the Hispanic infant mortality rate may not represent all Hispanic subgroups, such as Cubans, who have more favorable statistics regarding prenatal care and LBW newborns (Kochanek and Hudson, 1995).

One encouraging note is that the gap in mortality rates between all nonwhite races has been narrowing. Since the Indian Health Service assumed responsibility for the health of Native Americans, infant mortality for Native Americans has declined from 62.7 deaths per 1000 live births in the 1950s to 9.8 in the mid-1980s. This improvement, however, is primarily the result of declines in neonatal mortality. The postneonatal death rates for Native Americans remains more than twice as high as in the white race. This suggests that Native American infants leave the hospital healthy but go to unsafe environments, which decreases their chances of survival past the first year (Nakamura and others, 1991).

Childhood Mortality

For children older than 1 year of age, death rates have always been less than those for infants, as Table 1-5 shows. Children ages 5 to 14 years have the lowest rate of death. However, a sharp rise occurs during later adolescence, primarily from injuries, homicide, and suicide—all potentially preventable conditions that in 1992 were responsible for about 80% of deaths in teenagers and young adults 15 to 24 years old (Kochanek and Hudson, 1995). A general trend in racial differences that occurs in infant mortality is also apparent in childhood deaths for all ages and for both sexes. Whites have fewer deaths for all ages; for both whites and blacks, male deaths outnumber female deaths.

After 1 year of age there is a dramatic change in the causes of death, with injuries being the leading cause during childhood, adolescence, and young adulthood. In addition, violent deaths have been steadily increasing among young people ages 10 through 25 years, especially blacks and males (Rachuba, Stanton, and Howard, 1995). Homicide is the second leading cause of death in the 15- to 24-year age-group. Children 12 years of age and older tend to be killed by non–family members (acquaintances and gangs, typically of the same race) and most frequently by firearms. Suicide, a form of self-violence, is the third leading cause of death among teenagers and young adults 15 to 24 years old. White males in this age-group are especially at risk (see Suicide, Chapter 17.)

The causes of increased violence against children and self-inflicted violence are not fully understood. In young children the increase in homicide may represent more accurate identification of child abuse. In all cases the problem of child homicides is an extremely complex one, involving numerous social, economic, and other influences. Prevention lies in a better understanding of the social and psychologic factors that lead to the high rates of homicide and suicide. Nurses need to be especially aware of young people who are depressed, repeatedly in trouble with the criminal justice system, or associated with groups known to be violent. Prevention requires identification of these youngsters, as well as therapeutic intervention by qualified professionals.

The major declines in death rates during childhood have been in deaths caused by gastrointestinal diseases, infectious diseases, perinatal conditions, neoplasms, and injuries. The absence of infectious diseases as a leading cause of death is testimony to the role antibacterial agents and immunizations have played in the declining mortality rates. More effective treatment of severe infections has resulted in other disorders becoming more prominent in the list of leading killers. (Most notable among these are the neoplasms, although fewer children die from cancer than ever before. For example, see Leukemias, Chapter 26.) However, infectious disease may again play a prominent role in childhood mortality. Of particular concern is the increasing incidence of HIV infection in children. In 1992 HIV infection ranked as the seventh leading cause of death for children aged 1 to 14 years, and sixth for those 15 to 24 years of age. Although HIV infection was the seventh leading cause of death for 1- to 4-year-olds, the number of deaths due to this cause was relatively small—161 deaths, or 2% of deaths from all causes for that age-group. During 1994, 1768 cases of AIDS were reported in adolescents. Of these, 64% were exposed to HIV primarily through transfusions of clotting factor for hemophilia/coagulation disorder (Child Health, 1995).

TABLE 1-6. Mortality from leading types of injuries, United States, 1990 (rates per 100,000 population in each age-group)

| | AGE (YEARS) | | | |
TYPE OF ACCIDENT	UNDER 1	1-4	5-14	15-24
Males				
All causes	1083.1	52.4	28.5	147.4
Accidents (all types)	25.2	20.8	13.5	65.9
Motor vehicle	5.0 (2)*	6.9 (1)	7.0 (1)	49.5 (1)
Drowning†	2.2 (5)	5.0 (2)	2.1 (2)	4.4 (2)
Fires and burns	2.9 (4)	4.4 (3)	1.0 (3)	1.1 (5)
Firearms	—	—	1.0 (4)	2.4 (3)
Ingestion of food/object	4.6 (3)	0.8 (4)	—	—
Mechanical suffocation	6.7 (1)	0.6 (5)	—	—
Poisoning	—	—	—	1.5 (4)
Accidents as a percent of all deaths	2.3%	40%	47%	45%
Females				
All causes	855.5	41.0	19.3	49.0
Accidents (all types)	21.8	13.7	7.2	20.8
Motor vehicle	4.9 (2)	5.6 (1)	4.7 (1)	17.9 (1)
Drowning†	1.7 (5)	2.6 (3)	0.7 (3)	0.4 (4)
Fires and burns	2.7 (4)	2.9 (2)	0.8 (2)	0.5 (3)
Firearms	—	—	0.1 (4)	0.2 (5)
Ingestion of food/object	3.0 (3)	0.5 (4)	—	—
Mechanical suffocation	5.4 (1)	0.3 (5)	—	—
Poisoning	—	—	—	0.6 (2)
Accidents as a percent of all deaths	2.5%	34%	37%	42%

Modified from National Center for Health Statistics, Public Health Service, U.S. Department of Health and Human Services, as cited in *Accident Facts,* Chicago, 1993, National Safety Council.
*Indicates rank among the leading types of accidents.
†Exclusive of deaths in water transportation.

Injuries—The Leading Killer. Injuries cause more deaths and disabilities in children than do all causes of disease combined. As children grow older, the percentage of deaths from injuries increases (Table 1-6). Injuries have not shown the dramatic declines seen in other areas of childhood mortality because an injury has traditionally been regarded as an unavoidable accident or a behavioral problem, rather than a health problem. The term *accident* suggests a chaotic, random event that is "luck" or "chance"; the term *injury* is preferred because it connotes a sense of responsibility and control. In addition injury control, including research, has not received high priority or sufficient financial support. Research on injuries has not been based on a theoretic framework, as has been done with diseases. There is a need to view injuries and their prevention in terms of *host,* the affected person, *environment,* the time and place, and *agent,* the object that is the direct cause.

The pattern of deaths caused by unintentional injuries, especially from motor vehicles, drowning, and burns, is remarkably consistent in most Western societies, such as Canada. However, the United States far exceeds other countries in the number of violent deaths. The leading causes of deaths from injuries for each age-group according to sex are presented in Table 1-6. Fortunately, prevention strategies such as use of car restraints, bicycle helmets, and smoke detectors have resulted in a significant decrease in fatalities for children ages 1 to 19 years (Child Health, 1995). Currently, all states in the United States have enacted legislation requiring young children to be properly restrained in motor vehicles. Despite safety efforts, the overwhelming cause of death in children over 1 year of age is motor vehicle (MV)-related fatalities, including occupant, pedestrian, bicycle, and motorcycle deaths (Fig. 1-1). The majority of deaths from injuries occur in males. Even though the *percentage* of infants dying from motor vehicle (MV) injuries is small compared with the total number of deaths in that age-group, children under 1 year of age still have a high death rate from MV occupant deaths, primarily from failure to be properly restrained.

When deaths from injuries are compared according to sex and age, the causes of death differ. The developmental stage of the child partially determines the types of injuries that are most likely to occur at a specific age. A child between the ages of 1 and 4 years is equally likely to die as an occupant or as a pedestrian in MV injuries. However, children ages 5 to 9 years are more likely to die from pedestrian crashes, whereas adolescents are more likely to die from occupant crashes. Children ages 10 to 14 are at greatest risk of bicycling fatalities. The majority of bicycling deaths are from head injuries. Helmets can reduce the risk of head injury by 85%, but only a minority of children wear them (American Academy of Pediatrics, 1995).

Drowning and burns are the second and third leading causes of death in boys ages 1 to 14, but the order is reversed in girls (Fig. 1-2). Drowning continues to be a significant cause of death in older teenagers. In addition, firearms are a major cause of death in males but not in females (Fig. 1-3). During infancy aspiration or suffocation often ranks as the leading cause of death but is infrequent in older children (Fig. 1-4). More than half of all poisonings occur in children under 2 years of age (Fig. 1-5). By age 4 to 5 years, nonintentional poisonings are uncommon. Another increase occurs in the 15- to 24-year age-group, where it is the fourth leading cause of death from injury. Poisoning in this age-group is typically intentional and usually represents death from suicide

(especially in females) or drug abuse. Death from falls is seen primarily in children ages 1 to 14 years.

Analyzing deaths from specific types of injuries by age and sex is useful in identifying high-risk groups. When comparing deaths from injuries with other causes of childhood mortality, it is clear that preventing injuries offers the greatest promise for improving survival. Recent data indicates that advanced physical development imposes additional risks for 5- to 8-year-olds. Nurses certainly play a major role in providing anticipatory guidance to parents and older children regarding hazards during each age period (Christoffel and others, 1996).

Injury prevention is discussed in each chapter on health promotion of the various age-groups.

MORBIDITY

The prevalence of a specific illness in the population at a particular time is known as *morbidity statistics.* These are generally presented as rates per 1000 population because of their greater frequency of occurrence. Unlike mortality statistics, morbidity is very difficult to define and may denote acute illness, chronic disease, or disability. Unlike death rates, which are updated annually, morbidity statistics are revised much less frequently and do not necessarily represent the general population. The following discussion is intended to present an overview of illness in children from a variety of perspectives.

Childhood Morbidity

Acute illness may be defined as symptoms severe enough to limit activity or require medical attention. Respiratory illness accounts for about 50% of all acute conditions; about 11% are caused by infections and parasitic disease, and 15% are caused by injuries. The chief illness of childhood is the common cold (Pless, 1992).

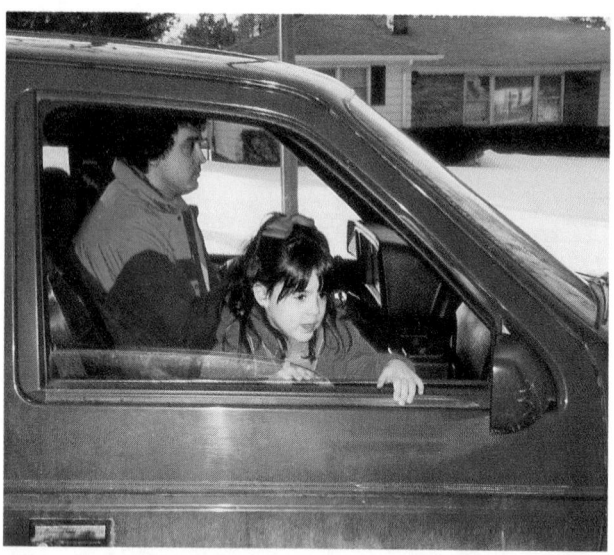

FIG. 1-1. Motor vehicle injuries are the leading cause of death in children over 1 year of age. The majority of the fatalities involve occupants who are unrestrained.

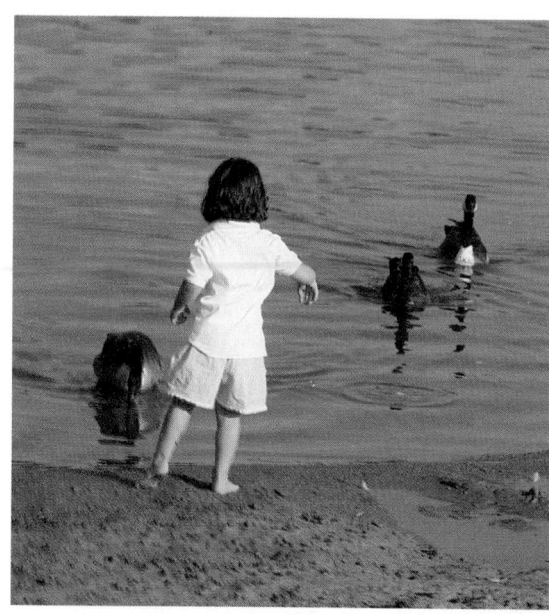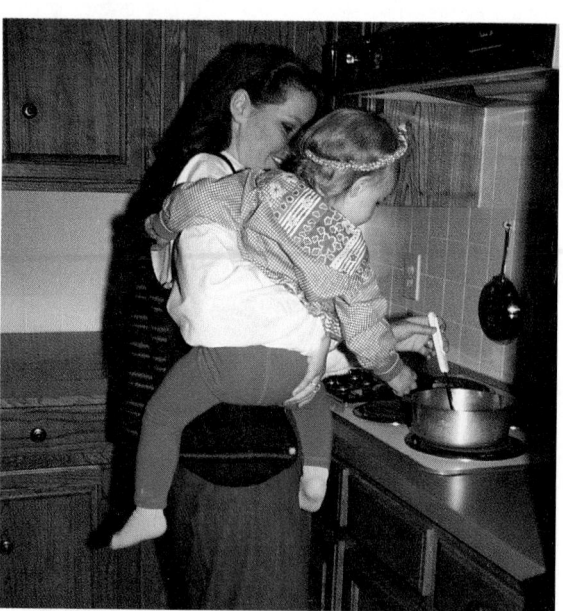

FIG. 1-2. A, Drowning is the second leading cause of death from injury in boys and the third in girls ages 1 to 14 years. It remains the second leading cause of death from injury for both sexes ages 15 to 24 years. **B,** Burns are the second leading cause of death from injury in girls and the third in boys ages 1 to 14 years.

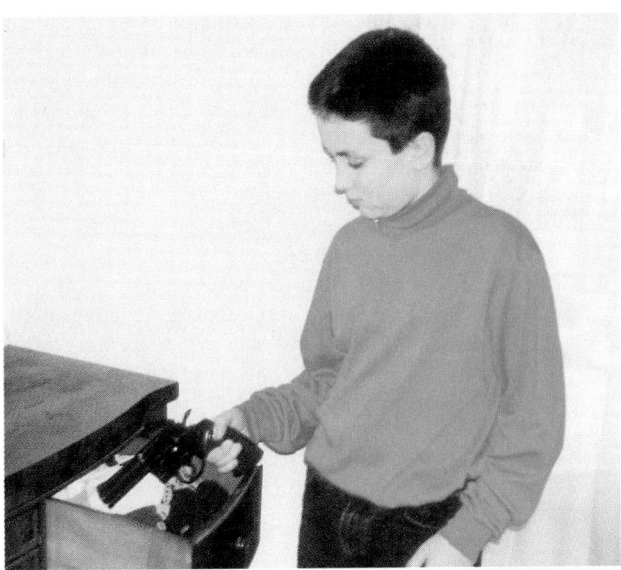

FIG. 1-3. Improper use of firearms is the fourth leading cause of death from injury in boys and girls ages 5 to 14 years and the third leading cause of death from injury in boys ages 15 to 24 years.

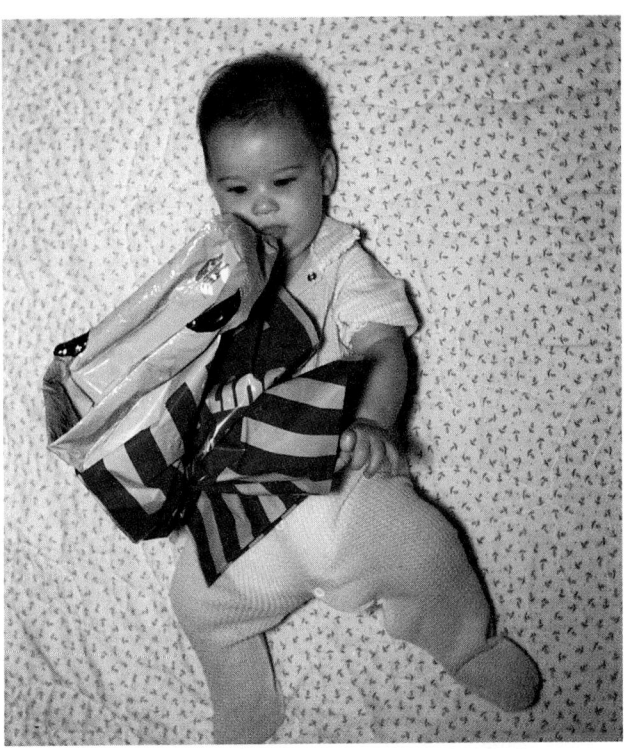

FIG. 1-4. Aspiration/suffocation is often the leading cause of death from injury in infants, especially boys.

The types of diseases that children contract during childhood vary according to age. For example, upper respiratory tract infection and enuresis tend to decrease with age, whereas other disorders, such as acne and headaches, tend to increase with age. Also, children who have had any type of problem are more likely to have that problem again than are children in the general population. Morbidity is not distributed randomly in children. Children from poor families tend to have more health problems than children from nonpoor families. This finding suggests the need for heightened efforts to improve access to health care for low-income children.

Recent concern has focused on groups of children who have increased morbidity—homeless children, children living in poverty, children of low birth weight, children with chronic illnesses, foreign-born adopted children, and children in daycare centers. A number of different factors account for these at-risk groups. A major cause is limited access to health care, especially for the homeless, the poverty stricken, and those with chronic health problems. Other reasons include improved survival of children with chronic health problems, particularly infants of very low birth weight. Children residing in certain at-risk environments, such as country of origin (for adopted children) and daycare centers, are more likely to have a variety of medical conditions, especially infections (American Academy of Pediatrics, 1991).

Injury-related morbidity is also significant. Almost 16 million children are seen in emergency rooms for their injuries—600,000 children are hospitalized, and about 30,000 youngsters suffer permanent disability from injuries each year (Division of Injury Control, 1990).

Probably the most important aspect of morbidity is the degree of disability it produces. *Disability* can be measured in days off from school or days confined to bed. It can be the result of an acute or chronic disorder. On an average a child loses 5.3 days per year because of injury or illness. Of all chil-

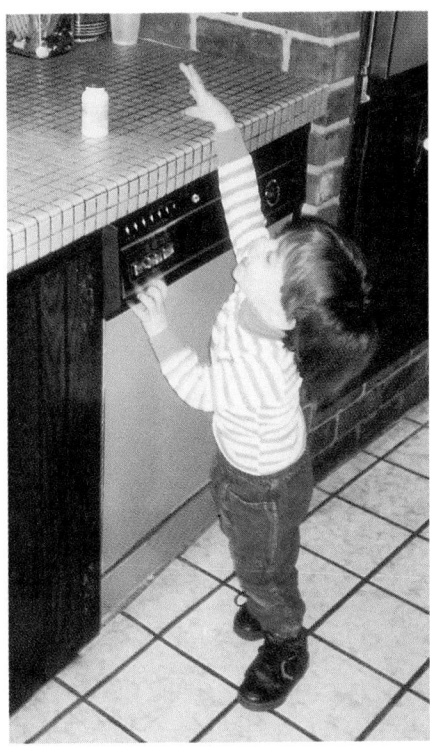

FIG. 1-5. Poisoning causes a considerable number of injuries in children under 4 years of age, but it is the fourth leading cause of death from injury (usually from suicide) in young people ages 15 to 24 years.

ASYNCPANO

dren under 17 years of age, more than 95% are not disabled in any way. About 2% have mild disability, another 2% have moderate disability, and 0.2% are severely disabled (Pless, 1992). (The incidence of chronic conditions is discussed in Chapter 18).

Although childhood is a time of relative health, it is the rare child who never becomes ill. Part of nurses' intervention is education of parents regarding the usual types of childhood illnesses and recognition of those symptoms requiring treatment. Future progress in decreasing childhood morbidity, as in childhood mortality, rests more on parent education than on miraculous discoveries such as antibiotics. Nurses play a vital role in advancing child care through health promotion.

The New Morbidity

In addition to disease and injury, children face other problems that can significantly alter their health. These include behavioral, social (family), and educational problems that are sometimes referred to as the *new morbidity.* Estimates on the incidence of these problems vary, but they represent at least 5% and as much as 25% to 30% of health problems in specific age-groups, social classes, and medical facilities. Although no conclusive characteristics have been identified for children with new-morbidity problems, some findings are significant in terms of defining a high-risk group. This group includes children (1) from the lowest socioeconomic strata, (2) ages 7 to 14 years, (3) of male gender, (4) from one-parent families, (5) with a presenting complaint of a chronic physical disorder, (6) with reading skills below grade level, and (7) with higher rates of school absenteeism (Gortmaker and others, 1990). As new "epidemics" such as violence, poverty, technology-dependent children, drug-addicted infants, and infection with HIV continue to emerge, nurses will need to continue professional education efforts to manage children's psychosocial problems effectively (American Academy of Pediatrics, 1993).

EVOLUTION OF CHILD HEALTH CARE IN THE UNITED STATES

Children in colonial America were born into a world with many hazards to their health and survival. Epidemics were common, and no control or treatment was known. Physicians were few, and only a small number had any formal training. Midwives also were untrained, basing their practice on past experiences. Books providing information on child care and feeding were scarce and, when available, were useful only to a minority of literate parents.

Medical care by physicians was limited to wealthy families who lived in or could travel to more developed cities. Children who lived on farms were mainly cared for by another family member or by a competent neighbor. Traveling medicine men, with their various forms of quackery, were common. Black slave children had only as much care as their owner was able or willing to provide. Native American children were treated for disease according to the tradition of each tribe, which was often a mixture of medicine, magic, and religion. With the colonization of America the tribes were exposed to many new, often fatal, diseases.

Statistics on childhood mortality during the colonial period are largely unavailable. Epidemic diseases were prevalent, however, and included smallpox, measles, mumps, chickenpox, influenza, diphtheria, yellow fever, cholera, and whooping cough, but the disease that surpassed all others as a cause of childhood death was dysentery. Sometimes entire families succumbed to this illness. Other diseases that were major contributors to childhood illness were the "slow epidemic" of tuberculosis, nutritional diseases, and injuries (Schmidt, 1976).

Although scientific knowledge was accumulating, especially from work done in Europe, there were no organized efforts in the United States to apply that knowledge to the care of the sick. It was not until the Industrial Revolution was well under way in the nineteenth century that the consequences of childhood illness and injury and the effects of child labor, poverty, and neglect became more widely recognized. The end of the nineteenth century is often regarded as the dark ages of pediatrics, and the first half of the twentieth century as the dawn of improved health care for children (Cone, 1976).

The study of pediatrics began in the last half of the 1800s, particularly under the influence of a Prussian-born physician, *Abraham Jacobi* (1830-1919), who is referred to as the *Father of Pediatrics.* With several other physicians he broke new ground in the scientific and clinical investigation of childhood diseases. One outstanding achievement was the establishment of "milk stations," where mothers could bring sick children for treatment and learn the importance of pure milk and its proper preparation.

The crusade for pure milk helped bring the dairy industry under legal control and led to the establishment of infant welfare stations. The remarkable decline in infant mortality since 1900 has been achieved through prevention and health-promoting measures such as improved sanitation and pasteurization of milk. Before these regulations existed, the unsanitary milk supply was a chief source of infantile diarrhea and bovine tuberculosis. Cows were often kept in filthy stables and fed garbage and distillery wastes. Milk from cows fed distillery wastes was reported to make infants "tipsy." Some of the cows were so diseased with tuberculosis that they had to be raised on cranes to be milked.

At about the same time, increasing concern developed for the social welfare of children, especially those who were homeless or employed as factory laborers. The work of one such reformer, *Lillian Wald* (1867-1940), had far-reaching effects on child health and nursing. She founded the Henry Street Settlement in New York City, which eventually provided nursing service, social work, and an organized program of social, cultural, and educational activities. Wald is regarded as the founder of public health or community nursing. She was instrumental in establishing the role of the first full-time school nurse, *Lina Rogers.* Soon other nurses were employed to teach parents and children about the prevention or need for treatment of minor skin conditions, malnutrition, and other impairments or illnesses identified in the school. An outgrowth of nursing involvement in school health was the development of pediatric courses and specialized clinical experience in schools of nursing.

As more causes of disease were identified, there was an emphasis on isolation and asepsis. In the early 1900s children with contagious diseases were isolated from adult patients. Parents were prohibited from visiting because they might transmit disease to and from the home. Even toys and personal articles of clothing were kept from the child. It was not until the 1940s and the famous works of Spitz and Robertson on institutionalized children that the effects of isolation and maternal deprivation were recognized. This brought forth a surge of interest in the psychologic health of children and resulted in changes for hospitalized children, such as rooming-in, sibling visitations, child life (play) programs, prehospitalization preparation, parent education, and hospital schooling.

Influenced by social reformers such as Lillian Wald, national leaders began to take action to improve children's living conditions. In 1909 President Theodore Roosevelt called the first *White House Conference on Children.* It focused on care of dependent children and attempted to address the deplorable working conditions of youngsters. As a result of this conference, the *U.S. Children's Bureau* was established in 1912. This marked the beginning of a period of studies of economic and social factors related to infant mortality, maternal deaths, and maternal and infant care in rural areas, all of which created the basis for stimulating better standards of care for mothers and children. This helped lead to the first Maternity and Infancy Act (Sheppard-Towner Act) in 1921, which provided grants to states to develop a Division of Maternal and Child Health (MCH) as a unit of the health department.

With the passage of *Title V of the Social Security Act (SSA)* in 1935, a federal-state partnership was established under the administration of the Children's Bureau. Title V included federal grants-in-aid to states, matched by state funds, for three types of work: *maternal and child health (MCH), Crippled Children's Services (CCS),* and *child welfare services.* The first programs provided by Title V were prenatal, postnatal, and child health clinics and training of personnel. The early emphasis of the CCS was on orthopedic care. With the recognition that a child's ability to function also could be limited by a chronic illness, state CCS programs became involved with children with developmental, behavioral, and educational problems and more recently with home care of children with complex medical conditions. This broadened concept was officially reflected in the 1985 passage of legislation that changed the name of the CCS to the *Program for Children with Special Health Needs (CSHN).*

Numerous other federal programs have been developed. Some that have had a major impact on maternal and child health include the following:

Medicaid. In 1965 Medicaid was created under Title XIX of the Social Security Act to reduce financial barriers to health care for the poor. It is the largest maternal-child health program. A major project under Medicaid is the Child Health Assessment Program (CHAP), which provides services for a large number of pregnant women and children. Not all poor children are eligible for Medicaid; financial eligibility varies considerably from state to state.

Aid to Families with Dependent Children (AFDC). AFDC was established by the Social Security Act of 1935 as a cash grant program to enable states to aid needy children without fathers.

MCH Services Block Grant. The MCH Services Block Grant provides health services to mothers and children, particularly those with low income or limited access to health services. Its primary purposes are to reduce infant mortality, reduce the incidence of preventable disease and handicapping conditions among children,

and increase the availability of prenatal, delivery, and postpartum care to eligible mothers.

Alcohol, Drug Abuse, and Mental Health Block Grant. Established by the Omnibus Budget Reconciliation Act of 1981, the block grant provides funds to states for (1) projects to support prevention, treatment, and rehabilitation related to substance abuse and (2) grants to community mental health centers for the identification, assessment, and treatment of severely mentally disturbed children and adolescents.

Social Services Block Grant. Established under Title XX of the Social Security Act, this block grant provides states with funds for child daycare, protective and emergency services, counseling, family planning, home-based services, information and referral, and adoption and foster care services.

Women, Infants, and Children (WIC). In 1974 the WIC Special Supplemental Food Program was started. It provides nutritious food and nutrition education to low-income, pregnant, postpartum, and lactating women and to infants and children up to age 5 years. Other nutrition programs include Food Stamps, National School Lunch Program, School Breakfast Program, and Child Care Food Program, which provides financial assistance for nutritious meals to children in daycare centers, family and group daycare homes, and Head Start centers.

Education for All Handicapped Children Act (P.L. 94-142). In 1975 P.L. 94-142 was passed to provide a free appropriate public education to all handicapped children from ages 3 to 21 and to provide for those supportive services (speech, counseling, and so on) that ensure the benefit of special education.

Education of the Handicapped Act Amendments of 1986 (P.L. 99-457). In 1986 P.L. 99-457 was passed to allow for the provision of federal funding to states to develop and implement a statewide, comprehensive, coordinated, and multidisciplinary program of early intervention services for handicapped infants and toddlers and their families.

Family and Medical Leave Act (FMLA). Signed into law in 1993, FMLA allows eligible employees to take up to 12 weeks of unpaid leave from their jobs every year to care for newborn or newly adopted children; to care for children, parents, or spouses who have serious health conditions; or to recover from their own serious health conditions. After the leave, the law entitles employees to return to their previous jobs or to equivalent jobs with the same pay, benefits, and other conditions.

Despite the number of federal and state programs available to assist children and families, there are serious barriers to health care in the United States, including (1) *financial barriers,* such as not having insurance or having insurance that does not cover certain services; (2) *system barriers,* such as having to travel great distances for health care or state-to-state variations in Medicaid benefits; and (3) *knowledge barriers,* such as not knowing about the need or value of prenatal or child health supervision or being unaware of the services that are available. The current thrust in health care initiative is to improve children's and families' access to health care.

One of the most drastic changes in health care delivery has been the establishment of a prospective payment system based on *diagnosis related groups (DRGs).* The DRG categories allow pretreatment (prospective) billing for almost all U.S. hospitals reimbursed by Medicare. With hospitals now financially responsible when Medicare patients exceed the allotted admission stay, more patients are being discharged early. This has created an immense need for home care and other sources of community-based services. The exact impact DRGs will have on pediatric care is uncertain, but because health care cost containment is a national priority, it is inevitable that some form of prospective payment will affect children. Nurses need to be aware of the changing economics and prepared to meet the challenges, especially those related to the movement of care to *health maintenance organizations (HMOs)*.

PEDIATRIC NURSING

PHILOSOPHY OF CARE

Nursing of infants and children is consistent with the *definition of nursing* as "the diagnosis and treatment of human responses to actual or potential health problems." The definition incorporates the four essential features of contemporary nursing practice:

1. Attention to the full range of human experiences and responses to health and illness without restriction to a problem-focused orientation
2. Integration of objective data with knowledge gained from an understanding of the patient or group's subjective experience
3. Application of scientific knowledge to the processes of diagnosis and treatment
4. Provision of a caring relationship that facilitates health and healing (American Nurses Association, 1995)

Family-Centered Care

The philosophy of *family-centered care* recognizes the family as the constant in a child's life and that service systems and personnel must support, respect, encourage, and enhance the strength and competence of the family (Johnson, McGonigel, and Kaufmann, 1989). Families are supported in their natural caregiving and decision-making roles by building on their unique strengths as individuals and families. Patterns of living at home and in the community are promoted. The needs of all family members, not just the child's, are considered (see box). The philosophy acknowledges diversity among family structures and backgrounds; family goals, dreams, strategies, and actions; and family support, service, and information needs (Ahmann, 1994).*

Two basic concepts in this process are enabling and empowerment. Professionals *enable* families by creating opportunities and means for all family members to display their present abilities and competencies and to acquire new ones that are necessary to meet the needs of the child and family. *Empowerment* describes the interaction of professionals with families in such a way that families maintain or acquire a sense of control over their family lives and attribute positive changes that result from helping behaviors that foster their own strengths, abilities, and actions (Dunst, Trivette, and Deal, 1988).

---

*Resources on family-centered care are available from the Association for Care of Children's Health, 7910 Woodmont Ave., Suite 300, Bethesda, MD 20814; (301) 654-6549. A facilitator's guide, *Recognizing Family-Centered Care,* and other publications are available from Project Copernicus, 2911 E. Biddle St., Baltimore, MD 21213; (410) 550-9700.

For additional information, please view "Family-Centered Care" in *Whaley and Wong's Pediatric Nursing Video Series,* St Louis, 1996, Mosby; (800) 426-4545.

THE KEY ELEMENTS OF FAMILY-CENTERED CARE

Incorporating into policy and practice the recognition that the *family is the constant* in a child's life while the service systems and support personnel within those systems fluctuate

Facilitating *family/professional collaboration* at all levels of hospital, home, and community care:
  care of an individual child
  program development, implementation, and evaluation
  policy formation

Exchanging complete and unbiased information between family members and professionals in a supportive manner at all times

Incorporating into policy and practice the recognition and *honoring of cultural diversity,* strengths, and individuality within and across all families, including *ethnic, racial, spiritual, social, economic, educational,* and *geographic diversity*

Recognizing and respecting *different methods of coping* and implementing comprehensive policies and programs that provide *developmental, educational, emotional, environmental, and financial support* to meet the diverse needs of families

Encouraging and facilitating *family-to-family support* and networking

Ensuring that *home, hospital,* and *community service* and *support systems* for children needing specialized health and developmental care and their families are *flexible, accessible, and comprehensive* in responding to diverse family-identified needs

Appreciating families as families and children as children, recognizing that they possess a wide range of strengths, concerns, emotions, and aspirations beyond their need for specialized health and developmental services and support

From Shelton TL, Stepanek JS: *Family-centered care for children needing specialized health and developmental services,* Bethesda, MD, 1994, Association for the Care of Children's Health.

The *parent-professional partnership* is a powerful mechanism for enabling and empowering families. Parents serve as respected equals with professionals* and have the right to decide what is important for themselves and their family; the professional's role is to support and strengthen the family's ability to nurture and promote its members' development in a way that is both enabling and empowering.

Partnerships imply the belief that partners are capable individuals who become more capable by sharing knowledge, skills, and resources in a manner that benefits all participants. Collaboration is viewed as a continuum. Families have the option of being anywhere along that continuum, depending on the strengths and needs of the child, the family, and the professionals who are involved (Shelton, Jeppson, and Johnson, 1987). The nurse can help *every* family, including those with a previous history of serious personal and/or family problems, to identify their strengths, build on them, and assume a comfortable level of participation (see Thinking Critically About . . . box). Although caring for the family is strongly emphasized throughout the text, it is also highlighted in features such as Cultural Awareness, Family Focus, and Family Home Care boxes.

---

*For information about parent-professional partnerships, a free pamphlet, *Equals in This Partnership,* is available from The National Center for Infants, Toddlers and Families, 34 15th Street NW, Washington, D.C., 20005-1013, (202)638-1144.

THINKING CRITICALLY ABOUT ...
Family-Centered Care

Although professionals readily accept the concept of family-centered care, they have been slow to implement practices that embody the "family as the patient." This lag has occurred in part because family-centered care requires a shift in orientation regarding provisions of services. The philosophy requires stretching beyond clinical practices that have become tradition because of their convenience to the institution and personnel (Ahmann, 1994).

Family-centered care requires viewing families as the center of care, with their input serving as the major determinant of the interventions provided. For example, exclusion policies are replaced with *family-based care,* such as parental and child *choice* regarding separation during procedures, open visiting hours, and no limitations on the ages or numbers of visitors, except per family request (Flint and Walsh, 1988). In fact, should the word "visitors" even be used? Family members certainly are not visitors to their child; nurses and other staff are!

In your practice, what policies can be considered family-based care? How can those that are not family-based care be changed? What reasons do staff give for preferring practices that exclude families? Compare the agency's policies with its mission statement and purpose. Sadly, you may find what Hostler (1992) reported that during visits to 30 leading hospitals in the U.S. not one single model of excellence in the implementation of family-centered care was found. Fortunately, models of family-centered care, such as the Nursing Mutual Participation Mode (Curley, 1988; Curley and Wallace, 1992), do exist and have documented benefits, such as (Curley and Wallace, 1992; Johnson, Jeppson, and Redburn, 1992):

- Families experience greater feelings of confidence and competence and less stress in caring for their children
- The dependence of families on professional caregivers decreases
- Costs of care decrease
- Professionals experience greater job satisfaction
- Both parents and providers are empowered to develop new skills and expertise

Atraumatic Care

Although tremendous advances have been made in pediatric care, much of what is done to children to cure illness and prolong life is traumatic, painful, upsetting, and frightening. Unfortunately, minimizing the trauma of medical interventions has not kept pace with the technologic advances. With knowledge of the stressors imposed on ill children and their families and armed with interventions shown to be safe and effective in eliminating or reducing the stressors, health professionals must direct their attention to providing care that is as atraumatic as possible.

Atraumatic care is the provision of therapeutic care in settings, by personnel, and through the use of interventions that eliminates or minimizes the psychologic and physical distress experienced by children and their families in the health care system. *Therapeutic care* encompasses the prevention, diagnosis, treatment, or palliation of chronic or acute conditions. *Setting* refers to whatever place that care is given—the home, the hospital, or any other health care setting. *Personnel* include anyone directly involved in providing therapeutic care. *Interventions* range from psychologic approaches, such as preparing children for procedures, to physical interventions, such as providing space for a parent to room in with a child. *Psychologic distress* may include anxiety, fear, anger, disappointment, sadness, shame, or guilt. *Physical distress* may range from sleeplessness and immobilization to the experience of disturbing sensory stimuli, such as pain, temperature extremes, loud noises, bright lights, or darkness. Simply, atraumatic care is concerned with the who, what, when, where, why, and how of any procedure performed on a child for the purpose of preventing or minimizing psychologic and physical stress (Wong, 1989).

The overriding goal in providing atraumatic care is *first, do no harm.* Three principles provide the framework for achieving this goal: (1) prevent or minimize the child's separation from the family; (2) promote a sense of control; and (3) prevent or minimize bodily injury and pain. Examples of providing atraumatic care include fostering the parent-child relationship during hospitalization, preparing the child before any unfamiliar treatment or procedure, controlling pain, allowing the child privacy, providing play activities for expression of fear and aggression, minimizing loss of control, and respecting cultural differences.

Throughout the text the concept of atraumatic care is an integral part of all discussions of nursing care. Selected examples are highlighted in Atraumatic Care boxes. Many other boxes and tables focusing on culture, family teaching, research, and critical thinking incorporate aspects of providing care as atraumatically as possible. Chapter 21, Family-Centered Care of the Child During Illness and Hospitalization, is organized according to the principles of providing atraumatic care.

Primary Nursing

Part of the trend in nursing practice, particularly in pediatrics, is a deeper commitment to patient accountability. One of the outgrowths of this has been the movement toward *primary nursing,* which involves 24-hour responsibility and accountability by one nurse for the care of a small group of patients. The primary nurse becomes the bedside nurse, with few if any duties delegated to other staff. If responsibilities are shared, it is usually with an associate primary nurse who maintains continuity of care when the primary nurse is not working.

One of the traditional problems with primary nursing has been providing consistency in scheduling the same nurse and associate. In addition, delegation of responsibilities to other members of the health care team has become common practice (see also Future Trends, p. 16). An approach that maintains consistency of care is to designate one primary nurse and as many associates as are needed to ensure that the same staff care for the child. This group forms the *primary core.* One nurse is assigned to the patient for each shift, and additional staff are assigned for these individuals' days off. By identifying the primary core for a specific period in advance, all the staff working with the child can plan care jointly, with the primary nurse maintaining overall responsibility.

The philosophy of primary care is supported throughout the discussion of nursing of children. In some instances the one-to-one relationship between child and nurse is emphasized because of its therapeutic benefit, such as in nonorganic failure to thrive. However, primary core nursing is universally a supportive intervention in pediatric nursing because it provides a consistent caregiver for the child and focuses on the family unit as an integral component in the planning and implementation of care.

Case Management*

Nursing case management is an extension of primary nursing (Weinstein, 1991). As a general concept, case management is a care delivery system that balances cost and quality and was created in response to pressure from payers to provide care in a more cost-effective manner. Although the movement to case management began in adult care, it was quickly adapted to pediatric care. Simultaneously, benefits to case management, such as improved patient/family satisfaction, decreased fragmentation of care, and the ability to describe and measure outcomes for a homogenous group of patients, became apparent.

Case management is not a new concept. It has been used in outpatient settings, primarily by assigning a case manager to a particular patient or group of patients. The new model includes a timeline for care as a component of the process. These timelines for care have a variety of names: critical paths, guidelines for care, case management plans, Caremaps,† coordinated care plans, or other titles that are agreed on within a specific agency. Regardless of the name given to the timeline, these are multidisciplinary plans that include all the components of care for an episode or multiple episodes of illness, as well as the outcomes that are expected as a result of delivering that care. They can be confined to inpatient care or can include the entire continuum of care, including home care (see also Chapter 20).

Concurrent with the movement to provide care in a systematic manner have been efforts by professional and government organizations to develop *clinical practice guidelines* for the care of an illness, disease, or related problem. Whereas timelines for care are usually developed within an institution and reflect local practice patterns, clinical guidelines are being developed on a national level that reflect the research that has been conducted relative to a specific disease or illness. A federal agency that is developing clinical guidelines is the **Agency for Health Care Policy and Research (AHCPR).**‡

As the movement for providing care based on guidelines continues, institutions will be challenged to incorporate clinical guidelines into the timelines for care that are developed locally. The result of this effort will mean that professionally developed clinical guidelines will be integrated into practice at the local level.

Because of the movement to provide care based on clinical guidelines, it is expected that in the future payment for health care will also be tied to clinical guidelines. This effort

will provide encouragement for care to be provided in the most cost-effective manner while ensuring that care is based on guidelines that reflect current research rather than traditional practice.

With the present efforts to improve the health care system in the United States and to provide universal health coverage while controlling costs, managed care has become a key model in health care reform. Nurses should take an active role in being part of the final plan and in creating opportunities for the profession to be a leader, not a follower, in the delivery of care (Hemphill and Biester, 1994).

ROLE OF THE PEDIATRIC NURSE

Therapeutic Relationship

The establishment of a therapeutic relationship is the essential foundation for providing quality nursing care (Price, 1993). Pediatric nurses need to be meaningfully related to children and their families and yet separate enough to distinguish their own feelings and needs. In a *therapeutic relationship,* caring, well-defined boundaries separate the nurse from the child and family. These boundaries are positive and professional, and promote the family's control over the child's health care (Barnsteiner and Gillis-Donovan, 1990). Both the nurse and the family are empowered, and open communication is maintained. In a *nontherapeutic relationship* these boundaries are blurred, and many of the nurse's actions may serve personal needs, such as a need to feel wanted and involved, rather than the family's needs.

Although relevant in all settings, a family-centered approach to nursing practice is most obvious in the home care arena. However, it is in the home care setting that nurses face the greatest challenge in determining the boundary between a collaborative relationship with the family and becoming part of the family system. Several factors challenge the maintenance of such clear boundaries: the informal home environment, the casual social conversations that occur with family members throughout the day, the participation by family members in care of the child, and the attempt by some families to reduce the stress of having a stranger in the home by incorporating the nurse as a member of the family.

Exploring whether relationships with patients are therapeutic or nontherapeutic can help nurses identify problem areas early in their interactions with children and families. Although questions for exploring types of involvement can be labeled negative or positive, no one action makes a relationship therapeutic or nontherapeutic. For example, nurses may spend additional time with the family but still recognize their own needs and maintain professional separateness. An important clue to nontherapeutic relationships is the staff's concerns about their peer's actions with the family.

Family Advocacy/Caring

Although the nurse is responsible to self, the profession, and the institution of employment, the primary responsibility is to the consumer of nursing services, the child and family. The nurse must work with members of the family, identifying *their* goals and needs, and plan interventions that best meet the defined problems. As an advocate, the nurse assists children and their families in making informed choices and acting in the child's best interest (Rushton, 1993). Advocacy involves

---

*Annette C. Bollig, MSN, RN, wrote this section.
†Caremap is a registered trademark of the Center for Case Management, Inc., South Natick, MA.
‡To order guidelines, contact AHCPR Publications Clearinghouse, PO Box 8547, Silver Spring, MD 20907; (800) 358-9295.

UNITED NATIONS' DECLARATION OF THE RIGHTS OF THE CHILD

All children need:
  To be free from discrimination
  To develop physically and mentally in freedom and dignity
  To have a name and nationality
  To have adequate nutrition, housing, recreation, and medical services
  To receive special treatment if handicapped
  To receive love, understanding, and material security
  To receive an education and develop his or her abilities
  To be the first to receive protection in disaster
  To be protected from neglect, cruelty, and exploitation
  To be brought up in a spirit of friendship among people

ensuring that families are aware of all available health services, informed adequately of treatments and procedures, involved in the child's care, and encouraged to change or support existing health care practices. The United Nations Declaration of the Rights of the Child (see box above) provides guidelines for nursing practice to ensure that every child receives optimum care. The nurse uses this knowledge to adapt care for the child's optimum physical and emotional well-being.

As nurses care for children and families, they must demonstrate *caring,* expressing compassion and empathy for others. Aspects of caring embody the concept of atraumatic care and the development of a therapeutic relationship with clients. Parents perceive caring as a sign of quality nursing care, which is often focused on the nontechnical needs of the child and family. Parents describe "personable" care as actions by the nurse, including acknowledging the parent's presence, listening, making the parent feel comfortable in the hospital environment, involving the parent and child in the nursing care, showing interest and concern for their welfare, showing affection and sensitivity to the parent and child, communicating with them, and individualizing the nursing care. Parents perceive "personable" nursing care as being integral to establishing a positive relationship (Price, 1993).

The nurse is aware of the needs of children and works with all caregivers to ensure that these fundamental requirements are met. This often necessitates that the nurse expand the boundaries of practice to less traditional settings. The nurse may be involved in education, political/legislative change, rehabilitation, screening, administration, and even engineering and architecture. Regardless of how removed from direct patient care individual nurses become, they continue to foster health care practices that promote the well-being of children by incorporating knowledge of child growth and development into particular roles of practice. For example, as an educator the nurse has the primary responsibility of helping others learn about and care for children. Their audience may be other nurses, parents, schoolteachers, other members of the health team, or the general public. In some states nurses are involved in mass media programs for immunization of all children.

Disease Prevention/Health Promotion

The trends toward health care have been prevention of illness and maintenance of health, rather than treatment of disease or disability. Nursing has kept pace with this change, especially in the area of child care. In 1965 specialized *pediatric nurse practitioner (PNP)* programs began to develop that have led to several specialized ambulatory or primary care roles for nurses. The thrust of these programs has been to educate nurses beyond the basic preparational stage in areas of child health maintenance so that all children can receive high-quality care (Lancaster and Lancaster, 1993). The practitioner programs have expanded to prepare school nurse, developmental, and oncology pediatric nurse practitioners. Although the curriculum varies, the course content generally includes history taking, physical diagnosis, growth and development, health education, pharmacology, counseling, common childhood problems, and planning care for individuals and groups. Most of these programs are now part of graduate nursing education.

The *clinical nurse specialist (CNS)* role has been developed in an attempt to provide expert nursing care. In addition, the CNS serves as a role model for the staff's clinical practice, as a researcher to validate nursing observations and interventions, as a change agent within the health care system, and as a consultant/teacher to the health care team (Naylor and Brooten, 1993). The clinical specialist is competent in providing nursing care during all stages of illness or wellness and functions in any of the settings where patients may be found—the hospital, home, community, clinic, or long-term facility. The CNS role has developed within each of the traditional specialty areas and includes subspecialties, such as cardiovascular, oncologic, and neurologic pediatric CNS. The educational preparation includes a graduate degree in nursing. Several graduate programs now combine the PNP and CNS roles. Although the title for the merged roles varies, these nurses are commonly called *advanced nurse practitioners (ANP or ARNP)* (Jackson, 1995).

Every nurse involved with child care must practice preventive health. Regardless of the identified problem, the role of the nurse is to plan care that fosters every aspect of growth and development. Based on a thorough assessment process, problems related to nutrition, immunizations, safety, dental care, development, socialization, discipline, or schooling frequently become obvious. Once the problem is identified, the nurse acts to intervene directly or to refer the family to other health persons or agencies.

The best approach to prevention is education and anticipatory guidance. In this book each chapter on health promotion includes sections on anticipatory guidance. An appreciation of the hazards or conflicts of each developmental period enables the nurse to guide parents regarding childrearing practices aimed at preventing potential problems. One of the most significant examples is safety. Because each age-group is at risk for special types of injuries, preventive teaching can help prevent most injuries, thus significantly lowering permanent disability and mortality from injuries in children.

Prevention also involves less obvious aspects of child care. Besides preventing physical disease or injury, the nurse's role is also to promote mental health. For example, it is not sufficient to administer immunizations without regard for the psychologic trauma associated with the procedure. Optimum health involves the practice of good medicine with a humane approach to health care; the nurse is often the one professional capable of ensuring "humanity."

Health Teaching

Health teaching is inseparable from family advocacy and prevention. Health teaching may be a direct goal of the nurse, such as during parenting classes, or may be indirect, such as helping parents and children understand a diagnosis or medical treatment, encouraging children to ask questions about their bodies, referring families to health-related professional or lay groups, supplying patients with appropriate literature, and providing anticipatory guidance.

Health teaching is often one area in which nurses need preparation and practice with competent role models, because it involves transmitting information at the child and family's level of understanding and desire for information. As an effective educator, the nurse focuses on giving appropriate health teaching with generous feedback and evaluation to promote learning.

Support/Counseling

Attention to emotional needs requires support and sometimes counseling. Frequently the role of child advocate or health teacher is supportive by the very nature of the individualized approach. Support can be offered in many ways, the most common of which include listening, touching, and physical presence. The last two are most helpful with children because they facilitate nonverbal communication.

Counseling involves a mutual exchange of ideas and opinions that provides the basis for mutual problem solving. It involves support, as well as teaching, techniques to foster expression of feelings or thoughts, and approaches to help the family cope with stress. Optimally, counseling not only helps to resolve a crisis or problem but also enables the family to attain a higher level of functioning, greater self-esteem, and closer relationships. Although counseling is often the role of nurses in more specialized areas, counseling techniques are discussed in various sections of this text to help students and nurses cope with immediate crises and refer families for additional professional assistance.

Restorative Role

The most basic of all nursing roles is the restoration of health through caregiving activities. Nurses are intimately involved with meeting the physical and emotional needs of children, including feeding, bathing, toileting, dressing, security, and socialization. Although they are responsible for instituting physicians' orders, they are also held singularly accountable for their own actions and judgments regardless of written orders.

A significant aspect of restoration of health is continual assessment and evaluation of physical status. Indeed, the concentrated focus throughout the text on physical assessment, pathophysiology, and scientific rationale for therapy is to assist the nurse in decision making regarding health status. The nurse must be aware of normal findings in order to identify and document deviations intelligently. In addition, the pediatric nurse never loses sight of the emotional and developmental needs of the individual child, which can significantly influence the course of the disease process.

Coordination/Collaboration

The nurse, as a member of the health team, collaborates and coordinates nursing services with the activities of other professionals. Working in isolation does not serve the child's best interest. First, the concept of "holistic care" can only be realized through a unified interdisciplinary approach. Second, being aware of individual contributions and limitations to the child's care, the nurse must collaborate with other specialists to provide for high-quality health services. Failure to recognize limitations can be nontherapeutic at best and destructive at worst. For example, the nurse who feels competent in counseling but who is really inadequate in this area may not only prevent the child from dealing with a crisis but may also impede future success with a qualified professional.

Even nurses who practice in isolated geographic areas widely separated from other health professionals cannot be considered independent. Every nurse works interdependently with the child and family, collaborating on needs and interventions so that the final care plan is one that truly meets the child's needs. Unfortunately, this is one aspect of collaboration and coordination that is lacking in health care planning. Often numerous disciplines work together to formulate a comprehensive approach without consulting with clients regarding their ideas or preferences. The nurse is in a vital position to include consumers in their care, either directly or indirectly, by communicating their thoughts to the health team.

Ethical Decision Making*

Ethical dilemmas arise when competing moral considerations underlie various alternatives. Parents, nurses, physicians, and other health care team members may reach different but morally defensible decisions by assigning different weight to the competing moral values. These competing moral values may include *autonomy,* the patient's right to be self-governing; *nonmaleficence,* the obligation to minimize or prevent harm; *beneficence,* the obligation to promote the patient's well-being, and *justice,* the concept of fairness (Erlen and Burns, 1992). Thus nurses must determine the most beneficial or least harmful action within the framework of societal mores, professional practice standards, the law, institutional rules, religious traditions, the family's value system, and the nurse's personal values.

When ethical conflicts occur, nurses may experience conflicting loyalties to their profession, colleagues, patients and families, institutions, and society. Moreover, the nurse's role in ethical decision making can be ambiguous. A nurse may be obliged to carry out procedures based on physician orders or hospital policy that are inconsistent with the patient's best interest. At times, members of the health care team do not seek the nurse's input or involvement, leaving the nurse with incomplete information about the clinical situation or without a voice in decision making.

The role of nurses as members of the health care team justifies their participation in collaborative ethical decision making. Nurses routinely use a systematic problem-solving method known as the *nursing process,* to resolve clinical problems. Each decision requires the nurse to collect pertinent physiologic and psychosocial data, assess relevant values held by the patient and family, and incorporate those data into a plan of care. Each of these activities is a crucial component of ethical decision making.

---

*Cindy Hylton Rushton, PhD, RN, C, FAAN, wrote this section.

Furthermore, because nurses spend the most time directly caring for the child, they are in a unique position to provide insight about the patient's condition and response to therapy. In addition, they assist families in dealing with their grief and stress and often interpret information regarding the child's condition, prognosis, and treatment options to help families make informed decisions. Because of their relationship to families, nurses are often able to represent the child's and parents' values, beliefs, and preferences, thus serving as an important liaison for communication between the family and other health team members.

The nurse can also use the professional code of ethics for guidance. A code of ethics provides one with means for professional self-regulation. The Code for Nurses by the American Nurses' Association focuses on the nurse's accountability and responsibility to the client and emphasizes the nursing role as an independent professional role that upholds its own legal liability (see box).

Nurses must prepare themselves systematically for collaborative ethical decision making. This can be accomplished through formal coursework, continuing education, contemporary literature, and working to establish an environment conducive to ethical discourse. Moreover, nurses must be knowledgeable about mechanisms for dispute resolution, case review by ethics committees, procedural safeguards, state statutes, and case law.

Nurses may face ethical issues regarding patient care, such as the use of lifesaving measures for very-low-birth-weight newborns or the terminally ill child's right to refuse treatment. They may struggle with questions regarding truthfulness, balancing their rights and their responsibilities in caring for children with AIDS, whistle-blowing, or resource allocation. Throughout the text such dilemmas are addressed in boxes titled "Thinking Critically About . . ." The conflicting ethical arguments are presented to help nurses clarify their value judgments when confronted with similar sensitive issues.

Research

Practicing nurses should contribute to research because they are the individuals observing human responses to health and illness. Unfortunately, few nurses systematically record or analyze such observations. For example, pediatric nurses devise innovative methods to encourage children to comply with treatments. Only if these interventions are clinically evaluated and shared with other nurses, especially through publications, can a body of knowledge on nursing practice develop.

Research also implies a questioning of *why* something is effective and *if* there is a better approach. Evaluation is essential to the nursing process, and research is one of the best ways to accomplish this. Therefore nurses need to be more involved in research and in applying research findings to their practice. Throughout the text, research relevant to nursing of children and families is incorporated as appropriate and is also highlighted in the Thinking Critically About . . . boxes. Research findings are presented to encourage nurses to base their practice on theoretic foundations, not tradition.

Health Care Planning

Up to this point the nurse's role has been viewed through the nucleus of a family. However, the nursing role is far more extensive and includes the community or society as a whole. Traditionally nurses have been involved in public health care, either on a continuous or an episodic basis. Rarely, however, have nurses been involved in health care planning, especially on a political or legislative level. Their role must also involve the decision-making body of government. As the largest health care profession, nursing needs to have a voice, especially as family/consumer advocate. This does not mean that the nurse must hold public office. Rather, it suggests knowledge and awareness of community needs, interest in government formulation of bills, support of politicians to ensure passage (or rejection) of significant legislation, and active involvement in groups dedicated to the welfare of children, such as professional nursing societies, parent-teacher organizations, parent support groups, religious organizations, and voluntary organizations.

Health care planning involves not only providing new services but also promoting the highest quality of existing ones. Nursing needs to ensure the excellence of its own profession through each individual member, who practices according to the Code of Nurses and standards of practice. A *standard of practice* is the level of performance that is expected of a professional. Pediatric nurses are obligated to follow the Standards of Maternal-Child Health Nursing (see box on p. 16) and specific standards for their specialty, such as pediatric on-

CODE FOR NURSES

1. The nurse provides services with respect for human dignity and the uniqueness of the client unrestricted by considerations of social or economic status, personal attributes, or the nature of health problems.
2. The nurse safeguards the client's right to privacy by judiciously protecting information of a confidential nature.
3. The nurse acts to safeguard the client and the public when health care and safety are affected by the incompetent, unethical, or illegal practice of any person.
4. The nurse assumes responsibility and accountability for individual nursing judgments and actions.
5. The nurse maintains competence in nursing.
6. The nurse exercises informed judgment and uses individual competence and qualifications as criteria in seeking consultation, accepting responsibilities, and delegating nursing activities to others
7. The nurse participates in activities that contribute to the ongoing development of the profession's body of knowledge.
8. The nurse participates in the profession's efforts to implement and improve standards of nursing.
9. The nurse participates in the profession's efforts to establish and maintain conditions of employment conducive to high-quality nursing care.
10. The nurse participates in the profession's effort to protect the public from misinformation and misrepresentation and to maintain the integrity of nursing.
11. The nurse collaborates with members of the health professions and other citizens in promoting community and national efforts to meet the health needs of the public.

American Nurses' Association, 1976, 1985. Reproduced with permission of the American Nurses' Association.

AMERICAN NURSES' ASSOCIATION STANDARDS OF MATERNAL AND CHILD HEALTH NURSING PRACTICE

Standard I: The nurse helps children and parents attain and maintain optimum health.

Standard II: The nurse assists families to achieve and maintain a balance between the personal growth needs of individual family members and optimum family functioning.

Standard III: The nurse intervenes with vulnerable clients and families at risk to prevent potential developmental and health problems.

Standard IV: The nurse promotes an environment free of hazards to reproduction, growth and development, wellness, and recovery from illness.

Standard V: The nurse detects changes in health status and deviations from optimum development.

Standard VI: The nurse carries out appropriate interventions and treatment to facilitate survival and recovery from illness.

Standard VII: The nurse assists clients and families to understand and cope with developmental and traumatic situations during illness, childbearing, childrearing, and childhood.

Standard VIII: The nurse actively pursues strategies to enhance access to and utilization of adequate health care services.

Standard IX: The nurse improves maternal and child health nursing practice through evaluation of practice, education, and research.

From American Nurses' Association: *Standards of Maternal and Child Health Nursing Practice,* Washington, DC, 1983, The Association. (As of this writing, unrevised and out of print.)

cology nursing or school nursing.* They should also be involved in making certain their colleagues implement the standards, through education, role modeling, and supervision.

Throughout the text the highest standards of nursing practice are continually reflected in the emphasis on thorough assessment, focus on scientific rationale as the basis for care, summary of nursing care goals and responsibilities, and comprehensive discussion of growth and development. Family-centered principles are continually evident in the consideration of dynamics affecting the child, parents, siblings, and extended members. The nurse is viewed as a vital component of the health care delivery system. Although nursing functions are clearly outlined, nursing responsibilities must be equally emphasized.

FUTURE TRENDS

The present shift in focus from treatment of disease to promotion of health is likely to further expand nurses' roles in ambulatory care, with prevention and health teaching receiving a major emphasis. As prospective payment becomes a certainty in pediatric care, the need for home care and commu-

---

*Available from the **Association of Pediatric Oncology Nurses,** 4700 W. Lake Avenue, Glenview, IL 60025-1485, (708) 375-4700, fax (708) 375-4777; and the **National Association of School Nurses,** Lamplighter Lane, PO Box 1300, Scarborough, ME 04074, (207) 883-2117.

nity health services will necessitate that nurses become more independent and highly skilled beyond the traditional care settings. Both these trends are illustrated throughout the book, with increased emphasis on prevention through anticipatory guidance, child health and family assessment, and discharge planning and home care. For example, a separate chapter on home care emphasizes the expanding role of the nurse into the community. As changing social policy shapes the expanding health care arena, the focus of nursing care is no longer what we *do for* families, but rather what we *do with* them (Plotnick and Presler, 1996). Therefore the philosophy of family-centered care is no longer an option, but a mandate.

Technologic advances will also influence pediatric nurses' roles. Increasing technical skills related to patient care, as well as the demand for computer knowledge in the work setting, are inevitable future trends. As more positions are created in the health care system that do not require a nursing background, such as "patient care educator" and unlicensed assistive personnel, nurses will be required to continually update their knowledge and prove their unique contribution. *Unlicensed assistive personnel (UAP)* "are individuals who are trained to function in an assistive role to the registered professional nurse in the provision of [student] care activities as delegated by and under the supervision of the registered professional nurse" (American Nurses Association, 1994).

Nursing ALERT When the RN determines that someone who is not licensed to practice nursing can safely provide a selected nursing activity or task for a patient and delegates that activity to the individual, the RN remains responsible and accountable for the care provided.

Changing demographics will also impact pediatric nursing. Although the actual number of children under age 18 years will increase from 64.3 million in 1990 to an estimated 78 million in 2020, their relative importance in terms of proportion of the total population will decrease from 26% to 24%. In other words, the adult population is growing faster than the pediatric population. Accompanying this trend is a decrease in younger children and an increase in older children, as well as a decrease in the white population with an increase in minority groups. For example, white births are expected to decline in the 1990s, black births are projected to rise, and the largest increases will occur in Hispanic (70%) and Asian (50%) births (Guyer and others, 1995). Such changes will impact the delivery of health care, with problems of adolescents and minority groups taking on more significance. As the elderly make up a larger percentage of the population, health care dollars will be split between the youngest and the oldest groups, with shrinking resources having to meet the needs of both. Nurses will need to keep abreast of developments in adolescent medicine and continually adapt their care to the cultural milieu in which they practice. An ever-present challenge will be cost containment without sacrificing quality care.

KEY POINTS

- "Healthy People 2000" sets the health care objectives for the 1990s and focuses on prevention as the method of achieving its goals.
- Although the infant mortality rate in the United States is at an all-time low, the United States lags significantly behind most other developed countries.
- Birth weight is the leading determinant of neonatal death in developed countries.
- Injuries are the leading cause of death in children over age 1 year, with the majority being caused by motor vehicle injuries.
- Childhood morbidity encompasses acute illness, chronic disease, and disability.
- Eighty percent of childhood illness is attributable to infections, with respiratory tract infections occurring two to three times as often as all other illnesses combined.
- The "new morbidity," or "pediatric social illness," refers to behavioral, social, and educational problems that can significantly alter a child's health.
- The study of pediatrics began in the last half of the 1800s under the influence of Abraham Jacobi, who is referred to as the Father of Pediatrics.
- The work of Lillian Wald, a social reformer, has had far-reaching effects on child health and nursing. She started visiting nurse services in New York City and was instrumental in establishing the role of the first full-time school nurse.
- Primary nursing involves care and accountability by one nurse for a small patient population.
- The philosophy of family-centered care recognizes the family as the constant in a child's life and that service systems and personnel must support, respect, encourage, and enhance the strength and competence of the family.
- The pediatric nurse's roles include a therapeutic relationship, family advocacy, disease prevention/health promotion, health teaching, support-counseling, coordination/collaboration, ethical decision making, research, and health care planning.
- With the shift in focus from treatment of disease to promotion of health, nurses' roles may expand in ambulatory care, with emphasis on prevention and health teaching.
- Changing demographics will result in greater significance of adolescents' and minority groups' problems and decreasing resources for health care.

REFERENCES

Ahmann E: Family-centered care: the time has come, *Pediatr Nurs* 20(1):52-53, 1994.

American Academy of Pediatrics, Committee on Early Childhood, Adoption and Dependent Care: Initial medical evaluation of an adopted child, *Pediatrics* 88(3):642-644, 1991.

American Academy of Pediatrics, Committee on Injury and Poison Prevention: Bicycle helmets, *Pediatrics* 95(4):609-610, 1995.

American Academy of Pediatrics, Committee on Psychosocial Aspects of Child and Family Health: The pediatrician and the "new morbidity," *Pediatrics* 92(5):731-733, 1993.

American Nurses Association: *Nursing's social policy statement,* Washington, DC, 1995, American Nurses Publishing.

American Nurses Association: *Registered professional nurses and unlicensed assistive personnel,* Washington, DC, 1994, American Nurses Publishing.

Barnsteiner J, Gillis-Donovan J: Being related and separate: a standard for therapeutic relationships, *MCN* 15(4):223-228, 1990.

Child health USA '94, Washington, DC, US Department of Health and Human Services, Public Health Service, Health Resources and Services Administration, Maternal and Child Health Bureau, DHHS, Pub No HRSA-MCH-95-1, July 1995.

Christoffel K and others: Psychosocial factors in childhood pedestrian injury: a matched case-control study, *Pediatrics* 97(1):33-42, 1996.

Cone TE Jr: Highlights of two centuries of American pediatrics, 1776-1976, *Am J Dis Child* 130:762-775, 1976.

Curley M: Effects of the nursing mutual participation model of care on parental stress in the pediatric intensive care unit, *Heart Lung* 17(6):682-688, 1988.

Curley M, Wallace J: Effects of the Nursing Mutual Participation Model of Care on parental stress in the pediatric intensive care unit—a replication, *Pediatr Nurs* 7(6):377-385, 1992.

Division of Injury Control, Center for Environmental Health and Injury Control, Centers for Disease Control: Childhood injuries in the United States, *Am J Dis Child* 144(6):627-646, 1990.

Dunst C, Trivette C, Deal A: *Enabling and empowering families,* Cambridge, MA, 1988, Brookline Books.

Erlen JA, Burns JA: Demystifying ethical decision making, *Orthop Nurs* 11(1):49-53, 1992.

Flint NS, Walsh M: Visiting policies in pediatrics: parents' perceptions and preferences, *J Pediatr Nurs* 3(4):237-246, 1988.

Gortmaker S and others: Chronic conditions, socioeconomic risks, and behavioral problems in children and adolescents, *Pediatrics* 85(3):267-276, 1990.

Guyer B and others: Annual summary of vital statistics—1994, *Pediatrics* 96(6):1029-1039, 1995.

Healthy people 2000—national health promotion and disease prevention objectives, GPO 017-001-00474-0, Washington, DC, 1991, US Public Health Service.

Hemphill NP, Biester DJ: Case management in a reformed health care system, *J Pediatr Nurs* 9(2):124-125, 1994.

Hostler S: Personal communication. Cited in Johnson BH, Jeppson ES, Redburn L: *Caring for children and families: guidelines for hospitals,* Bethesda, MD, 1992, Association for the Care of Children's Health.

Jackson PL: Opportunities and challenges for pediatric nurse practitioners, *Pediatr Nurs* 21(1):43-46, 1995.

Johnson BH, Jeppson ES, Redburn L: *Caring for children and families: guidelines for hospitals,* Bethesda, MD, 1992, Association for the Care of Children's Health.

Johnson BH, McGonigel M, Kaufmann R, eds: *Guidelines and recommended practices for the Individualized Family Service Plan,* Washington, DC, 1989, Association for the Care of Children's Health.

Khoury MJ, Erickson JD: Improved ascertainment of cardiovascular malformations in infants with Down's syndrome, Atlanta, 1968 through 1989: implications for the interpretation of increasing rates of cardiovascular malformations in surveillance systems, *Am J Epidemiol* 136(12):1457-1464, 1992.

Kochanek KD, Hudson BL: *Advance report of final mortality statistics: 1992.* Monthly vital statistics report 43(6), suppl, Hyattsville, MD, 1995, National Center for Health Statistics.

Lancaster J, Lancaster W: Nurse practitioners: health care providers whose time has come, *Fam Community Health* 16(2):1-8, 1993.

Mason JO, McGinnis JM: Healthy people 2000: an overview of the national health promotion and disease prevention objectives, *Public Health Rep* 105(5):441-446, 1990.

Mili F and others: Prevalence of birth defects among low–birth-weight infants, *Am J Dis Child* 145(11):1313-1318, 1991.

Naeye RL: Race and infant mortality, *Am J Dis Child* 147(10):1030-1031, 1993.

Nakamura RM and others: Excess infant mortality in an American Indian population, 1940-1990, *JAMA* 266(16):2244-2248, 1991.

Naylor MD, Brooten D: The roles and functions of clinical nurse specialists, *Image J Nurs Sch* 25(1):73-78, 1993.

Nursing: a social policy statement, Kansas City, MO, 1980, American Nurses' Association.

Pless I: *Morbidity and mortality among the young.* In Hoekelman RA and others, editors: *Primary pediatric care,* ed 2, St Louis, 1992, Mosby.

Plotnick J, Presler B: Rugged individualism and compassion: the foundation of public policy, *MCN* 21(1):20-33, 1996.

Price PJ: Parents' perceptions of the meaning of quality nursing care, *Adv Nurs Sci* 16(1):33-41, 1993.

Rachuba L, Stanton B, Howard D: Violent crime in the United States, *Arch Pediatr Adolesc Med* 149(9):953-960, 1995.

Rushton CH: Child/family advocacy: ethical issues, practical strategies, *Crit Care Med* 21(9):S387, 1993.

Schmidt WM: Health and welfare of colonial American children, *Am J Dis Child* 130:694-701, 1976.

Schoendorf KC and others: Mortality among infants of black as compared with white college-educated parents, *N Engl J Med* 326(23):1522-1526, 1992.

Swartz MK: The handgun as a consumer product, *J Pediatr Health Care* 8(6):288-290, 1994.

Thompson DG: Critical pathways in the intensive care and intermediate care nurseries, *MCN* 19(1):29-32, 1994.

Thompson R, Rivara F, Thompson D: A case-control study of the effectiveness of bicycle safety helmets, *N Engl J Med* 320:1361-1367, 1989.

Wegman ME: Annual summary of vital statistics—1993, *Pediatrics* 94(6):792-803, 1994.

Weinstein R: Hospital case management: the path to empowering nurses, *Pediatr Nurs* 17(3):289-293, 1991.

Wilcox AJ, Skjaerven R: Birth weight and perinatal mortality: the effect of gestational age, *Am J Public Health* 82(3):378-382, 1992.

Wong D: *Principles of atraumatic care.* In Feeg V, editor: *Pediatric nursing: forum on the future: looking toward the 21st century,* Pitman, NJ, 1989, Anthony J Jannetti.

BIBLIOGRAPHY

Mortality and Morbidity

Bass JL and others: Childhood injury prevention counseling in primary care settings: a critical review of the literature, *Pediatrics* 92(4):544-550, 1993.

Blum RW and others: American Indian—Alaska native youth health, *JAMA* 267(12):1637-1644, 1992.

Dannenberg AL, Vernick JS: A proposal for the mandatory inclusion of helmets with new children's bicycles, *Am J Public Health* 83(5):644-646, 1993.

Fingerhut LA, Jones C, Makuc D: *Firearm and motor vehicle injury mortality—variations by state, race, and ethnicity: United States, 1990-91,* Advance data from vital and health statistics, No 242, Hyattsville, MD, 1994, National Center for Health Statistics.

Hall JR and others: Traumatic death in urban children, revisited, *Am J Dis Child* 147(1):102-107, 1993.

Igoe JB: Healthy people 2000, *Pediatr Nurs* 16(6):584-586, 1990.

Jones NE: Childhood injuries: an epidemiologic approach, *Pediatr Nurs* 18(3):235-239, 1992.

Jones NE: Childhood residential injuries, *MCN* 18(3):168-172, 1993.

Kliegman RM: Perpetual poverty: child health and the underclass, *Pediatrics* 89(4):710-713, 1992.

Lenaghan P: Healthy people 2000, *J Emerg Nurs* 18(5):480-481, 1992.

Mandelbaum JL: Child survival: what are the issues? *J Pediatr Health Care* 6(3):132-137, 1992.

Sewell KH, Gaines SK: A developmental approach to childhood safety education, *Pediatr Nurs* 19(5):464-466, 1993.

Society of Pediatric Nurses (SPN): Policy statement on pediatric firearm injuries, *SPN News* 4(1):7, 1995.

Society of Pediatric Nurses (SPN): Policy statement on pediatric injury prevention, *SPN News* 4(1):6, 1995.

Yanhauer A: A classic study of infant mortality—1911-1915, *Pediatrics* 94(6):874-877, 1994.

Zadinsky JK, Boettcher JH: Preventability of infant mortality in a rural community, *Nurs Res* 41(4):223-227, 1992.

Evolution of Child Health Care

Arnold L and others: Lessons from the past, *MCN* 14(2):75-82, 1989.

Burns M, Thornam CB: Broadening the scope of nursing practice: federal programs for children, *Pediatr Nurs* 19(6):546-552, 1993.

Cone TE, Jr: *History of American pediatrics,* Boston, 1980, Little, Brown.

DeGraw C and others: Public law 99-457: new opportunities to serve young children with special needs, *J Pediatr* 113(6):971-974, 1988.

Farel A: Public health in early intervention: historic foundations for contemporary training, *Inf Young Child* 1(1):63-70, 1988.

Gale C: Inadequacy of health care for the nation's chronically ill children, *J Pediatr Health Care* 3(1):20-27, 1989.

Harvey B: New series of essays on pediatric history, *Pediatrics* 92(3):467-468, 1993.

Inglis AD: United States maternal and child health services, *Neonatal Network* 9(8):35-43, 1991.

Kilmon C, Poteet G: Child care needs of nursing personnel: the challenge for the future, *Pediatr Nurs* 6(3):369-374, 1988.

McMillan JA: What we must do for children in the 1990s, *Contemp Pediatr* 7(7):28-50, 1990.

Murphy M: What price success: can we afford "saved" babies? *J Pediatr Health Care* 3(6):285-286, 1989.

Oberg C: Medically uninsured children in the United States: a challenge to public policy, *Pediatrics* 85(5):824-833, 1990.

Velsor-Friedrich B: The federal government and child health, *J Pediatr Nurs* 5(1):56-58, 1990.

Williams BC, Miller CA: Preventive health care for young children: findings from a 10-country study and directions for United States policy, *Pediatrics* 89(5, suppl):983-998, 1992.

Pediatric Nursing

Barnsteiner JH and others: Defining and implementing a standard for therapeutic relationships, *J Holistic Nurs* 12(1):35-48, 1994.

Bell PL: Neonatal case management: a challenge for advanced practice nurses, *J Perinat Neonatal Nurs* 8(2):48-56, 1994.

Betz CL: Will nursing education respond to the changes in health care?, *J Pediatr Nurs* 10(2):81, 1995.

Bottorff JL: Nursing: a practice science of caring, *Adv Nurs Sci* 14(1):26-39, 1991.

Broome ME: A commentary on confronting the challenges, *Pediatr Nurs* 21(1):49-50, 1995.

Clochesy JM and others: Preparing advanced practice nurses for acute care, *Am J Crit Care* 3(4):255-259, 1994.

Delegation of school health services to unlicensed assistive personnel: A position paper of the National Association of State School Nurse Consultants, *J School Nurs* 11(4):13-16, 1995.

El-Sherif C: Nurse practitioners—where do they belong within the organizational structure of the acute care setting? *Nurs Pract* 20(1):62-65, 1995.

Engleman SG: From myths to a critical path: what happens when someone asks why? *J Pediatr Nurs* 10(1):69-71, 1995.

Feeg VD: The future of pediatric nursing: anticipating the health care needs of children, *Imprint* 37(4):70-77, 1990.

Fein EZ: Keeping expert nurses expert, *MCN* 19(6):305-308, 1994.

Fenton M, Brykezynski K: Qualitative distinctions and similarities in the practice of clinical nurse specialists and nurse practitioners, *J Profess Nurs* 9:313-326, 1993.

Fry-Revere S: Ethics consultation: an update on accountability issues, *Neonatal Intens Care* 7(4):58-64, 1994.

Harper DC: Advanced practice nursing: changes on the horizon, *Pediatr Nurs* 21(1):41-42, 1995.

Hinds PS: Crossing the lines of professionalism, *J Pediatr Oncol Nurs* 11(4):137, 1994.

Hylton Rushton C, Armstrong L, McEnhill M: Establishing therapeutic boundaries as patient advocates, *Pediatr Nurs* 22(3):185-189, 1996.

Jerome JM, Ferraro-McDuffie AR: Nurse self-awareness in therapeutic relationships, *Pediatr Nurs* 18(2):153-156, 1992.

Keefe MR: An integrated approach to incorporating research findings into practice, *MCN* 18(2):65-70, 1993.

Kolcaba KY: The art of comfort care, *Image J Nurs Sch* 27(4):287-289, 1995.

Kowalski K and others: The high-touch paradigm: a 21st-century model for maternal-child nursing, *MCN* 21(1):43-50, 1996.

McAliley LG and others: Therapeutic relations decision making: the rainbow framework, *Pediatr Nurs* 22(3):199-203, 210.

Miltenberger-Olsen G: *I am a nurse: a historical perspective,* Bixby, OK, 1995, Angel Wings Publishing.

Naylor M, Brooten D: The roles and functions of clinical nurse specialists, *Image J Nurs Sch* 25:73-78, 1993.

Pearson L: Annual update of how each state stands on legislative issues affecting advanced nursing practice, *Nurs Pract* 20(1):13-18, 1995.

Rushton CH, Infante MD: Keeping secrets: the ethical and legal challenges, *Pediatr Nurs* 21(5):479-482, 1995.

Shelton T, Stepanek J: *Family-centered care for children needing specialized health and developmental services,* Bethesda, MD, 1994, Association for the Care of Children's Health.

Totka JP: Exploring the boundaries of pediatric practice: nurse stories related to relationships, *Pediatr Nurs* 22(3):191-196, 1996.

Winslow EH: How patients define caring may surprise you, *Am J Nurs* 94(6):57-58, 1994.

Case Management

Crummette BD, Boatwright DN: Case management in inpatient pediatric nursing, *Pediatr Nurs* 17(5):469-73, 1991.

Davis B, Steele S: Case management for young children with special health care needs, *Pediatr Nurs* 17(1):15-20, 1991.

Elizondo AP: Nursing case management in the neonatal intensive care unit, Part 2: developing critical pathways, *Neonatal Network* 14(1):11-19, 1995.

Kaufman J: Case management services for children with special health care needs: a family-centered approach, *J Case Manag* 1(2):53-56, 1992.

Lewis CC and others: Care management for children who are medically fragile/technology-dependent, *Issues Compreh Pediatr Nurs* 15(2):73-91, 1992.

Lynam L: Case management and critical pathways: friend or foe? *Neonatal Network* 13(8):48-49, 1994.

Patterson J: The role of the nurse manager in a case management delivery system, *Pediatr Nurs* 17(3):282, 1991.

Smith LD: Continuity of care through nursing case management of the chronically ill child, *Clin Nurs Specialist* 8(2):65-68, 1994.

Steele S: Nurse and parent collaborative case management in a rural setting, *Pediatr Nurs* 19(6):612-615, 1993.

NURSING PROCESS IN CARE OF THE CHILD AND FAMILY

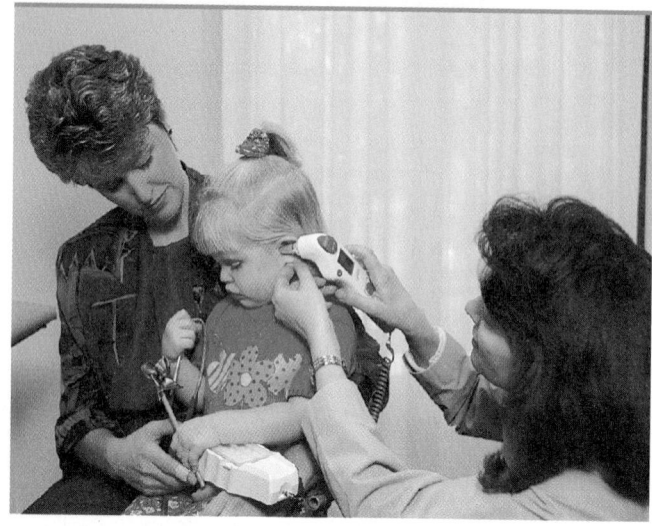

" $\mathcal{N}$ o procedure is so routine that critical thinking is not necessary to interpret the results. "

Donna L. Wong, author

RELATED TOPICS

LEARNING OBJECTIVES
On completion of this chapter the reader will be able to:

- Define critical thinking
- List the five steps of the nursing process
- Differentiate among different types of assessment: comprehensive, screening, and focused

- Define nursing diagnosis
- Differentiate among three domains of nursing practice: dependent, independent, and interdependent

- Describe the five steps in developing a goal/outcome
- Differentiate standard nursing care plan from individualized care plan

CRITICAL THINKING AND NURSING PROCESS*

A systematic thought process is essential to a profession. It assists the professional in meeting the needs of the client. Critical thinking is purposeful, goal-directed thinking that assists individuals to make judgments based on evidence rather than guesswork (Alfaro-LeFevre, 1995). It is based on the scientific method of inquiry, in which the nursing process also has its roots. Critical thinking and nursing process are considered crucial to professional nursing in that they comprise a holistic approach to problem solving.

Critical thinking is a complex developmental process based on rational and deliberate thought. Becoming a critical thinker provides a common denominator for knowledge that exemplifies disciplined and self-directed thinking. The knowledge is acquired, assessed, and organized by thinking. The cognitive skills used in high-quality thinking require intellectual discipline, self-evaluation, counter thinking, opposition, challenge, and support (Paul, 1993). Critical thinking transforms the ways in which individuals view themselves, understand the world, and make decisions (Chaffee, 1994).

Crucial dimensions of critical thought include the perfections of thought, the elements of thought, and the domains of thought. A logical connection develops between the elements and the problem at hand when thinking is clear, precise, accurate, relevant, consistent, and fair. Self-evaluation questions that enhance the development of critical thinking are listed in the box to the right (Paul, 1993).

In recognition of the importance of this skill, Critical Thinking Exercises have been added to this text. These exercises present a situation and the student is asked to use the skills of critical thinking to come to the best conclusion.

Christina Algiere Kasprisin, MS, RN, wrote this chapter.
*Pam DiVito-Thomas, MS, RN, wrote this section.

> ## CRITICAL THINKING SELF-EVALUATION QUESTIONS
>
> - What is the purpose of my thinking?
> - What precise questions am I trying to answer?
> - Within what point of view am I thinking?
> - What information am I using?
> - How am I interpreting that information?
> - What concepts or ideas are central to my thinking?
> - What conclusions am I coming to?
> - What am I taking for granted, what assumptions am I making?
> - If I accept the conclusions, what are the implications?
> - What would the consequences be if I put my thoughts into action?
>
> From Paul, R: *Critical thinking: what every person needs to survive in a rapidly changing world,* Rohnert Park, CA, 1993, Foundation for Critical Thinking.

The nursing process is the framework for the practice of professional nursing. It is a method of problem identification and problem solving that describes what the nurse actually does. The five-step model that is accepted as the nursing process is as follows: assessment, diagnosis (problem identification), planning (with outcome development), implementation, and evaluation. The second step of the nursing process, nursing diagnosis, is the naming of the child/family's problem in common nursing language. The American Nurses Association (ANA) has established Standards for Practice (use of the nursing process) and Standards of Professional Performance (professional behavior) (see box). In the Standards of Care the nursing diagnosis phase of the nursing process is separated into two steps: the nursing diagnosis and outcome identification. This model represents a six-step process. The **North American Nursing Diagnosis Association**

AMERICAN NURSES ASSOCIATION STANDARDS FOR PRACTICE

Standards of Care (Use of the Nursing Process)

Standard		
	I	**Assessment:** The nurse collects client health data.
	II	**Diagnosis:** The nurse analyzes assessment data in determining diagnoses.
	III	**Outcome Identification:** The nurse identifies expected outcomes individualized to the client.
	IV	**Planning:** The nurse develops a plan of care that prescribes interventions to attain expected outcomes.
	V	**Implementation:** The nurse implements the interventions identified in the plan of care.
	VI	**Evaluation:** The nurse evaluates the client's progress toward attainment of outcomes.

Standards of Professional Performance (Professional Behavior)

Standard		
	I	**Quality of Care:** The nurse systematically evaluates the quality and effectiveness of nursing practice.
	II	**Performance Appraisal:** The nurse evaluates his/her own nursing practice in relation to professional practice standards and relevant statutes and regulations.
	III	**Education:** The nurse acquires and maintains current knowledge in nursing practice.
	IV	**Collegiality:** The nurse contributes to the professional development of peers, colleagues, and others.
	V	**Ethics:** The nurse's decisions and actions on behalf of clients are determined in an ethical manner.
	VI	**Collaboration:** The nurse collaborates with the client, significant others, and health care providers in providing client care.
	VII	**Research:** The nurse uses research findings in practice.
	VIII	**Resource Utilization:** The nurse considers factors related to safety, effectiveness, and cost in planning and delivering client care.

From *Standards of Clinical Nursing Practice,* Washington, DC, 1991, American Nurses Association.

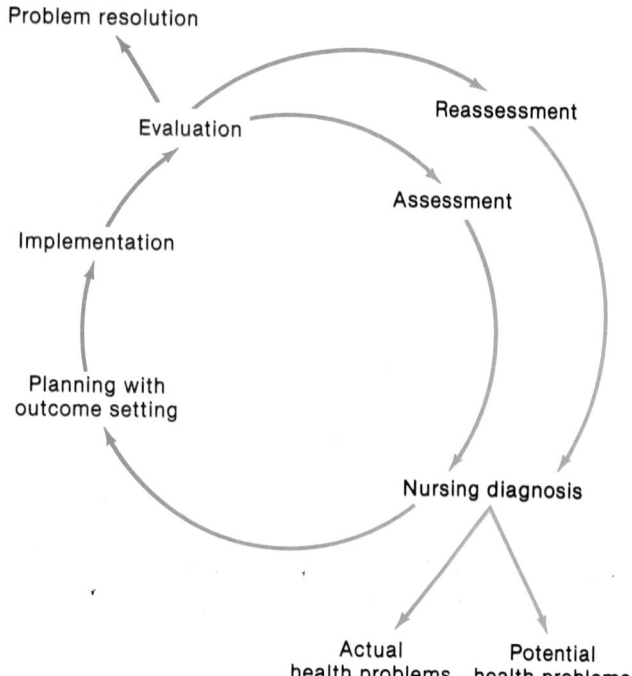

FIG. 2-1. Stages of the nursing process.

(NANDA)* is responsible for the clinical testing and approval of proposed nursing diagnoses.

The nursing process can be envisioned as a continuous cycle. The nurse continually assesses both the child and the family. The data gathered must be compared with the expected information. The nurse then proceeds with the plan of care or modifies it accordingly. When evaluation is performed, patient status is reassessed and a new cycle begins (Fig. 2-1). In pediatric nursing the nurse must be alert to specific nursing diagnoses for the child as well as for the family. In some instances the only problems identified may be those that apply to family members rather than to the pediatric patient. Such diagnoses include alterations in family process and in parenting. Consequently the family unit must always be viewed as the patient. However, in the nursing of adults, family members may be less directly involved in the patient's care.

ASSESSMENT

Nursing assessment is the foundation of the nursing process and the cornerstone of professional nursing practice. It is the deliberate and systematic collection of data from a variety of sources (see box above). All clients must be assessed from the physiologic, psychologic, cultural, spiritual, and environmental perspectives. This thorough assessment should be performed periodically on children and their families. The specific setting in which the nurse practices will influence how comprehensive the assessment will be, but all areas should be included (see also History Taking, Chapter 6). There are

*North American Nursing Diagnosis Association, 1211 Locust Street Philadelphia, PA 19107; (212)545-8105 or fax (215)545-8107.

SOURCES FOR DATA COLLECTION

Interview/health history:
  Child
  Family
  Significant individuals
Observation of social interactions
Developmental assessment
Physical assessment
Laboratory data
Consultation with other health professionals

---

three levels of assessment: comprehensive, screening, and focused.

A *comprehensive assessment* is one in which all areas are thoroughly assessed. When a comprehensive assessment is impractical or inappropriate, a *screening assessment* is indicated. This assessment supplies the data necessary to provide basic safe nursing care. For example, a screening assessment may be indicated for a newly admitted critically ill patient, because attention must be devoted to preserving and maintaining life. The comprehensive assessment can be deferred until the child's condition has stabilized. Another indication for screening is the ambulatory surgical patient who is comprehensively assessed by the referring health care provider before being admitted to the outpatient setting. If a suspected problem area is observed, an in-depth *focused assessment* for that area should be performed.

Most nurses find it helpful to base nursing process on a framework that facilitates the collection, organization, and use of data. That framework can be formatted in several different ways, and examples have included a systems approach focused on physiologic data, a format based on Maslow's hierarchy of needs, and assessments based on the work of nursing theorists such as Newman, Roy, and Orem. Regardless of the organizing framework, a nursing perspective must be used.

Both NANDA and Marjory Gordon (1995) have developed frameworks; NANDA bases its framework on 9 human response patterns, and Gordon bases hers on 11 functional health patterns (see box on p. 23 and Appendix G). In clinical practice the classification systems serve as a framework for organizing a nursing assessment and standardizing data collection. Additional research is needed to broaden the list of nursing diagnoses, especially for specialty areas such as pediatrics, and define a universally accepted taxonomy.

During the assessment period the nurse seeks information to describe and explain the strengths and difficulties of the child and family. The nurse must be able to communicate effectively with both the child and the family. Obtaining a complete assessment from a pediatric client presents numerous challenges. The very young child cannot answer questions and may not be able to localize signs and symptoms to aid in the physical examination. The older school-age child may be embarrassed and reluctant to give information with parents present. For these reasons the nurse must look for subtle changes in behavior that may indicate physical distress as well as the need for privacy. The preadolescent and adolescent should be interviewed both with and without the parents to

CLASSIFICATION SYSTEMS FOR NURSING DIAGNOSES

Human Response Patterns*

Exchanging—Mutual giving and receiving
Communicating—Sending messages
Relating—Establishing bonds
Valuing—The assigning of relative worth
Choosing—The selection of alternatives
Moving—Activity
Perceiving—The reception of information
Knowing—The meaning associated with information
Feeling—The subjective awareness of sensation or affect

Functional Health Patterns†

Health perception-health management pattern—Perceptions related to general health management and preventive practices
Nutritional-metabolic pattern—Intake of food and fluids related to metabolic requirements
Elimination pattern—Regularity and control of excretory functions, bowel, bladder, skin, and wastes
Activity-exercise pattern—Activity patterns that require energy expenditure and provide for rest
Sleep-rest pattern—Effectiveness of sleep and rest periods
Cognitive-perceptual pattern—Adequacy of language, cognitive skills, and perception related to required or desired activities; includes pain perception
Self-perception—Self-concept pattern—Beliefs and evaluation of self-worth
Role-relationship pattern—Family and social roles, especially parent-child relationships
Sexuality-reproductive pattern—Problems or potential problems with sexuality or reproduction
Coping-stress tolerance pattern—Stress tolerance level and coping patterns, including support systems
Value-belief pattern—Values, goals, or beliefs that influence health-related decisions and actions

*Modified from the North American Nursing Diagnosis Association: *Nursing diagnoses: definitions and classifications, 1995-1996,* Philadelphia, 1994, NANDA.
†Modified from Gordon M: *Manual of nursing diagnosis, 1995-1996,* St Louis, 1995, Mosby.

FORMULATING A NURSING DIAGNOSIS

Formulating a nursing diagnosis is the naming of a human response. It is a very client-centered, individualized process. Because the nursing diagnosis focuses on the response, often two individuals with the same medical diagnosis will have differing nursing diagnoses.

Both James T. and Brian L. are 16 years old and have eczema. James follows the medical regimen and in general is not affected by the appearance of his skin. In contrast, Brian, who also follows the medical regimen, is greatly distressed over his appearance. He is refusing to attend school and other events because of the eczema.

A possible nursing diagnosis for James might be—*impaired skin integrity related to lesions and inflammatory response.* His response to the eczema is to follow the plan of care. However, Brian is greatly bothered by the skin lesions. A potential diagnosis for Brian might be—*Impaired social interaction related to fear of embarrassment and negative reactions of others.*

NURSING DIAGNOSIS

Nursing diagnosis is a clinical judgment about individual, family, or community responses to actual or potential health problems/life processes. Nursing diagnosis provides the basis for selection of nursing interventions to achieve outcomes for which the nurse is accountable (NANDA, 1991). NANDA has identified three categories of nursing diagnoses: (1) actual, (2) high risk, and (3) wellness. As the second stage of the nursing process the nurse must now interpret and make decisions about the data gathered. The nurse then organizes or clusters the data into similar categories to identify significant areas.

Once the cues have been clustered, the nurse decides if a nursing diagnosis exists (see box above).

Nursing diagnoses do *not* describe everything that nursing does. Nursing practice consists of three dimensions: dependent, interdependent, and independent activities. The differences reside in the source of authority for the action (Hickey, 1990). *Dependent activities* are those areas of nursing practice that hold the nurse accountable for implementing the prescribed medical regimen. *Interdependent activities* are those areas of nursing practice in which medical and nursing responsibility and accountability overlap and require collaboration between the two disciplines. *Independent activities* are those areas of nursing practice that are the direct responsibility of the nurse. Nursing diagnoses should reflect the interdependent and independent dimensions of nursing (Fig. 2-2).

Collaborative problems (Carpenito, 1995) are patient issues that usually involve a collaborative approach to prevention, treatment, or intervention. Other disciplines, such as medicine, physical therapy, respiratory therapy, or nutritional therapy may be consulted. Often collaborative problems involve the structure and function of body organs and systems. By virtue of their education and training nurses are able to predict and prevent potential complications of many medical diagnoses.

determine the perspectives of all concerned. The teenager and the parent may have different opinions on how each is functioning. (For a detailed discussion of communication with parents and children, see Chapter 6.)

As the nurse proceeds through the assessment phase, combining interview skills with physical assessment, cues are identified. A *cue* is information that influences decisions. When a cue is given by the patient, the nurse can decide to collect additional information or to use the cue directly in diagnostic judgment. The initial nursing assessment is complete when (1) the nurse has baseline data about the child and family, (2) the health care needs are evaluated, (3) the areas that interfere with the child and family's functioning are identified, and (4) a statement is made about any problems that exist.

After the initial assessment is completed, all cues must be analyzed. The patient's response should be compared with the expected response considering cultural/ethnic and religious variables. Each piece of data should provide information relative to a judgment about the functioning of the client.

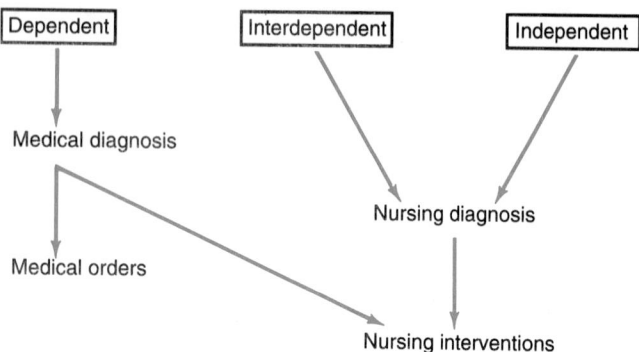

FIG. 2-2. Dimensions of professional nursing practice.

DIAGNOSTIC STATEMENT

The first part of the diagnostic statement for actual problems is the human response, how the individual responds to a state of illness or health. The etiology is the second part, which can be expressed as related or risk factors. Related factors identify the variables that contribute to the presence of the human response. These factors also direct the nursing interventions that will modify the response. Risk factors are items that are used to predispose an individual to an unhealthful event. Signs and symptoms may be used for the third part of the diagnostic statement usually preceded by the words "as evidenced by (aeb)" or separated by a "/".

Problem/Human Response

The nursing diagnosis is composed of three components: problem, etiology, and signs and symptoms (often referred to as **PES**). The first—the problem statement—describes the child's response to health pattern deficits in the child, family, or community. This is the patient's response to disturbances of life processes, patterns, functions, or development, including those occurring secondary to disease. This first portion of the diagnostic statement directs outcome development.

Not all children will have actual health problems. Some may have a potential health problem, which is a risk state requiring nursing intervention to prevent the development of an actual problem. Potential health problems indicate the presence of **risk factors** (signs indicating a potential health problem), which predispose a child and family to a dysfunctional health pattern and are limited to individuals at greater risk than the population as a whole. Intervention is directed toward reducing risk factors. To differentiate actual from potential health problems, the word *risk* is included in the nursing diagnosis statement (e.g., *Risk for infection*).

The statement of a nursing diagnosis may not be a "problem." The nurse may write a positive nursing diagnosis, such as a statement from the diagnostic categories noting that the patient has developed adaptive responses to a health problem that the nurse wishes to support or facilitate. *Anticipatory grieving* is an example of an adaptive response. *Dysfunctional grieving*, on the other hand, is a maladaptive response that the nurse would attempt to modify.

— *prolongd—goines into depression*

Etiology/Related or Contributing Factors

The second component of the PES format, the etiology, describes the physiologic, situational, and maturational factors that cause the problem or influence its development. The etiology may be behaviors of the patient, factors in the environment, or an interaction of both. The etiology is written using NANDA diagnostic categories (e.g., *Noncompliance related to powerlessness*). In using the PES format it is important that the nurse not link the problem statement and etiology with words that imply cause and effect. Etiologies are probable causes; using words that imply cause and effect can result in legal or professional difficulties. Although a direct cause-effect relationship may not be involved, the etiology does influence the problem. Therefore the phrase *related to* is used to indicate a relationship between the problem and its etiology.

Differentiating among various etiologies is critically important because *interventions to alter the health problem are directed toward the etiology*. This is a primary concept in understanding nursing diagnosis process and the PES format. For example, a problem statement of *Noncompliance in dietary restrictions* could have various etiologies, such as (1) knowledge deficit, (2) denial of illness, (3) low economic resources, or (4) cultural conflict. Interventions for a knowledge deficit would be very different from interventions for low economic resources.

Not only is differentiation between etiologies critically important, so is being *specific* about the etiology. For example, if the nursing diagnosis is *Noncompliance to dietary restrictions related to knowledge deficit,* the nurse might intervene in varying ways, depending on whether the knowledge deficit is associated with (1) an inability to read, (2) a lack of educational materials, or (3) a lack of practice in menu planning. When the etiology is a broad category such as knowledge deficit, the nurse must investigate further to clarify the origin of the etiology. If the knowledge deficit is an inability to read, then nonwritten patient education material may be needed. If the dietary alterations are complex, practice in menu planning may be necessary. For example, in one family with a child who had congestive heart failure, the origin of the knowledge deficit was an inability to plan meals that were low in sodium. The nursing interventions were directed at teaching the mother, as well as the grandmother (who cared for the child during the day), what foods to prepare and having them compile sample menus.

Although nursing interventions are directed at the etiology, the problem statement does *influence* interventions. For example, with the nursing diagnoses of *Social isolation related to impaired physical mobility, level 3,* and *Constipation related to impaired physical mobility, level 3,* the interventions are directed at the impaired mobility. However, the focus (or outcome) of mobilizing the patient is different. In the first nursing diagnosis, interventions address the movement of the patient into a social environment. Interventions for the second diagnosis address the need for more physical activity, a high-fiber diet, and increased fluids.

At times the etiology of the problem statement is unknown. The use of the term *unknown etiology* in the diagnostic statement alerts the nurse and other members of the nursing staff to perform further assessment for etiologic factors. The inclusion of signs and symptoms substantiates the identification of the problem (e.g., *Altered parenting related to unknown etiology: history of child abuse, delayed growth and development*). Just as the medical profession treats symptomatically for an unknown etiology, the nursing profession di-

rects care at the presenting signs and symptoms until an etiology is identified.

Signs and Symptoms/Defining Characteristics

The third component, signs and symptoms, refers to a cluster of cues and/or defining characteristics that are derived
from patient assessment and indicate actual health problems.
The defining characteristics are observable when the health
problem is present. When a defining characteristic is essential
for the diagnosis to be made, it is considered critical. These
critical defining characteristics help differentiate between diagnostic categories. For example, in deciding between the diagnostic categories related to family function and coping, the
defining characteristics are critical in choosing the most appropriate nursing diagnosis (see Family Focus box).

Defining characteristics are derived from initial and ongoing patient assessment and may be included in the signs and
symptoms to clarify problems and etiologies in the nursing
diagnosis. Signs and symptoms are usually documented with
assessment data and are not necessarily included in the nursing diagnosis statement. Signs and symptoms are included in
the nursing diagnosis statement only when needed for clarity, such as in the following example: *Ineffective individual
coping related to pain/refusing to move, apprehensive of anyone jarring bed, rapid pulse, irritable, improved behavior after analgesic administered.* The signs and symptoms clarify the
child's behavioral manifestations to the pain and the response
to pharmacologic intervention. This information is helpful in
directing nursing care; for example, it indicates that better
pain management is needed.

● ● ●

Throughout the text the nursing care plans incorporate
nursing diagnoses that relate to the specific condition or disorder. Because nursing diagnoses should only prescribe interventions that nurses can perform independently, nursing
interventions related to medical management are identified
by an asterisk.

PLANNING

Once the diagnoses and patient problems have been identified, a care plan is developed and ***expected outcomes*** (or goals)
are established, which are projected changes in a patient's
health status, clinical condition, or behavior that occur as a
result of nursing interventions. The ultimate objective of
nursing care is to convert the nursing diagnoses or clinical
problem into a desired health state. The goal or expected outcome must be established before the interventions can be developed.

Many factors are considered when the outcomes are developed. The outcome must be patient centered and individualized according to the capabilities and limitations of the
child and family. Unreasonable or unrealistic outcomes will
only ensure the care plan's failure. The ideal way to determine outcomes is in a conference with the family and child,
if appropriate, where all significant persons can agree on what
is to be done, learned, or experienced. The final test of the
projected outcome is that it must be observable and measurable, so that the care plan can be evaluated. The steps in
developing outcome statements are listed in the box on
p. 26.

FAMILY FOCUS
**Using Defining Characteristics
to Select an Appropriate
Nursing Diagnosis**

An 18-month-old only child is admitted with respiratory distress
and a presumptive diagnosis of epiglottitis. Initial nursing actions
are focused on the physiologic status of the child. As the condition stabilizes, family assessment data are gathered. The child's
immunizations are current, he is clean and well nourished, and
his developmental age is appropriate. The parents are present at
admission. Both are employed, and the child is cared for by the
maternal grandparents. The mother is distraught about the sudden onset of the respiratory distress. She states that earlier just
a "runny nose" was present. She asks appropriate questions and
seems to understand that epiglottitis is a sudden illness that typically follows symptoms of a cold. She asks what she can do to
make her child more comfortable and less fearful, and is able to
implement the suggestions. The father supports both the child
and the mother but assumes a more passive, "listening" role.

At least three nursing diagnoses that relate to family/parent
situations can be considered. The first step is to review the definition and defining characteristics for each and decide which is
most appropriate for this family:

Altered parenting—inability of nurturing figure to create an
environment that promotes optimum growth and develop-
ment of another human being
Selected defining characteristics:
Inattentive to infant/child needs
Inappropriate caretaking behaviors

Family coping: potential for growth—family member has
effectively managed adaptive tasks involved with client's
health challenge and is exhibiting desire and readiness for
enhanced health and growth in regard to self and in relation
to client
Selected defining characteristics:
Family member attempts to describe growth impact or
crisis on own values, priorities, goals, or relationships

Altered family process—inability of family system (household members) to meet needs of members, carry out family
functions, or maintain communication for mutual growth and
maturation
Selected defining characteristics:
Inability of family members to relate to each other for
mutual growth and maturation
Failure to send and receive clear messages
Inability to accept and receive help

Among these choices, the most appropriate nursing diagnosis is
Family coping: potential for growth. The parents are attentive to the
child's needs and appear to have appropriate caregiving skills. The
sudden illness of the child has disrupted the family's pattern, but
the mother demonstrates effective coping and the ability to learn
and implement new comforting skills. The other two diagnoses
require some maladaptive feature, which is not found in this situation.

DEVELOPING OUTCOME STATEMENTS

1. Focus on the problem statement of the nursing diagnosis.
2. Using measurable verbs, describe the desired patient's behavior or change in clinical status.
3. Add modifiers that describe what, where, how, and when.
4. Add the achievement time.
5. Examine the statement. Determine if it is measurable, realistic, and achievable.

Examples of Outcome Statements

Measurable Verbs	Modifiers	Achievement Time
Demonstrate	Correct handwashing technique	After watching film twice
Walk	Three times around the nurse's station	24 hours after surgery
Eat	Two high-fiber foods	Each meal
Administer	Correct insulin dose	By discharge
Drink	2000 ml fluids	Per day

Modified from Saint Francis Hospital: *Professional nursing project manual*, Tulsa, OK, 1991, Saint Francis Hospital.

While developing the appropriate outcomes, the nurse must determine the priorities of care. Foremost is the need to stabilize the child physiologically; then other problems may be addressed. The time interval that defines this nurse-patient relationship will influence what outcomes may be expected. *Long-term goals* are viewed as the desired health status for the child and family and require considerable time to be realized. *Short-term goals* can usually be met within hours or days and can be small steps toward the long-term goal or an end in themselves in certain health situations. Regardless of whether the goals are long or short term, nursing interventions should be goal directed. This enables the patient to receive the maximum benefit from nursing care.

Nursing Care Plans

The planning phase is the development of the nursing care plan—the identification of which nursing interventions will help achieve the identified outcome. The standard nursing care plans in this text provide guidelines for the care of children and families with a particular problem. *Standard care plans* are plans that are sufficiently broad to account for situations that may develop in patients with particular problems. For this reason, the care plans often have numerous nursing diagnoses. These possible nursing diagnoses can guide patient observation and data collection in monitoring the development of adverse reactions. *Individualized care plans* are plans that are concerned with only those diagnoses that apply to the particular patient situation. Consequently, in actual practice all the problems presented in a standard care plan may not occur. When a standard nursing care plan is used as a guide in developing an individualized care plan, the problems not pertinent to the situation are eliminated and the outcomes are individualized to the specific situations. The characteristics of standard and individualized nursing care plans are compared in Table 2-1.

Patient goals describe what the patient will be expected to do, such as "child will maintain adequate hydration." Patient goals reflect expected outcomes. The word *patient* refers to the child and all significant others, especially the family. This broad use of *patient* reflects the text's philosophy that "the family is the patient." However, because in pediatrics *patient* traditionally refers to the child, in the Nursing Care Plans the patient is specified in parentheses, e.g., "patient (family)," if the goal statement does not directly involve the child. *Nursing interventions,* at times referred to as nursing actions or nursing orders, are specific directives for nursing care that are carried out to help the particular patient move from the present state to the state described in the projected outcomes. The objective of the nursing intervention is to direct individualized care to a patient.

In developing nursing interventions, the nurse, child, and family are essential components in the planning process. Se-

---

TABLE 2-1. Characteristics of standard and individualized nursing care plans

	STANDARD CARE PLAN*	INDIVIDUALIZED CARE PLAN
Assessment	Information is specific only to problem	Information is specific to identified problem and to child and family
Nursing diagnosis	All probable nursing diagnoses with general etiologic factors are considered	Only nursing diagnoses specific to child and family are considered; cause of disease directs actual plan of care
Planning	Goals are broad and represent nursing goals and patient goals	Goals are specific and reflect patient outcomes
Implementation	Nursing interventions are broad and applicable to most patients with problem	Nursing interventions are specific and provide direction for nursing care of individual patient
Evaluation	Progress patient is *expected* to make is identified	Progress patient has actually made toward outcome is identified

*Describes format used in nursing care plans in the text that may differ from other types of standardized nursing care plans.

lected resource persons may be included, such as a clinical nurse specialist, child-life specialist, dietitian, physical therapist, social worker, chaplain, or physician.

There are a number of patient and family factors to consider in developing nursing interventions, including the following:

- Knowledge, skills, and abilities of the child and family
- Child's and family's perception of health
- Ethnic, cultural, and religious factors
- Access to needed resources and/or support people
- Financial resources
- Coping mechanisms currently used

In determining the nursing interventions, it is important to be aware of the impact that the problem will have on both the child and the family. The assessment data should be reviewed and discussed with the family to determine how much time and energy they can invest in health promotion activities. The child and family with a chronic disorder must value having the disorder under control. The child may see the benefits as increased time with peers or decreased hospitalizations. If control is valued, there is a greater likelihood that the desired behaviors will be incorporated into the child's lifestyle. The family's economic level must be taken into consideration; this includes any financial problems that may occur and any resources or assistance that can be used. Ethnic, cultural, and religious factors can also influence the outcome attainment. For example, in ethnic groups that use soy sauce routinely as a seasoning for food, adherence to a low-sodium diet may be very difficult.

There are nurse factors that will influence the translation of a nursing goal into a nursing intervention. These include creativity in finding ways to help a patient carry out a necessary activity and the ability of the rest of the staff to carry out the nursing interventions. For example, is the nursing intervention practical and able to be carried out within the time frame available? To meet the objective of providing individualized care to the patient and/or family, the intervention should be creative yet realistic. An essential component of implementing the care plan is the cooperation of all involved staff. The need for consistency in care planning is illustrated in the following example.

Many diverse factors influence nursing care. These include nurses' strongly held personal beliefs and their ethnic or cultural backgrounds. For example, philosophic differences among members of the nursing staff created many difficulties in planning care for a chronically ill child. He would stay up very late watching television and playing games with the night staff when the unit was quiet. As a result, he would sleep late in the morning, miss meals, and be too tired for the necessary physical and respiratory therapy. These difficulties were presented at a patient care conference (Fig. 2-3). At this time the nursing staff agreed to develop a contract with the patient, one that *all* would adhere to. A reasonable bedtime and awakening time were agreed on, and the patient received certain privileges for keeping to the schedule. For this patient the conference and the written care plan that was established provided the staff with the structure needed to change the child's behavior.

Nursing interventions depend on the causes of the nursing diagnosis or patient problem and the desired outcomes.

Nursing interventions should also be designed to direct observation and care to the medical diagnoses. The nurse may determine that vital signs need to be measured more frequently. A nursing order will ensure that this is interpreted and carried out with regard to the child's condition. To translate the nursing goal into a nursing intervention, the nurse must have data from the patient to answer these questions: What? When? How often? How long? Where? For example, if a nursing goal is to increase fluid intake, the interventions might state "increase fluid to at least 2000 ml in 24 hours. 1000 ml, 7-3; 800 ml, 3-11; 200 ml, 11-7. Child likes orange and apple juice, dislikes carbonated beverage. Offer fluids qh from 0900 to 2100."

The nurse generates and evaluates ideas for nursing interventions and selects those that have the greatest probability of success. Nursing interventions should not be focused on the symptoms of the disorder. Interventions at the symptom level may help temporarily but seldom solve the underlying problem. Routine interventions should not be used without considering individual patient needs and converting them to specific outcomes. The physician's orders should not be reworded.

Nursing interventions should be written for both patient and nurse behaviors. The most important interventions should be placed first, based on priority of patient needs. The interventions should be reviewed with the patient and family so that they can have a feeling of control. As nurses increase their knowledge about a client, nursing interventions, including collaboratory and coordinating activities, may need to be revised. Suggestions from dietitians, social workers, or physical therapists should be considered when writing nursing interventions. Education needs or referral to an outside agency are also incorporated into discharge planning.

Currently a national, multicenter study is in progress to identify nursing interventions (Iowa Intervention Project, 1995).

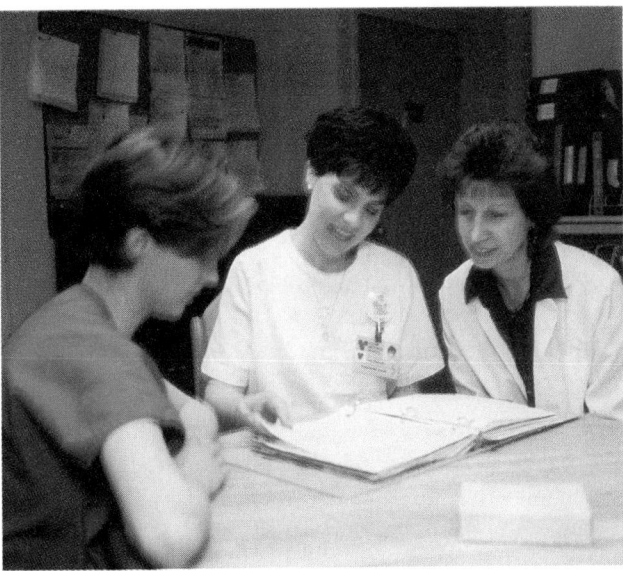

FIG. 2-3. A patient care conference is an effective strategy for planning individualized care for the child and family.

IMPLEMENTATION

Implementation is the actual delivery of nursing care to the patient. This phase of the nursing process puts the nursing and medical care plan into action. The nurse's activities are guided by the nursing and medical diagnoses, as well as by the patient's current status. For example, the nurse provides the patient with the assistance needed for activities of daily living, hygiene, and safety precautions.

The interventions performed span the dependent, interdependent, and independent domains of nursing practice. In the dependent domain the nurse implements the direction/ orders of the responsible practitioner. The interdependent and independent domains of nursing are usually governed by nursing interventions, but some practitioners may provide direction in the interdependent area. However, in all domains nursing judgment is necessary to determine if the order is appropriate for the patient. This involves both an assessment of the patient and an understanding of the intervention.

During the implementation phase the nurse should use each interaction with the child and family to continue assessing and reassessing nursing diagnoses and the care plan. Interventions such as baths, which require prolonged patient contact, are especially valuable for validating data with the patient.

The implementation of the care plan should be documented in the patient's permanent record. Interventions can be charted on the flow record, and the patient's response should be charted in the progress note. Once the nursing interventions have been implemented, they need to be continually assessed to provide feedback and to evaluate whether they need modification. Assessing the patient's progress toward the projected outcomes enables the nurse to evaluate the effectiveness of the orders. If the nursing interventions have been effective, the signs and symptoms used to diagnose the problem should be changed, outcomes should be achieved, and the patient should be moving toward the time when termination of the nurse-patient relationship will take place and discharge to the home setting or other health care facility will occur.

EVALUATION

The final step of the nursing process is evaluation. Although it sounds easy, evaluation is a very difficult process without measurable outcomes. Effectively evaluating a patient requires several steps (Hickey, 1990). First, criteria and standards are established that can be used to guide observations to determine patient progress in terms of the diagnoses and goals. For a child with nonorganic failure to thrive (NFTT), criteria might include a daily weight change. Second, the

---

> ### GUIDELINES FOR DOCUMENTATION OF NURSING CARE
>
> Initial assessments and reassessments
> Nursing diagnoses and/or patient care needs
> Interventions identified to meet the patient's nursing care needs
> Nursing care provided
> Patient's response to, and the outcomes of, the care provided
> Abilities of patient and/or, as appropriate, significant other(s) to manage continuing care needs after discharge

---

nurse observes the patient to determine what skills and knowledge have been mastered. This involves assessing feeding behaviors and parent-infant interactions. Third, these observed data are compared with the expected outcomes and the amount of progress recorded. For example, for a child with NFTT, actual weight gain is compared with an expected 1 ounce per day. Finally, a judgment is made about whether the patient outcome meets the established goal. If the patient is not achieving the expected outcomes, the plan must be assessed to determine what obstacles, if any, exist.

DOCUMENTATION

Although documentation is not one of the five steps of the nursing process, it is essential for evaluation. The nurse can assess and identify problems, plan, and implement without documentation; however, evaluation is best performed with written evidence of progress toward outcomes. The patient's medical record should include evidence of those elements listed in the box.

The nursing process has become an integral part of professional practice as identified by the ANA Standards of Practice. The **Joint Commission on Accreditation of Healthcare Organizations (JCAHO)** is actively involved in accrediting many health care providers. Currently hospitals, nursing homes, ambulatory services, and home health agencies can choose to be accredited by this group.

One of the focus areas for this accreditation process is the use of *continuous quality improvement (CQI)*. This process is an ongoing review of systems, problem identification, and resolution that allows the institution to establish and maintain quality care.

Currently the attention in health care is focused on patient outcomes. Criteria are established for what changes should occur in the patient as a result of the interaction with the health care team. At discharge the care is evaluated to ensure that the outcomes were met.

KEY POINTS

- Critical thinking is purposeful, goal-directed thinking based on rational and deliberate thought.
- The nursing process is the orderly, systematic method of determining the client's problems, making plans to solve them, initiating the plan or assigning others to implement it, and evaluating the extent to which the plan was effective in resolving the identified problems.
- Assessment is the deliberate and systematic collection of data.
- Problem identification is the analysis of assessment data to determine what areas of dysfunction or potential dysfunction exist.
- Nursing diagnoses are client problems that nurses, by virtue of their education and experience, are able and licensed to treat.
- Planning is the development of outcomes with interventions to meet them.
- Outcome development involves five steps: (1) focusing on the problem statement; (2) describing the patient's desired behavior after nursing care—with a measurable verb; (3) adding modifiers that describe what, where, how, and when; (4) setting the achievement time; and (5) reviewing the outcome to ensure that it is measurable, realistic, and achievable.
- Implementation is the actual delivery of nursing care to the child and family.
- Evaluation is the comparison of the child's status with the expected outcomes.

REFERENCES

Alfaro-Lefevre R: *Applying nursing process,* Philadelphia, 1995, Lippincott.

American Nurses Association: *Standards of clinical nursing,* Washington, DC, 1991, The Association.

Carpenito LJ: *Nursing diagnosis application to clinical practice,* ed 6, Philadelphia, 1995, Lippincott.

Carroll-Johnson RM, editor: *Classification of nursing diagnoses: proceedings of the Ninth Conference,* North American Nursing Diagnosis Association (NANDA), Philadelphia, 1991, Lippincott.

Chaffee J: A classic false dilemma: teaching vs. infusing critical thinking, *Educational Vision* 8-9, 1994.

Gordon M: *Manual of nursing diagnosis, 1995-1996,* St Louis, 1995, Mosby.

Hickey PW: *Nursing process handbook,* St Louis, 1990, Mosby.

Iowa Intervention Project: Validation and coding of the NIC taxonomy, *Image J Nurs Sch* 27(1):43-49, 1995.

Paul R: *Critical thinking: what every person needs to survive in a rapidly changing world,* Rohnert Park, CA, 1993, Foundation for Critical Thinking.

BIBLIOGRAPHY

Alspach J: The revised JCAHO nursing care standards: areas of emphasis, *Crit Care Nurs* 11(8):12-14, 1991.

Bulechek GM, McCloskey JC: *Nursing interventions: treatments for nursing diagnoses,* Philadelphia, 1985, Saunders.

Carlson JH and others: *Nursing diagnosis: a case study approach,* Philadelphia, 1991, Saunders.

Case B: Walking around the elephant: a critical-thinking strategy for decision making, *J Cont Ed Nurs* 25(8):101-109, 1994.

Christensen PJ, Kenney JW: *Nursing process: application of theories, frameworks, and models,* ed 4, St Louis, 1995, Mosby.

D'Argenio C: *Implementing nursing diagnosis-based practice,* Gaithersburg, MD, 1991, Aspen.

Fitzpatrick JJ: Conceptual basis for the organization and advancement of nursing knowledge: nursing diagnosis/taxonomy, *Nurs Diagn* 1(3):102-106, 1990.

Ford JS, Profetto-McGrath J: A model for critical thinking within the context of curriculum praxis, *J Nurs Ed* 33(8):341-344, 1994.

Gordon M: *Nursing diagnosis: process and application,* ed 3, St Louis, 1994, Mosby.

Gordon M and others: Clinical judgment: an integrated model, *Adv Nurs Sci* 16(4):55-70, 1994.

Iyer PW, Camp NH: *Nursing documentation: a nursing process approach,* ed 2 St Louis, 1995, Mosby.

Jennings BM: Patient outcomes research: seizing the opportunity, *Adv Nurs Sci* 14(2):59-72, 1991.

Kataoka-Yahiro M, Saylor C: A critical thinking model for nursing judgment, *J Nurs Ed* 33(8):351-356, 1994.

Kintgen-Andrews J: Critical thinking and nursing education: perplexities and insights, *J Nurs Ed* 30(4):152-157, 1991.

Levin R and others: Diagnostic content validity of nursing diagnoses, *Image J Nurs Sch* 21(1):40-44, 1989.

Lindsey AM: Identification and labeling of human responses, *J Prof Nurs* 6(3):143-150, 1990.

Lyons J, Hester N: Research-generated nursing diagnoses for healthy school-age children, *Issues Compr Pediatr Nurs* 10(3):149-159, 1987.

McFarland GK, McFarlane EA: *Nursing diagnosis and intervention: planning for patient care,* ed 2, St Louis, 1993, Mosby.

McLane A: Measurement and validation of diagnostic concepts: a decade of progress . . . review of nursing diagnosis research, *Heart Lung* 16(6):616-624, 1987.

McMurray A: Time to extend the "process"? *Austr J Adv Nurs* 6(4):40-43, 1989.

Mills WC: Nursing diagnosis: the importance of a definition, *Nurs Diagn* 2(1):3-8, 1991.

Mitchell GJ: Nursing diagnosis: an ethical analysis, *Image J Nurs Sch* 23(2):99-104, 1991.

Naylor MD and others: Measuring the effectiveness of nursing practice, *Clin Nurs Spec* 5(4):210-215, 1991.

North American Nursing Diagnosis Association: *Nursing diagnoses: definitions and classifications, 1995-1996,* Philadelphia, 1994, NANDA.

Pinkley CL: Exploring NANDA's definition of nursing diagnosis: linking diagnostic judgments with the selection of outcomes and interventions, *Nurs Diagn* 2(1):26-32, 1991.

Potter PA, Perry AG: *Fundamentals of nursing: concepts, process, and practice,* ed 3, St Louis, 1993, Mosby.

Tanner C: *Teaching clinical judgment.* In Fitzpatrick J, Taunton R, editors: *Annual Review of Nursing Research,* vol 5, New York, 1987, Wiley.

Tanner C and others: The phenomenology of knowing the patient, *Image J Nurs Sch* 25(4):273-280, 1993.

Waltz CF, Sylvia BM: Accountability and outcome measurement: where do we go from here? *Clin Nurs Spec* 5(4):202-203, 1991.

Warren JJ, Hoskins LM: The development of NANDA's nursing diagnosis taxonomy, *Nurs Diagn* 1(4):163-168, 1990.

White J: Patterns of knowing: review, critique, and update, *Adv Nurs Sci* 17(4):73-86, 1995.

SOCIAL, CULTURAL, AND RELIGIOUS INFLUENCES ON CHILD HEALTH PROMOTION

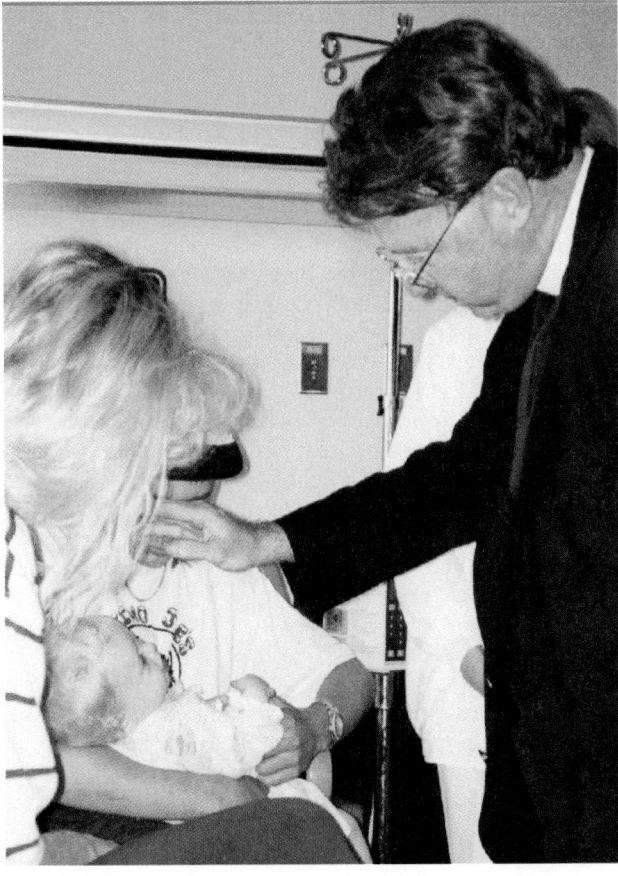

RELATED TOPICS

LEARNING OBJECTIVES
On completion of this chapter the reader will be able to:

- Define *culture, culture shock, ethnicity,* and *race*
- Describe the subcultural influences on child development in the areas of socialization, education, and aspiration
- Compare and contrast the advantages and disadvantages

encountered in the educational system by children from lower- and middle-class backgrounds
- Characterize family life in present-day America
- Identify four common diseases or disorders that affect certain ethnic or cultural groups

- Identify areas of potential conflict of values and customs for a nurse interacting with a family from a different cultural/ethnic group
- Describe three religious groups whose beliefs significantly affect their health practices

CULTURE

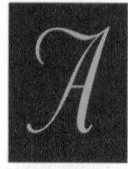 culture is a pattern of assumptions, beliefs, and practices that unconsciously frames or guides the outlook and decisions of a group of people (Buchwald and others, 1994). Culture differs from both race and ethnicity. *Race* is defined as a division of mankind possessing traits that are transmissible by descent and sufficient to characterize it as a distinct human type. One classification of race, based on skin color, is caucasoid (white), negroid (black), and mongoloid (yellow). *Ethnicity* is the affiliation of a set of persons who share a unique cultural, social, and linguistic heritage. *Socialization* is the process by which children acquire the beliefs, values, and behaviors of a given society in order to function within that group.

A culture is composed of individuals who share a set of values, beliefs, practices (language, dress, diet, health care), social relationships, law, politics, economics, and norms of behavior that is learned, integrative, social, and satisfying (Habayeb, 1995). Culture is not a surface veneer that covers a basic outlook shared by all human beings but an ingrained orientation to life that serves as a frame of reference for individual perception and judgment. People from one culture differ from those in other cultures in the ways they think, solve problems, perceive, and structure the world. Essentially, culture incorporates experiences of the past, influences thought and action in the present, and transmits these traditions to future group members. Adaptation is necessary, however, for the culture to survive in an ever-changing world. Consciously and unconsciously, the members abandon, modify, or assume new patterns to meet the needs of the group.

The culture in which children are reared determines the type of food they will eat, the language they will speak, the ideals of behavior they will follow, and the way they will conduct themselves in social roles. To be acceptable members of the culture, children must learn how the culture expects them to behave toward others in the group. In turn, they learn how they can expect others to behave toward them. This cultural understanding is typically established in children by age 5 years (Lynch, 1992).

Related to the large culture are many *subcultures,* those smaller groups within a culture that possess many characteristics of the larger culture while contributing their own particular values. Subcultural influences are discussed in more detail later in this chapter. *small group— some unique traits*

Cultures and subcultures contribute to the uniqueness of child members in such a subtle way and at such an early age that children grow up to feel that their beliefs, attitudes, values, and practices are the "correct" or "normal" ones; those of other cultures may be viewed as "deviant" or "wrong." A set of values learned in childhood is apt to characterize children's attitudes and behavior for life, guiding their long-range strivings and monitoring their short-range, impulsive inclinations. Thus every ongoing society socializes each succeeding generation to its cultural heritage.

The manner and sequence of the growth and development phenomenon are universal and fundamental features of all children; however, the variations in behavioral responses that children display to similar events are believed to be determined by cultures. Inborn temperament and modes of behavior that prompt children to behave in their own preferred and highly individual manner may be in harmony or in conflict with the culture. Such forces as heredity and maturation impose limits on the influence that parents and other social groups may bring to bear.

The culture fosters and reinforces those behaviors deemed desirable and appropriate; it attempts to suppress or extinguish those at conflict with cultural norms. Some cultures encourage aggressive behaviors in their children; others favor amiability and compliance. Some foster individual resourcefulness and competition; others emphasize cooperation and submission to group interest. Cultures may also differ in whether status in the group is based on age or on skill. Even children's play and their types of games are culturally determined. In some cultures children play in groups composed of members of the same sex; in others they play in mixed-sex groups. In some cultures team games predominate; in others most play is limited to individual games.

Standards and norms vary from culture to culture and location to location; a practice that is accepted in one area may meet with disapproval or create tension in another. The extent to which cultures tolerate divergence from the established norm varies among cultures and subcultural groups. Although conformity provides a degree of security, it is a decided deterrent to change.

SOCIAL ROLES

Much of children's self-concept is derived from their ideas about their social roles. Roles are cultural creations; therefore the culture prescribes patterns of behavior for persons in a variety of social positions. All persons who hold similar social positions have the obligation to behave in a particular manner. A role prohibits some behaviors and allows for others. Because it delineates and clarifies roles, the culture is a significant influence on the development of children's self-concept (i.e., the attitudes and beliefs they have about themselves).

A social group consists of a system of roles carried out in both primary and secondary groups. A *primary group* is characterized by intimate, continued face-to-face contact, mutual support of the members, and the ability to order or constrain a considerable proportion of individual members' behavior. Two such groups are the family and the peer group, both of which exert a great deal of influence on the child. Some communities (e.g., contemporary rural, religious, or ethnic communities) also exert a strong primary-group influence. All members know each other, most belong to the same subgroups, and all are concerned about each member's behavior. There is considerable support among the community members and little conflict of values. Relatives are likely to live close together, allowing young members ample opportunity to observe and absorb the practices and customs of the culture. Any member of the community feels justified in evaluating and censuring the conduct of another.

Secondary groups are groups that have limited, intermittent contact and in which there is generally less concern for members' behavior. These groups offer little in terms of support or pressure toward conformity except in rigidly limited

---

Laura L. Kuensting, MSN(R), RN, revised this chapter.

areas. Examples of secondary groups are professional associations and church organizations (also considered in relation to subgroups). The childrearing orientation in a secondary-group environment, such as urban communities, differs considerably from that of a primary-group community. An urban community is dynamic and rapidly changing; therefore many of the traditional behaviors and values do not meet its needs. Consequently, parents are often uncertain about what to teach their children. They may wish to rear their children with values consistent with their own, but the differences in experience between the generations are too great. As a result, they often grant their children autonomy in some areas of decision making early in the developmental process, and other secondary groups assume a greater influence. The children are exposed to an assortment of social groups with diverse sets of values and expectations. None of the groups is highly dominant in its influence; therefore the children are exposed to an eclectic set of values, some in agreement and some at conflict with the others. From these they must ultimately select those that they determine to be best for them and adopt them to form a consistent set of roles and behaviors to be incorporated into the self-concept.

Guilt and Shame Orientation

Conditioning children to feel either guilt or shame for misdeeds is a technique used by a culture to control social behavior—to internalize the norms and expectations of others. Some cultural groups value a well-developed conscience (superego) and condition their children to feel guilt following wrongdoing. Offenders get an uncomfortable physical feeling and want to purge themselves. Since guilt is based within the individual, successful conditioning produces self-regulated persons who punish themselves without their being caught in the act of wrongdoing.

In many cultural groups guilt is lacking and social controls are based on the use of shame. Offenders do not want anyone to see them when they have been found guilty of a wrongful deed. Sometimes children in these groups learn that anything is acceptable as long as one is not caught; the shame results when the forbidden act is found out by others.

Although both techniques are used by members of both primary- and secondary-group communities, shame is apt to be more successful in a primary-group community because most behaviors are quite public. In secondary-group communities it is less effective; persons are not as apt to be caught and, if caught, can withdraw and join a group that is unaware of the misdeed. Guilt probably has a greater influence on behavior in urban communities, although many authorities believe that the trend in urban North America is shifting away from a guilt orientation. Rapid changes in the North American culture leave parents unsure of their own values; therefore much of their function is abandoned to the school and peers. Peers are notorious for using shame as a disciplinary technique.

SUBCULTURAL INFLUENCES

Except in rare situations, children grow and develop in a blend of cultures and subcultures. In a large, complex society such as the United States, different groups have their own set of standards, values, and expectations within the collective ways of the large culture. Although many cultural differences are related to geographic boundaries, subcultures are not always restricted by location.

Children's membership in a cultural subgroup is, for the most part, involuntary. They are born into a family with a specific ethnic and/or racial heritage, socioeconomic level, and religious beliefs. Although in the complex North American society there are countless subcultures and considerable variation in the way of life, those subcultures that seem to exert the greatest influence on childrearing are ethnicity, social class, and occupational role. In addition, schools and peer-group subcultures are strong influences in the socialization of the child.

Ethnicity

As mentioned earlier, *ethnicity* is the classification of or affiliation with any of the basic groups or divisions of mankind or any heterogeneous population differentiated by customs, characteristics, language, or similar distinguishing factors. Ethnic differences extend to many areas and include such manifestations as family structure, language, food preferences, moral codes, and expression of emotion.

To establish their place in the group, children learn how to adhere to a mode of behavior that is in accordance with standards distinctive to the group and learn how they can expect others to behave toward them. They take their cues from observing and imitating those to whom they are exposed. For example, children of a racial minority form a perception of their role as a group member by observing the manner in which role models within the subgroup respond to treatment by people outside the subgroup. When they see group members display an attitude of inferiority, they assume this to be the appropriate behavior. These perceptions are then incorporated into their own self-concept.

In the United States the cross-cultural lines are becoming blurred as subcultures are assimilated and blended into the larger culture (Fig. 3-1). Although ethnic differences in childrearing are probably diminishing, they remain important. It is particularly difficult for persons to attempt to maintain an identity with a subculture while living and conforming to the requirements of the dominant culture. Universal customs and language used in commercial and educational systems are different from those of the minority culture. Often the values are in conflict. Consequently, children reared in this environment are confused about roles and values, and they usually adopt those of the more influential or higher-status culture. Youth, in particular, are influenced by the locally dominant group.

 Although ethnic groups differ in the behavioral and personal traits they value in their children, certain basic values appear to be shared. When parents from 24 different countries of origin were asked to rank the importance of 13 behavior and personality characteristics in children (e.g., "honesty," "having good manners"), there was strong agreement regarding those most valued (Johns, 1987).

The term *ethnocentrism* refers to the emotional attitude that one's own ethnic group is superior to others, that one's values, beliefs, and perceptions are the correct ones, and that the group's ways of living and behaving are the best way. Ethnic stereotyping or labeling stems from ethnocentric views of people (Friedman, 1990). Ethnocentrism implies that all

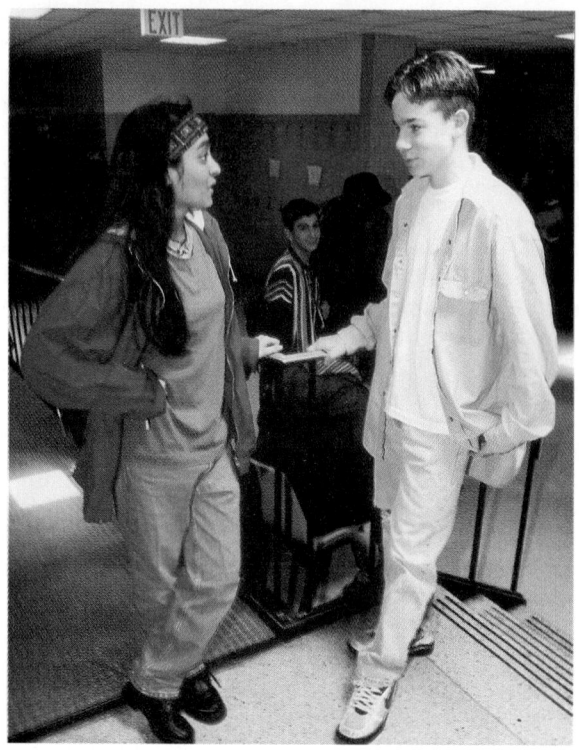

FIG. 3-1. Youngsters from different cultural backgrounds interact within the larger culture.

other groups are inferior and that their ways are not in the best interests of the group. This attitude strongly influences the ability of one person to evaluate the beliefs and behaviors of others objectively. This inherent viewpoint of individuals tends to bias their interpretation and understanding of the behavior of others.

Social Class/Occupation

Although there are exceptions, probably the greatest influence on childrearing practices and their consequences is the social class of the family into which a child is born. Differences in childrearing goals and practices, as well as in attitudes toward health, have been found to be greater between social classes than between races or ethnic groups. In North America social class and socioeconomic level are essentially synonymous and are most easily determined by occupation; for example, the upper middle class consists primarily of professional and business people, almost all with a college education. The working class includes employees in manufacturing, trades, and service occupations (such as barbers or hairdressers) who have a high school education. In the lower class, the breadwinners are typically unskilled laborers or unemployed families who may or may not be on public assistance (Elkin and Handel, 1989). Since children are reared differently by parents who vary in respect to these factors, social class can be expected to produce substantial variation in their upbringing.

Middle and Upper Class. Children from these classes live in an enriched environment that provides material comforts and broader opportunities. The parents are usually edu-

cated beyond high school and have occupations that require judgment, creativity, and resourcefulness. These attributes are fostered in their children. Other authority figures such as teachers with whom the children are routinely in contact are usually from a middle-class background and have activities and expectations for the children that are similar to those of the parents.

Most middle-class parents are future oriented, have higher educational and occupational aspirations for their children, and use long-range planning to meet these goals (Shaffer, 1985). Middle-class parents typically encourage their children to participate in activities that foster achievement, such as dancing lessons, athletics, and scouting, in the belief that this will make them well-rounded, self-directed adults.

In the area of discipline, middle-class parents are more apt to use manipulative techniques such as reasoning and drawing on the child's sense of guilt. They tend to scold and use isolation rather than physical punishment. There is more concern regarding the *intent* of the act than the *consequence* of the act.

It is believed that upper-class parents are more permissive and foster desirable behavior through positive reinforcement. However, much of the actual child care in upper-class families is delegated to surrogates, such as housekeepers, governesses, or private schools. The parent serves as an arbitrator between the children and the servants.

Lower and Working Class. The uncertainty of their life leads members of the lower classes to be present oriented; that is, to take advantage of gratification when possible. This orientation is distinctly different from that of most members of the middle class, who may be more willing to delay gratification to achieve a long-term goal.

Children in lower-class families encounter major educational disadvantages, reflected in the high incidence of academic failure and attendant dropout rate. Some of the major educational disadvantages many children from the lower social class encounter include the following:

- Parents are more likely to value the concrete and tangible rather than the abstract and are therefore less inclined to encourage these qualities in their children.
- Parents are less likely to read to the child or encourage educational play because of their own educational level.
- No role models may be available to support the value of education.
- Inadequate funding and/or poor quality of education may exist in neighborhood schools.
- Poor health and inadequate nutrition of the children is common.
- Parents are more likely to have limited communication skills, such as simple grammar, inability to express abstractions, and ethnic dialects, which hamper interactions with teachers from middle-class backgrounds.

Parents from lower and working classes are generally tradition oriented, stressing obedience and conformity to parental values and external regulations. The most frequently used form of discipline for undesirable behavior is physical punishment. Parents are usually less interested in the direction of children's activities than with conduct; they are more concerned that children stay out of trouble.

With better job security through unionization, unemployment compensation, and other welfare features, some segments of the lower classes are finding life more predictable.

concerned c̄ intent of behavior

[handwritten: no role models for education]

They are less apt to seize gratifications lest the opportunity vanish and are beginning to develop long-range goals, including an increased interest in education for their children. *[handwritten: no dad]*

Poverty *[handwritten: ares - 2 or 3 - 5 different kids worse off than lower class]*

A subcultural influence closely related to but different from social class is the condition known as poverty. It is a relative concept and is usually associated with the general standards of a population. The term *poverty* implies both visible and invisible impoverishment. *Visible poverty* refers to lack of money or material resources, which includes insufficient clothing, poor sanitation, and deteriorating housing. *Invisible poverty* refers to social and cultural deprivation such as limited employment opportunities, inferior educational opportunities, lack of or inferior medical services and health care facilities, and an absence of public services.

The very poor in the society who consistently exist on or below the poverty level live in a perpetual state of despair. Their limited skills give them no bargaining power in the job market, and the education needed to improve their status is beyond them. The poor desire better things for their children but are trapped in a circular pattern that perpetuates their life condition. Their powerlessness to control their fate or condition is a source of fatalism and resignation that is characteristic of the group in general. Optimism, when it is manifested, is more likely to be expressed in terms of luck or chance. This fatalistic attitude, which significantly impedes occupational and educational aspirations, also inhibits the poor from seeking health care or practicing preventive health care measures. For example, if someone is injured or killed in an automobile accident, it is usually considered bad luck, not something they could have prevented by wearing a seat belt. *[handwritten: tend to use more physical or corporal pun.]*

Factors Related to Poverty. Throughout the United States there are groups of people, geographically segregated, who constitute what are known as "pockets of poverty." These are seen in the dense urban areas, such as the ghettos, and many rural areas, especially those that are geographically isolated from the needed facilities and services. The nonurbanized regions identified as poverty areas in the United States are Appalachia, the deep South, the lower Southwest, and northern New England.

Certain ethnic or racial groups are overrepresented in the impoverished population. The most obvious of these are blacks, Latinos, and Native Americans.

Homelessness. One of the most pressing problems in the United States is the growing number of homeless families. Homeless individuals are those persons who lack resources and community ties necessary to provide for their own adequate shelter. In the past the homeless population traditionally included single adults, mostly men. Currently, the fastest growing segment of the homeless consists of families, most commonly single mothers with two or three children. Another group of homeless children are the "runaway" and "throwaway" adolescents. Over 90% of this group tend to come from minority ethnic groups and usually from troubled families, including mentally and physically abusive parents.

Lack of a permanent dwelling deprives children of the most basic necessities for proper growth and development. Children who are homeless suffer from physical and mental disorders that exceed those found in poor families who have a permanent residence (Bassuk and Rosenberg, 1990). Homelessness is particularly damaging for preschool children. Preschoolers in shelters exhibit slower development and more emotional-behavioral problems than do children from poor families with homes (Rescoria, Parker, and Stolley, 1991).

Migrant Families. One of the most disadvantaged groups is migrant farm workers and their children. The low position of these families on the economic scale and their mobile existence subject them to inadequate sanitation, substandard housing, social isolation, and lack of educational and medical facilities. This life-style is especially deleterious to the children. For example, children are apt to live in a number of localities and attend a variety of schools in the course of a year with no continuity in either education or health care. In addition, most migrant families have no health care insurance. Because both parents work in the fields, children receive little adult supervision; therefore, accident rates are high and meals are erratic. Except where prohibited by law, children are even recruited to work in the fields along with the adults. Some migrants have a home base to which they return at the end of a growing season; others travel continuously, migrating north in summer and south in winter.

Affluence

On the opposite end of the socioeconomic spectrum are the children of affluent members of society. Although they can live within the warmth of a positive family relationship, many of them appear to be just as deprived as poverty-stricken children. Wealth does not provide protection against many of life's problems and disappointments, especially in the area of parent-child relationships. Like their counterparts in the poverty groups, children of the affluent may suffer from discrimination, inadequate parenting, or unsatisfactory role models.

Children of the wealthy suffer most from lack of parental contact. There may be long separations from loving, caring parents because of social or business interests. Some have a cold, sometimes hostile parent, who is rarely available to them. Even their places of residence contribute to their isolation and loneliness. Paid parent surrogates, including servants, sports professionals (such as tennis or swimming instructors), and private school personnel, provide them with adult companionship and authority. During the early years many wealthy children form stronger attachments to these people than to their parents. However, as the children grow older, they become aware of class distinctions. They realize that they must separate from these early relationships to form bonds with individuals in their class. Parents may begin involving the older adolescent in the family business and in adult social activities. But for many young people a meaningful life with their family has come too late. They feel lonely, isolated, and unloved (Adams, 1991).

Many children from wealthy families, like those from poor families, seem to thrive and flourish, making positive contributions to their families and society. However, some grow up to display a lack of motivation or self-discipline, and boredom. They are suspicious of others, finding it difficult to believe they are liked for themselves and not for their money or position, and they do not trust others enough to enter into true friendships. Affluent children may also fail to acquire skills to handle responsibility and money.

Religion

Probably the most influential factor in shaping the culture of the United States is the Judeo-Christian faith. Many immigrants came to the country for religious freedom and established a religious and moral atmosphere that persists today. However, there are individual differences that are part of the general culture.

The religious orientation of the family dictates a code of morality and influences the family's attitudes toward education, male and female role identity, and beliefs regarding their ultimate destiny (Fig. 3-2). It may also determine the school that the children attend, the companions with whom they associate, and often their mate selection.

In a few instances, such as in the Mennonite and Amish communities, religion is the basis of a common way of life that determines where and how the children are reared.

Schools

Next to the family the schools exert the major force in providing continuity between generations by conveying a vast amount of culture from the older members to the young. In this way children are prepared to carry out the traditional social roles they are expected to assume as adults in society. School rules and regulations regarding attendance, authority relationships, and the system of sanctions and rewards based on achievement transmit to the child the behavioral expectations of the adult world of employment and relationships. School is often the only institution in which children systematically learn about the negative consequences of behaviors that deviate from social expectations. Teachers are expected to stimulate and guide the intellectual development of children and their sense of esthetics and to foster their capacity for creative problem solving. Through education individuals in the lower classes are offered the opportunity for further education and the capacity to move up in the social strata.

Traditionally the socialization process of school has begun when the child enters kindergarten or first grade. Today, with almost 60% of mothers of preschool children working outside the home, this socialization process begins much earlier for a significant number of children in a variety of child care settings.

Peer Cultures

Peer groups also have an impact on the socialization of children (Fig. 3-3). Peer relationships become increasingly important and influential as children proceed through school. In school, children have what can be regarded as a culture of their own. It is most apparent in the school and in the unsupervised play group. The play group presents this culture in a much purer form than does the school, which is partly produced by adults.

During their lives children are exposed to value systems such as those of the family, ethnic group, and social class. In peer-group interaction they are confronted with a variety of these sets of values. The values imposed by the peer group are especially compelling because children must accept and conform to them in order to be accepted as members of the group. When the peer values are not too different from those of family and teachers, the mild conflict created by these small differences serves to separate children from the adults in their lives and to strengthen the feeling of belonging to the peer group.

The kind of socialization provided by the peer group depends on the special subculture that develops from the background, interests, and capabilities of its members. Some groups support school achievement, others focus on athletic prowess, and still others are decidedly antithetic to educative goals. Scholastic achievement is strongly related to the value system of the peer groups. Many conflicts between teachers and students and between parents and students can be attributed to fear of rejection by peers. A conflict between what is expected from parents regarding academic achievement and

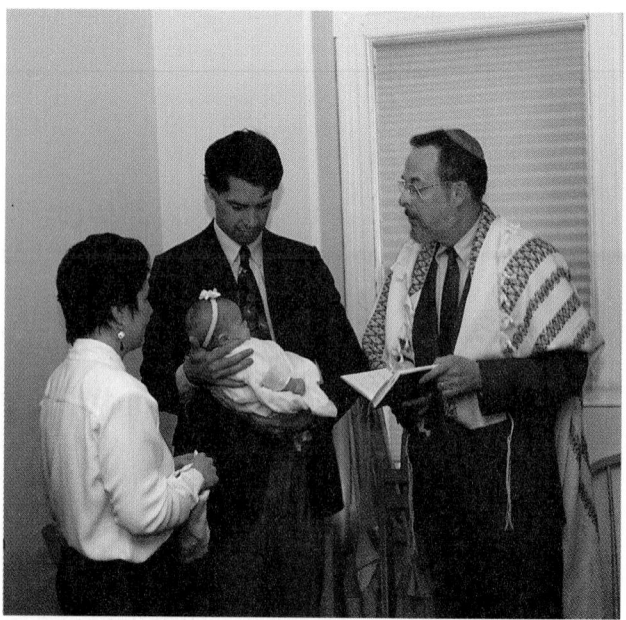

FIG. 3-2. Soon after an infant is born, many families have special religious ceremonies.

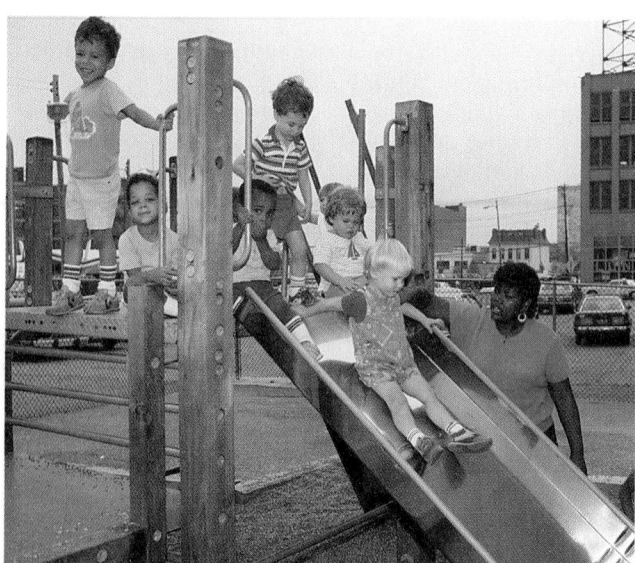

FIG. 3-3. Children from a variety of cultural and ethnic backgrounds begin to socialize in the child care setting.

what is expected from the peer culture is especially pronounced in high school.

Although it has neither the traditional authority of the parents nor the legal authority of the schools for teaching information, the peer group manages to convey a substantial amount of information to its members, especially about taboo subjects, such as sex and drugs. Through peer relationships, children learn ways to deal with dominance and hostility and to relate with persons in positions of leadership and authority. The peer subculture relieves boredom and provides recognition that individual members do not receive from teachers and other authority figures.

The peer-group culture has secrets, mores, and codes of ethics with which they promote feelings of group solidarity and detachment from adults. Traditions and folkways are transferred from "generation to generation" of schoolchildren and have a great influence over the behavior of all group members. There are age-related games and other activities, and as children move from one level to the next, folkways of the younger group are discarded as those of the older group are adopted. For example, a school-age child rides a bicycle to school; the high school student prefers to drive a car. As they advance, children are forward oriented only—they look forward with anticipation but look backward with contempt.

Biculture

Some children are exposed to the values, role relationships, and life-styles of two cultures—a virtual "straddling" of two cultures. Although sometimes observed in play groups, this background is usually not a significant factor until children enter school. Children of one culture must unlearn some of the established practices of the culture in order to become socialized in the other, especially in role relationships. For example, children from Hispanic and Asian cultures are taught to look away when scolded; in U.S. schools the teacher expects direct eye contact—"Look at me when I speak to you" (Sloat and Matsuura, 1990). Children learn new roles and social behavior more rapidly than their adult counterparts.

This biculture is particularly marked in language differences. The bilingual child is said to be at a disadvantage in school situations of the dominant culture, especially a culture in which there is controversy over bilingual education. Those supporting bilingual education adhere to the principle that children will understand more readily and perform more realistically (especially in testing situations) if learning is directed in their own language; others contend that children living in a dominant culture should adopt the ways of that culture, including language.

THE CHILD AND FAMILY IN NORTH AMERICA

North America is an aggregate of numerous cultures that are blended with the unique heritage of pioneering frontiersmen. The frontier background of the North American culture has contributed to the overall orientation to life and childrearing. There has always been a basic optimistic view of the world, a belief that things can be better and that the children can and will be better off than the parents. This hopeful outlook and a general future orientation, together with the possibility of upward social mobility, have created a pervasive overall attitude of optimism. Increasing development of self-confidence and autonomy in children is fostered and encouraged. Children are generally permitted a greater degree of freedom than in more tradition-oriented cultures, where individuals remain in one class for life.

Family life in North America is characterized by increasing geographic and economic mobility. There is less reliance on tradition, families are fragmented, and there is limited opportunity to transmit and acquire the traditional and accepted customs of a culture. Consequently, young adults rely to a greater extent on the professed experts, peers, and the mass media for acquisition of acceptable patterns of behavior, including childrearing practices. Conflicting information can be a source of confusion and frustration as parents attempt to determine the comparatively stable, essential components of the culture and transmit these to their children.

Children in North America grow up with a number of adults who differ from one another but who all provide input as role models, teachers, and standards for behavior. Most children live in some form of nuclear family located in sharply differentiated neighborhoods determined by income and ethnic status within a highly technical, largely urban society. Class differences in childrearing persist, but they are becoming less divergent as a result of the increased homogeneity of the culture.

Minority-Group Membership

The United States has more racial, ethnic, and religious minority groups than any other country. Ethnic minority groups are becoming increasingly important because it is anticipated that these groups will produce children at a faster rate than will the majority white population. Consequently, the minority population is increasing while the majority white population is decreasing. Blacks are the largest minority group, followed closely by Hispanics. By the year 2000 one in every four Americans will be black, Hispanic, or Asian (Fleming, 1989). (See Cultural Awareness box.)

One of the difficulties with including diverse groups of people under ethnic labels, such as black, Asian, or Hispanic, is that the groups can differ tremendously in their own cultural heritage. Just as the majority white population differs

 CULTURAL AWARENESS
Classification of Minority Groups

The definition of various minority groups is not universal. In the 1990 U.S. census form, *blacks* included persons identified, for example, as African- or Afro-American, Haitian, Jamaican, West Indian, or Nigerian. Persons of *Spanish/Hispanic* origin included Mexican, Mexican-American, Chicano, Puerto Rican, Cuban, Argentinean, Colombian, Costa Rican, Dominican, Ecuadoran, Guatemalan, Honduran, Nicaraguan, Peruvian, and Salvadoran persons, as well as persons from other Spanish-speaking countries or the Caribbean, or Central or South America. *Mexican-American* referred only to persons of Mexican origin or ancestry. In some writings the term *Latino* refers to individuals from Mexico and Central America (Friedman, 1990). *Asian* or *Pacific Islander* groups include Chinese, Japanese, Hawaiian, Filipino, Vietnamese, Korean, Asian Indian, Guamanian, and Samoan (Martin, 1992).

according to various subcultures, such as socioeconomic status and occupation, so do the minority groups.

Nursing ALERT Generalizations made about an ethnic group may not apply to certain groups and individuals.

When minority groups immigrate to another country, a certain degree of cultural/ethnic blending occurs through the process of *acculturation*—those gradual changes produced in a culture by the influence of another culture that cause one or both cultures to be more similar to the other. However, the changes occur to various degrees in different families and groups. At one time it was believed that the great diversity among the ethnic groups in the United States would result in a great "melting pot" where the differences among different cultures would eventually diminish to produce a homogeneous society. However, this does not appear to be the case. Many groups continue to identify with their traditional heritage while adapting to the ill-defined concept of the "American way."

Early in life children become aware of their racial or ethnic status and of the discriminatory attitudes of the majority culture toward their group. The direct effects of discrimination are anger and low self-esteem, which become manifest in a variety of behaviors. Inner conflicts and suppressed hostility that focus children's attention inward may be factors in the failure of many children to achieve in other areas.

Evidence indicates that changes in attitudes are slowly taking place in some groups and in some places. With growing awareness, interest, and understanding by increasing numbers of the majority group, which has accompanied the emergence of racial and ethnic pride, minority-group children are becoming more secure and confident in their racial or ethnic identity.

CULTURAL SHOCK

The term *cultural shock* describes the "feelings of helplessness and discomfort and a state of disorientation experienced by an outsider attempting to comprehend or effectively adapt to a different cultural group because of differences in cultural practices, values, and beliefs" (Leininger, 1978). This state occurs with both clients and health care providers who move from one cultural setting to another. It can happen to persons who immigrate to a new country (such as the Asian refugees) or persons from a subcultural group who must adjust to the ways of an unfamiliar subgroup (such as children entering the school subculture or consumers who enter the hospital subculture). Cultural shock is characterized by the inability to respond to or function in a new or strange situation.

Numerous factors influence reactions to a new environment. Language barriers, including dialects and jargon (such as medical language) specific to a subcultural group, inhibit effective communication. Habits and customs (such as different role behaviors or etiquette) and differences in attitudes and beliefs are puzzling to the stranger in the new environment. The outsider experiences an intense sense of isolation and feelings of loneliness and nonrelatedness. Nurses entering an unfamiliar cultural situation can reduce the cultural

---

CRITICAL THINKING EXERCISE
Reducing Cultural Shock

A woman from the Middle East is visiting her child who is hospitalized for a serious illness. Her husband left for home a short time ago to wash and change clothes. She speaks little English. You need to obtain consent from her for an emergency procedure. She is hesitant and refuses to sign the consent form. You:

1. document that the mother refuses to sign the consent form and inform the physician that the procedure cannot be done.
2. realize that she may be hesitant to sign for consent without her husband present because her culture requires the male to make the decisions for the welfare of the family members.
3. explain to her that you cannot help her child unless she signs for permission to do so.
4. realize that she may not understand what you're saying and try to find an interpreter.

The correct answer is two. In the Arab culture men typically make the decisions and wives are expected to support those decisions. Trying to find an interpreter or intimidating her to sign does not address the main issue of the Arab cultural tradition. Although in emergency cases treatment is often approved by the institution or state if a physician documents treatment is necessary and that any delay in treatment may jeopardize the health of the child, in this situation, contacting the father first is appropriate.

---

shock by becoming familiar with the cultural groups with which they work and by learning tolerance of the values, beliefs, and customs of these groups. (See Critical Thinking Exercise.)

Nursing ALERT Because American cultures and subcultures can be so diverse, it is essential that nurses be aware of and knowledgeable about the predominant groups in their work community and apply the knowledge in their practice.

CULTURAL/RELIGIOUS INFLUENCES ON HEALTH CARE
SUSCEPTIBILITY TO HEALTH PROBLEMS

Some groups of people are more susceptible than others to certain illnesses. An innate susceptibility is acquired through generations of evolutionary changes that take place within constrained or segregated populations. The proximity to disease, environmental factors, and the general physical status are significant factors associated with health problems.

Hereditary Factors

The genetic constitution of individuals as groups influences the degree to which they are susceptible to a specific disorder. It may be the result of an inherent lack of resistance to a disease organism, a trait that is an advantage in one environment but places the possessor at a disadvantage in another, or it may be the consequence of intermarriage within a relatively narrow range of geographic, ethnic, or religious restrictions.

A classic example of a geographic constraint is the common communicable disease rubeola (measles). The rubeola virus, or the populations that were continually exposed to it, became altered in such a way that the disease was considered to be a universal disease of childhood from which the majority of children suffered without ill effects. When other populations (e.g., the inhabitants of the Hawaiian Islands) were exposed to the virus by explorers and missionaries, they experienced a violent response that resulted in high mortality.

A number of conditions show ethnic or racial differences. For example, Tay-Sachs disease, characterized by early neurologic deterioration and mental retardation, affects primarily Ashkenasi Jewish families, particularly those of Northeastern European origin, whereas Sephardic Jewish families appear to be no more at risk for the disease than are other populations. The incidence of cystic fibrosis is highest in whites and almost nonexistent in Asians, and the rare affected blacks are usually in areas where there is apt to be mixed ancestry. A classic disorder of blacks, especially Africans, is sickle cell disease (see Chapter 26); however, the incidence of cardiovascular disease, pneumonia, and diabetes is also high among blacks. Native Americans have particularly high rates of tuberculosis, diarrhea, alcoholism, and suicide. Racial and ethnic differences are further considered in relation to diseases and defects as they are discussed throughout the book.

Common food items and drugs may cause health problems in certain ethnic groups. For example, persons of Mediterranean, African, Near Eastern, and Asian origin frequently have glucose-6-phosphate dehydrogenase (G-6-PD) deficiency. They may develop acute hemolytic anemia after they ingest fava (horse or broad) beans or certain drugs such as aspirin preparations, sulfonamides, or primaquine. Other groups, especially southern Europeans, Jews, Arabs, blacks, Asians, and Native Americans, have a deficiency of lactase, the enzyme needed to metabolize lactose. Ingestion of lactose can cause abdominal distention, flatus, and diarrhea. Unknowing but well-meaning health workers may be responsible for these symptoms in their clients when they prescribe foods or food supplements containing lactose as sources of nutrients.

Physical Characteristics.   Among racial groups there are observable differences in physical appearance. The most obvious are skin and hair coloring and texture. Skin color is determined by the amount of melanin pigment present in the skin. Persons from countries located near the equator have darkly pigmented skin, which serves to protect the skin from the year-round exposure to the sun's rays; persons from the northern countries have very light skin, which provides for maximum exposure to the sun's rays (necessary for vitamin D metabolism) during the short daylight hours. There can be wide variations in skin color between these two extremes in terms of geographic origin or from intermixing of dark and light skin color. As a consequence of the dark pigmentation, the detection of skin color changes (e.g., vasomotor alterations, cyanosis, jaundice) can be difficult and requires modification of assessment techniques (see Table 7-9).

Variations in the newborn are often related to racial or ethnic origin. For example, newborn infants of Asian and black parents are smaller than infants of white parentage, and bluish pigmented areas (mongolian spots) on the sacral region are a common observation on Oriental, black, Native American, and Mexican-American infants.

Evaluation of stature and body build reveals some racial tendencies. Children from Asian countries are commonly smaller, falling below the 10th percentile on weight and height charts used for children in the United States (Baze, 1991). This difference in stature can lead to misinterpretation of health status and capabilities. A small child may appear very intelligent for body size but be of average mental ability for age.

Socioeconomic Factors

The most overwhelming adverse influence on health is socioeconomic status. A higher percentage of lower-class individuals are suffering from some health problem at any one time than are those in any other group. The sum of all aspects of their situation contributes to and compounds health problems; this includes crowded living conditions and poor sanitation, which facilitate transfer of disease. Although all children are at risk for lead toxicity, there is a higher incidence of lead poisoning in children from lower-class families, where there is more ready access to lead in the environment (Centers for Disease Control, 1991).

In the lower classes children are less likely to be immunized against preventable diseases than are children in the upper and middle classes. Lack of funds or inaccessibility to health services inhibits treatment for any but severe illness or injury. Sometimes health care is inadequate because of ignorance. In some areas a disorder is so commonplace that it is looked on as unavoidable; it is not recognized as something that requires (or is amenable to) treatment. The parents may not have information regarding causes, treatment, outcome of the illness, or preventive measures.

Poverty.   A high correlation between poverty and the prevalence of illness has long been observed. Impoverished families suffer from poor nutrition; without medical insurance they have little if any preventive health care, inadequate health maintenance, and very limited access to medical treatment. One of the most significant health problems related to poverty is a high infant mortality rate. Day-to-day needs of food, clothing, and lodging take precedence over health care as long as the ailing person feels able to perform activities of daily living.

Poor families are denied access to many health institutions for emergency or other hospital care. Frequently they must travel long distances to service centers that are willing to assume their care. In an emergency they must find money for taxi fare, borrow an automobile, or seek other means of transportation. They must find care for dependents, such as other infants and small children, or have them accompany them when taking the ill child for care. Families tend to delay preventive care indefinitely unless health services are relatively accessible. They are more likely to consult folk practitioners or other persons within their community.

Poor nutrition accounts for many health problems in the lower classes. Lack of funds and knowledge results in a diet that may be seriously lacking in essential food substances, especially protein, vitamins, and iron. This inadequate diet often leads to nutritional deficiency disorders and growth retardation in children. In many the total intake is insufficient to support normal growth. Unstructured eating patterns and irregularly scheduled mealtimes can also contribute to erratic food intake and a proportionately larger consumption of non-nourishing snacks, which can result in excessive weight gain.

Because of deficient preventive care, dental problems are more prevalent. Lack of standard immunizations, together with reduced resistance from poor nutrition, renders the exposed children in poor segments of the population vulnerable to communicable diseases. Poor sanitation and crowded living conditions also contribute to the higher incidence and perpetuation of illness. In general, poor people become ill more frequently and remain ill for longer periods of time than do persons in the general population.

Homelessness. One of the most pressing problems in the United States is the growing number of homeless families. *Homeless individuals* are those persons who lack resources and community ties necessary to provide for their own adequate shelter. In the past the homeless population traditionally included single adults, mostly men. Currently, the fastest growing segment of the homeless population consists of families, constituting at least one third of the people without homes throughout the United States. The largest group includes single mothers from minority groups with two or three young children. The homeless two-parent family is mostly white with fewer children.

Many families are becoming homeless because of physical abuse, substance abuse, disagreements with the landlord, poor living conditions, job layoffs, low income, parental mental illness, domestic conflict, and unexpected family or economic crises. Most families move into homelessness gradually after family members and friends are no longer willing to provide housing (Davidhizar and Frank, 1992).

Another group of homeless children are the "runaway" and "throwaway" adolescents; in the United States this group numbers between 250,000 and 500,000. Many runaways are victims of physical and sexual abuse and leave home because of long-term family or school problems. Poor parent-child relationships, extreme family conflict, feelings of alienation from parents, inconsistency in supervision, and unpredictability in discipline are other factors often cited.

Lack of a permanent dwelling deprives children of the most basic necessities for proper growth and development. Homelessness disrupts a child's friendships and schooling. Homeless children suffer from physical and mental disorders that exceed those found in poor children who have a permanent residence (Bassuk and Rosenberg, 1990), and they are particularly vulnerable for early initiation of and sustained participation in substance-abuse behaviors (Wagner, Melragon, and Menke, 1993).

Migrant Families. Migrants generally suffer more illness, both acute and chronic, than does the general population. They are subject to unhealthy environments, poverty, and insufficient medical care; their health-seeking behavior in general is an illness- or injury-oriented recourse to medical care. The health problems of migrant children appear to be dental caries, upper respiratory tract infections, otitis media, scabies and lice, intestinal parasites, pesticide exposure, injuries, teenage pregnancy, and growth and development delay

(American Academy of Pediatrics, 1989). Affected persons will postpone seeking care for themselves or their children until physical pain or suffering is almost unbearable.

When medical care is provided to a migrant family, follow-up care is usually impossible because of their transient life-style. Compliance to medical therapies is primarily related to accessibility and availability. For example, medications provided by health workers are more likely to be taken than those that must be obtained at a pharmacy. In addition, medications are often discontinued following self-perceived recovery. Compliance is more likely if treatment regimens do not interfere with work or family responsibilities.

CUSTOMS AND FOLKWAYS

Nurses must be aware of the need to consider cultural differences in clients when providing health care. An understanding of the various beliefs regarding the causation of illness and disease, as well as traditional health practices, is essential to successful intervention. The more nurses know about the values, beliefs, and customs of other ethnic groups, the better able they are to meet the needs of these families and to gain their cooperation and compliance.

NURSING TIP Develop a cultural reference manual that includes a brief description of the culture, views on health, illness, diet, and other matters, and a list of interpreters, ethnic community services, or other sources for quick reference (Kuensting and Sanders, 1995).

Cultural Relativity

Although clinical characteristics of a disease or condition are essentially the same across cultures, how a child or family interprets or experiences it varies. Culture as an influence is one obvious explanation for variance. *Cultural relativity* is the concept that any behavior must be judged first in relation to the context of the culture in which it occurs. Nurses must first relate to the family's perceptions and interpretations of experiences from the family's background and cultural belief system before they can effectively intervene.

Some cultures, for example, may view a chronic illness or disability as affecting only particular aspects of a child's life, and the child as a whole is viewed as normal. In contrast, Chinese families more frequently describe the illness as having global effects on many aspects of the child's present and future life (Elfert, Anderson, and Lai, 1991). These contrasting views may result in a difference in goals and expectations parents have for their children.

In some cultures the child's gender may influence a family's perception of the implications of an illness or disability. For example, in the Arabic and Asian cultures the male child is held in higher esteem than the female child. This also holds true for some families of Jewish, Italian, Greek, and Indian origin. The male child may receive better health care and more food, because this is the child who will take care of his parents in their old age (Issacs, 1989).

Defining disease or signs and symptoms of illness is also influenced by culture. Some cultures, for example, perceive diarrhea as a cleansing of the body that is essential for health maintenance and illness prevention and/or cure. Furthermore, signs or symptoms resulting from diarrhea and ensuing dehydration, such as malaise, fever, anorexia, and irritability, may be viewed as separate illness entities.

Nurses can often recognize a family's health-related cultural perceptions and interpretations through discussion and observation. Implications of these perceptions should be explored and considered when effective culturally appropriate interventions are being planned.

Relationships with Health Care Providers

The manner of relating with health care providers differs considerably among cultural groups. One area of conflict to some nurses is the attitude toward time and waiting that is part of some cultures. For example, blacks are very flexible in their time orientation; a black family may be late for or miss appointments because other issues take precedence over the appointment, and they may not communicate this to the health agency. Hispanics, too, have a very relaxed view of time. Whereas the dominant culture in the United States says that "time flies," the Hispanic says, "time walks." The Japanese, on the other hand, consider time to be valuable and to be used wisely. They tend to be punctual for medical appointments and persistent in following prescribed regimens. A Vietnamese family will subordinate time to values considered to be more significant, such as propriety. They may be late for an appointment because of an overextended visit by a friend in their home. In general, Asian-Americans view the American focus on time as offensive. They spend hours getting to know people and view predetermined, abrupt endings as rude. Introductory small talk is considered good manners (Randall-David, 1989).

In many cultural groups the mother assumes the responsibility for health care; in others both parents are involved equally in relationships with health workers. A somewhat different approach is apparent in some of the Asian cultures. For example, the father in Vietnamese families, as unquestioned head of the family, is traditionally the family member who interacts with persons, including health care providers, outside the family unit (Fig. 3-4).

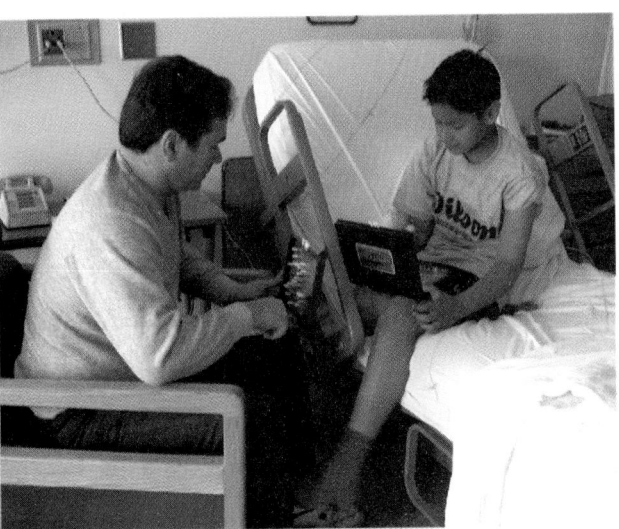

FIG. 3-4. A father with his hospitalized child.

In the Hispanic family the father, as head of the house, makes decisions regarding illness and treatment of family members, but the grandmother in the extended family is consulted regarding child care. Usually the family confers with other members before reaching a decision regarding treatment or hospitalization of a child. The Arab family also relies on others to give advice and guidance in a time of crisis. A Japanese father may appear to be passive and uninvolved but actually is involved according to his own cultural standards.

> **Nursing ALERT** In working with families, it is essential for nurses to identify key members. Failure to include these significant individuals in teaching can seriously hinder adherence to the plan of care.

Nurses should make themselves aware of any specific attitudes regarding the manner of approach to a child in a given culture. Navajo Indians do not like a stranger near their infants. It is feared that the stranger may "witch" the child and cause him or her harm. On the other hand, if a stranger, particularly a woman, lavishes attention on a Latino infant but fails to touch the child, he or she will develop symptoms of the "evil eye" (see p. 43). Vietnamese and Korean families may become upset if a newborn is admired at length for fear the evil spirits will overhear and desire the infant.

Some ethnic groups, such as the Amish, consider a child's admission to the hospital a family affair, with all members gathering to support and console the child and parents. In others, such as the Samoan family, the family is willing to relinquish the care of the child to the hospital authority without interference. Their visits with the child are short, although intense, but this behavior may be misinterpreted by the hospital staff as disinterest or abandonment.

Nurses who are members of a majority culture may encounter tension and distrust in a child from a minority culture as a result of the child's learned perception or relationships with other persons in the majority group. Based on these perceptions, minority children often suspect that nurses may have hostile feelings toward them and fear ill treatment. When such children are hospitalized, this feeling compounds the feelings of loneliness, helplessness, and retribution that accompany fearful happenings and separation from families. The reverse situation may be encountered by a nurse from a minority culture attempting to meet the needs of a child who has been conditioned to view the nurse's cultural or ethnic group as inferior.

Communication. Communication may be a source of distress and misunderstanding between persons from different ethnic groups, especially if the languages are different. Ideally, conversations with families who are unable to speak the dominant language are best conducted by a health care worker who speaks the language of the family. If this is not possible, it may be necessary to use an interpreter. However, use of an interpreter can be a source of misunderstanding if the interpreter is unfamiliar with medical terminology or if there are no corresponding words in the second language to express the ideas and concepts under discussion (see Communicating with Families Through an Interpreter, Chapter 6).

Some persons with poor or limited language comprehension may simply smile and nod in agreement if they do not understand the questions or directives. It is vital that the family fully understand all implications of a child's care and management before they sign permits for special procedures or assume responsibility for the child's care. It is not uncommon for a Vietnamese or a Japanese family to indicate "yes" when in fact they mean "no" in order to avoid social disharmony. They tend to use indirectness rather than confrontation and may become evasive when direct questioning makes them feel uncomfortable.

NURSING TIP *Helpful Communication Tools*

1. Have a series of audio and audiovisual recordings in several languages designed to greet and familiarize the family with the hospital.
2. In the event an interpreter is not available, develop a multilingual booklet containing illustrations of commonly used phrases and hospital routines.
3. Have legal consent forms and explanations of common diagnostic tests available in several languages.
4. Keep cards with common greetings, phrases, and names of body parts in the family's language with the patient's chart, for example, *miseries* (pain) and *locked bowels* (constipation) in blacks and *caida de la mollera* (fallen fontanel from dehydration), *susto* (fright), *dolor, duels,* or *lele* (pain), and *la diarrhea* (diarrhea) in Hispanics.

Nonverbal communication is a practiced art in many Native American tribes, and the members are highly sensitive to body language. They emphasize periods of silence to formulate thoughts in preparation for speech and often remain silent after listening to statements by others in order to properly assimilate what has been said. Interruption, interjection, or haste to arrive at abrupt conclusions is perceived as immature behavior.

The level of comfort with body space or distance from others varies among cultures. Anglos are generally comfortable at an arm's length, Hispanics tend to get closer, and Asians prefer a greater distance.

Eye contact is viewed differently in cultures. Although Anglos are advised to look people straight in the eye, it is not uncommon for persons in some ethnic groups to avoid eye contact and become uncomfortable when conversing with health workers. A Vietnamese patient may not look directly into the nurse's eyes, as a sign of respect. Some Native Americans will make eye contact during the initial greeting, but continued, unwavering eye contact is considered insulting and disrespectful. Asians may consider eye contact a sign of hostility or impoliteness.

Gestures also may have different meanings. For example, some Asians consider finger or foot pointing disrespectful. Native Americans consider vigorous handshaking a sign of aggression, whereas to Anglos the gesture is a sign of good will.

Families may be reluctant to question or otherwise initiate contact with health professionals. In the Asian cultures, for example, it is considered a sign of disrespect to question those who are viewed as persons of authority. A Japanese family may wait silently rather than ask or question. They believe that the health professionals know best and will meet their needs without being asked. It is also important to avoid criticism.

Criticism can cause Asians to "lose face," to feel ashamed, which is highly undesirable.

Families may have poor language comprehension. Many persons are able to read and write English better than they can speak or understand it. Also, the dominant language usually takes over in anxiety-provoking situations, even in persons who are able to communicate satisfactorily under ordinary circumstances.

Terms of address and use of first and last names vary among cultures and can create confusion. For example, in Asian cultures the family name is given first in respect for the family and the given name follows. Therefore all siblings in a family have the same first name. Ethiopians have a very complex system whereby women retain their last names after marriage and the paternal grandfather's name becomes the child's last name.

The expression of emotion also varies ethnically. In some cultures (e.g., Hispanic or Jewish) emotions are expressed openly and members are accustomed to sharing their sorrows and joys with family and friends. Conversely, Nordic and Asian groups are more restrained.

Health care providers generally ask questions and use handouts, booklets, and—particularly with children—dolls and pictures as communication aids. This is uncommon in some cultures. For example, Native American healers ask few questions and do not use forms. In some cultures it is inappropriate or considered taboo to look at the inside of the body, even in pictures, or to use dolls or puppets (Malach and Segel, 1990). Nurses need to consider both verbal and nonverbal communication techniques to interact effectively with children and their families from different cultures (see Guidelines for Culturally Sensitive Interactions, p. 110).

Food Customs

Food customs and symbolism are an integral part of various cultural, ethnic, and religious groups. Although in a large country such as the United States most persons have adopted the eclectic food habits that have evolved over countless generations, many ethnic and geographic food traditions and preferences are retained. Special holidays, ceremonies, and life experiences such as births, birthdays, weddings, and death are often marked by special food items or feasts. In many cultures specific food practices are followed during pregnancy in the belief that certain foods damage the developing fetus.

The distinctive food customs of ethnic groups are a product of their native environment, determined by availability. Fish is a staple food of persons living near the ocean, such as people from Japan, Polynesia, southern Europe, and Scandinavia. Fruit and vegetable preferences are directly related to the climate in which they grow naturally or can be cultivated. The types of grain that are ethnically associated are also those that grow best in the native lands. For example, rice is the staple grain of Asians. The diet of the Eskimo is predominantly fish and meat, depending on which is the most easily procured in the area. Even in the continental United States there are regional favorites, such as rice, hominy grits, and okra in the southern states. In some cultures food is highly spiced; in others foods tend to be bland. Table 3-1 lists the food items common to most cultures and can be used to select foods that most children know and like.

There are a number of restrictions related to food items.

TABLE 3-1. Foods common to most ethnic food patterns					
MEAT AND ALTERNATIVES	**MILK AND MILK PRODUCTS**	**GRAIN PRODUCTS**	**VEGETABLES**	**FRUITS**	**OTHERS**
Pork*	Milk	Rice	Carrots	Apples	Fruit juices
Beef	Ice cream	White bread	Cabbage	Bananas	
Chicken	Yogurt	Noodles, macaroni, spaghetti	Green beans	Oranges	
Eggs		Dry cereal	Greens (especially spinach)	Peaches	
Beans			Sweet potatoes or yams	Pears	
			Tomatoes		

From Endres JB, Rockwell RE: *Food, nutrition, and the young child,* St Louis, 1980, Mosby, p 180.
*May be restricted because of religious custom.

Some have a physiologic origin, such as lack of dairy foods in the diets of some persons of African or Asian ancestry in whom a hereditary lactase deficiency prevents digestion of foods containing lactose. Others have religious restrictions, such as kosher foods and food preparation of the Orthodox Jewish faith and the vegetarian diet of Seventh-Day Adventists (see Vegetarian Diets, Chapter 11).

Children in a strange environment, such as the hospital, feel much more comfortable when they are served familiar foods. Hospital food often tastes strange and bland. The family may be concerned that their child is not receiving foods appropriate to their culture and beliefs. Where possible, it is advisable to provide children's ethnic foods or allow families to bring favorite foods. Concern for differences in food habits and patterns projects an attitude of respect for the family's ethnic or religious heritage.

HEALTH BELIEFS AND PRACTICES

Health Beliefs

Beliefs related to the cause of illness and the maintenance of health are an integral part of the cultural heritage of families. Often inseparable from religious beliefs, they influence the way that families cope with health problems and the way that they respond to health care providers. Predominant among most cultures are beliefs related to natural forces, supernatural forces, and imbalance between forces.

Natural Forces.   The most common natural forces held responsible for ill health if the body is not adequately protected include cold air entering the body, impurities in the air, or other natural sources. For example, a Chinese mother may overdress her infant in an effort to keep cold wind from entering the child's body. The Chinese believe that cold weather, rain, and wind are responsible for "cold" conditions.

In the black culture natural phenomena such as phases of the moon, seasons of the year, and planet positions are believed to affect the body and its processes. Therefore health maintenance is strongly associated with the ability to read "the signs." Most Native Americans consider health to be a state of harmony with nature and the universe.

Supernatural Forces.   High on the list of causes of illness are forces beyond comprehension and logical explanation. Evil influences such as voodoo, witchcraft, or evil spirits are viewed in some cultures as causes of adverse health, especially those illnesses that cannot be explained by other means.

A health belief that is common among people from Latin American, Mediterranean, Near Eastern, some Asian, and some African societies is the concept of the *evil eye* (*mal ojo* is the Hispanic term). It is part of the concept of health as a state of balance; illness is a state of imbalance (see below). Strength and power are associated with the evil eye. Therefore, as long as an individual's strength and weakness remain in balance, he or she is unlikely to become a victim of the evil eye. Weaknesses are not necessarily physical. For example, an excess of some emotion, such as envy, can create a weakness. Infants and small children, because of immature development of their internal strength-weakness states, are especially vulnerable to the gaze of the evil eye. Consequently, the evil eye concept serves to rationalize an inexplicable onset of illness in children who display such symptoms as restlessness, crying, diarrhea, vomiting, and fever.

Although seldom expressed to health care providers, the belief that a witch can cast a spell over others at the request of someone who wishes them ill is found in Hispanic, African, and Australian aboriginal cultures. The victim is often tortured in effigy by pins driven into a doll at the location where the intended victim is to be hurt. "Voodoo deaths" have occurred from the victim's belief in the curse and may result from dehydration as the victim gives up the will to live and refuses to drink (Chidester, 1990).

Imbalance of Forces.   The concept of balance or equilibrium is widespread throughout the world. One of the most common imbalances supported by the Hispanic, Filipino, Chinese, and Arab cultures is that which exists between "hot" and "cold." This belief is reputedly derived from the Hippocratic theory of humoral pathology, which states that illness is caused by an imbalance of the four humors: phlegm, blood, black bile, and yellow bile. Hot and cold describe certain properties and conditions completely unrelated to temperature. Diseases, areas of the body, foods, and illnesses are classified as either "hot" or "cold." In Chinese health belief the forces are termed *yin (cold)* and *yang (hot).* To maintain health, these hot and cold forces must be kept in balance.

Illness is treated by restoring normal balance through the application of appropriate "hot" or "cold" remedies. A "cold" condition such as a respiratory disease is believed to be caused by exposure to cold weather, rain, or cold wind entering the body; it is treated by administration of "hot" foods, herbs, or drugs. Menstruation is considered to be a "hot" condition; therefore, women are cautioned against ingesting "hot" foods, which might increase menstrual flow or produce cramping. Ingesting too much of either "hot" or "cold" foods can also be interpreted as a cause of illness.

Health care workers who are aware of this belief are better able to understand why some persons refuse to eat certain foods. It is possible to help families devise a diet that contains the necessary balance of basic food groups prescribed by the medical subculture while conforming to the beliefs of the ethnic subculture.

The hot-cold food classification may have adverse effects. For example, newborn infants are often started on evaporated milk formulas. Evaporated milk is considered to be a "hot" food, whereas whole milk is viewed as a "cold" food. Infants tend to develop rashes, which are believed to be caused by "hot" foods; in such cases parents may decide to switch to whole milk. However, parents fear that it is dangerous to change too rapidly, so they often feed the child some type of neutralizing substance, which may create additional health problems. Such a problem might be averted if the family's preference is determined before discharge from the hospital and a formula prescribed that is agreeable to both the family and the practitioner.

Health Practices

There are numerous similarities among cultures regarding prevention and treatment of illness. All cultures have some types of home remedies that they apply before seeking help from other persons. Within the ethnic community folk healers who are endowed with the ability to "cure" maladies are sought for special situations and when home remedies are unsuccessful. There is the *curandero* (male) or *curandera* (female) of the Mexican-American community whose healing powers are believed to be a gift from God. The Asian consults a herbalist, knowledgeable in medicines, and/or an ethnic physician practiced in Asian therapies, including acupuncture, acupressure, and moxibustion (application of heat). Native Americans consult a variety of healers with specific skills and knowledge. Specialized medicine persons diagnose illness, provide nonsacred treatments (usually by way of massage and herbs), and care for souls. Other specialists perform sacred services or effect cures through spiritual means.

The folk healers are very powerful persons in their community. They "speak the language" of the family who seeks help and often combine their rituals and potions with prayer and entreaties to God. They also are able to create an atmosphere conducive to successful management. Furthermore, they exhibit a sincere interest in the family and their problem.

Some folk remedies are compatible with the medical regimen and can be used to reinforce the treatment plan. For example, most of the foods contraindicated for persons with peptic ulcers are "hot" foods and would be avoided because of their belief systems. Also, aspirin (a "hot" medication) is an appropriate therapy for "cold" diseases such as the common cold and arthritis. It is not uncommon to discover that a folk prescription has a scientific basis. However, numerous health remedies or preventive practices have no scientific basis, such as the use of garlic or *asafetida*, (a piece of rotten

flesh that looks like a dried sponge) that are worn around the neck to prevent contagious diseases. Also, the wearing of copper or silver bracelets to protect the wearer as he or she grows has no scientific basis. Practices that do no harm should be respected.

To overcome the effect of the evil eye usually requires specialized rituals conducted by the appropriate practitioner. For example, the Chicano curandera ascertains that the condition is truly the result of the evil eye by performing an assessment ritual and then, with a confirmed diagnosis, performs a curative ritual. Sometimes the faith in the folk practitioner results in a delay in obtaining needed medical treatment, although the practitioner will usually suggest medical care if his or her ministrations are unsuccessful.

Health practices of different cultures may also present problems in assessment and interpretation. For example, certain cultural practices or remedies can be misdiagnosed as evidence of "child abuse" by uninformed professionals (see box). It is important to explain why these and other familiar remedies may now be considered harmful. Families need to understand how such practices can place them in jeopardy with child protective services and to explore alternative measures that are more acceptable to the dominant culture (Hayes and Dreher, 1991).

Cultural health remedies that are detrimental to health include eating clay, excessive amounts of salt, or compounds that contain lead or mercury. A careful history can reveal these remedies, but it may require the collaboration of a folk healer to convince a user to stop the practice.

CULTURAL PRACTICES POSSIBLY CONSIDERED ABUSIVE BY THE DOMINANT CULTURE

Coining—A Vietnamese practice that may produce weltlike lesions on the child's back when a coin, held on edge, is repeatedly rubbed lengthwise on the oiled skin to rid the body of the disease

Cupping—An Old World practice (also practiced by the Vietnamese) of placing a container (e.g., tumbler, bottle, jar) containing steam against the skin surface to "draw out the poison" or other evil element. When the heated air within the container cools, a vacuum is created that produces a bruiselike blemish on the skin directly beneath the mouth of the container

Burning or **moxibustion**—A practice of some Southeast Asian groups where small areas of skin are burned to treat enuresis and temper tantrums

Forced kneeling—A child discipline measure of some Caribbean groups where a child is forced to kneel for a long period of time

Topical garlic application—A practice of Yemenite Jews in which crushed garlic cloves or garlic-petroleum jelly plaster is applied to the wrists to treat infectious disease; the practice can result in blisters or garlic burns

Traditional remedies that contain lead—*Greta* and *azarcon* (Mexico; used for digestive problems), *paylooah* (Southeast Asia; used for rash or fever), and *surma* (India; used as a cosmetic to improve eyesight)

Traditional remedy that contains mercury—*Azoque* (Spanish word for quicksilver; used to treat diarrhea).

Genital gestures and practices—Telugu-speaking people of central southern India touch and kiss the penis as a sign of greeting that honors the son over the daughter; the gestures are not erotic or sexual communications (Money, Prakasam, and Joshi, 1991).

[handwritten notes:] Bruises over bony prominences sign of healthy child. Pattern or shape — report

Haitian folk medicine considers it essential to rid the newborn of meconium to ensure neonatal survival. The newborn's first food is a *lok*, or purgative, prepared by cooking a mixture of castor oil, grated nutmeg, sour orange juice, garlic, unrefined sugar, and water. It may be administered several times until the color of the newborn's bowel movement changes from black to yellow. All other oral intake may be restricted until this occurs, which may result in dehydration (DeSantis, 1988).

Faith healing and religious rituals are closely allied with many folk-healing practices. Wearing of amulets, medals, and other religious relics believed by the culture to protect the individual and facilitate healing is a common practice. It is important for health workers to recognize the value of this practice and keep the items where the family has placed them or nearby. It offers comfort and support and rarely impedes medical and nursing care. If an item must be removed during a procedure, it should be replaced, if possible, when the procedure is completed. The reason for its temporary removal is explained to the family, and they are reassured that their wishes will be respected (see Family Focus box).

Nurses can be most effective by operating from a multicultural perspective. Adopting a multicultural perspective means using appropriate aspects of each health cultural orientation under consideration to develop culturally acceptable health care interventions.

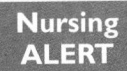

FAMILY FOCUS
On Cultural Awareness

I am a pediatric emergency nurse with a high regard for cultural diversities and a respect for healing practices and beliefs. I even made a manual for my emergency department that contains some of the information needed to help us to understand and communicate with subcultures in the urban community that we serve. Although I learned a great deal putting this manual together, it doesn't come close to the lesson I learned with the following experience:

A 15-month-old Bosnian female in status epilepticus was carried in by her parents. They were very frightened and spoke very little English. I learned that the child had received a measles, mumps, and rubella (MMR) immunization the day before. As I proceeded to unwrap her from the blanket she was in, I quickly assessed the A, B, Cs (airway, breathing, and circulation). I noticed that she was very warm (probably a febrile seizure) and a rag soaked in alcohol was tied around each thigh. Focusing on her potential airway compromise and trying to calm the parents, I proceeded to put an oxygen mask on her, undress her for a full assessment, and remove the alcohol rags. I spoke to the parents all the while in a calm, soothing voice. Once an IV was established and I gave her Ativan, the seizures stopped. So did the communication between her parents and me. I noticed that they would no longer give me eye contact, and the mother would not even speak to me after the seizures stopped. It wasn't until I was returning to the department from admitting her that I realized why they might have stopped communicating with me . . . I had removed the rags! Had I only thought to replace the rags or asked their permission to remove the rags, things may have been different.

Laura L. Kuensting, MSN(R), RN
Cardinal Glennon Children's Hospital
St. Louis, Missouri

Avoid directly criticizing traditional health cultural beliefs and practices as wrong or harmful or implying that biomedical measures are uniformly correct and effective, and the only way to prevent illness or treat sickness. Such criticisms usually result in rejection of both biomedical health care practitioners and their health teaching. When folk practices do not interfere with the welfare of the patient, they need not be discouraged. Often a compromise can be reached that accomplishes the goal of the nurse while maintaining the dignity and self-esteem of the child and family.

Folklore Related to Prenatal Influences

The processes of pregnancy and birth have been surrounded by strongly held beliefs and superstitions that involve taboos and prescriptions for behavior directed toward ensuring the well-being of the unborn child.

It has been a widespread belief that the appearance of the unborn child will be improved if the pregnant woman looks at beautiful people or things. The same concept in reverse has been used to explain birth defects. For example, if a pregnant woman was frightened by a rabbit, it was believed that her child would be born with a cleft (harelip) lip; a microcephalic infant was attributed to the mother's seeing a monkey during pregnancy; and the mother's viewing a person with missing limbs would cause the unborn child to be similarly affected. Activities such as a mother reaching her arms above her head, walking in circles, or tying knots were believed to cause the umbilical cord to be knotted or twisted around the neck of the fetus. Even the shape of birthmarks and other skin defects is sometimes believed to reflect maternal impressions. For example, eating strawberries by the mother is associated with nevi. Articles of apparel or adornment, food cravings, emotions such as fright and anger, undesirable thoughts, and the time and manner of announcing the pregnancy are all believed to influence the well-being of the unborn child.

In most instances these customs are relatively harmless and are not in conflict with sound health practices. However, in some situations conformity to cultural or subcultural beliefs may compromise the health and well-being of the mother or fetus (e.g., the practice of eating clay). Nurses and other health care workers must be understanding and take care to explore with the mother all the ramifications of the practice without creating undue stress and guilt.

Not all of these beliefs are unfounded. There is evidence that maternal emotions may indeed affect the fetus.

RELIGIOUS BELIEFS

Religion influences the life-style of most cultures. Among many groups illness, injury, or death is believed to be sent by God as a punishment for sin. Some may believe that health workers will be unable to help a person whom God is punishing and may express a fatalistic attitude toward treatment, stating it is "the will of God." Others view it as a test of strength, like the testing of Job in the Bible, and strive to remain faithful and overcome the conflicts.

Religious affiliation has implications for many health-related functions and procedures. It is comforting for the

Text continued on p. 51.

TABLE 3-2. Religious beliefs that affect nursing care

BELIEFS ABOUT BIRTH AND DEATH	BELIEFS ABOUT DIET AND FOOD PRACTICES	BELIEFS ABOUT MEDICAL CARE	COMMENTS
Adventist (Seventh-Day Adventist; Church of God)			
Birth: Opposed to infant baptism Baptism by immersion in adulthood *Death:* Desires baptism before death	Meat prohibited in some groups No alcohol, coffee, or tea	Some believe in divine healing and practice anointing with oil and use of prayer May desire communion or baptism when ill Believe in man's choice and God's sovereignty Some oppose hypnosis as therapy	Sabbath: Saturday for many Accept Bible literally
Baptist (27 Groups)			
Birth: Opposed to infant baptism Believers baptized by immersion as adults *Death:* Counsel and prayer with clergy, family, patient	Some groups discourage coffee, tea, and alcohol	"Laying on of hands" (some) May encounter resistance to some therapies, such as abortion Believe God functions through physician Some believe in predestination; may respond passively to care	Fundamentalist and conservative groups accept Bible as inspired word of God
Black Muslim			
Birth: No baptism *Death:* Carefully prescribed procedure for washing and shrouding dead	Prohibit alcohol, pork, and foods traditional among American blacks (e.g., corn bread, collard greens)	Faith healing unacceptable Always maintain personal habits of cleanliness	General adherence to Muslim tenets overlaid, in many instances, by antagonism to whites, especially Christians and Jews Do not indulge in activities (such as sleeping) more than is necessary to health
Buddhist Churches of America			
Birth: No infant baptism Infant presentation *Death:* Last rite chanting often practiced at bedside soon after death Priest should be contacted	No requirements or restrictions Some sects are strictly vegetarian Discourage use of alcohol and drugs	Illness believed to be a trial to aid development of soul; illness due to Karmic causes May be reluctant to have surgery or certain treatments on holy days Cleanliness believed to be of great importance Family may request Buddhist priest for counseling	Optimistic outlook; teach ways to overcome fears, anxieties, apprehension
Church of Christ Scientist (Christian Science)			
Birth: No baptism *Death:* No last rites	No requirements or restrictions	Deny the existence of health crisis; see sickness and sin as errors of mind that can be altered by prayer Oppose human intervention with drugs or other therapies; however, accept legally required immunizations Many adhere to belief that disease is a human mental concept that can be dispelled by "spiritual truth" to extent that they refuse all medical treatment	Many desire services of practitioner or reader; will sometimes refuse even emergency treatment until they have consulted a reader Unlikely to donate organs for transplant

Sources: Carpenito, 1992; Conley, 1990; Kozier and Erb, 1995; Spector, 1985; personal communications.

TABLE 3-2. Religious beliefs that affect nursing care—cont'd

BELIEFS ABOUT BIRTH AND DEATH	BELIEFS ABOUT DIET AND FOOD PRACTICES	BELIEFS ABOUT MEDICAL CARE	COMMENTS
Church of Jesus Christ of Latter Day Saints (Mormon)			
Birth: No baptism at birth Infant is "blessed" by church official at first opportunity after birth (in church) Baptism by immersion at 8 years	Prohibit tea, coffee, alcohol Encourage sparing use of meats Fasting for 24 hours on first Sunday each month (from after evening meal Saturday until evening meal Sunday)	Devout adherents believe in divine healing through annointment with oil and "laying on of hands" by church officials (elders) Medical therapy not prohibited	Married adults wear special undergarments May request Sacrament on Sunday while in hospital Financial support for sick available through well-funded welfare system Discourage cremation Discourage use of tobacco
Death: No special rites but may desire presence of church elders during any acute illness, when condition worsens, when undergoing risky or frightening tests or procedures, when feeling sick enough to die, or when dying			
Eastern Orthodox (Turkey, Egypt, Syria, Rumania, Bulgaria, Cyprus, Albania, etc.)			
Birth: Most believe in infant baptism by immersion 8 to 40 days after birth	Restrictions depend on specific sect	Anointment of the sick No conflict with medical science	Discourage cremation
Death: Last rites obligatory for impending death			
Episcopal (Anglican)			
Birth: Infant baptism mandatory; urgent if poor prognosis	Abstain from meat on fast days May fast on Wednesday, Friday, during Lent, and before Christmas Some fast for 6 hours before receiving Holy Communion	Some believe in spiritual healing Rite for anointing sick available but not mandatory	Religious icons very important Communion four times yearly: Christmas, Easter, June 30, and August 15; may be mandatory for some
Death: Last rites available but not mandatory			
Friends (Quakers)			
Birth: No baptism Infant's name recorded in official book	No requirements or restrictions Most practice moderation Avoid alcohol and illicit drugs	No special rites or restrictions	Believe in plain speech and dress Pacifists
Greek Orthodox			
Birth: Baptism considered important Performed 40 days after birth If not possible to baptize by sprinkling or immersion, church allows child baptism "in the air" by moving the child in the form of a cross as appropriate words are said	Church-prescribed fast periods—usually occur on Wednesday, Friday, and during Lent; consist of avoiding meat and (in some cases) dairy products If health compromised, priest may be contacted to convince family to forego fasting	Each health crisis handled by ordained priest; deacon may also serve in some cases Holy Communion administered in hospital Some may desire Sacrament of the Holy Unction performed by priest	Oppose euthanasia Believe every reasonable effort should be made to preserve life until termination by God Discourage autopsies that may cause dismemberment Prefer burial to cremation

Continued.

TABLE 3-2. Religious beliefs that affect nursing care—cont'd

BELIEFS ABOUT BIRTH AND DEATH	BELIEFS ABOUT DIET AND FOOD PRACTICES	BELIEFS ABOUT MEDICAL CARE	COMMENTS
Greek Orthodox, cont'd *Death:* Last rites, administration of Sacrament of Holy Communion Should be performed while dying person is still conscious			
Hindu *Birth:* No ritual *Death:* Special prescribed rites Priest pours water into the mouth of dead child, ties a thread around neck or wrist to signify blessing (should not be removed) Family washes body and is particular about who touches body	Many dietary restrictions Beef and veal not eaten Some strict vegetarians	Illness or injury believed to represent sins committed in previous life Accept most modern medical practices	Cremation preferred
Islam (Muslim/Moslem) *Birth:* No baptism *Death:* Patient must confess sins and beg forgiveness before death; family should be present Family washes and prepares body, then turns it to face Mecca Only relatives and friends may touch body	Prohibit all pork products and any meat that is not ritually slaughtered Daylight fasting practiced during ninth month of Muhammadan year (Ramadan) Strict Muslims do not use alcohol or mind-altering drugs	Faith healing not acceptable unless psychologic condition of patient is deteriorating; performed for morale Ritual washing after prayer; prayer takes place five times daily (on rising, midday, afternoon, early evening, and before bed); during prayer, face Mecca and kneel on prayer rug	Older Muslims often have a fatalistic view that may interfere with compliance to therapy May oppose autopsy
Jehovah's Witness *Birth:* No baptism *Death:* No last rites	Eat nothing to which blood has been added; can eat animal flesh that has been drained	Adherents are generally absolutely opposed to blood transfusions, including banking of own blood; individuals can sometimes be persuaded in emergencies May be opposed to use of albumin, globulin, factor replacement (hemophilia), vaccines	Often possible to obtain a court order appointing a hospital official as temporary guardian to consent to a child's transfusion when parents refuse consent Autopsy approved only as required by law

TABLE 3-2. Religious beliefs that affect nursing care—cont'd

BELIEFS ABOUT BIRTH AND DEATH	BELIEFS ABOUT DIET AND FOOD PRACTICES	BELIEFS ABOUT MEDICAL CARE	COMMENTS
Judaism (Orthodox and Conservative)			
Birth: No baptism Ritual circumcision of male infants on eighth day; performed by Mohel (ritual circumciser familiar with Jewish law and aseptic technique) Reform Jews favor ritual circumcision, but not as a religious imperative *Death:* Remains are ritually washed by members of the Ritual Burial Society Burial should take place as soon as possible	Numerous dietary kosher laws exist that may be influenced by local practices and family and cultural tradition Allowed only meat from animals that are vegetable eaters, are cloven hoofed, chew their cud, and are ritually slaughtered; fish that have scales and fins Prohibit any combination of meat and milk; milk products served first can be followed by meat in a few minutes, but milk may not be consumed for several hours after eating meat Fasting for 24 hours is part of Yom Kippur observance Matzo replaces leavened bread during Passover week	May resist surgical procedures during Sabbath, which extends from sundown Friday until sundown Saturday Seriously ill and pregnant women are exempt from fasting Illness is grounds for violating dietary laws (e.g., patient with congestive heart failure does not have to use kosher meats, which are high in sodium)	Oppose all forms of mutilation, including autopsy; body parts not donated or removed; amputated limbs, organs, or surgically removed tissues should be made available to family for burial Donation or transplantation of organs requires rabbinical consent May oppose prolongation of life after irreversible brain damage
Lutheran			
Birth: Baptize only living infants shortly after birth *Death:* Last rites optional	No requirements or restrictions	If grave prognosis, family may request anointing and blessing of sick or visit by church official	Accept scientific developments
Mennonite (Similar to Amish)			
Birth: No baptism in infancy Baptism during early or middle teens	No requirements or restrictions	No illness rituals Deep concern for dignity and self-determination of individual that would conflict with shock treatment or medical treatment affecting personality or will	
Methodist			
Birth: No baptism at birth; performed on children or adults *Death:* No ritual	No requirements or restrictions	Communion may be requested before surgery or similar crisis	Encourage donation of body or body parts to medical science
Nazarene			
Birth: Baptism optional *Death:* No last rites	No requirements or restrictions Alcohol prohibited	Church official administers communion and laying on of hands Adherents believe in divine healing but not exclusive of medical treatment	Cremation permitted

Continued.

TABLE 3-2. Religious beliefs that affect nursing care—cont'd

BELIEFS ABOUT BIRTH AND DEATH	BELIEFS ABOUT DIET AND FOOD PRACTICES	BELIEFS ABOUT MEDICAL CARE	COMMENTS
Pentecostal (Assembly of God, Four-Square) *Birth:* No baptism at birth Baptism by complete immersion after age of accountability *Death:* No last rites	Abstain from alcohol, eating blood, strangled animals, or anything to which blood has been added Some individuals may resist pork	No restrictions regarding medical care Deliverance from sickness is provided for in atonement; may pray for divine intervention in health matters and seek God in prayer for themselves and others when ill	Some insist illness is divine punishment; most consider it an intrusion of Satan Practice glossolalia (speaking in tongues)
Orthodox Presbyterian *Birth:* Infant baptism by sprinkling *Death:* Last rites not a sacramental procedure; scripture reading and prayer	No requirements or restrictions	Communion administered when appropriate and convenient Blood transfusion accepted when advisable Pastor or elder should be called for ill person Believe science should be used for relief of suffering	Full forgiveness granted for any illness connected with a sin
Roman Catholic *Birth:* Infant baptism by sprinkling mandatory; especially urgent in poor prognosis, when it may be performed by anyone *Death:* Rite for anointing of the sick is mandatory Family or patient may request anointing if prognosis is grave	Fasting and abstaining from meat mandatory on Ash Wednesday and Good Friday; fasting optional during Lent; no meat on Fridays during Lent as general rule Children and most hospital patients exempt from fasting (eating only one full meal and no eating between meals) Some older Catholics may adhere to older rule of no meat on Friday	Encourage anointing of sick, although this may be interpreted by older members of church as equivalent to the old terminology "extreme unction" or "last rites"; they may require careful explanation if reluctance associated with fear of imminent death Traditional church teaching does not approve of contraceptives or abortion	Family may request that major amputated limb be buried in consecrated ground Transplant accepted as long as loss of organ does not deprive donor of life or functional integrity of body Autopsy acceptable Religious articles, especially wearing medals, important and should be removed only when necessary and replaced as soon as possible
Russian Orthodox *Birth:* Baptism by priest only *Death:* Traditionally after death arms are crossed, fingers set in a cross	No meat or dairy products on Wednesday, Friday, and during Lent	Cross necklace is important and should be removed only when necessary and replaced as soon as possible Adherents believe in divine healing, but not exclusive of medical treatment	Opposed to autopsy, embalming, or cremation
Unitarian Universalist *Birth:* Some practice infant baptism; most consider it unnecessary *Death:* No ritual	No requirements or restrictions	Believe God helps those who help themselves Some may prefer not to have clergy visit them in hospital	Cremation preferred to burial

family of an ill child to have this need recognized and respected. Nurses need to determine if there are any special considerations, including dietary restrictions, related to spiritual practices that are important to the family. Family members are asked whether they want a clergy member present and whether they prefer hospital staff to call or prefer to do this on their own.

NURSING TIP Children will rarely voice a need for spiritual support. Listen closely for indirect references such as "God doesn't care what happens to people" (Clutter, 1991).

It is also important to determine the wishes of the family regarding baptism, rites or practices related to death, and other religious rituals (such as circumcision, communion, or use of amulets or icons). Religion, which offers families understanding and spiritual support, is a valuable asset to health care. Characteristics of selected religions with beliefs that affect health care are outlined in Table 3-2.

IMPORTANCE OF CULTURE AND RELIGION TO NURSES

To begin to understand and to deal effectively with families in a multicultural community or in a unicultural community that is different from one's own, nurses must be aware of their own attitudes and values regarding a way of life, including health practices. Nurses, too, are a product of their own cultural background. They also need to recognize that they are part of the "nursing culture." Nurses function within the framework of a professional culture with its own values and traditions and, as such, become socialized into their professional culture in their educational program and later in their work environments and professional associations (Friedman, 1990).

Frequently nurses and other health care workers are not aware of their own cultural values and how those values influence their thoughts and actions. Those who are aware of their own culturally founded behavior are more sensitive to cultural behavior in others. To recognize that a behavior may be characteristic of a culture rather than an "abnormal" behavior places nurses at an advantage in their relationships with families. When nurses respect the cultural differences of a family, they are better able to determine whether the behavior is distinctive to the individual or a characteristic of the culture.

Cultural standards and values, the family structure and function, and past experiences with health care influence a family's feelings and attitudes toward health, their children, and health care delivery systems. It is often difficult for nurses to be nonjudgmental and objective in working with families whose behaviors and attitudes differ from or conflict with their own. Being aware of one's own feelings and attitudes and respecting those of the family are essential to a helping relationship and achievement of nursing goals. Relying on one's own values and experiences for guidance can result only in frustration and disappointment. It is one thing to know what is needed to deal with a health problem; it is often quite another to implement a fruitful course of action unless nurses work within the cultural and socioeconomic framework of the family. (See Critical Thinking Exercise.)

CRITICAL THINKING EXERCISE
Cultural Practices

Knowledge of cultural practices in a locality can be as important as knowledge of communicable diseases. This knowledge:

1. is not valuable unless the nurse uses it to assess contributing cultural factors that may aid or hinder the care of the child and family.
2. is not helpful unless the nurse is part of the culture.
3. is valuable only in making nurses aware of diversities in care.
4. is learned only from reading about the traditional beliefs and practices of cultural groups.

The correct answer is one. Information about a culture is not valuable unless you apply the knowledge to the situation. A nurse does not need to be a part of a culture to be aware of differences and to respect its practices. Although cultural knowledge may be helpful in awareness of diversities in practices and care, putting the knowledge to use is the challenge and the goal. Information about cultures is learned from a variety of methods: observation, previous experience/interactions, television, journals, textbooks, travel, and so on.

It is beneficial to adapt ethnic practices to the health needs of the family rather than attempt to change long-standing beliefs. To aid their efforts to understand and respect the cultural beliefs of families, nurses should have a readily available resource file containing pertinent information about the cultural and subcultural characteristics of the community in which they practice (e.g., traditional practices related to infant feeding practices and the time and manner of weaning and toilet training). Bridging cultural gaps in delivery of health care to children requires the establishment of a close relationship with families and other influential persons in the community (such as the local folk healer) and periodic assessment of one's own attitudes and behaviors and those of other health workers toward people of other racial or ethnic origins.

Some characteristics of selected cultures are outlined in Table 3-3. Tables 3-2 and 3-3 are presented as beginning frameworks for practicing transcultural nursing. Nurses must assess the cultural and religious practices of families to identify how these practices are similar to and different from those of their own cultural and religious backgrounds. Guidelines for assessing cultural and religious practices of families are described on p. 124.

Nursing ALERT These generalizations are presented to help nurses learn the unique beliefs and practices of various groups and are not meant to be stereotypes of any group. It is critical to remember that no cultural group is homogeneous, every racial and ethnic group contains great diversity, and knowledge of a culture may not reflect an individual member's beliefs (Nance, 1995).

TABLE 3-3. Cultural characteristics related to health care of children

CULTURAL GROUP	HEALTH BELIEFS	HEALTH PRACTICES
Asian-Americans *Chinese*	A healthy body viewed as gift from parents and ancestors and must be cared for Health is one of the results of balance between the forces of *yin* (cold) and *yang* (hot), energy forces that rule the world Illness caused by imbalance Believe blood is source of life and is not regenerated *Chi* is innate energy Lack of *chi* and blood results in deficiency that produces fatigue, poor constitution, and long illness	Goal of therapy is to restore balance of *yin* and *yang* Acupuncturist applies needles to appropriate meridians identified in terms of *yin* and *yang* Acupressure and *tai chi* replacing acupuncture in some areas Moxibustion is application of heat to skin over specific meridians Wide use of medicinal herbs procured and applied in prescribed ways Folk healers are herbalist, spiritual healer, temple healer, fortune healer Meals may or may not be planned to balance hot and cold Milk intolerance relatively common Use of condiments (e.g., monosodium glutamate and soy sauce) may create difficulty with some diet regimens (e.g., low-salt diets)

Japanese	Three major belief systems:
	  Shinto religious influence
	    Humans inherently good
	    Evil caused by outside spirits
	    Illness caused by contact with polluting agents (e.g., blood, corpses, skin diseases)
	  Chinese and Korean influence
	    Health achieved through harmony and balance between self and society
	    Disease caused by disharmony with society and not caring for body
	  Portuguese influence
	    Upholds germ theory of disease
		Believe evil removed by purification
		Energy restored by means of acupuncture, acupressure, massage, and moxibustion along affected meridians
		Kampō medicine—use of natural herbs
		Believe in removal of diseased parts
		Trend is to use both Western and Oriental healing methods
		Care of disabled viewed as family's responsibility
		Take pride in child's good health
		Seek preventive care, medical care for illness
		May avoid some food combinations (e.g., milk and cherries, watermelon and crab) and believe pickled plums to have special properties

Vietnamese	Good health considered to be balance between *yin* (cold) and *yang* (hot) Believe person's life has been predisposed toward certain phenomena by cosmic forces Health believed to be result of harmony with existing universal order; harmony attained by pleasing good spirits and avoiding evil ones Belief in *am duc*, the amount of good deeds accumulated by ancestors Many use rituals to prevent illness Practice some restrictions to prevent incurring wrath of evil spirits	Family uses all means possible before using outside agencies for health care Fortune-tellers determine event that caused disturbance May visit temple to procure divine instruction Use astrologer to calculate cyclical changes and forces Regard health as family responsibility; outside aid sought when resources run out Certain illnesses considered only temporary (such as pustules, open wounds) and ignored Seek generalist health healers May use special diets to prevent illness and promote health Lactose intolerance prevalent
Filipinos	Believe God's will and supernatural forces govern universe Illness, accidents, and other misfortunes are God's punishment for violations of His will Widely accept "hot" and "cold" balance and imbalance as cause of health and illness	Some use amulets as a shield from witchcraft or as good luck pieces Catholics substitute religious medals and other items

Sources: Anderson and Fenichel, 1989; Bloch, 1983; Char, 1981; Chen-Louie, 1983; DeSantis, 1988; Ehling, 1981; Greathouse and Miller, 1981; Hashizume and Takano, 1983; Holland and Sweeney, 1985; Hollingsworth, Brown, and Brooten, 1980; Lacay, 1981; Monrroy, 1983; Orque, 1983a, 1983b; Randall-David, 1989; Sodetaini-Shebata, 1981.

FAMILY RELATIONSHIPS	COMMUNICATION	COMMENTS
Extended family pattern common Strong concept of loyalty of young to old Respect for elders taught at early age—acceptance without questioning or talking back Children's behavior a reflection on family Family and individual honor and "face" important Self-reliance and self-restraint highly valued; self-expression repressed Males valued more highly than females; women submissive to men in family	Open expression of emotions unacceptable Often smile when do not comprehend	Do not react well to painful diagnostic workup; are especially upset by drawing of blood Deep respect for their bodies and believe it best to die with bodies intact; therefore may refuse surgery Believe in reincarnation Older members fear hospitals; often believe hospital is a place to go to die Children sometimes breast-fed for up to 4 or 5 years*

Close intergenerational relationships
Family provides anchor
Family tends to keep problems to self
Value self-control and self-sufficiency
Concept of *haji* (shame) imposes strong control; unacceptable behavior of children reflects on family
Many adopt practices of contemporary middle class
Concern for child's missing school may result in sending to school before fully recovered from illness
	Issei—born in Japan; usually speak Japanese only
	Nisei, Sansei, and *Yonsei* have few language difficulties
	New immigrants able to read and write English better than able to speak or understand it
	Make significant use of nonverbal communication with subtle gestures and facial expression
	Tend to suppress emotions
	Will often wait silently
		Generational categories:
		  Issei—1st generation to live in U.S.
		  Nisei—2nd generation
		  Sansei—3rd generation
		  Yonsei—4th generation
		Issei and *Nisei*—tolerant and permissive childrearing until 5 or 6, then emphasis on emotional reserve and control
		Cleanliness highly valued
		Time considered valuable and used wisely
		Tendency to practice emotional control may make assessment of pain more difficult

Family is revered institution Multigenerational families Family is chief social network Children highly valued Individual needs and interests are subordinate to those of family group Father is main decision maker Women taught submission to men Parents expect respect and obedience from children	Many immigrants are not proficient in speaking and understanding English May hesitate to ask questions Questioning authority is sign of disrespect; asking questions considered impolite Use indirectness rather than forthrightness in expressing disagreement May avoid eye contact with health professionals as a sign of respect	Consider status more important than money Children taught emotional control Time concept more relaxed—consider punctuality less significant than other values (i.e., propriety) Place high value on social harmony
Family is highly valued, with strong family ties Multigenerational family structure common, often with collateral members as well Personal interests are subordinated to family interests and needs Members avoid any behavior that would bring shame on the family	Immigrants and older persons may not be able to speak or understand English	Tend to have a fatalistic outlook on life Believe time and providence will solve all

---

*Most Asian cultures consider the child 1 year old at the time of birth. Traditional Chinese custom adds 1 year on January 1 regardless of the birthday—a child born in December is 2 years old the next January.

Continued.

TABLE 3-3. Cultural characteristics related to health care of children—cont'd

CULTURAL GROUP	HEALTH BELIEFS	HEALTH PRACTICES
American Blacks	Illness classified as: Natural—affected by forces of nature without adequate protection (e.g., cold air, pollution, food and water) Unnatural—evil influences (e.g., witchcraft, voodoo, hoodoo, hex, fix, rootwork); symptoms often associated with eating Believe serious illness sent by God as punishment (e.g., parents punished by illness or death of child) Believe serious illness can be avoided May resist health care because illness is "will of God"	Self-care and folk medicine very prevalent Folk therapies usually religious in origin Attempt home remedies first; poorer people do not seek help until illness serious Usually seek help from: "Old lady"—woman in community with a common knowledge of herbs; consulted regarding pediatric care Spiritualist—has received gift from God for healing incurable diseases or solving personal problems; strongly based in Christianity Priest (voodoo priest/priestess)—most powerful healer Root doctor—meets need for herbs, oils, candles, and ointments Prayer is common means for prevention and treatment
Haitians*	Illnesses have a supernatural or natural origin Supernatural illnesses are caused by angry voodoo spirits, enemies, or the dead, especially deceased ancestors Natural illnesses are based on conceptions of natural causation: Irregularities of blood volume, flow, purity, viscosity, color and/or temperature (hot/cold) Gas (*gaz*) Movement and consistency of mother's milk Hot/cold imbalance in the body Bone displacement Movement of diseases Health is maintained by good dietary and hygienic habits	Health is a personal responsibility Foods have properties of "hot"/"cold" and "light"/"heavy" and must be in harmony with one's life cycle and bodily states Natural illnesses are treated by home remedies first Supernatural illness treated by healers: voodoo priest (*houngan*) or priestess (*mambo*), midwife (*fam saj*), and herbalist or leaf doctor (*dokte fey*) Amulets and prayer used to protect against illness due to curses or willed by evil people
Hispanic Americans *Mexican-Americans (Latinos, Chicanos, Raza-Latinos)*	Health beliefs have strong religious association Believe in body imbalance as a cause of illness, especially imbalance between *caliente* (hot) and *frio* (cold) or "wet" and "dry" Some maintain good health is a result of "good luck"—a reward for good behavior Illness prevented by performing properly, eating proper foods, and working proper amount of time; accomplished through prayer, wearing religious medals or amulets, and sleeping with relics at home Illness is a punishment from God for wrongdoing, forces of nature, and the supernatural	Seek help from *curandero* or *curandera*, especially in rural areas Curandero(a) receives his/her position by birth, apprenticeship, or a "calling" via dream or vision Treatments involve use of herbs, rituals, and religious artifacts Practice for severe illness—make promises, visit shrines, offer medals and candles, offer prayers Adhere to "hot" and "cold" food prescriptions and prohibitions for prevention and treatment of illness
Puerto Ricans	Subscribe to the "hot-cold" theory of causation of illness Believe some illnesses caused by evil spirits and forces	Infrequent use of health care systems Seek folk healers—use of herbs, rituals Consult spiritualist medium for mental disorders *Santeria* is system and practitioners are called *santeros* Treatments classified as "hot" or "cold"

*This section was written by Lydia DeSantis, PhD, RN.

FAMILY RELATIONSHIPS	COMMUNICATION	COMMENTS
Strong kinship bonds in extended family; members come to aid of others in crisis Less likely to view illness as a burden Augmented families common (unrelated persons living in same household) Place strong emphasis on work and ambition Sex-role sharing among parents Elderly members respected	Alert to any evidence of discrimination Place importance on nonverbal behavior May use nonstandard English or "black English" Use "testing" behaviors to assess personnel in health care situations before seeking active care Best to use simple, direct, but caring approach	High level of caution and distrust of majority group Social anxiety related to tradition of humiliation, oppression, and loss of dignity Will elect to retain dignity rather than seek care if values are compromised Strong sense of peoplehood High incidence of poverty Black minister a strong influence in black community Visits by family minister are sought, expected, and valued in helping to cope with illness and suffering
Maintenance of family reputation is paramount Lineal authority supreme; children in a subordinate position in family hierarchy Children valued for parental social security in old age and expected to contribute to family welfare at an early age Children viewed as "gifts from god" and treated with indulgence and affection	Recent immigrants and older persons may speak only Haitian creole May prefer family/friends to act as translators and confidants Often smile and nod in agreement when do not understand Quiet and gentle communication style and lack of assertiveness lead health care providers to falsely believe they comprehend health teaching and are compliant Will not ask questions if health care provider is busy or rushed	Will use biomedical and ethnomedical (folk) systems simultaneously Resistant to dietary and work restrictions Adherence to prescribed treatments directly related to perceived severity of illness
Traditionally men considered breadwinners and key decision makers in matters outside the home; women considered homemakers Males considered big and strong *(macho)* Strong kinship; extended families include *compadres* (godparents) established by ritual kinship Children valued highly and desired, taken everywhere with family Many homes contain shrines with statues and pictures of saints Elderly treated with respect	May use nonstandard English Most bilingual; many only speak Spanish May have a strong preference for native language and revert to it in times of stress May shake hands or engage in introductory embrace Interpret prolonged eye contact as disrespectful	High degree of modesty—often a deterrent to seeking medical care and open discussions of sex Youngsters often reluctant to share communal showers in schools Relaxed concept of time—may be late for appointments More concerned with present than with future and therefore may focus on immediate solutions rather than long-term goals Magicoreligious practices common May view hospital as place to go to die
Family usually large and home centered—the core of existence Father has complete authority in family—family provider and decision maker Wife and children subordinate to father Children valued—seen as a gift from God Children taught to obey and respect parents; corporal punishment to ensure obedience	May use nonstandard English Spanish speaking or bilingual Strong sense of family privacy—may view questions regarding family as impudent	Relaxed sense of time Pay little attention to *exact* time of day Suspicious and fearful of hospitals

Continued.

TABLE 3-3. Cultural characteristics related to health care of children—cont'd

CULTURAL GROUP	HEALTH BELIEFS	HEALTH PRACTICES
Cuban-Americans†	Prevention and good nutrition are related to good health	Diligent users of the medical model, in part because of aggressive public health practices on the island before and after the revolution Eclectic health-seeking practices, including preventive measures, extensive use of the medical model, and, in some instances, folk medicine of both religious and nonreligious origins; home remedies; in many instances seek assistance of *santeros* (Afro-Cuban healers) and spiritualists to complement medical treatment Nutrition is important; parents show overconcern with eating habits of their children and spend a considerable part of the budget on food; traditional Cuban diet is rich in meat and starch; consumption of fresh vegetables added in United States
Native Americans (numerous tribes)	Believe health is state of harmony with nature and universe Respect of bodies through proper management All disorders believed to have aspects of supernatural Violation of a restriction or prohibition thought to cause illness Fear of witchcraft May carry objects believed to guard against witchcraft Theology and medicine strongly interwoven	Medicine persons: Altruistic persons who must use powers in purely positive ways Persons capable of both good and evil—perform negative acts against enemies Diviner-diagnosticians—diagnose but do not have powers or skill to implement medical treatment Specialists—use herbs and curative but nonsacred medical procedures Medicine persons—use herbs and ritual Singers—cure by the power of their song obtained from supernatural beings; effect cures by laying on of hands

†This section was written by Mercedes Sandaval, PhD

KEY POINTS

- A culture is composed of individuals with a set of values, beliefs, practices, and information that is learned, integrative, social, and satisfying.
- Nurses have a responsibility to understand the influence of culture, race, and ethnicity on the development of social and emotional relationships, childrearing practices, and attitudes toward health.
- Socialization is the process by which children acquire the beliefs, values, and behaviors considered desirable or appropriate by the culture.
- A child's self-concept evolves from ideas about his or her social roles.
- Guilt and shame are two behaviors commonly conditioned in children to control social behavior.
- Important subcultural influences on children include ethnicity, social class, poverty, affluence, occupation, religion, schools, peers, and biculture.
- Membership in a minority group presents special challenges for children, although changes in societal attitudes are slowly taking place.
- Cultural shock refers to a person's feeling of helplessness and disorientation while trying to adapt to a different cultural group and its practices, values, and beliefs.
- A child's physical characteristics and susceptibility to health problems are strongly related to ethnic and cultural variations of hereditary and socioeconomic forces.
- Cultural beliefs related to the course of illness and maintenance of health may focus on natural forces, supernatural forces, or imbalance of forces.
- In planning and implementing patient care, nurses need to strive to adapt ethnic practices to the family's health needs rather than attempt to change longstanding beliefs.
- No cultural group is homogeneous, and every racial and ethnic group contains great diversity.

FAMILY RELATIONSHIPS	COMMUNICATION	COMMENTS
Strong family ties with mother and father kinships Children supported and assisted by parents long after becoming adults Elderly cared for at home	Most are bilingual (English/Spanish) except for segments of the senior population	In less than 30 years Cubans have been able to obtain a higher standard of living than other Hispanic groups in United States Have been able to retain many of their former social institutions: bilingual and private schools, clinics, social clubs, the family as an extended network of support, etc. Many do not feel discriminated against nor harbor feelings of inferiority with respect to Anglo-Americans or "mainstream" population
Extended family structure—usually includes relatives from both sides of family Elder members assume leadership roles	Most continue to speak their Indian language, as well as English Nonverbal communication	Time orientation—present Respect for age Going to hospital associated with illness or disease; therefore may not seek prenatal care, since pregnancy viewed as natural process Tend to take time to form an opinion of professionals

REFERENCES

Adams PJ: Effects of poverty and affluence. In Hendee WR: *The health of adolescents,* San Francisco, 1991, Jossey-Bass.

American Academy of Pediatrics: Health care for children of migrant families, *Pediatrics* 84(4):739-740, 1989.

Anderson P, Fenichel D: *Serving culturally diverse families of infants and toddlers with disabilities,* Washington, DC, 1989, National Center for Clinical Infant Programs.

Bassuk EL, Rosenberg L: Psychosocial characteristics of homeless children and children with homes, *Pediatrics* 85(3):257-261, 1990.

Baze S: Measuring physical growth. In Smith D, editor: *Comprehensive child and family nursing skills,* St Louis, 1991, Mosby.

Bloch B: Nursing care of black patients. In Orque MS, Bloch B, Monrroy LSA, editors: *Ethnic nursing care,* St Louis, 1983, Mosby.

Buchwald D and others: Caring for patients in a multicultural society, *Patient Care* 28(11):105-120, 1994.

Carpenito LJ: *Nursing diagnosis: application to clinical practice,* ed 4, Philadelphia, 1992, Lippincott.

Centers for Disease Control: *Preventing lead poisoning in young children,* Atlanta, GA, 1991, US Department of Health and Human Services.

Char EL: The Chinese American. In Clark AL, editor: *Culture and childrearing,* Philadelphia, 1981, FA Davis.

Chen-Louie T: Nursing care of Chinese American patients. In Orque MS, Bloch B, Monrroy LSA, editors: *Ethnic nursing care,* St Louis, 1983, Mosby.

Chidester D: *Patterns of transcendence: religion, death, and dying,* Belmont, CA, 1990, Wadsworth.

Clutter L: Fostering spiritual care for the child and family. In Smith D, editor: *Comprehensive child and family nursing skills,* St Louis, 1991, Mosby.

Conley L: Childbearing and childrearing practices in Mormonism, *Neonatal Network* 9(3):41-48, 1990.

Davidhizar R, Frank B: Understanding the physical and psychosocial stressors of the child who is homeless, *Pediatr Nurs* 18(6):559-562, 1992.

DeSantis L: Cultural factors affecting newborn and infant diarrhea, *J Pediatr Nurs* 3(6):391-398, 1988.

Ehling MB: The Mexican American (El Chicano). In Clark AL, editor: *Culture and childrearing*, Philadelphia, 1981, FA Davis.

Elfert H, Anderson J, Lai M: Parents' perceptions of children with chronic illness: a study of immigrant Chinese families, *J Pediatr Nurs* 6(2):114-120, 1991.

Elkin F, Handel G: *The child and society: the process of socialization*, New York, 1989, Random House.

Fleming J: Meeting the challenge of culturally diverse populations, *Pediatr Nurs* 15(6):566, 634, 1989 (guest editorial).

Friedman M: Transcultural family nursing: application to Latino and black families, *Pediatr Nurs* 5(3):214-222, 1990.

Greathouse B, Miller VG: The black American. In Clark AL, editor: *Culture and childrearing*, Philadelphia, 1981, FA Davis.

Hashizume S, Takano J: Nursing care of Japanese patients. In Orque MS, Bloch B, Monrroy LSA, editors: *Ethnic nursing care*, St Louis, 1983, Mosby.

Hayes J, Dreher C: Providing culturally sensitive care. In Smith D, editor: *Comprehensive child and family nursing skills*, St Louis, 1991, Mosby.

Holland S, Sweeney E: *Vietnamese children and families: the impact of culture*, Washington, DC, 1985, Association for Care of Children's Health.

Hollingsworth AO, Brown LP, Brooten DA: The refugees and childbearing: what to expect, *RN* 43(11):45-48, 1980.

Issacs P: Growth parameters and blood values in Arabic children, *Pediatr Nurs* 15(6):579-583, 1989.

Johns K: What parents value most in their children: evidence that country of origin makes little difference, *Sociology Soc Res* 71(3):238-242, 1987.

Kozier B, Erb G: *Fundamentals of nursing*, ed 5, Menlo Park, CA, 1995, Addison-Wesley.

Kuensting L, Sanders G, editors: *Cultural considerations*, Park Ridge, IL, 1995, Emergency Nurses Association.

Lacay G: The Puerto Rican in mainland America. In Clark AL, editor: *Culture and childrearing*, Philadelphia, 1981, FA Davis.

Leininger M: *Transcultural nursing*, New York, 1978, Wiley.

Lynch E: From cultural shock to cultural learning. In Lynch E, Hanson M, editors: *Developing cross-cultural competence*, Baltimore, 1992, Paul H Brookes.

Malach F, Segel N: Perspectives on health care delivery systems for American Indian families, *Child Health Care* 19(4):219-228, 1990.

Martin JA: Birth characteristics for Asian or Pacific Islander subgroups, 1992. Monthly vital statistics report; vol 43 no 10, suppl, Hyattsville, MD, 1995, National Center for Health Statistics.

Money J, Prakasam K, Joshi V: Transcultural developmental sexology: genital greeting versus child molestation, *Issues Child Abuse Accusations* 9(4):215-216, 1991.

Monrroy LSA: Nursing care of Raza/Latina patients. In Orque MS, Bloch B, Monrroy LSA, editors: *Ethnic nursing care*, St Louis, 1983, Mosby.

Nance TA: Intercultural communication: finding common ground, *JOGNN* 24(3):249-255, 1995.

Orque MS: Nursing care of Filipino American patients. In Orque MS, Bloch B, Monrroy LSA, editors: *Ethnic nursing care*, St Louis, 1983a, Mosby.

Orque MS: Nursing care of South Vietnamese patients. In Orque MS, Bloch B, Monrroy LSA, editors: *Ethnic nursing care*, St Louis, 1983b, Mosby.

Randall-David E: *Strategies for working with culturally diverse communities and clients*, Washington, DC, 1989, Association for the Care of Children's Health.

Rescoria L, Parker R, Stolley P: Ability, achievement, and adjustment in homeless children, *Am J Orthopsychiatry* 61(2):210-220, 1991.

Shaffer DC: *Developmental psychology: theory, research and application*, Monterey, CA, 1985, Brooks/Cole Publishing Co.

Sloat A, Matsuura, W: Intercultural communication. In Craft M, Denehy J, editors: *Nursing interventions for infants and children*, Philadelphia, 1990, WB Saunders.

Sodetaini-Shibata AE: The Japanese American. In Clark AL, editor: *Culture and childrearing*, Philadelphia, 1981, FA Davis.

Spector RE: *Cultural diversity in health and illness*, ed 2, New York, 1985, Appleton-Century Crofts.

Wagner J, Melragon B, Menke E: Homeless children: interdisciplinary drug prevention intervention, *J Child Adolesc Psychiatr Ment Health Nurs* 6(1):22-30, 1993.

BIBLIOGRAPHY

General

Ahmann E: "Chunky stew": appreciating cultural diversity while providing health care for children, *Pediatr Nurs* 20(3):320-322, 1994.

Anderson JM: Health care across cultures, *Nurs Outlook* 38(3):136-139, May/June, 1990.

Bauwens EE, Anderson S: Social and cultural influences on health care. In Stanhope M, Lancaster J, editors: *Community health nursing*, ed 3, St Louis, 1992, Mosby.

Buchwald D and others: Five vignettes of cross-cultural care, *Patient Care* 29(11):120-123, 1994.

Chan S: Early intervention with culturally diverse families of infants and toddlers with disabilities, *Inf Young Child* 3(2):78-87, 1990.

Choi ES, Hamilton RK: The effects of culture on mother-infant interaction, *JOGNN* 15:256-261, 1986.

Conatser C: Effect of wealth on approach to patient care, *J Assoc Pediatr Oncol Nurses* 3(2):14-19, 1986.

Culture and nursing practice: an applied view, *Holistic Nurs Pract* 6(3):entire issue, 1992.

Evans V: Sociodemographic trends toward the 21st century. In Feeg V, editor: *Pediatric nursing: forum on the future: looking toward the 21st century*, Pitman, NJ, 1989, Anthony J Jannetti.

Giger J, Davidhizar R: *Transcultural nursing: assessment and intervention*, ed 2, St Louis, 1995, Mosby.

Habayeb GL: Cultural diversity: a nursing concept not yet reliably defined, *Nurs Outlook* 43(5):224-227, 1995.

Juarez G: Controlling pain: when culture clashes with pain control, *Nursing* 25(5):90, 1995.

Kohn S: Dismantling sociocultural barriers to care, *Healthcare Forum J* 38(3):30-3, 1995.

Lenburg CB and others: *Promoting cultural competence in and through nursing education: a critical review and comprehensive plan for action*, Washington DC, 1995, American Academy of Nursing.

Meleis AI and others: *Diversity, marginalization and culturally competent health care: issues in knowledge development*, Washington DC, 1995, American Academy of Nursing.

Olness K: Cultural issues in primary pediatric care. In Hoekelman RA, editor: *Primary pediatric care*, ed 2, St Louis, 1992, Mosby.

Tripp-Reimer T, Afifi LA: Cross-cultural perspectives on patient teaching, *Nurs Clin North Am* 24(3):613-619, 1989.

Tripp-Reimer T, Brink PJ, Saunders JM: Cultural assessment: content and process, *Nurs Outlook* 32:78-82, 1984.

Tseng W, Hsu J: *Culture and family*, Binghamton, NY, 1990, Haworth Press.

Religion

Abbott DA, Berry M, Meredith WH: Religious beliefs and practice: a potential asset in helping families, *Fam Relations* 39(4):443-448, 1990.

Adams CE and others: The effects of religious beliefs on the health care practices of the Amish, *Nurs Pract* 11(3):58-67, 1986.

Carson V: *Spiritual dimensions of nursing practice*, Philadelphia, 1989, WB Saunders.

Conley L: Childbearing and childrearing practices in Mormonism, *Neonatal Network* 9(3):41-48, 1990.

Gershan JA: Judaic ethical beliefs and customs regarding death and dying, *Crit Care Nurse* 5(1):32-34, 1985.

Masulis K: When parents refuse treatment for their children . . . Jehovah's Witnesses, *J Christ Nurs* 4(2):10-12, 1987.

O'Rouke K: Pain relief: the perspective of Catholic tradition, *J Pain Symptom Manage* 7(8):485-491, 1992.

Roberson MHB: The influence of religious beliefs on health choices of Afro-Americans, *Top Clin Nurs* 7(3):57-63, 1985.

Shelly JA: Spiritual care: planting seeds of hope, *Crit Care Update* 9(2):7-15, 1982.

Sodestrom KE, Martinson IM: Patients' spiritual coping strategies: a study of nurse and patient perspectives, *Oncol Nurs Forum* 14(2):41-46, 1987.

Swan R: The law should protect all children . . . children in faith-healing sects, *J Christ Nurs* 4(2):40, 1987.

Thurkauf GE: Understanding the beliefs of Jehovah's Witnesses, *Focus Crit Care* 16(3):199-204, 1989.

Specific Ethnic Groups

Berne AS and others: A nursing model for addressing the health needs of homeless families, *Image J Nurs Sch* 22(1):8-13, 1990.

Bishop S: The mental health of children and families in rural America, *J Child Adolesc Psychiatr Ment Health Nurs* 3(3):77-78, 1990.

Cheadle A and others: Relationship between socioeconomic status, health status, and lifestyle practices of American Indians: evidence from a plains reservation population, *Pub Health Rep* 109(3):405-413, 1994.

Davis RE: The heart and soul of Puerto Rican community: caring and caregivers, *J Multicult Nurs* 1(2):21-27, 1994.

de Leon Siantz M: Correlates of maternal depression among Mexican-American migrant farmworker mothers, *Child Adolesc Psychiatr Ment Health Nurs* 3(1):9-13, 1990.

Desantis L: Infant feeding practices of Haitian mothers in South Florida: cultural beliefs and acculturation, *Matern Child Nurs J* 15:77-89, 1986.

Duque MC: Caring for Colombian children within the realm of health and disease, *J Pediatr Nurs* 9(3):213-216, 1994.

Egan MG: A family assessment challenge: refugee youth and foster family adaptation, *Top Clin Nurs* 7(3):64-69, 1985.

Foreman JT: *Susto* and the health needs of the Cuban refugee population, *Top Clin Nurs* 7(3):40-47, 1985.

Hansen M, Resick L: Health beliefs, health care, and rural Appalachian subcultures from an ethnographic perspective, *Fam Community Health* 13(1):1-10, 1990.

Marrio EB, Hall RR: Asian family traditions and their influence in transcultural health care delivery, *Child Health Care* 15(3):172-177, 1987.

Martinson IM: The challenge of culturally diverse pediatric clients. In Feeg V, editor: *Pediatric nursing: forum on the future: looking toward the 21st century,* Pitman, NJ, 1989, Anthony J Jannetti.

Mattson S, Lew L: Culturally sensitive prenatal care for Southeast Asians, *JOGNN* 21(1):48-54, 1992.

Pass CM: Psychological factors, childbearing, and black female adolescents, *J Pediatr Nurs* 1:247-259, 1986.

Powell D, Zambrana R, Silva-Palacios V: Designing culturally responsive parent programs: a comparison of low-income Mexican and Mexican-American mothers' preferences, *Fam Relations* 39(3):298-304, 1990.

Ramirez AG: A media-based acculturation scale for Mexican-Americans: application to public health education programs, *Fam Community Health* 9(3):63-71, 1986.

Rosenburg JA: Health care for Cambodian children: integrating treatment plans, *Pediatr Nurs* 12:118-125, 1986.

Rozendal N: Understanding Italian American cultural norms, *J Psychosoc Nurs Ment Health Serv* 25(2):29-35, 1987.

van Breda A: Health issues facing Native American children, *Pediatr Nurs* 15(6):575-577, 1989.

Wood D: Homeless children: their evaluation and treatment, *J Pediatr Health Care* 3(4):194-199, 1989.

FAMILY INFLUENCES ON CHILD HEALTH PROMOTION

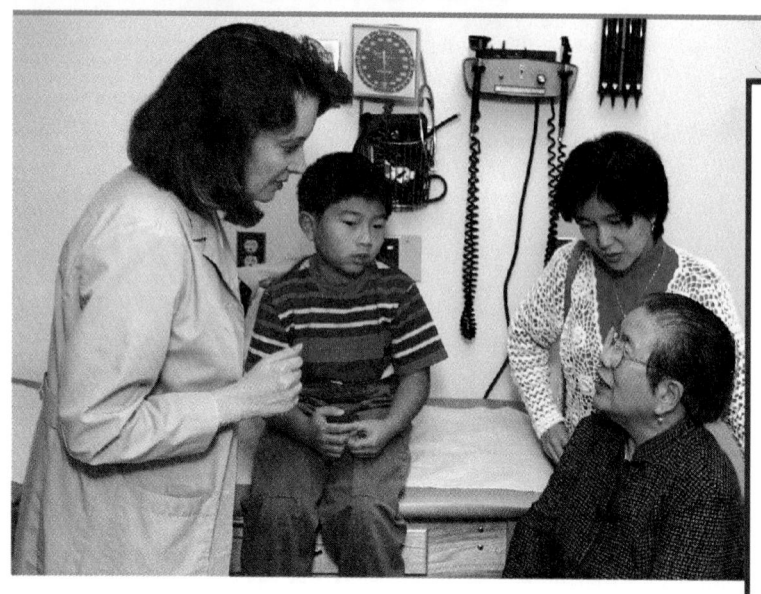

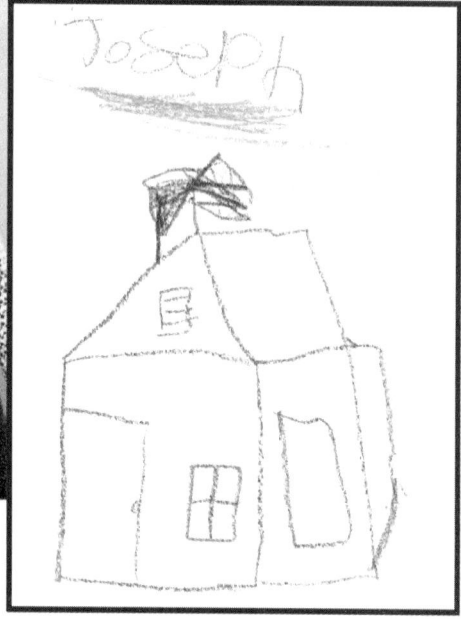

" *My family is important to me, because I'm the only child. They love me.* "

Joseph, age 8 years

RELATED TOPICS

GENERAL CONCEPTS

DEFINITION OF FAMILY

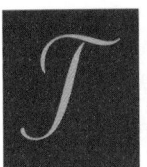
he term *family* has been defined in a number of ways and for a number of purposes according to the individual's own frame of reference, value judgment, or the discipline. For example, biology describes the family as fulfilling the biologic function of perpetuation of the species. Psychology emphasizes the interpersonal aspects of the family and its responsibility for personality development. Economics views the family as a productive unit providing for material needs, and sociology depicts it as the social unit that reacts with the larger society. Others define family in relation to the persons who make up the family unit; the most common type of relationships are *consanguineous* (blood relationships), *affinal* (marital relationships), and *family of origin* (family unit person is born into).

Traditionally a family has been conceptualized as a group, with the belief that both a mother and a father are needed to rear a child. Nearly all societies grant a very high rank to the married status, but in today's society a broad definition of the family is needed, such as "a group of people, living together or in close contact, who take care of one another and provide guidance for their dependent members." Most importantly for any given patient, "family" is whatever the client considers it to be (Patterson, 1995).

Nursing of infants and children is intimately involved with care of the child *and* the family. Consequently, nurses must be aware of the functions of the family, various types of family structures, and theories that provide a foundation for understanding the changes within a family and for directing family-oriented interventions.

FAMILY THEORIES

A *family theory* can be viewed as a "set of lenses" used to describe families and how the family unit responds to events both within and outside the family. Each family theory makes certain assumptions about the family and has inherent strengths and limitations. Most nurses use a combination of theories in their work with children and families. Commonly

used theories are family systems theory, family stress theory, and developmental theory.

Family Systems Theory

Family systems theory is derived from general systems theory, a science of "wholeness" that is characterized by interaction among the components of the system and between the system and the environment. *General systems theory* expanded scientific thought from a simplistic view of direct cause and effect (A causes B) to a more complex and interrelated theory (A influences B, but B also affects A). In family systems theory the family is viewed as a system that continually interacts with its members and the environment. The emphasis is on the *interaction* between the members, such that a change in one family member creates a change in other members, which in turn results in a new change in the original member. Consequently, a problem or dysfunction does not lie in any one member but rather in the type of interactions used by the family. Because it is the interactions, rather than individual members, that are viewed as the source of the problem, the family becomes the patient and the focus of care. Examples of the application of family systems theory to clinical problems are nonorganic failure to thrive and child abuse. According to family systems theory, the problem does not rest solely with the parent or child but in the type of interactions between the parent and child, as well as in a host of other factors that affect their relationship.

The family is viewed as a whole that is different from the sum of the individual members. For example, in a household of parents and one child there are not only three individuals, but also four interactive units that characterize the family system. These include three dyads (the marital relationship, the mother-child relationship, and the father-child relationship) and a triangle (the mother-father-child relationship). This concept of *nonsummativity*—"the whole is greater than the sum of its parts"—implies that, when working with a family the nurse must be aware of the relationships between family members. To effect positive change in a family, it is necessary to work with and through the several subsystems of the family.

Another important concept, *adaptability,* views the family as a highly adaptable unit. When problems exist within the family, change can be effected by altering the interaction or feedback messages that perpetuate disruptive behavior. *Feed-*

Caryn S. Hess, MS, RN, assisted in the revision of this chapter.

back refers to processes within the family that help identify strengths and needs and determine how well goals are being accomplished. Positive feedback initiates change, whereas negative feedback resists change. When the family system is disrupted, change can occur at any point in the system. Although family systems theorists may pursue the family history in trying to understand current family interaction and problem patterns, the emphasis is on what is occurring *now* in the family and on intervening to change that pattern. This focus allows for sometimes rapid and dramatic changes.

A major factor that influences a family's adaptability is its *boundary,* an imaginary but very real line that exists between the family and its environment. This boundary may be open or closed. An *open family* welcomes input into its system by accepting new ideas, information, resources, and opportunities. This type of family reaches out for help and uses the available support systems. In contrast, a *closed family* resists input by viewing change as threatening. The family is suspicious of any available support and strives to maintain the family system by avoiding outside influences. Knowledge of boundaries is critical when teaching or counseling families. Although open families are receptive to intervention, closed families typically resist assistance and more effort is required to gain their trust and acceptance.

Family Stress Theory

Family stress theory, first proposed by Reuben Hill (1949), is concerned with how families react to stressful events and suggests factors that promote adaptation to these events. Families encounter *stressors,* life events that affect the family unit and have the potential to produce change in the family's social system. Stressors may be predictable (e.g., parenthood) and unpredictable (e.g., illness or unemployment). These stressors are cumulative, involving simultaneous demands from work, family, and community life. Too many stressful events occurring within a relatively short period of time—usually 1 year—can overwhelm the family's ability to cope, thus placing the family system at risk for breakdown or its members at risk for physical and emotional health problems. When the family experiences too many stressors for it to cope adequately, a state of crisis ensues. For adaptation to occur under these circumstances, a change in family structure and/or interaction is necessary.

Family stress theory also encompasses certain capabilities the family can use to manage a crisis brought on by too many stressors. The *Typology Model of Adjustment and Adaptation* (McCubbin and McCubbin, 1989), a comprehensive family stress model, summarizes these capabilities through four components:

1. **Basic attributes** of the family—the family type—that explain how the family typically operates and behaves
2. **Resources** of individual family members, the family unit, and the community, including social support from extended family, friends, neighbors, and health professionals
3. **Perception** of how the family defines the situation, its impact, and their ability to manage
4. **Coping behaviors or strategies** that family members or the family unit can use to keep the family functioning as a unit, decrease an individual member's tension, anxiety, and distress, and increase understanding of the particular situation or problem

The Typology Model of Adjustment and Adaptation helps explain why families differ in their responses to stressors. For example, bringing their child with special needs to a treatment facility for therapy might be considered a crisis by a family without a car or money for public transportation, yet may only be defined as a minor inconvenience by another family with adequate and appropriate resources.

The Typology model has been further expanded to the *Resiliency Model of Family Stress, Adjustment and Adaptation.* This model emphasizes family adaptation and is designed to help professionals develop strategies for intervention based on a systematic diagnosis and evaluation of the family under stress (McCubbin and McCubbin, 1994).

Developmental Theory

Developmental theory is an outgrowth of several theories of development. Foremost among the developers is Duvall (1977), who described eight developmental tasks of the family throughout its life span (see box). The family is described

---

DUVALL'S DEVELOPMENTAL STAGES OF THE FAMILY

Stage I: Marriage and an Independent Home: The Joining of Families
Reestablish couple identity.
Realign relationships with extended family.
Make decisions regarding parenthood.

Stage II: Families with Infants
Integrate infants into the family unit.
Accommodate to new parenting and grandparenting roles.
Maintain the marital bond.

Stage III: Families with Preschoolers
Socialize children.
Parents and children adjust to separation.

Stage IV: Families with Schoolchildren
Children develop peer relations.
Parents adjust to their children's peer and school influences.

Stage V: Families with Teenagers
Adolescents develop increasing autonomy.
Parents refocus on midlife marital and career issues.
Parents begin a shift toward concern for the older generation.

Stage VI: Families as Launching Centers
Parents and young adults establish independent identities.
Renegotiate marital relationship.

Stage VII: Middle-Aged Families
Reinvest in couple identity with concurrent development of independent interests.
Realign relationships to include in-laws and grandchildren.
Deal with disabilities and death of older generation.

Stage VIII: Aging Families
Shift from work role to leisure and semiretirement or full retirement.
Maintain couple and individual functioning while adapting to the aging process.
Prepare for own death and dealing with the loss of spouse and/or siblings, and other peers.

Modified from Wright LM, Leahey M: *Nurses and families: a guide to family assessment and intervention,* Philadelphia, 1984, FA Davis.

as a small group, a semiclosed system of personalities that interacts with the larger cultural social system. As an interrelated system, changes do not occur in one part without a series of changes in other parts.

Developmental theory addresses family change over time by using Duvall's family life-cycle stages, based on the predictable changes in the structure, function, and roles of the family, with the age of the oldest child as the marker for stage transition. Thus the arrival of the first child marks the transition from stage I to stage II. As the first child grows and develops, the family enters subsequent stages. In every stage the family is faced with certain developmental tasks. At the same time, each member of the family must achieve individual developmental tasks as part of each family life-cycle stage.

Additions to family development theory reflect more inclusive and accurate versions of contemporary family life. New life-cycle norms have also been developed for divorced families, reconstituted families, low-income families, alcoholic families, and dual-earner families (Carter and McGoldrick, 1989). Developing norms for gay or lesbian families has been more difficult because of the absence of rituals or markers that typically delineate life-cycle stages.

Developmental theory can be applied to nursing practice in a number of ways. For example, the nurse can assess how well new parents are accomplishing the individual and family developmental tasks associated with transition to parenthood. New applications should emerge as more is learned about developmental stages for nonnuclear and nontraditional families.

FAMILY NURSING INTERVENTIONS

In working with children, nurses must include family members in their plan of care. In essence, the *patient is the family.* To discover family dynamics and the unit's strengths and weaknesses, a thorough family assessment is needed (see Chapter 6). The interventions nurses use with families depend on their theoretic model of the family. For example, in family systems theory the focus is on the interactions of the members rather than on an individual member. In this case using group dynamics to involve all members in the intervention process and being a skillful communicator are essential. Systems theory also presents an excellent opportunity for anticipatory guidance. Since each member of the family reacts to every stress experienced by that system, such as the birth of a child, nurses can intervene to help the family prepare for and cope with the change. Also, at each stress point there is the opportunity for change and learning because families are more open to interventions at this time (Brazelton, 1995).

In the family stress theory crisis intervention strategies are employed, and the chief focus is on helping members cope with the challenging event. In the developmental theory a primary nursing function is to provide anticipatory guidance that prepares members for transition to the next family stage.

Nurses use a variety of strategies when working with families (see box). It is important for nurses to be aware of their degree of professional competence in using family nursing interventions. An important nursing role is to recognize situations where referral to more specialized services is required. (See Critical Thinking Exercise.)

FAMILY FUNCTION AND STRUCTURE

Function refers to a special duty or performance required in the course of work or activity; it may also refer to the interactions of family members. *Structure* is a manner of organization or the arrangement of a number of parts that are interrelated in specified, recurring ways. The structure of a family may vary according to the composition of its component parts and according to its life-cycle. Both structure and function are altered and modified as the needs of the family change.

FAMILY NURSING INTERVENTIONS

Behavior modification
Contracting
Case management/coordination
Collaborative strategies
Counseling, including support, cognitive reappraisal, and reframing
Empowering families through active participation
Environmental modification
Family advocacy
Family crisis intervention
Networking, including use of self-help groups and social support
Providing information and technical expertise
Role modeling
Role supplementation
Teaching strategies, including stress management, life-style modifications, and anticipatory guidance

From Friedman MM: *Family nursing: theory and practice,* ed 3, Norwalk, CT, 1992, Appleton & Lange.

CRITICAL THINKING EXERCISE
Family Theories

As the school nurse you are working with a family that consists of a mother, father, and their 10-year-old son and 16-year-old daughter. The daughter, Jenny, has stopped going to school this week. Although she has had many conflicts with her parents, her relationship with her father is very strained. He recently took away her driving privileges because of curfew violations. Jenny says she is quitting school if she can not drive. Which of the following three family theories would you apply when working with this family?

1. Developmental theory
2. Family stress theory
3. Family system theory

The best answer is three. In family system theory the family is viewed as a system that continually interacts with its members. Family interactions rather than individual members are viewed as the source of the problems. Although developmental and family stress theories could be applied, the family is experiencing an interaction problem more than a developmental or stress-related problem.

FAMILY FUNCTION

Authorities agree that families serve society in many ways. They play a vital role in the economy because they produce and consume goods and services. They also are the basic unit for replacing dying members of the society. Furthermore, to maintain its continuity society must transmit its knowledge, customs, values, and beliefs to the young. Where children are not an economic necessity, their primary function is to receive and to give love. Although goals for socialization and childrearing practices differ from one culture to another, in most societies the family appears to have three major objectives in relation to children: caregiving, nurturing, and training.

FAMILY STRUCTURE

The *family structure,* or *family composition,* consists of individuals, each with a socially recognized status and position, who interact with one another on a regular, recurring basis in socially sanctioned ways. When members are gained or lost through events (e.g., marriage, divorce, birth, death, abandonment, incarceration), the family composition is altered and roles must be redefined or redistributed.

Traditionally the family structure refers to either nuclear or extended families. However, family composition has assumed new configurations in recent years, with the single-parent family and stepfamilies becoming prominent forms. It is not uncommon for children to belong to several different family groups during their lifetime.

Nuclear Family

The *nuclear,* or *conjugal, family* consists of a husband, a wife, and their children (natural or adopted) who live in a common household. This is the reproductive unit in which the marital tie (legally or otherwise sanctioned) is the chief binding force. A strongly functional nuclear family is the prototype of human relationships and the basic unit from which more complex family forms are composed. In some instances one or more additional persons (e.g., a relative, friend, foster child, or others) may reside in the same household. Some authorities classify childless couples as nuclear families because the conjugal alliance has the theoretic potential for reproduction.

The nuclear family is more characteristic of an urban, mobile society. It is free to move where there is better financial opportunity and concomitant improvement in other areas, such as social class and prestige. It is not economically bound to a geographic area or dependent on the cooperative efforts of other members. The family members are employed on an individual basis, and economic resources are in the form of money, which allows the family to purchase goods and services from others.

Although extended families residing in the same household are rapidly disappearing in North American society, the isolated nuclear family without relatives within easy visiting distance is uncommon. Most consanguineous family members maintain contact through visits, telephone calls, letters, and gift exchanges. Having no relatives readily available for advice and assistance with child care, parents in some nuclear families are more likely to turn to "experts" for childrearing guidance.

The majority of nuclear families are associated with an ex-

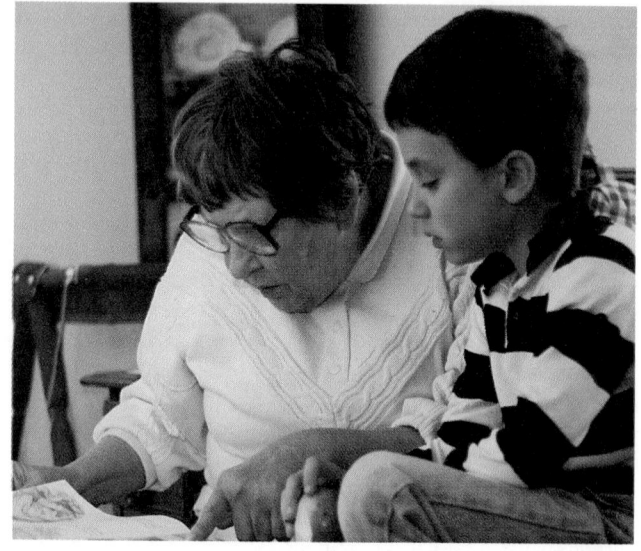

FIG. 4-1. Children benefit from interaction with grandparents even when they do not share the same household.

tended kinship network of nuclear families living in separate households but in close geographic proximity. This concept, sometimes referred to as a *modified extended family,* describes a meaningful aspect of daily existence that is reflected in frequent visiting and the exchange of services and financial aid. This family association meets the members' psychologic needs to a greater extent than do experts, friends, or organizations (Fig. 4-1). It is not uncommon for families to reject the opportunity for social or economic advancement rather than leave such kinship associations.

Affiliative Relationships.   Although the nuclear family is predominantly a legally sanctioned institution, in a number of families the attachment is only *affiliative* (i.e., nonmarital) *cohabitation.* These families consist primarily of two adults but may include children. The mother and father live together, often with children from previous relationships, and share family responsibilities. However, the family unit is less stable, and relationships are subject to change. Instability of the social environment in the home has been associated with juvenile delinquency, which appears to be related to the number of family constellations (changes in the adult members of the household) experienced during childhood. This is probably a reflection of repeated adjustment to a variety of authority figures with differing expectations.

Single-Parent Family

The *single-parent family* is not a new phenomenon. Throughout history, deaths from disease, childbirth, and wars have resulted in many one-parent families, although frequently remarriage occurs. The contemporary single-parent family, however, has emerged partially as a consequence of women's rights movements wherein more women (and men) have established separate households because of divorce, death, desertion, or illegitimacy. In addition, a more liberal attitude in the courts has made it possible for single persons, both male and female, to adopt children, whereas previously, rigid prerequisites specified that both a father and a mother

the family is whatever they decide it is.

must be present in the home. Although single-parent families are usually headed by the mother, it is becoming increasingly common for fathers to be awarded custody of dependent children in divorce settlements. A significant number of single-parent families result from a single mother who wishes to have a child but does not choose to have a husband. Also, unmarried mothers often choose to keep and raise their children rather than place them for adoption or marry, and are frequently absorbed into the extended family. With the increased psychologic independence of women as a whole and the increased acceptability of illegitimacy in society, more unmarried women are deliberately choosing mother-child families. The challenges of these single-parent families are discussed on p. 64.

Binuclear Family

The term *binuclear family* is used to describe the situation that allows parents to continue the parenting role while terminating the spousal unit. The degree of cooperation between households and the time the child spends with each can vary. In *joint custody* the court assigns divorcing parents equal rights and responsibilities to the minor child or children. These alternate family forms are efforts on the part of those concerned to view divorce as a process of reorganization and redefinition of a family rather than as a family dissolution. Joint custody and co-parenting are discussed further on p. 74 in relation to special parenting situations.

Reconstituted Family

Reconstituted families, also referred to as *stepfamilies,* are those in which one or both of the married adults have children from a previous marriage residing in the household. The term *blended families,* or *combined families,* more often refers to families composed of parents and the children each of them brings from a previous marriage. Most reconstituted families involve a mother, her children, and a stepfather. Reconstituted families are discussed further on p. 78.

Extended Family

The *extended family* combines nuclear families into larger units through the parent-child relationship. It consists of the nuclear family plus lineal or collateral relatives. Most often it is composed of two or more residential units of three or more generations affiliated through extension of the parent-child relationship (i.e., grandparents, parents, and grandchildren).

In the extended family childrearing is often a shared responsibility. Relatives are present and available to help young parents with household chores and child care activities. Daily lives of the children are organized around the needs and requirements of the family, with assigned tasks and obligations.

Extended family structure is more functional in areas where land is the basis of wealth and sustenance. Today the best examples of extended family units can be found among successful farmers, Native Americans, and certain recent immigrants. Extended families may form under conditions of either extreme poverty in order to pool resources or extreme wealth in order to consolidate resources.

Alternative Family Structures

Several other family structures exist that are much less common. The *polygamous family,* in which a spouse of either sex has more than one mate at the same time, is not legally sanctioned in the United States. In countries where it exists, polygamy is usually accorded a higher status than monogamy. It may be limited to ruling families or to high-status persons and tends to be practiced by a small segment of the population.

Another type of family structure that is relatively uncommon today is the *communal family.* The communal family emerged from a disenchantment with most contemporary life choices and is often seen in cults. Communal groups share common ownership of property and goods; in cooperatives there is private ownership of property, but certain goods and services are shared and exchanged cooperatively without monetary consideration. There is strong reliance on group members and material interdependence. The mother-child tie is strong during infancy and early childhood, but many parents are happy to relinquish older children to the care of others.

A *same-sex, homosexual,* or *gay/lesbian family* is one in which there is a common-law tie between two persons of the same sex who have children. Estimates of the number of children of gay or lesbian parents range from 6 to 14 million (Patterson, 1992). Although most children in gay/lesbian households are biologic from a former, legal marriage, there are other means by which homosexuals acquire children. For example, they may be foster or adoptive parents, lesbian mothers may conceive through artificial fertilization, or a gay male couple may become parents through use of a surrogate mother. Research indicates that the quality of parenting and home life of gay men and lesbians, whether they are single or in a partner relationship, is equivalent to that of nongay parents (Bozett, 1984; Harris and Turner, 1986; Turner, Scadden, and Harris, 1985). Because this family form is more common than most persons may realize, it is important for the nurse to understand that homosexual families are simply different from the heterosexual family form, not necessarily better or worse. The gay/lesbian family environment can be just as healthy as any other. According to reported research, children in gay/lesbian households are no more likely to be gay than are children reared in heterosexual households (Bozett, 1989; Gottman, 1990; Huggins, 1989; Paul, 1986). Nurses need to be nonjudgmental and to learn how to accept differences rather than demonstrate a homophobic prejudice that can have a detrimental effect on the nurse–child/family relationship. Moreover, the more knowledge of the child's family constellation and life-style nurses have, the greater benefit they can be to the gay or lesbian parent and the child. (See Critical Thinking Exercise on p. 66.)

Family Strengths

Increasing interest has been shown in the family characteristics that seem to help families function effectively. Experts suggest that there are about 12 major, nonmutually exclusive qualities of strong families (see box on p. 66). They caution that not all strong families are characterized by the presence of all 12 qualities, but that a combination of qualities appears to define strong families (Dunst, Trivette, and Deal, 1988). Knowledge of these factors guide the nurse at each step of the nursing process. The nurse is better able to predict the ways in which families may cope and respond to a stressful event, provide individualized support that builds on

CRITICAL THINKING EXERCISE
Family Structure

As the nurse, you are interviewing the mother of John, a school-age boy. The mother says their family consists of herself, her son, her lesbian partner, and two foster children. John's father lives in another state and has no contact with him. John has one grandparent who lives in another city in a nursing home. When planning care for John and his family, John's family should be considered to be which of the following?

1. Nuclear family of mother, father, and son
2. Single parent family of mother and son
3. Extended family of mother, father, grandparent, and son
4. Family members identified by the mother

The best answer is four. The family defines who are its members. In this situation, John's family consists of those people who live in his home at the present time. Traditionally family composition has referred to either nuclear or extended families. However, many alternative family structures such as John's occur. The nurse needs to recognize that not all families are traditional in their membership.

QUALITIES OF STRONG FAMILIES

1. A belief in and sense of *commitment* toward promoting the well-being and growth of individual family members, as well as that of the family unit
2. *Appreciation* for the small and large things that individual family members do well and *encouragement* to do better
3. Concentrated effort to spend *time* and do things together, no matter how formal or informal the activity or event
4. A sense of *purpose* that permeates the reasons and basis for "going on" in both bad and good times
5. A sense of *congruence* among family members regarding the value and importance of assigning time and energy to meet needs
6. The ability to *communicate* with one another in a way that emphasizes positive interactions
7. A clear set of *family rules, values,* and *beliefs* that establishes expectations about acceptable and desired behavior
8. A varied repertoire of *coping strategies* that promote positive functioning in dealing with both normative and non-normative life events
9. The ability to engage in *problem-solving* activities designed to evaluate options for meeting needs and procuring resources
10. The ability to be *positive* and see the positive in almost all aspects of their lives, including the ability to see crisis and problems as an opportunity to learn and grow
11. *Flexibility* and *adaptability* in the roles necessary to procure resources to meet needs
12. A *balance* between the use of internal and external family resources for coping and adapting to life events and planning for the future

From Dunst C, Trivette C, Deal A: *Enabling and empowering families: principles and guidelines for practice,* Cambridge, MA, 1988, Brookline Books.

family strengths and unique functioning style, and assist family members in obtaining appropriate resources.

FAMILY ROLES AND RELATIONSHIPS

Each individual has a position, or status, in the family structure and plays culturally and socially defined roles in interactions within the family group. Each family has its own traditions and values and sets its own standards for interaction within and outside the group. Each determines the experiences the children should have, those they are to be shielded from, and how each of these experiences meets the needs of family members. Where family ties are strong, social control is highly effective, and most members conform to their roles willingly and with commitment. Conflicts arise when people do not fulfill their roles in ways that meet other family members' expectations, either because they are unaware of the expectations or because they choose not to meet them.

PARENTAL ROLES

In all family groups the socially recognized status of father and mother exists with socially sanctioned roles that prescribe appropriate sexual behavior and childrearing responsibilities. The guides for behavior in these roles serve to control sexual conflict in society and provide for prolonged care of children. The degree to which parents are committed and the way they play their roles are influenced by their unique socialization experience.

Role definitions are changing as a result of the changing economy and the women's liberation movement. Women are achieving equality with men in education, more are entering the labor force, and the number of women who choose to

have fewer children or none at all is increasing. During childhood, particularly in the upper and middle classes, the trend is toward deemphasizing the basic male-female characteristics of aggression, dependence, and achievement. As the role of the woman changes, there must necessarily be a change in the complementary role of the man. Fathers are taking a more active role in childrearing and household activities, particularly in middle-class families. Marital roles remain most segregated in the lower classes. Redefinition of sex roles in the American family is taking place, but a cultural lag of the persisting traditional role definitions creates conflicts in many of these families.

ROLE LEARNING

Roles are learned through the socialization process. During all stages of development children learn and practice, through interaction with others and in their play, a set of social roles and something of the characteristics of other roles. They behave in patterned and more or less predictable ways because they learn roles that define mutual expectations in typical and recurring social relationships. Role conceptions are transmitted by socializing agents (parents, peers, authority figures) who use positive and negative sanctions to ensure conformity to their norms.

In some cultures the role behavior expected of children conflicts with desirable adult behavior. For example, in the United States children are expected to be submissive in childhood but dominant as adults. This conflict of expectations is known as *role discontinuity.* Other cultures value the same behaviors, such as courage and aggression, both in children and adults; this provides *role continuity.*

Role-structuring initially takes place within the family unit, where the children fulfill a set of roles and respond to the complementary roles of their parents and other family members. The roles of the children are shaped primarily by the parents, who apply direct or indirect pressures in an attempt to induce or force children into the desired patterns of behavior. Each set of parents has their own techniques, and each will determine the course that the process of socialization is to follow (see Limit-Setting and Discipline, p. 71).

Research indicates that birth order influences the role each sibling is assigned within the family (Hoopes and Harper, 1987). When children enter a particular family, they sense the physical, social, and emotional values associated with their own specific roles. They then develop characteristic response patterns to fulfill their roles. Each sibling position role is created to meet both the family's and the individual's needs. For example, firstborn children learn that their job assignment is to produce outcomes that meet with the family's approval and to enforce explicit family rules. Second-born children play a key role in maintaining open communication and clarifying messages among family members. Third-born children feel especially responsible for balance in the marital relationship. (See also box on p. 68.)

Children respond to life situations according to behaviors learned in reciprocal transactions. As they acquire important role-taking skills, their relationships with others change. They become proficient at understanding others as they acquire the ability to discriminate their own perspectives from those of others. Children who get along well with others and attain status in the peer group have well-developed role-taking skills.

FAMILY SIZE AND CONFIGURATION

The size and composition of the family directly influence child development. No two children grow in exactly the same environment, although identical twins most nearly approximate this. For example, in a nuclear family with two children—even of the same sex—one will live in a family with an older sibling, whereas the other will be reared in a family with a younger sibling. In a family where there is a 10-year age span among the children, one may be born to a 20-year-old mother and the other to a 30-year-old mother. For the child in each situation the environment is different.

Family Size

Parenting practices differ between small and large families. In small families more emphasis is placed on the individual development of the children. Parenting is intensive rather than extensive, and there is constant pressure to measure up to family expectations. Children's development and achievement are measured against that of other children in the neighborhood and social class. In small families there is more democratic participation by the children than in larger families.

Children in large families are able to adjust to a variety of changes and crises. There is more emphasis on the group and less on the individual (Fig. 4-2). Cooperation is essential, of-

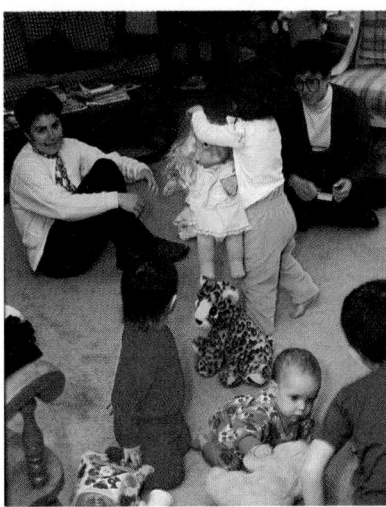

FIG. 4-2. Innumerable relationships and activities are possible in a large family.

ten because of economic necessity. The large number of persons sharing a limited amount of space requires a greater degree of organization, administration, and authoritarian control. The control is wielded by a dominant family member—a parent or an older child. Because the number of children reduces the intimate, one-to-one contact between the parent and any individual child, siblings may turn to each other to have their needs met. Individual children may adopt specialized roles in an attempt to gain recognition in the family.

Discipline is often administered by older siblings in large families. Siblings are usually better attuned to what constitutes misbehavior, and sibling disapproval or ostracism is frequently more meaningful than parental measures. Large families seem to generate a sense of security in the children fostered by sibling support and cooperation. However, adolescents from a large family are more peer oriented than family oriented.

Spacing of Children and Ordinal Position

Age differences between siblings affect the childhood environment, but to a lesser extent than does the sex of the siblings. The arrival of a sibling has the greatest impact on the older child, and a 2- to 4-year difference in age appears to be most threatening. When the older child is very young, the self-image is too immature to be threatened. At an older age the child is better able to understand the situation and therefore is less likely to see the newcomer as a threat, although the child does feel the loss of the only-child status. Studies reveal that there is more affection and less rivalry or hostility when children are spaced 4 or more years apart (Lobato, 1990).

In general, the narrower the spacing between siblings, the more the children influence one another, especially in emotional characteristics; the wider the spacing, the greater the influence of the parents. This is not to say that bonds are nonexistent between siblings with large age spans, nor that siblings with only a year or two difference in age will always feel a strong bond. However, high accessibility during these de-

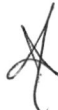

INFLUENCE OF ORDINAL POSITION ON CHILDREN

Firstborn Children

Are more achievement oriented
Are more dominant
Receive more physical punishment
Are allowed to show more aggression to siblings
Have stronger consciences, are more self-disciplined and inner directed
Are more socially anxious
Are prone to feelings of guilt
Identify more with parents than with peers
Are more conservative
Are subject to greater parental expectations
Begin to speak earlier in life
Demonstrate higher intellectual achievement
Plan better and experience fewer frustrations
Are likely to be most wanted

Middle Children

Have more demands made on them for household help
Are praised less often
Receive less of the parents' time
Learn to compromise and be adaptable
Are less stimulated toward achievement
Are more difficult to characterize because of a variety of positions in family

Youngest Children

Are less dependent than firstborn children
Are less tense, more affectionate, and more good-natured
Tend to identify more with peer group than with parents
Are more flexible in their thinking
Are popular with classmates
Have fewer demands placed on them for household help

Only Children

Resemble firstborn children
Are more mature and cultivated
Experience greater parental pressure for mature behavior and achievement
Demonstrate superiority in language facility
Rarely develop into stereotype of spoiled, selfish child
Often enjoy a rich fantasy life as a result of isolation

velopmentally formative years is the almost routine accompaniment of an influential sibling relationship. High-access siblings are generally close in age and the same gender, which promotes access to common life events. They often attend the same school, play with the same friends, date in the same circle, and share a common bedroom and clothing.

It has also been observed for some time that the birth position of children affects their personalities. Parents treat children differently, and sibling interactions are different depending on the children's position within the family. The major influences of ordinal position on children are presented in the accompanying box. However, children vary tremendously; these generalizations represent averages and do not apply in all situations.

Sibling Interaction

Most children have at least one brother or sister. Asked why they chose to have a second child, most parents give as their primary reason the fact that they did not want their firstborn to be an only child (Lobato, 1990). Right or wrong, many

people believe that children develop best within the company of other children.

Perhaps the sibling relationship's most unique feature is its duration. Likely the longest relationship one will share with another human being, the sibling relationship lasts through a lifetime, often 50 to 80 years, as compared with the child-parent relationship of approximately 30 to 50 years. Siblings spend long periods of time together and come to know each other—at their best and worst—extremely well.

Sibling Functions. Siblings exert power, exchange services, and express feelings in reciprocal ways that are often not revealed explicitly in the presence of parents. They see themselves in their brother or sister, experience life vicariously through their sibling's behavior, and begin to expand on their own possibilities. Siblings can also be touchstones for what the other would *not* like to be, and they tend to use each other as yardsticks for comparison. They are sounding boards for one another; they offer a safe forum for experimenting with new behaviors and roles before using either with parents or nonfamily peers.

Brothers and sisters provide each other with tangible services (e.g., lending money, clothing, toys, sports equipment, teaching a skill), help with childhood problems, provide support in dealing with parents or others outside the family, and may provide an introduction to a new friendship group. Children learn to negotiate and bargain, and sometimes to manipulate. Because siblings share approximately equal power, many opportunities arise for conflict and conflict resolution. They learn about sharing, competition, rivalry, and compromise. Siblings can also protect one another from parental-executive abuse of power and can form a coalition to deal with the issues of authority, power, and emotional support. Negotiating with parents is stronger when siblings act together rather than singly.

Siblings interpret the outside world for each other and perform genuine educative functions for the parents. A related function is pioneering, wherein one sibling initiates a process, thereby giving permission to the others to follow accordingly. Patterns may include breaking explicit family rules, taking new developmental pathways (such as leaving the family), or adopting different moral/political codes and life-styles.

Tattling can be an important lever in sibling interactions. On the other hand, there is often a conspiracy of silence among siblings, leaving the parents feeling isolated and excluded. A willingness to make and maintain each other's privacy often serves as a powerful bond of loyalty among the children. It is this loyalty that often distinguishes the relationship between siblings from that between friends.

More Active Sibling Relationships. Sibling relationships vary among cultures. Certain factors, however, may be giving the sibling relationship greater significance in North America than in the past. Shrinking family size, longer life spans, divorce and remarriage, geographic mobility, maternal employment and alternative sources of child care, competitive pressures, stress, and various forms of parental insufficiency may be propelling siblings into greater contact and emotional interdependence than ever before.

For example, siblings often join forces to confront the trauma of divorce. They frequently rely on each other for support when parents remarry. The large number of working mothers means that many young siblings today have large amounts of time when their relationship is not monitored by a personally committed adult. Often an older sibling is required to baby-sit, resulting in children spending more and more time together unsupervised. In a worried, mobile, small-family, high-stress, fast-paced, parent-absent society, children often turn to a sibling to meet their need for contact, constancy, and permanency.

Multiple Births

A deviation in early development that occurs with variable frequency is multiple births. Twins are not uncommon in the population, but triplets are rare and quadruplets or quintuplets are extremely unusual. In any of these situations the offspring can be of the like or unlike sex (i.e., derived from a single ovum, from multiple ova, or a combination of the two, which can involve one or more cell divisions). The cause of twinning is unknown, but the increase in the number of larger multiples (quintuplets, sextuplets) during recent years has been associated with fertility-enhancing techniques (ovulation-inducing drugs and assisted reproductive techniques such as in vitro fertilization) (Ventura and others, 1995). Twins are of two distinct types: identical, or monozygotic (MZ); and fraternal, or dizygotic (DZ) (see box). In the United States the overall twinning rate is approximately 1 in 80 pregnancies and consists of one third MZ and two thirds DZ twins.

A special kind of sibling relationship is observed in twins, although their tendencies to get along with each other and to quarrel are not too different from those of any other two siblings, especially if they are different-sex fraternal twins. Twins generally tend to work out a relationship that is reasonably satisfactory to both and demonstrate early independence from parental attention. They develop a remarkable capacity for cooperative play and considerable loyalty and generosity toward each other. It is not uncommon for them to evolve a private language between themselves that may interfere with development of the family language.

In a twinship, one member of the pair, to a greater or lesser extent, is more dominant, outgoing, and assertive than the other, often to the consternation of their parents. However, the seemingly more passive twin is able to accomplish as much and get his or her way as frequently as the more assertive twin.

Identical twins differ in their response to the tendency of some parents to treat twins exactly alike. The present philosophy is to determine the degree to which the children demonstrate an inclination toward togetherness. Some twins thrive best when they are constantly in each other's company; others prefer more individuality and separateness. The conservative approach is to allow the children to follow their natural inclinations. Early years of togetherness are often the basis of the children's security. To separate them too early may produce unnecessary stresses. The tendency is to foster individual differences as they are evidenced in order to ease the process of separation when it becomes advisable.

Parents of twins have numerous adjustments to make, from challenges in attachment and bonding (see Promote Parent-Infant Bonding (Attachment): Maternal Attachment, Chapter 8) to the stresses of the heavy workload and monetary expenses. The **National Organization of Mothers of Twins Clubs, Inc.,** * has local chapters throughout the United States and Canada to offer information and support to parents of twins and is highly recommended as a resource for all new parents of twins. The **Twins Foundation**†—an organization founded by a group of twins and designed to aid twins and other multiples—is recommended for older children.

CHARACTERISTICS OF TWINS

Monozygotic (MZ, Identical Twins)	Dizygotic (DZ, Fraternal Twins)
Result of one fertilized ovum that became separated early in development	Result of fertilization of two ova
Alike physically and genetically	Differ physically and genetically
Same sex	May be like or opposite sex
Frequency:	Frequency:
Occurs uniformly in all populations	Varies among races (highest—blacks, lowest—Asians, intermediate—whites)
Unaffected by maternal age	More common with advancing maternal age (maximum at age 35-39, then decreases rapidly)
Tendency unaffected by heredity	Marked familial tendency Expressed only in the female Fathers appear to transmit disposition toward double ovulation to daughters
Similar behavior	Dissimilar behavior; more sibling rivalry

PARENTING

MOTIVATION FOR PARENTHOOD

A dominant characteristic in all societies is that adults are expected to become parents and to be gratified by the experience. Pressures of tradition, sentiment regarding the state of motherhood, and religious exhortations to fulfill divine commands of fertility profoundly influence decision making, since conformity to social-role expectations is a strong influence in family planning.

Although many pregnancies are unplanned, there are numerous reasons why couples decide to initiate a pregnancy. Many consider children a normal part of marriage, others see them as proof of their adulthood, some desire heirs for the family name and fortune, and a few want to fulfill a parent's wish for grandchildren. Having a child in an attempt to save an unstable marriage is a poor reason that usually fails in its goal. However, in most instances the couple sincerely wish to become parents.

Factors that are likely to influence family size are social

---

*P.O. Box 23188, Albuquerque, NM 87192-1188; (505) 275-0955.
†P.O. Box 6043, Providence, RI 02904-6043; (401) 729-1000.

class, religion, race, type of conjugal-role relationships, and the social-psychologic aspects of sexual relations. Of course, how effectively the couple practices contraception may determine whether the family size remains as planned. Also, in the case of divorce and remarriage an individual may decide to have more children with the new spouse.

PREPARATION FOR PARENTHOOD

The basic goals of parenting are to promote the physical survival and health of the children, to foster the skills and abilities necessary to be a self-sustaining adult, and to foster behavioral capabilities for maximizing cultural values and beliefs. However, new parents approach parenthood with meager experience and scant knowledge, although no other task can compare, in overall consequences, with that of rearing a human being. Parents learn by trial and error, committing the same mistakes that have been committed by countless other parents, but they somehow manage to accomplish the task, becoming more skilled with each additional child. Tradition rather than rational planning furnishes the chief norms for childrearing. Experience in having been nurtured as a child is an essential component of successful parenting.

Their own parents are probably the only persons that parents observe intimately in the parental role; this results in a *generational continuity*—parents rear their own children in much the same way as they themselves were reared. Other essential skills and knowledge parents need in order to feel more comfortable in the parenting role include a basic understanding of childhood growth and development, bathing, feeding, use of play, and interpersonal communication skills. All this information is integrated throughout this text.

TRANSITION TO PARENTHOOD

Although there is disagreement as to whether or not the birth of a couple's first child should be labeled a crisis, the early weeks of an infant's life call for a couple to make drastic adjustments. Although the parents have anticipated and perhaps prepared for the child's arrival, birth means the sudden imposition of totally dependent care 24 hours a day for the new member of the family. It may very well be a crisis if the event is perceived as disturbing old habits and relationships and eliciting new responses. It requires role changes, destroys or significantly modifies former relationships, and means adjusting to new role realignments. Whereas previously the roles of a couple were husband and wife, they now become, in addition, father and mother. It is difficult to adjust to being parents, but it is a normal human experience and a tool for personal growth.

The birth of an infant is a highly significant event that alters the behavior of both mothers and fathers. No amount of preparation can truly and fully prepare prospective parents for the constant and immediate needs of an infant. Certain factors, however, influence the transition to the parental role. One factor in which the cultural trend has changed in recent years is parental age. The most satisfactory age for childbearing has been established as the years between 18 and 35. During this time parents are considered to be in optimum health, with a predicted life span that allows sufficient time and vigor to raise a family. However, the age at which parents begin their families has changed over the last few decades in the United States, with a substantial increase in the birth rate for

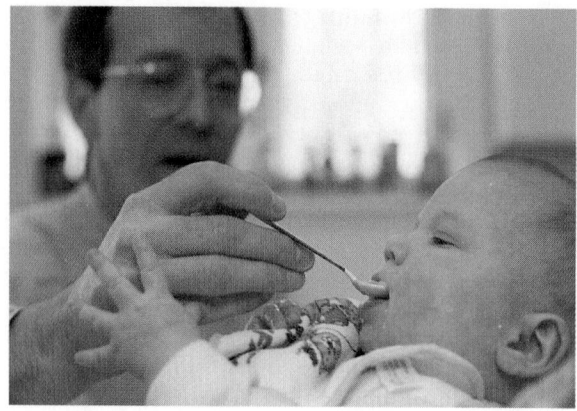

FIG. 4-3. Fathers who assume care of their children may feel more comfortable and successful in their parenting role than those who do not.

women 30 to 44 years of age and a slight decline for women ages 18 to 29 years (Ventura and others, 1995).

Other factors influencing the transition to the parental role include the following:

- First-time parents who have had parenting education experience less stress in the transition than do those who have not (Gage and Christensen, 1991).
- Parents with previous experience, such as another child, appear to be more relaxed and have less conflict in disciplinary relationships, and they are more aware of normal growth and development expectations.
- Fathers who are highly involved with their child often feel more comfortable and successful in the parenting role (Fig. 4-3).
- The amount of stress experienced by one or both parents may interfere with their ability to exhibit patience and understanding, or otherwise cope with their children's behavior.
- Special characteristics of the infant, such as a temperamentally difficult infant, can cause the parents to lose confidence and doubt their abilities. Also, an infant with special care needs, such as those associated with a disability, can be a significant source of added stress.
- Marital relationships can have a negative effect on parental transition, since marital tension or strife can alter caregiving routines and interfere with enjoyment of the infant. Conversely, parents who support and encourage one another serve as a positive influence on establishing a satisfying parental role. The best single predictor of postpartum marital adjustment is the couple's level of marital adjustment during pregnancy (Wallace and Gotlib, 1990).

Support Systems

Successful adaptation to the stress of transition to parenthood involves at least two types of family resources (McCubbin and McCubbin, 1989). First are the *internal resources* of the family, such as adaptability and integration. Changing from an orderly, predictable life to a relatively disordered, unpredictable one is a universal adaptation families must make. Rigid schedules are impossible to maintain, and former activities must be curtailed or abandoned. *Adaptation* is reflected in learning to be patient, becoming better organized, and becoming more flexible. *Integration* involves an attempt of the couple to continue some activities they engaged in before they became parents. In this way couples are able to maintain a sense of continuity and appreciate the importance of the husband-wife relationship.

The second kind of resource for coping with stress is the

use of *coping strategies* that strengthen the organization and functioning of the family. These include the use of community resources, the use of social support, and the adoption of a future orientation. Interpersonal supports that provide information, advice, and caretaking are derived from friends, relatives, and neighbors. Relationships with family, friends, and community are essential. For fathers, positive work relationships seem to be especially important; for mothers, activities with friends are important (Daniels and Moos, 1988). Arranging for time away from the child or children is also beneficial. Fathers can assume care of the family to allow the mother some time to herself at home or away from the home, even if just for an afternoon or evening. Adoption of a future orientation provides reassurance to parents that things will get better, that they will cope, and that it is realistic to plan for the time when they will be able to engage in self-fulfilling activities.

It is also reassuring to know that others experience ambivalent feelings toward parenthood and share the same difficulties and frustrations. Exchanging ideas and experiences with other parents provides an opportunity to voice concerns and to learn new ways of coping with the multiple problems of childrearing. Whether it is family, friends, or community resources, parents need persons to whom they can turn for advice, comfort, and assistance—persons with whom they can share the joys and difficulties of childrearing.

PARENTING BEHAVIORS

Parental Styles of Control

Although there are variations and degrees in parenting styles, they can generally be described as either authoritarian, permissive, or authoritative. *Authoritarian,* or *dictatorial,* parents try to control their children's behavior and attitudes through unquestioned mandates. They establish rules and regulations or a standard of conduct that they expect to be followed rigidly and unquestioningly. They value and reward absolute obedience, mute acceptance of their word, and unfailing respect for the family's principles and beliefs. They forcefully punish any behavior that is contrary to parental standards. Parental authority is exercised with little explanation and little involvement of the child in decision making. The message is: "Do it because I say so."

Punishment need not be corporal but may be stern withdrawal of love and approval. Careful training often results in rigidly conforming behavior in the children, who tend to be sensitive, shy, self-conscious, retiring, and submissive. They are more apt to be courteous, loyal, honest, and dependable but docile. These behaviors are more typically observed when parental arbitrary power assertion is accompanied by close supervision and a reasonable level of affection. If not, arbitrary power assertion is more likely to be associated with both defiant and antisocial behavior.

Permissive, or *laissez-faire,* parents exert little or no control over their children's actions. These well-meaning parents sometimes confuse permissiveness with license. They avoid imposing their own standards of conduct and allow their children to regulate their own activity as much as possible. These parents consider themselves to be resources for the children, not role models. If rules do exist, the parents explain the underlying reason, encourage the children's opinions, and consult them in decision-making processes. They employ lax, inconsistent discipline, do not set sensible limits, and do not prevent the children from upsetting the home routine. The parents rarely punish the children, since most behavior is considered acceptable. Consequently, the children, in effect, control the parents. Children of submissive parents are often disobedient, disrespectful, irresponsible, aggressive, and generally defiant of authority.

Authoritative, or *democratic,* parents combine some childrearing practices from both the foregoing extremes. They direct their children's behavior and attitudes by emphasizing the reason for rules and negatively reinforcing deviations. They respect the individuality of each of their children and allow them to voice their objections to family standards or regulations. Parental control is firm and consistent but tempered with encouragement, understanding, and security. Control is focused on the issue, not on withdrawal of love or the fear of punishment. These parents foster "innerdirectedness," a conscience that regulates behavior based on feelings of guilt or shame for wrongdoing, not on fear of being caught or punished. Parents' realistic standards and reasonable expectations produce children with high self-esteem who are self-reliant, assertive, inquisitive, content, and highly interactive with other children.

The most successful type of childrearing seems to be the authoritative method. Parents do not set rigid, arbitrary limits but maintain firm control, particularly in areas of parent-child disagreement. Permissiveness is tempered with reasonable and consistent setting of limits. Parental power is shared, and both parents provide leadership but listen to what the children think.

LIMIT-SETTING AND DISCIPLINE

In its broadest sense, *discipline* means to teach or refers to a set of rules governing conduct. In a narrower sense, it refers to the action taken to enforce the rules following noncompliance. *Limit-setting* refers to establishing the rules or guidelines for behavior. Generally, the clearer the limits that are set and the more consistently they are enforced, the less need there is for disciplinary action.

Therefore the initial goal for the family is for the nurse to help parents establish realistic and concrete "rules." Limit-setting and discipline are positive, necessary components of childrearing and serve several useful functions as they help children:

- Test their limits of control
- Achieve in areas appropriate for mastery at their level
- Channel undesirable feelings into constructive activity
- Protect themselves from danger
- Learn socially acceptable behavior

Children want and need limits. Unrestricted freedom is a tremendous threat to their security and safety. Through testing the limits imposed on them, children learn the extent to which they can manipulate their environment, as well as gain reassurance from knowing that others will be there to protect them from potential harm.

Minimizing Misbehavior

The goals of or reasons for misbehavior may include attention, power, defiance, and a display of inadequacy (the child

FAMILY HOME CARE
Minimizing Misbehavior

Set realistic goals for acceptable behavior and expected achievements.

Structure opportunities for small successes to lessen feelings of inadequacy.

Praise children for desirable behavior with attention and verbal approval.

Structure the environment to prevent unnecessary difficulties, (e.g., place fragile objects in inaccessible area).

Set clear and reasonable rules; expect the same behavior regardless of the circumstances, and if exceptions are made, clarify that the change is for one time only.

Teach desirable behavior through own example, such as using a quiet, calm voice rather than screaming.

Review expected behavior before special or unusual events, such as visiting a relative or having dinner in a restaurant.

Phrase requests for appropriate behavior positively, such as "Put the book down," rather than "Don't touch the book."

Call attention to unacceptable behavior as soon as it begins; use distraction to change the behavior or offer alternatives to annoying actions, such as a quiet toy for one that is excessively noisy.

Give advance notice or "friendly reminders," such as "When the TV program is over, it is time for dinner" or "I'll give you to the count of three and then we have to go."

Be attentive to situations that increase the likelihood of misbehaving, such as overexcitement or fatigue, or decreased personal tolerance to minor infractions.

Offer sympathetic explanations for not granting a request, such as "I am sorry I can't read you a story now, but I have to finish dinner. Then we can spend time together."

Keep any promises made to children.

Avoid outright conflicts; temper discussions with statements such as "Let's talk about it and see what we can decide together" or "I have to think about it first."

Provide children with opportunities for power and control.

GUIDELINES
Implementing Discipline

Consistency—Implement disciplinary action exactly as agreed on and for each infraction.

Timing—Initiate discipline as soon as child misbehaves; if delays are necessary, such as to avoid embarrassment, verbally disapprove of the behavior and state that disciplinary action will be implemented.

Commitment—Follow through with the details of the discipline, such as timing of minutes; avoid distractions that may interfere with the plan, such as telephone calls.

Unity—Make certain that all caregivers agree on the plan and are familiar with the details to prevent confusion and alliances between child and one parent.

Flexibility—Choose disciplinary strategies that are appropriate to child's age, temperament, and the severity of the misbehavior.

Planning—Plan discipline strategies in advance and prepare child if feasible, (e.g., explain use of time-out); for unexpected misbehavior, try to discipline when you are calm.

Behavior-orientation—Always disapprove of the behavior, not the child, with such statements as "That was a wrong thing to do. I am unhappy when I see behavior like that."

Privacy—Administer discipline in private, especially with older children who may feel ashamed in front of others.

Termination—Once the discipline is administered, consider child as having a "clean slate" and avoid bringing up the incident or lecturing.

misses classes because of a fear that he or she is unable to do the work). Children may also misbehave because the rules are not clear or consistently applied. Acting-out behavior, such as a temper tantrum, may represent uncontrolled frustration, anger, depression, or pain.

The best approach is to structure interactions with children so that unacceptable behavior is prevented or minimized. Although many parents devise strategies that are most effective for their child, general guidelines include those listed in the Family Home Care box.

General Guidelines for Implementing Discipline

Regardless of the type of discipline used, certain principles are essential in ensuring the efficacy of the approach (see Guidelines box). Many strategies, such as behavior modification, can only be implemented effectively when principles of consistency and timing are followed. A pattern of intermittent or occasional enforcement of limits actually prolongs the undesired behavior because children learn that if they are persistent, the behavior is permitted eventually. Delaying punishment weakens its intent, and practices such as telling the

child, "Wait until your father comes home," are not only ineffectual, but also convey negative connotations about the other parent.

Types of Discipline

To deal with misbehavior, parents need to implement appropriate disciplinary action. Numerous approaches are available, and some have definite advantages over others.

Reasoning involves explaining why an act is wrong and is usually appropriate for older children, especially when moral issues are involved. However, young children cannot be expected to "see the other side" because of their egocentrism. Children in the preoperative stage of cognitive development (toddlers and preschoolers) have a limited ability to distinguish between their point of view and those of others (Blum and others, 1995).

Sometimes children use the "reasoning" as a way of gaining attention. For example, they may misbehave in order for the parents to give them a lengthy explanation of the wrongdoing because negative attention is better than none. When children use this technique, parents may have to end the explanation by stating, "This is the rule, and this is how I expect you to behave. I won't explain it any further."

Unfortunately, reasoning is often combined with *scolding*, which sometimes takes the form of shame or criticism. For example, the parent may state, "You are a bad boy for hitting your brother." Children take such remarks seriously and personally, believing that *they* are bad.

Nursing ALERT When reprimanding children, focus only on the misbehavior, not on the child. Use of "I" messages rather than "you" messages expresses personal feelings without accusation or ridicule. For example, an "I" message attacks the behavior—"I am upset when Johnny is punched; I don't like to see him hurt"—not the child.

Positive and negative reinforcement is the basis of *behavior modification* theory—behavior that is rewarded will be repeated; behavior that is not, will be extinguished. Using *rewards* is a positive approach; by encouraging children to behave in specified ways, the tendency to misbehave is lessened. With young children, using paper stars is a very effective method. For older children the "token system" is appropriate, especially if a certain number yields a special reward, such as a trip to the movies or a new book. In planning a reward system, clearly explain the expected behaviors to the child and the rewards must be reinforcing. A chart should be used to record the stars or tokens, and every earned reward should be promptly given. Verbal approval should always accompany material rewards.

Consistently *ignoring* behavior will eventually extinguish or minimize the act. Although this approach sounds very simple, it is often difficult to implement consistently. Parents frequently "give in" and resort to previous patterns of discipline. Consequently, the behavior is actually reinforced because the child learns that persistence gains parental approval.

For ignoring to be effective, health professionals must devote a fair amount of time toward (1) explaining the approach in detail, (2) recording behavior before the extinction process is instituted to see if a problem exists and to compare results after ignoring is begun, (3) making certain that the parent's attention is the reinforcer, and (4) warning parents of a phenomenon called "response burst," which refers to an *increase* in the child's behavior soon after the process is initiated because the child is "testing" the parents to see if they are serious about the plan.

The strategy of *consequences* involves allowing children to experience the results of their misbehavior and includes three types:

1. **Natural**—Those that occur without any intervention, such as being late and missing dinner
2. **Logical**—Those that are directly related to the rule, such as not being allowed to play with another toy until the used ones are put away
3. **Unrelated**—Those that are imposed deliberately, such as no playing until homework is completed or the use of time-out

Natural or logical consequences are preferred but are effective only when they are meaningful to children. For example, the natural consequence of living in a messy room may do little to encourage cleaning up, but allowing no friends over until the room is neat can be very motivating! Withdrawing privileges is often an unrelated consequence. After the child experiences the consequence, the parent should refrain from any comment, because the usual tendency is for the child to try to place blame for imposing the rule.

Time-out is actually a refinement of the common practice of "sending the child to his or her room" and is a type of unrelated consequence. It is also based on the premise of removing the reinforcer (i.e., the satisfaction or attention the

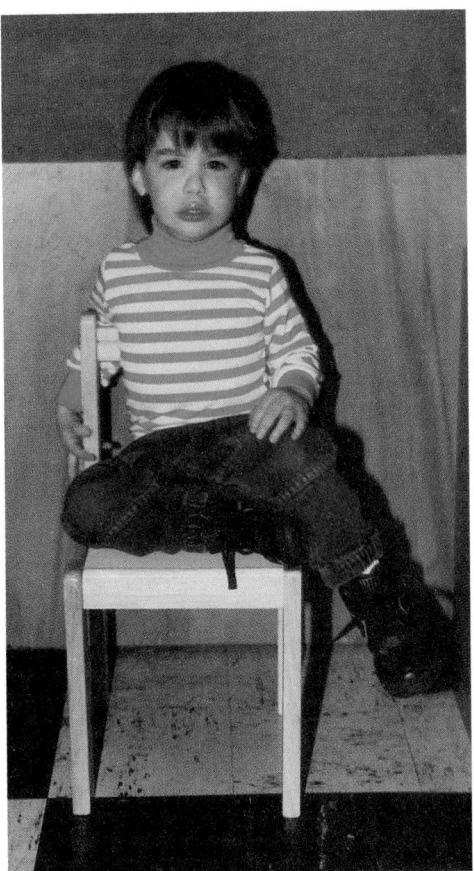

FIG. 4-4. Time-out is an excellent disciplinary strategy for young children.

child is receiving from the activity). When placed in an unstimulating and isolated place, children become bored and consequently agree to behave in order to reenter the family group (Fig. 4-4). Time-out avoids many of the problems of other disciplinary approaches, because no physical punishment is involved, no reasoning or scolding is given, and the parent is usually not present for all of the time-out, facilitating his or her ability to consistently apply the punishment. It also offers both the child and the parent a "cooling off" time. To be effective, time-out must be planned in advance (see Family Home Care box, p. 74).

Corporal or *physical punishment* most often takes the form of spanking. Based on the principles of aversive therapy, inflicting pain through spanking causes a dramatic short-term decrease in the behavior. However, there are some serious flaws in this approach: (1) it teaches children that violence is acceptable; (2) many times the spanking is the result of parental rage and may physically harm the child; and (3) children become "accustomed" to spanking, requiring more severe corporal punishment each time. Consequently, parents may use paddles, whips, or other objects, or they may eliminate a spanking because of their unwillingness to "hit the child harder," a practice that may prolong the behavior.

Spanking can result in severe physical injury and even death (Eichelberger, Beal, and May, 1991). Nevertheless, corporal punishment is often exempted from the category of assault, even when it produces specific injuries, which may be

FAMILY HOME CARE
Using Time-Out

Select an area for time-out that is safe, convenient, and unstimulating, but where the child can be monitored, such as the bathroom, hallway, or laundry room; avoid frightening areas such as a cellar or a dark closet.

Determine what behaviors warrant a time-out.

Make sure children understand the "rules" and how they are expected to behave.

Explain to children the process of time-out:

When they misbehave, they will be given *one* warning.

If they do not obey, they will be sent to the place designated for time-out.

They are to sit there for a specified period of time.

If they cry, refuse, or display any disruptive behavior, the time-out period will begin *after* they quiet down.

When they are quiet for the duration of the time, they can then leave the room.

A rule for the length of time-out is *1 minute per year of age*; use a kitchen timer with an audible bell to record the time rather than a watch.

Implement time-out in a public place by selecting a suitable area or explain to children that time-out will be spent immediately on returning home and mark their hand with a felt-tip pen as a reminder.

treated as "accidental" or "incidental" to discipline (Garbarino and others, 1992).

Even when corporal punishment does not involve serious physical damage to children, the psychologic impact may be great (Hyman and others, 1985). It can also interfere with effective parent-child interaction; children who receive corporal punishment are less likely to learn what they *should* do, because the focus is on what they *should not* do (Nelms, 1993). In addition, when the parent is not around, the misbehavior is likely to occur, for children have not learned to behave well for their own sake. Parental use of corporal punishment may also interfere with the child's development of moral reasoning.

The use of corporal punishment, a model of violent behavior, has been questioned more of late in conjunction with concern regarding increasing violence in contemporary society. Unfortunately, the practice continues to play a role in the public education of schoolchildren in many parts of the United States.

SPECIAL PARENTING SITUATIONS

Parenting is a demanding task under the most ideal circumstances, but when parents and children are faced with situations that deviate from what is considered to be the norm, the potential for family disruption is increased. Some of the issues that are encountered frequently are divorce, single parenthood, reconstituted families, adoption, and dual-career families. The problems associated with children of alcoholic parents, parents with physical disabilities, homeless parents,

or incarcerated parents are ones that are not addressed in the following discussions but may be topics that the reader may wish to investigate.

PARENTING THE ADOPTED CHILD

Adoption establishes the legal relationship of parent and child between persons who are not related by birth, with the same rights and obligations that exist between children and their biologic parents. In healthy families the ties of affection between the adoptive parents and their children are just as strong as biologic ties.

Although most adoptions are by couples who have been unable to have children of their own, many people—including single, divorced, and widowed persons—consider adoption for other reasons. There are some who feel a responsibility to provide a home for a child who needs one; others are able to have more children of their own but are seriously concerned about overpopulation and elect to increase their family through adoption; many are families who are finding "room for one more" with whom to share their love. Also, almost half the adoptable children in the United States are adopted by relatives, either stepparents or members of the extended family.

The Adoptive Family

Most problems faced by adoptive parents are no different from those encountered by biologic parents. All parents want to be good parents, but this desire is often intensified in adoptive parents. Adoptive parents have been portrayed as more apprehensive and insecure than biologic parents, and in need of more assistance. However, adoptive parents may feel the need for less assistance than biologic parents. This feeling is probably due to the adoptive parents' completely voluntary decision to become parents, the relatively long time they had to prepare for parenting, and the maturity associated with adopting (Edwards, 1987).

Unlike biologic parents who prepare for their child's birth with prenatal classes and the support of friends and relatives, adoptive parents have few sources of support and preparation for the new addition to their family (Koepke and others, 1991) (Fig. 4-5). Nurses who offer services to adoptive parents can provide the information, support, and reassurance needed to reduce parental anxiety regarding the adoptive process and refer them to parental support groups that provide guidance for adoptive parents. Such sources can be contacted through a state or county welfare office.

An initial concern that may be encountered by the adopting family is parent-infant attachment. Adoptive mothers have many of the same initial feelings for their infants and reactions to becoming parents as do birth mothers. Both adoptive and birth mothers react to the first moments with their infants with strong and varied emotions, ranging from happiness to distress. Research indicates that adoptive mothers are likely to develop emotional ties at much the same time that birth mothers do. Bonding will not be hindered by the lack of either a biologic relationship or immediate contact with their infants (Koepke and others, 1991).

The sooner infants enter their adoptive home, the better for purposes of parent-infant attachment. The more caregivers the infant has had before adoption, the more problems are likely to be encountered in attachment. The infant must

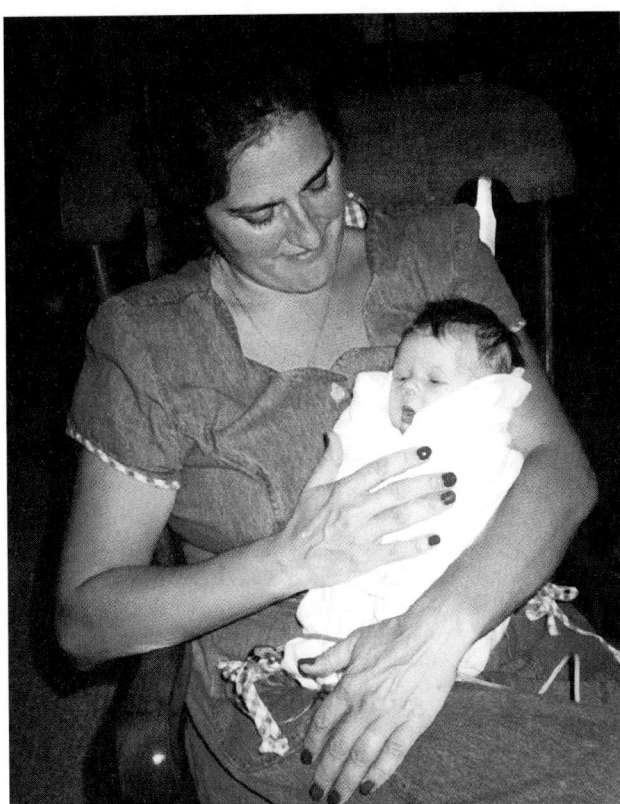

FIG. 4-5. Adoptive parents are often "instant parents." Both they and the child need time to learn about each other.

break the bond with the previous caregiver and form a new bond with the adoptive parents.

One of the difficulties of rearing adopted older children is helping them to deal with having had another set of parents. Children who are adopted after 2 years of age maintain an image of previous parenting persons. In addition to their biologic parents, the children may have lost siblings, grandparents, friends, and personal possessions. Often they have lived in several foster homes in which they formed attachments. They need time and assistance in working through the grief process that is an integral part of any loss. At the same time, they must adjust to a new household and relationships. Children who have experienced many losses and disappointments find adjustment more difficult and take a longer period of time to overcome fear of rejection and to develop affectionate ties to the new family. They grieve for those they left behind and may be afraid to love in case they must again move on.

Another area of special concern to adoptive parents is the task of telling children that they are adopted. Unfortunately, there are no clear-cut guidelines for parents to follow in determining precisely when children are ready for the information, and parents are naturally reluctant to present the child with such unsettling news. However, it is an important aspect of their parental responsibilities, and although they may be tempted to withhold the fact from the child, it is an essential component of the child's identity. Most authorities believe that children should be informed at a young enough age

that as they grow older, they do not remember a time when they did not know they were adopted (see Critical Thinking Exercise.)

Parents can anticipate some behavior changes following the disclosure—especially in children who are older. Children may use the fact of their adoption as a weapon to manipulate and threaten parents. There is the inevitable "My real mother would not treat me like this," or "You don't love me as much because I'm adopted." Statements such as these hurt parents and increase their feelings of insecurity, so that as parents they may become overly permissive. Adopted children need the same undemanding love as any other child, combined with firm discipline and limit-setting.

The adolescent years may also present special challenges. The normal confrontations of adolescents and parents may assume more painful aspects in adoptive families. Adolescents may use their adoption as a tool in defying parental authority or as a justification for aberrant behavior. As they attempt to master the task of identity formation, the feeling of abandonment by their biologic parents may come to awareness or may be intensified. During this time adopted children may feel the need to discover the identity of their biologic parents in order to define themselves and their identity—one of the major tasks of adolescent development. Sex differences in reacting to adoption may surface. It has been shown that girls may have more difficulty accepting their sexuality, since they may not be able to identify with a nonfertile female parent. It is important for parents to reassure their children that they understand the feelings of needing to search for one's identity.

Cross-Racial and International Adoption. Adoption of children of racial backgrounds different from that of the family is relatively commonplace. In addition to the problems faced by adopted children of any age, children of a cross-racial adoption must deal with their differentness. It is advised that parents who adopt such children do everything to preserve the adopted children's racial heritage.

Although the children are full-fledged members of an adopting family and citizens of the adopted country, those with a foreign appearance or other marked racial characteristics may create dilemmas outside the family. Strangers, or even relatives and friends, may make thoughtless comments and talk about the children as though they were not members of the family. It is vital that the family make it clear to others that this is their child and a cherished member of the family.

In international adoptions the medical information the parents receive may be quite complete or very sketchy (Hostetter and Johnson, 1989). Many internationally adopted children were born prematurely, and common health problems such as infant diarrhea and malnutrition may delay growth and development. Some children may have serious or multiple health problems. Many foreign-born children have not been immunized adequately (American Academy of Pediatrics, 1991). Cultural practices, such as constant holding rather than letting the child explore, may further affect the child's progress. On arrival, regardless of age, some internationally adopted children may experience temporary adjustment problems. In addition to giving advice on medical management, nurses should provide these parents with opportunities to discuss their feelings and situations.

PARENTING AND DIVORCE

Since the mid-1960s there has been a marked change in the stability of families that is reflected in increased rates of divorce, single-parenthood, and remarriage. In 1994 the divorce rate for the United States was 4.6 per 1000 total population (Singh and others, 1995). The divorce rate has changed very little since 1987. In the previous decade the rate increased almost yearly, with a peak in 1979. Although almost one half of all divorcing couples are childless, over 1 million children experience divorce each year, and most of the children are very young.

During a divorce, parents' coping abilities may be compromised. The parents may be much too preoccupied with their own feelings, needs, and life changes to be available and supportive to their children. Newly employed parents, usually mothers, are likely to leave children with new caregivers, in strange settings, or alone after school. The parent may also spend more time away from home, searching for or establishing new relationships. Sometimes, however, the adult feels frightened and alone and begins to depend on the child as a substitute for the absent partner. This dependence places an enormous burden on the child.

Common characteristics in the custodial household following separation and divorce include disorder, coercive types

of control, inflammable tempers in both parents and children, reduced parental competence, a greater sense of parental helplessness, poorly enforced discipline, and diminished regularity in enforcing household routines. Noncustodial parents also are seldom prepared for the role of visitor, may assume the role of recreational and "fun" parent, and may not have a residence suitable for children's visits. They may be concerned about maintaining the arrangement over the years to follow.

Impact of Divorce on Children

The results of numerous studies show that divorce has a profound effect on children. Long-term studies indicate that many youngsters suffer for years from psychologic and social difficulties associated with continuing and/or new stresses in the postdivorce family. A main outcome is heightened anxiety about forming enduring relationships as young adults (Wallerstein, 1991). Even when a divorce is amiable and open, children may recall parental separation with the same emotions felt by victims of a natural disaster: loss, grief, and vulnerability to forces beyond their control (Tuttle, 1992).

The impact of divorce on children depends on a variety of factors, including the age and sex of the children, the outcome of the divorce, and the quality of the parent-child relationship and parental care during the years following the divorce. Family characteristics appear to be more crucial to children's well-being than specific child characteristics, such as age or sex. The most important factor is continuing conflict between the divorced parents (Amato and Keith, 1991; Wallerstein and Johnston, 1990). Children cope better when parents adopt an attitude of "together for our child while separate for us" (Leung and Robson, 1990). High levels of ongoing family conflict are related to problems of social development, emotional stability, and cognitive skills for the child.

Complications sometimes associated with divorce include efforts on the part of one parent to subvert the child's loyalties to the other, abandonment to other caregivers, and adjustment to a stepparent. In the majority of divorce cases the mother receives custody of the child; this has an effect on the male child's identification with a father figure in addition to all the other ramifications of living in a family without a father or in a single-parent family. Many divorced mothers with young children move in with parents, other relatives, or friends in some kind of dependent or sharing arrangement.

Children may feel a sense of shame and embarrassment concerning the family situation. Such feelings cause children to see themselves as different, inferior, or unworthy of love, especially if they feel any responsibility for the family dissolution. Although the social stigma attached to divorce no longer produces the emotions it has in the past, it may still exist in some small towns and can reinforce children's negative self-image. The lasting effects of divorce depend on the children's and the parents' adjustment to the transition from an intact family to a single-parent family and, often, to a reconstituted family.

Although most studies have concentrated on the negative effects of divorce on youngsters, positive outcomes of divorce have been reported. A successful postdivorce family, either as a single-parent or as a reconstituted family, can improve the quality of life for adults and children. Living with conflict is resolved, and a better relationship with one or both parents may result. Children may also have less contact with a disturbed parent. Greater maturity, independence, and commitment to sustaining relationships are also positive outcomes (Wallerstein and Johnston, 1990). However, emotional adjustment is closely associated with the child's personal adjustment before the divorce (Demo and Acock, 1988).

Age- and Sex-Related Responses to Divorce.   Previously it was believed that divorce had a greater impact on younger children, but more recent observations indicate that divorce constitutes a major disruption for children in all age-groups. The feelings and behaviors of children may differ according to age (see box below) and sex, but all suffer stresses second only to the stress produced by the death of a parent.

Although considerable research has looked at sex differences in children's adjustments to divorce, the findings are not conclusive. In general, it appears that boys have more problematic behavior than girls after divorce. Also, postdivorce parenting difficulties tend to be greater with sons than with daughters and typically begin before the divorce (Shaw, Emery, and Tuer, 1993).

Telling the Children.   Parents are understandably hesitant to tell children about their decision to divorce. A vast majority of parents neglect to discuss with their preschool children either the divorce or the inevitable changes it brings. Without preparation, even children who remain in the family home are confused by the parental separation, and this confusion seems to overpower any soothing effects remaining in the home may have (Stirtzinger and Cholvat, 1990).

Most likely, the children are already experiencing vague, uneasy feelings that are more difficult to cope with than being told truthfully about the situation. If possible, the initial disclosure should include both parents and siblings, followed by later discussions with each child individually. Ample time should be set aside for the discussions, and they should take place during a period of calm, not after an argument. Parents who physically hold or touch their children provide them with a feeling of warmth that is reassuring. The discussions should include the reason for the divorce—minimizing blame—and reassurance that the divorce is not the fault of the children. Children may feel guilty, as though they have somehow failed or are being punished for misbehavior. They wonder what role they played in the divorce or failure to keep the family together.

Parents need not fear crying in front of the children; it gives the children permission to cry also. Children need to ventilate their feelings. They normally feel anger and resentment and should be allowed to communicate these feelings without punishment. They also have feelings of terror and

---

FEELINGS AND BEHAVIORS OF CHILDREN RELATED TO DIVORCE

Infancy

Effects of reduced mothering or lack of mothering
Increased irritability
Disturbance in eating, sleeping, and elimination
Interference with attachment process

Early Preschool Children (Ages 2-3 Years)

Frightened and confused
Blame themselves for the divorce
Fear of abandonment
Increased irritability, whining, tantrums
Regressive behaviors (e.g., thumb-sucking, loss of elimination control)
Separation anxiety

Later Preschool Children (Ages 3-5 Years)

Fear of abandonment
Blame themselves for the divorce; decreased self-esteem
Bewilderment regarding all human relationships
Become more aggressive in relationships with others (e.g., siblings, peers)
Engage in fantasy to seek understanding of the divorce

Early School-Age Children (Ages 5-6 Years)

Depression and immature behavior
Loss of appetite and sleep disorders
May be able to verbalize some feelings and understand some divorce-related changes
Increased anxiety and aggression
Feel abandoned by departing parent

Middle School-Age Children (Ages 6-8 Years)

Panic reactions
Feelings of deprivation—loss of parent, attention, money, and secure future
Profound sadness, depression, fear, and insecurity

Feelings of abandonment and rejection
Fear regarding the future
Difficulty expressing anger at parents
Intense desire for reconciliation of parents
Impaired capacity to play and enjoy outside activities
Decline in school performance
Altered peer relationships—become bossy, irritable, demanding, and manipulative
Frequent crying, loss of appetite, sleep disorders
Disturbed routine, forgetfulness

Later School-Age Children (Ages 9-12 Years)

More realistic understanding of divorce
Intense anger directed at one or both parents
Divided loyalties
Able to express feelings of anger
Ashamed of parental behavior
Feel the need for revenge; may wish to punish the parent they hold responsible
Feel lonely, rejected, and abandoned
Altered peer relationships
Decline in school performance
May develop somatic complaints
May engage in aberrant behavior such as lying, stealing
Temper tantrums
Dictatorial attitude

Adolescents (Ages 12-18 Years)

Able to disengage themselves from parental conflict
Feel a profound sense of loss—of family, childhood
Feelings of anxiety
Worry about themselves, parents, siblings
Express anger, sadness, shame, embarrassment
May withdraw from family and friends
Disturbed concept of sexuality
May engage in acting-out behaviors

abandonment and long for consistency and order in their lives. They need to know where they will live, who will take care of them, if they will be with their siblings, and if there will be enough money to live on. The children may also fear that if the parents stopped loving each other, they could stop loving them as well. Their need for assurance of love is tremendous at this time.

Custody and Parenting Partnerships

Traditionally when parents separated, the mother was given custody of the children. Now both parents and the courts are seeking alternatives. The present belief is that neither fathers nor mothers should be awarded custody automatically. Rather, custody should be awarded to the parent who is best able to provide for the children's welfare. In certain situations children experience severe stress when living or spending time with a parent. In most divorce cases the mother still receives custody of the child with visitation agreements for the father. However, more courts are now awarding custody to fathers. Men usually make more money and can offer more material benefits than many women are able to provide. The incidence of delinquent support payments to custodial mothers is a matter of universal knowledge and concern.

Often overlooked are the changes that may occur in the children's relationships with other relatives, especially grandparents. Grandparents on the noncustodial side are often kept from their grandchildren; those on the custodial side may be overwhelmed by their adult child's return to the household with grandchildren.*

Two other, less common, custody arrangements are divided custody and joint custody. *Divided,* or *split, custody* means that each parent is awarded custody of one or more of the children, thereby separating siblings. For example, sons might live with the father and daughters with the mother. Joint custody takes one of two forms. In *joint physical custody* the parents alternate the physical care and control of the children on a reasonably equitable basis while maintaining shared parenting responsibilities legally. This type of custody arrangement works well for families who live close to each other and whose occupations allow an active role in the care and rearing of the children. In *joint legal custody,* the children reside with one parent but both parents are the children's legal guardians and both participate in childrearing (Arditti, 1992).

Co-parenting offers substantial benefits for the family: children can be close to both parents, and life with each parent can be more normal as opposed to a disciplinarian mother and a recreational father. However, to be successful, the parents must place a high value on the commitment to provide as normal parenting as possible and be able to separate their marital conflicts from the parenting roles. No matter what type of custody arrangement is awarded, the primary consideration is the welfare of the children.

SINGLE-PARENTING

Single-parent status is acquired by means of divorce, separation, or death, or through birth or adoption of a child by a single person. Although divorce rates have stabilized, the number of single-parent households continues to rise. Today, one child in four lives in a single-parent family, with the majority of single parents being women (Center for the Study of Social Policy, 1993). It is estimated that at least half the children born during the 1980s will spend part of their time in a family headed by a divorced, separated, widowed, or never-married mother (Norton and Glick, 1986).

Managing shortages of money, time, and energy is a major concern of single parents. Studies repeatedly confirm the financial difficulties of single-parent families, particularly in the case of single mothers. (The average income of single-mother families is 60% that of single-father families; in addition, only 31% of mother-headed households receive any child support or alimony [Center for the Study of Social Policy, 1993].) In fact, the stigma of poverty may be more keenly felt than the discrimination associated with being a single parent (Richards, 1989). In addition, these families are often forced by their financial status to live in communities where inadequate housing and personal safety are concerns. When relocation is necessary, families may have to move away from friends and neighbors who have been sources of emotional support. Many single parents have trouble arranging for adequate child care, and care for sick children is especially difficult to obtain. Single mothers trying to balance work, chores, and child care may frequently give up personal activities, recreation, and even rest.

Fathers who have custody of their children have many of the same problems as divorced mothers. They feel overburdened by the responsibility, are depressed, and are concerned about their ability to cope with the emotional needs of their children, especially the needs of girls. They find it difficult at first to coordinate household tasks, school visits, and other activities associated with managing a household alone. Fathers often demand more assistance with household tasks and more independence from their children than custodial mothers do, and they are likely to make use of alternative caregiving and support systems.

Supports and resources for single-parent families include health care services that are open evenings and weekends, high-quality child care, respite child care to relieve parental exhaustion and burnout, and parent enhancement centers for advancing education and job skills, providing recreational activities, and offering parenting education. Groups for single-parent fathers and grandparents who are primary caregivers are also important (Strett, 1989). There is a need on the part of the parent for social contacts and a life separate from the children for the emotional growth of both parent and child. The single parent can find support and encouragement from **Parents Without Partners, Inc.,*** an organization designed to meet the needs of this increasingly important group.

PARENTING IN RECONSTITUTED FAMILIES

In the United States approximately half of all children in homes where parents have divorced will experience yet another major change in their lives within 3 years of a

---

*Grandparents, a newsletter for grandparents in divided families, is published by Scarsdale Family Counseling Service, 405 Harwood Building, Scarsdale NY 10583; (914) 723-3281.

*International Headquarters, 401 N. Michigan Avenue, Chicago, IL 60611-4267; (312) 644-6610.

Let relationships develop slowly and naturally. Don't expect too much too soon, from the children, from your spouse, or from yourself.

Don't criticize or belittle lost (or new) parents, or try to erase or replace them. Stepparents are additional parents.

Expect confused feelings, anxieties, competition for attention, bids for loyalty. Decide on standards of discipline and behavior and stick to them.

Communicate. Don't pretend everything is fine if it isn't. Look at problems squarely and deal with them openly.

If you need help, admit it and get it. Read a book, get counseling, join a support group, call a family meeting.

From Stein B: Yours, mine, and ours: a look at stepfamilies, *Growing Parent* 12(9):1-5, 1984.

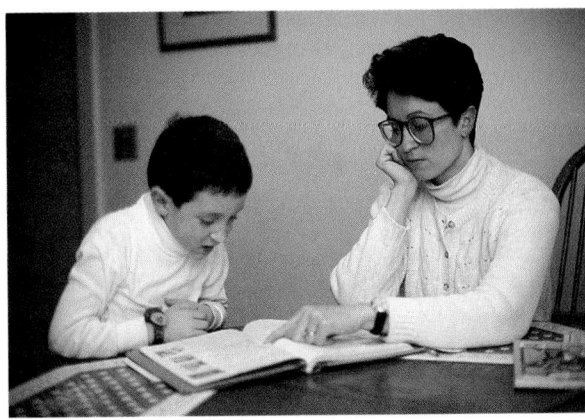

FIG. 4-6. Working mothers must accomplish numerous tasks as part of their busy day.

divorce—a return to a nuclear family and the sudden acquisition of a stepparent when the custodial parent remarries (Hetherington, Stanley-Hagen, and Anderson, 1989). The entry of a stepparent into a ready-made family requires adjustments for all the family members. Some obstacles to the role adjustments and family problem solving include disruption of previous life-styles and interaction patterns, complexity in the formation of new ones, and lack of social supports. Despite these problems, most children from divorced families want to live in a two-parent home.

The term "parenting coalition" has been suggested to describe the situation where there are more than two parents for a child, as in stepfamilies (Visher and Visher, 1989). This term implies the need for cooperation rather than competition between the biologic parents and the stepparents. Cooperative parenting relationships can allow more time for each set of parents to be alone to establish their own relationship. Under ideal circumstances, power conflicts between the two households can be reduced, and tension and anxiety can be lessened for all family members. In addition, the children's self-esteem can be increased, and there is a greater likelihood of continued contact with grandparents. The development of a parenting coalition requires time. Flexibility, mutual support, and open communication are critical in successful relationships in stepfamilies and stepparenting situations.

Unfortunately, stepfamilies usually do not seek help to prevent problems from arising. Typically, information and counseling are sought only when problems have surfaced and can no longer be ignored. A preventive rather than remedial approach to stepfamilies and stepparenting is needed (Ganong and Coleman, 1989) (see Family Focus box).

PARENTING IN DUAL-EARNER FAMILIES

No change in family life-style has had more impact than the large numbers of women entering the workplace. As women moved away from the traditional homemaker pattern, the numbers of dual-earner families increased dramatically. In 1993, 54% of mothers with children under 3 years of age were in the civilian labor force; 64% of women with children 3 to

5 years of age were employed (Children's Defense Fund, 1994). This trend is unlikely to diminish. As a result, the family is subjected to considerable stress as members attempt to meet the challenge of the often competing demands of occupational needs and those regarded as necessary for a rich family life.

Role definitions are frequently altered to arrange an equitable division of time and labor, as well as to resolve conflicts between earlier and later norms, especially those related to the traditional norms of the culture. Overload is a common source of stress in a dual-earner family, and social activities are significantly curtailed. Time demands and scheduling are major problems, and when there are children, the demands can be even more intense; dual-earner couples may increase the strain on themselves in order to avoid creating stress for their children, although there is no evidence to indicate that the dual-earner life-style, as such, is stressful to children. However, the stress experienced by the parents may affect the children indirectly.

Working Mothers

Even though working mothers have become the norm in the United States, disapproving attitudes from some health care workers and some child care books, lack of a national policy on child care, and "scripts" from their own childhood of being cared for by an at-home mother contribute to the torn and guilty feelings many working mothers experience (Balk and Christoffel, 1988). Fathers are taking a more active role in child care. By 1991 one of every five preschool children (under age 5) was cared for by the father while the mother worked outside the home (O'Connell, 1993).

The quality of child care is a persistent concern for all working parents. However, mothers are more likely than fathers to adjust their work schedule to accommodate child care needs. Even in families where the father is the primary caregiver while the mother is at work, 40% of mothers adjusted their work hours to meet child care needs, compared with 6% of fathers (O'Connell, 1993).

The mother's status as a working woman has not been found consistently to have either positive or negative effects on children's development and educational outcomes (Balk and Christoffel, 1988) (Fig. 4-6). Working women who scored high on measures of emotional well-being, sensitivity to and acceptance of their children, satisfaction with nonwork time, and positive feelings about their marriage were more likely to have securely attached infants, regardless of child care arrangements (Belsky, 1988). One consistent finding is that the "consequences of maternal employment" (mental health, marital satisfaction, children's well-being) are favorable when the woman's employment status is consistent with her and her partner's preferences about it (Spitzke, 1988). Also, the economic background of the family interacts with the effects of the type of child care and its psychologic outcomes (Friedman and others, 1994).

Nurses play an important role in helping families to find suitable sources of child care and to prepare children for this experience (see Alternate Child Care Arrangements, Chapter 10).

ACCOMMODATING CONTEMPORARY PARENTING SITUATIONS

During recent years both the private and government sectors have noted some of the problems contemporary families face. Many of these issues involve working parents. For example, perhaps one of the greatest stressors for the working single parent or dual-earner families is when a child becomes ill. Frequency of childhood illness, exclusion practices of most licensed child care programs, and employer's limited sick leave policies are contributing factors. While the preferred type of care for the sick child is that provided by the parents at home, families have a variety of options. These include in-home care by a trained provider other than the child's parent, care by a relative, on-site care in the child's usual program, and care in a separate, specialized group daycare setting for mildly ill children (Giebink, 1993). Sick child care in a group setting is becoming popular in many communities. Although standards and criteria for such settings have been established (Smith, Shillam, and Zimmerman, 1989), research is needed to determine outcomes for children.

Some employers have become more family focused and give parents time off to be with their sick children. Increasing numbers are also more generous in the amount of time they offer parents—fathers as well as mothers—to remain at home after the birth or adoption of a child. More flexible work schedules and family-oriented legislation can also ease the burden of managing family and work responsibilities (Arnold and Brecht, 1990). The passage of the *Family and Medical Leave Act (FMLA)* in 1993 set the stage for a greater focus on the issues that contemporary American families face. Under this law parents are guaranteed time away from work without pay and without jeopardizing their employment to care for their children in certain situations.

KEY POINTS

- Since there is no agreement about the definition of *family,* a family is what the client considers it to be.
- Three theories that have significant relevance and application to pediatric nursing are family system theory, developmental theory, and family stress theory.
- Although the traditional family structure has been nuclear or extended, in recent years other forms, such as the single-parent family, have emerged.
- Family size and positioning within the family structure have a strong impact on a child's development.
- Interpersonal skills and a basic understanding of childhood growth and development are two essential areas of focus for parents.
- Parents tend to predominate in one of three types of parental control: authoritarian, permissive, and authoritative.

- Three areas of special concern to adoptive families include the initial attachment process, the task of telling the children they are adopted, and identity formation during adolescence.
- Marital factors within the home significantly influence a child's development. The impact of divorce on a child depends on age and sex, outcome, and quality of the parent-child relationship and parental care following the divorce.
- Single-parenting and stepparenting create adjustment difficulties and add stress to the already-demanding parental role. Significant numbers of children will live in a single-parent or reconstituted family at some point.

REFERENCES

Amato PR, Keith B: Parental divorce and the well-being of children: a meta-analysis, *Psychol Bull* 110(1):26-46, 1991.

American Academy of Pediatrics, Committee on Early Childhood, Adoption and Dependent Care: Initial medical evaluation of an adopted child, *Pediatrics* 88(3):642-644, 1991.

Arditti J: Differences between fathers with joint custody and non-custodial fathers, *Am J Orthopsychiatry* 62(2):186-195, 1992.

Arnold L, Brecht M: Legislative issues affecting parenting: an overview of current policies, *J Perinat Neonat Nurs* 4(2):24-32, 1990.

Balk S, Christoffel K: Advising the working mother, *Contemp Pediatr* 5(9):56-85, 1988.

Belsky J: The "effects" of infant day care reconsidered, *Early Childhood Res Q* 3(3):235-272, 1988.

Blum NJ and others: Disciplining young children: the role of verbal instructions and reasoning, *Pediatrics* 96(2):336-341, 1995.

Bozett FW: Parenting concerns of gay fathers, *Top Clin Nurs* 6:60-71, 1984.

Bozett FW: Gay fathers: a review of the literature. In Bozett FW, editor: *Homosexuality and the family*, New York, 1989, Harrington Park.

Brazelton TB: Working with families: opportunities for early intervention, *Pediatr Clin North Am* 42(1):1-10, 1995.

Carter B, McGoldrick M: *The changing family life cycle: a framework for family therapy*, Needham Heights, MA, 1989, Allyn & Bacon.

Center for the Study of Social Policy: *Kids count*, Washington, DC, 1993, Annie E Casey Foundation.

Children's Defense Fund: *The State of America's Children 1994*, Washington, DC, 1994, CDF.

Daniels D, Moos R: Exosystem influences on family and child functioning, *J Soc Behav Pers* 3(4):113-133, 1988.

Demo D, Acock A: The impact of divorce on children, *J Marriage Fam* 50:619-648, 1988.

Dunst C, Trivette C, Deal A: *Enabling and empowering families: principles and guidelines for practice*, Cambridge, MA, 1988, Brookline Books.

Duvall ER: *Family development*, ed 5, Philadelphia, 1977, JB Lippincott.

Edwards J: Perceived needs of adoptive and biologic parents, *Issues Compr Pediatr Nurs* 10:223-234, 1987.

Eichelberger S, Beal D, May R: Hypovolemic shock in a child as a consequence of corporal punishment, *Pediatrics* 87(4):570-571, 1991.

Friedman SL and others: Effects of child care on psychological development: issues and future directions for research, *Pediatrics* 94 6(suppl 2):1069-1070, 1994.

Gage M, Christensen D: Parental role socialization and the transition to parenthood, *Fam Relations* 40(3):332-337, 1991.

Ganong L, Coleman M: Preparing for remarriage: anticipating the issues, seeking solutions, *Fam Relations* 38:28-33, 1989.

Garbarino J and others: *Children in danger: coping with the consequences of community violence*, San Francisco, 1992, Josey-Bass.

Giebink G: Care of the ill child in day-care settings, *Pediatrics* 91(1, pt 2):229-233, 1993.

Gottman J: Children of gay and lesbian parents. In Bozett FW, Sussman M, editors: *Homosexuality and family relations*, New York, 1990, Harrington Park.

Harris MB, Turner PH: Gay and lesbian parents, *J Homosex* 12:103-113, 1986.

Hetherington EM, Stanley-Hagan M, Anderson ER: Marital transitions: a child's perspective, *Am Psychol* 44(2):303-312, 1989.

Hill R: *Families under stress*, New York, 1949, Harper & Row.

Hoopes M, Harper J: *Birth order roles and sibling patterns in individual and family therapy*, Rockville, MD, 1987, Aspen.

Hostetter M, Johnson D: International adoption: an introduction for physicians, *Am J Dis Child* 143:325-332, 1989.

Huggins S: A comparative study of self-esteem of adolescent children of divorced lesbian mothers and divorced heterosexual mothers, *J Homosex* 18(1/2):123-135, 1989.

Hyman I and others: *Child abuse in the schools: community and judicial attitudes*. Paper presented at the 62nd annual meeting of the American Orthopsychiatric Association, New York, April 24, 1985.

Koepke J and others: Becoming parents: feelings of adoptive mothers, *Pediatr Nurs* 17(4):333-336, 1991.

Leung AK, Robson WL: Children of divorce, *J R Soc Health* 110(5):161-163, 1990.

Lobato D: *Brothers, sisters, and special needs*, Baltimore, MD, 1990, Paul H Brookes.

McCubbin MA, McCubbin HI: Families coping with illness: the resiliency model of family stress, adjustment, and adaptation. In Danielson CB, Bissel BH, Winstead-Fry P, editors: *Families, health, and illness*, St Louis, 1994, Mosby.

McCubbin M, McCubbin H: Theoretical orientation to family stress and coping. In Figley C, editor: *Treating families under stress*, New York, 1989, Brunner/Mazel.

Nelms B: Discipline: what do you recommend? *J Pediatr Health Care* 7(1):1-2, 1993.

Norton A, Glick P: One-parent families: a social and economic profile, *Fam Relations* 35:8-17, 1986.

O'Connell M: *Where's papa? Fathers' role in child care*, Washington, DC, 1993, Population Reference Bureau.

Patterson C: Children of lesbian and gay parents, *Child Dev* 63:1025-1042, 1992.

Patterson J: Promoting resilience in families experiencing stress, *Pediatr Clin North Am* 42(1):47-63, 1995.

Paul J: *Growing up with a gay, lesbian, or bisexual parent: an exploratory study of experiences and perceptions*, Unpublished doctoral dissertation, Berkeley, CA, 1986, University of California at Berkeley.

Richards L: The precarious survival and hard-won satisfaction of white single-parent families, *Fam Relations* 38:396-403, 1989.

Shaw DS, Emery RE, Tuer MD: Parental functioning and children's adjustment in families of divorce: a prospective study, *J Abnormal Child Psychology* 21(1):119-134, 1993.

Singh GK and others: Annual summary of births, marriages, divorces, and deaths: United States, 1994. Monthly vital statistics report 43:13. Hyattsville, MD, 1995, National Center for Health Statistics.

Smith K, Shillam P, Zimmerman F: Standards and criteria: group child care for sick children, *Pediatr Nurs* 15(6):600-602, 1989.

Spitzke G: Women's employment and family relations: a review, *J Marriage Fam* 50(3):595-618, 1988.

Stirtzinger R, Cholvat L: Preschool age children of divorce: transitional phenomena and the mourning process, *Can J Psychiatry* 35:506-514, 1990.

Strett R: Support services for single parents, *Early Childhood Update* 5:6, winter 1989.

Tuttle G: Divorce: how are the children coping? *Can Nurse* 88(11):13-16, 1992.

Visher E, Visher J: Parenting coalitions after remarriage: dynamics and therapeutic guidelines, *Fam Relations* 38:65-70, 1989.

Ventura SJ and others: Advance report of final natality statistics, 1993. Monthly vital statistics report 44:3, supp. Hyattsville, MD, 1995, National Center for Health Statistics.

Wallace P, Gotlib I: Marital adjustment during the transition to parenthood: stability and predictors of change, *J Marriage Fam* 52(1):21-29, 1990.

Wallerstein JS: The long-term effects of divorce on children: a review, *J Am Acad Child Adolesc Psychiatry* 30(3):349-360, 1991.

Wallerstein JS, Johnston JR: Children of divorce: recent findings regarding long-term effects and recent studies of joint and sole custody, *Pediatr Rev* 11(7):197-204, 1990.

BIBLIOGRAPHY

General

Aldous J: Family development and the life course: two perspectives on family change, *J Marriage Fam* 52(3):571-583, 1990.

Bornstein MH, editor: *Handbook of parenting,* vols 1-4, Hillsdale, NJ, 1995, Lawrence Erlbaum.

Cohen WI: Family-oriented pediatric care: taking the next step, *Pediatr Clin North Am* 42(1):11-20, 1995.

Friedman M: *Family nursing: theory and practice,* ed 3, Norwalk, CT, 1992, Appleton-Century-Crofts.

Gilliss CL and others, editors: *Toward a science of family nursing,* Menlo Park, CA, 1989, Addison-Wesley.

Green M: No child is an island: contextual pediatrics and the "new" health supervision, *Pediatr Clin North Am* 42(1):79-88, 1995.

Kune-Karrer BM, Taylor EH: Toward multiculturality: implications for the pediatrician, *Pediatr Clin North Am* 42(1):21-30, 1995.

Lavee Y, Olson D: Family types and response to stress, *J Marriage Fam* 53(3):786-788, 1991.

MacPhee M: The family systems approach and pediatric nursing care, *Pediatr Nurs* 21(5):417-423, 437, 1995.

Schor EL: The influence of families on child health: family behaviors and child outcomes, *Pediatr Clin North Am* 42(1):89-102, 1995.

Wright LM, Leahey M, editors: *Nurses and families: a guide to family assessment and intervention,* Philadelphia, 1984, FA Davis.

Family Constellations/Parenting

Bigner JJ, Jacobsen RB: Parenting behaviors of homosexual and heterosexual fathers, *J Homosex* 18(1/2):173-186, 1989.

Bozett FW: Gay fathers: a review of the literature, *J Homosex* 18(1/2):137-162, 1989.

Carter-Jessop L, Yoos L: Parental thinking: assessment and applications in nursing, *Matern Child Nurs J* 22(2):49-55, 1994.

Christophersen ER: Discipline, *Pediatr Clin North Am* 39:395-412, 1992.

Gellerstedt ME, leRoux P: Beyond anticipatory guidance: parenting and the family life cycle, *Pediatr Clin North Am* 42(1):65-78, 1995.

Howard BJ: Discipline in early childhood, *Pediatr Clin North Am* 38:1351-1396, 1991.

Patterson JM, Garwick AW: Levels of meaning in family stress theory, *Fam Proc* 33:287-304, 1994.

Visher JS, Visher EB: Beyond the nuclear family: resources and implications for pediatricians, *Pediatr Clin North Am* 42(1):31-46, 1995.

Special Parenting Situations

Anable KE: Children of divorce: ways to heal the wounds, *Clin Nurse Spec* 5(3):133-137, 1991.

Arditti JA: Noncustodial fathers: an overview of policy and resources, *Fam Relations* 39(4):460-465, 1990.

Benin M, Edwards D: Adolescents' chores: the differences between dual- and single-career families, *J Marriage Fam* 52(2):361-373, 1990.

Bray JH, Berger SH: Noncustodial father and paternal grandparent relationship in stepfamilies, *Fam Relations* 39(4):414-419, 1990.

Brazelton TB: Putting a child in day care: issues for working parents, *Pediatrics* 91(1, pt 2):271-272, 1993.

Bredekamp S: Day-care standards: need and impact, *Pediatrics* 91(1, pt 2):234-236, 1993.

Brubeck D, Beer J: Depression, self-esteem, suicide ideation, death anxiety, and GPA in high school students of divorced and non-divorced parents, *Psychol Rep* 71(3, pt I):755-763, 1992.

Caldwell BM: Impact of day care on the child, *Pediatrics* 91 (1, pt 2):225-228, 1993.

Christensen DH, Dahl CM, Rettig KD: Noncustodial mothers and child support: examining the larger context, *Fam Relations* 39(4):388-394, 1990.

Day care for early preschool children: implications for the child and family, *Am J Psychiatry* 150(8):1281-1287, 1993.

Depner CE, Bray JH: Modes of participation for noncustodial parents: the challenge for research, policy, practice and education, *Fam Relations* 39(4):378-381, 1990.

Dvoskin AG: Child custody. In Hoekelman RA and others, editors: *Primary pediatric care,* ed 2, St Louis, 1992, Mosby.

Fairchild MW, Zebal BH: Children of divorce. In Hoekelman RA and others, editors: *Primary pediatric care,* ed 2, St Louis, 1992, Mosby.

Ferreiro BW: Presumption of joint custody: a family policy dilemma, *Fam Relations* 39(4):420-426, 1990.

Garvin V, Leber D, Kalter N: Children of divorce: predictors of change following preventive intervention, *Am J Orthopsychiatry* 61(3):438-447, 1991.

Hajal F, Rosenberg D: The family life cycle in adoptive families, *Am J Orthopsychiatry* 61(1):78-85, 1991.

Healy JM Jr, Malley JE, Stewart AJ: Children and their fathers after parental separation, *Am J Orthopsychiatry* 60(4):531-543, 1990.

Johnston JR: Role diffusion and role reversal: structural variation in divorced families and children's functioning, *Fam Relations* 39(4):405-413, 1990.

Melnyk BM: Changes in parent-child relationships following divorce, *Pediatr Nurs* 17(4):337-341, 1991.

Menaghan D, Parcel T: Parental employment and family life: research in the 1980s, *J Marriage Fam* 52(4):1079-1098, 1990.

Nickman SL: Adoption and foster care. In Hoekelman RA and others, editors: *Primary pediatric care,* ed 2, St Louis, 1992, Mosby.

Richman JM, Chapman MV, Bowen GL: Recognizing the impact of marital discord and parental depression on children: a family-centered approach, *Pediatr Clin North Am* 42(1):167-180, 1995.

Schwartzberg AZ: The impact of divorce on adolescents, *Hosp Community Psychiatry* 43(6):634-637, 1992.

Shaw DS: The effects of divorce on children's adjustment: review and implications, *Behav Modif* 15(4):456-485, 1991.

Tiedje LB, Collins C: Combining employment and motherhood, *MCN* 14:9-14, 1989.

Tschann J and others: Family process and children's functioning during divorce, *J Marriage Fam* 51:431-444, 1990.

Volling B, Belsky J: Multiple determinants of father involvement during infancy in dual-earner and single-earner families, *J Marriage Fam* 53(2):461-474, 1991.

Wallerstein JS, Blakeslee S: *Second chances: men, women, and children a decade after divorce,* New York, 1989, Ticknor & Fields.

DEVELOPMENTAL INFLUENCES ON CHILD HEALTH PROMOTION

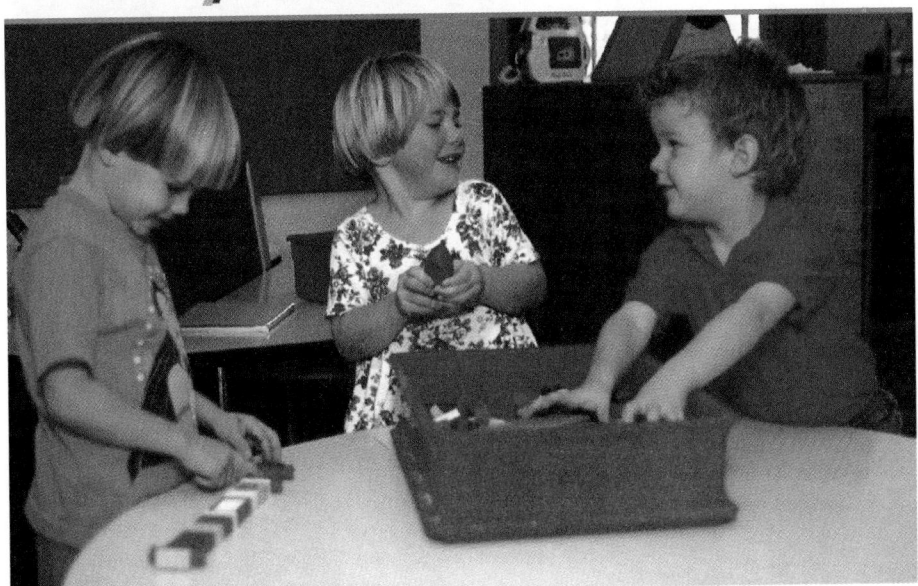

RELATED TOPICS

GROWTH AND DEVELOPMENT

FOUNDATIONS OF GROWTH AND DEVELOPMENT

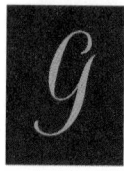 rowth and development, usually referred to as a unit, expresses the sum of the numerous changes that take place during the lifetime of an individual. The entire course is a dynamic process that encompasses several interrelated dimensions:

Growth—an increase in number and size of cells as they divide and synthesize new proteins; results in increased size and weight of the whole or any of its parts

Development—a gradual change and expansion; advancement from lower to more advanced stages of complexity; the emerging and expanding of the individual's capacities through growth, maturation, and learning

Maturation—an increase in competence and adaptability; aging; usually used to describe a qualitative change; a change in the complexity of a structure that makes it possible for that structure to begin functioning; to function at a higher level

Differentiation—processes by which early cells and structures are systematically modified and altered to achieve specific and characteristic physical and chemical properties; sometimes used to describe the trend of mass to specific; development from simple to more complex activities and functions

Stages of Development

Most authorities in the field of child development conveniently categorize child growth and behavior into approximate age stages or in terms that describe the features of an age-group. The age ranges of these stages are admittedly arbitrary and, because they do not take into account individual differences, cannot be applied to all children with any degree of precision. However, this categorization affords a convenient means to describe the characteristics associated with the majority of children at periods when distinctive developmental changes appear and specific developmental tasks must be accomplished. (A *developmental task* is a set of skills and competencies peculiar to each developmental stage that children must accomplish or master in order to deal effectively

 For additional information, please view "Growth and Development" in *Whaley and Wong's Pediatric Nursing Video Series,* St Louis, 1996, Mosby; (800) 426-4545.

with their environment.) It is also significant for nurses to know that there are characteristic health problems peculiar to each major phase of development. The sequence of descriptive age periods and subperiods that are used here and elaborated in subsequent chapters is listed in the accompanying box on p. 85.

Patterns of Growth and Development

There are definite and predictable patterns in growth and development that are continuous, orderly, and progressive. These patterns, or trends, are universal and basic to all human beings, but each human being accomplishes these in a manner and time unique to that individual.

Directional Trends. Growth and development proceed in regular, related directions or gradients and reflect the physical development and maturation of neuromuscular functions (Fig. 5-1). The first pattern is the *cephalocaudal,* or *head-to-tail,* direction. That is, the head end of the organism develops first and is very large and complex, whereas the lower end is small and simple and takes shape at a later period. The physical evidence of this trend is most apparent during the period before birth, but it also applies to postnatal behavior development. Infants achieve structural control of the head before they have control of the trunk and extremities, hold their back erect before they stand, use their eyes before their hands, and gain control of their hands before they have control of their feet.

Second, the *proximodistal,* or *near-to-far,* trend applies to the midline-to-peripheral concept. A conspicuous illustration is the early embryonic development of limb buds, which is followed by rudimentary fingers and toes. In the infant, shoulder control precedes mastery of the hands, the whole hand is used as a unit before the fingers can be manipulated, and the central nervous system develops more rapidly than the peripheral nervous system.

These trends or patterns are bilateral and appear symmetric—each side develops in the same direction and at the same rate as the other. For some of the neurologic functions, this symmetry is only external because of unilateral differentiation of function at an early stage of postnatal development. For example, by the age of approximately 5 years the child has demonstrated a decided preference for the use of one hand over the other, although previously either one had been used.

The third trend, *differentiation,* describes development

DEVELOPMENTAL AGE PERIODS

Prenatal period: Conception to birth
Germinal: Conception to approximately 2 weeks
Embryonic: 2 to 8 weeks
Fetal: 8 to 40 weeks (birth)
A rapid growth rate and total dependency make this one of the most crucial periods in the developmental process. The relationship between maternal health and certain manifestations in the newborn emphasizes the importance of adequate prenatal care to the health and well-being of the infant.

Infancy period: Birth to 12 months
Neonatal: Birth to 27 or 28 days
Infancy: 1 to approximately 12 months
The infancy period is one of rapid motor, cognitive, and social development. Through mutuality with the caregiver (parent), the infant establishes a basic trust in the world and the foundation for future interpersonal relationships. The critical first month of life, although part of the infancy period, is often differentiated from the remainder because of the major physical adjustments to extrauterine existence and the psychologic adjustment of the parent.

Early childhood: 1 to 6 years
Toddler: 1 to 3 years
Preschool: 3 to 6 years
This period, which extends from the time the children attain upright locomotion until they enter school, is characterized by intense activity and discovery. It is a time of marked physical and personality development. Motor development advances steadily. Children at this age acquire language and wider social relationships, learn role standards, gain self-control and mastery, develop increasing awareness of dependence and independence, and begin to develop a self-concept.

Middle childhood: 6 to 11 or 12 years
Frequently referred to as the "school age," this period of development is one in which the child is directed away from the family group and is centered around the wider world of peer relationships. There is steady advancement in physical, mental, and social development with emphasis on developing skill competencies. Social cooperation and early moral development take on more importance with relevance for later life stages. This is a critical period in the development of a self-concept.

Later childhood: 11 to 19 years
Prepubertal: 10 to 13 years
Adolescence: 13 to approximately 18 years
The tumultuous period of rapid maturation and change known as adolescence is considered to be a transitional period that begins at the onset of puberty and extends to the point of entry into the adult world—usually high school graduation. Biologic and personality maturation are accompanied by physical and emotional turmoil, and there is redefining of the self-concept. In the late adolescent period the young person begins to internalize all previously learned values and to focus on an individual, rather than a group, identity.

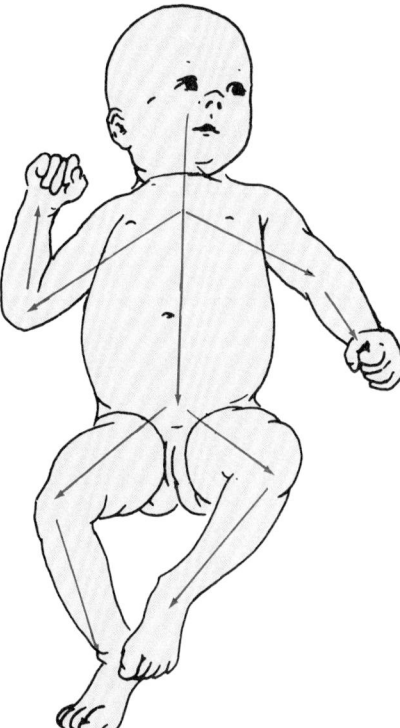

FIG. 5-1. Directional trends in growth.

from simple operations to more complex activities and functions. From very broad, global patterns of behavior, more-specific, refined patterns emerge. All areas of development (physical, mental, social, and emotional) proceed in this direction. Through the process of development and differentiation, early embryonal cells with vague, undifferentiated functions progress to an immensely complex organism composed of highly specialized and diversified cells, tissues, and organs. Generalized development precedes specific or specialized development; gross, random muscle movements take place before fine muscle control.

Sequential Trends. In all dimensions of growth and development there is a definite, predictable sequence, with each child normally passing through every stage. Children crawl before they creep, creep before they stand, and stand before they walk. Later facets of the personality are built on the early foundation of trust. The child babbles, then forms words and, finally, sentences; writing emerges from scribbling.

Developmental Pace. Although there is a fixed, precise order to development, it does not progress at the same rate or pace. There are periods of accelerated growth and periods of decelerated growth in both total body growth and the growth of subsystems. The rapid growth before and after birth gradually levels off throughout early childhood. Growth is relatively slow during middle childhood, markedly increases at the beginning of adolescence, and levels off in early adulthood. Each child grows at his or her own pace. Marked differences are observed between children as they reach and surmount developmental milestones.

 Research suggests that normal growth, in particular, height in infants, may occur in brief (possibly even 24-hour) bursts that punctuate long periods in which no measurable growth takes place (Lampl, 1992). Further, findings indicate a stuttering or *saltatory* pattern of growth that follows no regular cycle and can occur after "quiet" periods that last as long as 4 weeks. Mothers reported that their children were usually fussy and voraciously hungry a day or two before the growth spurt.

Sensitive Periods.   There are limited times during the process of growth when the organism will interact with a particular environment in a specific manner. Periods termed *critical, sensitive, vulnerable,* and *optimal* are those times in the lifetime of an organism when it is more susceptible to positive or negative influences.

The quality of interactions during these sensitive periods determines whether the effects on the organism will be beneficial or harmful. For example, physiologic maturation of the central nervous system is influenced by adequacy and timing of contributions from the environment, such as stimulation and nutrition. The first 3 months of prenatal life are sensitive periods for physical growth of the fetus.

Psychologic development also appears to have sensitive periods when an environmental event has maximal influence on the developing personality. For example, primary socialization occurs during the first year when the infant makes the initial social attachments and establishes a basic trust in the world. A warm relationship with a parent figure is fundamental to a healthy personality. The same concept might be applied to readiness for learning skills such as toilet training or reading. In these instances there appears to be an opportune time when the skill is best learned.

Individual Differences

Each child grows in his or her own unique and personal way. Great individual variation exists in the age at which developmental milestones are reached. The sequence is predictable; the exact timing is not. Rates of growth vary, and measurements are defined in terms of ranges to allow for individual differences. Some children are fast growers, others are moderate, and some are slower to reach maturity. Periods of fast growth, such as the pubescent growth spurt, may begin earlier or later in some children than in others. Children may grow fast or slowly during the spurt and may finish sooner or later than other children. Gender is an influential factor because girls seem to be more advanced in physiologic growth at all ages.

BIOLOGIC GROWTH AND PHYSICAL DEVELOPMENT

As children grow, their external dimensions change. These changes are accompanied by corresponding alterations in structure and function of internal organs and tissues that reflect the gradual acquisition of physiologic competence. Each part has its own rate of growth, which may be directly related to alterations in the size of the child (e.g., the heart rate). Skeletal muscle growth approximates whole body growth; brain, lymphoid, adrenal, and reproductive tissues follow distinct and individual patterns (Fig. 5-2). When there

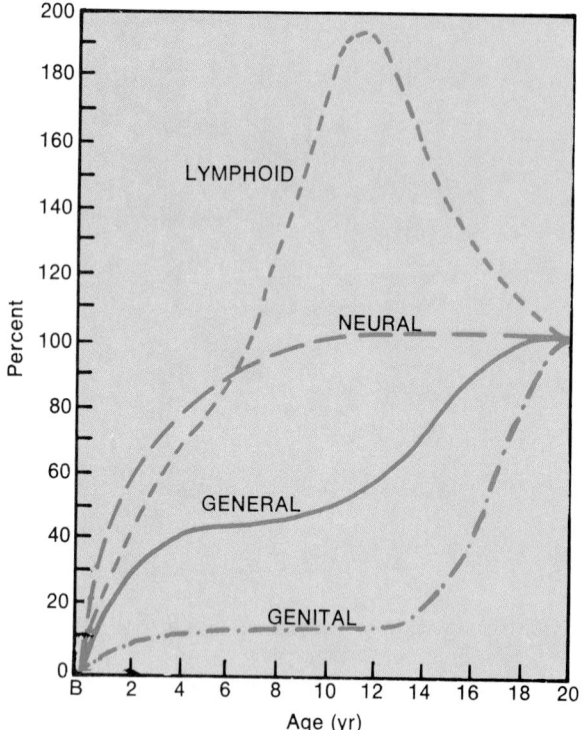

FIG. 5-2. Growth rates for the body as a whole and three types of tissues. *Lymphoid type:* thymus, lymph nodes, and intestinal lymph masses; *neural type:* brain, dura, spinal cord, optic apparatus, and head dimensions; *general type:* body as a whole, external dimension, and respiratory, digestive, renal, circulatory, and musculoskeletal systems. (From Harris JA and others: *The measurement of man,* Minneapolis, 1930, University of Minnesota Press.)

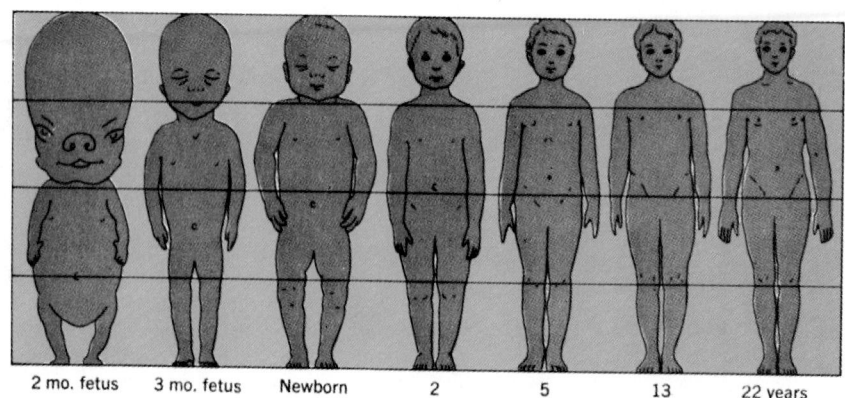

FIG. 5-3. Changes in body proportions from before birth to adulthood. (From Crouch JE, McClintic JR: *Human anatomy and physiology,* ed 2, New York, 1976, Wiley & Sons.)

has been a secondary cause of growth deficiency, such as severe illness or acute malnutrition, recovery from the illness or the establishment of an adequate diet will produce a dramatic acceleration of the growth rate that usually continues until the child's individual growth pattern is resumed.

External Proportions

Variations in the growth rate of different tissues and organ systems produce significant changes in body proportions during childhood. The cephalocaudal trend of development is most evident in total body growth as indicated by these changes (Fig. 5-3). During fetal development the head is the fastest growing body part, and at 2 months of gestation the head constitutes 50% of total body length. During infancy growth of the trunk predominates; the legs are the most rapidly growing part during childhood; in adolescence the trunk once again elongates. In the newborn infant the lower limbs are one third the total body length but only 15% of the total body weight; in the adult the lower limbs constitute one half of the total body height and 30% or more of the total body weight. As growth proceeds, the midpoint in head-to-toe measurements gradually descends from a level even with the umbilicus at birth to the level of the symphysis pubis at maturity.

Biologic Determinants of Growth and Development

The most prominent feature of childhood and adolescence is physical growth. Throughout development various tissues in the body undergo changes in growth, composition, and structure. In some tissues the changes are continuous (e.g., bone growth and dentition); in others significant alterations occur at specific stages (e.g., appearance of secondary sex characteristics). When these measurements are compared with standardized norms, a child's developmental progress can be determined with a high degree of confidence (Table 5-1).

Linear growth, or *height,* occurs almost entirely as a result of skeletal growth and is considered a stable measurement of general growth. Growth in height is not uniform throughout life but ceases when maturation of the skeleton is complete. The maximum growth in length occurs before birth, but the newborn continues to grow at a rapid, though slower, rate.

NURSING TIP Double the child's height at the age of 2 years to estimate how tall he or she may be as an adult.

TABLE 5-1. General trends in height and weight gain during childhood

AGE-GROUP	WEIGHT*	HEIGHT*
Infants *Birth-6 months*	Weekly gain: 140-200 g (5-7 oz) Birth weight doubles by end of first 4-7 months†	Monthly gain: 2.5 cm (1 inch)
6-12 months	Weight gain: 85-140 g (3-5 oz) Birth weight triples by end of first year	Monthly gain: 1.25 cm (½ inch) Birth length increases by approximately 50% by end of first year
Toddlers	Birth weight quadruples by age 2½ Yearly gain: 2-3 kg (4½-6½ lb)	Height at age 2 is approximately 50% of eventual adult height Gain during second year: about 12 cm (4¾ inches) Gain during third year: about 6-8 cm (2⅜-3¼ inches)
Preschoolers	Yearly gain: 2-3 kg (4½-6½ lb)	Birth length doubles by age 4 Yearly gain: 5-7.5 cm (2-3 inches)
School-Age Children	Yearly gain: 2-3 kg (4½-6½ lb)	Yearly gain after age 7: 5 cm (2 inches) Birth length triples by about age 13
Pubertal Growth Spurt *Females—10-14 years*	Weight gain: 7-25 kg (15-55 lb) Mean: 17.5 kg (38⅛ lb)	Height gain: 5-25 cm (2-10 inches); approximately 95% of mature height achieved by onset of menarche or skeletal age of 13 Mean: 20.5 cm (8¼ inches)
Males—11-16 years	Weight gain: 7-30 kg (15-65 lb) Mean: 23.7 kg (52⅛ lb)	Height gain: 10-30 cm (4-12 inches); approximately 95% of mature height achieved by skeletal age of 15 years Mean: 27.5 cm (11 inches)

*Yearly height and weight gains for each age-group represent averaged estimates from a variety of sources.
†Jung and Czajka-Narins, 1985.

At birth, *weight* is more variable than height and is, to a greater extent, a reflection of the intrauterine environment. The average newborn weighs from 3175 to 3400 g (7 to 7½ pounds). In general, the birth weight doubles by 4 to 7 months of age and triples by the end of the first year. By the end of the second year it usually quadruples. After this point the "normal" rate of weight gain, just as the growth in height, assumes a steady annual increase of approximately 2 to 2.75 kg (4⅖ to 6 pounds) per year until the adolescent growth spurt.

Both *bone age* determinants and state of *dentition* are used as indicators of development. Because both are discussed elsewhere, neither is elaborated here (see next section for bone age; see also Chapters 10 and 12 for dentition).

Skeletal Growth and Maturation

The most accurate measure of general development is *skeletal* or *bone, age,* the radiologic determination of osseous maturation. Skeletal age appears to correlate more closely with other measures of physiologic maturity (such as onset of menarche) than with chronologic age or height. This "bone age" is determined by comparing the mineralization of ossification centers and advancing bony form to age-related standards.

Bone formation begins during the second month of fetal life when calcium salts are deposited in the intercellular substance (matrix) to form calcified cartilage first and then true bone. There are some differences in this bone formation. In small bones the bone continues to form in the center and cartilage continues to be laid down on the surfaces. In long bones the ossification begins in the *diaphysis* (the long central portion of the bone) and continues in the *epiphysis* (the end portions of the bone). Between the diaphysis and the epiphysis, an *epiphyseal cartilage plate* unites with the diaphysis by columns of spongy tissue, the *metaphysis.* Active growth in length takes place in the epiphyseal growth plate. Interference with this growth site by trauma or infection can result in deformity.

The first centers of ossification appear in the 2-month-old embryo, and at birth the number is approximately 400, about half the number at maturity. New centers appear at regular intervals during the growth period and provide the basis for assessment of bone age. Postnatally the earliest centers to appear (at 5 to 6 months of age) are those of the capitate and hamate bones in the wrist. Therefore radiographs of the hand and wrist provide the most useful areas for screening to determine skeletal age, especially before age 6 years. These centers appear earlier in girls than in boys.

Neurologic Maturation

In contrast to other body tissues, which grow rapidly after birth, the nervous system grows proportionately more rapidly before birth. Two periods of rapid brain cell growth occur during fetal life: a dramatic increase in the number of neurons between 15 and 20 weeks of gestation and another increase at 30 weeks, which extends to 1 year of age. The rapid growth of infancy continues during early childhood and then slows to a more gradual rate during later childhood and adolescence.

It is believed that no new nerve cells appear after the sixth month of fetal life. Postnatal growth consists of increasing the amount of cytoplasm around the nuclei of existing cells, increasing the number and intricacy of communications with other cells, and advancing their peripheral axons to keep pace with expanding body dimensions. This allows for increasingly complex movement and behavior. Neurophysiologic changes also provide the foundation for language, learning, and behavior development. Neurologic or electroencephalographic development is sometimes used as an indicator of maturational age in the early weeks of life.

Lymphoid Tissues

Lymphoid tissues contained in the lymph nodes, thymus, spleen, tonsils, adenoids, and blood lymphocytes follow a growth pattern unlike that of other body tissues. These tissues are small in relation to total body size, but they are well developed at birth. They increase rapidly to reach adult dimensions by 6 years of age and continue to grow. At about age 10 to 12 years they reach a maximum development that is approximately twice their adult size. This is followed by a rapid decline to stable adult dimensions by the end of adolescence.

Development of Organ Systems

All tissues and organ systems undergo changes during development. Some are striking; others are more subtle. Many have implications for assessment and care. Because the major importance of these changes relates to their dysfunction, the developmental characteristics of various systems and organs are discussed throughout the book as they relate to these areas. Physical characteristics and physiologic changes that vary with age are included in age-group descriptions.

PHYSIOLOGIC CHANGES

Physiologic changes that take place in all organs and systems are discussed as they relate to dysfunction. Others, such as pulse and respiratory rates and blood pressure, are an integral part of physical assessment (see Chapter 7). In addition, there are changes in basic functions, including metabolism, temperature, and patterns of sleep and rest.

Metabolism

The rate of metabolism when the body is at rest (*basal metabolic rate,* or *BMR*) demonstrates a distinctive change throughout childhood. Highest in the newborn infant, the BMR closely relates to the proportion of surface area to body mass, which changes as the body increases in size. In both sexes the proportion decreases progressively to maturity. The BMR is slightly higher in boys at all ages and further increases during pubescence over that in girls.

The rate of metabolism determines the caloric requirements of the child. The basal energy requirement of infants is about 108 kcal/kg of body weight and decreases to 40 to 45 kcal/kg at maturity (Table 5-2). Water requirements remain at approximately 1.5 ml per calorie of energy expended throughout life. Children's energy needs vary considerably at different ages and with changing circumstances. The energy requirement to build tissue steadily decreases with age, following the general growth curve; however, energy needs vary with the individual child and may be considerably higher. For short periods (e.g., during strenuous exercise) and more prolonged periods (e.g., illness), the needs can be very high.

TABLE 5-2. Recommended daily requirements for calories and protein through adolescence*

AGE (YEARS)	ENERGY ALLOWANCE (KCAL/KG)	PROTEIN (G)
Infants		
0-½	108	13
½-1	98	14
Children		
1-3	102	16
4-6	90	24
7-10	70	28
Males		
11-14	55	45
15-18	45	49
Females		
11-14	47	46
15-18	40	44

*Data from Food and Nutrition Board: *Recommended daily allowances*, ed 10, Washington, DC, 1989, National Academy Press.

FYI Each degree of fever increases the basal metabolism 10% with a corresponding fluid requirement.

Temperature

Body temperature, reflecting metabolism, displays the same decrement from infancy to maturity (see inside back cover). Following the unstable regulatory ability in the neonatal period, heat production steadily declines as the infant grows into childhood. Individual differences of 0.5° to 1° F are normal, and occasionally a child normally displays an unusually high or low temperature. Beginning at approximately 12 years of age, the temperature in girls remains relatively stable, whereas in boys it continues to fall for a few years longer. Females maintain a temperature slightly above that of males throughout life.

Even with improved temperature regulation, infants and young children are highly susceptible to temperature fluctuations. Body temperature responds to changes in environmental temperature and is increased with active exercise, crying, and emotional upset. Infections can cause a higher and more rapid temperature increase in infants and young children than in older children. In relation to body weight, an infant produces more heat per unit than do children near maturity. Consequently, during active play or when heavily clothed, an infant or small child is likely to become overheated.

Sleep and Rest

Sleep, a protective function in all organisms, allows for repair and recovery of tissues following activity. As in most aspects of development, there is wide variation among individual children in the amount and distribution of sleep at various ages. As children mature, there is a change in the total time they spend in sleep and in the amount of time they spend in deep sleep.

Newborn infants sleep much of the time that is not occupied with feeding and other aspects of their care. As infants grow older, the total time spent in sleep gradually decreases, they remain awake for longer periods, and they sleep longer at night. During the latter part of the first year, most children sleep through the night and take one or two naps during the day. By the time they are 12 to 18 months old, most children have eliminated the second nap. After age 3 years the child has usually given up daytime naps except in those cultures in which an afternoon nap or siesta is customary. During ages 4 to 10 sleep time declines slightly and then increases somewhat during the pubertal growth spurt. The changes in length of sleep at different ages is shown in Fig. 5-4.

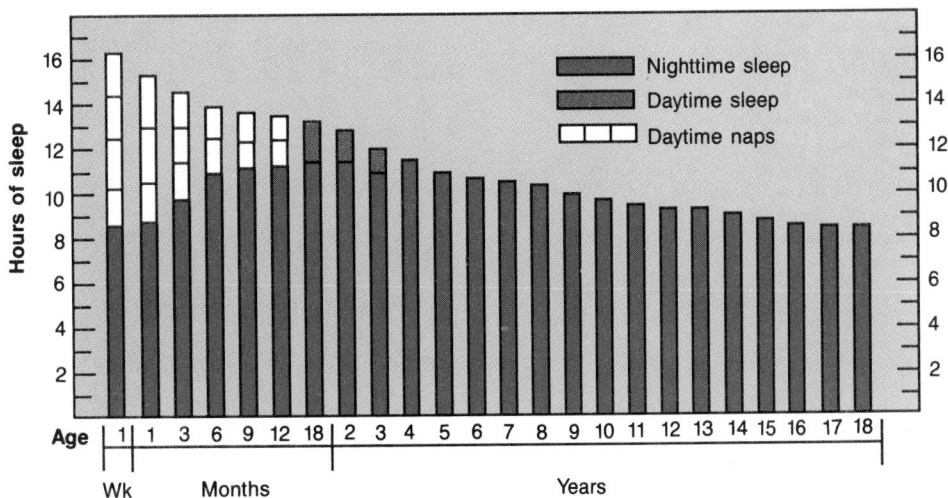

FIG. 5-4. Changes in number of hours of sleep with increasing age. (Modified from Ferber R: *Solve your child's sleep problems,* New York, 1985, Simon & Schuster.)

There is a change in the quality of sleep as children mature. The time spent in deep, restful sleep increases from 50% in infancy to 80% in the older child.

TEMPERAMENT

Defined as "the manner of thinking, behaving, or reacting characteristic of an individual" (Chess and Thomas, 1985), *temperament* refers to the way in which a person deals with life. From the time of birth, children exhibit marked individual differences in the way that they respond to their environment and the way others, particularly the parents, respond to them and their needs. A generic basis has been suggested for some differences in temperament. Nine characteristics of temperament have been identified through interviews with parents (see box). Temperament refers to behavioral tendencies, not to discrete behavioral acts. There are no implications of good or bad. Most children can be placed into one of three common categories based on their overall pattern of temperamental attributes:

   The easy child. Easy-going children are even-tempered, are regular and predictable in their habits, and have a positive approach to new stimuli. They are open and adaptable to change and display a mild to moderately intense mood that is typically positive. Approximately 40% of children fall into this category.

   The difficult child. Difficult children are highly active, irritable, and irregular in their habits. Negative withdrawal responses are typical, and they require a more structured environment. These children adapt slowly to new routines, people, or situations. Mood expressions are usually intense and primarily negative. They exhibit frequent periods of crying, and frustration often produces violent tantrums. This group comprises about 10% of children.

   The slow-to-warm-up child. Slow-to-warm-up children typically react negatively and with mild intensity to new stimuli and, unless pressured, adapt slowly with repeated contact. They respond with only mild but passive resistance to novelty or changes in routine. They are quite inactive and moody but show only moderate irregularity in functions. Fifteen percent of children demonstrate this temperament pattern.

Thirty-five percent of children either have some, but not all, of the characteristics of one of the categories or are inconsistent in their behavioral responses. Many normal children demonstrate this wide range of behavioral patterns.

Significance of Temperament

Observations indicate that children who display the difficult or slow-to-warm-up patterns are more vulnerable to behavior problems in early and middle childhood. However, any child can develop behavior problems if there is dissonance between the child's temperament and the environment. Demands for change and adaptation that are in conflict with children's capacities can become excessively stressful. However, authorities emphasize that it is not children's temperament patterns that place them at risk but the *degree of fit* between children and their environments, specifically their parents, that determines the degree of vulnerability. The greater the difference between the child's temperament and the ability of the parents to accept and deal with the behavior, the greater the likelihood of subsequent behavior problems. Because temperament is identified primarily by parental perceptions, a child described as difficult at one time may be perceived as easy at a later date (Wolk and others, 1992). (For example, see Failure to Thrive, Chapter 11.)

Child temperament appears to be a relevant factor in parental adjustment. Difficult child temperament has been directly related to maternal distress, discomfort in the role of parent, poor spousal relationships, and negative changes in way of life (Sheeber and Johnson, 1992).

Early identification of temperament provides a useful tool for caregivers in anticipating probable areas of difficulty or risk associated with development. For example, "difficult" children may be prone to colic in infancy, and active children require more vigilance to prevent injury. Also, school entry will require different approaches for children with different temperaments.

Several parental questionnaires have been devised to facilitate assessment of temperament. Nurses who employ these assessment tools are better able to help parents interpret their child's behavior and to provide anticipatory guidance regarding numerous aspects of childrearing.

DEVELOPMENT OF PERSONALITY AND MENTAL FUNCTION

Personality and cognitive skills develop in much the same manner as biologic growth—new accomplishments build on previously mastered skills. Many aspects depend on physical growth and maturation. This is not a comprehensive account of the multiple facets of personality and behavior development. Many aspects are integrated with the child's emotional and social development in later discussion of various age-groups. Table 5-3 summarizes some of the developmental theories.

ATTRIBUTES OF TEMPERAMENT

Activity—level of physical motion during activity, such as sleep, eating, play, dressing, and bathing

Rhythmicity—regularity in the timing of physiologic functions, such as hunger, sleep, and elimination

Approach-withdrawal—nature of initial responses to a new stimulus, such as people, situations, places, foods, toys, and procedures (*Approach* responses are positive and are displayed by activity or expression; *withdrawal* responses are negative expressions or behaviors.)

Adaptability—ease or difficulty with which the child adapts or adjusts to new or altered situations

Threshold of responsiveness (sensory threshold)—amount of stimulation, such as sounds or light, required to evoke a response in the child

Intensity of reaction—energy level of the child's reactions, regardless of quality or direction

Mood—amount of pleasant, happy, friendly behavior compared with unpleasant, unhappy, crying, unfriendly behavior exhibited by the child in various situations

Distractibility—ease with which a child's attention or direction of behavior can be diverted by external stimuli

Attention span and persistence—length of time a child pursues a given activity (*attention*) and the continuation of an activity in spite of obstacles (*persistence*)

TABLE 5-3. Summary of personality, cognitive, and moral development theories

STAGE/AGE	PSYCHOSEXUAL STAGES (FREUD)	PSYCHOSOCIAL STAGES (ERIKSON)	COGNITIVE STAGES (PIAGET)	MORAL JUDGMENT STAGES (KOHLBERG)
I Infancy *Birth to 1 year*	Oral-sensory	Trust vs mistrust	Sensorimotor (birth to 2 years)	
II Toddlerhood *1-3 years*	Anal-urethral	Autonomy vs shame and doubt	Preoperational thought, preconceptual phase (transductive reasoning, e.g., specific to specific) (2-4 years)	Preconventional (pre-moral) level Punishment and obedience orientation
III Early Childhood *3-6 years*	Phallic-locomotion	Initiative vs guilt	Preoperational thought, intuitive phase (transductive reasoning) (4-7 years)	Preconventional (pre-moral) level Naive instrumental orientation
IV Middle Childhood *6-12 years*	Latency	Industry vs inferiority	Concrete operations (inductive reasoning and beginning logic) (7-11 years)	Conventional level Good-boy, nice-girl orientation Law-and-order orientation
V Adolescence *12-18 years*	Genitality	Identity and repudiation vs identity confusion	Formal operations (deductive and abstract reasoning) (11-15 years)	Postconventional or principled level Social-contract orientation Universal ethical principle orientation (no longer included in revised theory)

THEORETIC FOUNDATIONS OF PERSONALITY DEVELOPMENT

According to Freud, all human behavior is energized by psychodynamic forces, and this psychic energy is divided among three components of personality: the id, the ego, and the superego. The *id*, the *unconscious mind*, is the inborn component that is driven by instincts. The id obeys the pleasure principle of immediate gratification of needs regardless of whether the object or action can actually do so. The *ego*, the *conscious mind*, serves the reality principle. It functions as the conscious or controlling self that is able to find realistic means for gratifying the instincts while blocking the irrational thinking of the id. The *superego*, the *conscience*, functions as the moral arbitrator and represents the ideal. It is the mechanism that prevents individuals from expressing undesirable instincts that might threaten the social order.

Psychosexual Development (Freud)

Freud considered the sexual instincts to be significant in the development of the personality. However, he used the term *psychosexual* to describe any *sensual pleasure.* During childhood certain regions of the body assume a prominent psychologic significance as the source of new pleasures and new conflicts gradually shifts from one part of the body to another at particular stages of development:

Oral stage (birth to 1 year). During infancy the major source of pleasure seeking is centered on oral activities such as sucking, biting, chewing, and vocalizing. Children may prefer one of these over the others, and the preferred method of oral gratification can provide some indication of the personality they develop.

Anal stage (1 to 3 years). Interest during the second year of life centers in the anal region as sphincter muscles develop and children are able to withhold or expel fecal material at will. At this stage the climate surrounding toilet training can have lasting effects on children's personalities.

Phallic stage (3 to 6 years). During the phallic stage the genitals become an interesting and sensitive area of the body. Children recognize differences between the sexes and become curious about the dissimilarities. This is the period around which the controversial issues of the Oedipus and Electra complexes, penis envy, and castration anxiety are centered.

Latency period (6 to 12 years). During the latency period children elaborate on previously acquired traits and skills. Physical and psychic energy are channeled into acquisition of knowledge and vigorous play.

Genital stage (age 12 and over). The last significant stage begins at puberty with maturation of the reproductive system and production of sex hormones. The genital organs become the major source of sexual tensions and pleasures, but energies are also invested in forming friendships and preparation for marriage.

Psychosocial Development (Erikson)

The most widely accepted theory of personality development is that advanced by Erikson (1963). Although built on Freudian theory, it is known as *psychosocial* development and emphasizes a healthy personality as opposed to a pathologic approach. Erikson also uses the biologic concepts of critical periods and epigenesis, describing key conflicts or core problems that the individual strives to master during critical periods in personality development. Successful completion or mastery of each of these core conflicts is built on the satisfactory completion or mastery of the previous core.

Each psychosocial stage has two components—the favorable and the unfavorable aspects of the core conflict—and progress to the next stage depends on resolution of this conflict. No core conflict is ever mastered completely but remains a recurrent problem throughout life. No life situation is ever secure. Each new situation presents the conflict in a new form. For example, when children who have satisfactorily achieved a sense of trust encounter a new experience (e.g., hospitalization) they must again develop a sense of trust in those responsible for their care in order to master the situation. Erikson's life span approach to personality development consists of eight stages; however, only the first five relating to childhood are included here:

Trust vs mistrust (birth to 1 year). The first and most important attribute to develop for a healthy personality is a basic *trust*. Establishment of basic trust dominates the first year of life and describes all the child's satisfying experiences at this age. Corresponding to Freud's oral stage, it is a time of "getting" and "taking in" through all the senses. It exists only in relation to something or someone; therefore, consistent, loving care by a mothering person is essential to development of trust. *Mistrust* develops when trust-promoting experiences are deficient or lacking, or when basic needs are inconsistently or inadequately met. Although shreds of mistrust are sprinkled throughout the personality, from a basic trust in parents stems trust in the world, other people, and oneself. The result is *faith* and *optimism*.

Autonomy vs shame and doubt (1 to 3 years). Corresponding to Freud's anal stage, the problem of *autonomy* can be symbolized by the holding on and letting go of the sphincter muscles. The development of autonomy during the toddler period is centered around children's increasing ability to control their bodies, themselves, and their environment. They want to do things for themselves, using their newly acquired motor skills of walking, climbing, and manipulating and their mental powers of selection and decision making. Much of their learning is acquired through imitating the activities and behavior of others. Negative feelings of *doubt* and *shame* arise when children are made to feel small and self-conscious, when their choices are disastrous, when others shame them, or when they are forced to be dependent in areas in which they are capable of assuming control. The favorable outcomes are *self-control* and *willpower*.

Initiative vs guilt (3 to 6 years). The stage of *initiative* corresponds to Freud's phallic stage and is characterized by vigorous, intrusive behavior, enterprise, and a strong imagination. Children explore the physical world with all their senses and powers. They develop a conscience. No longer guided only by outsiders, there is an inner voice that warns and threatens. Children sometimes undertake goals or activities that are in conflict with those of parents or others, and being made to feel that their activities or imaginings are bad produces a sense of *guilt*. Children must learn to retain a sense of initiative without impinging on the rights and privileges of others. The lasting outcomes are *direction* and *purpose*.

Industry vs inferiority (6 to 12 years). The stage of *industry* is the latency period of Freud. Having achieved the more crucial stages in personality development, children are ready to be workers and producers. They want to engage in tasks and activities that they can carry through to completion; they need and want real achievement. Children learn to compete and cooperate with others, and they learn the rules. It is a decisive period in their social relationships with others. Feelings of *inadequacy* and *inferiority* may develop if too much is expected of them or if they believe that they cannot measure up to the standards set for them by others. The ego quality developed from a sense of industry is *competence.*

Identity vs role confusion (12 to 18 years). Corresponding to Freud's genital period, the development of *identity* is characterized by rapid and marked physical changes. Previous trust in their bodies is shaken, and children become overly preoccupied with the way they appear in the eyes of others as compared with their own self-concept. Adolescents struggle to fit the roles they have played and those they hope to play with the current roles and fashions adopted by their peers, to integrate their concepts and values with those of society, and to come to a decision regarding an occupation. Inability to solve the core conflict results in *role confusion.* The outcome of successful mastery is *devotion* and *fidelity* to others and to values and ideologies.

THEORETIC FOUNDATIONS OF MENTAL DEVELOPMENT

The term *cognition* refers to the process by which developing individuals become acquainted with the world and the objects it contains. Children are born with inherited potentials for intellectual growth, but they must develop into that potential through interaction with the environment. By assimilating information through the senses, processing it, and acting on it, they come to understand relationships between objects and between themselves and their world. With cognitive development, children acquire the ability to reason abstractly, to think in a logical manner, and to organize intellectual functions or performances into higher-order structures. Language, morals, and spiritual development emerge as cognitive abilities advance.

Cognitive Development (Piaget)

Cognitive development consists of age-related changes that occur in mental activities. The best-known theory regarding children's thinking, and a more comprehensive developmental theory than those already described, was developed by the Swiss psychologist Jean Piaget (1969). According to Piaget, intelligence enables individuals to make adaptations to the environment that increase the probability of survival, and that through their behavior individuals establish and maintain equilibrium with the environment.

Piaget proposed three stages of reasoning: (1) intuitive, (2) concrete operational, and (3) formal operational. When they enter the stage of concrete logical thought at about age 7 years, children are able to make logical inferences, classify, and deal with quantitative relationships about concrete things. Not until adolescence are they able to reason abstractly with any degree of competence. Each stage is derived from and builds on the accomplishments of the previous stage in a continuous, orderly process. The course of intellectual development is both maturational and invariant and is divided into the following stages (ages are approximate):

Sensorimotor (birth to 2 years). The sensorimotor stage of intellectual development consists of six substages (see pp. 294 and 363) that are governed by sensations in which simple learning takes place. Children progress from reflex activity through simple repetitive behaviors to imitative behavior. They develop a sense of "cause-and-effect" as they direct behavior toward objects. Problem solving is primarily trial and error. They display a high level of curiosity, experimentation, and enjoyment of novelty and begin to develop a sense of self as they are able to differentiate themselves from their environment. They become aware that objects have *permanence*—that an object exists even though it is no longer visible. Toward the end of the sensorimotor period children begin to use language and representational thought.

Preoperational (2 to 7 years). The predominant characteristic of the preoperational stage of intellectual development is *egocentrism,* which in this sense does not mean selfishness or self-centeredness, but the inability to put oneself in the place of another. Children interpret objects and events, not in terms of general properties, but in terms of their relationships or their use to them. They are unable to see things from any perspective other than their own; they cannot see another's point of view, nor can they see any reason to do so (see Cognitive Development [Piaget], Chapter 13).

Preoperational thinking is concrete and tangible. Children cannot reason beyond the observable, and they lack the ability to make deductions or generalizations. Thought is dominated by what they see, hear, or otherwise experience. However, they are increasingly able to use language and symbols to represent objects in their environment. Through imaginative play, questioning, and other interacting, they begin to elaborate concepts and to make simple associations between ideas. In the latter stage of this period their reasoning is *intuitive* (e.g., the stars have to go to bed just as they do) and they are only beginning to deal with problems of weight, length, size, and time. Reasoning is also *transductive*—because two events occur together, they cause each other, or knowledge of one characteristic is transferred to another (e.g., all women with big bellies have babies).

Concrete operations (7 to 11 years). At this age thought becomes increasingly logical and coherent. Children are able to classify, sort, order, and otherwise organize facts about the world to use in problem solving. They develop a new concept of permanence—*conservation* (see Cognitive Development [Piaget], Chapter 16). That is, they realize that physical factors, such as volume, weight, and number, remain the same even though outward appearances are changed. They are able to deal with a number of different aspects of a situation simultaneously. They do not have the capacity to deal in abstraction; they solve problems in a concrete, systematic fashion based on what they can perceive. Reasoning is *inductive.* Through progressive changes in thought processes and relationships with others, thought becomes less self-centered. They can consider points of view other than their own. Thinking has become socialized.

Formal operations (11 to 15 years). Formal operational thought is characterized by adaptability and flexibility. Adolescents can think in abstract terms, use abstract symbols, and draw logical conclusions from a set of observations. For example, they can solve the following question: If A is larger than B, and B is larger than C, which symbol is the largest? (The answer is A.) They can make hypotheses and test them; they can consider abstract, theoretic, and philosophic matters. Although they may confuse the ideal with the practical, most contradictions in the world can be dealt with and resolved.

Language Development

Children are born with the mechanism and capacity to develop speech and language skills. However, they will not speak spontaneously. The environment must provide a means for them to acquire these skills. Speech requires intact physiologic structure and function (including respiratory, auditory, and cerebral) plus intelligence, a need to communicate, and stimulation.

The rate of speech development varies from child to child and is directly related to neurologic competence and cognitive development. Gesture precedes speech, and in this way a small child communicates satisfactorily. As speech develops, gesture recedes but never disappears entirely. At all stages of language development, children's comprehension vocabulary (what they understand) is greater than their expressed vocabulary (what they can say), and this development reflects a continuing process of modification that involves both the acquisition of new words and the expanding and refining of word meanings previously learned. By the time they begin to walk, children are able to attach a name to objects and persons.

The first parts of speech used are nouns, sometimes verbs (e.g., "go"), and combination words (such as "bye-bye"). Responses are usually structurally incomplete during the toddler period, although the meaning is clear. Next they begin to use adjectives and adverbs to qualify nouns, followed by adverbs to qualify nouns and verbs. Later, pronouns and gender words are added (such as "he" and "she"). By the time children enter school, they are able to use simple, structurally complete sentences that average five to seven words.

Moral Development (Kohlberg)

Children also acquire moral reasoning in a developmental sequence. Moral development, as described by Kohlberg (1968), is based on cognitive developmental theory and consists of the following three major levels, each of which has two stages:

Preconventional level. The preconventional level of moral development parallels the preoperational level of cognitive development and intuitive thought. Culturally oriented to the labels of good/bad and right/wrong, children integrate these in terms of the physical or pleasurable consequences of their actions. At first children determine the goodness or badness of an action in terms of its consequences. They avoid punishment and obey without question those who have the power to determine and enforce the rules and labels. They have no concept of the basic moral order that supports these consequences. Later children determine that the right behavior consists of that which satisfies their own needs (and sometimes the needs of others). Although elements of fairness, give and take, and equal sharing are evident, they are interpreted in a very practical, concrete manner without loyalty, gratitude, or justice.

Conventional level. At the conventional stage children are concerned with conformity and loyalty. They value the maintenance of family, group, or national expectations regardless of consequences. Behavior that meets with approval and pleases or helps others is considered to be good. One earns approval by being "nice." Obeying the rules, doing one's duty, showing respect for authority, and maintaining the social order is the correct behavior. This level is correlated with the stage of concrete operations in cognitive development.

Postconventional, autonomous, or principled level. At the postconventional level the individual has reached the cognitive stage of formal operations. Correct behavior tends to be defined in terms of general individual rights and standards that have been examined and agreed on by the entire society. Although procedural rules for reaching consensus become important with emphasis on the legal point of view, there is also emphasis on the possibility for changing law in terms of societal needs and rational considerations.

The most advanced level of moral development is one in which self-chosen ethical principles guide decisions of conscience. These are abstract and ethical but universal principles of justice and human rights with respect for the dignity of persons as individuals. It is believed that few persons reach this stage of moral reasoning.

Spiritual Development

Spiritual beliefs are closely related to the moral and ethical portion of the child's self-concept and, as such, must be considered as part of the child's basic needs assessment. Children need to have meaning, purpose, and hope in their lives. Also, the need for confession and forgiveness is present, even in very young children. Extending beyond religion (an organized set of beliefs and practices), spirituality affects the whole person: mind, body, and spirit (Clutter, 1991). Fowler (1974) has identified seven stages in the development of faith, four of which are closely associated with and parallel cognitive and psychosocial development in childhood:

Stage 0: Undifferentiated. This stage of development encompasses the period of infancy during which children have no concept of right or wrong, no beliefs, and no convictions to guide their behavior. However, the beginnings of a faith are established with the development of basic trust through their relationships with the primary caregiver.

Stage 1: Intuitive-projective. Toddlerhood is primarily a time of imitating the behavior of others. Children imitate the religious gestures and behaviors of others without comprehending any meaning or significance to the activities. During the preschool years children assimilate some of the values and beliefs of their parents. Parental attitudes toward moral codes and religious beliefs convey to children what they consider to be good and bad. Children still imitate behavior at this age and follow parental beliefs as part of their daily lives rather than through an understanding of their basic concepts.

Stage 2: Mythical-literal. Through the school-age years, spiritual development parallels cognitive development and is closely related to children's experiences and social interaction. Most have a strong interest in religion during the school-age years. The existence of a deity is accepted, and petitions to an omnipotent being are important and expected to be answered; good behavior is rewarded, and bad behavior is punished. Their developing conscience bothers them when they disobey. They have a reverence for thoughts and matters and are able to articulate their faith. They may even question its validity.

Stage 3: Synthetic-convention. As children approach adolescence, however, they become increasingly aware of spiritual disappointments. They recognize that prayers are not always answered (at least on their own terms) and may begin to abandon or modify some religious practices. They begin to reason, to question some of the established parental religious standards, and to drop or modify some religious practices.

Stage 4: Individuating-reflexive. Adolescents become more skeptical and begin to compare the religious standards of their parents with those of others. They attempt to determine which to adopt and incorporate into their own set of values. They also begin to compare religious standards with the scientific viewpoint. It is a time of searching rather than reaching. Adolescents are uncertain about many religious ideas but will not achieve profound insights until late adolescence or early adulthood.

DEVELOPMENT OF SELF-CONCEPT

The term *self-concept* includes all the notions, beliefs, and convictions that constitute an individual's self-knowledge and that influence that individual's relationships with others. It is not present at birth but develops gradually as a result of unique experiences within the self, with significant others, and with the realities of the world. However, an individual's self-concept may or may not reflect reality.

In infancy the self-concept is primarily an awareness of one's independent existence learned in part as a result of social contacts and experiences with others. The process becomes more active during toddlerhood as children explore the limits of their capacities and the nature of their impact on others. School-age children are more aware of differences among people, are more sensitive to social pressures, and become more preoccupied with issues of self-criticism and self-evaluation. During early adolescence children focus more on physical and emotional changes taking place and on peer acceptance. The self-concept is crystallized during later adolescence as young people organize their self-concept around a set of values, goals, and competencies acquired throughout childhood.

Body Image

A vital component of self-concept, *body image* refers to the subjective concepts and attitudes that individuals have toward their own bodies. It consists of the physiologic (the perception of one's physical characteristics), psychologic (values and attitudes toward the body, abilities, and ideals), and social nature of one's image of self (the self in relation to others). All three of the components interrelate with each other. Body image is a complex phenomenon that evolves and changes during the process of growth and development. Any actual or perceived deviation from the "norm" (no matter how this is interpreted) is cause for concern. The extent to which a characteristic, defect, or disease affects children's body image is influenced by the attitudes and behavior of those around them.

The significant others in their lives exert the most important and meaningful impact on children's body image. Labels that are attached to them (such as "skinny," "pretty," or "fat") or body parts (such as "ugly mole," "bug eyes," or "yucky skin") are incorporated into the body image. Because they lack the understanding of deviations from the physical standard or norm, children notice prominent differences in others and unwittingly make "rude" and often cruel remarks about such minor deviations as large or widely spaced front teeth, large or small eyes, moles, or extreme variations in height.

Infants receive input about their bodies through self-exploration and sensory stimulation from others. As they begin to manipulate their environment, they become aware of their bodies as separate from others. Toddlers learn to identify the various parts of their bodies and are able to use symbols to represent objects. Preschoolers become aware of the wholeness of their bodies and discover the genitals. Exploration of the genitals and the discovery of differences between the sexes become important. There is only a vague concept of internal organs and function (Selekman, 1983).

School-age children begin to learn about internal body structure and function and become aware of differences in body size and configuration. They are highly influenced by the cultural norms of society and current fads. Children whose bodies deviate from the norm are often criticized or ridiculed.

Adolescence is the age when children become most concerned about the physical self. The familiar body changes and the new physical self must be integrated into the self-concept. Adolescents face conflicts over what they see and what they visualize as the ideal body structure. Body image formation during adolescence is a crucial element in the shaping of identity, the psychosocial crisis of adolescence.

Self-Esteem

The term *self-esteem* refers to a personal, subjective judgment of one's worthiness derived from and influenced by the social groups in the immediate environment and individuals' perceptions of how they are valued by others. Self-esteem changes with development. Highly egocentric toddlers are unaware of any difference between competence and social approval. Preschool and early school-age children, on the other hand, are increasingly aware of the discrepancy between their competencies and the abilities of more advanced children. Being accepted by adults and peers outside the family group becomes more important to them. Positive feedback enhances their self-esteem; they are vulnerable to feelings of worthlessness and are anxious about failure.

As children's competencies increase and they develop meaningful relationships, their self-esteem rises. Their self-esteem is again at risk during early adolescence when they are defining an identity and sense of self in the context of their peer group. Unless children are continually made to feel incompetent and of little worth, a decrease in self-esteem during vulnerable times is only temporary. Children assess the following aspects of themselves in forming an overall evaluation of their self-esteem (Sieving and Zirbel-Donisch, 1990):

Competence: How adequate are my cognitive, physical, and social skills?

Sense of control: How well can I complete tasks needed to produce desired actions? Is someone or something specific vs luck or chance responsible for my successes and failures?

Moral worth: How closely do my actions and behaviors meet moral standards that have been set?

Worthiness of love and acceptance: How worthy am I of love and acceptance from parents, other significant adults, siblings, and peers?

Factors that influence the formation of a child's self-esteem include (1) the child's temperament and personality, (2) abilities and opportunities available to accomplish age-appropriate developmental tasks, (3) significant others, and (4) social roles assumed and the expectations of these roles (see also Psychosocial History, Chapter 6).

ROLE OF PLAY IN DEVELOPMENT

Through the universal medium of play children learn what no one can teach them. They learn about their world and how to deal with this environment of objects, time, space, structure, and people. They learn about themselves operating within that environment—what they can do, how to relate to things and situations, and how to adapt themselves to the demands society makes on them. Play is the *work* of the child. In play children continually practice the complicated, stressful processes of living, communicating, and achieving satisfactory relationships with other people.

CLASSIFICATION OF PLAY

From a developmental point of view, patterns of children's play can be categorized according to content and social character. In both there is an additive effect; each builds on past accomplishments, and some element of each is maintained throughout life. At each stage in development the new predominates.

CONTENT OF PLAY

The content of play involves primarily the physical aspects of play, although social relationships cannot be ignored. The content of play follows the directional trend of the simple to the complex:

Social-affective play. Play begins with social-affective play, wherein infants take pleasure in relationships with people. As adults talk, touch, nuzzle, and in various ways elicit a response from an infant, the infant soon learns to provoke parental emotions and responses with such behaviors as smiling, cooing, or initiating games and activities. The type and intensity of the adult behavior with children vary among cultures.

Sense-pleasure play. Sense-pleasure play is a nonsocial stimulating experience that originates from without. Objects in the environment—light and color, tastes and odors, textures and consistencies—attract children's attention, stimulate their senses, and give pleasure. Pleasurable experiences are derived from handling raw materials (water, sand, food), from body motion (swinging, bouncing, rocking), and from other uses of senses and abilities (smelling, humming; Fig. 5-5).

Skill play. Once infants have developed the ability to grasp and manipulate, they persistently demonstrate and exercise their newly acquired abilities through skill play, repeating an action over and over again. The element of sense-pleasure play is often evident in the practicing of a new ability, but all too frequently the determination to conquer the elusive skill produces pain and frustration (e.g., learning to ride a bicycle).

Unoccupied behavior. In unoccupied behavior children are not playful but focus their attention momentarily on anything that strikes their interest. Children daydream, fiddle with clothes or other objects, or walk aimlessly. This role differs from that of onlookers, who actively observe the activity of others.

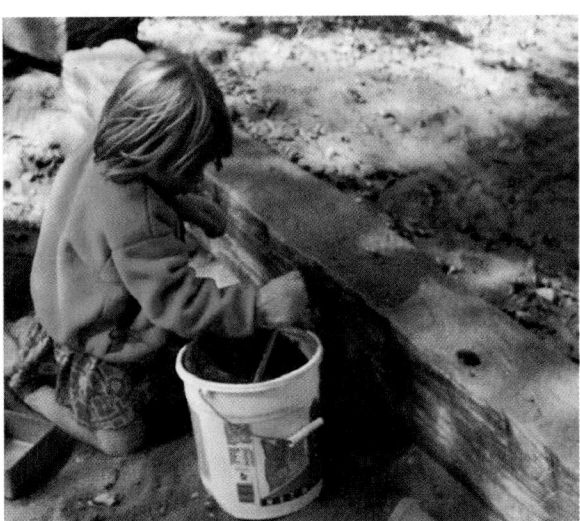

FIG. 5-5. Children derive pleasure from handling raw materials.

Dramatic, or pretend, play. One of the vital elements in children's process of identification is dramatic play, also known as symbolic or pretend play. It begins in late infancy (11 to 13 months) and is the predominant form of play in the preschool child. Once children begin to invest situations and people with meanings and to attribute affective significance to the world, they can pretend and fantasize almost anything. By acting out events of daily life, children learn and practice the roles and identities modeled by the members of their family and society. Children's toys, replicas of the tools of society, provide a medium for learning about adult roles and activities that may be puzzling and frustrating to them. Interacting with the world is one way children get to know it. The simple, imitative, dramatic play of the toddler, such as using the telephone, driving a car, or rocking a doll, evolves into more complex, sustained dramas of the preschooler, which extend beyond common domestic matters to the wider aspects of the world and the society, such as playing police officer, storekeeper, teacher, or nurse. Older children work out elaborate themes, act out stories, and compose plays (Fig. 5-6).

Games. Children in all cultures engage in games alone and with others. Solitary activity involving games begins as very small children participate in repetitive activities and progress to more complicated games that challenge their independent skills, such as solving puzzles, solitaire, and computer or video games. Very young children participate in simple, *imitative games,* such as pat-a-cake and peekaboo. Preschool children learn and enjoy *formal games* that begin with ritualistic, self-sustaining games, such as ring-around-a-rosy and London Bridge. With the exception of some simple board games, preschool children do not engage in *competitive games.* Preschoolers hate to lose and will try to cheat, want to change rules, or demand exceptions and opportunities to change their moves. School-age children and adolescents enjoy competitive games, including cards, checkers, chess, and physically active games such as baseball.

Social Character of Play

The play interactions of infancy are between the child and an adult. Children continue to enjoy the company of an adult but are increasingly able to play alone. As age advances, interaction with age-mates increases in importance and becomes an essential part of the socialization process. Through interaction, highly egocentric infants, unable to tolerate delay or interference, ultimately acquire concern for others and the ability to delay gratification or even to reject gratification at the expense of another. A pair of toddlers engage in considerable combat because their personal needs cannot tolerate delay or compromise. By the time they reach age 5 or 6 years, children are able to arrive at a compromise or make use of arbitration, usually after they have attempted but failed to gain their own way. Through continued interaction with peers and the growth of conceptual abilities and social skills, children are able to increase participation with others in the following types of play:

Onlooker play. During onlooker play children watch what other children are doing but make no attempt to enter into the play activity. There is an active interest in observing the interaction of others but no movement toward participating. Watching an older sibling bounce a ball is a common example of the onlooker role.

Solitary play. During solitary play children play alone with toys different from those used by other children in the same area. They enjoy the presence of other children but make no effort to get close to or speak to them. Their interest is centered on their own activity, which they pursue with no reference to the activities of the others.

Parallel play. During parallel activities children play independently but among other children. They play with toys like those the children around them are using, but as each child sees fit, neither influencing nor being influenced by the other children. Each plays beside, but not with, other children (Fig. 5-7). There is no group association. Parallel play is the characteristic play of toddlers, but it may also occur in other groups of any age. Individuals who are involved in a creative craft with each person separately working on an individual project are engaged in parallel play.

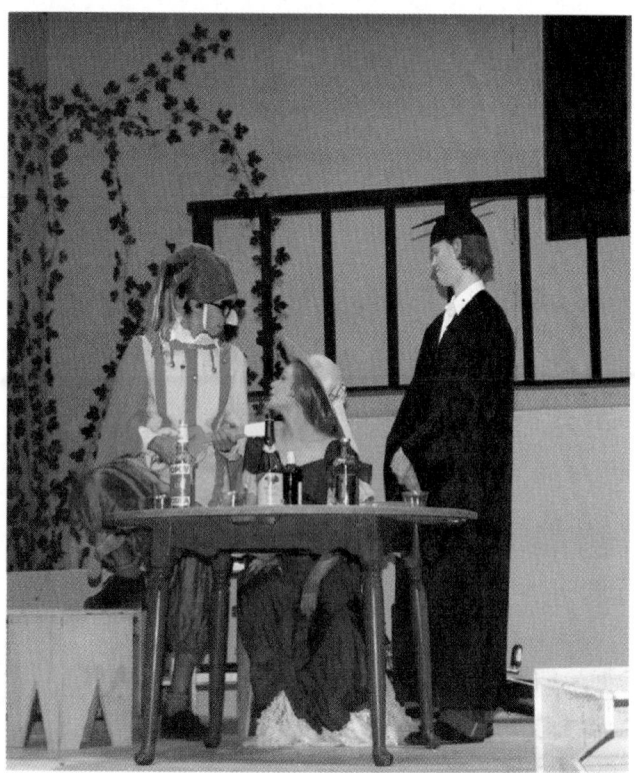

FIG. 5-6. Older children enjoy being in plays.

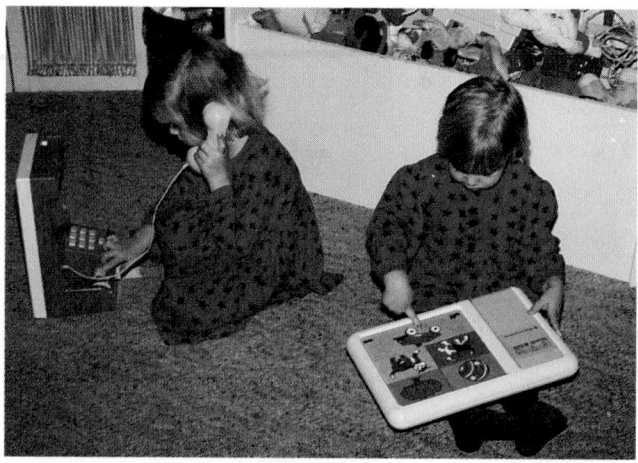

FIG. 5-7. Parallel play.

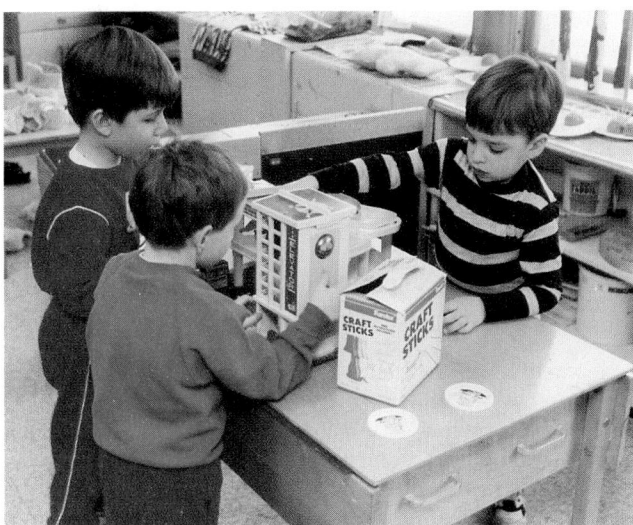

FIG. 5-8. Associative play.

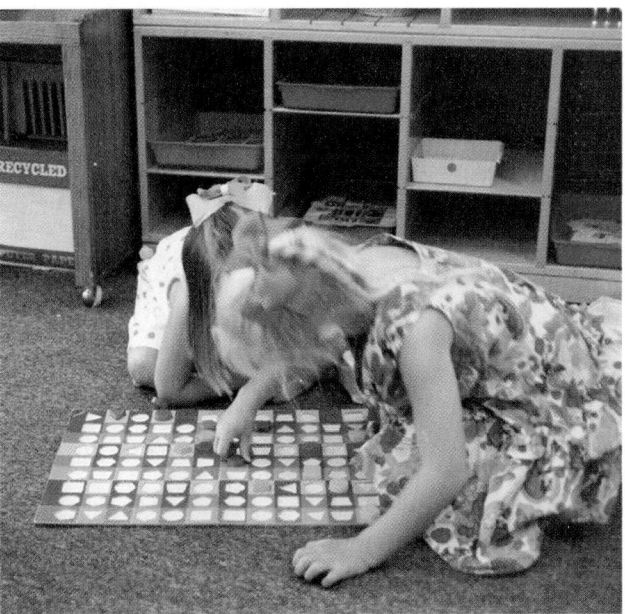

FIG. 5-9. Cooperative play.

Associative play. In associative play children play together and are engaged in a similar or even identical activity, but there is no organization, division of labor, leadership assignment, or mutual goal. Children borrow and lend play materials, follow each other with wagons and tricycles, and sometimes attempt to control who may or may not play in the group. Each child acts according to his or her own wishes; there is no group goal (Fig. 5-8). For example, two children play with dolls, borrowing articles of clothing from each other and engaging in similar conversation, but neither directs the other's actions or establishes rules regarding the limits of the play session. There is a great deal of behavioral contagion: when one child initiates an activity, the entire group follows the example.

Cooperative play. Cooperative play is organized, and children play in a group *with* other children (Fig. 5-9). They discuss and plan activities for the purposes of accomplishing an end—to make something, to attain a competitive goal, to dramatize situations of adult or group life, or to play formal games. The group is loosely formed, but there is a marked sense of belonging or not belonging. The goal and its attainment require organization of activities, division of labor, and playing roles. The leader-follower relationship is definitely established, and the activity is controlled by one or two members who assign roles and direct the activity of the others. The activity is organized to allow one child to supplement another's function in order to complete the goal.

FUNCTIONS OF PLAY

Sensorimotor Development

Sensorimotor activity is a major component of play at all ages and is the predominant form of play in infancy. Active play is essential for muscle development and serves a useful purpose as a release for surplus energy. Through sensorimotor play children explore the nature of the physical world. Infants gain impressions of themselves and their world through tactile, auditory, visual, and kinesthetic stimulation. Toddlers and preschoolers revel in body movement and exploration of things in space. With increasing maturity sensorimotor play becomes more differentiated and involved. Whereas very young children run for the sheer joy of body movement, older children incorporate or modify the motions into increasingly complex and coordinated activities such as races, games, roller skating, and bicycle riding.

Intellectual Development

Through exploration and manipulation children learn colors, shapes, sizes, textures, and the significance of objects. They learn the significance of numbers and how to use them, they learn to associate words with objects, and they develop an understanding of abstract concepts and spatial relationships, such as *up, down, under,* and *over.* Activities such as puzzles and games help them develop problem-solving skills. Books, stories, films, and collections expand knowledge and provide enjoyment as well. Play provides a means to practice and expand language skills. Through play children continually rehearse past experiences to assimilate them into new perceptions and relationships. Play helps children comprehend the world in which they live and distinguish between fantasy and reality.

Socialization

From very early infancy children show interest and pleasure in the company of others. Their initial social contact is with the mothering person, but through play with other children they learn to establish social relationships and solve the problems associated with these relationships. They learn to give and take, which is more readily learned from critical peers than from the more tolerant adults. They learn the sex role that society expects them to fulfill, as well as approved patterns of behavior and deportment. Closely associated with socialization is development of moral values and ethics. Children learn right from wrong, the standards of the society, and to assume responsibility for their actions.

Creativity

In no other situation is there more opportunity to be creative than in play. Children can experiment and try out their ideas in play through every medium at their disposal, including raw materials, fantasy, and exploration. Creativity is stifled by pressure toward conformity; therefore striving for peer approval may inhibit creative endeavors in the school-age or adolescent child. Creativity is primarily a product of solitary activity; yet creative thinking is often enhanced in group settings where listening to others' ideas stimulates further exploration of one's own ideas. Once children feel the satisfaction of creating something new and different, they transfer this creative interest to situations outside the world of play.

Self-Awareness

Beginning with active explorations of their bodies and awareness of themselves as separate from the mother, the process of self-identity is facilitated through play activities. Children learn who they are and their place in the world. They become increasingly able to regulate their own behavior, to learn what their abilities are, and to compare their abilities with those of others. Through play children are able to test their abilities, to assume and try out various roles, and to learn the effect their behavior has on others.

Therapeutic Value

Play is therapeutic at any age. It provides a means for release from the tension and stress encountered in the environment. In play children can express emotions and release unacceptable impulses in a socially acceptable fashion. Children are able to experiment and test fearful situations and can assume and vicariously master the roles and positions that they are unable to perform in the world of reality. Children reveal much about themselves in play. Through play children are able to communicate to the alert observer the needs, fears, and desires that they are unable to express with their limited language skills. Throughout their play children need the acceptance of adults and their presence to help them control aggression and to channel their destructive tendencies.

Moral Value

Although children learn at home and at school those behaviors considered right and wrong in the culture, the interaction with peers during play contributes significantly to their moral training. Nowhere is the enforcement of moral standards so rigid as in the play situation. If they are to be acceptable members of the group, children must adhere to the accepted codes of behavior of the culture—fairness, honesty, self-control, consideration for others, and so on. Children soon learn that their peers are less tolerant of violations than are adults and that to maintain a place in the play group they must conform to the standards of the group.

TOYS

The type of toys chosen by and/or provided for children can facilitate their development in the areas just described. Toys that are small replicas of the culture and its tools help them assimilate their culture. Toys that require pushing, pulling, rolling, and manipulating teach them about physical properties of the items and help to develop muscles and coordination. Rules and the basic elements of cooperation and organization are learned through board games.

Because they can be employed in a variety of ways, raw materials with which children can use their own creativity and imaginations are sometimes superior to ready-made items. For example, building blocks can be used to construct a variety of things, to count, and to learn shapes and sizes.

Toy Safety

Selection of toys and play equipment is a joint effort between parents and children, but evaluation of their safety is the responsibility of the adult. Government agencies do not inspect and police all toys on the market. Therefore adults who purchase, supervise purchases, or allow children to use play equipment need to evaluate such equipment for its safety, including toys that are gifts or those that are purchased by the children themselves (see Family Home Care box). They should also be alert to notices of toys determined to be defective and recalled by the manufacturers. Parents and health workers can obtain information on a variety of recalled products and can report potentially dangerous toys and child products to the **U.S. Consumer Product Safety Commission (CPSC)*** or, in Canada, the **Canadian Toy Testing Council.†**

SELECTED FACTORS THAT INFLUENCE DEVELOPMENT

HEREDITY

Inherited characteristics have a profound influence on development. The sex of the child, determined by random selection at the time of conception, directs both the pattern of growth and the behavior of others toward the child. In all cultures, attitudes and expectations are different with respect to the sex of the child. Sex plus other hereditary determinants strongly affects the end result of growth and the rate of progress toward it. There is a high correlation between parent and child with regard to traits such as height, weight, and rate of growth. Most physical characteristics, including shape and form of features, body build, and physical peculiarities, are inherited and can influence the way in which children grow and interact with their environment. Many dimensions of personality, such as temperament, activity level, responsiveness, and a tendency toward shyness, are believed to be inherited.

Differences in health and vigor of children may be attributed to hereditary traits. An inherited physical or mental disorder will alter or modify a child's physical and/or emotional growth and interactions. The extent to which disabling conditions interfere with the child's growth and well-being is considered in relation to numerous disabilities throughout the remainder of the book.

NEUROENDOCRINE FACTORS

It has been suggested there may be a growth center in the hypothalamic region responsible for maintaining genetically determined growth patterns. Some functional relationship is believed to exist between the hypothalamus and the endo-

---

*CPSC hotline: (800) 638-CPSC.
†22 Hamilton Ave. North, Ottawa, Ontario, Canada K1Y 1V6; (613) 729-7101.

FAMILY HOME CARE
Toy Safety*

Selection

Select toys that suit the skills, abilities, and interests of children.

Select toys that are safe for the specific child; look for a label that indicates the intended age-group. Toys that are safe for one age may not be safe for another.

For infants, toddlers, and all children who still mouth objects, avoid toys with small parts that may pose a fatal choking hazard or aspiration hazard. Toys in this category are usually labeled: "Not recommended for children under 3 years."

For infants avoid toys with strings or cords that are 7 inches or longer, since they may cause strangulation.

For all children under 8 years, avoid electric toys with heating elements.

For children under 5 years, avoid arrows or darts.

Check for safety labels such as "flame retardant" or "flame resistant."

Select toys durable enough to survive rough play; look for sturdy construction such as tightly secured eyes, nose, or any small parts.

Select toys light enough that they will not cause harm if one falls on a child.

Look for toys with smooth, rounded edges. Avoid toys with sharp edges that can cut or that have sharp points. Points on the inside of the toy can puncture if the toy is broken.

Avoid toys with any shooting or throwing objects that can injure eyes.

This includes toys into which other missiles, such as sticks or pebbles, might be used as substitutes for the intended projectiles.

Arrows and darts used by children should have blunt tips and be manufactured from resilient materials; make certain tips are securely attached.

Make certain that materials in toys are nontoxic.

Avoid toys that make loud noises that might be damaging to a child's hearing.

Even some squeaking toys are too loud when held close to the ear.

If selecting caps for cap guns, look for the label required by Federal law to be on boxes or packages of caps that states: "Warning—Do not fire closer than 1 foot to the ear. Do not use indoors."

Make certain that arrows or darts have soft tips, rubber suction cups, or other protective tips. Check to be certain that tips are secure.

If selecting a toy gun, be certain that the barrel or the entire gun is brightly colored to avoid being mistaken as a real gun.

Check toy instructions for clarity. They should be clear to an adult and, when appropriate, to the child.

Supervision

Maintain a safe play environment.

Remove and discard plastic wrappings on toys immediately; they could suffocate a child.

Remove large toys, bumper pads, and boxes from playpens; an adventuresome child can use such items as a means of climbing or falling out.

Set "ground rules" for play.

Supervise young children closely during play.

Teach children how to use toys properly and safely.

Instruct older children to keep their toys away from younger brothers, sisters, and friends.

Keep children who are playing with riding toys away from stairs, hills, traffic, and swimming pools.

Establish and enforce rules regarding protective gear.

Insist that children wear helmets when using bicycles, skateboards, or in-line skates.

Insist that children wear gloves and wrist, elbow, and knee pads when using skateboards or in-line skates.

Instruct children on electrical safety.

Teach children the proper way to unplug an electric toy—pull on the plug, not the cord.

Teach children to beware of electrical appliances and even electrically operated playthings; frequently children are unfamiliar with the hazards of electricity in association with water.

Teach children the safe use of utensils that under certain circumstances can cause injury—scissors, knives, needles, heating elements, or loops, long string, or cord.

Maintenance

Inspect old and new toys regularly for breakage, loose parts, and other potential hazards.

Look for jagged or sharp edges or broken parts that might constitute a choking hazard.

Check movable parts to make certain they are attached securely to the toys; sometimes pieces that are safe when attached to the toy become a danger when detached.

Examine all outdoor toys regularly for rust and weak or sharp parts that could become a danger to a child.

Check electrical cords and plugs for cracked or fraying parts.

Maintain toys in good repair, without signs of possible hazards such as sharp edges, splinters, weak seams, or rust.

Make repairs immediately, or discard out of reach of children.

Sand sharp wooden toys or splintered surfaces smooth.

Use only paint labeled "nontoxic" to repaint toys, toy boxes, or children's furniture.

Storage

Provide a safe place for children to store toys.

Select a toy chest or toy box that is ventilated, is free of self-locking devices that could trap a child inside, and has a lid designed not to pinch a child's fingers or fall on a child's head.

If containers other than toy chests are used for storage purposes, they should be fitted with spring-loaded support devices if they have a hinged lid to avoid entrapment and suffocation.

Teach children to store toys safely in order to prevent accidental injury from stepping, tripping, or falling on a toy.

Playthings meant for older children and adults should be safely stowed away on high shelves, in locked closets, or in other areas unavailable to younger children.

*Another helpful resource is *Toy safety: guidelines for parents* from American Academy of Pediatrics, Division of Publications, 141 Northwest Point Blvd, PO Box 927, Elk Grove Village, IL 60009-0927; (800) 433-9016.

crine system that influences growth. There is also evidence, based on observations of denervated skeletal muscles, that the peripheral nervous system may influence growth, because muscles deprived of nerve supply degenerate. Many of these effects are not sufficiently explained by disuse or diminished blood supply.

Probably all hormones affect growth in some fashion. Three hormones—growth hormone, thyroid hormone, and androgens—when given to persons deficient in these hormones, stimulate protein anabolism and thereby produce retention of elements essential for building protoplasm and bony tissue. It appears that each of the hormones that has a significant influence on growth manifests its major effect at a different period of growth (see Chapter 29).

NUTRITION

Nutrition is probably the single most important influence on growth. Dietary factors regulate growth at all stages of development, and their effects are exerted in numerous and complex ways. During the rapid prenatal growth period, faulty nutrition may influence development from the time of implantation of the ovum until birth. During infancy and childhood the demand for calories is relatively great, as evidenced by the rapid increase in both height and weight. At this time protein and caloric requirements are higher than at almost any period of postnatal development. As the growth rate slows with its concomitant decrease in metabolism, there is a corresponding reduction in caloric and protein requirements (see Table 5-2).

Growth is uneven during the periods of childhood between infancy and adolescence when there are plateaus and small growth spurts. The child's appetite will fluctuate in response to these variations until the turbulent growth spurt of adolescence, when adequate nutrition is extremely important but may be subjected to numerous emotional influences. Adequate nutrition is closely related to good health throughout life, and an overall improvement in nourishment is evidenced by the gradual increase in size and early maturation of children in this century.

INTERPERSONAL RELATIONSHIPS

Relationships with significant others play a critical role in development, particularly in emotional, intellectual, and personality development. Not only do the quality and quantity of contacts with other persons exert an influence on the growing child, but the widening range of contacts is essential to learning and the development of a healthy personality.

The mothering person is unquestionably the single most influential person during early infancy. This person is the one who meets the infant's basic needs of food, warmth, comfort, and love. He or she provides stimulation for the child's senses and facilitates his or her expanding capacities. Through this person, the child learns to trust the world and feel secure to venture in increasingly wider relationships.

It is generally the parents who are most influential in helping the child to assume sex-role identification. Parents define and reinforce acceptable sex-role behavior and provide sex-appropriate role models for the child. In the absence of a sex-role model in the family setting, the child may adopt some characteristics of the opposite-sex parent or sibling. Frequently the child identifies with a teacher or other significant person of the same sex.

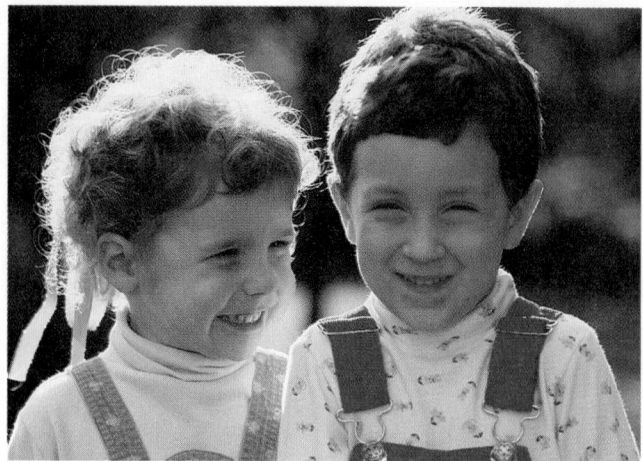

FIG. 5-10. Peers become increasingly important as children develop friendships outside the family group.

Siblings are children's first peers, and the way in which they learn to relate to each other affects later interactions with peers outside the family group. The sphere of persons from whom children seek approval widens to include other members of their family, their peers, and, to a lesser extent, other authority figures (e.g., teachers). The increasing importance of the peer group in determining the behavior of school-age children and adolescents is well documented (Fig. 5-10).

When children fail to have quality interpersonal relationships with "mothering" persons, they experience *emotional deprivation.* The most prominent feature of emotional deprivation, particularly during the first year, is developmental retardation. Much of the information regarding the adverse effects of interpersonal influences on development has been acquired through retrospective studies of gross deprivation and trauma. The most notable instances involved homeless infants who were placed in institutions for care. Those infants, who did not receive consistent mothering care, failed to gain weight even with an adequate diet; were pale, listless, and immobile; and were unresponsive to stimuli that usually elicit a response, such as smiling or cooing, in the normal infant. If emotional deprivation continues for a sufficient length of time, the child may not survive infancy.

Although the most remarkable examples of emotional deprivation were first recognized among infants in institutions, the term *masked deprivation* has been used to describe children reared in homes where there is a distorted parent-child relationship or otherwise disordered home environment. Infants do not thrive if the caregiving person is hostile, fearful of handling them, or indifferent to them and their needs. Such children exhibit poor growth even though they are apparently free of physical disease. Growth retardation in these children is believed to be caused by a psychologically induced endocrine imbalance that interferes with growth. These same infants and children display "catch-up" growth in a changed environment. (See Failure to Thrive, Chapter 11.)

SOCIOECONOMIC LEVEL

Evidence indicates that the socioeconomic level of children's families has a significant impact on growth and development.

At all ages children from upper- and middle-class families are taller than comparative children of families in the lower socioeconomic strata. The cause of these differences is less definite, although the poorer health and nutrition of lower socioeconomic levels are probably significant factors. Nutritious food sources (especially proteins) are scarce, and other factors (e.g., larger family size and irregularity in eating, sleeping, and exercise) may play a role.

Families from lower socioeconomic groups may lack the knowledge or resources needed to provide the safe, stimulating, and enriched environment that fosters optimum development for children. They may be unable to move from unsafe neighborhoods where drug traffic and drive-by shootings are the norm. The effects on the emotional development of children living under these conditions have been compared with those experienced by children living in war zones.

DISEASE
Altered growth and development is one of the clinical manifestations in a number of hereditary disorders. Growth impairment is particularly marked in skeletal disorders, such as the various forms of dwarfism and at least one of the chromosomal anomalies (Turner syndrome). Many of the disorders of metabolism, such as vitamin D–resistant rickets, the mucopolysaccharidoses, and the numerous endocrine disorders, interfere with the normal growth pattern. In other disorders the tendency is toward the upper percentile of height (e.g., Klinefelter syndrome and Marfan syndrome).

Many chronic illnesses that are associated with varying degrees of growth failure are congenital cardiac anomalies and respiratory disorders such as cystic fibrosis. Any disorder characterized by the inability to digest and absorb body nutrients will have an adverse effect on growth and development.

ENVIRONMENTAL HAZARDS
Hazards in the environment are a source of concern to health care providers and others interested in health and safety. Physical injuries are the most prevalent consequences of environmental dangers, and these are discussed extensively throughout the book as they apply in relation to age, specific hazards, and selected physical disabilities.

The harmful agents most often associated with health risks are chemicals and radiation. Water, air, and food contamination from a variety of origins are well documented. Significant sources of exposure are substances in the immediate environment, such as lead and asbestos, chemicals secreted in breast milk (especially prescribed drugs and nicotine), and contamination within well-insulated homes (especially from disinfectants or burning of substances that produce toxic fumes). Passive inhalation of tobacco smoke by infants and children is a hazard at all stages of development. The harmful effects of large doses of radiation are unquestioned, although the effects of low-dose or short-term radiation are debatable, as are the safe vs harmful dosage levels.

STRESS IN CHILDHOOD
Defined from both a physiologic and an emotional point of view, essentially *stress* is "an imbalance between environmental demands and a person's coping resources that . . . disrupts the equilibrium of the person" (Masten and others, 1988).

Although all children experience stress, some youngsters appear to be more vulnerable than others. Children's age, temperament, life situation, and state of health affect their vulnerability, reactions, and ability to handle stress. Also, the responses to a stressor can be behavioral, psychologic, or physiologic. It is impossible, unrealistic, and undesirable to protect children from stress, but providing them with interpersonal security helps them develop coping strategies for dealing with stress. The concept of an *emotional bank,* in which deposits, as well as withdrawals, can be made can help parents and caregivers maintain a proper perspective regarding the effects of stress and coping (Usdin, 1988). Children with a good, positive balance in the account can tolerate significant withdrawal experiences. For children with a low balance, even a minor withdrawal may bankrupt the account, causing it to be overdrawn.

Parents and other caregivers can try to recognize signs of stress in order to help children deal with stresses before they become overwhelming. Signs of stress take many forms but are typically the same ones seen in children who are abused (see Chapter 14) or depressed (see Chapter 17). If a number of stresses are imposed on children at the same time, the children are more vulnerable. When a succession of stresses produces an excessive stress load, children may experience a serious change in health and/or behavior.

It is most important that parents and persons working with children understand the nature of childhood stress and ways it can be recognized or anticipated. Caregivers must *listen* to children so they are aware of children's fears and concerns and must let them know that they are important and that what they say matters. Physical contact is comforting and reassuring to children. Simply holding, touching, or hugging children is both relaxing and comforting and facilitates communication. Spending unhurried time with children, family outings, vacations, and exposing children to positive influences help build children's strength and security. Supportive interpersonal relationships are essential to the psychologic well-being of children.

Coping
Coping refers to a special class of individual reactions to stressors—specifically, a reaction to a stressor that resolves, reduces, or replaces the affect state classified as stressful. *Coping strategies* are the specific ways in which children cope with stressors, as distinguished from *coping styles,* which are relatively unchanging personality characteristics or outcomes of coping (Ryan-Wenger, 1992). Children, like adults, respond to everyday stress by trying to change the circumstances or trying to adjust to circumstances the way they are. Any strategy that provides relaxation is effective in reducing stress, and most children have their own natural methods, such as withdrawal, physical activity, reading, listening to music, working on a project, or taking a nap. Some turn to parents to solve their problems, or they may develop socially unacceptable strategies, such as cheating, stealing, or lying.

Children can be taught stress-reduction techniques to use in coping. First, they must be helped to recognize signs of tension in themselves and then taught any of a variety of appropriate strategies—special exercises, relaxation and breathing, mental imagery, and numerous other simple activities. Also, parents and other caregivers can anticipate possible stress-provoking events and prepare children for coping by role playing a scenario or "talking it through" beforehand.

Most of the stress-reducing strategies discussed in Chapter 21 in relation to managing pain are effective for any stress situation.

Probably the most useful tool that children can learn is how to solve problems. When children can view any new situation as a problem to be solved and an opportunity to learn, they are not vulnerable to the control of others. It provides them with a sense of mastery over their own lives and reinforces the fact that they have within themselves the ability and information to handle whatever comes their way. Problem-solving skill gives them the confidence to know where and how to seek help when they need it.

INFLUENCE OF THE MASS MEDIA

Media can have an enormous influence on the developing child. Children may identify closely with people or characters portrayed in reading materials, movies, videos, and television programs and commercials. Today children tend to select media figures as their ideal role models, whereas in the past the majority of children chose their parents or parent surrogates as the people they most wanted to be like (Duck, 1990). This trend can be viewed as a grave concern or a magnificent opportunity to promote positive role models. There is no doubt that the communications media provide children with a means for extending their knowledge about the world in which they live and have contributed to narrowing the differences between classes.

Reading Materials

The oldest form of mass media, books, newspapers, and magazines, contribute to children's competence in almost every direction, as well as providing enjoyment. Recognition of the impact that reading matter used in the schools has on the value system and socialization processes has prompted re-evaluation of the content of textbooks in terms of the biased presentation of male and female role models, the sugar-coated view of life situations, and the biased history of minority groups.

Fairy tales, for generations the mainstay of young children's literature, for a time suffered condemnation as being sexist, overly violent in content, and riddled with unfavorable stereotypes, such as the wicked stepmother, dwarfs, and physical unattractiveness associated with evil. They are now believed to provide an excellent medium for explaining puzzling and important topics such as death, stepparents, and inner feelings and turmoils. Although they do not provide solutions, fairy tales confront children with emotional predicaments and offer suggestions for dealing with them.

Comic books and other pulp reading material have been popular in every generation, usually at the expense of literature provided by schools, libraries, and parents. Many children have nothing else to read. The easy reading, quick action, and adventure in brief episodes seem to fulfill a need for children who are striving to understand both aggression in others and their own impulses. Reading ability, intelligence, and school adjustment apparently have no relationship to the number and type of comic books read. Most comic books appear to be relatively harmless to the majority of children and may be beneficial. Comic books seem to have only a minor influence on acquisition of beliefs, values, and behaviors. The popularity of this medium has prompted some educators to encourage translations of literature into comic book form to stimulate students' interest in the classics.

Movies

Movies, although usually not closely bound to reality, often portray an assortment of socially approved behaviors. Such movies perhaps make a contribution to children's value systems and provide opportunities for desirable social learning. On the other hand, children, especially adolescents, flock to the "macho" movies and those in which the heroes resort to violent resolution of problems, such as the use of karate techniques and wild car chases. The carry-over of these influences into daily life and relationships may account, in part, for the increase in violent behavior of young persons.

Another concern is the number of "slasher" and R-rated movies available to children and teenagers in theaters, on cable television, and on videocassettes. The content of movies has changed markedly during the past few years, with mutilation as a major theme. For children who are unable to distinguish between reality and fantasy, these films play on their deepest fears, resulting in bedtime fears, nightmares, and a fearful view of the world (Schmitt, 1989).

Young children can be frightened by some movies considered to be safe for family viewing. For example, the villainous witches in *Snow White* and the *Wizard of Oz* can be terrifying figures. Also, some of the classic Disney movies such as *Snow White* and *Cinderella,* which depict stepmothers as evil, destructive persons, can have a negative effect on children-stepmother relationships or can be confusing to children who have developed a positive relationship with a stepmother. Parents who are aware of this possibility can use viewing such films as opportunities to open discussion, provide explanations, and explore difficult or troubling concepts or events.

 Children as young as 4 years can recognize that cartoons are "make-believe," but children as old as age 6 continue to assume that noncartoon features are at least roughly analogous to social reality (Downs, 1990).

Television

The medium with the most impact on children in North America today is television, which has become one of the most significant socializing agents in the lives of young children. The content of programs and commercials provides multiple sources for acquiring information, modeling behaviors, and observing value orientations. Besides producing a leveling effect on class differences in general information and vocabulary, TV exposes children to a wider variety of topics and events than they encounter in day-to-day life. Television always has time to talk to children and is a form of access to the adult world.

 The average child in the United States spends more time watching television than in any other activity except sleeping: 25 hours per week for children 2 to 5 years old, 22 hours for children 6 to 12 years old, and 23 hours for 12 to 17-year-olds. These figures do not include videocassette recorder (VCR) use (American Academy of Pediatrics, 1990).

Most researchers have concluded that protracted television viewing can have detrimental effects on children. Increased verbal and physical aggressive behavior, reduced persistence at problem solving, greater sex-role stereotyping, and reduced creativity have been reported repeatedly.

Excessive television viewing has also been linked to obesity and high blood cholesterol levels in children (Gortmaker, Dietz, and Cheng, 1990). The passive activity is frequently accompanied by eating—in many cases high-calorie snacks. Furthermore, children may expend tremendous mental energy processing the audiovisual messages from TV, which may be very exhausting and make them less likely to engage in physical activity later. Television viewing has a fairly profound effect of lowering the metabolic rate and may be a mechanism for the relationship between obesity and the amount of television viewing (Klesges, Shelton, and Klesges, 1993).

In a study to identify children at risk for heart disease, researchers found that more than half of the children with high cholesterol levels watched at least 2 hours of television each day. Using a family history of heart disease or high cholesterol as the screening indicator for cholesterol testing in children, researchers identified three out of four children with high cholesterol levels. When these families were also questioned about the time their children spent watching television, investigators were able to identify 90% of the children with high cholesterol levels by using 2 or more viewing hours as the risk factor (Goldsmith, 1990).

TV programs and commercials, like movies, contain many implicit and explicit messages that promote alcohol consumption, smoking, violence, and promiscuous or unsafe sexual activity. An area of increasing concern is Music Television (MTV), especially when heavy metal rock groups, whose lyrics and videos sensationalize violent sex, suicide, and satanism, are featured. Although no clear evidence documents a relationship between television viewing and sexual activity or the use of alcohol or tobacco, the frequency of adolescent pregnancy and sexually transmitted diseases, the prevalence of alcohol-related deaths among adolescents, and the popularity of smoking among youth represent major sources of concern and speculation.

On the positive side, television has been shown to be a positive influence on children's abilities to deal with a variety of social issues, such as divorce, the arrival of a new baby, discrimination, honesty, and helpfulness. Children who view educational programming (such as "Mister Rogers' Neighborhood" and "Sesame Street") for a long period of time become more affectionate, considerate, cooperative, and helpful toward their playmates. The ways that minority and ethnic characters are portrayed on television can have an impact on the way the majority culture views minority persons and on the self-image of minority children.

Many parents are concerned about the effects of television viewing on their children, and most would like information regarding its use (Benard-Bonnin and others, 1991). Parents need to supervise the amount and type of TV programs their children watch and to teach their children how to watch TV (see Family Home Care box).

 FAMILY HOME CARE
Television Viewing

Provide a positive role model by developing television substitutes such as reading, athletics, physical conditioning, and hobbies.

Construct a time chart of child's activities (homework, TV viewing, scheduled outside activities, playing with a friend).

Discuss with child what you both believe to be a balanced set of activities.

At the beginning of each week select appropriate programs from television schedules.

Allow child to select programs from this approved list.

Limit child's viewing to 2 hours or less per day.

Rule out TV at specific times (e.g., before breakfast or on school nights).

Make a list of alternative activities (e.g., riding a bicycle, reading a book, or working on a hobby).

Require that child choose to do something from this list before watching TV.

Watch programs with child.

Discuss program and commercial content with child:
  Distinguish between the real and the unreal.
  Correlate consequences with actions.
  Point out subtle messages.
  Explore alternatives to aggressive conflict resolution.
  Stress purpose of program (e.g., entertainment, education).
  Explain likes and dislikes.

Turn the TV off after the selected program is over.

Monitor cable and pay TV selections; use a lockbox if necessary.

Limit use of TV as a safe distraction to potentially stressful times (e.g., keeping the children occupied while the parent gets organized after a difficult day).

KEY POINTS

- Growth describes a change in quantity and occurs when cells divide and synthesize new proteins.
- Maturation, a qualitative change, describes the aging process or an increase in competence and adaptability.
- Differentiation refers to a biologic description of the processes by which early cells and structures are modified and altered to achieve specific and characteristic physical and chemical properties.
- Development involves change from a lower to a more advanced stage of complexity.
- The five major developmental periods are prenatal, infancy, early childhood, middle childhood, and later childhood (pubescence and adolescence).
- Growth and development proceed in predictable patterns of direction, sequence, and pace.
- The directional trends in growth and development are cephalocaudal, proximodistal, and mass to specific.
- Physical development includes increase in height and weight and changes in body proportion, dentition, and some body tissues.
- The three broad classifications of child temperament are the easy child, the difficult child, and the slow-to-warm-up child.
- The developmental theories most widely used in explaining child growth and development are Freud's psychosexual stages, Erikson's stages of psychosocial development, Piaget's stages of cognitive development, and Kohlberg's stages of moral development.
- Development of self-concept occurs through children's interactions and observations of their own experiences with others and with the environment.
- Play is one of the most important media through which children learn about themselves, others, and their environment.
- Factors influencing development include heredity, neuroendocrine factors, nutrition, interpersonal relationships, socioeconomic status, disease, stress, and mass media.

REFERENCES

American Academy of Pediatrics, Committee on Communications: Children, adolescents and television, *Pediatrics* 85(6):1119-1120, 1990.

Bernard-Bonnin A and others: Television and the 3- to 10-year-old child, *Pediatrics* 88(1):48-54, 1991.

Chess S, Thomas A: Temperamental differences: a critical concept in child health care, *Pediatr Nurs* 11:167-171, 1985.

Clutter L: Fostering spiritual care for the child and family. In Smith DP and others, editors: *Comprehensive child and family nursing skills*, St Louis, 1991, Mosby.

Downs A: Children's judgments of televised events: the real versus pretend distinction, *Percept Mot Skills* 70:779-782, 1990.

Duck J: Children's ideals: the role of real-life versus media figures, *Austr J Psychol* 42:19-29, 1990.

Erikson EH: *Childhood and society*, ed 2, New York, 1963, WW Norton.

Fowler JW: Toward a developmental perspective on faith, *Religious Educ* 69:207-219, 1974.

Goldsmith M: Youngsters dialing up cholesterol levels? *JAMA* 264(23):2976, 1990.

Gortmaker S, Dietz W, Cheng L: Inactivity, diet, and the fattening of America, *J Am Diet Assoc* 90(9):1247-1252, 1990.

Jung FE, Czajka-Narins DM: Birth weight doubling and tripling times: an updated look at the effects of birth weight, sex, race and type of feeding, *Am J Clin Nutr* 42:182-189, 1985.

Klesges R, Shelton M, Klesges L: Effects of television on metabolic rate: potential implications for childhood obesity, *Pediatrics* 91(2):281-286, 1993.

Kohlberg L: Moral development. In Sills DL, editor: *International encyclopedia of the social sciences*, New York, 1968, Macmillan.

Lampl M: Saltation and stasis: a model of human growth, *Science* 258(5083):801-803, 1992.

Masten A and others: Competence and stress in school children: moderating effects of individual and family qualities, *J Child Psychol Psychiatry* 29:747-764, 1988.

Piaget J: *The theory of stages in cognitive development*, New York, 1969, McGraw-Hill.

Ryan-Wenger N: A taxonomy of children's coping strategies: a step toward theory development, *Am J Orthopsychiatry* 62(2):256-263, 1992.

Schmitt BD: Nightmares on main street, *Am J Dis Child* 143:649, 1989 (editorial).

Selekman J: The development of body image in the child: a learned response, *Top Clin Nurs* 5(1):13-21, 1983.

Sheeber L, Johnson J: Child temperament, maternal adjustment, and changes in family life style, *Am J Orthopsychiatry* 62(2):178-185, 1992.

Sieving R, Zirbel-Donisch S: Development and enhancement of self-esteem in children, *J Pediatr Health Care* 4(6):290-296, 1990.

Usdin G: Investing in the "emotional bank" concept, *Child Teens Today* 8(6):7, 1988.

Wolk S and others: Factors affecting parents perceptions of temperament in early infancy, *Am J Orthopsychiatry* 62(1):71-82, 1992.

BIBLIOGRAPHY

Allen LH and others: The interactive effects of dietary quality on the growth and attained size of young Mexican children, *Am J Clin Nutr* 56(2):353-364, 1992.

Baillargeon R, DeVos J: Object permanence in young infants: further evidence, *Child Dev* 62(6):1227-1246, 1991.

Bantz DL, Siktberg L: Teaching families to evaluate age-appropriate toys, *J Pediatr Health Care* 7:111-114, 1993.

Brown MS and others: Type A behavior in children: what a pediatric nurse practitioner needs to know, *J Pediatr Health Care* 3:131-136, 1989.

Busen NH: Societal values: a cause of stress in children, *J Pediatr Health Care* 2:300-306, 1988.

Carey WB: Temperament: a tool for coping with problem behavior, *Contemp Pediatr* 6(1):139-153, 1989.

Chess S, Thomas A: Temperamental differences: a critical concept in child health care, *Pediatr Nurs* 11:167-171, 1985.

Chess S, Thomas A: *Temperament in clinical practice,* New York, 1986, Guilford Press.

Derksen DJ and others: Children and the influence of the media, *Prim Care* 21(4):747-758, 1994.

Dixon SD, Stein MT: *Encounters with children: pediatric behavior and development,* ed 2, St Louis, 1992, Mosby.

Fabes RA, Eisenberg N: Young children's coping with interpersonal anger, *Child Dev* 63(1):116-128, 1992.

Flavell JH and others: Young children's understanding of different types of beliefs, *Child Dev* 63(4):960-977, 1992.

Garmezy N, Rutter M, editors: *Stress, coping, and development in children,* New York, 1989, McGraw-Hill.

Grey M, Hayman LL: Assessing stress in children: research and clinical implications, *J Pediatr Nurs* 2:316-327, 1987.

Health L, Bresolin L, Rinaldi R: Effects of media violence on children: a review of the literature, *Arch Gen Psychiatry* 46(4):376-379, 1989.

Henry J, Giordano B: Introduction—assessment of growth in infants and children: normal and abnormal patterns, *J Pediatr Health Care* 5:289-290, 1992.

Hobbie C: Relaxation-techniques for children and young people, *J Pediatr Health Care* 3:83-87, 1989.

Holaday B and others: Vygotsky's zone of proximal development: implications for nurse assistance of children's learning, *Issues Compr Pediatr Nurs* 17(1):15-27, 1994.

Houldin A, Fullard W, Heverly M: Toddler temperament and the quality of the child-rearing environment, *Pediatr Nurs* 15(5):491-496, 544, 1989.

Jessee PO: Nurses, children, and play, *Issues Compr Pediatr Nurs* 15(4):261-269, 1992.

Klein J and others: Adolescents' risky behavior and mass media use, *Pediatrics* 92(1):24-31, 1993.

Levine MD, Carey WB, Crocker AC: *Developmental-behavioral pediatrics,* ed 2, Philadelphia, 1992, WB Saunders.

Lewis M, Alessandri SM, Sullivan MW: Differences in shame and pride as a function of children's gender and task difficulty, *Child Dev* 63(3):630-638, 1992.

Lillard AS: Pretend play skills and the child's theory of mind, *Child Dev* 64(2):348-371, 1993.

Marino BL: Studying infant and toddler play, *J Pediatr Nurs* 6(1):16-20, 1991.

Mebert CJ: Dimensions of subjectivity in parents' ratings of infant temperament, *Child Dev* 62(2):352-361, 1991.

Morrow JD: The eyes have it: visual attention as an index of infant cognition, *J Pediatr Health Care* 7:150-155, 1993.

Robinson TN and others: Does television viewing increase obesity and reduce physical activity? Cross-sectional and longitudinal analyses among adolescent girls, *Pediatrics* 91:273-280, 1993.

Rollins J: Meeting the child's developmental needs through play. In Smith DP and others, editors: *Comprehensive child and family nursing skills,* St Louis, 1991, Mosby.

Rollins J: Nurses as gangbusters: a response to gang violence in America, *Pediatr Nurs* 19(6):559-567, 1993.

Sahler OJZ: Theories and concepts of development as they relate to pediatric practice. In Hoekelman RA and others, editors: *Primary pediatric care,* ed 3, St Louis, 1997, Mosby.

Sameroff AJ and others: Stability of intelligence from preschool to adolescence: the influence of social and family risk factors, *Child Dev* 64(1):80-97, 1993.

Shapiro CM, Flanigan MJ: Function of sleep, *Br Med J* 306:383-385, 1993.

Sieving R, Zirbel-Donisch S: Development and enhancement of self-esteem in children, *J Pediatr Health Care* 4(6):290-296, 1990.

Smitherman C: The lasting impact of fetal alcohol syndrome and fetal alcohol effect on children and adolescents, *J Pediatr Health Care* 8:121-126, 1994.

Stein KF: Schema model of self-concept, *Image J Nurs Sch* 27(3):187-193, 1995.

St Peters M and others: Television and families: what do young children watch with their parents? *Child Dev* 62(6):1409-1423, 1991.

Strayer J: Children's concordant emotions and cognitions in response to observed emotions, *Child Dev* 64(1):188-201, 1993.

Thomas RM: *Comparing theories of child development,* ed 3, Belmont, CA, 1992, Wadsworth.

Chapter 6

COMMUNICATION AND HEALTH ASSESSMENT OF THE CHILD AND FAMILY

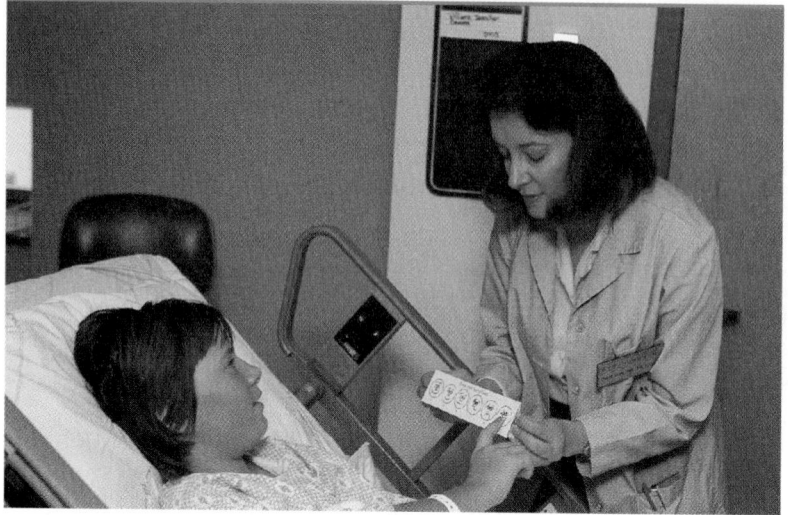

"A simple measurement scale using facial expressions helps children communicate the severity of their pain."

Donna L. Wong, author

RELATED TOPICS

COMMUNICATION

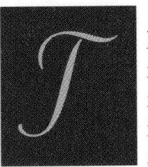he forms of communication may be verbal, nonverbal, or abstract. *Verbal communication* may involve language and its expression, vocalizations in the form of laughs, moans, or squalls, or the implications of what is not said in light of what has been said. *Nonverbal communication* is often called body language and includes gestures, movements, facial expressions, postures, and reactions. *Abstract communication* takes the form of play, artistic expression, symbols, photographs, and choice of clothing. Because it is possible to exert greater conscious control over verbal communication, it is a less reliable indicator of true feelings, especially with children.

Many factors influence the communication process. To be successful (gratifying), communication must be appropriate to the situation, properly timed, and clearly delivered. This implies that nurses understand and use techniques of effective communication, including listening. Verbal and nonverbal messages must be congruent; that is, two or more messages sent via different levels must not be contradictory.

VERBAL COMMUNICATION— THE POWER OF WORDS

Words shape reality, and thus they hold tremendous power. A person can change another's perception of reality by the choice of words that are used. For example, if the diagnosis of cancer is always referred to as a tumor, cyst, malignancy, or carcinoma, patients may never really know that they have cancer. Consequently, they may assume less responsibility for their care than if they were aware of the seriousness of the condition. By learning to recognize how patients and health professionals use language to manipulate reality, one can also learn how to change perceptions and communicate more effectively.

Avoidance Language

The most common way that people try to alter reality is by avoiding words that truly describe it. For example, euphemisms such as "passed on" are used instead of "death." Avoidance language indicates that a person wants to hide something, particularly feelings. As a rule, accepting a person's use of euphemisms only serves to perpetuate the fears and never helps the person deal with them. In contrast, use of straightforward, precise, descriptive language lends perspective to the situation and allows the person to discuss the fears. Most often, imagined fears are much worse than reality.

Distancing Language

People may use impersonal words, such as "it" or "others," to shield themselves from the painful reality of a situation. For example, parents may state that they know *someone* with a child who is slow, when they may actually be talking about personal fears regarding *their* child. By realizing that the parents may need to talk about this difficult subject, the nurse can provide sensitive statements that ease them into discussing their situation.

One of the dangers in supporting distancing language is that the person may effectively deny that a problem exists. To return to the previous example, if the issue of retardation is never approached directly but is allowed to be "someone else's problem," the parents may not be able to make decisions for special schools or individualized training.

Sometimes distancing is desirable because the topic may be too painful to discuss directly. The use of the third-person technique (p. 116) may be very therapeutic in allowing an individual the opportunity to indirectly approach a subject and receive feedback but still remain in control.

NONVERBAL COMMUNICATION— PARALANGUAGE

In addition to the spoken word, messages are also relayed through nonverbal means, or *paralanguage*—the pitch, pause, intonation, rate, volume, and stress apparent in speech. Young children become very adept at understanding paralanguage; long before they know the meaning of words, they sense anxiety or fear by the rise in pitch or the accelerated rate of the parent's voice. By careful observation of the spoken word, nurses can better understand the meaning of another's verbal message and more accurately control their own paralanguage.

Because most people do not exert conscious control over their paralanguage, it is a valuable clue to feelings and concerns. For example, *pausing* may signify a need to formulate thoughts, recall information, or fabricate a story. Frequent pauses often make the speaker sound unsure. Long pauses may mean that the individual needs more information.

Rate is another characteristic that gives unspoken messages. Talking too fast usually makes the speaker sound glib and insensitive. Talking slowly with a firm tone and appropriate pauses conveys authority. Therefore, a person is much more likely to "hear" instructions if the latter approach is used. Children in particular respond attentively to a slow, even, steady voice.

Confirming and Disconfirming Behaviors

People respond to each other through *confirming behaviors,* such as nodding the head, using direct eye contact, repeating or requesting clarification, and making appropriate comments, or *disconfirming behaviors,* such as tapping fingers or a foot, turning away from the speaker, avoiding eye contact, and interrupting (Heineken and Roberts, 1983). Because there is a reciprocal relationship between such behaviors, nurses need to use confirming behaviors to receive confirmation in return. This "mirroring" effect is particularly evident in children because of their sensitivity to nonverbal cues.

GUIDELINES FOR COMMUNICATION AND INTERVIEWING

The most widely used method of communicating with parents on a professional basis is the interview process. Unlike social conversation, interviewing is a specific form of goal-directed communication. As nurses converse with children and adults, they focus on the individuals to determine the kind of persons they are, their usual mode of handling problems, whether help is needed, and the way in which they react to counseling. Developing interviewing skills requires time and practice, but following some guiding principles can facilitate this process.

ESTABLISHING A SETTING FOR COMMUNICATION

Appropriate Introduction

Nurses should introduce themselves to, and ask the name of, each family member who is present (see Thinking Critically About . . . box). Address parents or other adults using their appropriate titles, such as "Mr." and "Mrs.," unless they specify a preferred name. Record the preferred name on the medical record. Using formal address or their preferred names, rather than using first names or "mom" or "dad," conveys respect and regard for the parents or other caregivers and the critical role they play in the lives of their children (Leff and Walizer, 1992).

At the beginning of the visit, include children in the interaction by asking them their name, age, and other information. Nurses often direct all questions to adults, even when children are old enough to speak for themselves. This serves to terminate one extremely valuable source of information: the patient. When the child is included, follow the general rules for communicating with children (p. 114).

THINKING CRITICALLY ABOUT . . .
Nurses' Form of Address

Language (and dress) convey information about age, class, status, education, role, and professional autonomy. Campbell-Heider and Hart (1993) contend that nurses' use of "Ms.," "Mr.," "Mrs.," "Nurse," or "Doctor" maintains a formality that suggests a professional status. In contrast, when nurses introduce themselves to families by their first names, they encourage a social relationship that is quickly enhanced with informal conversation, especially if it is about the nurse. Nurses may also assume a subordinate position when they address physicians as "Doctor" but the physicians use the nurses' first names. One study found that parents perceived nurses as "pleasant servants" and relied on physicians for important information about their child's progress (McBurney and Schultz, 1993). Could informal addresses by nurses contribute to this perception of them as "servants?"

With children we might argue that using first names is friendly and less threatening. But consider children's usual forms of address for professionals and adult relatives and friends. If first names are used, they are often preceded with "Doctor," "Miss," "Coach," or "Aunt." In many cultures respect for elders must include formal address.

Think about the form of address you use. Is it parallel with forms of address used by other professionals and families? Do nurses with doctorates use the title "Doctor?" Ask for their opinions and experiences regarding using the title. Try using more formal styles of address, such as "Ms." or "Nurse" with your surname, and note the reactions of others. Do you think professionalism and status are influenced by form of address?

Role Clarification and Explanation of the Interview

During the introduction it is also necessary to clarify the nurse's particular role in the health setting. For example, nurses performing interviews may be pediatric nurse practitioners, inpatient staff nurses, clinic nurses, office nurses, visiting nurses, or school nurses. A parent is much more likely to reveal personal information about the child and family if the relevance and importance of the interview are stressed. If this is not done, parents may refuse to elaborate on certain areas because they feel it has no bearing on the "problem." In addition, because more than one member of the health team may take a history during the course of a hospital admission, it is important to clarify the reason for each interview.

Another reason for role clarification is education of the health consumer. With expanded roles in nursing, it is not unusual for families to think that the examiner is a physician rather than a nurse. Role clarification is especially important because some parents may feel deceived if they later are made aware of the nurse's identity. The general consumer acceptance of pediatric nurse practitioners (PNPs) has been very favorable, so it is also important to acknowledge their expertise by emphasizing PNPs' role.

Preliminary Acquaintance

To make the family feel at ease and to develop rapport, begin the interview with some general conversation. The opening statements should be general but still informative. Comments such as "How have things been since your last visit?"

"Tell me about Johnny," or (to the child) "What do you think is going to happen today?" allow the parent or child to express the main concern in a casual, relaxed atmosphere.

The preliminary acquaintance conversation also reveals how responsive the informant may be to questions. For example, using open-ended statements, such as "Tell me about the baby," may lead the parent into a lengthy detailed discussion. In this case direct questions toward specific answers to avoid irrelevant remarks. At other times a parent may respond to open-ended questions with only minimal information, in which case continue to use open-ended questions rather than "yes" or "no" type questions.

Assurance of Privacy and Confidentiality

The place where the interview is conducted is almost as important as the interview itself. The physical environment should allow for as much privacy as possible, with distractions, such as interruptions, noise, or other visible activity, kept to a minimum. At times it may be necessary to turn off a television or radio. The environment should also have some play provision for young children to keep them occupied during the parent-nurse interview (Fig. 6-1). Parents who are constantly interrupted by their children are unable to concentrate fully on the questions asked of them and tend to give short answers to terminate the interview as quickly as possible. (See Critical Thinking Exercise.)

Confidentiality is another essential component of the initial phase of the interview. Since the interview is usually shared with other members of the health team or the teacher (as in the case of students), be certain to inform the parents of the confidential limits of the conversation. If there is concern regarding confidentiality in a situation, such as talking to a parent suspected of child abuse or a teenager contemplating suicide, deal with this directly and inform the person that in such instances confidentiality cannot be ensured.

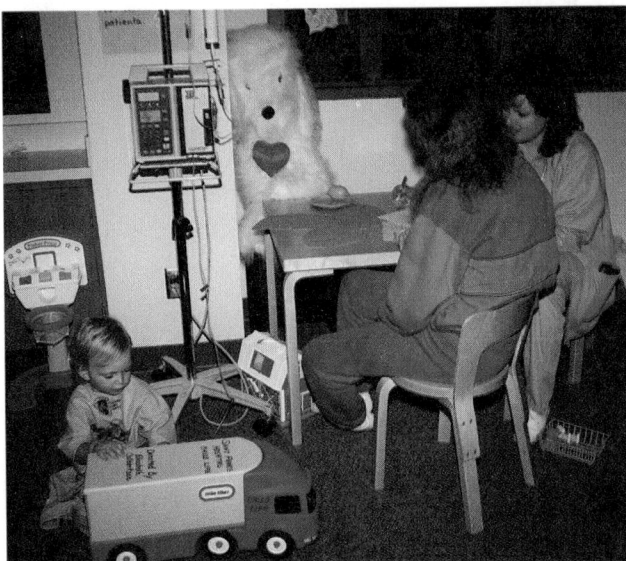

FIG. 6-1. Child plays while nurse interviews parent.

COMMUNICATING WITH FAMILIES

COMMUNICATING WITH PARENTS

Although the parent and child are separate and distinct individuals, relationships with the child are frequently mediated via the parent, particularly in the case of younger children. For the most part, information about the child is acquired by direct observation or is communicated to the nurse by the parents. Usually it can be assumed that because of the close contact with the child, the parent gives reliable information. Making an assessment of the child requires input from the child (verbal and nonverbal), information from the parent, and the nurse's own observations of the child and interpretation of the relationship between the child and the parent. Counseling and guidance must be directed to the caregiver of infants and small children; when children are old enough to be active participants in their own health maintenance, the parent becomes a collaborator in health care.

Encouraging the Parent to Talk

Interviewing parents not only offers the opportunity to determine the health and developmental status of the child, but also offers information about factors that influence the child's life. Whatever the parent sees as a problem should be a concern of the nurse. These problems are not always easy to identify. Nurses need to be alert for clues and signals by which a parent communicates worries and anxieties. Careful phrasing with broad open-ended questions such as "What is Jimmy eating now?" provides more information than several single-

---

CRITICAL THINKING EXERCISE

The Interview

During your interview with Ms. Gaines, 2½-year-old Jesse continually interrupts the conversation. Although Ms. Gaines has told her several times to be quiet, the interruptions continue. Frustrated, the mother states firmly, "If you don't be good, the nurse will give you a shot." Jesse begins to cry softly and hugs her mother's legs. Your most appropriate response is to:

1. State: "Ms. Gaines, don't threaten Jesse that way. Her behavior isn't bothering me."
2. Do nothing, because Jesse has become quiet.
3. State: "Jesse, nurses don't give needles because children are not being quiet. Here are paper and crayons to draw some pictures while your mom and I talk."
4. Hug Jesse and give her crayons and paper to draw.

The correct answer is three. The threat of injections or other painful or frightening procedures should never be used to gain a child's cooperation. You want to reassure Jesse about this, but at the same time reinforce the need for her to be quiet. Providing play materials helps keep her occupied.

Although the other responses may seem appropriate, they fail to remove the threat of a "shot" to Jesse. In particular, the first response can alienate your relationship with the parent. It also dismisses the issue that the interruptions do bother Ms. Gaines and most likely affect the quality of the interview.

answer questions such as "Is Jimmy eating what the rest of the family eats?"

Sometimes the parent will take the lead without prompting. At other times it may be necessary to direct another question on the basis of an observation such as "Connie seems unhappy today" or "How do you feel when David cries?" If the parent appears to be tired or distraught, consider asking, "What do you do to relax?" or "What help do you have with the children?" A comment such as "You handle the baby very well. What kinds of experience have you had with babies?" to new parents who appear comfortable with their first child gives positive reinforcement and provides an opening for any questions they might have regarding the care of the infant. Often all that is required to keep parents talking is a nod or saying "yes" or "uh-huh."

When attempting to elicit feelings and covert problem areas, avoid closed-ended questions that begin with "Does . . .," "Did . . .," or "Is . . .," which usually require only a single response. In addition, asking questions such as "Does your son have any problems at school?" subtly implies a lack of parental skills and evokes defensiveness. Instead, say, "What . . .," "How . . .," "Tell me about . . ." and to encourage elaboration with "You were saying . . .," "You say that . . .," or reflecting back a key word. Open-ended questions are nonthreatening and encourage description.

Directing the Focus

The ability to direct the focus of the interview while allowing for maximum freedom of expression is one of the most difficult goals in effective communication. One approach is the use of open-ended or broad questions, followed by guiding statements. For example, if the parent proceeds to list the other children by name, say, "Tell me their ages, too." If the parent continues to describe each child indepth, which is not the purpose of the interview, the nurse can redirect the focus by stating, "Lets talk about the other children later. You were beginning to tell me about Paul's activities at school." This approach conveys interest in the other children but focuses the assessment on the patient.

In the event that the parent has suggested that a problem exists with one of the other children, reintroduce this subject at the end of the interview to assess the need for further family follow-up. Saying to the parent, "Before, you were mentioning that your older son is having trouble in school. Tell me what you see as the problem," reintroduces this subject but only in terms of the possible problem.

Listening and Cultural Awareness

Listening is the most important component of effective communication. When listening is truly aimed at understanding the client, it is an active process that requires concentration and attention to all aspects of the conversation—verbal, nonverbal, and abstract. Major blocks to listening are environmental distraction and premature judgment.

The attitudes and feelings of the nurse are easily injected into an interview. Often nurses' perceptions of a parent's behavior are influenced by their own perceptions, prejudices, and assumptions, which may include racial, religious, and cultural stereotypes. What may be interpreted as passive hostility or disinterest in a parent may be shyness or an expression of anxiety. For example, in Western cultures eye contact and

directness are signs of paying attention. However, in many non-Western cultures, including that of Native Americans, directness, such as looking someone in the eye, is considered rude. Children are taught to avert their gaze and to look down when being addressed by an adult, especially one with authority (Sloat and Matsuura, 1990). Therefore judgments about "listening," as well as verbal interactions, need to be made with an appreciation of cultural differences (see Guidelines box and Chapter 3).

Although it is necessary to make some preliminary judgments, listen with as much objectivity as possible by clarifying meanings and attempting to see the situation from the parent's point of view. Effective interviewers use conscious control over their reactions, responses, and the techniques they use.

Minimum verbal activity with active listening facilitates parent involvement. It is tempting to spend time explaining, describing, and interpreting health information when the opportunity presents itself. However, it is possible to provide effective health education by timing the information prop-

GUIDELINES
Culturally Sensitive Interactions

Nonverbal Strategies

Invite family members to choose where they would like to sit or stand, allowing them to select a comfortable distance.

Observe interactions with others to determine which body gestures (e.g., shaking hands) are acceptable and appropriate. Ask when in doubt.

Avoid appearing rushed.

Be an active listener.

Observe for cues regarding appropriate eye contact.

Learn appropriate use of pauses or interruptions for different cultures.

Ask for clarification if nonverbal meaning is unclear.

Verbal Strategies

Learn proper terms of address.

Use a positive tone of voice to convey interest.

Speak slowly and carefully, not loudly, when families have poor language comprehension.

Encourage questions.

Learn basic words and sentences of family's language, if possible.

Avoid professional terms.

When asking questions, tell family why the questions are being asked, the way in which the information they provide will be used, and how it might benefit their child.

Repeat important information more than once.

Always give the reason or purpose for a treatment or prescription.

Use information written in family's language.

Offer the services of an interpreter when necessary (see p. 112).

Learn from families and representatives of their culture methods of communicating information without creating discomfort.

Address intergenerational needs (e.g., family's need to consult with others).

Be sincere, open, and honest and, when appropriate, share personal experiences, beliefs, and practices to establish rapport and trust.

erly and presenting only as much as is necessary at the moment.

Careful listening facilitates the use of clues, verbal leads, or signals from the interviewee to move the interview along. Frequent references to an area of concern, repetition of certain key words, and/or a special emphasis on something or someone serve as cues to the interviewer for the direction of inquiry. Concerns and anxieties are usually mentioned in a casual, offhand manner. Even though they are casual, they are important and deserve careful scrutiny to identify problem areas. For example, a parent who is concerned about a child's habit of bed-wetting may casually mention that the child's bed was "wet this morning."

Because the interview is almost always triangular—between the nurse, parent, and child—the parent may wish to convey information in such a way as to prevent the child from hearing it. This requires active listening on the part of the nurse to hear the unspoken message. The following example illustrates this point:

> During a routine health visit, the nurse performed a complete history and physical examination on a 4-year-old girl. The child was accompanied by her mother, who appeared to be a reliable, well-informed, and talkative informant. During the child's birth history, the mother gave all the information asked. However, during the family history, the mother stated to the nurse, "I had a hysterectomy 6 years ago." Because the nurse gave no indication of acknowledging the significance of this statement, the mother repeated it, only this time she stressed the "6 years." The nurse, who had not been listening as attentively as she should have, realized that the mother was telling her something very important. The mother raised her eyebrows and gently shook her head "no," warning the nurse not to explore this area too openly. The nurse correctly read the cues and stated, "Let's return to your health history later."
>
> At the completion of the physical examination, the nurse brought the child to the health center's playroom and took the opportunity to investigate this contradictory information of a "4-year-old child born to a woman with a hysterectomy 6 years ago." The mother revealed that the child was adopted. The mother was greatly concerned about the fact that the child was unaware of this and requested the nurse's advice.
>
> Fortunately, the nurse had "listened" carefully enough to realize the significance of this woman's concern and allowed her the opportunity to discuss it in private.

Listening is also helpful in assessing reliability. For example, the answers elicited at the beginning of the interview may differ from those at the end, when the parent feels more confident in revealing problems. It is important to identify any discrepancies and reintroduce those topics for further investigation.

Using Silence

Silence as a response is often one of the most difficult interviewing techniques to learn. It requires a sense of confidence and comfort on the part of the interviewer to allow the interviewee space in which to think without interruptions. Silence permits the interviewee to sort out thoughts and feelings and search for responses to questions. It also allows for sharing of feelings in which two or more people absorb the emotion to its depth.

Sometimes it is necessary to break the silence and reopen communication. Do this in a way that encourages the person to continue talking about what is considered important. Breaking a silence by introducing a new topic or by prolonged talking essentially terminates the interviewee's opportunity to use the silence. Suggestions for breaking the silence include statements such as "Is there anything else you wish to say?" "I see you find it difficult to continue; how may I help?" or "I don't know what this silence means. Perhaps there is something you would like to put into words but find difficult to say."

Being Empathic

Empathy is the capacity to understand what another person is experiencing from within that person's frame of reference; it is often described as the ability to put oneself in another's shoes. The essence of empathic interaction is accurately understanding another's feelings (Bellet and Maloney, 1991). Empathy differs from *sympathy,* which is *having* feelings or emotions in common with another person, rather than *understanding* those feelings. Sympathy is not therapeutic in the helping relationship, because it leads to feeling emotionally overinvolved, and potentially to professional burnout (Holden, 1990).

Of the different types of support, such as empathy, encouragement, or reassurance, empathy is the most beneficial but least used form (Wissow, Roter, and Wilson, 1994). Some individuals are naturally empathic; however, empathy can be learned by attending to the verbal and nonverbal language of the interviewee. *Neurolinguistic programming (NLP)* is concerned with the *manner* of accessing and understanding information and is an excellent method of increasing empathic communication. Although people may use all the following sensory modalities to communicate, usually one modality predominates: visual, auditory, or kinesthetic. The specific sensory mode is identified by observing the type of verbs, adjectives, and adverbs the person uses and then using this mode in responding to the individual. For example, if a person using the visual mode states, "I can't *see* why you have to perform these procedures on my child," a response using the same mode is, "What do you *see* as the reason for them?"

Defining the Problem

To arrive at a solution to a problem, the nurse and the parent must agree that a problem exists. Sometimes the parent may believe that there is a problem that the nurse is unable to see. For example, a mother was overly concerned about every small sniffle, sneeze, or cough in her infant, who had been carefully examined and found to be healthy with no evidence of a respiratory problem. On careful questioning, the nurse discovered that a previous child had died of pneumonia in infancy. Consequently the nurse was better able to understand the mother's concern and could help the mother deal with her special anxieties about her infant; the nurse could also teach her how to recognize any need for concern.

Occasionally the nurse identifies a problem that the parent denies exists. In this case pursue the situation and either find a way to deal with it or enlist the aid of other health team members. For example, the parents of a child with Down syndrome may refuse to believe that their child is different from any other child of the same age. They may say, "He is just a little slow," or "All the child needs to do is to try harder." A child with an obvious behavior problem may be described by the parents as "stubborn." Such statements may be clues that the parents have not progressed past the stage of denial in adjusting to the condition.

Solving the Problem

Once the problem is identified and agreed on by the parent and the nurse, they can begin to arrive at a solution. A parent who is included in the problem-solving process is more apt to follow through with a course of action. Such questions as "What have you tried so far?" or "What have you thought about doing?" provide leads for exploration and give the parents the feeling that their ideas and solutions are worthwhile. These can be followed by "What prevents you from trying that?" "That sounds like a good plan," and "You seem to be stumped. Have you considered trying this?" Such approaches encourage active participation and reinforce rather than belittle parents' efforts to solve their problems.

Sometimes the parents arrive at a solution that the nurse does not consider the best alternative. If it can be ascertained that it will do no harm and if the parents are convinced of its merits, it is usually best to allow them to continue with the plan. A course of action is more likely to be carried out when parents can reach their own conclusions. However, when parental decisions may be hazardous, nurses are obligated to discuss the risks with the family and try to reach a more beneficial solution. Whenever possible, decisions should be theirs, with the nurse serving as a *facilitator* in problem solving.

Providing Anticipatory Guidance

The ideal way to handle a situation is to deal with it *before* it becomes a problem. The best preventive measure is anticipatory guidance. Traditionally, anticipatory guidance has focused on providing families with information on normal growth and development, and nurturing childrearing practices. For example, one of the most significant areas in pediatrics is injury prevention. Beginning prenatally, parents need specific instructions on home safety. Because of the child's maturing developmental skills, home safety changes must be implemented early to minimize risks to the child.

Many normal developmental changes can disturb unprepared parents, such as a toddler's diminished appetite, negativism, altered sleeping patterns, and anxiety toward strangers. Such topics are discussed in the chapters on health promotion to provide the nurse with knowledge to counsel parents.

However, anticipatory guidance should extend beyond giving information to empowering families to use the information as a means of building competence in their parenting abilities. To achieve this level of anticipatory guidance, (Gorzka and others, 1991):

- Base interventions on needs identified by the family, not by the professional
- View the family as competent or as having the ability to be competent
- Provide opportunities for the family to achieve competence

Avoiding Blocks to Communication

A number of blocks to communication can adversely affect the quality of the helping relationship. Many of these blocks are initiated by the interviewer, such as giving unrestricted advice or forming prejudged conclusions. Another type of block occurs primarily with the interviewees and deals with information overload. When individuals are presented with too much information or information that is overwhelming,

---

BLOCKS TO COMMUNICATION

Socializing
Giving unrestricted and sometimes unasked-for advice
Offering premature or inappropriate reassurance
Giving overready encouragement
Defending a situation or opinion
Using stereotyped comments or cliches
Limiting expression of emotion by asking directed, closed-ended questions
Interrupting and finishing the person's sentence
Talking more than the interviewee
Forming prejudged conclusions
Deliberately changing the focus

Signs of Information Overload

Long periods of silence
Wide eyes and fixed facial expression
Constant fidgeting or attempting to move away
Nervous habits (e.g., tapping, playing with hair)
Sudden disruptions (e.g., asking to go to the bathroom)
Looking around
Yawning, eyes drooping
Frequently looking at a watch or clock
Attempting to change topic of discussion

---

they will often demonstrate signals of increasing anxiety or decreasing attention. Such signals should alert the interviewer to give less information or to clarify what has been said. Some of the more common blocks to communication, including signs of information overload, are listed in the box.

Communication blocks can be corrected by careful analysis of the interview process. One of the best methods for improving interviewing skills is audiotape and/or videotape feedback. With supervision and guidance, the interviewer can recognize the blocks and consciously avoid them.

Communicating with Families through an Interpreter

Sometimes communication is impossible because two people speak different languages. In this case it is necessary to obtain information through a third party, the interpreter. When an interpreter is used, the same guidelines for interviewing are used. Specific guidelines for using an adult interpreter are presented in the Guidelines box.

Communicating with families through an interpreter requires sensitivity to cultural, legal, and ethical considerations. For example, in some cultures using a child as an interpreter is considered an insult to an adult, because children are expected to show respect by not questioning their elders. In some cultures class differences between the interpreter and the family may cause the family to feel intimidated and less inclined to offer information. Therefore choose the translator carefully, and provide time for the interpreter and family to establish rapport.

Issues of legal and ethical concerns may also arise. For example, in obtaining informed consent through an interpreter, it is important that the family be fully informed of all aspects of the particular procedure that they are consenting to. Issues of confidentiality may arise when family members related to another patient are asked to interpret for the family, thus

GUIDELINES
Using an Interpreter

Explain to interpreter the reason for the interview and the type of questions that will be asked.

Clarify whether a detailed or brief answer is required and whether the translated response can be general or literal.

Introduce interpreter to family and allow some time before the actual interview so that they can become acquainted.

Communicate directly with family members when asking questions to reinforce interest in them and to observe nonverbal expressions, but do not ignore interpreter.

Pose questions to elicit only one answer at a time, such as "Do you have pain?" rather than "Do you have any pain, tiredness, or loss of appetite?"

Refrain from interrupting family member and interpreter while they are conversing.

Avoid commenting to interpreter about family members, since they may understand some English.

Be aware that some medical words, such as "allergy," may have no similar word in another language; avoid medical jargon whenever possible.

Respect cultural differences; it is often best to pose questions about sex, marriage, or pregnancy indirectly—ask about "child's father" rather than "mother's husband."

Allow time following the interview for interpreter to share something that he or she felt could not be said earlier; ask about interpreter's impression of nonverbal clues to communication and family members' reliability or ease in revealing information.

Arrange for family to speak with same interpreter on subsequent visits whenever possible.

revealing sensitive information that may be shared with other families on the unit.

When no one else is available to translate, children within the family are often asked to assume this role. In this situation it is important to stress *literal* translation of parent responses. To maximize correct translations, it may be necessary to interrupt the parent and ask the child to translate every few sentences. When using children as interpreters, ask questions directed at specific answers and assess the interpreted translation in terms of nonverbal expressions of communication.*

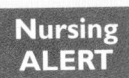

Nursing ALERT When using translated materials, such as a health history form, be sure the informant is literate in the foreign language.

COMMUNICATING WITH CHILDREN

Although the greatest amount of verbal communication may usually be carried out with the parent, do not exclude the child during the interview. Pay attention to infants and younger children through play or by occasionally directing questions or remarks to them. Include older children as active participants.

In communication with children of all ages, the nonverbal components of the communication process convey the most significant messages. It is difficult to disguise feelings, attitudes, and anxiety when relating to children. They are very alert to surroundings and attach meaning to every gesture and move that is made; this is particularly true of very young children.

Active attempts to make friends with children before they have had an opportunity to evaluate an unfamiliar person tend to increase their anxiety. A helpful tactic is to continue to talk to the child and parent but go about activities that do not involve the child directly, thus allowing the child to observe from a safe position. If the child has a special toy or doll, "talk" to the doll first. Ask simple questions such as "Does your teddy bear have a special name?" to ease the child into conversation. Other guidelines for communicating with children are presented in the Guidelines box on p. 114. Specific guidelines for preparing children for procedures, a common nursing function, are discussed in Chapter 22.

Communication Related to Development of Thought Processes

The normal development of language and thought offers a frame of reference for knowing how to communicate with children. Thought processes progress from concrete to functional and finally to abstract, formal operations.

Infancy. Because they are unable to use words, infants primarily use and understand nonverbal communication. Infants communicate their needs and feelings through nonverbal behaviors and vocalizations that can be interpreted by someone who is around them for a sufficient amount of time. Infants smile and coo when content and cry when distressed. Crying is provoked by unpleasant stimuli from inside or outside, such as hunger, pain, body restraint, or loneliness. Adults interpret this to mean that an infant needs something and consequently try to alleviate the discomfort and reduce tension. Crying (or the desire to cry) persists as a part of everyone's communication repertoire.

Infants respond to adults' nonverbal behaviors. They become quiet when they are cuddled, patted, or receive other forms of gentle, physical contact. They derive comfort from the sound of a voice, even though they do not understand the words that are spoken. Until infants reach the age at which they experience stranger anxiety, they readily respond to any firm, gentle handling and quiet, calm speech. Loud, harsh sounds and sudden movements are frightening.

Older infants' attentions are centered on themselves and their parents; therefore any stranger is a potential threat until proved otherwise. Holding out the hands and asking the child to "come" is seldom successful, especially if the infant is with the parent. If infants must be handled, simply pick them up firmly without gestures. Observe the position in which the parent holds the infant. Most infants have learned to prefer a particular position and manner of handling. In general, infants are more at ease upright than horizontal. Also, hold infants so that they can see their parents. Until they have developed the understanding that an object (in this case the parent) removed from sight can still be present, they have no way of knowing that the object is still there.

Early Childhood. Children under 5 years of age are egocentric. They see things only in relation to themselves and

*Interpreting services are also available through American Telephone and Telegraph (AT&T) by calling (800) 628-8486 or (800) 752-6096.

GUIDELINES
Communicating with Children

Allow children time to feel comfortable.

Avoid sudden or rapid advances, broad smiles, extended eye contact, or other gestures that may be seen as threatening.

Talk to the parent if child is initially shy.

Communicate through transition objects such as dolls, puppets, or stuffed animals before questioning a young child directly.

Give older children the opportunity to talk without the parents present.

Assume a position that is at eye level with child (Fig. 6-2).

Speak in a quiet, unhurried, and confident voice.

Speak clearly, be specific, use simple words, and short sentences.

State directions and suggestions *positively*.

Offer a choice only when one exists.

Be honest with children.

Allow them to express their concerns and fears.

Use a variety of communication techniques.

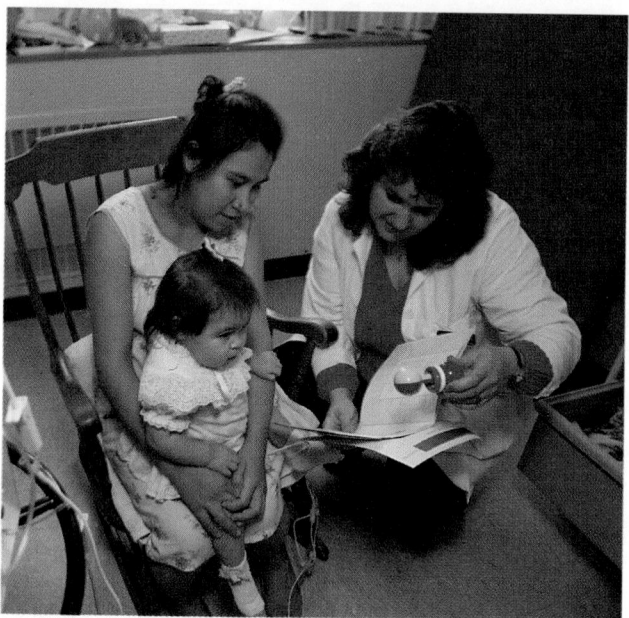

FIG. 6-2. Nurse assumes position at child's level.

from their point of view. Therefore focus communication on *them*. Tell them what they can do or how they will feel. Experiences of others are of no interest to them. It is futile to use another child's experience as an attempt to gain the cooperation of very small children. Allow them to touch and examine articles that will come in contact with them. A stethoscope bell will feel cold; palpating a neck might tickle. Although they have not yet acquired sufficient language skills to express their feelings and wants, toddlers are able to communicate effectively with their hands to transmit ideas without words. They push an unwanted object away, pull another person to show them something, point, and cover the mouth that is saying something they do not wish to hear.

Everything is direct and concrete to small children. They are unable to work with abstractions and interpret words literally. Analogies escape them because they are unable to separate fact from fantasy. For example, they attach literal meaning to such common phrases as "two-faced," "sticky fingers," or "coughing your head off." Children who are told they will get "a little stick in the arm" may not be able to envision an injection (Fig. 6-3). Therefore avoid using a phrase that might be misinterpreted by a small child (see Family Home Care box under Preparation for Procedures, Chapter 22).

Use language that is consistent with the child's developmental level. For example, in talking with a toddler, use simple, *short* sentences, repeat words that are *familiar* to the child, and limit descriptions to *concrete* explanations. Be certain that nonverbal messages are consistent with words and actions. For example, do not smile while doing something painful; children may think you enjoy hurting them.

Young children assign human attributes to inanimate ob-

jects. Consequently, they fear that objects may jump, bite, cut, or pinch all by themselves. Children do not know that these devices are unable to perform without human direction. To minimize their fear, keep unfamiliar equipment out of view until it is needed.

School-Age Years. Younger school-age children rely less on what they see and more on what they know when faced with new problems. They want explanations and reasons for everything but require no verification beyond that. They are interested in the functional aspect of all procedures, objects, and activities. They want to know why an object exists, why it is used, how it works, and the intent and purpose of its user. They need to know what is going to take place and why it is being done to *them* specifically. For example, to explain a procedure such as taking a blood pressure, show the child how squeezing the bulb pushes air into the cuff and makes the "silver" in the tube go up. Let the child operate the bulb. An explanation for the reason might be as simple as "I want to see how far the silver goes up when the cuff squeezes your arm." Consequently, the child becomes an enthusiastic participant.

School-age children have a heightened concern about body integrity. Because of the special importance and value they place on their body, they are overly sensitive to anything that constitutes a threat or suggestion of injury to it. This concern extends to their possessions also, so that they may appear to overreact to loss or threatened loss of treasured objects. Helping children to voice their concerns enables the nurse to provide reassurance and to implement activities that reduce their anxiety. For example, if a shy child dislikes being the center of attention, ignore that particular child by

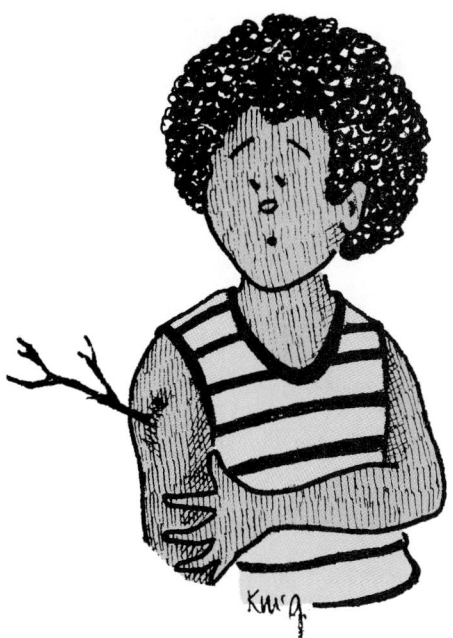

FIG. 6-3. A young child may take the expression "a little stick in the arm" literally.

talking and relating to other children in the family or group. When children feel more comfortable, they will usually interject personal ideas, feelings, and interpretations of events.

Older children have an adequate and satisfactory use of language. They still require relatively simple explanations, but their ability to think concretely can facilitate communication and explanation. Commonly they have sufficient experience with health and health workers to understand what is transpiring and generally what is expected of them.

Adolescence. As children move into adolescence, they fluctuate between child and adult thinking and behavior. They are riding a current that is moving them rapidly toward a maturity that may be beyond their coping ability. Therefore, when tensions rise, they may seek the security of the more familiar and comfortable expectations of childhood. Anticipating these shifts in identity allows the nurse to adjust the course of interaction to meet the needs of the moment. No single approach can be relied on consistently, and encountering cooperation, hostility, anger, bravado, and a variety of other behaviors and attitudes can be expected. It is as much a mistake to regard the adolescent as an adult with an adult's wisdom and control as it is to assume that the teenager has the concerns and expectations of a child.

Frequently adolescents are more willing to discuss their concerns with an adult outside the family, and they often welcome the opportunity to interact with a nurse. They are accepting of anyone who displays a genuine interest in them. However, adolescents are quick to reject persons who attempt to impose their values on them, whose interest is feigned, or who appear to have little respect for who they are and what they think or say.

As with all children, adolescents need to express their feelings. Generally, they talk quite freely when given an opportunity. However, what adolescents say cannot always be taken at face value. When emotional factors are involved, the feelings that are interjected into words are as significant as the words that are used. To give support, be attentive, try not to interrupt, and avoid comments or expressions that convey disapproval or surprise. Avoid prying and asking embarrassing questions, and resist any impulse to give advice. Frequently adolescents reveal their feelings or a source of concern or ask a question when they are involved in routine matters such as a physical assessment.

Teenagers characteristically have a language and culture all their own that further sets them apart. To avoid misinterpretation, clarify terms frequently. Occasionally adolescents refuse to answer or answer only in monosyllables. Usually this happens when they are opposed to the contact or do not yet feel safe enough to reveal themselves. In this instance confine discussions to irrelevant topics to reduce the element of threat until such time as they feel more secure. Be alert for signals indicating they are ready to talk. The major sources of concern for adolescents are attitudes and feelings toward sex, substance abuse, relationships with parents, peer-group acceptance, and developing a sense of identity.

Interviewing the adolescent presents some special situations. The first may be whether to talk with the adolescent alone, with the adolescent and parents together, or with each person individually. Of course, if the adolescent is alone, there is no question, except whether to suggest to the teenager that the parents may be interviewed at another time. If the parents and teenager are together, talking with the adolescent first has the advantage of immediately identifying with the young person, thus fostering the interpersonal relationship. However, talking with the parents initially may provide insight into the family relationship. In either case, give both parties an opportunity to be included in the interview. If time constraints are important, such as during history taking, clarify these at the onset to avoid appearing to "take sides" by talking more with one person than with the other.

Confidentiality is of great important when interviewing adolescents. Explain to parents and teenagers the limits of confidentiality, specifically that young persons' disclosures will not be shared unless they indicate a need for intervention, as in the case of suicidal behavior.

Another dilemma in interviewing adolescents is that two views of a problem frequently exist—the teenager's and the parents'. Clarification of the problem is a major task. However, providing both parties with an opportunity to discuss their perceptions in an open and unbiased atmosphere can, by itself, be therapeutic. Demonstrating positive communication skills can help families communicate more effectively (see Guidelines box on p. 117).

COMMUNICATION TECHNIQUES

In addition to such conventional interviewing methods as reflection and open-ended questions, a number of techniques encourage family members to express their thoughts and feelings in a less directive and confrontational manner. Several

CREATIVE COMMUNICATION TECHNIQUES WITH CHILDREN

Verbal Techniques

"I" Messages

Relate a feeling about a behavior in terms of "I."
Describe effect behavior had on the person.
Avoid use of "you."
  "You" messages are judgmental and provoke defensiveness.
  Example: "You" message—"You are being very uncooperative about doing your treatments."
  Example: "I" message—"I am concerned about how the treatments are going because I want to see you get better."

Third-Person Technique

Involves expressing a feeling in terms of a third person ("he," "she," "they").
Is less threatening than directly asking children how they feel because it gives them an opportunity to agree or disagree without being defensive.
  Example: "Sometimes when a person is sick a lot, he feels angry and sad because he cannot do what others can." Either wait silently for a response or encourage a reply with a statement such as "Did you ever feel that way?"
Approach allows children three choices: (1) to agree and, hopefully, express how they feel; (2) to disagree; or (3) to remain silent, in which case they probably have such feelings but are unable to express them at this time.

Facilitative Responding

Involves careful listening and reflecting back to patients the feelings and content of their statements.
Responses are empathic and nonjudgmental, and legitimize the person's feelings.
Formula for facilitative responses: "You feel _____ because _____."
  Example: If child states, "I hate coming to the hospital and getting needles," a facilitative response is, "You feel unhappy because of all the things that are done to you."

Storytelling

Uses the language of children to probe into areas of their thinking while bypassing conscious inhibitions or fears.
Simplest technique is asking children to relate a story about an event, such as "being in the hospital."
Other approaches:
  Show children a picture of a particular event, such as a child in a hospital with other people in the room, and ask them to describe the scene.
  Cut out comic strips, remove words, and have child add statements for scenes.

Mutual Storytelling

Reveals child's thinking and attempts to change child's perceptions or fears by retelling a somewhat different story (more therapeutic approach than storytelling).
Begins by asking child to tell a story about something, followed by another story told by the nurse that is similar to child's tale but with differences that help child in problem areas.
  Example: Child's story is about going to the hospital and never seeing his or her parents again. Nurse's story is also about a child (using different names but similar circumstances) in a hospital whose parents visit everyday, but in the evening after work until the child is better and goes home with them.

Bibliotherapy

Uses books in a therapeutic and supportive process.*
Provides children with an opportunity to explore an event that is similar to their own but sufficiently different to allow them to distance selves from it and remain in control.

General guidelines for using bibliotherapy are:
  Assess child's emotional and cognitive development in terms of readiness to understand the book's message.
  Be familiar with the book's content (intended message or purpose) and the age for which it is written.
  Read the book to the child if child is unable to read.
  Explore the meaning of the book with the child by having child:
    Retell the story
    Read a special section with the nurse or parent
    Draw a picture related to the story and discuss the drawing
    Talk about the characters
    Summarize the moral or meaning of the story

Dreams

Often reveal unconscious and repressed thoughts and feelings.
  Ask child to talk about a dream or nightmare.
  Explore with child what meaning dream could have.

"What If" Questions

Encourage child to explore potential situations and to consider different problem-solving options.
  Example: "What if you got sick and had to go the hospital?" Children's responses reveal what they know already and what they are curious about; provide opportunity for helping children learn coping skills, especially in potentially dangerous situations.

Three Wishes

Involves asking, "If you could have any three things in the world, what would they be?"
If child answers, "That all my wishes come true," ask child for specific wishes.

Rating Game

Uses some type of rating scale (numbers, sad to happy faces) to rate an event or feeling.
  Example: Instead of asking youngsters how they feel, ask how their day has been "on a scale of 1 to 10, with 10 being the best."

Word Association Game

Involves stating key words and asking children to say the first word they think of when they hear the word.
  Start with neutral words and then introduce more anxiety-producing words, such as "illness," "needles," "hospitals," and "operation."
  Select key words that relate to some event in child's life that is relevant.

Sentence Completion

Involves presenting a partial statement and having child complete it.
Some sample statements are following:
  The thing I like best (least) about school is _____.

  The best (worst) age to be is _____.

  The most (least) fun thing I ever did was _____.

  The thing I like most (least) about my parents is _____.

  The one thing I would change about my family is _____.

  If I could be anything I wanted, I would be _____.

  The thing I like most (least) about myself is _____.

*See Sources for Books for Bibliotherapy in Bibliography at end of chapter.

CREATIVE COMMUNICATION TECHNIQUES WITH CHILDREN—cont'd

Pros and Cons

Involves selecting a topic, such as "being in the hospital," and having child list "five good things and five bad things" about it.

Is an exceptionally valuable technique when applied to relationships, such as things family members like and dislike about each other.

Nonverbal Techniques

Writing

Is an alternative communication approach for older children and adults.

Specific suggestions include:

Keep a journal or diary.

Write down feelings or thoughts that are difficult to express.

Write "letters" that are never mailed (a variation is making up a "pen pal" to write to).

Keep an account of child's progress from both a physical and an emotional viewpoint.

Drawing

Is one of the most valuable forms of communication—both nonverbal (from looking at the drawing) and verbal (from child's story of the picture).

Children's drawings tell a great deal about them because they are projections of their inner selves.

Spontaneous drawing involves giving child a variety of art supplies and providing the opportunity to draw.

Directed drawing involves a more specific direction, such as "draw a person" or the "three themes" approach (state three things about child and ask child to choose one and draw a picture) (Fig. 6-4).

GUIDELINES FOR EVALUATING DRAWINGS:

Use spontaneous drawings and evaluate more than one drawing whenever possible.

Interpret drawings in light of other available information about child and family.

Interpret drawings as a whole rather than on specific details of the drawing.

Consider individual elements of the drawing that may be significant:

Sex of figure drawn first—Usually relates to child's perception of own sex role.

Size of individual figures—Expresses importance, power, or authority.

Order in which figures are drawn—Expresses priority in terms of importance.

Child's position in relation to other family members—Expresses feelings of status or alliance.

Exclusion of a member—May denote feeling of not belonging or desire to eliminate.

Accentuated parts—Usually express concern for areas of special importance (e.g., large hands may be a sign of aggression).

Absence of or rudimentary arms and hands—Suggest timidity, passivity, or intellectual immaturity; tiny, unstable feet may be an expression of insecurity, and hidden hands may mean guilt feelings.

Placement of drawing on the page and type of stroke—Free use of paper and firm, continuous strokes express security, whereas drawings restricted to a small area and lightly drawn in broken or wavering lines may be a sign of insecurity.

Erasures, shading, or cross-hatching—Expresses ambivalence, concern, or anxiety with a particular area.

Magic

Uses simple magic tricks to help establish rapport with child, encourage compliance with health interventions, and provide effective distraction during painful procedures.

Although "magician" talks, no verbal response from child is required.

Play

Is universal language and "work" of children.

Tells a great deal about children because they project their inner selves through the activity.

Spontaneous play involves giving child a variety of play materials and providing the opportunity to play.

Directed play involves a more specific direction, such as providing medical equipment or a dollhouse for focused reasons, such as exploring child's fear of injections or exploring family relationships.

 GUIDELINES
Communicating with Adolescents

Build a Foundation

Spend time together.

Encourage expression of ideas and feelings.

Respect their views.

Tolerate differences.

Praise good points.

Respect their privacy.

Set a good example.

Communicate Effectively

Give undivided attention.

Listen, listen, listen.

Be courteous, calm, and open-minded.

Try not to overreact. If you do, take a break.

Avoiding judging or criticizing.

Avoid the "third degree" of continuous questioning.

Choose important issues when taking a stand.

After taking a stand:

Think through all options.

Make expectations clear.

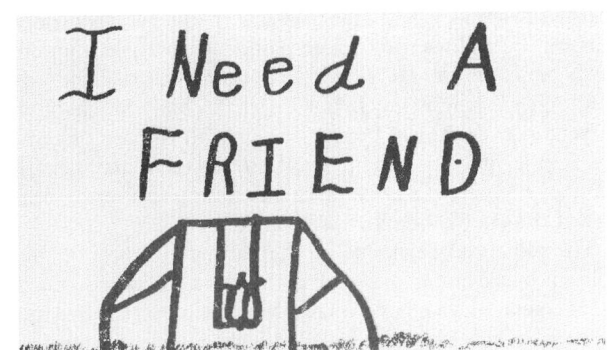

FIG. 6-4. Using the three themes approach, this child chose the theme, "the first day of school." The drawing and title reveal the child's loneliness and insecurity in a new setting.

approaches are projective—they present nonspecific material that enables individuals to externalize or project inner aspects of themselves to others.

A variety of verbal techniques can be used to encourage communication. Some of these techniques can be used to pose questions or explore concerns in a less threatening manner. Others can be presented as "word games," which are often well received by children. However, for many children and adults, talking about feelings is difficult and verbal communication may be more stressful than supportive. In such instances several nonverbal techniques can be used to encourage communication.

Both verbal and nonverbal techniques are described in the box on pp. 116-117. Because of the importance of play in communicating with children, play is discussed more extensively below. Any of the verbal or nonverbal techniques can give rise to strong feelings that surface unexpectedly. Be prepared to handle them or to recognize when issues go beyond your ability to deal with them. At that point, consider an appropriate referral.

Play

Play is a universal language of children. It is one of the most important forms of communication and can be an effective technique in relating to them. Clues about physical, intellectual, and social developmental progress can often be gleaned from the form and complexity of a child's play behaviors. Play requires a minimum of equipment or none at all. Therapeutic play is often used to reduce the trauma of illness and hospitalization (Chapter 21) and to prepare children for therapeutic procedures (Chapter 22).

Because their ability to perceive precedes their ability to transmit, small infants respond to activities that register on their senses. Patting, stroking, and other skin play convey messages. Repetitive actions, such as stretching infants' arms out to the side while they are lying on their back and then folding them across the chest or raising and revolving the legs in a bicycling motion, will elicit pleasurable sounds. Colorful items to catch the eye or interesting sounds such as a ticking clock, chimes, bells, or singing can be used to attract children's attention.

Older infants respond to simple games. The old game of peekaboo is an excellent means of initiating communication with infants while maintaining a "safe," nonthreatening distance. After this intermittent eye-to-eye contact, the nurse is no longer viewed as a stranger but as someone who is a friend. This can be followed by touch games. Clapping an infant's hands together for pat-a-cake or wiggling the toes for "this little piggy" delights an infant or small child. Much of the nursing assessment can be carried out with the use of games and simple play equipment while the infant remains in the safety of the parent's arms or lap. Talking to a foot or other part of the child's body is an effective tactic.

The nurse can capitalize on the natural curiosity of small children by playing games such as "Which hand do you take?" and "Guess what I have in my hand" or by manipulating items such as a flashlight or stethoscope. Finger games are very useful. More elaborate materials, such as puppets and replicas of familiar or unfamiliar items, serve as excellent means to communicate with small children. The variety and extent are limited only by the nurse's imagination.

Through play children reveal their perceptions of interpersonal relationships with their family, friends, or hospital personnel. Children may also reveal the wide scope of knowledge they have acquired from listening to others around them. For example, through needle play, children may disclose how carefully they have watched each procedure by precisely duplicating the technical skills. They may also reveal how well they remember those who performed procedures. One child who painstakingly reenacted every detail of a tedious medical procedure also played the role of the physician who had repeatedly shouted at her to be still for the long ordeal. Her anger at him was most evident during the play session and revealed the cause for her abrupt withdrawal and passive hostility toward the medical and nursing staff following the test.

Play sessions serve not only as assessment tools for determining children's awareness and perception of their illness but also as methods of intervention and evaluation. In the previous example, when the child revealed anger toward the physician, the nurse acted the part of the patient but this time did not accept the physician's harsh commands to stay still. Instead the nurse said to the physician all the things the child had wished she could say.

Subsequent play sessions can also be used to evaluate the child's progress. A change in the type of drawing or the theme of the play may indicate progression toward or away from the ability to deal with anxiety.

HISTORY TAKING

PERFORMING A HEALTH HISTORY

The format used for history taking may be (1) *direct*—the nurse asks for information via direct interview with the informant—or (2) *indirect*—the informant supplies the information by completing some type of questionnaire. The direct method is superior to the indirect approach or a combination of both. However, in view of time constraints, the direct approach is not always practical. If the direct approach cannot be used, review parents' written responses and question them regarding any unusual answers. The categories listed in the box encompass children's current and past health status and information about their psychosocial environment.

Identifying Information

Much of the identifying information may already be available from other recorded sources. However, if the parent and youngster seem anxious, use this opportunity to ask about such information to help them feel more comfortable.

Informant. One of the important elements of identifying information is the informant, the person(s) who furnished the information. Record (1) who the person is (child, parent, or other), (2) an impression of reliability and willingness to communicate, and (3) any special circumstances, such as the use of an interpreter or conflicting answers by more than one person.

Chief Complaint

The chief complaint is the specific reason for the child's visit to the clinic, office, or hospital. It may be viewed as the theme

OUTLINE OF A PEDIATRIC HEALTH HISTORY

Identifying Information

1. Name
2. Address
3. Telephone
4. Birthdate and place
5. Race/ethnic group
6. Sex
7. Religion
8. Date of interview
9. Informant

Chief Complaint (CC)—To establish the major *specific* reason for the child's and parents' seeking professional health attention

Present Illness (PI)—To obtain *all* details related to the chief complaint

Past History (PH)—To elicit a profile of the child's previous illnesses, injuries, or operations

1. Birth history (pregnancy, labor, and delivery, perinatal history)
2. Previous illnesses, injuries, or operations
3. Allergies
4. Current medications
5. Immunizations
6. Growth and development
7. Habits

Review of Systems (ROS)—To elicit information concerning any potential health problem

1. General
2. Integument
3. Head
4. Eyes
5. Ears
6. Nose
7. Mouth
8. Throat
9. Neck
10. Chest
11. Respiratory
12. Cardiovascular
13. Gastrointestinal
14. Genitourinary
15. Gynecologic
16. Musculoskeletal
17. Neurologic
18. Endocrine

Family Medical History—To identify the presence of genetic traits or diseases that have familial tendencies and to assess exposure to a communicable disease in a family member and family habits that may affect the child's health, such as smoking and other chemical use

Psychosocial History—To elicit information about the child's self-concept

Sexual History—To elicit information concerning the child's sexual concerns and/or activities and any pertinent data regarding adults' sexual activity that influence the child

Family History—To develop an understanding of the child as an individual and as a member of a family and a community

1. Family composition
2. Home and community environment
3. Occupation and education of family members
4. Cultural and religious traditions
5. Family function and relationships

Nutritional Assessment—To elicit information on the adequacy of the child's nutritional intake and need

1. Dietary intake
2. Clinical examination

GUIDELINES
Analyzing the Symptom: Pain

Type—Be as specific as possible. With young children, asking the parents how they know the child is in pain may help describe its type, location, and severity. For example, a parent may state, "My child must have a severe earache because she pulls at her ears, rolls her head on the floor, and screams. Nothing seems to help." Help older children describe the "hurt" by asking them if it is sharp, throbbing, dull, aching, or stabbing. Record whatever words they use in quotes.

Location—Be specific. "Stomach pains" is too general a description. Children can better localize the pain if they are asked to "point with one finger to where it hurts" or to "point to where Mommy or Daddy would put a Band-Aid." Determine if the pain radiates by asking, "Does the pain stay there or move? Show me with your finger where the pain goes."

Severity—Best determined by finding out how it affects the child's usual behavior. Pain that prevents a child from playing, interacting with others, sleeping, and eating is most often severe. Assess pain intensity using a rating scale, such as a numeric scale or faces scale (see Table 21-2).

Duration—Include the duration, onset, and frequency. Describe this in terms of activity and behavior, such as "pain lasted all night, because child refused to sleep and cried intermittently."

Influencing factors—Include anything that causes a change in the type, location, severity, or duration of the pain: (1) precipitating events (those that cause or increase the pain), (2) relieving events (those that lessen the pain, such as medications), (3) temporal events (times when the pain is relieved or increased), (4) positional events (standing, sitting, lying down), and (5) associated events (meals, stress, coughing).

Occasionally it is difficult to isolate one symptom or problem as the chief complaint because the parent may identify many. In this situation be as specific as possible when asking questions. For example, asking informants to state which *one* problem or symptom prompted them to seek help now may help them focus on the most immediate concern.

Present Illness

The history of the present illness* is a narrative of the chief complaint from its earliest onset through its progression to the present. Its four major components are: (1) the details of *onset*, (2) a complete *interval* history, (3) the *present* status, and (4) the reason for seeking help *now*. The focus of the present illness is on all factors relevant to the main problem, even if they have disappeared or changed during the onset, interval, and present.

Analyzing a Symptom. Because pain is often the most characteristic symptom denoting the onset of a physical problem, it is used as an example for analysis of a symptom. Assessment includes (1) type, (2) location, (3) severity, (4) duration, and (5) influencing factors (see Guidelines box; see also Pain Assessment, Chapter 21).

---

with the present illness as the description of the problem. The chief complaint is elicited by asking open-ended neutral questions, such as "What seems to be the matter?" "How may I help you?" or "Why did you come here today?" Avoid labeling-type questions, such as "How are you sick?" or "What is the problem?" since it is possible that the reason for the visit is not an illness or problem.

*The term *illness* is used in its broadest sense to denote any problem of a physical, emotional, or psychosocial nature. It is actually a history of the chief complaint.

Past History

The past history contains information relating to all previous aspects of the child's health status and concentrates on several areas that are ordinarily deleted in the history of an adult, such as birth history, detailed feeding history, immunizations, and growth and development. Since a great deal of data is included in this section, use a combination of open-ended and fact-finding questions. For example, begin interviewing for each section with an open-ended statement, such as "Tell me about your child's birth," in order to provide the informants with the opportunity to relate what they think is most important. Ask fact-finding questions related to specific details whenever necessary to focus the interview on certain topics.

Birth History. The birth history includes all data concerning (1) the mother's health during pregnancy, (2) the labor and delivery, and (3) the infant's condition immediately after birth. Since prenatal influences have significant effects on a child's physical and emotional development, a thorough investigation of the birth history is essential. Because parents may question what relevance pregnancy and birth have on the child's present condition, particularly if the child is past infancy, explain why such questions are included. An appropriate statement may be, "I will be asking you some questions about your pregnancy and . . . (refer to child by name) birth. Your answers will give me a more complete picture of his (or her) overall health."

Because emotional factors also affect the outcome of pregnancy and the subsequent parent-child relationship, investigate (1) concurrent crises during pregnancy and (2) prenatal attitudes toward the fetus. It is best to approach the topic of parental acceptance of pregnancy through indirect questioning. Asking parents if the pregnancy was planned is a leading statement because they may respond affirmatively for fear of criticism if the pregnancy was unexpected. Rather, encourage parents to disclose their true reactions by referring to specific facts relating to the pregnancy, such as the spacing between offspring, an extended or short interval between marriage and conception, or the concurrent experience of pregnancy and adolescence. The parent can choose to explore such statements with further explanations or, for the moment, may not be able to reveal such feelings. If the parent remains silent, refocus on this topic later in the interview.

Dietary History. Because parental concerns are common and nursing interventions are important in ensuring optimum nutrition, the dietary history is discussed in detail at the end of this chapter under Nutritional Assessment.

Previous Illnesses, Injuries, and Operations. When inquiring about past illnesses, begin with a general statement, such as "What other illnesses has your child had?" Since parents are most likely to recall serious health problems, ask specifically about colds, earaches, and childhood diseases, such as measles, rubella (German measles), chickenpox, mumps, pertussis (whooping cough), diphtheria, tuberculosis, scarlet fever, strep throat, tonsillitis, or allergic manifestations.

In addition to illnesses, ask about injuries that required medical intervention, operations, and any other reason for hospitalization, including the dates of each incident. It is important to focus on injuries such as accidental falls, poisonings, chokings, or burns, since this may be a potential area for parental guidance.

GUIDELINES
Taking an Allergy History

Ask the following questions:
Are you allergic to any medication or other product, such as latex (e.g., rubber gloves, balloons, catheters)? If yes, what are you allergic to and in what form?
What type of reaction did you have?
How soon after the therapy was started or you came in contact with the product did this occur?
How long ago did the reaction occur?
Who told you that it was an allergic reaction?
Have you taken this product or other drugs of similar class after this reaction occurred? If yes, did you experience similar problems?

Modified from Pau A, Morgan J, Terlingo A: Drug allergy documentation by physicians, nurses and medical students, *Am J Hosp Pharm* 46(3):570-573, 1989.

Allergies. Ask about commonly known allergic disorders, such as hay fever and asthma, as well as unusual reactions to drugs, food, latex products (see Spina bifida, Chapter 32) or other contact agents, such as poisonous plants, animals, household products, or fabrics. If asked appropriate questions, most people can give reliable information about drug reactions (see Guidelines box).

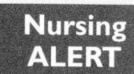
Nursing ALERT Information about allergic reactions to drugs or other products is essential. Failure to document a serious reaction places the child at risk if the agent is given.

Current Medications. Inquire about current drug regimens, including vitamins, antipyretics (especially aspirin), antibiotics, antihistamines, decongestants, or antitussives. List all medications, including name, dose, schedule, duration, and reason for administration. Not infrequently parents are unaware of the actual name of the drug. Whenever possible, ask parents to bring the containers with them to the next visit, or ask them for the name of the pharmacy and call for a list of all the child's recent prescription medications. However, this list will not include over-the-counter medications.

Immunizations. A record of all immunizations is essential. Since many parents are unaware of the exact name and date of each immunization, the most reliable source of information is a hospital, clinic, or private practitioner's record. All immunizations and "boosters" are listed, stating (1) the name of the specific disease, (2) the number of injections, (3) the dosage (sometimes lesser amounts are given if a reaction is anticipated), (4) the ages when administered, and (5) the occurrence of any reaction following the immunization.

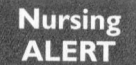
Nursing ALERT Inquire about previous administration of any horse or other foreign serum, recent administration of gamma globulin or blood transfusion, and anaphylactic reactions to neomycin or chicken eggs.

Growth and Development. The most important previous growth patterns to record are (1) approximate weight at 6 months, 1 year, 2 years, and 5 years of age; (2) approximate length at ages 1 and 4 years; and (3) dentition, including age of onset, number of teeth, and symptoms during teething. Developmental milestones include (1) age of holding up head steadily, (2) age of sitting alone without support, (3) age of walking without assistance, (4) age of saying first words with meaning, (5) present grade in school, (6) scholastic grades, and (7) interaction with other children, peers, and adults.

Use specific and detailed questions when inquiring about each developmental milestone. For example "sitting up" can mean many different activities, such as sitting propped up, sitting in someone's lap, sitting with support, sitting up alone but in a hyperflexed position for assisted balance, or sitting up unsupported with the back slightly rounded. A clue to misunderstanding of the requested activity may be an unusually early age of achievement (see Developmental Assessment, Chapter 7).

Habits. Habits are an important area to explore (see box). Parents frequently express concerns during this part of the history. Encourage their input by saying, "Please tell me any concerns you have about your child's habits, activities, or development." Investigate further any concerns that are expressed.

One of the most common concerns relates to sleep. Many children develop a normal sleep pattern, and all that is required during the assessment is a general overview of nighttime sleep and nap schedules. However, a number of children also develop sleep problems (see Sleep Problems, Chapters 10 and 13). When sleep problems occur, a more detailed sleep history is required in order to guide appropriate interventions.*

Habits related to use of chemicals apply primarily to older children and adolescents. If a youngster admits to smoking, drinking, or drug use, ask about the quantity and frequency. Questions such as "Have you ever had a drinking or drug problem?" or "When was the last time you had a drink or took drugs?" may yield more reliable data than questions such as "How much do you drink?" or "How often do you drink or take drugs?" Clarify that "drinking" includes all types of alcohol, such as beer and wine. When quantities such as a "glass" of wine or a "can" of beer are given, ask about the size of the container.

---

*A sleep history and a sleep chart for the family to record the child's daily sleep and wake activities is available in Wong DL: *Wong and Whaley's Clinical manual of pediatric nursing,* ed 4, St Louis, 1996, Mosby.

HABITS TO EXPLORE DURING HEALTH INTERVIEW

Behavior patterns, such as nail-biting, thumb-sucking, pica (habitual ingestion of nonfood substances), rituals ("security" blanket or toy), and unusual movements (head-banging, rocking, overt masturbation, and walking on toes)

Activities of daily living, such as hour of sleep and arising, duration of nighttime sleep and naps, type and duration of exercise, regularity of stools and urination, age of toilet training, and occurrences of daytime or nighttime bed-wetting

Unusual disposition, as well as response to frustration

Use or abuse of alcohol, drugs, coffee, or cigarettes

If older children deny use of chemical substances, inquire about past experimentation. Asking, "You mean you never tried to smoke or drink?" implies that the nurse expects some such activity, and the youngster may be more inclined to answer truthfully. Be aware of the confidential nature of such questioning, the adverse effect that the parents' presence may have on the adolescent's willingness to answer, and that self-report may not be an accurate account of chemical abuse.

Review of Systems

The review of systems is a specific review of each body system, similar to the order of the physical examination (see box on p. 122). Often the history of the present illness provides a complete review of the system involved in the chief complaint. Since asking questions about other body systems may appear unrelated and irrelevant to the parents or child, precede the questioning with an explanation of why the data are needed (similar to the explanation concerning the relevance of the birth history) and reassure the parents that the child's main problem has not been forgotten.

Begin the review of a specific system with a broad statement, such as "How has your child's general health been?" or "Has your child had any problems with his eyes?" If the parent states that there have been past problems with some body function, pursue this with an encouraging statement, such as "Tell me more about that." If the parent denies any problems, query for specific symptoms, such as "No headaches, bumping into objects, or squinting?" If the parent reconfirms the absence of such symptoms, record positive statements in the history, such as "Mother denies headaches, bumping into objects, or squinting." In this way, anyone who reviews the health history is aware of exactly what symptoms were investigated.

Family Medical History

The family medical history is used primarily for the purpose of discovering the potential existence of hereditary or familial diseases in the parents and child. In general, it is confined to first-degree relatives (parents, siblings, grandparents, and immediate aunts and uncles). Information for each family member includes age, marital status, state of health if living, cause of death if deceased, and any evidence of the following conditions: heart disease, hypertension, cancer, diabetes mellitus, obesity, congenital anomalies, allergy, asthma, seizures, tuberculosis, sickle cell disease, mental retardation, mental disorders such as depression or psychosis, emotional problems, syphilis, or rheumatic fever. Confirm the accuracy of the reported disorders by inquiring about the symptoms, course, treatment, and sequelae of each diagnosis.

Geographic Location. One of the important areas to explore when assessing the family health history is geographic location, including the birthplace and travel to different areas in or outside of the country, for identification of possible exposure to endemic diseases. Although the primary interest focuses on the child's temporary residence in various localities, also inquire about close family members' travel, especially during tours of military service or business trips. Children are especially susceptible to parasitic infestation in areas of poor sanitary conditions and to vector-borne diseases, such as those from mosquitoes or ticks in warm and humid or heavily wooded regions.

GUIDELINES FOR REVIEW OF SYSTEMS

General—overall state of health, fatigue, recent and/or unexplained weight gain or loss (period of time for either), contributing factors (change of diet, illness, altered appetite), exercise tolerance, fevers (time of day), chills, night sweats (unrelated to climatic conditions), frequent infections, general ability to carry out activities of daily living

Integument—Pruritus, pigment or other color changes, acne, eruptions, rashes (location), tendency for bruising, petechiae, excessive dryness, general texture, disorders or deformities of nails, hair growth or loss, hair color change (for adolescent, use of hair dyes or other potentially toxic substances, such as hair straighteners)

Head—headaches, dizziness, injury (specific details)

Eyes—visual problems (ask about behaviors indicative of blurred vision, such as bumping into objects, clumsiness, sitting very close to television, holding a book close to face, writing with head near desk, squinting, rubbing the eyes, bending head in an awkward position), cross-eye (strabismus), eye infections, edema of lids, excessive tearing, use of glasses or contact lenses, date of last optic examination

Nose—nosebleeds (epistaxis), constant or frequent running or stuffy nose, nasal obstruction (difficulty in breathing), alteration or loss of sense of smell

Ears—earaches, discharge, evidence of hearing loss (ask about behaviors, such as need to repeat requests, loud speech, inattentive behavior), results of any previous auditory testing

Mouth—mouth-breathing, gum bleeding, toothaches, toothbrushing, use of fluoride, difficulty with teething (symptoms), last visit to dentist (especially if temporary dentition is complete), response to dentist

Throat—sore throats, difficulty in swallowing, choking (especially when chewing food—may be from poor chewing habits), hoarseness, or other voice irregularities

Neck—pain, limitation of movement, stiffness, difficulty in holding head straight (torticollis), thyroid enlargement, enlarged nodes or other masses

Chest—breast enlargement, discharge, masses, enlarged axillary nodes (for adolescent female, ask about breast self-examination)

Respiratory—chronic cough, frequent colds (number per year), wheezing, shortness of breath at rest or on exertion, difficulty in breathing, sputum production, infections (pneumonia, tuberculosis), date of last chest x-ray examination, and skin reaction from tuberculin testing

Cardiovascular—cyanosis or fatigue on exertion, history of heart murmur or rheumatic fever, anemia, date of last blood count, blood type, recent transfusion

Gastrointestinal—(much of this in regard to appetite, food tolerance, and elimination habits has been asked elsewhere)—nausea, vomiting (not associated with eating, may be indicative of brain tumor or increased intracranial pressure), jaundice or yellowing skin or sclera, belching, flatulence, recent change in bowel habits (blood in stools, change of color, diarrhea, or constipation)

Genitourinary—pain on urination, frequency, hesitancy, urgency, hematuria, nocturia, polyuria, unpleasant odor to urine, force of stream, discharge, change in size of scrotum, date of last urinalysis (for adolescent, sexually transmitted disease, type of treatment; for male adolescent, ask about testicular self-examination)

Gynecologic—menarche, date of last menstrual period, regularity or problems with menstruation, vaginal discharge, pruritus, date and result of last Pap smear (include obstetric history as discussed under birth history when applicable); if sexually active, type of contraception, sexually transmitted disease and type of treatment

Musculoskeletal—weakness, clumsiness, lack of coordination, unusual movements, back or joint stiffness, muscle pains or cramps, abnormal gait, deformity, fractures, serious sprains, activity level

Neurologic—seizures, tremors, dizziness, loss of memory, general affect, fears, nightmares, speech problems, any unusual habits

Endocrine—intolerance to weather changes, excessive thirst and/or urination, excessive sweating, salty taste to skin, signs of early puberty

Psychosocial History

The traditional medical history includes a personal and social section that concentrates on children's personal status, such as school adjustment and any unusual habits, and the family and home environment. Since several personal aspects are covered under development and habits, and the social aspects are discussed in detail under Family Assessment, only those issues related to children's ability to cope and their general view of themselves in terms of self-concept are presented here (see Development of Self-Concept, Chapter 5).

Through observation obtain a general idea of how children handle themselves in terms of confidence in dealing with others, ability to answer questions and coping with new situations. Observe the parent-child relationship for the types of messages sent to children about their coping skills and self-worth. Do the parents treat the child with respect, focusing on strengths, or is the interaction one of constant reprimands, with emphasis on weaknesses and faults? Do the parents help the child learn new coping strategies or support the ones the child uses?

Messages about body image are also conveyed through the parent-child interaction. Do the parents label the child and body parts, such as "bad boy," "skinny legs," or "ugly scar"? Do the parents handle the child gently, using soothing touch to calm an anxious child, or do they treat the child roughly, using slaps or restraint to force compliance? If the child touches certain parts of the body, such as the genitals, do the parents make comments that suggest a negative connotation?

With older children, many of the communication strategies discussed earlier in the chapter are useful in eliciting more definitive information about their coping and self-concept. Children can write down five things they like and dislike about themselves. Sentence completion statements such as "The thing I like best (or worst) about myself is _____," "If I could change one thing about myself, it would be _____," or "When I am scared, I _____," can be used.

Sexual History

The sexual history is an essential component of adolescents' health assessment. The history uncovers areas of concern related to sexual activity, alerts the nurse to circumstances that may indicate screening for sexually transmitted diseases or testing for pregnancy, and provides information related to the need for sexual counseling, such as safe sex practices.

One approach toward initiating a conversation about sexual concerns is to begin with a history of peer interactions. Open-ended statements such as "Tell me about your social life," or "Who are your closest friends?" generally lead into a discussion of dating and sexual issues. To probe further, include questions about the adolescent's attitudes on such topics as sex education, "going steady," "living together," and premarital sex. Phrase questions to reflect concern rather than judgment or criticism of sexual practices.

In any conversation regarding sexual history, be aware of the language that is used in either eliciting or conveying sexual information. For example, avoid asking if the adolescent is "sexually active," since this term is broadly defined. "Are you having sex with anyone?" is probably the most direct and best understood question. Since homosexual experimentation may occur, refer to all sexual contacts in nongender terms, such as "anyone" or "partners," rather than "girlfriends" or "boyfriends."

A detailed account of sexual partners is needed if the patient has a history of, displays any of the symptoms of, or asks for treatment of a sexually transmitted disease. A difficult but necessary part of the interview is to determine the sites of possible infection. Since sexual diseases can be contracted at any of the body orifices, inform the adolescent that a sexually transmitted disease can be acquired without visible signs of disease at nongenital sites.

FAMILY ASSESSMENT

Assessment of the family, both its structure and function, is an important component of the history-taking process. Because the quality of the functional relationship between the child and family members is a major factor in emotional and physical health, family assessment is discussed separately and in greater detail apart from the more traditional health history.

Family assessment is the collection of data about the composition of the family and the relationships among its members. In its broadest sense *family* refers to all those individuals who are considered by the family member to be significant to the nuclear unit, including relatives, friends, and other social groups, such as the school and church. While family assessment is not family therapy, it can and frequently is therapeutic. Involving family members in discussing family characteristics and activities often stimulates productive discussion and insight into family dynamics and relationships.

Because of the time involved in performing an in-depth family assessment as presented here, be selective in deciding when knowledge of family function may facilitate nursing care. During brief contacts with families a full assessment is not appropriate, and screening with one or two questions from each category may reflect the health of the family system or the potential need for additional assessment. Indications for performing a comprehensive family assessment are children receiving comprehensive well-child care, experiencing major stressful life events (e.g., chronic illness, disability, parental divorce, or death of a family member), requiring extensive home care, who have developmental delays, who have had repeated accidental injuries and those with suspected child abuse, and with behavioral or physical problems that suggest family dysfunction as the cause.

ASSESSMENT OF FAMILY STRUCTURE

Family structure refers to the composition of the family—who lives in the home and those social, cultural, religious, and economic characteristics that influence the child's and family's overall psychobiologic health (see also Chapters 3

and 4). Since the information elicited in this part of the history is often the most personal and confidential, include it toward the end of the interview when rapport is well established.

The most common method of eliciting information on the family structure is to interview family members. The principal areas of concern (see box on p. 124) are (1) family composition, (2) home and community environment, (3) occupation and education of family members, and (4) cultural and religious traditions.

> **Nursing ALERT** In assessing family composition it is sometimes difficult to ascertain the status of the adult relationships. If the parent fails to mention the other parent, ask, "Where is the child's father (or mother)?" Avoid saying "husband" or "wife" because this assumes that only marital relationships exist.

Several structural assessment tools can be used to collect and record data about the family composition and environment. Like the interview method, such tools also provide information about relationships, although several additional methods should be used to assess family function.

A *sociogram* is a drawing of circles that indicates the significant persons in an individual's life; its use is appropriate for adults and children as young as 5 years of age. The person is given blank paper and a pencil with the instructions: "Draw a circle to represent you. Around the circle draw circles to represent the most significant persons in your life and label each. Draw the circles in proximity to your circle to represent closeness. For example, the person who is most significant is the circle closest to you." Family members can label the relationships as supportive with a plus sign or negative with a minus sign.

Not only is the sociogram a portrait of the person's significant relationships, it may also uncover unresolved relationships (Fig. 6-5). After completing the sociogram, encourage the family to explore their feelings further with questions such as the following:

- How would you change the circles to improve relationships?
- How do you think you could accomplish these changes?
- If one person in the circle were to change, what effect do you think that would have on others in the circle?

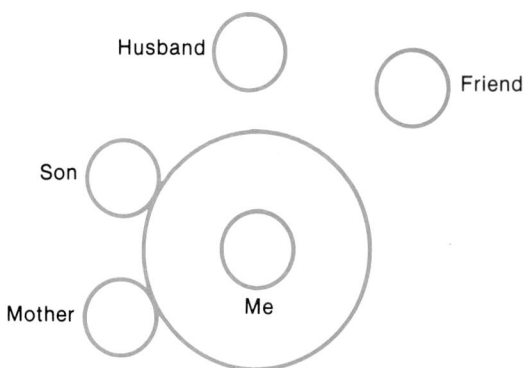

FIG. 6-5. Sociogram of mother with strong, unresolved grief feelings regarding loss of child.

FAMILY ASSESSMENT INTERVIEW

General Guidelines for Family Interview

Schedule the interview with the family at a time that is most convenient for all parties; include as many family members as possible; clearly state the purpose of the interview.

Begin the interview by asking each person's name and their relationship to each other.

Restate the purpose of the interview and the objective.

Keep the initial conversation general to put members at ease and to learn the "big picture" of the family.

Identify major concerns and reflect these back to the family to be certain that all parties perceive the same message.

Terminate the interview with a summary of what was discussed and a plan for additional sessions if needed.

Structural Assessment Areas

Family Composition

Immediate members of the household (names, ages, and relationships)

Significant extended family members

Previous marriages, separations, death of spouses, or divorces

Home and Community Environment

Type of dwelling/number of rooms/occupants

Sleeping arrangements

Number of floors, accessibility of stairs, elevators

Adequacy of utilities

Safety features (fire escape, smoke detector, guardrails on windows, use of car restraint)

Environmental hazards (e.g., chipped paint, poor sanitation, pollution, heavy street traffic)

Availability and location of health facilities, schools, play areas

Relationship with neighbors

Recent crises or changes in home

Child's reaction/adjustment to recent stresses

Occupation and Education of Family Members

Types of employment

Work schedules

Work satisfaction

Exposure to environmental/industrial hazards

Sources of income and adequacy

Effect of illness on financial status

Highest degree or grade level attained

Cultural and Religious Traditions

Religious beliefs and practices

Cultural/ethnic beliefs and practices

Language spoken in home

ASSESSMENT QUESTIONS INCLUDE THE FOLLOWING:

Does the family identify with a particular religious/ethnic group? Are both parents from that group?

How is religious/ethnic background part of family life?

What special religious/cultural traditions are practiced in the home (e.g., food choices and preparation)?

Where were family members born, and how long have they lived in this country?

What language does the family speak most frequently?

Do they speak/understand English?

What do they believe causes health or illness?

What religious/ethnic beliefs influence the family's perception of illness and its treatment?

What methods are used to prevent/treat illness?

How does the family know when a health problem needs medical attention?

Who is the person the family contacts when a member is ill?

Does the family rely on cultural/religious healers or remedies? If so, ask them to describe the type of healer or remedy.

Who does the family go to for support (clergy, medical healer, relatives)?

Does the family experience discrimination because of their race, beliefs, or practices? Ask them to describe.

Functional Assessment Areas

Family Interactions and Roles

Interactions refer to ways family members relate to each other

Chief concern is amount of intimacy and closeness among the members, especially spouses

Roles refer to behaviors of people as they assume a different status or position

OBSERVATIONS INCLUDE THE FOLLOWING:

Family members' responses to each other (cordial, hostile, cool, loving, patient, short-tempered)

Obvious roles of leadership vs submission

Support and attention shown to various members

ASSESSMENT QUESTIONS INCLUDE THE FOLLOWING:

What activities do the family perform together?

Whom do family members talk to when something is bothering them?

What are members' household chores?

Who usually oversees what is happening with the children, such as at school or concerning their health?

How easy or difficult is it for the family to change or accept new responsibilities for household tasks?

Power, Decision Making, and Problem Solving

Power refers to individual member's control over others in family; manifested through family decision making and problem solving

Chief concern is clarity of boundaries of power between parents and children

One method of assessment involves offering a hypothetical conflict or problem, such as a child failing school, and asking family how they would handle this situation

ASSESSMENT QUESTIONS INCLUDE THE FOLLOWING:

Who usually makes the decisions in the family?

If one parent makes a decision, can the child appeal to the other parent to change it?

What input do children have in making decisions or discussing rules?

Who makes and enforces the rules?

What happens when a rule is broken?

Communication

Concerned with clarity and directness of communication patterns

OBSERVATIONS INCLUDE THE FOLLOWING:

Who speaks to whom

If one person speaks for another or interrupts

If members appear disinterested when certain individuals speak

If there is agreement between verbal and nonverbal messages

Further assessment includes periodically asking family members if they understood what was just said and to repeat the message

ASSESSMENT QUESTIONS INCLUDE THE FOLLOWING:

How often do family members wait until others are through talking before "having their say?"

Do parents or older siblings tend to lecture and preach?

Do parents tend to talk "down" to the children?

Expression of Feelings and Individuality

Concerned with personal space and freedom to grow with limits and structure needed for guidance

Observing patterns of communication offers clues to how freely feelings are expressed

ASSESSMENT QUESTIONS INCLUDE THE FOLLOWING:

Is it OK for family members to get angry or sad?

Who gets angry most of the time? What do they do?

If someone is upset, how do other family members try to comfort this person?

Who comforts specific family members?

When someone wants to do something, such as try out for a new sport or get a job, what is the family's response (offer assistance, discouragement, or no advice)?

ASSESSMENT OF FAMILY FUNCTION

Family function is concerned with how the family behaves toward one another and with the quality of the relationships (see also Chapter 4). It is considered the most important component in determining "family health." Assessment of function requires more skill on the part of the interviewer than does assessment of structure and is best approached after structure is assessed. As in assessment of family structure, the more traditional method of eliciting information on family function is by interviewing family members. The principal areas of concern are discussed in the box on p. 124.

In addition to observing and interviewing the family to assess family function, several other methods are available and should be used as needed to obtain a comprehensive assessment. The following section discusses selected instruments that are reliable and valid but require little or no formal training and minimal time to administer.

The *Family APGAR (FAPGAR)* is a brief screening questionnaire designed to reflect a family member's satisfaction with the functional state of the family (Smilkstein, Ashworth, and Montano, 1982) (see Appendix A). The acronym APGAR is for Adaptation, Partnership, Growth, Affection, and Resolve (commitment). The acronym was chosen because it is familiar to health professionals, but it bears no relationship to the Apgar scoring system for newborns.

The questions in the box below can be used in the interview without the APGAR ratings to elicit similar types of information. It can be completed in about 5 minutes, can be used by families with traditional and alternative life-styles and from different cultures, and is appropriate for children age 10 years or older. Separate forms have been designed to assess relationships with friends and fellow workers, since these groups represent other significant sources of support.

The responses to the five questions are scored as follows: "Almost always"—2; "Some of the time"—1; and "Hardly ever"—0. Each score is totaled. Scores of 7 to 10 suggest a highly functional family; 4 to 6, a moderately dysfunctional family; and 0 to 3, a severely dysfunctional family. Also, a low score in any single item could signal family dysfunction. The family APGAR is not recommended for use with individuals from enmeshed (overly close) or "psychosomatic" families. Persons with health problems, such as asthma, atopic dermatitis, or irritable bowel syndrome, may report falsely high scores (Smilkstein, 1993).

Undoubtedly the richest environment for observing a child's development and interactions with family members is the home. Two tools that can be used to assess the child's home environment are the *Home Observation for Management of the Environment (HOME)* * *Inventory* (Caldwell

---

*The forms and an administration manual are available for a fee from the Center for Research on Teaching and Learning, College of Education, University of Arkansas at Little Rock, 2801 S. University Ave., Little Rock, AK 72204; (501) 569-3422.

FAMILY APGAR

Definition	Functions Measured by the Family APGAR	Relevant Open-Ended Questions
Adaptation is the use of intrafamilial and extrafamilial resources for problem solving when family equilibrium is stressed during a crisis.	How resources are shared, or the degree to which a member is satisfied with the assistance received when family resources are needed	How have family members aided each other in time of need? In what way have family members received help or assistance from friends and community agencies?
Partnership is the sharing of decision-making and nurturing responsibilities by family members.	How decisions are shared, or the member's satisfaction with mutuality in family communication and problem solving	How do family members communicate with each other about such matters as vacations, finances, medical care, large purchases, and personal problems?
Growth is the physical and emotional maturation and self-fulfillment that is achieved by family members through mutual support and guidance.	How nurturing is shared, or the member's satisfaction with the freedom available within the family to change roles and attain physical and emotional growth or maturation	How have family members changed during the past years? How has this change been accepted by family members? In what ways have family members aided each other in growing or developing independent life-styles? How have family members reacted to your desire for change?
Affection is the caring or loving relationship that exists among family members.	How emotional experiences are shared, or the member's satisfaction with the intimacy and emotional interaction that exists in the family	How have members of your family responded to emotional expressions, such as affection, love, sorrow, or anger?
Resolve is the commitment to devote time to other members of the family for physical and emotional nurturing. It also usually involves a decision to share wealth and space.	How time (and space and money) is shared, or the member's satisfaction with the time commitment that has been made to the family by its members	How do members of your family share time, space, and money?

Modified from Smilkstein G: The Family APGAR: a proposal for a family function test and its use by physicians, *J Fam Pract* 6(6):1231-1239, 1978.

and Bradley, 1984) and the *Home Screening Questionnaire (HSQ)** (Frankenburg and Coons, 1986). Both are divided into two age-groups—birth to 3 years of age and 3 to 6 years of age. HOME has an additional inventory for children ages 6 to 10 years. Forms are also available for children with moderate to severe disabilities in each of the three age-groups for visual, auditory, orthopedic, and cognitive impairments. The HOME assesses the quality and quantity of the social, emotional, and cognitive support that is available to children in their home environment, including low-income families and low–birth-weight children (Bradley and others, 1994).

Some of the HOME items require direct observation, whereas others necessitate questioning of the parents. Each item receives a "yes" or "no" response. The number of "yes" responses correlates with the amount of appropriate environmental stimulation. Any "no" responses indicate possible areas for intervention and counseling. Use of HOME requires about a 1-hour home visit with both the child and the major caregiver.

The HSQ was developed using HOME as a guide. The 0- to 3-year form consists of 30 items plus a checklist of toys available to the child in the home. The 3- to 6-year form has 34 items and a similar toy checklist. The questions are written at approximately a third- to sixth-grade reading level and, unlike the HOME, can be completed by the parents in any setting in about 15 to 20 minutes. Scoring directions are de-

---

*The forms and manual are available for a fee from Denver Developmental Materials, Inc., P.O. Box 6919, Denver, CO 80206-0919; (303) 355-4729 or (800) 419-4729.

tailed in the manual and are based on credits for different answers. For each age-group there is a minimum score for determining suspect or nonsuspect results.

NUTRITIONAL ASSESSMENT

DIETARY INTAKE

Knowledge of the child's dietary intake is a useful and practical component of a nutritional assessment. However, it is also one of the most difficult factors to assess. Individuals' recall of food consumption, especially amounts eaten, is frequently unreliable. In addition, people may be hesitant to reveal their eating patterns if they sense criticism from the nurse. People from different cultures may have difficulty adequately describing the types of food they eat. Despite these obstacles, a food intake record is essential. Several methods are available.

Regardless of the format used in recording food intake, every nutritional assessment should begin with a *dietary history.* The exact questions used to elicit a dietary history vary with the child's age. In general, the younger the child, the more specific and detailed the history should be. The box below provides a sample dietary history for children, and includes additional questions regarding infant feeding.

The broad overview elicited from the dietary history can be helpful in evaluating food frequency records (see box). It also is concerned with financial and cultural factors that in-

---

DIETARY HISTORY

What are the family's usual mealtimes?
Do family members eat together or at separate times?
Who does the family grocery shopping and meal preparation?
How much money is spent to buy food each week?
How are most foods prepared—baked, broiled, fried, other?
How often does the family or your child eat out?
   What kinds of restaurants do you go to?
   What kinds of food does your child typically eat at restaurants?
Does your child eat breakfast regularly?
Where does your child eat lunch?
What are your child's favorite foods, beverages, and snacks?
   What are the average amounts eaten per day?
   What foods are artificially sweetened?
   What are your child's snacking habits?
   When are sweet foods usually eaten?
   What are your child's toothbrushing habits?
What special cultural practices are followed? What ethnic foods are eaten?
What foods and beverages does your child dislike?
How would you describe your child's usual appetite (hearty eater, picky eater)?
What are your child's feeding habits (breast, bottle, cup, spoon, eats by self, needs assistance, any special devices)?
Does your child take vitamins or other supplements? Do they contain iron or fluoride?
Are there any known or suspected food allergies? Is your child on a special diet?
Has your child lost or gained weight recently?
Are there any feeding problems (excessive fussiness, spitting up, colic, difficulty sucking or swallowing)? Are there any dental problems or appliances, such as braces, that affect eating?

What types of exercise does your child do regularly?
Is there a family history of cancer, diabetes, heart disease, high blood pressure, or obesity?

Additional Questions for Infants
What was the infant's birth weight? When did it double? Triple?
Was the infant premature?
Are you breast-feeding or have you breast-fed your infant? For how long?
If you use a formula, what is the brand?
   How long has the infant been taking it?
   How many ounces does the infant drink a day?
Are you giving the infant cow's milk (whole, low-fat, skimmed)?
   When did you start?
   How many ounces does the infant drink a day?
Do you give your infant extra fluids (water, juice)?
If the infant takes a bottle to bed at nap or nighttime, what is in the bottle?
At what age did you start cereal, vegetables, meat or other protein sources, fruit/juice, finger food, table food?
Do you make your own baby food or use commercial foods, such as infant cereal?
Does the infant take a vitamin/mineral supplement? If so, what type?
Has the infant shown an allergic reaction to any food(s)? If so, list the foods and describe the reaction.
Does the infant spit up frequently, have unusually loose stools, or have hard, dry stools? If so, how often?
How often do you feed your infant?
How would you describe your infant's appetite?

FOOD FREQUENCY RECORD*					
FOOD GROUP	NUMBER OF SERVINGS (DAY, WEEK)	SERVING SIZE (IN CUP, TABLESPOON, OR OUNCE PORTIONS)	FOOD GROUP	NUMBER OF SERVINGS (DAY, WEEK)	SERVING SIZE (IN CUP, TABLESPOON, OR OUNCE PORTIONS)
Breads/Cereals/Rice/ Pasta Bread, tortilla Cooked pasta, rice, hot cereal Dry cereal (not presweetened) Crackers Muffins Other			**Milk/Cheese/Yogurt** Milk Cheese Yogurt Pudding Ice cream Other		
Vegetables Yellow or orange Green/leafy Other			**Other Protein Foods** Meat Fish Poultry Egg Peanut butter Legumes (dried beans, peas) Nuts Other		
Fruits/Juice Citrus (orange, grapefruit, strawberries, lemon, lime, tangerine) Noncitrus Other			**Fats/Oils/Sweets** Butter, oil, margarine, mayonnaise, salad dressing Soda, punch Cake/cookie, etc Candy Presweetened cereal		

*For comparison of actual intake with recommended intake, see Food Guide Pyramid, Fig. 11-1.

CULTURAL AWARENESS
Food Practices

Because cultural practices are very prevalent in food preparation, consider carefully the kinds of questions that are asked and the judgments made in regard to counseling. For example, some cultures, such as Hispanic, black, and Native American, include many vegetables, legumes, and starches in their diet that together provide sufficient essential amino acids, even though the actual amount of meat or dairy protein is low. (See Chapter 3 for cultural food practices.)

fluence food selection and preparation. (See Cultural Awareness box).

The most common and probably easiest method of assessing daily intake is the *24-hour recall*. The child or parent recalls every item eaten in the past 24 hours and the approximate amounts. The 24-hour recall is most beneficial when it represents a typical day's intake. Some of the difficulties with a daily recall are the family's inability to remember exactly what was eaten and inaccurate estimation of portion size. To increase accuracy of reporting portion sizes, the use of food models and additional questioning are recommended. In general, this method is most useful in providing *qualitative* information about the child's diet.

To improve the reliability of the daily recall, the family can complete a *food diary* by recording every food and liquid consumed for a certain number of days. A 3-day record consisting of 2 weekdays and 1 weekend day is representative for most people. Providing specific charts to record intake can improve compliance. The family should record items immediately after eating.

A *food frequency questionnaire* or *record* (see box) provides information about the number of times in a day, week, or month a child consumes items from the different food groups. In general, it provides a qualitative overview but has the advantage of avoiding recall based on a "typical" day. It can be especially useful when verifying a food history or diary.

CLINICAL EXAMINATION

A significant amount of information regarding nutritional deficiencies is elicited from a clinical examination, especially from assessing the skin, hair, teeth, gums, lips, tongue, and eyes. Hair, skin, and mouth are vulnerable because of the rapid turnover of epithelial and mucosal tissue. Table 6-1 summarizes clinical signs of possible nutritional deficiency or

TABLE 6-1. Clinical assessment of nutritional status

EVIDENCE OF ADEQUATE NUTRITION	EVIDENCE OF DEFICIENT OR EXCESS NUTRITION	DEFICIENCY/EXCESS*
General Growth		
Within 5th and 95th percentiles for height, weight, and head circumference	Below 5th or above 95th percentiles for growth	Protein, calories, fats, and other essential nutrients, especially A, pyridoxine, niacin, calcium, iodine, manganese, zinc
Steady gain with expected growth spurts during infancy and adolescence	Absence of or delayed growth spurts; poor weight gain	
Sexual development appropriate for age	Delayed sexual development	Excess vitamin A, D
Skin		
Smooth, slightly dry to touch	Hardening and scaling	Vitamin A
Elastic and firm	Seborrheic dermatitis	Excess niacin
Absence of lesions	Dry, rough, petechiae	Riboflavin
Color appropriate to genetic background	Delayed wound healing	Vitamin C
	Scaly dermatitis on exposed surfaces	Riboflavin, vitamin C, zinc
	Wrinkled, flabby	Niacin
	Crusted lesions around orifices, especially nares	Protein and calories
		Zinc
	Pruritus	Excess vitamin A, riboflavin, niacin
	Poor turgor	Water, sodium
	Edema	Protein, thiamin
		Excess sodium
	Yellow tinge (jaundice)	Vitamin B_{12}
		Excess vitamin A, niacin
	Depigmentation	Protein, calories
	Pallor (anemia)	Pyridoxine, folic acid, vitamin B_{12}, C, E (in premature infants), iron
		Excess vitamin C, zinc
	Paresthesia	Excess riboflavin
Hair		
Lustrous, silky, strong, elastic	Stringy, friable, dull, dry, thin	Protein, calories
	Alopecia	Protein, calories, zinc
	Depigmentation	Protein, calories, copper
	Raised areas around hair follicles	Vitamin C
Head		
Even molding, occipital prominence, symmetric facial features	Softening of cranial bones, prominence of frontal bones, skull flat and depressed toward middle	Vitamin D
Fused sutures after 18 months	Delayed fusion of sutures	Vitamin D
	Hard tender lumps in occiput	Excess vitamin A
	Headache	Excess thiamin
Neck		
Thyroid not visible, palpable in midline	Thyroid enlarged; may be grossly visible	Iodine
Eyes		
Clear, bright	Hardening and scaling of cornea and conjunctiva	Vitamin A
Good night vision	Night blindness	
Conjunctiva—pink, glossy	Burning, itching, photophobia, cataracts, corneal vascularization	Riboflavin
Ears		
Tympanic membrane—pliable	Calcified (hearing loss)	Excess vitamin D
Nose		
Smooth, intact nasal angle	Irritation and cracks at nasal angle	Riboflavin
		Excess vitamin A

*Nutrients listed are deficient unless specified as excess.

TABLE 6-1. Clinical assessment of nutritional status—cont'd

EVIDENCE OF ADEQUATE NUTRITION	EVIDENCE OF DEFICIENT OR EXCESS NUTRITION	DEFICIENCY/EXCESS*
Mouth		
Lips—smooth, moist, darker color than skin	Fissures and inflammation at corners	Riboflavin Excess vitamin A
Gums—firm, coral pink color, stippled	Spongy, friable, swollen, bluish red or black color, bleed easily	Vitamin C
Mucous membranes—bright pink, smooth, moist	Stomatitis	Niacin
Tongue—rough texture, no lesions, taste sensation	Glossitis Diminished taste sensation	Niacin, riboflavin, folic acid Zinc
Teeth—uniform white color, smooth, in-tact	Brown mottling, pits, fissures Defective enamel Caries	Excess fluoride Vitamin A, C, D, calcium, phosphorus Excess carbohydrates
Chest		
In infants, shape is almost circular	Depressed lower portion of rib cage	Vitamin D
In children, lateral diameter increases in proportion to anteroposterior diameter	Sharp protrusion of sternum	
Smooth costochondral junctions	Enlarged costochondral junctions	Vitamin C, D
Breast development—normal for age	Delayed development	See General Growth, above, especially zinc
Cardiovascular System		
Pulse and blood pressure (BP) within normal limits	Palpitations Rapid pulse	Thiamin Potassium Excess thiamin
	Arrhythmias	Magnesium, potassium Excess niacin, potassium
	Increased BP Decreased BP	Excess sodium Thiamin; excess niacin
Abdomen		
In young children, cylindric and promi-nent	Distended, flabby, poor musculature Prominent, large	Protein, calories Excess calories
Older children, flat	Potbelly, constipation	Vitamin D
Normal bowel habits	Diarrhea	Niacin Excess vitamin C
	Constipation	Excess calcium, potassium
Musculoskeletal System		
Muscles—firm, well-developed, equal strength bilaterally	Flabby, weak, generalized wasting Weakness, pain, cramps	Protein, calories Thiamin, sodium, chloride, potassium, phosphorus, magnesium Excess thiamin
	Muscle twitching, tremors Muscular paralysis	Magnesium Excess potassium
Spine—cervical and lumbar curves (double S curve)	Kyphosis, lordosis, scoliosis	Vitamin D
Extremities—symmetric; legs straight with minimum bowing	Bowing of extremities, knock-knees Epiphyseal enlargement Bleeding into joints and muscles, joint swelling, pain	Vitamin D, calcium, phosphorus Vitamin A, D Vitamin C
Joints—flexible, full range of motion, no pain or stiffness	Thickening of cortex of long bones with pain and fragility, hard tender lumps in extremities Osteoporosis of long bones	Excess vitamin A Calcium; excess vitamin D

Continued.

TABLE 6-1. Clinical assessment of nutritional status—cont'd		
EVIDENCE OF ADEQUATE NUTRITION	**EVIDENCE OF DEFICIENT OR EXCESS NUTRITION**	**DEFICIENCY/EXCESS***
Neurologic System		
Behavior—alert, responsive, emotionally stable	Listless, irritable, lethargic, apathetic (sometimes apprehensive, anxious, drowsy, mentally slow, confused)	Thiamin, niacin, pyridoxine, vitamin C, potassium, magnesium, iron, protein, calories
		Excess vitamin A, D, thiamin, folic acid, calcium
	Masklike facial expression, blurred speech, involuntary laughing	Excess manganese
Absence of tetany, convulsions	Convulsions	Thiamin, pyridoxine, vitamin D, calcium, magnesium
		Excess phosphorus (in relation to calcium)
Intact peripheral nervous system	Peripheral nervous system toxicity (unsteady gait, numb feet and hands, fine motor clumsiness)	Excess pyridoxine
Intact reflexes	Diminished or absent tendon reflexes	Thiamin, vitamin E

*Nutrients listed are deficient unless specified as excess.

excess. Few are diagnostic for a specific nutrient, and if suspicious signs are found, they must be confirmed with dietary and biochemical data. Generally, the clinical examination does not reveal children *at risk* for a deficiency or excess.

Anthropometry, an essential parameter of nutritional status is the measurement of height, weight, head circumference, proportions, skinfold thickness, and arm circumference in young children. Height and head circumference reflect past nutrition, whereas weight, skinfold thickness, and arm circumference reflect present nutritional status, especially of protein and fat reserves. Skinfold thickness is a measurement of the body's fat content because approximately one half of the body's total fat stores are directly beneath the skin. The upper arm muscle circumference is correlated with measurements of total muscle mass. Since muscle serves as the body's major protein reserve, this measurement is considered an index of the body's protein stores. Ideally growth measurements are recorded over a period of time, and comparisons are made regarding the *velocity* of growth based on previous and present values. Techniques for anthropomorphic measurement are discussed in Chapter 7.

Numerous *biochemical tests* are available for assessing nutritional status and include analysis of plasma, blood cells, urine, or tissues from liver, bone, hair, and fingernails. Many of these tests are complicated and are not performed routinely. Common laboratory procedures for nutritional status include measurement of hemoglobin, hematocrit, transferrin, albumin, creatinine, and nitrogen. Laboratory values for these tests and more specific nutrient measurements are given in Appendix E.

EVALUATION OF NUTRITIONAL ASSESSMENT

After collecting the data needed for a thorough nutritional assessment, evaluate the findings to plan appropriate counseling. From the data, assess if the child is (1) malnourished, (2) at risk for becoming malnourished, or (3) well nourished with adequate reserves.

Analyze the daily food diary for the variety and amounts of foods suggested in the Food Guide Pyramid (see Fig. 11-1). For example, if the list includes no vegetables, inquire about this rather than assume that the child dislikes vegetables, because it could be that none were served on that day. Also, evaluate the information in terms of the family's ethnic practices and financial resources. Encouraging increased protein intake with additional meat may be unfeasible for families on a limited budget or in conflict with food practices that use meat sparingly, such as in Asian meal preparation.

Compare findings from clinical examination and anthropometry with the data obtained from the dietary intake. For example, signs of anemia and a dietary record of iron-poor foods suggest laboratory analysis of hemoglobin, hematocrit, and transferrin. Refer any suspicious findings for further evaluation.

KEY POINTS

- Communication, the most important skill nurses must possess in the care of children, has verbal, nonverbal, and abstract components.
- To effectively establish a setting for communication, nurses must make an appropriate introduction, clarify their role and the purpose of the interview, and ensure privacy and confidentiality.
- When communicating with parents, nurses need to encourage parental involvement, listen carefully, use silence, and be empathic.
- Communication with children must reflect their developmental stage.
- Verbal communication techniques that have proved to be effective include the third-person technique, facilitative responding, storytelling, bibliotherapy, the use of "what if" questions, and other word games.
- Nonverbal communication with children may take the form of writing, drawing, magic, and play.

- The objectives of performing a health history are to identify pertinent information, determine the chief complaint, analyze the present illness, secure the past history, review biologic systems, and record a family medical history and child psychosocial and sexual history.
- Family assessment is the collection of data about family composition and relationships among its members; it also focuses on home and community environment, occupation and education, and cultural and religious traditions.
- The family function interview examines interaction and roles, power, decision making, problem solving, communication, and expression of feelings and individuality.
- Nutritional assessment is performed by determination of dietary intake, clinical examination, and biochemical analysis.

REFERENCES

Bellet PS, Maloney MJ: The importance of empathy as an interviewing skill in medicine, *JAMA* 266(13):1831-1832, 1991.

Bradley RH and others: A reexamination of the association between HOME scores and income, *Nurs Res* 43(5):260-266, 1994.

Caldwell B, Bradley R: *Home observation for measurement of the environment,* rev ed, Little Rock, AR, 1984, University of Arkansas.

Campbell-Heider N, Hart CA: Updating the nurse's bedside manner, *Image J Nurs Sch* 25(2):133-139, 1993.

Frankenburg W, Coons C: Home Screening Questionnaire: its validity in assessing home environment, *J Pediatr* 108(4):624-626, 1986.

Gorzka PA and others: Parenting: categories for anticipatory guidance, *J Child Adolesc Psychiatr Ment Health Nurs* 4(1):16-19, 1991.

Heineken J, Roberts FB: Confirming, not disconfirming: communicating in a more positive manner, *MCN* 8(1):78-80, 1983.

Holden RJ: Empathy: the art of emotional knowing in holistic nursing care, *Holistic Nurs Pract* 5(1):70-79, 1990.

Leff P, Walizer E: *Building the healing partnership,* Cambridge, MA, 1992, Brookline Books.

McBurney BH, Schultz C: Defining quality services in a general pediatric unit, *J Nurs Care Qual* 7(3):51-60, 1993.

Sloat A, Matsuura W: Intercultural communication. In Craft M, Denehy J, editors: *Nursing interventions for infants and children,* Philadelphia, 1990, WB Saunders.

Smilkstein G: Family APGAR analyzed, *Fam Med* 25(5):293-294, 1993 (letter to the editor).

Smilkstein G, Ashworth C, Montano D: Validity and reliability of the family APGAR as a test of family function, *J Fam Pract* 15(2):303-311, 1982.

Wissow LS, Roter DL, Wilson MEH: Pediatrician interview style and mother's disclosure of psychosocial issues, *Pediatrics* 93(2):289-295, 1994.

BIBLIOGRAPHY

Communication Strategies/Health Interview

Able-Boone H, Dokecki P, Smith M: Parent and health care provider communication and decision making in the intensive care nursery, *Child Health Care* 18(3):113-141, 1989.

Andrist L: Taking a sexual history and educating clients about safe sex, *Nurs Clin North Am* 23(4):959-973, 1988.

Baretich D, Stephenson P, Igoe J: Using art to understand children's perceptions of roles in physician's office visits, *Pediatr Nurs* 15(4):356-360, 1989.

Barnes LP: Strategies for using interviewing skills in patient teaching, *MCN* 19(6):311, 1994.

Barnsteiner JH, Gillis-Donovan J: Being related and separate: a standard for therapeutic relationships, *MCN* 15:223-228, 1990.

Boyle WE Jr, Hoekelman RA: The pediatric history. In Hoekelman RA and others, editors: *Primary pediatric care,* ed 3, St Louis, 1997, Mosby.

Brantly DK: Communicating with children: age-related techniques. In Smith D and others, editors: *Comprehensive child and family nursing skills,* St Louis, 1991, Mosby.

Brantly DK: Conducting an interview. In Smith D and others, editors: *Comprehensive child and family nursing skills,* St Louis, 1991, Mosby.

Brantly DK: Conducting the psychosocial assessment of the child. In Smith D and others, editors: *Comprehensive child and family nursing skills,* St Louis, 1991, Mosby.

Buchwald D and others: The medical interview across cultures, *Patient Care* 27(7):141-166, 1993.

Butz A, Alexander C: Use of health diaries with children, *Nurs Res* 40(1):59-61, 1991.

Byrnes K: Conducting the pediatric health history: a guide, *Pediatr Nurs* 22(2):135-137, 1996.

Cassell E, Coulehan J, Putnam S: Making good interview skills better, *Patient Care* 23(6):145-148, 1989.

Crowther, D: Metacommunications: a missed opportunity, *J Psychosoc Nurs* 29(4):13-16, 1991.

Denehy J: Communicating with children through drawings. In Craft M, Denehy J, editors: *Nursing interventions for infants and children,* Philadelphia, 1990, WB Saunders.

DiLeo JH: *Children's drawings as diagnostic aids,* New York, 1980, Brunner/Mazel.

DiLeo JH: *Interpreting children's drawings,* New York, 1983, Brunner/Mazel.

Dunst C, Trivette C, Deal A: *Enabling and empowering families: principles and guidelines for practice,* Cambridge, MA, 1988, Brookline Books.

Elizabath J: Form of address: an addition to history taking? *Br Med J* 298(6668):257, 1989.

Faber A, Mazlish E: *How to talk so kids will listen and listen so kids will talk,* New York, 1980, Avon Books.

Fochtman D: Therapeutic relationships, *J Pediatr Oncol Nurs* 8(1):1-2, 1991.

Freeman M: Therapeutic use of storytelling for older children who are critically ill, *Child Health Care* 20(4):208-215, 1991.

Garbarino J and others: *What children can tell us: eliciting, interpreting, and evaluating information from children,* San Francisco, 1989, Jossey-Bass.

Gaynard L, Goldberger J, Laidley L: The use of stuffed, body-outline dolls with hospitalized children and adolescents, *Child Health Care* 20(4):216-224, 1991.

Glascoe F, MacLean W, Stone W: The importance of parents' concerns about their children's behavior, *Clin Pediatr* 30(1):8-11, 1991.

Green M: Twenty interview questions that work, *Contemp Pediatr* 9(11):47-71, 1992.

Hahn K: Therapeutic storytelling: helping children learn and cope, *Pediatr Nurs* 13(3):175-178, 1987.

Hart R and others: *Therapeutic play activities for hospitalized children,* St Louis, 1992, Mosby.

Hauck MR: Cognitive abilities of preschool children: implications for nurses working with young children, *J Pediatr Nurs* 6(4):230-245, 1991.

Hudson C and others: Storytelling: a measure of anxiety in hospitalized children, *Child Health Care* 16(2):118-122, 1987.

Johnson B: Children's drawings as a projective technique, *Pediatr Nurs* 16(1):11-16, 1990.

Kramer N: Comparison of therapeutic touch and casual touch in stress reduction of hospitalized children, *Pediatr Nurs* 16(5):483-485, 1990.

Lynn M: Projective technique: a way of getting "hidden" information, part I, *J Pediatr Nurs* 1(6):58-60, 1986.

Messinger R, Davidson PN, Hoekelman RA: Communication with parents and patients. In Hoekelman RA and others, editors: *Primary pediatric care,* ed 3, St Louis, 1997, Mosby.

Nance TA: Intercultural communication: finding common ground, *JOGNN* 24(3):249-255, 1995.

O'Malley ME, McNamara ST: Children's drawings: a preoperative assessment tool, *AORN J* 57(5):1074-1089, 1993.

Rollins J: Childhood cancer: siblings draw and tell, *Pediatr Nurs* 16(1):21-27, 1990.

Stevens NV: Obtaining a health history. In Smith D and others, editors: *Comprehensive child and family nursing skills,* St Louis, 1991, Mosby.

Sunde ER, Mabe PA, Josephson A: Difficult parents: from adversaries to partners, *Clin Pediatr* 32(4):213-219, 1993.

Thompson SW: Communication techniques for allaying anxiety and providing support for hospitalized children, *J Child Adolesc Psychiatry Ment Health Nurs* 4(3):119-122, 1992.

Tiedman M, Simon K, Clatworthy S: Communicating through therapeutic play. In Craft M, Denehy J, editors: *Nursing interventions for infants and children,* Philadelphia, 1990, WB Saunders.

Tuffnell DJ and others: Use of translated written material to communicate with non–English-speaking patients, *Br Med J* 309(6960):992, 1994.

Vezeau T: Storytelling: a practitioner's tool, *MCN* 18:193-196, 1993.

Walker C: Use of art and play therapy in pediatric oncology, *J Pediatr Oncol Nurs* 6(4):121-126, 1989.

Winkelstein M: Fostering positive self-concept in the school-age child, *Pediatr Nurs* 15(3):229-233, 1989

Family Assessment

Birenbaum LK: Measurement of family coping, *J Pediatr Oncol Nurs* 8(1):39-42, 1991.

Bradley R, Caldwell B: Using the home inventory to assess the family environment, *Pediatr Nurs* 14(2):97-103, 1988.

Brantly DK: Conducting a psychosocial assessment of the family. In Smith D and others, editors: *Comprehensive child and family nursing skills,* St Louis, 1991, Mosby.

Coleman WL: The first interview with a family, *Pediatr Clin North Am* 42(1):119-130, 1995.

Danielson CB, Hamel-Bissell B, Winstead-Fry P: *Families, health, and illness,* St Louis, 1993, Mosby.

Donelly E: Family health assessment, *Home Health Nurse* 11(2):30-37, 1993.

Gilliss C and others: *Toward a science of family nursing,* Menlo Park, CA, 1989, Addison-Wesley.

Lapp C, Diemert C, Enestvedt R: Family-based practice: discussion of a tool merging assessment with intervention, *Fam Community Health* 12(4):21-28, 1990.

Lotas M and others: The HOME scale: the influence of socioeconomic status on the evaluation of the home environment, *Nurs Res* 41(6):338-341, 1992.

Martinson I: The challenge of culturally diverse pediatric clients. In *Pediatric nursing: forum on the future: looking toward the 21st century,* Pitman, NJ, 1989, Anthony J Jannetti.

McCubbin H, McCubbin M: Family system assessment in health care. In McCubbin H, Thompson A, editors: *Family assessment inventories for research and practice,* ed 2, Madison, WI, 1991, The University of Wisconsin–Madison.

Rosenbaum J: A cultural assessment guide: learning cultural sensitivity, *J Can Nurs Assoc* 87(4):32-33, 1991.

Speer J, Sachs B: Selecting the appropriate family assessment tool, *Pediatr Nurs* 11(5):349-355, 1985.

Touliatos J, Perlmutter B, Straus M, editors: *Handbook of family measurement techniques,* London, 1990, Sage Publications.

Wright L, Leahey M: *Nurses and families: a guide to family assessment and intervention,* Philadelphia, 1984, FA Davis.

Nutritional Assessment

American Academy of Pediatrics, Committee on Nutrition: *Pediatric nutrition handbook,* Elk Grove Village, IL, 1993, The Academy.

Basch C and others: Validation of mothers' reports of dietary intake by four- to seven-year-old children, *Am J Public Health* 80(11):1314-1317, 1990.

Benjamin D: Laboratory tests and nutritional assessment: protein-energy status, *Pediatr Clin North Am* 36(1):139-161, 1989.

Buzzard IM, Willet WC, editors: First international conference on dietary assessment methods: assessing diets to improve world health, *Am J Clin Nutr* 59(1, suppl): entire issue, 1994.

Kristal A and others: Development and validation of a food use checklist for evaluation of community nutrition interventions, *Am J Public Health* 80(11):1318-1322, 1990.

Liguori R: Assessing nutritional status. In Smith D and others, editors: *Comprehensive child and family nursing skills,* St Louis, 1991, Mosby.

Pipes PL, Trahms CM: *Nutrition in infancy and childhood,* ed 5, St Louis, 1995, Mosby.

Simko M, Cowell C, Hreha M: *Practical nutrition: a quick reference for the health care practitioner,* Rockville, MD, 1989, Aspen.

Sources of Books for Bibliotherapy

Association for the Care of Children's Health: *Books for children and teenagers about hospitalization, illness, and disabling conditions,* Washington, DC, 1987, The Association.

Berg PJ, Devlin MK, Gedaly-Duff V: Bibliotherapy with children experiencing loss, *Issues Compr Pediatr Nurs* 4:37-50, 1980.

Cohen L: "Here's something I want you to read," *RN* 55(10):56-59, 1992.

Cuddigan M, Hanson MB: *Growing pains: helping children deal with everyday problems through reading,* Chicago, 1988, American Library Association.

Dreyer S: *The Bookfinder 4: when kids need books,* Circle Pines, MN, 1989, American Guidance Service.

Fassler J: *Helping children cope: mastering stress through books and stories,* London, 1978, The Free Press.

Fosson A, Husband E: Bibliotherapy for hospitalized children, *South Med J* 77(3):342-346, 1984.

Oppenheim J, Brenner B, Boegehold B: *Choosing books for kids,* NY, 1986, Ballantine Books.

Wallace NE: Special books for special children, *Child Health Care* 12(1):34-36, 1983.

PHYSICAL AND DEVELOPMENTAL ASSESSMENT OF THE CHILD

Chapter 7

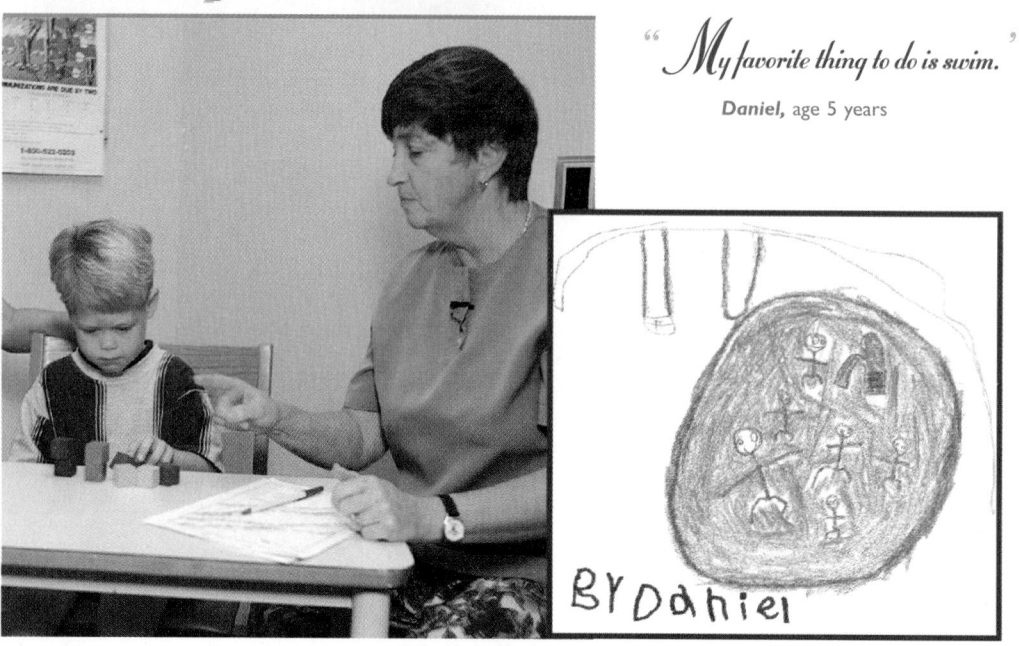

" *My favorite thing to do is swim.* "

Daniel, age 5 years

BY Daniel

RELATED TOPICS

GENERAL APPROACHES TOWARD EXAMINING THE CHILD

SEQUENCE OF THE EXAMINATION

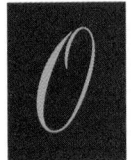Ordinarily the sequence for examining patients follows a head-to-toe direction. The main function of such a systematic approach is to provide a general guideline for assessment of each body area to minimize omitting segments of the examination. The standard recording of data also facilitates exchange of information among different professionals. The typical organization of a physical examination is indicated in the chapter outline. In examining children, this orderly sequence is frequently altered to accommodate the child's developmental needs, although the examination is recorded following the head-to-toe model. Using developmental and chronologic age as the main criteria for assessing each body system accomplishes several goals:

- Minimizes stress and anxiety associated with assessment of various body parts
- Fosters a trusting nurse-child-parent relationship
- Allows for maximum preparation of the child
- Preserves the essential security of the parent-child relationship, especially with young children
- Maximizes the accuracy and reliability of assessment findings

PREPARATION OF THE CHILD

Although the physical examination consists of painless procedures, to a child the use of a tight arm cuff, probes in the ears and mouth, pressing on the abdomen, and listening to the chest with a cold piece of metal can be considerably stressful. Therefore the same considerations discussed in Chapter 22 for preparing children for procedures are followed here. In addition to that discussion, general guidelines related to the examining process are presented in the box on p. 136. The physical examination should be as pleasant as possible, as well as educational. For example, the nurse can use a detailed drawing or anatomically correct doll to help preschoolers and older children learn about their bodies (Vessey, Braithwaite, and Weidmann, 1990). The "paper-doll" technique is a useful approach to teaching children about the part of the body that is being examined (Fig. 7-1). At the conclusion of the visit, the child can bring home the paper doll as a memento of the experience.

In most instances children cooperate best when their parents remain with them. There are occasions, however, when older children, particularly adolescents, prefer to be examined alone, such as during the genital examination. Frequently the child being examined is also accompanied by a sibling, who may be disruptive because of boredom. It is a helpful tactic to involve the sibling in the examination by allowing the child to hold the stethoscope or a tongue blade and praising the child for the "help" during the assessment.

Table 7-1 summarizes guidelines for positioning, preparing, and examining children at various ages. Because no child fits precisely into one age category, it may be necessary to vary the approach after a preliminary assessment of the child's developmental achievements and needs. Even when the best approach is used, many toddlers are uncooperative and unable to be consoled for much of the physical examination. However, some seem intrigued by the new surroundings and unusual equipment and respond more like preschoolers than toddlers. Likewise, some early preschoolers may require more of the "security measures" employed with younger children, such as continued parent-child contact, and less of the preparatory measures used with preschoolers, such as playing with the equipment before and during the actual examination (Fig. 7-2).

Although the variations in the general approaches are numerous, some of them are elaborated here because they are more common. For example, the suggested sequence may change considerably when the child is in pain or when obvious physical defects are present. In either situation examine the affected area last to minimize distress early in the examination and to focus on normal, healthy, or functioning body parts.

Positioning may also be altered because of physical distress. For example, the child who is having difficulty breathing may not be able to lie down; thus perform as much of the physical examination as possible with the child in a sitting or slightly reclining position, or complete the examination at another time.

PHYSICAL EXAMINATION

Although the approach to and sequence of the physical examination differ according to the child's age, the following discussion outlines the traditional model for physical assessment. Although the focus includes all pediatric age-groups, the reader is referred to Chapter 8 for a detailed discussion of a newborn assessment. Because the physical examination

GENERAL GUIDELINES FOR PERFORMING PEDIATRIC PHYSICAL EXAMINATION

Perform examination in appropriate, nonthreatening area.
　Have room well lit and decorated with neutral colors.
　Have room temperature comfortably warm.
　Place all strange and potentially frightening equipment out of sight.
　Have some toys, dolls, stuffed animals, and games available for child.
　If possible, have rooms decorated and equipped for different-age children.
　Provide privacy, especially for school-age children and adolescents.
Provide time for play and becoming acquainted.
Observe behaviors that signal child's readiness to cooperate:
　Talking to the nurse
　Making eye contact
　Accepting the offered equipment
　Allowing physical touching
　Choosing to sit on examining table rather than parent's lap
If signs of readiness are not observed, use the following techniques:
　Talk to parent while essentially "ignoring" child; gradually focus on child or a favorite object, such as a doll.
　Make complimentary remarks about child, such as appearance, dress, or a favorite object.
　Tell a funny story or play a simple magic trick.
　Have a nonthreatening "friend" available, such as a hand puppet to "talk" to child for the nurse (see Fig. 7-22, A)
If child refuses to cooperate, use the following techniques:
　Assess reason for uncooperative behavior; consider that a child who is unduly afraid may have had a previous traumatic experience.
　Try to involve child and parent in process.
　Avoid prolonged explanations about examining procedure.
　Use a firm, direct approach regarding expected behavior.
　Perform examination as quickly as possible.
　Have attendant gently restrain child.
　Minimize any disruptions or stimulation.
　　Limit number of people in room.
　　Use isolated room.
　　Use quiet, calm, confident voice.

Begin examination in a nonthreatening manner for young children or children who are fearful:
　Use those activities that can be presented as games, such as test for cranial nerves (see Table 7-12) or parts of developmental screening tests (p. 176).
　Use approaches such as "Simon says" to encourage child to make a face, squeeze a hand, stand on one foot, and so on.
　Use "paper-doll" technique.
　　Lay child supine on an examining table or floor that is covered with a large sheet of paper.
　　Trace around child's body outline.
　　Use body outline to demonstrate what will be examined, such as drawing a heart and listening with stethoscope before performing activity on child.
If several children in the family will be examined, begin with most cooperative child to provide modeling of desired behavior.
Involve child in examination process:
　Provide choices, such as sitting on table or in parent's lap.
　Allow child to handle or hold equipment.
　Encourage child to use equipment on a doll, family member, or examiner.
　Explain each step of the procedure in simple language.
Examine child in a comfortable and secure position:
　Sitting in parent's lap
　Sitting upright if in respiratory distress
Proceed to examine the body in an organized sequence (usually head to toe) with the following exceptions:
　Alter sequence to accommodate needs of different-age children (see Table 7-1).
　Examine painful areas last.
　In emergency situation, examine vital functions (airway, breathing, and circulation) and injured area first.
Reassure child throughout examination, especially about bodily concerns that arise during puberty.
Discuss findings with family at end of examination.
Praise child for cooperation during examination; give reward such as a small toy or sticker.

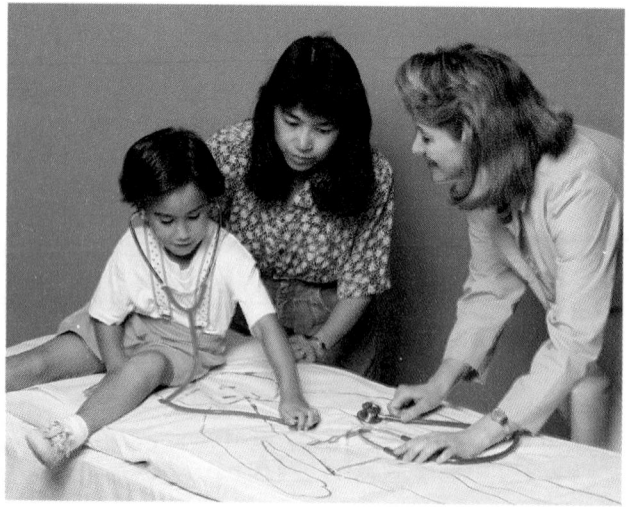

FIG. 7-1. Using paper-doll technique to prepare child.

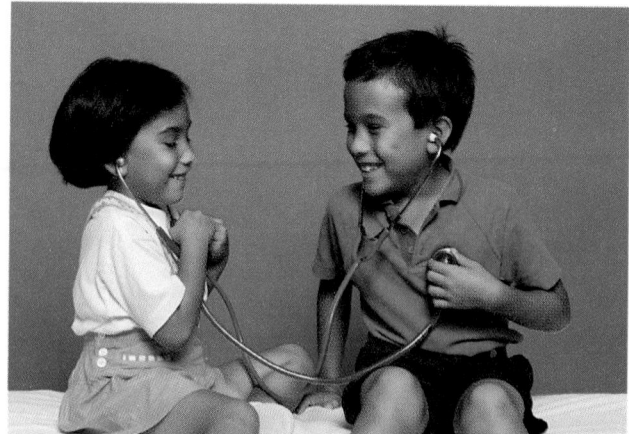

FIG. 7-2. Preparing children for physical examination.

TABLE 7-1. Age-specific approaches to physical examination during childhood

POSITION	SEQUENCE	PREPARATION
Infant Before sits alone: supine or prone, preferably in parent's lap; before 4 to 6 months: can place on examining table After sits alone: use sitting in parent's lap whenever possible If on table, place with parent in full view	If quiet, auscultate heart, lungs, abdomen Record heart and respiratory rates Palpate and percuss same areas Proceed in usual head-toe direction Perform traumatic procedures last (eyes, ears, mouth [while crying]) Elicit reflexes as body part examined Elicit Moro reflex last	Completely undress if room temperature permits Leave diaper on male Gain cooperation with distraction, bright objects, rattles, talking Smile at infant; use soft, gentle voice Pacify with bottle of sugar water or feeding Enlist parent's aid for restraining to examine ears, mouth Avoid abrupt, jerky movements
Toddler Sitting or standing on/by parent Prone or supine in parent's lap	Inspect body area through play: "count fingers," "tickle toes" Use minimal physical contact initially Introduce equipment slowly Auscultate, percuss, palpate whenever quiet Perform traumatic procedures last (same as for infant)	Have parent remove outer clothing Remove underwear as body part examined Allow to inspect equipment; demonstrating use of equipment usually ineffective If uncooperative, perform procedures quickly Use restraint when appropriate; request parent's assistance Talk about examination if cooperative; use short phrases Praise for cooperative behavior
Preschool Child Prefer standing or sitting Usually cooperative prone/supine Prefer parent's closeness	If cooperative, proceed in head-toe direction If uncooperative, proceed as with toddler	Request self-undressing Allow to wear underpants if shy Offer equipment for inspection; briefly demonstrate use Make up "story" about procedure: "I'm seeing how strong your muscles are" (blood pressure) Use paper-doll technique Give choices when possible Expect cooperation; use positive statements: "Open your mouth"
School-Age Child Prefer sitting Cooperative in most positions Younger child prefers parent's presence Older child may prefer privacy	Proceed in head-toe direction May examine genitalia last in older child Respect need for privacy	Request self-undressing Allow to wear underpants Give gown to wear Explain purpose of equipment and significance of procedure, such as otoscope to see eardrum, which is necessary for hearing Teach about body functioning and care
Adolescent Same as for school-age child Offer option of parent's presence	Same as older school-age child	Allow to undress in private Give gown Expose only area to be examined Respect need for privacy Explain findings during examination: "Your muscles are firm and strong" Matter-of-factly comment about sexual development: "Your breasts are developing as they should be" Emphasize normalcy of development Examine genitalia as any other body part; may leave to end

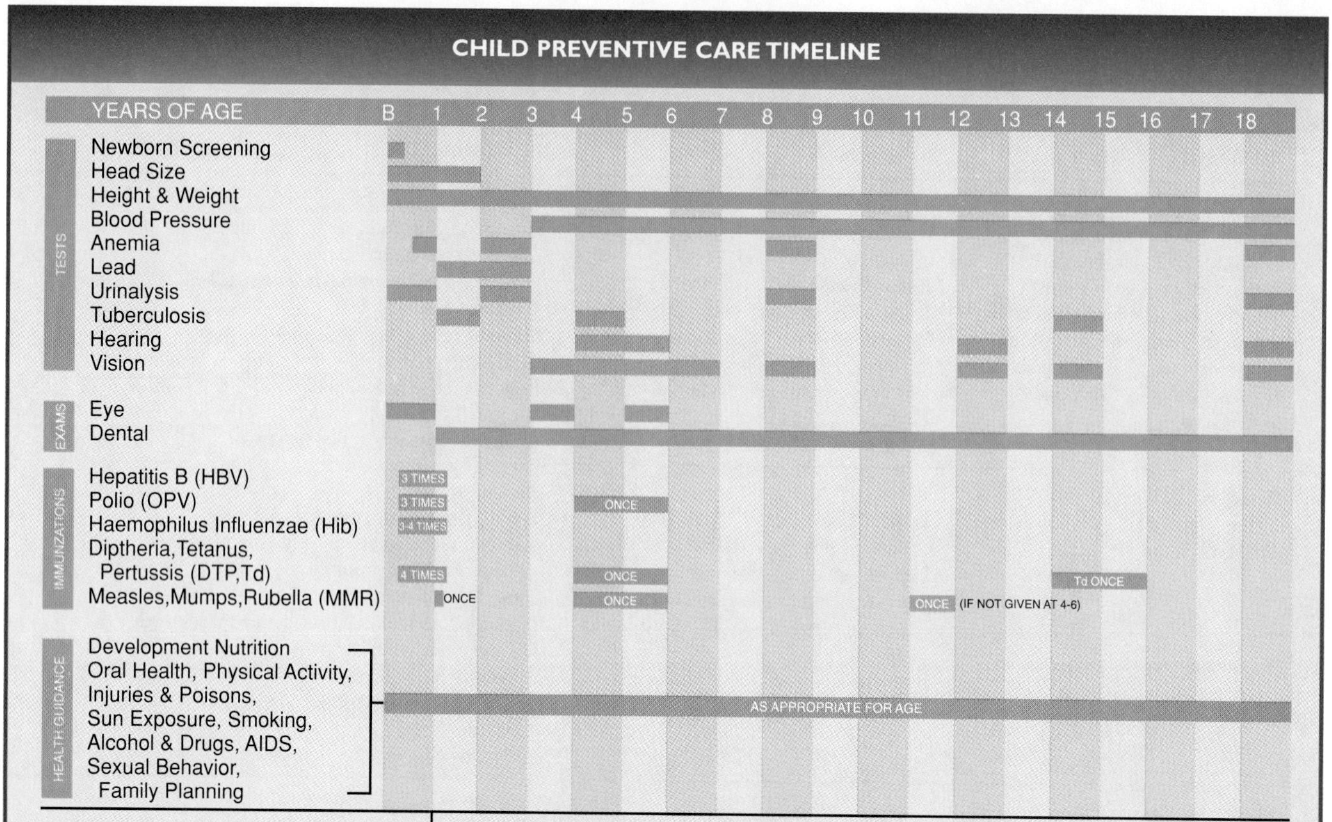

Key: Recommended by all major authorities.
Recommended by some major authorities.

Please note: Children with special risk factors may need more frequent and additional types of preventive care. Some examples:

RISK FACTOR	PREVENTIVE SERVICES NEEDED
Exposure to TB	TB test
Sexually active	Pap test (females); syphilis, gonorrhea, chlamydia tests
High-risk sexual behavoir	AIDS test, hepatitis immunization
Drug abuse	AIDS, TB tests, hepatitis immunization

From *Child health guide: put prevention into practice,* US Department of Health and Human Services, undated, pp. 20-21.

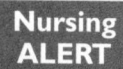

is a vital part of preventive pediatric care, a schedule for periodic health visits is given in the box.

GROWTH MEASUREMENTS

Measurement of physical growth in children is a key element in evaluation of their health status. Physical growth parameters include weight, height (length), skinfold thickness, arm circumference, and head circumference. Values for these growth parameters are plotted on percentile charts, and the child's measurements in percentiles are compared with those of the general population.

The most commonly used growth charts in the United States are from the ***National Center for Health Statistics (NCHS)*** and are available for boys and girls ages (see Appendix D):

- **Birth to 36 months**—records weight by age, recumbent length by age, weight for length, and head circumference by age
- **Two to 18 years**—records weight by age, stature by age
- **Prepubescence**—records weight for stature

Nursing ALERT The prepubescent charts are only appropriate for plotting values for prepubescent boys and girls, regardless of chronologic age, and not for any child showing signs of pubescence, such as breast budding, testicular enlargement, or growth of axillary or pubic hair.

Two sets of charts include data for children ages 2 to 3 years; the major difference between the two charts is that one set (birth to 36 months) is based on ***recumbent length,*** and the other set (2 to 18 years) uses ***stature*** (standing height). These two methods of measuring length are not equivalent. Measurements using recumbent length are greater by as much as 2 cm, or nearly 1 inch, in this age-group than measurements obtained using stature. Such a difference between measurements can lead to an erroneous conclusion of delayed growth if length is plotted during one visit and stature during the next visit on the birth to 36-month chart.

Nursing ALERT Plot only recumbent length on the birth to 36-month NCHS growth charts and stature on the 2- to 18-year growth charts.

The NCHS growth charts use the 5th and 95th percentiles as criteria for determining which children are outside the normal limits for growth. In general, those whose height or weight falls below the 5th percentile are considered underweight or small in stature; those whose measurements are above the 95th percentile are considered overweight or large in stature.

Overall evaluation of growth requires judgment in interpretation of growth percentiles. Generally, children whose

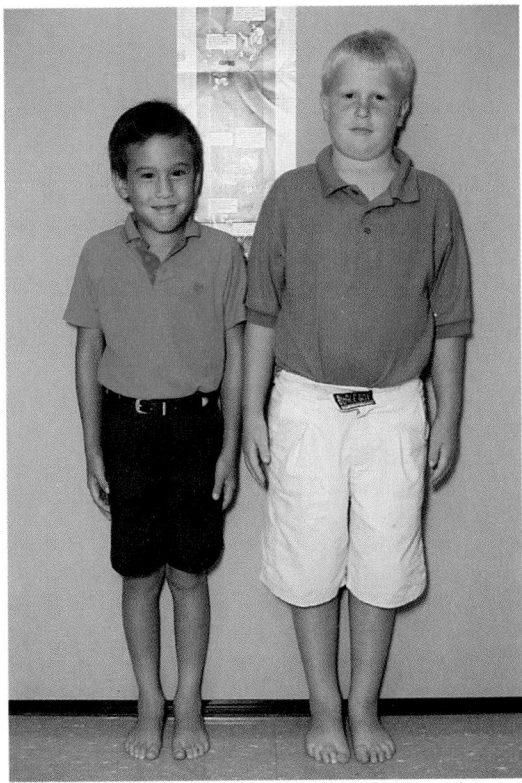

FIG. 7-3. These children of identical age (8 years) are markedly different in size. The child on the left, of Asian descent, is at the 5th percentile for height and weight. The child on the right is above the 95th percentile for height and weight. However, both children demonstrate normal growth patterns.

TABLE 7-2. Expected growth rates at various ages

AGE	EXPECTED GROWTH RATE (IN CM/YEAR)
1 to 6 months	18-22
6 to 12 months	14-18
2nd year	11
3rd year	8
4th year	7
5th to 10th years	5-6

From *Human growth and growth disorders: an update*, South San Francisco, 1989, Genentech.

height or weight falls below the 5th percentile or above the 95th percentile should be followed closely. However, small or large size may be genetic (Fig. 7-3) (see Cultural Awareness box). Comparing children's growth trends with those of their parents is essential in evaluating adequate growth. Since the NCHS charts used a sample of children who were mainly bottle-fed, the growth percentiles for breast-fed infants must be carefully interpreted.

Breast-fed infants grow slower than bottle-fed infants, especially during the second half of the first year. This slower growth is normal, although it may be at or below the 5th percentile (Dewey and others, 1995).

Children whose growth may be questionable include the following:

- Children whose height and weight percentiles are widely disparate (e.g., height in the 10th percentile and weight in the 90th percentile, especially with above-average skinfold thickness)
- Children who fail to show the expected growth rates in height and weight, especially during the rapid growth periods of infancy and adolescence (Table 7-2)
- Children who show a sudden increase, except during puberty, or a decrease in a previously steady growth pattern

Since growth is a continuous but uneven process, the most reliable evaluation lies in comparison of growth measurements over a prolonged time.

Length

The term *length* refers to measurements taken when children are supine (also referred to as *recumbent length*). Until children are 24 months old (36 months if the birth to 36-month chart is used), measure recumbent length. Because of the normally flexed position during infancy, fully extend the body by (1) holding the head in midline, (2) grasping the knees together gently, and (3) pushing down on the knees until the legs are fully extended and flat against the table. If using a measuring board, place the head firmly at the top of the board and the heels of the feet firmly against the footboard.

If such a measuring device is not available, measure length by placing the child on a paper-covered surface, marking the end points of the top of the head and the heels of the feet, and measuring between these two points (Fig. 7-4). For accurate measurement hold the writing utensil at a right angle to the table when marking the cephalic point; position the feet with the toes pointing directly to the ceiling when mark-

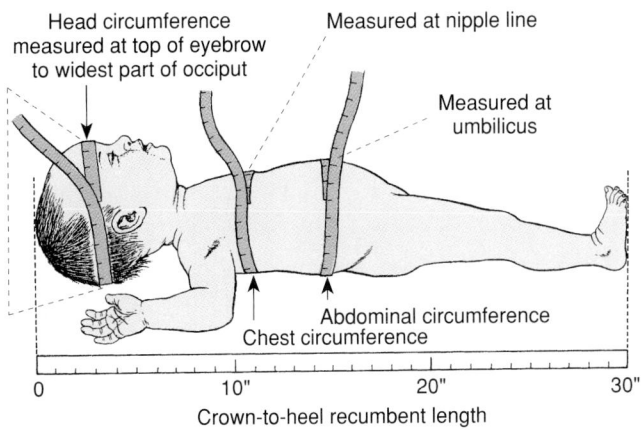

FIG. 7-4. Measurement of head, chest, and abdominal circumference and crown-to-heel (recumbent) length.

ing the heel point. Regardless of the method used, have someone assist in holding the child's head in midline while you extend the legs and take the measurements.

Height

The term *height* (or *stature*) refers to the measurement taken when children are standing upright. Measure height by having the child, with shoes removed, stand as tall and straight as possible, with the head in midline and the line of vision parallel to the ceiling or floor. Be sure the child's back is to the wall or other vertical flat surface, with the heels, buttocks, and back of the shoulders touching the wall and the medial malleoli touching if possible (Fig. 7-5). Check for and correct bending of the knees, slumping of the shoulders, or raising of the heels of the feet.

NURSING TIP Normally height is less if measured in the afternoon than in the morning. To minimize this variation, apply modest upward pressure under the jaw or the mastoid processes behind the ears.

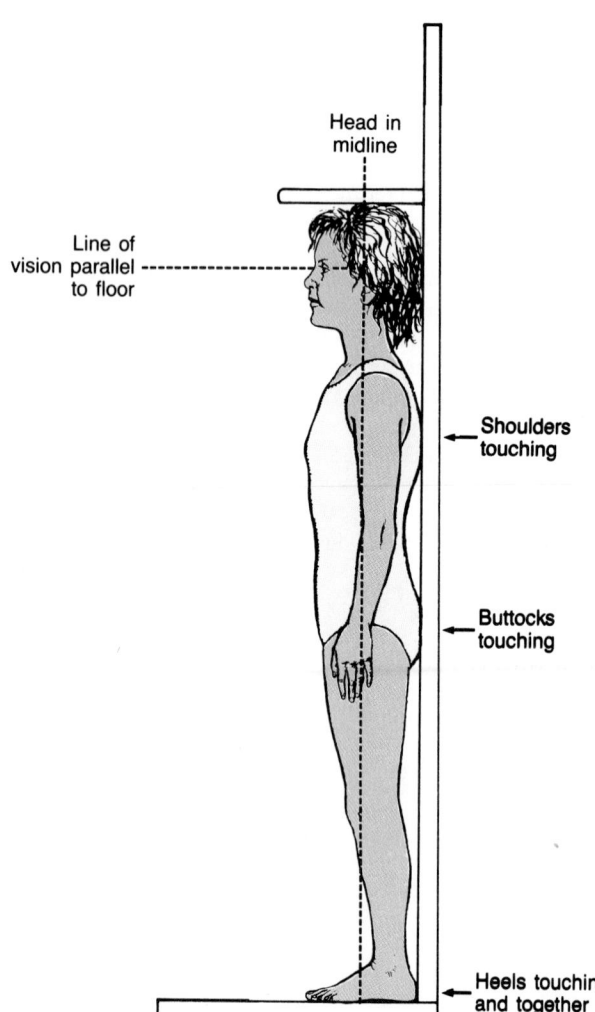

FIG. 7-5. Measurement of height. (Redrawn from *Human growth and growth disorders: an update,* South San Francisco, 1989, Genentech.)

For the most accurate measurement, use a wall-mounted unit (*stadiometer;* see Fig. 7-5). The movable measuring rod of platform scales is accurate only if it maintains a parallel position to the floor and rests securely on the topmost part of the head. To improvise a flat surface for measuring length, attach a paper or metal tape or yardstick to the wall, position the child adjacent to the tape, and place a three-dimensional object, such as a thick book or box, on top of the head. Rest the side of the object firmly against the wall to form a right angle. Measure length or stature to the nearest 1 mm or ⅛ inch.

Weight

Weight is measured with an appropriately sized beam balance scale, which measures weights to the nearest 10 g or ½ ounce for infants and 100 g or ¼ pound for children. Before the child is weighed, the scale is balanced by setting it at zero and noting if the balance registers exactly in the middle of the mark. If the end of the balance beam rises to the top or bottom of the mark, more or less weight, respectively, is added. Some scales are designed to allow for self-correction, but others need to be recalibrated by the manufacturer. Scales vary in their accuracy; infant scales tend to be more accurate than adult platform scales, and newer scales tend to be more accurate than older ones, especially at the upper levels of weight measurement. When precise measurements are needed, two nurses should take the weight independently, and if there is a discrepancy, a third reading should be taken (Burke, Roberts, and Maloney, 1988).

Take measurements in a comfortably warm room. When the birth to 36-month growth charts are used, children should be weighed nude. Older children are usually weighed while wearing their underpants or a light gown. However, always respect the privacy of all children. If the child must be weighed wearing some article of clothing or some type of special device, such as a prosthesis or an armboard for an intravenous device, note this when recording the weight. Children who are measured for recumbent length are usually weighed on an infant platform scale and placed in a lying-down or sitting position. When weighing children, place your hand lightly above the body of the infant to prevent the child from accidentally falling off the scale (Fig. 7-6, *A*) or stand close to the toddler, ready to prevent a fall (Fig. 7-6, *B*). For maximum asepsis, cover the scale with a clean sheet of paper between each child's measurement.

Skinfold Thickness and Arm Circumference

Measures of relative weight and stature cannot distinguish between adipose (fat) tissue or muscle. One convenient measure of body fat is *skinfold thickness,* which is increasingly recommended as a routine measurement (see also Anthropometry, Chapter 6). Skinfold thickness is measured with special calipers, such as the Lange calipers. The most common sites for measuring skinfold thickness are the triceps (most practical for routine clinical use), subscapula, suprailiac, abdomen, and upper thigh. For greatest reliability the exact procedure for measurement must be followed and the average of at least two measurements of one site recorded (see Guidelines box).

Arm circumference is an indirect measure of muscle mass. Measurement of arm circumference follows the same proce-

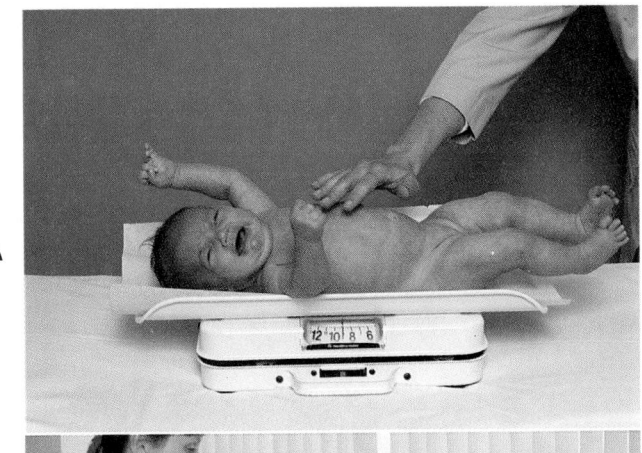

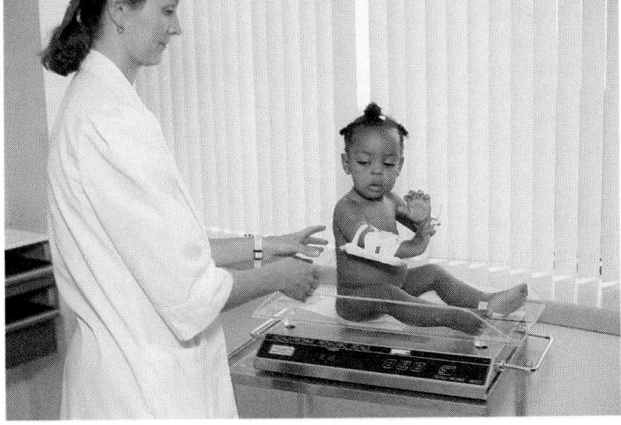

FIG. 7-6. **A,** Infant on scale. **B,** Toddler on scale. Note presence of nurse to prevent falls.

GUIDELINES
Measuring Triceps Skinfold Thickness

With child's right arm flexed 90 degrees at elbow, mark midpoint between acromion and olecranon on posterior aspect of arm.

With arm hanging freely, grasp a fold of skin between thumb and forefinger 1 cm above midpoint.

Gently pull fold away from underlying muscle and continue to hold until measurement is completed.

Place caliper jaws over skinfold at midpoint mark and follow directions for using the device.

Estimate reading to nearest 1 mm, 2 to 3 seconds after applying pressure.

Take measurements until duplicates agree within 1 mm.

ATRAUMATIC CARE
Reducing Young Children's Fears

Young children, especially preschoolers, fear intrusive procedures because of their poorly defined body boundaries. Therefore, avoid invasive procedures, such as measuring rectal temperature, whenever possible. Also, avoid using the word "take" when measuring vital signs, since young children interpret words literally and may think that their temperature or other function will be taken away. Instead, say, "I want to know how warm you are."

---

dure for skinfold thickness except measure the midpoint with a paper or steel tape. Place the tape vertically, along the posterior aspect of the upper arm to the acromial process and to the olecranon process; half the measured length is the midpoint. Percentiles for triceps skinfold and arm circumference in children are listed in Appendix D and may be used as reference data. However, the percentiles are not standards or norms, because values between the 5th and 95th percentiles are not ranges of normal.

Head Circumference

Measure head circumference in children up to 36 months of age and in any child whose head size is questionable. Measure the head at its greatest circumference, usually slightly above the eyebrows and pinna of the ears and around the occipital prominence at the back of the skull (see Fig. 7-4). Since head shape can affect the location of the maximum circumference, more than one measurement at points above the eyebrows may need to be taken to obtain the most accurate measure. Use a paper or metal tape because a cloth tape can stretch and give a falsely small measurement. For greatest accuracy, use devices with tenths of a centimeter because the percentile charts have only 0.5 cm increments.

Plot the head size on the appropriate growth chart under head circumference. Generally, head and chest circumferences are equal at about 1 to 2 years of age. During childhood chest circumference exceeds head size by about 5 to 7 cm (2 to 3 in). (For newborns see Physical Assessment, Chapter 8.)

PHYSIOLOGIC MEASUREMENTS

Physiologic measurements, key elements in evaluating physical status of vital functions, include temperature, pulse, respiration, and blood pressure. Compare each physiologic recording with normal values for that age-group (see inside back cover). In addition, compare the values taken on preceding health visits with present recordings. For example, a falsely elevated blood pressure reading may not indicate hypertension if previous recent readings have been within normal limits. The isolated recording may indicate some stressful event in the child's life.

As in most procedures carried out with children, older children and adolescents are treated much the same as are adults. However, special consideration must be given to preschool children (see Atraumatic Care box).

For best results in taking vital signs of infants, count respirations first, before the infant is disturbed, take the pulse next, and measure temperature last. If vital signs cannot be taken without disturbing the child, record the child's behavior (e.g., crying) along with the measurement.

Temperature

Temperature can be measured at several sites in the body via the oral, rectal, axillary, skin, or tympanic membrane route. Recent substitutes for the traditional mercury thermometer are the electronic thermometer, the tympanic membrane sen-

TABLE 7-3. Comparison of body temperature techniques

DESCRIPTION/PROCEDURE	COMMENTS
Mercury Glass Thermometer Heat causes mercury to expand and rise in glass tube	Only difference in selection of mercury thermometers is that rectal type has more rounded tip as compared with oral type, which has more slender, elongated tip Appropriate length of time mercury thermometer should remain in place for accurate measurement of temperature is controversial; a general rule is to leave thermometer in place about 3 minutes, or follow agency policy (see also Nursing Tip, p. 144)
Oral temperature Place under tongue in right or left posterior sublingual pocket, not in front of tongue; have child keep mouth closed without biting on thermometer	Sublingual site indicates rapid changes in core body temperature *better* than rectal site Several factors affect temperature of mouth, such as hot or cold beverages, smoking, open-mouth breathing, and ambient temperature Oxygen by mask lowers oral temperature, but clinical significance of difference is questionable
Axillary temperature Place under arm with tip in center of axilla and keep close to skin, not clothing; hold child's arm firmly against side (Fig. 7-7, *A*)	Recommended for children who object strongly to rectal temperature but for whom an oral temperature is not feasible Has advantage of avoiding intrusive procedure and eliminating risk of rectal perforation and possible peritonitis May be affected by poor peripheral perfusion (lower value) or use of radiant warmers or brown fat in cold-stressed neonates (higher value)

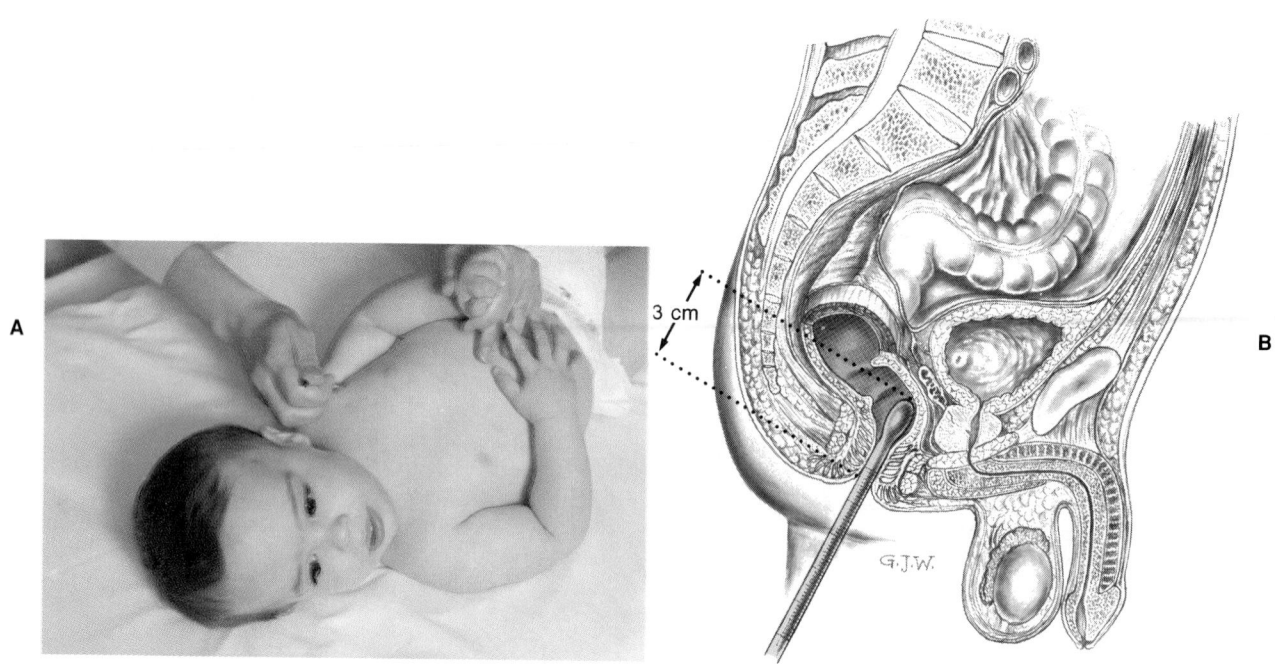

3 cm

FIG. 7-7. **A,** Position for taking axillary temperature. **B,** Cross section of rectum illustrates curve at approximately 3 cm from anus, where risk of perforation from thermometer is greatest in infants up to 3 months of age.

TABLE 7-3. Comparison of body temperature techniques—cont'd

DESCRIPTION/PROCEDURE	COMMENTS
Rectal temperature Place well-lubricated tip not more than 2.5 cm (1 inch) into rectum; securely hold thermometer close to anus May place child in side-lying, supine, or prone position (i.e., supine with knees flexed toward abdomen); cover penis, because procedure often stimulates urination A small child may be placed prone across parent's lap	Taken only when no other route or device can be used (e.g., in children whose mental age or temperament prevents cooperation and understanding instructions, agitated children, and those who have had oral or axillary injuries or surgery) Not recommended, because core temperature is not obtained unless thermometer is inserted to depth of at least 5 cm, which incurs risk of rectal perforation, especially in infants less than 3 months of age, since colon curves at depth of 3 cm (Fig. 7-7, *B*); also not recommended in anyone who has had rectal surgery, or in children with diarrhea or those receiving chemotherapy that affects mucosa Stool in rectum and less blood flow to area affects accuracy, especially in measuring changes in body temperature
Electronic Thermometer Senses temperature with electronic component called thermistor mounted at tip of plastic and stainless steel probe, which is connected to electronic recorder; temperature measurement appears on digital display within 60 seconds Place probe in mouth, axilla, or rectum as with mercury thermometer	Ideally suited to pediatric use because plastic sheath is unbreakable, and child's mouth can remain open when oral temperature is taken
Infrared Thermometry Infrared thermometer measures thermal radiation from axilla, ear canal opening, or tympanic membrane; temperature measurement appears on digital display in about 1 second **Tympanic membrane sensor** Insert covered probe tip gently in ear canal pointing toward midpoint between opposite eyebrow and sideburns (Terndrup and Rajk, 1992) For most accurate results, straighten ear canal for sensor to measure heat from drum, not sides of canal (see Fig. 7-20), take three measurements, and record highest reading Most models use "offsets" or internal calculations that transform ear temperature into supposedly equivalent oral or rectal temperatures	 Tympanic membrane is excellent site because both eardrum and hypothalamus (temperature-regulating center) are perfused by same circulation Sensor is unaffected by cerumen; presence of suppurative or nonsuppurative otitis media does not significantly affect measurement; ear against surface, i.e., mattress, may be higher in temperature than exposed ear; warm ambient temperature may increase aural temperature Procedure is well accepted by infants and children Because of difficulty with correct placement in young infants' ears, accuracy may be affected (Weiss, Poeltler, and Gocka, 1993)
Ear sensor (OTOTEMP) * Measures infrared heat energy radiating from canal opening, scans canal for highest temperature reading, and then calculates arterial temperature (correlates highly with core or internal body temperature) Insert hemispherical probe in ear opening; ear tug is not necessary	Available in two sizes; smaller size of LighTouch Pedi-Q is for smaller children Does not calculate offsets; therefore reading is only for arterial temperature (not equivalent to other sites)
Axillary sensor (Ototemp LighTouch Neonate) * Measures infrared heat energy radiating from axilla Touch covered probe to axilla, depress and release button, remove and read	Can be used on wet skin, in incubators, or under radiant heaters, warming pads, or other heat sources

*Manufactured by EXERGEN Corporation, 51 Water Street, Watertown, MA 02172, 1-800-422-3006, (617) 923-9900, FAX (617) 923-9911.

Continued.

TABLE 7-3. Comparison of body temperature techniques—cont'd

DESCRIPTION/PROCEDURE	COMMENTS
Digital Thermometer Consists of probe that connects to microprocessor chip, which translates signals into degrees and sends temperature measurement to digital display Used like oral mercury thermometer	More accurate and easier to read, but somewhat more expensive than mercury or plastic strip thermometer
Tempa-Dot Single-use disposable thermometer with specific chemical mixture in each circle that changes color to measure temperature in increments of two tenths of a degree Used like mercury thermometer; kept in mouth (1 minute), axilla (3 minutes), and rectum (3 minutes); color change is read 10-15 seconds after removing thermometer	Found to be accurate and reliable for children with and without fever, especially for temperature below 38° C (100.4° F) (Pontious and others, 1994a, 1994b) Easier to read than mercury or plastic strip thermometer Safer than glass thermometers (disposable and flexible) Read thermometer away from heat source (e.g., radiant warmer) If unused thermometer changes color from storage in warm area (above 35° C [95° F]), place in freezer for 1 hour, then at room temperature for 24 hours before using
Plastic Strip Thermometer (Thermograph) Changes color in response to sensed temperature changes Place strip on forehead until color change occurs; usually takes less than 15 seconds Some strips are used like oral mercury thermometer	Accuracy is variable; best used for screening Advantages for home use include simple instructions and minimal cost Can provide continuous measurement without disturbing child

sor, the Tempa-Dot, the plastic strip, and the digital thermometer. These devices offer the advantages of measuring temperature rapidly and/or avoiding oral or rectal intrusion (Table 7-3). Although the accuracy of these instruments differs, accuracy is decreased to a greater extent if correct technique is not used (Pontious and others, 1994b).

NURSING TIP When using a tympanic membrane sensor, first use an otoscope to visualize the eardrum. Once the drum is seen, note the type of ear tug and speculum placement in the ear. Use the same procedure for inserting the probe tip.

No universal agreement exists regarding the length of time mercury thermometers should be kept in place. Recommendations based on research are 7 minutes for an oral reading, 4 minutes for a rectal reading, and 5 minutes for an axillary reading. However, these times may vary widely within practice settings and may not represent clinically significant differences from temperature readings taken for shorter intervals.

NURSING TIP If in doubt about the optimum length of insertion time, reinsert the mercury thermometer after the first reading for a short time and recheck the scale for a rise. If the value is increased, reinsert the thermometer until the next reading is the same as the previous reading.

Normal body temperature registers 37.0° C (98.6° F) via the oral route. Traditionally it has been assumed that rectal temperatures are 1° F higher and axillary temperatures are 1° F lower than oral temperatures. However, it has been demonstrated that this difference is considerably less (Pontious

and others, 1994a). Because of these variations, chart the route along with the recorded temperature reading.

Whenever a child feels extra warm to the touch, measure the temperature even if it was normal only a short time before. Other signs of increased body temperature are flushed skin, increased respiratory and heart rate, malaise, and a "glassy look" to the eyes.

Pulse

A satisfactory pulse can be taken radially in children over 2 years of age. However, in infants and young children the apical impulse (heard through a stethoscope held to the chest at the apex of the heart) is more reliable. (See Fig. 7-29 for location of pulses.) Count the pulse for 1 full minute in infants and young children because of possible irregularities in rhythm. However, when frequent apical rates are needed, use shorter counting times (e.g., 15- or 30-second intervals). For

TABLE 7-4. Grading of pulses

GRADE	DESCRIPTION
0	Not palpable
+1	Difficult to palpate, thready, weak, easily obliterated with pressure
+2	Difficult to palpate, may be obliterated with pressure
+3	Easy to palpate, not easily obliterated with pressure (normal)
+4	Strong, bounding, not obliterated with pressure

greater accuracy, measure the apical rate while the child is asleep; record the child's behavior along with the rate. Pulses may be graded according to the criteria in Table 7-4. Compare radial and femoral pulses at least once during infancy to detect the presence of circulatory impairment, such as coarctation of the aorta. (See inside back cover for normal rates for pediatric age-groups.)

Respiration

Count the respiratory rate in the same manner as for the adult patient. However, in infants observe abdominal movements because respirations are primarily diaphragmatic. Since the movements are irregular, count them for 1 full minute for accuracy (see also p. 163). (See inside back cover for normal respiratory rates in children.)

Blood Pressure (BP)

BP measurement by noninvasive methods is part of a routine vital sign determination. BP should be measured annually in children 3 years of age through adolescence, and in children with symptoms of hypertension, children in emergency rooms and intensive care units, and high-risk infants (Report of the Second Task Force, 1987). Several authorities also recommend routine measurements in low-risk neonates (Seidel, Rosenstein, and Pathak, 1993).

Measurement Devices. The most common method of measuring BP uses *auscultation* and either a *mercury-gravity* or *aneroid sphygmomanometer.* Both types are reliable and accurate, but the mercury-gravity manometer does not require recalibration as does the aneroid type.

BP can also be measured using electronic devices that employ oscillometric or Doppler techniques. In *oscillometry,* pressure changes are transmitted through the arterial wall to the pressure cuff, and the oscillations are detected by a pressure-sensitive indicator. Oscillometers have digital readouts for systolic, diastolic, and *mean arterial pressures (MAP),* and pulse. The MAP is not the same as the mean BP (arithmetic average of systolic and diastolic pressures). Rather, it is a value somewhat lower than the arithmetic mean. BP readings using oscillometry, such as Dinamap, are generally higher and correlate better with direct radial artery values than measurements using auscultation (see Table 7-8). Oscillometry also eliminates common problems found with the auscultation method, such as deflating the cuff too rapidly, not hearing the softest sounds, and rounding numbers for the Korotoff sounds.

The *Doppler ultrasound* translates changes in ultrasound frequency caused by blood movement within the artery to audible sound by means of a transducer in the cuff. The Doppler is useful for systolic pressure measurement but is unreliable for diastolic pressure measurement. Oscillometric and Doppler instruments are very useful in measuring BP in infants and have largely replaced the flush method, which reflects only the mean BP, and the auscultatory method.

Selection of Cuff. No matter what type of noninvasive technique is used, the most important factor in accurately measuring BP is the use of an appropriately sized cuff (*cuff size* refers only to the inner inflatable bladder, not the cloth covering). Unfortunately, authorities disagree on the correct method for determining cuff size. The Report of the Second Task Force (1987) recommends cuff size based on *limb*

TABLE 7-5. Commonly available blood pressure cuffs

CUFF NAME*	BLADDER WIDTH (CM)	BLADDER LENGTH (CM)
Newborn	2.5-4.0	5.0-9.0
Infant	4.0-6.0	11.5-18.0
Child	7.5-9.0	17.0-19.0
Adult	11.5-13.0	22.0-26.0
Large arm	14.0-15.0	30.5-33.0
Thigh	18.0-19.0	36.0-38.0

From Report of the Second Task Force on Blood Pressure Control in Children—1987, *Pediatrics* 79(1):1-25, 1987.
*Cuff name does not guarantee that the cuff will be appropriate size for a child within that age range.

length (Table 7-5):

- Width sufficient to cover approximately 75% of upper arm between top of shoulder and olecranon
- Length sufficient to completely encircle circumference of limb with or without overlapping
- Enough room at antecubital fossa to place bell of stethoscope
- Enough room at upper edge of cuff to prevent obstruction of axilla

The American Heart Association (Frohlich and others, 1988) recommends a method based on *limb circumference* (Table 7-6):

- Width 40% to 50% of limb circumference; measured at upper arm midway between top of shoulder and olecranon
- Length sufficient to completely or nearly completely encircle circumference of limb without overlapping

Using limb length for selecting cuff width may produce satisfactory BP readings in children with average weight for height, but inaccurate readings in children with thick arms. Using limb circumference for selecting cuff width more accurately reflects direct arterial BP than using limb length, because this method takes into account the varying thickness of the arm and the amount of pressure required to compress the artery (Park and Guntheroth, 1989). For measurement sites other than the upper arms, the limb circumference guidelines can be used, although the shape of the limb (i.e., conical shape of the thigh) may prevent appropriate placement of the cuff and inaccurately reflect intraarterial BP.

Cuffs that are either too narrow or too wide affect the accuracy of BP measurements, although wide cuffs tend to affect BP readings less. If the cuff is too small, the reading on the device is falsely high. If the cuff is too large, the reading is falsely low.

Nursing ALERT In choosing cuff sizes, use an appropriately sized cuff. When the correct size is not available, use an oversized cuff rather than an undersized one or use another site that more appropriately fits the cuff size. Do not choose a cuff based on the name of the cuff (i.e., an "infant" cuff may be too small for some infants).

TABLE 7-6. Recommended bladder dimensions for blood pressure cuffs

ARM CIRCUMFERENCE AT MIDPOINT (CM)	CUFF NAME*	BLADDER WIDTH (CM)	BLADDER LENGTH (CM)
5-7.5	Newborn	3	5
7.5-13	Infant	5	8
13-20	Child	8	13
24-32	Adult	13	24
32-42	Wide adult	17	32
42-50	Thigh	20	42

From Frohlich ED and others: Recommendations for human blood pressure determination by sphygmomanometers: report of a special task force appointed by the Steering Committee, American Heart Association, *Circulation* 77:501A, 1988.
*Cuff name does not guarantee that the cuff will be appropriate size for a child within that age range.

TABLE 7-7. Differences in oscillometric systolic BP between arm and lower extremity sites in normal children

AGE-GROUP (YEARS)	SYSTOLIC BP × (MEAN ± SD)	
	ARM-THIGH	ARM-CALF
4-8	−7.1±6.8	−9.3± 7.4
9-16	−2.4±7.7	−5.0±26.9

From Park M, Lee D, Johnson GA: Oscillometric blood pressures in the arm, thigh, and calf in healthy children and those with aortic coarctation, *Pediatrics* 91(4):761-765, 1993.

When another site is used, BP measurements using non-invasive techniques may differ. Generally, systolic pressure in the lower extremities (thigh or calf) is greater than pressure in the upper extremities, and systolic BP in the calf is higher than that in the thigh. These differences are listed in Table 7-7 and apply to oscillometric measurements taken on the right extremities with the child supine and the cuff size based on the circumference method (Park, Lee, and Johnson, 1993).

Nursing ALERT Compare blood pressure in the upper and lower extremities at least once to detect abnormalities, such as coarctation of the aorta, in which the lower extremity pressure is less than the upper extremity pressure.

Measurement and Interpretation. Measuring and interpreting BP in infants and children requires additional attention to correct procedure because (1) limb sizes vary and cuff selection must accommodate the circumference; (2) excessive pressure on the antecubital fossa affects the Korotkoff sounds; (3) children easily become anxious, which can elevate BP; and (4) BP values change with age and growth. Larger children, especially in terms of height, have higher normal BPs than smaller children of the same age.

Although the technique of BP measurement in children is generally the same as that used for adults (see Guidelines box), some aspects of the procedure are especially important. Because children are easily upset by unfamiliar procedures, prepare them for BP measurement. For children of preschool age and above, explain each step of the procedure and tell them how the cuff will feel, such as a tight feeling or an arm hug. Use explanations such as "I want to see how strong your muscle is" or "Let's watch the silver rise in the tube."

Because the child should be quiet and relaxed during the procedure, measure BP before performing any anxiety-producing procedures. Infants and small children may be more quiet if the reading is taken while they are sitting in the parent's lap.

Use a pediatric stethoscope and bell for hearing BP sounds in small children and infants. If auscultation is not possible, obtain a systolic reading by palpation; measure the point at which the pulse at the radial or brachial artery reappears as the cuff is deflated.

The average BP readings at various ages throughout childhood using sphygmomanometry are listed on the inside back cover, and readings using oscillometry are listed in Table 7-8. A *normal* BP is defined as a systolic and diastolic BP less than the 90th percentile for age and sex. (See also Hypertension in Chapter 25.)

Nursing ALERT Published norms for BP, such as those on the inside back cover, are valid only if the same method of measurement (auscultation and limb length for cuff size) is used in clinical practice.

NURSING TIP Use the following quick formula for average *systolic BP* using auscultation:

1 to 7 years: age in years + 90

8 to 18 years: (2 × age in years) + 83

Use the following formula for average *diastolic BP* using auscultation:

1 to 5 years: 56

6 to 18 years: age in years + 52

GENERAL APPEARANCE

The general appearance of the child is a cumulative, subjective impression of the child's physical appearance, state of nutrition, behavior, personality, interactions with parents and nurse (also siblings if present), posture, development, and speech. Although general appearance is recorded in the beginning of the physical examination, it encompasses all the observations of the child during the interview and physical assessment.

Note the *facies,* the facial expression and appearance of the child. For example, the facies may give clues to children who are in pain; have difficulty breathing; feel frightened, discontented, or happy; are mentally deficient; or are acutely ill.

Observe the *posture, position,* and types of *body movement.* The child with hearing or vision loss may characteristically tilt the head in an awkward position to hear or see better. The child in pain may favor a body part. The child with low self-esteem or a feeling of rejection may assume a slumped, careless, and apathetic pose or posture. Likewise, a child with confidence, a feeling of self-worth, and a sense of security usually demonstrates a tall, straight, well-balanced posture. While observing such "body language," do not interpret too freely but rather record objectively.

Note the child's *hygiene* in terms of cleanliness; unusual body odor; the condition of the hair, neck, nails, teeth, and feet; and the condition of the clothing. Such observations are excellent clues to possible instances of neglect, inadequate financial resources, housing difficulties (e.g., no running water), or lack of knowledge concerning children's needs.

General appearance includes an overall impression of the child's state of *nutrition.* This impression is more than a statement describing body weight or stature, such as "slender and tall." It is an estimation of the quality, as well as the quantity, of nutritional intake. For example, two children can be of the same height and weight, yet one can appear overweight because of flabby, loose skin, whereas the other child appears strong, robust, and well built because of firm, well-defined musculature. Likewise, a small, slender child may be well nourished with no signs of chronic undernutrition, such as bony prominences, protuberant abdomen, flat buttocks, gaunt facies, and poor muscle tone with evidence of wasting.

GUIDELINES
Measuring Blood Pressure

Use an appropriately sized cuff.

Use same position, preferably sitting, and right arm for brachial artery site (Fig. 7-8, *A*).

Use alternate site as needed to accommodate available cuff sizes:

Use smaller size on forearm: place cuff above wrist and auscultate radial artery (Fig. 7-8, *B*).

Use larger size on thigh: place cuff above knee and auscultate popliteal artery (Fig. 7-8, *C*).

Use larger size on calf: place cuff above malleoli or at midcalf and auscultate posterior tibial or dorsal pedal artery (Fig. 7-8, *D*).

Position limb at level of heart.

Rapidly inflate cuff to about 20 mm Hg above point at which radial pulse disappears.

Release cuff pressure at a rate of about 2 to 3 mm Hg/sec during auscultation of artery.

Read mercury-gravity manometer at eye level.

Record systolic value as onset of a clear tapping sound (first Korotkoff sound).

Record diastolic pressure as:

Fourth Korotkoff sound (K4) (low-pitched, muffled sound) for children up to age 12 years

Fifth Korotkoff sound (K5) (disappearance of all sound) for children ages 13 to 18 years

Record also limb, position, cuff size, and method of measurement.

If using electronic monitor, follow manufacturer's instructions and guidelines for correct cuff size.

With oscillometric device (i.e., Dinamap), can use all four limb sites, but reserve the thigh for last, since it is the most uncomfortable.

Stabilize limb during cuff deflation, since movement interferes with the device's ability to measure BP accurately.

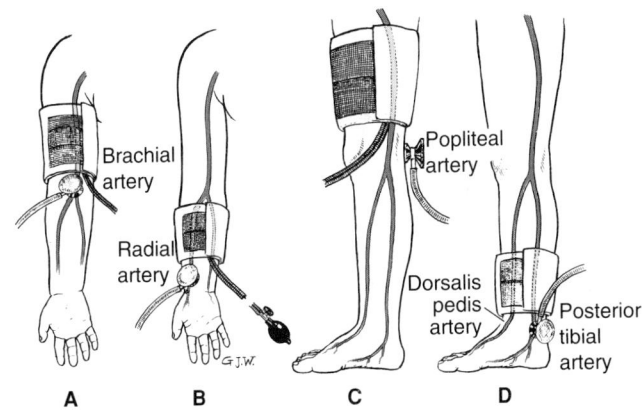

FIG. 7-8. Sites for measuring blood pressure. **A,** Upper arm. **B,** Lower arm or forearm. **C,** Thigh. **D,** Calf or ankle.

TABLE 7-8. Normative Dinamap BP values (systolic/diastolic, mean arterial pressure in parentheses)

AGE-GROUP	MEAN	90TH PERCENTILE	95TH PERCENTILE
Newborn (1-3 days)	65/41 (50)	75/49 (59)	78/52 (62)
1 month to 2 years	95/58 (72)	106/68 (83)	110/71 (86)
2-5 years	101/57 (74)	112/66 (82)	115/68 (85)

From Park M, Menard S: Normative oscillometric blood pressure values in the first 5 years in an office setting, *Am J Dis Child* 143(7):860-864, 1989.

Compare your impression of the nutritional state with the parents' history of feeding practices. Discrepancies between the two "impressions" may be a valuable area for nutritional counseling. For example, parents who believe that their child is too thin and eats too little, despite evidence of adequate growth and physical signs of proper nutrition, may find it helpful to keep a daily diary in order to calculate the child's cumulative food intake. Many parents are surprised at the quantity of food ingested, even though the amounts at each meal or snack are small.

Behavior includes the child's personality, level of activity, reaction to stress, requests, frustration, interactions with others (primarily the parent and nurse), degree of alertness, and response to stimuli. Some mental questions that serve as reminders for observing behavior include: What is the child's overall personality? Does the child have a long attention span or is he or she easily distracted? Can the child follow two or three commands in succession without the need for repetition? What is the youngster's response to delayed gratification or frustration? Is eye-to-eye contact used during conversation? What is the child's reaction to the nurse and family members? Is the child quick or slow to grasp explanations?

Development can be assessed by carefully observing the child, but verify your impressions with screening tests. Various tests for assessing development, speech, vision, and hearing are discussed later in this chapter and in Chapter 19.

Record an overall estimate of the child's speech development, motor skills, degree of coordination, and recent area of achievement under general appearance. For example, the following statement may apply to an 18-month-old child: "Motor development advanced for age; climbs, runs, jumps (most recent motor skill), manipulates small objects with ease; excellent coordination and balance; beginning to name many objects; uses two-word phrases; and enjoys 'talking' to self and others."

SKIN

Skin is assessed for color, texture, temperature, moisture, and turgor. Examination of the skin and its accessory organs primarily involves inspection and palpation. The normal *color* in light-skinned children varies from a milky-white and rose color to a deeply hued pink color. Dark-skinned children, such as those of Native American, Hispanic, or black descent, have inherited various brown, red, yellow, olive-green, and bluish tones in their skin. Oriental persons have skin that is normally of a yellow tone.

Several variations in skin color can occur, some of which warrant further investigation. The types of color change and their appearance in children with light or dark skin are summarized in Table 7-9.

Normally the skin *texture* of young children is smooth, slightly dry, not oily or clammy. Evaluate skin *temperature* by symmetrically feeling each part of the body and comparing upper areas with lower ones. Note any difference in temperature.

Determine *tissue turgor*, or the amount of elasticity in the skin, by grasping the skin on the abdomen between the thumb and index finger, pulling it taut, and quickly releasing it. Elastic tissue immediately assumes its normal position without residual marks or creases. In children with poor skin turgor the skin remains suspended or tented for a few sec-

onds before slowly falling back on the abdomen. Skin turgor is one of the best estimates of adequate hydration and nutrition.

Accessory Structures

Inspection of the accessory structures of the skin may be performed while the skin is being examined or when the scalp and extremities are being assessed.

Inspect the *hair* for color, texture, quality, distribution, and elasticity. Children's scalp hair is usually lustrous, silky, strong, and elastic. Genetic factors affect the appearance of hair. For example, the hair of black children is usually curlier and coarser than that of white children. Hair that is stringy, dull, brittle, dry, friable, and depigmented may suggest poor nutrition. Record any bald or thinning spots. Loss of hair in infants may indicate lying in the same position and may be a clue for counseling parents concerning the child's stimulation needs.

Inspect the hair and scalp for general cleanliness. Various ethnic groups condition their hair with oils or lubricants, which, if not thoroughly washed from the scalp, clog the sebaceous glands, causing scalp infections. Also examine the area for lesions, scaliness, evidence of infestation, such as lice or ticks, and signs of trauma, such as ecchymosis, masses, or scars.

In children who are approaching puberty, look for growth of secondary hair as a sign of normally progressing pubertal changes. Note precocious or delayed appearance of hair growth because, although not always suggestive of hormonal dysfunction, it may be of great concern to the early- or late-maturing adolescent.

Inspect the *nails* for color, shape, texture, and quality. Normally the nails are pink, convex, smooth, and hard but flexible (not brittle). The edges, which are usually white, should extend over the fingers. Dark-skinned individuals may have more deeply pigmented nail beds. Short, ragged nails are typical of habitual biting. Uncut, dirty nails are a sign of poor hygiene.

Each individual has a distinct set of handprints and footprints. The patterns, or *dermatoglyphics,* are unique to the individual and vary a great deal in detail and complexity. The palm normally shows three flexion creases (Fig. 7-9, *A*). In some situations, such as Down syndrome, the two distal hori-

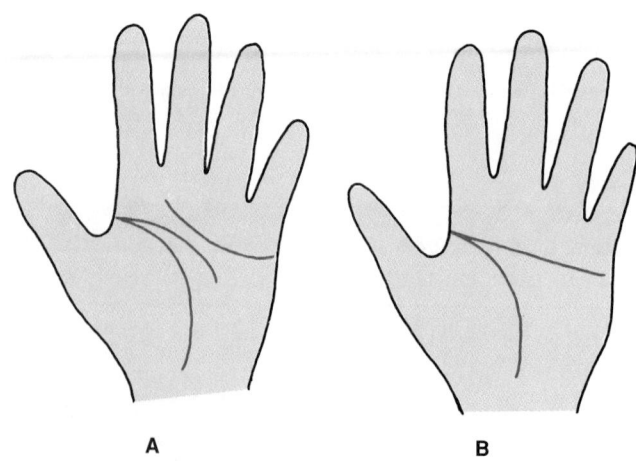

FIG. 7-9. Examples of flexion creases on palm. **A,** Normal. **B,** Transpalmar crease.

TABLE 7-9. Differences in color changes of racial groups

DESCRIPTION	APPEARANCE IN LIGHT SKIN	APPEARANCE IN DARK SKIN
Cyanosis A bluish tone through skin reflects reduced (deoxygenated) hemoglobin	Bluish tinge, especially in palpebral conjunctiva (lower eyelid), nail beds, earlobes, lips, oral membranes, soles, and palms	Ashen gray lips and tongue
Pallor Paleness may be a sign of anemia, chronic disease, edema, or shock	Loss of rosy glow in skin, especially face	Ashen-gray appearance in black skin More yellowish-brown color in brown skin
Erythema Redness may be result of increased blood flow from climatic conditions, local inflammation, infection, skin irritation, allergy, or other dermatoses or may be caused by increased numbers of red blood cells as a compensatory response to chronic hypoxia	Redness easily seen anywhere on body	Much more difficult to assess; rely on palpation for warmth or edema
Ecchymosis Large, diffuse areas, usually black and blue in color, are caused by hemorrhage of blood into skin; are typically result of injuries	Purplish to yellow-green areas; may be seen anywhere on skin	Very difficult to see unless in mouth or conjunctiva
Petechiae Same as ecchymosis except for size: small, distinct pinpoint hemorrhages 2 mm or less in size; can denote some type of blood disorder, such as leukemia	Purplish pinpoints most easily seen on buttocks, abdomen, and inner surfaces of the arms or legs	Usually invisible except in oral mucosa, conjunctiva of eyelids, and conjunctiva covering eyeball
Jaundice Yellow staining of the skin usually caused by bile pigments	Yellow staining seen in sclera of eyes, skin, fingernails, soles, palms, and oral mucosa	Most reliably assessed in sclera, hard palate, palms, and soles

zontal creases are fused to form a single horizontal crease, the *single palmar crease* or *transpalmar crease* (Fig. 7-9, *B*). If grossly abnormal lines or folds are observed, sketch a picture to describe them and refer the finding to a specialist for further investigation.

LYMPH NODES

Lymph nodes are usually assessed when the part of the body in which they are located is examined. Although the body's lymphatic drainage system is extensive, the usual sites for palpating accessible lymph nodes are shown in Fig. 7-10.

Palpate nodes by using the distal portion of the fingers and gently but firmly pressing in a circular motion along the regions where nodes are normally present. During assessment of the nodes in the head and neck, tilt the child's head upward slightly but without tensing the sternocleidomastoid or trapezius muscles. This position facilitates palpation of the *submental, submaxillary, tonsillar,* and *cervical nodes.* Palpate the *axillary nodes* with the arms relaxed at the side but slightly abducted. Assess the *inguinal nodes* with the child in the supine position. Note size, mobility, temperature, and tenderness, as well as reports by the parents regarding any visible change of enlarged nodes. In children small, non-

tender, movable nodes are usually normal. Tender, enlarged, warm lymph nodes generally indicate infection or inflammation close to their location. Report such findings for further investigation.

HEAD AND NECK

Observe the head for general *shape* and *symmetry.* A flattening of one part of the head, such as the occiput, may indicate that the child continually lies in this position. Marked asymmetry is usually abnormal and may indicate premature closure of the sutures (craniosynostosis).

Note *head control* in infants and *head posture* in older children. Most infants by 4 months of age should be able to hold the head erect and in midline when in a vertical position.

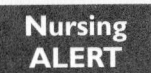 **Nursing ALERT**   Significant head lag after 6 months of age strongly indicates cerebral injury and is referred for further evaluation.

Evaluate range of motion by asking the older child to look in each direction (to either side, up, and down) or manually putting the younger child through each position. Limited

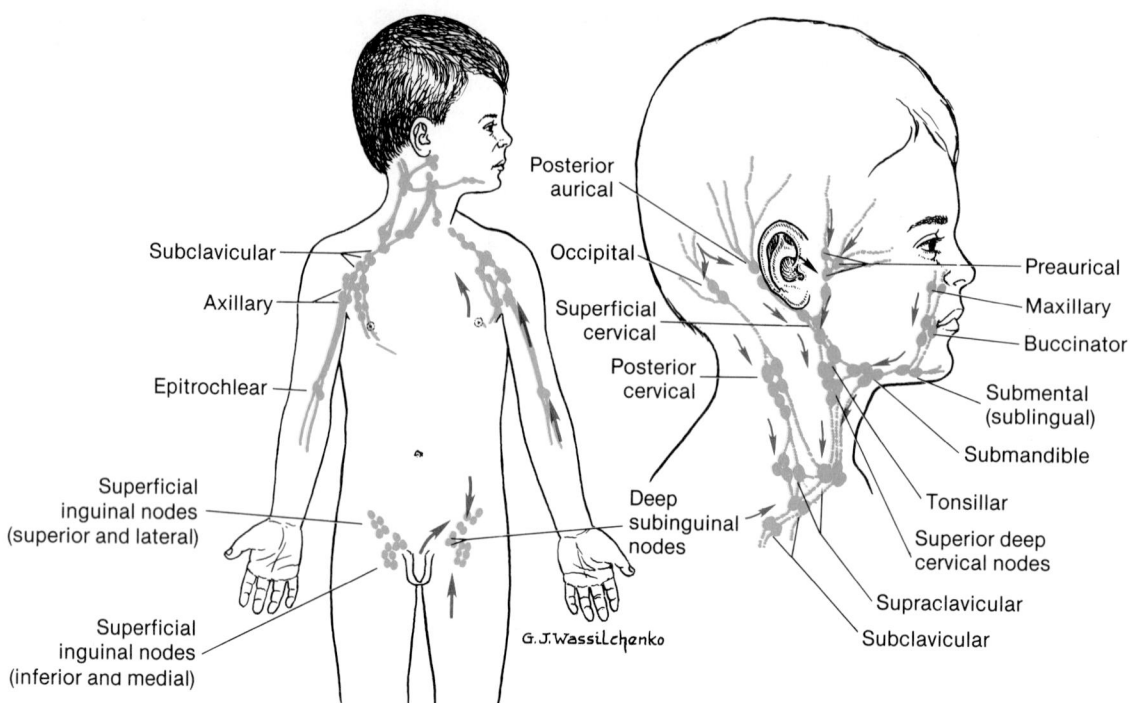

FIG. 7-10. Location of superficial lymph nodes. Arrows indicate directional flow of lymph.

range of motion may indicate *wryneck,* or *torticollis,* a result of injury to the sternocleidomastoid muscle, in which the child holds the head to one side with the chin pointing toward the opposite side.

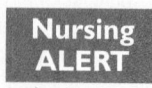

Nursing ALERT   Hyperextension of the head (opisthotonos) with pain on flexion is a serious indication of meningeal irritation and is referred for immediate medical evaluation.

Palpate the *skull* for patent sutures, fontanels, fractures, and swellings. Normally the posterior fontanel closes by the second month of life and the anterior fontanel fuses between 12 and 18 months of age. Early or late closure is noted, since either may be a sign of a pathologic condition. For a more detailed discussion of the cranial bones, see Chapter 8.

While examining the head, observe the *face* for symmetry, movement, and general appearance. Ask the child to "make a face" to assess symmetric movement and disclose any degree of paralysis. Note any unusual facial proportion, such as an unusually high or low forehead, wide- or close-set eyes, or a small, receding chin.

In addition to assessment of the head and neck for movement, inspect the neck for size and palpate it for associated structures. The neck is normally short with skinfolds between the head and shoulders during infancy; however, it lengthens during the next 3 to 4 years.

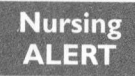

Nursing ALERT   If any masses are detected in the neck, report them for further investigation. Large masses can block the airway.

EYES

Inspection of External Structures

Inspect the *lids* for proper placement on the eye. When the eye is open, the upper lid should fall between the upper iris and the top portion of the pupil. When the eyes are closed, the lids should completely cover the cornea and sclera (Fig. 7-11).

Determine the general slant of the *palpebral fissures* or lids by drawing an imaginary line through the two points of the medial canthus and across the outer orbit of the eyes and aligning each eye on the line. Usually the palpebral fissures lie horizontally. However, in Orientals the slant is normally upward.

Also inspect the lining of the lids, the *palpebral conjunctiva.* To examine the lower conjunctival sac pull the lid down while the patient looks up. To evert the upper lid, hold the upper lashes and gently pull *down* and *forward* as the child looks down. Normally the conjunctiva appears pink and glossy. Vertical yellow striations along the edge are the *meibomian* or *sebaceous glands* near the hair follicle. Located in the inner or medial canthus and situated on the inner edge of the upper and lower lids is a tiny opening, the *lacrimal punctum.* Note any excessive tearing or inflammation of the lacrimal apparatus.

The *bulbar conjunctiva,* which covers the eye up to the limbus or junction of the cornea and sclera, should be transparent. The *sclera,* or white covering of the eyeball, should be clear. Tiny black marks in the sclera of heavily pigmented individuals are normal.

The *cornea,* or covering of the iris and pupil, should be clear and transparent. Record opacities because they can be signs of scarring or ulceration, which can interfere with vision. The best way to test for opacities is to illuminate the

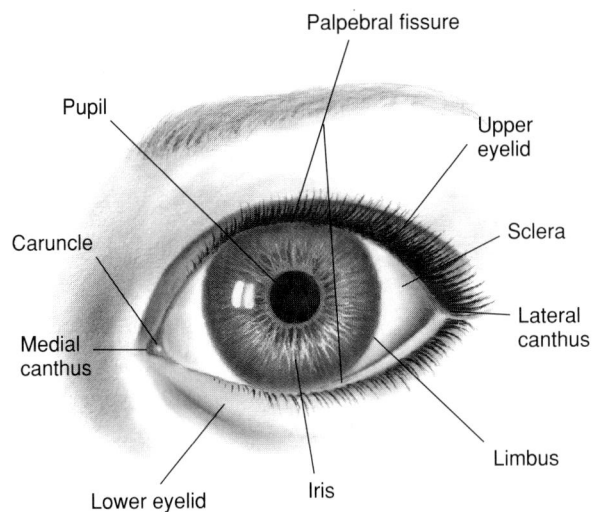

FIG. 7-11. External structures of eye.

ject is brought near the eye. Normal findings on examination of the pupils may be recorded as *PERRLA,* which means *pupils equal, round, react to light and accommodation.*

Inspect the *iris* for color, size, and clarity. Permanent eye color is usually established by 6 to 12 months of age. As the iris and pupil are inspected, look for the *lens.* Normally the lens is not visible through the pupil.

Inspection of Internal Structures

The ophthalmoscope permits visualization of the interior of the eyeball with a system of lenses and a high-intensity light. The lenses permit clear visualization of eye structures at different distances from the nurse's eye and correct visual acuity differences in the examiner and child. Use of the ophthalmoscope requires practice to know which lens setting produces the clearest image.

The ophthalmic and otic head are usually interchangeable on one "body" or handle, which encloses the power source, either disposable or rechargeable batteries. The nurse should practice changing the heads, which snap on and are secured with a quarter turn, and replacing the batteries and light bulbs. Nurses who are not directly involved in physical assessment are often responsible for ensuring that the equipment functions properly.

Preparing the Child.   The nurse can prepare the child for the ophthalmic examination by showing the child the instrument, demonstrating the light source and how it shines in the eye, and explaining the reason for darkening the room. For infants and young children who do not respond to such explanations, it is best to try to use distraction to encourage them to keep their eyes open. Forcibly parting the lids results in an uncooperative, watery-eyed child and a frustrated nurse. Usually, with some practice, the nurse can elicit a red

eyeball by shining a light at an angle (obliquely) toward the cornea.

Compare the *pupils* for size, shape, and movement. They should be round, clear, and equal. Test their *reaction to light* by quickly shining a source of light toward the eye and removing it. As the light approaches, the pupils should constrict; as the light fades, the pupils should dilate. Test *accommodation,* or the focusing ability of the eyes to produce clear vision at different distances, by having the child look at a bright, shiny object at a distance and quickly moving the object toward the face. The pupils should constrict as the ob-

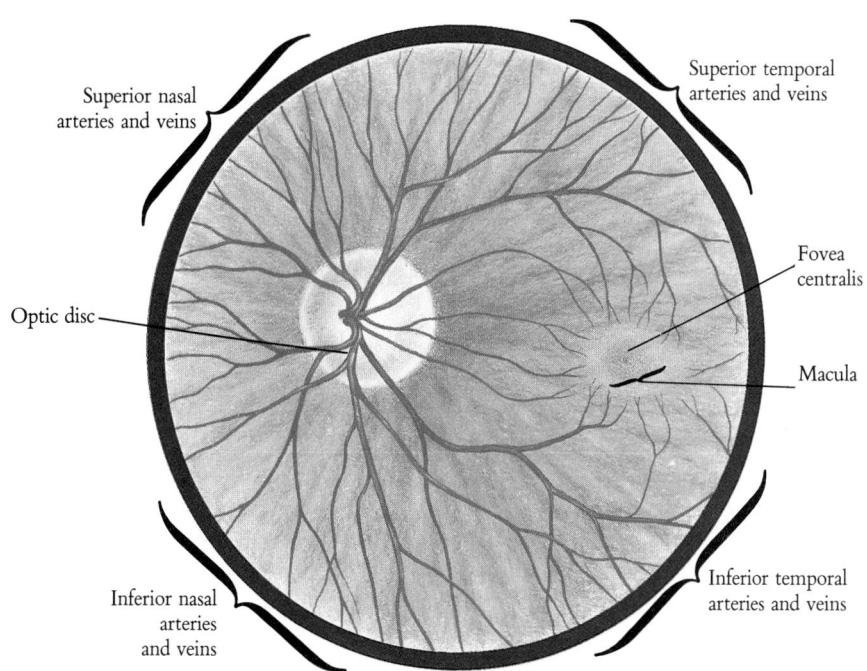

FIG. 7-12. Structures of fundus. (From Seidel HM and others: *Mosby's guide to physical examination,* ed 3, St Louis, 1995, Mosby.)

reflex almost instantly while approaching the child and may also gain a momentary inspection of the blood vessels, macula, or optic disc.

Funduscopic Examination. Fig. 7-12 shows the structures of the back of the eyeball, or the *fundus.* The fundus is immediately apparent as the *red reflex.* The intensity of the color increases in darkly pigmented individuals.

> **Nursing ALERT** A brilliant, uniform red reflex is an important sign because it virtually rules out almost all serious defects of the cornea, aqueous chamber, lens, and vitreous chamber. Any dark shadows or opacities are recorded because they indicate some abnormality in any of these structures.

As the ophthalmoscope is brought closer to the eye, the most conspicuous feature of the fundus is the **optic disc,** the area where the blood vessels and optic nerve fibers enter and exit from the eye. The color of the disc is creamy pink; it is lighter in color than the surrounding fundus. Normally it is round or vertically oval.

After the optic disc is located, the area is inspected for **blood vessels.** The central retinal artery and vein appear in the depths of the disc and emanate outward with visible branching. The *veins* are darker in color and about one fourth larger in size than the *arteries.* Normally the branches of the arteries and veins cross each other.

Other structures that may be seen are the *macula,* the area of the fundus with the greatest concentration of visual receptors, and, in the center of the macula, a minute glistening spot of reflected light called the *fovea centralis;* this is the area of most perfect vision.

Vision Testing

Several tests are available for assessing vision. This discussion focuses on four areas: (1) binocularity, (2) visual acuity, (3) peripheral vision, and (4) color vision. Refer to Chapter 19 for behavioral and physical signs that indicate visual impairment.

Binocularity. Normally, by the age of 3 to 4 months children achieve the ability to fixate on one visual field with both eyes simultaneously (binocularity). One of the most important tests for binocularity is alignment of the eyes to detect nonbinocular vision, or *strabismus.* In strabismus, or "cross-eye," one eye deviates from the point of fixation. If the malalignment is constant, the weak eye becomes "lazy," and the brain eventually suppresses the image produced by that eye. If strabismus is not detected and corrected by age 4 to 6 years, blindness from disuse, known as *amblyopia,* may result.

Two tests commonly used to detect malalignment are the corneal light reflex and the cover tests. In the *corneal light reflex test* (also called *red reflex gemini test* or *Hirschberg test*), shine a flashlight or the light of the ophthalmoscope directly into the patient's eyes from a distance of about 40.5 cm (16 inches). If the eyes are *orthophoric,* or normal, the light falls symmetrically within each pupil (Fig. 7-13, *A*). If the light falls off center in one eye, the eyes are malaligned. *Epicanthal folds,* excess folds of skin that extend from the roof of the nose to the inner termination of the eyebrow and that partially or completely overlap the inner canthus of the

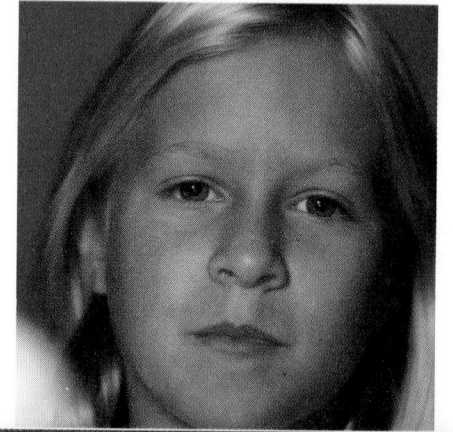

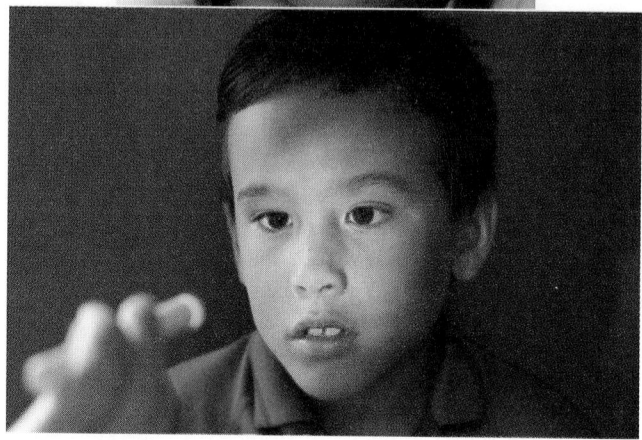

FIG. 7-13. A, Corneal light reflex test demonstrating orthophoric eyes. **B,** Pseudostrabismus. Inner epicanthal folds cause eyes to appear malaligned; however, corneal light reflexes fall perfectly symmetrically.

eye, may give a false impression of malalignment *(pseudostrabismus)* (Fig. 7-13, *B*). Epicanthal folds are often found in Oriental children.

In the *cover test,* one eye is covered, and the movement of the *uncovered* eye is observed while the child looks at a near (33 cm, or 13 in) or distant (50 cm, or 20 in) object. If the uncovered eye does not move, it is aligned. If the uncovered eye moves, a malalignment is present because when the stronger eye is temporarily covered, the weaker eye attempts to fixate on the object.

In the *uncover test* occlusion is shifted back and forth from one eye to the other, and movement of the *covered* eye is observed as soon as the occluder is removed while the child focuses on a point in front of him or her. If normal alignment is present, shifting the cover from one eye to the other will not cause the covered eye to move. If malalignment is present, the covered eye will move from its position when covered to a straight position when uncovered. This test takes more practice than the other cover test because the occluder must be moved back and forth quickly and accurately in order to see the eye move. Because deviations can occur at different ranges, it is important to perform the cover tests at both close and far distances.

NURSING TIP The cover test is usually easier to perform if the examiner uses his or her own hand rather than a card-type occluder (Fig. 7-14). Attractive occluders fashioned like an ice cream cone or happy-face lollipop cut from cardboard are also well received by young children.

Visual Acuity Testing in Children Beyond Infancy. The most common test for measuring visual acuity (the ability to see near and far objects clearly) is the ***Snellen Letter chart,*** which consists of lines of letters of decreasing size (see Appendix C). Each line is given a value; for example, line 7 is "20."

During testing children stand 20 feet from the chart (with heels at the 20-foot line) and read each line. If they can read line 7, they have 20/20 vision, the accepted standard for normal acuity. If they can read only line 2, they have 20/100 vision—they are able to see at a distance of 20 feet what people with 20/20 or normal eyesight can see at 100 feet.

Other letter or symbol screening tests are described in Table 7-10. Many of the tests that are suitable for preschoolers can also be used for difficult-to-test children, such as those with developmental delays. The ***Snellen symbol chart*** is frequently used to screen preschool children (see Appendix C). However, many young children have difficulty because of confusion in identifying the direction of the E, rather than inability to see the symbol clearly. To avoid this problem, the ***Blackbird Preschool Vision Screening System*** was developed by a nurse (Fig. 7-15). The screening system uses a modified E that resembles a bird and a story about the Blackbird to help engage children's attention. Testing is done with flash cards or a wall-mounted chart, and the children are instructed to indicate the direction of the bird's flight. Some have reported a higher percentage of children successfully tested with the Blackbird System than with the Snellen Ē (Sato-Viacrucis, 1985). The Blackbird System also contains guidelines for vision screening the noncommunicative, nonreaders, or non–English-speaking children to assist screeners with more difficult-to-test populations, and the ***Blackbird Storybook Home Eye Test*** is designed for parents to prescreen young children at home.

Although most chart tests are designed for testing at 20 feet, modifications can be made for testing at closer ranges because it is easier to engage children's attention at a closer range, and the charts require less space for the screening lane. Measurements at closer range are converted to the standard 20-foot scale by multiplying the two numbers by the number that converts the first one to 20. For example, 10/25 is equivalent to 20/50. When closer ranges are used, proper positioning of the child (e.g., with heels on the 10-foot mark) is essential. Because young children are active, their tendency to move or lean forward can affect the testing more at close distances than at farther ones. (See Critical Thinking Exercise on p. 155.)

There are no universal criteria for referring children when using Snellen charts. The ***National Society to Prevent Blindness*** (1988) recommends the following criteria for referral of children for a complete eye examination:

1. Three-year-old children with vision in either eye of 20/50 or less (inability to correctly identify one more than half the symbols on the 40-foot line) or a two-line difference in visual acuity between

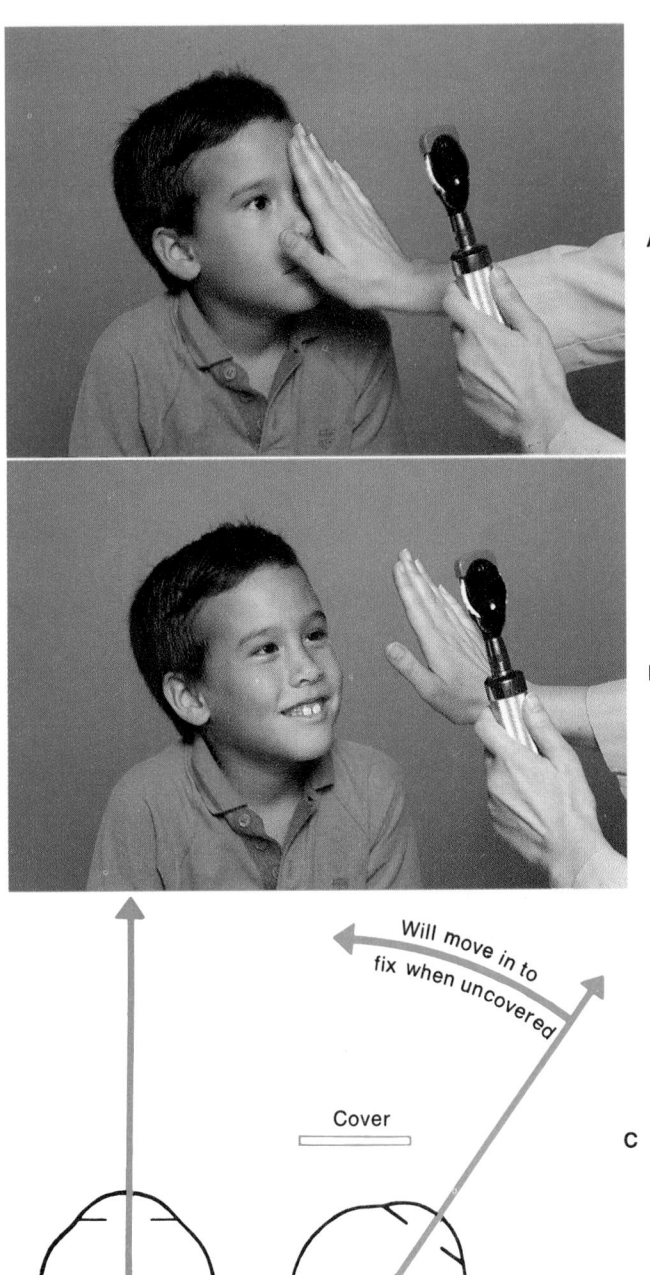

FIG. 7-14. Uncover test for strabismus. **A,** Eye is occluded, child is fixating on light source. **B,** If eye does not move when uncovered, eyes are aligned. **C,** Exophoria. As eye is uncovered, it shifts to fixate on object. (**C** from Prior JA, Silberstein JS, Stang JM: *Physical diagnosis: the history and examination of the patient,* ed 6, St Louis, 1981, Mosby.)

TABLE 7-10. Letter or symbol vision acuity tests

DESCRIPTION	COMMENTS*
Snellen Letter† Uses letters of the English alphabet for testing at 20 feet	Suitable for most children above the second grade who are familiar with reading the alphabet
Snellen E† Uses the capital letter E pointing in four directions; children "read" the chart by showing the direction of the letter E or using a large duplicate E to match the chart E at 20 feet	For illiterate or non–English-speaking people, preschool children, and grade 1 Preschool children often have difficulty with direction despite adequate vision
Home Eye Test for Preschoolers‡ Uses a large letter E for demonstration and an E chart for testing at 10 feet	Designed for use by parents for children ages 3 to 6 years
Blackbird Preschool Vision Screening System§ Uses a modified E to resemble a flying bird; children identify which way the bird is flying. Uses flash cards, story-telling, and disposable cardboard eyeglass occluders	Designed for children as young as 3 years
Blackbird Storybook Home Eye Test§ Similar to above	Designed for use by parents for children as young as 2½ years
HOTV or Matching Symbol† Uses the four letters H, O, T, and V on a chart for testing at 10 or 20 feet Child names the letters on the chart or matches them to a demonstration card	Suitable for children as young as 3 years Avoids the problem with image reversal and eye-hand coordination that can occur with the letter E
Faye Symbol Chart† Use pictures of a house, apple, and umbrella on a chart for testing at 10 feet	Suitable for children as young as 27 to 30 months
Denver Eye Screening Test (DEST)‖ Uses single cards for the letter E, one for demonstration and one for testing at 15 feet Also uses Allen Picture Cards (a tree, birthday cake, horse and rider, telephone, car, house, and teddy bear) for testing at 15 feet	Suitable for children 2½ years and older May be reliably used with cooperative children from the age of 24 months
DOT Test† Uses a series of different-sized dots; child points to one of the nine dots randomly positioned on a disk	Suitable for children as young as 24 months

*Ages for testing are based on published reports. Proper instruction of young children is essential for successful screening.
†Available from Good-Lite Co., 1540 Hannah Ave., Forest Park, IL 60130; (708) 366-3860.
‡Available from the National Society to Prevent Blindness, 500 E. Remington Rd., Schaumburg, IL 60173; (800) 331-2020.
§Available from Blackbird Vision Screening System, P.O. Box 277424, Sacramento, CA 95827; (800) 363-6884.
‖Available from Denver Developmental Materials, Inc., P.O. Box 6919, Denver, CO 80206-0919; (303) 355-4729.

the eyes in the passing range (e.g., 20/20 in one eye and 20/40 in the other eye)
2. All other ages and grades with vision in either eye of 20/40 or less (inability to correctly identify one more than half the symbols on the 30-foot line)
3. All children who consistently show any signs of possible visual disturbances, regardless of visual acuity (see Chapter 19).

Visual Acuity Testing in Infants and Difficult-to-Test Children. In newborns vision is tested mainly by checking for *light perception* by shining a light into the eyes and noting responses such as pupillary constriction, blinking, following the light to midline, increased alertness, or refusal to open the eyes after exposure to the light. Although the simple maneuver of checking light perception and eliciting the pupillary light reflex indicates that the anterior half of the visual apparatus is intact, it does not confirm that the infant can see. In other words, this test does not assess whether the brain receives the visual message and interprets the signals.

Another test of visual acuity is the infant's ability to fix on and follow a target. Although any brightly colored or pat-

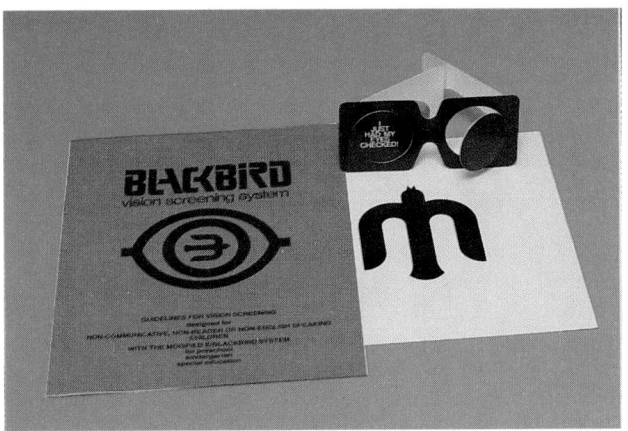

FIG. 7-15. Blackbird Vision Screening System. Note Blackbird symbol and special "eyeglass" occluder.

CRITICAL THINKING EXERCISE

Vision Screening

Your nursing class will be assisting with EPSDT (Early Periodic Screening, Diagnosis, and Treatment) screens for preschoolers. You are responsible for setting up the area for visual screening. You will need all of the following equipment *except*:

1. Snellen acuity charts
2. Pirate patches
3. Penlights
4. A paper or metal tape measure

The correct answer is one. The Snellen chart is inappropriate because it uses letters, and it cannot be assumed that preschoolers know their alphabet. The "Lazy E" acuity chart is not ideal, because preschoolers may not have the perceptual abilities needed to determine which direction the "legs" of the E are pointing. A picture acuity chart or the Blackbird System should be used with this population. Pirate patches serve as eye occluders and are needed for assessing acuity and alignment. Penlights are needed for assessing corneal light reflex and pupil reactivity. A nonstretchable tape measure is used to determine the correct distance for assessing acuity when using an eye chart.

Contributed by Judith A. Vessey, PhD, RN,C.

terned object can be used, the human face is excellent. Hold the infant upright while moving your face slowly from side to side.

Nursing ALERT If visual fixation and following are not present by 3 to 4 months of age, further ophthalmologic evaluation is needed.

Other signs that may indicate visual loss include fixed pupils, marked strabismus, constant nystagmus, setting-sun sign, and slow lateral movements. Unfortunately, it is very difficult to test each eye separately; the presence of such signs in one eye could indicate unilateral blindness.

Special tests are available for testing infants and other difficult-to-test children to assess acuity and/or confirm blindness. For example, in *visually evoked potentials,* the eyes are stimulated with a bright light or pattern, and electrical activity to the visual cortex is recorded through scalp electrodes. Acuity is assessed by using progressively smaller patterns.

Peripheral Vision.   In children who are old enough to cooperate, estimate *peripheral vision,* or the visual field of each eye, by having children fixate on a specific point directly in front of them as an object, such as a finger or a pencil, is moved from beyond the field of vision into the range of peripheral vision. Check each eye separately and for each quadrant of vision. As soon as children see the object, have them say "stop." At that point measure the angle from the anteroposterior axis of the eye (straight line of vision) to the peripheral axis (point at which the object is first seen). Normally children see about 50 degrees upward, 70 degrees downward, 60 degrees nasalward, and 90 degrees temporally. Limitations in peripheral vision may indicate blindness from damage to structures within the eye or to any of the visual pathways.

Color Vision.   Another important test is for color vision. It is estimated that 8% to 10% of white males and less than half that percentage of black males inherit the X-linked disorder known as *color vision deficit* (less acceptable term, *color blindness*). From 0.5% to 1% of white females are affected. Although the severity of impaired perception of color varies considerably, the two most common types are *protanomaly,* in which the child confuses gray with pink or pale blue with green, and *deuteranomaly,* in which the child confuses gray with pale purple or green. In most of these individuals the color vision deficit causes no major problems. However, some of the difficulties encountered by individuals with more severe deficits may be inability to distinguish amber or red traffic lights, failure to see a red brake light on the rear of a car, difficulty in distinguishing green traffic lights from certain types of incandescent street lamps, and a poor sense of color coordination of clothing. For school-age children the greatest difficulty lies in performance of academic skills that use color as a visual aid. Adolescents may be ineligible for certain vocational opportunities, such as electronics, photography, printing, interior decorating, pharmaceuticals, textiles, police work, and several types of military service.

The tests available for color vision include the *Ishihara test* and the *Hardy-Rand-Rittler (HRR) test.* Each consists of a series of cards (pseudoisochromatic) on which is printed a color field composed of spots of a certain "confusion" color. Against the field is a number or symbol similarly printed in dots but of a color likely to be confused with the field color by the person with a color vision deficit. As a result, the figure or letter is invisible to an affected individual but is clearly seen by a person with normal vision. By using the HRR test, which uses symbols rather than numbers, reliable testing can be done on children as young as 3 years of age (Kovalesky, 1985). Nurses administering the test must be familiar with the testing materials and should be able to inform the parents of the disorder's effects on practical areas of living, its genetic transmission, and its irreversibility.

EARS

Inspection of External Structures

The entire external earlobe is called the *pinna,* or *auricle,* and is located on each side of the head. Measure the *height* alignment of the pinna by drawing an imaginary line from the outer orbit of the eye to the occiput or most prominent protuberance of the skull. The top of the pinna should meet or cross this line. Low-set ears are commonly associated with renal anomalies or mental retardation. Measure the *angle* of the pinna by drawing a perpendicular line from the imaginary horizontal line and aligning the pinna next to this mark. Normally the pinna lies within a 10-degree angle of the vertical line (Fig. 7-16). If it falls outside this area, record the deviation and look for other anomalies.

Normally the pinna extends slightly outward from the skull. Except in newborn infants, ears that are flat against the head or protruding away from the scalp may indicate problems. Flattened ears in infants may suggest a frequent side-lying position and, just as with isolated areas of hair loss, may be a clue to investigating parents' understanding of the child's stimulation needs.

Inspect the *skin* surface around the ear for small openings, extra tags of skin, or sinuses. If a sinus is found, note this because it may represent a fistula that drains into some area of the neck or ear. Cutaneous tags represent no pathologic process but may cause parents concern in terms of the child's appearance.

Also assess the ear for *hygiene.* An otoscope is not necessary for looking into the external canal to note the presence of *cerumen,* a waxy substance produced by the ceruminous glands in the outer portion of the canal. Cerumen is usually yellow-brown and soft. If an otoscope is used and any discharge is seen, its color and odor are noted. Prevent transmitting potentially infectious material to the other ear or to another child through handwashing and using disposable specula or sterilizing reusable specula between each examination.

Inspection of Internal Structures

The head of the otoscope permits visualization of the tympanic membrane by use of a bright light, a magnifying glass,

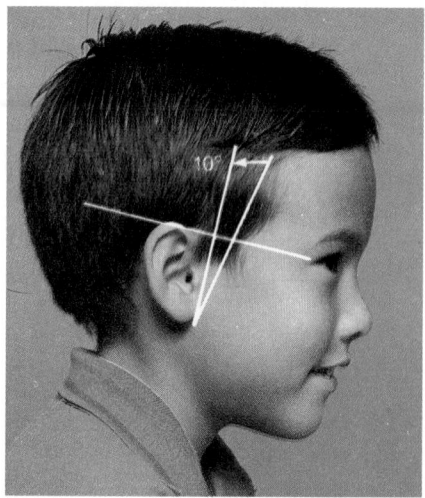

FIG. 7-16. Ear alignment.

and a speculum. Some otoscopes have an attachment for a pneumonic device to insert air into the canal to determine membrane compliance (movement). The speculum, which is inserted into the external canal, comes in a variety of sizes to accommodate different canal widths. The largest speculum that fits comfortably into the ear is used in order to achieve the greatest area of visualization. The lens, or magnifying glass, is movable, allowing the examiner to insert an object, such as a curette, into the ear canal through the speculum while still viewing the structures through the lens.

Positioning the Child. Before beginning the otoscopic examination, position the child properly and restrain if necessary. Older children usually cooperate and do not need restraint. However, prepare them for the procedure by allowing them to play with the instrument, demonstrating how it works, and stressing the importance of remaining still. A helpful suggestion is to let them observe you examining the parent's ear. Restraint is needed for younger children because the ear examination upsets them (see Atraumatic Care box).

As you insert the speculum into the meatus, move it around the outer rim to accustom the child to the feel of something entering the ear. If examining a painful ear, touch a nonpainful part of the affected ear, then examine the unaffected ear, and finally return to the painful ear. By this time the child is usually less fearful of anything causing discomfort to the ear and will cooperate more.

For their protection and safety, infants and toddlers must be restrained for the otoscopic examination. There are two general positions of restraint. In one the child is seated sideways in the parent's lap with one arm "hugging" the parent and the other arm at the side. The ear to be examined is toward the nurse. With one arm the parent holds the child's head firmly against his or her chest, and with the other arm "hugs" the child, thereby securing the child's free arm. The ear is examined using the same procedure for holding the otoscope as described later (Fig. 7-17, *A*).

The other position involves placing the child on the side, back, or abdomen with the arms at the side and the head turned so that the ear to be examined points toward the ceiling. Lean over the child and use the upper part of the body to restrain the arms and upper trunk movements, and the examining hand to stabilize the head. This position is practical for young infants or for older children who need minimal restraining, but it may not be feasible for other children who protest vigorously. For safety enlist the parent's or an assistant's help in immobilizing the head by firmly placing one hand above the ear and the other on the child's back or side, abdomen, or back (Fig. 7-17, *B*).

With cooperative children examine the ear with the child in a side-lying, sitting, or standing position. One disadvan-

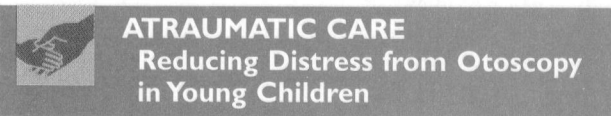

ATRAUMATIC CARE
Reducing Distress from Otoscopy in Young Children

Make examining the ear a game by explaining that you are looking for a "big elephant" in the ear. This kind of "fairy tale" is an absorbing distraction and usually elicits cooperation. After the ear has been examined, clarify that "looking for elephants" was only pretending and thank the child for letting you look in his or her ear.

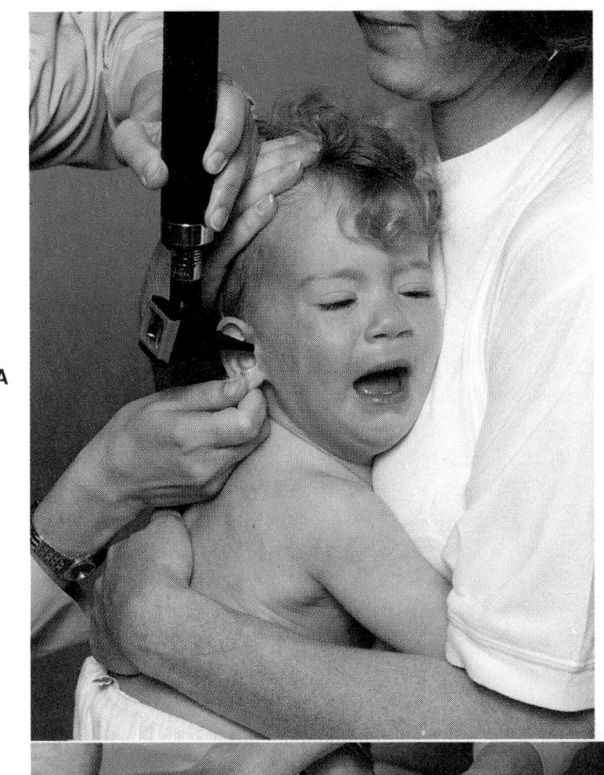

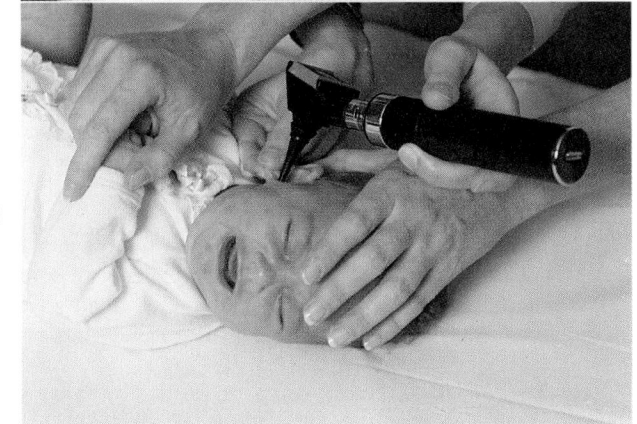

FIG. 7-17. Position for restraining child, **A,** and infant, **B,** during otoscopic examination.

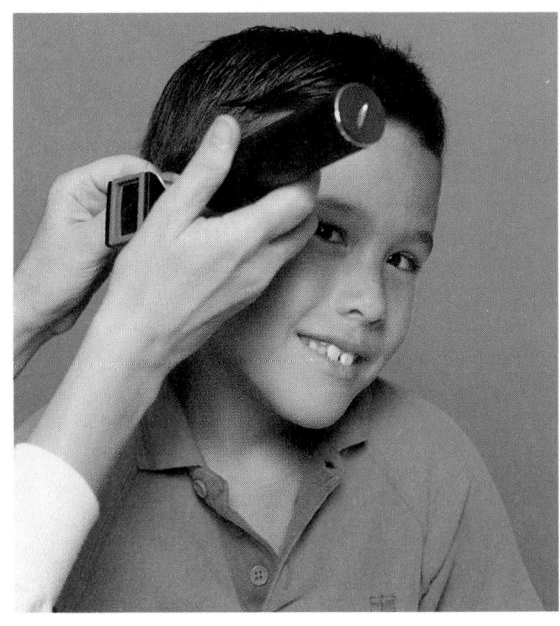

FIG. 7-18. Positioning head by tilting it toward opposite shoulder for full view of tympanic membrane.

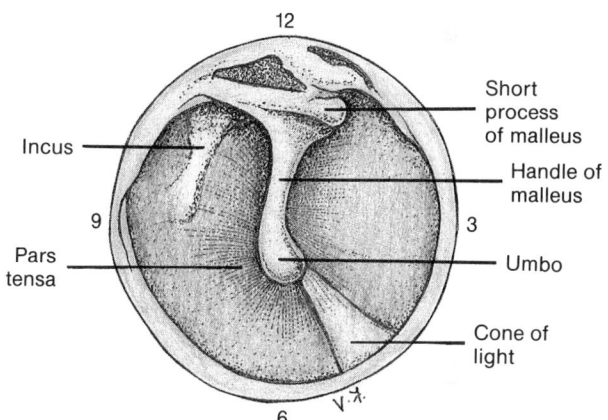

FIG. 7-19. Landmarks of tympanic membrane with "clock" superimposed. (Modified from Potter PA, Perry AG: *Basic nursing: theory and practice,* ed 2, St Louis, 1991, Mosby.)

tage to standing is that the child may "walk away" as the otoscope enters the canal. If the child is standing or sitting, tilt the head slightly toward the child's opposite shoulder to achieve a better view of the drum (Fig. 7-18).

With the thumb and forefinger of the free (usually nondominant) hand, grasp the auricle. For the two positions of restraint, hold the otoscope upside down at the junction of its head and handle with the thumb and index finger. Place the other fingers against the skull to allow the otoscope to move with the child in case of sudden movement. In examining a cooperative child, hold the handle with the otic head upright or upside down. Use the dominant hand to examine both ears or reverse hands for each ear, whichever is more comfortable.

Before using the otoscope, visualize the external ear and the tympanic membrane as being superimposed on a clock (see Fig. 7-19). The numbers become important geographic landmarks. Introduce the speculum into the meatus between the 3 and 9 o'clock positions in a *downward* and *forward* position. Because the canal is curved, the speculum does not permit a panoramic view of the tympanic membrane unless the canal is straightened. In infants the canal curves upward. Therefore, pull the pinna *down* and *back* to the 6 to 9 o'clock range to straighten the canal (Fig. 7-20, *A*).

With older children, usually those over 3 years of age, the canal curves downward and forward. Therefore pull the pinna *up* and *back* toward a 10 o'clock position (Fig. 7-20, *B*). If there is difficulty in visualizing the membrane, try repositioning the head, introducing the speculum at a different angle, and pulling the pinna in a slightly different direction. Do not

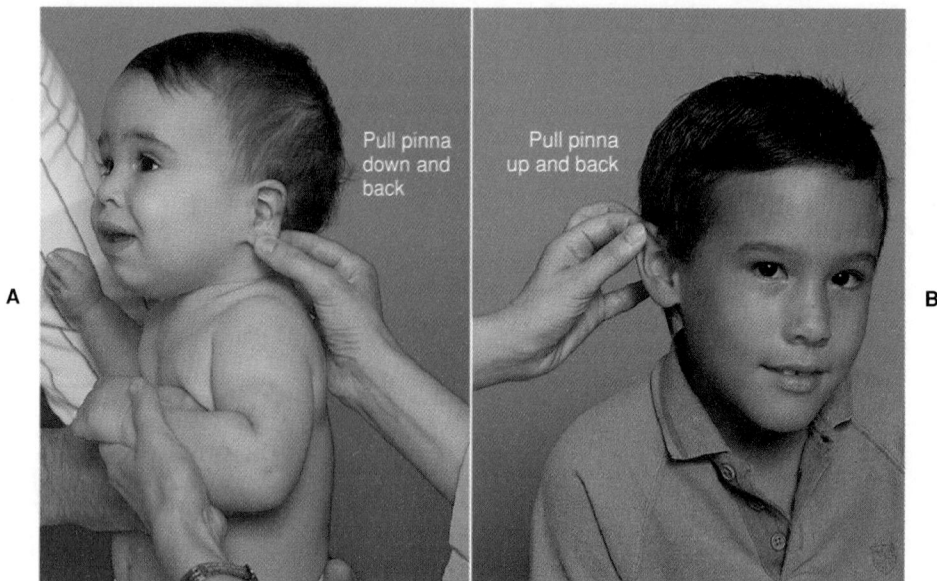

FIG. 7-20. Positioning of eardrum in infant, **A,** and in child over 3 years of age, **B.**

insert the speculum past the cartilaginous (outermost) portion of the canal, usually a distance of 0.60 to 1.25 cm (¼ to ½ inch) in older children. Insertion of the speculum into the posterior or bony portion of the canal causes pain.

In neonates and young infants the walls of the canal are pliable and floppy because of the underdeveloped cartilaginous and bony structures. Therefore the very small 2-mm speculum usually needs to be inserted deeper into the canal than in older children. Great care must be exercised not to damage the walls or drum. For this reason, only an experienced examiner should insert an otoscope into the ears of very young infants.

Otoscopic Examination. As you introduce the speculum into the external canal, inspect the walls of the canal, the color of the tympanic membrane, the light reflex, and the usual landmarks of the bony prominences of the middle ear.

The *walls* of the external auditory canal are pink, although they are more pigmented in dark-skinned children. Minute hairs are evident in the outermost portion, where cerumen is produced. Note signs of irritation, foreign bodies, or infection.

Foreign bodies in the ear are not uncommon in children and range from erasers to beans. Symptoms may include pain, discharge, and affected hearing. Soft objects, such as paper or insects, can be removed with forceps. Small, hard objects, such as pebbles, can be removed with a suction tip, a hook, or irrigation. However, irrigation is contraindicated if the object is vegetative matter, such as beans or pasta, which swells when in contact with fluid.

Nursing ALERT If there is any doubt about the type of object in the ear and the appropriate method to remove it, refer the child to the appropriate practitioner.

The *color* of the *tympanic membrane* is a translucent, light pearly pink or gray. Note marked erythema (which may indicate suppurative otitis media), a dull nontransparent grayish color (sometimes suggestive of serous otitis media), or ashen-gray areas (signs of scarring from a previous perforation). A black area usually suggests a perforation of the membrane that has not healed.

The characteristic tenseness and slope of the tympanic membrane cause the light of the otoscope to reflect at about the 5 or 7 o'clock position. The *light reflex* is a fairly well-defined cone-shaped reflection, which normally points away from the face.

The *bony landmarks* of the drum are formed by the *umbo,* or tip of the malleus bone. It appears as a small, round, opaque concave spot near the center of the drum. The *manubrium* (long process or handle) of the malleus appears to be a whitish line extending from the umbo upward to the margin of the membrane. At the upper end of the long process near the 1 o'clock position (in the right ear) is a sharp, knoblike protuberance, representing the *short process* of the malleus. Note the absence of the light reflex or loss or abnormal prominence of any of these landmarks.

Auditory Testing

Several types of hearing tests are available (Table 7-11). Some of them, such as audiometric testing, involve specialized equipment that measures the degree of hearing loss. Others, such as tests for the startle reflex in neonates, are rough estimations of perception of sound. The nurse must operate under a high index of suspicion for those children who may have conditions associated with hearing loss and who may have developed behaviors that indicate auditory impairment. Types of hearing loss, causes, clinical manifestations, and appropriate treatment are discussed in Chapter 19.

TABLE 7-11. Selected hearing and tympanic membrane compliance tests*

DESCRIPTION	COMMENTS
Clinical Hearing Tests In newborns elicit the startle reflex and observe other neonatal responses to loud noises, such as facial grimaces, blinking, gross motor movement, quiet if crying or crying if quiet, opening the eyes, or ceasing sucking activity. During infancy note child's reaction to a noise. Stand about 18 inches away from infant, to the side, and out of child's peripheral field of vision. With the room silent and infant sitting in parent's lap, distracted by some object, make a voice sound such as "ps" or "phth" (high-pitched) or "oo" (low-pitched), ring a bell or a rattle, or rustle tissue paper.	An objective sign of alerting to sound may be an increase in heart rate or respiratory rate. Absence of alerting behaviors suggests hearing loss. Eliciting the startle reflex is used only in infants from birth to 4 months. Test is usually inadequate for children beyond infancy because of their tendency to ignore sounds or be distracted.
Crib-O-Gram Neonatal screening tool that analyzes hearing responses by comparing the infant's motor activity before, during, and after a sound is introduced. A motion-sensitive transducer is placed beneath the mattress, and a microprocessor "reads" the infant's movements.	Both administration of the test and its scoring are totally automated. The test is repeated several times to increase reliability. A consistent change in activity that coincides with the test sound is scored as a pass. Neonates who are premature or ill may not respond to sound despite adequate hearing.
Tympanometry Measures tympanic membrane compliance (or mobility) and estimates middle ear air pressure. A soft rubber cuff is pressed over the external canal to produce an airtight seal; an automatic reading of air pressure registers on the machine.	Detects middle ear disease and abnormalities but does not indicate the degree of hearing loss or the interpretation of sound. Difficult to perform in young children because of inability to maintain an adequate seal or excessive movement by the child.
Conduction Tests *Rinne test*—Stem of tuning fork is placed against the mastoid bone until the sound ceases to be audible. Tuning fork is then moved so that the prongs are held near, but not touching, the auditory meatus. Child should again hear the sound *(Rinne positive).* If sound is not again audible *(Rinne negative),* some abnormality is interfering with the conduction of air through the external and middle chambers. *Weber test*—Stem of tuning fork is held in the midline of the head. Child should hear the sound equally in both ears *(Weber positive).* With air conductive loss, child will hear the sound better in the affected ear *(Weber negative).*	Requires the cooperation and ability of the child to signal when the sound is no longer audible and when it is again heard. Not useful for most children before preschool age. Frequently not suitable for young children because of their difficulty in discriminating between "better, more, or less."
Audiometry Electrical audiometer measures the threshold of hearing for pure-tone frequencies and loudness. A sound is transmitted to the child's ear and reduced until child indicates the sound is no longer heard; this procedure is repeated for several sounds covering the range found in conversation. In an air conduction audiogram the sounds are transmitted through earphones. In a bone conduction audiogram the sounds are passed through a plaque placed over the mastoid bone.	Provides valuable information regarding the severity of the hearing loss, the sound cycles involved, and the possible location of the defect. Requires specialized training of personnel, expensive equipment, and cooperation from the child in terms of confirming the perception of sound. For children ages 24 months to about 5 years, play audiometry can be used; it is based on behavior modification and involves reinforcement for correct response.

*Any child who is suspected of a hearing loss because of poor performance using screening tests is referred for special audiometric or BAER testing.

Continued.

TABLE 7-11. Selected hearing and tympanic membrane compliance tests—cont'd

DESCRIPTION	COMMENTS
Evoked Otoacoustic Emissions (EOAEs) Special OAE analyzer delivers a rapid series of clicks to the ear through a probe fitted with a tympanometry tip that is inserted closely in the external auditory canal. The presence of OAEs, defined as sound energy emitted by the cochlea that is believed to be generated by the movement of the outer hairs of the organ of Corti, is usually associated with normal or near-normal cochlear sensitivity; their absence indicates a hearing loss of at least 20-25 dB, provided there is no conductive dysfunction (Abdo, Feghali, and Stapells, 1993).	Preferred method of screening neonates for sensorineural hearing loss (ototoxicity and noise-induced hearing loss). Requires specialized equipment. Minimal training is required. Infants must be in a quiet sleep for testing. Results do not indicate severity of cochlear damage; should be followed by BAER (see below).
Brainstem-Auditory Evoked Response (BAER) Through electrode wires attached to the infant's or child's scalp, electrical or brain wave potentials generated within the auditory system are transmitted to a computer for analysis. Following repetitive acoustic stimulation, the waveforms from a normal sleeping or quiet infant consist of several peaks and valleys that reflect activations of neural structures of the brain.	Requires specialized training of personnel and expensive equipment.

NOSE

Inspection of External Structures

The nose is located in the middle of the face just below the eyes and above the lips. Compare its placement and alignment by drawing an imaginary vertical line from the center point between the eyes down to the notch of the upper lip. The nose should lie exactly vertical to this line, with each side exactly symmetric. Note its location, any deviation to one side, and asymmetry in overall size and in diameter of the nares (nostrils). The *bridge* of the nose is sometimes flat in Asian and black children. Observe the ***alae nasi*** for any sign of flaring, which indicates respiratory difficulty. Always report any flaring of the alae nasi. Fig. 7-21 illustrates the usual landmarks used in describing the external structures of the nose.

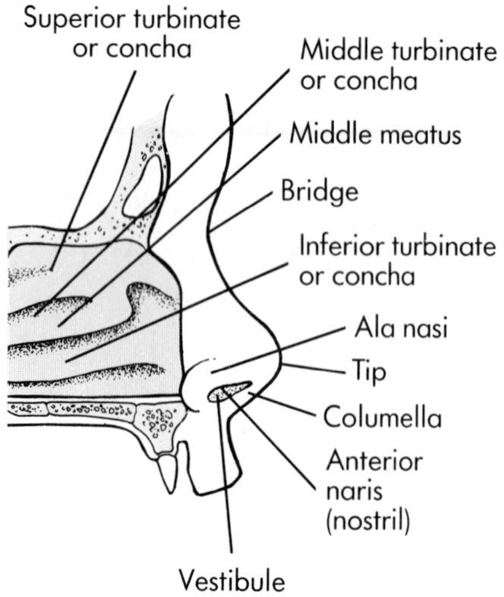

Inspection of Internal Structures

Inspect the ***anterior vestibule*** of the nose by pushing the tip upward, tilting the head backward, and illuminating the cavity with a flashlight or otoscope without the attached ear speculum.

Note the ***color*** of the ***mucosal lining,*** which is normally redder than the oral membranes, as well as any swelling, discharge, dryness, or bleeding. There should be no discharge from the nose.

On looking deeper into the nose, inspect the ***turbinates*** or ***concha,*** plates of bone that jut into the nasal cavity and are enveloped by mucous membrane. The turbinates greatly increase the surface area of the nasal cavity as air is inhaled. The spaces or channels between the turbinates are called ***meatus*** and correspond to each of the three turbinates. Normally the front end of the inferior and middle turbinate and the middle meatus are seen. They should be the same color as the lining of the vestibule.

Inspect the ***septum,*** which should divide the vestibules equally. Note any deviation, especially if it causes an occlusion of one side of the nose. A perforation may be evident within the septum. If this is suspected, shine the light of the otoscope into one naris and look for admittance of light through the perforation to the other nostril.

Since olfaction is an important function of the nose, testing for smell may be done at this point or as part of cranial nerve assessment (see Table 7-12 on p. 174).

MOUTH AND THROAT

With a cooperative child, almost the entire examination of the mouth and throat can be accomplished without the use of a tongue blade. Ask the child to open the mouth wide, to

Superior turbinate or concha
Middle turbinate or concha
Middle meatus
Bridge
Inferior turbinate or concha
Ala nasi
Tip
Columella
Anterior naris (nostril)
Vestibule

FIG. 7-21. External landmarks and internal structures of nose.

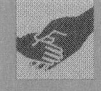

ATRAUMATIC CARE
Encouraging Opening the Mouth
for Examination

Perform the examination in front of a mirror.
Let child first examine someone else's mouth, such as the parent, the nurse, or a puppet (Fig. 7-22, A) and then examine child's mouth.
Instruct child to tilt the head back slightly, breathe deeply through the mouth, and hold the breath; this action lowers the tongue to the floor of the mouth without the use of a tongue blade.

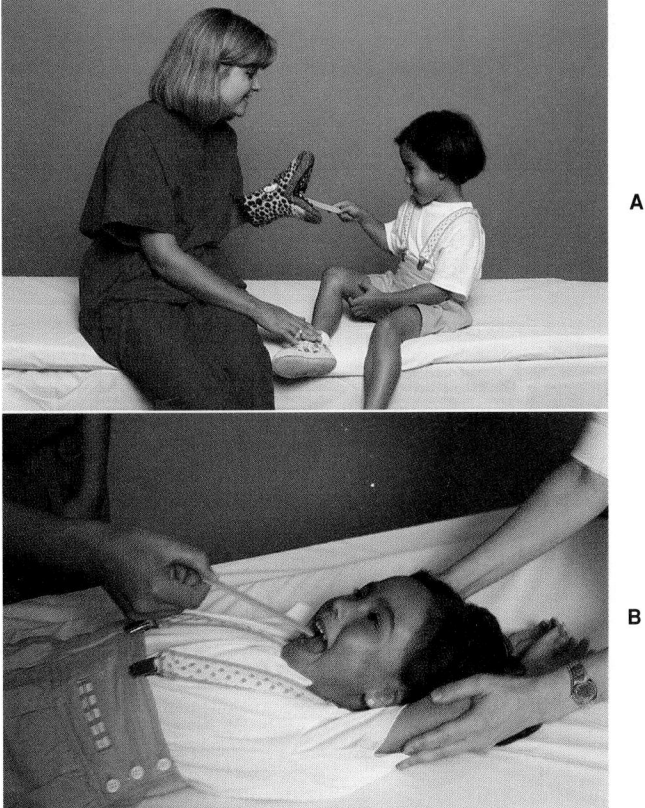

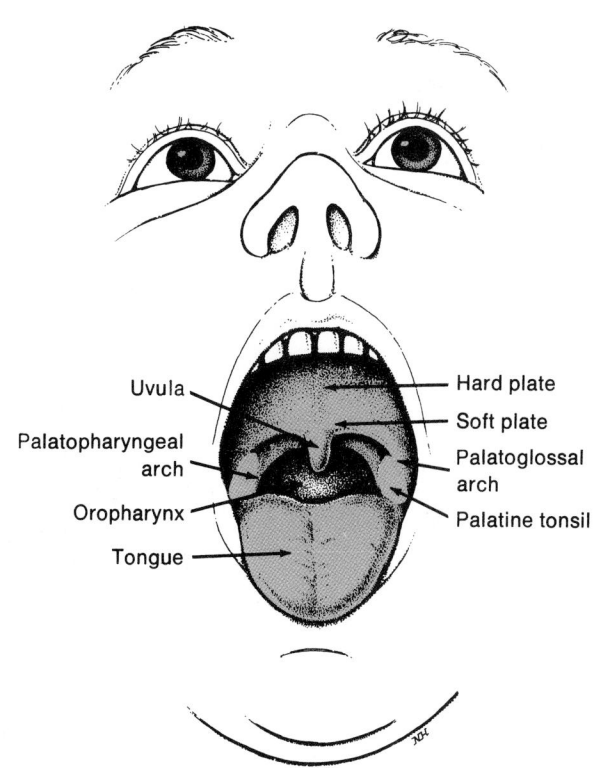

FIG. 7-22. **A,** Encouraging child to cooperate. **B,** Positioning child for examination of mouth.

move the tongue in different directions for full visualization, and to say "ahh," which depresses the tongue for full view of the back of the mouth (tonsils, uvula, and oropharynx). For a closer look at the buccal mucosa or lining of the cheeks, ask children to use their fingers to move the outer lip and cheek to one side (see also Atraumatic Care box).

Infants and toddlers, however, usually resist attempts to keep the mouth open. Because inspecting the mouth is an upsetting part of the examination, leave it to the end of the physical examination (along with examination of the ears) or do it during episodes of crying. However, the use of a tongue blade (preferably flavored) to depress the tongue is necessary. Place the tongue blade along the *side* of the tongue, not in the center back area where the gag reflex is elicited. Fig. 7-22, *B*, illustrates proper positioning of the child for the oral examination.

The major structure of the exterior of the mouth is the *lips.* The lips should be moist, soft, smooth, and pink, the color of a deeper hue than the surrounding skin. The lips should be symmetric when relaxed or tensed. Assess symmetry when the child talks or cries.

Inspection of Internal Structures

The major structures that are visible within the oral cavity and oropharynx are the mucosal lining of the lips and cheeks, gums or gingiva, teeth, tongue, palate, uvula, tonsils, and posterior oropharynx (Fig. 7-23). Inspect all areas lined with *mucous membranes* (inside the lips and cheeks, gingiva, underside of tongue, palate, and back of pharynx) for color, any areas of white patches or ulceration, bleeding, sensitivity, and moisture. The membranes should be bright pink, smooth, glistening, uniform, and moist.

Inspect the *teeth* for number in each dental arch, for hygiene, and for occlusion or bite (see also Teething, Chapter 10). Discoloration of tooth enamel with obvious plaque (whitish coating on the surface of the teeth) is a sign of poor dental hygiene and indicates a need for counseling. Brown spots in the crevices of the crown of the tooth or between the teeth may be caries (cavities). Chalky white to yellow or brown areas on the enamel may indicate fluorosis (excessive fluoride ingestion). Teeth that appear greenish black may be stained temporarily from ingestion of supplemental iron.

Examine the *gums (gingiva)* surrounding the teeth. The color is normally coral pink, and the surface texture is stippled, similar to the appearance of orange peel. In dark-skinned children, the gums are more deeply colored, and a brownish area is often observed along the gum line.

Uvula

Palatopharyngeal arch

Oropharynx

Tongue

Hard plate

Soft plate

Palatoglossal arch

Palatine tonsil

FIG. 7-23. Interior structures of mouth.

Inspect the *tongue* for the presence of papillae, small projections that contain several taste buds and give the tongue its characteristic rough appearance. Note the size and mobility of the tongue. Normally the tip of the tongue should extend to the lips or beyond.

The roof of the mouth consists of the *hard palate*, which is located near the front of the oral cavity, and the *soft palate*, which is located toward the back of the pharynx and which has a small midline protrusion called the *uvula*. Carefully inspect the palates to be sure that they are intact. The arch of the palate should be dome shaped. A narrow, flat roof or a high, arched palate affects the placement of the tongue and can cause feeding and speech problems. Test movement of the uvula by eliciting a gag reflex. It should move upward to close off the nasopharynx from the oropharynx.

Examine the oropharynx and note the size and color of the *palatine tonsils.* They are normally the same color as the surrounding mucosa, glandular, rather than smooth in appearance, and barely visible over the edge of the palatoglossal arches. The size of the tonsils varies considerably during childhood. However, report any swelling, redness, or white areas on the tonsils.

CHEST

Inspect the *chest* for size, shape, symmetry, movement, breast development, and the presence of the bony landmarks formed by the ribs and sternum. The *rib cage* consists of twelve ribs and the sternum, or breast bone, located in the midline of the trunk (Fig. 7-24). The *sternum* is composed of three main parts. The *manubrium,* the uppermost portion, can be felt at the base of the neck at the *suprasternal notch.* The largest segment of the sternum is the *body,* which forms the *sternal angle (angle of Louis)* as it articulates with the manubrium. At the end of the body is a small, movable process called the *xiphoid.* The angle of the costal margin as it attaches to the sternum is called the *costal angle* and is normally about 45 to 50 degrees. These bony structures are important landmarks in the location of ribs and intercostal spaces.

Intercostal spaces (ICS) are the spaces between the ribs. They are numbered according to the rib directly *above* the space. For example, the space immediately below the second rib is the second intercostal space.

The *thoracic cavity* is also divided into segments by drawing imaginary lines on the chest and back. Fig. 7-25 illustrates the anterior, lateral, and posterior divisions.

Measure the *size* of the chest by placing the measuring tape around the rib cage at the nipple line (see Fig. 7-4). For greatest accuracy take two measurements, one during inspiration and the other during expiration, and record the average. Chest size is important mainly in comparison with its relationship to head circumference, which is discussed on p. 139. Always report marked disproportions because most are caused by abnormal head growth, although some may be the result of altered chest shape, such as *barrel chest* (chest is round) or *pigeon chest* (sternum protrudes outward).

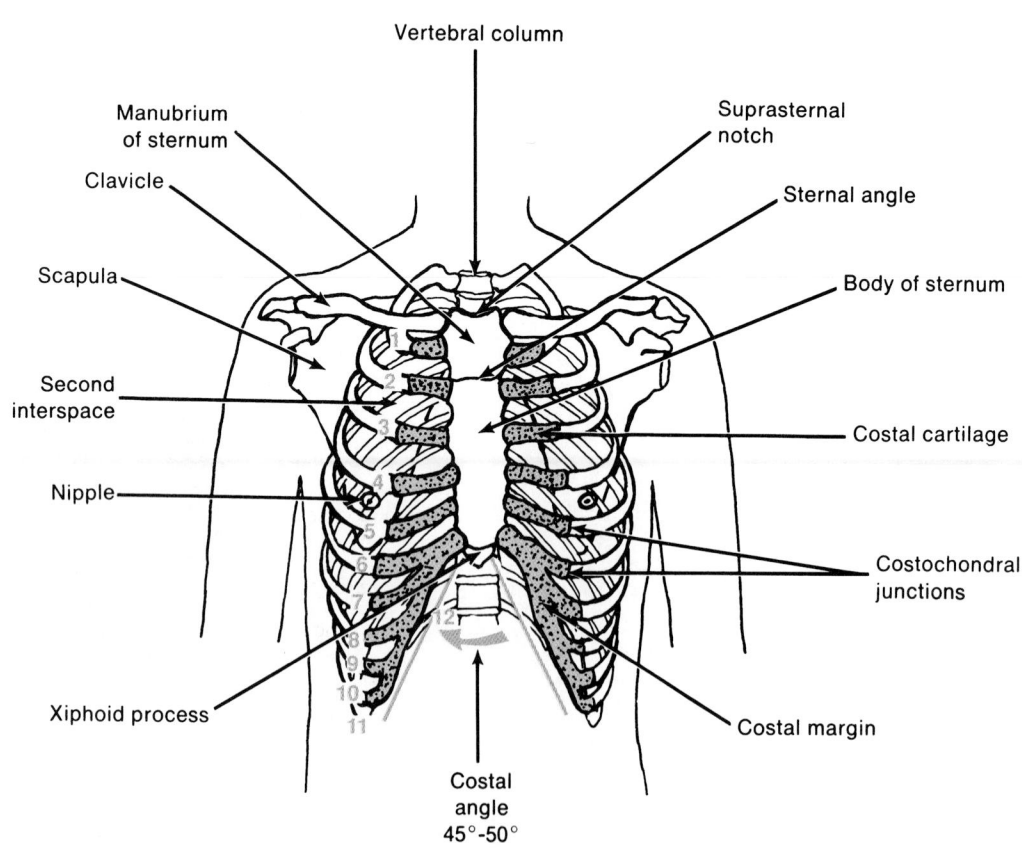

FIG. 7-24. Rib cage.

During infancy the *shape* of the chest is almost circular, with the anteroposterior (front-to-back) diameter equaling the transverse or lateral (side-to-side) diameter. As the child grows, the chest normally increases in the transverse direction, causing the anteroposterior diameter to be less than the lateral diameter. Note the *angle* made by the lower costal margin and the sternum, and palpate the junction of the ribs to the costal cartilage (costochondral junction) and sternum, which should be fairly smooth.

Movement of the chest wall should be symmetric bilaterally and coordinated with breathing. During inspiration, the chest rises and expands, the diaphragm descends, and the costal angle increases. During expiration, the chest falls and decreases in size, the diaphragm rises, and the costal angle narrows (Fig. 7-26). In children under 6 or 7 years of age, respiratory movement is principally abdominal or diaphragmatic. In older children, particularly females, respirations are chiefly thoracic. In either type, the chest and abdomen should rise and fall together. Always report any asymmetry of movement.

While inspecting the skin surface of the chest, observe the position of the *nipples*, as well as any evidence of *breast development*. Normally the nipples are located slightly lateral to the midclavicular line between the fourth and fifth ribs. Note symmetry of nipple placement and normal configuration of a darker pigmented areola surrounding a flat nipple in the prepubertal child.

Pubertal breast development usually begins in girls between 10 and 14 years of age (see Chapter 16). Record early (precocious) or delayed breast development, as well as evidence of any other secondary sexual characteristics. In males *breast enlargement (gynecomastia)* may be caused by hormonal or systemic disorders, but more commonly it is a result of adipose tissue from obesity or a transitory body change during early puberty. In either situation investigate the child's feelings regarding breast enlargement.

In adolescent females who have achieved sexual maturity, palpate the breasts for evidence of any masses or hard nodules. Use this opportunity to discuss the importance of routine self-breast examination. Emphasize that most palpable masses are benign to decrease any fear or concern that results when a mass is felt.

LUNGS

The *lungs* are situated inside the thoracic cavity, with one lung on each side of the sternum. Each lung is divided into an *apex*, which is slightly pointed and rises above the first rib; a *base*, which is wide and concave and rides on the dome-shaped diaphragm; and a body, which is divided into *lobes*. The right lung has three lobes: the upper, middle, and lower. The left lung has only two lobes, the upper and lower, because of the space occupied by the heart (Fig. 7-27).

Inspection of the lungs primarily involves observation of respiratory movements, which are discussed above.

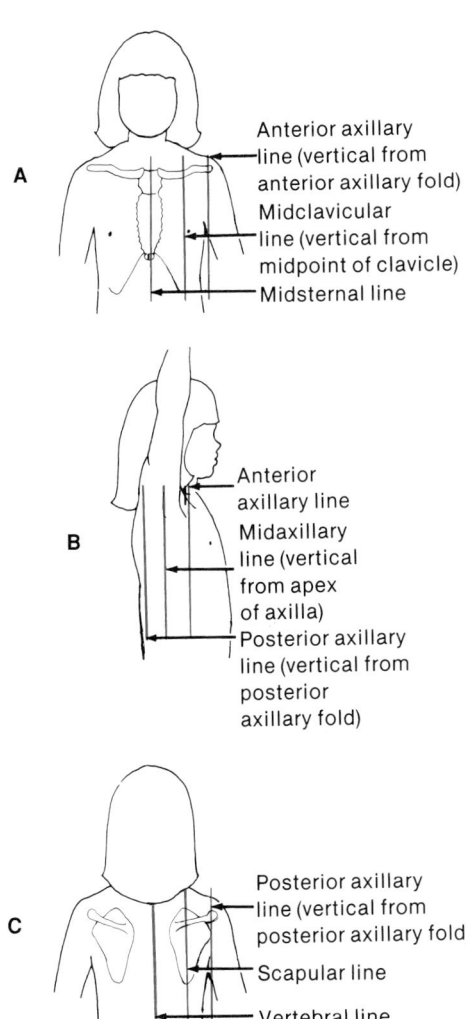

FIG. 7-25. Imaginary landmarks of chest. **A,** Anterior. **B,** Right lateral. **C,** Posterior.

Anterior axillary line (vertical from anterior axillary fold)
Midclavicular line (vertical from midpoint of clavicle)
Midsternal line

Anterior axillary line
Midaxillary line (vertical from apex of axilla)
Posterior axillary line (vertical from posterior axillary fold)

Posterior axillary line (vertical from posterior axillary fold)
Scapular line
Vertebral line

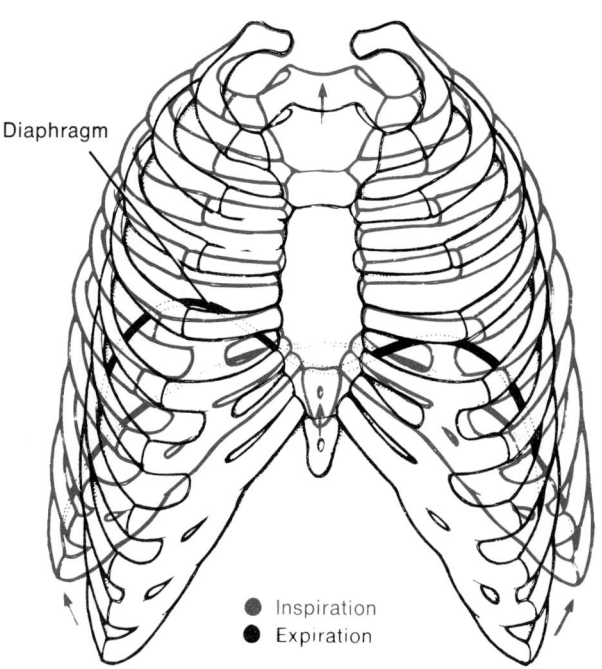

Diaphragm

Inspiration
Expiration

FIG. 7-26. Movement of chest during respiration.

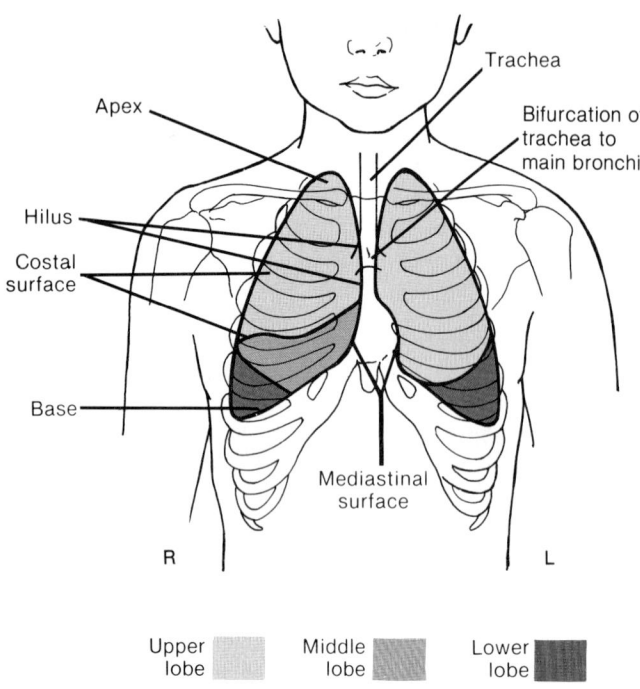

FIG. 7-27. Location of lobes of lungs within thoracic cavity.

Evaluate respirations for rate (number per minute), rhythm (regular, irregular, or periodic), depth (deep or shallow), and quality (effortless, automatic, difficult, or labored). Note the character of breath sounds, such as noisy, grunting, snoring, or heavy.

Evaluate respiratory movements by placing each hand flat against the back or chest with the thumbs in midline along the lower costal margin of the lungs. The child should be sitting during this procedure and, if cooperative, should take several deep breaths. During respiration your hands will move with the chest wall. Assess the amount and speed of respiratory excursion and note any asymmetry of movement.

Experienced examiners may percuss the lungs. The anterior lung is percussed from apex to base, usually with the child in the supine or sitting position. Each side of the chest is percussed in sequence in order to compare the sounds. When the posterior lung is percussed, the procedure and sequence are the same, although the child should be sitting. Resonance is heard over all the lobes of the lungs that are not adjacent to other organs. Any deviation from the expected sound is recorded and reported.

Auscultation

Auscultation involves using the stethoscope to evaluate breath sounds (see Guidelines box). Breath sounds are best heard if the child inspires deeply (see Atraumatic Care box). In the lungs breath sounds are classified as vesicular, bronchovesicular, or bronchial (see box).

Absent or *diminished breath sounds* are always an abnormal finding warranting investigation. Fluid, air, or solid masses in the pleural space all interfere with the conduction of breath sounds. Diminished breath sounds in certain segments of the lung can alert the nurse to pulmonary areas that may benefit from chest physiotherapy. Increased breath sounds following pulmonary therapy indicate improved passage of air through the respiratory tract.

Various pulmonary abnormalities produce *adventitious sounds* that are not normally heard over the chest. These sounds occur in addition to normal or abnormal breath sounds. They are classified into two main groups: *crackles,* which result from the passage of air through fluid or moisture, and *wheezes,* which are produced as air passes through narrowed passageways, regardless of the cause, such as exudate, inflammation, spasm, or tumor. Considerable practice with an experienced tutor is necessary to differentiate the

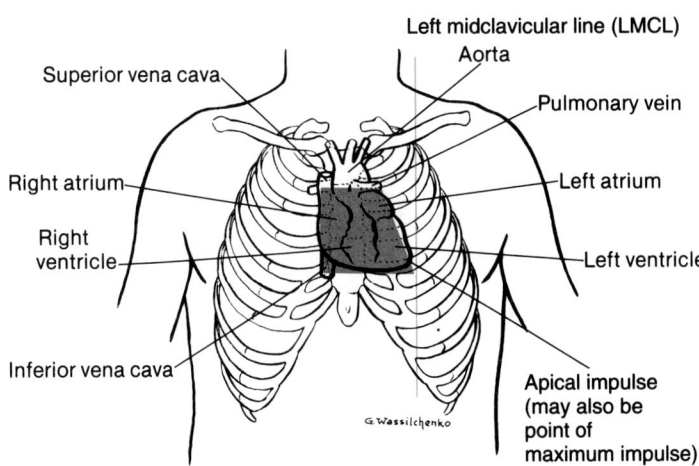

FIG. 7-28. Position of heart within thorax.

various types of lung sounds. Often it is best to describe the type of sound heard in the lungs rather than trying to label it. Always report any abnormal sounds for further medical evaluation.

HEART

The heart is situated in the thoracic cavity between the lungs in the mediastinum and above the diaphragm (Fig. 7-28). About two thirds of the heart lies within the left side of the rib cage, with the other third on the right side as it crosses the sternum. The heart is positioned in the thorax like a trapezoid:

Vertically along the right sternal border (RSB) from the second to the fifth rib

Horizontally (long side) from the lower right sternum to the fifth rib at the left midclavicular line (LMCL)

Diagonally from the left sternal border (LSB) at the second rib to the LMCL at the fifth rib

Horizontally (short side) from the RSB and LSB at the second intercostal space (ICS)—base of the heart

Inspection is best done with the child sitting in a semi-Fowler position. Look at the anterior chest wall from an angle, comparing both sides of the rib cage with each other. Normally they should be symmetric. In children with thin chest walls, a pulsation may be visible. Because comprehensive evaluation of cardiac function is not limited to the heart, also consider other findings such as the presence of all pulses (especially the femoral pulses) (Fig. 7-29), distended neck veins, clubbing of the fingers, peripheral cyanosis, edema, blood pressure, and respiratory status.

Use palpation to determine the location of the *apical impulse (AI)*, the most lateral cardiac impulse that may correspond to the apex. The AI is found:

- Just lateral to the left MCL and fourth ICS in children <7 years of age
- At the left MCL and fifth ICS in children >7 years of age

Although the AI gives a general idea of the size of the heart (with enlargement, the apex is lower and more lateral), its normal location is quite variable, making it a rather unreliable indicator of heart size.

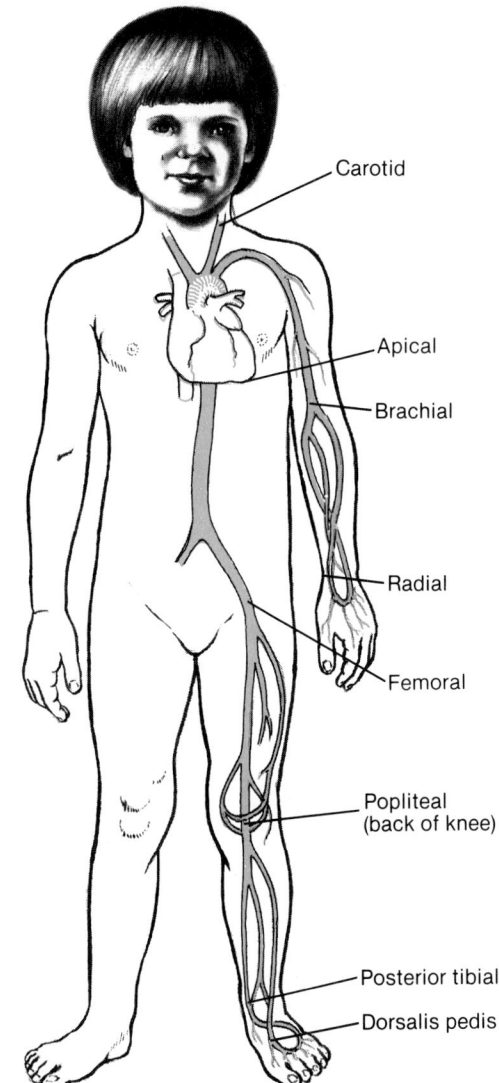

FIG. 7-29. Location of pulses.

The *point of maximum intensity (PMI)*, as the name implies, is the area of most intense pulsation. Usually the PMI is located at the same site as the AI, but it can occur elsewhere. For this reason, the two terms should not be used synonymously.

Assess *capillary filling time*, an important test for peripheral circulation, by pressing the skin lightly on a central site, such as the forehead, or a peripheral site, such as the top of the hand, to produce a slight blanching. The time it takes for the blanched area to return to its original color is the *capillary refill time*.

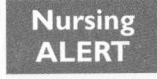 Capillary refill should be brisk—in less than 2 seconds; prolonged refill may be associated with poor systemic perfusion, as well as a cool ambient temperature.

Auscultation

Origin of Heart Sounds. The heart sounds are produced by the opening and closing of the valves and the vibration of blood against the walls of the heart and vessels. Normally two sounds—S_1 and S_2—are heard, which correspond respectively to the familiar "lub dub" often used to describe the sounds. S_1 is caused by closure of the *tricuspid* and *mitral valves* (sometimes called the *atrioventricular valves*). S_2 is the result of closure of the *pulmonic* and *aortic valves* (sometimes called *semilunar valves*). Normally the split of the two sounds in S_2 is distinguishable and widens during inspiration. *Physiologic splitting* is a significant normal finding.

Nursing ALERT	"Fixed splitting," in which the split in S_2 does not change during inspiration, is an important diagnostic sign of atrial septal defect.

Two other heart sounds—S_3 and S_4—may be produced. S_3 is normally heard in some children; S_4 is rarely heard as a normal heart sound; usually it indicates the need for further cardiac evaluation.

Another important category of heart sounds is *murmurs*, sounds that are produced by vibrations within the heart chambers or in the major arteries from the back-and-forth flow of blood. The description and classification of murmurs are skills that require considerable practice and training. Consult with an experienced practitioner whenever a murmur is identified or suspected.

Differentiating Normal Heart Sounds. Fig. 7-30 illustrates the approximate anatomic position of the valves within the heart chambers. Note that the anatomic location of valves does not correspond to the area where the sounds are heard best. The auscultatory sites are located in the direction of the blood flow through the valves.

Normally S_1 is louder at the apex of the heart in the mitral and tricuspid area, and S_2 is louder near the base of the heart in the pulmonic and aortic area. Listen to each sound by inching down the chest. The following areas should also be auscultated for sounds, such as murmurs, which may radiate to these sites: sternoclavicular area above the clavicles and manubrium, area along the sternal border, area along the left midaxillary line, and area below the scapulae.

NURSING TIP To distinguish between S_1 or S_2 heart sounds, simultaneously palpate the carotid pulse with the index and middle finger and listen to the heart sounds; S_1 is synchronous with the carotid pulse.

Auscultate the heart with the child in at least two positions: sitting and reclining. If adventitious sounds are detected, further evaluate them with the child standing, sitting and leaning forward, and lying on the left side. For example, atrial sounds such as S_4 are heard best with the person in a recumbent position and usually fade if the person sits or stands.

Evaluate heart sounds for (1) *quality* (should be clear and distinct, not muffled, diffuse, or distant); (2) *intensity*, especially in relation to the location or auscultatory site (should not be weak or pounding); (3) *rate* (should be the same as the radial pulse); and (4) *rhythm* (should be regular and

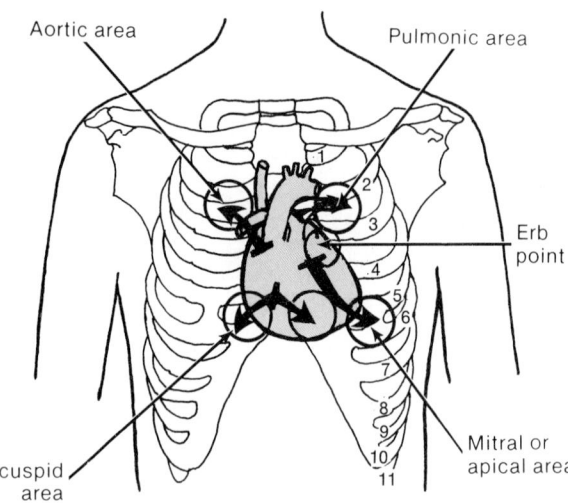

FIG. 7-30. Direction of heart sounds for anatomic valve sites and areas (circled) for auscultation.

even). A particular arrhythmia that occurs normally in many children is *sinus arrhythmia*, in which the heart rate increases with inspiration and decreases with expiration. Differentiate this rhythm from a truly abnormal arrhythmia by having children hold their breath. In sinus arrhythmia, cessation of breathing causes the heart rate to remain steady.

ABDOMEN

Examination of the abdomen involves inspection, followed by auscultation and then palpation. Perform palpation last because it may distort the normal abdominal sounds. Knowledge of the anatomic placement of the abdominal organs is essential to differentiate normal, expected findings from abnormal ones (Fig. 7-31).

For descriptive purposes the abdominal cavity is divided into four quadrants by drawing a vertical line midway from the sternum to the pubic symphysis and a horizontal line across the abdomen through the umbilicus. Each section is named as follows:

- Left upper quadrant (LUQ)
- Left lower quadrant (LLQ)
- Right upper quadrant (RUQ)
- Right lower quadrant (RLQ)

Inspection

Inspect the *contour* of the abdomen with the child erect and supine. Normally the abdomen of infants and young children is quite cylindric and, in the erect position, fairly prominent because of the physiologic lordosis of the spine. In the supine position the abdomen appears flat. A midline protrusion from the xiphoid to the umbilicus or pubic symphysis is usually *diastasis recti*, or failure of the rectus abdominis muscles to join in utero. In a healthy child a midline protrusion is usually a variation of normal muscular development.

Nursing ALERT	A tense, boardlike abdomen is a serious sign of paralytic ileus and intestinal obstruction.

The *skin* covering the abdomen should be uniformly taut, without wrinkles or creases. Sometimes silvery, whitish striae ("stretch marks") are seen, especially if the skin has been stretched as in obesity. Superficial veins are usually visible in light-skinned, thin infants, but distended veins are an abnormal finding.

Observe *movement* of the abdomen. Normally chest and abdominal movements are synchronous. In infants and thin children *peristaltic waves* may be visible through the abdominal wall; they are best observed by standing at eye level to and across from the abdomen. Always report this finding.

Examine the *umbilicus* for size, hygiene, and evidence of any abnormalities, such as hernias. The umbilicus should be flat or only slightly protruding. If a herniation is present, palpate the sac for abdominal contents and estimate the approximate size of the opening. *Umbilical hernias* are common in infants, especially in black children.

Hernias may exist elsewhere on the abdominal wall (Fig. 7-32). An *inguinal hernia* is a protrusion of peritoneum through the abdominal wall in the inguinal canal. It occurs mostly in males, is frequently bilateral, and may be visible as a mass in the scrotum. To locate a hernia, slide the little finger into the external inguinal ring at the base of the scrotum and ask the child to cough. If a hernia is present, it will hit the tip of the finger.

NURSING TIP If the child is too young to cough, have the child blow up a balloon or laugh to raise the intraabdominal pressure sufficiently to demonstrate the presence of an inguinal hernia.

A *femoral hernia*, which occurs more frequently in girls, is felt or seen as a small mass on the anterior surface of the thigh just below the inguinal ligament in the femoral canal (a potential space medial to the femoral artery). Feel for a hernia by placing the index finger of your right hand on the child's right femoral pulse (left hand for left pulse) and the middle ring finger flat against the skin toward the midline. The ring finger lies over the femoral canal, where the herniation occurs. Palpation of hernias in the pelvic region is often part of the examination of genitalia.

Auscultation

The most important finding to listen for is *peristalsis*, or *bowel sounds*, which sound like short metallic clicks and gurgles. Their frequency per minute should be recorded (e.g., 5 bowel sounds per minute). Bowel sounds may be stimulated by stroking the abdominal surface with a fingernail. Report absence of bowel sounds or hyperperistalsis because either usually denotes an abdominal disorder.

Palpation

Two types of palpation are performed: superficial and deep. In *superficial palpation* lightly place your hand against the skin and feel each quadrant, noting any areas of tenderness,

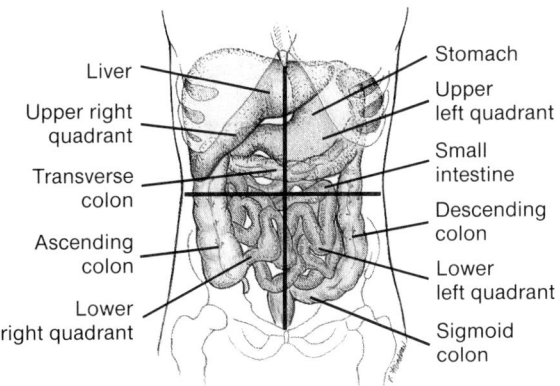

FIG. 7-31. Location of structures in abdomen. Cross rules divide cavity into quadrants. (From Potter PA, Perry AG: *Basic nursing: theory and practice,* ed 3, St Louis, 1995, Mosby.)

Liver
Upper right quadrant
Transverse colon
Ascending colon
Lower right quadrant
Stomach
Upper left quadrant
Small intestine
Descending colon
Lower left quadrant
Sigmoid colon

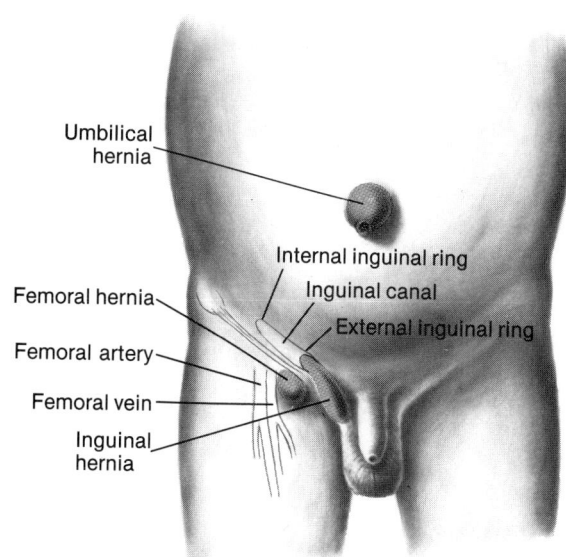

FIG. 7-32. Location of hernias.

Umbilical hernia
Internal inguinal ring
Inguinal canal
External inguinal ring
Femoral hernia
Femoral artery
Femoral vein
Inguinal hernia

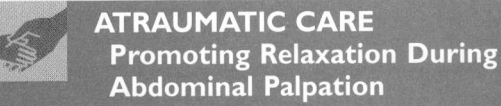

ATRAUMATIC CARE
Promoting Relaxation During Abdominal Palpation

Position child comfortably, such as in a semireclining position in the parent's lap, with knees flexed.
Warm the hands before touching the skin.
Use distraction, such as telling stories or talking to child.
Teach child to use deep breathing and to concentrate on an object.
Give infant a bottle or pacifier.
Begin with light, superficial palpation and gradually progress to deeper palpation.
Palpate any tender or painful areas last.
Have child hold the parent's hand and squeeze it if palpation is uncomfortable.
Use the nonpalpating hand to comfort child, such as placing the free hand on the child's shoulder while palpating the abdomen.
To minimize sensation of tickling during palpation:
    Have children "help" with palpation by placing their hand over the palpating hand.
    Have them place their hand on the abdomen with the fingers spread wide apart, and palpate between their fingers.

muscle tone, and superficial lesions, such as cysts. Because superficial palpation is often perceived as tickling, several techniques can be used to minimize this sensation and provide relaxation (see Atraumatic Care box on p. 167). Admonishing the child to stop laughing only draws attention to the sensation and decreases cooperation.

Deep palpation is used for palpating organs and large blood vessels and for detecting masses and tenderness that were not discovered during superficial palpation. Palpation usually begins in the lower quadrants and proceeds upward to avoid missing the edge of an enlarged liver or spleen. Except for palpating the liver, successful identification of other organs, such as the spleen, kidney, and part of the colon, requires considerable practice with tutored supervision. Report any questionable mass.

The lower edge of the *liver* is sometimes felt in infants and young children as a superficial mass 1 to 2 cm (0.4 to 0.8 inch) below the right costal margin (the distance is sometimes measured in fingerbreadths). Normally the liver descends during inspiration as the diaphragm moves downward. Do not mistake this downward displacement as a sign of liver enlargement.

| 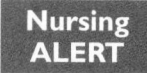 **Nursing ALERT** | If the liver is palpable 3 cm below the right costal margin or the spleen is palpable more than 2 cm below the left costal margin, these organs are enlarged—a finding that is always reported for further medical investigation. |

Palpate the *femoral pulses* by placing the tips of two or three fingers (index, middle, and/or ring) along the inguinal ligament about midway between the iliac crest and pubic symphysis. Feel both pulses simultaneously to make certain that they are equal and strong (Fig. 7-33).

| **Nursing ALERT** | Absence of femoral pulses is a significant sign of coarctation of the aorta and is referred for medical evaluation. |

GENITALIA

Examination of genitalia conveniently follows assessment of the abdomen while the child is still supine. In adolescents inspection of the genitalia may be left to the end of the examination. The best approach is to examine the genitalia matter-of-factly, placing no more emphasis on this part of the assessment than on any other segment. It helps to relieve children's and parents' anxiety by telling them the results of the findings, for example, "Everything looks fine here."

If it is necessary to ask questions, such as about discharge or difficulty in urinating, respect the child's privacy by covering the lower abdomen with the gown or underpants. To prevent embarrassing interruptions, keep the door or curtain closed and post a "do not disturb" sign. Have a drape ready to cover the genitalia if someone enters the room.

In examining the genitalia, wear gloves whenever touching body substances. It might be helpful for the adolescent to know that wearing gloves also prevents skin-to-skin contact.

The genital examination is an excellent time for eliciting questions of concern about body functioning or sexual activity. Also use this opportunity to increase or reinforce the child's knowledge of reproductive anatomy by naming each body part and explaining its function. For males, this part of the health assessment is an opportune time to teach self-testicular examination.

Male Genitalia

Note the external appearance of the glans and shaft of the penis, the prepuce, the urethral meatus, and the scrotum (Fig. 7-34). The *penis* is generally small in infants and young boys until puberty, when it begins to increase in both length and width. In an obese child the penis often looks abnormally small because of the folds of skin partially covering it at the base. Be familiar with normal pubertal growth of the external male genitalia in order to compare the findings with the expected sequence of maturation (see Chapter 16).

Examine the *glans* (head of the penis) and *shaft* (portion between the perineum and prepuce) for signs of swelling, skin lesions, inflammation, or other irregularities. Any of these signs may indicate underlying disorders, especially sexually transmitted diseases.

The *urethral meatus* is carefully inspected for location and evidence of discharge. Normally it is centered at the tip of the glans.

Hair distribution is also noted. Normally before puberty no pubic hair is present. Soft downy hair at the base of the

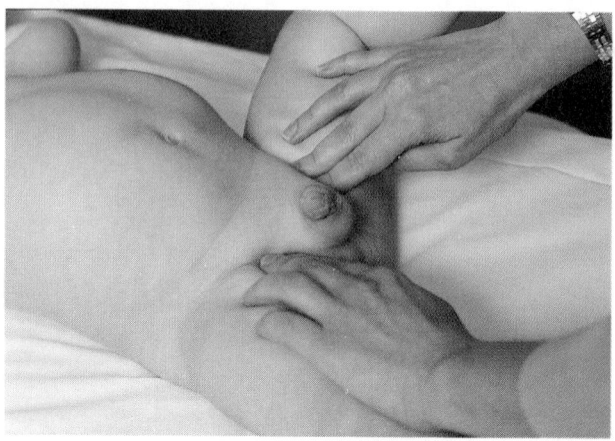

FIG. 7-33. Palpating for femoral pulses.

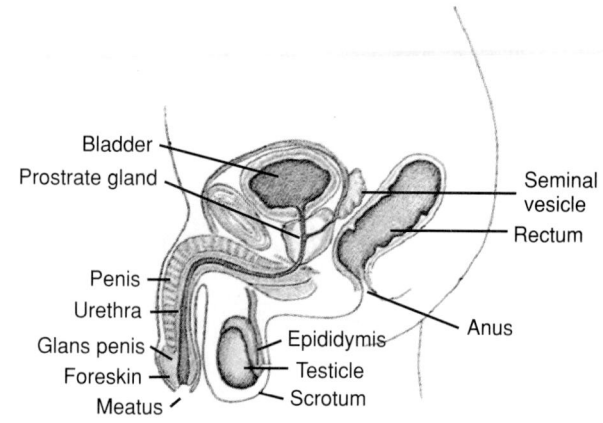

FIG. 7-34. Major structures of genitalia in uncircumcised postpubertal male. (From Potter PA, Perry AG: *Basic nursing: theory and practice,* ed 3, St Louis, 1995, Mosby.)

penis is an early sign of pubertal maturation. In older adolescents hair distribution is diamond-shaped from the umbilicus to the anus.

The location and size of the *scrotum* are noted. The scrota hang freely from the perineum behind the penis, and the left scrotum normally hangs lower than the right. In infants the scrota appear large in relation to the rest of the genitalia. The skin of the scrotum is loose and highly rugated (wrinkled). During early adolescence the skin normally becomes redder and coarser. In dark-skinned children the scrota are usually more deeply pigmented.

Palpation of the scrotum includes identification of the testes, epididymis, and, if present, inguinal hernias. The two *testes* are felt as small ovoid bodies about 1.5 to 2 cm (0.6 to 0.8 inch) long—one in each scrotal sac. They do not enlarge until puberty, when they approximately double in size.

When palpating for the presence of the testes avoid stimulating the *cremasteric reflex,* which is stimulated by cold, touch, emotional excitement, or exercise. This reflex pulls the testes higher into the pelvic cavity. Several measures are useful in preventing the cremasteric reflex during palpation of the scrotum. First, warm the hands. Second, if the child is old enough, examine him in a tailor or "Indian" position, which stretches the muscle, preventing its contraction (Fig. 7-35, *A*). Third, block the normal pathway of ascent of the testes by placing the thumb and index finger over the upper part of the scrotal sac along the inguinal canal (Fig. 7-35, *B*). If there is any question concerning the existence of two testes, place the index and middle fingers in a scissors fash-

ion to separate the right and left scrotum. If after using these techniques the testes have not been palpated, feel along the inguinal canal and perineum to locate masses that may be undescended testes. Although undescended testes may descend at any time during childhood and are checked at each visit, failure to palpate testes is reported.

Female Genitalia

The examination of female genitalia is limited to inspection and palpation of external structures. If a vaginal examination is required, an appropriate referral is made unless the nurse is qualified to perform the procedure. A convenient position for examination of the genitalia involves placing the young child supine on the examining table or in a semireclining position on the parent's lap with the feet supported on your knees as you sit facing the child. Divert the child's attention from the examination by instructing her to try to keep the soles of her feet pressed against each other. Separate the labia majora with the thumb and index finger and retract outward in order to expose the labia minora, urethral meatus, and vaginal orifice.

Examine the female genitalia for size and location of the structures of the *vulva* or *pudendum* (Fig. 7-36). The *mons pubis* is a pad of adipose tissue over the symphysis pubis. At puberty the mons is covered with hair, which extends along the labia. The usual pattern of female *hair distribution* is an inverted triangle. The appearance of soft downy hair along the labia majora is an early sign of sexual maturation.

Note the size and location of the *clitoris*. It is a small erec-

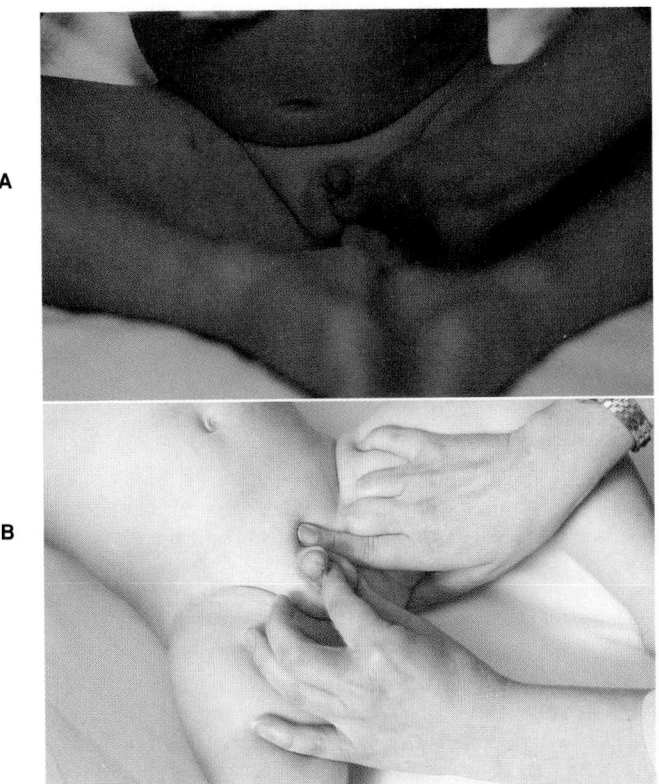

FIG. 7-35. A, Preventing cremasteric reflex by having child sit in "tailor" position. **B,** Blocking inguinal canal during palpation of scrotum for descended testes.

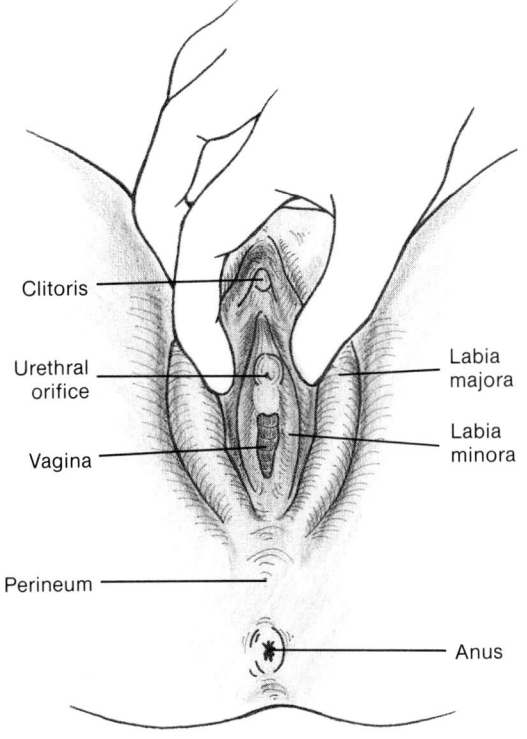

FIG. 7-36. External structures of genitalia in postpubertal female. Labia are spread to reveal deeper structures. (From Potter PA, Perry AG: *Basic nursing: theory and practice,* ed 3, St Louis, 1995, Mosby.)

tile organ located at the anterior end of the labia minora. It is covered by a small flap of skin, the *prepuce.*

The *labia majora* are two thick folds of skin running posteriorly from the mons to the posterior commissure of the vagina. Internal to the labia majora are two folds of skin called the *labia minora.* Although the labia minora are usually prominent in the newborn, they gradually atrophy, which makes them almost invisible until their enlargement during puberty.

The inner surface of the labia should be pink and moist. Note the size of the labia and any evidence of fusion, which may suggest male scrota. Normally no masses are palpable within the labia.

The *urethral meatus* is located posterior to the clitoris and is surrounded by Skene glands and ducts. Although not a prominent structure, the meatus appears as a small V-shaped slit. Note its location, especially if it opens from the clitoris or inside the vagina. Gently palpate the glands, which are common sites of cysts and sexually transmitted lesions.

The *vaginal orifice* is located posterior to the urethral meatus. Its appearance varies depending on individual anatomy and sexual activity. Ordinarily examination of the vagina is limited to inspection. In virgins a thin crescent-shaped or circular membrane, called the *hymen,* may cover part of the vaginal opening. In some instances it completely occludes the orifice. After rupture, small rounded pieces of tissue called *caruncles* remain. Although an imperforate hymen denotes lack of penile intercourse, a perforate one does not necessarily indicate sexual activity (see also Sexual Abuse, Chapter 14).

Nursing ALERT In females who have been circumcised, the genitalia will appear different. Do not show surprise or disgust, but note the appearance and discuss the procedure with the young woman (see also Cultural Awareness box on p. 206).

Surrounding the vaginal opening are *Bartholin glands,* which secrete a clear, mucoid fluid into the vagina for lubrication during intercourse. Palpate the ducts for cysts. Also note the discharge from the vagina, which is usually clear or white.

ANUS

Following examination of the genitalia, the anal area is easily examined, although the child should be placed on the abdomen. Note the general firmness of the *buttocks* and symmetry of the *gluteal folds.* Assess the tone of the anal sphincter by eliciting the *anal reflex.* Gently scratching the anal area results in an obvious quick contraction of the external anal sphincter.

BACK AND EXTREMITIES

Spine

The general *curvature* of the spine is noted. Normally the back of a newborn is rounded or C-shaped from the thoracic and pelvic curves. The development of the cervical and lumbar curves approximates development of various motor skills, such as cervical curvature with head control, and gives the older child the typical double-S curve.

Marked curvatures in posture are abnormal (see Fig. 31-18). *Scoliosis,* lateral curvature of the spine, is an important childhood problem, especially in females. Although scoliosis may be identified by observing and palpating the spine and noting a sideways displacement, more objective tests include:

1. With the child standing erect, clothed only in underpants (and bra if older girl), observe from behind, noting asymmetry of the shoulders and hips.
2. With the child bending forward so that the back is parallel to the floor, observe from the side, noting asymmetry or prominence of the rib cage.

A slight limp, a crooked hemline, or complaints of a sore back are other signs and symptoms of scoliosis.

Inspect the *back,* especially along the spine, for any tufts of hair, dimples, or discoloration. *Mobility* of the vertebral column is easily assessed in most children because of their propensity for constant motion during the examination. However, mobility can be tested by asking the child to sit up from a prone position or to do a modified sit-up exercise.

Movement of the cervical spine is an important diagnostic sign of neurologic problems, such as meningitis. Normally movement of the head in all directions is effortless.

Nursing ALERT Hyperextension of the neck and spine, or *opisthotonos,* which is accompanied by pain when the head is flexed, is always referred for immediate medical evaluation.

Extremities

Inspect each extremity for symmetry of length and size; refer any deviation for orthopedic evaluation. Count the fingers and toes to be certain of the normal number. This is so often taken for granted that an extra digit *(polydactyly)* or fusion of digits *(syndactyly)* may go unnoticed.

Inspect the arms and legs for *temperature* and *color,* which should be equal in each extremity, although the feet may normally be colder than the hands.

Assess the *shape* of bones. Several variations of bone shape may be observed in children. Although many of them cause parents concern, most are benign and require no treatment. *Bowleg,* or *genu varum,* is lateral bowing of the tibia. It is clinically present when the child stands with the medial malleoli (rounded prominence on either side of the ankle) opposite each other and the space between the knees is greater than approximately 5 cm (2 inches) (Fig. 7-37). Toddlers are usually bow-legged after beginning to walk until all their lower back and leg muscles are well developed. Unilateral or asymmetric bowlegs that are present beyond the age of 2 to 3 years, particularly in black children, may represent pathologic conditions requiring further investigation.

Knock-knee, or *genu valgum,* appears as the opposite of bowleg, in that the knees are close together but the feet are spread apart. It is determined clinically by using the same method as for genu varum but by measuring the distance between the malleoli, which normally should be less than 7.5 cm (3 inches) (Fig. 7-38). Knock-knee is normally present in children from about 2 to 7 years of age. Knock-knee that is excessive, asymmetric, accompanied by shortened stature, or evident in a child nearing puberty requires further evaluation.

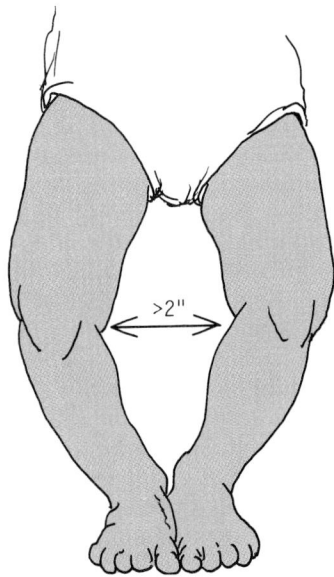

FIG. 7-37. Bowleg.

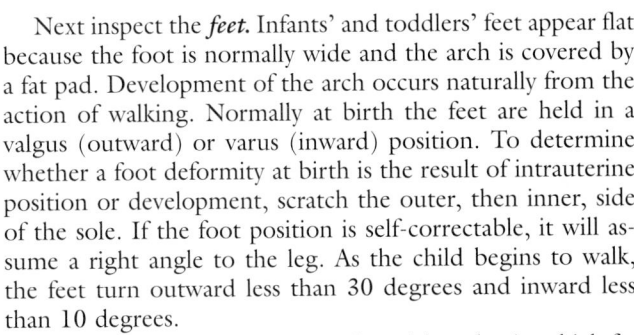

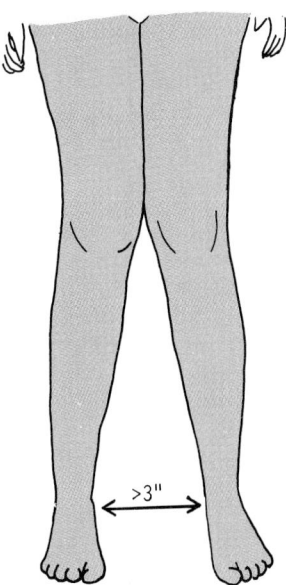

FIG. 7-38. Knock-knee.

Next inspect the *feet.* Infants' and toddlers' feet appear flat because the foot is normally wide and the arch is covered by a fat pad. Development of the arch occurs naturally from the action of walking. Normally at birth the feet are held in a valgus (outward) or varus (inward) position. To determine whether a foot deformity at birth is the result of intrauterine position or development, scratch the outer, then inner, side of the sole. If the foot position is self-correctable, it will assume a right angle to the leg. As the child begins to walk, the feet turn outward less than 30 degrees and inward less than 10 degrees.

Toddlers have a "toddling" or broad-based gait, which facilitates walking by lowering the center of gravity. As the child reaches preschool age, the legs are brought closer together. By school age the walking posture is much more graceful and balanced.

The most common gait problem in young children is *pigeon toe,* or *toeing in,* which usually results from torsional deformities, such as internal tibial torsion (abnormal rotation or bowing of the tibia). Tests for tibial torsion include measuring the thigh-foot angle, which requires considerable practice for accuracy.

Elicit the *plantar* or *grasp reflex* by exerting firm but gentle pressure with the tip of the thumb against the lateral sole of the foot from the heel upward to the little toe and then across to the big toe. The normal response in children who are walking is flexion of the toes. *Babinski sign,* dorsiflexion of the big toe and fanning of the other toes, is normal during infancy but abnormal after about 1 year of age or when locomotion begins (see Fig. 8-9).

Joints

Evaluate the joints for *range of motion.* Normally this requires no specific testing if the nurse has been observant of the child's movements during the examination. However, the hips should be routinely investigated in infants for congenital dislocation. Signs of congenital hip dislocation are discussed in Chapter 31. Report any evidence of joint immobility or hyperflexibility.

Palpate the joints for *heat, tenderness,* and *swelling.* These signs, as well as redness over the joint, warrant further investigation.

Muscles

Note symmetry and quality of muscle development, tone, and strength. Observe *development* by looking at the shape and contour of the body in both a relaxed and a tensed state. Estimate *tone* by grasping the muscle and feeling its firmness when it is relaxed and contracted. A common site for testing tone is the biceps muscle of the arm. Children are usually willing to "make a muscle" by clenching their fist.

Estimate *strength* by having the child use an extremity to push or pull against resistance, as in the following examples:

Arm strength. Child holds the arms outstretched in front of the body and tries to raise the arms while downward pressure is applied.

Hand strength. Child shakes hands with nurse and squeezes one or two fingers of the nurse's hand.

Leg strength. Child sits on a table or chair with the legs dangling and tries to raise the legs while downward pressure is applied.

Note symmetry of strength in the extremities, hands, and fingers, and report evidence of paresis or weakness.

NEUROLOGIC ASSESSMENT

The assessment of the nervous system is the broadest and most diverse part of the examining process, since every human function, both physical and emotional, is controlled by neurologic impulses. Much of the neurologic examination has already been discussed, such as assessment of behavior, sensory testing, and motor functioning. The following focuses on a general appraisal of cerebellar functioning, deep tendon reflexes, and the cranial nerves.

TESTS FOR CEREBELLAR FUNCTION

Finger-to-nose test. With child's arm extended, ask child to touch the nose with the index finger with eyes open and then closed.

Heel-to-shin test. While standing, have child run the heel of one foot down the shin or anterior aspect of the tibia of the other leg, both with eyes opened and then closed.

Romberg test. With eyes closed, have child stand with heels together; falling or leaning to one side is abnormal and is called *Romberg sign.*

Cerebellar Functioning

The cerebellum controls balance and coordination. Much of the assessment of cerebellar functioning is included in observing the child's posture, body movements, gait, and development of fine and gross motor skills. Tests such as balancing on one foot and the heel-to-toe walk assess balance. Test *coordination* by asking the child to reach for a toy, button clothes, tie shoes, or draw a straight line on a piece of paper, provided the child is old enough to do these activities. Coordination can also be tested by any sequence of rapid successive movements, such as quickly touching each finger with the thumb of the same hand.

Several tests for cerebellar function are described in the accompanying box and can be performed as games. When the Romberg test is done, stay beside the child if there is a possibility that the child may fall. School-age children should be able to perform these tests, although, in the finger-to-nose test, preschoolers normally can only bring the finger within 5 to 7.5 cm (2 to 3 inches) of the nose. Difficulty in performing these exercises indicates poor sense of position (especially with the eyes closed) and incoordination (especially with the eyes opened).

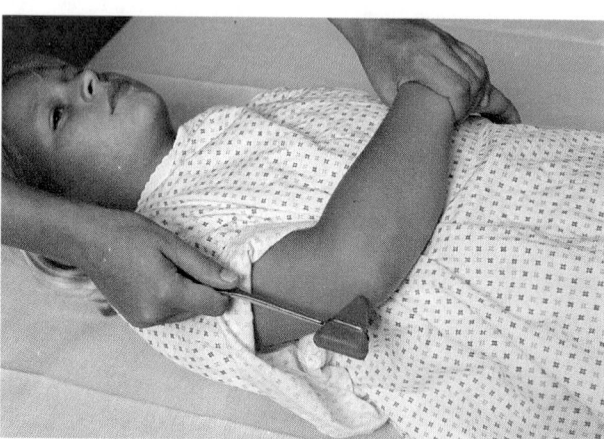

FIG. 7-39. Testing for triceps reflex. Child is placed supine, with forearm resting over chest, and triceps tendon is struck. Alternate procedure: child's arm is abducted, with upper arm supported and forearm allowed to hang freely. Triceps tendon is struck. Normal response is partial extension of forearm.

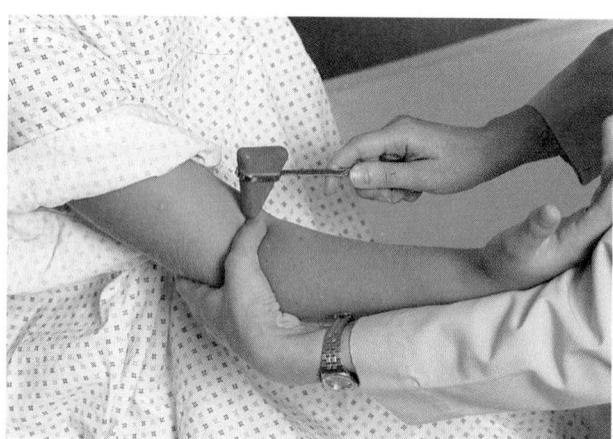

FIG. 7-40. Testing for biceps reflex. Child's arm is held by placing partially flexed elbow in examiner's hand with thumb over antecubital space. Examiner's thumbnail is struck with hammer. Normal response is partial flexion of forearm.

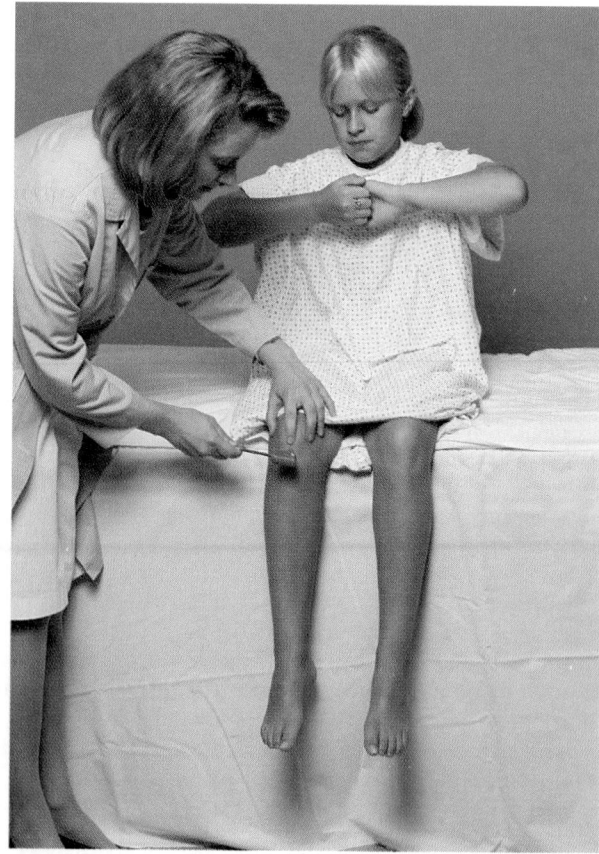

FIG. 7-41. Testing for patellar, or knee jerk, reflex, using distraction. Child sits on edge of examining table (or on parent's lap) with lower legs flexed at knee and dangling freely. Patellar tendon is tapped just below kneecap. Normal response is partial extension of lower leg.

Reflexes

Testing reflexes is an important part of the neurologic examination. Persistence of primitive reflexes (see Chapter 8), loss of reflexes, or hyperactivity of deep tendon reflexes is usually the result of a cerebral insult.

Elicit reflexes by using the rubber head of the reflex hammer, flat of the finger, or side of the hand. If the child is easily frightened by equipment, use your hand or finger. Although testing reflexes is a simple procedure to perform, the child may inhibit the reflex by unconsciously tensing the muscle. To avoid tensing, distract younger children with toys or talk to them. Older children can concentrate on the exercise of grasping their two hands in front of them and trying to pull them apart. This diverts their attention away from the testing and causes involuntary relaxation of the muscles.

Deep tendon reflexes are stretch reflexes of a muscle. The most common deep tendon reflex is the *knee jerk,* or *patellar reflex* (this is sometimes called the *quadriceps reflex*). The reflexes normally elicited are described in Figs. 7-39 to 7-42. Report any diminished or hyperreflexic response for further evaluation.

Cranial Nerves

Assessment of the cranial nerves is an important area of neurologic assessment (Table 7-12). With young children present the tests as games to encourage trust and security at the beginning of the examination. Or include the cranial nerve test when each "system" is examined, such as tongue movement and strength, gag reflex, swallowing, and position of the uvula during examination of the mouth.

DEVELOPMENTAL ASSESSMENT

One of the most essential components of a complete health appraisal is assessment of developmental functioning. *Screening procedures* are designed to identify quickly and reliably those children whose developmental level is below normal for their age and who therefore require further investigation. They also provide a means of recording objective measurements of present developmental functioning for future reference. Since the passage of P.L. 99-457, the Education of the Handicapped Act Amendments of 1986, much greater emphasis is placed on developmental assessment of children with disabilities, and nurses can play a vital role in providing this service. All the procedures discussed in this section can be administered in a variety of settings—home, school, daycare center, hospital, practitioner's office, or clinic.

DENVER II

The most widely used developmental screening tests for young children have been the series of tests developed by Dr. William Frankenburg and his colleagues in Denver, Colorado. The oldest and best known, the *Denver Developmental Screening Test (DDST)* and its revision, the *DDST-R,* have been revised, restandardized, and renamed the *Denver-II.* Before administering the Denver II, the examiner should be trained by, and receive a certificate from, a master instructor who has been trained by the Denver faculty.* The Denver II differs from the DDST in items, test form, interpretation, and referral (see Appendix C). The previous total of 105 items has been increased to 125, including an increase from 21 DDST to 39 Denver II language items. Previous items that were difficult to administer and/or interpret have been either modified or eliminated. Many items that were previously tested by parental report now require observation by the examiner.

Each item was evaluated to determine if significant differences exist on the basis of sex, ethnic group, maternal education, and place of residence. Items for which clinically significant differences exist were replaced, or if retained, are discussed in the Technical Manual. When evaluating children delayed on one of these items, the examiner can look up norms for the subpopulations to consider if the delay may be caused by sociocultural or environmental differences.

The items on the test form are arranged in the same format as the DDST-R. The norms for the distribution bars were updated with the new standardization data but retain the 25th, 50th, 75th, and 90th percentile divisions. The test form contains a place to rate the child's behavioral characteristics

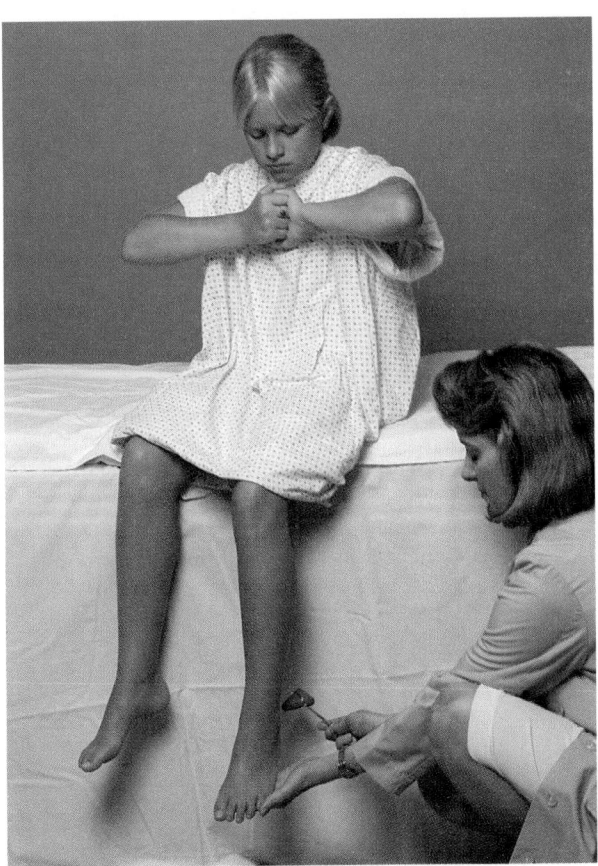

FIG. 7-42. Testing for Achilles reflex. The child should be in the same position as for the knee jerk reflex. Foot is supported lightly in examiner's hand, and Achilles tendon is struck. Normal response is plantar flexion of foot (foot pointing downward).

---

*Forms and complete instructions are available from Denver Developmental Materials, Inc., P.O. Box 6919, Denver, CO 80206-9019; (303) 355-4729, 1-800-419-4729. The DDST and DDST-R are no longer available because they have been replaced by the DENVER II.

TABLE 7-12. Assessment of cranial nerves

DISTRIBUTION/FUNCTION	TEST
I—Olfactory Nerve Olfactory mucosa of nasal cavity Smell	With eyes closed, have child identify odors such as coffee, alcohol from a swab, or other smells; test each nostril separately
II—Optic Nerve Rods and cones of retina, optic nerve Vision	Check for perception of light, visual acuity, peripheral vision, color vision, and normal optic disc

III—Oculomotor Nerve
Extraocular muscles (EOM) of eye:
   Superior rectus (SR)—moves eyeball up and in
   Inferior rectus (IR)—moves eyeball down and in
   Medial rectus (MR)—moves eyeball nasally
   Inferior oblique (IO)—moves eyeball up and out
Pupil constriction and accommodation
Eyelid closing
	Have child follow an object (toy) or light in the six cardinal positions of gaze (see Fig. 7-43)
	
	Perform PERRLA
	Check for proper placement of lid

IV—Trochlear Nerve Superior oblique muscle (SO)—moves eye down and out	Have child look down and in (Fig. 7-43)
V—Trigeminal Nerve Muscles of mastication Sensory: face, scalp, nasal and buccal mucosa	Have child bite down hard and open jaw; test symmetry and strength With child's eyes closed, see if child can detect light touch in the mandibular and maxillary regions Test corneal and blink reflex by touching cornea lightly (approach from the side so that child does not blink before cornea is touched)
VI—Abducens Nerve Lateral rectus (LR) muscle—moves eye temporally	Have child look toward temporal side (Fig. 7-43)
VII—Facial Nerve Muscles for facial expression Anterior two thirds of tongue (sensory)	Have child smile, make funny face, or show teeth to see symmetry of expression Have child identify a sweet or salty solution; place each taste on anterior section and sides of protruding tongue; if child retracts tongue, solution will dissolve toward posterior part of tongue
VIII—Auditory, Acoustic, or Vestibulocochlear Nerve Internal ear Hearing/balance	Test hearing; note any loss of equilibrium or presence of vertigo
IX—Glossopharyngeal Nerve Pharynx, tongue Posterior one third of tongue (sensory)	Stimulate posterior pharynx with a tongue blade; child should gag Test sense of sour or bitter taste on posterior segment of tongue
X—Vagus Nerve Muscles of larynx, pharynx, some organs of gastrointestinal system, sensory fibers of root of tongue, heart, lung, and some organs of gastrointestinal system	Note hoarseness of voice, gag reflex, and ability to swallow Check that uvula is in midline; when stimulated with a tongue blade, should deviate upward and to stimulated side
XI—Accessory Nerve Sternocleidomastoid and trapezius muscles of shoulder	Have child shrug shoulders while applying mild pressure; with examiner's hands placed on shoulders, have child turn head against opposing pressure on either side; note symmetry and strength
XII—Hypoglossal Nerve Muscles of tongue	Have child move tongue in all directions; have child protrude tongue as far as possible; note any midline deviation Test strength by placing tongue blade on one side of tongue and having child move it away

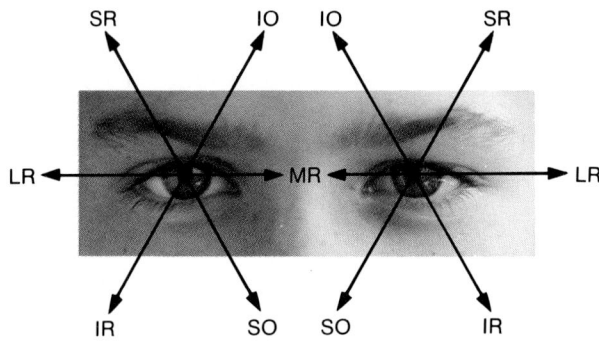

FIG. 7-43. Testing cardinal positions of gaze.

(compliance, interest in surroundings, fearfulness, and attention span).

To determine relative areas of advancement and areas of delay, sufficient items should be administered to establish the basal and ceiling levels in each sector. By scoring appropriate items as "pass," "fail," "refusal," or "no opportunity," and relating such scores to the age of the child, each item can be interpreted as described in the accompanying box. To identify cautions, all items intersected by the age line are administered. To screen solely for developmental delays, only the items located totally to the *left* of the child's age line are administered. Criteria for referral are based on the availability of resources in the community (also see the box).

Research on the Denver II's validity and accuracy is in its beginning stages. One study found that most children with even subtle developmental problems were identified. However, almost half of the children without developmental problems received suspect scores, resulting in a high rate of overreferrals (Glascoe and others, 1992). To minimize overreferrals, a decision for referral depends not only on the results of the Denver II, but also on the practitioner's clinical judgment after considering the child's developmental history; general health status; social, cultural, and emotional environment; and the availability of local resources for diagnosis and treatment (Frankenburg, 1994a).

Although it is not the purpose of this discussion to detail the instruction manual, some points concerning preparation, administration, and interpretation of the Denver II are important to stress. Before beginning the screen, ask if the child was born prematurely and correctly calculate the adjusted age. Up to 24 months of age, allowances are made for infants born prematurely by subtracting the number of weeks of missed gestation from their present age and testing them at the adjusted age. For example, a 16-week-old infant who was born 4 weeks early is tested at a 12-week adjusted age level. Explain to the parents and child, if appropriate, that the screenings are *not* intelligence tests but a method of showing what the child can do at a particular age. Emphasize that the child is *not* expected to perform each item on the test.

Tell the parent before the screening begins that the results of the child's performance will be explained after all the items have been concluded. It is the nurse's responsibility to properly inform parents of any testing or screening procedure before its administration so that they are fully aware of its purpose and intent.

Prepare toddlers and preschoolers for the procedure by presenting it as a game. Frequently the Denver II is an excellent way to begin a health appraisal because it is nonthreatening, requires no painful or unfamiliar procedures, and capitalizes on the child's natural activity of play. Because children are easily distracted, perform each item quickly and present only one toy from the kit at a time. After that toy's purpose is concluded, such as building a tower of blocks or identifying its color, replace the toy in the bag and take out another one. Other temporary factors that may interfere with the child's performance include fatigue, illness, fear, hospitalization, separation from the parent, or general unwillingness to perform the activities. In addition, undiagnosed mental retardation, hearing loss, vision loss, neurologic impairment, or a familial pattern of slow development greatly influences the child's performance.

Following completion of the Denver II, ask the parent if the child's performance was typical of behavior at other times. If the parent replies affirmatively and the child's cooperation was satisfactory, explain the results, emphasizing all successful items first, then those items failed but which the child was not expected to pass, and finally those items that were delays. If the parent replies that the child's performance was not typical of usual behavior, it is best to defer any scoring or discussion of results, especially if the refusals yield a suspect score. In this situation reschedule testing for a time when the child is more likely to cooperate.

In explaining a normal score, focus on how well the child performed and reinforce the parents' efforts in satisfactorily stimulating their child. In addition to assessing the child's present developmental level, the Denver II can be used to guide parents toward those activities that are appropriate, although not necessarily expected, for the child's age. By testing for items to the right of the age line (ones the child is not expected to perform), children with advanced development, who may be gifted, can be identified.

In explaining delays, carefully note the parent's response, especially casual acceptance, such as "He'll catch up," or questions, such as "Does this mean my child is retarded?" Be aware of personal anxieties during these situations and refrain from giving glib reassurances, such as "I'm sure he will do better the next time." Rather, respond honestly to parents' questions, yet with appropriate flexibility and concern, stressing the need for further developmental testing.

REVISED PRESCREENING DEVELOPMENTAL QUESTIONNAIRE (R-PDQ)

The R-PDQ is a revision of the original PDQ (Frankenburg, Fandal, and Thornton, 1987). Advantages of the R-PDQ include the addition and arrangement of items to be more age-appropriate, simplified parent scoring, and easier comparison with Denver Developmental Screening Test (DDST) norms for professionals. The R-PDQ is a parent-answered prescreen consisting of 150 questions from the DDST, although only a subset of questions are asked for each age-group. The form may need to be read to parents and caregivers who are less educated.

Four different forms are available and are selected based on age: orange (0 to 9 months), purple (9 to 24 months), gold (2 to 4 years), and white (4 to 6 years) (see Appendix C). The caregiver answers the questions until (1) three "NOs" are circled (they do not have to be consecutive) or (2) all the questions on both sides of the form have been answered. Scoring is based on the number of delays (see box on p. 175). Children who have no delays are considered to

be developing normally. If a child has one delay, the caregiver is provided with age-appropriate developmental activities to pursue with the child and a rescreen with the R-PDQ is done 1 month later. If on rescreening a child has one or more delays, the Denver II is administered as soon as possible. If a child has two or more delays on the first screening with the R-PDQ, the Denver II is administered as soon as possible.

DEVELOPMENTAL SCREENING AND INTERPRETATION

Although screening tests are an effective method of applying the knowledge of children's expected rate of development to a large segment of the population, they are only as successful as the individual's expertise in administering them. Because many of the screening tests are devised to be used by paraprofessionals, there are inherent risks in screening if such individuals are not properly trained or supervised. For example, false-positives can label the child as developmentally delayed and cause problems that otherwise might not have existed. False-negatives can prevent children with problems from receiving the help they need.

Nurses administering developmental screening or supervising paraprofessionals' testing need to assess the child's "whole picture" and not rely solely on any screening procedure. Development, like growth and health, is a dynamic process. Tests such as the Denver II should be used as part of *developmental surveillance,* a continuous comprehensive primary health care approach that includes the parents as partners with professionals (Frankenburg, 1994b). Evaluation of the child's total well-being is the result of evaluating data from a comprehensive health and family history, physical examination, and developmental screening.

KEY POINTS

- The most common approach to examining children follows a head-to-toe sequence.
- Growth measurements during the physical examination focus on length, height, weight, skinfold thickness, and arm and head circumference. Assessment of growth is measured against standard growth charts to determine a child's status in comparison with other children of the same age.
- Measurements of temperature, pulse, respiration, and blood pressure constitute the physiologic approach to assessment.
- The general appearance of a child is a cumulative, subjective impression of physical appearance, state of nutrition, behavior, personality, interactions with parents and nurse, posture, development, and speech.

- Assessment of the skin, which primarily involves inspection and palpation, focuses on color, texture, temperature, moisture, and turgor. The nurse needs to be aware of both physiologic and ethnic factors that may affect these areas.
- In assessment of the lymph nodes, the nurse examines, by palpation, the part of the body in which the glands are located.
- The head is inspected for shape, symmetry, mobility, and head control.
- Examination of the eyes includes placement and alignment, inspection of external and internal structures, and vision testing.

- Ears are examined for placement and alignment, inspection of external and internal structures, and auditory testing.
- The lungs are examined by methods of inspection, palpation, percussion, and auscultation.
- Auscultation is the most important procedure for examining the heart.
- Abdominal assessment follows an orderly sequence of inspection, auscultation, and palpation, since palpation may distort normal abdominal sounds.

- Examination of the genitalia may provoke anxiety in the child, and the nurse must avoid any transference of anxiety.
- Neurologic assessment addresses behavior; motor, sensory, and cerebellar functioning; reflexes; and cranial nerves.
- The Denver II, a major revision and a restandardization of the DDST, differs from the DDST in items included in the test, the test form, and the interpretation of scoring.

REFERENCES

Abdo MH, Feghali JG, Stapells DR: Transient evoked otoacoustic emissions: clinical applications and technical considerations, *Int J Pediatr Otorhinolaryngol* 25:61-71, 1993.

Burke S, Roberts C, Maloney R: Infant and child weights: reliability and validity of scales, *Issues Compr Pediatr Nurs* 11(4):241-249, 1988.

Dewey KG and others: Growth of breast-fed infants deviates from current reference data: a pooled analysis of U.S., Canadian, and European data sets, *Pediatrics* 96(3):495-503, 1995.

Frankenburg WK: Preventing developmental delays: is developmental screening sufficient? I. Developmental screening and the Denver II, *Pediatrics*, 93(4):586-589, 1994a.

Frankenburg WK: Preventing developmental delays: is developmental screening sufficient? II. Partners in health care, *Pediatrics* 93(4):589-593, 1994b.

Frankenburg WK, Fandal A, Thornton S: Revision of Denver Prescreening Developmental Questionnaire, *J Pediatr* 110(4):653-657, 1987.

Frohlich E and others: Recommendations for human blood pressure determination by sphygmomanometers: report of a special task force appointed by the Steering Committee, American Health Association, *Circulation* 77:501A, 1988.

Glascoe FP and others: Accuracy of the Denver-II in developmental screening, *Pediatrics* 89:1221-1225, 1992.

Kovalesky A: *Nurses' guide to children's eyes,* New York, 1985, Grune & Stratton.

National Society to Prevent Blindness: *Guide to testing distance visual acuity,* Schaumburg, IL, 1988, The Society.

Park JK, Guntheroth WG: Accurate blood pressure measurement in children, *Am J Noninvas Cardiol* 3:297-309, 1989.

Park M, Lee D, Johnson GA: Oscillometric blood pressures in the arm, thigh, and calf in healthy children and those with aortic coarctation, *Pediatrics* 91(4):761-765, 1993.

Pontious S and others: Accuracy and reliability of temperature measurement in the emergency department by instrument and site in children, *Pediatr Nurs* 20(1):58-63, 1994a.

Pontious S and others: Accuracy and reliability of temperature measurement by instrument and site, *J Pediatr Nurs* 9(2):114-123, 1994b.

Report of the Second Task Force on blood pressure control in children—1987, *Pediatrics* 79(1):1-25, 1987.

Sato-Viacrucis K: The evolution of the Snellen E to the Blackbird, *School Nurse,* pp 18-19, Spring 1985.

Seidel HM, Rosenstein BJ, Pathak A: *Care of the full term newborn,* St Louis, 1993, Mosby.

Terndrup TE, Rajk J: Impact of operator technique and device on infrared emission detection tympanic thermometry, *J Emerg Med* 10:683-687, 1992.

Vessey J, Braithwaite K, Wiedmann M: Teaching children about their internal bodies, *Pediatr Nurs* 16(1):29-33, 1990.

Weiss ME, Poeltler D, Gocka I: Infrared tympanic thermometry for neonatal temperature assessment, *JOGNN* 23(9):798-804, 1993.

BIBLIOGRAPHY

Physical Assessment

Barber N, Kilmon C: Reactions to tympanic temperature measurement in an ambulatory setting, *Pediatr Nurs* 15(5):477-481, 1989.

Barness LA: *Manual of pediatric physical diagnosis,* ed 6, St Louis, 1991, Mosby.

Beach PS, McCormick DP: Editorial comment: clinical applications of ear thermometry, *Clin Pediatr* 30(4, suppl):3-4, 1991.

Betts PR, Voss LD, Bailey BJR: Measuring the heights of very young children, *Br Med J* 304:1351-1352, 1992.

Bowers A, Thompson J: *Clinical manual of health assessment,* ed 4, St Louis, 1992, Mosby.

Church JL, Baer KJ: Examination of the adolescent: a practical guide, *J Pediatr Health Care* 1(2):65-72, 1987.

Combs JT: Two useful tools for exploring the middle ear, *Contemp Pediatr* 10(11):60-75, 1993.

Crouch ER Jr, Crouch ER: Pediatric vision screening: Why? When? What? How? *Contemp Pediatr* 8:9-30, 1991.

Cunningham DR: Auditory screening. In Hoekelman RA and others, editors: *Primary pediatric care,* ed 2, St Louis, 1992, Mosby.

Davis K: The accuracy of tympanic temperature measurement in children, *Pediatr Nurs* 19(3):267-272, 1993.

Donham J: Rales and rhonchi: why do we use these terms? *Focus Crit Care* 11(5):20-22, 1984.

Erickson RS and others: Accuracy of infrared ear thermometry and traditional temperature methods in young children, *Heart Lung* 23(3):181-195, 1994.

Gemberling C: The adolescent gynecologic examination: an overview, *J Pediatr Health Care* 1(3):141-151, 1987.

Greene J: Making adolescent space in a pediatric office, *Pediatr Nurs* 15(4):402-404, 1989.

Gundy JH: The pediatric physical examination. In Hoekelman RA and others, editors: *Primary pediatric care,* ed 2, St Louis, 1992, Mosby.

Haddock BJ, Merrow DL, Swanson MS: The falling grace of axillary temperatures, *Pediatr Nurs* 22(2):121-125, 1996.

Henry JJ: Routine growth monitoring and assessment of growth disorders, *J Pediatr Health Care* 6(5):291-301, 1992.

Hinton A, Moore-Gillon V: Recent advances: otorhinolaryngology, *Br Med J* 309:651-654, 1994.

Johnson A, Stayte M, Wortham C: Vision screening at 8 and 18 months, *Br Med J* 299:545-549, 1989.

Killam P: Orthopedic assessment of young children: developmental variations, *Nurse Pract* 14(7):27-28, 1989.

Kronmiller J: Oral soft tissue abnormalities in children, *Pediatr Nurs* 13(3):161-165, 1987.

Lieber MT, Taub AS: Common foot deformities and what they mean for parents, *MCN* 13(1):47-50, 1988.

Linley JF: Screening children for common orthopedic problems, *Am J Nurs* 87(10):1312-1316, 1987.

Martyn K and others: Comparison of axillary, rectal and skinbased temperature assessment in preschoolers, *Nurse Pract* 13(4):31-36, 1988.

Mason KJ: Pediatric orthopaedics: developmental norms, *Orthop Nurs* 8(4):45-50, 1989.

Neinstein L and others: Comfort of male adolescents during general and genital examination, *J Pediatr* 115(3):494-497, 1989.

Olk D: Quieting the disruptive sibling, *Contemp Pediatr* 6(10):116, 1989.

Orlando M, Frank T: Audiometer and audioscope hearing screening compared with threshold test in young children, *J Pediatr* 110(2):261-263, 1987.

Pandit JC: Testing acuity of vision in general practice: reaching recommended standard, *Br Med J* 309(6966):1408, 1994.

Petersen-Smith A and others: Comparison of aural infrared with traditional rectal temperatures in children from birth to age three years, *J Pediatr* 125(1):83-85, 1994.

Phillips S, Bohannon W, Heald F: Teenagers' choices regarding the presence of family members during the examination of genitalia, *J Adolesc Health Care* 4(4):245-249, 1986.

Pickering TG: Blood pressure measurement and detection of hypertension, *Lancet* 344(8914):31-35, 1994.

Pinyerd BJ: Assessment of infant growth, *J Pediatr Health Care* 6(5):302-308, 1994.

Roche A, Guo S, Moore W: Weight and recumbent length from 1 to 12 mo of age: reference data for 1-mo increments, *Am J Clin Nutr* 49:599-607, 1989.

Roche A and others: Head circumference reference data: birth to 18 years, *Pediatrics* 79:(5):706-712, 1987.

Sanet R, Ellis G: What is the most effective vision screening tool to use with preschool-age children in early childhood programs? *School Nurse* 6:27-31, 1990.

Schubiner H: Preventive health screening in adolescent patients, *Prim Care* 16(1):211-230, 1989.

Schuman AJ: Taking the pain—and fear—out of office visits, *Contemp Pediatr* 8(4):81-87, 1991.

Seidel H and others: *Mosby's guide to physical examination,* ed 3, St Louis, 1995, Mosby.

Stata K: Improving hearing screening programs in the elementary school, *School Nurse* 4(3):16-19, 1988.

Strahlman ER: Vision screening. In Hoekelman RA and others, editors: *Primary pediatric care,* ed 3, St Louis, 1997, Mosby.

Sullivan L: How effective is preschool vision, hearing, and developmental screening? *Pediatr Nurs* 14(3):181-183, 1988.

Tolmas HC: Adolescent pelvic examination: an effective practical approach, *Am J Dis Child* 145(11):1269-1284, 1991.

Tsesis VA: Creating the virtual office, *Contemp Pediatr* 12(2):103-109, 1995.

Unti SM: The critical first year: history, physical examination, and general developmental assessment, *Pediatr Clin North Am* 41(5):859-873, 1994.

Wasserman RC: Screening for vision problems in pediatric practice, *Pediatr Rev* 13(1):4-5, 1992.

Wells N and others: Does tympanic temperature measure up? *MCN* 20(2):95-100, 1995.

Wong DL: The paper-doll technique, *Pediatr Nurs* 7(6):39-40, 1981.

Wong DL: From sites to sensors: taking infants' temperatures, *Am J Nurs* 89(3):321, 1989.

Developmental Assessment

Adesman AR: Is the Denver II Developmental Test worthwhile? *Pediatrics* 90(6):1009-1010, 1992 (letter to the editor).

Allen MC, Alexander GR: Gross motor milestones in preterm infants: correction for degree of prematurity, *J Pediatr* 116(6):955-959, 1990.

Casey PH, Swanson M: A pediatric perspective of developmental screening in 1993, *Clin Pediatr* 32(4):209-212, 1993.

Casey PH and others: Developmental intervention: a pediatric clinical review, *Pediatr Clin North Am* 33(4):899-923, 1986.

Dworkin P: British and American recommendations for developmental monitoring: the role of surveillance, *Pediatrics* 84(6):1000-1010, 1989.

Dworkin P: Developmental screening—expecting the impossible? *Pediatrics* 83(4):619-621, 1989.

Finney JW, Weist MD: Behavioral assessment of children and adolescents, *Pediatr Clin North Am* 39(3):369-378, 1992.

First LR, Palfrey JS: The infant or young child with developmental delay, *N Engl J Med* 330(7):478-483, 1994.

Frankenburg W: Does Denver II produce meaningful results? *Pediatrics* 90(3):478-479, 1992 (reply to the editor).

Frankenburg WK, Chen J, Thornton S: Common pitfalls in the evaluation of developmental screening tests, *J Pediatr* 113(5):1110-1113, 1988.

Frankenburg WK, Thornton S: A child development program for a busy office practice, *Contemp Pediatr* 6(2):90-106, 1989.

Glascoe F, Byrne K: Is the Denver II Developmental Test worthwhile? *Pediatrics* 90(6):1010-1011, 1992 (reply to the editor).

Meisels SJ: Can developmental screening tests identify children who are developmentally at risk? *Pediatrics* 83(4): 578-585, 1989.

Ouden LD and others: Is it correct to correct? Developmental milestones in 555 "normal" preterm infants compared with term infants, *J Pediatr* 118(3):399-404, 1991.

Squires JK, Nickel R, Bricker D: Use of parent-completed developmental questionnaires for child-find and screening, *Infants Young Child* 3(2):46-57, 1990.

Steele SM: Assessing developmental delays in preschool children, *J Pediatr Health Care* 2(3):141-145, 1988.

Wade GH: Update on the Denver II, *Pediatr Nurs* 18(2):140-141, 1992.

Chapter 8

HEALTH PROMOTION OF THE NEWBORN AND FAMILY

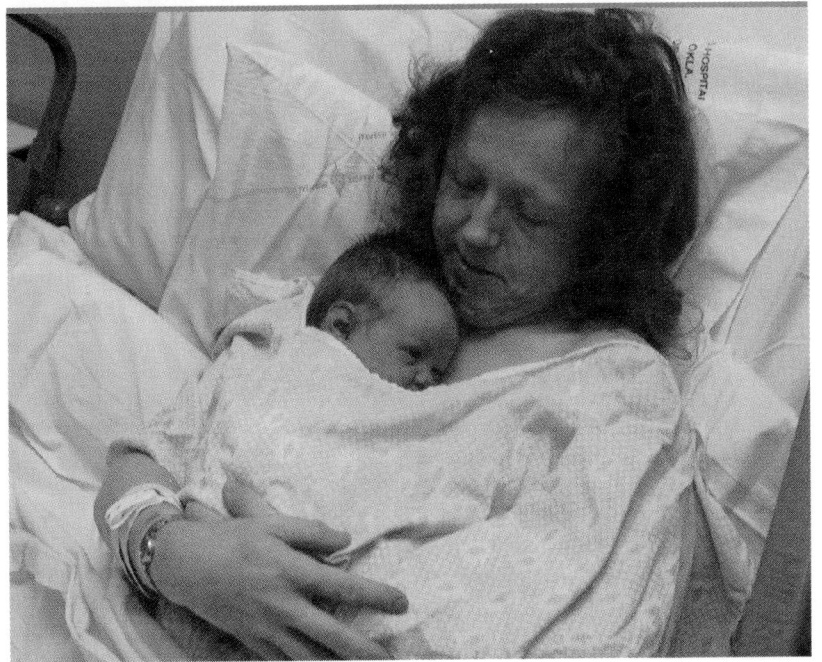

" *The [kangaroo care] is great! Look how he calmed down. Maybe this would have helped with my son who had colic.* "

Cheryl, mother of newborn Alexander

RELATED TOPICS

LEARNING OBJECTIVES
On completion of this chapter the reader will be able to:

- Identify the principal cardiorespiratory changes that occur during transition to extrauterine life
- Identify the immature physiologic functioning of each

body system and its significance to nursing care of the newborn
- Perform an initial and transitional assessment of the newborn based on the Apgar score and periods of reactivity

- Perform a newborn physical assessment based on recognition of expected normal findings
- Outline a nursing care plan for the newborn in the nursery
- Assess and promote parent-infant attachment behaviors

ADJUSTMENT TO EXTRAUTERINE LIFE

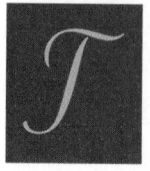he most profound physiologic change required of the neonate is transition from fetal or placental circulation to independent respiration. The loss of the placental connection means the loss of complete metabolic support, especially the supply of oxygen and the removal of carbon dioxide. The normal stresses of labor and delivery produce alterations of placental gas exchange patterns, acid-base balance in the blood, and cardiovascular activity in the infant. Factors that interfere with this normal transition or that increase fetal *asphyxia* (a condition of hypoxemia, hypercapnia, and acidosis) will affect the fetus's adjustment to extrauterine life.

IMMEDIATE ADJUSTMENTS

Respiratory System

The most critical and immediate physiologic change required of the newborn is the onset of breathing. The stimuli that help initiate the first respiration are primarily chemical and thermal. *Chemical factors* in the blood (low oxygen, high carbon dioxide, and low pH) initiate impulses that excite the respiratory center in the medulla. The primary *thermal stimulus* is the sudden chilling of the infant who leaves a warm environment and enters a relatively cooler atmosphere. This abrupt change in temperature excites sensory impulses in the skin that are transmitted to the respiratory center.

The significance of *tactile stimulation* is questionable. Probably descent through the birth canal and normal handling during delivery have some effect on initiation of respiration. Slapping the infant's feet or buttocks has no beneficial effect. However, it can waste precious time in the event of respiratory difficulty and can cause additional damage if cerebral trauma has occurred.

The initial entry of air into the lungs is opposed by the surface tension of the fluid that filled the fetal lungs and the alveoli. However, fetal lung fluid is removed by the lymphatic vessels and pulmonary capillaries. Some fluid is also removed during the normal forces of labor and delivery. As the chest emerges from the birth canal, fluid is squeezed from the lungs through the nose and mouth. Following complete delivery of the chest, a brisk recoil of the thorax occurs. Air enters the upper airway to replace the lost fluid. In cesarean birth the chest is not compressed and the newborn may need additional respiratory support.

In the alveoli the surface tension of the fluid is reduced by *surfactant,* a substance produced by the alveolar epithelium that coats the alveolar surface. The effect of surfactant in facilitating breathing is discussed in relation to respiratory distress syndrome (see Chapter 9).

Circulatory System

Equally important as the initiation of respiration are the circulatory changes that allow blood to flow through the lungs. These changes, which occur more gradually, are the result of pressure changes in the lungs, heart, and major vessels. The transition from fetal circulation to postnatal circulation involves the functional closure of the fetal shunts: the foramen ovale, the ductus arteriosus, and eventually the ductus venosus. (For a review of fetal circulation, see Chapter 25.)

Once the lungs are expanded, the inspired oxygen dilates the pulmonary vessels, which decreases pulmonary vascular resistance and consequently increases pulmonary blood flow. As the lungs receive blood, the pressure in the right atrium, right ventricle, and pulmonary arteries decreases. At the same time there is a progressive rise in systemic vascular resistance from the increased volume of blood through the placenta at cord clamping. This increases the pressure in the left side of the heart. Because blood flows from an area of high pressure to one of low pressure, the circulation of blood through the fetal shunts is reversed.

The most important factor controlling ductal closure is the increased oxygen concentration of the blood. Secondary factors are the fall in endogenous prostaglandins and acidosis. The foramen ovale closes functionally at or soon after birth. The ductus arteriosus is closed functionally by the fourth day. Anatomic closure takes considerably longer. Failure of the ducts to close results in congenital heart defects (see Chapter 25).

Because of the reversible flow of blood through the ducts during the early neonatal period, functional murmurs are occasionally heard. In conditions such as crying or straining, the increased pressure shunts unoxygenated blood from the right side of the heart across the ductal opening, causing transient cyanosis.

PHYSIOLOGIC STATUS OF OTHER SYSTEMS

Thermoregulation

Next to establishing respiration, heat regulation is most critical to the newborn's survival. Although the newborn's ca-

---

David Wilson, MS, RNC, revised this chapter.

pacity for heat production is adequate, several factors predispose the newborn to excessive heat loss:

1. The newborn's large surface area facilitates heat loss to the environment, although this is partially compensated for by the newborn's usual position of flexion, which decreases the amount of surface area exposed to the environment.
2. The newborn's thin layer of subcutaneous fat provides poor insulation for conservation of heat.
3. The newborn's mechanism for producing heat is different from that of the adult, who can increase heat production through shivering. The chilled neonate cannot shiver but produces heat through *nonshivering thermogenesis,* which involves increased metabolism and oxygen consumption.

The principal thermogenic sources are the heart, liver, and brain. However, there is an additional source unique to the newborn known as *brown adipose tissue (BAT),* or *brown fat.* Brown fat, which owes its name to its larger content of mitochondrial cytochromes, has a greater capacity for heat production through intensified metabolic activity than does ordinary adipose tissue. Heat generated in brown fat is distributed to other parts of the body by the blood, which is warmed as it flows through the layers of this tissue. Superficial deposits of brown fat are located between the scapulae, around the neck, in the axillae, and behind the sternum. Deeper layers surround the kidneys, trachea, esophagus, some major arteries, and adrenals. The location of brown fat may explain why the nape of the neck often feels warmer than the rest of the infant's body.

Although newborns' ability to conserve heat is usually a matter of concern, they also can have difficulty dissipating heat in an overheated environment, which increases the risk of hyperthermia.

Hemopoietic System

The *blood volume* of the newborn depends on the amount of placental transfer of blood. The blood volume of the full-term infant is about 80 to 85 ml/kg of body weight. Immediately after birth the total blood volume averages 300 ml, but depending on how long the infant is attached to the placenta, as much as 100 ml can be added to the blood volume. Blood values for the newborn are listed in Appendix E.

Fluid and Electrolyte Balance

Changes occur in the *total body water volume,* extracellular fluid volume, and intracellular fluid volume during the transition from fetal to postnatal life. At birth the total weight of the infant is 73% fluid, as compared with 58% in the adult. The infant has a proportionately higher ratio of extracellular fluid than the adult and consequently has a higher level of total body sodium and chloride and a lower level of potassium, magnesium, and phosphate.

A very important aspect of fluid balance is its relationship to other systems. Besides the rate of fluid exchange being seven times greater in the infant than in the adult, the infant's *rate of metabolism* is twice as great in relation to body weight. As a result twice as much acid is formed, leading to more rapid development of acidosis. In addition the immature kidneys cannot sufficiently concentrate urine to conserve body water. These three factors make the infant more prone to problems of dehydration, acidosis, and possible overhydration.

Gastrointestinal System

The ability of the newborn to digest, absorb, and metabolize foodstuff is adequate but limited in certain functions. Enzymes are adequate to handle the proteins and simple carbohydrates (monosaccharides and disaccharides), but deficient production of pancreatic amylase impairs utilization of complex carbohydrates (polysaccharides). Deficiency of pancreatic lipase limits absorption of fats, especially with ingestion of foods with high saturated fatty acid content, such as cow's milk.

The liver is the most immature of the gastrointestinal organs. The activity of the enzyme *glucuronyl transferase* is reduced, which affects the conjugation of bilirubin with glucuronic acid and contributes to the physiologic jaundice of the newborn. The liver is also deficient in forming plasma proteins. The decreased plasma protein concentration probably plays a role in the edema usually seen at birth. Prothrombin and other coagulation factors are also low. The liver stores less glycogen at birth than later in life. Consequently the newborn is prone to hypoglycemia, which may be prevented by early and effective feeding, especially breast-feeding.

Some salivary glands are functioning at birth, but the majority do not begin to secrete saliva until about the age of 2 to 3 months, when drooling is frequent. Stomach capacity is limited to about 90 ml; thus the infant requires frequent small feedings. The colon also has a small volume; the newborn may have a bowel movement after each feeding. Because newborns who breast-feed have more frequent feedings, they may have more frequent stools than infants who bottle-feed. However, the pattern may change after the first few weeks.

The infant's intestine is longer in relation to body size than that in the adult. Therefore there are a larger number of secretory glands and a larger surface area for absorption as compared with the adult's intestine. There are rapid peristaltic waves and simultaneous nonperistaltic waves along the entire esophagus. These waves, combined with an immature relaxed cardiac sphincter, make regurgitation a common occurrence. Progressive changes in the stooling pattern indicate a properly functioning gastrointestinal tract (see box).

CHANGE IN STOOLING PATTERNS OF NEWBORNS

Meconium

Infant's first stool; composed of amniotic fluid and its constituents, intestinal secretions, shed mucosal cells, and possibly blood (ingested maternal blood or minor bleeding of alimentary tract vessels).

Passage of meconium should occur within the first 24 to 48 hours, although it may be delayed up to 7 days in very-low-birth-weight infants (Verma and Dhanireddy, 1993).

Transitional Stools

Usually appear by third day after initiation of feeding; greenish brown to yellowish brown, thin, and less sticky than meconium; may contain some milk curds.

Milk Stool

Usually appears by fourth day.

In *breast-fed infants* stools are yellow to golden, are pasty in consistency, and have an odor similar to that of sour milk.

In *formula-fed infants* stools are pale yellow to light brown, are firmer in consistency, and have a more offensive odor.

Renal System

All structural components are present in the renal system, but there is a functional deficiency in the kidney's ability to concentrate urine and to cope with conditions of fluid and electrolyte stress, such as dehydration or a concentrated solute load.

Total volume of urine per 24 hours is about 200 to 300 ml by the end of the first week. However, the bladder voluntarily empties when stretched by a volume of 15 ml, resulting in as many as 20 voidings per day. The first voiding should occur within 24 hours. The urine is colorless and odorless and has a specific gravity of about 1.020.

Integumentary System

At birth all the structures within the skin are present, but many of the functions of the integument are immature. The two layers of the skin, the epidermis and dermis, are loosely bound to each other and are very thin. Slight friction across the epidermis, such as from rapid removal of adhesive tape, can cause separation of these layers and blister formation. The transitional zone between the cornified and living layers of the epidermis is effective in preventing fluid from reaching the skin surface.

The *sebaceous glands* are very active late in fetal life and in early infancy because of the high levels of maternal androgens. They are most densely located on the scalp, face, and genitalia and produce the greasy vernix caseosa that covers the infant at birth. Plugging of the sebaceous glands causes milia.

The *eccrine glands,* which produce sweat in response to heat or emotional stimuli, are functional at birth, and palmar sweating on crying reaches levels equivalent to those of anxious adults by 43 weeks of gestation. Observing palmar sweating is helpful in assessing pain. The eccrine glands produce sweat in response to higher temperatures than those required in adults, and the retention of sweat may result in miliaria. The *apocrine glands* remain small and nonfunctional until puberty.

The growth phases of hair follicles usually occur simultaneously at birth. During the first few months the synchrony between hair loss and regrowth is disrupted, and there may be overgrowth of hair or temporary alopecia. Boys' hair grows faster than girls' hair, and in both sexes scalp hair growth is slower at the crown.

Because the amount of *melanin* is low at birth, newborns are lighter skinned than they will be as children. Consequently they are more susceptible to the harmful effects of the sun.

Musculoskeletal System

At birth the *skeletal system* contains larger amounts of cartilage than of ossified bone, although the process of ossification is fairly rapid during the first year. The nose, for example, is predominantly cartilage at birth and is frequently flattened by the force of delivery. The six skull bones are relatively soft and are separated only by membranous seams. The sinuses are incompletely formed in the newborn.

Unlike the skeletal system, the *muscular system* is almost completely formed at birth. Growth in size of muscular tissue is caused by hypertrophy, rather than hyperplasia, of cells.

Defenses Against Infection

The infant is born with several defenses against infection. The first line of defense is the *skin* and *mucous membranes,* which protect the body from invading organisms. The second line of defense is the *cellular elements* of the immunologic system, which produce several types of cells capable of attacking a pathogen. The *neutrophils* and *monocytes* are phagocytes, which means they can engulf, ingest, and destroy foreign agents. *Eosinophils* also probably have a phagocytic property, since they increase in number in the presence of foreign protein. The *lymphocytes* (T- and B-cells) are capable of being converted to other cell types, such as monocytes and antibodies. Although the phagocytic properties of the blood are present in the infant, the inflammatory response of the tissues to localize an infection is immature.

The third line of defense is the formation of specific *antibodies* to an antigen. Exposure to various foreign agents is necessary for antibody production to occur. Infants are generally not capable of producing their own immunoglobulins (Ig) until the beginning of the second month of life, but they receive considerable passive immunity in the form of IgG from the maternal circulation and from human milk (see p. 208). They are protected against most major childhood diseases, including diphtheria, measles, poliomyelitis, infectious hepatitis, and rubella for about 3 months, provided the mother has developed antibodies to these illnesses.

Endocrine System

Ordinarily the endocrine system of the newborn is adequately developed, but its functions are immature. For example, the posterior lobe of the pituitary gland produces limited quantities of *antidiuretic hormone (ADH),* or *vasopressin,* which inhibits diuresis. This renders the young infant highly susceptible to dehydration.

The effect of maternal *sex hormones* is particularly evident in the newborn. The labia are hypertrophied, and the breasts may be engorged and secrete milk (witch's milk) from the first few days of life to as long as 2 months of age. Female newborns may have *pseudomenstruation* (more often seen as a milky secretion than actual blood) from a sudden drop in progesterone and estrogen levels.

Neurologic System

At birth the nervous system is incompletely integrated but sufficiently developed to sustain extrauterine life. Most neurologic functions are *primitive reflexes*. The *autonomic nervous system* is crucial during transition, because it stimulates initial respirations, helps maintain acid-base balance, and partially regulates temperature control.

Myelination of the nervous system follows the cephalocaudal-proximodistal (head-to-toe—center-to-periphery) laws of development and is closely related to observed mastery of fine and gross motor skills. *Myelin* is necessary for rapid and efficient transmission of some, but not all, nerve impulses along the neural pathway. The tracts that develop myelin earliest are the sensory, cerebellar, and extrapyramidal tracts. This accounts for the acute senses of taste, smell, and hearing in the newborn, as well as the perception of pain. All *cranial nerves* are present and myelinated except for the optic and olfactory nerves.

Sensory Functions

The newborn's sensory functions are remarkably well developed and have a significant effect on growth and development, including the attachment process.

Vision. At birth the eye is structurally incomplete. The *fovea centralis* is not yet completely differentiated from the macula. The *ciliary muscles* are also immature, limiting the ability of the eyes to accommodate and focus on an object for any length of time. The infant can track and follow objects. The *pupils* react to light, the blink reflex is responsive to a minimal stimulus, and the corneal reflex is activated by a light touch. *Tear glands* usually do not begin to function until 2 to 4 weeks of age.

The newborn has the ability to focus momentarily on a bright or moving object that is within 20 cm (8 inches) and in the midline of the visual field. In fact, the infant's ability to fixate on coordinated movement is greater during the first hour of life than during the succeeding several days. Visual acuity is reported to be between 20/100 and 20/400, depending on the vision measurement techniques.

The infant also demonstrates visual preferences: medium colors (yellow, green, pink) over bright (red, orange, blue) or dim colors; black-and-white contrasting patterns, especially geometric shapes and checkerboards; large objects with medium complexity rather than small, complex objects; and reflecting objects over dull ones.

Hearing. Once the amniotic fluid has drained from the ears, the infant probably has *auditory acuity* similar to that of an adult. The neonate reacts to a loud sound of about 90 decibels with a startle reflex. The newborn's response to sounds of low frequency versus those of high frequency differs; the former, such as the sound of a heartbeat, metronome, or lullaby, tends to decrease an infant's motor activity and crying, whereas the latter elicits an alerting reaction. There is also an early sensitivity to the sound of human voices, although not specifically speech sounds. For example, infants younger than 3 days of age can discriminate the mother's voice from that of other females. As early as age 2 weeks the infant may stop crying to listen to the sound of a voice.

The internal and middle *ear* are large at birth, but the external canal is small. The mastoid process and the bony part of the external canal have not yet developed. Consequently the tympanic membrane and facial nerve are very close to the surface and can be easily damaged.

Smell. Newborns react to strong odors such as alcohol or vinegar by turning their heads away. Breast-fed infants are able to smell breast milk and will cry for their mothers when the breasts are engorged and leaking. Infants are also able to differentiate the breast milk of their mother from the breast milk of other women by smell. Maternal odors are believed to influence the attachment process and successful breast-feeding.

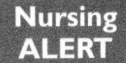

Nursing ALERT Unnecessary routine washing of the breast may interfere with establishment of early breast-feeding (Varendi, Porter, and Winberg, 1994).

Taste. The newborn has the ability to distinguish between tastes. Various types of solutions elicit differing gustofacial reflexes. A tasteless solution elicits no facial expression; a sweet solution elicits an eager suck and a look of satisfaction; a sour solution causes the usual puckering of the lips; and a bitter liquid produces an angry, upset expression. Newborns prefer glucose and water to sterile water. During early childhood the taste buds are distributed mostly on the tip of the tongue.

Touch. At birth the infant is able to perceive tactile sensation in any part of the body, although the face (especially the mouth), hands, and soles of the feet seem to be most sensitive. There is increasing documentation that touch and motion are essential to normal growth and development. Gentle patting of the back or rubbing of the abdomen usually elicits a calming response from the infant. However, painful stimuli, such as a pinprick, will elicit an angry, upsetting response.

NURSING CARE OF THE NEWBORN AND FAMILY

❖ Assessment

The newborn requires thorough, skilled observation to ensure a satisfactory adjustment to extrauterine life. Physical assessment following delivery can be divided into four phases: (1) the initial assessment using the Apgar scoring system, (2) transitional assessment during the periods of reactivity, (3) assessment of gestational age, and (4) periodic assessment through systematic physical examination. In addition, the nurse must be aware of those behaviors that signal successful attachment between the infant and parents. Awareness of the expected normal findings during each assessment process helps the nurse recognize any deviation that may prevent the infant from progressing uneventfully through the early postnatal period. With increasingly shorter labor, delivery, recovery, and postpartum admission, the accomplishment of thorough newborn assessment and parent teaching has become a challenge.

TABLE 8-1. Infant evaluation at birth—Apgar Scoring System

SIGN	0	1	2
Heart rate	Absent	Slow, <100	>100
Respiratory effort	Absent	Irregular, slow	Good, strong cry
Muscle tone	Limp	Some flexion of extremities	Well flexed
Reflex irritability	No response	Grimace	Cry, sneeze
Color	Blue, pale	Body pink, extremities blue	Completely pink

Initial Assessment: Apgar Scoring

The most frequently used method to assess the newborn's immediate adjustment to extrauterine life is the ***Apgar scoring system.*** The score is based on observation of heart rate, respiratory effort, muscle tone, reflex irritability, and color (Table 8-1). Each item is given a score of 0, 1, or 2. Evaluations of all five categories are made at 1 and 5 minutes after birth and are repeated until the infant's condition stabilizes. Total scores of 0 to 3 represent severe distress, scores of 4 to 6 signify moderate difficulty, and scores of 7 to 10 indicate absence of difficulty in adjusting to extrauterine life. The Apgar score is affected by the degree of prematurity, maternal sedation or analgesia, and neuromuscular disorders.

The Apgar score reflects the general condition of the infant at 1 and 5 minutes based on the five parameters described above. The Apgar score is not a tool, however, that stands on its own to either interpret past events or predict future events linked to the infant's eventual neurologic or physical status. In addition, the Apgar score is not used to determine the newborn's need for resuscitation at birth (American Academy of Pediatrics, 1990a).

Clinical Assessment of Gestational Age

Assessment of gestational age is an important criterion because perinatal morbidity and mortality are related to gestational age and birth weight. A frequently used method of de-

NEUROMUSCULAR MATURITY

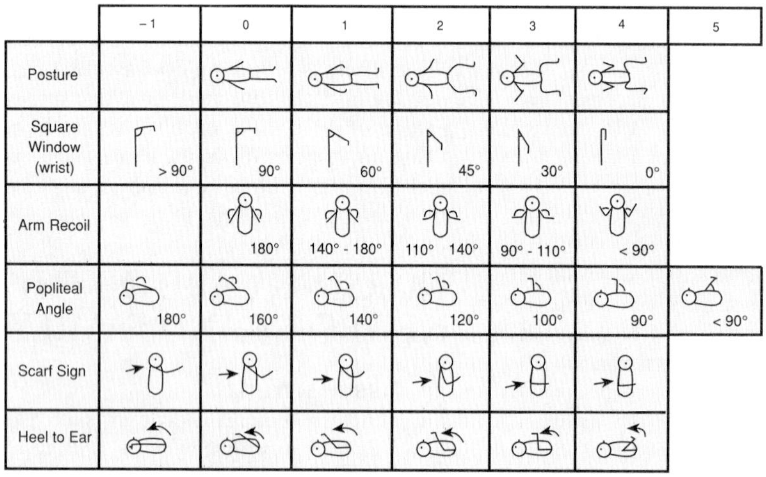

A

PHYSICAL MATURITY

	-1	0	1	2	3	4	5
Skin	sticky friable transparent	gelatinous red, translucent	smooth pink, visible veins	superficial peeling &/or rash, few veins	cracking pale areas rare veins	parchment deep cracking no vessels	leathery cracked wrinkled
Lanugo	none	sparse	abundant	thinning	bald areas	mostly bald	
Plantar Surface	heel-toe 40-50 mm: -1 <40 mm: -2	>50 mm no crease	faint red marks	anterior transverse crease only	creases ant. 2/3	creases over entire sole	
Breast	imperceptible	barely perceptible	flat areola no bud	stippled areola 1-2 mm bud	raised areola 3-4 mm bud	full areola 5-10 mm bud	
Eye/Ear	lids fused loosely: -1 tightly: -2	lids open pinna flat stays folded	sl. curved pinna; soft; slow recoil	well-curved pinna; soft but ready recoil	formed & firm instant recoil	thick cartilage ear stiff	
Genitals (male)	scrotum flat, smooth	scrotum empty faint rugae	testes in upper canal rare rugae	testes descending few rugae	testes down good rugae	testes pendulous deep rugae	
Genitals (female)	clitoris prominent labia flat	prominent clitoris small labia minora	prominent clitoris enlarging minora	majora & minora equally prominent	majora large minora small	majora cover clitoris & minora	

MATURITY RATING

score	weeks
-10	20
-5	22
0	24
5	26
10	28
15	30
20	32
25	34
30	36
35	38
40	40
45	42
50	44

FIG. 8-1. A, New Ballard Scale for newborn maturity rating. Expanded scale includes extremely premature infants and has been refined to improve accuracy in more mature infants. (From Ballard JL and others: New Ballard Score, expanded to include extremely premature infants, *J Pediatr* 119:418, 1991.)

termining gestational age is the simplified *Assessment of Gestational Age* by Ballard, Novack, and Driver (1979) (Fig. 8-1, *A*). The Ballard scale, an abbreviated version of the *Dubowitz scale,* can be used to measure gestational ages of infants between 35 and 42 weeks (Dubowitz and Dubowitz, 1977). It assesses six external physical and six neuromuscular signs. Each sign has a number score, and the cumulative score correlates with a maturity rating of from 26 to 44 weeks of gestation.

The *New Ballard Scale,* a revision of the original scale, can be used with newborns as young as 20 weeks of gestation. The tool has the same physical and neuromuscular sections but includes −1 and −2 scores that reflect signs of extremely premature infants, such as fused eyelids; imperceptible breast tissue; sticky friable transparent skin; no lanugo; and square-window (flexion of wrist) angle of greater than 90 degrees (see Fig. 8-1, *A,* and the description of the tests in the box). The examination of infants with a gestational age

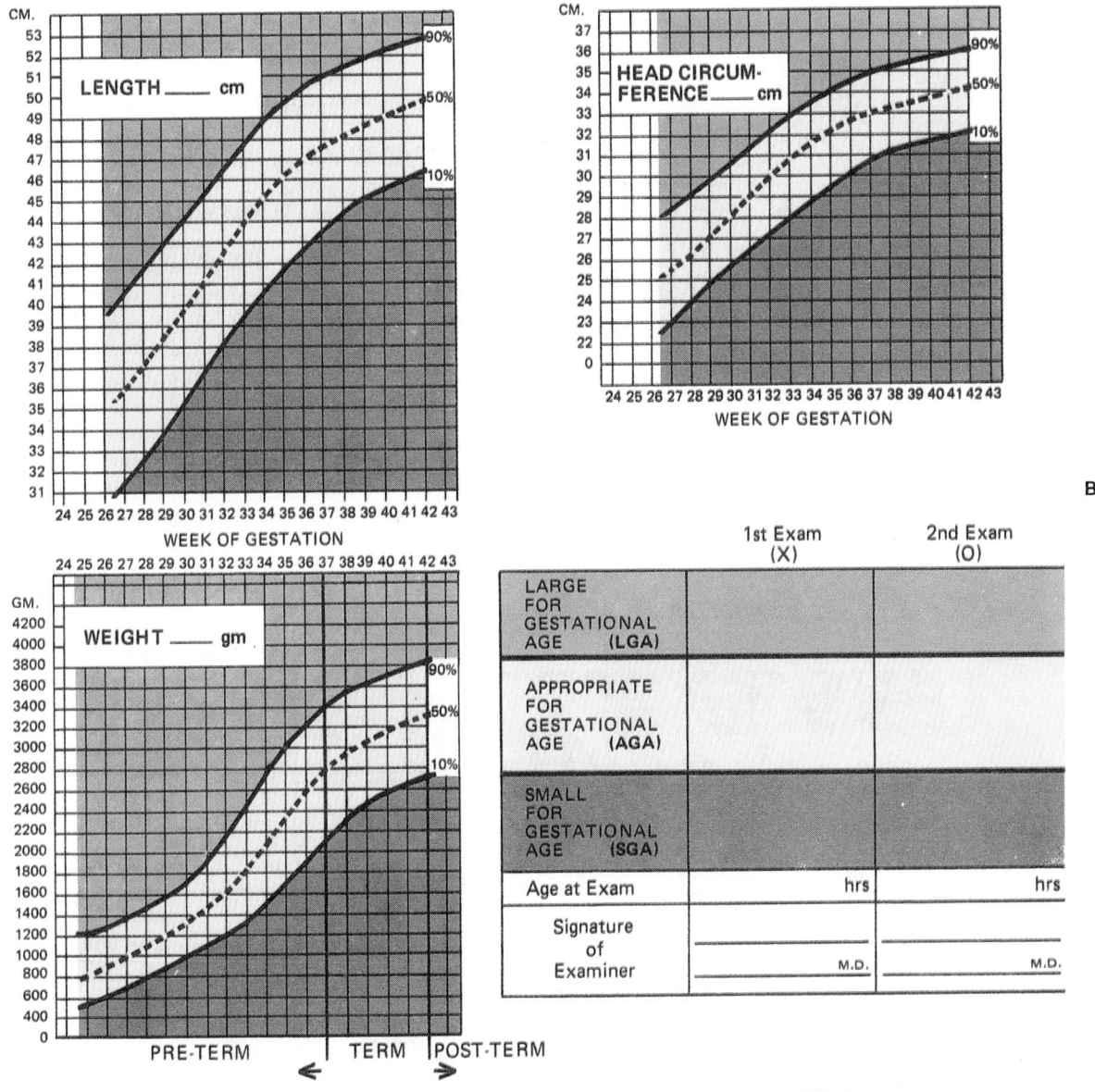

FIG. 8-1, cont'd. B, Newborn classification based on maturity and intrauterine growth. (Modified from Lubchenko LC, Hansman C, Boyd E: Intrauterine growth in length and head circumference as estimated from live births at gestational ages from 26 to 42 weeks, *J Pediatr* 37:403, 1966; Battaglia FC, Lubchenko LD: A practical classification of newborn infants by weight and gestational age, *J Pediatr* 71:159, 1967.)

TESTS USED IN ASSESSING GESTATIONAL AGE

Posture. With infant quiet and in a supine position, observe degree of flexion in arms and legs. Muscle tone and degree of flexion increase with maturity. Full flexion of the arms and legs = 4.

Square window. With thumb supporting back of arm below wrist, apply gentle pressure with index and third fingers on dorsum of hand without rotating infant's wrist. Measure angle between base of thumb and forearm. Full flexion (hand lies flat on ventral surface of forearm) = 4.

Arm recoil. With infant supine, fully flex both forearms on upper arms, hold for 5 seconds; pull down on hands to fully extend and rapidly release arms. Observe rapidity and intensity of recoil to a state of flexion. A brisk return to full flexion = 4.

Popliteal angle. With infant supine and pelvis flat on a firm surface, flex lower leg on thigh and then flex thigh on abdomen. While holding knee with thumb and index finger, extend lower leg with index finger of other hand. Measure degree of angle behind knee (popliteal angle). An angle of less than 90 degrees = 5.

Scarf sign. With infant supine, support head in midline with one hand; use other hand to pull infant's arm across the shoulder so that infant's hand touches shoulder. Determine location of elbow in relation to midline. Elbow does not reach midline = 4.

Heel to ear. With infant supine and pelvis flat on a firm surface, pull foot as far as possible up toward ear on same side. Measure distance of foot from ear and degree of knee flexion (same as popliteal angle). Knees flexed with a popliteal angle of less than 90 degrees = 4.

of 26 weeks or less should be performed at a postnatal age of less than 12 hours. For infants with a gestational age of at least 26 weeks, the examination can be performed up to 96 hours after birth. The scale overestimates gestational age by 2 to 4 days in infants younger than 37 weeks of gestation, especially at gestational ages of 32 to 37 weeks (Ballard and others, 1991).

Weight Related to Gestational Age. The weight of the infant at birth also correlates with the incidence of perinatal morbidity and mortality. Because many infants who weigh less than 2500 g (5½ pounds) are not premature by gestational age, there is often confusion in distinguishing between preterm and small-for-gestational-age infants; fetal growth, gestational age, and fetal maturity are closely related but are not synonymous. Maturity implies functional capacity—the degree to which the neonate's organ systems are able to adapt to the requirements of extrauterine life. Therefore gestational age is more closely related to fetal maturity than is birth weight. Because heredity influences a newborn's size, noting the size of other family members is part of the assessment process.

Classification of infants at birth by both *birthweight* and *gestational age* provides a more satisfactory method for predicting mortality risks and providing guidelines for management of the neonate than estimating gestational age or birth weight alone. The infant's birth weight, length, and head circumference are plotted on standardized graphs that identify normal values for gestational age (Fig. 8-1, *B*). The infant whose weight is *appropriate for gestational age (AGA)* (between 10th and 90th percentile) can be presumed to have grown at a normal rate regardless of the time of birth—preterm, term, or postterm. The infant who is *large for gestational age (LGA)* (above 90th percentile) can be presumed to have grown at an accelerated rate during fetal life; the *small-for-gestational-age (SGA)* infant (below 10th percentile) can be assumed to have grown at a retarded rate during intrauterine life. Fig. 8-2 illustrates the disparity between birth weights of three preterm infants of the same gestational

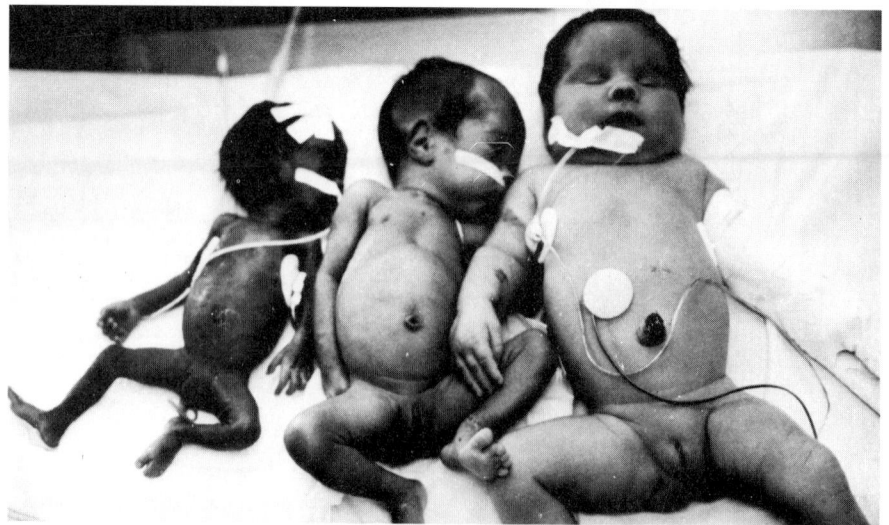

FIG. 8-2. Three infants, same gestational age, weight 600, 1400, and 2750 g, respectively, from left to right. (From Korones SB: *High-risk newborn infants: the basis for intensive nursing care*, ed 4, St Louis, 1986, Mosby.)

age of 32 weeks. The infant with a birth weight of 600 g has over a 50% mortality, the infant weighing 1400 g has a 25% to 50% mortality, and the infant weighing 2750 g has less than a 4% mortality. Therefore birth weight influences mortality—the lower the birth weight and gestational age, the higher the mortality.

General Measurements.   Several important measurements of the newborn have significance when compared with each other as well as when recorded over time on a graph. For the full-term infant, average *head circumference* is between 33 and 35.5 cm (13 to 14 inches). Head circumference may be somewhat less, immediately after birth, because of the molding process that occurs during a normal vaginal delivery. Usually by the second or third day the skull is normal in size and contour.

Chest circumference is 30.5 to 33 cm (12 to 13 inches). Head circumference is usually about 2 to 3 cm (about 1 inch) greater than chest circumference. Because of the molding of the head during delivery, these measurement may initially appear equal.

Head circumference may also be compared with *crown-to-rump* length, or sitting height. Crown-to-rump measurements are usually 31 to 35 cm (12.5 to 14 inches) and are approximately equal to head circumference. The relationship of the head and crown-to-rump measurements is more reliable than that of the head and chest. In a recent study Severn (1994) noted that neonatal head circumference and crown-to-rump length provide a more accurate means for identifying infants at risk; head circumference was shown to be equal to or up to 1 cm more than crown-to-rump length in 62% of the infants examined and determined to be normocephalic.

Head-to-heel length is also measured. Because of the usual flexed position of the infant, it is important to extend the leg completely when measuring total body length. The average length of the newborn is 48 to 53 cm (19 to 21 inches) (Fig. 8-3).

Body weight is taken soon after birth because weight loss occurs fairly rapidly. Normally the neonate loses about 10% of the birth weight by 3 to 4 days of age because of loss of excessive extracellular fluid and meconium, as well as limited food intake, especially in breast-fed infants. The birth weight is usually regained by the tenth day of life. Most newborns weigh 2700 to 4000 g (6 to 9 pounds), the average weight being about 3400 g (7.5 pounds). Accurate birth weights and lengths are important because they provide a baseline for assessment of future growth.

Another category of measurements is vital signs. *Axillary temperatures* are taken because insertion of a thermometer into the rectum can cause perforation of the mucosa (see Fig. 7-7, *B*). Core body temperature varies according to the periods of reactivity but is usually 36.5° to 37.5° C (97.7° to 99.5° F). Skin temperature is slightly lower than core body temperature. Therefore, axillary temperature may be less than rectal temperature, although the difference is small (as little as 0.2° F) between axillary and rectal sites. Because brown adipose tissue is located in the axillary pocket, axillary readings may be elevated whenever nonshivering thermogenesis (NST) occurs. However, axillary readings may be normal in cold-stressed infants where NST is not triggered or is overwhelmed (Bliss-Holtz, 1993).

There is also controversy regarding the accuracy of tympanic membrane sensors for measuring temperature. However, in a comparison of axillary and tympanic membrane temperature measurements in neonates, the use of tempanic membrane readings was helpful in determining the infants' thermal state (Bliss-Holtz, 1993). The accuracy of monitoring term and preterm infants' axillary temperature with one particular electronic thermometer (IVAC 2080) in the predictive mode has also been established (Weiss and Richards, 1994). There is no universal agreement on placement times for glass thermometers, although 3 to 5 minutes is adequate (Bliss-Holtz, 1989; Haddock, Vincent, and Merrow, 1986).

Pulse and *respirations* also vary according to the periods of reactivity and the infant's behaviors but are usually in the range of 120 to 140 beats/min and 30 to 60 breaths/min, respectively. Both are counted for a full 60 seconds to detect irregularities in rate or rhythm. Heart rate is taken apically with a stethoscope.

Measurement of *blood pressure* is recommended; it provides useful baseline data and may indicate cardiac problems. Blood pressure is most easily and accurately assessed using oscillometry (Dinamap), although the device is less reliable when mean arterial pressure is below 40 mm Hg (Chia and others, 1990) (Fig. 8-4). Routine BP measurement on healthy full-term neonates is not recommended because it is a poor predictor of hypertension later in life (American Academy of Pediatrics, 1993a). The average oscillometric systolic/diastolic pressure is 65/41 at 1 to 3 days of age (Park and Menard, 1989). Compare BP in the upper and lower extremities, which should be equal.

| **Nursing ALERT** | Systolic pressure in the calf that is 6 to 9 mm Hg less than systolic pressure in the upper arm is a sign of coarctation of the aorta and is reported for further evaluation (Park and Lee, 1989). |

A suggested schedule for monitoring vital signs is on the newborn's admission to the nursery and then once every 8 hours until discharge (American Academy of Pediatrics and American College of Obstetricians and Gynecologists, 1992).

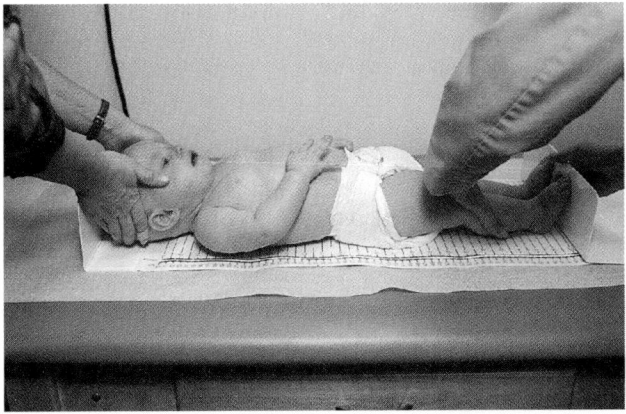

FIG. 8-3. Measurement of infant length.

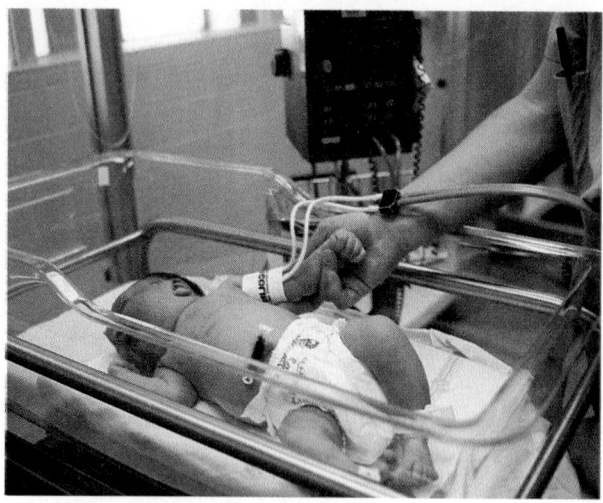

FIG. 8-4. Measurement of blood pressure using oscillometry.

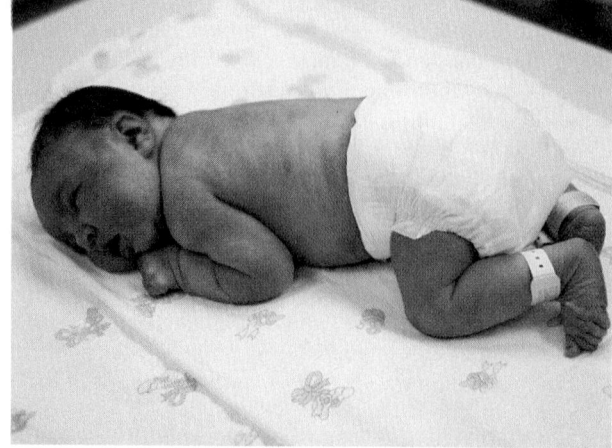

FIG. 8-5. Flexion position of neonate.

However, this schedule may vary according to institutional policy. Any change in the infant, such as in color, muscle tone, or behavior, necessitates more frequent monitoring.

General Appearance. Before each body system is assessed, it is important to describe the general *posture* and behavior of the newborn. The overall appearance yields valuable clues to the physical status of the infant.

In the full-term neonate the posture is one of complete *flexion* as a result of in utero position (Fig. 8-5). Most infants are born in a vertex presentation with the head flexed and the chin resting on the upper chest, the arms flexed with the hands clenched, the legs flexed at the knees and hips, and the feet dorsiflexed. The vertebral column is also flexed. It is important to recognize any deviation from this very characteristic fetal position.

The infant's *behavior* is carefully noted, especially the degree of alertness, drowsiness, and irritability, which are common signs of neurologic problems. Some questions to mentally ask when assessing behavior include the following:

- Is the infant awakened easily by a loud noise?
- Is the infant comforted by rocking, sucking, or cuddling?
- Do there seem to be periods of deep and light sleep?
- When awake, does the infant seem satisfied after a feeding?
- What stimuli elicit responses from the infant?
- When disturbed, how much does the infant protest?

Skin. The *texture* of the newborn's skin is velvety smooth and puffy, especially about the eyes, the legs, the dorsal aspect of the hands and the feet, and the scrotum or labia. Skin *color* depends on racial and familial background and varies greatly among newborns. In general, the white infant is usually pink to red; the black newborn may appear a pinkish or yellowish brown. Infants of Hispanic descent may have an olive tint or a slight yellow cast to the skin. Infants of Oriental descent may be a rosy or yellowish tan. The color of Native American newborns depends on the tribe and can vary from a light pink to a dark, reddish brown. By the second or third day the skin turns to its more natural tone and is drier and flakier. Several other color changes that may be noted on the skin are described later in this chapter, in Table 8-4.

Head. General observation of the *contour* of the head is important, since molding occurs in almost all vaginal deliveries. In a vertex delivery the head is usually flattened at the forehead, with the apex rising and forming a point at the end of the parietal bones and the posterior skull or occiput dropping abruptly. The usual, more oval contour of the head is apparent by 1 to 2 days after birth. The change in shape occurs because the bones of the cranium are not fused, allowing for overlapping of the edges of these bones to accommodate to the size of the birth canal during delivery. Such molding does not occur in infants born by cesarean section.

Six bones—the frontal, occipital, two parietals, and two temporals—make up the cranium. Between the junction of these bones are bands of connective tissue called *sutures.* At the junction of the sutures are wider spaces of unossified membranous tissue called *fontanels.* The two most prominent fontanels in infants are the *anterior fontanel,* formed by the junction of the sagittal, coronal, and frontal sutures, and the *posterior fontanel,* formed by the junction of the sagittal and lambdoid sutures (Fig. 8-6, *A*).

NURSING TIP The location of the suture is easily remembered because the coronal suture "crowns" the head and the sagittal suture "separates" the head.

The skull is palpated for all patent sutures and fontanels, noting size, shape, molding, or abnormal closure. The sutures feel like cracks between the skull bones, and the fontanels feel like wider *soft spots* at the junction of the sutures. These are palpated by using the tip of the index finger and running it along the ends of the bones (Fig. 8-6, *B*).

The anterior fontanel is diamond shaped and measures 4 to 5 cm (about 2 inches) at its widest point (from bone to bone, rather than from suture to suture). The posterior fontanel is easily located by following the sagittal suture toward the occiput. The posterior fontanel is triangular, usually measuring between 0.5 and 1 cm (less than ½ inch) at its widest part. The fontanels should feel flat, firm, and well demarcated against the bony edges of the skull. Frequently pulsations are visible at the anterior fontanel. Coughing, crying, or lying down may temporarily cause the fontanels to bulge and become more taut.

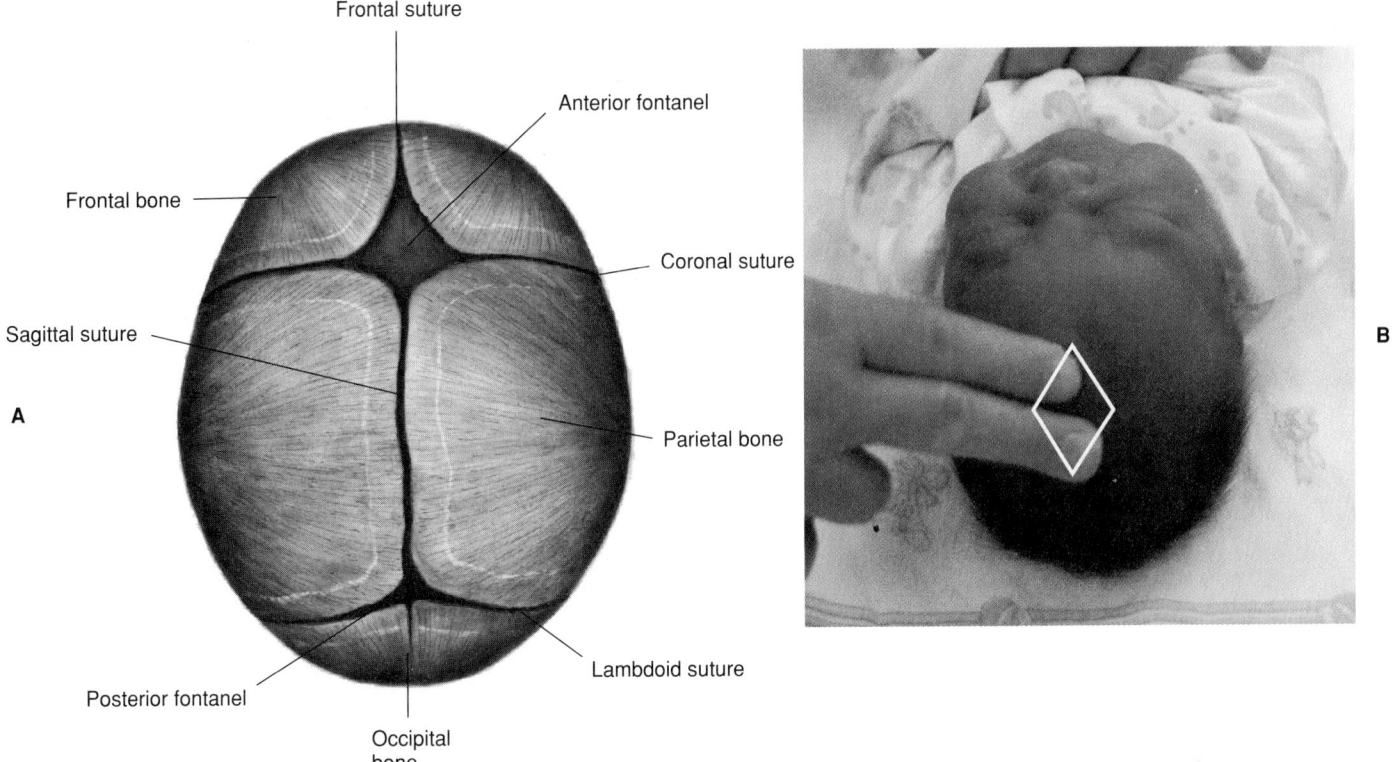

FIG. 8-6. **A,** Location of sutures and fontanels. **B,** Palpating anterior fontanel.

> **Nursing ALERT** Always record and report a widened, tense, bulging fontanel (sign of increased intracranial pressure) and a markedly sunken, depressed fontanel (sign of dehydration).

The degree of **head control** is assessed. Although **head lag** is normal in the newborn, the degree of ability to control the head in certain positions should be recognized. If the supine infant is pulled from the arms into a semi-Fowler position, marked head lag and hyperextension are noted (Fig. 8-7, *A*). However, as the infant is brought forward into a sitting position, the infant will attempt to control the head in an upright position. As the head falls forward onto the chest, many infants will attempt to right it into the erect position. Also, if the infant is held in ventral suspension (i.e., held prone above and parallel to the examining surface), the infant will hold the head in a straight line with the spinal column (Fig. 8-7, *B*). When lying on the abdomen, the newborn has the ability to lift the head slightly, turning it from side to side.

> **Nursing ALERT** Report evidence of excessive head lag and observe for other signs of neurologic deficit.

Eyes. Since newborns tend to have their eyes tightly closed, it is best to begin the examination of the eyes by observing the lids for edema, which is normally present for the first 2 days after delivery. The eyes are observed for symmetry. *Tears* may be present at birth, but purulent discharge from the eyes shortly after birth is abnormal.

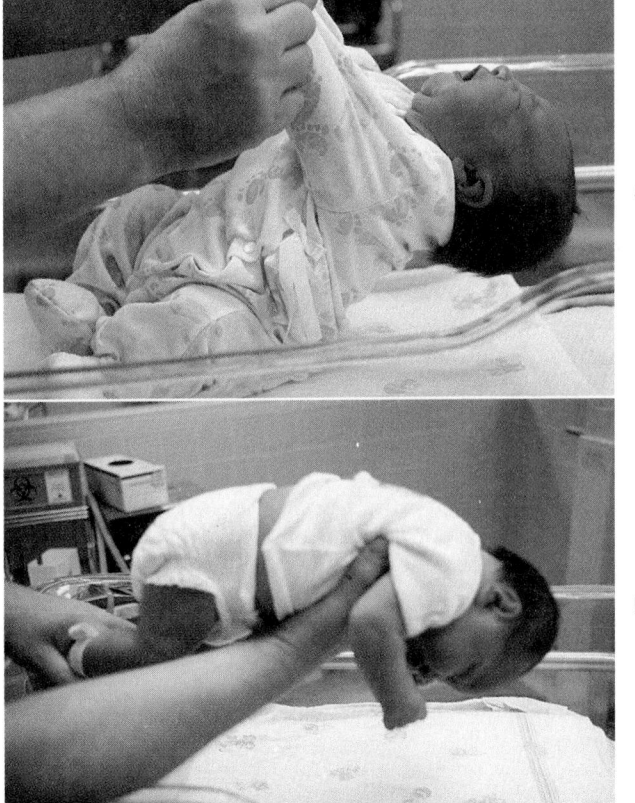

FIG. 8-7. Head control in infant. **A,** Inability to hold head erect when pulled to sitting position. **B,** Ability to hold head erect when placed in ventral suspension.

Nursing ALERT
Report purulent discharge, which may signify **ophthalmia neonatorum** (infectious conjunctivitis of the newborn).

To visualize the surface structures of the eye, the infant is held supine and the head is gently lowered. The eyes will usually open, similar to the mechanism of a doll's eyes. The *sclera* should be white and clear.

The cornea is examined for the presence of any opacities or haziness. The *corneal reflex* is normally present at birth but is generally not elicited unless brain or eye damage is suspected. The pupil will usually respond to light by constricting. The pupils are normally malaligned. A searching *nystagmus* or *strabismus* is common. The color of the iris is noted. Most light-skinned newborns have slate gray or dark blue eyes, whereas dark-skinned infants have brown eyes.

A funduscopic examination is quite difficult to perform because of the infant's tendency to keep the eyes tightly closed. However, a *red reflex* should be elicited.

Nursing ALERT
Always record and report absence of the red reflex. It may indicate the presence of retinal hemorrhages or congenital cataracts.

Ears. The ears are examined for position, structure, and auditory function. The top of the pinna should lie in a horizontal plane to the outer canthus of the eye (see Fig. 7-16). The pinna is often flattened against the side of the head from pressure in utero. An otoscopic examination is ordinarily not performed, because the *canals* are filled with vernix caseosa and amniotic fluid, making visualization of the *tympanic membrane* difficult.

Auditory ability is assessed by making a sharp, loud noise close to the infant's head and noting the presence of the *startle reflex* (see Table 8-2) or twitching of the eyelids. Nurses should be aware of newborns considered at risk for hearing loss so that early testing can be performed (see Hearing Impairment, Chapter 19).

Nursing ALERT
Always report the absence of any behavioral response to a sudden noise, an indication of congenital deafness.

Nose. The nose is usually flattened after birth, and bruises are common. Patency of the *nasal canals* can be assessed by holding the hand over the infant's mouth and one canal and noting the passage of air through the unobstructed opening. If nasal patency is questionable, it is reported, because most newborns are obligatory nose breathers. Sneezing and thin white mucus are common, but a thick, bloody nasal discharge without sneezing may suggest the *snuffles* of congenital syphilis.

Nursing ALERT
Always report flaring of the nares, because it is a serious sign of air hunger from respiratory distress.

Mouth and Throat. An external defect of the mouth, such as cleft lip, is readily apparent; however, the internal structures require careful inspection. The palate is normally highly arched and somewhat narrow. Rarely, teeth may be present. A common finding is **Epstein pearls,** small, white, epithelial cysts along both sides of the midline of the hard palate. They are insignificant and disappear in several weeks.

The *frenulum* of the upper lip is a band of thick, pink tissue that lies under the inner surface of the upper lip and extends to the maxillary alveolar ridge. It is particularly evident when the infant yawns or smiles. It disappears as the maxilla grows.

The *sucking reflex* is elicited by placing a nipple or non-latex gloved finger in the infant's mouth. The infant should exhibit a strong, vigorous suck. The *rooting reflex* is obtained by stroking the cheek and noting the infant's response of turning toward the stimulated side and sucking (Fig. 8-8).

The *uvula* can be inspected while the infant is crying and the chin is depressed. However, it may be retracted upward and backward during crying. Tonsillar tissue is generally not seen in the newborn. *Natal teeth,* teeth present at birth, as opposed to *neonatal teeth,* which erupt during the first month of life), are seen infrequently and erupt chiefly at the position of the lower incisors. They are reported because they are frequently found with developmental abnormalities and syndromes, including cleft lip and palate. Most natal teeth are loosely attached. However, current thinking suggests preserving them until they exfoliate naturally (McDonald and Avery, 1994), unless breast-feeding is impaired from the neonate biting the breast.

Neck. Since the newborn's neck is short and covered with folds of tissue, adequate assessment of the neck requires allowing the head to fall gently backward in hyperextension while the back is supported in a slightly raised position. Observe for range of motion, shape, and any abnormal masses, and palpate and compare each clavicle for possible fractures.

Chest. The *shape* of the newborn's chest is almost cir-

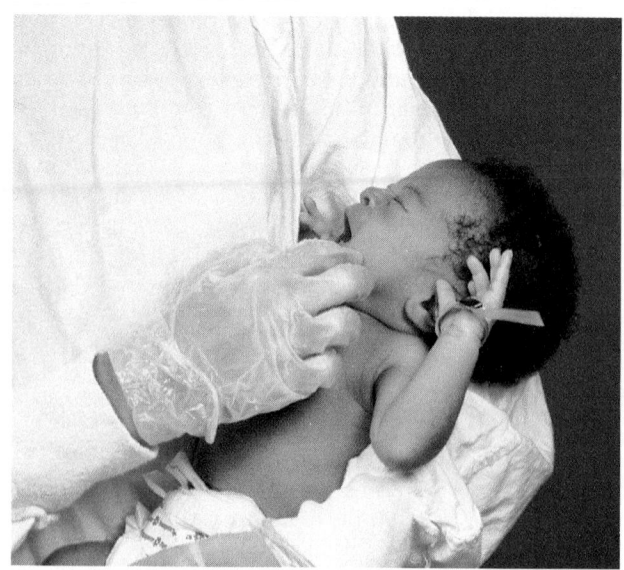

FIG. 8-8. Eliciting rooting reflex. (From Seidel HM and others: *Mosby's guide to physical examination,* ed 3, St Louis, 1995, Mosby.)

cular because the anteroposterior and lateral diameters are equal. The ribs are very flexible, and slight intercostal retractions are normally seen on inspiration. The xiphoid process is commonly visible as a small protrusion at the end of the sternum. The sternum is generally raised and slightly curved.

The breasts are inspected for size, shape, and nipple formation, location, and number. Breast enlargement appears in many newborns of either sex by the second or third day and is caused by maternal hormones. Occasionally a milky substance, sometimes called "witch's milk," is secreted by the infant's breasts by the end of the first week. *Supernumerary nipples* may be found on the chest or even in the axilla.

Lungs. The normal *respirations* of the newborn are irregular and abdominal, and the rate is between 30 and 60 breaths/min. Periods of *apnea* less than 15 seconds in duration are considered normal. After the initial forceful breaths required to initiate respiration, subsequent breaths should be easy and fairly regular in rhythm. Occasional irregularities occur in relation to crying, sleeping, and feeding.

Auscultation is best performed when the infant is quiet. Bronchial breath sounds should be equal bilaterally. Any differences in auscultatory findings between symmetric sites is reported. *Crackles* soon after birth indicate areas of atelectasis, which represent the normal transition of the lungs to extrauterine life. However, persistence of crackles or presence of wheezing is also reported.

Heart. *Heart rate* is auscultated and may range from 100 to 180 beats/min shortly after birth and, when the infant's condition has stabilized, from 120 to 140 beats/min. The *point of maximum intensity (PMI)* may be palpated and is usually found in the fourth to fifth intercostal space, medial to the left midclavicular line. The PMI gives some indication of the location of the heart, which may be displaced in conditions such as congenital diaphragmatic hernia or pneumothorax. *Dextrocardia,* an anomaly wherein the heart is on the right side of the body, is reported, since the abdominal organs may also be reversed, with associated circulatory abnormalities.

NURSING TIP Because auscultation of neonatal breath sounds and heart tones is often difficult for the untrained ear, practice auscultating one parameter at a time. Close your eyes and mentally block out the extraneous sounds heard, such as room noise or neonatal movement; offer the newborn a pacifier. Auscultation of a murmur and decreased air movement in specific lung fields requires patience and practice; it may require auscultating the heart tones or breath sounds for 1 to 3 minutes each.

Abdomen. The normal *contour* of the abdomen is cylindric and usually prominent with visible veins. Bowel sounds are heard a few hours after birth. Visible peristaltic waves may be observed in thin newborns but should not be seen in well-nourished infants.

The *umbilical cord* is inspected to determine the presence of two arteries, which look like papular structures, and one vein, which has a larger lumen than the arteries and a thinner vessel wall. At birth the cord appears bluish white and moist. After clamping, it begins to dry and appears a dull, yellowish brown. It progressively shrivels in size and turns greenish black.

Palpation is done after inspection of the abdomen. The *liver* is normally palpable 1 to 3 cm (about ½ to 1 inch) below the right costal margin. The tip of the *spleen* can sometimes be felt, but a palpable spleen more than 1 cm below the left costal margin suggests enlargement and warrants further investigation. Although both *kidneys* should be palpated, this maneuver requires considerable practice. When felt, the lower half of the right kidney and the tip of the left kidney are 1 to 2 cm above the umbilicus.

During examination of the lower abdomen, it is particularly important to palpate for *femoral pulses,* which should be strong and equal bilaterally.

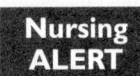 **Nursing ALERT** Absence of the femoral pulses may indicate coarctation of the aorta, a congenital heart defect. Absent or weak femoral pulses are always reported for further evaluation.

Female Genitalia. Normally the *labia minora, labia majora,* and *clitoris* are edematous, especially following a breech delivery. However, the labia and clitoris must be carefully inspected to identify any evidence of ambiguous genitalia or other abnormalities. Normally in a female the urethral opening is located behind the clitoris.

Virtually all female newborns have hymens, and this fact should be noted on the chart for future reference in case of concern regarding sexual abuse. A *hymenal tag* is occasionally visible from the posterior opening of the vagina. It is composed of tissue from the hymen and the labia minora. It usually disappears in several weeks. Generally, the vaginal vault is not inspected.

Vaginal discharge may be noted during the first week of life. This pseudomenstruation is a manifestation of the abrupt decrease of maternal hormones and usually disappears by 2 to 4 weeks. Fecal discharge from the vaginal opening indicates a rectovaginal fistula and is always reported. Vernix caseosa may be present in large amounts between the labia.

Male Genitalia. The *penis* is inspected for the location of the urethral opening, which is located at the tip. However, the opening may be totally covered by the prepuce, or foreskin, which covers the glans penis. A tight prepuce is a very common finding in the newborn. It should not be forcefully retracted, except to locate the urinary opening. *Smegma,* a white cheesy substance, is commonly found around the glans penis, under the foreskin. Small, white, firm lesions called *epithelial pearls* may be seen at the tip of the prepuce. An erection is common in the newborn.

The *scrotum* may be large, edematous and pendulous in the full-term neonate, especially in the infant born in breech position. It is more deeply pigmented in dark-skinned races. A noncommunicating *hydrocele* commonly occurs unilaterally and disappears within a few months. Always palpate the scrotum for the presence of *testes* (see Chapter 7). In small newborns, particularly premature infants, the undescended testes may be palpable within the inguinal canal. Absence of the testes may also be a sign of ambiguous genitalia, especially when accompanied by a small scrotum and penis. *Inguinal hernias* may or may not be manifested immediately after birth. A hernia is more easily detected when the infant is crying. Palpable *lymph nodes* are most commonly found in the inguinal area.

Back and Anus. The *spine* is inspected with the infant prone. The shape of the spine is gently rounded, with none of the characteristic S-shaped curves seen later in life. Any abnormal openings, masses, dimples, or soft areas are noted. With the infant still prone, symmetry of the gluteal folds is carefully noted. Any evidence of asymmetry is reported, and tests for congenital hip dislocation are performed by trained (or skilled) examiners (see Chapter 31).

Passage of meconium from the anal opening indicates anal patency. If an imperforate anus is suspected and is not readily obvious, a small catheter should be inserted into the anal opening.

Nursing ALERT Do not use a gloved finger or rectal thermometer to test for anal patency because of the risk of mucosal perforation; also, the smaller diameter of the thermometer may pass through even a severely stenotic anus. Always report failure to pass meconium by 48 hours.

Extremities. The extremities are examined for symmetry, range of motion, and reflexes. The fingers and toes are counted, and supernumerary digits *(polydactyly)* or fusion of digits *(syndactyly)* is noted. A partial syndactyly between the second and third toes is a common variation seen in otherwise normal infants. The nail beds should be pink, although slight blueness is evident in acrocyanosis.

The palms of the hands should have the usual creases (see Fig. 7-9). The full-term newborn usually has creases covering the entire sole of the foot. The soles of the feet are flat with prominent fat pads.

Range of motion of the extremities should be observed throughout the entire examination. The hips are rotated to identify a congenital dislocation. With the infant supine, the legs should be flexed *gently* at the hips and knees and abducted to almost 175 degrees. Limitation in abduction often indicates dislocation. Symmetry is noted when the infant moves, particularly when a Moro reflex is elicited.

Muscle tone should also be assessed. By attempting to extend a flexed extremity, the nurse determines if tone is equal bilaterally. Extension of any extremity is usually met with resistance, and when released, the extremity returns to its previous flexed position. *Hypotonia* suggests some degree of hypoxia, neurologic disorder, or Down syndrome. *Asymmetry* of muscle tone may indicate a degree of paralysis from brain damage or nerve damage. Failure to move the lower limbs suggests a spinal cord lesion or injury. *Tremors, twitches,* and *myoclonic jerks* characterize neonatal seizures or may indicate neonatal narcotic withdrawal syndrome. Quivering or momentary tremors are usually normal.

Two reflexes are elicited. The first is the *grasp reflex.* Touching the palms of the hands or soles of the feet near the base of the digits causes flexion or grasping (Fig. 8-9, *A*). The other is the *Babinski reflex.* Stroking the outer sole of the foot upward from the heel across the ball of the foot causes the big toe to dorsiflex and the other toes to hyperextend (Fig. 8-9, *B*).

Neurologic System. Assessing neurologic status is a critical part of the physical assessment of the newborn. Much of the neurologic examination takes place during examination of body systems, such as eliciting localized reflexes and observing posture, muscle tone, head control, and movement. However, several important mass (total body) reflexes also need to be elicited (Table 8-2). They are usually left to the end of the examination because they may disturb the infant and interfere with auscultation.

Transitional Assessment: Periods of Reactivity

The newborn exhibits behavioral and physiologic characteristics that may at first appear to be signs of stress. However, during the initial 24 hours, changes in heart rate, respiration, motor activity, color, mucus production, and bowel activity occur in an orderly, predictable sequence that is normal and indicates lack of stress.

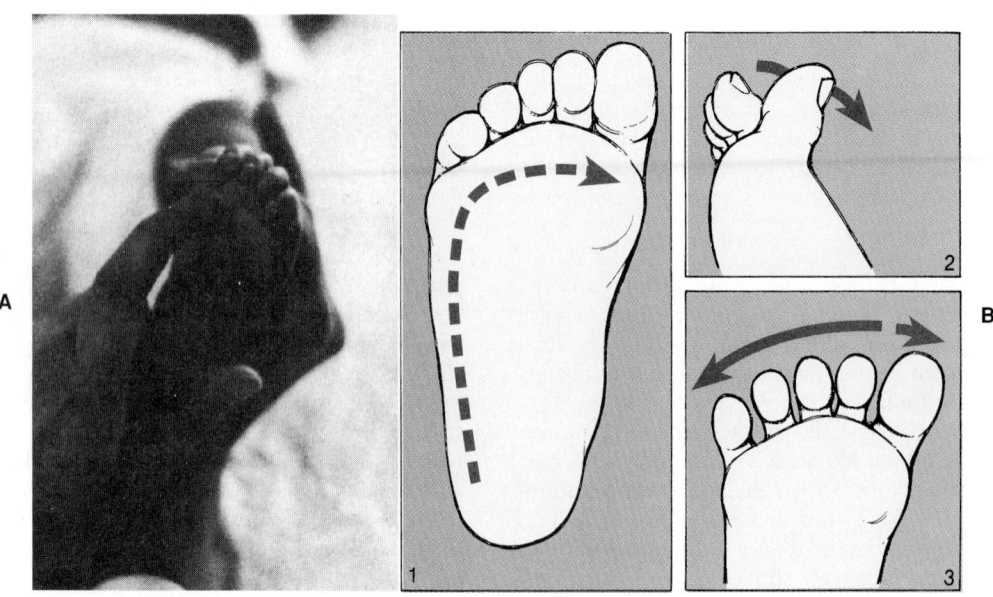

FIG. 8-9. A, Plantar or grasp reflex. **B,** Babinski reflex. *1,* Direction of stroke. *2,* Dorsiflexion of big toe. *3,* Fanning of toes.

For 6 to 8 hours after birth, the newborn is in the *first period of reactivity.* During the first 30 minutes the infant is very alert, cries vigorously, may suck the fist greedily, and appears very interested in the environment. At this time the neonate's eyes are usually open, suggesting that this is an excellent opportunity for mother, father, and child to see each other. Because the newborn has a vigorous suck, this is also an opportune time to begin breast-feeding. The infant will usually grasp the nipple quickly, satisfying both mother and infant. This is particularly important for nurses to remember, because after this initially highly active state the infant may be quite sleepy and uninterested in sucking. Physiologically the respiratory rate during this period is as high as 80 breaths/min, rales may be heard, heart rate reaches 180 beats/min, bowel sounds are active, mucous secretions are increased, and temperature may decrease.

After this initial stage of alertness and activity, the infant enters the *second stage* of the first reactive period, which generally lasts 2 to 4 hours. Heart and respiratory rates decrease, temperature continues to fall, mucus production decreases, and urine or stool is usually not passed. The infant is in a state of sleep and relative calm. Any attempt at stimulation usually elicits a minimal response. Because of the continued decrease in body temperature, undressing or bathing is avoided during this time.

The *second period of reactivity* begins when the infant awakes from this deep sleep; it lasts about 2 to 5 hours, and provides another excellent opportunity for child and parents to interact. The infant is again alert and responsive, heart and respiratory rates increase, the gag reflex is active, gastric and respiratory secretions are increased, and passage of meconium frequently occurs. This period is usually over when the amount of respiratory mucus has decreased. Following this stage is a period of stabilization of physiologic systems and a vacillating pattern of sleep and activity.

Behavioral Assessment

Another important area of assessment is observation of behavior. Infants' behavior helps shape their environment, and their ability to react to various stimuli affects how others relate to them. The principal areas of behavior for newborns are sleep, wakefulness, and activity, such as crying.

One method of systematically assessing the infant's behavior is the use of the *Brazelton Neonatal Behavioral Assessment Scale (BNBAS)* (Brazelton, 1996). The BNBAS is an interactive examination that assesses the infant's response to 28 items organized according to the clusters in the box above. It is generally used as a research or diagnostic tool and requires special training.

In addition to its use as an initial and ongoing tool to assess neurologic and behavioral responses, the scale can be used as an assessor of initial parent-child relationships, as a preventive instrument that identifies the caregiver as one who may benefit from a role model, and as a guide to help parents to focus on their infant's individuality and to develop a deeper attachment to their child. Studies demonstrate that by showing parents the unique characteristics of their infant, a more positive perception of the infant develops, with increased interaction between infant and parent (Beal, 1989).

Patterns of Sleep and Activity. Newborns begin life with a systematic schedule of sleep and wakefulness that is initially evident during the periods of reactivity. Following

---

CLUSTERS OF NEONATAL BEHAVIORS IN BRAZELTON NEONATAL BEHAVIORAL ASSESSMENT SCALE

Habituation—Ability to respond to and then inhibit responding to discrete stimulus (light, rattle, bell, pinprick) while asleep

Orientation—Quality of alert states and ability to attend to visual and auditory stimuli while alert

Motor performance—Quality of movement and tone

Range of state—Measure of general arousal level or arousability of infant

Regulation of state—How infant responds when aroused

Autonomic stability—Signs of stress (tremors, startles, skin color) related to homeostatic (self-regulating) adjustment of the nervous system

Reflexes—Assessment of several neonatal reflexes

---

this initial period it is not unusual for the infant to sleep almost constantly for the next 2 to 3 days in order to recover from the exhausting birth process.

The infant's sleep comprises five distinct states, which are summarized in Table 8-3. *State* refers to an interaction between the infant and the environment in which the infant's behaviors form a continuum from arousal to consciousness. The cycle of these sleep states is highly variable and is based on the number of hours an infant sleeps per day, which may range anywhere from 10½ to 23 hours, with an average of 16½ hours. States of sleep and periods of activity are highly influenced by environmental stimuli. As early as the immediate postbirth period, state is influenced by type of care. The sleep of infants in mothers' rooms is significantly more quiet, and they cry less than infants in the nursery. It is especially important for parents to understand these states and the methods effective in altering them. An aware infant exhibits more motor activity before feeding than after. Feeding usually terminates the state of crying when hunger is the cause. Usually swaddling or wrapping an infant snugly in a blanket both promotes sleep and maintains body temperature. Intermittent, vertical rocking promotes more bright-alert behavior, whereas continuous, horizontal rocking induces more drowsy behavior.

Cry. The newborn should begin extrauterine life with a strong, lusty cry. The sounds produced by crying can be described as hunger, anger, pain, and "bid for attention" cries. Discomfort (pain) sounds initially consist of gasps and cries in which the consonant *H* is clearly distinguishable. The duration of crying is as highly variable in each infant as is the duration of sleep patterns. Some newborns may cry as little as 5 minutes or as much as 2 hours or more per day.

Behavioral states can be influenced by environmental stimuli. Feeding usually terminates the crying when hunger is the cause. However, an awake infant exhibits more motor activity before feeding than after. Swaddling or wrapping an infant snugly in a blanket promotes sleep and maintains body temperature. Rocking the infant reduces crying and induces quiet alertness or sleep.

Assessment of Attachment Behaviors

One of the most important areas of assessment is careful observation of those behaviors that are thought to indicate the formation of emotional bonds between the newborn and

TABLE 8-2. Assessment of reflexes in the newborn

REFLEXES	EXPECTED BEHAVIORAL RESPONSES
Localized	
Eyes	
Blinking or corneal reflex	Infant blinks at sudden appearance of a bright light or at approach of an object toward cornea; persists throughout life
Pupillary	Pupil constricts when a bright light shines toward it; persists throughout life
Doll's eye	As head is moved slowly to right or left, eyes lag behind and do not immediately adjust to new position of head; disappears as fixation develops; if persists, indicates neurologic damage
Nose	
Sneeze	Spontaneous response of nasal passages to irritation or obstruction; persists throughout life
Glabellar	Tapping briskly on glabella (bridge of nose) causes eyes to close tightly
Mouth and throat	
Sucking	Infant begins strong sucking movements of circumoral area in response to stimulation; persists throughout infancy, even without stimulation, such as during sleep
Gag	Stimulation of posterior pharynx by food, suction, or passage of a tube causes infant to gag; persists throughout life
Rooting	Touching or stroking the cheek along side of mouth causes infant to turn head toward that side and begin to suck; should disappear at about age 3-4 months, but may persist for up to 12 months (see Fig. 8-8)
Extrusion	When tongue is touched or depressed, infant responds by forcing it outward; disappears by age 4 months *Prevent from choking*
Yawn	Spontaneous response to decreased oxygen by increasing amount of inspired air; persists throughout life
Cough	Irritation of mucous membranes of larynx or tracheobronchial tree causes coughing; persists throughout life; usually present after first day of birth
Extremities	
Grasp	Touching palms of hands or soles of feet near base of digits causes flexion of hands and toes (see Fig. 8-9, *A*): palmar grasp lessens after age 3 months, to be replaced by voluntary movement; plantar grasp lessens by 8 months of age
Babinski	Stroking outer sole of foot upward from heel and across ball of foot causes toes to hyperextend and hallux to dorsiflex (see Fig. 8-9, *B*); disappears after age 1 year
Ankle clonus	Briskly dorsiflexing foot while supporting knee in partially flexed position results in one to two oscillating movements ("beats"); eventually no beats should be felt
Mass	
Moro	Sudden jarring or change in equilibrium causes sudden extension and abduction of extremities and fanning of fingers, with index finger and thumb forming a **C** shape, followed by flexion and adduction of extremities; legs may weakly flex; infant may cry (Fig. 8-10); disappears after age 3-4 months, usually strongest during first 2 months
Startle	A sudden loud noise causes abduction of the arms with flexion of elbows; hands remain clenched; disappears by age 4 months
Perez	While infant is prone on a firm surface, thumb is pressed along spine from sacrum to neck; infant responds by crying, flexing extremities, and elevating pelvis and head; lordosis of the spine, as well as defecation and urination, may occur; disappears by age 4-6 months
Asymmetric tonic neck	When infant's head is turned to one side, arm and leg extend on that side, and opposite arm and leg flex (Fig. 8-11); disappears by age 3-4 months, to be replaced by symmetric positioning of both sides of body
Trunk incurvation (Galant) reflex	Stroking infant's back alongside spine causes hips to move toward stimulated side; disappears by age 4 weeks
Dance or step	If infant is held so that sole of foot touches a hard surface, there is a reciprocal flexion and extension of the leg, simulating walking (Fig. 8-12); disappears after age 3-4 weeks, to be replaced by deliberate movement
Crawl	When placed on abdomen, infant makes crawling movements with arms and legs; disappears at about age 6 weeks (Fig. 8-13)
Placing	When infant is held upright under arms and dorsal side of foot is briskly placed against hard object, such as table, leg lifts as if foot is stepping on table; age of disappearance varies

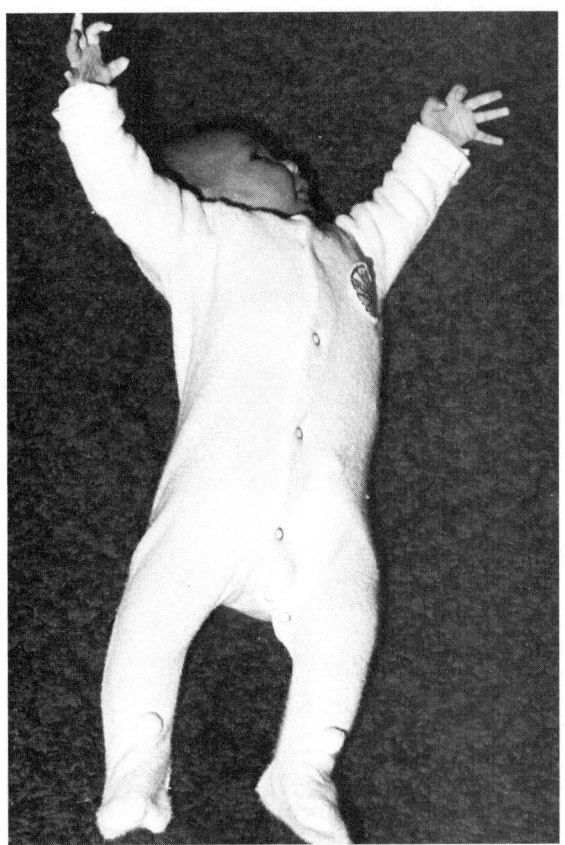

FIG. 8-10. Moro reflex.

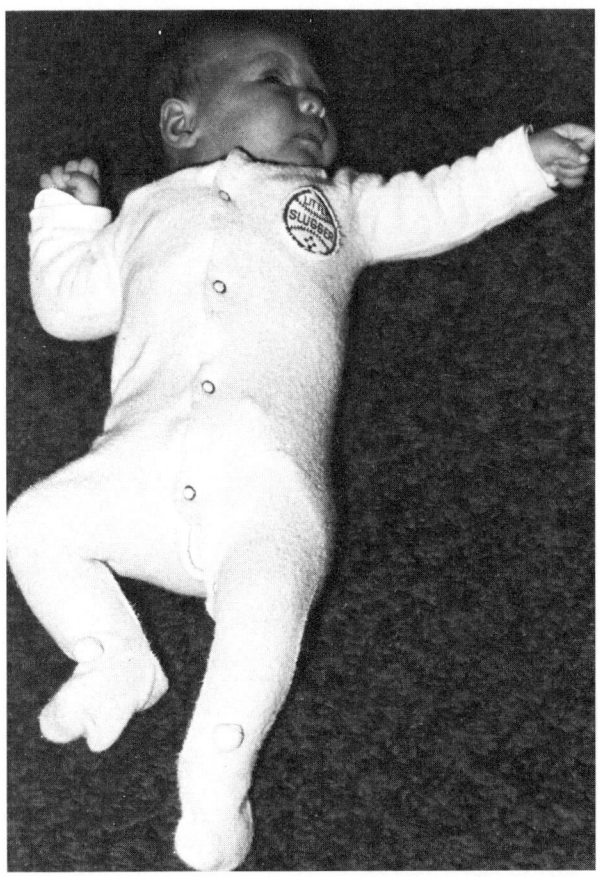

FIG. 8-11. Tonic neck reflex.

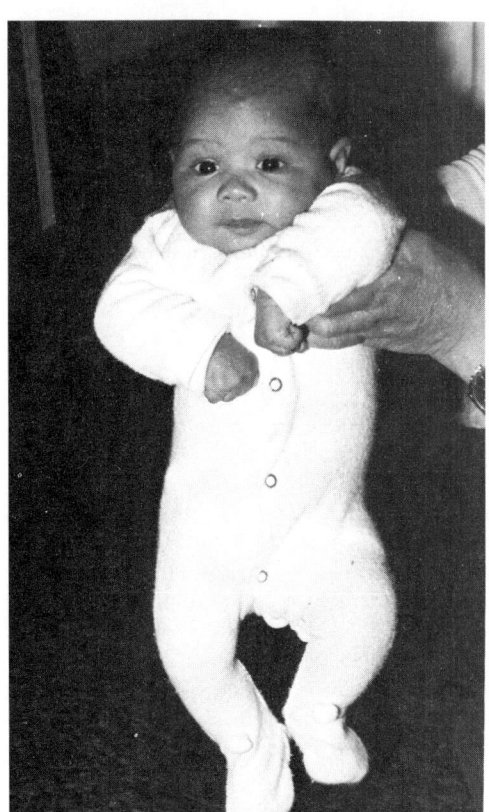

FIG. 8-12. Dance reflex.

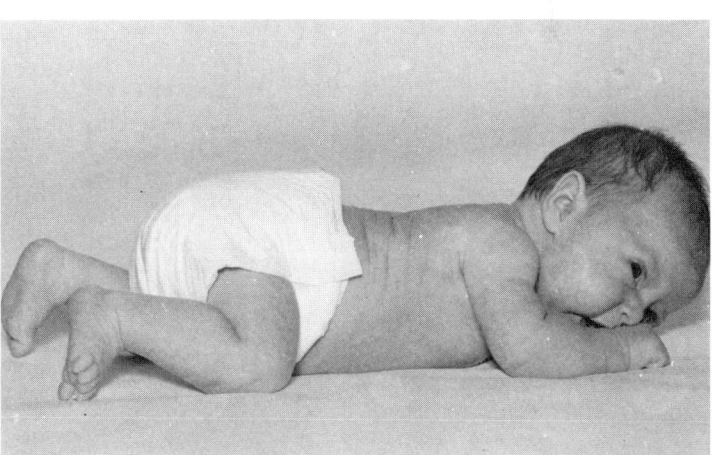

FIG. 8-13. Crawl reflex.

TABLE 8-3. States of sleep and activity

STATE/BEHAVIOR*	DURATION	IMPLICATIONS FOR PARENTING
Regular Sleep Closed eyes Regular breathing No movement except for sudden bodily jerks	4-5 hours/day, 10-20 minutes/sleep cycle	External stimuli do not arouse infant Continue usual house noises Leave infant alone if sudden loud noise awakens infant and child cries
Irregular Sleep Closed eyes Irregular breathing Slight muscular twitching of body	12-15 hours/day, 20-45 minutes/sleep cycle	External stimuli that did not arouse infant during regular sleep may minimally arouse child Periodic groaning or crying is usual; do not interpret as an indication of pain or discomfort
Drowsiness Eyes may be open Irregular breathing Active body movement	Variable	Most stimuli arouse infant Pick infant up during this time rather than leaving in crib
Alert Inactivity Responds to environment by active body movement and staring at close-range objects	2-3 hours/day	Satisfy infant's needs such as hunger Place infant in area of home where activity is continuous Place toys in crib or playpen Place objects within 17.5-20 cm (7-8 inches) of infant's view
Waking and Crying May begin with whimpering and slight body movement Progresses to strong, angry crying and uncoordinated thrashing of extremities	1-4 hours/day	Remove intense internal or external stimuli Stimuli that were effective during alert inactivity are usually ineffective Rock and swaddle to decrease crying

*Some classifications divide the fifth state into two states: alert with activity and crying.

GUIDELINES
Assessing Attachment Behavior

When the infant is brought to the parents, do they reach out for the child and call the child by name?

Do the parents speak about the child in terms of identification—whom the infant looks like; what appears special about their child over other infants?

When parents are holding the infant, what kind of body contact is there—do parents feel at ease in changing the infant's position; are fingertips or whole hands used; are there parts of the body they avoid touching or parts of the body they investigate and scrutinize?

When the infant is awake, what kinds of stimulation do the parents provide—do they talk to the infant, to each other, or to no one; how do they look at the infant—direct visual contact, avoidance of eye contact, or looking at other people or objects?

How comfortable do the parents appear in terms of caring for the infant? Do they express any concern regarding their ability or disgust for certain activities, such as changing diapers?

What type of affection do they demonstrate to the newborn, such as smiling, stroking, kissing, or rocking?

If the infant is fussy, what kinds of comforting techniques do the parents use, such as rocking, swaddling, talking, or stroking?

family, especially the mother. Such behaviors include the *en face position;* undressing and touching the infant; smiling, kissing, and talking to the infant; and holding, rocking and cradling the child close to the body (see Guidelines box at left). However, because assessment is closely related to interventions that promote attachment (e.g., encouraging these behaviors in parents), the major portion of assessing attachment behaviors is discussed on p. 210.

Physical Assessment

An essential aspect of the care of the newborn is a thorough physical assessment that includes estimation of gestational age and physical examination to identify normal characteristics and existing abnormalities. These initial and ongoing assessments are critical to establishing baseline data for planning, implementing, and evaluating care and are a nursing priority in caring for the newborn. The discussion of physical examination focuses on normal findings and variations from the norm that require little or no intervention. The reader is encouraged to review the material in Chapter 7 for further discussions of examination techniques. General guidelines for conducting a physical examination are presented in the Guidelines box. Table 8-4 summarizes physical examination of the newborn.

Text continued on p. 201.

TABLE 8-4. Summary of physical assessment of the newborn

USUAL FINDINGS	COMMON VARIATIONS/MINOR ABNORMALITIES	POTENTIAL SIGNS OF DISTRESS/MAJOR ABNORMALITIES
General Measurements *Head circumference*—33-35 cm (13-14 inches); about 2-3 cm (1 inch) larger than chest circumference *Chest circumference*—30.5-33 cm (12-13 inches) *Crown-to-rump length*—31-35 cm (12.5-14 inches); approximately equal to head circumference *Head-to-heel length*—48-53 cm (19-21 inches) *Birth weight*—2700-4000 g (6-9 pounds)	Molding after birth may decrease head circumference Head and chest circumferences may be equal for first 1-2 days after birth Loss of 10% of birth weight in first week; regained in 10-14 days	Head circumference <10th or >90th percentile Birth weight <10th or >90th percentile
Vital Signs *Temperature* Axillary—36.5°-37° C (97.9°-98° F)	Crying may increase body temperature slightly Radiant warmer will falsely increase axillary temperature	Hypothermia Hyperthermia
Heart rate Apical—120-140 beats/min	Crying will increase heart rate; sleep will decrease heart rate During first period of reactivity (6 to 8 hours), rate can reach 180 beats/min	Bradycardia—Resting rate below 80-100 beats/min Tachycardia—Rate above 160-180 beats/min Irregular rhythm
Respirations 30-60 breaths/min	Crying will increase respiratory rate; sleep will decrease respiratory rate During first period of reactivity (6 to 8 hours), rate can reach 80 breaths/min	Tachypnea—Rate above 60 breaths/min Apnea >15 seconds
Blood pressure Oscillometric—65/41 mm Hg in arm and calf	Crying and activity will increase BP Placing cuff on thigh may agitate infant; thigh BP may be higher than arm or calf BP by 4-8 mm Hg	Oscillometric systolic pressure in calf 6-9 mm Hg less than in upper extremity (sign of coarctation of aorta)
General Appearance *Posture*—Flexion of head and extremities, which rest on chest and abdomen	*Frank breech*—Extended legs, abducted and fully rotated thighs, flattened occiput, extended neck	Limp posture, extension of extremities
Skin At birth, bright red, puffy, smooth Second to third day, pink, flaky, dry Vernix caseosa Lanugo Edema around eyes, face, legs, dorsa of hands, feet, and scrotum or labia *Acrocyanosis*—Cyanosis of hands and feet *Cutis marmorata*—Transient mottling when infant is exposed to decreased temperature	Neonatal jaundice after first 24 hours Ecchymoses or petechiae caused by birth trauma *Milia*—Distended sebaceous glands that appear as tiny white papules on cheeks, chin, and nose *Miliaria or sudamina*—Distended sweat (eccrine) glands that appear as minute vesicles, especially on face *Erythema toxicum*—Pink papular rash with vesicles superimposed on thorax, back, buttocks, and abdomen; may appear in 24 to 48 hours and resolve after several days *Harlequin color change*—Clearly outlined color change as infant lies on side; lower half of body becomes pink, and upper half is pale	Progressive jaundice, especially in first 24 hours Cracked or peeling skin Generalized cyanosis Pallor Mottling Grayness Plethora Hemorrhage, ecchymoses, or petechiae that persist *Sclerema*—Hard and stiff skin Poor skin turgor Rashes, pustules, or blisters *Café-au-lait spots*—Light brown spots *Nevus flammeus*—Port-wine stain

Continued.

TABLE 8-4. Summary of physical assessment of the newborn—cont'd

USUAL FINDINGS	COMMON VARIATIONS/MINOR ABNORMALITIES	POTENTIAL SIGNS OF DISTRESS/MAJOR ABNORMALITIES
Skin—cont'd	*Mongolian spots*—Irregular areas of deep blue pigmentation, usually in sacral and gluteal regions; seen predominantly in newborns of African, Native American, Asian, or Hispanic descent *Telangiectatic nevi ("stork bites")*—Flat, deep pink localized areas usually seen in back of neck	
Head *Anterior fontanel*—Diamond shaped, 2.5-4.0 cm (1-1.75 inches) (see Fig. 8-6) *Posterior fontanel*—Triangular, 0.5-1 cm (0.2-0.4 inch) Fontanels should be flat, soft, and firm Widest part of fontanel measured from bone to bone, not suture to suture	Molding following vaginal delivery Third sagittal (parietal) fontanel Bulging fontanel because of crying or coughing *Caput succedaneum*—Edema of soft scalp tissue *Cephalhematoma* (uncomplicated)—Hematoma between periosteum and skull bone	Fused sutures Bulging or depressed fontanels when quiet Widened sutures and fontanels *Craniotabes*—Snapping sensation along lambdoid suture that resembles indentation of ping-pong ball
Eyes Lids usually edematous Color—Slate gray, dark blue, brown Absence of tears Presence of red reflex Corneal reflex in response to touch Pupillary reflex in response to light Blink reflex in response to light or touch Rudimentary fixation on objects and ability to follow to midline	Epicanthal folds in Oriental infants Searching nystagmus or strabismus *Subconjunctival (scleral) hemorrhages*—Ruptured capillaries, usually at limbus	Pink color of iris Purulent discharge Upward slant in non-Orientals Hypertelorism (3 cm or greater) Hypotelorism Congenital cataracts Constricted or dilated fixed pupil Absence of red reflex Absence of pupillary or corneal reflex Inability to follow object or bright light to midline Blue sclera Yellow sclera
Ears Position—Top of pinna on horizontal line with outer canthus of eye Startle reflex elicited by a loud, sudden noise Pinna flexible, cartilage present	Inability to visualize tympanic membrane because of filled aural canals Pinna flat against head Irregular shape or size Pits or skin tags	Low placement of ears Absence of startle reflex in response to loud noise Minor abnormalities may be signs of various syndromes, especially renal
Nose Nasal patency Nasal discharge—Thin white mucus Sneezing	Flattened and bruised	Nonpatent canals Thick, bloody nasal discharge Flaring of nares (alae nasi) Copious nasal secretions or stuffiness (may be minor)
Mouth and Throat Intact, high-arched palate Uvula in midline Frenulum of tongue Frenum of upper lip Sucking reflex—Strong and coordinated Rooting reflex Gag reflex Extrusion reflex Absent or minimal salivation Vigorous cry	*Natal teeth*—Teeth present at birth; benign but may be associated with congenital defects *Epstein pearls*—Small, white epithelial cysts along midline of hard palate	Cleft lip Cleft palate Large, protruding tongue or posterior displacement of tongue Profuse salivation or drooling *Candidiasis (thrush)*—White, adherent patches on tongue, palate, and buccal surfaces Inability to pass nasogastric tube Hoarse, high-pitched, weak, absent, or other abnormal cry

TABLE 8-4. Summary of physical assessment of the newborn—cont'd

USUAL FINDINGS	COMMON VARIATIONS/MINOR ABNORMALITIES	POTENTIAL SIGNS OF DISTRESS/MAJOR ABNORMALITIES
Neck Short, thick, usually surrounded by skinfolds Tonic neck reflex	*Torticollis* (wry neck)—Head held to one side with chin pointing to opposite side	Excessive skinfolds Resistance to flexion Absence of tonic neck reflex Fractured clavicle
Chest Anteroposterior and lateral diameters equal Slight sternal retractions evident during inspiration Xiphoid process evident Breast enlargement	Funnel chest (pectus excavatum) Pigeon chest (pectus carinatum) Supernumerary nipples Secretion of milky substance from breasts ("witch's milk")	Depressed sternum Marked retractions of chest and intercostal spaces during respiration Asymmetric chest expansion Redness and firmness around nipples Wide-spaced nipples
Lungs Respirations chiefly abdominal Cough reflex absent at birth, present by 1-2 days Bilateral equal bronchial breath sounds	Rate and depth of respirations may be irregular, periodic breathing Crackles shortly after birth	Inspiratory stridor Expiratory grunt Retractions Persistent irregular breathing Periodic breathing with repeated apneic spells Seesaw respirations (paradoxical) Unequal breath sounds Persistent fine crackles Wheezing Diminished breath sounds Peristaltic sounds on one side, with diminished breath sounds on same side
Heart *Apex*—Fourth to fifth intercostal space, lateral to left sternal border S_2 slightly sharper and higher in pitch than S_1	*Sinus arrhythmia*—Heart rate increases with inspiration and decreases with expiration Transient cyanosis on crying or straining	*Dextrocardia*—Heart on right side Displacement of apex, muffled Cardiomegaly Abdominal shunts Murmurs Thrills Persistent cyanosis Hyperactive precordium
Abdomen Cylindric in shape *Liver*—Palpable 2-3 cm below right costal margin *Spleen*—Tip palpable at end of first week of age *Kidneys*—Palpable 1-2 cm above umbilicus *Umbilical cord*—Bluish white at birth with two arteries and one vein *Femoral pulses*—Equal bilaterally	Umbilical hernia *Diastasis recti*—Midline gap between recti muscles *Wharton's jelly*—unusually thick umbilical cord	Abdominal distention Localized bulging Distended veins Absent bowel sounds Enlarged liver and spleen Ascites Visible peristaltic waves Scaphoid or concave abdomen Green umbilical cord Presence of only one artery in cord Urine or stool leaking from cord Palpable bladder distention following scanty voiding Absent femoral pulses Cord bleeding or hematoma

Continued.

TABLE 8-4. Summary of physical assessment of the newborn—cont'd

USUAL FINDINGS	COMMON VARIATIONS/MINOR ABNORMALITIES	POTENTIAL SIGNS OF DISTRESS/MAJOR ABNORMALITIES
Female Genitalia Labia and clitoris usually edematous Urethral meatus behind clitoris Vernix caseosa between labia Urination within 24 hours	*Pseudomenstruation*—Blood-tinged or mucoid discharge Hymenal tag	Enlarged clitoris with urethral meatus at tip Fused labia Absence of vaginal opening Meconium from vaginal opening No urination within 24 hours Masses in labia Ambiguous genitalia
Male Genitalia Urethral opening at tip of glans penis Testes palpable in each scrotum Scrotum usually large, edematous, pendulous, and covered with rugae; usually deeply pigmented in dark-skinned ethnic groups Smegma Urination within 24 hours	Urethral opening covered by prepuce Inability to retract foreskin *Epithelial pearls*—Small, firm, white lesions at tip of prepuce Erection or priapism Testes palpable in inguinal canal Scrotum small	*Hypospadias*—Urethral opening on ventral surface of penis *Epispadias*—Urethral opening on dorsal surface of penis *Chordee*—Ventral curvature of penis Testes not palpable in scrotum or inguinal canal No urination within 24 hours Inguinal hernia Hypoplastic scrotum *Hydrocele*—Fluid in scrotum Masses in scrotum Meconium from scrotum Discoloration of testes Ambiguous genitalia
Back and Rectum Spine intact, no openings, masses, or prominent curves Trunk incurvation reflex Anal reflex Patent anal opening Passage of meconium within 48 hours	Green liquid stools in infant under phototherapy Delayed passages of meconium in very-low-birth-weight neonates	Anal fissures or fistulas Imperforate anus Absence of anal reflex No meconium within 36 hours Pilonidal cyst or sinus Tuft of hair along spine Spina bifida (any degree)

Extremities
Ten fingers and toes
Full range of motion
Nail beds pink, with transient cyanosis immediately after birth
Creases on anterior two thirds of sole
Sole usually flat
Symmetry of extremities
Equal muscle tone bilaterally, especially resistance to opposing flexion
Equal bilateral brachial pulses
	Partial syndactyly between second and third toes
	Second toe overlapping into third toe
	Wide gap between first (hallux) and second toes
	Deep crease on plantar surface of foot between first and second toes
	Asymmetric length of toes
	Dorsiflexion and shortness of hallux
		Polydactyly—Extra digits
		Syndactyly—Fused or webbed digits
		Phocomelia—Hands or feet attached close to trunk
		Hemimelia—Absence of distal part of extremity
		Hyperflexibility of joints
		Persistent cyanosis of nail beds
		Yellowing of nail beds
		Sole covered with creases
		Transverse palmar (simian) crease
		Fractures
		Decreased or absent ROM
		Dislocated or subluxated hip
		   Limitation in hip abduction
		   Unequal gluteal or leg folds
		   Unequal knee height (Allis or Galeazzi sign)
		   Audible click on abduction (Ortolani sign)
		Asymmetry of extremities
		Unequal muscle tone or range of motion

TABLE 8-4. Summary of physical assessment of the newborn—cont'd

USUAL FINDINGS	COMMON VARIATIONS/MINOR ABNORMALITIES	POTENTIAL SIGNS OF DISTRESS/MAJOR ABNORMALITIES
Neuromuscular System Extremities usually maintain some degree of flexion Extension of an extremity followed by previous position of flexion Head lag while sitting, but momentary ability to hold head erect Able to turn head from side to side when prone Able to hold head in horizontal line with back when held prone	Quivering or momentary tremors	*Hypotonia*—Floppy, poor head control, extremities limp *Hypertonia*—Jittery, arms and hands tightly flexed, legs stiffly extended, startles easily Asymmetric posturing (except tonic neck reflex) *Opisthotonic posturing*—Arched back Signs of paralysis Tremors, twitches, and myoclonic jerks Marked head lag in all positions

GUIDELINES
Physical Examination of the Newborn

Provide a normothermic and nonstimulating examination area.
Undress only body area examined to prevent heat loss.
Proceed in an orderly sequence (usually head to toe) with the following exceptions:
Observe infant's attitude and position of flexion first to avoid disturbing him/her
Perform all procedures that require quiet next, such as auscultating the lungs, heart, and abdomen.
Perform disturbing procedures, such as testing reflexes, last.
Measure head, chest, and length at same time to compare results.
Proceed quickly to avoid stressing infant.
Check that equipment and supplies are working properly and are accessible.
Comfort infant during and after the examination if upset.
Talk softly.
Hold infant's hands against chest.
Swaddle and hold.
Give pacifier or nonlatex gloved finger to suck.

❖ Nursing Diagnoses
A number of nursing diagnoses are prominent in the nursing care of the newborn and family, and others specific to individual cases become evident. The most common nursing diagnoses are outlined in the Nursing Care Plan on pp. 214-216.

❖ Planning
The goals for the newborn and family are as follows:

1. Infant will maintain a patent airway.
2. Infant will maintain a stable body temperature.
3. Infant will experience no infections or injuries.
4. Infant will receive optimum nutrition.
5. Family will exhibit attachment behavior.
6. Family will be prepared for discharge and home care.

❖ Implementation
Maintain a Patent Airway
Establishing a patent airway is a primary objective in the delivery room and is the responsibility of the attending nurses and practitioners. However, maintaining a patent airway continues to be a priority goal in the nursery with attention to proper positioning of the infant to facilitate drainage of secretions, especially after feeding (see Fig. 8-17). The **American Academy of Pediatrics** recommends the supine or side-lying position during sleep for healthy newborns. Infants with breathing problems or excessive vomiting should sleep prone. This recommendation is based on the possible association between sleeping prone and sudden infant death syndrome (Infant sleep position and sudden infant death syndrome, 1994) (see Chapter 11). A bulb syringe is kept near the infant and is used if suctioning is required. Used bulb syringes should probably be replaced every 24 hours in the hospital and boiled for 10 minutes before reuse in the home to eliminate bacterial contamination.*

Nursing ALERT To avoid aspiration of amniotic fluid or mucus, clear the pharynx first, then the nasal passages. Compress the bulb *before* insertion to prevent forcing secretions into the bronchi.

If more forceful removal of secretions is required, mechanical suction is used. The use of the proper-size catheter and correct suctioning technique is essential to prevent mucosal damage and edema. Gentle suctioning is necessary to prevent reflex bradycardia, laryngospasm, and cardiac arrhythmias from vagal stimulation. Oropharyngeal suctioning is performed for 3 to 5 seconds with sufficient time between suctioning to allow the infant to reoxygenate.

In some nurseries the stomach is routinely lavaged to remove amniotic fluid and mucous, which may cause abdomi-

*Home care instructions for using a bulb syringe are available in Wong DL: *Wong and Whaley's Clinical manual of pediatric nursing,* ed 4, St Louis, 1996, Mosby.

nal distention and interfere with the establishment of respiration. Passing a catheter to the stomach also rules out esophageal atresia. Vital signs are closely monitored, and any indication of respiratory distress is immediately reported.

> **Nursing ALERT**
>
> Signs of respiratory distress include tachypnea, grunting, flaring alae nasi, intercostal retractions, stridor, abnormal breath sounds, cyanosis, or pallor.

Maintain Stable Body Temperature

Conserving the newborn's body heat is an essential nursing goal. It requires an understanding of the causes of heat loss: evaporation, radiation, conduction, and convection. Nursing care is based on preventing these from occurring.

At birth a major cause of heat loss is *evaporation,* the loss of heat through moisture. The amniotic fluid that bathes the infant's skin favors evaporation. Heat loss through evaporation is minimized by rapidly drying the skin and hair with a warmed towel and placing the infant in a heated environment.

Another major cause of heat loss is *radiation,* the loss of heat to cooler solid objects in the environment that are not in direct contact with the infant. Loss of heat through radiation increases as these solid objects become colder and closer to the infant. The temperature of ambient or surrounding air in the incubator essentially has no effect on loss of heat through radiation. This is a critical point to remember when attempting to maintain a constant temperature for the infant, because even though the temperature of the ambient air is optimal, the infant can become hypothermic. The use of radiant heating devices such as heat lamps or phototherapy lights with an incubator may cause overheating of the infant, since infants cannot effectively dissipate radiant heat through the Plexiglas wall of the incubator. For this same reason, an incubator should not be exposed to direct sunlight (Thomas, 1994).

An example of radiant heat loss is the placement of the incubator close to a cold window, drafty doorway, or air-conditioning unit. The cold from either source will cool the walls of the incubator and, subsequently, the body of the neonate. To prevent this, the infant is placed as far away as possible from walls, windows, and ventilating units. If heat loss continues to be a problem, a radiant warmer or warming lamp may be placed over the infant or infant and mother.

Heat loss can also occur through conduction and convection. *Conduction* involves loss of heat from the body because of direct contact of skin with a cooler solid object. This can be minimized by placing the infant on a padded, covered surface and providing insulation through clothes and blankets rather than by placing the infant directly on a hard table. Placing the newborn very close to the mother, such as in her arms or on her abdomen, is physically beneficial in terms of conserving heat, as well as fostering maternal attachment.

Convection is similar to conduction, except that heat loss is aided by surrounding air currents. For example, placing the infant in the direct flow of air from a fan or air-conditioner vent will cause rapid heat loss through convection. Transporting the neonate in a crib with solid sides reduces airflow around the infant.

Protect From Infection and Injury

The most important practice for preventing cross-infection is thorough handwashing of all individuals involved in the infant's care (see Thinking Critically About . . . box). Several other procedures to prevent infection include eye care, umbilical care, bathing, and care of the circumcision. Vitamin K is administered to protect against hemorrhage. In addition, several safety measures are practiced, particularly in terms of proper identification, and screening tests are used to detect various disorders.

Identification. Proper identification of the newborn is absolutely essential. The nurse must verify that two identifying bands are securely fastened, usually on both ankles, and verify the information (name, sex, mother's admission number, date, and time of birth) against the birth records and the child's actual sex. Some institutions have more sophisticated methods of infant identification, such as a color photograph kept in the medical record, storage of blood for DNA genotyping, and/or electronic surveillance systems for infant security (Butz and others, 1993). Foot printing or finger printing is *not* currently recommended for newborn identification (American Academy of Pediatrics and American College of Obstetricians and Gynecologists, 1992).

The nurse needs to discuss safety issues with the mother the first time the infant is brought to her. A written copy of the safety instructions should also be given to the parent. Parents are instructed to look at name badges of nurses and hospital personnel who come to take infants and not to relinquish their infants to anyone without proper identification. Some hospitals have systems of color-coded badges or symbols that are changed daily to decrease the likelihood of infant abduction. Mothers are also advised not to leave the infant alone in the crib while they shower; rather, they should ask to have the infant returned to the nursery if a family member is not present in the room. The nurse should document in the chart that these instructions were given.

Eye Care. Prophylactic eye treatment against *ophthalmia neonatorum,* infectious conjunctivitis of the newborn, includes the use of (1) silver nitrate (1%) solution, (2) erythromycin (0.5%) ophthalmic ointment or drops, or (3) tetracycline (1%) ophthalmic ointment or drops (preferably in

> **THINKING CRITICALLY ABOUT . . .**
> **Gowning**
>
> A common ritual in many newborn nurseries is the use of cover gowns and "scrub" clothes to prevent infection. However, several studies have shown that this practice is ineffective and costly (Birenbaum and others, 1990; Rush and others, 1990; Thigpen, 1991). Some believe that "gowning" reinforces the use of handwashing; however, research does not support this assumption. Rather, when gowns were used, fewer care providers entered the unit (Donowitz, 1986). Benefits to discontinuing the practice of gowning may include saving staff time in procedures and the cost of laundering and stocking gowns (Pelke and others, 1994). One could speculate that the inconvenience of using gowns may even affect care if it discourages staff from visiting patients. What are the gowning policies in your agency and what reasons are given for their use?

GUIDELINES
Ophthalmia Neonatorum
Prophylaxis

1. Clean the eyelids with sterile cotton and sterile water if needed.
2. Separate lids and apply 2 drops or a 1 to 2 cm (½ inch) ribbon of ointment in each conjunctival sac.
3. Massage lids to ensure spread of the medication.
4. Wipe excess medication from eye with sterile cotton 1 minute after application.
5. Do not rinse eyes with sterile normal saline.

single-dose ampules or tubes) (see Guidelines box). The drug of choice until recently was either erythromycin or tetracycline because both were thought to afford protection against *Chlamydia trachomatis,* the major cause of ophthalmia neonatorum in the United States. Although silver nitrate is effective against gonococcal conjunctivitis, it was thought to be ineffective against *Chlamydia* and can cause a severe chemical conjunctivitis (American Academy of Pediatrics and American College of Obstetricians and Gynecologists, 1992). However, there is accumulating evidence that neither erythromycin nor tetracycline significantly reduces the incidence of chlamydial conjunctivitis and that silver nitrate may be more effective than erythromycin (Zanoni, Isenberg, and Apt, 1992). Although eye prophylaxis is mandatory in the United States, health care facilities are free to choose specific drugs. Effective prophylaxis may be better directed at treating maternal chlamydial infection.

Since studies on maternal attachment emphasize that in the first hour of life a newborn has a greater ability to focus on coordinated movement than at any other time during the next several days and since eye contact is very important in the development of maternal-infant bonding, the routine administration of silver nitrate or antibiotics can be postponed for up to 1 hour. However, there must be some kind of checklist to ensure that the drug is given within this time.

Vitamin K Administration. Shortly after birth, vitamin K is administered as a single intramuscular dose of 0.5 to 1 mg to prevent hemorrhagic disease of the newborn (see Chapter 9). Normally vitamin K is synthesized by the intestinal flora. However, since the infant's intestine is sterile at birth and since breast milk contains low levels of vitamin K, the supply is inadequate for at least the first 3 to 4 days. The major function of vitamin K is to catalyze the synthesis of prothrombin in the liver, which is needed for blood clotting and coagulation. The vastus lateralis muscle is the preferred injection site because of the absence of other well-developed muscle masses.

Hepatitis B (HBV) Vaccine Administration. To decrease the incidence of HBV in children and its serious consequences, cirrhosis and liver cancer, in adulthood, the first of three doses of HBV vaccine is recommended between birth and 2 days of age for uninfected newborns. It is recommended at birth for neonates whose mothers are positive for HBV surface antigen (HBsAg). The injection is given in the vastus lateralis muscle. This muscle is used because this site

is associated with a better immune response than the dorsogluteal area (a muscle typically not used in infants in the United States) (American Academy of Pediatrics, 1994b). (See also Immunizations, Chapter 10.)

Premature infants born to HBsAg-negative women should be vaccinated just before hospital discharge, provided the infant weighs 2000 g or more, or that the vaccination be delayed until 2 months of age if the infant weighs less than 2000 gs. Infants born to HBsAg-positive mothers should be immunized shortly after birth with HBV vaccine and hepatitis B immune globulin regardless of gestational age or birth weight (American Academy of Pediatrics, 1994b).

Newborn Screening for Disease. A number of genetic disorders can be detected in the newborn period. There is no national policy in the United States; therefore the extent of neonatal screening is determined by state laws and voluntary guidelines. Most states require screening for phenylketonuria (PKU), hypothyroidism, galactosemia, and sickle cell disease (see Chapters 9 and 26).

The American Academy of Pediatrics (1995) also recommends routine prenatal and perinatal human immunodeficiency virus (HIV) counseling and testing for all pregnant women and their newborns. Benefits of early identification of HIV-infected infants are aggressive nutritional supplementation; appropriate changes in their immunization schedule; monitoring and evaluating of immunologic, neurologic, and neuropsychologic functions for possible changes caused by antiretroviral therapy and initiation of special educational needs; evaluation for the need of other therapies, such as immunoglobulin for the prevention of bacterial infections; tuberculosis screening and treatment; and management of communicable disease exposures. As a result of virologic diagnostic techniques such as HIV culture, polymerase chain reaction (PCR), and immune complex-dissociated p24 antigen, diagnosis of HIV infection can be made in almost 50% of infants at birth and 95% or more of infants by 1 to 3 months of age.

The nurse's responsibility is to educate parents regarding the importance of screening and to collect appropriate specimens at the recommended time, preferably after 24 hours of age (Coody and others, 1993). However, with early discharge, adequate screening for PKU requires a follow-up screen within 3 weeks (American Academy of Pediatrics, 1992). Accurate screening depends on good-quality blood spots (see Atraumatic Care box on p. 204) on approved filter paper forms. The blood should completely saturate the filter paper spot on one side only. The paper should not be handled, placed on wet surfaces, or contaminated with substances, such as coffee or tea.

Bathing. Bath time can be an opportunity for the nurse to accomplish much more than general hygiene. It is an excellent time for observations of the infant's behavior, such as irritability, state of arousal, alertness, and muscular activity. Bathing is done after the vital signs have stabilized. There is no need to immediately wash a newborn, except to remove blood from the face and head. Cleansing only grossly soiled areas with soap and water rather than giving a daily bath does not increase infection rates in the hospital. As part of infection control, nurses should wear gloves when in contact with body substances such as amniotic fluid or vernix.

ATRAUMATIC CARE
Heel Punctures

Repeated heel lancing may be needed to obtain sufficient blood for the spot test. The use of automated lancet devices, such as Tenderfoot,* has been found to cause less pain and require fewer punctures than using manual lance blades (Blain-Lewis, 1992; Paes and others, 1993). EMLA, a topical anesthetic, also significantly reduces the pain of heel puncture (Fitzgerald, Millard, and McIntosh, 1989). Giving infants a plain pacifier or a sucrose solution during the procedure decreases the amount of crying (Campos, 1993; Haouari and others, 1995), but less behavioral upset may not indicate less physiologic stress.

*Manufactured by International Technidyne, Inc., Edison, NJ.

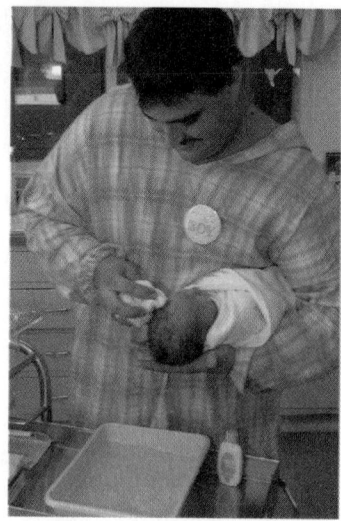

FIG. 8-14. Bath time is an excellent opportunity for parents to learn about their newborn.

Bath time provides an opportunity for the nurse to involve the parents in the care of their child, to teach correct hygiene procedures, and to learn about their infant's individual characteristics (Fig. 8-14). The appropriate types of bathing supplies and the need for safety in terms of water temperature and supervision of the infant at all times during the bath are stressed. For example, if sponges are used, they need to dry thoroughly between each use (may require a clothes dryer) to prevent growth of organisms.

Parents are encouraged to examine every finger and toe of their infant during bathing. Frequently normal variation such as Epstein pearls, mongolian spots, or "stork bites" cause parents much worry because they are unaware of the insignificance of such findings. Minor birth injuries may appear as major defects to them. Explaining how these occurred and when they will disappear reassures parents of their infant's normalcy. Common variations are discussed further in Chapter 9.

One of the most important considerations in skin cleansing is preservation of the skin's "acid mantle," which is formed from the uppermost horny layer of the epidermis, sweat, superficial fat, metabolic products, and external substances such as amniotic fluid, microorganisms, and cosmetics. The infant's skin surface has a pH of about 5 soon after birth, and the bacteriostatic effects of this pH are significant. Consequently, only plain warm water should be used for the bath. If a cleanser is needed, Dove is gentle and effective. Alkaline soaps such as Ivory, oils, powder, and lotions are not used, because they alter the acid mantle, thus providing a medium for bacterial growth. Talcum powder has the added risk of aspiration if it is applied too close to the infant's face. A safer alternative is a cornstarch-based powder (see also Diaper Dermatitis, Chapter 30).

Bathing should be done in the nursery after the vital signs have stabilized. Cleansing proceeds in the cephalo-caudal direction. A washcloth is used and turned so that a clean part touches the skin with each stroke. The eyes are carefully wiped from the inner to the outer aspect of the lid. The face is cleansed next. The nares are carefully inspected for any crusted secretions. The scalp is usually wiped, although it is sometimes necessary to shampoo the hair. Shampooing is best accomplished by positioning the infant's head over a small basin, lathering the scalp with a mild soap, and rinsing by pouring water from a small vessel over the head into the ba-

sin. The rest of the body should be covered during this procedure, and the head should be dried quickly to prevent heat loss from evaporation. The ears are cleaned with the twisted end of a washcloth, not with a cotton-tipped swab, which, if inserted into the canal, can damage the ear.

The rest of the body is washed in a similar manner. However, certain areas such as the folds of the neck, the axillae, and creases at joints need special attention. Vernix caseosa easily accumulates in the folds of the neck; therefore, the area should be thoroughly washed and dried. Vigorous scrubbing in order to remove vernix is not recommended, because it may disrupt the acid mantle of the skin.

The genitalia of both sexes require careful cleansing. Cleansing of the vulva is done in a front-to-back direction. The bath is a perfect opportunity to stress this part of hygiene to the mother, both for the infant's and for her own protection against urinary tract infection.

Cleansing the male genitalia involves washing the penis and scrotum. Sometimes smegma needs to be removed by wiping around the glans. The foreskin is not retracted, because it is normally tight in newborns.

Nursing ALERT   If an infant is not to be circumcised, the parents are taught how to cleanse under and around the foreskin by *retracting it gently only as far as it will go* and returning it to its normal position. Leaving the prepuce in a retracted position constricts the blood vessels supplying the glans penis, causing edema.

The buttocks and anal area are thoroughly cleansed of any fecal material. As with the rest of the body, the area is dried to prevent a warm, moist environment that fosters growth of bacteria.

A diaper is applied after the bath. It should fit snugly around the thighs and abdomen to prevent urine from leaking. In males cloth diapers should be folded with extra thickness in the front to provide greater absorbency. In females the placement of the extra fold depends on whether the infant is prone or supine. Diapers are fastened with the back side overlapping the front side to allow full flexion of the hips.

The nurse should discuss the choice of cloth or disposable diapers with parents. In the United States the most commonly used diapers are disposable paper diapers and either home-laundered or commercially laundered cloth diapers. A number of factors—cost, convenience, skin care benefits, infection control, and environmental concerns—influence the relative merits of these three diaper types. In general, home-laundered diapers are the least expensive when home labor cost is not included. Once home labor cost is included, the price difference between disposable diapers, diaper service reusable diapers, and home-laundered diapers is quite small, although paper diapers tend to cost the most. Disposable diapers are the most convenient, although a diaper service eliminates the need to shop for replacement diapers.

Disposable diapers with absorbent gelling material (AGM) have benefits related to preserving healthy skin, preventing diaper dermatitis (see Chapter 30), and controlling spread of infection because of their better containment of urine and feces.

The most controversial issue surrounding the discussion of disposable vs cloth diapers has been their effect on the environment. Disposable diapers are discarded as solid waste in landfills, whereas waste from laundered diapers is disposed of as treated sewage. The main differences between solid waste and treated sewage are cost and possibly sanitation, with solid waste being more expensive. However, the manufacture and disposal of cloth and paper diapers affect energy resources and the environment differently. Paper diapers consume more raw materials and generate more solid waste. Cloth diapers, especially home-laundered ones, use more water and energy and create more water and air pollution (Wong and others, 1992).

Care of the Umbilicus. Because the umbilical stump is an excellent medium for bacterial growth, various methods of cord care are practiced, such as the topical application of triple dye (a solution of brilliant green, proflavine hemisulfate, and crystal violet), bacitracin ointment, or povidone-iodine. Regardless of the type of treatment, the diaper is placed below the cord to avoid irritation and wetness on the site.

- Average separation time of 14 days using triple dye daily during hospitalization; average time of 10 days using povidone-iodine applied daily until cord separation; average separation time of 7 days using only a dry gauze dressing
- Delayed separation in infants with hyperbilirubinemia and septicemia, in infants delivered by cesarean section, in infants born prematurely, and in the second-born of twins

It takes a few more weeks for the cord base to heal completely following cord separation. During this time care consists of keeping the cord clean and dry and may include wiping the base with alcohol.

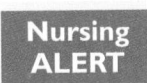 **Nursing ALERT** Instruct parents to report any signs of cord infection, such as presence of erythema and malodorous, purulent discharge, to their health care professional.

Circumcision. Circumcision, the surgical removal of the foreskin on the glans penis, is usually done in the hospital, although it is not a common practice in most countries. Despite the frequency of the procedure in the United States, there is much controversy regarding the benefits and risks (see box). In light of these arguments, parents must be allowed an *informed* consent regarding circumcision. Ideally, prospective parents should have an opportunity to examine all the facts and to decide for themselves (including choosing options for pain control and deciding whether or not they observe the procedure) without unnecessary pressure from health care professionals.

 Nursing ALERT Studies have shown conclusively that infants react to stimuli, such as pain. Therefore, nurses must consider their participation in a surgical procedure that involves no anesthesia to be a barbaric practice. Some anesthesia/analgesia is better than none. (See Atraumatic Care box.)

RISKS AND BENEFITS OF NEONATAL CIRCUMCISION

Risks	Benefits
Complications: Hemorrhage Infection Dehiscence (separation of approximated edges of skin) Meatitis (from loss of protective foreskin) Adhesions Concealed penis Urethral fistula Meatal stenosis Pain in unanesthetized infants (long-term consequences unknown, but short-term stresses include increased heart rate, behavior changes, prolonged crying, increased cortisol levels, and decreased blood oxygenation)	Prevention of penile cancer and posthitis (inflammation of prepuce) Decreased incidence of balanitis (inflammation of glans) and, possibly, urinary tract infection in infant males, as well as some sexually transmitted diseases later in life Prevention of complications associated with later circumcision Preservation of male's body image that is consistent with peers (in countries where procedure is common)

ATRAUMATIC CARE
Anesthesia to the Surgical Site

To reduce the pain of circumcision, a local dorsal penile nerve block (DPNB) can be administered at the base of the penis or into the foreskin at the level of the corona (Masciello, 1990). For maximum anesthesia, a waiting time of 5 minutes is needed for lidocaine and 3 minutes for chloroprocaine (Spencer and others, 1992). Buffering the lidocaine with 8.4% sodium bicarbonate in a 10:1 ratio, adding bupivacaine (a long-lasting anesthetic), and using a 30-gauge needle for the intradermal injection can reduce the pain associated with DPNB (Christoph and others, 1988; Rabinowitz and Hulbert, 1995). EMLA* cream (eutectic mixture of local anesthetics) provides a noninvasive form of local anesthesia (Benini and others, 1993).

*Manufactured by Astra Pharmaceuticals; for product information call (800) 228-EMLA.

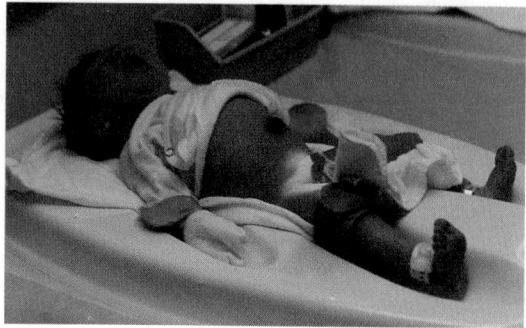

FIG. 8-15. *Proper positioning of infant in circumstraint.*

Circumcision is usually performed in the nursery. It should not be performed immediately after delivery because of the neonate's unstabilized physiologic status and increased susceptibility to stress. Preoperative nursing care includes allowing the infant nothing by mouth before the procedure to prevent aspiration of vomitus (about 2 hours), checking for a signed consent form, and adequately restraining the infant, usually on a special board (Fig. 8-15). All the equipment used for the procedure, such as gloves, instruments, dressings, and draping towels, must be sterile.

The procedure involves freeing the foreskin from the glans penis by using a scalpel, Gomco or Mogen (see Cultural Awareness box) clamp, or Plastibell. In the *Gomco technique* the foreskin is clamped and removed; the clamp crushes the nerve endings and blood vessels, promoting hemostasis. In the *Plastibell procedure* the foreskin is removed using a plastic ring and a string tied around the foreskin like a tourniquet. The excess foreskin is trimmed. In about 5 to 8 days the plastic ring separates and falls off.

As soon as the procedure is completed, the infant is released from the restraints and comforted. If the parents were not present during the procedure, they are informed of the infant's status and reunited with their son.

Care of the circumcision depends on the type of procedure. If a clamp was used, a petrolatum gauze dressing may be applied loosely to prevent adherence to the diaper. If the Plastibell was applied, no special dressing is required. Since the area is tender, the diaper is applied loosely to prevent friction against the penis; the first void is recorded.

NURSING TIP To check for the first void in disposable diapers made of absorbent gelling material, pinch the crotch of the diaper for a "clumpy, doughy" feeling, because these diapers will feel dry despite voiding.

Normally on the second day a yellowish white exudate forms as part of the granulation process. This is not a sign of infection and is not forcibly removed. As healing progresses, the exudate disappears. Parents are cautioned to report any evidence of bleeding, unusual swelling, or absence of voiding to the practitioner.

Provide Optimum Nutrition

Selection of a feeding method is one of the major decisions faced by parents. In general, there are three acceptable choices: human milk, commercially prepared cow's milk formula, and modified evaporated cow's milk. There are signifi-

CULTURAL AWARENESS
Circumcision

In the Jewish culture circumcision is performed during a highly significant ceremony called a *berith,* or *brit,* which takes place on the eighth day of life. A specially trained professional known as a *mohel* stretches the prepuce over the glans, pulling it though a slit in a shield (usually a Mogen clamp) and cutting it with a knife. The traditional technique is not sterile, and bleeding is controlled by tight bandaging around the penis (Cohen and others, 1992). The infant may be given some sweet wine before the procedure. Blankets instead of straps are usually used to restrain the infant to a board, and the parents are present (Trochtenberg, 1990).

Female circumcision (mutilation) is also practiced, particularly in Africa, the Middle East, and Southeast Asia—and in immigrants from these countries to the United States, Australia, Canada, and Europe. In the most extensive operation (excision or infibulation) the clitoris, labia minora, and medial aspects of labia majora are removed. The remaining labia majora are sewn closed, except for a small opening for urine and menses (McCleary, 1994). Anesthesia is used very rarely. In African and Asian cultures, female circumcision is used to prove virginity and to reduce sexual pleasure, thus promoting fidelity. The World Health Organization condemns all forms of female genital mutilation (Female genital mutilation, 1994).

cant nutritional, economic, and psychologic advantages and differences among these methods (see box on p. 207). Nurses need to be aware of the types of feeding to help parents choose the method that best meets their needs (see also Chapter 10).

Comparison of Human Milk and Cow's Milk. Although this discussion focuses on the differences between cow's milk and human milk, whole cow's milk is not recommended for infants less than 12 months of age. There are significant nutritional differences between human milk and whole cow's milk. Cow's milk contains much more available protein (3.5 g/dl) than human milk (0.7 g/dl), but more than the infant requires. The type of protein also differs. Human milk contains more whey proteins, especially lactalbumin, a more complete protein than casein protein. The higher percentage of casein in cow's milk results in the formation of large, hard curds. Human milk is more easily digested because of the presence of soft, flocculent curds. Therefore, stomach emptying time is more rapid with human milk, necessitating more frequent feedings. Human milk also contains a higher amount of cystine, an amino acid essential during the first few weeks of life, because the enzyme cystathionase, which converts methionine to cystine, is very low in newborns. Taurine, a conditionally essential amino acid (necessary under certain conditions, such as fetal development and early infancy), is also present in larger amounts in human milk. Taurine is involved in fat metabolism, retinal development, and auditory maturation.

Cow's milk and human milk both provide 20 kcal/ounce, but human milk contains a higher amount of lactose, a disaccharide that is converted into the monosaccharides glucose and galactose. Galactose is essential for the formation of galactolipids, which are necessary for the growth of the central nervous system.

ADVANTAGES OF HUMAN MILK VS COW'S MILK

Human Milk:

Contains adequate (not excessive) protein; has greater quantities of certain amino acids, including cystine and taurine

Contains more lactalbumin (produces easily digested curds) than casein (produces large, hard curds)

Contains more lactose, which in the gut stimulates growth of microorganisms, which synthesize some B vitamins and produce organic acids that may retard growth of harmful bacteria

Contains more monounsaturated fatty acids, which enhance absorption of fat and calcium

Contains adequate (not excessive) minerals with exception of fluoride (low in both)

Amounts of iron and zinc are low but more readily absorbed

Contains less calcium and phosphorus but a more favorable ratio of the minerals, which prevents excessive calcium excretion

Contains adequate amounts of vitamins A, B complex, and E; vitamin C content depends on maternal intake; vitamin D is low but more readily absorbed (vitamins C, D, and E are low in cow's milk, but K is higher)

Contains growth modulators that modify growth or maturation

Offers several immunologic benefits: contains various immunoglobulins (Ig), especially IgA; macrophages, granulocytes, T- and B-cell lymphocytes, and other factors that inhibit bacterial growth

Has laxative effect

Is economical, readily available, and sanitary

Has psychologic benefits of close bond between infant and mother during feeding

---

Although the amount of fat in both types of milk is similar, the type of fat differs. Human milk contains more monounsaturated fatty acids, especially linoleic acid, whereas cow's milk has more polysaturated fatty acids. Human milk has smaller fat globules than cow's milk, which enables the infant to absorb human milk fat more efficiently. In addition, the fat content of human milk varies during the feeding and with time of day. It is highest toward the end of feeding and at midday (Lawrence, 1994).

The mineral content of cow's milk is considerably greater than that of human milk, with the exception of iron and fluoride. Although the amount of iron is low in both types of milk, the iron in human milk is much better absorbed by the infant. Another difference is the amount of calcium and phosphorus, minerals especially needed by the rapidly growing infant. Cow's milk contains more of these minerals but a lower calcium-to-phosphorus ratio (1.5 to 1). Because of the infant's immature regulatory mechanisms, calcium is excreted, resulting in hypocalcemia, which may cause tetany. Human milk contains a smaller amount but more balanced proportion of these minerals, with a higher calcium-to-phosphorus ratio (2 to 1). Both types of milk contain adequate amounts of zinc, a mineral identified as essential to the human. However, the zinc in human milk is more readily absorbed. Both types of milk are low in fluoride, and supplementation is recommended (see Fluoride, Chapter 12).

Both human and cow's milk provide adequate amounts of vitamins A and B complex. Vitamin C is low in cow's milk but higher in human milk, assuming the mother's intake is adequate. Vitamin D is low in human milk but adequate, depending on the mother's intake and the infant's exposure to sunlight. Cow's milk and its preparations are usually fortified with vitamin D. Human milk contains only one fourth the amount of vitamin K as cow's milk, requiring supplementation at birth.

Although commercial cow's milk formulas are modified to closely resemble the nutritional content of human milk, other significant advantages to human milk exist. The presence of growth modulators, such as epidermal growth factor (EGF), appear to stimulate DNA synthesis and intestinal tract maturation. Human milk contains high levels of lysozyme activity and immunoglobulin A (IgA) and affords protection against several bacterial and viral diseases, especially those of the respiratory (including otitis media) and gastrointestinal systems. Human milk may protect against development of food allergies and enhances the active immune response to *Haemophilus influenzae* type B vaccine. In addition, human milk contains numerous other host defense factors, such as macrophages, granulocytes, and T- and B-lymphocytes.

There is preliminary evidence that human milk increases the child's intelligence, especially when fed to premature infants. Human milk may contain factors, such as long-chain lipids and hormones, that influence brain growth and maturation (Lanting and others, 1994). Other physiologic benefits of human milk are its laxative effect and less irritation of the skin from stools. Nonphysiologic advantages are discussed under Breast-feeding (p. 208).

Nursing ALERT Do not use microwaving to defrost frozen human milk. High-temperature microwaving (72° C to 98° C [162° to 208° F]) significantly destroys the anti-infective factors. The safety of low-temperature microwaving (20° to 53° C [68° to 127° F]) is questionable (Quan and others, 1992).

Evaporated Milk and Commercially Prepared Formulas. The analysis of human and cow's milk shows that whole cow's milk is unsuitable for infant nutrition. It must be diluted to meet the lowered protein requirement, but when dilute, it does not meet the caloric or fat requirement. Modified evaporated milk or commercially prepared formula is chosen as a substitute.

In the United States a very small percentage of infants are fed *evaporated milk formula.* However, it has many advantages over whole milk. It is readily available in cans, needs no refrigeration if unopened, is less expensive than commercial formula, provides a softer, more digestible curd, and contains more lactalbumin and a higher calcium-to-phosphorus ratio. A common rule for preparing evaporated milk formula is diluting the 13-ounce can of milk with 17 ounces of water and adding 1 to 2 tablespoons of sugar or corn syrup.

Evaporated milk must not be confused with condensed milk, which is a form of evaporated milk with 45% more sugar. Because of its high carbohydrate concentration and disproportionately low fat and protein content, condensed milk is not used for infant feeding. Likewise, skim milk must not be used because it is deficient in caloric concentration, significantly increases the renal solute load and water demands, and deprives the body of essential fatty acids.

Commercially prepared formulas are milk-based formulas that have been modified to closely resemble the nutritional content of human milk. However, they are not an exact substitute. For example, human milk has more cholesterol and saturated fatty acids than commercial formula. Total cholesterol levels are higher in breast-fed infants, although they decrease once weaning begins. If human milk provides optimum infant nutrition, some have questioned whether the lower cholesterol and higher polyunsaturated fats in commercial formula are sufficient (Kallio and others, 1992).

Commercial formulas are available in three preparations: (1) a ready-to-use form in cans or bottles, (2) a concentrated liquid form that is diluted with an equal amount of water, and (3) a powdered form that must be prepared according to the manufacturer's directions. One consideration in the use of commercially prepared formulas is their cost. Families should do comparison shopping, since one preparation can be considerably more expensive than another.

Breast-Feeding. *Human milk* is the preferred form of nutrition for the full-term infant. Unfortunately, the incidence of breast-feeding in the United States has been declining since its peak in 1982, when about 60% of mothers breast-fed their newborns. Although the incidence of breast-feeding decreased among all groups of women, the greatest decline occurred in women who were black, younger in age, low-income, poorly educated, enrolled in the Women, Infants, and Children (WIC) program, or parents of a low–birth-weight infant. Some believe that the increasingly early discharge of new mothers from hospitals, more aggressive marketing of infant formulas to the public, and increased number of employed mothers have contributed to the decline (Freed, 1993).

In addition to the physiologic qualities of human milk, the most outstanding psychologic benefit of breast-feeding is the close maternal-child relationship. The infant is nestled very close to the mother's skin, can hear the rhythm of her heartbeat, feel the warmth of her body, and sense a peaceful security. The mother has a very close feeling of union with her child and feels a sense of accomplishment and satisfaction as the infant sucks milk from her.

Human milk is the most economical form of feeding. It is always available, ready to serve at room temperature, and free of contamination. Although human milk is not sterile, healthy full-term infants can tolerate varying amounts of nonpathogenic and pathogenic organisms. The protection against infection can provide additional cost savings in terms of fewer medical visits and less time lost from work for the employed mother.

Breast-feeding may also offer protection against obesity and atherosclerosis, although the evidence is inconclusive. Breast-fed infants, especially beyond 2 to 3 months of age, tend to grow at a satisfactory but slower rate than bottle-fed infants (Dewey and others, 1991).

Contraindications to breast-feeding include (Lawrence, 1994):

- Hepatitis C virus (HCV) in mother
- Serious, debilitating maternal disease, such as heart disorder or advanced cancer
- Active tuberculosis not under treatment in mother
- Human immunodeficiency virus (HIV)
- Galactosemia in the infant

- Cytomegalovirus (CMV)—primary risk is to infants receiving CMV-infected donor milk, not to infected mother's infant who already has CMV

Mastitis is usually not a contraindication if the discomfort is tolerable. Rarely, "breast milk jaundice" may require temporary cessation of breast-feeding (see Chapter 9).

Breast-feeding can also be used with twin births (Sollid and others, 1989). If both twins are full term, they can begin feedings immediately after birth (Fig. 8-16). Simultaneous feeding promotes the rapid production of milk needed for both infants and makes the milk that would normally be lost in the let-down reflex available to one of the twins. When only one infant is hungry, the mother should feed singly. She should also alternate breasts when feeding each infant and avoid favoring one breast for one infant. The sucking patterns of infants vary, and each infant needs the visual stimulation and exercise that alternating breasts provides.

Probably the greatest disadvantage of breast-feeding to many mothers is the perceived inconvenience of loss of freedom and independence. Being committed to feeding the infant every 2 to 3 hours can be overwhelming, especially to women with multiple responsibilities. Many women resume their careers shortly after their pregnancy and prefer to use bottle-feeding. However, breast-feeding and employment are possible, especially with the use of breast pumping. Although breast-feeding is the preferred form of infant feeding, mothers' decisions regarding their preferences must be supported and respected.

Successful breast-feeding probably depends more on the mother's desire to breast-feed, satisfaction with breast-feeding, and available support systems than on any other factors. Contrary to popular belief, breast-feeding is not instinctive. Mothers need support, encouragement, and assistance during their postpartum hospital stay and at home to enhance their opportunities for success and satisfaction. The follow-

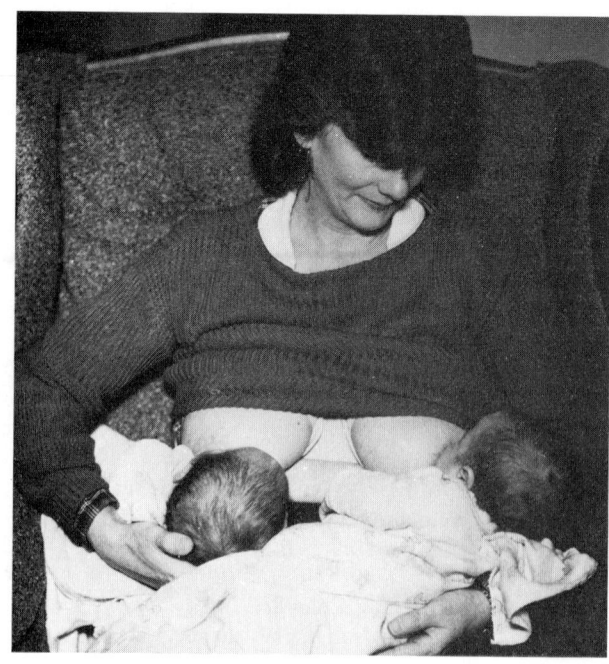

FIG. 8-16. Simultaneous breast-feeding of twins.

ing hospital interventions promote breast-feeding (Kurinij and Shiono, 1991):

- Routines, such as frequent and early breast-feeding, especially during the first hour of life; immediate skin-to-skin contact, rooming-in, feeding on demand, and careful control of drugs
- Direct modeling of the importance of breast-feeding by staff, such as implementing demand nursing with no formula supplementation and decreased emphasis on infant formula products
- Increased information and support to mothers, especially phone follow-up
- Nurses play a very significant role in the breast-feeding decision and must make themselves available to families for guidance and support. Several excellent books (Lawrence, 1994) and organizations, such as **LaLeche League,*** are available as resources for professionals and breast-feeding mothers.

Bottle-Feeding.   Bottle-feeding generally refers to the use of bottles for feeding commercial or evaporated milk formula rather than using the breast, although in some instances human milk may be expressed and fed with a bottle. Bottle-feeding is an acceptable method of feeding. However, nurses should not assume that new parents automatically know how to bottle-feed their infant. These parents also need support and assistance in meeting their infant's needs.

NURSING TIP An angled bottle is preferable to a straight bottle, because it encourages more physiologic positioning of the infant, improves the infant's comfort level, and decreases the need for burping (Farber, Van Fossen, and Koontz, 1995).

Providing newborns with nutrition is only one aspect of the feeding. Holding them close to the body while rocking or cuddling them helps to ensure the emotional component of feeding. Like breast-fed infants, bottle-fed infants need to be held on either side of the lap to expose them to different stimuli. The feeding should not be hurried. Even though they may suck vigorously for the first 5 minutes and seem to be

*P.O. Box 1209, Franklin Park, IL 60131-8209; (800) LA-LECHE. In Canada: 495 Main St., Winchester, Ontario, Canada K0C 2K0; (613) 448-1842.

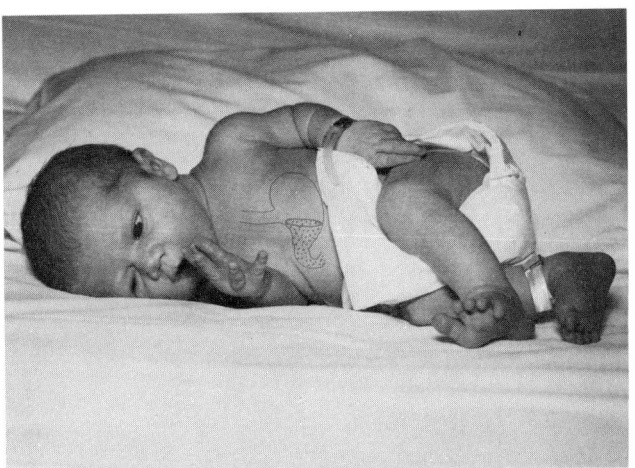

FIG. 8-17. Right-side–lying position after feeding.

satisfied, they are allowed to continue sucking. Infants need at least 2 hours of sucking a day. If there are six feedings per day, then about 20 minutes of sucking at each feeding provides for oral gratification.

After feedings infants are positioned on the right side to permit the feeding to flow toward the lower end of the stomach and to allow any swallowed air to rise above the fluid and through the esophagus (Fig. 8-17). This position prevents regurgitation and distention. To maintain the side-lying position, a pillow can be placed snugly behind the infant's back.

Propping the bottle is discouraged for the following reasons:

1. It denies the infant the important component of close human contact.
2. The infant may aspirate formula while sleeping.
3. It may facilitate the development of middle ear infections. As the infant lies flat and sucks, milk that has pooled in the pharynx becomes a suitable medium for bacterial growth. Bacteria then enter the eustachian tube, which leads to the middle ear, causing acute otitis media.
4. It encourages continuous pooling of formula in the mouth, which can lead to bottle caries when the teeth erupt (see Chapter 12).

Preparation of Formula.   The two traditional ways of preparing formula are the terminal heat method (all the utensils and formula are boiled together for 25 minutes) and the aseptic method (the equipment is boiled separately, after which the formula is poured into the bottles). Because of improved sanitary conditions in developed countries, neither of these methods is essential. The clean technique is satisfactory, including using a dishwasher. Persons preparing the formula wash their hands well and then wash all the equipment used to prepare the formula, including the cans of formula or evaporated milk. The formula is prepared and bottled immediately before each feeding. Warming the formula is optional, although many parents prefer to warm it before feeding. Any milk remaining in the bottle after the feeding is discarded, since it is an excellent medium for bacterial growth. Opened cans of formula are covered and refrigerated until the next feeding.

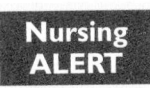
Nursing ALERT   Warming bottles in the microwave oven is not recommended because of the risk of burns from bottles exploding or from the hot temperature of the fluid.

Recommendations for labeling infant formulas require that the directions for preparation and use of the formula include pictures and symbols for nonreading individuals. In addition, manufacturers are translating the directions into foreign languages, such as Spanish and Vietnamese, to prevent misunderstanding and errors in formula preparation.

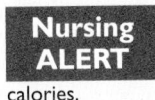
Nursing ALERT   Impress on families that the proportions *must not be altered*—neither diluted to extend the amount of formula nor concentrated to provide more calories.

Feeding Schedules.   Ideally, feeding schedules should be determined by the infant's hunger. *Demand feedings* involve feeding infants when they signal readiness. *Scheduled feedings* are arranged at predetermined intervals. Some hospitals routinely feed infants every 4 hours. Although this is satisfactory for bottle-fed infants, it hinders the breast-feeding process. Since breast-fed infants tend to be hungry every 2 to 3 hours because of the easy digestibility of the milk, they should be fed on demand.

Supplemental feedings should *not* be offered to breast-fed infants before lactation is well established, because these feedings may satiate the infant and may cause nipple preference. Supplemental water is not needed in breast-fed infants, even in hot climates (Sachdev and others, 1991). Satiated infants suck less vigorously at the breast, and milk depends on the breast being emptied at each feeding. If milk is allowed to accumulate in the ducts, causing breast engorgement, ischemia results, suppressing the activity of the acini, or milk-secreting cells. Consequently, milk production is reduced. In addition, the process of sucking from a bottle is different from breast-nipple compression. The relatively inflexible rubber nipple prevents the tongue from its usual rhythmic action. Infants learn to put the tongue against the nipple holes to slow down the more rapid flow of fluid. When infants use these same tongue movements during breast-feeding, they may push the human nipple out of the mouth and may not grasp the areola properly (Lawrence, 1994).

Usually by 3 weeks of age lactation and a feeding schedule are well established. Bottle-fed infants retain about 2 to 3 ounces of formula at each feeding and are fed about six times a day. The quantity of formula consumed is based on the caloric need of 108 kcal/kg; therefore, a newborn who weighs 3 kg requires 324 kcal/day. Since commercial formula has 20 kcal/oz, about 16 ounces (480 ml) will provide the daily caloric requirement. Breast-fed infants may feed as frequently as 10 to 12 times a day. Larger infants are able to retain increased amounts because of greater stomach capacity; as a result, they generally sleep through the night sooner than smaller infants or breast-fed infants.

Feeding Behavior. Five fairly distinct behavioral stages occur during successful feeding (O'Grady, 1971). Recognizing these steps can assist nurses in identifying potential feeding problems caused by improper feeding techniques. *Prefeeding behavior,* such as crying or fussing, demonstrates the infant's level of arousal and degree of hunger. To encourage the infant to grasp the breast properly, it is preferable to begin feeding during the quiet alert state, before the infant becomes upset. *Approach behavior* is indicated by sucking movements or the rooting reflex. *Attachment behavior* includes those activities that occur from the time the infant receives the nipple and sucks (sometimes more pronounced during initial attempts at breast-feeding). *Consummatory behavior* consists of coordinated sucking and swallowing. Persistent gagging might indicate unsuccessful consummatory behavior. *Satiety behavior* is observed when infants let the parent know that they are satisfied, usually by falling asleep.

Promote Parent-Infant Bonding (Attachment)

The process of parenting is based on a mutual relationship between parent and infant. Although the words "bonding" and "attachment" are sometimes referred to as separate phenomena, with *bonding* representing the development of

emotional ties from parent to infant and *attachment* representing the emotional ties from infant to parent, in this discussion the words are used interchangeably to denote both processes.

As more is learned about the complexity of neonates and about their potential for influencing and shaping their environments, particularly their interaction with significant others, it is apparent that promoting positive parent-child relationships necessitates an understanding of factors involved in identifying behavioral steps in attachment, variables that enhance or hinder this process, and methods of teaching parents ways to develop a stronger relationship with their children, especially by recognizing potential problems.

Infant Behavior. Nurses must appreciate the individuality and uniqueness of each infant. According to the infant's temperament, the infant will change and shape the environment, which will undoubtedly influence future development. Obviously, an infant who sleeps 20 hours a day will be exposed to fewer stimuli than the infant who sleeps 16 hours a day. In turn, each infant is likely to effect a different response from parents. The infant who is quiet, undemanding, and passive may receive much less attention than the infant who is responsive, alert, and active. Behavioral characteristics such as irritability and consolability can influence the ease of transition to parenthood and the parent's perception of the infant.

Nurses can positively influence the attachment of parent and child. The first step is recognizing individual differences and explaining to parents that such characteristics are normal. For example, some people believe that infants sleep throughout the day, except for feedings. For some newborns this may be true, but for many it is not. Understanding that the infant's wakefulness is part of biologic rhythm and not a reflection of inadequate parenting can be crucial in promoting healthy parent-child relationships. Another aspect of helping parents involves supplying guidelines on how to enhance the infant's development during awake periods. Placing the child in a crib to stare at the same mobile every day is not particularly exciting, but carrying the infant into each room as one does daily chores can be fascinating. Simple suggestions can make life very stimulating for the infant and much more pleasurable and gratifying for the parents (see box).

Maternal Attachment. Research has suggested that there is a *maternal sensitive period* immediately and for a

---

HOW TO MAKE THE INFANT'S WORLD MORE EXCITING*

Infant prefers animated and auditory objects.

Infant enjoys novelty, quickly tires of seeing same objects; mobile should be changed frequently.

Infant prefers to look at medium-intensity colors and contrasting colors, such as black and white.

Infant likes geometric shapes and checkerboards; prefers patterns over straight lines.

Contrasting lights and reflective surfaces such as mirrors are especially interesting.

But most of all, nothing is as fascinating as the human face and voice!

*Objects should be placed about 20 cm (8 inches) away from infant.

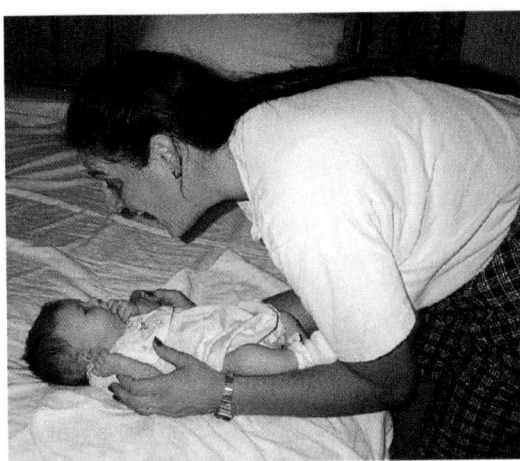

FIG. 8-18. *En face* position between parent and infant can be significant in attachment process.

short time after birth, when parents have a unique ability to attach to their infants (Klaus, Kennell, and Klaus, 1995). Mothers demonstrate a predictable and orderly pattern of behavior during the development of the attachment process. When mothers are presented with their nude infants, they begin examining the infant with their fingertips, concentrating on touching the extremities, and then proceed to massage and encompass the trunk with their entire hands. Assuming the *en face position,* in which the mother's and the infant's eyes meet in visual contact in the same vertical plane, is significant in the formation of affectional ties (Fig. 8-18). Although similar patterns of touching have been observed, additional studies demonstrate different patterns for mothers. Consequently, nurses must exercise caution in interpreting behaviors such as touching.

Several studies have attempted to substantiate the long-term benefits of providing parents with opportunities to optimally bond with their infant during the initial postpartum period. Although there has been some evidence that increased parent-child contact encourages prolonged breast-feeding and may minimize the risks of parenting disorders, conclusions about the long-term effects of such early intervention on parenting and child development must be viewed tentatively and cautiously. In addition, some authorities claim that the emphasis on bonding has been unjustified and may lead to guilt and fear in those parents who did not receive early contact with their infant. There is also concern over the literal interpretation of "sensitive" or "critical" to imply that without early contact optimum bonding cannot occur or, conversely, that early contact alone is sufficient to ensure competent parenting.

Certainly, it should be stressed to parents that while early bonding may be valuable, it does not represent an "all or none" phenomenon. Throughout the child's life there will be multiple opportunities for the development of parent-child attachment. Bonding is a complex process that develops gradually and is influenced by numerous factors, only one of which is the type of initial contact between the newborn and parent.

Another component of successful maternal attachment is the concept of *reciprocity* (Brazelton, 1974). As the mother responds to the infant, the infant must respond to the mother by some signal such as sucking, cooing, eye contact, grasping, or molding (conforming to the other's body during close physical contact). The first step is *initiation,* in which interaction between infant and parent begins. Next is *orientation,* which establishes the partners' expectation of each other during the interaction. Following orientation is *acceleration* of the attention cycle to a peak of excitement. The infant reaches out and coos, both arms jerk forward, the head moves backward, the eyes dilate, and the face brightens. After a short time *deceleration* of the excitement and *turning away* occur, in which the infant's eyes shift away from the mother's and the child grasps his or her own shirt. During this cycle of nonattention, repeated verbal or visual attempts to reinitiate the infant's attention are ineffective. This deceleration and turning away probably prevent the infant from being overwhelmed by excessive stimuli. In a good interaction both partners have synchronized their attention-nonattention cycles. Parents or other caregivers who do not allow the infant to turn away and who continually attempt to maintain visual contact encourage the infant to turn off the attention cycle and thus prolong the nonattention phase.

Although this description of reciprocal interacting behavior is usually observed in the infant by 2 to 3 weeks of age, nurses can use this information to teach parents how to interact with their infant. Recognizing the attention vs nonattention cycles and understanding that the latter is not a rejection of the parent helps parents develop competence in parenting.

Paternal Engrossment.   Fathers also show specific attachment behaviors to the newborn. This process of *paternal engrossment,* forming a sense of absorption, preoccupation, and interest in the infant, includes (1) visual awareness of the newborn, especially focusing on the beauty of the child, (2) tactile awareness, often expressed in a desire to hold the infant, (3) awareness of distinct characteristics with emphasis on those features of the infant that resemble the father, (4) perception of the infant as perfect, (5) development of a strong feeling of attraction to the child that leads to intense focusing of attention on the infant, (6) experiencing a feeling of extreme elation, and (7) feeling a sense of deep self-esteem and satisfaction. These responses are greatest during the early contacts with the infant and are intensified by the neonate's normal reflex activity, especially the grasp reflex and visual alertness. In addition to behavioral reactions, fathers also demonstrate physiologic responses such as increased heart rate and blood pressure during interactions with their newborns.

The process of engrossment has significant implications for nurses. It is imperative to recognize the importance of early father–infant contact in releasing these behaviors. Fathers need to be encouraged to express their positive feelings, especially if such emotions are contrary to the cultural belief that fathers should remain stoic. If this is not clarified, fathers may feel confused and attempt to suppress the natural sensations of absorption, preoccupation, and interest in order to conform with societal expectations.

Mothers also need to be aware of the responses of the father toward the newborn, especially since one of the consequences of paternal preoccupation with the infant is less overt attention toward the mother. If both parents are able to share their feelings, each can appreciate the process of attachment toward their child and will avoid the unfortunate conflict of being insensitive and unaware of the other's needs. In addition, a father who is encouraged to form a relationship with his newborn is less likely to feel excluded and abandoned once the family returns home and the mother directs her attention toward caring for the infant.

Ideally the process of engrossment should be discussed with parents before the delivery, such as in prenatal classes, to reinforce the father's awareness of his natural feelings toward the expected child. Focusing on the future experience of seeing, touching, and holding one's newborn may also help expectant fathers become more comfortable in accepting their paternal feelings toward the unborn child. This in turn can assist them in being more supportive toward the mother, especially as the labor and delivery event draws near.

At the infant's birth the nurse can play a vital role in helping the father to release or express engrossment by assessing the neonate in front of the couple; pointing out normal characteristics, especially the grasp reflex, encouraging identification through consistent referral to the child by name; encouraging the father to cuddle, hold, talk to, or feed the infant; and demonstrating whenever necessary the soothing powers of caressing, stroking, and rocking the child (Fig. 8-19). Fathers are encouraged to be with the mother during labor and delivery and to spend time alone with the mother and newborn after delivery. Whenever possible, the father should "room in" with the mother.

The nurse observes for the same indications of affection toward the child from the father as those expected in the mother, such as visual contact in the en face position and embracing the infant close to the body. When present, such behaviors are reinforced. If such responses are not obvious, the nurse needs to assess the father's feelings regarding this birth, cultural beliefs that may prevent his expression of emotions, and other factors in order to help him facilitate a positive attachment during this critical period.

Siblings.   Although the attachment process has been discussed almost exclusively in terms of the parents and infants, it is essential that nurses be aware of other family members, such as siblings and members of the extended family, who need preparation for the acceptance of this new child. Young children in particular need sensitive preparation for the birth to minimize sibling jealousy.

There is an increasing trend to allow siblings to visit the mother on the postpartum unit and to hold the newborn (Fig. 8-20). Another trend has been siblings witnessing the birth. Unlike sibling visitation, the evidence supporting this practice is much more controversial and conflicting. Children exhibit different degrees of involvement in the birth process. Young children often fall asleep toward the end of delivery. Some reported benefits include children's increased knowledge of the birth process, less regressive behavior following the birth, and more mothering and caregiving behavior toward the infant. Some practitioners add facilitated family bonding and assimilation of the newborn into the family as positive outcomes (Stanford and others, 1992). Parents whose children attended the birth have echoed these same benefits and have expressed their desire to repeat the experience should another pregnancy occur. Despite these positive findings, opponents believe that allowing children to observe a delivery could lead to emotional difficulties (Sugar, 1991), although there is no research to support this contention. As research mounts, birthing centers that allow siblings at the birth are developing more definitive guidelines, such as an age requirement of at least 4 to 5 years, the presence of a supportive person for the sibling only, and an adequate sequence of preparation in which parents explore all options for preparing their other children.

From observations during sibling visitation there is evidence that sibling attachment occurs. However, the en face position is assumed much less often among the newborn and siblings than between mother and newborn, and when this position is used, it is brief. Siblings focus more on the head

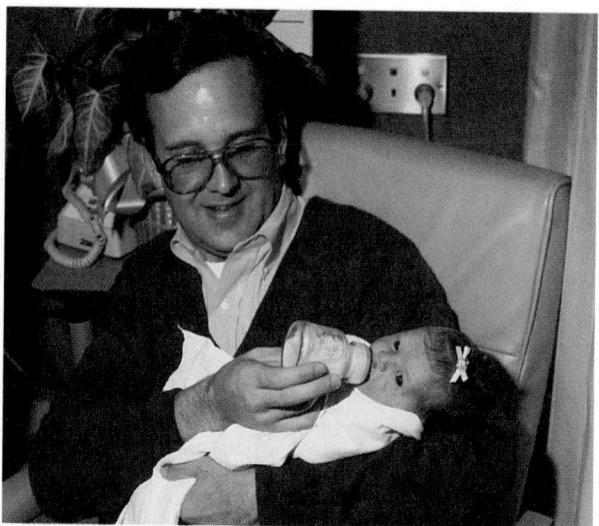

FIG. 8-19. A desire to hold the infant and participate in caregiving activities is an indication of paternal engrossment.

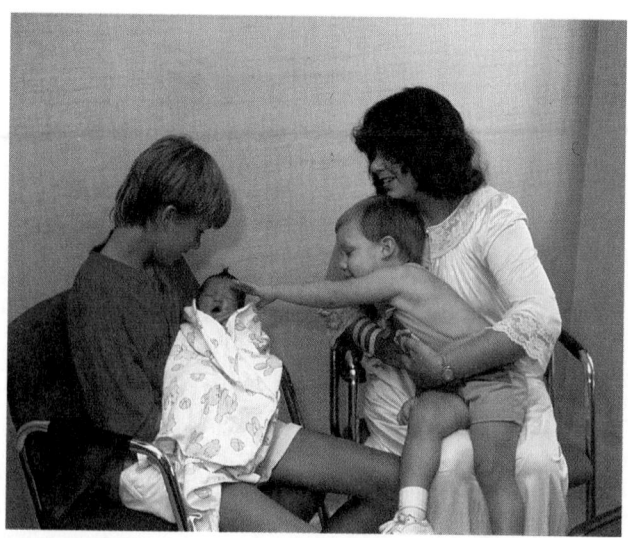

FIG. 8-20. Sibling visitation shortly after birth can be significant in the attachment process.

or face than on touching or talking to the infant. The siblings' verbalizations are focused less on attracting the infant's attention and more on addressing the mother about the newborn. Children who have established a prenatal relationship with the fetus have demonstrated more attachment behaviors, supporting the suggestion of encouraging prenatal acquaintance. Additional research is needed to establish theories on sibling bonding as have been constructed for parental bonding.

Minimal research is available on bonding and multiple births, and even less is known about paternal engrossment and sibling attachment. In regard to maternal-twin bonding, the conclusions of different authors vary. Some report that mothers bond equally to each twin at the time of birth, even if one twin is ill (Abbink, 1982). Others suggest that mothers of twins may take months or even years to form individual attachments to each child and even longer if the twins are identical.

Nurses can be instrumental in promoting bonding of multiple births. The most important principle is to assist the parents in recognizing the individuality of the children, especially in monozygotic (identical) twins. The mother should visit with each newborn, including a sick infant, as much as possible after birth. Rooming-in and breast-feeding are encouraged. Any characteristics that are unique to each child are emphasized, and each infant is called by name, rather than calling them "the twins." Asking the family questions such as "How do you tell Sally and Amy apart?" and "In what ways are Sally and Amy different and similar?" helps point out their individual characteristics (Anderson and Anderson, 1990). The Brazelton Neonatal Behavioral Assessment Scale (BNBAS) can be used to illustrate these differences and to stress effective strategies for dealing with multiple personalities at the same time.

Another area of attachment that has received minimal attention is maternal bonding of multiparous mothers. Research suggests that there are several additional tasks to "taking on" a second child. These include the following (Walz, 1983):

- Promoting acceptance and approval of the second child
- Grieving and resolving the loss of an exclusive dyadic relationship with the first child
- Planning and coordinating family life to include a second child
- Reformulating a relationship with the first child
- Identifying with the second child by comparing with the first child for physical and psychologic characteristics
- Assessing one's affective capabilities in providing sufficient emotional support and nurturance simultaneously to two children

Employed mothers who have a second child report fewer concerns regarding general aspects of separation from their child and the effect of separation on the child, but similar concerns regarding separation due to employment. It appears that although experience may decrease some concerns, it may not minimize others.

Prepare for Discharge and Home Care

With increasingly shorter maternity admissions, as well as a trend toward *mother-infant care,* also called *dyad* or *couplet care,* discharge planning, referral, and home visiting have become important components of comprehensive care. First-time, as well as "experienced," parents benefit from guidance and assistance with the infant's care, such as breast- or for-

mula feeding, and with the family's integration of a new member, particularly sibling adjustment.

To assess and meet these needs, teaching must begin early, ideally *before the birth.* Not only is the admission time short (typically 24 to 48 hours), but also mothers are in the *taking-in phase,* where they demonstrate passive and dependent behaviors. Therefore, on the first postpartum day women may not be able to absorb large amounts of information (Ament, 1990). Rather, this time may be better spent highlighting essential aspects of care, such as infant feeding, rather than teaching infant bathing with a return demonstration. Parents can also be given a list of mother and infant care topics as part of the nursing admission history to choose issues they wish to review.

Many concerns exist regarding early discharge, especially lack of support for breast-feeding, delayed diagnosis of jaundice, and incomplete screening for phenylketonuria and congenital hypothyroidism (Charles and Prystowsky, 1995). To better meet the needs of mothers being discharged soon after delivery, some institutions have implemented programs to provide early follow-up postpartum care at no additional cost to the mother (Weinberg, 1994).

With family structures changing, it is essential that nurses identify the primary caregiver, which may not be the mother but a father, grandparent, or baby-sitter (Carlson, 1993). Also, nurses should not assume that terminology associated with mother-infant care is understood. Words relating to the anatomy (e.g., "meconium," "labia," "edema," and "genitalia") and to breast-feeding (e.g., "areola," "colostrum," and "let-down reflex") may be unfamiliar to mothers. Mothers with other children do not necessarily understand more words, and young age and less education decrease comprehension (DiFlorio, 1991).

An essential area of discharge counseling is the safe transportation of the newborn home from the hospital. Ideally this information should also be provided *before* delivery to allow parents an opportunity to purchase a suitable infant car restraint.

When purchasing a car restraint, parents should consider cost and convenience. The convertible-type seats are more expensive initially but cost less than two separate systems. Convenience is a major factor, because a cumbersome restraint may be used less and improperly. Before buying a restraint, it is best to try out different models. For example, some types are too large for subcompact cars. Asking friends about the advantages and disadvantages of their restraints is helpful, but borrowing their car seat or purchasing a used one can be dangerous. Parents should use only a restraint that has directions for use and a certification label stating that it complies with Federal Motor Vehicle Safety standards (both should be on the seat). They should not use a restraint that has been involved in a crash. Some service clubs and hospitals have loan programs for restraints. Information about approved models and other aspects of car restraints is available from several organizations and sources.*

---

*American Academy of Pediatrics, 141 Northwest Point Blvd., P.O. Box 927, Elk Grove Village, IL 60007, (800) 433-9016; and local division of traffic safety or **National Highway Traffic Safety Administration Auto Safety Hotline,** (800) 424-9393. Guidelines for car seat safety are available in Wong DL: *Wong and Whaley's Clinical manual of pediatric nursing* ed 4, St Louis, 1996, Mosby.

NURSING CARE PLAN
The Normal Newborn and Family

NURSING DIAGNOSIS: Ineffective airway clearance related to excess mucus, improper positioning

PATIENT GOAL I: Will maintain a patent airway

• **NURSING INTERVENTIONS/RATIONALES**

Suction mouth and nasopharynx with bulb syringe as needed
  Compress bulb before insertion and aspirate pharynx, then nose, *to prevent aspiration of fluid*
With mechanical suction, limit each suctioning attempt to 5 seconds with sufficient time between attempts *to allow reoxygenation*
Position infant on right side after feeding *to prevent aspiration*
Position infant supine or on side during sleep as recommended by American Academy of Pediatrics
Perform as few procedures as possible on infant during first hour and have oxygen ready for use if respiratory distress should develop
Take vital signs according to institutional policy and more frequently if necessary
  Observe for signs of respiratory distress and report any of the following immediately:
    Tachypnea
    Grunting, stridor
    Abnormal breath sounds
    Flaring alae nasi
    Cyanosis or pallor
Keep diapers, clothing, and blankets loose enough *to allow maximum lung (abdominal) expansion and to avoid overheating*
Clean nares of any crusted secretions during bath or when necessary
Check for patent nares

• **EXPECTED OUTCOMES**

Airway remains patent
Breathing is regular and unlabored
Respiratory rate is within normal limits (see inside back cover for normal limits)

NURSING DIAGNOSIS: High risk for altered body temperature related to immature temperature control, change in environmental temperature

PATIENT GOAL I: Will maintain stable body temperature

• **NURSING INTERVENTIONS/RATIONALES**

Wrap infant snugly in a warmed blanket
Place infant in a preheated environment (under radiant warmer or next to mother)
Place infant on a padded, covered surface

*Dependent nursing action.

Take infant's temperature on arrival at nursery or mother's room; proceed according to hospital policy regarding method and frequency of monitoring
Maintain room temperature between 24° and 25.5° C (75° to 78° F) and humidity about 40% to 50%
Give initial bath according to hospital policy
  Prevent chilling of infant during bath
  Postpone bath if there is any question regarding stabilization of body temperature
  Dress infant in a shirt and diaper and swaddle in a blanket or cover with blanket
Provide infant with a head covering if heat loss is a problem, *since large surface area of head favors heat loss*
Keep infant away from drafts, air conditioning vents, or fans
Place infant in a recessed cubicle with high-enough walls to *shield from cross-ventilation*
Warm all objects used to examine or cover infant (e.g., place them under radiant warmer)
Uncover only one area of body for examination or procedures
Postpone circumcision until after temperature stabilizes or use radiant warmer during procedure
Be alert to signs of hypothermia or hyperthermia

• **EXPECTED OUTCOME**

Infant's temperature remains at optimum level (36.5° to 37.5° C [97.7° to 99.5° F])

NURSING DIAGNOSIS: High risk for infection or inflammation related to deficient immunologic defenses, environmental factors, maternal disease

PATIENT GOAL I: Will exhibit no evidence of infection

• **NURSING INTERVENTIONS/RATIONALES**

Wash hands before and after caring for each infant
Wear gloves when in contact with body secretions
Use of cover gowns is controversial *because studies show they do not decrease infection rates but do increase costs*
Make certain appropriate eye prophylaxis has been carried out
Check eyes daily for evidence of inflammation or discharge
Keep infant from potential sources of infection (e.g., persons with respiratory or skin infections, improperly prepared food sources, other unclean items)
Clean vulva in posterior direction *to prevent fecal contamination of vagina or urethra;* stress this to parents
While cleaning penis, do not retract foreskin; gently wipe away smegma
Maintain asepsis during circumcision
*If infant has been circumcised, cover area with a petrolatum jelly gauze (if ordered)
Check for voiding after circumcision; disposable diaper may feel dry when wet, but crotch area of diaper will feel "clumpy" or "doughy" and heavy
Keep umbilical stump clean and dry
Place diapers below umbilical stump
Assess cord daily for odor, color, and drainage
*Apply antibacterial agent and/or alcohol to cord as ordered
*Administer hepatitis B vaccine (HBV) in vastus lateralis

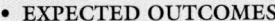

NURSING CARE PLAN
The Normal Newborn and Family—cont'd

- **EXPECTED OUTCOMES**

Infant exhibits no evidence of infection or inflammation
Eyes remain clear with no evidence of irritation
Genital area is free of irritation
Cord appears dry, surrounding area free of infection
Infant receives HBV vaccine

> **NURSING DIAGNOSIS:** High risk for trauma related to physical helplessness

PATIENT GOAL 1: Will be clearly and correctly identified

- **NURSING INTERVENTIONS/*RATIONALES***

Make certain infant is properly identified *for placement with correct mother*
 Ensure that identification (ID) band(s) are properly and securely placed
 Check infant's ID band often *to ensure correct infant identity*
Discuss safety issues with parents, especially mother, *to prevent "switching" of infants and possible kidnapping*
Observe staff's ID badge and give infant only to properly identified personnel
Never leave infant alone in crib or room

- **EXPECTED OUTCOMES**

Infant is clearly and correctly identified
Parents observe safety practices
ID band remains in place

PATIENT GOAL 2: Will have no physical injury

- **NURSING INTERVENTIONS/*RATIONALES***

Avoid using rectal thermometer *because of risk of rectal perforation*
Never leave infant unsupervised on a raised surface without sides
Always close diaper pins (if used) and place them away from infant's body
Keep pointed or sharp objects away from infant
Keep own fingernails short and trimmed; avoid jewelry that can scratch infant
Employ appropriate methods of handling and transporting infant

- **EXPECTED OUTCOME**

Infant remains free of physical injury

PATIENT GOAL 3: Will exhibit no evidence of bleeding

- **NURSING INTERVENTIONS/*RATIONALES***

*Administer vitamin K intramuscularly, using vastus lateralis muscle as site of injection
Check circumcision site; assess for any oozing *that may indicate bleeding tendencies*

---
*Dependent nursing action.

- **EXPECTED OUTCOME**

Infant exhibits no evidence of bleeding

> **NURSING DIAGNOSIS:** Altered nutrition: less than body requirements (high risk) related to immaturity, parental knowledge deficit

PATIENT GOAL 1: Will receive optimum nutrition

- **NURSING INTERVENTIONS/*RATIONALES***

Assess strength of suck and coordination with swallowing *to identify possible problem affecting feeding*
Offer initial intake according to parent's preference, hospital policy, and practitioner's protocol
Prepare for demand feeding of breast-fed infants; night feedings determined by condition and preferences of mother
Offer bottle-fed infants 2 to 3 ounces of formula every 3 to 4 hours or on demand
Support and assist breast-feeding mothers during initial feedings and more frequently if necessary
Avoid routine water or supplemental feedings for breast-feeding infants because they may *decrease the desire to suck and cause nipple preference*
Encourage father or other support person to remain with mother to help her and infant with positioning, relaxation, and reinforcement
Encourage father or other support person to participate in bottle-feeding
Place infant on right side after feeding *to prevent aspiration*
Observe stool pattern

- **EXPECTED OUTCOMES**

Infant demonstrates strong suck
Infant retains feedings
Infant receives an adequate amount of nutrients (specify amount and frequency of feedings)
Infant loses less than 10% of birth weight

> **NURSING DIAGNOSIS:** Altered family processes related to maturational crisis, birth of term infant, change in family unit

PATIENT (FAMILY) GOAL 1: Will exhibit parent-infant attachment behaviors

- **NURSING INTERVENTIONS/*RATIONALES***

As soon after delivery as possible encourage parents to see and hold infant; place newborn close to face of parents *to establish visual contact*
Ideally, perform eye care after initial meeting of infant and parents, within 1 hour after birth *when infant is alert and most likely to visually relate to parent*
Identify for parents specific behaviors manifested by infant (e.g., alertness, ability to see, vigorous suck, rooting behavior, and attention to human voice)
Discuss with parents their expectations of fantasy child vs real child if indicated

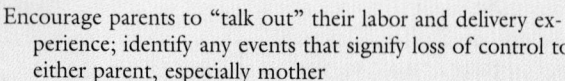

NURSING CARE PLAN
The Normal Newborn and Family—cont'd

Encourage parents to "talk out" their labor and delivery experience; identify any events that signify loss of control to either parent, especially mother

Identify behavioral steps in attachment process and evaluate those aspects that could be considered positive and those that may represent inadequate or delayed parenting

Encourage family to call for infant frequently if not rooming-in

Observe and assess reciprocity of cues between infant and parent *to identify behaviors that may need strengthening*

Assist parents in recognizing attention-nonattention cycles and in understanding their significance

Assess variables affecting development of attachment through observing infant and parent and interviewing each parent or other significant caregiver

• **EXPECTED OUTCOMES**

Parents establish contact with infant immediately or soon after birth

Parents demonstrate attachment behaviors, such as touch, eye contact, naming and calling infant by name, talking to infant, participating in caregiving activities

Parents recognize attention-nonattention cycles

PATIENT (SIBLING) GOAL 2: Will demonstrate adjustment/attachment behaviors toward newborn

• **NURSING INTERVENTIONS/*RATIONALES***

Allow to visit and touch newborn when feasible

Explain physical differences in newborn, such as bald head, umbilical stump and clamp, circumcision, *to lessen any fear siblings might have*

Explain to siblings realistic expectations regarding newborn's abilities and needs
    Requires complete care
    Is not a playmate

Encourage siblings to participate in care at home *to make them feel part of the experience*

Encourage parents to spend individual time with other children at home *to reduce feelings of jealousy toward new sibling*

• **EXPECTED OUTCOME**

Siblings express interest in newborn and realistic expectations for their age

PATIENT (FAMILY) GOAL 3: Will be prepared for discharge and home care

• **NURSING INTERVENTIONS/*RATIONALES***

Discuss with parents correct preparation of formula:
    Stress that proportions must not be altered to dilute or concentrate the formula
    Discourage microwaving of bottles *to avoid burns*

Encourage use of support persons, such as lactation specialist or members of La Leche League, for assistance with breast-feeding

Instruct in other aspects of newborn care:
    Bathing
    Umbilical and circumcision care
    Recognize states of activity for optimum interaction (see Table 8-3)

Encourage participation in parenting classes, if offered

Discuss importance and proper use of federally approved car restraints
    If infant is small, advise parents to use rolled blankets and towels in crotch area to *prevent slouch and along sides to minimize lateral movement,* but never use padding underneath or behind infant, *since it creates slackness in harness, leading to possible ejection from seat in a crash*
    Refer to organizations that may rent car restraints

If parent-infant attachment is at risk, refer to appropriate agencies (social services, family and child services, at-risk programs)

• **EXPECTED OUTCOMES**

Family demonstrates ability to provide care for infant

Family keeps appointments for follow-up care

Infant rides home in federally approved car restraint

Family members avail themselves of needed services

In the United States and Canada all states and provinces have mandated the use of child restraints (Brady-Fryer and Gent, 1993). Therefore hospitals and birthing centers should have policies regarding the safe discharge of a newborn in a car safety seat and provisions for parents to learn to use the device correctly (American Academy of Pediatrics, 1990b). Parents are more likely to use a restraint correctly and consistently if the proper use of one is demonstrated and its necessity is stressed.

Although federal safety standards do not specify the *minimum* weight of an infant and the appropriate type of restraint,

newborns weighing 2 kg (4 pounds, 8 ounces) receive relatively good support in convertible seats with a seat back-to-crotch strap height of 14 cm (5½ inches) or less. Rolled blankets and towels may be needed by the crotch to prevent slouching and can be placed along the sides to minimize lateral movements. Seats with shields (large padded surfaces in front of the child) and armrests (found on some other models) are unacceptable because of their proximity to the infant's face and neck (Bull and others, 1989). (For a discussion of appropriate car restraints for premature infants see p. 243, and for infants see Motor Vehicle Injuries in Chapters 10 and 12.)

Nursing ALERT

Padding is never placed underneath or behind the infant, because it creates slack in the harness, leading to the possibility of the child's ejection from the seat in the event of a crash. In vehicles with passenger-side air bags, the rear-facing safety seat must be placed in the backseat to avoid injury to the infant from the released air bag forcing the safety seat against the vehicle seat (Air-bag-associated fatal injuries, 1995).

❖ Evaluation

The effectiveness of nursing interventions is determined by continual reassessment and evaluation of care based on the following observational guidelines and expected outcomes:

1. Observe infant's color and respiratory patterns.
2. Monitor axillary temperature regularly; observe for signs of chilling, such as respiratory distress.
3. Observe for any evidence of infection, especially at the umbilicus or site of circumcision; check identification bands; check medical record for documentation of prophylactic eye treatment, vitamin K injection, HBV vaccine, and screening tests.
4. Monitor daily weight.
5. Observe interactions between infant and family members; interview family regarding their feelings about the newborn.
6. Observe parents' ability to provide care for infant; interview parents regarding any concerns about infant's care at home.
7. Observe parents' correct use of car restraint on discharge.

Expected outcomes:
See Nursing Care Plan, pp. 214-216.

KEY POINTS

- Transition from fetal or placental circulation to independent respiration is the most important physiologic change required of the newborn.
- Chemical and thermal factors help initiate the neonate's first respiration.
- Circulatory changes in the neonate result from shifts in pressure in the heart and major vessels and from functional closures of the fetal shunts.
- The newborn's large surface area, thin layer of subcutaneous fat, and unique mechanism for producing heat predispose the newborn to excessive heat loss.
- The infant's high rate of metabolism is closely correlated with the rate of fluid exchange, which is seven times greater in the infant than in the adult.
- The skin and mucous membranes, the reticuloendothelial system, and antibodies are the first, second, and third lines of defense against infection.
- Apgar scoring, the initial assessment of the newborn, focuses on heart rate, respiratory effort, muscle tone, reflex irritability, and color.
- Physical assessment of the newborn includes assessment of clinical gestational age, general measurements, general appearance, head-to-toe assessment, and parent-infant attachment, or bonding.

- Neurologic assessment focuses on localized reflexes and posture, muscle tone, head control, and movement and is best accomplished during the general physical examination.
- Behavioral assessment of newborns with the Brazelton Neonatal Behavioral Assessment Scale examines responses to seven categories: habituation, orientation, motor performance, range of state, regulation of state, autonomic regulation, and reflexes.
- Physical care for the newborn includes maintaining a patent airway, maintaining a stable body temperature, protecting from infection and injury, and providing optimum nutrition.
- Although the attachment, or bonding, process primarily affects infants and parents, siblings also play an important role.
- With short maternity admissions, teaching needs to begin before birth and continue after discharge with telephone and/or home follow-up.
- An essential aspect of discharge teaching is ensuring the newborn's safe transportation home in a federally approved, backward-facing car restraint.

REFERENCES

Abbink C: Bonding as perceived by mothers of twins, *Pediatr Nurs* 8(6):411-413, 1982.

Air-bag-associated fatal injuries to infants and children riding in front passenger seats—United States, *MMWR* 44(45):845-846, 1995.

Ament LA: Maternal tasks of the puerperium reidentified, *JOGNN* 19(4):330-335, 1990.

American Academy of Pediatrics: *Textbook of neonatal resuscitation,* Elk Grove Village, IL, 1990a, The Academy.

American Academy of Pediatrics, Committee on Accident and Poison Prevention: Safe transportation of newborns from the hospital, *Pediatrics* 86(3):486-487, 1990b.

American Academy of Pediatrics, Committee on Fetus and Newborn: Routine evaluation of blood pressure, hematocrit, and glucose in newborns, *Pediatrics* 92(3):474-476, 1993.

American Academy of Pediatrics, Committee on Infectious Diseases: *1994 Redbook: Report of the Committee on Infectious Diseases,* ed 23, Elk Grove Village, IL, 1994a, The Academy.

American Academy of Pediatrics, Committee on Infectious Diseases: Update on timing of hepatitis B vaccination for premature infants and for children with lapsed immunizations, *Pediatrics* 94(3):403-404, 1994b.

American Academy of Pediatrics, Provisional Committee on Pediatric AIDS: Perinatal human immunodeficiency virus testing, *Pediatrics* 95(2):303-307, 1995.

American Academy of Pediatrics, Task Force on Circumcision: Report of the Task Force on Circumcision, *Pediatrics* 84(4):388-391, 1989b.

American Academy of Pediatrics and American College of Obstetricians and Gynecologists: *Guidelines for perinatal care,* ed 3, Elk Grove Village, IL, 1992, The Academy.

Anderson A, Anderson B: Toward a substantive theory of mother-twin attachment, *MCN* 15(6):373-377, 1990.

Ballard JL, Novak KK, Driver M: A simplified score for assessment of fetal maturation of newly born infants, *J Pediatr* 95(5):769-774, 1979.

Ballard JL and others: New Ballard Score, expanded to include extremely premature infants, *J Pediatr* 119:417-423, 1991.

Beal J: The effect on father-infant interaction of demonstrating the Neonatal Behavioral Assessment Scale, *Birth* 16(1):18-22, 1989.

Benini F and others: Topical anesthesia during circumcision in newborn infants, *JAMA* 270(7):850-853, 1993.

Birenbaum HJ and others: Gowning on a postpartum ward fails to decrease colonization in the newborn infant, *Am J Dis Child* 144(9):1031-1033, 1990.

Blain-Lewis N: Comparative studies of bruising and healing after heelstick, *Neonatal Intensive Care* 5(5):18-21, 1992.

Bliss-Holtz J: Determination of thermoregulatory state in full-term infants, *Nurs Res* 42(4):204-207, 1993.

Brady-Fryer B, Gent M: Kids and car seats, *Can Nurse* 89(2):23-25, 1993.

Brazelton TB: Mother-infant reciprocity. In Klaus M and others, editors: *Maternal attachment and mothering disorders,* New Brunswick, NJ, 1974, Johnson & Johnson Baby Products.

Brazelton TB and Nugent JK: Neonatal behavioural assessment scale, London, 1996 MacKeith Press.

Bull M and others: Special children, special car seats, *Contemp Pediatr* 6(11):122-136, 1989.

Butz AM and others: Newborn identification: compliance with AAP guidelines for perinatal care, *Clin Pediatr* 32(2):111-113, 1993.

Campos RG: Soothing neonates' response to a stressful procedure, *Neonatal Network* 12(6):93, 1993.

Carlson GE: When grandmothers take care of grandchildren, *MCN* 18(4):206-207, 1993.

Charles S, Prystowsky B: Early discharge, in the end: maternal abuse, child neglect, and physician harassment, *Pediatrics* 96(4):746-747, 1995.

Chessare JB: Circumcision: is the risk of urinary tract infection really the pivotal issue? *Clin Pediatr* 31(2):100-104, 1992.

Chia F and others: Reliability of the Dinamap noninvasive monitor in the measurement of blood pressure of ill Asian newborns, *Clin Pediatr* 29(5):262-267, 1990.

Christoph R and others: Pain reduction in local anesthetic administration through pH buffering, *Ann Emerg Med* 17(2):117-120, 1988.

Cohen HA and others: Postcircumcision urinary tract infection, *Clin Pediatr* 31(6):322-324, 1992.

Coody D and others: Early hospital discharge and the timing of newborn metabolic screening, *Clin Pediatr* 32(8):463-466, 1993.

Dewey K and others: Adequacy of energy intake among breast-fed infants in the DARLING study: relationships to growth velocity morbidity, and activity levels, *J Pediatr* 119(4):538-547, 1991.

DiFlorio I: Mothers' comprehension of terminology associated with the care of a newborn baby, *Pediatr Nurs* 17(2):193-196, 1991.

Donowitz LG: Failure of the overgown to prevent nosocomial infection in a pediatric intensive care unit, *Pediatrics* 77:35-38, 1986.

Dubowitz LMS, Dubowitz V: *Gestational age of the newborn,* Menlo Park, CA, 1977, Addison-Wesley.

Farber SD, Van Fossen RL, Koontz SW: Quantitative and qualitative video analysis of infants feeding: angled- and straight-bottle feeding systems, *J Pediatr* 126(6):S118-124, 1995.

Female genital mutilation, *AAP News* 10(2):3, 1994.

Fitzgerald M, Millard C, McIntosh N: Cutaneous hypersensitivity following peripheral tissue damage in newborn infants and its reversal with topical anaesthesia, *Pain* 39:31-36, 1989.

Freed GL: Time to teach what we preach, *JAMA* 269(2):243-245, 1993.

Haddock, B, Vincent P, Merrow D: Axillary and rectal temperatures of full-term neonates: are they different? *Neonatal Network* 5(1):36-40, 1986.

Haouari N and others: The analgesic effect of sucrose in full-term infants: a randomized controlled trial, *Br Med J* 310:1498-1500, 1995.

Infant sleep position and sudden infant death syndrome (SIDS) in the United States: joint commentary from the American Academy of Pediatrics and selected agencies of the federal government, *Pediatrics* 93(5):820, 1994.

Kallio MJT and others: Exclusive breast-feeding and weaning: effect on serum cholesterol and lipoprotein concentrations in infants during the first year of life, *Pediatrics* 89(4):663-666, 1992.

Klaus MH, Kennell JH, Klaus PH: *Bonding: building the foundations of secure attachment and independence,* Menlo Park, CA, 1995, Addison Wesley.

Kurinij N, Shiono P: Early formula supplementation of breast-feeding, *Pediatrics* 88(4):745-750, 1991.

Lanting CI and others: Neurological differences between 9-year-old children fed breast-milk or formula-milk as babies, *Lancet* 344(8933):1319-1322, 1994.

Lawrence R: *Breastfeeding: a guide for the medical profession,* ed 4, St Louis, 1994, Mosby.

Masciello AL: Anesthesia for neonatal circumcision: local anesthesia is better than dorsal penile nerve block, *Obstet Gynecol* 75:834-838, 1990.

McCleary PH: Female genital mutilation and childbirth: a case report, *Birth* 21(4):221-223, 1994.

McDonald RE, Avery DR: *Dentistry for the child and adolescent,* ed 6, St Louis, 1994, Mosby.

O'Grady R: Feeding behavior in infants, *Am J Nurs* 71(4):736-739, 1971.

Paes B and others: A comparative study of heel-stick devices for infant blood collection, *Am J Dis Child* 147(3):346-348, 1993.

Park M, Lee D: Normative arm and calf blood pressure values in the newborn, *Pediatrics* 83(2):240-243, 1989.

Park M, Menard S: Normative oscillometric blood pressure values in the first 5 years in an office setting, *Am J Dis Child* 143(7):860-864, 1989.

Pelke S and others: Gowning does not affect colonization or infection rates in a neonatal intensive care unit, *Arch Pediatr Adolesc Med* 148:1016-1020, 1994.

Quan R and others: Effects of microwave radiation on antiinfective factors in human milk, *Pediatrics* 89(4):667-669, 1992.

Rabinowitz R, Hulbert WC: Newborn circumcision should not be performed without anesthesia, *Birth* 22(1):45-46, 1995.

Rush J and others: A randomized controlled trial of a nursery ritual: wearing cover gowns to care for healthy newborns, *Birth* 17(1):25-30, 1990.

Sachdev H and others: Water supplementation in exclusively breast-fed infants during summer in the tropics, *Lancet* 337(8747):929-933, 1991.

Severn CB: Head circumference–crown-rump length: practical measurements for neonatal screening, *Neonat Intens Care* 7(4):52-7, 1994.

Sollid D and others: Breast-feeding multiples, *J Perinat Neonat Nurs* 3(1):46-65, 1989.

Spencer D and others: Dorsal penile nerve block in neonatal circumcision: chloroprocaine versus lidocaine, *Am J Perinatol* 9(3):214-218, 1992.

Stanford J and others: Letting children observe deliveries, *N Engl J Med* 326(16):1085-1086, 1992.

Sugar M: Letting children observe deliveries, *N Engl J Med* 325(14):1048, 1991 (letter to the editor).

Thigpen JL: Responding to research: realistic use of scrub clothes and cover gowns, *Neonatal Network* 9(5):41-44, 1991.

Thomas K: Thermoregulation in neonates, *Neonatal Network* 13(2):15-22, 1994.

Trochtenberg DS: Neonatal circumcision, *N Engl J Med* 323(17):1206, 1990 (letter to the editor).

Varendi H, Porter RH, Winberg J: Does the newborn baby find the nipple by smell?, *Lancet* 344(8928):989-990, 1994.

Verma A, Dhanireddy R: Passage of first stool in very low birth-weight infants, *Pediatr Notes* 17(4):1, 1993.

Walz BL: Maternal tasks of taking on a second child in the post-partum period, *Matern Child Nurs J* 12(3):185-216, 1983.

Weinberg S: An alternative to meet the needs of early discharge: the tender beginnings postpartum visit, *MCN* 19:339-342, 1994.

Weiss ME, Richards MT: Accuracy of electronic axillary temperature measurement in term and preterm neonates, *Neonatal Network* 13(8):35-40, 1994.

Wong DL and others: Diapering choices: a critical review of the issues, *Pediatr Nurs* 18(1):41-54, 1992.

Zanoni D, Isenberg S, Apt L: A comparison of silver nitrate with erythromycin for prophylaxis against ophthalmia neonatorum, *Clin Pediatr* 31(5):295-298, 1992.

BIBLIOGRAPHY

Physiologic Status of the Newborn/Assessment of the Neonate

Abrams L and others: Effect of peripheral IV infusion on neonatal axillary temperature measurement, *Pediatr Nurs* 15(6):630-632, 1989.

Allen MC, Capute AJ: Tone and reflex development before term, *Pediatrics* 85(suppl):393-399, 1990.

Becker PT, Lederman RP, Lederman E: Neonatal measures of attention and early cognitive status, *Res Nurs Health* 12:381-388, 1989.

Blackburn S: *Assessment of risk in the newborn: neonatal growth and maturity,* ed 2, White Plains, NY, 1990, March of Dimes Birth Defects Foundation.

Blackburn S: Renal function in the neonate, *J Perinat Neonatal Nurs* 8(1):37-47, 1994.

Bruno JP: Systemic neonatal assessment and intervention, *MCN* 20(1):21-24, 1995.

Dodd V: Gestational age assessment, *Neonatal Network* 15(1):27-36, 1996.

Fanaroff A, Martin R, editors: *Neonatal-perinatal medicine,* ed 5, St Louis, 1992, Mosby.

Haddock BJ, Merrow DL, Vincent PA: Comparisons of axillary and rectal temperatures in the preterm infant, *Neonatal Network* 6(5):67-71, 1988.

Hurwitz S: Skin lesions in the first year of life, *Contemp Pediatr* 10(1):110-128, 1993.

Jepson H, Talashek M, Tichy A: The Apgar score: evolution, limitations, and scoring guidelines, *Birth* 18(2):83-92, 1991.

Johnson KJ, Bhatia P, Bell EF: Infared thermometry of newborn infants, *Pediatrics* 87(1):34-38, 1991.

Kellogg ND, Parra JM: Linea vestibularis: a previously undescribed normal genital structure in female neonates, *Pediatrics* 87(6):926-929, 1991.

Kenner C: Measuring neonatal assessment, *Neonatal Network* 9(4):17-22, 1990.

Medoff-Cooper B, Ray W: Neonatal sucking behaviors, *Image J Nurs Sch* 27(3):195-200, 1995.

Moss G and others: Routine examination in the neonatal period, *Br Med J* 302(6781):878-879, 1991.

Parker S and others: Jitteriness in full-term neonates: prevalence and correlates, *Pediatrics* 85(1):17-23, 1990.

Tappero E, Honeyfield M, editors: *Physical assessment of the newborn,* Petaluma, CA, 1993, NICU Ink Book Pub.

Nursing Care of the Neonate: General

American Academy of Pediatrics, Committee on Genetics: Issues in newborn screening, *Pediatrics* 89(2):345-349, 1992.

Barnes LP: Infant care: teaching the basics, *MCN* 19(1):47, 1994.

Blackburn ST, Loper DL: *Maternal, fetal, and neonatal physiology,* Philadelphia, 1992, WB Saunders.

Braveman P and others: Early discharge of newborns and mothers: a critical review of the literature, *Pediatrics* 96(4):716-726, 1995.

Cetta F, Lambert G, Ros S: Newborn chemical exposure from over-the-counter skin care products, *Clin Pediatr* 30(5):286-289, 1991.

Coffman S, Levitt MJ, Deets C: Personal and professional support for mothers of NICU and healthy newborns, *JOGNN* 20(5):406-415, 1991.

Dextradeur CC, Godfrey TM: A badge of security, *MCN* 16(3):175-176, 1991.

Hanvey L: Values in maternal and newborn care, *Can Nurse* 86(9):22-24, 1990.

Kendig JW: Care of the normal newborn, *Pediatr Rev* 13(7):262-268, 1992.

Kenner C, Brueggemeyer A, Gunderson LP: *Comprehensive neonatal nursing,* Philadelphia, 1993, WB Saunders.

Kessel W and others: Early discharge: in the end, it is clinical judgment, *Pediatrics* 96(4):739-742, 1995.

O'Hara MA: Ophthalmia neonatorum, *Pediatr Clin North Am* 40(4):715-725, 1993.

Seidel HM, Rosenstein BJ, Pathak A: *Primary care of the newborn,* St Louis, 1993, Mosby.

Spadt SK, Sensenig KD: Infant kidnapping: it can happen in any hospital, *MCN* 15(1):52-54, 1990.

Weiss M, Armstrong M: Postpartum mothers; preferences for nighttime care of the neonate, *JOGNN* 29(4):290-295, 1991.

Circumcision

Fergusson DM, Lawton JM, Shannon FT: Neonatal circumcision and penile problems: an 8-year longitudinal study, *Pediatrics* 81(4):537-541, 1988.

Gordon A, Collin J: Save the normal foreskin, *Br Med J* 6869(306):1-2, 1993.

Lund MM: Perspectives on newborn male circumcision, *Neonatal Network* 9(3):7-12, 1990.

Myron AV, Maguire DP: Pain perception in the neonate: implications for circumcision, *J Prof Nurs* 7(3):188-195, 1991.

Omer-Hashi KH: Commentary: Female genital mutilation: perspectives from a Somalian midwife, *Birth* 21(4):224-226, 1994.

Williams N, Chel J, Kapila L: Why are children referred for circumcision? *Br Med J* 6869(306):28, 1993.

Nutrition

Cronenwett L and others: Single daily bottle use in the early weeks postpartum and breast-feeding outcomes, *Pediatrics* 90(5):760-766, 1992.

Danner S: How do we influence the breastfeeding decision? *Birth* 18(4):227-228, 1991.

Dewey K and others: Maternal versus infant factors related to breast milk intake and residual milk volume: the DARLING study, *Pediatrics* 87(6):829-837, 1991.

Dix D: Why women decide not to breastfeed, *Birth* 18(4):222-225, 1991.

Fomon SJ: *Nutrition of normal infants,* St Louis, 1993, Mosby.

Frantz K: Keep breastfeeding simple, keep it easy, keep it fun, *Birth* 18(4):228-229, 1991.

Freed G, Fraley K, Schanler R: Attitudes of expectant fathers regarding breast-feeding, *Pediatrics* 90(2):224-227, 1992.

Gamble D, Morse J: Fathers of breastfed infants: postponing and types of involvement, *JOGNN* 22(4):358-365, 1993.

Grossman LK and others: The effect of postpartum lactation counseling on the duration of breast-feeding in low-income women, *Am J Dis Child* 144(4):471-474, 1990.

Howie PW and others: Protective effect of breast feeding against infection, *Br Med J* 300:11-16, 1990.

Kearney MH, Cronenwett L: Breastfeeding and employment, *JOGNN* 20(6):471-480, 1991.

Lawrence PB: Breast milk: best source of nutrition for term and preterm infants, *Pediatr Clin North Am* 41(5):925-941, 1994.

Lawrence R: The clinician's role in teaching proper infant feeding techniques, *J Pediatr* 126(6):S112-117, 1995.

Maccagno-Smith R, Young M: Breastfeeding the sleepy infant, *Can Nurse* 89(2):20-22, 1993.

Mathew OP: Science of bottle feeding, *J Pediatr* 119(4):511-519, 1991.

Minchin MK: Positioning for breastfeeding, *Birth* 16(2):67-73, 1989.

Moore E, Bianchi-Gray M, Stephens L: A community hospital-based breastfeeding counseling service, *Pediatr Nurs* 17(4):383-389, 1991.

NAPNAP position statement . . . breast-feeding *J Pediatr Health Care* 7(6):289, 1993.

Nice FJ: Can a breast-feeding mother take medication without harming her infant? *MCN* 14:27-31, 1989.

Oberlander T and others: Short-term effects of feed composition on sleeping and crying in newborns, *Pediatrics* 90(5):733-740, 1992.

Queen P, Lang C. *Handbook of pediatric nutrition,* Gaithersburg, MD, 1993, Aspen.

Rentschler DD: Correlates of successful breast-feeding, *Image J Nurs Sch* 23(3):151-154, 1991.

Shrago L, Bocar D: The infant's contribution to breastfeeding, *JOGNN* 19(3):209-215, 1990.

Family/Parent-Infant Bonding (Attachment)

American Academy of Pediatrics, Committee on Fetus and Newborn: Postpartum (neonatal) sibling visitation, *Pediatrics* 76(4):650, 1985.

Beal JA: Methodological issues in conducting research on parent-infant attachment, *J Pediatr Nurs* 6(1):11-15, 1991.

Coffman S: Parent and infant attachment: review of nursing research 1981-1990, *Pediatr Nurs* 18(4):421-425, 1992.

Driscoll JW: Maternal parenthood and the grief process, *J Perinat Neonat Nurs* 4(2):1-10, 1990.

Eyer D: *Mother-infant bonding: a scientific fiction,* New Haven, CT, 1992, Yale University Press.

Farel AM and others: Interaction between high-risk infants and their mothers: the NCAST as an assessment tool, *Res Nurs Health* 14(2):109-118, 1991.

Fortier JC and others: Adjustment to a newborn, *JOGNN* 20(1):73-79, 1991.

Fuller JR: Early patterns of maternal attachment, *Health Care Women Int* 11(4);433-446, 1990.

Gaffney KF: New directions in maternal attachment research, *J Pediatr Health Care* 2(4):181-188, 1988.

Gullicks J, Crase S: Sibling behavior with a newborn: parents' expectations and observations, *JOGNN* 22(5):438-446, 1993.

Lobar SL, Phillips S: A clinical assessment strategy for maternal acquaintance-attachment behaviors, *Issues Compr Pediatr Nurs* 15(4):249-260, 1992.

Mercer RT, Ferketich SL: Predictors of parental attachment during early parenthood, *J Adv Nurs* 15:268-280, 1990.

Novak J, Novak R: Facilitating fathering. In Craft M, Denehy J: *Nursing interventions for infants and children,* Philadelphia, 1990, WB Saunders.

Palkovitz R: Changes in father-infant bonding beliefs across couples' first transition to parenthood, *Matern Child Nurs J* 29(3,4):141-154, 1992.

Porter LS, Sobong LC: Differences in maternal perception of the newborn among adolescents, *Pediatr Nurs* 16(1):101-104, 1990.

Pressler J: Promoting attachment. In Craft M, Denehy J: *Nursing interventions for infants and children,* Philadelphia, 1990, WB Saunders.

Short JD: Interdependence needs and nursing care of the new family, *Issues Compr Pediatr Nurs* 17:1-14, 1994.

Tomlinson PS: Verbal behavior associated with indicators of maternal attachment with the neonate, *JOGNN* 19(1):76-77, 1989.

Weingarten CT: Married mothers' perceptions of their premature or term infants and the quality of their relationships with their husbands, *JOGNN* 19(1):64-73, 1990.

Weiss ME, Armstrong M: Postpartum mothers' preferences for nighttime care of the neonate, *JOGNN* 20(4):290-295, 1990.

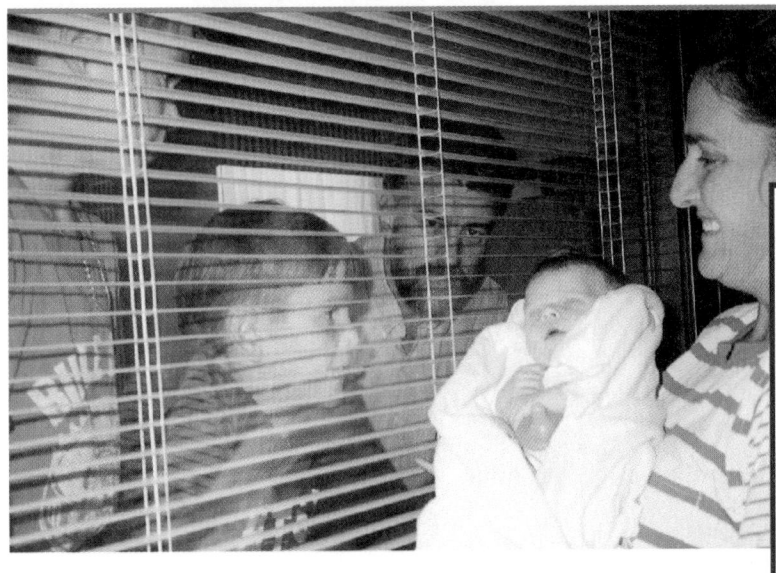

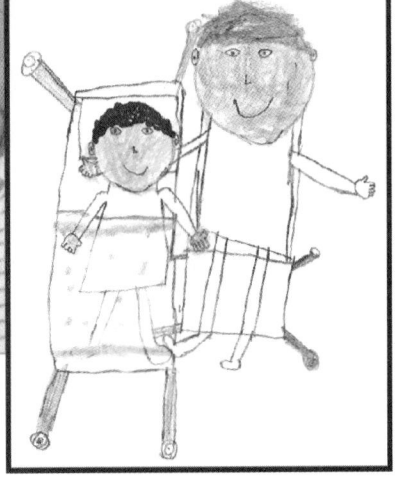

" *I've had joy, pride, and still some fear — not knowing how she would be after her critical start in life.* "

Bruce, father of
Anna, newborn with
Beta Strep infection

RELATED TOPICS

Administration of medications, Ch. 22
Assessment (newborn), Ch. 8
Cognitive impairment, Ch. 19
Collection of specimens, Ch. 22
Congenital adrenogenital hyperplasia, Ch. 29
Diaper dermatitis, Ch. 30
Family-centered home care, Ch. 20
Impact of chronic illness, disability, or death on the child and
   family, Ch. 18

Infant mortality, Ch. 1
Infection control, Ch. 22
Pain assessment; pain management, Ch. 21
Preparation for discharge and home care, Ch. 21
Procedures for maintaining respiratory function, Ch. 22
Procedures related to alternative feeding techniques, Ch. 22
Promotion of parent-infant bonding (attachment), Ch. 8

LEARNING OBJECTIVES
On completion of this chapter the reader will be able to:

- Recognize common deviations from normal in the newborn
- Perform a systematic assessment of an ill newborn
- Outline a general plan of care for a high-risk infant

- Discuss the role of the nurse in facilitating positive parent-child relationships
- Contrast characteristics of premature and full-term infants
- Discuss the rationale for screening newborns and for

genetic counseling when a newborn has a hereditary condition
- Modify a general care plan to meet the needs of an infant with a specific high-risk health deviation

BIRTH INJURIES

SOFT TISSUE INJURY

arious types of soft tissue injury may be sustained during the process of birth, primarily in the form of bruises and/or abrasions secondary to dystocia. Soft tissue injury usually occurs when there is some degree of disproportion between the presenting part and the maternal pelvis (cephalopelvic disproportion). The use of forceps to facilitate a difficult vertex delivery may produce discoloration or abrasion of the same configuration as the forceps on the sides of the neonate's face. Petechiae or ecchymoses may be observed on the presenting part after a breech or brow delivery. The sudden release of pressure on the head can produce scleral hemorrhages and/or generalized petechiae over the face and head after a difficult or precipitous delivery. Petechiae and ecchymoses may also appear on the head, neck, and face of an infant born with a nuchal cord, giving the infant's face a cyanotic appearance. Rarely, lacerations occur during cesarean section.

These traumatic lesions generally fade spontaneously within a few days, without treatment. However, petechiae may be a manifestation of an underlying bleeding disorder and are evaluated. Nursing care is primarily directed toward assessing the injury and providing an explanation and reassurance to the parents.

HEAD TRAUMA

Trauma to the head and scalp that occurs during the birth process is usually benign but occasionally results in more se-

rious injury. Injuries that produce serious trauma, such as intracerebellar hemorrhage and subdural hematoma, are discussed in relation to neurologic disturbances (see Chapter 28). Skull fractures are discussed in association with other fractures sustained during the process of birth.

Caput Succedaneum

The most commonly observed scalp lesion is *caput succedaneum,* a vaguely outlined area of edematous tissue situated over the portion of the scalp that presents in a vertex delivery (Fig. 9-1). The swelling consists of serum or blood, or both, accumulated in the tissues *above* the bone, and it often extends beyond the bone margins. The swelling may be associated with overlying petechiae or ecchymoses. No specific treatment is needed, and the swelling subsides within a few days.

Cephalhematoma

A *cephalhematoma* is formed when blood vessels rupture during a difficult labor or delivery, producing bleeding into the area *between* the bone and its periosteum. The boundaries of the cephalhematoma are sharply demarcated and do not extend beyond the limits of the bone (Fig. 9-1). A cephalhematoma may involve one or both parietal bones. Less frequently the occipital and rarely the frontal bones are affected. The swelling is usually minimal at birth but increases in size on the second or third day. Blood loss is usually not significant.

No treatment is indicated for uncomplicated cephalhematoma, and most lesions are absorbed within 2 weeks to 3 months. Lesions that result in severe blood loss to the area or that involve an underlying fracture require further evaluation and appropriate therapy.

David Wilson, MS, RNC, revised this chapter.

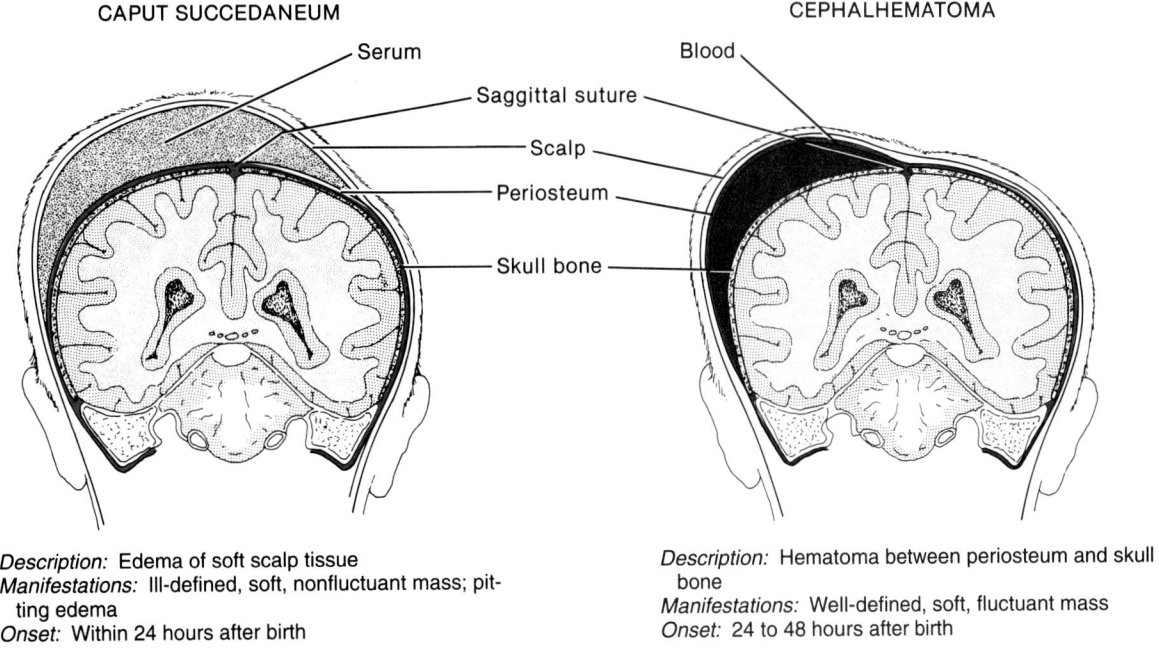

CAPUT SUCCEDANEUM — CEPHALHEMATOMA

Description: Edema of soft scalp tissue
Manifestations: Ill-defined, soft, nonfluctuant mass; pitting edema
Onset: Within 24 hours after birth

Description: Hematoma between periosteum and skull bone
Manifestations: Well-defined, soft, fluctuant mass
Onset: 24 to 48 hours after birth

FIG. 9-1. Comparison of caput succedaneum and cephalhematoma. (Modified from Bobak IM, Jensen MD: *Maternity and gynecologic care: the nurse and the family,* ed 5, St Louis, 1993, Mosby.)

Nursing Considerations

Nursing care is directed toward assessment and observation of the scalp injuries and vigilance in observing for possible associated complications such as infection, subdural hematoma, or intraventricular hemorrhage. Because these injuries resolve spontaneously, parents need reassurance of their usually benign nature.

FRACTURES

Fracture of the *clavicle,* or *collarbone,* is the most frequent birth injury. It is often associated with difficult vertex or breech delivery of infants who are large for gestational age. *Crepitus* (the crackling sound produced by the rubbing together of fractured bone fragments) is often heard and/or felt on further examination, and radiographs usually reveal a complete fracture with overriding of the fragments.

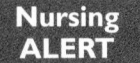 The newborn with a fractured clavicle may have no symptoms, but suspect a fracture if an infant has limited use of the affected arm, malposition of the arm, asymmetric Moro reflex, focal swelling or tenderness, or cries in pain when the arm is moved. Eliciting the scarf sign (extending arm across chest toward opposite shoulder) for assessment of gestational age is contraindicated if a fractured clavicle is suspected.

Fractures of *long bones,* such as the femur or the humerus, are difficult to detect by radiographic examination. Although osteogenesis imperfecta is a rare finding, a newborn infant with a fracture should be assessed for other evidence of this congenital disorder.

Fractures of the neonatal *skull* are uncommon. The bones, which are less mineralized and more compressible than bones in older infants and children, are separated by membranous seams that allow sufficient alteration in the head contour so that it adjusts to the birth canal during delivery. Skull fractures usually follow prolonged, difficult delivery or forceps extraction. Most fractures are linear, but some may be visible as depressed indentations resembling a Ping-Pong ball.

Nursing Considerations

Frequently no intervention may be prescribed other than maintaining proper body alignment, careful dressing and undressing of the infant, and handling and carrying that support the affected bone. For example, if the infant has a fractured clavicle, it is important to support the upper and lower back rather than pull the infant up from under the arms. Occasionally, for immobilization and relief of pain, the arm on the side of the fractured clavicle may be fixed on the body by pinning the sleeve to the shirt or by application of a triangular sling or a figure-8 bandage.

Linear skull fractures usually require no treatment. A Ping-Pong–type fracture may require decompression by surgical intervention. The infant is carefully observed for signs of neurologic complications. The parents of infants with a fracture of any bone should be involved in caring for the infant during hospitalization as part of discharge planning for care at home.

PARALYSES

Facial Paralysis

Pressure on the facial nerve during delivery may result in injury to cranial nerve VII. Clinical manifestations are primarily loss of movement on the affected side, such as inability to completely close the eye, slight drooping of the corner of the

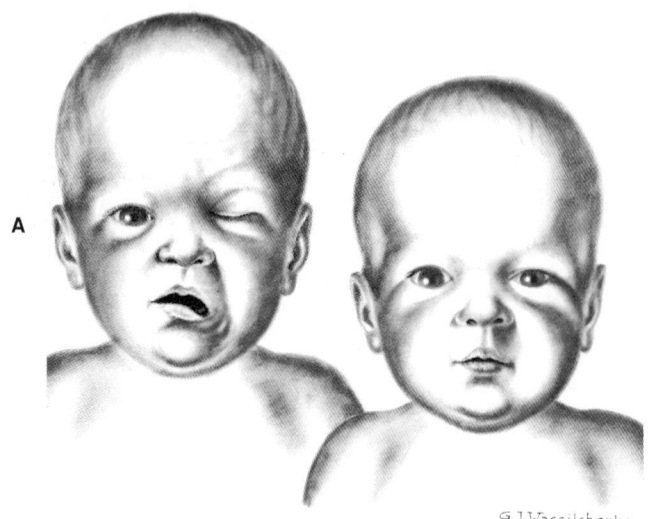

FIG. 9-2. A, Paralysis of right side of face 15 minutes after forceps delivery. Absence of movement on affected side is especially noticeable when infant cries. **B,** Same infant 24 hours later.

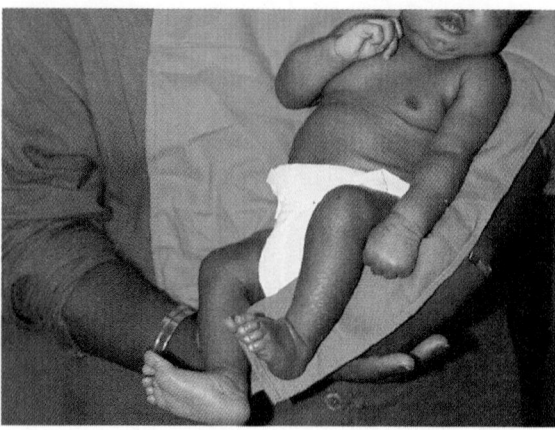

FIG. 9-3. Left-sided brachial plexus (Erb) palsy. Note extended, internally rotated arm and pronated wrist on affected side.

mouth, and absence of wrinkling of the forehead (Fig. 9-2). The paralysis is most noticeable when the infant cries. No medical intervention is necessary; the paralysis usually disappears spontaneously in a few days, but it may take as long as several months.

Brachial Palsy

Plexus injury results from forces that alter the normal position and relationship of the arm, shoulder, and neck. *Erb palsy (Erb-Duchenne paralysis),* caused by damage to the upper plexus, is usually a result of stretching or pulling away of the shoulder from the head. The less-common lower plexus palsy, or *Klumpke palsy,* results from severe stretching of the upper extremity while the trunk is relatively less mobile.

The clinical manifestations of *Erb palsy* are related to the paralysis of the affected extremity and muscles. The arm hangs limp alongside the body. The shoulder and arm are adducted and internally rotated. The elbow is extended and the forearm is pronated with the wrist and fingers flexed (Fig. 9-3). In lower plexus palsy the muscles of the hand are paralyzed with consequent wrist drop and relaxed fingers. In severe forms of brachial palsy, the entire arm is paralyzed and hangs limp and motionless at the side.

Treatment of an affected arm is aimed at preventing contractures of the paralyzed muscles and maintaining correct placement of the humeral head within the glenoid fossa of the scapula. Complete recovery from stretched nerves usually takes 3 to 6 months. However, avulsion of the nerves (complete disconnection from the spinal cord) results in permanent damage. For those injuries that do not improve spontaneously, surgical intervention may be needed (Brucker, 1991).

Phrenic Nerve Paralysis

Phrenic nerve paralysis resulting in diaphragmatic paralysis sometimes occurs in conjunction with brachial palsy. Respiratory distress is the most common and important sign of injury. Because injury to this nerve is usually unilateral, the lung on the affected side does not expand and respiratory efforts are ineffectual. Breathing is primarily thoracic and cyanosis is a prominent sign. Pneumonia is a frequent secondary complication.

Nursing Considerations

Nursing care of the infant with facial nerve paralysis involves aiding the infant to suck and assisting the parent with feeding techniques. Breast-feeding is not contraindicated, but the mother will need additional assistance in helping the infant to grasp and compress the areola. If the lid of the eye on the affected side does not close completely, artificial tears can be instilled daily to prevent drying of the conjunctiva and injury to the sclera and cornea. The lid is often taped shut to prevent injury.

Nursing care of the newborn with brachial palsy is concerned primarily with proper positioning of the affected arm. In upper arm paralysis the arm is abducted 90 degrees with external rotation at the shoulder, 90-degree flexion at the elbow, full supination of the forearm, and slight extension of the wrist so that the palm of the hand is turned toward the face. The position may be maintained with intermittent splinting. The arm should also receive passive range-of-motion exercises daily to maintain muscle tone and function.

When dressing the infant, give special preference to the affected arm. Begin undressing with the unaffected arm, and begin redressing with the affected arm to prevent unnecessary manipulation and stress on the paralyzed muscles. Parents are taught to use the "football" position to hold the infant and to avoid picking up the child from under the axilla or by pulling on the arms.

The infant with phrenic nerve paralysis requires the same nursing care as any infant with respiratory distress. As with other birth injuries, emotional needs of the family are similar to those discussed for soft tissue injury. Also, because of the extended treatment for some paralyses, follow-up care is essential.

COMMON PROBLEMS IN THE NEWBORN

ERYTHEMA TOXICUM NEONATORUM

Erythema toxicum neonatorum, also known as *flea-bite dermatitis* or *newborn rash,* is a benign, self-limiting eruption of unknown cause that usually appears within the first 2 days of life. The lesions are firm, 1 to 3 mm, pale yellow or white papules and/or pustules on an erythematous base; they resemble flea bites. The rash appears most commonly on the face, proximal extremities, trunk, and buttocks, but it may be located anywhere on the body except the palms and soles. The rash is more obvious during crying episodes. There are no systemic manifestations, and successive crops of lesions heal without pigmentation. The rash usually lasts about 5 to 7 days. The etiology is unknown. However, a smear of the pustule will show numerous eosinophils and a relative absence of neutrophils. When the diagnosis is questionable, bacterial, fungal, or viral, cultures should be obtained (Hurwitz, 1993). Although no treatment is necessary, parents are usually concerned about the rash and need to be reassured of its benign and transient nature.

CANDIDIASIS

Candida infections, also known as *candidiasis* or *moniliasis,* are not uncommon in the newborn. *Candida albicans,* the usual organism responsible, may cause disease in any organ system. It is a yeastlike fungus (it produces yeast cells and spores) that can be acquired from a maternal vaginal infection during delivery, by person-to-person transmission (especially poor handwashing technique), or from contaminated hands, bottles, nipples, or other articles. Mucocutaneous, cutaneous, and disseminated candidiasis infections are all observed in this age-group. It is usually a benign disorder in the neonate, often confined to the oral and diaper regions.

Candidal Diaper Dermatitis

The warm, moist atmosphere created in the diaper area provides an optimal environment for candidal growth. The dermatitis appears in the perianal area, inguinal folds, and lower abdomen. The affected area is intensely erythematous with a sharply demarcated, scalloped edge, frequently with numerous satellite lesions that extend beyond the larger lesion (Fig. 9-4). The usual source of infection is through the gastrointestinal tract when organisms are swallowed from the birth canal during delivery. It may also appear 2 to 3 days following an oral infection.

Therapy consists of applications of an anticandidal ointment, such as nystatin or clotrimazole (see also Diaper dermatitis, Chapter 30). Sometimes the infant is also given an oral antifungal preparation to eliminate any gastrointestinal source of infection (see following discussion.)

Oral Candidiasis

Oral candidiasis *(thrush)* is characterized by white, adherent patches on the tongue, palate, and inner aspects of the cheeks (Fig. 9-5). It is often difficult to distinguish from coagulated milk. The infant may refuse to suck because of pain in the mouth, but this is uncommon.

> **Nursing ALERT** Candidiasis can be distinguished from coagulated milk when attempts to remove the patches with a tongue blade are unsuccessful, usually resulting in bleeding from the scraped surfaces.

The condition tends to be acute in the newborn, and chronic in infants and young children, and to appear when the oral flora is altered as a result of antibiotic therapy. Although the disorder is usually self-limiting, spontaneous resolution may take as long as 2 months, during which time lesions may spread to the larynx, trachea, bronchi, and lungs and along the gastrointestinal tract. Thrush is treated with good hygiene, application of a fungicide, and correction of any underlying disturbance. The source of infection, usually the mother, should be treated to prevent reinfection.

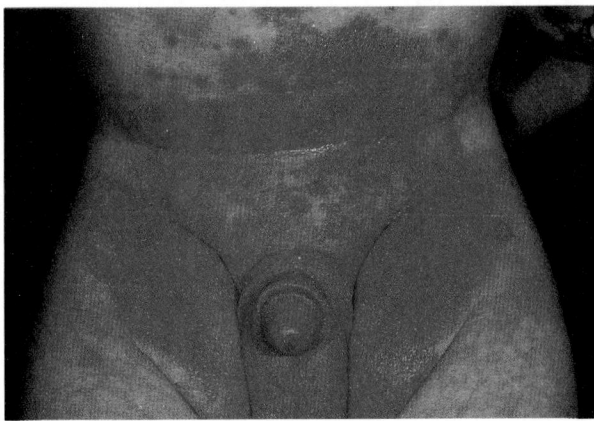

FIG. 9-4. Candida dermatitis. (From Habif TP: *Clinical dermatology: a color guide to diagnosis and therapy,* ed 2, St Louis, 1990, Mosby.)

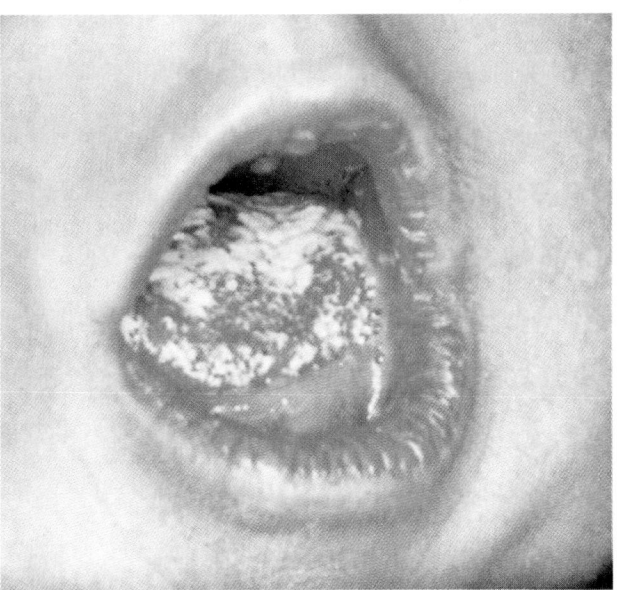

FIG. 9-5. Oral candidiasis (thrush). (From *Variations and minor departures in infants,* Evansville, IN, 1978, Mead Johnson & Co.)

Topical application of 1 ml nystatin (Mycostatin) over the surfaces of the oral cavity four times a day or every 6 hours is usually sufficient to prevent spread of the disease or prolong its course. Several other drugs may be used, including amphotericin B (Fungizone), clotrimazole (Lotrimin, Mycelex), fluconazole (Diflucan), or miconazole (Monistat, Micatin) given intravenously, orally, or topically. These agents have replaced the use of gentian violet solution. Therapy should be continued for at least 2 days after lesions disappear to prevent relapse (Levin and Wong, 1994).

Nursing Considerations
Nursing care is directed toward preventing spread of the infection and correct application of the prescribed topical medication. For candidiasis in the diaper area, the caregiver is taught to keep the diaper area clean and to apply the medication to affected areas as prescribed.

Oral nystatin is applied after feedings. The medication is distributed over the surface of the oral mucosa and tongue with an applicator, and the remainder of the dose is deposited in the mouth to be swallowed by the infant to treat any gastrointestinal lesions.

Other measures to control thrush, in addition to good hygienic care, include rinsing the infant's mouth with plain water after each feeding before applying the medication and boiling reusable nipples and bottles for at least 20 minutes after thorough washing (spores are heat-resistant). Pacifiers should be boiled for at least 20 minutes once daily, and the nipples of breast-feeding mothers should also be treated to prevent reinfection. Infants with candidal diaper dermatitis can introduce the yeast into the mouth from contaminated hands. Therefore placing clothes over the diaper can prevent this cycle of self-infection. The intravenous administration of amphotericin B must be closely monitored to prevent tissue damage and phlebitis.

"BIRTHMARKS"
Discolorations of the skin are very common findings in the newborn infant (see discussion on skin assessment of the newborn, Chapter 8). Most, such as mongolian spots or telangiectatic nevi, involve no therapy other than reassurance to parents of the benign nature of these discolorations. Some can be a manifestation of a disease that suggests further examination of the child and other family members (e.g., the multiple light brown *café-au-lait spots* that often characterize the autosomal-dominant hereditary disorder neurofibromatosis and are common findings in Albright syndrome).

Darker and/or more extensive lesions demand further scrutiny, and excision of the lesion is recommended when feasible or when excisional biopsy is performed. These lesions include the reddish brown solitary nodule that appears on the face or upper arm and usually represents a spindle and epithelioid cell nevus *(juvenile melanoma)*; the *giant pigmented nevus* (or *bathing trunk nevus*); the dark brown to black, irregular plaque that is at risk of transformation to malignant melanoma; and the dark brown or black macules that become more numerous with age *(junctional or compound nevi)*.

Vascular malformations are permanent lesions that are present at birth. Any vascular structure, capillary, vein, artery, or lymphatics, may be involved. The most common vascular

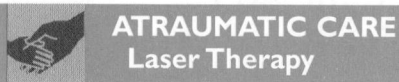

malformation is the *congenital capillary*, or *"port-wine,"* variety. The lesions are pink, red, or purple "stains" of the skin that often thicken, darken, and proportionately enlarge as the child grows.

Port-wine stains may also be associated with structural malformations, such as glaucoma and/or leptomeningial angiomatosis (tumor of blood or lymph vessels in the piaarachnoid) *(Sturge-Weber syndrome)* or bony and/or muscular overgrowth *(Klippel-Trenaunay-Weber syndrome)*. Children with port-wine stains on the eyelids, forehead, and cheeks, or on extremities should be monitored for these syndromes with periodic ophthalmologic examination, neurologic imaging, and measurement of extremities.

The treatment of choice for port-wine stains is the use of the flashlamp-pumped pulsed dye laser. A series of treatments are usually needed (see Atraumatic Care box). The treatments can significantly lighten or completely clear the lesions with almost no scarring or pigment change.

Hemangiomas are tumors that involve only capillaries. They may or may not be visible at birth, enlarge during the first year, and tend to resolve spontaneously. *Strawberry hemangiomas* are red, rubbery nodules with a rough surface. Usually, no treatment is needed unless they interfere with function, such as breathing, feeding, or vision. Unfortunately, if treatment is needed, surgery usually results in scarring.

Nursing Considerations
Birthmarks, especially those on the face, are upsetting to parents. Families need an explanation of the type of lesion, its significance, and possible treatment. They can benefit from seeing photographs of other infants before and after treatment for port-wine stains or from the passage of time for hemangiomas. If laser therapy is performed, parents are instructed to keep the infant's fingernails trimmed to prevent trauma to the area. The infant should be kept out of the sun for several weeks and then protected with a sunscreen of at least SPF 15. Parents are also cautioned to avoid disturbing (scraping) a hemangioma as this may cause bleeding and infection at the site.

NURSING CARE OF THE HIGH-RISK NEWBORN AND FAMILY
IDENTIFICATION OF HIGH-RISK NEWBORNS
The *high-risk neonate* can be defined as a newborn, regardless of gestational age or birth weight, who has a greater than average chance of morbidity or mortality because of condi-

tions or circumstances that are superimposed on the normal course of events associated with birth and the adjustment to extrauterine existence. The high-risk period encompasses human growth and development from the time of viability up to 28 days following birth and includes threats to life and health that occur during the prenatal, perinatal, and postnatal periods.

Classification of High-Risk Newborns

High-risk infants are most often classified according to birth weight, gestational age, and predominant pathophysiologic problems. The more common problems related to physiologic status are closely associated with the state of maturity of the infant and usually involve chemical disturbances (e.g., hypoglycemia, hypocalcemia) and consequences of immature organs and systems (e.g., hyperbilirubinemia, respiratory distress, hypothermia).

CLASSIFICATION OF HIGH-RISK INFANTS

Classification According to Size

Low-birth-weight (LBW) infant—An infant whose birth weight is less than 2500 g regardless of gestational age

Very-very-low-birth-weight (VVLBW) or extremely-low-birth-weight (ELBW) infant—An infant whose birth weight is less than 1000 g

Very-low-birth-weight (VLBW) infant—An infant whose birth weight is less than 1500 g

Moderately-low-birth-weight (MLBW)—An infant whose birth weight is 1501 to 2500 g

Appropriate-for-gestational-age (AGA) infant—An infant whose weight falls between the 10th and 90th percentiles on intrauterine growth curves

Small-for-date (SFD) or small-for-gestational-age (SGA) infant—An infant whose rate of intrauterine growth was slowed and whose birth weight falls below the 10th percentile on intrauterine growth curves

Intrauterine growth retardation (IUGR)—Found in infants whose intrauterine growth is retarded (sometimes used as a more descriptive term for the SGA infant)

Large-for-gestational-age (LGA) infant—An infant whose birth weight falls above the 90th percentile on intrauterine growth charts

Classification According to Gestational Age

Premature (preterm) infant—An infant born before completion of 37 weeks of gestation, regardless of birth weight

Full-term infant—An infant born between the beginning of the 38 weeks and the completion of the 42 weeks of gestation, regardless of birth weight

Postmature (postterm) infant—An infant born after 42 weeks of gestational age, regardless of birth weight

Classification According to Mortality

Live birth—Birth in which the neonate manifests any heartbeat, breathes, or displays voluntary movement, regardless of gestational age

Fetal death—Death of the fetus after 20 weeks of gestation and before delivery, with absence of any signs of life after birth

Neonatal death—Death that occurs in the first 27 days of life; early neonatal death occurs in the first week of life; late neonatal death occurs at 7 to 27 days

Perinatal mortality—Describes the total number of fetal and early neonatal deaths per 1000 live births

Postnatal death—Death that occurs at 28 days to 1 year

Formerly, weight at birth was considered to reflect a reasonably accurate estimation of gestational age. That is, if infants' birth weights exceeded 2500 g (5½ pounds), they were considered to be mature. However, intrauterine growth rates are not the same for all infants, and other factors (e.g., heredity, placental insufficiency, and maternal disease) influence intrauterine growth and birth weight. The classification system in the box encompasses birth weight, gestational age, and neonatal outcome. The lowest perinatal mortality is found in the full-term infant who weighs between 3000 and 4000 g (Fanaroff and Martin, 1992). (See Fig. 8-2 for size comparison of newborn infants.)

❖ Assessment

At birth the newborn is given a cursory, yet thorough, assessment to determine any apparent problems and identify those that demand immediate attention. This examination is primarily concerned with the evaluation of cardiopulmonary and neurologic functions. The assessment includes the assignment of an Apgar score (see Chapter 8) and an evaluation for any obvious congenital anomalies, or evidence of neonatal distress. Delivery rooms are equipped with a special resuscitation area where infants with evidence of distress are stabilized and evaluated before being transported to the NICU for therapy and more extensive assessment (see Clinical Assessment of Gestational Age, Chapter 8).

Maintaining detailed, ongoing records of all activities and observations is an important responsibility of nurses in the intensive care setting. Knowledge about and operation of complex pieces of equipment and mechanical devices are inherent in the care of the ill neonate. However, sophisticated monitoring and life-support systems cannot replace the vigilance and constant scrutiny of the infants by experienced personnel.

Systematic Assessment

A thorough systematic physical assessment (see Guidelines box on p. 228) is an essential component in the care of the high-risk infant. Subtle changes in feeding behavior, activity, color, or vital signs often indicate an underlying problem. The preterm infant, especially the VLBW infant, is ill equipped to withstand prolonged physiologic stress and may expire within minutes of exhibiting abnormal symptoms if the underlying pathologic process is not corrected. The alert nurse is aware of subtle changes and reacts promptly to implement interventions that will promote optimum functioning in the high-risk neonate. Changes in the infant's status are noted through ongoing observations of the infant's adaptation to the extrauterine environment.

Observational assessments of the high-risk infant are made according to the infant's acuity; the critically ill infant requires close observation and assessment of respiratory function, including continuous pulse oximetry and frequent evaluation of blood gases. Accurate documentation of the infant's status is an integral component of nursing care. With the aid of continuous, sophisticated cardiopulmonary monitoring, nursing assessments and daily care may be coordinated to allow for minimal handling of the infant (especially the VLBW or ELBW infant) to decrease the effects of environmental stress.

GUIDELINES
Physical Assessment

General Assessment

Using electronic scale, weigh daily, or more often if ordered.

Measure length and head circumference periodically.

Describe general body shape and size, posture at rest, ease of breathing, presence and location of edema.

Describe any apparent deformities.

Describe any signs of distress: poor color, mouth open, head bobbing, grimace, furrowed brow.

Respiratory Assessment

Describe shape of chest (barrel, concave), symmetry, presence of incisions, chest tubes, or other deviations.

Describe use of accessory muscles: nasal flaring or substernal, intercostal, or subclavicular retractions.

Determine respiratory rate and regularity.

Auscultate and describe breath sounds: stridor, crackles, wheezing, wet diminished sounds, areas of absence of sound, grunting, diminished air entry, equality of breath sounds.

Determine whether suctioning is needed.

Describe cry if not intubated.

Describe ambient oxygen and method of delivery; if intubated, describe size of tube, type of ventilator and settings, and method of securing tube.

Determine oxygen saturation by pulse oximetry and partial pressure of oxygen, and transcutaneous carbon dioxide (tcP_{CO_2}).

Cardiovascular Assessment

Determine heart rate and rhythm.

Describe heart sounds, including any murmurs.

Determine the point of maximum intensity (PMI), the point where the heartbeat sounds and palpates loudest (a change in the point of maximum intensity may indicate a mediastinal shift).

Describe infant's color (may be of cardiac, respiratory, or hematopoietic origin): cyanosis, pallor, plethora, jaundice, mottling.

Assess color of nail beds, mucous membranes, lips.

Determine blood pressure. Indicate extremity used and cuff size; check each extremity at least once.

Describe peripheral pulses, capillary refill (<2 to 3 seconds), peripheral perfusion (mottling).

Describe monitors, their parameters, and whether alarms are in "on" position.

Gastrointestinal Assessment

Determine presence of abdominal distention: increase in circumference, shiny skin, evidence of abdominal wall erythema, visible peristalsis, visible loops of bowel, status of umbilicus.

Determine any signs of regurgitation, and time related to feeding; character and amount of residual if gavage-fed; if nasogastric tube in place, describe type of suction, drainage (color, consistency, pH, guaiac).

Describe amount, color, consistency, and odor of any emesis.

Palpate liver margin.

Describe amount, color, and consistency of stools; check for occult blood and/or reducing substances if ordered or indicated by appearance of stool.

Describe bowel sounds: presence or absence (must be present if feeding).

Genitourinary Assessment

Describe any abnormalities of genitalia.

Describe amount (as determined by weight), color, pH, labstick findings, and specific gravity of urine (to screen for adequacy of hydration).

Check weight (the most accurate measure for assessment of hydration).

Neurologic-Musculoskeletal Assessment

Describe infant's movements: random, purposeful, jittery, twitching, spontaneous, elicited; level of activity with stimulation; evaluate based on gestational age.

Describe infant's position or attitude: flexed, extended.

Describe reflexes observed: Moro, sucking, Babinski, plantar reflex, and other expected reflexes.

Determine level of response and consolability.

Determine changes in head circumference (if indicated); size and tension of fontanels, suture lines.

Determine pupillary responses in infant >32 weeks of gestation.

Temperature

Determine skin and axillary temperature.

Determine relationship to environmental temperature.

Skin Assessment

Describe any discoloration, reddened area, signs of irritation, blisters, abrasions, or denuded areas, especially where monitoring equipment, infusions, or other apparatus come in contact with skin; also check and note *any* skin preparation used (e.g., povidone-iodine tape).

Determine texture and turgor of skin: dry, smooth, flaky, peeling, etc.

Describe any rash, skin lesion, or birthmarks.

Determine whether intravenous infusion device is in place and observe for signs of infiltration.

Describe parenteral infusion lines: location, type (arterial, venous, peripheral, umbilical, central, peripheral central venous); type of infusion (medication, saline, dextrose, electrolyte, lipids, total parenteral nutrition); type of infusion pump and rate of flow; type of needle (butterfly, catheter); appearance of insertion site.

Monitoring Physiologic Data

High-risk neonates are placed in a controlled thermal environment and monitored for heart rate, respiratory activity, and temperature. Monitoring devices are equipped with an alarm system that indicates when the vital signs are above or below preset limits. However, it is essential to check the infant's heartbeat and respirations, and compare these with the monitor reading.

The placement of electrodes is a continual nursing problem because of the lack of flat areas on the neonate's chest and the limited space for alternating sites, the size of the electrodes, and irritation from the paste or tape. Electrodes for cardiac monitors can often be applied to the back or the upper arms to provide relief for chest areas; nonadhesive limb electrodes eliminate possible skin irritation from tape. Hydro-

TABLE 9-1. Blood pressure ranges in different weight groups of healthy premature infants*

BIRTH WEIGHT (g)	SYSTOLIC (mm Hg)	DIASTOLIC (mm Hg)
501-750	50-62	26-36
751-1000	48-59	23-36
1001-1250	49-61	26-35
1251-1500	46-56	23-33
1501-1750	46-58	23-33
1751-2000	48-61	24-35

Modified from Hegyi T and others: Blood pressure ranges in premature infants. I. The first hours of life, *J Pediatr* 124(4):630, 1994.
*Defined as infants without a history of maternal hypertension, Apgar scores of less than 3 at 1 minute and less than 6 at 5 minutes, pneumothorax, hematocrit <0.32, serum pH <7.1, use of dopamine, infusion of erythrocytes or colloid, mechanical ventilation, or cardiopulmonary resuscitation.

gel electrodes* are gentler to the skin and are easily removed by lifting an edge from the skin and moistening with plain water to release the adhesive. If the same electrode is reapplied to the skin, the hydrogel should be rinsed with plain water to remove accumulated sodium from perspiration, which can eventually irritate the skin. It is important to follow the manufacturer's directions for care and handling of electrodes to avoid malfunction or burns to sensitive skin.

Blood pressure (BP) is monitored routinely in the sick neonate by either internal or external means. Direct recording with arterial catheters is often employed but carries the risks inherent in any procedure in which a catheter is introduced into an artery. An umbilical venous catheter may also be used to monitor the neonate's central venous pressure. Oscillometry (Dinamap) or Doppler transcutaneous apparatus are simple, effective means for detecting alterations in systemic BP (hypotension or hypertension). Normal BP ranges for healthy premature infants are listed in Table 9-1.

In the NICU frequent laboratory examinations and their interpretation are integral parts of the ongoing assessment of infants' progress. Accurate intake and output records are kept on all infants. An accurate output can be obtained by collecting urine in a plastic urine collection bag specifically made for premature infants (see Urine Specimens, Chapter 22) or by weighing the diapers, the simplest and least traumatic means of measuring urinary output. The preweighed wet diaper is weighed on a gram scale, and the gram weight of the urine is converted directly to milliliters (e.g., 25 g = 25 ml).

NURSING TIP When small volumes of urine are measured, superabsorbent disposable diapers, especially when kept closed, give more accurate measurements than cloth diapers because they are less affected by evaporative losses (Fox, 1992).

*One manufacturer is Sentry Medical Products, 17171 Murphy Ave, Irvine, CA 92714; (800) 854-6004 or (800) 966-1118 (in California).

Plastic collecting devices can be used when it is necessary to collect urine for laboratory examination. Since the volume normally voided is insufficient to float the standard urometer, a refractometer requiring only a single drop of urine is sometimes used. A drop of urine can be aspirated with a syringe from the wet diaper or from cotton balls placed in the diaper.

Blood examinations are a necessary part of the ongoing assessment and monitoring of the sick newborn's progress. The tests most often performed are blood glucose, bilirubin, calcium, hematocrit, and blood gases. Samples may be obtained from the heel, by venipuncture, by arterial puncture, or by an indwelling catheter in an umbilical vein, umbilical artery, or peripheral artery.

NURSING TIP Wrapping the foot in a warm, damp washcloth or disposable diaper is a simple way to create adequate vasodilation for a heel stick. Commercial warm packs are also available but should be used with extreme caution in ELBW and VLBW infants to prevent burns.

When numerous blood samples must be drawn, it is important to maintain an accurate record of the amount of blood being removed, especially in ELBW and VLBW infants, who can ill afford to have their blood supply depleted during the acute phase of their illness. To obtain frequent samples for monitoring arterial blood gas levels without repeated arterial punctures, pulse oximetry, transcutaneous oxygen ($tcPo_2$), and/or carbon dioxide ($tcPco_2$), are used.

❖ Nursing Diagnoses
The nursing diagnoses that represent general guides for nursing intervention are found in the Nursing Care Plan on pp. 244-248. Since a number of health problems accompany the high-risk infant, other conditions and complications are discussed later in this chapter and elsewhere in the book.

❖ Planning
The nursing care plan for the high-risk infant depends to a large extent on the diagnosis of the health problem that places the infant at risk. However, the following are basic goals for all high-risk infants:

1. Infant will exhibit adequate oxygenation.
2. Infant will maintain stable body temperature.
3. Infant will exhibit no evidence of nosocomial infection.
4. Infant will receive adequate hydration and nutrition.
5. Infant will maintain skin integrity.
6. Infant will exhibit normal increased intracranial pressure and no evidence of intraventricular hemorrhage (unless pre-existing condition).
7. Infant will experience no pain or a reduction of pain.
8. Infant receives appropriate developmental care.
9. Family receives appropriate support, including preparation for home care or for infant's death.

❖ Implementation

Respiratory Support
The primary objective in the care of high-risk infants is to establish and maintain respiration. Many infants require supplemental oxygen and assisted ventilation. Infants with or

without these supportive treatments are positioned to maximize oxygenation. Oxygen therapy is provided on the basis of the infant's requirements and illness (see Respiratory Distress Syndrome, p. 259, and Oxygen Therapy, Ch. 22).

Thermoregulation

After, or concurrent with, the establishment of respiration, the most crucial need of high-risk infants is the application of external warmth. To delay or prevent the effects of cold stress, infants are placed in a heated environment immediately after birth; they remain there until they are able to maintain thermal stability (balance heat production and conservation with heat dissipation). This is especially important for the preterm infant, whose very high skin surface relative to body mass promotes heat loss.

The naked or diapered infant is placed in the controlled microenvironment of an incubator. A Plexiglas top affords a clear view of the infant from all aspects (Fig. 9-6). There is easy access through portholes that minimize temperature and oxygen loss and a large door that provides a more extensive approach. Maximum accessibility is provided by an open unit with an overhead radiant warming system (Fig. 9-7).

Since overheating produces an increase in oxygen and calorie consumption, the infant is also jeopardized if he or she becomes hyperthermic. A *neutral thermal environment* is one that permits the infant to maintain a normal core temperature, with minimum oxygen consumption and calorie expenditure. The very small infant, especially one with a meager subcutaneous fat layer, can control body heat loss or gain only within a very limited range of environmental tempera-

ture. Recent studies indicate that optimum thermoneutrality cannot be predicted for every high-risk infant's needs. Guidelines for providing an optimum thermal environment suggest maintaining the infant's axillary temperature within a range of 36.5° to 37.5° C (97.7° to 99.5° F) (Thomas, 1994).

Consumption of oxygen is minimal at an abdominal skin temperature of 36.5° C (97.7° F). When abdominal skin temperature increases or decreases, the oxygen consumption increases. The range of abdominal skin temperature that produces a neutral thermal environment is 36° to 36.5° C (96.8° to 97.6° F).

The consequences of cold stress that produce additional hazards to the neonate are (1) hypoxia, (2) metabolic acidosis, and (3) hypoglycemia. Increased metabolism in response to chilling creates a compensatory increase in oxygen and calorie consumption. If available oxygen is not increased to accommodate this need, arterial oxygen tension is decreased. This is further complicated by a smaller lung volume in relation to the metabolic rate, which creates diminished oxygen in the blood and concurrent pulmonary disorders.

The three methods for maintaining a neutral thermal environment are by the use of an incubator (Fig. 9-6), a radiant warming panel (Fig. 9-7), and an open bassinet with cotton blankets. The dressed infant under blankets can maintain a temperature within a wider range of environmental temperatures; however, the close observations required by a high-

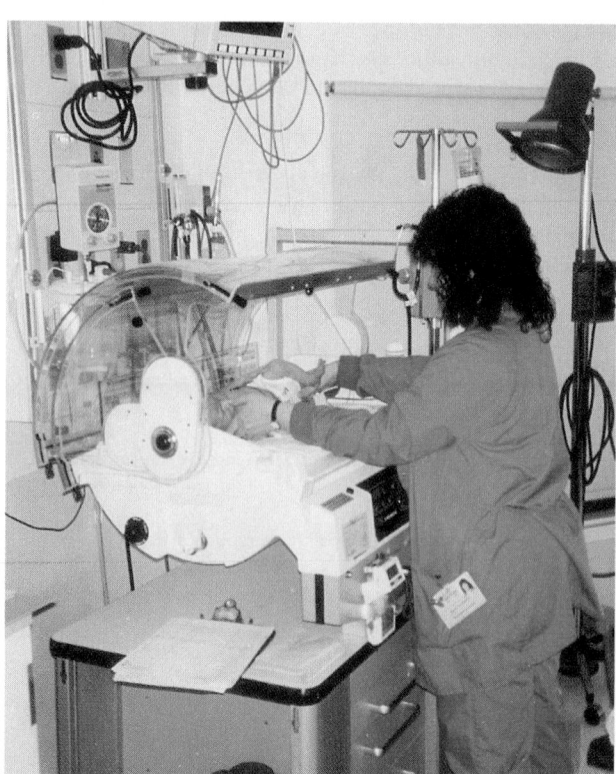

FIG. 9-6. Nurse caring for infant in incubator.

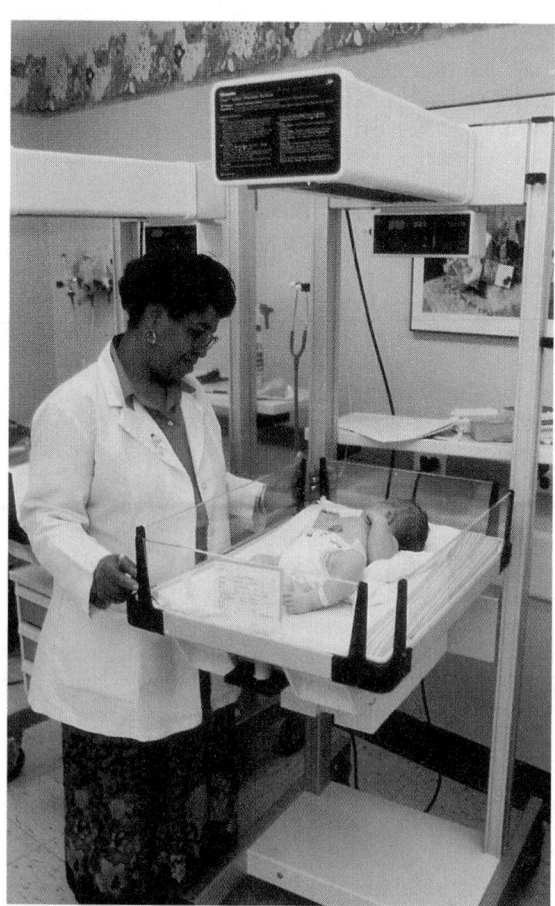

FIG. 9-7. Infant under overhead warming unit.

risk infant are best accomplished if the infant remains partially unclothed. The incubator should always be prewarmed before placing an infant in it. The use of *double-walled incubators* significantly improves the infant's ability to maintain a desirable temperature and reduce energy expenditure related to heat regulation. The infant is clothed and warmly wrapped in blankets when removed from the warm environment of the incubator for feeding or cuddling. Inside or outside the incubator, head coverings are effective in preventing heat loss. A fabric-insulated cap is more effective than one fashioned from stockinette (Blackburn and Loper, 1992).

An effective means for maintaining the desired range of temperature in the infant is by way of a *manually adjusted* or *automatically controlled (servocontrolled) incubator.* The latter mechanism, when set at the upper and lower limits of the desired circulating air temperature range, adjusts automatically in response to signals from a thermal sensor attached to the abdominal skin. If the infant's temperature drops, the warming device is triggered to increase heat output. The servocontrol is usually set to a desired skin temperature between 36° and 36.5° C (96.8° to 97.7° F).

Disadvantages are always inherent in any mechanical device; therefore an important part of nursing assessment is to compare the infant's temperature with the temperature in the incubator. For example, if the infant's temperature fluctuates in response to sepsis, the servocontrolled mechanism would respond by decreasing or increasing the ambient air temperature. Therefore a critical observation could be easily overlooked. A plastic bubble wrap or sheet may be used to decrease *insensible water loss* and preserve heat in ELBW and VLBW infants.

> **Nursing ALERT**
> When using a servocontrolled incubator, evaluate trends of increased or decreased ambient air temperature in response to fluctuations in the infant's body temperature to rule out sepsis or other dysfunction. (See Critical Thinking Exercise.)

Protection from Infection

Protection from infection is an integral part of all newborn care, but preterm and sick neonates are particularly susceptible. Frequent and meticulous handwashing between handling different infants and equipment is the foundation of a preventive program. This includes *all* persons who come in contact with infants and their equipment.

> **Nursing ALERT**
> The increased use of gloves for standard precautions does not eliminate the need for careful handwashing between high-risk neonates and between areas considered "dirty" (i.e., diapers) and "clean" (i.e., bottle feeding or IV drug administration).

Personnel with infectious disorders are either barred from the unit until they are no longer infectious or are required to wear suitable shields, such as masks or gloves, to reduce the likelihood of contamination. Standard precautions as a method of infection control are instituted in all nursery areas to protect the infants and staff (see Chapter 22). In some areas special clothing furnished by the institution is worn by

---

ᑕRITICAL THINKING EXERCISE

Thermoregulation

A 24-day-old 3-pound preterm infant in a servocontrolled incubator has consistently lost 30 to 50 g over the last 2 days following 2 weeks of adequate weight gain with gavage feedings. In addition, the environmental temperature in the incubator has steadily increased by 5° C while the infant's axillary temperature has ranged from 36.4° to 36.5° C (97.5° to 97.7° F). The incubator is located near a doorway of the NICU leading to an outer hallway; there is heavy traffic through this doorway. Other vital signs have remained consistently stable, and the incubator has been verified by engineers to be functioning properly. A possible explanation for the infant's increased environmental temperature control and appropriate intervention is:

1. Servocontrol is not effective in maintaining the temperature of an infant of this size; use air temperature control.
2. Air drafts from the doorway traffic and single-walled incubator increase radiant heat loss; a double-walled incubator should be used. An alternative is to use a cloth incubator cover and move the incubator away from the doorway.
3. The infant's larger body surface is creating conductive heat loss; wrap the infant snugly in a cotton blanket inside the incubator.
4. The infant more than likely has suffered damage to the central nervous system, such as an intraventricular hemorrhage, causing subsequent thermal instability; monitor the infant for signs of seizure activity.

The correct answer is two. Air drafts created by air vents and doors and staff traffic can cause radiant heat loss from the infant's warm body surface to the cooled exterior single wall of the incubator, subsequently increasing the demand for environmental temperature to maintain the infant's core body temperature.

This increased metabolic demand for energy leaves fewer calories available for growth.

Options one and three are not factual statements. Option four is unlikely, primarily because of the infant's age and stable vital signs.

---

everyone working in the unit. Fresh scrub dresses or suits are put on before entering the unit and are changed any time they become contaminated. When personnel leave the unit, the scrub clothing is protected by a cover gown that is removed and then discarded in the laundry hamper before the wearer reenters the unit. However, the benefit of "gowning" to control infection is not supported by research (Pelke and others, 1994).

The sources of infection rise in direct relationship to the number of persons and pieces of equipment coming in contact with the infants. Equipment used in the care of infants is cleaned on a regular basis as per the manufacturer's recommendations or institutional protocol; this includes cleaning of cribs, mattresses, incubators, radiant warmers, cardiorespiratory monitors, pulse oximeters, and Dinamap monitors after they are with one infant and before they are used with another. Since organisms thrive best in water, plumbing and humidifying equipment are particularly hazardous. Disposable equipment used for water-related therapies, such as nebulizers and plastic oxygen tubing, is changed regularly.

Hydration

It is not uncommon for high-risk infants to receive supplemental parenteral fluids to supply additional calories, electrolytes, and/or water. Adequate hydration is particularly important in preterm infants because their extracellular water content is higher (70% in full-term infants and up to 90% in preterm infants), their body surface is larger, and the capacity for osmotic diuresis is limited in preterm infants' underdeveloped kidneys. Therefore these infants are highly vulnerable to water depletion.

Parenteral fluids may be given to the high-risk neonate via several routes depending on the nature of the illness, the duration and type of fluid therapy, and institutional (or NICU) preference. Common routes of fluid infusion include peripheral, peripherally inserted central venous, surgically inserted central venous or arterial, and, at times, umbilical venous or umbilical arterial catheterization. The preferred sites for intravenous (IV) infusions in neonates are peripheral veins on the dorsal surfaces of hands or feet. Alternative sites are scalp veins and antecubital veins. Special precautions and frequent observations (at least once every hour) must accompany the use of peripheral lines with hypertonic solutions (dextrose 10% to 15%) and hyperalimentation. If peripheral sites are exhausted by long-term therapy, percutaneous central venous lines or a venous cutdown (usually inserted in the saphenous or antecubital vein) may be employed.

NURSING TIP A small armboard for the hand may be made by cutting a tongue blade in half (lengthwise) and padding it with gauze.

Nursing ALERT Nurses should be constantly alert for signs of infiltration (such as redness, edema, or color change of tissue, blanching at site) and for signs of overhydration (weight gain over 30 g/24 hr, periorbital edema, tachypnea, tachycardia, and moist crackles on lung auscultation).

Infants who are ELBW, tachypneic, receiving phototherapy, or in a radiant warmer have increased insensible water losses, which require appropriate fluid adjustments. Nurses must monitor fluid status by daily (or more frequent) weights, accurate intake and output of all fluids, including medications and blood products, specific gravity, dipstick measurements of urine, and evaluation of serum electrolyte levels. ELBW infants will often require more frequent monitoring of these parameters because of their inordinate fluid loss, immature renal function, and propensity to dehydration or overhydration. Intolerance of even dextrose 5% is not uncommon in the ELBW infant, with subsequent glycosuria and osmotic diuresis. Alterations in behavior, alertness, and/or activity level in these infants receiving intravenous fluids may signal an electrolyte imbalance, hypoglycemia, or hyperglycemia; the nurse is also observant for tremors or seizures in the VLBW or ELBW infant, since this may be a sign of hyponatremia or hypernatremia.

A common problem observed in infants who have an um-bilical catheter in place is vasoconstriction of peripheral vessels that can seriously impair circulation. The response is triggered by arterial vasospasm caused by the presence of the catheter, the infusion of fluids, or injection of medication. Blanching of the buttocks, genitalia, or legs or feet is an indication of vasospasm. The problem is recognized promptly and reported to the practitioner.

Nursing ALERT Circulatory effects are observed first in the toes but may extend to include the legs and buttocks. The toes first flush and then turn a mulberry color, and if the condition is not corrected, there may be serious complications involving the loss of a limb.

Nutrition

Optimum nutrition is critical in the management of LBW preterm infants, but there are difficulties in providing for their nutritional needs. The various mechanisms for ingestion and digestion of foods are not fully developed, and the more immature the infant, the greater the problem. In addition, the nutritional requirements of this group of infants are not known with certainty.

An infant's need for rapid growth and daily maintenance must be met in the presence of several anatomic and physiologic disabilities. Although some sucking and swallowing activities are demonstrated before birth and in preterm infants, coordination of these mechanisms does not occur until approximately 32 to 34 weeks of gestation, and they are not fully synchronized until 36 to 37 weeks. Initial sucking is not accompanied by swallowing, and esophageal contractions are uncoordinated. The gag reflex may not be developed until 36 weeks of gestation. Consequently, infants are highly prone to aspiration and its attendant dangers.

The amount and method of feeding are determined by the size and condition of the infant. Nutrition can be provided by either the parenteral or the enteral route or by a combination of the two. Infants who are ELBW, VLBW, and/or critically ill are often fed exclusively by the parenteral route because of their inability to digest and absorb enteral nutrition. Illness factors resulting in hypoxia and major organ immaturity further preclude the use of enteral feeding until the infant's condition is stabilized; necrotizing enterocolitis has been associated with enteral feedings in acutely ill or distressed infants (see section on necrotizing enterocolitis in this chapter).

Although the timing of the first feeding has been a matter of controversy, most authorities now believe that early feeding, usually within 3 to 6 hours after birth (provided that the infant is medically stable), reduces the incidence of complicating factors such as hypoglycemia, dehydration, and the degree of hyperbilirubinemia. The feeding regimen employed varies from institution to institution. The initial enteral feeding is usually not attempted until infants have adapted to extrauterine existence as evidenced by adequate oxygenation, evidence of GI motility, including passage of meconium, and stable cardiopulmonary status.

Total parenteral nutritional support of acutely ill infants may be accomplished quite successfully with commercially available intravenous solutions specifically designed to meet the infant's nutritional needs, including protein, amino acids, trace minerals, vitamins, carbohydrates (dextrose), and fat (lipid emulsion). Daily monitoring of weight, electrolytes, renal function, calcium, triglycerides (or lipoprotein), and hydration status is carried out to ensure adequate therapy.

Nipple Feeding. Vigorous infants can be fed from a nipple with little difficulty, whereas weaker preterm infants will require alternative methods. Sterile water may be offered first. The amount to be fed is determined largely by the infant's weight and tolerance of previous feeding and is increased by small increments until a satisfactory caloric intake is ensured. Sometimes supplementary calories are needed in the form of dietary additives, such as Lipomul* (which provides vegetable fat and carbohydrates), MCT oil† (which provides fat in the form of medium-chain triglycerides), Polycose, and human milk fortifier or formula with increased caloric density.

The rate of increase that is well tolerated varies from one infant to another, and determining this rate may be a nursing responsibility. Preterm infants require more time and patience to feed as compared with full-term infants, and the oral-pharyngeal mechanism may be stressed by an attempt to feed too rapidly. It is important not to tire the infants or overtax their capacity to retain the feedings. When infants require a prolonged time period (arbitrarily over 30 to 45 minutes) to complete a feeding, gavage feeding may be considered for the next time (see Critical Thinking Exercise).

---

*Roberts Pharmaceutical Corp., Eatontown, NJ.
†Mead Johnson & Co., Evansville, IN.

CRITICAL THINKING EXERCISE
Infant Feeding

The mother of a 4-pound, 36-week preterm infant who has only recently started nipple feeding expresses concern that the feeding takes 25 to 30 minutes and that the infant has one or two apneic episodes during feedings. The infant is gaining approximately 20 to 30 g per day, and axillary temperature has been 36.6° C (97.9° F) throughout the day. To assist the mother in understanding aspects of feeding a preterm infant, your best response should be to:

1. Suggest that the mother let the experienced nurse feed the infant until the mother learns to feed correctly.
2. Recommend that the mother use a softer, pliable nipple to allow the infant to feed faster.
3. Encourage the mother to continue feeding the infant, with frequent rest periods or pauses.
4. Explain to the mother that the infant will require all feedings to be given by gavage, since the infant is so small and has apnea.

The correct answer is three. It is not uncommon for preterm infants to experience apnea with nipple feedings. Frequent short breaks in feeding allow for swallowing and breathing to occur.

Option two is incorrect—a soft nipple is not desirable, and expediency in feeding is not always the major goal. Since the infant is demonstrating adequate weight gain, there is no reason to gavage feed or suspect pathologic apnea as suggested in option four. Option one is incorrect because it discounts the mother's involvement in the care of her infant.

Tolerance related to the infant's ability to nipple feed should be based on an evaluation of respiratory status, heart rate, and oxygen saturation; variations from normal may indicate stress and fatigue (Davis, 1992). The preterm infant will experience difficulty coordinating sucking, swallowing, and breathing, with resultant apnea, bradycardia, and decreased oxygen saturation. The preterm infant's ability to suck on a pacifier does not indicate complete readiness for nipple feeding or ability to coordinate the above-mentioned activities without some degree of stress; a gradual introduction of nippling in the preterm infant is based on careful evaluation of his or her ability to maintain adequate cardiopulmonary functions while nippling. When infants are unable to tolerate bottle-feedings, intermittent feedings by gavage are instituted until they gain enough strength and coordination to use the nipple.

> **Nursing ALERT** Poor feeding behaviors such as apnea, bradycardia, cyanosis, pallor, and decreased oxygen saturation in any infant who has previously fed well may indicate an underlying illness.

The nipple used should be relatively firm and stable. A high-flow, pliable nipple, although it requires less energy to use, may provide a flow rate that is too rapid for some preterm infants to manage without risk of aspiration. A firmer nipple facilitates a more "cupped" tongue configuration and allows for a more controlled, manageable flow rate.

The infant is positioned in the feeder's arms or placed semiupright in the lap (Fig. 9-8), and is held with the back curved slightly to simulate the position assumed naturally by most full-term newborns. Stroking the infant's lips, cheeks, and tongue before feeding helps promote oral sensitivity. In-

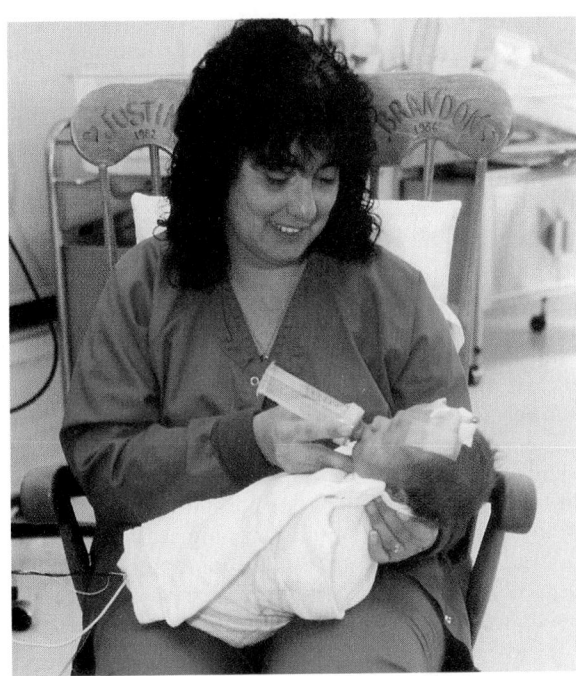

FIG. 9-8. Position for nipple feeding the premature infant.

ward and upward support to the infant's cheeks and a slightly upward lift to the chin are provided by the fingers to assist nipple compression during feeding.

Bottle-feedings are continued if infants are able to tolerate the feedings and take the required amount. The infant is best fed when fully alert. Drowsy infants feed more slowly, and liquid is more likely to fill the relaxed pharynx before the infant swallows, causing choking. Preterm infants are often slow feeders, requiring patience, frequent rest periods, and burping (or bubbling).

Nursing ALERT An increase in gastric residuals, abdominal distention, bilious vomiting, temperature instability, apneic episodes, and bradycardia may indicate early necrotizing enterocolitis (NEC) and are reported to the practitioner.

Breast-Feeding. Studies indicate that even small preterm infants are able to breast-feed if the infant has adequate sucking and swallowing reflexes and there are no other contraindications, such as respiratory complications, or concurrent illness. There is evidence supporting breast-feeding in VLBW infants, especially those with bronchopulmonary dysplasia who experienced less oxygen desaturation than bottle-fed neonates of the same weight and age (Bier and others, 1994). Mothers who wish to breast-feed their preterm infants are encouraged to pump their breasts until their infants are sufficiently stable to tolerate breast-feeding. Appropriate guidelines for the storage of expressed mother's milk (EMM) should be followed to decrease the risk of milk contamination and destruction of its beneficial properties. Premature infants are able to breast-feed when they (Gardner, O'Donnell, and Weisman, 1993):

- Experience wakeful periods and awaken before feedings
- Exhibit coordinated suck, swallow, and gag reflexes
- Have supplemental oxygen supplied by flow-by or nasal cannula
- Have adequate thermal support provided by swaddler, hat, or overhead radiant warmer

Time, patience, and dedication on the part of the mother and the nursing staff are needed to help high-risk infants with breast-feeding. The process is begun slowly—beginning with one feeding daily and gradually increasing the feedings as the infant tolerates them. Infants should not be placed on an empty breast to feed, since the infant will become exhausted, and nonnutritive sucking (NNS) does not stimulate milk production. The infant will become frustrated and refuse to feed without the reward of milk. Supplementary bottle feeding is inefficient, since the baby expends energy and calories to feed twice. Feeding more often, supplementing by gavage feeding, or using a training nipple is more energy and calorically efficient. Breast-feeding of the preterm infant often requires additional guidance by a lactation consultant; continued support and encouragement by the nursing staff is essential to breast-feeding preterm infants. In addition, postdischarge breast-feeding often requires further guidance, counseling, and support by nursing staff (Davis, 1992; Meier and others, 1993).

Gavage Feeding. Gavage feeding is a safe means of meeting the nutritional requirements of infants who are less than 32 weeks of gestation or infants who weigh less than 1500 g. These infants are usually too weak to suck effectively, are unable to coordinate swallowing, and lack a gag reflex. Gavage feedings may be provided by continuous drip regulated via infusion pump or by intermittent bolus feedings. For infants learning to nipple feed and who become excessively tired, are listless, or become cyanotic, intermittent gavage feeding is used as an energy-conserving technique.

A 15-inch (37.5 cm) size 5 or 8 French feeding tube is used to instill the formula, and the usual methods for determining correct placement are employed (see Chapter 22 for technique). Although the more relaxed cardiac sphincter makes passage of the tube easier, there may be changes in heart rate and blood pressure in response to vagal stimulation. The procedure is best accomplished when an infant is in a prone or a right side-lying position with the head slightly elevated. It is preferable to insert the tube through the mouth rather than the nares. Nasal insertion obstructs nose breathing and may irritate the delicate nasal mucosa. Passage through the mouth also provides an opportunity to observe the sucking response. However, because of less stimulation of the gag reflex, nasal tube gavage may be used in certain situations, such as in older preterm infants who need supplementation after nipple feeding but who fight, gag, and vomit with oral tube management.

The stomach is aspirated, the contents measured, and the aspirate returned as part of the feeding. The amount of the aspirate depends on the length of time since the previous feeding or concurrent illness. Whether or not the amount of the aspirate is deducted from the total feeding varies among units. Some advocate deducting to avoid overdistending the stomach. For example, if a feeding is 25 ml and the aspirate is 5 ml, the aspirate is returned plus 20 ml of feeding for a total of 25 ml. In other units the amount is determined on an individual basis.

The formula is allowed to flow by gravity, and the length of time varies. *This procedure is not used as a timesaving method for the nurse.* Complications of indwelling tubes include obstructed nares, mucous plugs, purulent rhinitis, epistaxis, infection, and possible stomach perforation.

The nurse needs to observe premature infants closely for behaviors that indicate readiness for bottle-feedings. These include (1) a strong, vigorous suck; (2) coordination of sucking and swallowing; (3) a gag reflex; (4) sucking on the gavage tube, hands, or pacifier; and (5) rooting and wakefulness before and sleeping after feedings. When these behaviors are noted, infants can be challenged with nipple feedings introduced slowly.

The infant may be held during gavage feedings by the caregiver or parent. Oxygen may be supplied via nasal cannula to facilitate handling. It is not recommended that the infant be removed from a primary source of oxygen, such as a hood or tent, for feedings, since this decreases oxygen availability. Flow-by oxygen may be given for brief episodes of desaturation, but this is inadequate for the duration of feedings, either by gavage or nipple. Also, NNS on a pacifier helps infants associate the sucking with the feeling of satiety. Oxygen by nasal cannula is often used as the infant's condition permits to allow greater parental contact and optimize oxygenation. (See discussion on skin-to-skin contact or kangaroo care in this chapter.)

Feeding Resistance

Any feeding technique that bypasses the mouth precludes the opportunity for the affected child to practice sucking and swallowing, or the opportunity to experience normal hunger and satiation cycles. Infants may demonstrate aversion to oral feedings by such behaviors as averting the head to the presentation of the nipple, extruding the nipple by tongue thrust, gagging, or even vomiting. Other observations include disinterest in or active resistance to oral play, diminished spontaneity and motivation, and shallow interpersonal relationships, probably related to the absence of some early incorporative patterns of normal oral experiences. The longer the period of nonoral feeding, the more severe the feeding problems, especially if this period occurs during the time when the infant progresses from reflexive to learned and voluntary feeding actions. Infancy is the period during which the mouth is the primary instrument for reception of stimulation and pleasure.

Infants who are identified as being at risk for feeding resistance should be provided with regular oral stimulation such as stroking the oral area from cheeks to lips, touching the tongue, placing some of the feeding on the lips and tongue, and associating feeding with pleasurable activities (holding, talking, making eye contact). Those who exhibit feeding aversion should begin a stimulation program to overcome resistance and acquire the ability to take nourishment by the oral route. Since management requires long-term commitment, successful implementation of a plan for oral stimulation depends on maximum parental involvement and provision of consistent nurses.

Energy Conservation

One of the major goals of care for the high-risk infant is conservation of energy. Much of the care described in this section is directed toward this end (e.g., disturbing the infant as little as possible, maintaining a neutral thermal environment, employing gavage feeding, promoting oxygenation, and judiciously implementing any caregiving activities that increase oxygen and caloric consumption). When the infant is not required to expend energy to cope with efforts to breathe, eat, or alter the body temperature, this energy can be used for growth and development. Diminishing noise levels and bright lights also promote rest (see also Infant Stress, p. 236, and Developmental Intervention, p. 237).

The prone position is optimum for most preterm infants and results in improved oxygenation, better-tolerated feedings, and more organized sleep-rest patterns. Infants exhibit less physical activity and energy expenditure when they are placed in the prone position (Fox and Molesky, 1990). Others appear to prefer a flexed side-lying posture. Prolonged supine positioning for preterm infants is not desirable, because they appear to lose their sense of equilibrium when supine and use vital energy in attempts to recover balance by postural changes. However, in light of the American Academy of Pediatrics' recommendation for the supine sleeping position for healthy full-term infants, position preferences should be discussed with the practitioner for home care.

Skin Care

The skin of premature infants is characteristically immature relative to that of full-term infants. Because of its increased sensitivity and fragility, no alkaline-based soap is used that might destroy the "acid mantle" of the skin. The increased permeability of the skin facilitates absorption of ingredients. All skin products (e.g., alcohol or povidone-iodine) are used with caution, and the skin is rinsed with water afterward, since these substances may cause severe irritation and chemical burns in LBW infants.

The skin is easily excoriated and denuded; therefore care must be taken to avoid damage to the delicate structure. The total skin is less thick than that of full-term infants and has fewer elastic fibers; also, there is less cohesion between the thinner skin layers. Adhesives used after heel sticks or to secure monitoring equipment or intravenous infusions may excoriate the skin or adhere to the skin surface so well that the skin can be separated from understructures and pulled away with the tape (epidermal stripping). The use of skin barriers protects healthy skin and helps excoriated skin heal.

It is unsafe to use scissors to remove dressings or tape from the extremities of very small and immature infants, because it is easy to snip off tiny extremities or nick loosely attached skin. Solvents used to remove tape are avoided because they tend to dry and burn the delicate skin. Guidelines for skin care are listed in the Guidelines box on p. 236.

During skin assessment of preterm infants, nurses are also alert to the subtle signs that indicate zinc deficiency, a problem sometimes seen in infants who have inadequate parenteral intake of zinc. Breakdown usually occurs in the areas around the mouth, buttocks, fingers, and toes. In VLBW infants it may also occur in the creases of the neck, wrists, ankles, and around wounds. Zinc deficiency is most likely to appear in infants with sepsis, those experiencing nasogastric losses, or those who have had surgery. Any suspicious lesions are reported to the practitioner so the condition may be evaluated.

Administration of Medications

Administration of therapeutic agents, such as drugs, ointments, intravenous infusions, and oxygen, requires judicious handling and meticulous attention to details. The computation, preparation, and administration of drugs in minute amounts often require collaboration between nurses, physicians, and pharmacists to reduce the chance of error. In addition, the immaturity of an infant's detoxification mechanisms and inability to demonstrate symptoms of toxicity (e.g., signs of auditory nerve involvement from ototoxic drugs such as gentamycin) complicate drug therapy and require that nurses be particularly alert for signs of adverse reaction. (See Administration of Medication, Chapter 22.)

Nurses should be aware of the hazards of administering bacteriostatic and hyperosmolar solutions to infants. Benzyl alcohol, a common preservative in bacteriostatic water and saline, has been shown to be toxic to newborns and should not be used to flush intravenous catheters or to dilute or reconstitute medications. It is recommended that medications with preservatives such as benzyl alcohol be avoided whenever possible. Nurses must read labels carefully to detect the presence of preservatives in any medication to be administered to an infant.

Hyperosmolar solutions present a potential danger to preterm infants. Hyperosmolar solutions given orally to infants can produce clinical, physiologic, and morphologic alter-

GUIDELINES
Neonatal Skin Care

General Skin Care

Cleanse skin with plain warm water. Use bland, nonalkaline soaps or cleansers only when necessary, such as for removal of stool.

Provide daily cleansing of eye, oral, and diaper areas, and any areas of skin breakdown.

Apply moisturizing agents to skin after cleansing with warm water to retain moisture and rehydrate skin. Cleanse skin gently of any old oil or cream before applying a new layer, except in diaper area (see Diaper Dermatitis, Chapter 29).

When safflower oil is applied, some essential fatty acids may be absorbed in addition to softening skin as a moisturizer.

Use pressure-relieving or reducing mattress to prevent pressure areas (see also Maintaining Healthy Skin, Chapter 22).

Use of Adhesives on Skin

Use minimal tape/adhesive. Evaluate need for all tape/adhesive used. Chart amount and placement of all tape used.

Use a protective, pectin-based or hydrocolloid skin barrier between skin and all tape/adhesives. Place on all areas where tape/adhesives are used, such as for securing chest tubes, nasogastric tubes, dressings, extremities to IV board, monitor leads, endotracheal tubes, and temperature probe (cut "keyhole" for temperature probe in barrier or place circular patch of skin barrier over probe).

Place pectin-based or hydrocolloid skin barriers directly over excoriated skin. Leave barrier undisturbed until it begins to peel off. With wet, oozing excoriations, dust site with a small amount of stoma powder (as used in ostomy care), brush excess away, and apply skin barrier. Hold barrier in place for several minutes to allow barrier to soften and mold to the skin surface.

Use transparent elastic film dressings to secure and protect central lines and peripheral arterial line insertion sites, as well as over open skin lesions. Leave dressing in place until it begins to peel off, usually within 5 to 7 days.

Alternate electrode placement and avoid standard adhesive, gelled electrode. Use limb electrodes rather than standard chest electrodes or use hydrogel or synthetic karaya gel electrodes. Assess skin thoroughly underneath electrodes. Remove and rotate electrodes minimally every 24 hours, or more frequently if skin injury is noted.

Remove adhesives with warm water-soaked gauze or a small amount of bland, diluted soap, rather than alcohol or adhesive removers. To remove a skin barrier, slowly and gently peel away from skin, holding barrier in one hand and supporting skin underneath with other hand. If needed, soak off with warm water. Do not use bonding agents such as tincture of benzoin or commercial swabs.

Avoid using scissors to remove tape or dressings to prevent cutting skin or amputating digits.

Use of Substances on Skin

Evaluate all substances that come in contact with infant's skin.

Avoid or limit use of the following substances that have potential for percutaneous absorption and systemic effects:

Adhesive removers	Isopropyl alcohol
Boric acid	Neomycin ointment
Chlorhexidene	Povidone iodine
Chlorophenol	Salicylic acid
Epinephrine	Steroids
Estrogen	Tincture of benzoin
Hexachlorophene	Silver sulfadiazine cream
Hydrogen peroxide	

If any of the above agents are used, chart amount and frequency of application.

Before using any topical agent, analyze components of preparation and:

Use sparingly and only when necessary.

Confine use to smallest possible area.

Whenever possible and appropriate, wash off with water.

Monitor infant carefully for signs of toxicity and systemic effects.

Use of Thermal Devices

Be cautious when using heat lamps because of increased potential for burns. If needed, measure actual temperature of exposed skin every 15 minutes.

When using heating pads (Aqua-K pads):

Change infant's position every 15 minutes initially and then every 1 to 2 hours.

Preset temperature of heating pads <40° C (104° F).

When using preheated transcutaneous electrodes:

Avoid use on infants <1000 g.

Set at lowest possible temperature (<44° C [111.2° F]) and secure with plastic wrap.

Use pulse oximetry rather than transcutaneous monitoring whenever possible.

When prewarming heels before phlebotomy, avoid temperatures >40° C.

Warm ambient humidity, direct away from infant, use aerosolized sterile water, and maintain ambient temperature so as not to exceed 40° C.

Document use of all heating devices.

Use of Fluid Therapy/Hemodynamic Monitoring

Be certain fingers or toes are visible whenever extremity is used for IV or arterial line.

Secure catheter or needle with transparent dressing/tape to promote easy visualization of site.

Assess site hourly for signs of ischemia, infiltration, and inadequate perfusion (check capillary refill).

Check that any restraints (e.g., armboards) are secured safely and not restricting circulation or movement (check for pressure areas).

Modified from Malloy MB, Perez-Woods R: Neonatal skin care: prevention of skin breakdown, *Pediatr Nurs* 17(1):41-48, 1991.

---

ations, the most serious of which is necrotizing enterocolitis. Medications (oral or parenteral) should be sufficiently diluted to prevent complications related to hyperosmolality.

Infant Stress

Preterm infants are subject to stress just as other human beings are, but are biologically deficient in their capacity to cope with or adapt to environmental stresses. Stress affects hypothalamus function, causing adverse effects on growth, heat production, and neurologic mechanisms. Interventions designed to reduce stress in infants produce improvement in sleeping behavior and growth (see Developmental Intervention and Care, which follows). Nurses can have a profound influence in creating a nonstressful environment by modifying behaviors and environmental factors that produce infant

SIGNS OF STRESS OR FATIGUE IN NEONATES

Autonomic Stress
Acrocyanosis
Deep, rapid respirations
Regular, rapid heart rate

Changes in State
Dull or sleep states
Crying or fussy
Glassy-eyed or strained alertness

Behavioral Changes
Unfocused and uncoordinated eyes
Limp arms and legs
Flaccid shoulders dropped back
Hiccoughs
Sneezes
Yawning
Straining, having a bowel movement

From Als H: Toward a synactive theory of development: promise for the assessment and support of infant and individuality, *Infant Ment Health J* 3:229-243, 1982.

stress in the NICU; for example, gentle handling, correct positioning, and reduction of noxious stimuli (pain relief) help to reduce stress. Alert observation of evidence of stress and providing appropriate intervention help to reduce disorganized behavior (see box for signs of stress).

Developmental Intervention and Care

Much attention has been focused on the effects of early intervention, or its lack, on both normal and preterm infants. Findings indicate that infants are able to respond to a greater variety of stimuli than was previously thought, and that the atmosphere and activities of the NICU are overstimulating. Consequently, infants in the NICU are subjected to *inappropriate* stimulation that may be harmful. For example, the noise level that results from monitoring equipment, alarms, and general unit activity have been correlated with the incidence of intracranial hemorrhage, especially in the ELBW or VLBW infant. Personnel should reduce noise-generating activities, such as closing doors (including incubator portholes), listening to loud radios or talking loudly, and handling equipment (e.g., trash containers). Nursing care activities, such as taking vital signs, changing the infant's position, weighing, and changing diapers, while essential to the care of the high-risk neonate, have been shown to be associated with frequent periods of hypoxia, oxygen desaturation, and elevated intracranial pressure (Peters, 1992). The more immature the infant, the less able he or she is to habituate to a single procedure, such as taking an oscillometric BP, without becoming overstimulated.

Twenty-four-hour surveillance of sick infants implies maximum visibility and often continuous bright lights. However, many units establish a night-day sleep pattern by either darkening the room, if the infants' conditions allow it, covering cribs with blankets, or placing eye patches over the infant's eyes at night. Infants may have scheduled rest periods during which the lights are dimmed, cribs or incubators are covered with blankets, and the infants are not disturbed for handling of any kind.

The present approach to developmental intervention is to tailor the interaction to the developmental level and tolerance of each infant. During the early stages of development (especially before 33 weeks of gestation), stimulation produces uncoordinated, random activity, such as jerky limb extension, hyperflexion, and irregular vital signs. At this stage infants need to have minimum environmental stimulation. They are handled with slow, controlled movements (some infants are unstable if moved abruptly), and their random movements are controlled with limbs held close to their bodies during turning or other position changes. Additional containment measures include support with blanket rolls, when medically feasible. A nest constructed by placing blanket rolls underneath the bed sheet helps infants in maintaining an attitude of flexion when prone or side-lying.

Although it must be individually adjusted, skin contact and short periods of gentle massage can be helpful to reduce stress. Regular passive skin-to-skin contact *(kangaroo care)* between parents and LBW infants helps alleviate stress. The parent wears a loose-fitting, open-front top that provides a modified marsupial-like pocket carrier for the infant. The undressed (except for diaper) infant is placed in a vertical position on the parent's bare chest, which permits direct eye contact, skin-to-skin sensations, and close proximity. Skin-to-skin contact between parent and infant, in addition to being a safe and effective method for VLBW infant-parent acquaintance, has been shown to have a positive healing effect for the mother with a high-risk pregnancy. Additional benefits of skin-to-skin care include earlier contact with mechanically ventilated infants, maintenance of neonatal thermal stability, increased feeding vigor, maintenance of organized behavioral state, decreased unnecessary activity and minimal untoward effects of being held (Gale, Franck, and Lund, 1993; Ludington-Hoe and others, 1994).

When infants have reached sufficient developmental organization and stability (especially between 34 and 36 weeks of gestation), interventions are designed and implemented to support their growing abilities. Nurses become adept at learning to read infants' behavioral clues (see box) and supplying appropriate interventions. Clues include both approach and avoidance behaviors. Approach behaviors that are supported and enhanced include tongue extension, handclasp, hand-to-mouth movements, sucking, looking, and cooing. Signs of stress or fatigue that signal the infant's need for "time-out" are described in the box on p. 238 and in the Critical Thinking Exercise on p. 238.

An intervention program for convalescing infants must be individualized and include parents early during the infant's hospitalization; teaching the parents to be responsive to the infant's individual cues is an important function of the NICU nurse. When infants are recovering and are free of support systems, medically stable, and on room air or smaller amounts of oxygen, they are assessed to document their behavioral styles. An effective program may be designed to provide limited sensory stimulation involving one or two senses or multisensory experiences that include tactile, visual, auditory, vestibular, olfactory, and gustatory stimuli. The objective of any intervention program is to avoid stressing infants—overstimulation is as detrimental as understimulation.

When the condition of an infant is sufficiently advanced to begin developmental intervention, some activities are individualized according to each infant's cues, temperament,

BEHAVIORAL MANIFESTATIONS OF DEVELOPMENTAL ORGANIZATION

Motor Stability Behaviors

Smooth, well-modulated posture and well-modulated tone
Synchronous smooth movements with efficient motoric strategies:
 Hand clasping
 Foot clasping
 Finger folding
 Hand-to-mouth maneuvers
 Grasping
 Suck searching and sucking
 Handholding
 Tucking (arms and legs flexed and kept close to body)

State Stability and Attention Regulation Behaviors

Clear, robust sleep states
Rhythmic, robust crying
Good self-quieting or consolability
Robust, focused, shiny-eyed alertness with intent or animated facial expressions, including:
 Frowning
 Cheek softening
 Mouth pursing to "ooh" face
 Cooing
 Attentional smiling

Data from Lawhon G: Management of stress in premature infants. In Angelini DJ, Whelan Knapp CW, Gives KM, editors: *Perinatal/neonatal nursing: a clinical handbook,* Boston, 1986, Blackwell Scientific Publications.

CRITICAL THINKING EXERCISE
Developmental Care

You are getting ready to feed a 4-week-old infant born at 28 weeks of gestation. While taking vital signs, you notice that the infant's color is pink but slightly mottled; he is yawning, extending his arms and legs, and splaying his fingers. Oxygen saturation by pulse oximetry indicates reading within the lower range of normal for this infant. You recognize these behaviors as manifestations of neonatal:

1. Preterm behavior
2. Subtle seizures
3. Stress
4. Onset of infection

The correct answer is three. Neonates who are preterm may exhibit these signs and others (see box on p. 237) when they are not able to habituate to external stimuli, including routine handling. Alone, these signs do not indicate subtle seizure activity or infection. They are normal preterm behaviors, but only to signal the infant's need for "time out."

state, behavioral organization, and particular needs. Intervention periods are short (e.g., 1 to 2 minutes of visual stimulation, 2 to 3 minutes of voices, and 5 minutes of quiet music). One type of intervention at a time is applied to document the infant's tolerance and response (see Guidelines box). The types and duration of any stimuli are adjusted on an individual basis, and the parents are involved as early as possible in learning about their infant's particular developmental needs.

Developmental care of the preterm neonate is an ongoing process in the NICU and is incorporated into the daily care given to each infant. The nurse, aware of the preterm infant's developmental needs, temperament, and newborn state, as well as environmental conditions that adversely affect the infant, plans nursing care accordingly to enhance optimum physical, psychosocial, and neurologic development. This task is often difficult to accomplish when invasive treatments or interventions are required to essentially stabilize the critically ill neonate.

Neonatal Pain

It has long been believed that the nerve pathways of newborn infants are not sufficiently myelinated to transmit painful stimuli, that the infant does not possess sufficiently integrated cortical function to interpret or recall pain experiences, and that the risk of anesthesia is too great to justify any possible benefit of pain relief (Anand and Hickey, 1987; McLaughlin and others, 1993). Nurses have been found to hold similar beliefs and to give significantly higher pain intensity ratings to full-term as opposed to preterm neonates. Consequently, invasive procedures (including some types of surgery) are performed on infants without anesthesia.

This traditional view has been refuted by a number of research studies, which indicate that infants, both preterm and full term, perceive and react to pain in much the same manner as children and adults. Evidence indicates that pain pathways, cortical and subcortical centers needed for pain perception, and neurochemical systems associated with pain transmission and modulation are intact and functional in the neonate. Slower conduction speed of unmyelinated fibers is offset by shorter interneuron distances traveled by the impulse (Anand and McGrath, 1993).

Physiologic responses in neonates to painful stimuli have been well documented by numerous studies. The summary of these observations indicates that painful stimuli cause a global stress response in infants undergoing surgery with minimal or no analgesia. This response is evidenced by cardiorespiratory changes (marked increases in heart rate and blood pressure, and decreased $tcPo_2$ or oxygen saturation), palmar sweating, increased intracranial pressure, and hormonal (release of catecholamines, growth hormone, glucagon, cortisol, other corticosteroids, and aldosterone and by hyperglycemia), and metabolic changes (increased plasma lactate, pyruvate, ketone bodies, and some fatty acids). With adequate analgesia and anesthesia infants experience less of a stress response and less postoperative mortality and morbidity (Anand and Hickey, 1992). Pain control during procedures can shorten periods of oxygen desaturation (Pokela, 1994).

Infants should receive appropriate analgesia or anesthesia for potentially painful procedures. Local or systemic pharmacologic agents are available to permit anesthesia or analgesia to neonates and are indicated for those undergoing surgical procedures (American Academy of Pediatrics, 1987; Burrows and Berde, 1993).

Other effects of pain may include increased wakefulness and irritability, as well as alterations in feeding, vomiting, loss of appetite, and loss of interest in or energy for sucking. Interruptions in sleep-wake patterns, behavioral states, and

GUIDELINES
Developmental Interventions

General Guidelines
Individualize interventions for each infant.
Offer only during periods of alertness.
Begin one type of stimulus at a time.
Provide intervention for short periods.
Space periods according to infant's tolerance.
Continually assess infant's response to developmental interventions.
Titrate interventions according to infant's cues.
Terminate stimulation if infant displays evidence of overstimulation (see box on p. 237).

Visual
Place photographs of parents and siblings in visual range (19 to 22 cm) in *en face* position.
Provide black-and-white mobiles with varied hanging shapes.
Initiate eye contact; repeat as tolerated.
Alternate holding black-and-white pattern still and moving it across infant's visual field.

Tactile
Stroke skin slowly and gently in head-to-toe direction; begin with trunk and move to more sensitive areas, such as face.
Provide alternate textures (e.g., sheepskin, satin, velvet).
Provide boundaries, foot bracing, blankets.

Auditory
Play tape of parents' and siblings' voices.
Softly play classical music, recording of womb sounds, or music box.
Speak with a variety of voice inflections; alternate adult and baby talk.
Call infant by name at each interaction.

Vestibular
Place on water bed with oscillations and waves per minute determined on an individual basis; alternate oscillations with rest periods (may not be acceptable intervention in some units).
Rock in chair.
Place in sling (hammock) and rock.
Provide passive range-of-motion exercises to knee and hip joints.
Close infant's fist around cloth toy.
Lift head to upright position, tip to right and then to left, stopping at midline (only with stable, more mature infants).
Slowly change position during handling.

Olfactory
Pass open container of breast milk or formula under nose.
Pass mother's perfume under nose.

Gustatory
Place infant's hand or a pacifier in mouth when sucking movements are observed or during gavage feeding.
Place 1 or 2 drops of milk in infant's mouth with each tube feeding.

parent-infant interactions also occur and may interfere with recovery from surgery.

Assessment of pain in the preverbal child is difficult, especially in the neonate, because most evaluative tools and verbal responses do not apply. Evaluation must be based on physiologic changes and behavioral observations. Although behaviors including vocalizations, facial expressions, body movements, and general state are common to all infants, they vary with different situations. Crying associated with pain is more intense and sustained. Facial expression is the most consistent and specific characteristic. The facial features include eye squeeze, brow bulge, open mouth, and taut tongue (see Fig. 21-3) (Grunau, Johnston, and Craig, 1990). Most infants respond with increased body movements; however, the infant may be experiencing pain even when lying quietly with eyes closed. The preterm infant's response to pain may be behaviorally blunted or absent. An infant who receives a muscle-paralyzing agent such as vecuronium during surgery will also be incapable of mounting a behavioral or visible pain response.

Nursing assessment for evidence of pain is indicated any time the infant suffers tissue damage. Observable manifestations identified as indicators of acute pain in neonates are listed in the box on p. 240. In addition, several pain measurement scales attempt to quantify pain by assigning numeric values to categories such as movement, facial expression, cry, vital signs, and state of arousal (Barrier and others, 1989; Lawrence and others, 1993; Stevens, 1994; Krechel and Bildner,

1995). Further research on the validity and reliability of such scales is needed to support their clinical use.

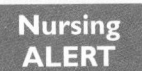 When in doubt about pain in infants, base your decision on the following rule: Whatever is painful to an adult or child is painful to an infant, unless proved otherwise.

Nonpharmacologic measures used to alleviate pain are discussed extensively in Chapter 21. Those employed to reduce discomfort in the neonatal intensive care unit (NICU) include repositioning, swaddling, containment, cuddling, rocking, music, reducing environmental stimulation, tactile comfort measures, and nonnutritive sucking. However, nonpharmacologic measures may not be sufficient to decrease physiologic distress, even if behavioral responses, such as crying, are lessened. In premature infants, additional stimulation, such as stroking, may *increase* physiologic distress.

Morphine and fentanyl are the most widely used opioid analgesics for pharmacologic management of neonatal pain. Continuous intravenous infusion of opioids provides effective and safe pain control (Farrington and others, 1993). Other methods of relieving pain are with epidural/intrathecal infusion, local and regional nerve blocks, and topical anesthetics (Choonara, 1992; Yaster and others, 1994). With the increasing use of opioids and other sedating drugs, such as midazo-

MANIFESTATIONS OF ACUTE PAIN IN THE NEONATE

Physiologic Responses

Vital signs: observe for variations
  Increased heart rate
  Increased blood pressure
  Rapid, shallow respirations
Oxygenation
  Decreased transcutaneous O_2 saturation (tcPo$_2$)
  Decreased arterial O_2 saturation (Sao$_2$)
Skin: observe color and character
  Pallor or flushing
  Diaphoresis
  Palmar sweating
Other observations
  Increased muscle tone
  Dilated pupils
  Decreased vagal nerve tone
  Increased intracranial pressure
  Laboratory evidence of metabolic or endocrine changes
    Hyperglycemia
    Lowered pH
    Elevated corticosteroids

Behavioral Responses

Vocalizations: observe quality, timing, and duration
  Crying
  Whimpering
  Groaning
Facial expression: observe characteristics, timing, orientation of eyes and mouth (see Fig. 21-3)
  Grimaces
  Brow furrowed
  Chin quivering
  Eyes tightly closed
  Mouth open and squarish
Body movements and posture: observe type, quality, and amount of movement or lack of movement; relationship to other factors
  Limb withdrawal
  Thrashing
  Rigidity
  Flaccidity
  Fist clenching
Changes in state: observe sleep, appetite, activity level
  Changes in sleep/wake cycles
  Changes in feeding behavior
  Changes in activity level
  Fussiness, irritability
  Listlessness

lam (Versed), for continuous pain control in neonates, nurses must be alert to signs of withdrawal if the drug is stopped abruptly. To avoid withdrawal, the dosage should be gradually reduced over a period of several days (Franck and Vilardi, 1995) (see Pain Management, Chapter 21).

Parents are often concerned that their infants are suffering pain during procedures. Nurses need to address these concerns and encourage the parents to speak with the professionals involved. Parents have the right to withhold consent for invasive procedures performed without adequate analgesia or anesthesia and are entitled to honest answers from those responsible for the infant's care. When permissible, they can also help provide comfort measures for the infant. It is important that parents are aware that nurses are sensitive to the infant's pain and are reassured that the infant will not suffer.

Family Support and Involvement

Often, professional health workers are so absorbed in the life-saving physical aspects of care that the emotional needs of infants and their families are ignored. The significance of early parent-child interaction and infant stimulation has been documented by reliable research, and nurses, aware of these infant and family needs, must incorporate activities that facilitate family interaction into the nursing care plan.

The birth of a preterm infant is an unexpected and stressful event for which families are emotionally unprepared. They find themselves simultaneously coping with their own needs, the needs of their infant, and the needs of their families (especially when there are other children). To compound the situation, the precarious nature of their infant's condition engenders an atmosphere of apprehension and uncertainty. They are faced with multiple crises and overwhelming feelings of responsibility, expense, and frustration.

All parents have some anxieties about the outcome of a pregnancy, but following a premature birth the concern is heightened about both the viability and the intactness of their infant. Mothers see their infant only briefly before the newborn is removed to the intensive care unit or even to another hospital, leaving them with just the recollection of the infant's very small size and unusual appearance. They usually feel alone or lost in the maternity ward, belonging neither with mothers who have lost their infants nor with those who delivered healthy, full-term infants. The staff and physicians are often guarded in discussing the infant's condition; mothers are continually expecting to hear that their infant has died, and they are sensitive to the anxieties of other mothers and staff members. Going home without their infant only serves to compound their feelings of disappointment, failure, and deprivation.

When an infant is to be transported from the hospital, the parents need a description of the new facility. They need to know the location, reputation, and nature of the facility and the care that the infant is expected to receive. The name of the infant's physician and the telephone number of the nursery is given to them, and unfamiliar terms, such as "neonatologist," "ventilator," "infusion," and "incubator," are explained. Explanations are kept simple, and parents are given the opportunity to ask questions. If booklets are available that describe the facility, they are given to the family.

Perhaps most important of all, the parents, especially the mother, should have some contact with the infant before the transport. To be able to see, touch, and (if possible) hold their infant facilitates the attachment process. Often a photograph, or even a videotape, of their infant can serve as a bond until the parents are able to travel to the regional facility. When possible, it is often advisable to transfer the mother to the same institution as her infant.

Parents need to be informed of their infant's progress and reassured that the infant is receiving proper care. They need to understand the smallest aspects of the infant's condition and treatment. Parents need a realistic assessment of the situation that is honest and direct. Using nonmedical terminology, moving at a pace that is comfortable for parents to assimilate the information, and avoiding lengthy technical explanations facilitate communication with family members. Tasks that must be accomplished by parents during their infant's care are presented in the box.

TASKS OF PARENTS OF A HIGH-RISK INFANT

Work through the events surrounding labor and delivery.
Acknowledge that the infant's life is endangered and that the infant might die, and begin the grief process.
Confront and recognize feelings of inadequacy and guilt in not delivering a healthy child.
Adapt to the neonatal intensive care environment.
Resume parental relationships with infant and initiate the care-giving role, *or*
Adapt to the loss in the event of neonatal death.

Modified from Siegel R, Gardner SL, Merenstein GB: Families in crisis: theoretical and practical considerations. In Merenstein GB, Gardner SL: *Handbook of neonatal intensive care,* ed 3, St Louis, 1993, Mosby.

Facilitating Parent-Infant Relationships. Because of their physiologic instability, infants are separated from their mothers immediately and surrounded by a complex, impenetrable barrier of glass windows, mechanical equipment, and special caregivers. There is increasing evidence to indicate that the emotional separation that accompanies the physical separation of mothers and infants interferes with the normal maternal-infant attachment process discussed in Chapter 8. Maternal attachment is a cumulative process that begins before conception, is strengthened by significant events during pregnancy, and matures through maternal-infant contact during the neonatal period.

When an infant is sick, the necessary physical separation appears to be accompanied by an emotional estrangement on the part of parents that may seriously damage the capacity for parenting their infant. This detachment is further hampered by the tenuous nature of the infant's condition. When survival is in doubt, parents may be reluctant to establish a relationship with their infant. They prepare themselves for the death of the infant while continuing to hope for recovery. This anticipatory grief (Chapter 18) and hesitancy to embark on a relationship are evidenced by behaviors such as delay in giving the infant a name, reluctance in visiting the nursery, or when they do visit, focusing on equipment and treatments rather than on their infant, and hesitancy to touch or handle the infant when they are provided with the opportunity.

Comprehensive management of high-risk newborns includes encouraging and facilitating parental involvement rather than isolating parents from their infant and associated care. This is particularly important in relation to mothers; to reduce the effects of physical separation, mothers are united with their newborn at the earliest opportunity. Preparing the parents to see their infant for the first time is a nursing responsibility.

Before the first visit, the parents should be prepared for their infant's appearance, the equipment that is attached to the child, and some indication of the general atmosphere of the unit. The initial encounter with the intensive care unit is a stressful experience, and the frightening array of people, equipment, and activity is likely to be overwhelming. A book of photographs or pamphlets describing the NICU environment (infants in incubators or under radiant warmers, monitors, mechanical ventilators, and intravenous equipment) provides a useful and nonthreatening introduction to the NICU.

Parents should be encouraged to visit their infant as soon as possible. Even if they saw the infant at the time of transport or shortly after birth, the infant may have changed considerably, especially if there are a number of medical and equipment requirements associated with the infant's hospitalization. At the bedside the nurse should explain the function of each piece of equipment and the role it plays in facilitating recovery. When possible, some items related to therapy can be removed; for example, phototherapy can be temporarily discontinued and eye patches removed to permit eye-to-eye contact.

Parents appreciate the support of a nurse during the initial visit with their infant, but they may also appreciate some time alone with the infant for a short while. It is important during the early visits to emphasize positive aspects of their infant's behavior and development so that parents can focus on their infant as an individual rather than on the equipment that surrounds the child. The nurse may describe the infant's spontaneous behaviors during care, such as grasp, swallowing, and movement, or make comments about the infant's biologic functions. Most institutions have open visiting policies so that parents and siblings may visit their infant as often as they wish.

Parents vary greatly in the degree to which they are able to interact with their infant. Some may wish to touch or hold their infant during the first visit, whereas others may not feel comfortable enough even to enter the nursery. These reactions depend on a variety of prenatal and postnatal factors, such as the parity of the mother and her preparation before birth; the size, condition, and physical appearance of the infant; and the type of treatment the infant is receiving. It is essential to recognize that the individualized pacing and quality of the interactions are more important than early onset of these interactions. Parents may not be receptive to early and extended infant contact, since they need time to adjust to the impact of an infant with birth problems and must be helped to grieve before acceptance of their infant can take place.

The parents' inability to focus on their infant is a clue for the nurse to assist the parents in expressing feelings of guilt, anxiety, helplessness, inadequacy, anger, and ambivalence. Nurses can help parents deal with these distressing feelings and recognize that they are normal responses shared by other parents. It is important to point out and reinforce the positive aspects of parents' behavior and interactions with their infant.

Most parents feel shaky and insecure about initiating interaction with their infant. Nurses can sense parents' level of readiness and offer encouragement in these initial efforts. Parents of premature infants follow the same acquaintance process as do parents of term infants. They may quickly proceed through the process or may require several days or even weeks to complete the process. Parents begin by touching their infant's extremities with their fingertips and poking the infant tenderly, and then proceed to caresses and fondling (Fig. 9-9). Touching is the first act of communication between parents and child. Parents need to be prepared for their infant's exaggerated and generalized startle responses to a touch so that they will not interpret these as negative reactions to their overtures. It may be necessary to limit tactile stimuli when the infant is critically ill and labile, but the nurse can offer other options—speaking softly or sitting at the bedside.

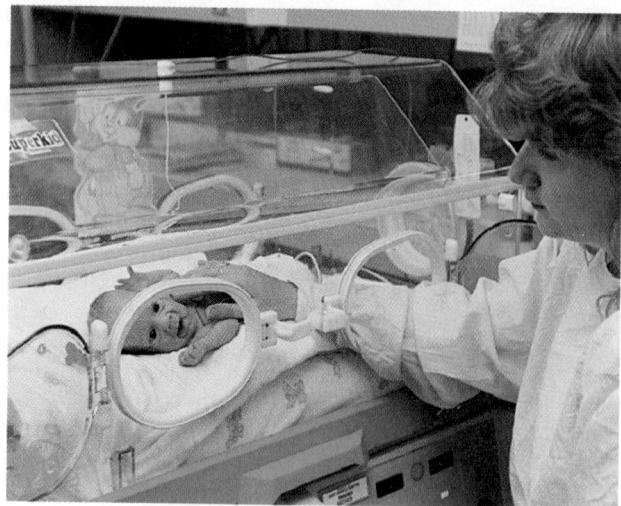

FIG. 9-9. Encouraging interaction of mother and her premature infant in intensive care unit facilitates mother-infant attachment process.

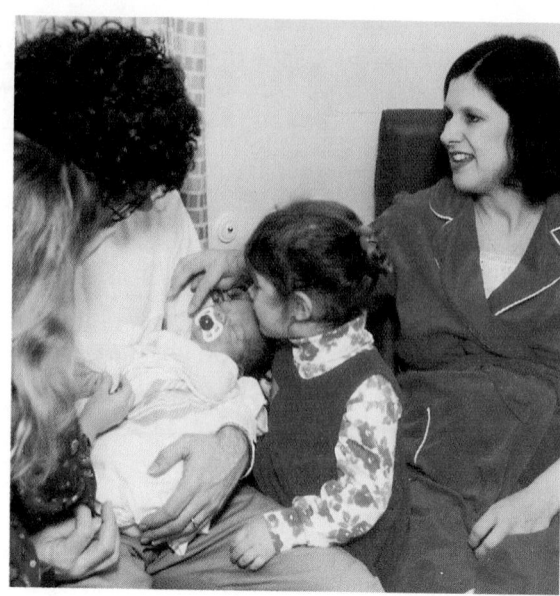

FIG. 9-10. Big sister gets acquainted with the new baby.

Parents of acutely ill preterm infants may express feelings of helplessness and lack of control. Involving the parent in some type of caregiving activity, no matter how minor it may seem to the nurse, enables the parent to "take on" a more active role. Examples of such caregiving for the acutely ill infant who cannot be held and is seemingly not responding positively include moistening the infant's lips with a small amount of sterile water on a cotton-tipped swab or slipping the diaper from under the infant when it is wet or soiled. Parents may also become involved by reading a children's storybook or nursery rhymes in a soft, soothing voice. Some families tape record the parents' voices telling or reading stories and play the tapes when the infant is able to cope with such stimuli. Feeding schedules are discussed, and parents are encouraged to visit at times when they can become involved in the care of their infant.

Parents need guidance in their relationships with their infant and assistance in their efforts to meet their infant's physical and developmental needs. The nursing staff must help parents understand that their preterm infant offers few behavioral rewards and show them how to accept small rewards from their infant. The infant's reactions and behaviors are explained to parents, who take their infant's jerky, rejective behavior personally. They need reassurance that these behaviors are not a reflection on their parenting skills. Parents are taught to recognize their infant's cues regarding stimulation, handling, and other interaction, especially aversive behaviors that indicate a need for rest. Nurses need to include parents in planning their infant's care and sensory stimulation materials, such as a music box or recording.

Above all, nurses must encourage and reinforce parents during their caregiving activities and interactions with their infant in order to promote healthy parent-child relationships. It is also helpful for the parents to have contact and communication with the infant's primary nurse and associate primary nurse. This decreases the amount of different information given to parents and often instills confidence that while the parents cannot be at their infant's bedside 24 hours a day, there are competent and caring nurses whom they may call

to inquire about the infant's status. Periodic parent conferences involving the primary practitioner, primary nurse, and associate primary nurse serve to clarify misunderstandings or problems related to the infant's condition. Other members of the NICU health care team, such as the perinatal social worker or surgeon, may become involved as necessary. The importance of facilitating the parental-infant attachment process cannot be overemphasized, since studies indicate that lack of early attachment in premature infants may contribute to problems such as child abuse later on.

Siblings. In the past, concerns about sibling visitation in the NICU focused on fears of infection and disruption of nursing routines. These fears have not been substantiated, and sibling visits are now part of the normal operation of most NICUs (Fig. 9-10). Children must be prepared for the unfamiliar NICU atmosphere, especially the sounds and sights of unfamiliar equipment and the physical appearance of the neonate. Contact with the infant helps siblings deal with the reality rather than the bizarre fantasies that are characteristic of young children. It also helps to bond the family as a unit.

Support Groups. Parents need to feel that they are not alone. Parent support groups have been of immeasurable value to families of infants in the NICU. Some groups consist of parents who have infants in the hospital who share the same anxieties and concerns. Other groups include parents who have had infants in the NICU and who have dealt with the crisis effectively. The groups are usually under the leadership of a staff person and involve physicians, nurses, and social workers, but it is the parents who can offer other parents something that no one else can provide.

One national organization that evolved from a local parent's group, **Parent Care, Inc.,*** provides information, referrals, and support to parents and professionals concerned

---

*1010 South Union St., Alexandria, VA 22314; (703) 836-4678.

with the care of high-risk infants. It also publishes a national newsletter and a resource directory that provide information on items useful to parents, such as "preemie" clothing, and hosts local and national conferences. Information can be obtained by contacting or forming a local group. The **Family Resource Coalition*** is a North American network of family support programs designed to help families of preterm infants.

Discharge Planning and Home Care

Parents become very apprehensive and excited as the time for discharge approaches. They have many concerns and insecurities regarding the care of their infant. They fear the child may still be in danger, that they will be unable to recognize signs of distress or illness in their infant, and that the infant may not yet be ready for discharge. Nurses need to begin early to assist parents in acquiring or increasing their skills in the care of their infant. Appropriate instruction must be provided and sufficient time allowed for the family to assimilate the information and learn the continuing special care requirements. Where rooming-in or other live-in arrangements are available, parents can stay for a few days and nights and assume the care of their infant under the supervision and support of the nursery staff.

There should be appropriate medical and nursing follow-up and referrals to services that can benefit the family, including developmental follow-up. Parents of preterm infants should also be given adequate information about immunizations with other discharge planning information (Langkamp and Langhough, 1993). Public health agencies provide nursing supervision, counseling, and referral for nursing visits. With the ever-increasing trend toward early discharge, many hospital-based and privately owned home health care agencies become involved in the follow-up and care of the NICU "graduate" in the home (see Chapter 20). Organized support groups are part of many communities, including those discussed previously, those designed for parents of infants who require special care because of specific defects or disabilities, and those for parents of multiple births. Some manufacturers provide for the special needs of such infants. For example, premature size disposable diapers are available from the manufacturers of Pampers.†

Car seat safety is an essential aspect of discharge planning, and infants less than 37 weeks of gestation should have a period of observation in an appropriate car seat to monitor for possible apnea, bradycardia, and decreased SaO_2. Several models can be adapted for small infants with the placement of blanket rolls on each side of the infant to support the head and trunk. For adequate support without slumping, the seat-back-to-crotch strap distance must be 14 cm (5½ inches) or less. LBW infants are best transported lying prone in infant-only child safety seats with harnesses designed to fit small bodies or well supported in a car bed restraint (Mini Swinger‡). The American Academy of Pediatrics (1996) has published guidelines for the safe transportation of premature infants. (See Chapters 8 and 10 for discussions of infant car restraints.)

Knowing that members of the staff (especially the primary nurse) are available for telephone or personal contact when the parents take the infant home provides a measure of security to anxious parents. Most NICU facilities maintain a policy of open communication between staff and parents both during the infant's hospitalization and following discharge. It is the responsibility of the NICU staff to make certain that parents are prepared to care for their infant—emotionally and physically.

Problems that may arise in the high-risk newborn include overfeeding, underfeeding, and difficulty separating the child from the parent. To help parents deal with the stress of home care for the infant, nurses can help families to discuss their fears and anxieties, which are exaggerated in parents of preterm infants, and encourage the family to create a normal routine in caring for the infant. Parents need to learn the normal developmental delays expected of premature infants and the importance of setting disciplinary limits and schedules. Continued explanations and clarification of the infant's true health status and ongoing support of the parents' efforts are important aspects of follow-up care.

Neonatal Loss

The precarious nature of many high-risk infants makes death a very real and ever-present possibility. Although infant mortality has been reduced sharply with improved technology, the mortality rate is still greatest in the neonatal period of life. Nurses in the NICU are the persons who must prepare the parents for an inevitable death and facilitate a family's grieving process after an expected or an unexpected death.

To help the parents understand that the death is a reality, it is important that the parents are encouraged to hold their infant before death and if possible be present at the time of death so that their infant can die in their arms if they choose. Many who deny the need to hold the infant later regret the decision. Parents should be provided with an opportunity to see, touch, hold, caress, examine, and talk to their infant privately after death, and to bathe their infant if they desire as a final act of caring. If parents are hesitant about seeing their dead infant, it is advisable to keep the body in the unit for a few hours, since many parents change their minds after the initial shock of the death.

Parents may need to see and hold the infant more than once: the first time to say "hello" and the last time to say "goodbye." If parents wish to see the infant after the body has been taken to the morgue, the infant should be retrieved, wrapped in a blanket, and taken to the mother's room or other private place. The nurse should stay with the parents and provide them an opportunity for private time alone with their dead infant.

A photograph of the infant taken before or after death is highly desirable. The parents may not wish to see the photograph at the time of death, but the chance to refer to it later will help make their infant seem more real, which is a part of the normal grief process. A photograph of their infant being held by the hand or touched by an adult offers a more positive image than a morgue-type photograph. Many NICUs have a grief or memory packet made up for the grieving parents, which may include the infant's handprints and foot-

*230 N. Michigan Ave., Suite 1625, Chicago, IL 60601.
†Proctor & Gamble; (800) 543-4932; in Ohio: (800) 582-2623.
‡Distributed by Shinn and Associates, 2154 Commons Parkway, Okemos, MI 48864; (517) 349-5575.

Text continued on p. 248.

Nursing Care Plan
The High-Risk Infant*

NURSING DIAGNOSIS: Ineffective breathing pattern related to pulmonary and neuromuscular immaturity, decreased energy, and fatigue

PATIENT GOAL 1: Will exhibit adequate oxygenation

- **NURSING INTERVENTIONS/RATIONALES**

Position for optimum air exchange
  Place prone when feasible, *since this position results in improved oxygenation, better-tolerated feedings, and more organized sleep-rest patterns*
  Place supine with neck slightly extended and nose pointing to ceiling in "sniffing" position *to prevent any narrowing of airway*
Avoid neck hyperextension *because it reduces diameter of trachea*
Observe for deviations from desired functioning; recognize signs of distress—grunting, cyanosis, nasal flaring, apnea
Suction *to remove accumulated mucus from nasopharynx, trachea, and endotracheal tube*
Suction only as necessary based on assessment (e.g., auscultation of chest, evidence of decreased oxygenation, increased infant irritability)
Never suction routinely, since it *may cause bronchospasm, bradycardia due to vagal nerve stimulation, hypoxia, and increased intracranial pressure (ICP), predisposing infant to intraventricular hemorrhage (IVH)*
Use proper suctioning technique *because improper suctioning can cause infection, airway damage, pneumothoraces, and IVH*
Use two-person suction technique *because assistant can provide immediate hyperoxygenation before and after catheter insertion*
†Carry out percussion, vibration, and postural drainage as prescribed *to facilitate drainage of secretions*
Avoid using Trendelenburg position, *since it can contribute to increased ICP and reduced lung capacity from gravity pushing organs against diaphragm*
  During diaper changes, raise infant slightly under hips and not by raising feet and legs
Use semiprone or side-lying position *to prevent aspiration in infant with excessive mucus or who is being fed*
Observe for signs of respiratory distress—nasal flaring, retractions, tachypnea, apnea, grunting, cyanosis, low oxygenation saturation (SaO_2)
Carry out regimen prescribed for supplemental oxygen therapy (maintain ambient O_2 concentration at minimum FIo_2 level based on arterial blood gases and Sao_2)
Maintain neutral thermal environment *to conserve utilization of O_2*
Closely monitor blood gas measurements and Sao_2 readings
Apply and manage monitoring equipment correctly (i.e., cardiac or oxygen)

Demonstrate understanding of function of respiratory support apparatus
  Mechanical ventilation apparatus
  Insufflation bags with masks and/or endotracheal tube adaptor
  Oxygen hoods/tents
  Humidifier warmers
Observe and assess infant's response to ventilation and oxygenation therapy

- **EXPECTED OUTCOMES**

Airway remains patent
Breathing provides adequate oxygenation and CO_2 removal
Respiratory rate and pattern is within appropriate limits for age and weight (specify)
Arterial blood gases and acid-base balance are within normal limits for postconceptional age
Tissue oxygenation is adequate

NURSING DIAGNOSIS: Ineffective thermoregulation related to immature temperature control and decreased subcutaneous body fat

PATIENT GOAL 1: Will maintain stable body temperature

- **NURSING INTERVENTIONS/RATIONALES**

Place infant in incubator, radiant warmer, or warmly clothed in open crib *to maintain stable body temperature*
Monitor axillary temperature in unstable infants (use skin probe or air temperature control; check function of servo-controlled mechanism when used)
Regulate servocontrolled unit or air temperature control as needed *to maintain skin temperature within accepted thermal range*
Use plastic heat shield as appropriate *to decrease heat loss*
Monitor for signs of hyperthermia—redness, flushing, diaphoresis (rarely)
Check temperature of infant in relation to ambient temperature and temperature of heating unit *to detect radiant heat loss*
Avoid situations that might predispose infant to heat loss, such as exposure to cool air, drafts, bathing, or cold scales
Monitor serum glucose values *to ensure euglycemia*

- **EXPECTED OUTCOME**

Infant's axillary temperature remains within normal range for postconceptional age

---

NURSING DIAGNOSIS: High risk for infection related to deficient immunologic defenses

PATIENT GOAL 1: Will exhibit no evidence of nosocomial infection

- **NURSING INTERVENTIONS/RATIONALES**

Ensure that all caregivers wash hands before and after handling infant *to minimize exposure to infective organisms*

---

*Relates primarily to low-birth-weight infant with weight of 1500 to 2500 g.
†Dependent nursing action.

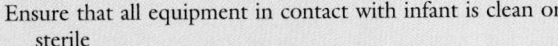

NURSING CARE PLAN
The High-Risk Infant—cont'd

Ensure that all equipment in contact with infant is clean or sterile

Prevent personnel with upper respiratory tract or communicable infections from coming into direct contact with infant

Isolate other infants who have infections according to institutional policy

Instruct health care workers and parents in infection control procedures

*Administer antibiotics as ordered

Ensure strict asepsis and/or sterility with invasive procedures and equipment such as peripheral IV therapy, lumbar punctures, and arterial/venous catheter insertion

- **EXPECTED OUTCOME**

Infant exhibits no evidence of nosocomial infection

> **NURSING DIAGNOSIS:** Altered nutrition: less than body requirements (high risk) related to inability to ingest nutrients because of immaturity and/or illness

PATIENT GOAL 1: Will receive adequate nourishment, with caloric intake to maintain positive nitrogen balance, and exhibit appropriate weight gain

- **NURSING INTERVENTIONS/***RATIONALES*

*Maintain parenteral fluid or total parenteral nutrition therapy as ordered

Monitor for signs of intolerance to total parenteral therapy, especially protein and glucose

Assess readiness to nipple feed, especially ability to coordinate swallowing and breathing

Nipple feed infant if strong sucking, swallowing, and gag reflexes are present (usually at gestational age of 34 to 35 weeks) *to minimize risk of aspiration*

Follow unit protocol for advancing volume and concentration of formula *to avoid feeding intolerance*

Use orogastric feeding if infant tires easily or has weak sucking, gag, or swallowing reflexes, *because nipple feeding may result in weight loss*

Assist mothers with expressing breast milk *to establish and maintain lactation until infant can breast-feed*

Assist mothers with breast-feeding when feasible and desirable

- **EXPECTED OUTCOMES**

Infant receives an adequate amount of calories and essential nutrients

Infant demonstrates a steady weight gain (approximately 20 to 30 g/day) once past acute phase of illness

> **NURSING DIAGNOSIS:** High risk for fluid volume deficit or excess related to immature physiologic characteristics of preterm infant and/or immaturity or illness

PATIENT GOAL 1: Will exhibit adequate hydration status

- **NURSING INTERVENTIONS/***RATIONALES*

Monitor fluid and electrolytes closely with therapies that increase insensible water loss (IWL) (e.g., phototherapy, radiant warmer)

Implement strategies to minimize IWL such as plastic covering, increased ambient humidity

Ensure adequate parenteral/oral fluid intake

Assess state of hydration (e.g., skin turgor, blood pressure, edema, weight, mucous membranes, urine specific gravity, electrolytes, fontanel)

Regulate parenteral fluids closely *to avoid dehydration, overhydration, or extravasation*

Avoid administering hypertonic fluids (e.g., undiluted medications, concentrated glucose infusions) *to prevent excess solute load on immature kidneys and fragile veins*

Monitor urinary output and laboratory values *for evidence of dehydration or overhydration* (adequate urinary output 1-2 ml/kg/hr)

- **EXPECTED OUTCOME**

Infant exhibits evidence of fluid homeostasis

> **NURSING DIAGNOSIS:** High risk for impaired skin integrity related to immature skin structure, immobility, decreased nutritional state, invasive procedures

PATIENT GOAL 1: Will maintain skin integrity

- **NURSING INTERVENTIONS**

See Guidelines box on neonatal skin care, p. 236

- **EXPECTED OUTCOME**

Skin remains clean and intact with no evidence of irritation or injury

> **NURSING DIAGNOSIS:** High-risk for injury from increased intracranial pressure (ICP) related to immature central nervous system and physiologic stress response

PATIENT GOAL 1: Will exhibit normal ICP (unless increased ICP is related to infant's illness) and no evidence of intraventricular hemorrhage (IVH) (unless preexisting condition)

- **NURSING INTERVENTIONS/***RATIONALES*

Decrease environmental stimulation *because stress responses, especially increased blood pressure, increase risk of elevated ICP*

---
*Dependent nursing action.

Continued.

NURSING CARE PLAN
The High-Risk Infant—cont'd

Establish a routine that provides for undisturbed sleep/rest periods *to eliminate or minimize times of stress*

Use minimal handling and handle or disturb infant only when absolutely necessary

Keep extra diapers under buttocks to facilitate changing soiled diapers; raise infant's hips, not feet and legs

Organize (cluster) care during normal waking hours as much as possible *to minimize sleep disruption and frequent intermittent noise*

Close and open drapes and dim lights *to allow for day/night schedule*

Cover incubator with cloth and place "do not disturb" sign nearby *to decrease light and alert others to infant's rest period*

Refrain from loud talking or laughing

Remain calm

Limit number of visitors and staff near infant at one time

Explain meaning of unfamiliar sounds

Keep equipment noise to minimum

Turn alarms as low as safely possible

Attend to alarms and telephones immediately

Place bedside equipment, such as ventilator or IV pump, away from head of bed

Turn outflow valve from ventilator away from infant's ear

Perform treatments requiring equipment at one time

Turn off bedside equipment that is not in use, such as suction and oxygen

Avoid loud, abrupt noises, such as discarding items in trash can, dropping items, placing items on top of incubator, closing doors and drawers, heavy traffic

Turn off any radios or televisions

May place soft earmuffs on infant

Assess and manage pain using pharmacologic and nonpharmacologic methods

Recognize signs of physical stress and overstimulation *to institute appropriate interventions promptly*

Avoid hypertonic medications and solutions *because they increase cerebral blood flow*

Elevate head of bed or mattress between 15 and 20 degrees *to decrease ICP*

Maintain adequate oxygenation *because hypoxia increases cerebral blood flow and ICP* (see interventions under nursing diagnosis of ineffective breathing pattern on p. 244)

Avoid any sudden turning of head to side, *which restricts carotid artery blood flow and adequate oxygenation to brain*

- **EXPECTED OUTCOME**

Infant exhibits no evidence of increased ICP or IVH

NURSING DIAGNOSIS: Pain related to procedures, diagnosis, treatment

PATIENT GOAL 1: Will experience no pain or reduction of pain

- **NURSING INTERVENTIONS/*RATIONALES***

Recognize that infants, regardless of gestational age, feel pain

Differentiate between clinical manifestations of pain and stress/fatigue (see p. 237)

Use nonpharmacologic pain measures appropriate to infant's age and condition: repositioning, swaddling, containment, cuddling, rocking, music, reducing environmental stimulation, tactile comfort measures (stroking, patting), and nonnutritive sucking (pacifier)

Encourage parents to provide comfort measures when possible

Administer analgesics around the clock *to provide continuous pain relief*

Monitor for side effects of opioids, especially respiratory depression and withdrawal, *to prevent and/or request treatment*

Assess effectiveness of nonpharmacologic and pharmacologic pain measures *because some comfort measures, (e.g., stroking) may increase premature infant's distress and drugs or dosages may need to be adjusted*

Convey an attitude of sensitivity and compassion for infant's discomfort

Discuss with family their concerns about infant's pain

Encourage family to speak with health practitioner about their concerns

- **EXPECTED OUTCOME**

Infant exhibits no or minimal signs of pain

NURSING DIAGNOSIS: Altered growth and development related to preterm birth, unnatural NICU environment, separation from parents

PATIENT GOAL 1: Will attain normal growth and development potential

- **NURSING INTERVENTIONS/*RATIONALES***

Provide optimum nutrition *to ensure steady weight gain and brain growth*

Provide regular periods of undisturbed rest *to decrease unnecessary O$_2$ use and caloric expenditure*

Provide age-appropriate developmental intervention

Recognize signs of overstimulation (flaccidity, yawning, staring, active averting, irritability, crying) *so that infant is allowed to rest and stress is reduced*

Promote parent-infant interaction, *since it is essential for normal growth and development*

- **EXPECTED OUTCOMES**

Infant exhibits a steady weight gain once past the acute phase of illness

Infant is exposed only to appropriate stimuli

NURSING DIAGNOSIS: Altered family processes related to situational/maturational crisis, knowledge deficit (birth of a preterm and/or ill infant), interruption of parental attachment process

NURSING CARE PLAN
The High-Risk Infant—cont'd

PATIENT (FAMILY) GOAL 1: Will be informed of infant's progress

• **NURSING INTERVENTIONS/*RATIONALES***

Prioritize information *to help parents understand most important aspects of care, signs of improvement, or deterioration in infant's condition*

Encourage parents to ask questions about child's status

Answer questions, facilitate expression of concern regarding care and prognosis

Be honest; respond to questions with correct answers *to establish trust*

Encourage mother and father to visit and/or call unit often *so they are informed of infant's progress*

Emphasize positive aspects of infant's status *to encourage sense of hope*

• **EXPECTED OUTCOME**

Parents express feelings and concerns regarding infant and prognosis, and demonstrate understanding and involvement in care

PATIENT (FAMILY) GOAL 2: Will exhibit positive attachment behaviors

• **NURSING INTERVENTIONS/*RATIONALES***

Encourage parents' visit as soon as possible *so that attachment process is initiated*

Encourage parents to:
   Visit infant frequently
   Address infant by name
   Touch, hold, and caress infant as appropriate for infant's physical condition
   Become actively involved in infant's care
   Bring clothing to dress infant as soon as condition permits

Reinforce parents' endeavors, *to increase their self-confidence*

Be alert to signs of tension and stress in parents

Enable parents to spend time alone with infant

Help parents interpret infant's responses; comment regarding any positive response and signs of overstimulation or fatigue

Help parents by demonstrating infant care techniques and offer support

Identify resources (e.g., transportation, baby-sitting) *to enable parents to visit*

• **EXPECTED OUTCOMES**

Parents visit infant soon after birth and at frequent intervals

Parents relate positively with infant (e.g., call infant by name, look at and touch infant)

Parents provide care for infant and demonstrate an attitude of comfort in relationships with infant

Parents identify signs of stress or fatigue in infant

PATIENT (SIBLINGS) GOAL 3: Will exhibit positive attachment behaviors

• **NURSING INTERVENTIONS/*RATIONALES***

Encourage siblings to visit infants when feasible

Explain environment, events, appearance of infant, and why infant cannot come home *to prepare them for visiting*

Provide photos of infant or other items if siblings are unable to visit

Encourage siblings to make pictures or bring other small items, such as a letter, for infant and place in incubator or crib

• **EXPECTED OUTCOMES**

Siblings visit infant in NICU or nursery

Siblings exhibit an understanding of explanations (specify)

Siblings receive infant-related items (specify)

PATIENT (FAMILY) GOAL 4: Will be prepared for home care

• **NURSING INTERVENTIONS/*RATIONALES***

Assess readiness of family (especially mother or other primary caregiver) to care for infant in home setting *to facilitate parents' transition to home with infant*

Teach necessary infant care techniques and observations

Encourage parent(s), when possible, to spend one or two nights in a hospital predischarge room before discharge with infant *to foster confidence in caring for infant at home*

Reinforce follow-up medical care

Refer to appropriate agencies or services *so that needed assistance is provided*

Encourage and facilitate involvement with parent support group or refer to appropriate support group(s) *for ongoing support*

Offer family opportunity to learn infant cardiopulmonary resuscitation and response to choking incident

• **EXPECTED OUTCOMES**

Family demonstrates ability to provide care for infant

Family members state how and when to contact available services

Family members recognize importance of follow-up medical care

---

NURSING DIAGNOSIS: Anticipatory grieving related to unexpected birth of high-risk infant, grave prognosis, and/or death of infant

---

PATIENT (FAMILY) GOAL 1: Will acknowledge possibility of child's death and demonstrate healthy grieving behaviors

• **NURSING INTERVENTIONS/*RATIONALES***

Provide family with the opportunity to hold their infant before death and, if possible, be present at the time of death

Support family's decision for terminating life support

Continued.

NURSING CARE PLAN
The High-Risk Infant—cont'd

Arrange for or perform appropriate baptism rite for infant

Provide family with the opportunity to see, touch, hold, caress, examine, and talk to their infant privately before and after death

Keep infant's body available for a few hours *to give family members who are hesitant an opportunity to see deceased infant if they change their minds*

Provide photographs taken before and after infant's death for family *to refer to at a later time to make infant real*

Take photograph of infant being held or touched by an adult; avoid morgue-type photograph *because it depersonalizes child*

Provide other tangible remembrances of child's death (e.g., name tags, identification band, lock of hair, footprints, blanket)

Encourage family to name infant if they have not done so

Identify resources to assist with funeral arrangements *to facilitate parental grieving*

- **EXPECTED OUTCOME**

Family discusses the reality of the death and conveys an attitude of realization

PATIENT (FAMILY) GOAL 2: Will receive adequate emotional and physical support

- **NURSING INTERVENTIONS/*RATIONALES***

Be available to family *to provide support*

Provide appropriate religious support (e.g., clergy)

Discuss infant's illness and death with family

Talk with family openly and honestly about funeral arrangements

Have information available regarding inexpensive services in the community

Inform family of all options available *so that they can make informed decisions*

Provide opportunity for family to call the unit if they have any questions regarding infant's illness and death

May contact family after the death *to assess coping and status of grieving process*

Refer family to appropriate support group(s) *for ongoing support*

- **EXPECTED OUTCOMES**

Family grieves for infant's death appropriately

Family demonstrates appropriate (culturally and socially influenced) grieving behaviors over infant's death

---

prints, a lock of hair, the bedside name card, and, as appropriate to the family's religious beliefs, a certificate of baptism. In some units special knitted clothing is made by hospital volunteer groups and donated for dressing the infant postmortem. Other tangible mementos of the child can be provided, such as name tags, armbands, and locks of hair shaved for intravenous insertion or other procedures. Naming the deceased infant is an important step in the grieving process; some parents may hesitate to give the newborn a name that had been chosen during the pregnancy for their special "baby." However, having a tangible person for whom to grieve is an important component of the grieving process.

At least one nurse who is familiar to the family should be present during the discussion about a dead or dying infant. The nurse should talk with parents openly and honestly about funeral arrangements, since few of them have had experience with this aspect of death. Many funeral homes now offer inexpensive arrangements for these special cases. Someone from the NICU should take the responsibility for acquiring this type of information. It is often helpful to parents for the NICU to have a list of local funeral homes, services offered, and a price for the service offered. Families need to be informed of options available, but it is preferable to encourage a funeral because the ritual provides an opportunity for parents to feel the support of friends and relatives. Issues regarding an autopsy or organ donation (when appropriate) are approached in a multidisciplinary fashion (primary practitioner and primary nurse) with respect, tact, and consideration of the family's wishes.

Before the parents leave the hospital, they are given the telephone number of the unit (if they do not have it) and invited to call any time they have any further questions. Many intensive care units make it a point to contact the parents following a neonatal death to assess the parents' coping mechanisms, evaluate the grieving process, and provide support as needed. Parents experiencing neonatal loss may retain vivid memories of the experience for many years, including memories of specific nursing care received (Calhoun, 1994). Several organizations are available to offer support and understanding to families who have lost a newborn, including **The Compassionate Friends,** * **SHARE (Source of Help in Airing & Resolving Experiences),**† and **AMEND (Aiding Mothers & Fathers Experiencing Neo-Natal Death).**‡ (See also Chapter 18 for further discussion of the family and the grief process.)

Baptism. Since many Christian parents wish to have their child baptized if death is anticipated or a decided possibility, this becomes a nursing responsibility. Whenever pos-

---

*P.O. Box 3696, Oak Brook, IL 60522-3696; (708) 990-0100. In Canada: 685 William Ave., Winnipeg, Canada, R3E 022.

†St. John's Hospital, 800 Carpenter, Springfield, IL 62769; (217) 544-6464, Ext. 5275.

‡Contact Maureen Connelly, 4324 Berrywick Terrace, St. Louis, MO 63128; (314) 487-7582.

sible, it is most desirable that a representative of the parents' faith (i.e., a Roman Catholic priest or a Protestant minister) perform such a ritual. When death is imminent, a practitioner can perform the baptism by simply pouring a few drops of water on the infant's forehead (a medicine dropper is a convenient means) while repeating the words, "I baptize you in the name of the Father and the Son and of the Holy Spirit." When the faith of the parents is uncertain, a conditional baptism can be carried out by saying, "If you are capable of receiving baptism, I baptize you in the name of the Father and of the Son and of the Holy Spirit." Parents are informed at an appropriate time of the infant's baptism.

❖ Evaluation

The effectiveness of nursing interventions is determined by continual reassessment and evaluation of care based on the following observational guidelines and expected outcomes:

1. Take vital signs and perform respiratory assessments at time intervals based on infant's condition and needs; observe infant's respiratory efforts and response to therapy; check functioning of equipment; review laboratory test results.
2. Measure abdominal skin and axillary temperatures at specified intervals.
3. Observe infant's behavior and appearance for evidence of sepsis.
4. Assess for hydration; assess and measure fluid intake; observe infant during feeding; measure amount of formula or parenteral intake; weigh daily.
5. Observe infant's skin for signs of irritation and breakdown.
6. Observe infant for evidence of increased intracranial pressure or signs of intraventricular hemorrhage.
7. Observe infant's physiologic and behavioral response to pain and to pain-relief interventions.
8. Observe infant's response to developmental care.
9. Observe parental interaction with infant; interview family regarding their feelings, concerns, and readiness for home care.
10. Assess family and observe their behaviors during and after the death of their infant.

Expected outcomes:
See Nursing Care Plan, pp. 244-248.

HIGH RISK RELATED TO DYSMATURITY

PRETERM INFANTS

Prematurity accounts for the largest number of admissions to an NICU. Not only does the immaturity place infants at risk for neonatal complications (e.g., hyperbilirubinemia and respiratory distress syndrome, which is highest in the preterm infant), but also for other high-risk factors (e.g., congenital abnormalities in association with prematurity).

The cause of prematurity is not known in most instances. The incidence of prematurity is lowest in the middle to high socioeconomic classes, in which pregnant women are generally in good health, are well nourished, and receive prompt and comprehensive prenatal care; the incidence is highest in the low socioeconomic class, in which a combination of deleterious circumstances is present. Other factors, such as multiple pregnancies, preeclampsia, and placental problems that interrupt the normal course of gestation prior to completion of fetal development, are responsible for a large number of preterm births.

The outlook for preterm infants is largely, but not entirely, related to the state of physiologic and anatomic immaturity of the various organs and systems at the time of birth. Infants born at term have advanced to a state of maturity sufficient to allow a successful transition to the extrauterine environment. Infants born prematurely must make the same adjustments but with functional immaturity proportional to the stage of development reached at the time of birth. The degree to which infants are prepared for extrauterine life can be predicted to some extent by weight and estimated gestational age (see Assessment of Clinical Gestational Age, Chapter 8).

Diagnostic Evaluation

Preterm infants have a number of characteristics that are distinctive at various stages of development. Identification of these characteristics provides valuable clues to the gestational age and hence to the physiologic capabilities of infants. The general, outward physical appearance changes as the fetus progresses to maturity. Characteristics of skin, general attitude (or posture) when supine, appearance of hair, and amount of subcutaneous fat provide cues to a newborn's physical development. Observation of spontaneous, active movements and response to stimulation and passive movement contributes to the assessment of neurologic status. The appraisal is made as soon as possible after admission to the nursery, since much of the observation and management of infants depends on this information (Fig. 9-11).

On inspection, preterm infants are very small and appear scrawny because they lack or have only minimal subcutaneous fat deposits, with a disproportionately large head in relation to the body, which reflects the cephalocaudal direction of growth. The skin is bright pink (often translucent, depending on the degree of immaturity), smooth, and shiny (may be edematous), with small blood vessels clearly visible underneath the thin epidermis. The fine lanugo hair is abundant over the body (depending on gestational age) but is sparse, fine, and fuzzy on the head. The ear cartilage is soft and pliable, and the soles and palms have minimal creases, resulting in a smooth appearance. The bones of the skull and the ribs feel soft, and the eyes may be closed. Male infants have few scrotal rugae, and the testes are undescended; the labia and clitoris are prominent in females.

In contrast to full-term infants' overall attitude of flexion and continuous activity, preterm infants are often inactive and listless although this varies with gestational age at birth and illness factors. The extremities maintain an attitude of extension and remain in any position in which they are placed. Reflex activity is only partially developed—sucking is absent, weak, or ineffectual; swallowing, gag, and cough reflexes are absent or weak; and other neurologic signs are absent or diminished. Physiologically immature, preterm infants are unable to maintain body temperature, have limited ability to excrete solutes in the urine, and have increased susceptibility to infection. A pliable thorax, immature lung tissue, and an immature regulatory center lead to periodic breathing, hypoventilation, and frequent periods of apnea. They are more susceptible to biochemical alterations such as hyperbilirubinemia and hypoglycemia, and they have a higher extracellu-

Posture—The preterm infant lies in a "relaxed attitude," limbs more extended; the body size is small, and the head may appear somewhat larger in proportion to the body size. The term infant has more subcutaneous fat tissue and rests in a more flexed attitude.

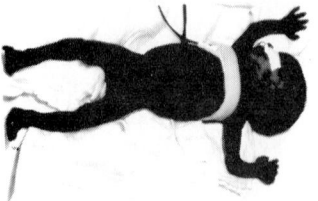 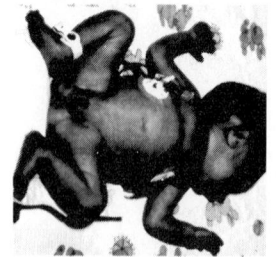

Ear—The preterm infant's ear cartilages are poorly developed, and the ear may fold easily; the hair is fine and feathery, and lanugo may cover the back and face. The mature infant's ear cartilages are well formed, and the hair is more likely to form firm separate strands.

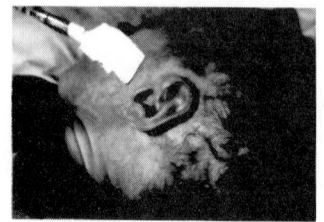 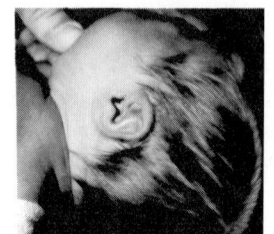

Sole of foot—The sole of the foot of the preterm infant appears more turgid and may have only fine wrinkles. The mature infant's sole (foot) is deeply creased.

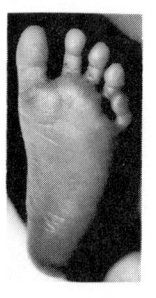 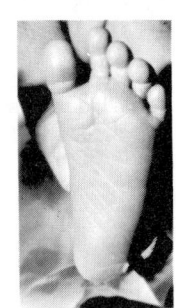

Female genitalia—The preterm female infant's clitoris is prominent, and labia majora are poorly developed and gaping. The mature female infant's labia majora are fully developed, and the clitoris is not as prominent or is completely covered.

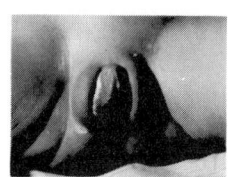 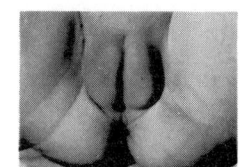

Male genitalia—The preterm male infant's scrotum is undeveloped and not pendulous; minimal rugae are present, and the testes may be in the inguinal canals or in the abdominal cavity. The term male infant's scrotum is well developed, pendulous, and rugated, and the testes are well down in the scrotal sac.

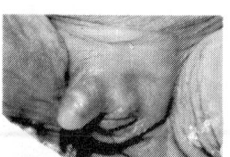 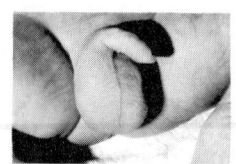

Scarf sign—The preterm infant's elbow may be easily brought across the chest with little or no resistance. The mature infant's elbow may be brought to the midline of the chest, resisting attempts to bring the elbow past the midline.

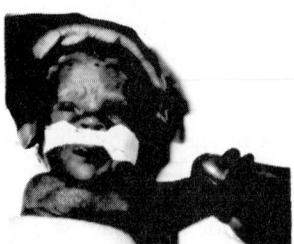 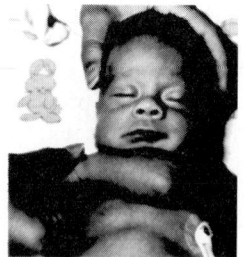

FIG. 9-11. Clinical and neurologic examinations comparing preterm and full-term infants.

NEUROLOGIC EVALUATION

PRETERM   **TERM**

Grasp reflex—The preterm infant's grasp is weak; the term infant's grasp is strong, allowing the infant to be lifted up from the mattress.

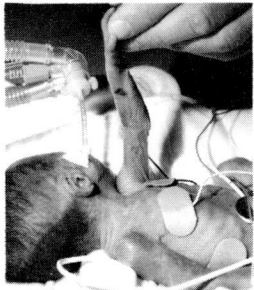
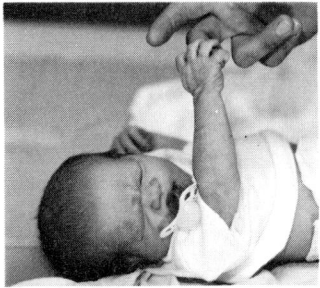

Heel-to-ear maneuver—The preterm infant's heel is easily brought to the ear, meeting with no resistance. This maneuver is not possible in the term infant, since there is considerable resistance at the knee.

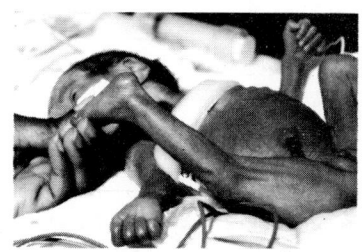
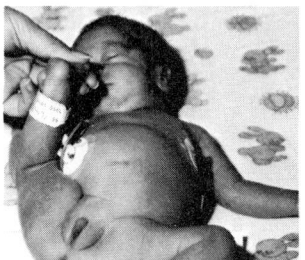

FIG. 9-11, cont'd. Clinical and neurologic examinations comparing preterm and full-term infants.

lar water content that renders them more vulnerable to fluid and electrolyte derangements. Preterm infants will exchange fully half their extracellular fluid volume every 24 hours as compared with one seventh of the volume in adults.

The soft cranium is subject to characteristic nonintentional deformation, or "preemie head," caused by positioning from one side to the other on a mattress. The head looks disproportionately longer from front to back, is flattened on both sides, and lacks the usual convexity seen at the temporal and parietal areas. This positional molding is frequently a concern to parents and may influence the parents' perception of the infant's attractiveness and their responsiveness to the infant. Positioning the infant on a waterbed mattress can reduce or minimize cranial molding.

Therapeutic Management

When delivery of a preterm infant is anticipated, the intensive care nursery is alerted, and a pediatrician, ideally a neonatologist, is present for the delivery. Infants who do not require resuscitation are transferred immediately to the NICU in a heated incubator where they are weighed, and intravenous lines, oxygen therapy, and other therapeutic interventions are initiated as needed. Resuscitation is conducted in the delivery area until infants can be safely transported to the NICU. Subsequent care is determined by the status of the infant. The general care of the preterm infant differs from that of the full-term infant primarily in the areas of respiratory support, temperature regulation, nutrition, susceptibility to infection, activity intolerance, and other consequences of physical immaturity.

Nursing Considerations

The nursing care, like the therapeutic management, is individualized for each infant. See appropriate discussions under Nursing Care of High-Risk Newborn and Family for additional details of care.

POSTMATURE INFANTS

Infants born of a gestation that extends beyond 42 weeks as calculated from the mother's last menstrual period (or by gestational age assessment) are considered to be postmature, or postterm, regardless of birth weight. This constitutes 3.5% to 15% of all pregnancies. The cause of delayed birth is unknown. Some infants are appropriate for gestational age but show the characteristics of progressive placental dysfunction. These infants, often called postmature infants, display the characteristics of infants who are 1 to 3 weeks of age, such as absence of lanugo, little if any vernix caseosa, abundant scalp hair, and long fingernails. Frequently the skin is cracked, parchmentlike, and desquamating. A common finding in postmature infants is a wasted physical appearance that reflects intrauterine deprivation. Depletion of subcutaneous fat gives them a thin, elongated appearance. The little vernix caseosa that remains in the skinfolds may be stained a deep yellow or green, which is usually an indication of meconium in the amniotic fluid.

There is a significant increase in fetal and neonatal mortality in postterm infants as compared with those born at term. They are especially prone to fetal distress associated with the decreasing efficiency of the placenta, macrosomia, congenital anomalies, and meconium aspiration syndrome.

The greatest risk occurs during the stresses of labor and delivery, particularly in infants of *primigravidas,* women delivering their first child. Cesarean section or induction of labor is usually recommended when infants are significantly overdue. Nursing care of the postterm infant, as well as therapeutic management, is individualized according to each infant's needs.

HIGH RISK RELATED TO PHYSIOLOGIC COMPLICATIONS

HYPERBILIRUBINEMIA

The term *hyperbilirubinemia* refers to an excessive accumulation of bilirubin in the blood and is characterized by *jaundice,* or *icterus,* a yellowish discoloration of the skin and other organs. Hyperbilirubinemia is a common finding in the newborn and in most instances is relatively benign. However, it can also indicate a pathologic state.

Hyperbilirubinemia may result from increased unconjugated or conjugated bilirubin. The unconjugated form (Table 9-2) is the type most commonly seen in newborns. The following discussion is limited to unconjugated hyperbilirubinemia.

Pathophysiology

Bilirubin is one of the breakdown products of hemoglobin that results from red blood cell (RBC) destruction. When RBCs are destroyed, the breakdown products are released into the circulation, where the hemoglobin splits into two fractions: heme and globin. The globin (protein) portion is used by the body, and the heme portion is converted to *unconjugated bilirubin,* an insoluble substance bound to albumin.

In the liver the bilirubin is detached from the plasma protein and, in the presence of the enzyme *glucuronyl transferase,* is conjugated with glucuronic acid to produce a highly soluble substance, *conjugated bilirubin glucuronide,* which is then excreted into the bile. In the intestine bacterial action reduces the conjugated bilirubin to urobilinogen and stercobilin, the pigment that gives stool its characteristic color.

TABLE 9-2. Comparison of major types of unconjugated hyperbilirubinemia

	PHYSIOLOGIC JAUNDICE	BREAST-FEEDING ASSOCIATED JAUNDICE (EARLY ONSET)	BREAST MILK JAUNDICE (LATE ONSET)	HEMOLYTIC DISEASE
Cause	Immature hepatic function plus increased bilirubin load from RBC hemolysis	Poor milk intake related to fewer calories consumed by infant before mother's milk is well established; enterohepatic shunting	Possible factors in breast milk that prevent bilirubin conjugation Less frequent stooling	Blood antigen incompatibility causes hemolysis of large numbers of RBCs Liver unable to conjugate and excrete excess bilirubin from hemolysis
Onset	After 24 hours (preterm infants, prolonged)	Second-fourth day	Fifth-seventh day	During first 24 hours (levels increase faster than 5 mg/dl/day)
Peak	72-90 hours	Third-fifth day	Tenth-fifteenth day	Variable
Duration	Declines on fifth-seventh day		May remain jaundiced for 3-12 weeks	
Therapy	Phototherapy if bilirubin levels increase significantly (rise in bilirubin greater than 5 mg/dl/day)	Frequent (10-12 times/day) breast-feeding Phototherapy for bilirubin 17-22 mg/dl in healthy term infants	Increase frequency of breast-feeding; use no supplementation such as glucose water; cessation of breast-feeding no longer recommended. Temporary discontinuation of breast-feeding for up to 24 hours; if bilirubin levels decrease, breast-feeding can resume May include home phototherapy with uninterrupted breast-feeding	*Postnatal*—Phototherapy; if severe, exchange transfusion *Prenatal*—Transfusion (fetus) Prevent sensitization (Rh incompatibility) of Rh-negative mother with RhoGAM

Most of the reduced bilirubin is excreted through the feces; a small amount is eliminated as urobilinogen in the urine.

Normally the body is able to maintain a balance between the destruction of RBCs and the use or excretion of by-products. However, when developmental limitations or a pathologic process interferes with this balance, bilirubin accumulates in the tissues to produce jaundice. The following are possible causes of hyperbilirubinemia in the newborn:

- Physiologic (developmental) factors (prematurity)
- Association with breast-feeding or breast milk
- Excess production of bilirubin (e.g., hemolytic disease, biochemical defects, bruises)
- Disturbed capacity of the liver to secrete conjugated bilirubin (e.g., enzyme deficiency, bile duct obstruction)
- Combined overproduction and undersecretion (e.g., sepsis)
- Some disease states (e.g., hypothyroidism, galactosemia, infant of a diabetic mother)
- Genetic predisposition to increased production (Native Americans, Asians)

The most common cause of neonatal hyperbilirubinemia is the relatively mild and self-limited *physiologic jaundice,* which generally appears around the third day of life and is caused by normal neonatal physiologic processes (Blackburn, 1995). However, hyperbilirubinemia may also be a result of a disease process such as hemolytic disease of the newborn or moderate to severe infection.

Diagnostic Evaluation

The degree of jaundice is determined by serum bilirubin measurements. Normal values of unconjugated bilirubin are 0.2 to 1.4 mg/dl. In the newborn, levels must exceed 5 mg/dl before jaundice or icterus is observable (see box). The definition of hyperbilirubinemia, whether due to physiologic or pathologic causes includes one or all of the following:

- Appearance of jaundice within 24 hours of birth
- Persistent jaundice after 1 (term neonate) or 2 (preterm) weeks
- Total serum bilirubin levels greater than 12 to 13 mg/dl
- Increase in serum bilirubin >5 mg/dl/day
- Direct bilirubin >1.5 to 2 mg/dl

Noninvasive monitoring of bilirubin via cutaneous reflectance measurements *(transcutaneous bilirubinometry)* allows for repetitive estimations of bilirubin. These devices work well on dark- and light-skinned infants and correlate fairly well with serum determinations of bilirubin level in full-term infants. Once phototherapy has been initiated, transcutaneous bilirubinometry is no longer useful as a screening tool.

Complications. Unconjugated bilirubin is highly toxic to neurons; therefore an infant with severe jaundice is at risk of developing *bilirubin encephalopathy* (interchangeably referred to as *kernicterus*), a syndrome of severe brain damage resulting from the deposition of unconjugated bilirubin in brain cells. Kernicterus describes the yellow staining of the brain cells that may result in bilirubin encephalopathy. The damage occurs when the serum concentration reaches toxic levels, regardless of cause. There is evidence that a fraction of unconjugated bilirubin crosses the blood-brain barrier in neonates with physiologic hyperbilirubinemia. When certain pathologic conditions exist in addition to elevated bilirubin levels, there is an increase in the blood-brain barrier's permeability to unconjugated bilirubin and, thus, potential irreversible damage. The exact level of serum bilirubin required to cause damage is as yet unknown.

Therapeutic Management

The primary goals in the treatment of neonatal hyperbilirubinemia are to prevent bilirubin encephalopathy and, as in any blood group incompatibility, to reverse the hemolytic process (see p. 256). The main form of treatment involves the use of phototherapy. Exchange transfusion is generally used for reducing dangerously high bilirubin levels that occur with hemolytic disease.

The pharmacologic management of hyperbilirubinemia with phenobarbital has centered primarily on the infant with hemolytic disease and is most effective when given to the mother several days before delivery. Phenobarbital essentially increases bilirubin conjugation and excretion in the liver. The use of phenobarbital in either the antenatal or the postnatal period, however, has not proved to be as effective as other treatments in reducing bilirubin. Bilirubin production in the newborn can be decreased by inhibiting heme oxygenase, an enzyme needed for heme breakdown (to biliverdin), with metalloporphyrins, especially tin-protoporphyrin and tin-mesoporphyrin. The use of these agents provides a preventive approach to hyperbilirubinemia; however, this procedure is not widely used.

Full-term infants with jaundice may also benefit from early initiation of feedings and frequent breast-feeding. These preventive measures are aimed at promoting increased intestinal motility, decreasing enterohepatic shunting (process whereby urobilinogen in the small intestine is converted back into unconjugated bilirubin and reenters the circulation, thus increasing bilirubin levels), and establishing normal bacterial flora in the bowel to effectively enhance the excretion of unconjugated bilirubin.

Phototherapy consists of the application of fluorescent light on the infant's exposed skin. Light promotes bilirubin excretion by *photoisomerization,* which alters the structure of bilirubin to a soluble form (lumirubin) for easier excretion. For phototherapy to be effective, the infant's skin must be fully exposed to an adequate amount of the light source.

An alternative to traditional phototherapy "bililights" is the *fiberoptic blanket* or *panel* (Wallaby,* Biliblanket†), which consists of a light-generating illuminator, a bundle of plastic fibers affixed to a panel that distributes the energy, and a soft, disposable, light-permeable cover to protect the infant. The blanket delivers therapeutic light consistently and con-

---

CLINICAL MANIFESTATIONS OF HYPERBILIRUBINEMIA

Jaundice—yellowish discoloration of skin
  Bright yellow or orange—unconjugated (indirect)
  Greenish, muddy yellow—conjugated (direct)
Intensity of jaundice
  Unrelated to degree of bilirubinemia
  Determined by serum bilirubin measurements

---

*Fiberoptic Medical Products, Inc., Allentown, PA.
†Ohmeda, Columbia, MO.

tinuously to the infant and achieves the same photoisomer-ization as conventional phototherapy (Schuman and Karush, 1992). The fiberoptic blanket is especially suited for home phototherapy. The portable blanket permits more infant-parent interaction, as well as better temperature control because the infant can be covered, and eliminates the need for eye patches (if eyes are not exposed to light source) and placing the lights at the correct distance.

Prognosis. Early recognition and treatment of hyper-bilirubinemia prevent severe brain damage (bilirubin enceph-alopathy). Impaired neurologic outcome is directly related to the serum bilirubin concentration. The main handicap is cerebral palsy, but sequelae may include clumsiness, hypotonia, and sensorineural hearing loss.

Nursing Considerations

❖ Assessment

Part of the routine physical assessment includes observing for evidence of jaundice at regular intervals. Jaundice is most reliably assessed by observing the infant's skin color from head to toe and the color of the sclera and mucous membranes. Applying direct pressure to the skin, especially over bony prominences such as the tip of the nose or the sternum, causes blanching and allows the yellow stain to be more pronounced. For dark-skinned infants the color of the sclera, conjunctiva, and oral mucosa is the most reliable indicator. Also, bilirubin (especially at high levels) is not uniformly distributed in skin. The nurse observes the infant in natural daylight for a true assessment of color.

> **Nursing ALERT**
>
> Evidence of jaundice that appears before the infant is 24 hours of age is an indication for assessing serum bilirubin levels.

The transcutaneous bilirubin meter is a useful screening device and is used to detect neonatal jaundice in full-term infants. However, phototherapy reduces the accuracy of the instrument; therefore its value is limited to the initial assessment. Blood samples are also taken for measurement of bilirubin in the laboratory.

> 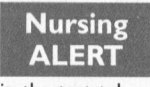 **Nursing ALERT**
>
> While blood is drawn, the bilirubin lights are turned off, and the blood is transported in a covered tube to avoid a false reading from bilirubin destruction in the test tube.

With increasingly shorter postpartum hospital stays, jaundice may appear after discharge. Therefore a careful history from the parents may reveal significant familial patterns of hyperbilirubinemia (older siblings of the infant). Other considerations in assessment include the ethnic origin of the family (e.g., higher incidence in Asian infants), type of delivery (e.g., induction of labor), and infant characteristics such as weight loss after birth, gestational age, sex, and presence of any bruising. The method of feeding and frequency of feeding are assessed.

> ### NURSING DIAGNOSES: INFANT WITH HYPERBILIRUBINEMIA
>
> High risk for altered body temperature related to use of phototherapy
> High risk for fluid volume deficit related to phototherapy
> Altered family processes related to situational crisis, prolonged hospitalization of infant

❖ Nursing Diagnoses

Based on the nursing assessment, a number of nursing diagnoses may be evident (see box above). Some are the same as for any high-risk infant; others may be related to concomitant health problems, such as prematurity or sepsis.

❖ Planning

The goals for the infant with hyperbilirubinemia and the family are as follows:

1. Infant will receive appropriate therapy if needed to reduce serum bilirubin levels.
2. Infant will experience no complications from therapy.
3. Family will receive emotional support.
4. Family will be prepared for home phototherapy (if prescribed).

❖ Implementation

Basic nursing care of the child with hyperbilirubinemia differs from that of any newborn infant only in management of specific therapy (see Nursing Care of the Newborn and Family, Chapter 8, and Nursing Care of the High-Risk Newborn and Family, p. 226).

Prevention of physiologic and breast-feeding jaundice may be possible with early introduction of feedings and frequent nursing. Every effort is made to provide an optimum thermal environment to reduce metabolic needs.

Phototherapy. The infant who receives phototherapy is placed nude under the light source and repositioned frequently to expose all body surface areas to the light. Once phototherapy has been initiated, frequent (every 4 to 12 hours) serum bilirubin levels are necessary because visual assessment of jaundice is no longer considered valid. Several precautions are instituted to protect the infant during phototherapy. The infant's eyes are shielded by an opaque mask to prevent exposure to the light (Fig. 9-12). The eye shield should be properly sized and correctly positioned to cover the eyes completely but prevent any occlusion of the nares. The infant's eyelids are closed before the mask is applied, since the corneas may become excoriated if they come in contact with the dressing. On each nursing shift the eyes are checked for evidence of discharge, excessive pressure on the lids, or corneal irritation. Eye shields are removed during feedings, and this opportunity is taken to provide visual and sensory stimulation. (See also Family Focus box.)

Minor side effects of phototherapy include loose, greenish stools; transient skin rashes; hyperthermia; increased metabolic rate; dehydration; electrolyte disturbances, such as hypocalcemia; and priapism. To prevent or minimize these effects, the temperature is monitored to detect early signs of hypothermia or hyperthermia and the skin is observed for evi-

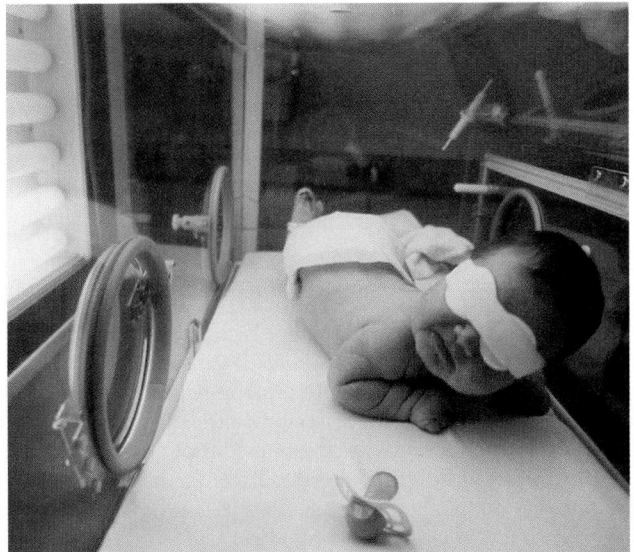

FIG. 9-12. Infant under phototherapy unit. Note that the eyes are shielded and a diaper is used to contain the diarrheal stools.

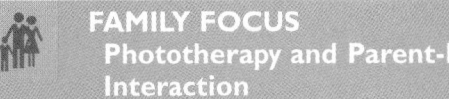

FAMILY FOCUS
Phototherapy and Parent-Infant Interaction

The traditional use of phototherapy has evoked concerns regarding a number of psychobehavioral issues, including parent-infant separation, potential social isolation, decreased sensorineural stimulation, altered biologic rhythms, altered feeding patterns, and activity changes. Parental anxiety is greatly increased, particularly at the sight of the newborn blindfolded and under special lights. The interruption of breast-feeding for phototherapy is a potential deterrent to successful maternal-infant attachment and interaction. Because research has demonstrated that bilirubin catabolism occurs primarily within the first several hours of the initiation of phototherapy, there is increased support for the removal of the infant from treatment for feeding and holding. Intermittent phototherapy may be just as effective as continuous therapy when used correctly. The benefits of stopping phototherapy for parental feeding and holding outweigh concerns related to the clearance of bilirubin (Blackburn and Loper, 1992).

dence of dehydration and drying, which can lead to excoriation and breakdown. Oily lubricants or lotions are not used on the skin in order to prevent increased tanning, or a "frying" effect. Full-term infants receiving phototherapy may require additional fluid volume to compensate for insensible and intestinal fluid loss. Because phototherapy enhances the excretion of unconjugated bilirubin through the bowel, loose stools may indicate accelerated bilirubin removal. Frequent stooling can cause perianal irritation; therefore meticulous skin care, especially keeping the skin clean and dry, is essential.

Once phototherapy is permanently discontinued, there is often a subsequent increase in the serum bilirubin level, often called the "rebound effect"; this is usually transient and resolves without resuming therapy.

Family Support. Parents need reassurance concerning their infant's progress. All the procedures are explained to familiarize them with the benefits and risks. For example, they need to be reassured that the naked infant who is under the bilirubin light is warm and comfortable. Parents may associate the use of eye shields with "blindness"; they are reassured that eye shields are for protection only. Eye shields are removed when the parents are visiting to facilitate the attachment process, and the parents can be reassured that the neonate is accustomed to darkness after months of intrauterine existence and benefits a great deal from auditory and tactile stimulation (see Family Focus box).

One of the most important nursing interventions is recognition of breast-feeding jaundice. Lack of familiarity among health professionals has caused many newborns prolonged hospitalization, termination of breast-feeding, and unnecessary phototherapy. Care of the new mother may include supporting successful and frequent breast-feeding. Parents also need reassurance of the benign nature of the jaundice and encouragement to resume breast-feeding if tempo-

rary cessation is prescribed. Unfortunately jaundice increases the risk of breast-feeding being discontinued and development of the *vulnerable child syndrome,* the belief of parents that their child has suffered a "close call" and is vulnerable to serious injury (see Critical Thinking Exercise on p. 256).

Discharge Planning and Home Care. With short hospital stays, mothers and infants may be discharged before evidence of jaundice is present. It is very important for the nurse to discuss signs of jaundice with the mother, because any clinical symptoms will probably appear at home.

If home phototherapy is instituted, the hospital or home health care nurse is usually responsible for teaching family members and assessing their abilities to implement the treatment safely. General guidelines for home care preparation and education are discussed in Chapters 20 and 21. Written instructions and supervision of care, especially application of eye shields, if needed, are essential. The minor side effects of phototherapy are reviewed, and parents may need instruction in taking axillary temperatures,* and recording times and amounts of feedings and the number of wet diapers and stools. Regardless of how benign the disorder or the therapy, these parents need support and understanding. Siblings also benefit from an explanation of the therapy to allay fears or misconceptions.

In jaundice associated with breast-feeding, follow-up blood studies are usually required to assess the progress of the jaundice. If temporary cessation of breast-feeding is prescribed, mothers should be taught to pump the breasts every 3 to 4 hours to maintain lactation; the expressed milk is frozen for use after breast-feeding is resumed.

❖ Evaluation

The effectiveness of nursing interventions is determined by continual reassessment and evaluation of care based on the

---

*Home care instructions for measuring temperature are available in Wong DL: *Wong and Whaley's Clinical manual of pediatric nursing,* ed. 4, St. Louis, 1996, Mosby.

following observational guidelines and expected outcomes:

1. Observe skin color; review bilirubinometric and/or laboratory findings.
2. Observe for signs of neurologic impairment (see box on p. 228).
3. Check placement of eye shields; observe skin for signs of dehydration; take temperature.
4. Interview family members and observe parent-infant interactions.

Expected outcomes:

1. Signs of hyperbilirubinemia diminish and/or disappear.
2. Infant displays no evidence of neurologic complications.
3. Infant exhibits no signs of adverse effects of phototherapy: eyes remain free of irritation, infant remains well hydrated, temperature remains below 38° C (100.4° F).
4. Family members demonstrate an understanding of the disease and its therapy; they interact with infant appropriately.

See Nursing Care Plan, The Newborn with Hyperbilirubinemia.*

---

*In Wong DL: *Wong and Whaley's Clinical manual of pediatric nursing,* ed 4, St Louis, 1996, Mosby.

HEMOLYTIC DISEASE OF THE NEWBORN (HDN)

Hyperbilirubinemia occurring within the first 24 hours of life is most often the result of HDN, an abnormally rapid rate of RBC destruction. This RBC destruction stimulates the production of RBCs, which, in turn, provides increasing numbers of cells for hemolysis. Major causes of increased erythrocyte destruction are isoimmunization (primarily Rh) and ABO incompatibility.

Blood Group Incompatibility

The membranes of human blood cells contain a variety of *antigens,* also known as *agglutinogens,* substances capable of producing an immune response if recognized by the body as a foreign substance. It is the reciprocal relationship between antigens on RBCs and antibodies in the plasma that causes *agglutination* (clumping) to take place. In other words, antibodies in the plasma of one blood group (except the AB group, which contains no antibodies) will produce agglutination when mixed with antigens of a different blood group. In the ABO blood group system the antibodies occur naturally. In the Rh system the person must be exposed to the Rh antigen before significant antibody formation takes place to cause a sensitivity response *(isoimmunization).*

Rh Incompatibility (Isoimmunization). The Rh blood group consists of several antigens, but for simplicity, only the terms *Rh-positive* (presence of antigen) and *Rh-negative* (absence of antigen) are used in this discussion (see Autosomal Inheritance Patterns, Appendix B). The presence or absence of the naturally occurring Rh factor determines the blood type.

Ordinarily no problems are anticipated when the Rh blood types are the same in both mother and fetus or if the mother is Rh-positive and the infant is Rh-negative. Difficulty may arise when the blood of the mother is Rh-negative and that of the infant is Rh-positive. Although the maternal and fetal circulations are separate, sometimes fetal RBCs (with antigens foreign to the mother) gain access to the maternal circulation through minute breaks in the placental vessels. The mother's natural defense mechanism responds to these alien cells by producing anti-Rh antibodies.

Under normal circumstances, this process of isoimmunization has no effect on the fetus during the first pregnancy with an Rh-positive fetus because the initial sensitization to Rh antigens rarely occurs before the onset of labor. However, as larger amounts of fetal blood are transferred to the maternal circulation during placental separation, maternal antibody production is stimulated. During a subsequent pregnancy with an Rh-positive fetus, these previously formed maternal antibodies to Rh-positive blood cells enter the fetal circulation, where they attack and destroy fetal erythrocytes (Fig. 9-13). Since the disease begins in utero, the fetus attempts to compensate for the progressive hemolysis by accelerating the rate of erythropoiesis. As a result, immature RBCs (erythroblasts) appear in the fetal circulation; hence the term *erythroblastosis fetalis.*

There is wide variability in the development of maternal sensitization to Rh-positive antigens. Sensitization may occur during the first pregnancy if the woman had previously received an Rh-positive blood transfusion. No sensitization may occur in situations in which a strong placental barrier pre-

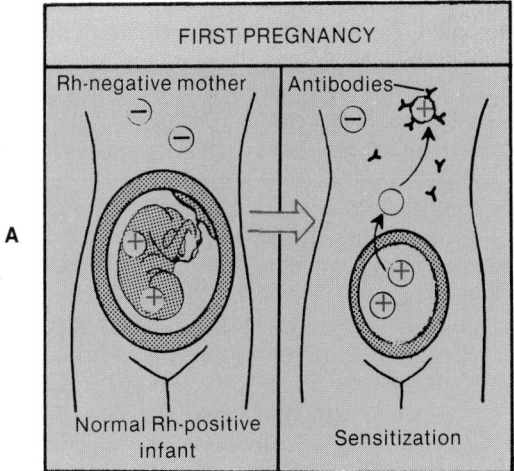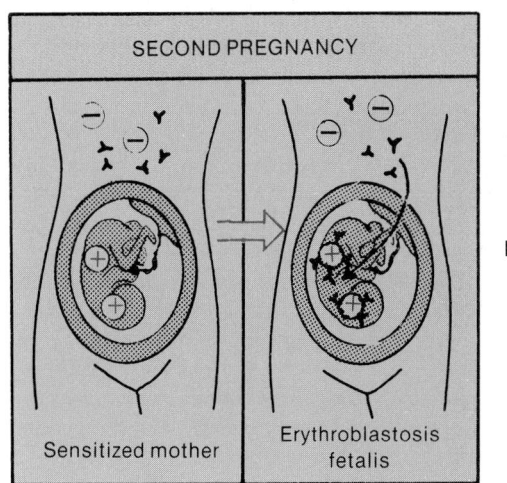

FIG. 9-13. Development of maternal sensitization to Rh antigens. **A,** Fetal Rh-positive erythrocytes enter maternal system. Maternal anti-Rh antibodies are formed. **B,** Anti-Rh antibodies cross placenta and attack fetal erythrocytes.

vents transfer of fetal blood into the maternal circulation. In about 10% to 15% of sensitized mothers there is no hemolytic reaction in the newborn.

In the most severe form of erythroblastosis fetalis, *hydrops fetalis,* the progressive hemolysis causes fetal hypoxia, cardiac failure, generalized edema (anasarca), and effusions into the pericardial, pleural, and peritoneal spaces. The fetus may be delivered stillborn or in severe respiratory distress. However, the use of intravascular (via an umbilical artery or vein) blood transfusion has improved the outcome of affected fetuses (Vomund and Witter, 1994).

ABO Incompatibility. Hemolytic disease may also occur when the major blood group antigens of the fetus are different from those of the mother. The major blood groups are A, B, AB, and O. The most common blood group incompatibility in the neonate is between a mother with O blood group and an infant with A or B blood group (see Table 9-3 for possible ABO incompatibilities). Naturally occurring anti-A or anti-B antibodies already present in the maternal circulation cross the placenta and attack the fetal RBCs, causing hemolysis. Usually the hemolytic reaction is less severe than in Rh incompatibility. Although the traditional thinking has been that the number of pregnancies is insignificant in the severity of ABO incompatibility, evidence suggests that the risk of hyperbilirubinemia is greater for subsequent offspring, especially if the first newborn had hyperbilirubinemia.

Clinical Manifestations

Jaundice appears shortly after birth (during the first 24 hours) and serum levels of unconjugated bilirubin rise rapidly. Most newborns with HDN are not jaundiced at birth. However, hepatosplenomegaly may be evident. If the fetus is severely affected, signs of anemia (notably, marked pallor) and hypovolemic shock are apparent at birth.

Diagnostic Evaluation

Diagnosis of isoimmunization before delivery can be made through amniocentesis and analysis of bilirubin levels in amniotic fluid. Increasing bilirubin levels indicate progressive fetal hemolysis and may indicate the need for an intrauterine transfusion or immediate termination of the pregnancy. A new method using polymerase chain reaction determines the RhD genotype of amniotic cells. If the fetus is found to be Rh-negative, no further testing is needed. Erythroblastosis fetalis caused by Rh incompatibility can also be assessed by evaluating rising anti-Rh antibody titers in the maternal circulation *(indirect Coombs test)* or by testing the optical density of amniotic fluid (delta 00450 test), since bilirubin discolors the fluid.

The disease in the newborn is suspected on the basis of the timing and appearance of jaundice (see Table 9-2) and can be confirmed postnatally by detecting antibodies attached to the circulating erythrocytes of affected infants *(direct Coombs test).* The Coombs test is routinely performed on cord blood samples from infants born to Rh-negative mothers.

Therapeutic Management

The primary aim of therapeutic management of isoimmunization is prevention. Postnatal therapy may involve phototherapy or exchange transfusion depending on the severity of hemolysis and the increase in serum bilirubin levels. Although

TABLE 9-3. Potential maternal-fetal ABO incompatibilities

MATERNAL BLOOD GROUP	INCOMPATIBLE FETAL BLOOD GROUP
O	A or B
B	A or AB
A	B or AB

phototherapy may control bilirubin levels in mild cases, the hemolytic disease may continue, causing severe hyperbilirubinemia and anemia if left untreated. Phototherapy may be the only treatment required for some infants with ABO incompatibility.

Prevention of Rh Isoimmunization.   The administration of *Rho immune globulin (RhIG)*, a human gamma globulin concentrate of anti-D, to all *unsensitized* Rh-negative mothers after delivery or abortion of an Rh-positive infant or fetus prevents the development of maternal sensitization to the Rh factor. The injected anti-Rh antibodies are thought to destroy (by subsequent phagocytosis and agglutination) fetal RBCs passing into the maternal circulation before they can be recognized by the mother's immune system. Since the immune response is blocked, anti-D antibodies and memory cells, which produce the primary and secondary immune responses, respectively, are not formed. The inhibition of memory cell formation is especially important because these cells provide long-term immunity by initiating a rapid immune response once the antigen is reintroduced.

To be effective, RhIG, such as RhoGAM, must be administered to unsensitized mothers within 72 hours (but possibly as long as 3 to 4 weeks) after the first delivery or abortion and repeated after subsequent ones. The administration of RhIG at 26 to 28 weeks of gestation further reduces the risk of Rh immunization. RhIG is not effective against existing Rh-positive antibodies in the maternal circulation.

> **Nursing ALERT**   RhIG is administered intramuscularly, not intravenously, only to Rh-negative women with a negative Coombs test—never to the infant or father.

Exchange Transfusion.   Exchange transfusion, in which the infant's blood is removed in small amounts (usually 5 to 10 ml at a time) and replaced with compatible blood (such as Rh-negative blood), is a mode of therapy for treatment for severe hyperbilirubinemia that is unresponsive to phototherapy. Exchange transfusion removes the sensitized erythrocytes, lowers the serum bilirubin level to prevent bilirubin encephalopathy, corrects the anemia, and prevents cardiac failure. Indications for exchange transfusion may include a positive direct Coombs test, hemoglobin concentration of cord blood below 12 g/dl, and a bilirubin level of 20 mg/dl in the full-term infant who is less than 24 hours old. However, some authorities advocate delaying exchange transfusions in full-term infants until the bilirubin levels are considerably higher (Newman and Maisels, 1992, Gartner, 1994). An infant born with hydrops fetalis or signs of cardiac failure as a result of HDN is a candidate for immediate exchange transfusion with fresh whole blood.

For exchange transfusion, fresh whole blood is typed and cross-matched to the mother's serum. The amount of donor blood used is usually double the blood volume of the infant, which is about 85 ml/kg body weight but is limited to no more than 500 ml. The two-volume exchange transfusion replaces approximately 85% of the neonate's blood.

An exchange transfusion is a sterile surgical procedure. A catheter is inserted into the umbilical vein and threaded into the inferior vena cava. Depending on the infant's weight, 5 to 10 ml of blood is withdrawn within 15 to 20 seconds, and the same volume of donor blood is infused over 60 to 90 seconds. If the blood has been citrated (addition of citrate phosphate dextrose adenine to prevent coagulation), calcium gluconate may be given after infusion of each 100 ml of donor's blood to prevent hypocalcemia.

Intrauterine Transfusion.   Infants of mothers already sensitized are sometimes treated by intrauterine transfusion, which consists of infusing blood into the peritoneal cavity or the umbilical vein of the fetus. The need for therapy is based on determinations of the optical density of amniotic fluid (via amniocentesis) as an index of the bilirubin concentration and degree of hemolysis.

Prognosis.   The severe anemia of isoimmunization may result in stillbirth, shock, congestive heart failure, poor feeding, or poor weight gain. Severe hyperbilirubinemia left untreated may result in bilirubin encephalopathy. Complications from exchange transfusion are uncommon. Despite the availability of an effective preventive measure, Rh HDN continues to cause significant morbidity and mortality in the United States.

Nursing Considerations

The initial nursing responsibility is recognizing hyperbilirubinemia. The possibility of hemolytic disease can be anticipated from the prenatal and perinatal history. Prenatal evidence of incompatibility and a positive Coombs test are cause for increased vigilance for early signs of jaundice in an infant.

If an exchange transfusion is needed, the nurse prepares the infant and the family and assists the practitioner with the procedure. Documentation of blood volumes exchanged, including the amount of blood withdrawn and infused, the time of each procedure, and the cumulative record of the total volume exchanged, are kept. Vital signs, monitored electronically, are evaluated frequently and correlated with removal and infusion of blood. If signs of cardiac or respiratory problems occur, the procedure is stopped temporarily and resumed once the infant's cardiorespiratory function stabilizes. The nurse also observes for signs of transfusion reaction.

> **Nursing ALERT**   Signs of exchange transfusion reaction include the following:
> Tachycardia or bradycardia
> Respiratory distress
> Dramatic change in blood pressure
> Temperature instability
> Rash

Throughout the procedure the infant requires attention to thermoregulation. Hypothermia increases oxygen and glucose consumption, causing metabolic acidosis. Not only do these consequences hinder the infant's overall physical ability to withstand the long procedure, but they also inhibit the binding capacity of albumin and bilirubin and the hepatic enzymatic reactions, thus increasing the risk of kernicterus. Conversely, hyperthermia damages the donor erythrocytes, elevating the free potassium content and predisposing the infant to cardiac arrest.

The procedure is performed under a radiant warmer. However, the infant is usually covered with sterile drapes that may prevent the radiant heat from sufficiently warming the skin. The blood is also warmed (using specially designed devices, never microwave ovens) before infusion.

After the procedure is completed, the nurse inspects the umbilical site for evidence of bleeding. The catheter may remain in place for use during repeated exchanges, if indicated.

Family Support.   Parents frequently feel guilty because they think they have caused the blood incompatibility. Parents should never be made to feel responsible or negligent. They are encouraged to verbalize and express their thoughts. Actions that were taken to prevent any problems, such as frequent antepartum examinations and blood tests, should be referred to and praised.

METABOLIC COMPLICATIONS

The stressed newborn infant is subject to a variety of complications related to physiologic function. Prominent among these are fluid and electrolyte derangements, hypoglycemia, and hypocalcemia. These complications often occur concurrently with or as a secondary result of other neonatal disorders and may therefore be difficult to differentiate from other conditions. The major characteristics of hypoglycemia and hypocalcemia are outlined in Table 9-4.

RESPIRATORY DISTRESS SYNDROME (RDS)

Respiratory distress is a name applied to respiratory dysfunction in neonates and is primarily a disease related to develop-

TABLE 9-4. Metabolic abnormalities		
	HYPOGLYCEMIA	HYPOCALCEMIA
Definition	Blood glucose concentration significantly lower than that in the majority of infants of the same age and weight	Abnormally low levels of calcium in circulating blood
Types	Early transitional neonatal: large or normal-size infants who appear to suffer from hyperinsulinism Classic transient neonatal: infants who suffered intrauterine malnutrition that depleted glycogen and fat stores Secondary: a response to perinatal stresses that increase infant's metabolic needs relative to glycogen stores Recurrent, severe: caused by an enzymatic or metabolic-endocrine defect	Early onset: appears in first 48 hours, appears in preterm infants who experienced perinatal hypoxia Late onset, cow's milk–induced hypocalcemia (neonatal tetany): apparent after first 3-4 days (high phosphorus/calcium ratio of cow's milk depresses parathyroid activity, reducing serum calcium levels)
Clinical Manifestations	Vague, often indistinguishable from other newborn conditions Cerebral signs: jitteriness, tremors, twitching, weak or high-pitched cry, lethargy, limpness, apathy, convulsions, and coma Other: cyanosis, apnea, rapid irregular respirations, sweating, eye rolling, poor feeding Signs often transient but recurrent	Early onset: jitteriness, apnea, cyanotic episodes, edema, high-pitched cry, abdominal distention Late onset: twitching, tremors, seizures
Laboratory Diagnosis	Plasma glucose concentrations less than 40 mg/dl in the first 24 hours, or less than 50 mg/dl thereafter	Serum calcium less than 7 mg/dl Ionized calcium less than 1.007 to 1.27 mmol/L
Treatment	Intravenous glucose administration Preventive: early feeding in normoglycemic infants	Early onset: increased milk feedings, administration of calcium supplements (sometimes) Late onset: Administration of calcium gluconate orally or intravenously (slowly); vitamin D
Nursing	See Nursing Care of the High-Risk Newborn and Family, p. 226 Identify infants with hypoglycemia Reduce environmental factors that predispose to hypoglycemia (e.g., cold, stress, respiratory distress) Employ proper feeding techniques Administer glucose as prescribed	See Nursing Care of the High-Risk Newborn and Family, p. 226 Identify infants with hypocalcemia Administer calcium as prescribed Observe for signs of acute hypercalcemia (e.g., vomiting, bradycardia) Manipulate environment to reduce stimuli that might precipitate a seizure or tremors (e.g., picking up infant suddenly, sudden jarring of crib)

mental delay in lung maturation. The terms *respiratory distress syndrome (RDS)* and *hyaline membrane disease (HMD)* are most often applied to the severe lung disorder that is not only responsible for more infant deaths than any other disease but also carries the highest risk in terms of long-term respiratory and neurologic complications (see Chapter 23 for a discussion of adult RDS). It is seen almost exclusively in preterm infants. The disorder is rare in infants of narcotic-addicted mothers or infants who have been subjected to chronic intrauterine stress (e.g., maternal preeclampsia or hypertension). Respiratory distress of a nonpulmonary origin in neonates may also be caused by sepsis, exposure to cold, airway obstruction (atresia), intraventricular hemorrhage, hypoglycemia, metabolic acidosis, acute blood loss, and drugs. Pneumonia in the neonatal period is respiratory distress caused by bacterial or viral agents and may occur alone or as a complication of RDS.

Pathophysiology

Preterm infants are born before the lungs are able to serve as efficient organs for gas exchange. This appears to be a critical factor in the development of RDS. Although the precise cause is still undetermined, several features in the development of the disorder are established, and there are a number of interdependent relationships that complicate the situation.

At the time of birth, infants must initiate breathing and then keep the previously fluid-filled lungs inflated with air. Most full-term infants successfully accomplish these adjustments; preterm infants with respiratory distress are unable to do so. Although numerous factors are involved, the central factor responsible for this adaptation is normal development of the surfactant system.

Surfactant is a surface-active phospholipid secreted by the alveolar epithelium. Acting much like a detergent, this substance reduces surface tension of fluids that line the alveoli and respiratory passages, resulting in uniform expansion and maintenance of lung expansion at low intraalveolar pressure. Immature development of these functions produces conse-

quences that seriously compromise respiratory efficiency. Deficient surfactant production causes unequal inflation of alveoli on inspiration and collapse of alveoli on end expiration. Without surfactant, infants are unable to keep their lungs inflated and therefore exert a great deal of effort to reexpand the alveoli with each breath. As a result, infants use more oxygen to expend this energy than they take in, which rapidly leads to exhaustion. With increasing exhaustion they are able to open fewer and fewer alveoli. This inability to maintain lung expansion produces widespread atelectasis.

Inadequate pulmonary perfusion and ventilation produce hypoxemia and hypercapnia. Prolonged hypoxemia activates anaerobic glycolysis, which produces increased amounts of lactic acid. An increase in lactic acid causes metabolic acidosis; inability of the atelectatic lungs to blow off excess carbon dioxide produces respiratory acidosis. Lowered pH causes further vasoconstriction. With deficient pulmonary circulation and alveolar perfusion, the Pao_2 continues to fall, the pH falls, and materials needed for surfactant production are not circulated to the alveoli.

Diagnostic Evaluation

The diagnosis of RDS is made on the basis of clinical manifestations (see box) and radiographic studies. The extent of respiratory and metabolic acidosis is determined by blood gas analysis. Criteria for visually evaluating the degree of respiratory distress are illustrated in Fig. 9-14.

Therapeutic Management

The treatment of RDS is largely supportive and includes all the general measures required for any preterm infant, as well as those instituted to correct imbalances. The supportive measures that are most crucial to a favorable outcome are (1) maintain adequate ventilation and oxygenation with either an oxygen hood or mechanical ventilation, (2) maintain acid-base balance, (3) maintain a neutral thermal environment, (4) maintain adequate tissue perfusion and oxygenation, (5) prevent hypotension, (6) maintain adequate hydration and electrolyte status, and (7) surfactant replacement therapy. Nipple and gavage feedings are contraindicated in any situation that creates a marked increase in respiratory rate because of the greater hazards of aspiration. In addition, administering formula to the infant with transient hypoxia places the infant at risk for necrotizing enterocolitis. Nutrition is provided by parenteral therapy during the acute stage of the disease.

Surfactant may be administered at birth as a preventive and/or prophylactic treatment of RDS or later on in the course of RDS as a rescue treatment. Surfactant is administered via the endotracheal tube (ET) directly into the infant's trachea. Once surfactant is absorbed, there is usually an increase in respiratory compliance requiring adjustment of ventilator settings to decrease MAP and prevent overinflation or hyperoxemia.

The goals of oxygen therapy are to provide adequate oxygen to the tissues, prevent lactic acid accumulation resulting from hypoxia, and at the same time avoid the potentially deleterious effects of oxygen barotrauma. Numerous methods have been devised to improve oxygenation (see Table 9-5). All require that the gas be warmed and humidified before entering the respiratory tract. If the infant does not require mechanical ventilation, oxygen can be supplied to a plastic hood

---

CLINICAL MANIFESTATIONS OF RDS

Respiratory Signs and Symptoms:

Tachypnea (up to 80 to 120 breaths/min) initially
Dyspnea
Pronounced intercostal and/or substernal retractions (Fig. 9-14)
Fine inspiratory rales
Audible expiratory grunt
Flaring of the external nares
Cyanosis and/or pallor

As the Disease Progresses:

Apnea
Flaccidity
Inertness
Unresponsiveness
Diminished breath sounds

Severe Disease Associated With:

Shocklike state
Diminished cardiac return and bradycardia
Low arterial blood pressure

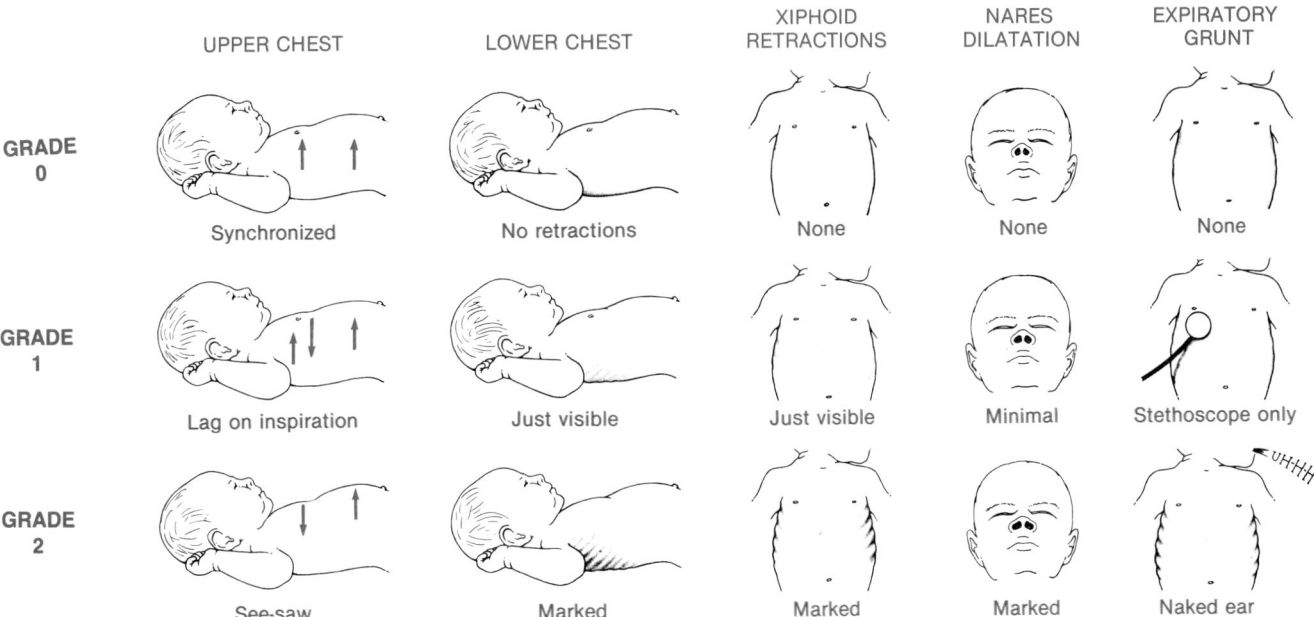

	UPPER CHEST	LOWER CHEST	XIPHOID RETRACTIONS	NARES DILATATION	EXPIRATORY GRUNT
GRADE 0	Synchronized	No retractions	None	None	None
GRADE 1	Lag on inspiration	Just visible	Just visible	Minimal	Stethoscope only
GRADE 2	See-saw	Marked	Marked	Marked	Naked ear

FIG. 9-14. Criteria for evaluating respiratory distress. (Modified from Silverman WA, Andersen DH: Controlled clinical trial of effects of water mist on obstructive respiratory signs, death rate, and necropsy findings among premature infants, *Pediatrics* 17:1-9, 1956.)

placed over the infant's head to supply variable concentrations of humidified oxygen (see Oxygen Therapy, Chapter 22). If oxygen saturation of the blood cannot be maintained at a satisfactory level and the carbon dioxide level ($Paco_2$) rises, infants will require ventilatory assistance.

Prevention. The most successful approach to prevention of RDS is prevention of premature delivery, especially in elective early delivery and cesarean section. Improved methods for assessing the maturity of the fetal lung by amniocentesis, although not a routine procedure, allow a reasonable prediction of adequate surfactant formation (see Diagnostic Evaluation). Since estimation of a date of delivery can be miscalculated by as much as 1 month, these tests are particularly valuable when scheduling elective cesarean section. An aggressive approach using tocolysis (such as ritadrine and terbutaline administration) to delay delivery and maternal administration of corticosteroids to induce surfactant production appears to reduce the incidence of RDS in preterm infants.

Prognosis

RDS is a self-limiting disease, and following a period of deterioration (approximately 48 hours) and in the absence of complications, affected infants begin to improve by 72 hours. Often heralded by the onset of diuresis, this improvement has been attributed primarily to increased production and greater availability of surface-active material.

Infants with RDS who survive the first 96 hours have a reasonable chance of recovery. However, complications of RDS include those described as complications of oxygen therapy: patent ductus arteriosus and congestive heart failure, intraventricular hemorrhage, bronchopulmonary dysplasia (BPD), retinopathy of prematurity, necrotizing enterocolitis, and neurologic sequelae.

Surfactant replacement therapy may improve the survival rate and reduce the severity of RDS. Treated infants may also have fewer respiratory complications.

Nursing Considerations

❖ Assessment

The most essential nursing function is to observe and assess the infant's response to therapy. Since oxygen concentration and ventilation parameters are prescribed according to the infant's blood gas measurements and pulse oximetry readings, and because an infant's status can change rapidly, continuous monitoring and close observation are mandatory.

Changes in oxygen concentration are based on these observations. The amount of oxygen administered, expressed as the fraction of inspired air (Fio_2), is determined on an individual basis according to pulse oximetry and/or direct or indirect measurement of arterial oxygen concentration. Capillary samples, collected from the heel (see Chapter 22 for procedure), are useful for pH and $Paco_2$ determinations but *not* for oxygenation status. Continuous pulse oximetry readings are recorded at least hourly. Blood sam-

---

NURSING DIAGNOSES: INFANT WITH RDS

Ineffective breathing pattern related to surfactant deficiency, alveolar instability, and pulmonary immaturity
Ineffective breathing pattern related to decreased energy
Impaired gas exchange related to immature alveolar structure
Impaired gas exchange related to inability to maintain lung expansion
High risk for trauma (brain tissue) related to hypoxemia and hypercapnia

pling is necessary 15 to 30 minutes after ventilator changes for the acutely ill infant and generally every 2 to 4 hours for sick infants.

❖ Nursing Diagnoses

Many of the diagnoses associated with any high-risk infant are appropriate for the infant with RDS. Diagnoses that are more specifically related to respiratory distress are listed in the box on p. 261.

❖ Planning

The major goals for the infant with respiratory distress are the same as for any high-risk infant (such as infant and family support) with special emphasis on respiratory needs:

1. Infant will exhibit optimum air exchange.
2. Infant will exhibit desired respiratory, cardiac, thermoregulatory, neurologic, and metabolic function (unless preexisting conditions are present).

❖ Implementation

Mucus may collect in the respiratory tract as a result of the infant's pulmonary condition. Secretions interfere with gas flow and predispose the infant to obstruction of the passages, including the ET tube. Suctioning should be performed only when necessary, based on individual infant assessment, which includes auscultation of the chest, evidence of decreased oxygenation, excess moisture in the ET tube, or increased infant irritability. Some centers use preoxygenation and hyperinflation to maintain adequate oxygenation and prevent associated complications.

> **Nursing ALERT**
>
> Suctioning is not an innocuous procedure (may cause bronchospasm, bradycardia due to vagal nerve stimulation, hypoxia, and increased intracranial pressure [ICP], predisposing the infant to intraventricular hemorrhage) and should *never* be carried out on a routine basis. Improper suctioning technique can also cause infection, airway damage, or even pneumothoraces.

When nasopharyngeal passages, the trachea, or the ET tube is being suctioned, the catheter should be inserted gently but quickly no further than the tip of the ET tube, and then intermittent suction is applied as the catheter is withdrawn. It is imperative that the time the airway is obstructed by the catheter be limited to no more than 5 seconds because continuous suction removes air from the lungs along with the mucus. It is recommended that the "two-person" suctioning procedure be used on infants who are acutely ill and who do not tolerate any procedure without profound decreases in oxygen saturation, decreased BP, and heart rate. The object of suctioning an artificial airway is to maintain patency of that airway, not the bronchi. Suction applied beyond the ET tube can cause traumatic lesions of the trachea. The Fio_2 should be increased by 10% before suctioning to compensate for a decrease in Fio_2 during the procedure (see Chapter 22).

> **Nursing ALERT**
>
> The pulse oximeter is observed before, during, and after the suctioning to provide an ongoing assessment of oxygenation status and to prevent hypoxemia.

Removal of secretions can be further facilitated by positioning and application of percussion and vibration to the thoracic wall. However, the Trendelenburg position should not be used with preterm infants, since it can contribute to increased ICP. Percussion and vibration are poorly tolerated in most ELBW and VLBW infants, often resulting in hypoxia, rib fractures, bruising, and further atelectasis. Chest physiotherapy should be carefully evaluated according to the infant's condition and with consideration of benefit/risk factors.

The most advantageous positions for facilitating an infant's open airway are on the side with the head supported in alignment by a small folded blanket or, when on the back, positioned to keep the neck slightly extended. With the head in the "sniffing" position, the trachea is opened at its maximum; hyperextension reduces the tracheal diameter in neonates. The supported side-lying position can also be used effectively.

Nursing responsibilities with surfactant administration include assistance in the delivery of the product, collection and monitoring of arterial blood gases, scrupulous monitoring of oxygenation with pulse oximetry, and assessment of the infant's tolerance of the procedure. Suctioning is usually delayed for an hour or so (depending on the type of surfactant and unit protocol) to allow for maximum effects to occur.

Inspection of the skin is part of routine infant assessment. Position changes and use of water pillows are helpful in guarding against skin breakdown.

Mouth care is especially important when infants are receiving nothing by mouth, and the problem is often aggravated by the drying effect of oxygen therapy. Drying and cracking can be prevented by good oral hygiene using sterile water. Irritation to the nares or mouth that occurs from appliances used to administer oxygen may be reduced by the use of a water-soluble ointment.

The nursing care of an infant with RDS is a demanding role; meticulous attention must be placed on subtle changes in the infant's oxygenation status. The importance of atten-

> ## Critical Thinking Exercise
> ### Respiratory Distress Syndrome
>
> A 32-week preterm infant requires mechanical ventilation for the treatment of RDS as a result of surfactant deficiency. The nurse is aware of problems associated with prematurity and RDS, such as hypoglycemia. Problems for which you are particularly vigilant in light of the use of mechanical ventilation with this infant and the knowledge of pathology include:
>
> 1. Meconium aspiration
> 2. Transient tachypnea
> 3. Air leaks
> 4. Persistent pulmonary hypertension
>
> *The correct answer is three. Infants who are preterm and lack adequate surfactant have immature alveoli and increased surface tension that predispose them to the development of air leaks during mechanical ventilation. The other three options are neonatal respiratory conditions usually unrelated to RDS of the type where surfactant deficiency is the major pathology.*

tion to detail cannot be overemphasized, particularly in regard to medication administration.

❖ Evaluation

The effectiveness of nursing interventions is determined by continual reassessment and evaluation of care based on the following observational guidelines and expected outcomes:

1. Perform frequent respiratory assessment (see assessment guidelines, p. 261).
2. Observe infant's behavior; weigh daily or as prescribed, take vital signs, and observe for signs of sepsis and respiratory complications (atelectasis, pneumothorax, pneumonia; see Critical Thinking Exercise).

Expected outcomes:

1. Respiratory rate and pattern is within appropriate limits for age and weight.
2. Tissue oxygenation is adequate; arterial blood gases and acid-base balance are within appropriate limits for postconceptional age.

See also Nursing Care Plan: The Infant with Respiratory Distress Syndrome* and Nursing Care Plan: The High Risk Infant, p. 244.

RESPIRATORY COMPLICATIONS

The newborn infant is vulnerable to a variety of pulmonary complications, some requiring oxygen therapy (Table 9-5). For example, the preterm infant is subject to periods of ap-

*In Wong DL: *Wong and Whaley's Clinical manual of pediatric nursing,* ed 4, St Louis, 1996, Mosby.

nea, and prenatal distress often causes the fetus to pass meconium, which may be aspirated before or during birth. Oxygen therapy, although lifesaving, is not without its hazards. Positive pressure introduced by mechanical apparatus has created an increase in the incidence of ruptured alveoli and subsequent **pneumothorax** and **bronchopulmonary dysplasia (chronic or respiratory lung disease). Retinopathy of prematurity (retrolental fibroplasia)** is observed almost exclusively in preterm infants and is also related to oxygen therapy and prematurity (see Table 9-6).

CARDIOVASCULAR COMPLICATIONS

The most serious cardiovascular disorders of the newborn are the congenital heart defects. Other conditions that occur in the newborn period are usually related to prematurity (e.g., anemia, patent ductus arteriosus) or other diseases (e.g., respiratory distress). Hemorrhagic disease of the newborn is related to physiologic characteristics of the newborn and is preventable. Some of these disorders are outlined in Table 9-7.

CEREBRAL COMPLICATIONS

Cerebral injury in newborn infants is not an uncommon observation. Newborn infants are particularly vulnerable to ischemic injury caused by variable (both increased and decreased) cerebral blood flow subsequent to asphyxia, and preterm infants, with a fragile cerebrovascular network, are highly prone to periventricular or intraventricular hemorrhage. Intracranial hemorrhage as a result of either trauma or hypoxia is a com-

---

TABLE 9-5. Common methods for assisted ventilation in neonatal respiratory distress

METHOD	DESCRIPTION	HOW PROVIDED
Common Methods		
Continuous positive airway pressure (CPAP) or continuous distending pressure (CDP)	Provides constant distending pressure to airway in spontaneously breathing infant	Nasal prongs Nasopharyngeal tubes Endotracheal tube
Positive end-expiratory pressure (PEEP)*	Provides increased end-expiratory pressure during expiration and between mandatory breaths that prevents alveolar collapse; maintains residual airway pressure	Endotracheal intubation and either volume-limited or pressure-limited ventilator
Intermittent mandatory ventilation (IMV)*	Allows infant to breathe spontaneously at own rate but provides mechanical cycled respirations and pressure at regular preset intervals	Endotracheal intubation and ventilator
Alternative Methods		
High-frequency ventilation (HFV)		
High-frequency positive-pressure ventilation (HFPPV)	Low-complaint circuit provides high gas flow through circuit: operates at rates between 60 and 150 breaths/min	Conventional infant ventilators; endotracheal tube
High-frequency oscillation (HFO)	Application of high-frequency, low-volume, sine-wave flow oscillations to airway at rates between 480 to 1200 breaths/min	Variable-speed piston pump (or loudspeaker, fluidic oscillator); endotracheal tube
High-frequency jet ventilation (HFJV)	Uses a separate, parallel, low-complaint circuit and injector port to deliver small pulses or jets of fresh gas deep into airway at rates between 250 and 900 breaths/min	May be used alone or with low-rate IMV; endotracheal tube

*Also referred to as conventional ventilation (vs HFV).

TABLE 9-6. Respiratory complications

DESCRIPTION	CLINICAL MANIFESTATIONS	TREATMENT	NURSING CONSIDERATIONS
Meconium Aspiration Syndrome (MAS)			
Aspiration of amniotic fluid containing meconium into fetal or newborn trachea in utero or at first breath	Meconium stained at birth Tachypnea Hypoxia Hyperventilation (early) Hypoventilation (later)	Suction hypopharynx at birth Intubate and suction trachea Treat for respiratory distress Prevent acidosis	See nursing care of infant with RDS, p. 261
Apnea of Prematurity			
Lapse of spontaneous breathing for 20 seconds or longer, that may or may not be followed by bradycardia, oxygen desaturation, and color change	Persistent apneic spells	Observe for apnea Check for thermal stability Administer theophylline or caffeine as ordered	Provide continuous electronic monitoring (respiratory and heart rates) Observe for presence of respirations Observe color Provide gentle tactile stimulation Suction nose and oropharynx if still apneic Apply artificial ventilation with bag-valve-mask and with sufficient pressure to lift rib cage Assess for and manage any precipitating factors (e.g., temperature, humidity, distention, ambient oxygen) Observe for signs of theophylline or caffeine toxicity: tachycardia (rate greater than 180 to 190 beats/min) and (later) vomiting, restlessness, irritability
Pneumothorax			
Presence of extraneous air in pleural space as a result of alveolar rupture	Tachypnea or apnea Grunting, flaring nares Retractions Absent or diminished breath sounds Shift in point of maximum intensity of heart sounds Bradycardia/cyanosis	Evacuate trapped air from pleural space through needle aspiration and/or chest tubes and water-seal drainage	Maintain close vigilance of infants with respiratory distress and/or those on assisted ventilation Provide appropriate care of chest drainage apparatus Keep emergency needle aspiration setup at bedside
Bronchopulmonary Dysplasia (BPD)			
Pathologic process related to alveolar damage from lung disease, prolonged exposure to high peak inspiratory pressures, and immature alveoli and respiratory tract	Dyspnea Barrel chest Inability to wean from mechanical ventilation following course of RDS (surfactant deficiency) Wheezing	Support respiratory efforts Prevent and/or control respiratory or systemic infections Supplemental oxygen in hospital/home	Provide opportunities for additional rest during feedings Observe for signs of fluid overload Assist with home oxygen therapy as needed Susceptibility to upper respiratory tract infections and frequent hospitalization for respiratory dysfunction Provide increased caloric density (feedings) with medium-chain triglycerides and glucose polymers

TABLE 9-7. Cardiovascular complications

DESCRIPTION	CLINICAL MANIFESTATIONS	THERAPEUTIC MANAGEMENT	NURSING CONSIDERATIONS
Patent Ductus Arteriosus (PDA) See Chapter 25	Decreased Po_2 Increased Pco_2 Recurrent apnea Bounding peripheral pulses Systolic or continuous murmur	Regulate parenteral fluids Provide respiratory support Administer indomethacin or perform ductal ligation	See Nursing Care of the High-Risk Newborn and Family, p. 226
Persistent Pulmonary Hypertension of the Newborn (PPHN) Severe pulmonary hypertension and large right-to-left shunt through foramen ovale and ductus arteriosus	Hypoxia Marked cyanosis Tachypnea with grunting and retractions Decreased peripheral pulses and prolonged capillary refill	Regulate fluids Provide supplemental oxygen and assisted ventilation Administer vasodilators Maintain acid-base balance	See Nursing Care of the High-Risk Newborn and Family, p. 226; Respiratory Distress Syndrome, p. 261 Organize nursing care to reduce stress to infant, especially noxious stimuli that cause increased oxygen demands Decrease physical manipulation and disturbance
Anemia Loss of blood from hemorrhage during delivery	Pallor Apnea Tachycardia Diminished activity Respiratory distress: grunting, nasal flaring, intercostal retractions	Transfuse with packed RBCs or erythropoietin factor for severe anemia	Monitor amount of blood drawn for tests Administer iron supplements as prescribed
Polycythemia/Hyperviscosity Syndrome Venous hematocrit 65% or greater owing to twin-to-twin or mother-to-fetus transfusion or increased RBC production	High incidence of: Cardiovascular symptoms (PPHN, cyanosis, apnea) Seizures Hyperbilirubinemia Gastrointestinal abnormalities	Implement partial exchange transfusion Provide appropriate therapy for associated problems	See Nursing Care of the High-Risk Newborn and Family, p. 226; Hyperbilirubinemia, p. 252
Hemorrhagic Disease of the Newborn Bleeding disorder resulting from transient deficiency of vitamin K–dependent blood factors	Oozing blood from umbilicus or circumcision Bloody or black stools Hematuria Ecchymoses	Administer prophylactic vitamin K	Administer vitamin K via intramuscular route
Retinopathy of Prematurity (ROP) Replacement of retina by fibrous tissue and blood vessels	Progressive vascular growth of retina Eventual blindness if not treated	Arrest proliferation process—cryotherapy Use supplemental oxygen judiciously and monitor oxygen blood levels carefully	See Nursing Care of the High-Risk Newborn and Family, p. 226 Monitor blood oxygen concentration

TABLE 9-8. Cerebral complications

DESCRIPTION	CLINICAL MANIFESTATIONS	THERAPEUTIC MANAGEMENT	NURSING CONSIDERATIONS
Hypoxic-Ischemic Brain Injury Nonprogressive neurologic (brain) impairment caused by intrauterine or postnatal asphyxia resulting in hypoxemia and/or cerebral ischemia	Appears within first 24 hours after hypoxic episode Seizures Abnormal muscle tone (usually hypotonia) Disturbance of sucking and swallowing Apneic episodes Stupor or coma	Provide supportive care Provide adequate ventilation Maintain cerebral perfusion Prevent cerebral edema Treat underlying cause Administer anticonvulsants	See Nursing Care of the High-Risk Newborn and Family, p. 226 Observe for signs that indicate cerebral hypoxia Monitor ventilatory and intravenous therapy Observe for and manage seizures Support family Provide guidelines for family management of neurologic damage
Periventricular/Intraventricular Hemorrhage (PVH/IVH) Hemorrhage into and around ventricles caused by ruptured vessels as a result of an event that increases cerebral blood flow to area	Sudden deterioration in condition Tense, bulging anterior fontanel Neurologic signs: Twitching Stupor Apnea Seizures Evident on ultrasonography and/or tomography	Supportive care: Provide ventilatory support Maintain oxygenation Regulate fluid and electrolytes, acid-base balance Suppress or prevent seizures	See Nursing Care of the High-Risk Newborn and Family, p. 226 Prevent increased cerebral blood pressure Avoid events that may increase/decrease cerebral blood flow (e.g., pain, unnecessary stimulation, endotracheal suctioning, hypoxia, hyperosmolar drugs, rapid volume expansion) Elevate head of bed 20 to 30 degrees, keep head in midline Support family
Intracranial Hemorrhage Subdural Subarachnoid Intracerebellar	Sudden decrease in hematocrit See Chapter 28 Change in sensorium Poor feeding	See Chapter 28	Same as for PVH/IVH

mon complication of preterm birth. Fragility and increased permeability of capillaries and prolonged prothrombin time predispose the preterm infant to trauma when delicate structures are subjected to the forces of labor. The more common cerebral complications are outlined in Table 9-8.

The highest incidence of abnormal neurologic findings occurs in infants with intracranial hemorrhage and very low birth weight. Major neurologic defects, such as cerebral palsy, hydrocephalus, seizures, and mental retardation, are usually diagnosed in the first 2 years of life. Less severe deficits, such as learning disorders, hyperactivity, and fine and gross motor incoordination may not be diagnosed until preschool or even school age. In survivors, cerebral palsy is the most common neurologic defect (see Chapter 32).

NEONATAL SEIZURES

Seizures in the neonatal period are usually the clinical manifestation of a serious underlying disease. Therefore, although not life-threatening as an isolated entity, seizures constitute a medical emergency because they signal a disease process that may produce irreversible brain damage. Consequently, it is imperative to recognize a seizure and its significance so that the cause, as well as the seizure, can be treated.

The causes of neonatal seizures include the following:

Metabolic disorders such as hypoglycemia and hypocalcemia
Toxic and electrolyte disturbances such as hypernatremia, hyponatremia, narcotic withdrawal, and bilirubin encephalopathy
Prenatal or postnatal infections, such as bacterial meningitis, sepsis, herpes simplex, and cytomegalic virus disease

Trauma at birth, such as severe hypoxia and intracranial hemorrhage

Congenital malformations, such as hydrocephaly and central nervous system agenesis

Miscellaneous disorders, such as degenerative diseases

The features of neonatal seizures are different from those observed in the older infant or child. The well-organized, generalized tonic-clonic seizures seen in older children are rare in the infant, especially the preterm infant. The seizures may be subtle and barely discernible or grossly apparent (see box).

Diagnostic Evaluation

Early evaluation and diagnosis of seizures is urgent. In addition to a careful physical examination, the pregnancy and family histories are investigated for familial and prenatal causes. Blood is drawn for glucose and electrolyte examination, and cerebrospinal fluid is obtained for examination for gross blood, cell count, protein, glucose, and culture. Electroencephalography may help identify subtle seizures but is less helpful in establishing a diagnosis. Other diagnostic procedures, such as computed tomography, echoencephalography, and magnetic resonance imaging (MRI), may be indicated.

CLINICAL MANIFESTATIONS OF NEWBORN SEIZURES OR TREMORS

Types of Seizures

Subtle seizures—signs may appear alone or in combination
 Clonic horizontal eye deviation
 Repetitive blinking or fluttering of eyelids
 Twitching
 Drooling
 Sucking or other oral-buccal-lingual movements
 Arm movements resembling rowing or swimming
 Leg movements described as pedaling or bicycling
 Apnea (common)

Generalized tonic seizures:
 Usually manifest as extensions of all four limbs, similar to decerebrate rigidity
 Upper limbs are maintained in stiffly flexed position resembling decorticate rigidity
 Appear more frequently in premature infants
 Commonly associated with intraventricular hemorrhage

Multifocal clonic seizures:
 Rhythmic jerking movements, about 1 to 3 per second
 May migrate randomly from one part of the body to another
 Simultaneous involvement of separate areas
 Convulsive movements may start at different times and at different rates

Myoclonic seizures:
 Single or multiple flexion jerks of limbs
 Often indicate a metabolic etiology

Jitteriness or Tremulousness

Repetitive shaking of an extremity or extremities
Observed with crying, may occur with changes in sleeping state, or may be elicited with stimulation
Relatively common in newborn
Mild jitteriness may be considered normal during first 4 days of life; occurs frequently after use of extracorporeal membrane oxygenation (ECMO)
Can be distinguished from seizures by several characteristics:
 Not accompanied by ocular movement as are seizures
 Dominant movement in jitteriness is tremor
 Seizure movement is clonic jerking that cannot be stopped by flexion of affected limb
 Jitteriness is highly sensitive to stimulation; seizures are not

---

Therapeutic Management

Treatment is directed toward prevention of cerebral damage and involves correction of metabolic derangements, respiratory and cardiovascular support, and suppression of the seizure activity. The underlying cause is treated (e.g., glucose infusion for hypoglycemia, calcium for hypocalcemia, and antibiotics for infection). If needed, respiratory support is provided, and antiepileptics may be administered, especially when the other measures fail to control the seizures. Phenobarbital is the drug of choice given intravenously or orally (if enteral feedings are tolerated) and is used if seizures are severe and persistent. Other drugs that may be employed are phenytoin (Dilantin), lorazepam, and diazepam (Valium).

Nursing Considerations

The major nursing responsibilities in the care of infants with seizures are to recognize when the infant is having a seizure so that therapy can be instituted, to carry out the therapeutic regimen, and to observe the response to the therapy and any further evidence of seizures or other symptomatology. Assessment and other aspects of care are the same as for all high-risk infants.

NURSING TIP A simple test to rule out pathology in neonatal tremors in full-term, stable newborns is to stimulate sucking. The test consists of placing a pacifier or the examiner's gloved finger in the mouth of the infant, who is lying supine with both hands free. The test indicates a tremor if the activity stops instantly with sucking and returns after the finger or pacifier is removed (Linder and others, 1989).

Parents need to be informed of their infant's status, and the nurse should reinforce and clarify the explanations of the practitioner. The infant's behaviors need to be interpreted for the parents, and the infant's responses to the treatment must be anticipated and their significance explained. Parents are encouraged to visit their infant and perform the parenting activities consistent with the plan of care. Seizures are a frightening phenomenon, and they generate a great deal of anxiety and fear, which is easily compounded by the justifiable concern of the staff. Providing support and guidance to the parents is an important nursing function.

HIGH RISK RELATED TO INFECTIOUS PROCESSES

SEPSIS

Sepsis, or *septicemia,* refers to a generalized bacterial infection in the bloodstream. Neonates are susceptible to infection because they have diminished nonspecific and specific immunity. Because of the infant's poor response to infectious agents, there is usually no local inflammatory reaction at the portal of entry to signal an infection, and the resulting symptoms tend to be vague and nonspecific. Consequently, diagnosis and treatment may be delayed. Because of their immature immune systems, infants are more vulnerable to bacterial invasion, which tends to be more serious and less likely to remain localized.

Sepsis in the neonatal period can be acquired prenatally

or during labor from infected amniotic fluid, across the placenta from the maternal bloodstream, or by direct contact with maternal tissues during the neonate's passage through the birth canal. Postnatal infection is acquired by cross-contamination from other infants, personnel, or objects in the environment, primarily lifesaving apparatus such as mechanical ventilators and indwelling venous and arterial catheters used for infusions, blood sampling, and monitoring of vital signs. Neonatal sepsis is most common in the infant at risk, particularly the preterm infant and the infant born after a difficult or traumatic labor and delivery.

Diagnostic Evaluation

Systemic infections are characterized by very subtle, vague, nonspecific, and almost imperceptible physical signs. Some of the usual manifestations observed in newborn sepsis are listed in the box below. Because sepsis is so easily confused with other neonatal disorders, the definitive diagnosis is established by laboratory and radiographic examination. Repeated blood cultures and analysis of potential primary sources of infection, such as the umbilicus, nasal-oral-pharyngeal cavity, ear canals, skin lesions, cerebrospinal fluid, stool, and urine,

---

CLINICAL MANIFESTATIONS OBSERVED IN NEONATAL SEPSIS

General Signs
Infant generally "not doing well"
Poor temperature control—hypothermia (common), hyperthermia (rare)

Circulatory System
Pallor, cyanosis, or mottling
Cool, clammy skin
Hypotension
Edema
Abnormal heartbeat—bradycardia, tachycardia, arrhythmia

Respiratory System
Irregular respirations, apnea, or tachypnea
Cyanosis
Grunting
Dyspnea
Retractions

Central Nervous System
Diminished activity—lethargy, hyporeflexia, coma
Increased activity—irritability, tremors, seizures
Full fontanel
Increased or decreased tone
Abnormal eye movements

Gastrointestinal System
Poor feeding
Vomiting, increased stomach residual after feeding
Diarrhea or decreased stool
Occult blood in stool
Abdominal distention
Hepatomegaly

Hematopoietic System
Jaundice
Pallor
Purpura, petechiae, ecchymoses
Splenomegaly
Bleeding

---

identify specific organisms. Direct (conjugated) hyperbilirubinemia is frequently seen in infants with sepsis, particularly of gram-negative origin. Blood studies may show signs of anemia, leukocytosis, or leukopenia. Leukopenia is usually an ominous sign because it is frequently associated with high mortality.

Therapeutic Management

Early recognition and diagnosis and institution of vigorous therapeutic measures are essential to increasing the chance for survival and reducing the likelihood of permanent neurologic damage. Treatment consists of circulatory support, respiratory support, aggressive administration of antibiotics, immunotherapy, and possibly transfusions with polymorphonuclear leukocytes.

Supportive therapy usually involves administration of oxygen if respiratory distress or cyanosis is evident, careful regulation of fluids, correction of electrolyte or acid-base imbalance, and isolation of the infant in an incubator. Blood transfusions may be needed to correct anemia or shock, and electronic monitoring of vital signs and regulation of the thermal environment are mandatory.

Prognosis. The newborn with sepsis is usually quite ill. The prognosis varies from patient to patient with the causative organism, and complications, but with early recognition, vigorous antibiotic therapy, and supportive therapy, mortality is less than 50% (Askin, 1995).

Nursing Considerations

Nursing care of the infant with sepsis is similar to the care of any high-risk infant. In addition, recognition of the existing problem is of paramount importance; it is usually the nurse who frequently observes and assesses the infant and who recognizes that "something is wrong" with the child. Awareness of the potential modes of transmission enables the nurse to identify those infants more at risk for developing sepsis.

Much of the care of the infant involves the medical treatment directed at illness. Knowledge of the side effects of the specific antibiotic and proper regulation and administration of the drug via the intravenous route are mandatory.

Part of the total care of the infant with sepsis is to decrease any additional physiologic or environmental stress. This includes providing an optimum, thermoregulated environment and anticipating potential problems such as dehydration or hypoxia. Another aspect of caring for the infant with sepsis involves observation for signs of meningitis, a frequent sequela of septicemia.

A severe complication of sepsis is shock, which is caused by the release of toxins within the bloodstream. Signs of shock are often difficult to distinguish from those of sepsis, such as rapid, irregular respirations and pulse. However, blood pressure usually falls in shock; therefore this measurement should be a part of the infant's routine vital signs.

NECROTIZING ENTEROCOLITIS (NEC)

NEC is an acute inflammatory disease of the bowel with increased incidence in preterm and other high-risk infants, but it is most common in those who weigh less than 2000 g. Three factors appear to play an important role in its development: intestinal ischemia, colonization by pathogenic bacteria, and excess substrate (formula) in the intestine.

Pathophysiology

The precise cause of the disorder is still speculative, although it appears to occur in an infant whose gastrointestinal tract has suffered a vascular compromise somehow related to an episode of hypoxia or sepsis, or after an exchange transfusion. The reduced blood supply to the intestines causes damage and death to mucosal cells lining the bowel wall. The intestines are unable to secrete protective mucus; therefore, the unprotected bowel wall is invaded by gas-forming bacteria, producing *pneumatosis intestinalis* (presence of air in the submucosal or subserosal surfaces of the colon), a consistent and diagnostic finding.

There is a consistent relationship between the development of NEC and enteric feeding of hypertonic formula, but it is unclear whether this is a result of the formula imposing a stress on an ischemic bowel or serving as a medium for bacterial growth.

Diagnostic Evaluation

The diagnosis of NEC is made from observations of physical signs and laboratory and radiographic findings (see box).

Therapeutic Management

Treatment of confirmed NEC consists of discontinuing all oral feedings and starting intravenous fluids, correcting fluid and electrolyte imbalances and hypoxia, instituting abdominal decompression via nasogastric suction, and administering systemic antibiotics.

Prognosis. Early recognition and prompt treatment improve the chances for successful medical management. If there is progressive deterioration under medical management or evidence of perforation, surgical resection and anastomosis are carried out. Extensive involvement may necessitate establishment of an ileostomy, jejunostomy, or colostomy.

Nursing Considerations

Nursing responsibilities begin with early recognition of the disease. Because the signs are similar to those observed in many other disorders of the newborn, nurses must be con-

---

CLINICAL MANIFESTATIONS OF NEC

Nonspecific Clinical Signs
Lethargy
Poor feeding
Hypotension
Vomiting
Apnea
Decreased urine output
Unstable temperature
Jaundice

Specific Signs
Distended (often shiny) abdomen
Blood in the stools or gastric contents
Gastric retention
Localized abdominal wall erythema or induration
Bilious vomitus

---

stantly aware of the possibility of this disease and alert to indications of its early development.

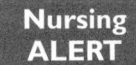 **Nursing ALERT** Observe for indications of early development of NEC by checking the abdomen frequently for distention (measuring abdominal girth, measuring residual gastric contents before feedings, and listening for the presence of bowel sounds) and performing all routine assessments for high-risk neonates.

When the disease is suspected, the nurse assists with diagnostic procedures and implements the therapeutic regimen. Vital signs, including blood pressure, are monitored for changes that indicate impending sepsis or cardiovascular shock. To avoid pressure on the distended abdomen and to facilitate observation, the infant is usually left undiapered and positioned on the side or supine.

Conscientious attention to nutritional and hydration needs is essential, and antibiotics are administered as prescribed. The time at which oral feedings are reinstituted varies considerably. Sterile water or electrolyte solution is given initially and followed by dilute human milk (if available) or elemental predigested formula. The concentration is gradually increased as tolerated until the infant is again taking full-strength feedings. Nonnutritive sucking is provided.

The infant who requires surgery is given the same careful care and observation as any infant with abdominal surgery, including colostomy care.* Throughout the management of the infant with NEC the nurse is continually alert to signs of complications, such as sepsis, disseminated intravascular coagulation, hypoglycemia, and other metabolic derangements.

BULLOUS IMPETIGO

Bullous impetigo *(impetigo neonatorum)* is a superficial skin infection most often caused by *Staphylococcus aureus.* It is characterized by the eruption of bullous vesicular lesions on previously untraumatized skin. The lesions may appear on any body surface and sometimes become widespread, but the usual distribution involves the buttocks, perineum, trunk, and face. They vary in size from a few millimeters to several centimeters in diameter, contain turbid fluid, and are easily ruptured. The bullae rupture in 1 to 2 days, leaving a superficial red, moist, denuded area with very little crusting.

Warm saline compresses applied to the lesions are followed by gentle cleansing and application of a topical antibiotic several times a day. Systemic antibiotics and corticosteroids are sometimes administered to small infants and those with widespread lesions. Recovery is usually rapid and uneventful.

Nursing Considerations

Once the diagnosis is suspected, the infant is isolated until therapy is instituted to prevent spread of the infection to other infants. Persons who have come in contact with the infant are investigated to determine a possible source of the infecting organism. Other infants in the nursery are scrutinized for early detection of any signs of infection. Parents and other

---

*Home care instructions on caring for the child with a colostomy are available in Wong DL: *Wong and Whaley's Clinical manual of pediatric nursing,* ed 4, St Louis, 1996, Mosby.

visitors are instructed regarding precautions for prevention of infection, especially thorough handwashing.

HIGH RISK RELATED TO MATERNAL FACTORS

INFANTS OF DIABETIC MOTHERS (IDMs)

Before insulin therapy, few diabetic women were able to conceive; for those who did, the mortality rate for both mother and infant was high. As a result of effective control of maternal diabetes and an increased understanding of fetal disorders, the morbidity and mortality of IDMs have been significantly reduced.

The severity of the maternal diabetes affects infant survival. Severity of maternal diabetes is determined by the duration of the disease before pregnancy, the age of onset, the extent of vascular complications, and abnormalities of the current pregnancy, such as pyelonephritis, diabetic ketoacidosis, pregnancy-induced hypertension, and noncompliance. The single most important factor influencing fetal well-being is the euglycemic status of the mother. It has been found that reasonable metabolic control started before conception and continued during the first weeks of pregnancy can prevent malformations in an IDM.

Pathophysiology

Hypoglycemia is defined as a blood sugar level below 40 mg/dl in the first 24 hours, or below 40 to 50 mg/dl thereafter regardless of gestational age. In the IDM hypoglycemia may appear a short time after birth and is associated with increased insulin activity in the blood. It is recommended that any neonate regardless of gestational or chronologic age with a plasma glucose value less than 20 to 25 mg/dl be treated with intravenous glucose (Cornblath and Schwartz, 1993). It has been demonstrated that IDMs have hypertrophy and hyperplasia of the pancreatic islet cells and that they are actually in a transient state of hyperinsulinism.

During fetal life high maternal blood sugar levels provide a continual stimulus to the fetal islet cells for insulin production. This sustained state of hyperglycemia promotes fetal insulin secretion that ultimately leads to excessive growth and deposition of fat, which probably accounts for the infants who are large for gestational age (LGA). When the glucose supply is removed abruptly at the time of birth, the continued production of insulin soon depletes the blood of circulating glucose, creating a state of hyperinsulinism and hypoglycemia within ½ to 4 hours. Precipitous drops in blood glucose levels can cause serious neurologic damage or death.

CLINICAL MANIFESTATIONS OF IDMs
Large for gestational age
Very plump and full faced
Liberal coat of vernix caseosa
Plethora
Listlessness and lethargy

All infants of these mothers with poor disease control have a characteristic appearance (see box). Although they are large, these infants are often born prematurely—either because of an elective early delivery or for other reasons.

Therapeutic Management

The most effective management appears to be careful observation of all IDMs in the special care nursery, with early feeding of breast milk or formula, if tolerated. Critically ill infants require intravenous infusions. Frequent determinations of blood glucose levels are needed for the first 2 days of life to assess the degree of hypoglycemia present at any given time.

Prognosis. If hypoglycemia is left untreated, it can cause rapid, irreversible central nervous system damage. With treatment most infants do well and recover completely. However, there is an increase in congenital anomalies, such as heart defects, in this group, as well as a high susceptibility to hypoglycemia, hypocalcemia, hyperbilirubinemia, and RDS. No satisfactory explanation has been accepted for all the abnormalities in these infants, although a number of complications may be related to the prematurity factor.

Nursing Considerations

Nursing care of IDMs requires observation for signs of complications to which they are more susceptible than other neonates. Hypoglycemia is the most immediate and consistent threat to these infants; therefore, feedings are initiated early and the infant is observed for central nervous system signs such as hyperirritability, tremors, and jitteriness during the early hours of life. Other complications that occur with increased frequency in IDMs are polycythemia, hyperbilirubinemia, sepsis, and respiratory distress syndrome. Vigilance is needed to detect signs that indicate development of any of these neonatal problems.

NARCOTIC-ADDICTED INFANTS

Narcotics, which have a low molecular weight, readily cross the placental membrane and enter the fetal system. When the mother is a habitual user of narcotics, in particular heroin or methadone, the unborn child becomes passively addicted to the drug, which places such infants at risk during the early neonatal period. *Neonatal abstinence syndrome (NAS)* describes the behaviors exhibited by the infant exposed to substances in utero that cause withdrawal.

Diagnostic Evaluation

Most passively addicted infants of drug-dependent mothers appear normal at birth but begin to exhibit signs of drug withdrawal within 12 to 24 hours if the mother has been taking only heroin. If she has been taking methadone, the signs appear somewhat later, anytime from 1 or 2 days to a week or more after birth. The manifestations become most pronounced between 48 and 72 hours of age and may last anywhere from 6 days to 8 weeks, depending on the severity of the withdrawal.

The clinical manifestations of withdrawal in the neonate, which are predominantly those of autonomic nervous system hyperirritability, may persist for 3 or 4 months. The most common acute signs are outlined in the box on p. 271. Although infants undergoing withdrawal suck avidly on fists and display an exaggerated rooting reflex, they are poor feeders.

SIGNS OF NARCOTIC WITHDRAWAL IN THE NEONATE

Irritability	Sweating
Tremors	Jitteriness
Shrill cry	Tachypnea (>60/min)
Hypertonicity	Sneezing
Frantic sucking of hands	Vomiting
Poor feeding	Temperature instability
Hyperactivity	Diarrhea
Decreased sleep	Seizures

Not all infants of heroin-addicted mothers will show signs of withdrawal. Because of irregular and varying degrees of drug use, quality of drug, and mixed drug usage by the mother, some infants display mild or variable manifestations. Most manifestations are the vague, nonspecific signs characteristic of all infants in general; therefore it is important to differentiate between drug withdrawal and other disorders before specific therapy is instituted. Often other states (e.g., hypocalcemia, hypoglycemia, or sepsis) coexist with the drug withdrawal.

Infants who do not display the signs of fetal alcohol syndrome but are born to mothers who are also heavy alcohol drinkers have significantly more tremors, hypertonia, restlessness, excessive mouthing movements, crying, and inconsolability than infants of addicted mothers who do not consume alcohol during pregnancy. An added concern regarding narcotic users is that many of the mothers often use other drugs, such as tranquilizers, sedatives, narcotics, amphetamines, phencyclidine (PCP), and other psychotropic agents.

Therapeutic Management

The treatment of the passively addicted infant initially consists of modulating the environment to decrease external stimuli. Drug therapies include parenteral and/or oral administration of phenobarbital, chlorpromazine, diazepam, paregoric, clonidine, or methadone (Franck and Vilardi, 1995).

Prognosis. The prognosis for drug-exposed infants depends on the type and amount of drug(s) taken by the mother and the stage(s) of fetal development in which the drug was taken. Overall mortality of infants born to narcotic-addicted mothers is increased, but with early recognition and treatment the morbidity and mortality associated with drug withdrawal are decreased.

Infants of narcotic-addicted mothers exhibit poor brain and body growth at birth. They have chronic feeding problems, irritability, abnormal neurologic responses, abnormal parent-infant interactions, developmental and cognitive delays, learning disabilities, and behavioral problems, including attention deficit–hyperactivity disorder.

Nursing Considerations

When possible, the nursery personnel are alerted to the likelihood of a drug-addicted infant. If the mother has had good prenatal care, the practitioner is aware of the problem and therapy has been instituted before delivery. However, a number of mothers deliver their infants without the benefit of adequate care, and the addiction is unknown to health care personnel at the time of delivery. The degree of narcosis or withdrawal is closely related to the amount of drug the mother has habitually taken, the length of time she has been taking of the drug, and the drug level of the mother at the time of delivery. The most severe symptoms are observed in the infants of mothers who have taken large amounts of drugs over a long period. In addition, the nearer to the time of delivery that the mother takes the drug, the longer it takes for the child to develop withdrawal and the more severe are the manifestations. The infant may not exhibit withdrawal symptoms until 7 to 10 days after delivery.

Once the presence of NAS is identified in an infant, nursing care is directed toward reducing the stimuli (such as dimmed lights and decreased noise levels) that might trigger hyperactivity and irritability, providing adequate nutrition and hydration and promoting maternal-infant relationships. Irritable and hyperactive infants have been found to respond to comforting, movement, and close contact. Wrapping infants snugly, as well as rocking and holding them tightly, limits their ability to self-stimulate. Arranging nursing activities to reduce the amount of disturbance helps to decrease exogenous stimulation.

Hyperactive infants must be protected from skin abrasions on the knees, toes, and cheeks that are caused by rubbing on bed linens when lying on their abdomens. Monitoring and recording the activity level and its relationship to other activities, such as feeding and preventing complications, are important nursing functions.

A valuable aid to anticipating problems in newborns is recognizing drug addiction in the mothers. Unless the mothers are enrolled in a methadone rehabilitation program, they seldom risk calling attention to their habit by seeking prenatal care. Consequently, infants and mothers are exposed to the additional hazards of obstetric and medical complications. Moreover, the nature of heroin addiction makes the user susceptible to disorders such as infection (hepatitis, human immunodeficiency virus [HIV]), foreign body reaction, and the hazards of inadequate nutrition and premature birth. Methadone treatment does not prevent withdrawal reaction in neonates, but the clinical course may be modified. Also, the intensive psychologic support of mothers is a factor in the treatment and reduction of perinatal mortality. Experience has indicated that mothers are usually anxious and depressed, lack confidence, have poor self-images, and have difficulty with interpersonal relationships. They may have a psychologic need for the pregnancy and an infant.

COCAINE EXPOSURE

Cocaine, the number one illicit drug used in the United States, has multiple modes of use. However, use of the relatively inexpensive and easily administered "crack" form is increasing alarmingly, especially among women. Because crack vaporizes at relatively low temperatures, it is smoked and absorbed in large quantities through the pulmonary vasculature. The drug readily crosses the placenta, placing the fetus at risk.

Cocaine is a CNS stimulant and peripheral sympathomimetic, and the effects on the fetus are secondary to maternal effects—increased BP, decreased uterine blood flow, and increased vascular resistance. Consequently, the fetus suffers decreased blood flow and oxygenation because of placental and fetal vasoconstriction. The difficulties encountered by cocaine-exposed infants are compounded when the mother is taking the drug in conjunction with other illicit drugs. Prenatal exposure to cocaine has been implicated as a risk for SIDS in infancy.

Infants may appear normal, or they may show neurologic problems at birth that may continue during the neonatal period and beyond. Two types of behavior may emerge as a result of cocaine effects on fetal development: neurobehavioral depression or excitability. The behaviors of the depressed infant include lethargy, poor suck, hypotonia, weak cry, and difficulty in arousing. The behaviors of the excitable neonate may include a high-pitched cry, hypertonicity, rigidity, irritability, inability to be consoled, and an intolerance to a change in routine. Other behaviors may include frequent startling, poor awake state, sleeping difficulties, and persistent primitive reflexes. Some infants develop late onset of symptoms (2-8 weeks). They may become irritable and hypertonic, experience sleep-awake disruptions, and demonstrate an inability to tolerate change; they may also be slightly febrile.

Sequelae of prenatal cocaine exposure include smaller head circumference, lower birth length, and lower birth weight. The head growth may be one of the best predicators of long-term development (Chasnoff and others, 1992). Long-term sequelae for newborns exposed to cocaine in utero include lower language and cognitive scores than a control group (Griffith, Azuma, and Chasnoff, 1994).

Therapeutic Management
Treatment of these infants is similar to that for narcotic-addicted infants—identification, reduction of external stimuli, supportive treatment aimed at alleviating symptoms, and, at times, sedation.

Nursing Considerations
Nursing care of cocaine-exposed infants is the same as that for narcotic-addicted infants. Since they have increased flexor tone, these infants respond to swaddling in a semi-flexed position. Effects of the drug from breast milk and topical cocaine applications to nipples have been reported; therefore mothers should be cautioned regarding this hazard to their infants. Referral to early intervention programs, including child health care, parental drug treatment, individualized developmental care, and parenting education, is essential in promoting the optimum outcome for these children.

MATERNAL INFECTIONS
The range of pathologic conditions produced by infectious agents is large, and the difference between the maternal and fetal effects caused by any one agent is also great. Some maternal infections, especially during early gestation, can result in fetal loss or malformations because the ability of the fetus to handle infectious organisms is limited and the fetal immunologic system is unable to prevent the dissemination of infectious organisms to the various tissues.

Not all prenatal infections produce teratogenic effects. Further, the clinical picture of disorders caused by transplacental transfer of infectious agents is not always well defined. One group of microbial agents can cause remarkably similar manifestations, and it is not uncommon to test for all when a prenatal infection is suspected. This is the so-called TORCHS complex, an acronym for:

T	Toxoplasmosis
O	Other (e.g., hepatitis)
R	Rubella
C	Cytomegalovirus infection
H	Herpes simplex
S	Syphilis

To determine the causative agent in a symptomatic infant, tests are performed to rule out each of these infections. The "O" category may involve testing for several viral infections (e.g., hepatitis B, varicella zoster, measles, mumps, human immunodeficiency virus [HIV], human papillomavirus, human parvovirus, and listeriosis). Bacterial infections are not included in the TORCHS workup, because they are usually identified by clinical manifestations and readily available laboratory tests. Gonococcal conjunctivitis (ophthalmia neonatorum) and chlamydial conjunctivitis have been significantly reduced by prophylactic measures at birth (see Chapter 8). The major maternal infections, their possible teratogenic effects, and specific nursing considerations are outlined in Table 9-9.

Nursing Considerations
One of the major goals in care of infants suspected of having an infectious disease is identification of the causative organism. Until the diagnosis is established, standard precautions are implemented according to institutional policy. In suspected cytomegalovirus and rubella infections, pregnant personnel are cautioned to avoid contact with the infant. Herpes simplex is easily transmitted from one infant to another; therefore risk of cross-contamination is reduced or eliminated by wearing gloves for patient contact. The hospital infection control department provides guidelines for the type and duration of precautions. Careful handwashing is the most important nursing intervention in reducing the spread of any infection.

Specimens need to be obtained for laboratory examinations, and the infant and parents need to be prepared for diagnostic procedures. When possible, long-term disabilities are prevented by early evaluation and implementation of therapy. The family is taught any special handling techniques needed for the care of their infant and signs of complications or possible sequelae. If sequelae are inevitable, the family will need assistance in determining how they can best cope with the problems, such as assistance with home care, referral to appropriate agencies, or placement in an institution for care.

The major goal of nursing care is prevention of these disorders with provision of adequate prenatal care for the expectant mother and precautions regarding exposure to teratogenic infections.

CONGENITAL ABNORMALITIES*

Congenital anomalies, or *birth defects,* can arise at any stage of prenatal development and show wide variability in etiologic factors as well as in type, extent, and frequency of defects. About 2 to 3% of all births are associated with a major anomaly, mental retardation, or genetic disease. An even greater number of children will begin to exhibit manifesta-

---

*Donna P. Smith, MS, RN, revised this section to p. 276, 280-281.

TABLE 9-9. Infections acquired from mother before, during, or after birth

FETAL OR NEWBORN EFFECT	COMMENTS AND NURSING CONSIDERATIONS*

Human Immunodeficiency Virus (HIV)
No significant difference between infected and uninfected infants at birth in some instances
Embryopathy reported by some observers:
    Depressed nasal bridge
    Mild upward or downward obliquity of eyes
    Long palpebral fissures with blue sclerae
    Patulous lips
    Ocular hypertelorism
    Prominent upper vermilion border
	Transmitted transplacentally; during delivery; in breast milk
	Recommended treatment: use of zidovudine (ZDV) to HIV-infected pregnant women and their infants, and use of chemoprophylaxis against *Pneumocystis carinii* pneumonia (PCP) in the HIV-exposed infants; drug of choice is trimethoprim and sulfamethoxazole (TMP-SMX, Bactrim, Septra)
	Documented routine HIV education and routine testing with consent for all pregnant women in the United States is recommended (American Academy of Pediatrics, 1995)

Chickenpox (Varicella-Zoster Virus [VZV]) First-trimester exposure—congenital varicella syndrome: limb dysplasia, microcephaly, cortical atrophy, chorioretinitis, cataracts, cutaneous scars, other anomalies, auditory nerve palsy, mental retardation	Transmitted: first trimester (fetal varicella syndrome); intrapartum (infection) Treatment: exposed infants—varicella-zoster immune globulin (VZIG) to infants born to mothers with onset of disease within 5 days before or 2 days after delivery (7 days before and 7 days after in United Kingdom) Isolation precautions 21 days after birth (if hospitalized) Prevention: universal immunization of all children with VZV vaccine
Chlamydia Infection (*Chlamydia Trachomatis*) Conjunctivitis, pneumonia	Transmitted: last trimester or intrapartum Apply prophylactic medication to eyes at time of birth Treatment: antibiotics
Coxsackievirus (Group B) Poor feeding, vomiting, diarrhea, fever; cardiac enlargement, arrhythmias, congestive heart failure; lethargy, seizures, meningeal involvement	Transmitted: first trimester or late in pregnancy
Cytomegalovirus (CMV) Microcephaly, cerebral calcifications, chorioretinitis Jaundice, hepatosplenomegaly Petechial or purpuric rash Neurologic sequelae: seizure disorders, sensorimotor deafness, mental retardation	Transmitted: throughout pregnancy Affected individuals excrete virus Virus detected in urine by electron microscopy Avoid kissing affected child Pregnant women should avoid close contact with known cases Treatment: antimetabolites, antiviral agent
Erythema Infectiosum (Parvovirus B19) Fetal hydrops and death from anemia and heart failure, early exposure Anemia from later exposure No teratogenic effects established Ordinarily, low risk of ill effect to fetus	Transmitted: transplacentally First-trimester infection most serious effects Pregnant health care workers should not care for patients who might be highly contagious (e.g., child with sickle cell anemia, aplastic crisis) Routine exclusion of pregnant women from workplace where disease is occurring is not recommended
Gonococcal Disease (*Neisseria Gonorrhoeae*) Ophthalmitis Neonatal gonococcal arthritis, septicemia, meningitis	Transmitted: last trimester or intrapartum Apply prophylactic medication to eyes at time of birth Obtain smears for culture Treatment: penicillin
Hepatitis B Virus (HBV) May be asymptomatic Acute hepatitis, changes in liver function	Transmitted: transplacentally, contaminated maternal secretions during delivery Treatment: hepatitis B immune globulin to all infants of HB$_S$AG-positive mothers Prevention: universal immunization of all infants with HBV vaccine (see Immunizations, Chapter 10)

*Isolation precautions depend on institutional policy (see Infection Control, Chapter 22).

Continued.

TABLE 9-9. Infections acquired from mother before, during, or after birth—cont'd

FETAL OR NEWBORN EFFECT	COMMENTS AND NURSING CONSIDERATIONS*
Herpes, Neonatal (Herpes Simplex Virus) Cutaneous lesions: vesicles at 6 to 10 days old; may be no lesions Disseminated disease resembles sepsis Visceral involvement: granulomas Early nonspecific signs: fever, lethargy, poor feeding, irritability, vomiting May include hyperbilirubinemia, seizures, flaccid or spastic paralysis, apneic episodes, respiratory distress, lethargy, or coma	History of genital infection in mother/partner in 50% of cases Transmitted: intrapartum either ascending and/or direct contact, especially primary infection Cesarean sections sometimes a preventive measure for mothers with active lesions Vaginal delivery of infants of mothers with recurrent infection thought to be at lower risk Suggest infants room-in with mother in private room
Listeriosis (Listeria) Acquired in late pregnancy: stillborn or acutely ill; may die within an hour after birth Late onset: septicemia; meningitis	Transmitted: transplacentally or by aspiration of secretions at birth Segregate infants until cultures are negative
Lyme Disease (Borrelia Burgdorferi) Stillbirth Congenital defects reported: congenital heart disease, syndactyly, cortical blindness Prematurity Rash	Transmitted: transplacentally Immediate treatment of affected pregnant women with appropriate antibiotic Advise pregnant women to avoid tick exposure in endemic areas
Rubella, Congenital (Rubella Virus) Eye defects: cataracts (unilateral or bilateral), microphthalmia, retinitis, glaucoma CNS signs: microcephaly, seizures, severe mental retardation Congenital heart defects: patent ductus arteriosus Auditory: high incidence of delayed hearing loss Intrauterine growth retardation Hyperbilirubinemia, spinal fluid abnormalities, thrombocytopenia, hepatomegaly	Transmitted: first trimester, early second trimester Pregnant women should avoid contact with all affected persons, including infants with rubella syndrome Emphasize vaccination of all unimmunized prepubertal children, susceptible adolescents, and adult females of childbearing age Caution women against pregnancy for at least 3 months after vaccination
Syphilis, Congenital (Treponema Pallidum) Copper-colored maculopapular cutaneous lesions (after seventh day), mucous membrane patches, hair loss, nail exfoliation, snuffles (syphilitic rhinitis), profound anemia, poor feeding, pseudoparalysis of one or more limbs, dysmorphic teeth (older child)	Transmitted: transplacentally, usually after eighteenth week of pregnancy Most severe form of syphilis Strict isolation of infant Treatment: penicillin
Toxoplasmosis (Toxoplasma Gondii) Hydrocephaly, cerebral calcifications, chorioretinitis (classic triad) Microcephaly, seizures, mental retardation, deafness Encephalitis, myocarditis, hepatosplenomegaly, anemia, jaundice, diarrhea, vomiting, purpura	Transmitted: throughout pregnancy Predominant host for organism is cats May be transmitted through cat feces, poorly cooked or raw infected meats Caution pregnant women to avoid contact with cat feces (e.g., emptying cat litter boxes) Treatment: sulfonamides, pyrimethamine

tions of a genetic disorder at later stages of development (see box). A few congenital defects are clearly caused by a single gene defect, some are associated with chromosome abnormalities, and others are produced by intrauterine environment factors. However, many of the more common defects (e.g., pyloric stenosis, central nervous system malformations, and congenital heart disease) appear to be consistent with multifactorial inheritance. Therefore, it is important to recognize that whereas some defects are strictly inherited, in many cases events specific to the pregnancy are responsible.

The types of malformations that can result from genetic or prenatal environmental causes can be *major structural abnormalities* with serious medical, surgical, or quality-of-life consequences, or they can be *minor anomalies* or *normal variants* with no serious consequences, such as a sacral dimple, an extra nipple, or an umbilical hernia. Malformations can occur in isolation, such as congenital heart defect, or multiple anomalies may be present. A recognized pattern of malformations due to a single specific cause is called a *syndrome,* such as Down syndrome or fetal alcohol syndrome.

ASSESSMENT CLUES TO GENETIC DISORDERS*

Major or minor birth defects (anomalies) and dysmorphic features—Cardiac defect, ear or eye abnormalities, micrognathia, forehead prominence, hairline low-set on forehead or nape of neck, wide-set eyes, epicanthal folds, low-set ears

Growth abnormalities—Short stature, overgrowth, asymmetric growth, intrauterine growth retardation

Skeletal abnormalities—Limb abnormalities, asymmetry, scoliosis, hyperextensible joints, hypotonic or hypertonic muscle tone, pectus excavatum, finger or joint abnormalities

Vision or hearing problems—Coloboma, cat's eye, hearing loss, vision loss

Metabolic disorders—Unusual odor of breath, urine, or stool

Sexual development abnormalities—Ambiguous genitalia, small penis, delayed onset of puberty, primary amenorrhea, precocious sexual development, large testicles

Skin disorders—Unusual pigmentation, café-au-lait spots, dry and scaly skin, skin tumors

Recurrent infection or immune deficiency—Ear infections, pneumonia

Developmental and speech delays or loss of milestones:

    Cognitive delays—Learning disabilities, mild to severe mental retardation

    Behavioral disorders—Hyperactivity, attention deficit disorder, autistic-like behavior, aggressive behavior

*Suggests genetic etiology if two or more findings are present.

Neural tube defects, cleft lip and/or cleft palate, deafness, congenital heart defects, and mental retardation are examples of anomalies that can occur in isolation or as part of a syndrome or association and that can be caused by either single-gene or chromosome abnormalities, or prenatal environmental factors.

CHROMOSOMAL ABERRATIONS

An *aberration* is defined as a deviation from that which is normal or typical. *Chromosomal aberrations* are deviations in either structure or number of chromosomes, and the consequences in either situation can usually be readily observed in the affected individual. A *structural aberration* involves loss, addition, rearrangement, or exchange of some of the genes of a chromosome. Deviations in chromosomal number involve the gain or loss of a chromosome and are designated with the suffix *-somy*. A cell that contains one less than the normal number of chromosomes (46) is called a *monosomy* because of the loss of one member of a chromosome pair; a cell containing one more than the normal number of chromosomes that results from the addition of an extra member to a normal pair is called a *trisomy*. Most chromosomal abnormalities result from abnormal cell division during germ cell formation or early cell division in the zygote. Others are caused by a *translocation* in which a segment of one chromosome breaks off and attaches to another chromosome. In a balanced translocation, that is, when no genetic material is gained or lost, the individual is usually normal in appearance and function. However, the translocation can be passed to

TABLE 9-10. Common autosomal aberrations

SYNDROME	CHROMOSOMAL ABNORMALITY AND NOMENCLATURE	AVERAGE INCIDENCE (LIVE BIRTH)*	MAJOR CLINICAL MANIFESTATIONS
Cri du chat	Deletion of short arm of No. 5 chromosome—46,XY,5p−	1:50,000	Distinctive weak, high-pitched, mewlike cry resembling the cry of a cat; small head; hypertelorism; failure to thrive; severe mental retardation—profound with age
Trisomy 13 (Patau)	Trisomy of No. 13 chromosome—47,XY,+13	1:4000-15,000	Multiple anomalies, including cleft lip and palate (frequently bilateral); ear malformations; microphthalmia; polydactyly; eye defects; mental retardation; early death
Trisomy 18 (Edwards)	Trisomy of No. 18 chromosome—47,XY,+18	1:3500-8000	Deformed and low-set ears; micrognathia; rocker-bottom feet; overlapping (index over third) fingers; prominent occiput; hypertelorism; failure to thrive and early death; mental retardation
Trisomy 21 (Down)	Trisomy of No. 21 chromosome—47,XY,+21 (trisomy); 46,XY +14;21 (translocation); 46,XY/47,XY,21+ (mosaic)	1:700†	Brachycephaly with flat occiput; inner epicanthal folds; small ears, nose, and mouth with protruding tongue; muscular hypotonia; broad, short hands with stubby fingers and transverse palmar crease; broad, stubby feet with wide space between big and second toes; cardiac defects; mental retardation; variable life expectancy

*Data from Nora JJ, Fraser FC: *Medical genetics: principles and practice*, ed 3, Philadelphia, 1989, Lea & Febiger.
†Risk related to maternal age: age 30 years = 1:1500; age 35 years = 1:300; age 40 years = 1:100; age 45 years = 1:25.

offspring in an unbalanced form, resulting in spontaneous abortion or a child with birth defects. Therefore, referral for genetic counseling is a special consideration for individuals found to have a translocation. Trisomies are the chromosomal aberrations encountered most frequently by health workers.

Both numeric and structural abnormalities of autosomes and sex chromosomes account for a variety of disorders of infancy and childhood. A few are associated with a group of characteristics that clearly indicate the precise chromosomal anomaly (Table 9-10). The most common is Down syndrome, which is usually caused by a trisomy of chromosome 21 (see Chapter 19 for a further discussion of Down syndrome). The other known viable autosomal trisomies involve chromosomes 18 and 13 and triploidy, which is a trisomy of every pair. Abnormalities of sex chromosomes are discussed in Chapter 17.

TABLE 9-11. Congenital effects of maternal ingestion of alcohol and smoking

FETAL OR NEWBORN EFFECTS	COMMENTS AND NURSING CONSIDERATIONS
Alcohol (Fetal Alcohol Syndrome [FAS])	
Facial features: hypoplastic maxilla, micrognathia, hypoplastic philtrum, short palpebral fissures	Exact quantity of alcohol needed to produce teratogenic effects in fetus is not known
Neurologic: mental retardation, motor retardation, microcephaly, hypotonia, hearing disorders	Recognized as the leading cause of mental retardation, outranking Down syndrome and spina bifida
Growth: prenatal growth retardation, persistent postnatal growth lag	Women with histories of heavy drinking should be counseled regarding risks to fetus
Behavior: irritability (infant), hyperactivity (child)	Provide mother with resources for treatment to decrease or eliminate alcoholic intake
Children and adults who demonstrate cognitive, behavioral, and psychosocial problems without the facial dysmorphia and growth retardation are referred to as having *fetal alcohol effects (FAE)*	
Maternal Tobacco Smoking	
Fetal growth retardation Increased perinatal deaths Increased spontaneous abortions	Women should be counseled regarding risks to fetus
Postnatal: growth and intellectual and emotional developmental deficits Increased risk of sudden infant death syndrome (SIDS)	Provide with resources to help eliminate smoking

DEFECTS CAUSED BY CHEMICAL AGENTS

The relationship of the fetal and maternal circulations allows for the interchange of chemical substances across the placental membrane. Many drugs have been suspected of producing congenital malformations, and some have been definitely implicated. Some of the most recognized teratogenic drugs include alcohol, tobacco, antiepileptic medications, isotretinoin (Accutane), lithium, cocaine, and diethylstilbestrol (Table 9-11).

The extent to which chemical agents affect the unborn child depends on the interplay of several factors—the nature of the agent and its accessibility to the fetus, the gestational age at which exposure occurred, the level and duration of the dosage, and the genetic makeup of the fetus. For example, chemicals administered between 15 and 90 days' of gestation may produce an effect if the tissue for which it has an affinity is in the process of differentiation at that time.

 One drug recognized for its carcinogenic effect is *diethylstilbestrol.* Large doses of this hormone given to pregnant women to prevent abortion cause adenocarcinoma of the vagina in a significant proportion of the female offspring when they reach adolescence and early adulthood.

Nursing Considerations

Expectant mothers are cautioned against ingesting any medication without first consulting a practitioner. To help ensure that fewer women will inadvertently take some chemical that might be harmful to the fetus, labels on medications are now required to include information regarding the possible teratogenic effects of the drug. All women of childbearing age should be educated regarding the effects of chemicals, especially alcohol, on the unborn fetus. The **Association of Birth Defect Children,** * offers help and information to families with children with defects caused by maternal exposure to drugs, chemicals, radiation, and other environmental agents.

INBORN ERRORS OF METABOLISM (IEMs)

IEMs constitute a large number of inherited diseases caused by the absence or deficiency of a substance essential to cellular metabolism, usually an enzyme. When the normal metabolic process is interrupted as a result of a missing enzyme, an accumulation of substances precedes the interruption, the end product of the process is absent, or the process takes an alternate metabolic pathway. The consequence is illness.

CONGENITAL HYPOTHYROIDISM (CH)

CH may have a number of etiologies and can be either permanent or transient. However, no matter what the cause, the manifestations (see box on p. 277) and management are similar. In some conditions the thyroid deficiency is severe and

---

*827 Irma Ave, Orlando, FL 32803; (800) 313-ABDC.

POSSIBLE MANIFESTATIONS OF CONGENITAL HYPOTHYROIDISM

At Birth	Before 3 Months of Age	Older Child
Gestation >42 weeks	Umbilical hernia	Short stature
Birth weight >4 kg (8.8 lb)	Mottled and dry skin	Infantile proportions persist; length of trunk long relative
Widened posterior fontanel	Constipation	to legs
Hypothermia, 95° F or less	Large tongue	Decreased metabolic rate; weight gain, often leading to
Peripheral cyanosis	Hoarse	obesity
Respiratory distress	Cold to touch	Infantile facial features of myxedema
Edema	Excessive sleepiness	Short forehead
Prolonged physiologic jaundice	Difficulty feeding related to lethargy	Wide, puffy eyes; wrinkled eyelids
Abdominal distention	Minimal crying	Broad, short, upturned nose
Vomiting		Large, protruding tongue
Delayed passage of meconium		Hair often dry, brittle, or lusterless, extending far down
Feeding difficulties		onto forehead
Hypoactivity		Dentition delayed and usually defective
		Intellectual deficit of varying degrees

manifestations develop early; in others the symptoms may be delayed for months or years.

CH occurs in approximately 1 of every 4000 newborns (American Academy of Pediatrics, 1993). Infants with Down syndrome have a much higher rate of either permanent or transient forms of the disorder. Also, a higher incidence of other congenital abnormalities has been observed in infants with CH.

Diagnostic Evaluation

Diagnosis is aimed at early identification of the disorder to prevent the serious effects on mental development resulting from delayed treatment. Neonatal screening consists of an initial filter paper blood spot thyroxine (T_4) measurement followed by measurement of thyroid-stimulating hormone (TSH) in specimens with low T_4 values. Tests are routine and mandatory in most areas of the United States. Although a heel-stick blood sample for the spot test is best obtained between 2 and 6 days of age, specimens are usually taken within the first 24 to 48 hours as part of a concurrent screen for other metabolic defects. Early screening can result in overdiagnosis (false-positives) but is preferable to missing the diagnosis. Screening results that show a low level of T_4 and a high level of TSH indicate CH.

Therapeutic Management

Treatment involves lifelong thyroid hormone replacement therapy as soon as possible after diagnosis to abolish all signs of hypothyroidism and reestablish normal physical and mental development. The drug of choice is synthetic levothyroxine sodium (Synthroid or Levothroid). Regular measurement of thyroxine levels is important in ensuring optimum treatment. Bone age surveys are also performed to ensure optimum growth.

Prognosis. If treatment is started shortly after birth, normal physical growth and intelligence are possible (Casado de Frias and others, 1993). The most significant factor adversely affecting eventual intelligence appears to be inadequate treatment, which may be related to noncompliance.

Nursing Considerations

The most important nursing objective is early identification of the disorder. Nurses caring for neonates must be certain that screening is performed, especially in infants who are discharged early or are born at home. Although the screening test is very specific, some children may not be identified, and nurses in ambulatory settings for well-infant care need to be aware of the earliest signs of the disorder. Parental remarks about an unusually "quiet and good" baby coupled with any of the early physical manifestations should lead the nurse to suspect hypothyroidism and refer the child for specific tests. Unfortunately, many parents harbor guilt about their impressions of the infant before the diagnosis because the child's inactivity may not have alerted them to a problem, with the result that treatment was delayed.

Once the diagnosis is confirmed, parents need an explanation of the disorder and the necessity of lifelong treatment. The importance of compliance with the drug regimen must be emphasized for the child to achieve normal growth and development (Miculan, Turner, and Paes, 1993). Since the drug is tasteless, it can be crushed and added to formula, water, or food. If a dose is missed, twice the dose should be given the next day. Parents also need to be aware of signs indicating overdose, such as rapid pulse, dyspnea, irritability, insomnia, fever, sweating, and weight loss. Ideally they should know how to count the pulse and be instructed to withhold a dose and consult their practitioner if the pulse rate is above a certain value. Signs of inadequate treatment are fatigue, sleepiness, decreased appetite, and constipation.

If the diagnosis was delayed past early infancy, the chance of permanent mental retardation is great. Such parents need the same guidance in caring for their child as do others who have an offspring with cognitive impairment (see Chapter 19). They need an opportunity to discuss their feelings regarding late recognition of the disorder. Although treatment will not reverse the intellectual deficit, it may prevent further damage. Genetic counseling is important, especially if the disorder is caused by an inborn error of thyroid hormone synthesis, an autosomal-recessive trait.

PHENYLKETONURIA (PKU)

PKU, a genetic disease inherited as an autosomal-recessive trait (see Appendix B), is caused by absence of the enzyme needed to metabolize the essential amino acid, *phenylalanine*. The disorder is detected in 1:10,000 to 15,000 live births and primarily affects white children, with the incidence

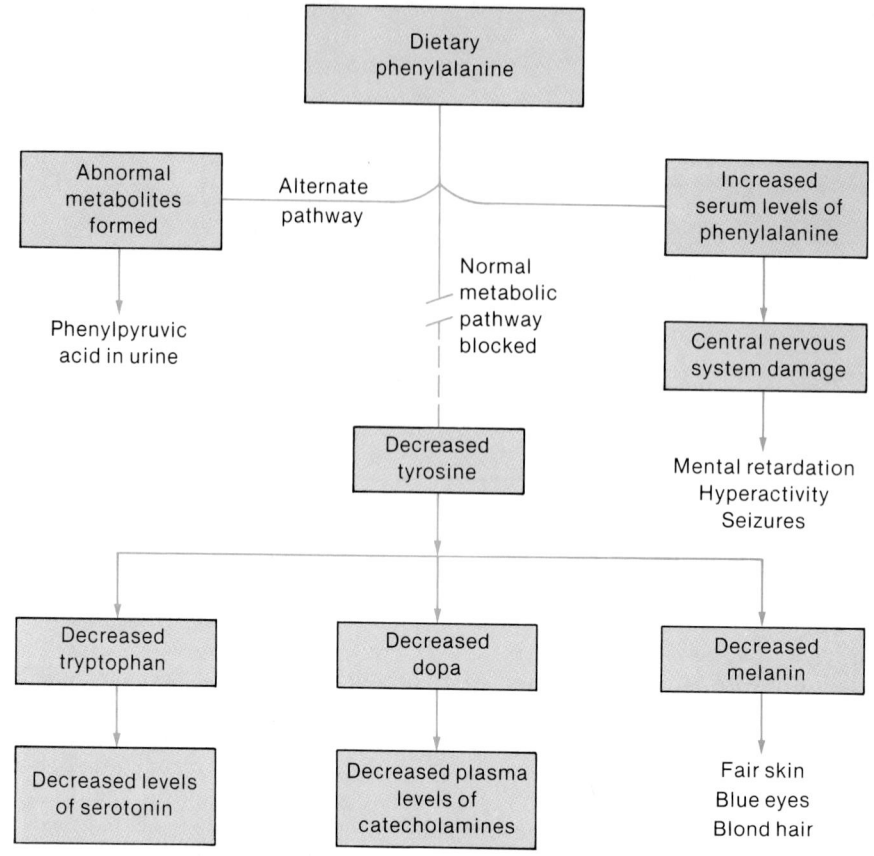

FIG. 9-15. Metabolic error and consequences in phenylketonuria.

highest in those living in the United States or Northern Europe. It is very rare in the African, Jewish, and Japanese populations.

Classic PKU is at one end of a spectrum of conditions known as *hyperphenylalaninemia.* Since rarer forms are the result of a deficiency of other enzymes and are diagnosed and treated differently, the following discussion of PKU is limited to the severe, classic form.

Pathophysiology

In PKU the hepatic enzyme *phenylalanine hydroxylase,* which normally controls the conversion of phenylalanine to tyrosine, is absent. This results in the accumulation of phenylalanine in the bloodstream and urinary excretion of abnormal amounts of its metabolites, the phenyl acids (Fig. 9-15). One of these phenyl ketones, *phenylpyruvic acid,* gives urine the characteristic musty odor associated with this disease and is responsible for the term *phenylketonuria.*

Amino acids produced by metabolism of phenylalanine are absent in PKU. One of these, *tyrosine,* is needed to form the pigment melanin and the hormones epinephrine and thyroxine. Decreased melanin production results in similar phenotypes of most children with phenylketonuria—blond hair, blue eyes, and fair skin that is particularly susceptible to eczema and other dermatologic problems. Children of genetically darker skin color may have red or brown hair.

Accumulation of phenylalanine and presumably the de-

creased levels of the neurotransmitters dopamine and tryptophan affect the normal development of the brain and central nervous system. Mental retardation occurs *before* the metabolites are detected in the urine and will progress if ingested phenylalanine levels are not lowered.

Diagnostic Evaluation

The objective in diagnosing PKU or treating the affected patient is to prevent mental retardation. All the tests for PKU are based on the detection of increasing phenylalanine levels in the blood or characteristic metabolites in the urine. The most commonly used test for screening newborns for PKU is the *Guthrie blood test.* When this test is performed reliably, serum phenylalanine levels greater than 4 mg/dl (normal = 2 mg/dl) can be detected.

 The *Guthrie test* is a bacterial inhibition assay for phenylalanine in the blood. *Bacillus subtilis,* present in the culture medium, grows if the blood contains an excessive amount of phenylalanine.

The screening test is most reliable if the blood sample is taken after the infant has ingested a source of protein. However, because of early discharge from the hospital, the American Academy of Pediatrics and American College of Obstetricians and Gynecologists (1992) recommend that (1) the test be performed on all newborns before they leave the nursery, regardless of age, and (2) a repeat blood specimen be obtained by the third week of life from all infants in whom the initial specimen was taken within the first 24 hours of life. There has been recent concern however, that a significantly large number of infants are *not* rescreened for PKU after early discharge and are at risk for missed or delayed diagnosis of PKU, particularly in states without laws mandating rescreening (Sinai and others, 1995).

Therapeutic Management

Treatment for the infant with PKU is dietary. Since the genetic enzyme is intracellular, systemic administration of phenylalanine hydroxylase is of no value. Phenylalanine cannot be eliminated, because it is an essential amino acid for tissue growth. Therefore dietary management must meet two criteria: (1) meet the child's nutritional need for optimum growth, and (2) maintain phenylalanine levels within a safe range.

The diet is calculated to allow 20 to 30 mg of phenylalanine per kilogram of body weight per day, which should maintain serum phenylalanine levels between 2 and 8 mg/dl. Significant brain damage usually occurs when levels are greater than 10 to 15 mg/dl. At levels less than 2 mg/dl the body begins to catabolize its protein stores, resulting in growth retardation. The daily amounts are individualized for each child and require frequent changes based on appetite, growth and development, and blood phenylalanine and tyrosine levels.

Since all natural food proteins contain about 15% phenylalanine, specially prepared milk substitutes, such as Lofenalac,* Pro-Phree,† or Phenex-1,† are prescribed for the infant. These products are made from specially treated enzymatic casein hydrolysate, which provides only 0.4% phenylalanine (28.5 mg/8 ounces). They also contain minerals and vitamins to provide a balanced nutritional formula. Tyrosine and several other amino acids are supplied in the formula. Because of the low phenylalanine content of breast milk, total or partial breast-feeding may be possible with close monitoring of phenylalanine levels; partial supplementation with a phenylalanine-free formula may be required in some cases to provide adequate calories and nutrients (Lawrence, 1994). Diet substitutes for older children, such as Phenyl-Free* and Phenex-2,† contain no phenylalanine and allow for greater exchanges with natural low-phenylalanine foods in the diet, leading to a more normal diet.

A low-phenylalanine diet is begun as soon as possible after birth and maintained through adolescence. To evaluate the effectiveness of dietary treatment, frequent monitoring of blood phenylalanine and tyrosine levels is necessary. Since phenylalanine levels greater than or equal to 20 mg/dl in mothers with PKU affect the normal embryologic development of the fetus, the low-phenylalanine diet must be resumed *before* pregnancy in affected women (Koch and others, 1993). These women should also be counseled about the risk that their child might have phenylketonuria (approximately 1 in 120), and reproductive options should be discussed.

Prognosis. Although early treatment of infants with PKU greatly improves their chances for achieving normal cognitive development, the outcome is not as favorable as previously thought. Even with adequate dietary control, a high percentage of children exhibit some degree of intellectual impairment. There is evidence of slower language acquisition and, in the school years, a higher frequency of learning and behavior problems, especially hyperactivity, anxiety, and poor concentration.

Nursing Considerations

The principal nursing considerations involve teaching the family regarding the dietary restrictions. Although the treatment may sound simple, the task of maintaining such a strict dietary regimen is very demanding, especially for older children and adolescents. Foods with low phenylalanine levels, such as vegetables, fruits, juices, and some cereals, breads, and starches, must be measured to provide the prescribed amount of phenylalanine. Most high-protein foods, such as meat and dairy products, are either eliminated or restricted to small amounts. The sweetener aspartame (NutraSweet, Equal) should be avoided because it is converted to phenylalanine in the body. However, small amounts, such as a single 12-ounce serving of diet cola, do not significantly raise phenylalanine levels.

During infancy, maintaining the diet presents few problems. Solid foods, such as cereal, fruits, and vegetables, are introduced as usual to the infant. As the child gets older decreased appetite and refusal to eat may reduce intake of the calculated phenylalanine requirement. During the school years, the need for independence and peer pressure may deter the child from eating the prescribed foods or abstaining from high-protein foods. Limitations of this diet are best illustrated by an example: a quarter-pound hamburger may be equal to a 2-day phenylalanine allowance for a school-age child. Illness and growth spurts will increase the body's need for this essential amino acid.

The assistance of a registered nutritionist is essential. Parents need a basic understanding of the disorder and practical suggestions regarding food selection and preparation.* Meal planning is based on an exchange list, and as soon as children are old enough, usually by early preschool, they should be involved in the daily calculation, menu planning, and formula preparation. A system of goal setting, self-monitoring, contracts, and rewards can promote compliance in adolescents.

Preparation of the formula can present some difficulties. It tends to be lumpy and has a distinctive odor and taste that has been described as similar to potato but more bitter. A blender or mixer dissolves the powder more easily, but this is inconvenient when traveling. Although the taste is virtually impossible to camouflage, adding orange Tang, fruit-flavored powdered punch, or strawberry or chocolate Quik helps to vary the flavor somewhat without greatly altering the phenylalanine content. The chocolate-flavored formula can be heated and served as hot cocoa or frozen into popsicles.

Family Support. In addition to the problem related to a child with a chronic disorder (see Chapter 18), the par-

---

*Mead Johnson & Co., Evansville, IN.
†Ross Laboratories, Columbus, OH.

*A helpful resource is *Low-Protein Cookery for Phenylketonuria*, edited by V. Schuett (1988); available from the University of Wisconsin Press, 114 N. Murray St., Madison, WI 53715; (608) 262-8782.

[handwritten note: health screening done on all infants need to be repeated]

ents have the burden of knowing that they are carriers of the defect and must make serious decisions regarding future children. Prenatal testing is now available to detect the presence of the defective gene in heterozygotes. Genetic counseling is especially important for an affected child, who theoretically has a 50% chance of bearing an affected offspring (see Genetic Counseling).

GALACTOSEMIA

Galactosemia is a rare autosomal-recessive disorder affecting approximately 1:50,000 births. It involves an inborn error of carbohydrate metabolism in which the hepatic enzyme *galactose-1-phosphate uridine transferase (UDP-galactose transferase)* is absent. The enzyme is one of three needed for the conversion of galactose to glucose. There is considerable genetic variability in enzyme deficiency, with some children having partial transferase activity.

As galactose accumulates in the blood, several organs are affected. Hepatic dysfunction leads to cirrhosis, resulting in jaundice in the infant by the second week of life. The spleen subsequently becomes enlarged as a result of portal hypertension. Cataracts are usually recognizable by 1 or 2 months of age; cerebral damage, manifested by the symptoms of lethargy and hypotonia, is evident soon afterward. Infants with galactosemia appear normal at birth, but within a few days after ingesting milk, which has a high lactose content, they begin to vomit and lose weight. Drowsiness, nausea, and diarrhea also occur. Death during the first month of life is not infrequent in untreated infants.

Diagnostic Evaluation

Diagnosis is made on the basis of galactosuria, increased levels of galactose in the blood, or decreased levels of UDP-galactose transferase activity in erythrocytes. Newborn screening for this disease is required in many states. Heterozygotes can also be identified, since heterozygotic individuals have significantly lower levels of the essential enzyme.

Therapeutic Management

Treatment of galactosemia consists of eliminating all milk and lactose-containing foods, including breast milk. During infancy, lactose-free formulas are used, with soy-protein formula being the feeding of choice.

Prognosis. Follow-up studies of children treated from birth or within the first 2 months of life after symptoms appear have found long-term complications, such as ovarian dysfunction, abnormal speech, cognitive impairment, growth retardation, and motor delay (Waggoner and Buist, 1993). These findings have revealed that eliminating sources of galactose does not significantly improve the outcome. New therapeutic strategies, such as replacing depleted metabolites or using gene replacement therapy, are needed to improve the prognosis for these children (Segal, 1993).

Nursing Considerations

Nursing interventions are similar to those for PKU, except that dietary restrictions are easier to maintain because many more foods are allowed. However, reading food labels very carefully for the presence of any form of lactose, especially dairy products, is mandatory. Many drugs, such as penicillin, contain lactose as filler and must also be avoided. Unfortu-

nately, lactose is an unlabeled ingredient in pharmaceuticals. (See also Family Support for PKU, p. 279.)

GENETIC EVALUATION AND COUNSELING

Genetic counseling is a communication process concerned with the human problems associated with the occurrence, or risk of occurrence, of a genetic disorder in a family. Nurses in the field of infant and child care continually encounter genetic diseases and families in which there is a risk that a disorder may be transmitted to or occur in an offspring. It is a responsibility of nurses to be alert to situations in which persons could benefit from genetic counseling (see Guidelines box), to become familiar with facilities in their areas where genetic counseling is available, and to learn the basic principles of heredity and types of genetic testing (Table 9-12). In this way they will be able to direct individuals and families to take advantage of needed services and to be active participants in the counseling process.

The success of counseling is measured by the way in which the family members use the information presented to them. Maintaining contact with the family or referring the family to an agency that can provide a sustained relationship, usually the public health agency in their locality, is one of the most important aspects of the counseling process. In a disorder that requires conscientious diet management, such as PKU, it is important to make certain that the family understands and follows the advice. Children born later must be carefully observed to ensure early detection of symptoms in the event that they have also inherited the disorder.

PSYCHOLOGIC ASPECTS OF GENETIC DISEASE

It requires time and understanding to deal with the emotional tension and anxiety generated in families who are faced with the prospect of a genetic disorder. Knowledge of and the ability to deal with the range of psychologic responses and all their ramifications (such as the grief reaction, guilt, anger, and coping mechanisms) are essential components of the nursing role in genetic counseling.

GUIDELINES
Referral Regarding Genetic Counseling

Individuals with a family history of hereditary diseases or birth defects
Known balanced translocation carriers or parents who have previously had a fetus or child with a chromosome abnormality
Couples with a history of multiple miscarriages, stillbirths, or infertility
Individuals at risk for ethnic-related disorders
Pregnant women exposed to teratogenic agents
Pregnant women of advanced maternal age (≥35 years)
Disorders in which pregnancy could threaten maternal or fetal life or health

TABLE 9-12. Types of genetic testing

TEST/METHOD	SPECIMEN	INDICATION	COMMENTS
Chromosome analysis (karyotyping)	Blood, skin, amniocytes, bone marrow	Detection of chromosome abnormality, sex determination, cancer classification	Almost 100% accuracy for whole or partial chromosome abnormality; will not detect microdeletions/duplication (submicroscopic chromosome segments) single-gene defects or multifactorial disorders
Fluorescence in situ hybridization (FISH)	Blood, skin, amniocytes, bone marrow	Detection of microdeletion/duplications of chromosome segments (not visible by chromosome analysis)	Still considered investigational but very promising as a technique that is a cross between chromosome analysis and single-gene DNA tests
Direct DNA mutation detection (polymerase chain reaction [PCR], southern blot, gene sequencing)	Blood, skin, amniocytes	Detection of gene mutation(s) in affected individual for diagnosis, in unaffected carrier, or presymptomatic diagnosis	Gene location must be mapped and disease producing mutations must be characterized; can test single individual
Indirect DNA linkage studies (restriction length fragment polymorphions [RLFPs], microsatellites, genetic markers)	Blood	Prediction of carrier, or presymptomatic status based on inheritance of same chromosomal segment as known affected individual	Must test several family members including 1-2 confirmed affected individuals for testing to be valid
Biochemical	Blood, skin, amniotic fluid, muscle biopsy, urine, stool	Detection of metabolic pathway errors, enzyme defects, neural tube/ventral wall detects	Results may be difficult to interpret if partial pathway error or modified substrate is present

It is important to stress that there is nothing shameful about an inherited or congenital defect and to emphasize any appropriate remedy. The threat of a hereditary "taint" often creates intrafamily strife, hostility, and marital disharmony, sometimes to the point of family disintegration. Relatives frequently cease reproduction after the diagnosis of a hereditary defect in a member, or the decision to reproduce may be postponed indefinitely on the basis of a disorder in a relative, even a remote one, of a prospective partner. Although people may understand the situation on an intellectual level, they may still harbor fears on an emotional level. A vital part of the nurse's role in genetic counseling is that of a sympathetic and supportive listener.

KEY POINTS

- Health problems of the newborn infant may result from hereditary conditions or from prenatal, natal, or postnatal environmental factors.
- Birth injuries are usually those affecting soft tissues, bones, or nervous tissues.
- High-risk neonates are those newborn infants, regardless of gestational age or birth weight, who have a greater than average chance of morbidity or mortality because of conditions or circumstances that are superimposed on the normal course of events associated with birth and adjustment to extrauterine life.

- Newborns feel pain, and adequate pain control, especially during surgery, can reduce morbidity and mortality.
- Nurses must be sensitive to pain in the neonate, be alert for signs of pain, and intervene appropriately.
- Appropriate developmental intervention for infants in the intensive care unit facilitates their growth and maturation.
- Parents are encouraged to interact with their high-risk infant and gradually assume care of the infant when the infant's condition allows and the parents feel comfortable in doing so.

- Hyperbilirubinemia is a common problem in the newborn that results from red blood cell breakdown that exceeds the ability of the immature liver to metabolize and excrete.
- Because of their immature physical status, preterm infants need special attention to promote respiratory efforts, maintain body temperature, conserve energy, prevent infection, and provide nutrition.
- Preterm infants are subject to a number of complications, including apnea, infection, anemia, respiratory distress syndrome, and intraventricular hemorrhage.
- Sepsis is a serious condition with nonspecific manifestations that render it difficult to distinguish from other conditions in the newborn infant.

- Maternal prenatal conditions are responsible for high-risk health problems in some newborn infants, especially maternal diabetes, physical dependency on drugs, some infections, and ingestion of certain chemical substances.
- Testing of newborns, as well as their mothers prenatally or perinatally, for human immunodeficiency virus (HIV) is recommended.
- The inborn errors of metabolism for which newborns are routinely screened are congenital hypothyroidism, phenylketonuria, and galactosemia.

REFERENCES

American Academy of Pediatrics: Perinatal human immunodeficiency virus testing, *Pediatrics* 95(2):303-307, 1995.

American Academy of Pediatrics, Committee on Fetus and Newborn, Committee on Drugs, Section on Anesthesiology, and Section on Surgery: Neonatal anesthesia, *Pediatrics* 80:446, 1987.

American Academy of Pediatrics, Committee on Genetics: Newborn screening for congenital hypothyroidism: recommended guidelines, *Pediatrics* 91(6):1203-1209, 1993.

American Academy of Pediatrics, Committee on Injury and Poison Prevention and Committee on Fetus and Newborn: Safe transportation of premature and low birth weight infants, *Pediatrics* 97(5):758-60, 1996.

American Academy of Pediatrics and American College of Obstetricians and Gynecologists: *Guidelines for perinatal care,* ed 3, Elk Grove Village, IL, 1992, The Academy and College.

Anand K, Hickey P: Halothane-morphine compared with high-dose sufentanil for anesthesia and postoperative analgesia in neonatal cardiac surgery, *N Engl J Med* 326(1):1-9, 1992.

Anand KJ, Hickey P: Pain and its effects in the human neonate and fetus, *N Engl J Med* 317:1321-1329, 1987.

Anand KJ, McGrath PJ: *Pain in neonates,* New York, 1993, Elsevier.

Askin DF: Bacterial and fungal infections in the neonate, *JOGNN* 24(7):635-643, 1995.

Barrier G and others: Measurement of post-operative pain and narcotic administration in infants using a new clinical scoring system, *Intensive Care Med* 15:S37-39, 1989.

Bier JAB and others: Breast-feeding of very low birth weight infants, *J Pediatr* 123(5):773-778, 1994.

Blackburn S: Hyperbilirubinemia and neonatal jaundice, *Neonatal Network* 14(7):15-25, 1995.

Blackburn ST, Loper DL: *Maternal, fetal, and neonatal physiology: a clinical perspective,* Philadelphia, 1992, WB Saunders.

Brucker J: Brachial plexus birth injury, *J Neurosci Nurs* 23(6):374-380, 1991.

Burrows FA, Berde CB: Optimal pain relief in infants and children, *Br Med J* 307(6908):815-816, 1993.

Calhoun LK: Parents' perceptions of nursing support following neonatal loss, *J Perinat Neonat Nurs* 8(2):57-66, 1994.

Casado de Frias E and others: Evolution of height and bone age in primary congenital hypothyroidism, *Clin Pediatr* 32(7):426-432, 1993.

Chasnoff IJ and others: Cocaine/polydrug use in pregnancy: two-year follow-up, *Pediatrics* 89:284-289, 1992.

Choonara I: Management of pain in newborn infants, *Semin Perinatol* 16(1):32-40, 1992.

Cornblath M, Schwartz R: Hypoglycemia in the neonate, *J Pediatr Endocrinol* 6(2):113-129, 1993.

Davis M: Fluids, electrolytes and nutrition in the low-birth-weight infant, *NAACOG Clin Issues Perinat Womens Health Nurs* 3(1):45-61, 1992.

Fanaroff AA, Martin RJ: *Neonatal-perinatal medicine: diseases of the fetus and infant,* ed 5, St Louis, 1992, Mosby.

Farrington EA and others: Continuous intravenous morphine infusion in postoperative newborn infants, *Am J Perinatol* 10(1):84, 1993.

Fox MD: Measurement of urine output volume: accuracy of diaper weights in neonatal environments, *Neonatal Network* 11(3):11-18, 1992.

Fox MD, Molesky MG: The effects of prone and supine positioning on arterial oxygen pressure, *Neonatal Network* 8:25-29, 1990.

Franck L, Vilardi J: Assessment and management of opioid withdrawal in ill neonates, *Neonatal Network* 14(2):39-48, 1995.

Gale G, Franck L, Lund C: Skin-to-skin (kangaroo) holding of the intubated premature infant, *Neonatal Network* 12(6):49-57, 1993.

Gardner SL, O'Donnell JP, Weisman LE: Breastfeeding the sick neonate. In Merenstein GB, Gardner SL, editors: *Handbook of neonatal intensive care,* ed 3, St Louis, 1993, Mosby.

Gartner LM: Neonatal jaundice, *Pediatr Rev* 15(11):422-432, 1994.

Griffith DR, Azuma SD, Chasnoff IJ: Three-year outcomes of children exposed prenatally to drugs, *J Am Acad Child Adolesc Psychiatr* 33(1):20-27, 1994.

Grunau RVE, Johnston CC, Craig KD: Neonatal facial and cry responses to invasive and noninvasive procedures, *Pain* 42(3):295-305, 1990.

Hegyi T and others: Blood pressure ranges in premature infants. I. The first hours of life, *J Pediatr* 124(4):627-633, 1994.

Hurwitz S: Skin lesions in the first year of life, *Contemp Pediatr* 10(1):110-128, 1993.

Koch R and others: The North American collaborative study of maternal phenylketonuria (PKU), *Int Pediatr* 8(1):89-96, 1993.

Krechel SW, Bildner J: CRIES: A new neonatal postoperative pain measurement score. Initial testing of validity and reliability, *Paediatr Anaesth* 5:53-61, 1995.

Langkamp DL, Langhough R: What do parents of preterm infants know about diphtheria, tetanus, and pertussis immunizations? *Am J Perinatol* 10(3):187, 1993.

Lawrence J and others: The development of a tool to assess neonatal pain, *Neonatal Network* 12(6):59-66, 1993.

Lawrence RA: *Breastfeeding: a guide for the medical profession,* ed 4, St Louis, 1994, Mosby.

Levin RH, Wong AF: Antifungal agents and their renal implications in the neonate, *J Perinat Neonatal Nurs* 8(1):59-73, 1994.

Linder N and others: Suckling stimulation test for neonatal tremor, *Arch Dis Child* 64:44-46, 1989.

Ludington-Hoe SM and others: Kangaroo care: research results, and practice implications and guidelines, *Neonatal Network* 13(1):19-27, 1994.

McLaughlin CR and others: Neonatal pain: a comprehensive survey of attitudes and practices, *J Pain Symptom Manage* 8(1):7-16, 1993.

Meier PP and others: Breastfeeding support services in the neonatal intensive care unit, *JOGNN* 22(4):338-347, 1993.

Miculan J, Turner S, Paes B: Congenital hypothyroidism: diagnosis and management, *Neonatal Network* 12(6):25-42, 1993.

Newman TB, Maisels MJ: Evaluation and treatment of jaundice in the term newborn: a kinder, gentler approach, *Pediatrics* 89(5):809-818, 1992.

Pelke S and others: Gowning does not affect colonization or infection rates in a neonatal intensive care unit, *Arch Pediatr Adolesc Med* 148:1016-1020, 1994.

Peters KL: Does routine care complicate the physiologic status of the premature neonate with respiratory distress syndrome? *J Perinat Neonat Nurs* 6(2):67-84, 1992.

Pokela M: Pain relief can reduce hypoxemia in distressed neonates during routine treatment procedures, *Pediatrics* 93(3):379-383, 1994.

Schuman AJ, Karush G: Fiberoptic vs conventional home phototherapy for neonatal hyperbilirubinemia, *Clin Pediatr* 31(6):345-352, 1992.

Segal S: The challenge of galactosemia, *Int Pediatr* 8(1):125-132, 1993.

Sherwood RA: The use of topical anesthesia in removal of port-wine stains in children, *J Pediatr* 122(5—2):S36-41, 1993.

Sinai LN and others: Phenylketonuria screening: effect of early newborn discharge, *Pediatrics* 96(4):605-608, 1995.

Stevens BJ: Personal communication, 1994.

Strauss RP, Resnick SD: Pulsed dye laser therapy for port-wine stains in children: psychosocial and ethical issues, *J Pediatr* 122(4):505-510, 1993.

Thomas K: Thermoregulation in neonates, *Neonatal Network* 13(2):15-22, 1994.

Vomund SL, Witter SE: Advanced techniques for the treatment of severe isoimmunization, *MCN* 19:18-23, 1994.

Waggoner DD, Buist N: Long-term complications in treated galactosemia, *Int Pediatr* 8(1):97-100, 1993.

Wertz DC, Fanos JH, Reilly PR: Genetic testing for children and adolescents: who decides? *JAMA* 272(11):875-880, 1994.

Yaster M and others: Local anesthetics in the management of acute pain in children, *J Pediatr* 124(2):165-176, 1994.

BIBLIOGRAPHY

Birth Injuries/Dermatologic Problems

Ashinoff R, Geronemus RG: Effect of the topical anesthetic EMLA on the efficacy of pulsed dye laser treatment of port-wine stains, *J Dermatol Surg Oncol* 16(11):1008-1011, 1990.

Bett BJ: Congenital giant pigmented nevi, *Dermatol Nurs* 6(5):307-312, 1994.

Eichenfield LF, Honig PJ: Difficult diagnostic and management issues in pediatric dermatology, *Pediatr Clin North Am* 38(3):687-710, 1991.

Feigin FD, Adcock LM, Miller DJ: Postnatal bacterial infections. In Fanaroff A, Martin R, editors: *Neonatal-perinatal medicine,* ed 5, St Louis, 1992, Mosby.

Goldman MP, Fitzpatrick RE, Ruiz-Esparza J: Treatment of port-wine stains (capillary malformation) with the flashlamp-pumped pulsed dye laser, *J Pediatr* 122(1):71-77, 1993.

Kimble C: Neonatal petechiae: strategies for nursing interventions, *Dermatol Nurs* 8(1):24-28, 1994.

Mangurten HH: Birth injuries. In Fanaroff A, Martin R, editors: *Neonatal-perinatal medicine,* ed 5, St Louis, 1992, Mosby.

Reese V and others: Association of facial hemangiomas with Dandy-Walker and other posterior fossa malformations, *J Pediatr* 122(3):379-384, 1993.

Silverman RA: Hemangiomas and vascular malformations, *Pediatr Clin North Am* 38(4):811-834, 1991.

Tappero EP, Honeyfield ME: *Physical assessment of the newborn: a comprehensive approach to the art of physical examination,* Petaluma, CA, 1993, NICU Ink.

Nursing Care of the High-Risk Infant

Alberti AM: Advancing the scope of practice of primary nurses in the NICU, *J Perinat Neonat Nurs* 5(3):44-50, 1991.

Allen MC: The high-risk infant, *Pediatr Clin North Am* 40(3):479-488, 1993.

Auerbach KG, Walker M: When the mother of a premature infant uses a breast pump: what every NICU nurse needs to know, *Neonatal Network* 13(4):23-29, 1994.

Bass JL, Mehta KA, Camara J: Monitoring premature infants in car seats: implementing the American Academy of Pediatrics policy in a community hospital, *Pediatrics* 91(6):1137-1141, 1993.

Beachy P, Deacon J, editors: *Core curriculum for neonatal intensive care nursing,* Philadelphia, 1993, WB Saunders.

Bier JAB and others: Breast-feeding of very low birth weight infants, *J Pediatr* 123(5):778, 1993.

Blackburn ST, Loper DL: *Maternal, fetal, and neonatal physiology: a clinical perspective,* Philadelphia, 1992, WB Saunders.

Brooten D, editor: Low-birth-weight neonates, *NAACOG Clin Issues Perinat Womens Health Nurs* 3(1), 1992.

Chally PS: Moral decision making in neonatal intensive care, *JOGNN* 21(6):475-482, 1992.

Crawford NG, Pruss AM: Preventing neonatal hepatitis B infection during the perinatal period, *JOGNN* 22(6):491-497, 1993.

Gennaro S, Bakewell-Sachs S: Discharge planning and home care for low-birth-weight infants, *NAACOG Clin Issues Perinat Womens Health Nurs* 3(1):29-146, 1992.

Gennaro S, Brooten D, Bakewell-Sachs S: Postdischarge services for low-birth-weight infants, *JOGNN* 20(1):29-36, 1991.

Gordon M, Montgomery LA: Minimizing epidermal stripping in the very low birth weight infant: integrating research and practice to affect infant outcome, *Neonatal Network* 15(1):37-44, 1996.

Kennedy C, Lipsitt L: Temporal characteristics of non-oral feedings and chronic feeding problems in premature infants, *J Perinat Neonat Nurs* 7(3):77-85, 1993.

Kenner C and others: *Comprehensive neonatal nursing: a physiologic perspective,* Philadelphia, 1993, WB Saunders.

Kinneer MD, Beachy P: Nipple feeding premature infants in the neonatal intensive-care unit: factors and decisions, *JOGNN* 22(2):147-155, 1994.

Klaus MH, Fanaroff AA: *Care of the high-risk neonate,* ed 4, Philadelphia, 1993, WB Saunders.

Letko MD: Detecting and preventing infant hearing loss, *Neonatal Network* 11(5):33-38, 1992.

Lotas MJ: Effects of light and sound in the neonatal intensive care unit environment on the low-birth-weight infant, *NAACOG Clin Issues Perinat Womens Health Nurs* 3(1):34-44, 1992.

MacDonald NE: Minimizing the risks of neonatal HSV, *Emerg Med* 25(7):98-101, 1993.

Malloy-McDonald MB: Skin care for high-risk neonates, *J WOCN* 22(4):177-182, 1995.

Merenstein GB, Gardner SL: *Handbook of neonatal intensive care,* ed 3, St Louis, 1993, Mosby.

Pickler RH, Higgins KE, Crummette BD: The effect of nonnutritive sucking on bottle-feeding stress in preterm infants, *JOGNN* 22(3):230-234, 1992.

Robertson AF, Bhatia J: Feeding premature infants, *Clin Pediatr* 32(1):36-44, 1993.

Shogan MG, Schumann LL: The effect of environmental lighting on the oxygen saturation of preterm infants in the NICU, *Neonatal Network* 12(5):7-13, 1993.

Tsang RC and others, editors: *Nutritional needs of the preterm infant: scientific basis and practical guidelines,* Baltimore, 1993, Williams & Wilkins.

Walker M: Breastfeeding the premature infant, *NAACOG Clin Issues Perinat Womens Health Nurs* Philadelphia, 1992, JB Lippincott.

Wilson D: Neonatal IVs: practical tips, *Neonatal Network* 11(2):49-53, 1992.

Zwick MB: Decreasing environmental noise in the NICU through staff education, *Neonatal Intensive Care* 6(2):16-19, 1993.

Infant Pain

Anand KJS: Neonatal stress responses to anesthesia and surgery, *Clin Perinatol* 17(1):207-214, 1990.

Bell SG: The national pain management guideline: implications for neonatal intensive care, *Neonatal Network* 13(3):9-17, 1994.

Bloch EC: Update on anesthesia management for infants and children, *Surg Clin North Am* 72(6):1207-1221, 1992.

Broome M, Tanzillo H: Differentiating between pain and agitation in premature neonates, *J Perinat Neonat Nurs* 4(1):53-62, 1990.

Budreau G, Kleiber C: Clinical indications of infant irritability, *Neonatal Network* 9(5):23-30, 1991.

Butler NC: The issue of medically caused pain in infants: ACCH members should be involved, *Child Health Care* 18(2):70-74, 1989.

Caron E, Maguire D: Current management of pain, sedation, and narcotic physical dependency of the infant on ECMO, *J Perinat Neonat Nurs* 4(1):63-74, 1990.

Cunningham N: Ethical perspectives on the perception and treatment of neonatal pain, *J Perinat Neonat Nurs* 4(1):75-83, 1990.

Davis DH, Calhoon M: Do preterm infants show behavioral responses to painful procedures? In Funk SG and others, editors: *Key aspects of comfort: management of pain, fatigue, and nausea,* New York, 1989, Springer.

Fitzgerald M: Pain and analgesia in the newborn, *Arch Dis Child* 64:441-443, 1989.

Franck LS: Pain in the nonverbal patient: advocating for the critically ill neonate, *Pediatr Nurs* 15(1):65, 1989.

Gordon P: Assessing and managing agitation in a critically ill infant, *MCN* 15(1):26-32, 1990.

Johnston CC, Stevens B: Pain assessment in newborns, *J Perinat Neonat Nurs* 4(1):41-52, 1990.

Maguire D, Maloney P: A comparison of fentanyl and morphine use in neonates, *Neonatal Network* 7(1):27-32, 1988.

Mainous RO: Research utilization: Pharmacologic management of neonatal pain, *Neonatal Network* 14(4):71-74, 1995.

Marshall RE: Neonatal pain associated with caregiving procedures, *Pediatr Clin North Am* 36(4):885-903, 1989.

Penticuff JH: Infant suffering and nurse advocacy in neonatal intensive care, *Nurs Clin North Am* 24(4):987-997, 1989.

Rogers MC: Do the right thing: pain relief in infants and children, *N Engl J Med* 326(1):55-56, 1991.

Developmental Intervention and Care

Affonso D and others: Reconciliation and healing from mothers through skin-to-skin contact provided in an American Tertiary Level Intensive Care Nursery, *Neonatal Network* 12(3):25-32, 1993.

Barba LA, King DJ, Walker CL: Infant definitive care unit: developmental care for the hospitalized NICU graduate, *Neonatal Network* 11(7):35-42, 1992.

Cusson RM, Lee AL: Parental interventions and the development of the preterm infant, *JOGNN* 23(1):60-68, 1993.

Fleisher BE: Individualized developmental care for very-low-birth-weight premature infants, *Clin Pediatr* 34:523-529, 1995.

Gale G, Franck L, Lund C: Skin-to-skin (kangaroo) holding of the intubated premature infant, *Neonatal Network* 12(6):49-51, 1993.

Lotas MJ: Effects of light and sound in the neonatal intensive care unit environment on the low-birth-weight infant, *NAACOG Clin Issues Perinat Womens Health Nurs* 3(1):34-44, 1992.

Victor L and Persoon J: Implementation of kangaroo care: A parent-health care team approach to practice change, *Crit Care Nurs Clin North Am* (4):891-895, 1994.

White-Traut RC and others: Environmental influences on the developing premature infant: theoretical issues and applications to practice. *JOGNN* 23(5):393-401, 1994.

Whitley S, Cowan M: Developmental intervention in the newborn intensive care unit, *NAACOG Clin Issues Perinat Women Health Nurs* 2(1):84-90, 1991.

Parental Involvement

Baker JG: Parents as partners in the NICU, *Neonatal Network* 14(1):9-10, 1995.

Bass LS: What do parents need when their infant is a patient in the NICU? *Neonatal Network* 10(4):25-33, 1991.

Calhoun LK: Parents' perceptions of nursing support following neonatal loss, *J Perinatol Neonat Nurs* 8(2):57-66, 1994.

Cusson RM and Lee AL: Parental Interventions and the development of the preterm infant, *JOGNN* 23(1):60-68, 1994.

Edwards LD, Saunders RB: Symbolic interactionism: a framework for the care of parents of preterm infants, *J Pediatr Nurs* 5:123-128, 1990.

Gennaro S and others: Concerns of mothers of low birthweight infants, *Pediatr Nurs* 16(5):459-462, 1990.

Griffin T: Nurse barriers to parenting in the special care nursery, *J Perinatol Neonat Nurs* 4(2):56-67, 1990.

Haut C, Peddicord K, O'Brien E: Supporting parental bonding in the NICU: a care plan for nurses, *Neonatal Network* 13(8):19-25, 1994.

Hamelin K, Ramachandran C: Kangaroo care, *Can Nurse* 89(6):15-18, 1993.

Harrison LL, Woods S: Early parental touch and preterm infants, *JOGNN* 20(4):299-306, 1991.

Haut C, Peddicord K, O'Brien E: Supporting parental bonding in the NICU: a care plan for nurses, *Neonatal Network* 13(8):19-25, 1994.

Jarrett MH: Parent partners: a parent-to-parent support program in the NICU Part II: program implementation, *Pediatr Nurs* 22(2):142-144, 1996.

Jellinek J and others: Facing tragic decisions with parents in the neonatal intensive care unit: clinical perspectives, *Neonatal Intensive Care* 5(3):24-29, 1992.

Kenner C: Caring for the NICU parent, *J Perinat Neonat Nurs* 4(3):78-87, 1990.

Krahn GL, Hallum A, Kime C: Are there good ways to give "bad news"? *Pediatrics* 91(3):578-582, 1993.

Lindsay JK and others: Creative caring in the NICU: parent-to-parent support, *Neonatal Network* 12(4):37-44, 1993.

McGettigan MC and others: Psychological aspects of parenting critically ill neonates, *Clin Pediatr* 33(1):77-81, 1994.

Page-Lieberman J, Hughes CB: How fathers perceive perinatal death, *MCN* 15(5):320-323, 1990.

Ryan P, Cote-Arsenault D, Sugarman L: Facilitating care after perinatal loss, *JOGNN* 29(5):385-389, 1991.

Sexton PR, Stephen SB: Postpartum mothers' perceptions of nursing interventions for perinatal grief, *Neonatal Network* 9(5):47-51, 1991.

Welch ID: Miscarriage, stillbirth, or newborn death: starting a healthy grieving process, *Neonatal Network* 9(8):53-57, 1991.

Neonatal Loss

Brown Y: Perinatal death and grieving, *Can Nurs* 87(8):26-29, 1991.

Evans ML, Englebardt SP: Evaluation of a multidisciplinary perinatal bereavement program, *Neonatal Network* 8(4):31-35, 1990.

Harrigan R and others: Perinatal grief: response to the loss of an infant, *Neonatal Network* 12(5):25-31, 1993.

Jellinek MS and others: Facing tragic decisions with parents in the neonatal intensive care unit: clinical perspectives, *Pediatrics* 89(1):119-122, 1992.

Kimble DL: Neonatal death: a descriptive study of fathers' experiences, *Neonatal Network* 9(8):45-50, 1991.

Leon IG: Perinatal loss: a critique of current hospital practices, *Clin Pediatr* 31(6):366-374, 1992.

Primeau MR, Lamb JM: When a baby dies: rights of the baby and parents, *JOGNN* 24(3):206-208, 1995.

Hyperbilirubinemia, Hypoglycemia, and Hypocalcemia

Ahlfors CE: Criteria for exchange transfusion in jaundiced newborns, *Pediatrics* 93(3):488-494, 1994.

Cole MD: New factors associated with the incidence of hypoglycemia: a research study, *Neonatal Network* 10(4):47-50, 1991.

Gartner LM: Neonatal jaundice, *Pediatrics in Review* 15(11):422-432, 1994.

George P, Lynch M: Ohmeda biliblanket vs Wallaby phototherapy system for the reduction of bilirubin levels in the home-care setting, *Clin Pediatr* 33(1):178-180, 1994.

Karp TB, Butler LA: Glucose metabolism in the neonate: the short and sweet of it, *Neonatal Network* 14(8):17-23, 1995.

Kenner C, Brueggemeyer A, Gunderson LP: *Comprehensive neonatal nursing: a physiologic perspective,* Philadelphia, 1993, WB Saunders.

Maisels MJ, Kring E: Risk of sepsis in newborns with severe hyperbilirubinemia, *Pediatrics* 90(5):741-743, 1992.

Meropol SB et al: Home phototherapy: use and attitudes among community pediatricians, *Pediatrics* 91(1):97-99, 1993.

Tan KL: Comparison of the efficacy of fiberoptic and conventional phototherapy for neonatal hyperbilirubinemia, *J Pediatr* 125(4):607-612, 1994.

Respiratory, Cardiovascular, and Cerebral Complications

Angeles DM: Pathophysiology and nursing management of persistent pulmonary hypertension of the newborn, *MCN* 17(6):314-321, 1992.

Annibale DJ: Evaluating the strength of medical literature: indomethacin in the neonatal intensive care unit, *Neonatal Intensive Care* 7(3):22-28, 1994.

Avila K, Mazza LV, Morgan-Trujillo L: High-frequency oscillatory ventilation: a nursing approach to bedside care, *Neonatal Network* 13(5):23-30, 1994.

Boeckling AC: Exogenous surfactant therapy for premature infants, *J Perinat Neonat Nurs* 6(2):59-66, 1992.

Carroll P: Clinical application of pulse oximetry, *Pediatr Nurs* 19(2):150-151, 1993.

Conte VH: Bronchopulmonary dysplasia. In Jackson PL, Vessey JA: *Primary care of the child with a chronic condition,* ed 2, St Louis, 1996, Mosby.

Doran L: Periventricular leukomalacia, *Neonatal Network* 11(4):7-13, 1992.

Florentino-Pineda I and others: Subgaleal hemorrhage in the newborn infant associated with silicone elastomer vacuum extractor, *J Perinat* 14(2):95-100, 1994.

Green A, Giattina K: Adenosine administration for neonatal SVT, *Neonatal Network* 12(5):15-18, 1993.

Greenspan JS: Liquid ventilation: a developing technology, *Neonatal Network* 12(4):23-28, 1993.

Grobman DW, Foley MM: Surfactant replacement therapy in newborns with hyaline membrane disease, *Crit Care Nurs Clin North Am* 4(3):515-520, 1992.

Haney C, Allingham T: Nursing care of the neonate receiving high-frequency jet ventilation, *JOGNN* 21(3):187-195, 1992.

Harvey K: Pulse oximetry: implications for practice, *JOGNN* 21(1):35-41, 1992.

Howard-Glenn L: Transition to home: discharge planning for the oxygen-dependent infant with bronchopulmonary dysplasia, *J Perinat Neonat Nurs* 6(2):85-94, 1992.

Klein MD, Whittlesey GC: Extracorporeal membrane oxygenation, *Pediatr Clin North Am* 41(2):365-384, 1994.

Mathew OP: Patient-triggered ventilation in the newborn, *Clin Pediatr* 34:597-602, 1995.

Paul KE: Recognition, stabilization, and early management of infants with critical congenital heart disease presenting in the first days of life, *Neonatal Network* 14(5):13-20, 1995.

Phelps DL: Retinopathy of prematurity, *Pediatr Clin North Am* 40(4):705-714, 1993.

Pramanik AK, Holtzman RB, Merritt TA: Surfactant replacement therapy for pulmonary diseases, *Pediatr Clin North Am* 40(5):913-936, 1993.

Prullage S, Milichar C: Stabilization and transportation of infant with PPHN, *Neonatal Network* 12(7):45-51, 1993.

Rikard D: Nursing care of the neonate receiving prostaglandin E therapy, *Neonatal Network* 12(4):17-22, 1993.

Sinski A, Corbo J: Surfactant replacement in adults and children with ARDS—an effective therapy? *Crit Care Nurs* 12:54, 1994.

Van Meurs KP and others: Congenital diaphragmatic hernia: long-term outcome in neonates treated with extracorporeal membrane oxygenation, *J Pediatr* 122(6):893-899, 1993.

Weinstein S, Stolar CJH: Newborn surgical emergencies: congenital diaphragmatic hernia and extracorporeal membrane oxygenation, *Pediatr Clin North Am* 40(6):1315, 1993.

Werner NP: Congestive heart failure: pathophysiology and management throughout infancy, *J Perinat Neonat Nurs* 7(3):59, 1993.

Infections

Green A: Intravenous immunoglobulin for neonates, *MCN* 16:208-211, 1991.

Hess DL: Chlamydia in the neonate, *Neonatal Network* 12(3):9-12, 1993.

Lott JW, Kenner C: Keeping up with neonatal infections: designer bugs, part I, *Matern Child Nurs* 19(4):207-213, 1994.

Mulligan MJ, Stiehm ER: Neonatal hepatitis B infection: clinical and immunologic considerations, *J Perinatol* 14(1):2-8, 1994.

Parker LA: Necrotizing enterocolitis, *Neonatal Network* 14(6):17-26, 1995.

Wilson RE: Ostomy care for infants with necrotizing enterocolitis, *J WOCN* 21(5):190-194, 1994.

Witek-Janusek L, Cusack C: Neonatal sepsis: confronting the challenge, *Crit Care Nurs Clin North Am* 6(2):405-412, 1994.

High Risk Related to Maternal Factors

Barabach LM, Glzaer G, Norris SC: Maternal perception and parent-infant interaction of vulnerable cocaine-exposed couplets, *J Perinat Neonat Nurs* 6(3):76-84, 1992.

Benson MS: Management of infants born to women infected with the human immunodeficiency virus, *J Perinat Neonat Nurs* 7(4):79-89, 1994.

Brooks-Gunn J, McCarton C, Hawley T: Effects of in utero drug exposure on children's development, *Arch Pediatr Adolesc Med* 148:33-39, 1994.

Dreher M, Nugent K, Hudgins R: Prenatal marijuana exposure and neonatal outcomes in Jamaica: an ethnographic study, *Pediatrics* 93(2):254-260, 1994.

Dusick AM and others: Risk of intracranial hemorrhage and other adverse outcomes after cocaine exposure in a cohort of 323 very low birth weight infants, *J Pediatr* 122(3):438-445, 1993.

Forrest DC: The cocaine-exposed infant. I. Identification and assessment, *J Pediatr Health Care* 6(1):3-7, 1994.

Forrest DC: The cocaine-exposed infant. II. Intervention and teaching, *J Pediatr Health Care* 6(1):7-11, 1994.

Jorgensen KM: The drug-exposed infant, *Crit Care Nurs Clin North Am* 4(3):481-485, 1992.

Kuehne EA, Reilly M: Prenatal cocaine exposure. In Jackson PL, Vessey JA, editors: *Primary care of the child with a chronic condition,* ed 2, St Louis, 1996, Mosby.

Mayes LC and others: Neurobehavioral profiles of neonates exposed to cocaine prenatally, *Pediatrics* 91(4):778-783, 1993.

Samson LF: Infants of diabetic mothers: current perspectives, *J Perinat Neonat Nurs* 6(1):61-70, 1992.

Youngkin EQ: Sexually transmitted diseases: current and emerging concerns, *JOGNN* 24(8):743-758, 1995.

Zuckerman B, Frank D: "Crack kids": not broken, *Pediatrics* 89(2):337-339, 1992.

Inborn Errors of Metabolism

Acosta PB, Wright L: Nurses' role in preventing birth defects in offspring of women with phenylketonuria, *JOGNN* 21(4):270-276, 1992.

Alemzadeh R and others: Is there compensated hypothyroidism in infancy? *Pediatrics* 90(2):207-211, 1992.

Berlin CA, Roth KS: All children are special: the child with PKU, *Clin Pediatr* 32(5):316-319, 1993.

Berry HK and others: Valine, isoleucine, and leucine: a new treatment for phenylketonuria, *Am J Dis Child* 144(5):539-543, 1990.

Buist N and others: Towards improving the diet for hyperphenylalaninemia and other metabolic disorders, *Int Pediatr* 8(1):80-88, 1993.

Cockburn F and others: Maternal phenylketonuria: diet, dangers and dilemmas, *Int Pediatr* 7(1):67-74, 1992.

Davidson A: Management and counseling of children with inherited metabolic disorders, *J Pediatr Health Care* 6(3):146-153, 1992.

Gleason LA and others: A treatment program for adolescents with phenylketonuria, *Clin Pediatr* 31(6):331-335, 1992.

Hufnal-Miller CA and others: Enteral theophylline and necrotizing enterocolitis in the low-birthweight infant, *Clin Pediatr* 32(11):647-653, 1993.

Irons M: Screening for metabolic disorders: how are we doing? *Pediatr Clin North Am* 40(5):1073-1086, 1993.

Ittmann PI, Bozynskin ME: Toxic epidermal necrolysis in a newborn infant after exposure to adhesive remover, *J Perinatol* 13(6):476-477, 1993.

Legido A and others: Treatment variables and intellectual outcome in children with classic phenylketonuria, *Clin Pediatr* 32(7):417-432, 1993.

Mazzocco M and others: Cognition and thyrosine supplementation among school-aged children with phenylketonuria, *Am J Dis Child* 146(11):1261-1264, 1992.

Miculan J, Turner S, Paes BA: Congenital hypothyroidism: diagnosis and management, *Neonatal Network* 12(6):25-30, 1993.

Segal S: The enigma of galactosemia, *Int Pediatr* 7(1):75-82, 1992.

Smith I, Beasley M, Ades A: Intellectual progress and quality of phenylalanine control in early treated children with phenylketonuria, *Int Pediatr* 6(1):52-55, 1991.

Wright L, Brown A, Davidson-Mundt A: Newborn screening: the miracle and the challenge, *J Pediatr Nurs* 7(1):26-42, 1992.

Yule KA: Phenylketonuria. In Jackson PL, Vessey JA, editors: *Primary care of the child with a chronic condition,* ed 2, St Louis, 1996, Mosby.

Genetics and Genetic Counseling

American Academy of Pediatrics, Committee on Genetics: Folic acid for the prevention of neural tube defects, *Pediatrics* 92(3):493-494, 1993.

Aylsworth AS: Genetic counseling for patients with birth defects, *Pediatr Clin North Am* 39(2):229-253, 1992.

Bianchi DW: The subtle signs of genetic disease in the newborn infant, *Genetic Resource* 8(2):5-8, 1994.

Carey JC: Health supervision and anticipatory guidance for children with genetic disorders (including specific recommendations for trisomy 21, trisomy 18, and neurofibromatosis I), *Pediatr Clin North Am* 39(1):25-53, 1992.

Cohen MM, Rosenblum-Vos LS, Prathaker G: Human cytogenetics: a current overview, *Am J Dis Child* 147:1159-1166, 1993.

Day S, Brunson G, Wang W: A successful education program for parents of infants with newly diagnosed sickle cell disease, *J Pediatr Nurs* 7(1):52-57, 1992.

D'Alton ME, DeCherney AH: Prenatal diagnosis, *N Engl J Med* 328(2):114-120, 1993.

Hobus I and others: Factors influencing whether or not couples seek genetic counseling: an explorative study in a paediatric surgical unit, *Clin Genet* 47:47-52, 1995.

Korf B: Molecular medicine: molecular diagnosis, *New Engl J Med* 332(18):1218-1220, 1995.

Milunsky A, editor: *Genetic disorders and the fetus,* ed 3, Baltimore, 1992, Johns Hopkins University Press.

Prows CA: Utilization of genetic knowledge in pediatric nursing practice, *J Pediatr Nurs* 7(1):58-62, 1992.

Robinson A, Linden MG: *Clinical genetics handbook,* ed 2, Boston, 1993, Blackwell Scientific Publications.

Williams JK: New genetic discoveries increase counseling opportunities, *MCN* 18:218-222, 1993.

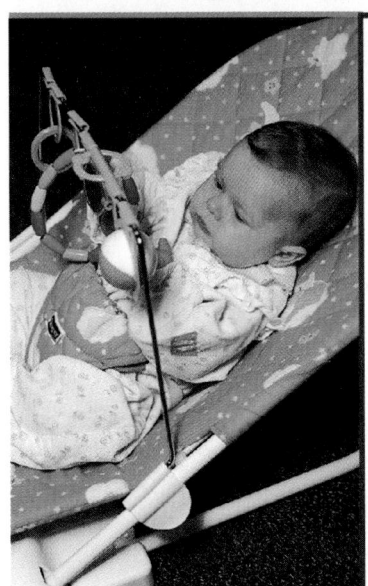

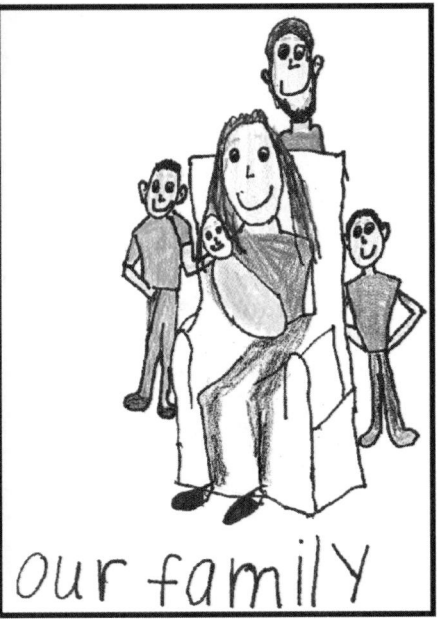

our family

" *I like having a baby sister. She plays peek-a-boo and laughs a lot.*"

3-month-old Anna's older brother, Daniel, age 9 years

RELATED TOPICS

PROMOTING OPTIMUM GROWTH AND DEVELOPMENT

BIOLOGIC DEVELOPMENT

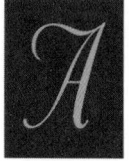At no other time in life are physical changes and developmental achievements so dramatic as during infancy. All major body systems undergo progressive maturation, and there is concurrent development of skills that increasingly allows infants to respond to and cope with the environment. Acquisition of these fine and gross motor skills occurs in an orderly head-to-toe and center-to-periphery (cephalo-caudal-proximodistal) sequence.

Proportional Changes

During the first year *growth* is very rapid, especially during the initial 6 months. Infants gain 680 g (1.5 pounds) a month until age 5 months, when the birth weight has at least doubled. An average weight for a 6-month-old child is 7.26 kg (16 pounds). Weight gain slows during the second 6 months. By 1 year of age the infant's birth weight has tripled, for an average weight of 9.75 kg (21.5 pounds). Infants who are breast-fed beyond 4 to 6 months of age typically gain less weight than those who are bottle-fed (Dewey and others, 1993).

Height increases by 2.5 cm (1 inch) a month during the first 6 months and also slows during the second 6 months. Increases in length occur in sudden spurts, rather than in a slow gradual pattern (Lampl, Veldhuis, and Johnson, 1992). Average height is 65 cm (25½ inches) at 6 months and 74 cm (29 inches) at 12 months. By 1 year the birth length has increased by almost 50%. The increase in length occurs mainly in the trunk, rather than in the legs, and contributes to the characteristic physique of the infant (see Fig. 5-3).

Head growth is also rapid. During the first 6 months head circumference increases approximately 1.5 cm (0.6 inch) a month but decreases to only 0.5 cm (0.2 inch) monthly during the second 6 months. The average size is 43 cm (17 inches) at 6 months and 46 cm (18 inches) at 12 months. By 1 year head size has increased by almost 33%. Closure of the cranial sutures occurs, with the posterior fontanel fusing by 6 to 8 weeks of age and the anterior fontanel closing by 12 to 18 months of age.

The expanding head size reflects the growth and differentiation of the *nervous system.* By the end of the first year the brain has increased in weight about two and one half times. The maturation of the brain is exhibited in the dramatic developmental achievements of infancy (see Table 10-2). The primitive reflexes are replaced by voluntary, purposeful movement. As myelinization occurs, the righting reflexes appear, as does the protective parachute reflex (Fig. 10-1), in which the hands and fingers extend forward, as in a protective response during a fall, when the infant is suddenly thrust downward while being held horizontally.

The *chest* assumes a more adult contour, with the lateral diameter becoming larger than the anteroposterior diameter. The chest circumference approximately equals the head circumference by the end of the first year. The *heart* grows less rapidly than does the rest of the body. Its weight is usually doubled by 1 year of age, in comparison with body weight, which triples during the same period. The size of the heart is still large in relation to the chest cavity; its width is about 55% of the width of the chest.

Maturation of Systems

Most organ systems change and grow during infancy. The *respiratory* rate slows somewhat (see inside back cover) and is relatively stable. Respiratory movements continue to be abdominal. Several factors predispose the infant to more severe and acute respiratory problems. The close proximity of the trachea to the bronchi and its branching structures rapidly transmits an infectious agent from one anatomic location to another.

Although the lumen of the trachea and bronchi enlarges during infancy, it remains small in comparison with the total size of the lung, maintaining high resistance to the volume of air inspired. The small airways are easily blocked by edema, mucus, or a foreign body. The flexible rib cage has less elastic recoil, and during respiratory distress, the work of breathing is increased. The short, straight eustachian tube closely communicates with the ear, allowing infection to ascend from the pharynx to the middle ear. In addition, the inability of the immune system to produce *immunoglobulin A* (IgA) in the mucosal lining provides less protection against infection in infancy than during later childhood.

The *heart* rate slows (see inside back cover) and frequently

David Wilson, MS, RNC, revised this chapter.

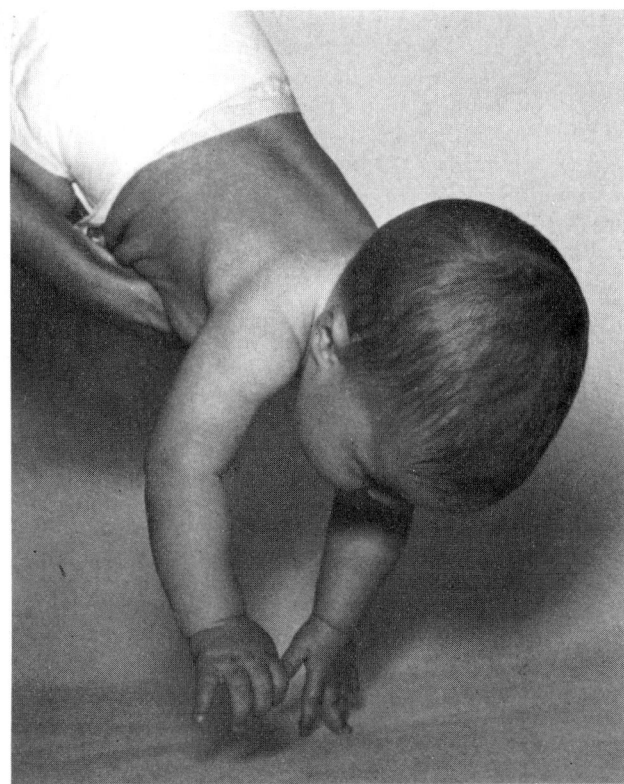

FIG. 10-1. Parachute reflex.

displays *sinus arrhythmia* (rate increases with inspiration and decreases with expiration). Blood pressure also changes during infancy (see inside back cover). Systolic pressure rises during the first 2 months as a result of the increasing ability of the left ventricle to pump blood into the systemic circulation. Diastolic pressure decreases during the first 3 months and then gradually rises to values close to those at birth. Fluctuations in blood pressure occur during varying states of activity and emotion.

Significant *hemopoietic changes* occur during the first year (see Appendix E). *Fetal hemoglobin (HgF)* is the primary hemoglobin for the first 2 to 3 months, with adult hemoglobin steadily increasing through the first half of infancy. Fetal hemoglobin results in a shortened survival of red blood cells (RBCs) and thus a decreased number of RBCs. A common result at 2 to 3 months of age is *physiologic anemia*. High levels of HgF are thought to depress the production of *erythropoietin,* a hormone released by the kidney that stimulates RBC production.

Maternal iron stores are present for the first 5 to 6 months and then gradually diminish, which also accounts for lowered hemoglobin levels toward the end of the first 6 months. The occurrence of physiologic anemia is not affected by an adequate supply of iron. However, when erythropoiesis is stimulated, iron supplies are necessary for formation of hemoglobin.

The *digestive processes* are immature at birth. Saliva is secreted in small amounts, but the majority of all digestive processes do not begin functioning until age 3 months, when drooling is common because of the poorly coordinated swallowing reflex. The enzyme *ptyalin* (also called *amylase*) is present in small amounts but usually has little effect on the foodstuff because of the small amount of time the food stays in the mouth. Digestion in the stomach consists primarily of the action of hydrochloric acid and rennin, an enzyme that acts specifically on the casein in milk to form curds, which are coagulated semisolid particles of milk. The curds cause the milk to be retained in the stomach long enough for digestion to occur.

Digestion also takes place in the duodenum, where pancreatic enzymes and bile begin to break down protein and fat. Secretion of the pancreatic enzyme *amylase,* which is needed for digestion of complex carbohydrates, is deficient until about the fourth to sixth month of life. *Lipase* is also limited, and infants do not achieve adult levels of fat absorption until 4 to 5 months of age. *Trypsin* is secreted in sufficient quantities to catabolize protein into polypeptides and some amino acids.

The immaturity of the digestive processes is evident in the appearance of stools. During infancy solid foods, such as peas, carrots, corn, and raisins, are passed incompletely broken down in the feces. An excess quantity of fiber disposes the child to loose, bulky stools. Breast-fed infants have twice as many stools as formula-fed infants.

Throughout infancy the stomach enlarges to accommodate a greater volume of food. By the end of the first year the infant is able to tolerate three meals a day and a before-bedtime feeding (breast or bottle), and may have one or two bowel movements daily. However, with any type of gastric irritation, the infant is vulnerable to diarrhea, vomiting, and dehydration (see Chapter 24).

Paralleling the ability of the gastrointestinal system to digest and absorb more complex foodstuff is the process of tooth eruption. *Tooth eruption* occurs in a fairly orderly sequence beginning at about 6 to 7 months of age (see discussion of teething on p. 307).

The *liver* is the most immature of all the gastrointestinal organs throughout infancy. The ability to conjugate bilirubin and to secrete bile is achieved after the first couple of weeks of life. However, the capacities for *gluconeogenesis,* formation of plasma protein and ketones, storage of vitamins, and deaminization of amino acids remain relatively immature for the first year of life.

The *immunologic system* undergoes numerous changes during the first year. The newborn receives significant amounts of maternal IgG, which confers immunity for about 3 months against antigens to which the mother was exposed. During this time the infant begins to synthesize IgG, and about 40% of adult levels are reached by 1 year of age. Significant amounts of IgM are produced at birth, and adult levels are reached by 9 months of age. The production of IgA is much more gradual, and maximum levels are not attained until puberty.

During infancy *thermoregulation* becomes more efficient as the ability of the skin to contract and muscles to shiver in response to cold increases. The peripheral capillaries respond to change in ambient temperature to regulate heat loss. In response to cold the capillaries constrict, conserving core body temperature and decreasing potential evaporative heat loss from the skin surface. In response to heat the capillaries dilate, decreasing internal body temperature through evaporation, conduction, and convection. Shivering *(shivering thermogenesis)* causes the muscles and muscle fibers to contract, generating metabolic heat, which is distributed throughout the body. Accumulation of adipose tissue during the first 6 months serves to insulate the body against heat loss.

At birth 75% of the infant's *body weight* is water and there is an excess of extracellular fluid (ECF). As the percentage of body water decreases, so does the amount of ECF—from 40% at term to 20% in adulthood. The high proportion of ECF, which is composed of blood plasma, interstitial fluid, and lymph, predisposes the infant to a more rapid loss of total body fluid and consequently dehydration.

The immaturity of the *renal structures* also predisposes the infant to dehydration. Complete maturity of the kidney occurs during the latter half of the second year, when the cuboidal epithelium of the glomeruli becomes flattened. Before this time the filtration capacity of the glomeruli is reduced. Urine is voided frequently and has a low specific gravity (1.000 to 1.010).

Auditory acuity is at adult levels during infancy. Visual acuity begins to improve, and binocular fixation is established. *Binocularity,* or the fixation of two ocular images into one cerebral picture *(fusion),* begins to develop by 6 weeks of age and should be well established by age 4 months. *Depth perception (stereopsis)* begins to develop by age 7 to 9 months but may exist earlier as an innate safety mechanism against accidental falling.

Fine Motor Behavior

Fine motor behavior includes the use of the hands and fingers in the prehension (grasp) of an object. Grasping occurs during the first 2 to 3 months as a reflex and gradually becomes voluntary. At 1 month the hands are predominantly closed and by 3 months are mostly open. By this time in-

fants demonstrate a desire to grasp an object, but they "grasp" it more with the eyes than with the hands. If a rattle is placed in the hand, the infant will actively hold onto it. By 4 months the infant regards both a small pellet and the hands and looks from the object to the hands and back again. By 5 months the infant is able to voluntarily grasp an object.

Gradually the palmar grasp (using the whole hand) is replaced with a pincer grasp (using the thumb and index finger). By 8 to 9 months the infant uses a crude pincer grasp but by 11 months has progressed to a neat pincer grasp (Fig. 10-2).

By 6 months infants have increased manipulative skill. They hold their bottle, grasp feet and pull them to the mouth, and feed themselves a cracker. By 7 months they transfer objects from one hand to the other, use one hand for grasping, and hold a cube in each hand simultaneously. They enjoy banging objects and will explore the movable parts of a toy.

By 10 months the pincer grasp is sufficiently established to enable infants to pick up a raisin and other finger foods. They can deliberately let go of an object and will offer it to someone. By 11 months they put objects into a container and like to remove them. By 1 year infants try to build a tower of two blocks but fail.

Gross Motor Development

Head Control. The full-term newborn can momentarily hold the head in midline and parallel when the body is suspended ventrally and can lift and turn the head from side to side when prone (see Fig. 8-7). This is not the case when the infant is lying prone on a pillow or soft surface; infants do not have the head control to lift their head out of the depression of the object and therefore risk suffocation (see Sudden Infant Death Syndrome, Chapter 11). However, marked head lag is evident when the infant is pulled from a lying to a sitting position. By 3 months of age infants can hold their

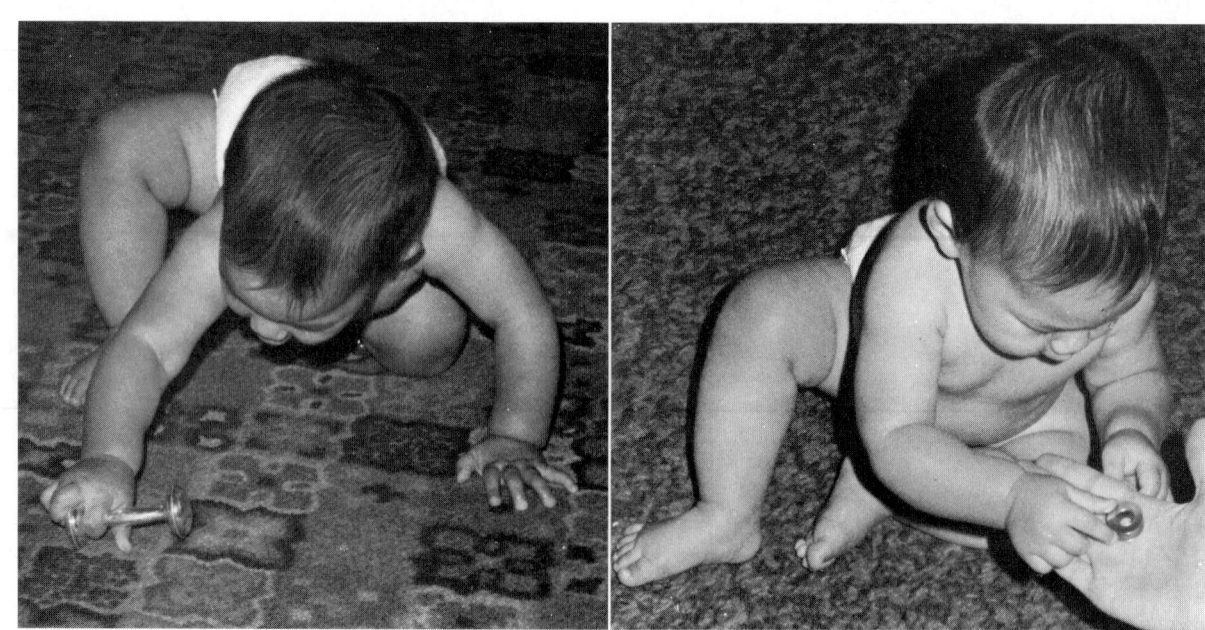

FIG. 10-2. A, Crude pincer grasp at 8 to 10 months. **B,** Neat pincer grasp at 10 to 11 months.

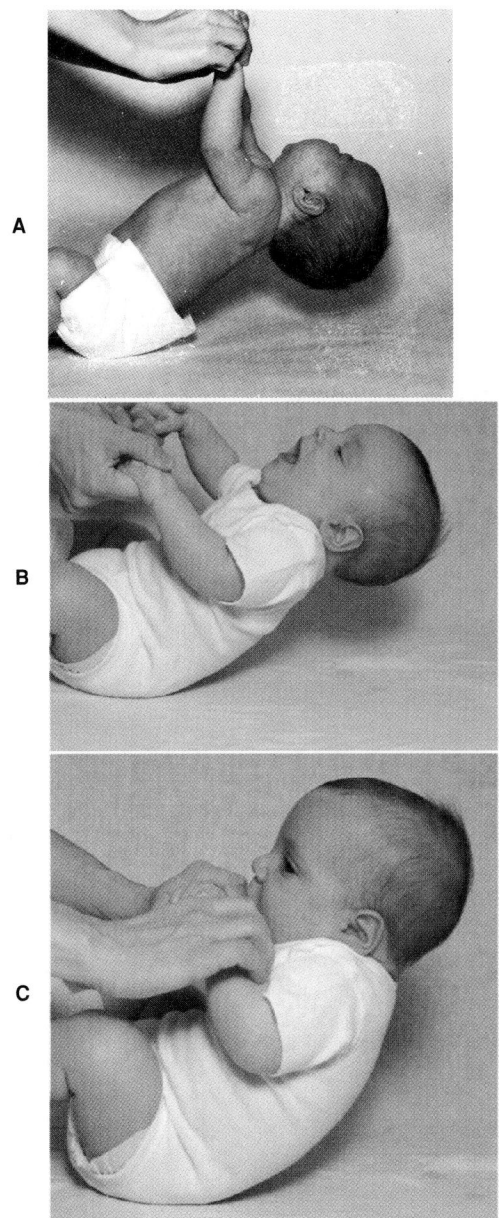

FIG. 10-3. Head control while pulled to sitting position. **A,** Complete head lag at 1 month. **B,** Partial head lag at 2 months. **C,** Almost no head lag at 4 months.

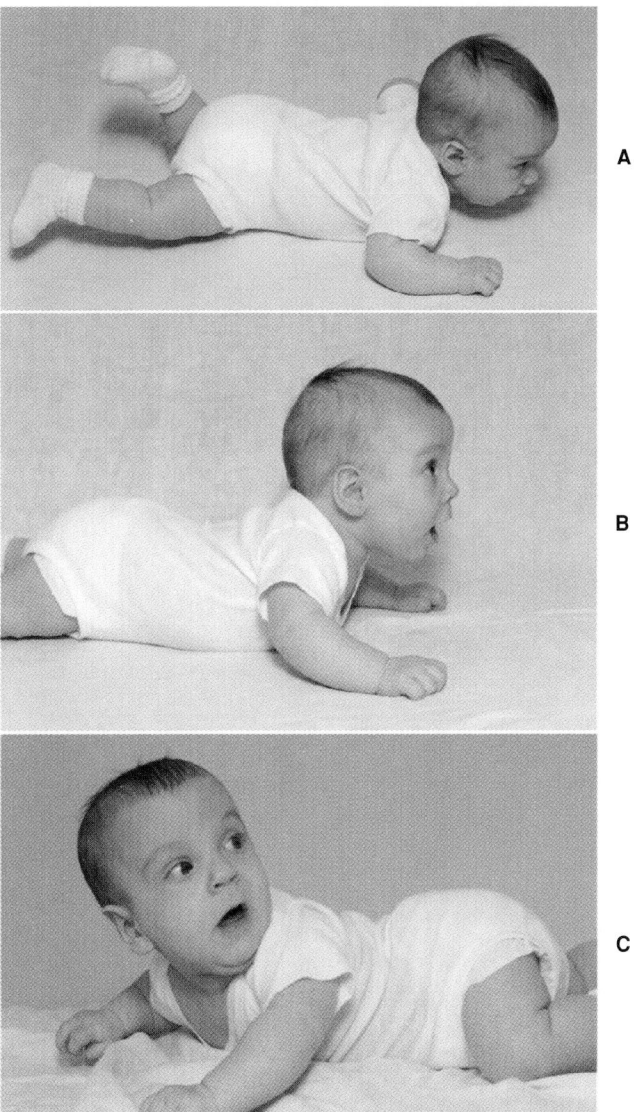

FIG. 10-4. Head control while prone. **A,** Infant momentarily lifts head at 1 month. **B,** Infant lifts head and chest 90 degrees and bears weight on forearms at 4 months. **C,** Infant lifts head, chest, and upper abdomen and can bear weight on hands at 6 months. Note how this position facilitates turning from abdomen to back.

head well beyond the plane of the body, and by 4 months of age they can lift the head and front portion of the chest about 90 degrees above the table, bearing their weight on the forearms. Only slight head lag is evident when the infant is pulled from a lying to a sitting position, and by 4 to 6 months head control is well established (Figs. 10-3 and 10-4).

| **Nursing ALERT** | Any child who displays head lag at 6 months of age should have a developmental/neurologic evaluation. |

Rolling Over. Newborns may roll over accidentally because of their rounded back. The ability to willfully turn from the abdomen to the back occurs at 5 months and from the back to the abdomen at 6 months. It is noteworthy that the parachute reflex (see Fig. 10-1), which elicits a protective response to falling, appears at 7 months.

Sitting. The ability to sit follows progressive head control and straightening of the back as shown in Fig. 10-5. For the first 2 to 3 months the back is uniformly rounded. The convex cervical curve forms at about 3 to 4 months when head control is established. The convex lumbar curve appears when the child begins to sit, at about age 4 months. As the spinal column straightens, the infant can be propped in a sitting position. By age 7 months infants can sit alone, leaning

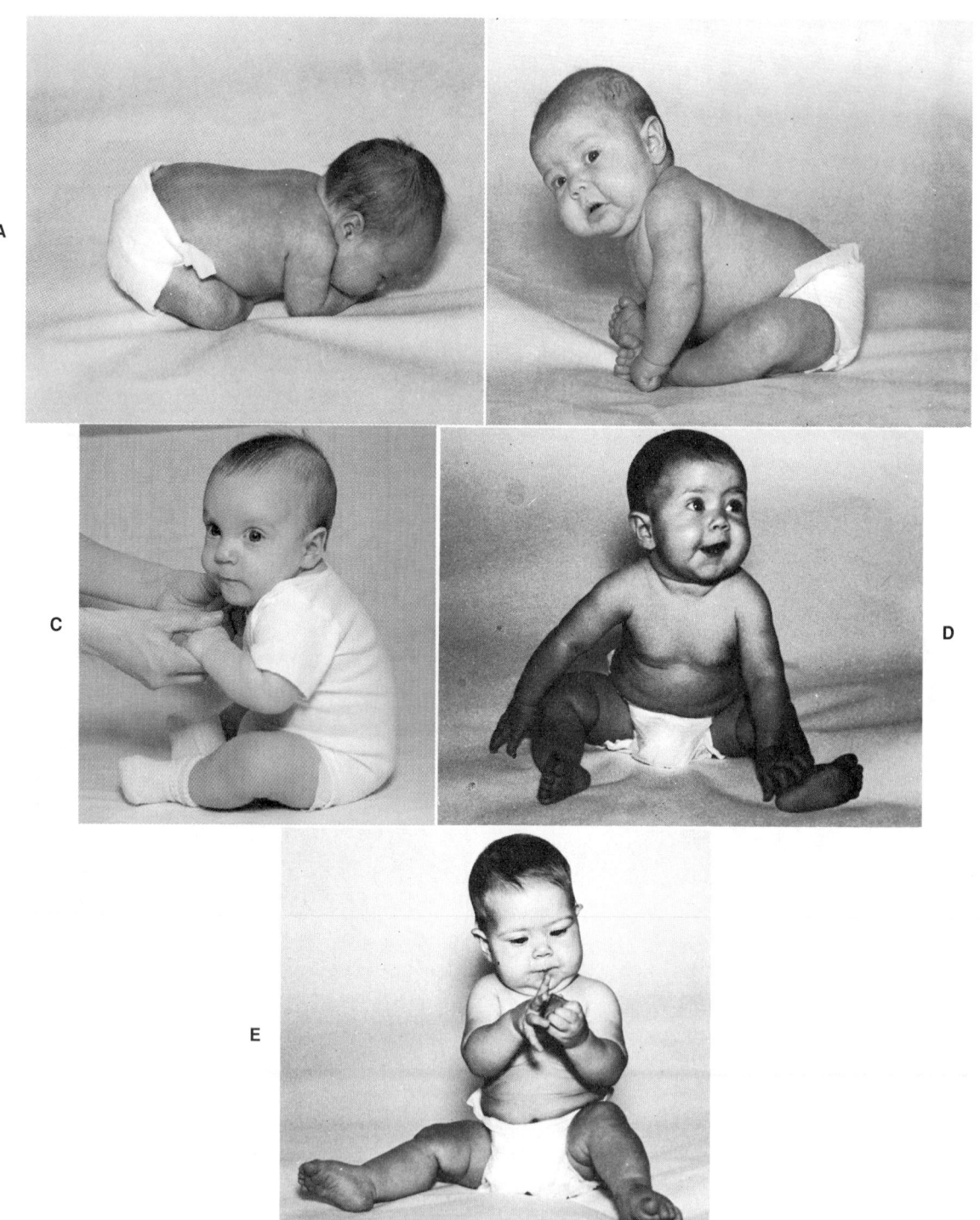

FIG. 10-5. Development of sitting. **A,** Back is completely rounded, and infant has no ability to sit upright at 1 month. **B,** Back is still rounded, but infant can sit up momentarily with some head control at 2 months. **C,** Back is rounded only in lumbar area, and infant is able to sit erect with good head control at 4 months. **D,** Infant can sit alone, leaning on hands for support, at 7 months. **E,** Infant sits without support at 8 months. Note the transferring of objects that occurs at 7 months.

forward on their hands for support. By age 8 months they can sit well unsupported and begin to explore their surroundings in this position rather than in a lying position. By 10 months they can maneuver from a prone to a sitting position.

Locomotion.   Locomotion involves acquiring the ability to bear weight, propel forward on all four extremities, stand upright with support, and finally walk alone (Fig. 10-6). Following a *cephalocaudal* pattern, infants 4 to 6 months old have increasing coordination in their arms. Initial locomotion results in infants propelling themselves backward by pushing with the arms. By 6 to 7 months infants are able to bear all their weight on their legs, with assistance. *Crawling* (propelling forward with belly on floor) progresses to *creeping* on hands and knees (with belly off floor) by 9 months. At this time they stand while holding onto furniture and can pull themselves to the standing position but are unable to maneuver back down, except by falling. By 11 months they walk

while holding onto furniture or with both hands held, and by 1 year they may be able to walk with one hand held. A number of infants attempt their first independent steps by their first birthday.

PSYCHOSOCIAL DEVELOPMENT

Developing a Sense of Trust (Erikson)

Erikson's phase I (birth to 1 year) is concerned with *acquiring a sense of trust* while overcoming a sense of *mistrust.* The trust that develops is a trust of self, of others, and of the world. Infants "trust" that their feeding, comfort, stimulation, and caring needs will be met. The crucial element for the achievement of this task is the *quality* of both the parent (caregiver)—child relationship and the care the infant receives. The provision of food, warmth, and shelter by itself is inadequate for the development of a strong sense of self. The infant and parent must jointly learn to satisfactorily meet their

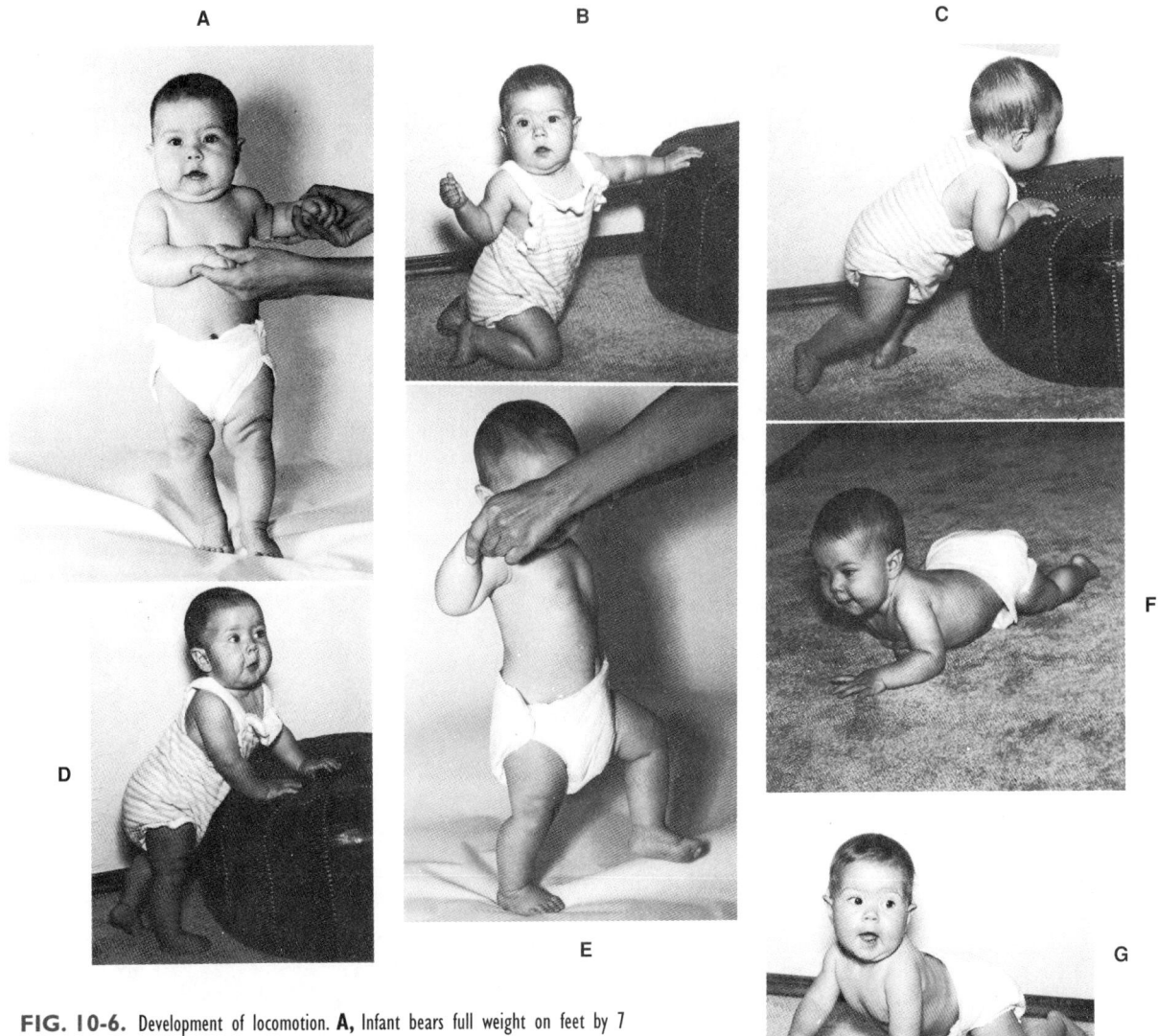

FIG. 10-6. Development of locomotion. **A,** Infant bears full weight on feet by 7 months. **B,** Infant can maneuver from sitting to kneeling position. **C,** Infant can pull self to standing position and **D,** can stand holding onto furniture at 9 months. **E,** While standing, infant takes deliberate step at 10 months. **F,** Infant crawls with abdomen on floor and pulls self forward, and then, **G,** creeps on hands and knees at 9 months.

needs in order for mutual regulation of frustration to occur. When this synchrony fails to develop, mistrust is the eventual outcome.

Failure to learn "delayed gratification" leads to mistrust. It can result from too much or too little frustration. If parents always meet their children's needs before the children signal their readiness, infants will never learn to test their ability to control the environment. If the delay is prolonged, infants will experience constant frustration and eventually mistrust others in their efforts to satisfy them. Therefore, consistency of care is essential.

The trust acquired in infancy is foundational for all the succeeding phases. It allows infants a feeling of physical comfort and security, which assists them in experiencing unfamiliar, unknown situations with a minimum of fear. Erikson has divided the first year of life into two oral/social stages. During the first 3 to 4 months, food intake is the most important social activity in which the infant engages. The newborn can tolerate little frustration or delay of gratification. Primary *narcissism* (total concern for oneself) is at its height.

However, as bodily processes such as vision, motor movements, and vocalization are better controlled, infants use more advanced behaviors to interact with others. For example, rather than crying, infants may put their arms up to signify a desire to be held.

The next social modality involves a mode of reaching out to others through *grasping.* Initially grasping is reflexive, but even as a reflex it has a powerful social meaning for the parents. The reciprocal response to the infant's grasping is the parents' holding on and touching. There is pleasurable tactile stimulation for both the child and the parents.

Tactile stimulation is extremely important in the total process of acquiring trust. The degree of mothering skill, the quantity of food, or the length of sucking does not determine the quality of the experience. Rather, it is the total nature of the quality of the interpersonal relationship that influences the infant's formulation of trust.

During the second stage, the more active and aggressive modality of *biting* occurs. Infants learn that they can hold onto what is their own and can more fully control their environment. During this stage infants may be confronted with one of their first conflicts. If they are breast-feeding, they quickly learn that biting causes withdrawal of the nipple and anxiety in the mother. Yet biting also brings internal relief from teething discomfort and a sense of power or control.

This conflict may be solved in a variety of ways. The mother may wean the infant from the breast and begin bottle-feeding, or the infant may learn to bite substitute "nipples," such as a pacifier, and retain pleasurable breast-feeding. The successful resolution of this conflict strengthens the mother-child relationship because it occurs at a time when infants are recognizing mother as the most significant person in their life.

COGNITIVE DEVELOPMENT

The Sensorimotor Phase (Piaget)

The theory most frequently used to explain *cognition,* or the ability to know, is that of Piaget. The period of birth to 24 months is termed the sensorimotor phase and is composed of six stages; however, inasmuch as this discussion is concerned with ages birth to 12 months, only the first four stages are discussed. The last two stages occur during the toddler period of 12 to 24 months and are discussed in Chapter 12.

During the sensorimotor phase the infant progresses from reflex behavior to simple repetitive acts to imitative activity. Three crucial events take place during this phase.

The first event involves *separation;* infants learn to separate themselves from other objects in the environment. They realize that others besides themselves control the environment and that certain readjustments must take place for mutual satisfaction to occur. This coincides with Erikson's concept of the formation of trust and mutual regulation of frustration.

The second major accomplishment is achieving the concept of *object permanence,* or the realization that objects that leave one's visual field still exist. A typical example of the development of object permanence is when infants are able to pursue objects they observe being hidden under a pillow or behind a chair (Fig. 10-7). This skill develops at approximately 9 to 10 months of age, which also corresponds to the time of increased locomotion skills.

The last major intellectual development of this period is the ability to use *symbols* or *"mental representation."* The use of symbols allows the infant to think of an object or situation without actually experiencing it. The recognition of symbols is the beginning of understanding time and space.

The four stages of Piaget's theory of cognitive development that affect infants are as follows:

Stage I: Use of reflexes. The first stage, from birth to 1 month, is identified by the *use of reflexes.* At birth the infant's individuality and temperament are expressed through the physiologic reflexes of sucking, rooting, grasping, and crying. The repetitious nature of the reflexes, along with the continuing myelinization of the brain, are the beginning of associations between an act and a sequential response. When infants cry because of hunger, a nipple is put in the mouth, and they suck, feel satisfaction, and sleep.

Stage II: Primary circular reactions. This stage marks the beginning of the replacement of reflexive behavior with voluntary acts.

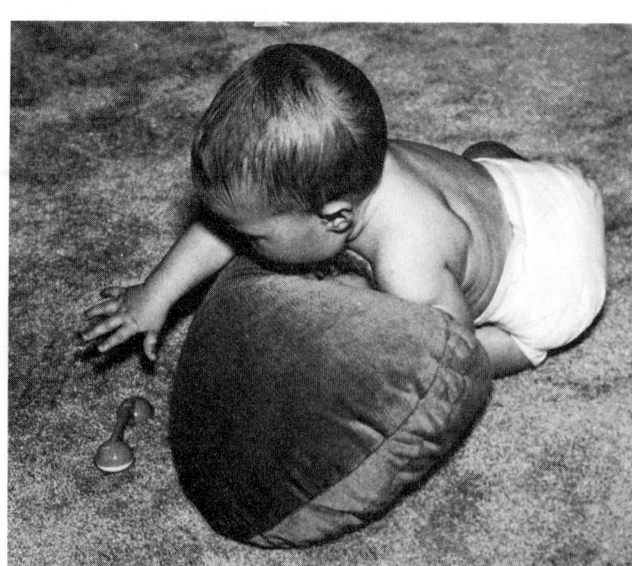

FIG. 10-7. Nine-month-old infant actively searches for object hidden behind pillow.

During this period from 1 to 4 months, activities such as sucking or grasping become deliberate acts that elicit certain responses. Infants incorporate and adapt their reactions to the environment and recognize the stimulus that produced a response. Previously they would cry until the nipple was brought to the mouth. Now they associate the nipple with the sound of the parent's voice. They accommodate this new piece of information and adapt by ceasing to cry when they hear the voice, before they receive the nipple.

Stage III: Secondary circular reactions. The third stage is a continuation of the previous one and lasts until 8 months of age. In this stage the circular primary reactions are intentionally repeated and prolonged for the response that results. Grasping and holding now become shaking, banging, and pulling. Shaking is performed to hear a noise, not solely for the pleasure of shaking. The quality and quantity of an act become evident. "More" or "less" shaking produces different responses. Causality, time, deliberate intention, and one's separateness from the environment begin to develop.

Three new processes of human behavior—imitation, play, and affect—occur. *Imitation* requires the differentiation of behaviors. By the second half of the first year, the infant can imitate sounds and simple gestures. *Play* becomes evident as the infant takes pleasure in performing a mastered act. Many of the infant's waking hours are absorbed in sensorimotor play. *Affect,* an outward manifestation of emotion and feeling, is seen as the infant develops.

Object permanence begins to develop at this time. During the first 6 months infants believe that an object exists only for as long as they can visually perceive it. In other words, out of sight, out of mind. When the object continues to be present or remembered even though it is beyond the range of perception, affect to external objects is evident. Object permanence is a critical component of parent-child attachment and is seen in the development of stranger anxiety at 6 to 8 months of age (p. 296).

Stage IV: Coordination of secondary schemata and its application to new situations. During the fourth sensorimotor stage, infants use previous behavioral achievements primarily as the foundation for adding new intellectual skills to their expanding repertoire. This stage from 9 to 12 months is largely transitional. Increasing motor skills allow for greater exploration of the environment. The child begins to discover that hiding an object does not mean that it is gone and that removing an obstacle will reveal the object (see Fig. 10-7). This marks the beginning of intellectual reasoning. Furthermore, they can experience an event by *observing* it, and they begin to associate symbols with events, such as "bye-bye" with "Daddy goes to work," but the classification is purely their own. Unlike the second stage, where the infant learned from the type of interaction between objects or individuals, in this stage the child learns from the object itself. Intentionality is further developed in that now infants will actively attempt to remove a barrier to their desired (or undesired) action. If something is in their way, they will attempt to climb over it or push it away. Previously an obstacle would cause them to give up any further attempt to achieve their desired goal.

DEVELOPMENT OF BODY IMAGE

The development of body image parallels sensorimotor development. Infants' kinesthetic and tactile experiences are the first perceptions of their body, and the mouth is the principal area of pleasurable sensations. Other parts of the body are primarily objects of pleasure—the hands and fingers to suck and the feet to play with. As physical needs are met, they feel comfort and satisfaction with their body. Verbal and nonverbal (touch) messages conveyed by the caregivers reinforce these feelings. For example, when infants smile, they receive emotional satisfaction from others who smile back.

The development of object permanence is basic to the de-

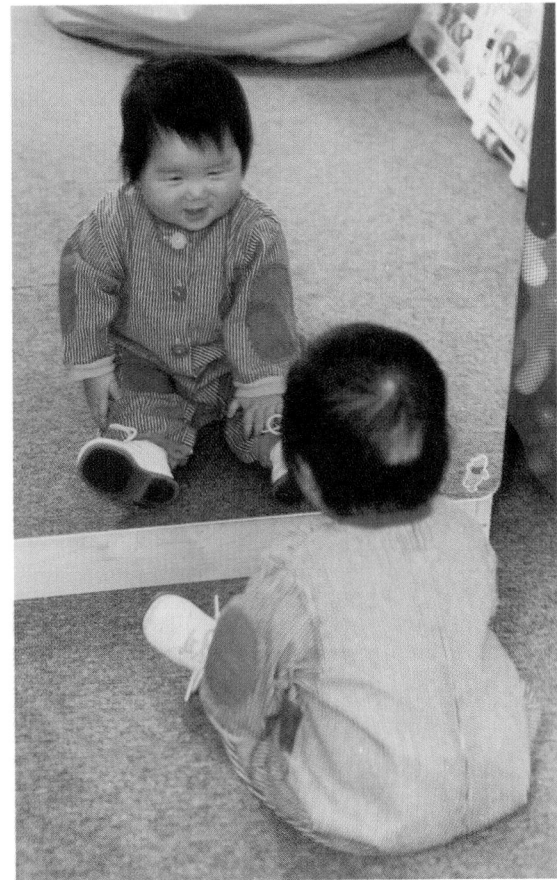

FIG. 10-8. Nine-month-old infant enjoying own image in mirror.

velopment of self-image. By the end of the first year infants recognize that they are distinct from their parents. At the same time, there is increasing interest in their image, especially in the mirror (Fig. 10-8). As motor skills develop, they learn that parts of the body are useful; for example, the hands bring objects to the mouth and the legs help them move to different locations. All of these achievements transmit messages to them about themselves. It is therefore important to transmit positive messages to infants about their bodies.

SOCIAL DEVELOPMENT

Infants' social development is initially influenced by their reflexive behavior, such as the grasp, and eventually depends primarily on the interaction between them and the principal caregivers. *Attachment* to the parent is increasingly evident during the second half of the first year. In addition, tremendous strides are made in communication and personal-social behavior. Whereas crying and reflexive behavior are methods to meet one's needs in the neonatal period, the social smile is an early step in social communication. This has a profound effect on family members and is a tremendous stimulus for evoking continued responses from others. By 4 months infants laugh aloud.

Play is a major socializing agent and provides stimulation needed to learn from and interact with the environment. By age 6 months infants are very personable. They play games such as peekaboo when their head is hidden in a towel; they signal their desire to be picked up by extending their arms; and they show displeasure when a toy is removed or their face is washed.

Attachment

Several components are crucial in the process of attachment. Some of them, such as the maternal sensitive period and paternal engrossment, are discussed in Chapter 8 and emphasize the importance of the first hour and days of life. The following is a discussion of attachment after the neonatal period. Although the word "mother" is frequently used, it does not refer exclusively to the biologic mother but to the consistent caregiver with whom the child relates more than anyone else. In light of the changing social climate, this may very well be the father. Studies on father-child attachment demonstrate that similar stages occur as with mother attachment, and that fathers are more involved in child care when mothers are employed (although mothers continue to do the majority of infant care) (Jones and Heermann, 1992).

During infancy attachment progresses with the child assuming an increasingly significant role. Two components of cognitive development are required for attachment: (1) the ability to discriminate the mother from other individuals and (2) the achievement of object permanence. Both these processes prepare the infant for an equally important aspect of attachment—separation from the parent.

During the formation of attachment to the parent, the infant progresses through four distinct but overlapping stages. For the first few weeks infants respond indiscriminately to anyone. Attachment is facilitated by eye contact during feedings and being held close to the caregiver's body. Beginning at about 8 to 12 weeks of age, infants cry, smile, and vocalize more to the mother than to anyone else but continue to respond to others, whether familiar or not. At about age 6 months infants show a distinct preference for the mother. They follow her more, cry when she leaves, enjoy playing with her more, and feel most secure in her arms. About 1 month after showing attachment to the mother, many infants begin attaching to other members of the family, most often the father.

Infants acquire other developmental behaviors that influence the attachment process. These include (1) differential crying, smiling, and vocalization (more to mother than to anyone else); (2) visual-motor orientation (looking more at mother even if she is not close); (3) crying when mother leaves the room; (4) approach through locomotion (crawling, creeping, or walking); (5) clinging (especially in presence of a stranger); and (6) exploring away from mother while using her as a secure base.

Stranger Anxiety. As infants develop the ability to differentiate among individuals, they learn to identify their mother or other primary caregiver from other individuals by 5 to 6 months of age. This cognitive awareness results in a preference for "mother" and is demonstrated by behaviors typical of stranger anxiety, such as clinging to the parent, crying, and turning away from the stranger (Fig. 10-9).

Family members, such as grandparents, often describe this behavior as an indication that the child is "spoiled." This is not the case. This process results from improving cognitive

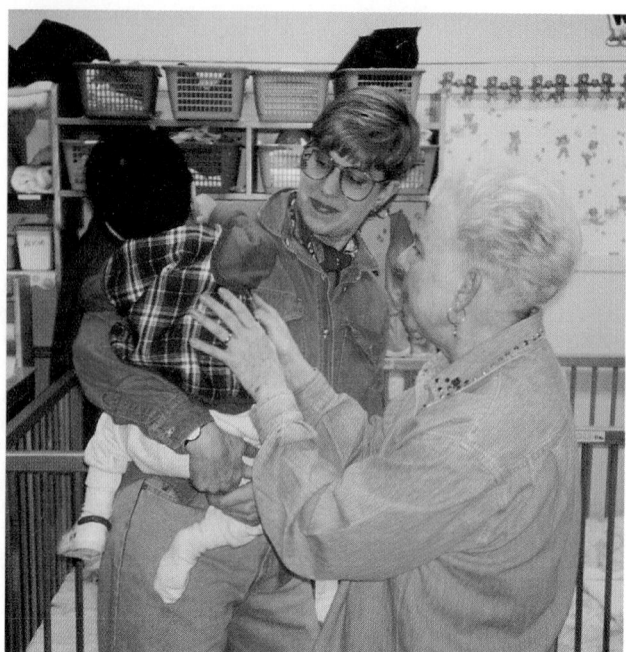

FIG. 10-9. Behaviors related to fear of strangers include clinging to the parent and turning away from the stranger.

development and peaks at 8 months of age. Because object permanence is just beginning to develop, infants may not notice the mother's absence if they are absorbed in an activity. However, when they realize her absence, they protest. From this point onward they become very alert to her activities and whereabouts.

Along with stranger anxiety, the child develops an anxiety related to separation from mother. This manifests itself by later infancy and lasts throughout early toddlerhood. By 11 to 12 months infants are able to anticipate the mother's imminent departure by watching her behaviors and begin to protest *before* she leaves. At this point many parents learn to postpone alerting the child to their departure until just before leaving.

Language Development

The infant's first means of verbal communication is crying. They learn to signal displeasure before pleasure. Many parents state that they can distinguish between different types of crying and from these messages are able to interpret the infant's needs. However, crying can be a source of acute distress for parents, especially the unconsolable crying of colic (see Chapter 11). Parents benefit from an explanation of the variability of crying among infants and assurance that periods of "unexplained fussiness" are normal. Some parents may need guidance in consoling techniques, such as holding, swaddling, massaging, caressing, rocking, walking, or stimulating sucking. During the end of the first year infants cry for attention, from fear, especially stranger fear, and from frustration, usually in response to their developing but inadequate motor skills.

Vocalizations heard during crying eventually become some

FAMILY FOCUS
Child's Developing Language Skills

During the acquisition of new language skills the child temporarily may give up other recently learned sounds or words. This is often distressing for parents, who have waited in anticipation for the words "dada" or "mama," since these sounds are frequently replaced by other vocalizations and may not be repeated for several weeks. Nurses should reassure parents that the child will again say these special words, and with increased meaning.

Nursing ALERT Be alert to parent reports about maternal postpartum depression and infant crying because these concerns may indicate a stressed mother-infant relationship (Miller, Barr, and Eaton, 1993).

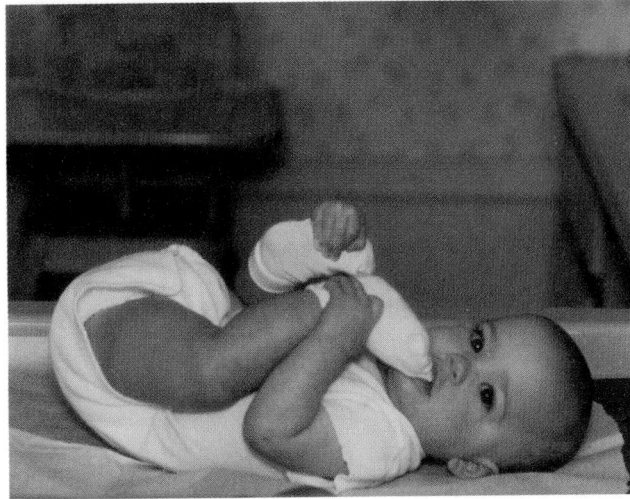

FIG. 10-10. During early infancy body parts are primarily objects of pleasure for the child.

syllables and words (e.g., the "mama" heard during vigorous crying). Infants vocalize as early as 5 to 6 weeks of age by making small throaty sounds. By 2 months they make single vowel sounds, such as *ah, eh,* and *uh.* By 3 to 4 months the consonants *n, k, g, p,* and *b* are added, and infants coo, gurgle, and laugh aloud. By 8 months they imitate sounds, add the consonants *t, d,* and *w,* and combine syllables, such as "dada," but they do not ascribe meaning to the word until 10 to 11 months of age (see Family Focus box). By 9 to 10 months they comprehend the meaning of the word "no" and obey simple commands. By age 1 year they can say three to five words with meaning.

Play

Play mirrors all the developmental tasks and allows children to experiment safely with their newly learned skills. Play during infancy represents the various social and cognitive modalities proposed by Erikson and Piaget. From shortly after birth, the senses of hearing and touch are the only ones fully developed. Therefore stimulation is geared to them. Being held or rocked and listening to a musical mobile are ideal at this time.

Infants' activity is primarily narcissistic, revolving around their own body. At 2 months of age infants will look at their extended hand as if it were an unfamiliar object. At about age 6 months infants play with their feet and find fingers excellent nipple substitutes (Fig. 10-10). During this time the ability to grasp is well under voluntary control, and everything is reached for and brought to the mouth for inquisitive exploration. When the pincer grasp is mastered, infants are absorbed with growing independence, refusing to allow others to feed them.

Play reflects infants' social development and their increasing awareness of the environment. From birth to age 3 months the infant's response to the environment is global and largely undifferentiated. Play is dependent; pleasure is demonstrated by a quieting attitude (age 1 month), later by a smile (age 2 to 3 months), and then by a squeal (age 3 to 4 months). By age 3 to 6 months infants show more discriminate interest in the stimuli presented to them and begin to play alone with a rattle or soft stuffed toy or to play with someone else. There is much more interaction during play. By 4 months of age they laugh aloud, show preference for

certain toys, and are excited when food or a favorite object is brought to them.

By 6 months to 1 year of age, play is more sophisticated and involves sensorimotor skills. Actual games are played, such as peekaboo, pat-a-cake, verbal repetition, and imitation of simple gestures in response to demonstration. Play is much more selective, not only in terms of specific toys but also in terms of "playmates." Although play is solitary or one-sided, infants choose with whom they will interact. At 6 to 8 months of age they usually refuse to play with strangers until they begin to know them. Parents are definite favorites and infants know how to attract their attention.

Stimulation is as important for developmental growth as food is for biologic growth. Knowledge of developmental milestones allows nurses to guide parents regarding proper play for infants. It is not sufficient to place a mobile over a crib and toys in a playpen for a child's optimum social, emotional, and intellectual development. Play must provide interpersonal contact, as well as recreational and educational stimulation. Infants need to be *played with,* not merely allowed to *play.* Although the type of play infants engage in is called *solitary,* this is a figurative, not literal, term to denote one-sided play. The kind of toys given to the child is much less important than the quality of personal interaction that occurs.

Table 10-1 lists play activities that are appropriate for the developmental level of the infant in view of motor, language, and personal-social achievements. Although the activities are grouped according to the major mode of stimulation provided, there is overlap in many instances. In addition, play activities suggested for one age-group may be appropriate for an older age-group but are generally inappropriate for a younger age-group. The most important component of play is safety.

TEMPERAMENT

The infant's temperament or behavioral style influences the kind of interaction that occurs between the child and parents

TABLE 10-1. Play during infancy

AGE (MONTHS)	VISUAL STIMULATION	AUDITORY STIMULATION	TACTILE STIMULATION	KINETIC STIMULATION
Suggested Activities				
Birth-1	Look at infant at close range Hang bright, shiny object within 20-25 cm (8-10 inches) of infant's face and in midline Hang mobiles with black-and-white contrast designs	Talk to infant, sing in soft voice Play music box, radio, television Have ticking clock or metronome nearby	Hold, caress, cuddle Keep infant warm May like to be swaddled	Rock infant, place in cradle Use carriage for walks
2-3	Provide bright objects Make room bright with pictures or mirrors on walls Take infant to various rooms while doing chores Place infant in infant seat for vertical view of environment	Talk to infant Include in family gatherings Expose to various environmental noises other than those of home Use rattles, wind chimes	Caress infant while bathing, at diaper change Comb hair with a soft brush	Use infant swing Take in car for rides Exercise body by moving extremities in swimming motion Use cradle gym
4-6	Place infant in front of unbreakable mirror Give brightly colored toys to hold (small enough to grasp)	Talk to infant, repeat sounds infant makes Laugh when infant laughs Call infant by name Crinkle different papers by infant's ear Place rattle or bell in hand	Give infant soft squeeze toys of various textures Allow to splash in bath Place nude on soft furry rug and move extremities	Use swing or stroller Bounce infant in lap while holding in standing position Support infant in sitting position, let infant lean forward to balance self Place infant on floor to crawl, roll over, sit
6-9	Give infant large toys with bright colors, movable parts, and noisemakers Place unbreakable mirror where infant can see self Play peekaboo, especially hiding face in a towel Make funny faces to encourage imitation Give ball of yarn or string to pull apart	Call infant by name Repeat simple words such as "dada," "mama," "bye-bye" Speak clearly Name parts of body, people, and foods Tell infant what you are doing Use "no" only when necessary Give simple commands Show how to clap hands, bang a drum	Let infant play with fabrics of various textures Have bowl with foods of different size and textures to feel Let infant "catch" running water Encourage "swimming" in large bathtub or shallow pool Give wad of sticky tape to manipulate	Hold upright to bear weight and bounce Pick up, say "up" Put down, say "down" Place toys out of reach; encourage infant to get them Play pat-a-cake
6-12	Show infant large pictures in books Take infant to places where there are animals, many people, different objects (shopping center) Play ball by rolling it to child, demonstrate "throwing" it back Demonstrate building a two-block tower	Read infant simple nursery rhymes Point to body parts and name each one Imitate sounds of animals	Give infant finger foods of different textures Let infant mess and squash food Let infant feel cold (ice cube) or warm objects; say what temperature each is Let infant feel a breeze (fan blowing)	Give large push-pull toys Place furniture in a circle to encourage cruising Turn in different positions
Suggested Toys				
Birth-6	Nursery mobiles Unbreakable mirrors See-through crib bumpers Contrasting colored sheets	Music boxes Musical mobiles Crib dangle bells Small-handled clear rattle	Stuffed animals Soft clothes Soft or furry quilt Soft mobiles	Rocking crib/cradle Weighted or suction toy Infant swing (wind-up)

TABLE 10-1.	Play during infancy—cont'd			
AGE (MONTHS)	VISUAL STIMULATION	AUDITORY STIMULATION	TACTILE STIMULATION	KINETIC STIMULATION
Suggested Toys—cont'd				
6-12	Various colored blocks Nested boxes or cups Books with rhymes and bright pictures Strings of big beads Simple take-apart toys Large ball Cup and spoon Large puzzles Jack-in-the box	Rattles of different sizes, shapes, tones, and bright colors Squeaky animals and dolls Records with light, rhythmic music	Soft, different-textured animals and dolls Sponge toys, floating toys Squeeze toys Teething toys Books with textures and objects, such as fur and zipper	Push-pull toys Baby swing (wind-up) Activity box for crib

and other family members (see general discussion of temperament in Chapter 5). In assessing a child's temperament, it is the parents' perception of the child and the degree of *fit* between their expectations and the child's actual temperament that are important. The more dissonance or lack of harmony between the child's temperament and the parent's ability to accept and deal with the behavior, the more risk for subsequent parent-child conflicts.

The *Infant Temperament Questionnaire (ITQ)* (Carey and McDevitt, 1978) can be used as a screening tool with parents. The questionnaire focuses on nine temperament variables, but the 95 questions relate specifically to activities such as sleep, feeding, play, diapering, and dressing. The scores from the ITQ help identify the child's temperamental style.

With knowledge of the infant's temperament, nurses are better able to (1) provide parents with background information that will help them see their child in a better perspective, (2) offer a more organized picture of their child's behavior and possibly reveal distortions in their perceptions of the behavior, and (3) guide parents regarding appropriate childrearing techniques (Chess and Thomas, 1985).

Childrearing Practices Related to Temperament

Most parents realize that their infant is born with unique characteristics, and few parents of difficult infants need to be told of the challenge of caring for them. However, very few parents are aware of the significance of the temperamental characteristics and of constructive approaches to dealing with them. The following are examples of interventions that promote more positive parenting of infants with different temperament styles.

Difficult children may respond better to scheduled feedings and structured caregiving routines than demand feedings and frequent changes in daily routines. These children sleep less and may need more structured approaches to bedtime to prevent bedtime problems. "Highly distractible children" may require additional soothing measures such as swinging, rocking, or being carried in a pack that the parent wears across the chest or back. Children with "high activity" levels require vigilant watching, and parents need to take extra precautions in safeguarding the home. These children

FAMILY FOCUS
Difficult Temperament and Preterm Infants

Parents typically rate preterm, low-birth-weight infants as being more difficult than full-term infants. Parents are often concerned that the difficult temperament is permanent and results from the many negative and painful hospital experiences. The family can be reassured that although these infants may be difficult to parent for the first 6 months of corrected age (chronologic age minus amount of prematurity), no particular perinatal event is responsible. Also, over time the infants tend to become less difficult (Gennaro, Medoff-Cooper, and Lotas, 1992).

benefit from increased opportunities for gross motor activity to constructively channel their energy.

The *slow-to-warm up child* may demonstrate more stranger fear than other children and may require more gradual and frequent preparation for new situations, such as substitute child care. Even the *easy child* can present problems in that the parents may need reminders to feed the child who sleeps for prolonged intervals and rarely cries. They may have to "retrain" the child because of the ease of developing troublesome habits, such as keeping the child up late or sleeping with the youngster.

Appropriate counseling based on awareness of the child's temperament can greatly enhance the quality of interaction between parents and infant. Even just letting parents know that "difficult" traits are innate can relieve feelings of guilt and incompetence (see Family Focus box).

• • •

A summary of growth and development during infancy is presented in Table 10-2. Although all milestones are important, some represent essential integrative aspects of development that lay the foundation for the achievement of more advanced skills. These essential milestones are designated by a bullet (•) in the chart. The table represents the *average* monthly age at which various skills are attained. It must be remembered that although the sequence is the same, the rate will vary among children.

Text continued on p. 306.

TABLE 10-2. Growth and development during infancy

AGE (MONTHS)	PHYSICAL	GROSS MOTOR	FINE MOTOR
1	Weight gain of 150 to 210 g (5 to 7 ounces) weekly for first 6 months Height gain of 2.5 cm (1 inch) monthly for first 6 months Head circumference increases by 1.5 cm (½ inch) monthly for first 6 months Primitive reflexes present and strong Doll's eye reflex and dance reflex fading Obligatory nose breathing (most infants)	• Assumes flexed position with pelvis high but knees not under abdomen when prone (at birth, knees flexed under abdomen) • Can turn head from side to side when prone, lifts head momentarily from bed (see Fig. 10-4, *A*) Has marked head lag, especially when pulled from lying to sitting position (see Fig. 10-3, *A*) Holds head momentarily parallel and in midline when suspended in prone position Assumes asymmetric tonic neck reflex position when supine When held in standing position, body limp at knees and hips In sitting position back is uniformly rounded, absence of head control (see Fig. 10-5, *A*)	Hands predominantly closed Grasp reflex strong Hand clenches on contact with rattle
2	Posterior fontanel closed Crawling reflex disappears	• Assumes less flexed position when prone—hips flat, legs extended, arms flexed, head to side Less head lag when pulled to sitting position (see Fig. 10-3, *B*) Can maintain head in same plane as rest of body when held in ventral suspension When prone, can lift head almost 45 degrees off table When held in sitting position, head is held up but bobs forward (see Fig. 10-5, *B*) Assumes asymmetric tonic neck reflex position intermittently	Hands frequently open Grasp reflex fading
3	• Primitive reflexes fading	Able to hold head more erect when sitting, but still bobs forward Has only slight head lag when pulled to sitting position Assumes symmetric body positioning Able to raise head and shoulders from prone position to a 45- to 90-degree angle from table; bears weight on forearms When held in standing position, able to bear slight fraction of weight on legs Regards own hand	• Actively holds rattle but will not reach for it Grasp reflex absent Hands kept loosely open Clutches own hand; pulls at blankets and clothes

• Milestones that represent essential integrative aspects of development that lay the foundation for the achievement of more advanced skills.
*Degree of visual acuity varies according to vision measurement procedure used.

SENSORY	VOCALIZATION	SOCIALIZATION/COGNITION
• Able to fixate on moving object in range of 45 degrees when held at a distance of 20-25 cm (8-10 inches) Visual acuity approaches 20/100* Follows light to midline Quiets when hears a voice	Cries to express displeasure Makes small throaty sounds Makes comfort sounds during feeding	Is in sensorimotor phase—stage I, use of reflexes (birth-1 month), and stage II, primary circular reactions (1-4 months) Watches parent's face intently as she or he talks to infant
Binocular fixation and convergence to near objects beginning When supine, follows dangling toy from side to point beyond midline Visually searches to locate sounds Turns head to side when sound is made at level of ear	• Vocalizes, distinct from crying Crying becomes differentiated Coos Vocalizes to familiar voice	• Demonstrates social smile in response to various stimuli
• Follows object to periphery (180 degrees) • Locates sound by turning head to side and looking in same direction Begins to have ability to coordinate stimuli from various sense organs	• Squeals aloud to show pleasure Coos, babbles, chuckles Vocalizes when smiling "Talks" a great deal when spoken to Less crying during periods of wakefulness	Displays considerable interest in surroundings Ceases crying when parent enters room Can recognize familiar faces and objects, such as feeding bottle Shows awareness of strange situations

Continued.

TABLE 10-2. Growth and development during infancy—cont'd

AGE (MONTHS)	PHYSICAL	GROSS MOTOR	FINE MOTOR
4	Drooling begins • Moro, tonic neck, and rooting reflexes have disappeared	• Has almost no head lag when pulled to sitting position (see Fig. 10-3, *C*) • Balances head well in sitting position (see Fig. 10-5, *C*) Back less rounded, curved only in lumbar area Able to sit erect if propped up Able to raise head and chest off surface to angle of 90 degrees (see Fig. 10-4, *B*) Assumes predominant symmetric position • Rolls from back to side	• Inspects and plays with hands; pulls clothing or blanket over face in play Tries to reach objects with hand but overshoots Grasps object with both hands Plays with rattle placed in hand, shakes it, but cannot pick it up if dropped Can carry objects to mouth
5	Beginning signs of tooth eruption Birth weight doubles	No head lag when pulled to sitting position When sitting, able to hold head erect and steady Able to sit for longer periods when back is well supported Back straight When prone, assumes symmetric positioning with arms extended • Can turn over from abdomen to back When supine, puts feet to mouth	• Able to grasp objects voluntarily Uses palmar grasp, bidextrous approach Plays with toes Takes objects directly to mouth Holds one cube while regarding a second
6	Growth rate may begin to decline Weight gain of 90 to 150 g (3 to 5 ounces) weekly for next 6 months Height gain of 1.25 cm (½ inch) monthly for next 6 months • Teething may begin with eruption of two lower central incisors • Chewing and biting occur	When prone, can lift chest and upper abdomen off table, bearing weight on hands (see Fig. 10-4, *C*) When about to be pulled to a sitting position, lifts head Sits in high chair with back straight Rolls from back to abdomen When held in standing position, bears almost all of weight Hand regard absent	Resecures a dropped object Drops one cube when another is given Grasps and manipulates small objects Holds bottle Grasps feet and pulls to mouth
7	Eruption of lower central incisors	When supine, spontaneously lifts head off table • Sits, leaning forward on both hands (see Fig. 10-5, *D*) When prone, bears weight on one hand Sits erect momentarily Bears full weight on feet (see Fig. 10-6, *A*) When held in standing position, bounces actively	• Transfers objects from one hand to the other (see Fig. 10-5, *E*) Has unidextrous approach and grasp Holds two cubes more than momentarily Bangs cube on table Rakes at a small object

• Milestones that represent essential integrative aspects of development that lay the foundation for the achievement of more advanced skills.

SENSORY	VOCALIZATION	SOCIALIZATION/COGNITION
Able to accommodate to near objects Binocular vision fairly well established Can focus on a 1.25 cm (½-inch) block Beginning eye-hand coordination	Makes consonant sounds *n, k, g, p, b* • Laughs aloud Vocalization changes according to mood	Is in stage III, secondary circular reactions Demands attention by fussing; becomes bored if left alone Enjoys social interaction with people Anticipates feeding when sees bottle or mother if breast-feeding Shows excitement with whole body, squeals, breathes heavily Shows interest in strange stimuli Begins to show memory
Visually pursues a dropped object Is able to sustain visual inspection of an object Can localize sounds made below the ear	Squeals Makes vowel cooing sounds interspersed with consonant sounds (e.g., *ah-goo*)	Smiles at mirror image Pats bottle or breast with both hands More enthusiastically playful, but may have rapid mood swings Is able to discriminate strangers from family Vocalizes displeasure when object taken away Discovers parts of body
Adjusts posture to see an object Prefers more complex visual stimuli Can localize sounds made above the ear Will turn head to the side, then look up or down	• Begins to imitate sounds • Babbling resembles one-syllable utterances—*ma, mu, da, di, hi* Vocalizes to toys, mirror image Takes pleasure in hearing own sounds (self-reinforcement)	Recognizes parents; begins to fear strangers Holds arms out to be picked up Has definite likes and dislikes Begins to imitate (cough, protrusion of tongue) Excites on hearing footsteps Laughs when head is hidden in a towel • Briefly searches for a dropped object (object permanence beginning) Frequent mood swings—from crying to laughing with little or no provocation
• Can fixate on very small objects Responds to own name Localizes sound by turning head in a curving arch Beginning awareness of depth and space Has taste preferences	• Produces vowel sounds and chained syllables—*baba, dada, kaka* Vocalizes four distinct vowel sounds "Talks" when others are talking	• Increasing fear of strangers; shows signs of fretfulness when mother disappears Imitates simple acts and noises Tries to attract attention by coughing or snorting Plays peekaboo Demonstrates dislike of food by keeping lips closed Exhibits oral aggressiveness in biting and mouthing Demonstrates expectation in response to repetition of stimuli

Continued.

TABLE 10-2. Growth and development during infancy—cont'd

AGE (MONTHS)	PHYSICAL	GROSS MOTOR	FINE MOTOR
8	Begins to show regular patterns in bladder and bowel elimination Parachute reflex appears (see Fig. 10-1)	• Sits steadily unsupported (see Fig. 10-5, *E*) Readily bears weight on legs when supported; may stand holding onto furniture Adjusts posture to reach an object	Has beginning pincer grasp using index, fourth, and fifth fingers against lower part of thumb Releases objects at will Rings bell purposely Retains two cubes while regarding third cube Secures an object by pulling on a string Reaches persistently for toys out of reach
9	Eruption of upper central incisors may begin	Creeps on hands and knees Sits steadily on floor for prolonged time (10 minutes) Recovers balance when leans forward but cannot do so when leaning sideways • Pulls self to standing position and stands holding onto furniture (see Fig. 10-6, *B-D*)	• Uses thumb and index finger in crude pincer grasp (see Fig. 10-2) Preference for use of dominant hand now evident Grasps third cube Compares two cubes by bringing them together
10	Labyrinth-righting reflex is strongest—when infant is in prone or supine position, is able to raise head	Can change from prone to sitting position Stands while holding onto furniture, sits by falling down Recovers balance easily while sitting While standing, lifts one foot to take a step (see Fig. 10-6, *E*)	Crude release of an object beginning Grasps bell by handle
11	Eruption of lower lateral incisors may begin	When sitting, pivots to reach toward back to pick up an object • Cruises or walks holding onto furniture or with both hands held	Explores objects more thoroughly (e.g., clapper inside bell) Has neat pincer grasp (see Fig. 10-2, *B*) Drops object deliberately for it to be picked up Puts one object after another into a container (sequential play) Able to manipulate an object to remove it from tight-fitting enclosure
12	• Birth weight tripled • Birth length increased by 50% Head and chest circumference equal (head circumference 46.5 cm [18½ inches]) Has total of six to eight deciduous teeth Anterior fontanel almost closed Landau reflex fading Babinski reflex disappears Lumbar curve develops; lordosis evident during walking	• Walks with one hand held Cruises well • May attempt to stand alone momentarily; may attempt first step alone Can sit down from standing position without help	Releases cube in cup Attempts to build two-block tower but fails Tries to insert a pellet into a narrow-necked bottle but fails Can turn pages in a book, many at a time

SENSORY	VOCALIZATION	SOCIALIZATION/COGNITION
	Makes consonant sounds *t*, *d*, and *w* Listens selectively to familiar words Utterances signal emphasis and emotion Combines syllables, such as *dada*, but does not ascribe meaning to them	Increasing anxiety over loss of parent, particularly mother, and fear of strangers Responds to word "no" Dislikes dressing, diaper change
Localizes sounds by turning head diagonally and directly toward sound Depth perception increasing	Responds to simple verbal commands Comprehends "no-no"	Parent (mother) is increasingly important for own sake Shows increasing interest in pleasing parent Begins to show fears of going to bed and being left alone Puts arms in front of face to avoid having it washed
	• Says "dada," "mama" with meaning Comprehends "bye-bye" May say one word (e.g., "hi," "bye," "no")	Inhibits behavior to verbal command of "no-no" or own name Imitates facial expressions, waves bye-bye Extends toy to another person but will not release it • Develops object permanence Repeats actions that attract attention and cause laughter Pulls clothes of another to attract attention Plays interactive games such as pat-a-cake Reacts to adult anger, cries when scolded Demonstrates independence in dressing, feeding, locomotive skills, and testing of parents Looks at and follows pictures in a book
	Imitates definite speech sounds	Experiences joy and satisfaction when a task is mastered Reacts to restrictions with frustration Rolls ball to another on request Anticipates body gestures when a familiar nursery rhyme or story is being told (e.g., holds toes and feet in response to "This little piggy went to market") Plays game up-down, "so big," or peekaboo Shakes head for "no"
Discriminates simple geometric forms (e.g., circle) Amblyopia may develop with lack of binocularity Can follow rapidly moving object Controls and adjusts response to sound; listens for sound to recur	• Says three to five words besides "dada," "mama" Comprehends meaning of several words (comprehension always precedes verbalization) Recognizes objects by name Imitates animal sounds Understands simple verbal commands (e.g., "Give it to me," "Show me your eyes")	Shows emotions such as jealousy, affection (may give hug or kiss on request), anger, fear Enjoys familiar surroundings and explores away from parent Is fearful in strange situation; clings to parent May develop habit of "security blanket" or favorite toy Has increasing determination to practice locomotor skills • Searches for an object even if it has not been hidden, but searches only where object was last seen

COPING WITH CONCERNS RELATED TO NORMAL GROWTH AND DEVELOPMENT

Separation and Stranger Fear

During infancy a number of fears can appear. However, the fear that causes parents most concern is related to the child's fear of strangers and separation. Although erroneously interpreted by some as a sign of undesirable, antisocial behavior, stranger fear and separation anxiety are important components of a strong, healthy parent-child attachment. However, this period can present difficulties for parent and child. Parents may be more hesitant to leave the child with others because the older infant protests violently against having a baby-sitter. To accustom the infant to new people, parents are encouraged to have close friends or relatives visit often. This provides for other persons with whom the child is comfortable and who can give parents time for themselves.

Infants also need opportunities to experience strangers safely. Usually toward the end of the first year, infants begin to venture away from the parent and demonstrate curiosity about strangers. If allowed to explore at their own rate, many infants will eventually "warm up." If parents hold the child away from their face, the infant can observe while maintaining close physical contact. The best approach for the stranger (who may be the nurse) is to talk to the parent, talk softly, meet the child at eye level (to appear smaller), maintain a safe distance from the infant, and avoid sudden, intrusive gestures, such as holding the arms out and smiling broadly.

Parents also may wonder whether they should encourage the child's clinging, dependent behavior, especially if there is pressure from others who view this as "spoiling." Parents need to be reassured that such behavior is healthy, desirable, and necessary for the child's optimum emotional development. If parents can reassure the infant of their presence, the infant will learn to realize that they are still there even if not physically present. Talking to infants when leaving the room, allowing them to hear one's voice on the telephone, and using transitional objects, such as a favorite blanket or toy, reassures them of the parent's continued presence.

Alternate Child Care Arrangements

For many parents, especially working mothers, locating safe and competent child care facilities for the infant is an increasingly difficult problem—one that is compounded by the number of mothers working outside the home. Over the past 30 years there has been a marked shift in child care arrangements, with fewer children being cared for at home and more children being cared for in group centers or other settings.

The basic types of care are in-home care, in either the parent's or another caregiver's home, and center-based care, usually in a daycare center. *In-home care* may consist of a full-time baby-sitter who lives in the home, a full-time baby-sitter who comes to the home, cooperative arrangements such as exchange baby-sitting, and family daycare. A licensed *family daycare home* typically provides care and protection for up to five children for part of a 24-hour day. *Center-based group care* usually refers to a daycare facility that provides care for six or more children, for 6 or more hours in a 24-hour day. *Work-based group care* is another option that is becoming increasingly popular as employers recognize the benefit of

quality and convenient child care to their employees. *Sick-child care* may also be available for times the youngster is ill. Such programs are often located in community hospitals (Landis and Chang, 1991).

Nurses may provide guidance to parents in selecting suitable, well-qualified facilities or individuals to care for their child. The decision to leave an infant in another's care often engenders doubt and guilt in the parent, despite reassurance that the provision of competent, loving care by someone other than the parent is not detrimental to the child's future development. Therefore any assistance is often appreciated.

Guidelines for selecting child care facilities are discussed in Chapter 13 under Preschool or Daycare Experience. The same conscientious attention should be applied to locating competent baby-sitters. References from other employers are essential, and there is no substitute for observing the interaction between the individual and the child. Although very young infants need little if any preparation for the introduction of a new caregiver, older infants may benefit from a gradual placement to reduce stranger anxiety. At all times the parent should have the right to visit the child, and regular conferences should be established to review the child's progress.

Limit-Setting and Discipline

As infants' motor skills advance and mobility increases, parents are faced with the need to set safe limits (see discussion of nurse's role in injury prevention on p. 330). Although there are numerous disciplinary techniques, some are more

---

CRITICAL THINKING EXERCISE
Thumb-Sucking

During a well-child visit you observe that Mrs. Lopez persistently takes the thumb out of her 10-month-old daughter, Maria's, mouth. You ask if she has concerns about the thumb-sucking. She replies, "Of course. Her teeth are coming in so nice and straight and I don't want the thumb to make them crooked." An appropriate response is:

1. "Sucking on a thumb or pacifier is very common in young children, especially in infants. It satisfies their need to suck and helps them to comfort themselves. Sometimes, making an issue of the sucking can cause it to last longer."
2. "Thumb-sucking is perfectly normal and children stop when they are ready. So don't worry about it."
3. "If thumb-sucking continues when most of her teeth are in, it will make them crooked. But we don't need to worry about it now."
4. "You are right to be concerned. Let her suck longer on the bottle to satisfy her sucking needs."

The correct answer is one. The response provides factual information in a nonjudgmental manner that invites further discussion. Options two and three are partly correct in regard to thumb-sucking but offer premature reassurance. Option four is incorrect and at 10 months of age, infants should be relying less, not more, on bottle-feeding, which can lead to excessive intake of milk, juice, or other sweetened beverages in place of solid foods and to dental caries (see Weaning, p. 311, and Dental health, p. 313).

appropriate for this age than others. Parents can begin discipline using a negative voice and stern eye contact. When the child engages in unacceptable activity, play should be stopped and a firm voice should be used. Corporal punishment is not recommended. Although parents may be concerned with starting discipline during infancy, it is important to stress that the earlier effective disciplinary methods are employed, the easier it is to continue these approaches. The most important components of discipline are consistency and appropriateness. The same behaviors must consistently be acknowledged in the same way, and the degree of limit-setting must be appropriate to the child's developmental level (see Limit-Setting and Discipline, Chapter 4).

Thumb-Sucking and Use of Pacifier

Sucking is the infant's chief pleasure, and it may not be satisfied by breast- or bottle-feeding. It is such a strong need that infants who are deprived of sucking, such as those with a cleft lip repair, will suck on their tongue. Some newborns are born with sucking pads on their fingers from in utero sucking activity. Several benefits of nonnutritive sucking have been documented, such as increased weight gain in preterm infants, decreased crying, and increased behavioral organization (Pickler and Frankel, 1995).

Problems arise when parents are concerned about sucking of fingers, thumb, or pacifier and attempt to restrain this natural tendency. Before offering advice, nurses should investigate the parents' feelings and base guidance on this information (see Critical Thinking Exercise).

During infancy and early childhood there is no need to restrain nonnutritive sucking. Malocclusion may occur if thumb-sucking persists past 4 years of age or when the permanent teeth erupt. There is probably less dental displacement with the use of a pacifier than with the use of a hard, rigid finger. Pacifiers may be relinquished earlier than thumbs because they are less readily available. If the child uses a pacifier, safety considerations in purchasing one must be stressed (see p. 322).

 Some evidence suggests that the early introduction of a pacifier (during first month) may shorten the duration of breast-feeding. Possible explanations include less stimulation of the breasts and less milk production or a sign that breast-feeding difficulties already exist (Victora and others, 1993).

To decrease dependence on nonnutritive sucking in young infants, sucking pleasure can be increased by prolonging feeding time. A small-holed, firm nipple causes stronger sucking and slower feeding. Also, the parent's excessive use of the pacifier to calm the child should be explored. It is not unusual for parents to place a pacifier in the infant's mouth as soon as crying begins, thus reinforcing a pattern of distress-relief.

Thumb-sucking reaches its peak at 18 to 20 months of age and is most prevalent when the child is hungry or tired. Persistent thumb-sucking in a listless, apathetic child always warrants investigation. It may be a sign of an emotional problem between parent and child or of boredom, isolation, and lack of stimulation.

Teething

One of the more difficult periods in the infant's (and parents') life is the eruption of the deciduous (primary) teeth, often referred to as *teething*. The age of tooth eruption shows considerable variation among children, but the order of their appearance is fairly regular and predictable (Fig. 10-11). The first primary teeth to erupt are the lower central incisors, which appear at approximately 6 to 8 months of age. These are followed closely by the upper central incisors.

NURSING TIP A quick guide to assessment of deciduous teeth during the first 2 years is: *age of the child in months* − 6 = *number of teeth*. For example: 8 months of age − 6 = 2 teeth at this age.

Teething is a physiologic process, and as the crown of the tooth breaks through the periodontal membrane, some discomfort may be experienced. Some children show minimal evidence of teething, such as drooling, increased finger-sucking, or biting on hard objects. Others are very irritable, have difficulty sleeping, and refuse to eat. Generally, signs of illness such as fever, vomiting, or diarrhea are not symptoms of teething but of illness. However, as many parents report, a low-grade temperature is common in the 4- to 19-day period before and on the day of tooth eruption (Jaber, Cohen, and Mor, 1992).

Cold is soothing. Giving the child a frozen teething ring or an ice cube securely wrapped in a washcloth helps to relieve the inflammation. Several nonprescription topical anes-

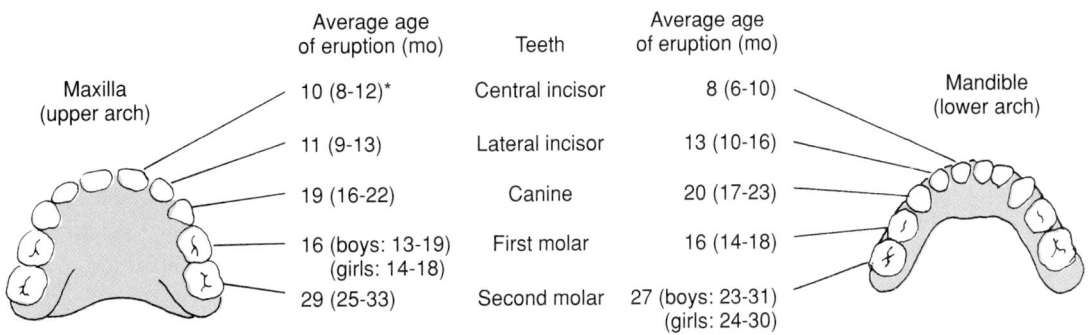

FIG. 10-11. Sequence of eruption of primary teeth. *Range represents ± 1 standard deviation or 67% of subjects studied. (Data from McDonald RE, Avery DR: *Dentistry for the child and adolescent,* ed 6, St Louis, 1994, Mosby.)

thetic ointments are available, such as Baby Ora-Jel. If these are used, parents are advised to apply them correctly. In the event of persistent irritability that affects sleeping and feeding, systemic analgesics, such as acetaminophen, can be given judiciously. Parents should know that this is a temporary measure.

> **Nursing ALERT** Teething powders or procedures such as cutting or rubbing the gums with aspirin are not used to reduce teething pain, because ingestion or aspiration of the powder, infection or irritation of the tissue, or aspiration of the aspirin can occur.

Infant Shoes

Many parents are unaware of the types of shoes that are appropriate for the older infant and buy expensive infant shoes because of misleading advertising claims. Inflexible shoes that have hard soles can be detrimental by delaying walking, aggravating intoeing and outtoeing, and impeding the development of supportive foot muscles. Counseling parents regarding footwear should begin when infants are 6 months old, well before they are standing or walking.

When children begin walking, the main reason for wearing shoes is *protection.* To provide protection, the shoe should retain its fit, be made of durable material with a smooth interior and few construction seams to irritate the skin, and be soft and flexible, especially in the toe area. A high-top shoe is not necessary for support but may be helpful in keeping the foot in the shoe.

A good shoe conforms to the shape of the foot, with a rounded toe area and sufficient toe room. During weight bearing, there should be at least the space of half the width of the thumbnail, or 1.25 cm (½ inch), between the end of the longest toe and the shoe. Roomy and square-toed socks also allow for growth and alignment. Inexpensive but well-constructed sneakers or soft-leather moccasin-type shoes are adequate for walking infants.

Even if the shoes are fitted properly, frequent changes are needed to accommodate the infant's rapidly growing feet. Shoe size changes at approximately 3-month intervals from 12 to 36 months of age; during this time the child's foot should be measured every 3 months. Curled toes when shoes are removed and redness and irritation of the skin on the bottom of the toes indicate the need for a larger size.

PROMOTING OPTIMUM HEALTH DURING INFANCY

NUTRITION

The First 6 Months

The decision to breast- or bottle-feed the infant is highly individual and is discussed in Chapter 8. This section is primarily concerned with nutrition during infancy.

Human milk is the most desirable and complete diet for the infant for the first 6 months. The normal infant receiving breast milk from a well-nourished mother needs no specific vitamin and mineral supplements, with the exception of iron by 4 to 6 months of age (when fetal iron stores are depleted) (Calvo, Galindo, and Aspres, 1992; Position statement, 1992). Supplements of 400 IU of vitamin D daily may be indicated if the mother's vitamin D intake is inadequate. Some authorities also suggest supplements if the infant does not benefit from adequate exposure to ultraviolet light (American Academy of Pediatrics, Committee on Nutrition, 1995.)

Employed mothers can continue breast-feeding with guidance and encouragement. Most mothers find that a program of breast-pumping when away from home and bottle-feeding of breast milk, with or without supplemental formula feedings, is successful. Milk can be expressed by hand or pump and safely refrigerated for up to 24 hours. After that time freezing is suggested. In addition to efficient breast-pumping, these mothers also cite the need for child care by a trusted agency or individual and support and assistance from significant others. Like all breast-feeding mothers, these women must have proper nutrition and rest for lactation. With a schedule of work and child care, careful planning is required to successfully manage the demands of both responsibilities.

An acceptable alternative to breast-feeding is commercial iron-fortified formula. Like human milk it supplies all the nutrients needed by the infant for the first 6 months. After 6 months, the only supplementation required for formula or human milk is fluoride (0.25 mg) if the local water supply is not fluoridated or if the infant is given ready-to-feed formula, in which fluoridated tap water is not used.

Commercially prepared vitamin/iron preparations with or without fluoride are available to meet the specific needs of the infant (see Fluoride, Chapter 12). Unmodified whole cow's milk, low-fat cow's milk, and imitation milks are not acceptable as a major source of nutrition for infants because of their altered ability to be digested, increased risk of contamination, and lack of components needed for appropriate growth. Whole milk may cause occult gastrointestinal bleeding and iron deficiency anemia in infants.

> **Nursing ALERT** Whole milk should not be introduced to infants until after 1 year of age (American Academy of Pediatrics, Committee on Nutrition, 1995).

The amount of formula per feeding and the number of feedings per day vary among infants. In general, the number of feedings decreases from six at 1 month of age to four to five at 6 months. Regardless of the number of feedings, the total amount of formula ingested should not exceed 32 ounces (960 ml) per day. Parents should be cautioned concerning the excessive use of juices and nonnutritive drinks such as Kool-aid during this period.

The addition of solid foods before 4 to 6 months of age is not recommended, although mothers may receive conflicting advice from other women (e.g., their mothers), who cared for children during the era of early introduction of solids. During the early months solid foods are not compatible with the ability of the gastrointestinal tract and nutritional needs of the infant. Feeding solids to young infants exposes them to food antigens that may produce food-protein allergy. In addition, the infant is not ready developmentally. The extrusion (protrusion) reflex is strong and pushes food out of the mouth, and infants instinctively suck when given food. Because of their limited range-of-motor abilities, infants are unable to deliberately push food away or avoid feeding. Therefore, early introduction of solids is a type of forced feeding, which may lead to excessive weight gain.

The Second 6 Months

During the second half of the first year human milk or formula continues to be the primary source of nutrition. If breast-feeding is discontinued, commercial iron-fortified formula should be substituted. Formulas specially marketed for older infants offer no advantages for infants.

The major change in feeding habits is the addition of solid foods to the infant's diet. Physiologically and developmentally, the infant is in a transition period at 4 to 6 months of age. By this time the gastrointestinal tract has matured sufficiently to handle more complex nutrients and is less sensitive to potentially allergenic foods. Tooth eruption is beginning and facilitates biting and chewing. The extrusion reflex has disappeared, and swallowing is more coordinated to allow the infant to accept solids easily. Head control is well developed, permitting infants to sit with support and purposely turn their head away to communicate disinterest in food. Voluntary grasping and improved eye-hand coordination gradually allow infants to pick up "finger" foods and feed themselves. Their increasing sense of independence is evident in their desire to hold their own bottle and try to "help" during feeding.

Selection and Preparation of Solid Foods

The choice of foods to introduce first is variable but should be based on the reasons for feeding, such as supplying nutrients not found in formula or breast milk. Infant cereal is generally introduced first because of its high iron content (7 mg of iron per 3 tablespoons of dry cereal). There are several types of commercially prepared infant cereals, such as rice, barley, oatmeal, and high-protein cereals, but rice is usually suggested as an initial food because of its easy digestibility and low allergenic potential.

Infant cereal is mixed with formula until whole milk is given. If the infant is breast-fed, the cereal is mixed with expressed breast milk or water. After 6 months of age, fruit juices can be mixed with the dry cereal; the vitamin C content of the juice enhances the absorption of iron in the cereal. Because of their benefit as a source of iron, infant cereals should be continued until the child is 18 months of age.

Fruit juice can be offered for its rich source of vitamin C and as a substitute for milk for one feeding a day. Large quantities of certain juices, such as apple, pear, prune, sweet cherry, peach, and grape are avoided because they may cause abdominal pain, diarrhea, or bloating in some children (American Academy of Pediatrics, Committee on Nutrition, 1991). Because vitamin C is naturally destroyed by heat, juice is not warmed. Containers of juice are always kept covered and refrigerated to prevent further vitamin loss.

Nursing ALERT Offer fruit juice from a cup, rather than a bottle, to prevent the development of "nursing" caries (see Low-Cariogenic Diet, Chapter 12).

The addition of other foods is arbitrary. A common sequence is strained fruits followed by vegetables and finally meats. If foods are introduced early, citrus fruits, meats, and eggs are still delayed until after 6 months of age because of their potential to result in allergy. At 6 months foods such as a cracker or zwieback can be offered as a type of finger and teething food. By 8 to 9 months junior foods and nutritious finger foods, such as a firmly cooked vegetable, raw pieces of fruit (except grapes), or cheese, can be given. By 1 year well-cooked table foods are served.

Commercially prepared baby foods are the most commonly used types of food served to infants in the United States. They are convenient and contain no added salt or sugar, but are relatively expensive. An alternative is preparing baby foods at home, which is a simple and inexpensive process. Fruits and vegetables can be steamed in a small amount of water and pureed in a blender or food processor. Many of them, such as ripe banana, can be mashed fine with a fork. Fruits such as apples or pears require little or no water in the cooking process. Vegetables such as carrots, potatoes, or string beans require additional water in the cooking and blending process. Preferably, home-prepared infant foods should be fresh or frozen, because canned foods, other than those prepared for infants, may have excessive sodium or sugar or be a source of lead from the container.

 There is no evidence that the addition of salt to foods such as peas, increases the infants acceptance of the new food (Sullivan and Birch, 1994).

Introduction of Solid Foods

When the spoon is first introduced to infants, they are likely to push away and appear dissatisfied. Some patience and skill are required to overcome this initial response, especially if the extrusion reflex is still present. A small-bowled, straight, and long-handled spoon, similar to a demitasse spoon, allows a small portion of food to be placed toward the back of the tongue. If food is placed on the front of the tongue and pushed out, it is simply scooped up and refed to the infant. As children become accustomed to the spoon, they will more eagerly accept the food and will eventually open their mouth in anticipation (or keep it closed in dislike). Since the first introduction of food is a new experience, the spoon feeding should be attempted before or after ingestion of a small amount of breast milk or formula to associate this new experience with a pleasurable and satisfying experience. Trying to introduce a new food *after* the entire milk feeding is usually useless, since the infant is satiated and has no inclination to try something new.

After several spoon feedings, new food can be introduced at the beginning of a meal. It is best to introduce many new foods during the first year, when the infant is more likely to eat them because of a hearty appetite resulting from a rapid growth rate.

Each new food is introduced at intervals of 4 to 7 days to allow for identification of food allergies. New foods are offered in small amounts, from 1 teaspoon to 1 to 2 tablespoons. As the amount of solid food increases, the quantity of milk is decreased to less than a liter a day to prevent overfeeding.

FAMILY HOME CARE
Introducing Solid Foods to Infants*

Introduce solids when infant is hungry.

Begin spoon feeding by pushing food to back of tongue because of infant's natural tendency to thrust the tongue forward.

Use a small spoon with a straight handle; begin with 1 or 2 teaspoons of food; gradually increase to a couple of tablespoons per feeding.

Introduce one food at a time, usually at intervals of 4 to 7 days to allow for identification of food allergies.

As the amount of solid food increases, decrease the quantity of milk to prevent overfeeding.

Do not introduce foods by mixing them with formula in the bottle.

---

*A recommended resource is *Starting solids: a guide for parents and child care providers,* available from the National Association of Pediatric Nurse Associates and Practitioners (NAPNAP), 1101 Kings Highway North, Suite 206, Cherry Hill, NJ 08034-1931.

FAMILY HOME CARE
Guidelines for Microwave Heating of Refrigerated Infant Formula

Prior to heating
- Heat only 4 oz or more
- Heat only *refrigerated* formula
- Always *stand* the bottle up
- Always leave bottle top *uncovered* to allow heat to escape

Heating instructions (full power)
- 4-oz bottles
  Heat for no more than 30 seconds
- 8-oz bottles
  Heat for no more than 45 seconds

Serving instructions
- Always replace nipple assembly; *invert* 10 times (vigorous shaking is unnecessary)
- Formula should be cool to the touch; formula warm to the touch may be too hot to serve
- Always *test* formula; place several drops on tongue or on top of the hand (not the inside wrist)

From Sigman-Grant M, Bush G, Anantheswaran, R: Microwave heating of infant formula: a dilemma resolved, *Pediatrics* 90(3):414, 1992.

Food should not be mixed in the bottle and fed through a nipple with a large hole. This deprives the child of the pleasure of learning new tastes and developing a discriminating palate. It can also cause problems with poor chewing of food later in life, since this experience would be lacking. A summary of the principles that govern the introduction of new foods is given in the Family Home Care box above.

Nursing ALERT   Although microwaving of bottles and baby food is not recommended, it remains a common practice. Guidelines have been developed for microwave heating of refrigerated formula and these should be given to the family (see Family Home Care box to the right).

The infant's first tries at self-feeding or cup feeding are sloppy experiences. Finger foods such as soft fruits or vegetables are just as good playthings as food; they can be squeezed, smeared, squashed, and thoroughly painted on oneself, others, and the surrounding environment. However, all of this is part of learning, and mastery follows many accidents.

If parents find this experience distressing, a few suggestions may prove helpful. The feeding area should have a floor that can be easily wiped and is relatively far from walls, upholstered furniture, or drapes. A hand-held portable vacuum is helpful in cleaning up crumbs. Messes are confined to one area if the child is seated in a high chair rather than allowed to crawl or walk around while drinking or eating. Infants should be expected to get themselves covered with food; therefore a large bib (plastic can be wiped easily but needs to be removed after feeding) should be used, as well as washable clothes that are easily removed. High chairs can be thoroughly cleaned in a shower. Outdoor dining provides an excellent opportunity for practicing with a cup, spoon, or fingers because accidents are simple to hose or sweep away. Children cannot be pressured into eating neatly or developing table manners before manipulative skill is acquired.

Preventing Obesity

The most prevalent nutritional disorder in the United States is overeating, and prevention begins early. From the infant's first feeding parents should allow their children to regulate the amount of formula they desire. No attempt should be made to encourage infants to finish the last drop or, later in childhood to clean their plate. A parent may misinterpret an infant's crying as a hunger cue and offer an unnecessary bottle, which the infant may take to satisfy a different need thus often conditioning the child to eat (or suck) when a need other than hunger is unmet. Young inexperienced parents may offer food as a cure-all for unmet needs that they do not understand.

Often, eating habits are controlled by the sociocultural background of the family, rather than by their knowledge of well-balanced nutrition. Common myths such as "a fat baby is a healthy baby" are difficult to dispel. In some cultures overweight infants are regarded as a sign of good mothering, and any suggestion regarding altering the child's weight is threatening to the parent. Understanding cultural values is important in effecting change through counseling.

If too much formula or milk is the problem, several strategies can be used to reduce the intake, although the nurse must caution parents not to overly restrict food/formula intake. A commercial formula, Advance,* is also available, which provides 20% fewer calories than regular formula or whole cow's milk. The other strategies are to substitute water for a bottle of formula or use a nipple with a smaller hole to prolong sucking with less intake. The objective is not for the infant to lose weight but to slow weight gain until the weight is appropriate for age and height.

---

*Manufactured by Ross Laboratories, Columbus, OH.

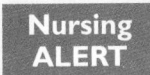 **Nursing ALERT** Dietary fat should not be restricted. Substituting skim or low-fat milk is unacceptable, because the essential fatty acids are inadequate and the solute concentration of protein and electrolytes, such as sodium, is too high.

The selection of solid foods is also an important aspect of controlling obesity. Approximately 20% of commercial baby foods contain less than 50 kcal/100 g, whereas another 20% contain more than 100 kcal/100 g. Choosing low-calorie foods can significantly lower the daily caloric intake without actually decreasing the total quantity of food. The use of sweet foods is kept to a minimum by not adding additional sugar to the formula or cereal and avoiding finger foods such as cookies. Other foods rich in calories that should be restricted in serving size rather than eliminated include butter, cream, ice cream, pudding, and chocolate.

Parents are encouraged to interpret the infant's signals of discomfort and intervene in ways other than through feeding. Crying, fussiness, and sucking do not necessarily indicate hunger. Rocking, stroking, holding, and offering a toy or a pacifier may be more appropriate than automatically responding with food.

Weaning

Defined as the process of giving up one method of feeding for another, *weaning* usually refers to relinquishing the breast or bottle for a cup. In Western societies this is generally regarded as a major task for infants and is frequently seen as a potentially traumatic experience. It is psychologically significant because the infant is required to give up a major source of oral pleasure and gratification.

There is no one time for weaning that is best for every child, but most infants show signs of readiness during the second half of the first year. They have learned that good things come from a spoon. Their increasing desire for freedom of movement may lessen their desire to be held close for feedings. They are acquiring more control over their actions and can easily manipulate a cup to their lips (even if it is held upside down!). Imitation becomes a powerful motivator by age 8 or 9 months, and they enjoy using a cup or glass as others do.

Weaning should be gradual, with one bottle- or breast-feeding being replaced at a time. The last feeding to be discontinued is usually the nighttime one. If breast-feeding is terminated before 5 or 6 months of age, weaning should be to a bottle to provide for the infant's continued sucking needs. If breast-feeding is discontinued later, especially by 12 to 14 months, weaning can be directly to a cup (Baby bottle, 1993).

SLEEP AND ACTIVITY

Sleep patterns vary among infants, and active infants typically sleep less than placid children. Generally, by 3 to 4 months of age most infants have developed a nocturnal pattern of sleep that lasts from 9 to 11 hours. The total daily sleep is about 15 hours. The number of naps per day varies, but by the end of the year infants may take one or two naps. Breast-fed infants usually sleep for less prolonged periods, especially during the night, than do bottle-fed infants. Because of the trend toward breast-feeding, sleep norms such as those described above, which were based primarily on bottle-fed infants, may no longer be relevant. Because of the possible association between the prone position and risk of sudden infant death syndrome (see Chapter 11), infants should be placed supine or side lying until they roll over on their own.

Most infants are naturally active and need no encouragement to be mobile. However, problems can arise when devices such as playpens, strollers, commercial swings, and walkers are used excessively. These restrict movement and prevent infants from exploring and developing gross motor skills. Contrary to popular belief, walkers do not enhance coordination and are dangerous if tipped over or placed near stairs. The American Academy of Pediatrics, Committee on Injury and Poison Prevention (1995) recommends a ban on the sale of infant walkers.

 Nursing ALERT Formal infant exercise programs do not provide any long-term benefit to normal infants, and the possibility for damage to the infant's skeletal system exists. For these reasons, such programs are not recommended (American Academy of Pediatrics, 1988).

Sleep Problems

Concerns regarding sleep are common during infancy. Sometimes they are as basic as parents' questioning if the infant needs additional sleep. In this case it is best to investigate the reason for their concern, stressing the individual needs of each child. Infants who are active during wakeful periods and who are growing normally are sleeping a sufficient amount of time.

However, there are a number of more serious concerns that require intervention. Sleep disturbances of physiologic origin are rare with the exception of colic, which is discussed in Chapter 11. The more common sleep disturbances are a learned pattern or developmental characteristic of some infants (Table 10-3). Although many families may report sleep problems that are typical of these patterns, interventions are offered *only* when the pattern is disruptive to the family (see Cultural Awareness box).

However, when a sleeping problem is presented, a careful assessment is essential. Charting sleep habits both before and after interventions is also an important strategy.* Questions

*A sleep history and a 2-week sleep record for families is available in Wong DL: *Wong and Whaley's Clinical manual of pediatric nursing,* ed 4, St Louis, 1996, Mosby.

TABLE 10-3. Selected sleep disturbances during infancy and early childhood

DISORDER/DESCRIPTION	MANAGEMENT
Nighttime Feeding* Child has a prolonged need for middle-of-night bottle- or breast-feeding Child goes to sleep at the breast or with a bottle Awakenings are frequent (may be hourly) Child returns to sleep after feeding; other comfort measures (e.g., rocking or holding) are usually ineffective	Increase daytime feeding intervals to 4 hours or more (may need to be done gradually) Offer last feeding as late as possible at night; may need to gradually reduce amount of formula or length of breast-feeding Offer no bottles in bed Put to bed *awake* When child is crying, check at progressively longer intervals each night; reassure child but do not hold, rock, take to parent's bed, or give bottle or pacifier
Developmental Night Crying Child aged 6-12 months with undisturbed nighttime sleep now awakes abruptly; may be accompanied by nightmares	Reassure parents that this is temporary phase Enter room immediately to check on child but keep reassurances *brief* Avoid feeding, rocking, taking to parent's bed, or any other routine that may initiate trained night crying
Trained Night Crying* (Inappropriate Sleep Associations) Child typically falls asleep in place other than own bed, e.g., rocking chair or parent's bed, and is brought to own bed while asleep; upon awakening, cries until usual routine is instituted, e.g., rocking	Put child in own bed when *awake* If possible, arrange separate sleeping area from other family members When child is crying, check at progressively longer intervals each night; reassure child but do not resume usual routine
Refusal to Go to Sleep* Child resists bedtime and comes out of room repeatedly Nighttime sleep may be continuous, but frequent awakenings and refusal to return to sleep may occur and become a problem if parent allows child to deviate from usual sleep pattern	Evaluate if hour of sleep is too early (child may resist sleep if not tired) Assist parents in establishing consistent before-bedtime routine and enforcing consistent limits regarding child's bedtime behavior If child persists in leaving bedroom, close door for progressively longer periods Use reward system with child to provide motivation
Nighttime Fears Child resists going to bed or wakes during the night because of fears Child seeks parent's physical presence and with parent nearby, falls asleep easily, unless fear is overwhelming	Evaluate if hour of sleep is too early (child may fantasize when nothing to do but think in dark room) Calmly reassure the frightened child; keeping a nightlight on may be helpful Use reward system with child to provide motivation to deal with fears Avoid patterns that can lead to additional problems, e.g., sleeping with child or taking child to parent's room If child's fear is overwhelming, consider desensitization, e.g., progressively spending longer periods of time alone; consult professional help for protracted fears Distinguish between nightmares and sleep terrors (confused partial arousals) (see Sleep problems, Chapter 13)

Modified from Ferber R: Behavioral "insomnia" in the child, *Psychiatr Clin North Am* 10(4):641-653, 1987.
*Guidelines for parents in dealing with these sleep problems are in Wong DL: *Wong and Whaley's Clinical manual of pediatric nursing,* ed 4, St Louis, 1996, Mosby.

regarding the frequency and duration of waking, the usual bedtime routine, the number of nighttime feedings, the perceived problem (e.g., how much disruption the behavior generates), and the attempted interventions are important in planning effective approaches designed for the specific sleep problem. A common suggestion given for any type of sleep problem—"let the child cry until falling asleep"—is very difficult to implement and is inappropriate for certain conditions. Once the parents relent and console the child, they have only reinforced the crying.

An equally effective and more atraumatic approach to night crying, known as *graduated extinction,* is to let the child cry for progressively longer times between *brief* parental interventions that consist only of reassurance, not rocking, holding, or using the bottle or pacifier. For example, the parents may check on the child every 5 minutes during the first night and progressively extend this interval by 5 minutes on successive nights (Ferber, 1985).

Families who cannot tolerate the unexpected crying spells while everyone else is asleep can try the two-step approach. Graduated extinction is used during naps and at bedtime until the parents retire. If the child cries during the night, the parents use comforting measures. However, once the child is partially trained, step 2 is initiated—the use of graduated extinction at all times (Schmitt, 1992).

The best way to prevent sleep problems is to encourage parents to establish bedtime rituals that do not foster problematic patterns. One of the most constructive is placing infants *awake* in their own crib. When infants are accustomed to falling asleep somewhere else, such as in their parent's arms, and then being transferred to their crib, they awaken in unfamiliar surroundings and are unable to fall asleep until the routine is repeated (Anders, Halpern, and Hua, 1992). Also, the bed should be used for sleeping only—not as a playpen. It is advisable not to hang playthings over or on the bed; in this way the child associates the bed with sleep—not with activity. Although these interventions described above and in Table 10-3 are usually successful, it is much easier to prevent the problem with appropriate counseling during the early months of the infant's life.

DENTAL HEALTH

Good dental hygiene begins as soon as the primary teeth erupt. The teeth and gums are initially cleaned by wiping them with a damp cloth; toothbrushing is too harsh for the tender gingiva. The infant can be stabilized by cradling with one arm and using the free hand to cleanse the teeth. Oral hygiene can be made pleasant by singing or talking to the infant. There are no clear guidelines as to when toothbrushing should begin. However, it is generally recommended that, as more teeth erupt and the infant adjusts to the routine of cleaning, a small, soft-bristled toothbrush can be used. Water is preferred to toothpaste, which the infant will swallow, and if fluoridated, will ingest excessive amounts (Nowak, 1993).

Fluoride, an essential mineral for building caries-resistant teeth, is needed beginning at 6 months of age if the infant does not receive water with an adequate fluoride content. The American Academy of Pediatrics, Committee on Nutrition (1995) no longer recommends fluoride supplementation from birth to 6 months. Also, the fluoride dosage has been decreased from earlier recommendations because of an increased occurrence of dental fluorosis from excessive fluoride ingestion (see Table 12-2).

Dietary considerations are also important because habits begun during infancy tend to continue into later years. Foods with concentrated sugar are used sparingly (if at all) in the infant's diet. The practice of coating pacifiers with honey or using commercially available hard-candy pacifiers is discouraged. Besides being cariogenic, honey also may cause infant botulism, and parts of the candy pacifier can be aspirated (See p. 322). Parents need to be counseled regarding the detrimental effects of frequent and prolonged bottle- or breast-feeding during sleep, when the sweet milk or other fluid, such as juice, bathes the teeth, producing **nursing caries.** (See also Chapter 12 for a more extensive discussion of dental care, including nursing caries.)

IMMUNIZATIONS

One of the most dramatic advances in pediatrics has been the decline of infectious diseases over the past 60 years because of the widespread use of immunization for preventable diseases. Although many of the presently available immunizations can be given to individuals of any age, the recommended primary schedule begins during infancy and, with the exception of boosters, is completed during early childhood. Therefore the discussion of childhood immunizations for diphtheria, tetanus, pertussis or acellular pertussis (DTP or DTaP); polio; measles, mumps, rubella (MMR); *Haemophilus influenzae* type b (Hib); hepatitis B virus (HBV); and chickenpox (varicella zoster virus [VZV]) is included under health promotion during infancy. Selected vaccines that are generally reserved for children considered at high risk for the disease are discussed here and as appropriate throughout the text. (See also Communicable Diseases, Chapter 14, for a discussion of several of the diseases for which vaccines are available.)

Unfounded fears regarding side effects of vaccines, especially DTP, have also had an impact on immunization rates and vaccine production. Concerns about DTP vaccine causing sudden infant death syndrome (SIDS) and pertussis vaccine resulting in permanent neurologic damage have caused many families to bring lawsuits against vaccine producers, causing a drastic increase in vaccine costs and at one time prompting some manufacturers to stop vaccine production. The Institute of Medicine (IOM) (1993) found no evidence for diphtheria and tetanus toxoids causing encephalopathy, infantile spasms, or SIDS. They did find a relationship between DTP vaccination and acute encephalopathy occurring within 7 days of the vaccination. This association occurs rarely—at a rate of 0 to 10.5/million immunizations—and probably occurs in children with an underlying neurologic disorder.

Practitioners are required to fully inform families of the risks and benefits of the vaccines. The U.S. Public Health Service has developed a series of vaccine information pamphlets (VIPs) for the DTP, MMR, and polio vaccines. Health professionals need to be aware of the importance of providing parents with sufficient time to read the information, discussing the vaccines to determine caregivers' understanding of the information, addressing parents' concerns, and dispelling unfounded fears. Since nurses frequently administer vaccines during health supervision visits, they may have the responsibility for adequately informing parents of the nature, prevalence, and risks of the disease; the type of immunization product to be used; expected benefits; the risk of side effects; and the need for accurate immunization records. Referring to immunizations as "baby shots" and limiting the discussion to vague statements about the vaccines are unacceptable practices.

Schedule for Immunizations

In the United States two organizations—the Advisory Committee on Immunization Practices (ACIP) of the U.S. Public

Health Service Centers for Disease Control and Prevention (CDC) and the Committee on Infectious Diseases of the American Academy of Pediatrics (AAP)—govern the recommendations for immunization policies and procedures. In Canada, recommendations are from the **National Advisory Committee on Immunization** under the authority of the Minister of National Health and Welfare. The policies of each committee are recommendations, not rules, and they change as a result of advances in the field of immunology. Nurses need to keep informed of the latest advances and changes in policy.

The recommended age for beginning primary immunizations of infants is at birth (Table 10-4). Children born prematurely should receive the *full dose* of each vaccine at the appropriate chronologic age. If the infant is hospitalized, OPV is initiated after discharge to prevent transmission of OPV in the nursery. Recommended schedules for children not immunized during infancy are included in Table 10-5.

TABLE 10-4. Recommended childhood immunization schedule United States, July-December 1996

Vaccines are listed under the routinely recommended ages. Bars indicate range of acceptable ages for vaccination. Shaded bars indicate *catch-up vaccination:* at 11-12 years of age, hepatitis B vaccine should be administered to children not previously vaccinated, and Varicella Zoster Virus vaccine should be administered to children not previously vaccinated who lack a reliable history of chickenpox.

AGE ▶ VACCINE ▼	BIRTH	1 MO	2 MOS	4 MOS	6 MOS	12 MOS	15 MOS	18 MOS	4-6 YRS	11-12 YRS	14-16 YRS
Hepatitis B[1,2]	Hep B-1		Hep B-2		Hep B-3					Hep B[2]	
Diphtheria, Tetanus, Pertussis[3] *whooping cough*			DTP	DTP	DTP	DTP[3] (DTaP at 15+ m)			DTP or DTaP	Td	
H. influenzae type b[4]			Hib	Hib	Hib[4]	Hib[4]					
Polio[5]			OPV[5]	OPV	OPV				OPV		
Measles, Mumps, Rubella[6]						MMR			MMR[6] or	MMR[6]	
Varicella Zoster Virus vaccine[7]						Var				Var[7]	

Approved by the Advisory Committee on Immunization Practices (ACIP), the American Academy of Pediatrics (AAP), and the American Academy of Family Physicians (AAFP).
From *Pediatrics* 98(1):158-160, 1996.
[1]*Infants born to HBsAg-negative mothers* should receive 2.5 μg of Merck vaccine (Recombivax HB) or 10 μg of SmithKline Beecham (SB) vaccine (Engerix-B). The second dose should be administered ≥ 1 mo after the first dose.
Infants born to HBsAg-positive mothers should receive 0.5 mL Hepatitis B Immune Globulin (HBIG) within 12 hr of birth, and either 5 μg of Merck vaccine (Recombivax HB) or 10 μg of SB vaccine (Engerix-B) at a separate site. The second dose is recommended at 1-2 mos of age and the third dose at 6 mos of age.
Infants born to mothers whose HBsAg status is unknown should receive either 5 μg of Merck vaccine (Recombivax HB) or 10 μg of SB vaccine (Engerix-B) within 12 hr of birth. The second dose of vaccine is recommended at 1 mo of age and the third dose at 6 mos of age.
[2]Adolescents who are 11-12 yrs of age and who have not previously received 3 doses of hepatitis B vaccine should initiate or complete the series. The second dose should be administered at least 1 mo after the first dose, and the third dose should be administered at least 4 mos after the first dose and at least 2 mos after the second dose.
[3]DTP4 may be administered at 12 mos of age, if at least 6 mos have elapsed since DTP3. DTaP (diphtheria and tetanus toxoids and acellular pertussis vaccine) is licensed for the fourth and/or fifth vaccine dose(s) for children ages ≥15 mos and may be preferred for these doses in this age group. Td (tetanus and diphtheria toxoids, adsorbed, for adult use) is recommended at 11-12 yrs of age if at least 5 yrs have elapsed since the last dose of DTP, DTaP, or DT.
[4]Three *H. influenzae* type b (Hib) conjugate vaccines are licensed for infant use. If PRP-OMP (PedvaxHIB [Merck]) is administered at 2 and 4 mos of age, a dose at 6 mos is not required. After completing the primary series, any Hib conjugate vaccine may be used as a booster.
[5]Oral poliovirus vaccine (OPV) is recommended for routine infant vaccination. Inactivated poliovirus vaccine (IPV) is recommended for persons with a congenital or acquired immune deficiency disease or an altered immune status as a result of disease or immunosuppressive therapy, as well as their household contacts, and is an acceptable alternative for other persons. The primary 3-dose series for IPV should be given with a minimum interval of 4 wks between the first and second doses and 6 mos between the second and third doses.
[6]The second dose of MMR is routinely recommended at 4-6 yrs of age or at 11-12 yrs of age, but may be administered at any visit, provided at least 1 mo has elapsed since receipt of the first dose.
[7]Varicella zoster virus vaccine (Var) can be administered to susceptible children any time after 12 months of age. Unvaccinated adolescents who are 11-12 yrs of age and who lack a reliable history of chickenpox should be vaccinated.

Tables 10-6 and 10-7 describe immunization schedules for Canadian children. Children who began primary immunization at the recommended age but who fail to receive all the doses do not have to begin the series again, but receive only the missed doses. In situations when there is doubt that the child will return for immunization according to the optimum schedule, HBV, DTP, OPV, MMR, and Hib vaccines can be administered simultaneously. However, parenteral vaccines are given in separate syringes in different injection sites (American Academy of Pediatrics, 1994).

Recommendations for Routine Immunizations

Hepatitis B Virus (HBV). HBV, a potentially fatal viral infection that eventually causes cirrhosis or liver cancer during adulthood, is an important pediatric disease because HBV infections occurring during childhood and adolescence can lead to these consequences. Up to 90% of infants infected perinatally and 25% to 50% of children infected before age 5 years will become HBV carriers. In addition, the incidence of HBV infection increases rapidly during adolescence (American Academy of Pediatrics, 1992). Despite the availability of a safe, effective vaccine, new cases have increased about 50% during the last decade. Past immunization strategies targeted several high-risk groups, including health care workers and others in contact with blood and body fluids, recipients of certain blood products (such as those with hemophilia), heterosexuals with multiple partners, sexually active homosexual and bisexual males, intravenous drug abusers, immigrants from countries where HBV is widespread, and children born to mothers who are HBV surface antigen (HBsAg) positive. To improve immunization rates, current recommendations include immunizations for all newborns, as well as several high-risk groups (Centers for Disease Control

TABLE 10-5. Recommended immunization schedule for children not immunized in the first year of life in the United States

RECOMMENDED TIME/AGE	IMMUNIZATION(S)[a,b]	COMMENTS
Younger Than 7 Years		
First visit	DTP, Hib, HBV[c], MMR, OPV, VZV	If indicated, tuberculin testing may be done at same visit
		If child is 5 years of age or older, Hib is not indicated
Interval after first visit:		
1 month	DTP, HBV	OPV may be given if accelerated poliomyelitis vaccination is necessary, such as for travelers to areas where polio is endemic
2 months	DTP, Hib,[c] OPV	Second dose of Hib is indicated only in children whose first dose was received when younger than 15 months
≥8 months	DTP or DTaP,[d] HBV, OPV	OPV is not given if the third dose was given earlier
4-6 years (at or before school entry)	DTP or DTaP,[d] OPV	DTP or DTaP is not necessary if the fourth dose was given after the fourth birthday; OPV is not necessary if the third dose was given after the fourth birthday
11-12 years	MMR	At entry to middle school or junior high school
10 years later	Td	Repeat every 10 years throughout life
7 Years and Older[e,f]		
First visit	HBV,[g] OPV, MMR, Td, VZV	After the 13th birthday, 2 doses of VZV are required 4 to 8 weeks apart
Interval after first visit:		
2 months	HBV,[g] OPV, Td	OPV may also be given 1 month after the first visit if accelerated poliomyelitis vaccination is necessary
8-14 months	HBV,[g] OPV, Td	OPV is not given if the third dose was given earlier
11-12 years	MMR	At entry to middle school or junior high
10 years later	Td	Repeat every 10 years throughout life

From American Academy of Pediatrics: *Report of the Committee on Infectious Diseases,* ed 23, Elk Grove Village, IL, 1994, The Academy. American Academy of Pediatrics, Committee on Infectious Diseases: Recommendations for the use of live attenuated varicella vaccine, *Pediatrics* 95(5):791-796, 1995.

[a]Abbreviations for vaccines are on p. 313. If all needed vaccines cannot be administered simultaneously, priority should be given to protecting the child against those diseases that pose the greatest immediate risk. In the United States these diseases for children younger than 2 years usually are measles and *Haemophilus influenzae* type b infection; for children older than 7 years, they are measles, mumps, and rubella (MMR).

[b]DTP or DTaP, HBV, Hib, MMR, VZV, and OPV can be given simultaneously at separate sites if failure of the patient to return for future immunizations is a concern.

[c]Any licensed Hib conjugate vaccine may be used.

[d]DTaP is not currently licensed for use in children younger than 15 months of age and is not recommended for primary immunization (i.e., first 3 doses) at any age.

[e]If person is 18 years or older, routine poliovirus vaccination is not indicated in the United States.

[f]Minimal interval between doses of MMR is 1 month.

[g]Priority should be given to hepatitis B immunization of adolescents.

TABLE 10-6. Routine primary immunization schedule for infants and children in Canada

AGE	IMMUNIZATION AGAINST				
2 months	Diphtheria	Pertussis	Tetanus	Poliomyelitis	*Haemophilus influenzae* b[1]
4 months	Diphtheria	Pertussis	Tetanus	Poliomyelitis	*Haemophilus influenzae* b
6 months	Diphtheria	Pertussis	Tetanus	Poliomyelitis[2]	*Haemophilus influenzae* b
12 months	Measles	Mumps	Rubella		
18 months	Diphtheria	Pertussis	Tetanus	Poliomyelitis	*Haemophilus influenzae* b
4-6 years	Diphtheria	Pertussis	Tetanus	Poliomyelitis	
14-16 years	Diphtheria[3]		Tetanus[3]	Poliomyelitis[2]	

From National Advisory Committee on Immunization: *Canadian immunization guide,* ed 4, Canada, 1993, Authority of the Minister of National Health and Welfare, Health Protection Branch, Laboratory Centre for Disease Control.
Notes:
1. Hib schedule shown is for HbOC or PRP-T vaccine. If PRP-OMP is used, give at 2, 4, and 12 months of age.
2. Omit this dose of OPV if used exclusively.
3. Td (tetanus and diphtheria toxoid), a combined adsorbed "adult-type" preparation for use in persons ≥7 years of age, contains less diphtheria toxoid than preparations given to younger children and is less likely to cause reactions in older persons. Repeat every 10 years throughout life.

TABLE 10-7. Routine immunization schedules for children not immunized in early infancy in Canada

TIMING	IMMUNIZATION AGAINST				
For Children 7 Years of Age and Younger					
First visit	Diphtheria	Pertussis	Tetanus	Poliomyelitis	*Haemophilus influenzae* b[1]
	Measles[4]	Mumps[4]	Rubella[4]		
2 months later	Diphtheria	Pertussis	Tetanus	Poliomyelitis	*Haemophilus influenzae* b[5]
2 months later	Diphtheria	Pertussis	Tetanus	Poliomyelitis[2]	
6-12 months later	Diphtheria	Pertussis	Tetanus	Poliomyelitis	*Haemophilus influenzae* b[5]
4-6 years[6]	Diphtheria	Pertussis	Tetanus	Poliomyelitis	
14-16 years	Diphtheria[3]	Tetanus[3]	Poliomyelitis[2]		
For Children 7 Years of Age and Older					
First visit	Diphtheria[3]		Tetanus[3]	Poliomyelitis	
	Measles	Mumps	Rubella		
2 months later	Diphtheria[3]		Tetanus[3]	Poliomyelitis	
6-12 months later	Diphtheria[3]		Tetanus[3]	Poliomyelitis	
10 years later	Diphtheria[3]		Tetanus[3]		

From National Advisory Committee on Immunization: *Canadian immunization guide,* ed 4, Canada, 1993, Authority of the Minister of National Health and Welfare, Health Protection Branch, Laboratory Centre for Disease Control.
Notes:
1-3. See Table 10-6.
4. Delay until subsequent visit if child is <12 months of age.
5. Recommended schedule and number of doses depend on the product used and the age of the child when vaccination is begun. Not required past age 5.
6. Omit these doses if the previous doses of DTP and polio were given after the fourth birthday.

and Prevention, 1994). The American Academy of Pediatrics (1994) also encourages the routine immunization of all adolescents against HBV when feasible.

The vaccine is given intramuscularly in the vastus lateralis in neonates, but may be given in the deltoid muscle during later infancy. Regardless of age, the dorsogluteal site is avoided because it has been associated with low antibody seroconversion rates, indicating a reduced immune response (Zuckerman, Cockcroft, and Zuckerman, 1992). It can be safely administered simultaneously at a separate site with DTP, MMR, and Hib vaccines. Dosage depends on the child's age and type of vaccine used (see Table 10-5).

Diphtheria. Diphtheria vaccine is commonly administered intramuscularly (1) in combination with tetanus and pertussis vaccines (DTP or DTaP) or DTP and Hib vaccines for children younger than 7 years of age, (2) in a combined vaccine with tetanus (DT) for children younger than 7 years of age who have some contraindication for receiving pertussis vaccine, (3) in smaller doses (15% to 20% of that in DTP or DT) with tetanus vaccine (Td) for use in children age 7 years and older, or (4) as a single antigen when combined antigen preparations are not indicated. Although the diphtheria vaccine does not produce absolute immunity, when

TABLE 10-8. Guide to tetanus prophylaxis in routine wound management, 1991

HISTORY OF ADSORBED TETANUS TOXOID (DOSES)	CLEAN, MINOR WOUNDS		ALL OTHER WOUNDS*	
	TD†	TIG	TD†	TIG
Unknown or < three	Yes	No	Yes	Yes
≥ Three‡	No§	No	No‖	No

From Recommendations of the Immunization Practices Advisory Committee (ACIP): Diphtheria, tetanus, and pertussis: recommendations for vaccine use and other preventive measures, *MMWR* 40(RR-10):1-28, 1991.
*Such as, but not limited to, wounds contaminated with dirt, feces, soil, and saliva; puncture wounds; avulsions; and wounds resulting from missiles, crushing, burns, and frostbite.
†For children < 7 years old; DTP (DT, if pertussis vaccine is contraindicated) is preferred to tetanus toxoid alone. For persons ≥ 7 years of age, Td is preferred to tetanus toxoid alone.
‡If only three doses of *fluid* toxoid have been received, then a fourth dose of toxoid, preferably an adsorbed toxoid, should be given.
§Yes, if > 10 years since last dose.
‖Yes, if > 5 years since last dose. (More frequent boosters are not needed and can accentuate side effects.)

given according to the recommended scheduled protective antitoxin persists for 10 years or more.

Tetanus.   Three forms of tetanus vaccine—tetanus toxoid, tetanus immune globulin (TIG) (human), and tetanus antitoxin (usually horse serum)—are available. Tetanus toxoid is used for routine primary immunization, usually in one of the combinations listed above, and provides protective antitoxin levels for 10 years or more.

For wound management, passive immunity is available with TIG or animal-source antitoxin. However, because the risk of severe reaction, such as anaphylactic shock or serum sickness, is always greater to the foreign substances of animal serum, the choice is TIG. In persons with a history of two previous doses of tetanus toxoid, a booster dose of the toxoid can be given. When tetanus toxoid and TIG are given concurrently, separate syringes and different intramuscular sites are used. Table 10-8 of the recommended procedure for tetanus prophylaxis in wound management.

Pertussis.   Pertussis vaccine is recommended for all children 6 weeks through 6 years of age (up to the seventh birthday) who have no neurologic contraindications to its use. It is not given to children 7 years or older because the risk of receiving the vaccine increases as the incidence, severity, and fatality of the disease decrease.

Currently two forms of pertussis vaccine are available for intramuscular administration in the United States. The **whole-cell pertussis vaccine** is prepared from inactivated cells of *Bordetella pertussis* and contains multiple antigens. In contrast, the **acellular pertussis vaccine** contains one or more immunogens derived from the **B. pertussis** organism. The highly purified acellular vaccine is associated with fewer local and systemic reactions than those occurring with the whole-cell vaccine in children of similar age. The whole-cell pertussis vaccine is used for the first three immunizations, usually given at 2, 4, and 6 months of age with diphtheria and tetanus. The acellular vaccine (DTaP [ACEL-IMUNE]) is licensed for use only as the fourth and fifth doses for children who have been immunized previously with at least three doses of the DTP vaccine (American Academy of Pediatrics, 1993a).

Polio.   The trivalent form of **oral poliovirus (OPV)** (developed by Sabin) is recommended for all children younger than 18 years of age who have no specific contraindications

to its use, regardless of the number of administrations of **inactivated poliovirus vaccine (IPV)** (developed by Salk) they have received. OPV is used in the United States because the live virus can be shed to contacts, who become immunized through this exposure. However, OPV has caused vaccine-associated paralysis in both recipients and contacts.

Because of the greater risk of vaccine-associated paralysis in children with immunodeficiency diseases, IPV is the vaccine of choice for immunocompromised children and any close contacts because it has no reported history of causing vaccine-associated paralysis. However, IPV has the disadvantage of being given by subcutaneous injection and producing less immunity. In the United States an enhanced-potency form of IVP is used.*

A recent change in the immunization schedule is that the third dose of polio vaccine can now be given at 6 months, along with the third doses of DTP and *H. influenzae* vaccines. This change is hoped to increase polio protection at an earlier age.

Measles.   Because of the presence of maternal antibodies, measles (rubeola) virus vaccine was usually delayed until 15 months of age for infants who live in communities where the disease is not prevalent. However, it can now be given at 12 to 15 months of age. During the course of measles outbreaks, the vaccine can be given any time after 6 months of age, followed by a second inoculation after age 12 months.

Because of continued outbreaks of measles among unvaccinated preschool-age children and among vaccinated school-age children and college students, a second measles immunization is recommended before school entry at 4 to 6 years or at 11 to 12 years of age. It is given subcutaneously with mumps and rubella (MMR).

Mumps.   Mumps virus vaccine is recommended for children at 12 to 15 months of age and is typically given in combination with measles and rubella. It should not be administered to infants younger than 12 months because persisting maternal antibodies can interfere with the immune response. It is administered subcutaneously in the combined MMR vaccine.

---

*As of this writing the CDC Advisory Panel has recommended that the first two doses of the enhanced-potency form of IPV be administered, followed by two doses of IPV.

Rubella. Rubella is a relatively mild infection in children, but in a pregnant woman it presents serious risks to the developing fetus. Therefore the aim of rubella immunization is actually protection of the unborn child rather than the recipient of the immunization.

Rubella immunization is recommended for all children at 12 to 15 months of age and is administered in a combined form with measles and mumps vaccine. Increased emphasis should also be placed on vaccinating all unimmunized prepubertal children and susceptible adolescents and adult women in the childbearing age-group.

Because the live attenuated virus may cross the placenta and present a risk to the developing fetus, rubella vaccine is not given to any pregnant woman. Although this is standard practice, current evidence from women who received the vaccine while pregnant and delivered unaffected offspring indicates that the risk to the fetus is negligible (Centers for Disease Control and Prevention, 1994). In addition, there is no reported danger of administering rubella vaccine to a child if the mother is pregnant. It is administered subcutaneously in the combined MMR vaccine.

Haemophilus Influenzae Type b (Hib). Hib conjugate vaccines provide protection against a number of serious infections caused by Hib, especially bacterial meningitis, epiglottitis, bacterial pneumonia, septic arthritis, and sepsis. (Hib is not associated with the viruses that cause influenza, or "flu.")

The following Hib conjugate vaccines are currently available:

- Diphtheria toxoid conjugate (PRP-D) (ProHIBit)
- Diphtheria CRM_{197} protein conjugate (PRP-HbOC) (Hib-TITER)
- Meningococcal protein conjugate (PRP-OMP) (Pedvax HIB)
- PRP conjugate with tetanus toxoid (PRP-T) (ActHIB and Omni-HIB)
- HibTITER is also combined in a vaccine with DTP (Tetramune).

These conjugate vaccines connect Hib to a nontoxic form of another organism, such as meningococcal protein or diphtheria protein. There is *no* antibody response to these nontoxic proteins, but they significantly improve the antibody response to Hib, especially in infants.

HbOC or PRP-T is recommended at 2, 4, and 6 months of age, with a booster at 12 to 15 months. Only two doses of PRP-OMP are required—at ages 2 to 6 months, administered at least 2 months apart with a booster at 12 to 15 months. PRP-D is not licensed for use in infants under 12 months. When possible, the Hib conjugate vaccine used at the first vaccination should be used for all subsequent vaccinations in the primary series. When either a Hib vaccine or Tetramune is used, the vaccine is administered by intramuscular injection (IM) using a separate syringe and at a separate site from any concurrent vaccinations.

Children under age 2 years who develop a Hib-related illness still need to be immunized; the vaccine is not recommended for children over age 5 years except for those with chronic conditions that affect their immune function.

Varicella. The live virus varicella zoster (VZ) or chickenpox vaccine is recommended for all children between 12 and 18 months of age and all older susceptible children, up to age 12 years. The dose is 0.5 ml, given subcutaneously,

with one dose for children 12 months to 12 years and two doses for youngsters after the thirteenth birthday. The vaccine must be kept frozen in the lyophilized form (stable particles that readily go into solution) and used immediately after being reconstituted to ensure maximum response.

A small number of immunized children may develop chickenpox. However, the disease is mild; children have fewer lesions and less itching, fever, or headache, and more than half have no symptoms other than the rash. The contagiousness of the infection is also significantly reduced (American Academy of Pediatrics, Committee on Infectious Diseases, 1995).

Recommendations for Selected Immunizations

Several additional vaccines are recommended for children at high risk for particular diseases. Most of these children have chronic disorders or impaired immune systems that make them more susceptible to certain infections than the general population. Selected immunizations are presented in Table 10-9. Others, such as the rabies vaccine, are discussed elsewhere in this text.

Reactions

Vaccines for routine immunizations are among the safest and most reliable drugs available. However, minor side effects do occur following many of the immunizations, and rarely a serious reaction may result from the vaccine.

With inactivated antigens, such as DTP, side effects are most likely to occur within a few hours or days of administration and are usually limited to local tenderness, erythema, and swelling at the injection site; low-grade fever; and behavioral changes (drowsiness, fretfulness, eating less, prolonged or unusual cry). Local reactions tend to be less severe when the deltoid site is used rather than the vastus lateralis and when a needle of sufficient length to deposit the vaccine in the muscle is used (see Atraumatic Care box on p. 322). Rarely, more severe reactions may occur. Especially with pertussis these may include loss of consciousness, convulsions, persistent inconsolable crying episodes, generalized or focal neurologic signs, fever (temperature at or above 40.5° C [105° F]), and systemic allergic reactions.

Nursing ALERT Recommend prophylactic use of acetaminophen at time of DTP immunization and every 4 to 6 hours for a total of 3 doses.

Advise parents to notify practitioner *immediately* of any unusual side effects.

Reactions to DTP tend to be more severe if they occurred with a previous immunization.

Hib vaccine is one of the safest vaccines available but may be associated with low-grade fever and mild local reactions at the site of injection, which resolve rapidly. Fever (temperature more than 38.5° C [101.3° F]) may rarely occur. HBV is equally well tolerated.

Unlike the inactivated antigens, live attenuated virus vaccines such as MMR and OPV multiply for days or weeks, and unfavorable reactions and "vaccine-associated" disorders can occur for a period of 30 to 60 days. However, they are usu-

TABLE 10-9. Recommendations for selected nonmandated vaccines

DESCRIPTION	ADMINISTRATION/PRECAUTIONS
Influenza Virus Vaccine Affords protection against strains of influenza Recommended for children age 6 months and older with chronic disorders of cardiovascular or pulmonary systems, including asthma, whose severity warranted regular medical care or hospitalization during preceding year; other eligible children include those with diabetes mellitus, renal dysfunction, anemia, immunosuppression, human immunodeficiency virus (HIV) infection, or those on long-term aspirin therapy (because of risk of developing Reye syndrome after influenza infection)	Administered in fall, preferably November; repeated yearly Intramuscular injection; 2 doses of split vaccine at least 4 weeks apart for children age 12 years or younger; 1 dose of split or whole vaccine for children over 12 years of age Contraindicated in persons with anaphylactic hypersensitivity to eggs May be given simultaneously with other childhood immunizations but at separate site
Pneumococcal Polysaccharide Vaccine (Pneumovax; PNU-IMUNE) Affords protection against 23 types of *Streptococcus pneumoniae* Recommended for children age 2 years and older with sickle cell disease, functional or anatomic asplenia, nephrotic syndrome, human immunodeficiency virus (HIV) infection, and Hodgkin's disease before beginning cytoreduction therapy	Subcutaneous or intramuscular injection Revaccination is not recommended Should be deferred during pregnancy
Meningococcal Polysaccharide Vaccine (Menomune) Affords protection against *Neisseria meningitidis;* sero-groups A, C, Y, and W-135 Recommended for children 2 years and older with terminal complement deficiencies and anatomic or functional asplenia	Subcutaneous injection Duration of protection unknown Safety during pregnancy not established
Hepatitis A Virus Vaccine (HAVRIX, Vaqta) Affords protection against hepatitis A virus Recommended for children ages 2 years and older who are at high risk for contracting hepatitis A: travelers to hepatitis A endemic areas; military personnel; ethnic and geographic populations with cyclic hepatitis A epidemics, such as Native American and Alaskan communities; homosexuals; IV-drug users and noninjection street-drug users; chronic liver disease patients; individuals with occupational risk of exposure, such as child care and institutional workers, as well as primate-animal handlers; and laboratory workers who handle live hepatitis A virus	HAVRIX: Intramuscular injection, 2 doses, 1 month apart, any time between 2 to 18 years; booster dose should be given 6 to 12 months after the second dose Vaqta: Requires only one injection between ages 2 and 17 years, followed by a booster dose 6 to 12 months later.

ally mild, although reactions to rubella tend to be more troublesome in older children and adults. The varicella vaccine produces minimal reactions, especially during adolescence. Adolescents may experience pain, tenderness, or redness at injection site and a mild vaccine-associated maculopapular or varicellaform rash at the injection site or elsewhere.

Contraindications/Precautions

Nurses need to be aware of the reasons for withholding immunizations—both for the child's safety in terms of avoiding reactions and for the child's maximum benefit from receiving the vaccine. Unfounded fears and lack of knowledge regarding contraindications can needlessly prevent a child from having protection from life-threatening diseases. The contraindications and precautions to the usual childhood vaccines are presented in Table 10-10.

Administration

The principal precautions in administering immunizations include proper storage of the vaccine to protect its potency and

institution of recommended procedures for injection. The nurse must be familiar with the manufacturer's directions for storage and reconstitution of the vaccine. For example, if the vaccine is to be refrigerated, it should be stored on a center shelf, not on the door where frequent temperature decreases from opening the refrigerator can alter the vaccine's potency. For protection against light the vial can be wrapped in aluminum foil. Periodic checks are established to ensure that no vaccine is used after its expiration date.

The DTP vaccines contain the adjuvant alum to retain the antigen at the injection site and prolong the stimulatory effect. Because subcutaneous or intracutaneous injection of the adjuvant can cause local irritation, inflammation, or abscess formation, attention to excellent intramuscular injection technique must be used (see Atraumatic Care box on p. 322).

The total series requires a number of injections, and every attempt is made to rotate the sites and administer the injections as painlessly as possible (see discussion on intramuscular injections in Chapter 22). When two or more injections are given at separate sites, the order of injections is arbitrary.

TABLE 10-10. Contraindications and precautions to vaccinations[a]

TRUE CONTRAINDICATIONS AND PRECAUTIONS	NOT CONTRAINDICATIONS (VACCINES MAY BE ADMINISTERED)
General for All Vaccines (DTP/DTaP, OPV, IPV, MMR, Hib, Hepatitis B, VZV)	
Contraindications	*Not contraindications*
Anaphylactic reaction to a vaccine contraindicates further doses of that vaccine	Mild to moderate local reaction (soreness, redness, swelling) following a dose of an injectable antigen
Anaphylactic reaction to a vaccine constituent contraindicates the use of vaccines containing that substance	Mild acute illness with or without low-grade fever
Moderate or severe illnesses with or without a fever	Current antimicrobial therapy
	Convalescent phase of illnesses
	Prematurity (same dosage and indications as for full-term infants)
	Recent exposure to an infectious disease
	History of penicillin or other nonspecific allergies or family history of such allergies
Diphtheria, Tetanus, Pertussis or Acellular Pertussis (DTP/DTaP)	
Contraindications	*Not contraindications*
Encephalopathy within 7 days of administration of previous dose of DTP	Temperature of <40.5° C (105 F) following a previous dose of DTP
	Family history of seizures[c]
Precautions[b]	Family history of sudden infant death syndrome
Fever of ≥40.5° C (105° F) within 48 hours after vaccination with a prior dose of DTP	Family history of an adverse event following DTP administration
Collapse or shocklike state (hypotonic-hyporesponsive episode) within 48 hours of receiving a prior dose of DTP	
Seizures within 3 days of receiving a prior dose of DTP[c]	
Persistent, inconsolable crying lasting ≥3 hours within 48 hours of receiving a prior dose of DTP	
Oral Polio (OPV)[d]	
Contraindications	*Not contraindications*
Infection with HIV or a household contact with HIV	Breast-feeding
Known altered immunodeficiency (hematologic and solid tumors; congenital immunodeficiency; and long-term immunosuppressive therapy)	Current antimicrobial therapy
Immunodeficient household contact	Diarrhea
Precaution[b]	
Pregnancy	
Inactivated Polio (IPV)	
Contraindication	
Anaphylactic reaction to neomycin or streptomycin	
Precaution[b]	
Pregnancy	

From Centers for Disease Control and Prevention: General recommendations on immunization: recommendations of the Advisory Committee on Immunization Practices (ACIP), *MMWR* 43(RR-1):24-25, 1994 and American Academy of Pediatrics: Committee on Infectious Diseases: Recommendations for the use of live attenuated varicella vaccine, *Pediatrics* 95(5):791-796, 1995.

[a]This information is based on the recommendations of the Advisory Committee on Immunization Practices (ACIP) and those of the Committee on Infectious Diseases (Red Book Committee) of the American Academy of Pediatrics (AAP). Sometimes these recommendations vary from those contained in the manufacturer's package inserts. For more detailed information, providers should consult the published recommendations of the ACIP, AAP, and the manufacturer's package inserts.

[b]The events or conditions listed as precautions, although not contraindications, should be carefully reviewed. The benefits and risks of administering a specific vaccine to an individual under the circumstances should be considered. If the risks are believed to outweigh the benefits, the vaccination should be withheld; if the benefits are believed to outweigh the risks (e.g., during an outbreak or foreign travel), the vaccination should be administered. Whether and when to administer DTP to children with proven or suspected underlying neurologic disorders should be decided on an individual basis. It is prudent on theoretic grounds to avoid vaccinating pregnant women. However, if immediate protection against poliomyelitis is needed, OPV is preferred, although IPV may be considered if full vaccination can be completed before the anticipated imminent exposure.

[c]Acetaminophen given before administering DTP and thereafter every 4 hours for 24 hours should be considered for children with a personal or family history of seizures in siblings or parents.

[d]No data exist to substantiate the theoretic risk of a suboptimal immune response from the administration of OPV and MMR within 30 days of each other.

[e]Persons with a history of anaphylactic reactions following egg ingestion should be vaccinated only with caution. Protocols have been developed for vaccinating such persons and should be consulted.

TABLE 10-10. Contraindications and precautions to vaccinations[a]—cont'd

TRUE CONTRAINDICATIONS AND PRECAUTIONS	NOT CONTRAINDICATIONS (VACCINES MAY BE ADMINISTERED)
Measles, Mumps, Rubella (MMR)[d]	
Contraindications	*Not contraindications[d]*
Anaphylactic reactions to egg ingestion and to neomycin[e]	Tuberculosis or positive PPD skin test
Pregnancy	Simultaneous TB skin testing[f]
Known altered immunodeficiency (hematologic and solid tumors, congenital immunodeficiency, and long-term immunosuppressive therapy)	Breast-feeding
	Pregnancy of mother of recipient
	Immunodeficient family member or household contact
	Infection with HIV
Precautions[b]	Nonanaphylactic reactions to eggs or neomycin
Recent immune globulin administration	
Immune globulin products and MMR should not be given simultaneously; if unavoidable, give at different sites and revaccinate or test for seroconversion in 3 months; if IG is given first, MMR should not be given for at least 3 to 6 months, depending on the dose; if MMR is given first, IG should not be given for 2 weeks	
Haemophilus Influenzae Type B (Hib)	
Contraindication	*Not a contraindication*
Nonidentified	History of Hib disease
Hepatitis B Virus (HBV)	
Contraindication	*Not a contraindication*
Anaphylactic reaction to common baker's yeast	Pregnancy
Varicella-Zoster Virus (VZV)	
Contraindications	*Not contraindications*
Immunocompromised individuals, such as those with congenital immunodeficiency, blood dyscrasias, leukemia, lymphoma, symptomatic HIV infection, and malignancy for which they are receiving immunosuppressive therapy	Presence of immunodeficient or HIV-seropositive family member
Asymptomatic HIV infection	Children receiving only inhaled steroids
Individuals who are receiving high doses of systemic corticosteroids (2 mg/kg/d or more of prednisone, or its equivalent or 20 mg/d of prednisone if their weight is > 10 kg) for > 1 month (interval of 1 month or more after discontinuation of steroid use is probably sufficient to safely administer vaccine)	Pregnancy of family member
Pregnancy	Nonanaphylactoid reactions, such as contact dermatitis, to neomycin
Anaphylactoid reaction to neomycin	
Precautions	
Immunization should be considered when child with acute lymphocytic leukemia has been in continuous remission for at least 1 year and has lymphocyte count over $700/\mu L$ and platelet count over $100\,000/\mu L$ 24 hours before vaccination	
Children with no history of varicella who are receiving systemic steroids for conditions such as nephrosis and asthma may be immunized if not otherwise immunosuppressed, assuming that they are receiving <2 mg/kg/d of prednisone or its equivalent (or <20 mg/d if their weight is >10 kg)	
When postpubertal females are immunized, pregnancy should be avoided for 1 month after immunization.	
May be considered for VZV-susceptible nursing mother, if risk for exposure to natural VZV is high	
Should not be administered within at least 5 months after receipt of any form of immune globulin or other blood product	
Salicylates should not be administered for 6 weeks after varicella vaccine because of the association between Reye syndrome, natural varicella, and salicylates	

[f]Measles vaccination may temporarily suppress tuberculin reactivity. If testing cannot be done the day of MMR vaccination, the test should be postponed for 4 to 6 weeks.

To minimize local reactions from DTP vaccines:

Select a needle of adequate length (1 inch in infants) to deposit the antigen deep in the muscle mass

Inject into the vastus lateralis or ventrogluteal muscle; the deltoid may be used in children 18 months or older except for HBV deltoid may be used during later infancy

Use an air bubble to clear the needle after injecting the vaccine (theoretically beneficial but unproved)

To minimize pain*:

Apply the topical anesthetic EMLA to the injection site for a minimum of 1 hour, preferably for up to 2 hours for greater penetration

In preschool children use distraction, such as telling the child to "take a deep breath and blow and blow and blow until I tell you to stop"

Note: Changing the needle on the syringe after drawing up the vaccine and before injecting it has not be shown to be effective in decreasing local reactions

*See also Pain Management, Chapter 21.

Some practitioners suggest injecting the less painful one first. Some believe this is DTP, whereas others suggest the MMR or Hib vaccine. Still others advocate injecting at two sites simultaneously (requires two operators). Research is needed to determine which sequence is least painful. Since allergic reactions can occur after injection of vaccines, appropriate precautions are taken (see Anaphylaxis, Chapter 25).

Another important nursing responsibility is accurate documentation. Each child should have an immunization record for parents to keep, especially for families who move frequently. The following information is documented on the medical record: day, month, and year of administration; manufacturer and lot number of vaccine; and the name, address, and title of the person administering the vaccine. Additional data to record are the site and route of administration and evidence that the parent or legal guardian gave informed consent before the immunization was administered. Any adverse reactions after the administration of any vaccine is reported to the *Vaccine Adverse Event Reporting System (VAERS).**

INJURY PREVENTION

Injuries are a major cause of death during infancy, especially for children 6 to 12 months old. Constant vigilance, awareness, and supervision are essential as the child gains increased locomotor and manipulative skills that are coupled with an insatiable curiosity about the environment. Table 10-11 lists the major developmental achievements of each period during infancy and the appropriate injury prevention plan.

Aspiration of Foreign Objects

Asphyxiation by foreign material in the respiratory tract, combined with mechanical suffocation, is the leading cause of fatal injury in children younger than 1 year of age. The size,

*For information call (800) 822-7967.

shape, and consistency of foods or objects are important determinants of fatal obstruction. For example, small spheric or cylindric and pliable objects (less than 3.2 cm, or 1¼ inches) are more likely to completely obstruct the airway. Unfortunately, common household items can be deadly to infants.

As soon as infants have the ability to find their mouth, they are vulnerable to aspiration of small objects, such as those left within reach or removable parts of objects that may on initial inspection appear safe. All *toys* must be carefully inspected for potential danger. Rattles, for example, have small beads in them to produce noise. A broken or cracked rattle can be dangerous because the beads can easily be aspirated while the infant has the toy in the mouth. Stuffed animals are another potentially dangerous toy if any of the parts, such as the eyes or nose, are removable buttons or plastic pieces. An active infant can grab a low-hanging mobile and quickly chew off a small piece. As soon as the infant crawls or plays on the floor, the floor must be kept free of any small articles that can be picked up and swallowed, such as coins.

When infant *clothes* are purchased, the type of closure is important. A front button can easily be pulled off and swallowed. Safety pins for diapers are kept closed and away from the dressing table. Even though a young infant may not search for them, practicing this good habit from the beginning prevents future injuries.

Food items are the second most common cause of aspiration, and the most frequent offenders are hot dogs, candy, nuts, and grapes. When new foods are given to the child, nuts, hard candies, marshmallows, large amounts of peanut butter, or fruits with pits or seeds are avoided. When traveling, especially in airplanes, or entertaining, snack foods such as peanuts and popcorn are kept away from young children. If given to young children, hot dogs must be cut into small, irregular pieces rather than served whole or sliced into sections, because their size (diameter), round shape, and consistency allow for complete occlusion of the airway. Perhaps the most dangerous food is dried beans, which, if aspirated, enlarge when they come in contact with the wet mucosa and block the airway.

Pacifiers can also be dangerous because the entire object may be aspirated if it is small or the nipple and shield may become detached from the handle and become lodged in the pharynx. Improvised pacifiers, such as those commonly made in hospitals from a padded nipple, also present dangers. The nipple may separate from the plastic collar and be aspirated. In addition, parents may continue to offer this pacifier to the infant at home. To prevent the hazards of improvised pacifiers, hospitals should use only safe commercial types. Candy pacifiers pose dangers because the candy portion can dislodge from the circular base and be aspirated. To be safe, pacifiers should have (Nowak, 1993) (Fig. 10-12):

- Sturdy, one-piece construction with material that is nontoxic, flexible, and firm but not brittle
- An easily grasped handle
- A mouthguard that cannot be separated from the nipple, has two ventilating holes, and is too large to be aspirated
- No detachable ribbon or string
- A label warning against tying the pacifier around the infant's neck

Using a syringe to accurately measure and dispense oral liquid medications to young children has become common

TABLE 10-11. Injury prevention during infancy

Age: Birth-4 Months

Major Developmental Accomplishments

Involuntary reflexes, such as the crawling reflex, may propel infant forward or backward and the startle reflex may cause the body to jerk

May roll over

Increasing eye-hand coordination and voluntary grasp reflex

Injury prevention

Aspiration

Not as great a danger to this age-group, but should begin practicing safeguarding early (see under 4-7 months)

Never shake baby powder directly on infant; place powder in hand and then on infant's skin; store container closed and out of infant's reach

Hold infant for feeding; do not prop bottle

Know emergency procedures for choking*

Use pacifier with one-piece construction and loop handle

Suffocation/Drowning

Keep all plastic bags stored out of infant's reach; discard large plastic garment bags after tying in a knot

Do not cover mattress with plastic

Use a firm mattress and loose blankets; no pillows

Make sure crib design follows federal regulations and mattress fits snugly†

Position crib away from other furniture and away from radiators

Avoid sleeping in bed with infant

Do not tie pacifier on a string around infant's neck

Remove bibs at bedtime

Never leave infant alone in bath

Do not leave infant under 12 months alone on adult or youth mattress

Falls

Always raise crib rails

Never leave infant on a raised, unguarded surface

When in doubt as to where to place child, use the floor

Restrain child in infant seat and never leave child unattended while the seat is resting on a raised surface

Avoid using a high chair until child can sit well with support

Poisoning

Not as great a danger to this age-group, but should begin practicing safeguards early (see under 4-7 months)

Burns

Install smoke detectors in home

Use caution when warming formula in microwave oven; always check temperature of liquid before feeding

Check bathwater

Do not pour hot liquids when infant is close by, such as sitting on lap

Beware of cigarette ashes that may fall on infant

Do not leave infant in the sun for more than a few minutes; keep exposed areas covered

Wash flame-retardant clothes according to label directions

Use cool-mist vaporizers

Do not leave child in parked car

Check surface heat of car restraint before placing child in seat

Motor vehicles

Transport infant in federally approved, rear-facing car seat that is not placed near an air bag safety device*

Do not place infant on the seat or in lap

Do not place child in a carriage or stroller behind a parked car

Bodily damage

Avoid sharp, jagged objects

Keep diaper pins closed and away from infant

Age: 4-7 Months

Major developmental accomplishments

Rolls over

Sits momentarily

Grasps and manipulates small objects

Resecures a dropped object

Has well-developed eye-hand coordination

Can focus on and locate very small objects

Mouthing is very prominent

Can push up on hands and knees

Crawls backward

Injury prevention

Aspiration

Keep buttons, beads, syringe caps, and other small objects out of infant's reach

Keep floor free of any small objects

Do not feed infant hard candy, nuts, food with pits or seeds, or whole or circular pieces of hot dog

Exercise caution when giving teething biscuits, because large chunks may be broken off and aspirated

Do not feed infant while child is lying down

Inspect toys for removable parts

Keep baby powder, if used, out of reach

Avoid storing large quantities of cleaning fluid, paints, pesticides, and other toxic substances

Discard used containers of poisonous substances

Do not store toxic substances in food containers

Discard used button-sized batteries; store new batteries in safe area

Know telephone number of local poison control center (usually listed in front of telephone directory)

Suffocation

Keep uninflated balloons out of reach

Remove all crib toys that are strung across crib or playpen when child begins to push up on hands or knees or is 5 months old

Falls

Restrain in a high chair

Keep crib rails raised to full height

Poisoning

Make sure that paint for furniture or toys does not contain lead

Place toxic substances on a high shelf or in locked cabinet

Hang plants or place on high surface rather than on floor

---

*Home care instructions for care of the choking infant and for use of child safety seats are available in Wong DL: *Wong and Whaley's Clinical manual of pediatric nursing,* ed 4, St Louis, 1996, Mosby.

†Information available from **U.S. Consumer Product Safety Commission;** (800) 638-CPSC.

Continued.

TABLE 10-11. Injury prevention during infancy—cont'd

Burns	*Bodily damage*
Keep faucets out of reach	Give toys that are smooth and rounded, preferably made of
Place hot objects (cigarettes, candles, incense) on high surface	wood or plastic
Limit exposure to sun; apply sunscreen	Avoid long, pointed objects as toys
Motor vehicles	Avoid toys that are excessively loud
See under Birth-4 months	Keep sharp objects out of infant's reach

Age: 8-12 Months

Major developmental accomplishments

Crawls/creeps	Throws objects
Stands, holding onto furniture	Is able to pick up small objects; has pincer grasp
Stands alone	Explores by putting objects in mouth
Cruises around furniture	Dislikes being restrained
Walks	Explores away from parent
Climbs	Increasing understanding of simple commands and phrases
Pulls on objects	

Injury prevention

Aspiration	*Falls*
Keep lint and small objects off floor, furniture, and out of reach of children	Fence stairways at top and bottom if child has access to either end†
Take care in feeding solid table food to ensure that very small pieces are given	Dress infant in safe shoes and clothing (soles that do not "catch" on floor, tied shoelaces, pant legs that do not touch floor)
Do not use beanbag toys or allow child to play with dried beans	Avoid using infant walkers
See also under 4-7 months	Ensure that furniture is sturdy enough for child to pull self to standing position and cruise
Suffocation/drowning	*Poisoning*
Keep doors of ovens, dishwashers, refrigerators, coolers, and front-loading clothes washers and dryers closed at all times	Administer medications as a drug, not as a candy
If storing an unused appliance, such as a refrigerator, remove the door	Do not administer medications unless so prescribed by a practitioner
Supervise contact with inflated balloons; immediately discard popped balloons and keep uninflated balloons out of reach	Replace medications and poisons immediately after use; replace caps properly if a child-protector cap is used
Fence swimming pools	Have syrup of ipecac in home; use only if advised
Always supervise when near any source of water, such as cleaning buckets, drainage areas, toilets	*Burns*
Keep bathroom doors closed	Place guards in front of or around any heating appliance, fireplace, or furnace
Eliminate unnecessary pools of water	Keep electrical wires hidden or out of reach
Keep one hand on child at all times when in tub	Place plastic guards over electrical outlets; place furniture in front of outlets
	Keep hanging tablecloths out of reach (child may pull down hot liquids or heavy or sharp objects)

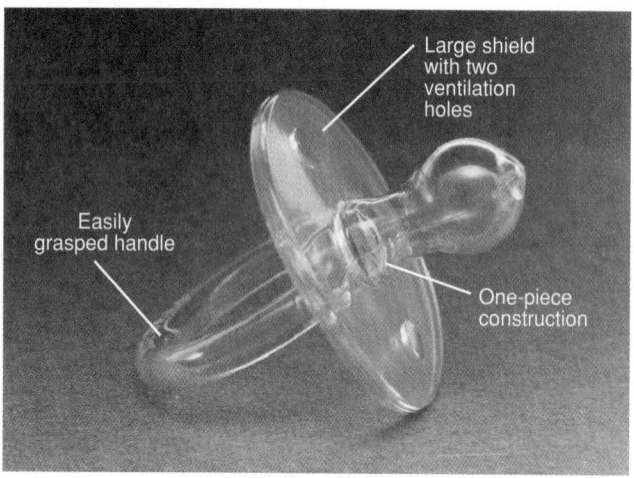

Large shield with two ventilation holes

Easily grasped handle

One-piece construction

FIG. 10-12. Design of safe pacifier.

practice. However, the *syringe cap* is a potential aspiration hazard. As a precaution, keep parts of medication devices out of the reach of children and be certain the cap is removed before dispensing medication.

Even safety devices can be dangerous. To prevent tampering, items (such as baby food jars) may be covered with a plastic oversleeve. The *tear-down strip* can be aspirated and is very difficult to locate because it is clear.

Another hazardous substance if aspirated is *baby powder,* which is usually a mixture of talc (hydrous magnesium silicate) and other silicates. Although the use of talc has been discouraged, it is a common baby care product and can cause severe and often fatal aspiration pneumonia. One of the factors involved in talc aspiration is the similar appearance of baby powder containers and nursing bottles. Talc containers often become favorite playthings and are placed in the mouth. Improper use of powder by sprinkling it directly on the skin creates a cloud of talc dust that is easily inhaled. Parents are advised of the danger of baby powder and are discouraged from using it. If they prefer to use a powder, a cornstarch preparation can be substituted (see Diaper Dermatitis, Chapter 30). Whenever a powder is used, it is placed in the hand and then applied to the skin, never shaken directly from the container to the skin. The container is kept closed and immediately stored in a safe place, especially away from curious toddlers, who often imitate caregiving activities and may accidentally shake it on the infant.

Suffocation

Mechanical suffocation includes suffocation by covering of the airway (i.e., mouth and nose), by pressure on the throat and chest, and by exclusion of air, such as by refrigerator entrapment. Nonfood items cause the majority of deaths in young children. *Latex balloons,* whether partially inflated, uninflated, or popped, are the leading cause of pediatric choking deaths from children's products (Holida, 1993). They should be kept away from infants and young children. Even the practice of inflating latex gloves to amuse children in health care settings may pose a danger.

Nursing ALERT	Encourage adults to do the following: Blow up balloons for children Supervise children's balloon play

Pick up and dispose of broken balloon pieces
Warn older children of dangers of chewing or sucking on balloons
Substitute Mylar balloons for latex balloons

In addition, the accessibility of plastic linings of diapers used on the infant and/or on dolls is especially dangerous to young children.

The *bed* or *crib* poses a number of hazards. An infant who is placed in a bed under blankets and sheets that are tucked in can be caught under them and be unable to wriggle free. Baby pillows filled with plastic foam beads that make them resemble small bean bags are dangerous; very young infants are suffocated when the pillow contours to the face and blocks the airway. There are potential dangers in adults sleeping with a small infant because of the possibility of their rolling over and smothering the child.

Infant strangulation may occur if the infant's head becomes caught between the crib slats and mattress or objects close to the crib. Suffocation deaths are not confined to cribs; ill-fitting mattresses in adult or youth beds, bunk beds, and waterbeds have also been reported. According to federal regulation the distance between crib slats should not be more than 2⅜ inches (about 6 cm), roughly the width of three adult fingers. Mattresses and bumper pads should fit snugly against the slats. A general rule is that if two adult fingers can be placed between the mattress and crib or bed side, the mattress is too small. A temporary solution is to place large, rolled towels in the space to create a snug fit.

Corner post extensions on cribs are another source of strangulation. Children have died when their clothing caught on raised corner posts as they climbed out of the crib. Voluntary manufacturing standards state the corner post extensions should not exceed 1/16 inch. However, the safety of *any* extension is questionable. Decorative extensions need to be

removed from cribs. Ideally, information regarding correct crib design should be given prenatally before parents have purchased or borrowed a crib.*

Mesh-sided playpens and cribs can result in death if the sides are left in the lowered position. Infants have suffocated when they fell off the edge of the mattress and the head or chest was compressed between the floorboard and mesh side. Parents should be advised of this danger and encouraged to *always* keep the sides locked securely in the up position whenever the child is in the playpen or crib.

The crib should be positioned away from large furniture, because children who crawl out of the crib may become caught between the two objects. Cribs should also be located away from windows, where drape or blind cords can become wrapped around the infant's neck.

Another cause of suffocation is *plastic bags.* Large plastic bags used over garments are very lightweight and can easily and quickly be wrapped around the head of an active infant or pressed against the face. Pillows and mattresses should not be covered with plastic for this reason. Older infants may play with a plastic bag and accidentally pull it over their heads. Because plastic is nonporous, suffocation takes place in a matter of minutes.

Cords either near the infant or tied around the infant's neck can potentially cause strangulation. Bibs are removed at bedtime, and objects such as pacifiers are never hung on a string around the infant's neck. This is a common practice in some cultures that can be remedied by attaching a *short* string tied to a pacifier and pinning the string on the child's shirt.

Toys that have strings attached, such as a telephone, or toys that are tied to cribs or playpens can be hazards because the string can become wrapped around the child's neck or the child can become entrapped in the toy. As a precaution, all cords should be less than 30 cm (12 inches) long. Crib toys should be hung high enough that the infant cannot become entangled in them or should no longer be used once the child is able to reach them.

Restraining straps, if applied too loosely or left unfastened, can be a hazard. For example, a child may slide off a high chair beneath the tray and become strangled on the loose strap. All straps should be fastened securely.

Motor Vehicle Injuries

Automobile injuries are the leading cause of accidental death in children older than 1 year of age. However, a significant number of infants are injured or die from improper restraint within the vehicle, most often from riding on the lap of another occupant. All infants must be secured in a federally approved restraint rather than held or placed on the seat of the car. There is no safe alternative.

Infant restraints are designed either as an infant-only model (Fig. 10-13) or as a convertible infant-toddler model. Either restraint is a semi-reclined seat that faces the *rear* of the car. A rear-facing car seat provides the very best protection for the disproportionately heavy head and the weak neck

---

*The booklet *It Hurts When They Cry* gives basic information on hazards, safety features, and proper use of nursery furniture and equipment. It is available at no charge from **U.S. Consumer Product Safety Commission,** Publication Request, Washington, DC 20207; (800) 638-2772. Additional free information is available from the **Danny Foundation,** 3158 Danville Blvd; P.O. Box 680, Alamo, CA 94507; (800) 83-DANNY.

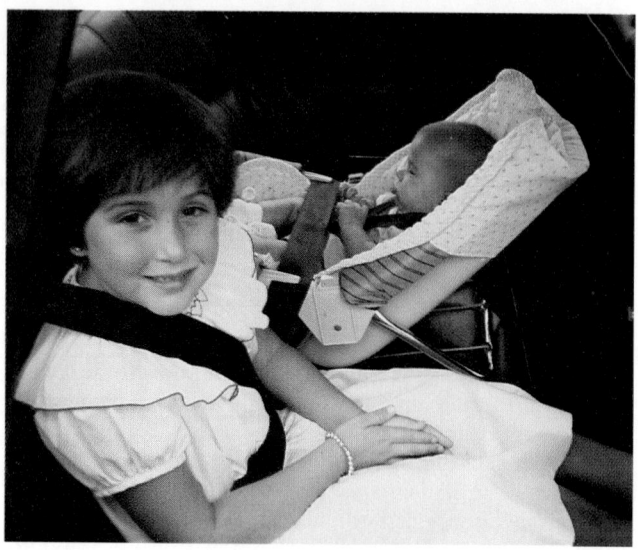

FIG. 10-13. Federally approved infant car restraint. Note placement in middle of back seat and use of car lap/shoulder belt for older child.

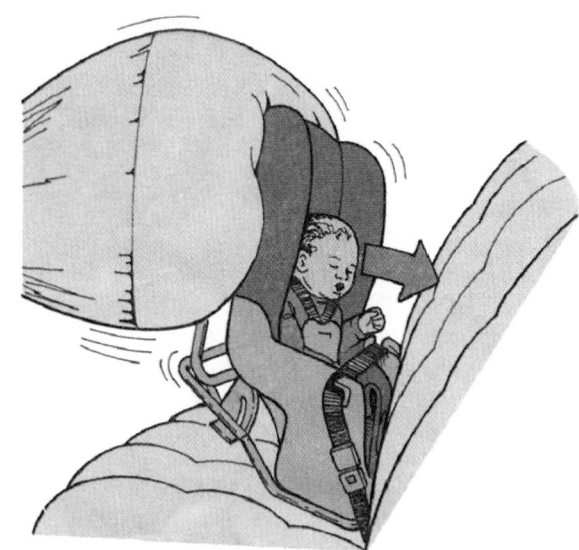

FIG. 10-14. An air bag could strike a child safety seat, seriously injuring the infant. (Redrawn from Health Alert, *AAP News* 10(4):22, 1994.)

of a young child. This position minimizes the stress on the neck by spreading the forces of a frontal crash over the entire back, neck, and head; the spine is supported by the back of the car seat. If the seat were faced forward, the head would whip forward because of the force of the crash, creating enormous stress on the neck.

> **Nursing ALERT** Infants should face the rear from birth to 20 pounds and as close to 1 year of age as possible.

The restraint is anchored to the vehicle with the car seat belt and has a harness system for restraining the infant. Some harness systems require a clip to keep the shoulder straps correctly positioned. Although many infant restraints can be recliners, they are only used in the car in the position specified by the manufacturer.

Generally, the middle of the back seat is considered the safest area of the car. However, an infant restraint may be positioned in the front seat, where the driver can observe the infant without having to turn around, provided that the seatbelt can be locked into position. Parents should check the car's vehicle owner's manual, because additional hardware may be needed.

> **Nursing ALERT** Rear-facing infant safety seats must not be placed in the front seats of cars equipped with an airbag on the passenger side. If an infant seat is placed in the passenger seat with an air bag, the child could be seriously injured if the air bag is released, since rear-facing infant seats extend closer to the dashboard (Air-bag associated fatal injuries, 1995) (Fig. 10-14).

For restraints to be effective, they must be used properly. Dressing the infant in an outfit with sleeves and legs allows the harness to securely hold the child in the seat. A small blanket or towel rolled tightly can be placed on either side of the head to minimize movement and keep the infant's hips against the back of the seat. Padding between the infant's legs and crotch is added to prevent slouching. Thick, soft padding is not placed under the infant or behind the back because during the impact the padding will compress, leaving the harness straps loose. (For further discussion of restraints see Chapter 12.)

Falls

Falls are most common after 4 months of age when the infant has learned to roll over, but they can occur at any age. Newborns are normally active, assume a flexed position, and have crawling reflexes that can propel them forward. The best advice is never to place a child unattended on a raised surface that has no type of guardrails. When in doubt, the safest place is the floor. Even though young infants cannot climb over a partially raised crib rail, it is best to form a habit of raising the rail all the way, because someday that infant will be able to climb out. Crib sides should have a latching device that cannot be easily released. The welds attaching the crib corner locks to the corner posts should not be cracked or broken. If the welds are damaged, the bedspring could fall to the floor. Ideally, cribs should be placed on carpeted, not hard, floors.

Another danger area for falling is a *changing table,* which is usually high and narrow. Although these tables have a restraining belt, children should never be left unattended, even when restrained. The best way to avoid having to leave is to arrange the area with all necessary articles within easy reach so that the child is always in full sight of the caregiver. It only takes a fraction of a second for an infant to fall off. During the latter half of the first year, infants usually resist dressing and diapering and may be difficult to manage. If there is danger that the child is strong enough to resist restraining, the infant should be changed on a safer surface, such as a clean floor.

Infant seats, high chairs, walkers, and *swings* present additional opportunities for falls. If the infant seat is placed on a table, the child should never be left unrestrained or unattended. The same rule is essential for other baby equipment, particularly when the child has learned to crawl and to stand up. Small infants can slip through a high chair if a protective harness is not used. The danger of falls from being unrestrained applies to shopping carts as well (Tully, 1993). High chairs are designed for older infants who can sit well and who are tall enough to have the tray at the level of their chest or abdomen. Infant walkers are responsible for a number of different types of injuries that occur because the walker tipped over or fell down stairs. Parents need to be warned of these dangers and encouraged to keep a constant vigil on their child's activities. The American Academy of Pediatrics Committee on Injury and Poison Prevention (1995) does not recommend the use of walkers.

Once infants are mobile, they should not be allowed to crawl unsupervised on any raised surface, near stairs, or near any water reservoir. Gates should be used at the *bottom* and *top* of *stairs,* because both present dangers to the crawling and climbing infant. However, certain types of gates can present hazards. Freestanding enclosures constructed of crisscrossed wood slats that expand and contract can trap the head or neck when children attempt to climb over them. If these types of gates are used, they must be securely fastened to prevent mobility of the slats.

As children begin to pull themselves to a standing position, *heavy objects,* such as unsturdy furniture or any freestanding item (e.g., wrought iron fish tank stands or concrete birdbath), can be extremely dangerous if pulled down on top of the child. To prevent injury from furniture tipping over, TVs should be placed on lower furniture, as far back as possible. Angle braces or anchors can secure furniture to walls.

Sometimes even when the environment is made safe, infants may literally trip over their own feet from *clothing.* Slippery socks; hard, slick soles on shoes or rubber soles that can catch, especially on a carpet; and long pants or pajama bottoms can easily upset a child's balance. Such dangers need to be pointed out to parents, especially when infants are taking their first steps.

Poisoning

Poisoning is one of the major causes of death in children younger than 5 years of age. The highest incidence occurs in those in the 2-year-old group, with the second highest incidence occurring in 1-year-old children. Infants who do not crawl are relatively free from danger of poisonous agents by virtue of immobility. However, once locomotion begins, danger from poisoning is present almost everywhere. There are more than 500 toxic substances in the average home, and about a third of all poisonings occur in the kitchen.

The major reason for ingestion of poisons is *improper storage.* To protect the infant, toxic agents should not be placed on a low shelf, table, or floor. Drugs that are kept in a purse pose additional dangers; if the purse is given to infants to play with, they may open it and ingest the drug. Another unrecognized hazard is during diaper changes when infants are near many toxic substances such as ointments, creams, oils, and talc. Parents may even hand infants a potentially poisonous object to quiet them. Such dangers need to be stressed to parents, and toys need to be kept at diapering areas to minimize risks.

Plants are another source of poisoning for infants. Plants are frequently placed on the floor, and the leaves or flowers are attractive and easy to pull off. More than 700 species of plants are known to have caused illness or death.

Another danger is ingestion of *button-sized batteries* that are used in devices such as hearing aids, calculators, watches, and cameras. Because they are bright and shiny, they are attractive to children. However, they can cause severe morbidity, even death, if lodged in the esophagus. The strong alkali in a battery can leak and cause a severe caustic burn. As a precaution small batteries must be safely stored and discarded where young children cannot easily retrieve them.

Not all poisonings result from ingestion—*inhalation* is another possible route, such as inhaling chlorine vapors from household cleaning or pool supplies. Recent concern has addressed passive cocaine toxicity in young children exposed to freebase cocaine ("crack") smoking by adults. Children should be protected from environments where these toxins exist (for a discussion of passive cigarette smoking, see Chapter 23).

The only sure way to prevent poisoning is to remove toxic agents, which means placing them high out of the infant's reach. However, because crawling infants soon become climbing toddlers, it is best to keep all toxic agents, especially drugs, in a locked cabinet. Special plastic hooks can be attached to the inside of cabinet doors to keep them securely closed (see Fig. 10-15). Firm thumb pressure is required to unlatch the hook, and small children are usually unable to manipulate them. Locks are best, but for frequently used cleaning agents, such as those often kept under a kitchen sink, hooks are a practical alternative.

With several hundred toxic substances in each house, locking up all potentially toxic substances could present a problem; however, careful planning can help. A large surplus of

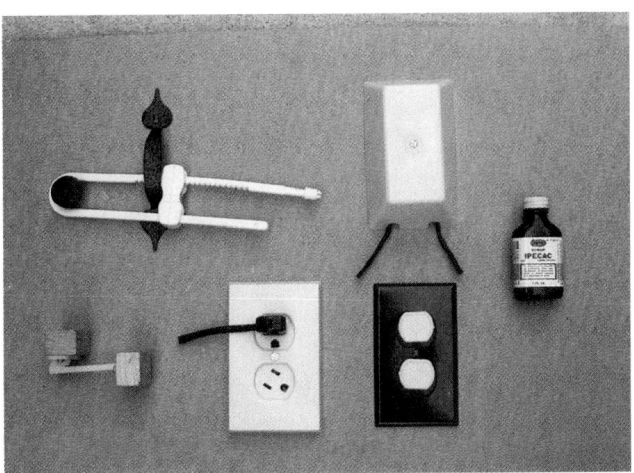

FIG. 10-15. Safety demonstration board. *Clockwise from lower left:* Cabinet latches, shock guard for electrical outlet, syrup of ipecac, and two types of outlet covers (white cover is passive device that automatically covers outlet when plug is removed).

cleaning agents, furniture polishes, laundry additives, paints, insecticides, and solvents should be avoided.

Used poison containers should be promptly discarded and not used to store another poison without adequately marking the package. Any potentially hazardous substance should not be stored in any type of food container. A popular container used to store toxic liquids is a soda bottle. A child who is unaware of the dangerous contents is a vulnerable victim for poisoning. Parents should know the location of local poison control centers and call them in the event of a suspected poisoning. Emergency measures for poisoning are discussed in Chapter 14.

Burns

Burns such as scalding from water that is too hot, excessive sunburn, and burns from house fires, electrical wires, sockets, and heating elements such as radiators, registers, and floor furnaces cause a significant number of deaths and many more injuries in infants. The infant's skin is particularly sensitive to irritation, and the mechanisms for temperature preception are not completely developed. As a general precaution, all homes should have smoke alarms installed near the bedroom areas.

Scald burns from **hot tap water** can be prevented by lowering the hot water heater to a safe temperature of 49° C (120° F). In addition, the bathwater should be checked before the infant is immersed in it. Scalds can also occur from bathing infants in the kitchen sink when the garbage disposal, occluded with debris, causes the draining dishwasher effluent to back up into the sink. The temperature of the effluent from a dishwasher is typically that of the maximum water temperature of the household water heater, but many dishwashers are equipped with heating elements that heat water to a temperature that is even higher. As a precaution, instruct caregivers to avoid bathing small children in the kitchen sink while the dishwasher is running.

If formula or food is warmed in a **microwave oven,** it must be checked before feeding because the container may remain cool while the contents are hot. Another danger is explosion of the bottle from the buildup of steam. Because of these dangers, microwaving infant formula or food should be avoided or done using the guidelines on p. 310. The handles of cooking utensils should be turned toward the back of the stove. When the infant is underfoot, pouring hot liquids and cooking with hot oil are avoided. Hanging tablecloths are also placed out of the infant's reach to prevent pulling hot items off the table.

Sunburn can be a source of a first- or second-degree burn. Exposure to direct sunlight should be avoided. When infants are in the sun, the body, especially the face and head, should be covered. Sunscreen can be used on older infants (see Sunburn, Chapter 30). Although black-skinned infants burn less readily, their thin skin can become sunburned and needs protection.

Electrical outlets should be covered with protective plastic caps that prevent the child from sucking on the outlet or putting objects such as hairpins into it (see Fig. 10-15). Live wires are placed out of reach so that curious infants cannot chew on them and break the rubber coating (Fig. 10-16). Infants should not be allowed to play near television sets, stereo units, or other appliances, whether these units are on or off; infants cannot determine when the appliance is safe.

Any **heat-producing element** should have a guard placed in front of it. Fireplaces should be well screened because they are very appealing and within easy access. Small portable heaters should be placed on a high surface. Floor furnaces should have barrier gates to prevent children from crawling or walking over them. Burning cigarettes, candles, and incense are kept out of reach, and infants should not be held by a smoking adult, because falling ashes are a hazard, especially to the eyes. Heated-mist vaporizers are a source of burns and should not be used. If humidity is needed, only cool mist vaporizers are safe.

By law, all infant sleepwear must be flame retardant. Unfortunately, this does not apply to all **infant clothing.** Flame-retardant fabric must never be viewed as the ultimate protection against burns. Repeated washings reduces the flame-retardant properties, and the use of soap or bleach destroys the protection. Inasmuch as detergent should be used for washing flame-retardant clothing, infants who are sensitive to such agents are unprotected when their clothing is washed even with a mild soap. If sleepwear is home sewn, parents are advised to look for specially treated flame-retardant fabric.

Another type of thermal injury occurs when children are exposed to excessive heat during confinement in poorly ventilated **vehicles.** The practice of leaving the windows open a couple of inches is not protective. The nurse should caution parents never to leave children in parked cars, especially when the automobile is in direct sunlight.

Children can also be burned by overheated metal hardware and vinyl seats in cars parked in the sun. As a precaution the surface heat of car restraints should be determined before placing children in them. Covering the restraints and hardware (such as metal latches on seat belts) may be necessary to prevent skin burns. An additional safeguard is buying a light-colored restraint, which absorbs less heat.

Drowning

Drowning in this age-group can occur in only inches of water. Consequently, infants should never be left unsupervised in a bathtub, hot tub, or near a source of water such as a swimming pool, lake, toilet, or bucket. Organized swimming

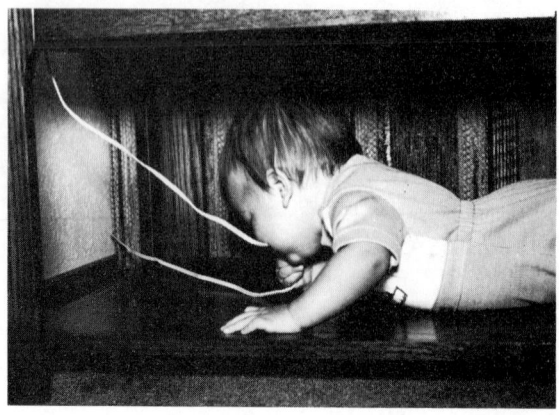

FIG. 10-16. Crawling infants can find hazardous electrical wires even in "hidden" areas.

FAMILY HOME CARE
Child Safety Home Checklist

Safety: Fire, Electrical, Burns

- ☐ Guards in front of or around any heating appliance, fireplace, or furnace (including floor furnace)*
- ☐ Electrical wires hidden or out of reach*
- ☐ No frayed or broken wires; no overloaded sockets
- ☐ Plastic guards or caps over electrical outlets, furniture in front of outlets*
- ☐ Hanging tablecloths out of reach, away from open fires*
- ☐ Smoke detectors tested and operating properly
- ☐ Kitchen matches stored out of child's reach*
- ☐ Large, deep ashtrays throughout house (if used)
- ☐ Small stoves, heaters, and other hot objects (cigarettes, candles, coffee pots, slow cookers) placed where they cannot be tipped over or reached by children
- ☐ Hot water heater set at 49° C (120° F) or lower
- ☐ Pot handles turned toward back of stove, center of table
- ☐ No loose clothing worn near stove
- ☐ No cooking or eating hot foods or liquids with child standing nearby or sitting in lap
- ☐ All small appliances, such as iron, turned off, disconnected, and placed out of reach when not in use
- ☐ Cool, not hot, mist vaporizer used
- ☐ Fire extinguisher available on each floor and checked periodically
- ☐ Electrical fuse box and gas outlet accessible
- ☐ Family escape plan in case of a fire practiced periodically; fire escape ladder available on upper-level floors
- ☐ Telephone number of fire or rescue squad and address of home with nearest cross street posted near phone

Safety: Suffocation and Aspiration

- ☐ Small objects stored out of reach*
- ☐ Toys inspected for small removable parts or long strings*
- ☐ Hanging crib toys and mobiles placed out of reach
- ☐ Plastic bags stored away from young child's reach, large plastic garment bags discarded after tying in knots*
- ☐ Mattress or pillow not covered with plastic or in manner accessible to child*
- ☐ Crib design according to federal regulations [crib slats less than 2⅜ inches (6 cm) apart] with snug-fitting mattress*†
- ☐ Crib positioned away from other furniture or windows*
- ☐ Portable playpen gates up at all times while in use*
- ☐ Accordion-style gates not used*
- ☐ Bathroom doors kept closed and toilet seats down*
- ☐ Faucets turned off firmly*
- ☐ Pool fenced with locked gate
- ☐ Proper safety equipment at poolside
- ☐ Electric garage door openers stored safely and garage door adjusted to rise when door strikes object
- ☐ Doors of ovens, trunks, dishwashers, refrigerators, and front-loading clothes washers and dryers kept closed*
- ☐ Unused appliance, such as a refrigerator, securely closed with lock or doors removed*
- ☐ Food served in small noncylindric pieces*
- ☐ Toy chests without lids or with lids that securely lock in open position*

- ☐ Buckets and wading pools kept empty when not in use*
- ☐ Clothesline above head level
- ☐ At least one member of household trained in basic life support (CPR), including first aid for choking‡

Safety: Poisoning

- ☐ Toxic substances, including batteries, placed on a high shelf, preferably in locked cabinet
- ☐ Toxic plants hung or placed out of reach*
- ☐ Excess quantities of cleaning fluid, paints, pesticides, drugs, and other toxic substances not stored in home
- ☐ Used containers of poisonous substances discarded where child cannot obtain access
- ☐ Telephone number of local poison control center and address of home with nearest cross street posted near phone
- ☐ Syrup of ipecac in home containing two doses per child
- ☐ Medicines clearly labeled in childproof containers and stored out of reach
- ☐ Household cleaners, disinfectants, and insecticides kept in their original containers, separate from food and out of reach
- ☐ Smoking in areas away from children

Safety: Falls

- ☐ Nonskid mats, strips, or surfaces in tubs and showers
- ☐ Exits, halls, and passageways in rooms kept clear of toys, furniture, boxes, or other items that could be obstructive
- ☐ Stairs and halls well lighted, with switches at both top and bottom
- ☐ Sturdy handrails for all steps and stairways
- ☐ Nothing stored on stairways
- ☐ Treads, risers, and carpeting in good repair
- ☐ Glass doors and walls marked with decals
- ☐ Safety glass used in doors, windows, and walls
- ☐ Gates on top and bottom of staircases and elevated areas, such as porch, fire escape*
- ☐ Guardrails on upstairs windows with locks that limit height of window opening and access to areas such as fire escape*
- ☐ Crib side rails raised to full height; mattress lowered as child grows*
- ☐ Restraints used in high chairs, walkers, or other baby furniture; preferably walkers not used*
- ☐ Scatter rugs secured in place or used with nonskid back
- ☐ Walks, patios, and driveways in good repair

Safety: Bodily Injury

- ☐ Knives, power tools, and unloaded firearms stored safely or placed in locked cabinet
- ☐ Garden tools returned to storage racks after use
- ☐ Pets properly restrained and immunized for rabies
- ☐ Swings, slides, and other outdoor play equipment kept in safe condition
- ☐ Yard free of broken glass, nail-studded boards, other litter
- ☐ Cement birdbaths placed where young child cannot tip them over*

*Safety measures are specific for homes with young children. All safety measures should be implemented in homes where children reside and visit frequently, such as those of grandparents or baby-sitters.

†Federal regulations are available from U.S. Consumer Product Safety Commission; (800) 638-CPSC.

‡Home care instructions for infant cardiopulmonary resuscitation and infant/child choking are available in Wong DL: *Wong and Whaley's Clinical manual of pediatric nursing*, ed 4, St Louis, 1996, Mosby.

instruction is not recommended for children under 4 years of age, because it may lead to a false sense of security. No infant can be expected to learn the elements of water safety or to react appropriately in an emergency. Therefore all young children need to be considered at risk when near water (American Academy of Pediatrics, Committee on Injury and Poison Prevention, 1993). Infants and toddlers are also at increased risk of infection and convulsions from swallowing large amounts of water.

Bodily Damage

Injuries can occur in numerous ways. Sharp, jagged-edged objects can cause wounds in the skin. Long-pointed articles, such as the common toothpick or fork, can be poked into the eye or ear, causing serious damage. Such articles should be safely stored away from the infant's reach; forks are best avoided for self-feeding until the child has mastered the spoon, usually by age 18 months.

In addition to hazards such as aspiration from toys, small articles can be placed in the ear or nose, and excessive noise from toys can result in sensorineural hearing loss. Although toys with the highest noise levels are model airplanes, air guns, toy cap guns, and firecrackers, even common squeaking toys used by young children may be harmful if placed close to the ear.

Even clothes and hair can present dangers to infants who cannot call attention to the problem. For example, constriction injuries can occur from excessively tight bands on socks, as well as fibers of hair or thread wrapped tightly around appendages, usually toes or fingers.

Another frequently unrecognized danger to infants is animal attacks. Helpless infants, as newcomers to the home, can provoke jealously in animals, especially dogs and cats. However, unprovoked attacks by ferrets and roosters have also been reported. Parents must be constantly vigilant to protect the child from household pets and farm animals (see Animal Bites, Chapter 30).

Nurse's Role in Injury Prevention

When the potential environmental dangers to which infants are vulnerable are considered, the task of preventing these injuries only begins to be appreciated. Nurses must be aware of the possible causes of injury in each age-group in order for *anticipatory* preventive teaching to occur. For example, the guidelines for injury prevention during infancy presented in Table 10-11 should be discussed *before* the child reaches the susceptible age-group. Preventive teaching ideally occurs during pregnancy. Inasmuch as two thirds of all injuries to children occur in the home, the importance of safety cannot be overemphasized. The Family Home Care box on p. 329 summarizes a home safety checklist that can be presented to parents to increase their awareness of danger areas in the home and assist them in implementing safety devices and practices *before* their absence can inflict injury on infants. In addition, displays such as a safety demonstration board (see Fig. 10-15) can be helpful in familiarizing parents with inexpensive, commercial devices that can be used in the home to prevent injuries.

NURSING TIP To help parents appreciate the dangers present in their home to young children, suggest that they get eye level with the floor to survey the environment from a child's view.

Injury prevention requires protection of the child and education of the caregiver. Nurses in ambulatory care settings, health maintenance centers, or visiting nurse agencies are in a most favorable position for injury education. This does not exclude nurses in inpatient facilities, who could use visiting times as an excellent opportunity for discussing this topic.

One approach to teaching injury prevention is to relate why children in various age-groups are prone to specific types of injuries. Stressing prevention is just as important as emphasizing the *why* of the injury. However, injury prevention must also be practical. Asking parents for their ideas leads to realistic suggestions that can be followed. For instance, bathroom cleaning agents, cosmetics, and personal care items can be placed on a top shelf in the linen closet, and towels or sheets can be stored on the lower shelves and floor.

If an injury has occurred, the nurse should not be too quick to admonish the parent. Injuries do not always indicate neglect. It is a difficult task to watch children carefully without overprotecting or unnecessarily confining them. Small falls help children learn the dangers of heights. Touching a hot object once can emphasize to the child the pain of

FAMILY HOME CARE
Guidance During Infant's First Year

First 6 Months

Understand each parent's adjustment to newborn, especially mother's postpartal emotional needs.

Teach care of infant and assist parents to understand his or her individual needs and temperament and that the infant expresses wants through crying.

Reassure parents that infant cannot be spoiled by too much attention during the first 4 to 6 months.

Encourage parents to establish a schedule that meets needs of child and themselves.

Help parents understand infant's need for stimulation in environment.

Support parents' pleasure in seeing child's growing friendliness and social response, especially smiling.

Plan anticipatory guidance for safety.

Stress need for immunization.

Prepare for introduction of solid foods.

Second 6 Months

Prepare parents for child's "stranger anxiety."

Encourage parents to allow child to cling to them and avoid long separation from either.

Guide parents concerning discipline because of infant's increasing mobility.

Encourage use of negative voice and eye contact rather than physical punishment as a means of discipline.

Encourage showing most attention when infant is behaving well, rather than when infant is crying.

Teach injury prevention because of child's advancing motor skills and curiosity.

Encourage parents to leave child with suitable caregiver to allow some free time.

Discuss readiness for weaning.

Explore parents' feelings regarding infant's sleep patterns.

a burn. Allowing children to explore while maintaining consistent, age-appropriate limits is sound advice.

Parents need to remember that infants and young children cannot anticipate danger or understand when it is or is not present. A dead electrical wire may present no actual harm, but if the child is allowed to play with it, a poor behavior is enforced and will be practiced when the child encounters a live wire. Although it is always wise to explain why something is dangerous, it must be remembered that small children need to be physically removed from the situation.

It is not easy to teach safety, supervise closely, and refrain from saying "no" a hundred times a day. Parents become acutely aware of this dilemma as soon as the infant learns to crawl. Preventing injuries to children is usually the first reason for limit-setting and discipline, but limits are also set to prevent damage to valuable household objects. When small children are in the home, dangerous objects must be removed or guarded and valuable articles placed out of reach.

When children are taught the meaning of "no," they should also be taught what "yes" means. Children should be praised for playing with suitable toys, their efforts at behaving or listening should be reinforced, and recreational toys that are innovative and creative should be provided for them. Infants love to tear paper and avidly pursue books, magazines, or newspapers left on the floor. Instead of always scolding them for destroying a valued book, child-safe books (such as those constructed of fabric) can be kept available for them to play with. If they enjoy pots and pans, a cabinet can be arranged with safe utensils for them to explore.

One additional factor must be stressed concerning injury prevention and education. Children are imitators; they copy what they see and hear. *Practicing safety teaches safety,* which applies to parents and their children and to nurses and their clients. Saying one thing but doing another confuses children and can lead to difficulties as the child grows older.

ANTICIPATORY GUIDANCE— CARE OF FAMILIES

Childrearing is no easy task; it presents challenges to new parents as well as to "seasoned" parents. With society's changing roles and mores, combined with a highly mobile population, there is little stability for traditional role models and time-honored methods of raising children. As a result, parents look more to professionals for guidance. Nurses are in an advantageous position to render assistance and suggestions. Every phase of a child's life has its particular traumas—toilet training for toddlers, unexplained fears for preschoolers, or identity crises for adolescents. For parents of an infant some challenges center around dependency, discipline, increased mobility, and safety. Major areas for parental guidance during the first year are listed in the Family Home Care box on p. 330.

KEY POINTS

- Biologic development of the child encompasses sensory changes, including binocularity and depth perception; maturation of biologic systems; fine motor development; and gross motor development.
- Erikson's theory of psychosocial development (birth to 1 year) is concerned with acquiring a sense of trust while overcoming a sense of mistrust.
- Piaget's theory of cognitive development, as it applies to the infant, focuses on the sensorimotor phase, which includes the use of reflexes, primary circular reactions, secondary circular reactions, and coordination of secondary schemata and their application to new situations.
- Development of body image begins in infancy; by 1 year of age infants recognize that they are distinct from their parents.
- Social development of the infant is guided by attachment, language development, personal-social behavior, and participation in play.
- Temperament is an important indicator of the kind of interaction that occurs between the child and parents and siblings.
- Parents are faced with many concerns, including infant fears, child care, limit-setting and discipline, thumb-sucking and pacifier use, teething, and choice of infant shoes.
- Breast milk or formula is the most desirable food for the infant during the first 6 months, followed by gradual introduction of solid food during the second 6 months. Whole milk is not recommended until after 12 months.
- Fluoride supplements (after 6 months) and appropriate dietary intake promote good dental hygiene.
- Infants may be prone to sleep disturbances, and the nurse should instruct the parents, after careful assessment, in adjusting the infant's schedule.
- Recommended routine immunizations include those for diphtheria, tetanus, pertussis, polio, measles, mumps, rubella, *Haemophilus influenzae* type b, hepatitis B virus, and varicella.
- Recommended immunizations for selected groups of children are influenza virus, pneumococcal, meningococcal, and hepatitis A virus vaccines.
- Because injuries are a major cause of death during infancy, parents should be alerted to motor vehicle, aspiration, suffocation, burn, drowning, falling, poisoning, and bodily injuries.

REFERENCES

Air-Bag-Associated Fatal Injuries to Infants and Children Riding in Front Passenger Seats—United States, *MMWR* 44(45):845-846, 1995.

American Academy of Pediatrics, Committee on Infectious Diseases: *1994 Red Book: report of the Committee on Infectious Diseases,* ed 23, Elk Grove Village, IL, 1994, The Academy.

American Academy of Pediatrics, Committee on Infectious Diseases: *Haemophilus influenzae* type b conjugate vaccines: recommendations for immunization with recently and previously licensed vaccines, *Pediatrics* 92(3):480-488, 1993a.

American Academy of Pediatrics, Committee on Infectious Diseases: Recommendations for the use of live attenuated varicella vaccine, *Pediatrics* 95(5):791-795, 1995.

American Academy of Pediatrics, Committee on Infectious Diseases: Universal hepatitis B immunization, *Pediatrics* 89(4):795-800, 1992.

American Academy of Pediatrics, Committee on Injury and Poison Prevention: Drowning in infants, children and adolescents, *Pediatrics* 92(2):292-294, 1993.

American Academy of Pediatrics, Committee on Injury and Poison Prevention: Injuries associated with infant walkers, *Pediatrics* 95(5):778-780, 1995.

American Academy of Pediatrics, Committee on Nutrition: Fluoride supplementation for children, *Pediatrics* 95(5):777, 1995.

American Academy of Pediatrics, Committee on Nutrition: Policy statement: the use of fruit juice in the diets of young children, *AAP News* 7(2):11, 1991.

American Academy of Pediatrics, Committee on SportsMedicine: Infant exercise programs, *Pediatrics* 82(5):800, 1988.

American Public Health Association and American Academy of Pediatrics: *Caring for our children: national health and safety performance standards: guidelines for out-of-home child care programs,* Washington, DC, 1992, The Association.

Anders TF, Halpern LF, Hua J: Sleeping through the night: a developmental perspective, *Pediatrics* 90(4):554-560, 1992.

Baby bottle tooth decay, *Pediatr Dent* 15(7):27, 1993 (special issue—reference manual).

Bell LM and others: Potential impact of linking an emergency department and hospital-affiliated clinics to immunize preschool-age children, *Pediatrics* 93(1):99-103, 1994.

Blasco PA: Normal and abnormal motor development, *Pediatr Rounds* 1(2):1-6, 1992.

Brazelton T: Parent-infant cosleeping revisited, *Ab Initio* 2(1):1-7, 1990.

Calvo EB, Galindo AC, Aspres NB: Iron status in exclusively breast-fed infants, *Pediatrics* 90(3):375-379, 1992.

Carey WB, McDevitt SC: Revision of the infant temperament questionnaire, *Pediatrics* 61(5):735-739, 1978.

Centers for Disease Control and Prevention: General recommendations on immunization: recommendations of the Advisory Committee on Immunization Practices (ACIP), *MMWR* 43(RR-1):1-38, 1994.

Chess S, Thomas A: Temperamental differences: a critical concept in child health care, *Pediatr Nurs* 11(3):167-171, 1985.

Dewey KG and others: Breast-fed infants are leaner than formula-fed infants at 1 year of age: the DARLING study, *Am J Clin Nutr* 57(2):140-145, 1993.

Ferber R: Solve your child's sleep problems, New York, 1985, Simon & Schuster.

Gennaro S, Medoff-Cooper B, Lotas M: Perinatal factors and infant temperament: a collaborative approach . . . common variables of three studies examined, *Nurs Res* 41(6):375-377, 1992.

Holida DL: Latex balloons: they can take your breath away, *Pediatr Nurs* 19(1):39-43, 68, 1993.

Institute of Medicine: Adverse events associated with childhood vaccines, Washington, DC, 1993, National Academy Press.

Jaber L, Cohen IJ, Mor A: Fever associated with teething, *Arch Dis Child* 67(2):233-234, 1992.

Jones L, Heermann J: Parental division of infant care: contextual influences and infant characteristics, *Nurs Res* 41(4):228-234, 1992.

Lampl M, Veldhuis JD, Johnson ML: Saltation and stasis: a model of human growth, *Science* 258(5083):801-803, 1992.

Landis SE, Chang A: Child care options for ill children, *Pediatrics* 88(4):705-718, 1991.

Miller A, Barr R, Eaton W: Crying and motor behavior of six-week-old infants and postpartum maternal mood, *Pediatrics* 92(4):551-558, 1993.

Nowak AJ: What pediatricians can do to promote oral health, *Contemp Pediatr* 10(4):90-106, 1993.

Pickler R, Frankel H: The effect of non-nutritive sucking on preterm infants' behavioral organization and feeding performance, *Neonatal Network* 14(2):83, 1995.

Position statement: infant feeding, *Clin Pediatr* 31(8):510, 1992.

Schachter F and others: Cosleeping and sleep problems in Hispanic-American urban young children, *Pediatrics* 84(3):522-530, 1989.

Schmitt BD: The "two-step" approach to infant sleep problems, *Contemp Pediatr* 9(11):37-38, 1992.

Sullivan SA, Birch LL: Infant dietary experience and acceptance of solid foods, *Pediatrics* 93(2):271-277, 1994.

Tully S: Injuries to children in shopping carts, *AAP News* 9(6):11, 1993.

Victora CG and others: Use of pacifiers and breastfeeding duration, *Lancet* 341(8842):404-406, 1993.

Wong DL: Guiding parents in selecting daycare centers, *Pediatr Nurs* 12(3):181-187, 1986.

Zuckerman JN, Cockcroft A, Zuckerman AJ: Site of injection for vaccination, *Br Med J* 305(6862):1158, 1992.

BIBLIOGRAPHY

Growth and Development

Belfer M: Body image: impacts and distortions. In Levine M and others, editors: *Developmental-behavioral pediatrics,* ed 2, Philadelphia, 1992, WB Saunders.

Erikson E: *Childhood and society,* ed 2, New York, 1963, WW Norton.

Friendly DS: Developmental of vision in infants and young children, *Pediatr Clin North Am* 40(4):693-703, 1993.

Garmezy N, Rutter M, editors: *Stress, coping, and development in children,* New York, 1989, McGraw-Hill.

Knobloch H, Stevens F, Malone AF: *Manual of developmental diagnosis,* Hagerstown, PA, 1980, Harper & Row.

Maier H: *Three theories of child development,* ed 3, New York, 1988, Harper & Row.

Marino B: Assessments of infant play: applications to research and practice, *Issues Compr Pediatr Nurs* 11(4):227-240, 1988.

Piaget J: *The construction of reality in the child,* New York, 1975, Ballantine Books.

Seligman S: Emotional and social development in infancy and early childhood, *Early Child Update* 5(4):1-2, 1989.

Singhi P, Radhika S: Kiss: a developmental milestone or a culture-determined skill? *Am J Dis Child* 146(6):663-664, 1992.

Vaughan III VC: Assessment of growth and development during infancy and early childhood, *Pediatr Rev* 13(3):88-97, 1992.

Attachment/Temperament/Parenting

Briss PA and others: A nationwide study of the risk of injury associated with day care center attendance, *Pediatrics* 93(3):364-368, 1994.

Calkins SD, Fox NA: The relations among infant temperament, security of attachment, and behavioral inhibition at twenty-four months, *Child Dev* 63(6):1456-1472, 1992.

Coffman S and others: Infant-mother attachment: relationships to maternal responsiveness and infant temperament *J Pediatr Nurs* 10(1):9-18, 1995.

Coffman S and others: Temperament and interactive effects: mothers and infants in a teaching situation, *Issues Compr Pediatr Nurs* 15:169-182, 1992.

Graham MV: Parental sensitivity to infant cues: similarities and differences between mothers and fathers, *J Pediatr Nurs* 8(6):376-384, 1993.

Harris E, Weston D, Lieberman A: Quality of mother-infant attachment and pediatric health care use, *Pediatrics* 84(2):248-254, 1989.

Isabella RA: Origins of attachment: maternal interactive behavior across the first year, *Child Dev* 64(2):605-621, 1993.

Koniak-Griffin D, Rummell M: Temperament in infancy: stability, change, and correlates, *Matern Child Nurs J* 17(1):25-40, 1988.

Wasserman R and others: Infant temperament and school age behavior: 6-year longitudinal study in the pediatric practice, *Pediatrics* 85(5):801-807, 1990.

Wong DL and others: Diapering choices: a critical review of the issues, *Pediatr Nurs* 18(1):41-54, 1992.

Concerns Related to Growth and Development

For bibliography on day care, see Chapter 13.

Castiglia P: Thumb sucking, *J Pediatr Health Care* 2(6):322-323, 1988.

Clutter L: Helping parents prepare for travel and vacations with children, *Pediatr Nurs* 14(3):211-215, 1988.

Friman PC: Concurrent habits: what would Linus do with his blanket if his thumb-sucking were treated? *Am J Dis Child* 144(12):1316-1318, 1990.

Glendon M: If the shoe fits . . . wear it, *Pediatr Nurs* 13(4):230-271, 1987.

Solomon R, Martin K: Can you spoil an infant? A primary care survey, *Am J Dis Child* 144(4):426-427, 1990.

Nutrition

Finberg L: How good a food for humans is cow's milk? *Am J Dis Child* 146(12):1432, 1992.

Fomon SJ: *Nutrition of normal infants,* St Louis, 1993, Mosby.

Forsyth JS and others: Relation between early introduction of solid food to infants and their weight and illnesses during the first two years of life, *Br Med J* 306(6892):1572-1576, 1993.

Fuchs GL and others: Iron status and intake of older infants fed formula vs cow milk with cereal, *Am J Clin Nutr* 58:343-348, 1993.

Lawrence RA: *Breast feeding: a guide for the medical profession,* ed 4, St Louis, 1994, Mosby.

Lawrence R: The clinician's role in teaching proper infant feeding techniques. *J Pediatrics* 126:5112-7, 1995.

McCain GC: Promotion of preterm infant nipple feeding with non-nutritive sucking, *J Pediatr Nurs* 10(1):3-8, 1995.

Nemethy M, Clore E: Microwave heating of infant formula and breast milk, *J Pediatr Health Care* 4(3):131-135, 1990.

Pinilla T, Birch LL: Help me make it through the night: behavioral entrainment of breast-fed infant's sleep patterns, *Pediatrics* 91(2):436-444, 1993.

Pipes PL, Trahms CM: *Nutrition in infancy and childhood,* ed 5, St. Louis, 1993, Mosby.

Schmitt BD: When weaning is delayed, *Contemp Pediatr* 7(6):67-68, 1990.

Sigman-Grant M, Bush G, Anantheswaran R: Microwave heating of infant formula: a dilemma resolved, *Pediatrics* 90(3):412-415, 1992.

Snow LS, Fry ME: Formula feeding in the first year of life, *Pediatr Nurs* 16(5):442-446, 1990.

Sullivan PB: Cows' milk induced intestinal bleeding in infancy, *Arch Dis Child* 68(2):240-245, 1993.

Weigley ES: Changing patterns in offering solids to infants. *Pediatr Nurs* 16(5):439-441, 1990.

Worobey J, Lewis M: Behavioral differences in response to stress between breast- and bottle-fed infants, *Top Clin Nutr* 7(3):48-55, 1992.

Sleep and Activity

Adair R and others: Reduced night waking in infancy: a primary care intervention, *Pediatrics* 89(4):585-588, 1992.

Adams L, Rickert V: Reducing bedtime tantrums: comparison between positive routines and graduated extinction, *Pediatrics* 84(5):756-761, 1989.

Balsmeyer B: Sleep disturbances of the infant and toddler, *Pediatr Nurs* 16(5):447-452, 1990.

Bardossi K: Getting kids to bed: How tough is too tough? *Contemp Pediatr* 8(1):97-105, 1991.

Horne J: Sleep and its disorders in children, *J Child Psychol Psychiatry* 33(3):473-487, 1992.

Jaffa T and others: Sleep disorders in children, *Br Med J* 306(6878):640-643, 1993.

Scher A and others: Toddlers' sleep and temperament: reporting bias or a valid link? A research note, *J Child Psychol Psychiatry* 33(7):1249-1254, 1992.

Schmitt BD: How to help the trained night feeder, *Contemp Pediatr* 9(11):41-49, 1992.

Schmitt BD: When your child refuses to go to bed, *Contemp Pediatr* 6(7):70-71, 1989.

Dental Health

For bibliography, see Chapter 12.

Immunizations

Abbotts B, Osborn LM: Immunization status and reasons for immunization delay among children using public health immunization clinics, *Am J Dis Child* 147:965-968, 1993.

Ad Hoc Working Group for the Development of Standards for Pediatric Immunization Practices: Standards for pediatric immunization practices, *JAMA* 269(14):1817-1822, 1993.

Adams WG and others: Decline of childhood *Haemophilus influenzae* type b (Hib) disease in the Hib vaccine era, *JAMA* 269(2):221-226, 1993.

American Academy of Pediatrics Committee on Practice and Ambulatory Medicine: Implementation of the immunization policy (S94-26), *Pediatrics* 96(2):360-361, 1995.

Brown J and others: Missed opportunities in preventive pediatric health care: immunizations or well-child care visits? *Am J Dis Child* 147(10):1081-1084, 1993.

Caulfield M: Hepatitis B: a disease needing a vaccine or a vaccine needing a disease? *Clin Pediatr* 32(7):443-444, 1993.

Centers for Disease Control and Prevention: Standards for pediatric immunization practices, *MMWR* 42(RR-5):1-13, 1993a.

Centers for Disease Control and Prevention: Use of vaccines and immune globulin in persons with altered immunocompetence: recommendations of the Advisory Committee on Immunization Practices (ACIP), *MMWR* 42(RR-4):1-18, 1993b.

Golden GS: The national childhood vaccine injury act: an update, *Contemp Pediatr* 10:96-105, 1993.

Gorelick MH, Baker MD: Epiglottitis in children, 1979 through 1992: effects of *Haemophilus influenzae* type b immunization, *Arch Pediatr Adolesc Med* 148(1):47-50, 1994.

Peter G: Childhood immunizations, *New Engl J Med* 327(25):1794-1800, 1992.

Schoendorf KC and others: National trends in *Haemophilus influenzae* meningitis mortality and hospitalization among children, 1980 through 1991, *Pediatrics* 93(4):663-668, 1994.

Szilagyi PG and others: Missed opportunities for childhood vaccinations in office practices and the effect on vaccination status, *Pediatrics* 91(1):1-7, 1993.

Zanga JR: Should there be a universal childhood vaccination against hepatitis B? II. A rebuttal, *Pediatr Nurs* 19(5):451-452, 1993.

Zell ER and others: Low vaccination levels of U.S. preschool and school-age children, *JAMA* 271(11):833-839, 1994.

Injury Prevention

For additional citations, see Chapters 1 and 12.

Agran PF, Winn DG, Castillo DN: On-lap travel: still a problem in motor vehicles, *Pediatrics* 90(1):27-29, 1992.

Botash A: Syringe caps: an aspiration hazard, *Pediatrics* 90(1):92-3, 1992.

Children and waterbeds, *Pediatr Nurs* 17(6):577, 1991 (letter and reply).

Coppens N: Parental responses to children in unsafe situations, *Pediatr Nurs* 16(6):571-574, 1990.

Gielen AC, Collins B: Community-based interventions for injury prevention, *Fam Community Health* 15(4):1-11, 1993.

Gunn WJ and others: Injuries and poisonings in out-of-home child care and home care, *Am J Dis Child* 145(7):779-781, 1991.

Health alert: Air bag/child seat warning label, *AAP News* 10(4):22, 1994.

Jones NE: Prevention of childhood injuries. II. Recreational injuries, *Pediatr Nurs* 18(6):619-621, 1992.

Ramsey K, Goldbach R, Stephenson S: Near fatal aspiration of a candy pacifier, *Pediatrics* 84(1):126-127, 1989.

Sheridan R, Sheridan M, Tompkins R: Dishwasher effluent burns in infants, *Pediatrics* 91(1):142-143, 1993.

Stewart DD: Child passenger safety: current technical issues for advocates and professionals, *Fam Community Health* 15(4):12-27, 1993.

Turner WT, Snow CW, Poteat GM: Accidental injuries among children in day care centers and family day care homes: brief report, *Child Health Care* 22(1):73-79, 1993.

Chapter 11

HEALTH PROBLEMS OF INFANTS

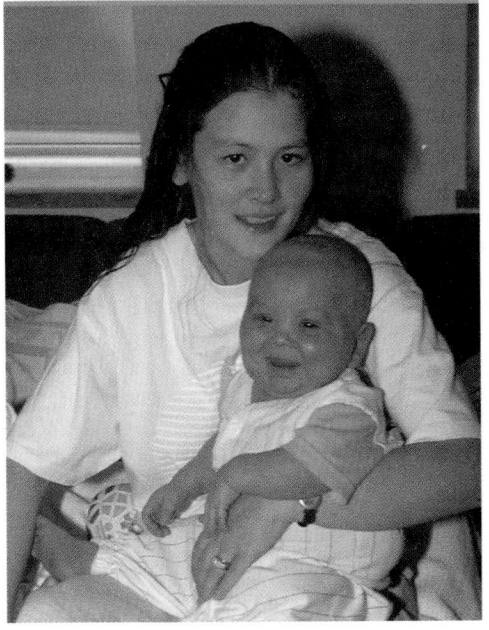

" *It's been 3 months since the cord blood transplant, and look at him now! Miracles do happen.* "

Linda, mother of
Randy, age 11
months, leukemia

RELATED TOPICS

LEARNING OBJECTIVES
On completion of this chapter the reader will be able to:

- Identify children at increased risk of developing nutritional disturbances
- Outline a nutritional counseling plan for vitamin or mineral deficiency and excess
- Outline a dietary plan for parents when the infant is sensitive to milk
- List measures that can be used to alleviate colic
- Plan nursing care that meets the physical and emotional needs of the nonorganic failure-to-thrive child and parent
- Provide nursing care that meets the immediate and long-term
needs of the family who has lost a child from sudden infant death syndrome
- Identify the stresses and needs of the family whose child is home monitored for apnea
- Identify characteristics of children with autism

NUTRITIONAL DISTURBANCES

VITAMIN DISTURBANCES

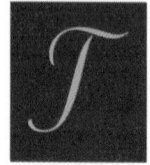

True vitamin disturbances are rare in the United States. Subclinical deficiencies are commonly seen, however, especially in lower socioeconomic groups, where dietary intake may be unbalanced. Vitamin deficiencies of the fat-soluble vitamins A and D may occur in malabsorptive disorders. Certain groups are at risk for vitamin D–deficient rickets: (1) children born of and breast-fed by mothers who are vitamin D deficient; (2) individuals who are exposed to minimal sunlight because of clothing, housing in areas of high pollution, or dark skin pigmentation; (3) adherence to vegetarian diets that are low in sources of vitamin D; and (4) use of milk products, such as yogurt or raw cow's milk, that are not supplemented with vitamin D, as the primary source of milk. Children may also be at risk secondary to disorders or their treatment. For example, children receiving high doses of salicylates as therapy for rheumatoid arthritis may have impaired vitamin C storage.

Recent studies indicate that vitamin A deficiency correlates with increased morbidity and mortality in children with measles. Complications from diarrhea and infections were increased, as was morbidity, in infants and children with vitamin A deficiency (Fawzi and others, 1993).

Of equal if not greater concern is the overuse of vitamins. An excessive dose of a vitamin is generally defined as 10 or more times the recommended dietary allowance (RDA), although the fat-soluble vitamins, especially A and D, tend to cause toxic reactions at lower doses. With the addition of vitamins to commercially packaged foods, the potential for hypervitaminosis has escalated, especially when vitamin supplements are used injudiciously. Hypervitaminoses of A and D present the greatest problems, because the fat-soluble vitamins are stored in the body and a much lower excess dose causes toxicity. However, it is now well documented that the water-soluble vitamins, B complex and C, can also cause toxicity. One vitamin supplement that is recommended for all women of childbearing age is a daily dose of 0.4 mg of folic acid, the usual RDA. Folic acid taken before conception and during early pregnancy can reduce the risk of neural tube defects, such as spina bifida, by at least 50% (Knowledge, 1995).

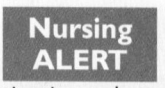 Educate childbearing adolescent females about the need for folic acid to prevent neural tube birth defects. It is most easily obtained from a daily multivitamin supplement.

Deficiencies and excesses of vitamins A, B complex, C, D, E, and K are summarized in Table 11-1, and the RDAs are listed in Appendix F. General nursing considerations are discussed below, and specific interventions are presented in the table.

David Wilson, MS, RNC, revised this chapter.

MINERAL DISTURBANCES

A number of minerals are essential nutrients. *Macrominerals* refer to those with daily requirements greater than 100 mg and include calcium, phosphorus, magnesium, sodium, potassium, chloride, and sulfur. *Microminerals,* or *trace elements,* have daily requirements less than 100 mg and include several essential minerals and those whose exact role in nutrition is still unclear. The greatest concern with minerals is deficiency, especially of iron, calcium, and zinc.

The regulation of mineral balance in the body is a complex process. Dietary extremes of mineral intake can cause a number of mineral interactions that can result in unexpected deficiencies or excesses. For example, excessive amounts of one mineral, such as zinc, can result in a deficiency of another mineral, such as copper, even if sufficient amounts of copper are ingested. Deficiencies can also occur when various substances in the diet interact with minerals. For example, iron, zinc, and calcium can form insoluble complexes with phytates and/or oxalates (found in plant proteins), which impair the bioavailability of the mineral. This type of interaction is important in vegetarian diets because plant foods, such as soy, are high in phytates.

 Contrary to popular belief, spinach is not a rich source of iron or calcium, because of its oxalate content.

Deficiencies and excesses of selected macrominerals and microminerals are summarized in Table 11-2, and the recommended RDAs are listed in Appendix F. General nursing considerations are discussed below, and specific interventions are presented in the table.

VEGETARIAN DIETS

Vegetarian diets can potentially cause nutritional deficiencies in children. The stricter the vegetarian diet, the more difficult it becomes to ensure adequate nutrition for infants and children. The major types of vegetarianism are the following:

Lacto-ovovegetarians, who exclude meat from their diet but eat milk and eggs and sometimes fish
Lactovegetarians, who exclude meat and eggs but drink milk
Pure vegetarians (vegans), who eliminate any food of animal origin, including milk and eggs
Zen macrobiotics, who are even more restrictive than pure vegetarians in that cereals, especially brown rice, are the mainstay of the diet.

Many individuals who are concerned about healthful diets subscribe to vegetarian diets that are not typified by the above categories. Therefore, during nutritional assessment it is necessary to list exactly what the diet includes and excludes.

The lacto-ovovegetarian diet is associated with the least deficiencies, although protein intake needs to be monitored. The lactovegetarian diet may also be low in protein, as well as iron. The major deficiencies in the stricter vegetarian diets are inadequate protein for growth, inadequate calories for energy and growth, poor digestibility of many of the natural, unprocessed foods, especially for infants, and deficiencies of vitamin B_{12}, niacin, thiamine, riboflavin, vitamin D, iron, calcium, and zinc. In the United States strict vegetarian diets

Text continued on p. 344.

TABLE 11-1. Vitamins and their nutritional significance

PHYSIOLOGIC FUNCTIONS/ SOURCES	RESULTS OF DEFICIENCY OR EXCESS	NURSING CONSIDERATIONS
Vitamin A (Retinol)*	**Deficiency**	
Functions	Night blindness	Encourage foods rich in vitamin A, such as whole cow's milk
Necessary component in formation of pigment rhodopsin (visual purple)	Keratinization (hardening and scaling) of epithelium	As milk consumption decreases, encourage foods rich in vitamin A
Formation and maintenance of epithelial tissue	Xerophthalmia (hardening and scaling of cornea and conjunctiva)	Ensure adequate intake in preterm infants
Normal bone growth and tooth development	Phrynoderma (toad skin)	Advise parents of safe use of supplements in child with measles
Needed for growth and spermatogenesis	Drying of respiratory, gastrointestinal, and genitourinary tracts	
Involved in thyroxine formation	Defective tooth enamel	
Antioxidant	Retarded growth	
	Impaired bone formation	
Sources	Decreased thyroxine formation	
Natural form —liver, kidney, fish oils, milk and nonskimmed milk products, egg yolk		
	Excess	
Provitamin A (carotene) —carrots, sweet potatoes, squash, apricots, spinach, collards, broccoli, cabbage, artichokes	*Early signs* —irritability, anorexia, pruritus, fissures at corners of nose and lips	Emphasize correct use of vitamin supplements and potential hazards of excess
	Later signs —hepatomegaly, jaundice, retarded growth, poor weight gain, thickening of the cortex of long bones with pain and fragility, hard tender lumps in extremities and occiput of the skull	Investigate child's dietary habits to calculate approximate intake; if excessive, remove supplemental source (e.g., daily feeding of liver)
	May cause birth defects from excessive maternal intake	
	NOTE: Overdose results from ingestion of large quantities of the vitamin only, not the provitamin; large amounts of carotene (carotenemia) cause yellow or orange discoloration of the skin (not the sclera, urine, or feces as in jaundice), but none of the above symptoms	Advise parents of the benign nature of carotenemia; treatment is avoidance of excess pigmented fruits or vegetables, especially carrots; skin color returns to normal in 2 to 6 weeks
Vitamin B₁ (Thiamin)†	**Deficiency**	*Vitamin B complex*
Functions	*Gastrointestinal* —anorexia, constipation, indigestion	Encourage foods rich in B vitamins
Coenzyme (with phosphorus) in carbohydrate metabolism	*Neurologic* —apathy, fatigue, emotional instability, polyneuritis, tenderness of calf muscles, partial anesthesia, muscle weakness, paresthesia, hyperesthesia, decreased or absent tendon reflexes, convulsions, and coma (in infants)	Stress proper cooking and storage techniques to preserve potency, such as minimum cooking of vegetables in small amount of liquid; storage of milk in opaque container
Needed for healthy nervous system		Advise against fad diets that severely restrict groups of food, such as vegetarianism (vegans or macrobiotics)
Sources	*Cardiovascular* —palpitations, cardiac failure, peripheral vasodilation, edema	Explore need for vitamin supplements when dieting or when using goat milk exclusively for infant feeding (deficient in folic acid) or when the breastfeeding mother is a strict vegetarian (vitamin B₁₂)
Pork, beef, liver, legumes, nuts, whole or enriched grains and cereals, green vegetables, fruits, milk, brown rice		
	Excess	
	Headache	
	Irritability	
	Insomnia	Emphasize correct use of vitamin supplements and potential hazards of excesses
	Rapid pulse	
	Weakness	

*Fat soluble.
†Water soluble.

Continued.

TABLE 11-1. Vitamins and their nutritional significance—cont'd

PHYSIOLOGIC FUNCTIONS/ SOURCES	RESULTS OF DEFICIENCY OR EXCESS	NURSING CONSIDERATIONS
Vitamin B$_2$ (Riboflavin)†		
Functions	*Deficiency*	Same as vitamin B complex
Coenzyme (with phosphorus) in carbohydrate, protein, and fat metabolism	Ariboflavinosis	
Maintains healthy skin, especially around mouth, nose, and eyes	*Lips* —cheilosis (fissures at corners of lips), perlèche (inflammation at corners of lips)	
	Tongue —glossitis	
Sources	*Nose* —irritation and cracks at nasal angle	
Milk and its products, eggs, organ meat (liver, kidney, and heart), enriched cereals, some green leafy vegetables,‡ legumes	*Eyes* —burning, itching, tearing, photophobia, corneal vascularization, cataracts	
	Skin —seborrheic dermatitis, delayed wound healing and tissue repair	
	Excess	
	Paresthesia, pruritus	
Niacin (Nicotinic Acid, Nicotinamide)†		
Functions	*Deficiency*	Same as vitamin B complex
Coenzyme (with riboflavin) in protein and fat metabolism	Pellagra	If used as hypolipidemic agent, stress safe dosage to prevent child's accidental ingestion
Needed for healthy nervous system, skin, and normal digestion	*Oral* —stomatitis, glossitis	
May lower cholesterol	*Cutaneous* —scaly dermatitis on exposed areas	
	Gastrointestinal —anorexia, weight loss, diarrhea, fatigue	
Sources	*Neurologic* —apathy, anxiety, confusion, depression, dementia	
Meat, poultry, fish, peanuts, beans, peas, whole or enriched grains except corn and rice	Death	
Milk and its products are sources of tryptophan (60 mg of tryptophan = 1 mg of niacin)	*Excess*	
	Release of vasodilator, histamine (flushing, decreased blood pressure, increased cerebral blood flow; aggravates asthma)	
	Dermatologic problems (pruritus, rash, hyperkeratosis, acanthosis nigricans)	
	Increased gastric acidity (aggravates peptic ulcer disease)	
	Hepatotoxicity	
	Increased serum uric acid levels	
	Elevated plasma glucose levels	
	Certain cardiac arrhythmias	
Vitamin B$_6$ (Pyridoxine)†		
Functions	*Deficiency*	Same as vitamin B complex
Coenzyme in protein and fat metabolism	Scaly dermatitis, weight loss, anemia, retarded growth, irritability, convulsions, peripheral neuritis	Stress proper cooking and storing techniques to preserve potency
Needed for formation of antibodies, hemoglobin		Cook food covered in small amount of water
Needed for utilization of copper and iron	*Excess*	Do not soak food in water
Aids in conversion of tryptophan to niacin	Peripheral nervous system toxicity (unsteady gait, numb feet and hands, clumsiness of hands, sometimes perioral numbness)	Store in light-resistant container
Sources	May cause peptic ulcer disease or seizures	
Meats, especially liver and kidney, cereal grains (wheat and corn), yeast, soybeans, peanuts, tuna, chicken, salmon		

†Water soluble.
‡Green leafy vegetables include spinach, broccoli, kale, turnip greens, mustard greens, collards, dandelion greens, and beet greens.

TABLE 11-1. Vitamins and their nutritional significance—cont'd

PHYSIOLOGIC FUNCTIONS/ SOURCES	RESULTS OF DEFICIENCY OR EXCESS	NURSING CONSIDERATIONS

Folic Acid (Folacin; Reduced Form is Called Folinic Acid or Citrovorum Factor)†

Functions

Coenzyme for single-carbon transfer (purines, thymine, hemoglobin)

Necessary for formation of red blood cells

Sources

Green leafy vegetables, cabbage, asparagus, liver, kidneys, nuts, eggs, whole grain cereals, legumes, bananas

Deficiency

Macrocytic anemia, bone marrow depression, glossitis, intestinal malabsorption

Excess

Rare because megadoses not available over the counter

May cause insomnia and irritability

Same as vitamin B complex

Stress proper cooking and storing techniques to preserve potency

   Cook food covered in small amount of water

   Do not soak food in water

   Store in light-resistant container

Women of childbearing age should supplement to prevent neural tube defects

---

Vitamin B_{12} (Cobalamin)†

Functions

Coenzyme in protein synthesis; indirect effect on formation of red blood cells (particularly on formation of nucleic acids and folic acid metabolism)

Needed for normal functioning of nervous tissue

Sources

Meat, liver, kidney, fish, shellfish, poultry, milk, eggs, cheese, nutritional yeast, sea vegetables

Deficiency

Pernicious anemia

(One form of deficiency from absence of intrinsic factor in gastric secretions)

General signs of severe anemia

Lemon-yellow tinge to skin

Spinal cord degeneration

Delayed brain growth

Excess

Excess is rare

Same as vitamin B complex

Vitamin C (Ascorbic Acid)†

Functions

Essential for collagen formation

Increases absorption of iron for hemoglobin formation

Enhances conversion of folic acid to folinic acid

Affects cholesterol synthesis and conversion of proline to hydroxyproline

Probably a coenzyme in metabolism of tyrosine and phenylalanine

May play role in hydroxylation of adrenal steroids

May have stimulating effect on phagocytic activity of leukocytes and formation of antibodies

Antioxidant agent

Sources

Citrus fruits, strawberries, tomatoes, potatoes, melon, cabbage, broccoli, cauliflower, spinach, papaya, mango

Deficiency

Scurvy

Skin —dry, rough, petechiae; perifollicular hyperkeratotic papules (raised areas around hair follicles)

Musculoskeletal —bleeding muscles and joints, pseudoparalysis from pain, swelling of joints, costochondral beading (scorbutic rosary)

Gums —spongy, friable, swollen, bleed easily, bluish red or black color, teeth loosen and fall out

General disposition —irritable, anorexic, apprehensive, in pain, refuses to move, assumes semi-froglike position when supine (scorbutic pose)

Signs of anemia

Decreased wound healing

Increased susceptibility to infection

Excess

Diarrhea

Increased excretion of uric acid and acidification of urine (may cause urate precipitation and formation of oxalate stones)

Hemolysis

Impaired leukocytosis activity

Damage to beta cells of pancreas and decreased insulin production

Reproductive failure

"Rebound scurvy" from withdrawal of large amounts

Encourage foods rich in vitamin C

Investigate infant's diet for sources of vitamin, especially when cow's milk is principal source of nutrition

Stress proper cooking and storing techniques to preserve potency

   Wash vegetables quickly; do not soak in water

Cook vegetables in covered pot with minimum water and for short time; avoid copper or cast iron cookware

Do not add baking soda to cooking water

Use fresh fruits and vegetables as soon as possible; store in refrigerator

Store juice in airtight, opaque container

Wrap cut fruit or eat soon after exposing to air

In caring for child with scurvy:

   Position for comfort and rest

   Handle very gently and minimally

   Administer analgesics as needed

   Prevent infection

   Provide good oral care

   Provide soft, bland diet

   Emphasize rapid recovery when vitamin is replaced

Emphasize correct use of vitamin supplement and potential hazards of excess

Identify groups at risk for vitamin C supplements: those with thalassemia; those on anticoagulant or aminoglycoside antibiotic therapy

---

†Water soluble.

Continued.

TABLE 11-1. Vitamins and their nutritional significance—cont'd

PHYSIOLOGIC FUNCTIONS/ SOURCES	RESULTS OF DEFICIENCY OR EXCESS	NURSING CONSIDERATIONS
Vitamin D₂ (Ergocalciferol) and D₃ (Cholecalciferol)*		
Functions	*Deficiency*	
Absorption of calcium and phosphorus and decreased renal excretion of phosphorus	Rickets	Encourage foods rich in vitamin D, especially fortified cow's milk
	Head —craniotabes (softening of cranial bones, prominence of frontal bones), deformed shape (skull flat and depressed toward middle), delayed closure of fontanels	In breast-fed infants encourage use of vitamin D supplements if maternal diet inadequate or infant exposed to minimal sunlight
Sources		In caring for child with rickets:
Direct sunlight	*Chest* —rachitic rosary (enlargement of costochondral junction of ribs), Harrison groove (horizontal depression in lower portion of rib cage), pigeon chest (sharp protrusion of sternum)	Maintain good body alignment
Cod liver oil, herring, mackerel, salmon, tuna, sardines		Reposition frequently to prevent decubiti and respiratory infection
Enriched food sources —milk, milk products, enriched cereals, margarine, breads, many breakfast drinks		Handle very gently and minimally
	Spine —kyphosis, scoliosis, lordosis	Prevent infection
	Abdomen —potbelly, constipation	Institute seizure precautions
	Extremities —bowing of arms and legs, knock-knee, saber shins, instability of hip joints, pelvic deformity, enlargement of hip joints, enlargement of epiphysis at ends of long bones	Have 10% calcium gluconate available in case of tetany
		Observe for possibility of overdose from supplements
	Teeth —delayed calcification, especially of permanent teeth	If prescribed, supervise proper use of orthopedic splints or braces
	Rachitic tetany —seizures	
	Excess	Same as vitamin A; may include low-calcium diet during initial therapy
	Acute —vomiting, dehydration, fever, abdominal cramps, bone pain, convulsions, and coma	
	Chronic —lassitude, mental slowness, anorexia, failure to thrive, thirst, urinary urgency, polyuria, vomiting, diarrhea, abdominal cramps, bone pain, pathologic fractures	
	Calcification of soft tissue —kidneys, lungs, adrenal glands, vessels (hypertension), heart, gastric lining, tympanic membrane (deafness)	
	Osteoporosis of long bones	
	Elevated serum levels of calcium and phosphorus	
Vitamin E (Tocopherol)*		
Functions	*Deficiency*	
Production of red blood cells and protection from hemolysis	Hemolytic anemia from hemolysis caused by shortened life of red blood cells, especially in premature infants, and focal necrosis of tissues	Initiate early feeding in premature infants; may need supplementation
Muscle and liver integrity		
Coenzyme factor in tissue respiration	Causes infertility in rats, but not in humans (does *not* increase human male virility or potency)	
Minimizes oxidation of polyunsaturated fatty acids and vitamins A and C in intestinal tract and tissues		
Possible role in treatment and prevention of bronchopulmonary dysplasia and retinopathy of prematurity is under investigation	*Excess*	
	Little is known; less toxic than other fat-soluble vitamins	

*Fat soluble.

TABLE 11-1. Vitamins and their nutritional significance—cont'd

PHYSIOLOGIC FUNCTIONS/ SOURCES	RESULTS OF DEFICIENCY OR EXCESS	NURSING CONSIDERATIONS
Vitamin E (Tocopherol)—cont'd *Sources* Vegetable oils, wheat germ oil, milk, egg yolk, muscle meats, fish, whole grains, nuts, legumes, spinach, broccoli		
Vitamin K* *Functions* Catalyst for production of prothrombin and blood-clotting factors II, VII, IX, and X by the liver *Sources* Pork, liver, green leafy vegetables (spinach, kale, cabbage)‡, tomatoes, egg yolk, cheese	*Deficiency* Hemorrhage *Excess* Hemolytic anemia in individuals who are deficient in glucose-6-phosphate dehydrogenase	Administer prophylactically to all newborns Other indications include intestinal disease, lack of bile, prolonged antibiotic therapy; may be used in management of blood-clotting time when anticoagulants such as warfarin (Coumadin) and dicumarol (bishydroxycoumarin), which are vitamin K antagonists, are used

*Fat soluble.
‡Green leafy vegetables include spinach, broccoli, kale, turnip greens, mustard greens, collards, dandelion greens, and beet greens.

TABLE 11-2. Minerals and their nutritional significance

PHYSIOLOGIC FUNCTIONS/ SOURCES	RESULTS OF DEFICIENCY OR EXCESS	NURSING CONSIDERATIONS
Calcium* *Functions* Bone and tooth development and maintenance (in combination with phosphorus) Muscle contractions, especially the heart Blood clotting Absorption of vitamin B_{12} Enzyme activation Nerve conduction Integrity of intracellular cement substances and various membranes *Sources* Dairy products, egg yolk, sardines, canned salmon with bones, dark green leafy vegetables (except spinach), soybeans, dried beans, and peas	*Deficiency* Rickets Tetany Impaired growth, especially of bones and teeth *Excess* Drowsiness, extreme lethargy Impaired absorption of other minerals (iron, zinc, manganese) Calcium deposits in tissues (renal failure)	Encourage foods rich in calcium, especially dairy products Caution that oxalates in leafy vegetables (spinach), oxalates in chocolates, and a high phosphorus intake (especially from carbonated beverages) can decrease calcium absorption Discourage use of whole cow's milk in newborns because the phosphorus-to-calcium ratio favors excretion of calcium Advise against fad diets, especially those that restrict dairy products Emphasize correct use of calcium-supplement, especially the possible interaction between megadoses of calcium and resulting deficiency states of other minerals
Chloride* *Functions* Acid-base and fluid balance Enzyme activation in saliva Component of hydrochloric acid in stomach *Sources* Salt, meat, eggs, dairy products, many prepared and preserved foods	*Deficiency* Acid-base disturbances (hypochloremic alkalosis, dehydration); occurs mostly in combination with sodium loss *Excess* Acid-base disturbance	Deficiency and excess are unusual; most diets supply adequate chloride (usually in combination with sodium) Disease states such as excessive vomiting can necessitate chloride replacement

TABLE 11-2. Minerals and their nutritional significance—cont'd

PHYSIOLOGIC FUNCTIONS/ SOURCES	RESULTS OF DEFICIENCY OR EXCESS	NURSING CONSIDERATIONS
Fluorine† *Functions* Formation of caries-resistant teeth Strong bone development *Sources* Fluoridated water and foods or beverages prepared with fluoridated water; fish, tea, commercially prepared chicken for infants	*Deficiency* Increased susceptibility to tooth decay *Excess* Fluorosis (mottling and/or pitting of enamel) Severe bone deformities	In areas with optimally fluoridated water, encourage sufficient intake to supply recommended amount of fluoride (see p. 373) In areas of unfluoridated water or when ready-to-use formula, bottled water, or breast milk is used, stress the importance of fluoride supplements In areas with excess fluoride in the water, consider the use of bottled water in drinking and possibly cooking to reduce the fluoride intake to safe levels Fluoride has the narrowest range of safe and adequate intake; therefore stress the importance of storing supplements in a safe area
Iodine† *Functions* Production of thyroid hormone Normal reproduction *Sources* Seafood, kelp, iodized salt, sea salt, enriched bread, milk (from dairy processing)	*Deficiency* Goiter (enlarged thyroid from decreased thyroxine formation) *Excess* Unknown from food sources; may occur from ingestion of iodine preparations, such as saturated solutions of potassium iodide (SSKI)	Encourage use of iodized salt for individuals living far from the sea If iodine preparations are in the home, stress the importance of safe storage
Iron† *Functions* Formation of hemoglobin and myoglobin Essential part of several enzymes and proteins	*Deficiency* Anemia (Chapter 26)	Encourage foods rich in iron Discourage excessive milk consumption, especially more than 1 L per day (milk is a very poor source of iron) If iron supplements are prescribed, teach parents factors that affect absorption (see box below)

FACTORS THAT AFFECT IRON ABSORPTION

Increase

Acidity (Low pH)—Administer iron between meals (gastric hydrochloric acid)

Ascorbic Acid (Vitamin C)—Administer iron with juice, fruit, or multivitamin preparation
Vitamin A
Calcium
Tissue need
Meat, fish, poultry
Cooking in cast iron pots

Decrease

Alkalinity (High pH)—Avoid any antacid preparation

Phosphates—Milk is unfavorable vehicle for iron administration

Phytates—Found in cereals

Oxalates—Found in many fruits and vegetables (plums, currants, green beans, spinach, sweet potatoes, tomatoes)

Tannins—Found in tea, coffee
Tissue saturation
Malabsorptive disorders
Disturbances that cause diarrhea or steatorrhea
Infection

---

*Macrominerals—required intake >100 mg/day.
†Microminerals or trace elements—required intake <100 mg/day.

TABLE 11-2. Minerals and their nutritional significance—cont'd

PHYSIOLOGIC FUNCTIONS/ SOURCES	RESULTS OF DEFICIENCY OR EXCESS	NURSING CONSIDERATIONS
Phosphorus*		
Functions	*Deficiency*	Dietary deficiency is uncommon, although prolonged use of antacids can produce deficiency, in which case supplementation is recommended
Bone and tooth development (in combination with calcium)	Weakness, anorexia, malaise, bone pain	
Involved in numerous chemical reactions, including protein, carbohydrate, and fat metabolism	*Excess*	To preserve calcium-to-phosphorus ratio in newborns, discourage use of whole cow's milk
Acid-base balance	Produces secondary calcium deficiency from disturbed calcium-to-phosphorus ratio	
Sources		
Dairy products, eggs, meat, poultry, legumes, carbonated beverages		
Potassium*		
Functions	*Deficiency*	Dietary deficiency and excess are unlikely, although disease states such as prolonged nausea and vomiting or the use of diuretics can result in hypokalemia; in such instances encourage replacement with supplements of rich food sources, such as bananas
Acid-base and fluid balance (major extracellular fluid areas)	Cardiac arrhythmias	
Nerve conduction	Muscular weakness	
Muscular contraction, especially the heart	Lethargy	
Release of energy	Kidney and respiratory failure	
	Heart failure	
Sources	*Excess*	
Bananas, citrus fruit, dried fruits, meat, fish, bran, legumes, peanut butter, potatoes, coffee, tea, cocoa	Cardiac arrhythmias	
	Respiratory failure	
	Mental confusion	
	Numbness of extremities	
Sodium*		
Functions	*Deficiency*	Deficiency intake is very rare, but losses secondary to nausea, vomiting, excessive sweating, and use of diuretics can occur and require replacement
Acid-base and fluid balance (major extracellular fluid cation)	Dehydration	
Cell permeability; absorption of glucose	Hypotension	
Muscle contraction	Convulsions	
	Muscle cramps	Encourage parents to limit excessive use of salt in preparing foods and to limit commercial foods with high sodium content, such as smoked meats
Sources	*Excess*	
Table salt, seafood, meat, poultry, numerous prepared foods	Edema	
	Hypertension	
	Intracranial hemorrhage	
Zinc†		
Functions	*Deficiency*	Encourage food sources rich in zinc, especially protein
Component of about 100 enzymes	Loss of appetite	
Synthesis of nucleic acids and protein in immune system and coagulation	Diminished taste sensation	Caution that fiber, phytates, oxalates, tannins (in tea or coffee), iron, and calcium adversely affect zinc absorption
Release of vitamin A from liver	Delayed healing	
Improved wound healing with vitamin C	*Skin lesions* —erythematous, crusted lesions around body orifices	
	Alopecia	Recognize groups at risk for zinc deficiency, such as vegetarians and Mexican-Americans, whose diets may have restricted or low meat content and high fiber, phytate content; and patients with malabsorption syndromes
Sources	Diarrhea	
Seafood (especially oysters), meat, poultry, eggs, wheat, legumes	Growth failure	
	Retarded sexual maturity	
	Excess	Emphasize correct use of zinc supplements and the possible interaction with other minerals
	Vomiting and diarrhea	
	Malaise, dizziness	
	Anemia, gastric bleeding	
	Impaired absorption of calcium and copper	

*Macrominerals—required intake >100 mg/day.
†Microminerals or trace elements—required intake <100 mg/day.

are common among members of Black Muslim or Seventh Day Adventist faiths.

Nursing Considerations

Identification of nutrient imbalance (or the potential for imbalance) is the initial nursing goal and requires assessment based on a dietary history and physical examination for signs of deficiency or excess (see Nutritional Assessment, Chapter 6). Once assessment data are collected, this information is evaluated against standard intakes to identify areas of concern. The most widely used standard is the *Recommended Dietary Allowances (RDAs),* developed by the **National Academy of Sciences, Food and Nutrition Board** (see Appendix F). The RDAs are not average requirements but recommendations intended to meet the physiologic needs of almost every healthy person. To meet the needs of those with the highest requirements, the RDAs will exceed most people's requirements. Therefore, children consuming less than the RDAs are not necessarily consuming an inadequate diet, but they are more likely at risk for deficiency than those who are consuming nutrients in amounts equal to the RDAs.

Several organizations have published dietary advice for the public. Most well-known are the Dietary Guidelines for Americans, which encourage eating a variety of foods, maintaining ideal body weight, consuming adequate starch and fiber, and limiting intake of fat, cholesterol, sugar, salt, and alcohol. Another source is the *Food Guide Pyramid* (Fig. 11-1), which replaces the basic four food groups that have traditionally been used to convey nutrition information to the public and applies to children as young as 2 years of age.

The number of servings and serving sizes are important components of the Food Guide Pyramid. Suggested serving sizes for the five food groups are listed in the box. Young children need the same variety of foods as older children but may need less than the 1600 calories provided by the suggested minimum number of servings in each food group. To meet their caloric needs, adjustments are made by using the minimum number of servings and smaller serving sizes. However, it is important that children have the equivalent of at least 2 cups of milk a day. Adolescents, who require increased calories for growth, should have 3 cups of milk a day and may require the maximum number of suggested servings. Current recommendations for fat intake for children over 2 years of age are that no more than 30% of calories should come from fat and the remainder of calories should come

---

FOOD GUIDE PYRAMID: SAMPLE SERVING SIZES

Bread, Cereal, Rice, and Pasta Group
1 slice of bread
1 ounce of ready-to-eat cereal
½ cup of cooked cereal, rice, or pasta

Vegetable Group
1 cup of raw leafy vegetable
½ cup of other vegetable, cooked or chopped raw
¾ cup of vegetable juice

Fruit Group
1 medium apple, banana, or orange
½ cup of chopped, cooked, or canned fruit
¾ cup of fruit juice

Milk, Yogurt, and Cheese Group
1 cup of milk or yogurt
1½ ounces of natural cheese
2 ounces of processed cheese

Meat, Poultry, Fish, Dry Beans, Eggs, and Nuts Group
2-3 ounces of cooked lean meat, poultry, or fish
½ cup of cooked dry beans, 1 egg, or 2 tablespoons of peanut butter count as 1 ounce of lean meat

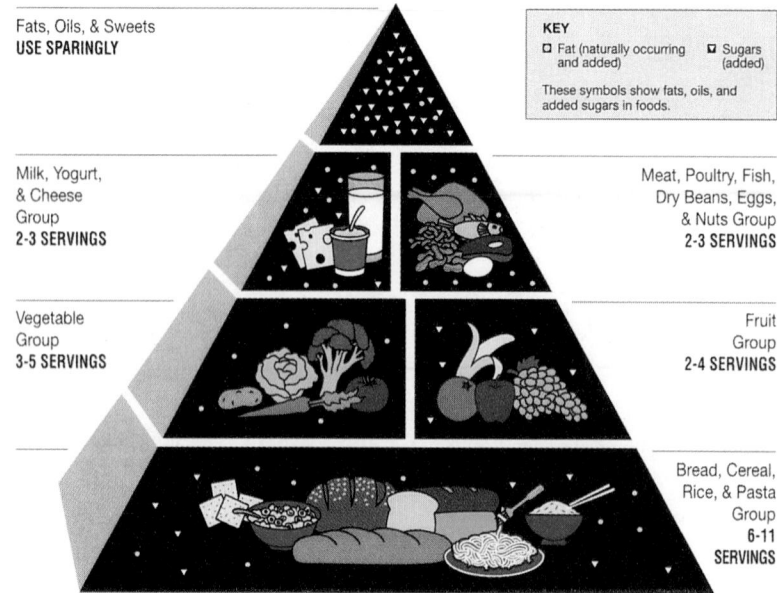

FIG. 11-1. Food Guide Pyramid: a guide to daily food choices. (Courtesy, U.S. Department of Agriculture, 1992).

from carbohydrates and protein (see also Hyperlipidemia [Hypercholesterolemia], Chapter 25).

Since one of the best assurances of nutritional adequacy is eating a variety of foods, families need guidelines for selecting foods that provide essential nutrients without exceeding energy requirements. With a varied and well-balanced diet most children do not need vitamin or mineral supplements. Unfortunately, there are no restrictions on the availability of toxic doses of vitamins or minerals. Nurses need to inform families of the potential dangers from excess vitamins or minerals. The idea that "more is better" is probably best dispelled by a simple explanation of the body's inability to use more than the needed requirement.

Achieving a nutritionally adequate vegetarian diet (with the exception of the strictest diets) is not difficult, but it requires careful planning and knowledge of nutrient sources. For children the lacto-ovovegetarian diet is nutritionally adequate; however, the vegan diet requires supplementation with vitamins D and B_{12} for children ages 2 to 12 years. Most authorities indicate that human breast milk or iron-fortified modified cow's milk (formula) is adequate for the first 6 months; breast-feeding may continue for up to 1 year of age. Although not required to meet nutritional requirements, iron-fortified rice cereal may be introduced after 4 months. The introduction of other solids is nutritionally unnecessary until 12 months and each should only be introduced one at a time. Iron-fortified cereal, in combination with breast milk or formula, is an adequate source of nutrition in the first year of life. The use of vitamin C juices with foods high in iron will further improve iron absorption. However, breast milk from vegetarian mothers can be deficient in vitamin B_{12}; supplementation of both mother and child is advisable. If cow's or human milk or commercial infant formula is not given, fortified soy milk is recommended. A variety of foods should be gradually introduced during the early years to ensure a more well-balanced intake.

Nursing ALERT When solid foods are introduced, the safety and digestibility of the selections must be considered. Raw fruits with seeds, vegetables, and nuts are hazardous for young children because of the danger of aspiration. Beans, grain cereals, and vegetables should be served well cooked and mashed during infancy.

To ensure sufficient protein in the diet, foods with *incomplete proteins* (those that do not have all the essential amino acids) must be eaten at the same meal with other foods that supply the missing amino acids. The three basic combinations of foods consumed by vegetarians that generally provide the appropriate amounts of essential amino acids are the following:

Grains (cereal, rice, pasta) and *legumes* (beans, peas, lentils, peanuts)
Grains and *milk products* (milk, cheese, yogurt)
Seeds (sesame, sunflower) and *legumes*

PROTEIN AND ENERGY MALNUTRITION (PEM)

Malnutrition continues to be a major health problem in the world today, particularly in children under 5 years of age. The lack of food, however, is not always the primary cause for malnutrition. In many developing and underdeveloped nations, *diarrhea* is a major factor in malnutrition. Additional factors are bottle-feeding (in poor sanitary conditions); inadequate knowledge of proper child care practices; parental illiteracy; economic and political factors; and simply the lack of food (David and Lobo, 1995a). The most extreme forms of malnutrition, or protein energy malnutrition, are kwashiorkor and marasmus.

Kwashiorkor

Kwashiorkor is a severe deficiency of energy with an adequate supply of calories. Taken from the Ghan language, the word means "the sickness the older child gets when displaced from the breast by another child" and aptly describes the syndrome that develops in the first child, usually between 1 and 4 years of age, when weaned from the breast once the second child is born. A diet consisting mainly of starch grains or tubers provides adequate calories in the form of carbohydrates but an inadequate amount of high-quality proteins.

The child with kwashiorkor has thin, wasted extremities and a prominent abdomen from edema (ascites). The edema often masks the severe muscular atrophy, making the child appear less debilitated than he or she actually is. The skin is scaly and dry and has areas of depigmentation. Several dermatoses may be evident, partly resulting from the vitamin deficiencies. Permanent blindness often results from the severe lack of vitamin A. Mineral deficiencies are common, especially iron, calcium, and zinc. The hair is thin, dry, coarse, and dull. Depigmentation is common, and patchy alopecia may occur.

Diarrhea frequently occurs from a lowered resistance to infection and subsequent gastroenteritis, anorexia, and malabsorption. Gastrointestinal disturbances include reversible fatty infiltration of the liver and atrophy of the acinar cells of the pancreas. Behavioral changes are evident as the child grows progressively irritable, lethargic, withdrawn, and apathetic. Fatal deterioration may be caused by recurrent diarrhea, infection, or circulatory failure.

Marasmus

Marasmus results from a low intake of both calories and protein. It is a common occurrence in developing countries during times of drought, especially in cultures where adults eat first; the remaining food is often insufficient in quality and quantity for the children.

Marasmus is usually a syndrome of physical and emotional deprivation and is not confined to geographic areas where food supplies are inadequate. It may be seen in children with failure to thrive, where the cause is not solely nutritional but primarily emotional.

Marasmus is characterized by gradual wasting and atrophy of body tissues, especially of subcutaneous fat. The child appears to be very old, with flabby and wrinkled skin, unlike the child with kwashiorkor, who appears more rounded from the edema. Fat metabolism is less impaired than in kwashiorkor, so that deficiency of fat-soluble vitamins is usually minimal or absent.

The child is fretful, apathetic, withdrawn, and so lethargic that prostration frequently occurs. Intercurrent infection with debilitating diseases, such as tuberculosis, parasitosis, and dysentery, is common.

Therapeutic Management

The treatment of PEM includes providing a diet with quality proteins, carbohydrates, vitamins, and minerals. When PEM occurs as a result of diarrhea, three management goals are identified: (1) rehydration with an oral rehydration solution (ORS) that also replaces electrolytes; (2) medications such as antibiotics and antidiarrheals; and (3) provision of adequate nutrition either by breast-feeding or a proper weaning diet. When the child is too ill to tolerate oral fluids, intravenous administration of fluids and electrolytes will be required to prevent death (David and Lobo, 1995b).

Nursing Considerations

Provision of essential physiologic needs, such as rest, individually tailored activity, and protection from infection, is paramount. Since children are usually weak and withdrawn, they depend on others for feeding. Hygiene may be distressing because of the poor integrity of the skin, and decubiti are a constant threat. Appropriate developmental stimulation should be provided also.

The larger problem is the prevention of these conditions through education concerning the importance of proper nutrition, whether breast-feeding or bottle-feeding when being weaned to semisolid foods. Since children with marasmus may suffer from emotional starvation as well, care should be consistent with care of the child with failure to thrive (p. 350).

FOOD SENSITIVITY

Food sensitivity is a general term that includes any type of adverse reaction to food or food additives. Food sensitivities can be divided into two broad categories:

> Food allergy or hypersensitivity—reactions involving immunologic mechanisms, usually immunoglobulin E (IgE); the reactions may be immediate or delayed and mild or severe, such as an anaphylactic reaction
>
> Food intolerance—reactions involving known or unknown nonimmunologic mechanisms; lactose intolerance is an example of a reaction that looks like allergy but is caused by deficiency of the enzyme lactase

Food allergy is caused by exposure to *allergens,* usually proteins (but not the smaller amino acids) that are capable of inducing IgE antibody formation ("sensitization") when ingested. *Sensitization* refers to the initial exposure of an individual to an allergen, resulting in an immune response; subsequent exposure induces a much stronger response that is clinically apparent. Consequently, food hypersensitivity typically occurs after the food has been ingested one or more times, but it can occur with the first ingestion because of transplacental sensitization in utero or because of sensitization to the substance passed through breast milk (Wilson, Self, and Hamburger, 1990). The most common food allergens are listed in the accompanying box.

Food allergies can develop at any time but are common during infancy, because the immature intestinal tract is more permeable to proteins than the mature intestinal tract, thus increasing the likelihood of an immune response. Allergies in general demonstrate a genetic component: children who have one parent with allergy have a 50% or greater risk of developing allergy; children who have both parents with allergy

---

HYPERALLERGENIC FOODS/SOURCES

Milk*: Ice cream, butter, margarine (if it contains dairy products), yogurt, cheese, pudding, baked goods, wieners, bologna, canned creamed soups, instant breakfast drinks, powdered milk drinks, milk chocolate

Eggs*: Mayonnaise, creamy salad dressing, baked goods, egg noodles, some cake icing, meringue, custard, pancakes, french toast, root beer

Wheat*: Almost all baked goods, wieners, bologna, pressed or chopped cold cuts, gravy, pasta, some canned soups

Legumes: Peanuts,* peanut butter or oil, beans, peas, lentils

Nuts*: Some chocolates, candy, baked goods, cherry soda (may be flavored with a nut extract), walnut oil

Fish or shellfish*: Cod liver oil, pizza with anchovies, Caesar salad dressing, any food fried in same oil as fish

Soy*: Soy sauce, teriyaki or worcestershire sauce, tofu, baked goods using soy flour or oil, soy nuts, soy infant formulas or milk, soybean paste, tuna packed in vegetable oil, many margarines

Chocolate: Cola beverages, cocoa, chocolate-flavored drinks

Buckwheat: Some cereals, pancakes

Pork, chicken: Bacon, wieners, sausage, pork fat, chicken broth

Strawberries, melon, pineapple: Gelatin, syrups

Corn: Popcorn, cereal, muffins, cornstarch, corn meal, corn bread, corn tortilla

Citrus fruits: Orange, lemon, lime, grapefruit; any of these in drinks, gelatin, juice, or medicines

Tomatoes: Juice, some vegetable soups, spaghetti, pizza sauce, and catsup

Spices: Chili, pepper, vinegar, cinnamon

*Most common allergens.

---

have up to a 100% risk of developing allergy. Allergy with a hereditary tendency is referred to as *atopy.*

Although the reason is unknown, many children "outgrow" their food allergies. Children with several food allergies may develop tolerance to each food at different times. The most common allergens, such as soy, are outgrown less readily than other food allergens. Because of the tendency to lose the hypersensitivity, allergic foods should be reintroduced into the diet after a period of abstinence (usually a year or more) to evaluate if the food can be safely added to the diet. Because of the incidence and severity of peanut allergy it is recommended that children under 3 years of age not ingest peanuts or peanut products.

There is evidence that food allergies can be prevented. The protective role of exclusive breast-feeding and avoidance of hyperallergenic foods is controversial, but most authorities often recommend such interventions with a family history of allergy.

Cow's Milk Allergy

Cow's milk allergy is a multifaceted disorder representing adverse systemic and local gastrointestinal reactions to cow's milk protein (see box). The diagnosis is initially made from the history, although the practitioner needs a high index of suspicion, since the timing and type of clinical manifestations vary greatly. Cow's milk allergy may be manifested as colic (see discussion on p. 348) or sleeplessness in an otherwise healthy infant.

COMMON CLINICAL MANIFESTATIONS OF COW'S MILK SENSITIVITY		
Gastrointestinal	**Respiratory**	**Other Signs and Symptoms**
Diarrhea	Rhinitis	Eczema
Vomiting	Bronchitis	Excessive crying
Colic	Asthma	Pallor (from anemia
Abdominal pain	Wheezing	secondary to
	Sneezing	chronic blood loss
	Coughing	in gastrointestinal
	Chronic nasal dis-	tract)
	charge	

FAMILY HOME CARE
Controlling Symptoms of Lactose Intolerance

In infants substitute soy-based formula for cow's milk formula or human milk.
Limit milk consumption to one glass at a time.
Drink milk with other foods rather than alone.
Eat hard cheese, cottage cheese, or yogurt instead of drinking milk.
Use enzyme tablets (Lactaid, Lactrase, Dairy Ease) to predigest the lactose in milk or supplement the body's own lactase (add tablets to milk or sprinkle on dairy products such as ice cream).
Eat small amounts of dairy foods daily to help colonic bacteria adapt to ingested lactose.

Diagnostic Evaluation. A number of diagnostic tests may be performed, including stool analysis for blood (both frank and occult bleeding can occur from the colitis), serum IgE levels, skin-prick testing, and radioallergosorbent test (RAST) (measures IgE antibodies to specific allergens in serum by radioimmunoassay). Both skin testing and RAST help identify the offending food, but the results are not always conclusive.

The most definitive diagnostic strategy is elimination of milk, followed by challenge testing after improvement of symptoms. Challenge testing involves reintroducing small quantities of milk in the diet to detect resurgence of symptoms; at times challenge testing involves the use of a placebo so that the parent is unaware of or "blind" to the timing of allergen ingestion.

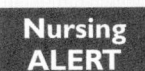

Careful observation of the child is required during a challenge test because of the possibility of anaphylactic reaction.

Therapeutic Management. Treatment of cow's milk allergy is elimination of all dairy products. For infants fed cow's milk formula, this primarily involves changing the formula to a casein or whey hydrolysate milk formula, in which the protein has been broken down (or "predigested") into its amino acids through enzymatic hydrolysis. Soy-based formula is not recommended, because as many as 20% of these infants are also allergic to soy. Goat's milk is not an acceptable substitute because it cross-reacts with cow's milk protein and is deficient in folic acid. Infants who are breast-fed but have symptoms of cow's milk hypersensitivity are treated by eliminating all dairy products from the lactating mother's diet. These women will require vitamin D and calcium supplementation to prevent deficiency. Infants are maintained on the dairy-free diet for 1 or 2 years, at which time very small quantities of milk are reintroduced.

Nursing Considerations. The principal nursing objectives are identification of potential milk allergy and appropriate counseling of parents regarding substitute formulas. The protein hydrolysate formulas are less palatable than milk-based formulas. Consequently, reluctance to accept the new formula may be a problem. This can be overcome by introducing the formula gradually over a few days using 1 ounce of new formula to 7 ounces of old formula, then 2 to 6 ounces, then 3 to 4, and as needed. Parents also need to be

reassured that the infant will receive complete nutrition from the new formula and will suffer no ill effects from the absence of cow's milk.

Once solid foods are started, parents need guidance in avoiding all associated milk products (see box on p. 346). Carefully reading all food labels helps avoid using prepared foods containing milk products.

Lactose Intolerance

Lactose intolerance refers to at least two different entities that involve a deficiency of the enzyme lactase, which is needed for the digestion of lactose. *Congenital lactose intolerance* appears soon after birth when the diet contains lactose from milk. Causes of lactose intolerance are attributed to disorders such as acquired immunodeficiency syndrome (AIDS) or gastrointestinal infections such as rotavirus and giardiasis. *Late-onset lactose intolerance* is similar to the congenital type but is manifested later in life. Ethnic groups with a high incidence of lactose intolerance include Orientals, southern Europeans, Arabs, Jews, and blacks. The principal manifestations include diarrhea, abdominal pain, distention, and flatus shortly after ingesting milk products.

In older children lactose intolerance may be diagnosed on the basis of the history and improvement following a lactose-free diet. In infants the hydrogen-breath test is frequently used. Undigested carbohydrate, such as lactose, in the colon causes gas production by bacteria. Breath samples are analyzed for the amount of hydrogen.

Treatment of lactose intolerance is elimination of offending dairy products or the use of enzyme replacement. In infants soy-based formula can be substituted for cow's milk formula or human milk. Some children are able to tolerate small amounts of lactose. Pretreated milk (with microbial-derived lactase) may improve lactose absorption. Since dairy products are a major source of calcium and vitamin D, supplementation of these nutrients is needed to prevent deficiency. Yogurt contains inactive lactase enzyme, which is activated by the temperature and pH of the duodenum; this lactase activity substitutes for the lack of endogenous lactase. Fresh yogurt may be tolerated better than frozen yogurt.

Nursing Considerations. Nursing care is similar to the interventions discussed for cow's milk allergy: explaining the dietary restrictions to the family; identifying alternate sources of calcium, such as yogurt, and ways of controlling the symptoms (see Family Home Care box on p. 347); stressing the importance of calcium and vitamin D supplementation; and discussing hidden sources of lactose, such as its use as a bulk agent in certain medications. Parents are advised to check with the pharmacist regarding this possibility when obtaining medication.

FEEDING DIFFICULTIES

REGURGITATION AND "SPITTING UP"

The return of small amounts of food after a feeding is a common occurrence during infancy. It should not be confused with actual vomiting, which can be associated with a number of disturbances, both insignificant and serious (see Chapter 24). For clarification the following terms are defined:

Spitting up—dribbling of unswallowed formula from the infant's mouth immediately after a feeding
Regurgitation—return of undigested food from the stomach, usually accompanied by burping

The insignificance of regurgitation or spitting up should be explained to parents, especially to those who are concerned. It can be reduced by some simple measures, such as frequent burping during and after feeding, minimal handling at feeding and after, and positioning of the child on the right side with the head slightly elevated after feeding. The inconvenience of spitting up is managed with the use of absorbent bibs on the infant and protective cloths on the parent.

Sometimes, frequent dribbling of formula causes excoriation of the corners of the mouth, chin, and neck. Keeping the area dry prevents skin breakdown but can be difficult to maintain. Helpful suggestions include applying a thin film of petrolatum or A and D ointment to the affected areas after cleansing and using absorbent nonplastic-lined terrycloth bibs that are changed frequently.

PAROXYSMAL ABDOMINAL PAIN (COLIC)

Colic is generally described as paroxysmal abdominal pain or cramping that is manifested by loud crying and drawing the legs up to the abdomen. Other definitions include variables such as duration of cry greater than 3 hours a day and parental dissatisfaction with the child's behavior. Colic is more common in young infants under the age of 3 months than in older infants, and infants with "difficult" temperaments are more likely to be colicky. Despite the obvious behavioral indications of pain, the child tolerates the formula well, gains weight, and thrives.

Among the theories that have been investigated as potential causes are too rapid feeding, overeating, swallowing excessive air, improper feeding technique (especially in positioning and burping), and emotional stress or tension between parent and child. Although all of these may occur, there is no evidence that one factor is consistently present. In some infants colic may be a sign of cow's milk allergy or intoler-

ance, and eliminating cow's milk products from the infant's diet and the diet of lactating mothers can reduce the symptoms. Parental smoking has also been associated with colic.

Therapeutic Management

Management of colic should begin with an investigation of diagnosable causes, such as cow's milk allergy. If a sensitivity to cow's milk is strongly suspected, a trial substitution of another formula, such as a casein hydrolysate (Nutramigen), is warranted. Soy formulas are avoided because of the possibility of sensitivity to soy protein as well. When no specific cause can be found, the supportive measures discussed under Nursing Considerations are employed.

The use of drugs, including sedatives, antispasmodics, antihistamines, and antiflatulents, such as simethicone, is sometimes recommended. The most commonly used sedatives are phenobarbitol and hydroxyzine hydrochloride (Atarax). The antispasmodic dicyclomine hydrochloride (Bentyl) is not recommended for infants under 6 months of age because of rare instances of death.

Nursing Considerations

The initial step in managing colic is to take a thorough, detailed history of the usual daily events. Areas that should be stressed include the following: (1) diet of the breast-feeding mother; (2) time of day when attacks occur; (3) relationship of the attacks to feeding time; (4) presence of specific family members during attacks, and habits, such as smoking by family members; (5) activity of the mother or usual caregiver before, during, and after the crying; (6) characteristics of the cry (duration, intensity); and (7) measures used to relieve the crying and their effectiveness. Of special emphasis is a careful assessment of the feeding process via *demonstration* by the parent.

If milk sensitivity is suspected, bottle-fed infants and breast-feeding mothers should follow a milk-free diet (see box on p. 346) for a minimum of 5 days in an attempt to reduce symptoms in the infant. Mothers should be cautioned that some nondairy creamers may contain calcium caseinate, a cow's milk protein. If this approach is helpful, lactating mothers may need calcium supplements to meet the body's requirement. Bottle-fed infants may improve with the same dietary modifications as for the child with cow's milk allergy (see p. 347).

More often than not, no change is required in feeding practices. When no cause can be identified, it is preferable to determine the time of the onset of crying and attempt to manipulate the circumstances associated with it. For example, some infants have episodes of colic around the family's dinner time, when all household members are home and the mother is preoccupied with cooking. The overstimulating, more tense atmosphere may upset the infant. Encouraging someone else to prepare dinner or the mother to prepare dinner earlier in the day and feed the infant in a more quiet area of the house may help reverse the environmental conditions that may have provoked the attack of colic. Other approaches for relieving colic are listed in the Family Home Care box. Parents are encouraged to try as many of these approaches as possible, because not all are effective for every infant (see also the Family Focus box and Critical Thinking Exercise).

FAMILY HOME CARE
Relieving Colic

Place infant prone over a covered hot-water bottle, heated towel, or covered heating pad.

Massage abdomen.

Change infant's position frequently; walk with child's face down and body across the parent's arm, with the hand under the abdomen applying gentle pressure (Fig. 11-2).

Use a front carrier for transporting infant.

Swaddle tightly with a soft, stretchy blanket.

Place in a wind-up swing.

Take for car rides or outside for a change in environment.

Use a commercial device* in the crib that simulates the vibration and sound of a car ride.

Provide smaller, frequent feedings; burp during and after feedings using the shoulder position, and place in an upright seat after feedings.

Introduce a pacifier for added sucking.

In breast-fed infants, mother should avoid all milk products for a trial period.

If household members smoke, avoid smoking near infant; preferably confine smoking activity to outside of home.

If nothing reduces the crying, place infant in crib and allow to cry; periodically hold and comfort child and put down again.

*Sweet Dreems, Inc., Sleep Tight Order Department, 4710 E. Walnut St., Westerville, Ohio 43081; (800) NO COLIC ([800] 662-6542).

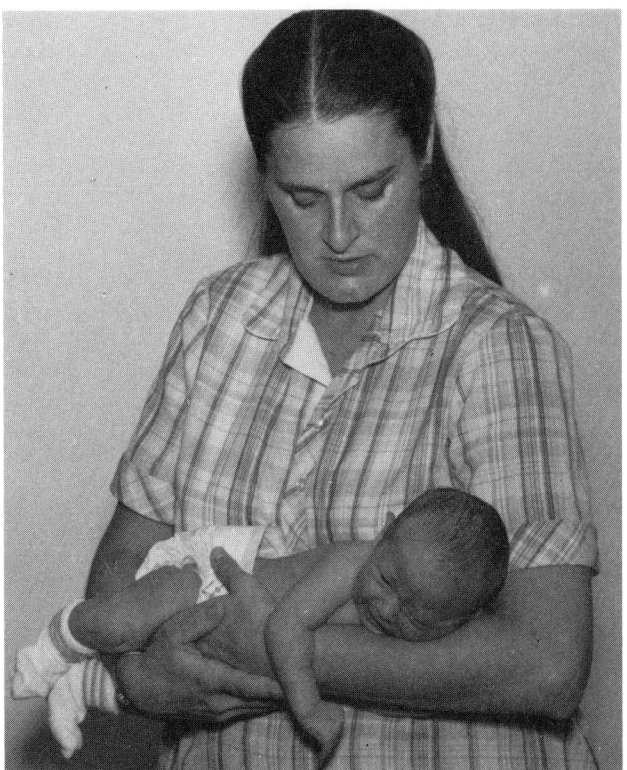

FIG. 11-2. The "colic carry" may be comforting to an infant with colic.

CRITICAL THINKING EXERCISE
Colic

During a routine clinic visit you notice that the mother of a 2-month-old infant appears very tired, gets easily confused answering simple questions, and casually mentions that the infant cries much more than her first child did and for no apparent reason. You direct the focus of the interview on the infant's behavior preceding the crying spells; feeding habits, including dietary history; and patterns of sleep. The mother suspects that the infant has colic. The best response to this mother is:

1. "Well, Dr. Smith will be in shortly, and you can discuss this with her."
2. "You must feel a little frustrated about this situation; can you tell me more about your concerns that maybe you have done something wrong with this child?"
3. "Colic is a complex problem for which there are few solutions other than giving the child medications and tolerating the crying the best way possible."
4. "We have some pamphlets on colic in the lobby; after you see the doctor, be sure to pick one up and read it at home."

The correct answer is two. This allows the mother time to express her feelings about the colicky infant, as well as her own fears about childrearing and possible inadequacies, and opens the door for a discussion of some solutions to the problem. The other options end the discussion and suggest that the mother or another health professional is responsible for a solution.

FAMILY FOCUS
Colic

Although colic is considered a minor ailment, the presence of a colicky, crying, irritable infant can have an intense emotional impact on parent-child attachment and family relationships. Parents, especially mothers, often relate histories of a daily routine that is laden with feelings of frustration, anger, despair, and helplessness. A vicious circle ensues in which the parent's own anxiety may be transferred to the infant, further increasing the tension, irritability, and crying.

One of the most important areas of nursing concern is the support of parents during the colic period. It should be stressed that despite the crying and obvious pain, the infant is doing well. Colic disappears spontaneously, usually by 3 months of age, although guarantees should never be given, because it may continue for much longer. The parent, especially the mother, should be encouraged to leave the house and arrange for some free time. Most important, it should be emphasized that colic does not indicate poor or inadequate parenting. Parents' negative feelings toward the infant and insecurities regarding their parenting abilities are normal. Parents are encouraged to talk about such feelings, since active listening may do more to relieve the colic syndrome than offering stereotyped advice, remedies, and glib statements such as, "Don't worry about it; your child will eventually outgrow the colicky spells."

FAILURE TO THRIVE (FTT)

FTT is a sign of inadequate growth resulting from inability to obtain and/or use calories required for growth. FTT has no universal definition, although one of the more common parameters is a weight (and sometimes height) that falls below the 5th percentile for the child's age. Some authorities prefer the 3rd percentile as a criterion, but the widely used National Center for Health Statistics growth charts include only the 5th, not the 3rd, percentile in their measurements. Growth measurements alone are not used to diagnose children with FTT. Rather, the finding of a persistent deviation from an established growth curve is cause for concern.

Three general categories of failure to thrive are the following:

Organic failure to thrive (OFTT)—result of a physical cause, such as congenital heart defects, neurologic lesions, microcephaly, chronic renal failure, gastroesophageal reflux, malabsorption syndrome, endocrine dysfunction, cystic fibrosis, or acquired immunodeficiency syndrome (AIDS).

Nonorganic failure to thrive (NFTT)—has a definable cause that is unrelated to disease. NFTT is most often the result of psychosocial factors, such as inadequate nutritional information by the parent; deficiency in maternal care or a disturbance in maternal-child attachment; or a disturbance in the child's ability to separate from the parent, leading to food refusal to maintain attention.

Idiopathic failure to thrive—unexplained by the usual organic and environmental etiologies but may also be classified as NFTT. Both categories of NFTT account for the majority of cases of FTT.

Traditionally the category of NFTT has implied a disturbance in the parent-child interaction. However, this is not always the case. Many other factors can lead to inadequate feeding of the infant, such as the following:

Poverty—lack of funds to buy sufficient food; may dilute formula to extend available supply

Health beliefs—use of fad diets; excessive concern with preventing conditions such as obesity, hypercholesterolemia, or nursing caries

Inadequate nutritional knowledge—cultural confusion of newly arrived immigrants who are unaware of appropriate food selections in American markets; parents with cognitive impairment

Family stress—overwhelming involvement with another chronically ill child; any number of other stresses (financial, marital, excessive parenting and employment responsibilities, depression, chemical abuse, acute grief)

Feeding resistance—result of nonoral nutritional therapy early in life

Insufficient breast milk—result of a number of different causes (fatigue, illness, poor release of milk, insufficient glandular tissue, lack of maternal confidence)

In these instances parent education and provision of necessary supports (financial or psychosocial) are successful in correcting the reason for the malnutrition. Dealing with families in which a child has NFTT because of a parent-child disturbance is much more difficult and is the focus of the nursing care discussion on p. 351.

Diagnostic Evaluation

Diagnosis is initially made from evidence of growth retardation. If FTT is recent, the weight, but not the height, is below accepted standards (usually the 5th percentile); if FTT is long-standing, both weight and height are depressed, indicating chronic malnutrition. Additional diagnostic procedures include a complete health and dietary history, physical examination for evidence of organic causes, developmental assessment, and a family assessment. Other tests are selected *only* as indicated to rule out organic problems. To prevent the overuse of diagnostic procedures, NFTT should be considered *early* in the differential diagnosis.

Therapeutic Management

Regardless of the cause of FTT, the treatment is directed at reversing the malnutrition. The goal is to provide sufficient calories to support "catch-up" growth—a rate of growth greater than the expected rate for age. Any coexisting medical problems are treated.

In most cases of NFTT a multidisciplinary team of physician, nurse, dietitian, child-life specialist, and social worker or mental health professional is needed to deal with the multiple psychologic problems. Efforts are made to relieve any additional stresses on the family, such as referrals to welfare agencies or supplemental food programs.

Prognosis

The prognosis for NFTT is related to the cause. If the parents have simply been ignorant of the infant's needs, teaching may remedy the child's limited caloric intake and permanently reverse the growth failure. Inadequate or decreased feeding periods by the infant's primary caretaker is often observed as the cause of NFTT in conjunction with family disorganization. When the family dysfunction is extensive, the prognosis is uncertain. Factors related to poor prognosis are severe feeding resistance, lack of awareness in and cooperation from the parent(s), low family income, low maternal educational level, and early age of onset of NFTT. Many of these children are below normal in intellectual development, have poorer language development and less well developed reading skills, attain lower social maturity, and have a higher incidence of behavioral disturbances. Such findings indicate that a long-term plan is needed for the optimum development of these children.

Nursing Considerations

❖ Assessment

Nurses play a critical role in the diagnosis of NFTT through their assessment of the child, parents, and family interaction. Knowledge of the characteristics of children with NFTT and their families is essential in helping identify these children and hastening the confirmation of a correct diagnosis (see box). Accurate assessment of initial weight and height and daily weight, as well as recording of all food intake, is vital. The feeding behavior of the child is documented, as well as the parent-child interaction during feeding, other caregiving activities, and play. (See also Nutritional Assessment, Chapter 6.) The approximate developmental age should be assessed on admission by administering an appropriate developmental test. Only after objective measurements are available is a plan of care for stimulation outlined.

The nursing admission history and ongoing assessment should also focus on the following characteristics that have been identified in many of these children and their parents.

The Child. Besides the obvious signs of malnutrition and delayed development, children with NFTT (see box) may interact differently from children with OFTT. They display

CLINICAL MANIFESTATIONS OF NONORGANIC FAILURE TO THRIVE

Growth failure—below 5th percentile in weight only or weight and height
Developmental retardation—social, motor, adaptive, language
Apathy
Poor hygiene
Withdrawn behavior
Feeding or eating disorders, such as vomiting, anorexia, pica, rumination
No fear of strangers (at age when stranger anxiety is normal)
Avoidance of eye contact
Wide-eyed gaze and continual scan of the environment ("radar gaze")
Stiff and unyielding or flaccid and unresponsive
Minimal smiling

intense interest in inanimate objects, such as a toy, but much less interest in social interactions. They are vigilant of people at a distance but become increasingly distressed as they come closer. They dislike being touched or held and avoid face-to-face contact. However, when held, they protest briefly on being put down and are apathetic when left alone.

Frequently there is a history of difficult feeding, vomiting, sleep disturbance, and excessive irritability. Habit patterns such as crying during feedings, vomiting, hoarding food in the mouth, ruminating after feeding, refusal to switch from liquids to solids, and aversion behavior, such as turning from food or spitting food, become attention-seeking mechanisms to prolong the attention received at mealtime. In addition, chronic reduction in calories can lead to appetite depression, which compounds the problem.

A feature of many children with NFTT is their irregularity (low rhythmicity) in activities of daily living. Some of these children typify the "difficult" temperament pattern. However, another type is the passive, sleepy, lethargic infant who does not wake up for feedings. Parents who have been advised of "demand feeding schedules" may be unsure of whether to wake the child or let the child sleep. Because of their inexperience and lack of guidance, parents may develop a pattern of infrequent feeding that is inadequate to meet the infant's nutritional needs. Such a pattern is particularly detrimental with the breast-feeding infant, in whom frequent nursing is essential to an adequate milk supply. Such characteristics in a child do not necessarily result in NFTT. Rather, a complex set of variables is significant, such as the degree of *fit* between the child's temperament and that of the parents. Since the personalities of infants can have definite effects on the parent-child attachment process, identifying such situations of disharmony may be one approach toward prevention and anticipatory guidance.

The Parents. Some parents are at increased risk for attachment problems because of (1) isolation and social crisis, (2) inadequate support systems, and (3) poor parenting as a child. Other factors that should be considered are lack of education; physical and mental health problems, such as retardation, depression, or drug dependence; immaturity, especially in adolescent parents; and lack of commitment to parenting, such as giving higher priority to career goals. Frequently these parents and their families are under stress and in multiple chronic emotional, social, and financial crises.

❖ Nursing Diagnoses

A number of nursing diagnoses are prominent in the nursing care of the child with NFTT. The most common nursing diagnoses are outlined in the Nursing Care Plan on NFTT. If an organic cause is found, additional nursing diagnoses may be related to care specific for that disorder, such as heart disease.

❖ Planning

Planning needs to begin as soon as possible on admission. The priority nursing goal is providing the infant with sufficient nutrients for growth. More specific nursing care depends on the identified cause of FTT. If an organic etiology is confirmed, care is related primarily to management of the disorder. If the problem is one of inadequate knowledge regarding child feeding, parental education is required. When serious psychosocial factors are involved, hospitalization is needed and additional interventions are required to meet the needs of both the child and the family. The following are goals for the hospitalized child with NFTT and family:

1. Child will experience weight gain.
2. Child will demonstrate positive response to developmental stimulation.
3. Family will demonstrate ability to provide appropriate care to child.
4. Family will receive adequate support and home services.

❖ Implementation

Because part of the difficulty between parent and child is dissatisfaction and frustration, the child should have a consistent primary nurse for all three shifts (Fig. 11-3). Only the same nurse caring for the child over a period of time can learn to perceive the child's cues and reverse the cycle of dissatisfaction, especially in the area of feeding. Because these children are not ill with any physical disorder but debilitated from general malnutrition, they should be placed in a room with noninfectious children of a similar age.

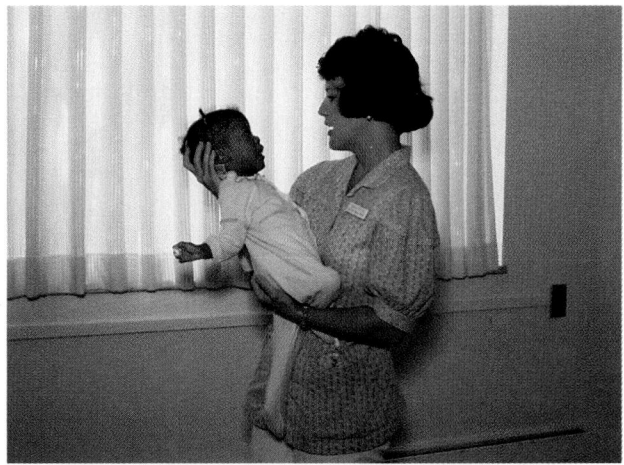

FIG. 11-3. A consistent nurse is important in developing trust in infants with nonorganic failure to thrive.

Because many of these children are responding to stimuli that have led to the negative feeding patterns, the first goal is to structure the feeding environment to encourage eating. Initially staff members may need to feed these children to assess thoroughly the difficulties encountered during the feeding process and to devise strategies that eliminate or minimize such problems. General guidelines for the feeding process are outlined in the Guidelines box.

Foods appropriate to the child's age are selected. To increase caloric intake, supplements, such as Polycose or powdered milk, can be added to foods, and powdered commercial formula can be prepared to yield 24 cal/oz rather than 20 cal/oz.

Besides attending to the physical needs of the child, the nurse must plan care for appropriate developmental stimulation. Once an approximate developmental age is established, a planned program of play is begun. Ideally a child-life specialist is involved to implement and supervise the stimulation program. Every effort is made to teach the parent how to play and interact with the child.

GUIDELINES
Feeding Children with Nonorganic Failure to Thrive

Provide a primary core of staff to feed the child. The same nurses are able to learn the child's cues and respond consistently.

Provide a quiet, unstimulating atmosphere. A number of these children are very distractible, and their attention is diverted with minimal stimuli. Older children do well at a feeding table; younger children should always be held.

Maintain a calm, even temperament throughout the meal. Negative outbursts may be commonplace in this child's habit formation. Limits on eating behavior definitely need to be provided, but they should be stated in a firm, calm tone. If the nurse is hurried or anxious, the feeding process will not be optimized.

Talk to the child by giving directions about eating. "Take a bite, Lisa" is appropriate and directive. The more distractible the child, the more directive the nurse should be to refocus attention on feeding. Positive comments about feeding are actively given.

Be persistent. This is perhaps one of the most important guidelines. Parents often give up when the child begins negative feeding behavior. Calm perseverance through 10 to 15 minutes of food refusal will eventually diminish negative behavior. Although forced feeding is avoided, "strictly encouraged" feeding is essential.

Maintain a face-to-face posture with the child when possible. Encourage eye contact and remain with the child throughout the meal.

Introduce new foods slowly. Often these children have been exclusively bottle-fed. If acceptance of solids is a problem, begin with pureed food and, once accepted, advance to junior and regular solid foods.

Follow the child's rhythm of feeding. The child will set a rhythm when the previous conditions are met.

Develop a structured routine. Disruption in their other activities of daily living has great impact on feeding responses, so bathing, sleeping, dressing, and playing, as well as feeding, are structured. The nurse should feed the child in the same way and place as often as possible. The length of the feeding should also be established (usually 30 minutes).

Nursing care of these children involves a "systems" approach. In other words, for the entire family to become healthy, each member must be helped to change. Care of the parents is aimed at helping them increase their feelings of self-esteem through positive, successful parenting skills. Initially this necessitates providing an environment in which they feel welcomed and accepted. Because these parents are often distrustful of authority figures, it may take some time before they develop any trust toward the nurse. One approach is to empathize with the parent about the difficulties of childrearing. For example, the nurse may state that many parents find adjusting to parenthood a trying time or that the demands of caring for an infant can become overwhelming.

Teaching infant care techniques to the parents is begun through *example* and *demonstration,* not by lecturing. As the nurse perceives the infant's cues, these are emphasized to the parents. For example, during a feeding the nurse might comment that the infant is still hungry because the child sucks vigorously and looks at the nurse. When the infant is satisfied, the nurse points out that the infant is signaling this by releasing the strong suck, closing the eyes, and breathing deeply and more slowly. By example, the child is gently placed in the crib for a nap.

At the same time, the parents are offered an opportunity to care for the infant without having demands made on them. For example, the nurse suggests that at the next feeding one of the parents offer the child the bottle. Whenever the parents participate, they are praised and encouraged to continue caring for the child.

Plans are made to continue these interventions at home. A public health or home health referral is made, and if a foster grandparent was included, this person should also visit the family. Social agencies that can provide financial or housing assistance to lessen the stress of everyday life are also contacted.

❖ Evaluation

The effectiveness of nursing interventions is determined by continual reassessment and evaluation of care based on the following observational guidelines and expected outcomes:

1. Record weight and caloric intake daily; document child's reaction to feeding environment; review notes to see if changes were made as necessary to improve eating and if consistent group of nurses fed child.
2. Perform developmental screening tests as needed.
3. Document parents' relationship with child, staff and other supportive individuals. Note length of time parents visit, appointments kept with referral services, and any requests for help.
4. Keep a record of all client teaching and note if outcome behaviors are met.

Expected outcomes:

1. Child gains weight (specify; usually a minimum of 1-2 oz/day).
2. Child displays a positive response to interventions (e.g., social smile).
3. Family demonstrates ability to provide appropriate care to child.
4. Family experiences reduction of anxiety and follows through on programs and activities.

See also Nursing Care Plan:
    The Child with Nonorganic Failure to Thrive.*

---

*In Wong DL: *Wong and Whaley's Clinical manual of pediatric nursing,* ed 4, St Louis, 1996, Mosby.

DISORDERS OF UNKNOWN ETIOLOGY

SUDDEN INFANT DEATH SYNDROME (SIDS)

SIDS is defined as the sudden death of an infant under 1 year of age that remains unexplained after a complete postmortem examination, including an investigation of the death scene and a review of the case history. It is the leading cause of death in children between the ages of 1 month and 1 year and claims the lives of 7000 infants annually. Table 11-3 summarizes the major epidemiologic characteristics of SIDS.

Etiology

Numerous theories have been proposed regarding the etiology of SIDS; however, the cause is unknown. The most compelling hypothesis is that SIDS is related to a brainstem abnormality in the neurologic regulation of cardiorespiratory control. Abnormalities include prolonged sleep apnea, increased frequency of brief inspiratory pauses, excessive periodic breathing, and impaired arousal responsiveness to increased carbon dioxide or decreased oxygen. However, sleep apnea is not the cause of SIDS. The vast majority of infants with apnea do not die, and only a minority of SIDS victims have documented apparent life-threatening events (ALTEs) (see Apnea of Infancy, p. 355). A theory that has been disproved associated SIDS with diphtheria, tetanus, and pertussis vaccines. The role of maternal smoking or exposure to second-hand smoke in the home has been postulated yet no conclusive evidence has pointed to these as the single cause of SIDS.

Studies from countries other than the United States link sleep habits with an increased risk of SIDS. Sleeping in the prone position may cause oropharyngeal obstruction or affect the thermal balance or arousal state. Whether sleeping in the prone position is in itself a risk factor or whether it depends on some other condition, such as sleeping on soft bedding, is unknown. Another theory is that SIDS may be caused by rebreathing of CO_2. Infants sleeping prone may be unable to move their heads to the side, thus increasing the risk of suffocation and lethal rebreathing (Kemp and others, 1993).

> **Nursing ALERT** Such findings have important implications for practices that may reduce the risk of SIDS, such as encouraging supine or side-lying sleeping positions, avoiding soft, moldable mattresses and pillows, and avoiding overheating during sleep. The American Academy of Pediatrics recommends the supine or side-lying sleep position for healthy infants (Infant sleep position, 1994). Infants with breathing problems or excessive vomiting should continue to sleep prone on a firm surface, mattress, or bedding.

Although the etiology is unknown, autopsies reveal consistent pathologic findings, such as pulmonary edema and intrathoracic hemorrhages, that confirm the diagnosis of SIDS. Consequently, all infants suspected of dying of SIDS should be autopsied, and these findings shared with the parents as soon as possible after the death.

> Postmortem findings in SIDS and accidental suffocation are practically the same. Also, not all communities have medical examiners to perform autopsies. Consequently, some deaths may or may not be correctly identified as SIDS. Therefore mortality can vary in different regions.

Children at Risk for SIDS

Certain groups of children are at increased risk for SIDS. These groups include the following:

1. Infants with one or more severe ALTEs requiring cardiopulmonary resuscitation (CPR) or vigorous stimulation
2. Preterm infants who continue to have pathologic apnea at the time of hospital discharge
3. Siblings of two or more SIDS victims
4. Infants with certain types of diseases or conditions, such as central hypoventilation

FACTORS	OCCURRENCE
Incidence	1.4:1000 live births
Peak age	2 to 4 months; 95% occur by 6 months
Sex	Higher percentage of males affected
Time of death	During sleep
Time of year	Increased incidence in winter; peak in January
Racial	Greater incidence in Native Americans and blacks, followed by whites, Asians, and Hispanics
Socioeconomic	Increased occurrence in lower socioeconomic class
Birth	Higher incidence in: Premature infants, especially infants of low birth weight Multiple births* Neonates with low Apgar scores Infants with central nervous system disturbances and respiratory disorders such as bronchopulmonary dysplasia Increasing birth order (subsequent siblings as opposed to firstborn child) Infants with a recent history of illness
Sleep habits	Prone position; use of soft bedding; overheating (thermal stress)
Feeding habits	Lower incidence in breast-fed infants
Siblings	May have greater incidence
Maternal	Young age; cigarette smoking, especially during pregnancy; substance abuse (heroin, methadone, cocaine)

TABLE 11-3. Epidemiology of SIDS

*Although a rare event, simultaneous death of twins from SIDS can occur.

Home monitoring and/or the use of respiratory stimulant drugs is recommended for these groups of children. No diagnostic tests exist to predict which infants, including those in the above groups, will survive or die, and home monitoring is no guarantee of survival. At the present time strategies to prevent SIDS are best directed at decreasing known or suspected risk factors, such as mothers seeking adequate prenatal care and avoiding cigarette smoking and drug abuse both before and after the child's birth (see also Nursing Alert). In addition, adherence to the guidelines for nonprone sleeping in healthy term infants is a positive step for the prevention of SIDS.

Whether subsequent siblings of the SIDS infant are at increased risk for SIDS is unclear. Even if the increased risk is correct, families have a 99% chance that their subsequent child will *not* die of SIDS. Home monitoring is not recommended for this group of children, but is often used by practitioners.

Nursing Considerations

Loss of a child from SIDS presents several crises with which the parents must cope. In addition to grief and mourning for the death of their child, the parents must face a tragedy that was extremely sudden, unexpected, and unexplained. The psychologic intervention for the family must deal with these additional variables. This discussion focuses primarily on the objectives of care for families experiencing SIDS, rather than on the process of grief and mourning, which is explored in Chapter 18.

One approach toward delineating the nursing care plan for these families is to base it on the usual sequence of events that occurs after the infant is found. This approach encompasses the different areas in which nurses may be involved with the family.

Finding the Infant. Usually it is the mother who finds the child dead in the crib. Typically the child is in a disheveled bed, with blankets over the head, and huddled into a corner. Frothy, blood-tinged fluid fills the mouth and nostrils, and the infant may be lying face down in the secretions, suggesting that he or she bled to death. The diaper is wet and full of stool, which is consistent with a cataclysmic type of death. The hands may be clutching the sheets, as if the child were in distress before death. The initial appearance of the child combined with the shock of such an unexpected event adds to the horror that the parents must face.

Frequently the mother is alone and must deal with her initial shock, panic, grief, questions of the other siblings, and the decision of where to find help. The first persons to arrive may be the police and ambulance attendants. Hopefully they will handle the situation by asking few questions; giving *no* indication of wrongdoing, abuse, or neglect; making sensitive judgments concerning the resuscitation efforts for the child; and comforting the members of the family as much as possible. These individuals should be properly informed about SIDS in order to recognize its characteristic signs and tell parents that their child probably died of a disease called sudden infant death syndrome, which cannot be predicted or prevented. A compassionate, sensitive approach to the family during the very first few minutes can help spare them some of the overwhelming guilt and anguish that frequently follow this type of death.

Arriving at the Emergency Room. The first contact that nurses typically have with these families is in the emergency room, when the infant is seen by a physician in order to be pronounced dead. Usually there is no attempt at resuscitation. During the time in the emergency room several aspects warrant special consideration. Parents are asked only factual questions, such as when they found the infant, how he or she looked, and who they called for help. Any remarks that may suggest responsibility, such as why didn't they go in earlier, didn't they hear the infant cry out, was the head buried in a blanket, or were the other siblings jealous of this child, are avoided.

The events that took place when help arrived are discussed. If resuscitation was attempted, the infant may have fractured ribs, internal bleeding, and traumatic bruising, which can simulate physical abuse. Also, if statements were made that were misguided, such as "This looks like suffocation," they can be corrected before parents harbor them in their minds as indications of their guilt. The discussion of an autopsy should be presented at this time, emphasizing that a diagnosis cannot be confirmed until the postmortem examination is completed. Instructions about the autopsy and funeral arrangements may need to be repeated or put in writing. If the mother was breast-feeding, she needs information about abrupt discontinuation of lactation.

Another important aspect of compassionate care for these parents is allowing them to say good-bye to their child. Before they go into the examining room, any blood or emesis is removed from the child, the body is covered partially with a sheet or blanket, and the room is put in order, especially if instruments and equipment were used. These are the parents' last moments with their child, and they should be as quiet, meaningful, peaceful, and undisturbed as possible. The child's belongings are packaged for the parents to take home if they wish. Because the parents leave the hospital without their infant, it is helpful to accompany them to the car or arrange for someone else to take them home.

Returning Home. When the parents return home, they should be visited by a competent, qualified professional as soon after the death as possible. Printed material that contains excellent information about SIDS (available from the national organizations*) should be provided.

During the initial visit the parents are helped to gain an intellectual understanding of the disease. The nursing objectives are to assess what the parents have been told, what they think happened, and how they have explained this to the other siblings, other family members, and friends.

Some parents are able to discuss their feelings openly, and the nurse supports this coping skill. However, others may be reluctant to express their grief, and the nurse may help these parents bring their feelings out into the open.

---

*Sudden Infant Death Syndrome Clearinghouse, 8201 Greensboro Dr., Suite 600, McLean, VA 22102, (703) 821-8955; **American Sudden Infant Death Syndrome (SIDS) Institute**, 275 Carpenter Dr., Suite 100, Atlanta, GA 30328, (800) 232-SIDS (in Georgia, [800] 847-SIDS); **The Sudden Infant Death Syndrome Alliance**, 10500 Little Patuxent Parkway, Suite 420, Columbia, MD 21044, (800) 221-SIDS.

The nurse can encourage the expression of emotions by asking about crying and feeling sad, angry, or guilty. It is an attempt to provoke a display of emotion, not just an admission of a feeling. During this session the parents should be helped to explore their usual coping mechanisms and, if these are ineffectual, to investigate new approaches. For example, one parent may refrain from discussing the death for fear of upsetting the other parent, but each may need to hear how the other feels.

The number of visits and plans for subsequent intervention need to be flexible. For example, the siblings may initially appear accepting of the explanation and well adjusted but may later refuse to go to sleep or ask questions about graves or funerals, indicating their need for further help in dealing with the death. Parents facing the question of a subsequent child will need support. Both the birth of a subsequent child and the survival of that child, especially past the age of death of the previous child, are important transitional stages for parents.

Because the mourning process may take *at least* a year for completion of acceptance and social reorganization, nurses should call on the family periodically to evaluate their progress. Many families receive much solace and support from talking to other parents who have lost a child to SIDS.

APNEA OF INFANCY (AOI)

AOI generally refers to pathologic apnea in infants of more than 37 weeks' gestation. The clinical presentation of AOI is an *apparent life-threatening event (ALTE)* (previously referred to by the inaccurate and misleading expression, "near-miss SIDS") that is described as:

- Frightening to the observer, who fears the child died or would have died without vigorous intervention
- Some combination of:
    Apnea—cessation of breathing for 20 seconds or more
    Color change—cyanosis or pallor, but sometimes plethora
    Marked change in muscle tone—usually extreme limpness
    Choking or gagging

AOI can be a symptom of many disorders, including sepsis, seizures, upper airway abnormalities, gastroesophageal reflux, hypoglycemia or other metabolic problems, impaired regulation of breathing during sleep or feeding, or a result of intentional poisoning by a caregiver. However, in about half the cases no cause is identified. Infants with a history of ALTEs are at increased risk for SIDS, but these children constitute less than 7% of all SIDS victims. A diagnosis of AOI is made when no identifiable cause for the ALTE is found (Keens and Ward, 1993).

Diagnostic Evaluation

The most widely used test is continuous recording of cardiorespiratory patterns (cardiopneumogram or pneumocardiogram). Four-channel (or multi-channel pneumogram) pneumocardiograms monitor heart rate, respirations (chest impedance), nasal airflow, and oxygen saturation. A more sophisticated test, polysomnography ("sleep test"), also records brain waves, eye and body movements, esophageal manometry, and end-tidal carbon dioxide measurements. However, none of these tests can predict risk. Some children with normal results may still have subsequent apneic episodes.

Therapeutic Management

Treatment usually involves continuous home monitoring of cardiorespiratory rhythms and/or the use of methylxanthines (respiratory stimulant drugs, such as theophylline or caffeine). Therapeutic levels are typically 6 to 10 or 13 μg/ml of theophylline and 10 to 20 μg/ml of caffeine. The criteria for discontinuing the monitoring is based on the infant's clinical condition. A general guideline for discontinuation is when infants with ALTEs have gone 2 or 3 months without significant numbers of episodes requiring intervention.

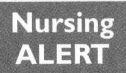

Nursing ALERT The concentration of theophylline required for apnea is less than that required for bronchodilation.

Nursing Considerations

The diagnosis of AOI engenders great anxiety and concern in parents, and the institution of home monitoring presents additional physical and emotional burdens. If monitoring is required, the nurse can be a major source of support to the family in terms of education about the equipment, observation of the infant's status, and immediate intervention during apneic episodes, including cardiorespiratory resuscitation (CPR) (see Critical Thinking Exercise). To help the family cope with the numerous procedures they must learn, ad-

---

CRITICAL THINKING EXERCISE
Home Apnea Monitoring

A family has just brought their newborn home on an apnea monitor. The diagnosis is apnea of prematurity. You are the nurse making the first home visit. You should expect to find all of the following except:

1. The parent appears knowledgeable about monitor use, responses to alarms, and CPR
2. The infant's respiratory status is stable and color is good
3. The monitor is plugged into an extension cord
4. The family appears anxious

The correct answer is three. No medical equipment should be plugged into extension cords. If necessary, furniture and equipment should be rearranged so that an appropriate outlet can be used. Regarding the other answers, parents should be well trained in caring for the child on an apnea monitor before being sent home. The nurse should usually only need to review procedures. However, if parents do not have the necessary information and skills, training should be a priority on the first home visit. Anxiety is common for the first 4 to 8 weeks of home apnea monitoring. An infant with a diagnosis of apnea of prematurity should appear healthy and should not evidence respiratory distress. Signs to the contrary necessitate immediate contact with the family's practitioner.

equate preparation before discharge and written instructions are essential.*

Several types of home monitors are available, and most hospitals select the model that the infant will use at home. Nurses, especially those involved in the care at home, must become familiar with the equipment, including its advantages and disadvantages. Safety is a major concern, since monitors can cause electrical burns and electrocution. The following precautions are recommended:

1. Remove leads from infant when not attached to monitor.
2. Unplug power cord from electrical outlet when cord is not plugged into monitor.
3. Use safety covers on electrical outlets to discourage children from inserting objects into a socket.

Siblings should also be supervised when near the infant and taught that the monitor is not a toy. Other safety practices include informing local utility and rescue squads of the home monitoring in case of an emergency. Telephone numbers for these services should be posted near all telephones in the home.

Caregivers need detailed information regarding proper attachment of the electrodes to the infant's chest with impedance monitors that detect chest movement. The electrodes are placed in the midaxillary line, at a space one or two fingerbreadths below the nipple (Fig. 11-4). Adhesive electrodes

---

*Home care instructions for apnea monitoring and CPR are available in Wong DL: *Wong and Whaley's Clinical manual of pediatric nursing*, ed 4, St Louis, 1996, Mosby. Educational materials may also be obtained from the American SIDS Institute.

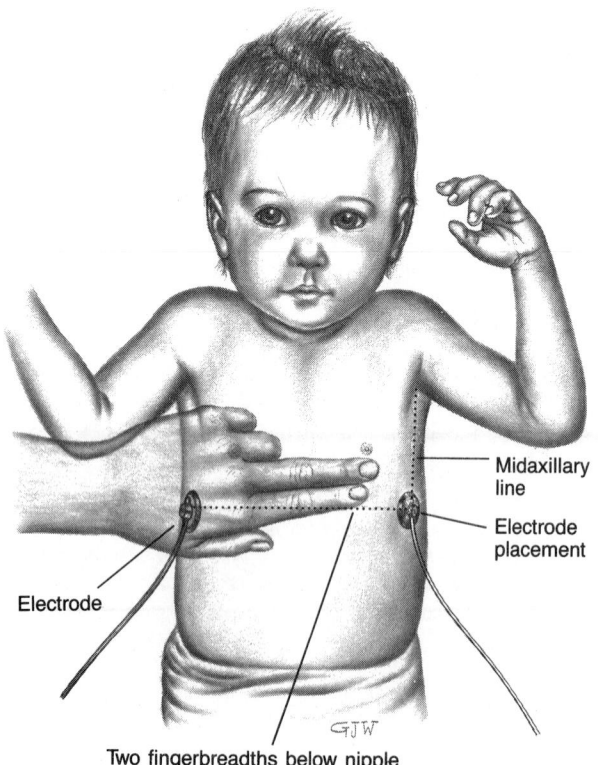

FIG. 11-4. Electrode placement for apnea monitoring. In small infants one fingerbreadth may be used.

are attached directly to the skin. For home use, electrodes attached to a belt that is placed around the child's trunk are preferred. The belt is positioned so that the electrodes contact the skin in the same area as shown in Fig. 11-4. Newer-technology monitors have memory chips that allow for event recording; this may prove to be an effective tool in evaluating the use of the monitor and reported frequency of alarms (Ahmann, Meny, and Fink, 1992).

Monitors are effective only if they are used. They do not prevent death but alert the caregiver to the ALTE in time to intervene. The need to use the monitor and to respond appropriately to alarms must be stressed. Noncompliance can result in the infant's death.

> **Nursing ALERT** If the infant is apneic, gently stimulate the trunk by patting or rubbing it. If the infant is prone, turn to the back and flick the feet. If there is still no response, begin CPR. Never vigorously shake the child. No more than 15 to 30 seconds are spent on stimulation before implementing CPR.

Family Support. Although AOI is not a chronic illness, many of the stresses observed during the monitoring period are characteristic of those of families with chronically ill children. Parents report increased stress, including concern for the child's survival, fear of incompetency in assuming home responsibility, inadequate respite care, social isolation, constant work, and fatigue. Siblings are affected, as well as the affected child, who may be characterized as "spoiled" and have developmental delays. To deal with these potential effects, nurses need to employ the same interventions as those discussed for children with chronic illness (see Chapter 19 and be aware of the need for referral when difficulties are suspected.

To lessen the continuous responsibility of monitoring, other family members, such as grandparents, should be taught how to manipulate the equipment, read and interpret the signals, and administer CPR. They are encouraged to stay with the infant for regular periods to allow parents respite. Support groups of other families who have successfully completed monitoring can also be of benefit. Since baby-sitters are difficult to locate, support group members or nursing students may be potential sources of qualified caregivers.

AUTISM

Autism, a complex developmental disorder accompanied by severe and usually permanent intellectual and behavioral deficits, is manifested during infancy and early childhood. It occurs in 1:2500 children, is about four times more common in males than in females (although females are more severely affected), and is not related to socioeconomic level, race, or religion.

Etiology

The etiology of autism is an unsolved and controversial question. However, considerable evidence supports a biologic cause. Individuals with autism may have abnormal electroencephalograms, seizures, delayed development of hand dominance, persistence of primitive reflexes, metabolic abnormalities (elevated blood serotonin), and cerebellar vermal hypoplasia (part of the brain involved in regulating motion and some aspects of memory).

There is also strong evidence for a genetic basis that in twins is consistent with an autosomal recessive pattern of inheritance. Twin studies demonstrate a very high concordance (96%) for monozygotic (identical) twins and a 24% concordance for dizygotic (nonidentical) twins. In addition, between 5% and 16% of males with autism are positive for the fragile X chromosome (see Fragile X Syndrome, Chapter 19).

Clinical Manifestations/Diagnostic Evaluation

Children with autism demonstrate several peculiar and bizarre characteristics, primarily in social interactions, communication, and behavior. The clinical manifestations typically seen in children with autism are described in the accompanying box. The majority of children with autism are mentally retarded, with scores typically in the moderate to severe range. More females than males tend to have very low intelligence scores. Despite relatively severe mental retardation, some children with autism (known as *savants*) excel in particular areas, such as art, music, memory, mathematic calculation, or perceptual skills, such as puzzle building.

Prognosis

Autism is a severely disabling condition. Only about 1% to 2% of the autistic population ultimately achieve independence, with the majority requiring lifelong supervision. Aggravation of psychiatric symptoms occurs in about half the children during adolescence, with girls having a tendency for

CLINICAL MANIFESTATIONS OF AUTISM

Social Relations and Behavior
Extreme interpersonal isolation
Intense, abnormal concern for preservation of sameness
Unyielding to cuddling and holding
Do not respond to verbal stimulation
Bizarre attachment to mechanical objects
Odd repetitive behaviors, such as flicking a light switch on and off
Difficult to manage; passive or irritable
Frequent temper tantrums and/or self-destructive behavior

Development
Mental retardation, usually severe
May have advanced gross motor skills
Normal to hyperactive
May have exceptional ability (e.g., memory)
Poor suck and feeding responses

Language
Echolalia or parrot speech (automatic repetition of words spoken to them)
Pronominal reversal (tendency to use "you" for "I")
Literal, concrete use of words (e.g., "in" to mean "door")

Sensory/Perceptual Processes
Sensory deficits even though vision and hearing intact
Act as if deaf, yet may be overly sensitive to sound
Hyposensitive or hypersensitive to pain
Have aversion to touch

continued deterioration. The prognosis is most favorable for children with communicative speech development by age 6 years and an intelligence quotient above 50 at the time of diagnosis. Early recognition of behaviors associated with autism is critical in order to implement appropriate interventions and family involvement.

Nursing Considerations

Therapeutic intervention for the child with autism is a specialized area involving professionals with advanced training. While numerous therapies have been employed, the most promising results have been through highly structured and intensive behavioral modification programs. In general, the objective is to increase social awareness of others, teach verbal communication, and decrease unacceptable behavior. However, the vast majority of these children need assistance and supervision throughout adulthood, although early diagnosis and early educational treatment positively influence the child's future development.

When these children are hospitalized, the parents are essential to planning care and ideally should stay with the child as much as possible. Decreasing stimulation by using a private or semiprivate room, avoiding extraneous auditory and visual distraction, and encouraging the parents to bring in possessions the child is attached to may lessen the disruptiveness of hospitalization. Since physical contact often upsets these children, minimum holding may be necessary to avoid behavioral outbursts.

Care must be taken when performing procedures on, administering medicine to, or feeding these children, since they are either fussy eaters who may willfully starve themselves or gag to prevent eating, or they are indiscriminate hoarders, swallowing any available edible or inedible items, such as a thermometer. Their disturbing sleep patterns may also pose problems in a hospital setting. A thorough assessment of the child's usual routine and activities can help maintain an environment that is more manageable and conducive to physical recovery.

A key principle in working with these children is establishing trust. They need to be introduced slowly to new situations, with visits with staff caregivers kept short whenever possible. Because these children have difficulty organizing their behavior and redirecting their energy, they need to be told directly what to do. Communication should be at the child's developmental level, brief, and concrete. Only one request is given at a time, such as "sit on bed."

Family Support. Autism, like so many other chronic conditions, involves the entire family and often becomes "a family disease." Unfortunately, the psychogenetic theory, popular in the 1960s especially among psychoanalysts, had portrayed the parents as detached, refrigerator-type individuals. Although the psychogenetic theory is unsupported by current findings, the theory has caused many public misconceptions about these families and greatly intensified many parents' guilt. Nurses can help alleviate the guilt and shame often associated with this disorder by stressing what is known from a biologic standpoint, as well as how little is known about the cause of autism.

Parents need expert counseling early in the course of the disorder and should be referred to the **Autism Society of**

America (ASA).* ASA is the most efficient clearinghouse for information about education, treatment programs and techniques, and facilities such as camps and group homes. There is also a siblings group called **SHARE (Siblings Helping Persons with Autism Through Resources and Energy).**

*7910 Woodmont Ave, Suite 650, Bethesda, MD 20814

As much as possible, the family is encouraged to care for the child in the home. With the help of family support programs in many states, families are often able to provide home care and assist with the educational services the child needs. As the young person approaches adulthood, the family may require assistance in locating a long-term care facility for the affected adult (see also Chapter 19).

KEY POINTS

- Common nutritional disturbances of infancy may result from vitamin and mineral deficiency or excess, some types of vegetarian diets, protein and calorie malnutrition, and food intolerance.
- Malnutrition refers to poor or inadequate nutrition and may result from undernutrition or overnutrition. Common manifestations of undernutrition in the infant include iron deficiency anemia, vitamin deficiencies, and failure to thrive. Manifestations of overnutrition are hypervitaminosis and obesity.
- Mineral disturbances may be caused by mineral-mineral interactions and mineral-diet interactions.
- Vegetarians may be classified into four groups: lactoovovegetarians, lactovegetarians, pure vegetarians, and zen macrobiotics.
- Protein-energy malnutrition may occur as a complication of underlying disease, lack of parental education about infant nutrition, inappropriate management of food allergy, or incorrect preparation of formula.
- Food intolerance encompasses food allergies and food sensitivities, the most serious of which are cow's milk allergy and lactose intolerance.

- Treatment of colic may involve change in feeding practices, correction of a stressful environment, and support of the parent.
- Failure to thrive may be classified as organic, resulting from some physical cause, or nonorganic, resulting from psychosocial factors involving the child and caregiver (e.g., maternal deprivation), environmental causes (e.g., inadequate parental knowledge of child feeding), or unexplained causes.
- Sudden infant death syndrome is the leading cause of death in children between the ages of 1 month and 1 year.
- The primary nursing responsibility in care associated with sudden infant death and other conditions of unknown etiology is emotional support of the family.
- Children with apnea of infancy receive home monitoring to alert the family to an apparent life-threatening event.
- Autism is a lifelong developmental disorder that is characterized by severe cognitive and social retardation, bizarre behavior, and gross language deficits.

REFERENCES

Ahmann E, Meny RG, Fink RJ: Use of home apnea monitors, *JOGNN* 21(5):394-399, 1992.

David S, Lobo ML: Childhood diarrhea and malnutrition in Pakistan, Part I: Incidence and prevalence, *J Pediatr Nurs* 10(2):131-137, 1995a.

David S, Lobo ML: Childhood diarrhea and malnutrition in Pakistan, Part II: Treatment and management, *J Pediatr Nurs* 10(3):204-209, 1995b.

Fawzi WW and others: Vitamin A supplementation and child mortality: a meta-analysis, *JAMA* 269(7):898-903, 1993.

Infant sleep position and sudden infant death syndrome (SIDS) in the United States: joint commentary from the American Academy of Pediatrics and selected agencies of the federal government, *Pediatrics* 93(5):820, 1994.

Keens TG, Ward SLD: Apnea spells, sudden death, and the role of the apnea monitor, *Pediatr Clin North Am* 40(5):897-911, 1993.

Kemp JS and others: Unintentional suffocation by rebreathing: a death scene and physiologic investigation of a possible cause of sudden infant death, *J Pediatr* 122(6):874-880, 1993.

Knowledge and use of folic acid by women of childbearing age—United States, 1995, *MMWR* 44(38):716-718, 1995.

Wilson N, Self T, Hamburger R: Severe cow's milk–induced colitis in an exclusively breast-fed neonate, *Clin Pediatr* 29(2):77-80, 1990.

BIBLIOGRAPHY

Vitamin and Mineral Disturbances/Protein Energy Malnutrition

Graham SM, Arvela OM, Wise GA: Long-term neurologic consequences of nutritional vitamin B_{12} deficiency in infants, *J Pediatr* 121(5):710-714, 1992.

Hendrickse RG: Kwashiorkor: the hypothesis that incriminates aflatoxins, *Pediatrics* 88(2):376-379, 1991.

Herrera MG and others: Vitamin A supplementation and child survival, *Lancet* 340:267-271, 1992.

Jelliffe DB, Jelliffe EFP: Causation of kwashiorkor: toward a multifactorial consensus, *Pediatrics* 90(1):110-113, 1992.

NIH Consensus Development Panel on Optimal Calcium Intake, *JAMA* 272(24):1942-1948, 1994.

Raiha NCR, Axelsson IE: Protein nutrition during infancy: an update, *Pediatr Clin North Am* 42(4):745-761, 1995.

Sills IN and others: Vitamin D deficiency rickets: reports of its demise are exaggerated, *Clin Pediatr* 33:491-493, 1994.

Udall JN Jr, Greene HL: Vitamin update, *Pediatr Rev* 13(5):185-194, 1992.

Vegetarian Diets

Dagnelie P and others: High prevalence of rickets in infants on macrobiotic diets, *Am J Clin Nutr* 51:202-208, 1990.

O'Connell J and others: Growth of vegetarian children: the farm study, *Pediatrics* 84(3):475-481, 1989.

Sanders TAB, Reddy S: Vegetarian diets and children, *Am J Clin Nutr* 59(suppl):1176s-1181s, 1994.

Trahms CM: Vegetarian diets for children. In Pipes PL, Trahms CM: *Nutrition in infancy and childhood,* ed 5, St Louis, 1993, Mosby.

Food Sensitivity

Bock SA, Sampson HA: Food allergy in infancy, *Pediatr Clin North Am* 41(5):1047-67, 1994.

Castiglia PT: Lactose intolerance, *J Pediatr Health Care* 8(1):36-38, 1994.

Mudd KE, Noone SA: Management of severe food allergy in the school setting, *J School Nurs* 11(3):30-33, 1995.

Preventing food allergy fatalities, *Emerg Med* 25(7):119-123, 1993.

Sampson HA and others: Anaphylactic reactions to foods, *N Engl J Med* 327:380-384, 1992.

Yellis MB: Breast milk and facilitation of gastrointestinal development and maturation, *Gastroenterol Nurs* 18(1):11-15, 1995.

Colic

Barr RG and others: The crying of infants with colic: a controlled empirical description, *Pediatrics* 90(1):14-21, 1992.

Hill DJ and others: Charting infant distress: an aid to defining colic, *J Pediatr* 121(5):755-758, 1992.

Jacobson D, Melvin N: A comparison of temperament and maternal bother in infants with and without colic, *J Pediatr Nurs* 10(3):181-187, 1995.

MacPhee M, Mori C, Goldson E: Change in the hospital setting: adopting a team approach for nonorganic failure-to-thrive, *J Pediatr Nurs* 9(4):218-225, 1994.

Treem WR: Infant colic: a pediatric gastroenterologist's perspective, *Pediatr Clin North Am* 41(5):1121-1138, 1994.

Weizman Z and others: Efficacy of herbal tea preparation in infantile colic, *J Pediatr* 122(4):650-652, 1993.

Failure to Thrive

Bithoney WG, Dubowitz H, Egan H: Failure to thrive/growth deficiency, *Pediatr Rev* 13(12):453-459, 1992.

Bithoney WG, Rathbun J: Failure to thrive. In Levine MD and others, editors: *Developmental-behavioral pediatrics,* ed 2, Philadelphia, 1992, WB Saunders.

Kelleher KJ and others: Risk factors and outcomes for failure to thrive in low birth weight preterm infants, *Pediatrics* 91(5):941-948, 1993.

Klein M: The home health nurse clinician's role in the prevention of nonorganic failure to thrive, *J Pediatr Nurs* 5(2):129-135, 1990.

Maggioni A, Lifshitz F: Nutritional management of failure to thrive, *Pediatr Clin North Am* 42(4):791-809, 1995.

Sudden Infant Death Syndrome/Apnea of Infancy

Bignall J: Decline in sudden infant deaths, *Lancet* 341:887, 1993.

Freed GE and others: Sudden infant death syndrome prevention and an understanding of selected clinical issues, *Pediatr Clin North Am* 41(5):967-990, 1994.

Hunt CE: Infant sleeping position: back to the bench, *Arch Pediatr Adolesc Med* 148(2):131-133, 1994.

Hunziker U, Barr R: Increased carrying reduces infant crying: a randomized controlled trial, *Pediatrics* 77(5):641-648, 1986.

Infant sleep position and sudden infant death syndrome (SIDS) in the United States: joint commentary from the American Academy of Pediatrics and selected agencies of the federal government, *Pediatrics* 93(5):820, 1994.

O'Donnell J: Theophylline misadventures: Part I, *Neonatal Network* 13(2):35-43, 1994.

Schoendorf KC, Kiely JL: Relationship of sudden infant death syndrome to maternal smoking during and after pregnancy, *Pediatrics* 90(6):905-908, 1992.

Spinner S and others: Recent advances in home apnea monitoring, *Neonatal Network* 14(8):39-46, 1995.

Stevens MS: Parents coping with infants requiring home cardiorespiratory monitoring, *J Pediatr Nurs* 9(1):2-12, 1994.

Whitaker S: The art and science of home infant apnea monitoring in the 1990s, *JOGNN* 24(1):84-89, 1995.

Autism

Baerg KL: Effective communication with autistic children, *Rehabil Nurs* 16(2):88-90, 1991.

Christian WP: Childhood autism. In Levine M and others, editors: *Developmental-behavioral pediatrics,* ed 2, Philadelphia, 1992, WB Saunders.

Denckla MB, James LS: An update on autism: a developmental disorder, *Pediatrics* 87(5, suppl):751-796, 1991.

Mulick JA, Jacobson JW, Kobe FH: Anguished silence and helping hands: autism and facilitated communication, *Skeptical Inquirer* 17(3):270-280, 1993.

Stone WL and others: Early recognition of autism: parental reports vs clinical observation, *Arch Pediatr Adolesc Med* 148:174-179, 1994.

Tuchman R, Gilman J: Pharmacotherapy of pervasive developmental disorders, *Int Pediatr* 8(2):211-218, 1993.

Zimmerman AW, Frye VH, Potter NT: Immunological aspects of autism, *Int Pediatr* 8(2):199-204, 1993.

Chapter 12

HEALTH PROMOTION OF THE TODDLER AND FAMILY

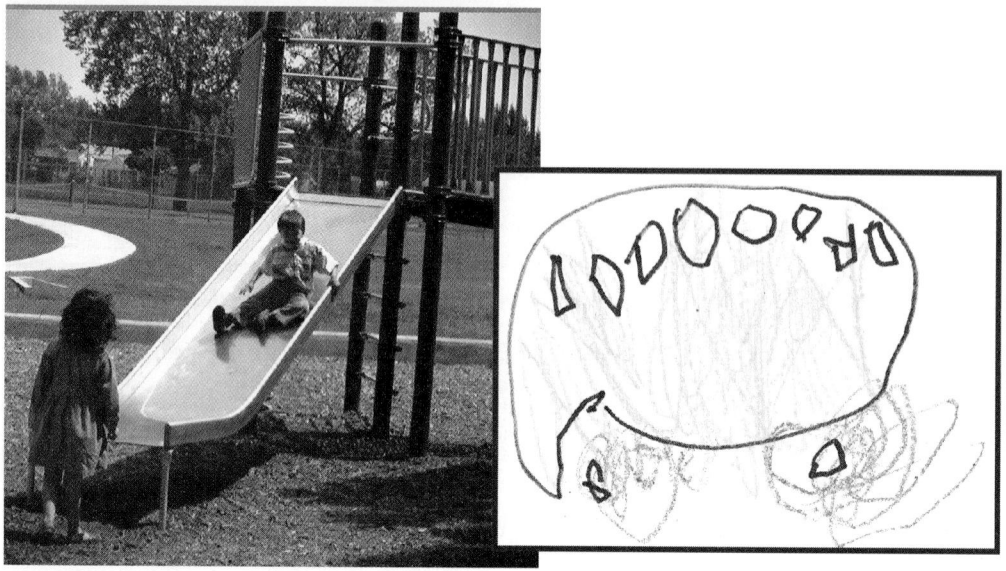

"I like to play with cars. This drawing is a van. I have to put them all away before I go to bed."

Daniel, age 3 years

RELATED TOPICS

PROMOTING OPTIMUM GROWTH AND DEVELOPMENT

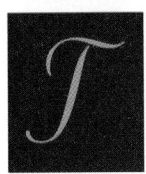he term *terrible twos* has often been used to describe the toddler years, the period from 12 to 36 months of age. It is a time of intense exploration of the environment as children attempt to find out how things work and how to control others through temper tantrums, negativism, and obstinacy. Although this can be a challenging time for parents and child as each learns to know the other better, it is an extremely important period for developmental achievement and intellectual growth.

BIOLOGIC DEVELOPMENT

Proportional Changes

Growth slows considerably during toddlerhood. The average *weight* gain is 1.8 to 2.7 kg (4 to 6 pounds) per year. The average weight at 2 years is 12 kg (27 pounds). The birth weight is quadrupled by 2½ years of age. The rate of increase in height also slows. The usual increment is an addition of 7.5 cm (3 inches) per year and occurs mainly in elongation of the legs rather than the trunk. The average *height* of a 2-year-old is 86.6 cm (34 inches). In general, adult height is about twice the 2-year-old child's height. Accurate measurement of height and weight during the toddler years should reveal a steady growth curve that is *steplike* in nature rather than linear (straight), which is characteristic of the growth spurts during the early childhood years.

The rate of increase in *head circumference* slows somewhat by the end of infancy, and head circumference is usually equal to chest circumference by 1 to 2 years of age. The usual total increase in head circumference during the second year is 2.5 cm (1 inch). Then the rate of increase slows until at age 5 years the increase is less than 1.25 cm (½ inch) per year. The anterior fontanel closes between 12 and 18 months of age.

Chest circumference continues to increase in size and exceeds head circumference during the toddler years. Its shape also changes as the transverse, or lateral, diameter exceeds the anteroposterior diameter. After the second year the chest circumference exceeds the abdominal measurement, which, in addition to the growth of the lower extremities, gives the child a taller, leaner appearance. However, the toddler retains a squat, "pot-bellied" appearance because of the less well developed abdominal musculature and short legs (Fig. 12-1). The legs retain a slightly bowed or curved appearance during the second year from the weight of the relatively large trunk.

Sensory Changes

Visual acuity of 20/20 is achieved during the toddler years, although 20/40 is considered acceptable. Full binocular vision is well developed, and any evidence of persistent strabismus requires professional attention as early as possible to prevent amblyopia. Depth perception continues to develop but, because of the child's lack of motor coordination, falls from heights continue to be a persistent danger.

The senses of *hearing, smell, taste,* and *touch* become increasingly well developed, coordinated with each other, and associated with other experiences. All the senses are used to explore the environment. Toddlers will visually inspect an object by turning it over; they may taste it, smell it, and touch it several times before they are satisfied with their investigation. They will shake it to see if it makes noise and vigorously test its durability.

Another example of the integrated function of the senses is the toddler's development of specific *taste preferences*. The child is much less likely than infants to try a new food because of its appearance or smell, not just its taste.

Maturation of Systems

Most of the physiologic systems are relatively mature by the end of toddlerhood. Volume of the *respiratory tract* and growth of associated structures continue to increase during early childhood, lessening some of the factors that predisposed the child to frequent and serious infections during infancy. The internal structures of the ear and throat continue to be short and straight, and the lymphoid tissue of the tonsils and adenoids continues to be large. As a result, otitis media, tonsillitis, and upper respiratory tract infections are common.

The respiratory and heart rates slow, and the blood pressure increases (see inside back cover). Respirations continue to be abdominal. Under conditions of moderate variation in temperature, the toddler rarely has the difficulties of the

Laurie Doerner, MSN, RN, revised this chapter.

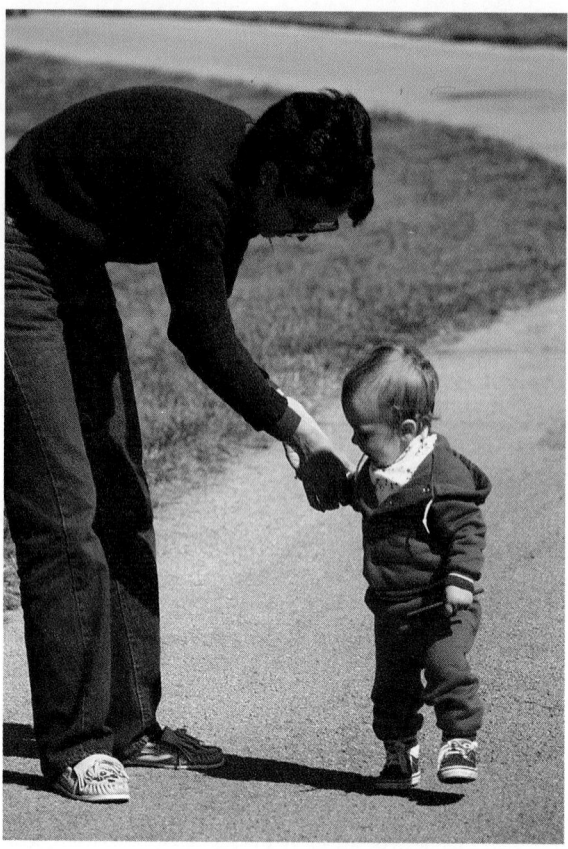

FIG. 12-1. Typical toddling gait.

young infant in maintaining ***body temperature.*** The mature functioning of the renal system serves to conserve fluid under times of stress, decreasing the risk of dehydration.

The ***digestive processes*** are fairly complete by the beginning of toddlerhood. The acidity of the gastric contents continues to increase and has a protective function, since it is capable of destroying many types of bacteria. Stomach capacity increases to allow for the usual schedule of three meals a day.

One of the more prominent changes of the gastrointestinal system is the voluntary control of elimination. With complete myelination of the spinal cord, control of the anal and urethral sphincters is gradually achieved. The physiologic ability to control the sphincters probably occurs somewhere between ages 18 and 24 months. Bladder capacity also increases considerably. By 14 to 18 months of age the child is able to retain urine for up to 2 hours or longer.

The ***defense mechanisms*** of the skin and blood, particularly phagocytosis, are much more efficient in toddlers than in infants. The production of antibodies is well established. However, many young children demonstrate a sudden increase in colds and minor infections when entering preschool or other group situations, such as daycare, because of their exposure to pathogens.

Gross and Fine Motor Development

The major ***gross motor skill*** during the toddler years is the development of locomotion. By 12 to 13 months of age toddlers walk alone using a wide stance for extra balance and by

18 months they try to run but fall easily. Between 2 and 3 years of age refinement of the upright, biped position is evident in improved coordination and equilibrium. At age 2, toddlers can walk up and down stairs, and by age 2½ years they can jump, using both feet, stand on one foot for a second or two, and manage a few steps on tiptoe. By the end of the second year they can stand on one foot, walk on tiptoe, and climb stairs with alternate footing.

Fine motor development is demonstrated in increasingly skillful manual dexterity. For example, by age 12 months toddlers are able to grasp a very small object but are unable to release it at will. At 15 months they can drop a pellet into a narrow-necked bottle. Casting or throwing objects and retrieving them become almost obsessive activities at about 15 months. By 18 months of age toddlers can throw a ball overhand without losing their balance.

Mastery of gross and fine motor skills is evident in all phases of the child's activity, such as play, dressing, language comprehension, response to discipline, social interaction, and proneness to injuries. Activities occur less in isolation and more in conjunction with other physical and mental abilities to produce a purposeful result. For example, the toddler walks to reach a new location, releases a toy to pick it up or to choose a new one, and scribbles to look at the image produced. The possibilities of the exploration, investigation, and manipulation of the environment—and its hazards—are endless.

PSYCHOSOCIAL DEVELOPMENT

Toddlers are faced with the mastery of several important tasks. If the need for basic trust has been satisfied, they are ready to give up dependence for control, independence, and autonomy. Some of the specific tasks to be dealt with include the following:

- Differentiation of self from others, particularly the mother
- Toleration of separation from parent
- Ability to withstand delayed gratification
- Control over bodily functions
- Acquisition of socially acceptable behavior
- Verbal means of communication
- Ability to interact with others in a less egocentric manner

Mastery of these goals is only begun during late infancy and the toddler years, and such tasks as developing interpersonal relationships with others may not be completed until adolescence. However, crucial foundations for successful completion of such developmental tasks are laid during these early formative years.

Developing a Sense of Autonomy (Erikson)

According to Erikson, the developmental task of toddlerhood is acquiring a sense of ***autonomy*** while overcoming a sense of ***doubt*** and ***shame.*** As infants gain trust in the predictability and reliability of their parents, environment, and interaction with others, they begin to discover that their behavior is their own and that it has a predictable, reliable effect on others. However, although they realize their will and control over others, they are confronted with the conflict of exerting autonomy and relinquishing the much-enjoyed dependence on others. Exerting their will has definite negative consequences, whereas retaining dependent, submissive behavior is generally rewarded with affection and approval. However, continued dependency creates a sense of doubt regarding their potential capacity to control their actions. This doubt is compounded by a sense of shame for feeling this urge to revolt against others' will and a fear that they will exceed their own capacity for manipulating the environment.

Just as the infant has the social modalities of grasping and biting, the toddler has the newly gained modality of holding on and letting go. To hold on and let go is evident with the use of the hands, mouth, eyes, and, eventually, the sphincters, when toilet training is begun. These social modalities are expressed constantly in the child's play activities, such as casting or throwing objects; taking objects out of boxes, drawers, or cabinets; holding on tighter when someone says, "No, don't touch"; and spitting out food as taste preferences become very strong.

Several characteristics, especially negativism and ritualism, are typical of toddlers in their quest for autonomy. As toddlers attempt to express their will, they often act with **negativism,** the persistent negative response to requests. The words "no" or "me do" can be the sole vocabulary. Emotions become very strongly expressed, usually in rapid mood swings. One minute toddlers can be engrossed in an activity, and the next minute they might be violently angry because they are unable to manipulate a toy or open a door. If scolded for doing something wrong, they can have a temper tantrum and almost instantaneously pull at the parent's legs to be picked up and comforted. Often these swift changes are difficult for parents to understand and cope with. Many parents find the negativism exasperating and, instead of dealing constructively with it, give into it, which further threatens children in their search for learning acceptable methods of interacting with others (see Negativism, p. 371).

In contrast to negativism, which frequently disrupts the environment, **ritualism,** the need to maintain sameness and reliability, provides a sense of comfort. Toddlers can venture out with security when they know that familiar people, places, and routines still exist. One can easily understand why change, such as hospitalization, represents such a threat to these children. Without the comfortable rituals, there is little opportunity to exert autonomy. Consequently, dependency and regression occur (see Regression, p. 371).

Erikson focuses on the development of the **ego,** which may be thought of as reason or common sense, during this phase of psychosocial development. There is a struggle as the child deals with the impulses of the **id** and attempts to tolerate frustration and learn socially acceptable ways of interacting with the environment. The **ego** is evident as the child is able to tolerate delayed gratification.

There is also a rudimentary beginning of the **superego,** or conscience, which is the incorporation of the morals of society and the process of acculturation. With the development of the ego, children further differentiate themselves from others and expand their sense of trust within themselves. But as they begin to develop awareness of their own will and capacity to achieve, they also become aware of their ability to fail. This ever-present awareness of potential failure creates doubt and shame. Successful mastery of the task of autonomy necessitates opportunities for self-mastery while withstanding the frustration of necessary limit-setting and delayed gratification. Opportunities for self-mastery are present in appropriate play activities, toilet training, the crisis of sibling rivalry, and successful interactions with significant others.

COGNITIVE DEVELOPMENT

Sensorimotor and Preconceptual Phase (Piaget)

The period from 12 to 24 months of age is a continuation of the final two stages of the sensorimotor phase. During this time the cognitive processes develop rapidly and at times seem similar to those of mature thinking. However, reasoning skills are still quite primitive and need to be understood to effectively deal with the typical behaviors of a child of this age.

Tertiary Circular Reactions.   In the fifth stage (13 to 18 months of age), the child uses active experimentation to achieve previously unattainable goals. Newly acquired physical skills are increasingly important for the function they serve rather than for the acts themselves. The child incorporates the old learning of secondary circular reactions with new skills and applies the combined knowledge to new situations, with emphasis on the results of the experimentation. In this way there is the beginning of rational judgment and intellectual reasoning. During this stage there is further differentiation of oneself from objects. This is evident in the child's increasing ability to venture away from the parent and to tolerate longer periods of separation.

Awareness of a causal relationship between two events is apparent. After flipping a light switch, toddlers are aware that a reciprocal response occurs. However, they are not able to transfer that knowledge to new situations. Therefore, every time they see what appears to be a light switch, they must reinvestigate its function. Such behavior demonstrates the beginning of categorizing data into distinct classes, subclasses, and so on. There are innumerable examples of this type of behavior as toddlers continuously explore the same object each time it appears in a new place.

Because classification of objects is still rudimentary, the appearance of an object denotes its function. For example, if the child's toys are stored in a paper bag or large container, that toy receptacle is no different from the garbage pail or laundry basket. If allowed to turn over the toy receptacle, the child will just as quickly do the same to other similar containers because, in the child's mind, there is no difference. Expecting the child to judge which receptacles are permissible to explore and which are not is inappropriate for this age-group. Instead, the forbidden object, such as the garbage pail, should be placed out of reach.

The discovery of objects as objects leads to the awareness of their spatial relationships. Children are able to recognize different shapes and their relationship to each other. For example, they can fit slightly smaller boxes into each other (nesting) and can place a round object into a hole, even if the board is turned around, upside down, or reversed. Children are also aware of space and the relationship of their body to dimensions such as height. They will stretch, stand on a low stair or stool, and pull a string to reach an object.

Object permanence has also advanced. Although they still cannot find an object that has been invisibly displaced or moved from under one pillow to another without their seeing the change, toddlers are increasingly aware of the existence of objects behind closed doors, in drawers, and under tables. Parents are usually acutely aware of this developmental achievement and find high places and locked cabinets the only places inaccessible to toddlers.

Invention of New Means Through Mental Combinations. From ages 19 to 24 months the child is in the final sensorimotor stage. During this stage the child completes the more primitive, autistic thought processes of infancy and is prepared for the more complex mental operations that occur during the phase of preoperational thought. One of the most dramatic achievements of this stage is in the area of object permanence. Children will now actively search for an object in several potential hiding places. In addition, they can infer a cause when only experiencing the effect. They can infer that an object was hidden in any number of places even if they only saw the original hiding place.

Imitation displays deeper meaning and understanding. There is greater symbolization to imitation. The child is acutely aware of others' actions and attempts to copy them in gestures and in words. *Domestic mimicry* (imitating household activities) and sex-role behavior become increasingly common during this period and during the second year. Identification with the parent of the same sex becomes apparent by the second year and represents the child's intellectual ability to differentiate different models of behavior and to imitate them appropriately (Fig. 12-2).

The conception of time is still embryonic, but children have some sense of timing in terms of anticipation, memory, and the limited ability to wait. They may listen to the command, "Just a minute," and behave appropriately. However, their sense of timing is exaggerated—1 minute can seem like an hour. Toddlers' limited attention spans also indicate their sense of immediacy and concern for the present.

Preconceptual Phase. At approximately 2 years of age the child enters the preconceptual phase of cognitive development, which lasts until about age 4. The preconceptual phase is a subdivision of the preoperational phase, which spans ages 2 to 7 years. The preconceptual phase is primarily one of transition that bridges the purely self-satisfying behavior of infancy and the rudimentary socialized behavior of latency. *Preoperational thought* implies that children cannot think in terms of *operations*—the ability to manipulate objects in relation to each other in a logical fashion. Rather, toddlers think primarily on the basis of their perception of an event. Problem solving is based on what they see or hear directly rather than on what they recall about objects and events. Several characteristics are unique to preoperational thought (see box on p. 365).

Within the second year the child increasingly uses language symbolically and is concerned with the "why" and "how" of things. For example, a pencil is "something to write with" and food is "something to eat." However, such mental symbolization is closely associated with prelogical reasoning. For instance, a needle is "something that hurts." Such painful experiences take on new significance because memory is associated with the specific event and fears are likely to develop, such as resistance to people who wear white uniforms or rooms that look like the practitioner's office. Because of the vulnerability of these early years, it is essential to prepare children for new experiences, whether it is a new baby-sitter or a visit to the dentist.

SPIRITUAL DEVELOPMENT

Toddlers have only a vague idea of God and religious teachings because of their immature cognitive processes. However, routines such as saying prayers before meals or at bedtime can be very important and comforting. Near the end of toddlerhood, when children use preoperational thought, there is some advancement of their understanding of God. Religious teachings, such as reward or fear of punishment (heaven or hell) and moral development (see discussion in Chapter 5), may influence their behavior.

DEVELOPMENT OF BODY IMAGE

As in infancy, the development of body image closely parallels cognitive development. With increasing motor ability toddlers recognize the usefulness of body parts and gradually learn their respective names. They also learn that certain parts of the body have various meanings; for example, during toilet training the genitals become significant and cleanliness is emphasized. By 2 years of age there is recognition of sexual differences and reference to self by name and then by pronoun.

Once they begin preoperational thought, toddlers can use symbols to represent objects, but their thinking may lead to inaccuracies. For example, if someone who is pregnant is called "fat," they will describe all "fat" women as having babies. There is a beginning recognition of words used to describe physical appearance, such as "pretty," "handsome," or "big boy." Such expressions eventually influence how children view their own bodies.

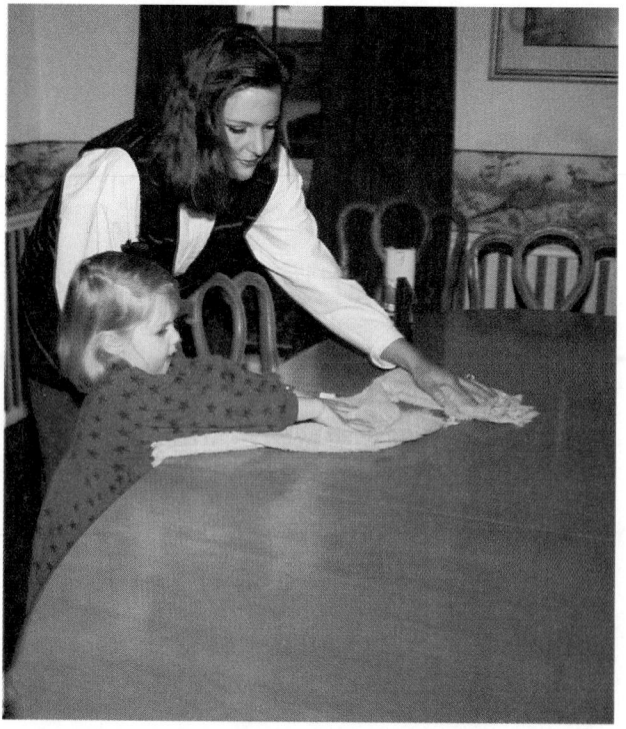

FIG. 12-2. Domestic mimicry and sex-role behavior are common during toddlerhood.

CHARACTERISTICS OF PREOPERATIONAL THOUGHT

Egocentrism—Inability to envision situations from perspectives other than one's own
Example: If a person is positioned between the toddler and another child, the toddler, who is facing the person, will explain that both children can see the middle person's face. The young child is unable to realize that the other person views the middle person from a different perspective, the back.
Implication: Avoid moralizing about "why" something is wrong if it requires an understanding of someone else's feelings or opinion. Telling a child to stop hitting because hitting hurts the other person is often ineffective because, to the aggressor, it feels good to hit someone else. Instead, emphasize that hitting is not allowed.
Transductive—Reasoning from the particular to the particular
Example: Child refuses to eat a food because something previously eaten did not taste good.
Implication: Accept child's reasoning; offer refused food at different time.
Global organization—Changing any one part of the whole changes the entire whole
Example: Child refuses to sleep in room because location of bed is changed.
Implication: Accept child's reasoning; use same bed position or introduce change slowly.
Centration—Focusing on one aspect rather than considering all possible alternatives
Example: Child refuses to eat a food because of its color, even though its taste and smell are acceptable.
Implication: Accept child's reasoning.
Animism—Attributing lifelike qualities to inanimate objects
Example: Child scolds stairs for making child fall down.
Implication: Join child in the "scolding." Keep frightening objects out of view.
Irreversibility—Inability to undo or reverse the actions initiated physically

Example: When told to stop doing something, such as talking, child is unable to think of positive activity.
Implication: State requests or instructions *positively* (e.g., "Be quiet."
Magical—Believing that thoughts are all-powerful and can cause events
Example: Child wishes someone died; then if the person dies, child feels at fault because of the "bad" thought that made the death happen.
Calling children "bad" because they did something wrong makes children feel as if they are bad.
Implication: Clarify that thoughts do not make things happen and that child is not responsible
Use "I" messages rather than "you" messages to communicate thoughts, feelings, expectations, or beliefs without imposing blame or criticism. Emphasize that the act is bad, not the child.
Inability to conserve—Inability to understand the idea that a mass can be changed in size, shape, volume, or length without losing or adding to the original mass (instead, children judge what they see by the immediate perceptual clues given to them)
Example: If two lines of equal length are presented in such a way that one appears longer than the other, child will state that one line is longer even if child measures both lines with a ruler or yardstick and finds that each has the same length.
Implication: Change the most obvious perceptual clue to reorient child's view of what is seen. For example, give medicine in a small medicine cup, rather than a large cup, since child will imagine that the large vessel contains more liquid. If child refuses the medicine in the small cup, pour it into a large cup, because the liquid will appear to be less in a tall, wide container.
Give a large flat cookie rather than a thick small one, or do the reverse with meat or cheese; child will usually eat larger size of favorite food and smaller size of less favorite food.

Although there has been little research done on body-image development in young children, it is evident that body integrity is poorly understood and that intrusive experiences are threatening. For example, toddlers forcefully resist procedures such as examining the ear or mouth and taking a rectal temperature. Toddlers also have unclear body boundaries and may associate nonviable parts, such as feces, with essential body parts. This can be seen in a toddler who is upset by flushing the toilet and watching the stool disappear.

Nurses can assist parents in fostering a positive body image in their child by encouraging them to avoid negative labels, such as "skinny arms" or "chubby legs"—self-perceptions that can last a lifetime. Body parts, especially those related to elimination and reproduction, should be called by their correct names. Respect for the body should be practiced.

DEVELOPMENT OF SEXUALITY

Just as toddlers explore their environment, they also explore their bodies and find that touching certain body parts is pleasurable. Genital fondling (masturbation) can occur and involves manual stimulation, as well as posturing movements (especially in young girls) such as tightening of the thighs or mechanical pressure applied to the pubic or suprapubic area (Lidster and Horsburgh, 1994). Other demonstrations of sensual activities include rocking, swinging, and hugging

people and toys. Parental reactions to toddlers' sexual behavior will influence the children's own attitudes and should be accepting rather than critical.

Children in this age-group are learning vocabulary associated with anatomy, elimination, and reproduction. Certain associations between words and functions become significant and can influence future sexual attitudes. For example, if parents refer to the genitals as dirty, especially in the context of elimination, this association between "genitals" and "dirty" may be transferred to sexual functions.

Sex-role differences become obvious to children and are evident in much of their imitative play. Early attitudes are formed about affectional behaviors between adults from observing parental and other adult sexual/sensual activities. (See also Sex Education, Chapter 13.)

SOCIAL DEVELOPMENT

A major task of the toddler period is differentiation of self from significant others, usually the mother. The differentiation process consists of two phases: *separation,* the children's emergence from a symbiotic fusion with the mother, and *individuation,* those achievements that mark children's assumption of their individual characteristics in the environment. Although the process begins during the latter half of infancy, the major achievements occur during the toddler years.

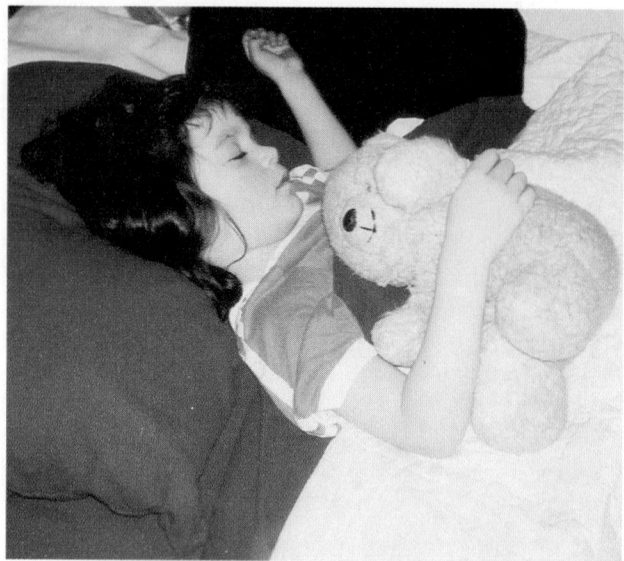

FIG. 12-3. Transitional objects, such as a warm and fuzzy stuffed animal, are sources of security to a toddler.

Toddlers have an increased understanding and awareness of object permanence and some ability to withstand delayed gratification and tolerate moderate frustration. As a result, toddlers react differently to strangers than do infants. The appearance of unfamiliar persons does not represent such a significant threat to their attachment to mother. They have learned from experience that parents exist when physically absent. Repetition of events such as going to bed without the parents but waking to find them there again reinforces the reliability of such brief separations. Consequently, toddlers are able to venture away from their parents for brief periods of time because of the security of knowing that the parents will be there when they return.

Transitional objects, such as a favorite blanket or toy, provide security for children, especially when they are separated from parents, dealing with a new stress, or just fatigued (Fig. 12-3). Security objects often become so important to toddlers that they refuse to have them taken away. Such behavior is normal; there is no need to discourage this tendency. During separations, such as daycare, hospitalization, or even staying overnight with a relative, transitional objects should be provided to minimize any feelings of fear or loneliness.

Learning to tolerate and master brief periods of separation is an important developmental task of children in this age-group. In addition, it is a necessary component of parenting, since brief periods of separation allow parents to recoup their energy and patience and to minimize directing their irritations and frustrations at the children.

Language Development

The most striking characteristic of language development during early childhood is the increasing level of comprehension. Although the number of words acquired—from about 4 at 1 year of age to approximately 300 at age 2 years—is notable, *the ability to comprehend and understand speech is much greater than the number of words the child can say.* This is particularly evident in bilingual families, where the vocabulary may be delayed, but comprehension in either language is appropriate.

At age 1 year the child uses one-word sentences or holophrases. The word "up" can mean "pick me up" or "look up there." For the child the one word conveys the meaning of a sentence, but to others it may mean many things or nothing. At this age about 25% of the vocalizations are intelligible. By the age of 2 years the child uses multiword sentences by stringing together two or three words, such as the phrases, "mama go bye-bye" or "all gone," and approximately 65% of the speech is understandable.

Personal-Social Behavior

One of the most dramatic aspects of development in the toddler is personal-social interaction. Parents frequently wonder why their manageable, docile, lovable infant has turned into a determined, strong-willed, volatile-tempered little tyrant. In addition, the tyrant of the terrible twos can swiftly and unpredictably revert back to the adorable infant. All of this is part of "growing up" and is evident in such areas as dressing, feeding, playing, and establishing self-control.

Toddlers are developing skills of independence, which are evident in all areas of behavior. By 15 months children feed themselves, drink well from a covered cup, and manage a spoon, with considerable spilling. By 24 months they use a spoon well and by 36 months may be using a fork. Between ages 2 and 3 years they eat with the family and like to help with chores such as setting the table or removing dishes from the dishwasher, but they lack table manners and may find it difficult to sit through the family's entire meal.

In dressing, toddlers also demonstrate strides in independence. The 15-month-old child helps by putting the arm or foot out for dressing and pulls shoes and socks off. The 18-month-old child removes gloves, helps with pullover shirts, and may be able to unzip. By age 2 years the toddler removes most articles of clothing and puts on socks, shoes, and pants without regard for right or left and back or front. Help is still needed to fasten clothes.

Play

Play magnifies the toddler's physical and psychosocial development. Interaction with people becomes increasingly important. The solitary play of infancy progresses to *parallel play*—the toddler plays alongside, not with, other children. Although sensorimotor play is still prominent, there is much less emphasis on the exclusive use of one sensory modality. The toddler inspects the toy, talks to the toy, tests its strength and durability, and invents several uses for it. Imitation is one of the most distinguishing characteristics of play and enriches children's opportunity to engage in fantasy. With less emphasis on sex-stereotyped toys, play objects such as dolls, carriages, dollhouses, dishes, cooking utensils, child-sized furniture, trucks, and dress-up clothes are suitable for both sexes (Fig. 12-4).

Increased locomotive skills make push-pull toys, straddle trucks or cycles, a small, low gym and slide, varied-size balls, and rocking horses appropriate for the energetic toddler. Finger paints, thick crayons, chalk, blackboard, paper, and puzzles with large, simple pieces use the child's developing fine motor skills. Interlocking blocks in varied sizes

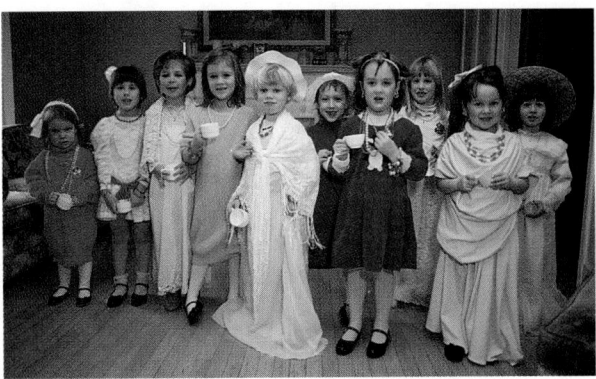

FIG. 12-4. Young children enjoy dressing up.

GUIDELINES
Assessing Toilet Training Readiness

Physical Readiness
Voluntary control of anal and urethral sphincters, usually by 18 to 24 months of age
Ability to stay dry for 2 hours; decreased number of wet diapers; waking dry from nap
Regular bowel movements
Gross motor skills of sitting, walking, and squatting
Fine motor skills to remove clothing

Mental Readiness
Recognizes urge to defecate or urinate
Verbal or nonverbal communicative skills to indicate when wet or has urge to defecate or urinate
Cognitive skills to imitate appropriate behavior and follow directions

Psychologic Readiness
Expresses willingness to please parent
Able to sit on toilet for 5 to 10 minutes without fussing or getting off
Curiosity about adults' or older sibling's toilet habits
Impatience with soiled or wet diapers; desire to be changed immediately

Parental Readiness
Recognizes child's level of readiness
Willing to invest the time required for toilet training
Absence of family stress or change, such as a divorce, moving, new sibling, or imminent vacation

and shapes provide hours of fun and, during later years, are useful objects for creative and imaginative play.

Talking is a form of play for the toddler, who enjoys musical toys such as play phonographs, "talking" dolls and animals, and play telephones. Appropriate children's television programs are excellent for children in this age-group, who learn to associate words with visual images. Toddlers also enjoy "reading" stories from a picture book and imitating the sounds of animals.

Tactile play is also important for the exploring toddler. Water toys, a sandbox with pail and shovel, finger paints, soap bubbles, and clay provide excellent opportunities for free creative and manipulative recreation. Adults sometimes forget the fascination of feeling slippery cream, such as whipped cream or pudding, catching airy bubbles, squeezing and reshaping clay, or smearing paints. These types of unstructured activities are as important as educational play to allow children freedom of expression.

Selection of appropriate toys must involve safety factors, especially in relation to size and sturdiness. The oral activity of toddlers makes them at risk for aspirating small objects or ingesting toxic substances. Parents need to be especially vigilant of toys played with in other children's homes or those of older siblings. Toys are a potential source of serious bodily damage to toddlers, who may have the physical strength to manipulate them but not the knowledge to appreciate their danger (see Family Home Care box: Toy Safety, Chapter 5).

SUMMARY OF GROWTH AND DEVELOPMENT DURING TODDLERHOOD

Table 12-1 summarizes the major features of growth and development for the age-groups of 15, 18, 24, and 30 months.

COPING WITH CONCERNS RELATED TO NORMAL GROWTH AND DEVELOPMENT

Toilet Training

One of the major tasks of toddlerhood is toilet training. Voluntary control of the anal and urethral sphincters is achieved

sometime after the child is walking, probably between ages 18 and 24 months. However, complex psychophysiologic factors are required for readiness. The child must be able to recognize the urge to let go and hold on and be able to communicate this sensation to the parent. In addition, there is probably some necessary motivation in the desire to please the parent by holding on, rather than pleasing oneself by letting go.

Usually physiologic and psychologic readiness is not complete until 18 to 24 months of age. By this time the child has mastered the majority of essential gross motor skills, can communicate intelligibly, is less in conflict with self-assertion and negativism, and is aware of the ability to control the body and please the parent. One of the most important responsibilities of nurses is to help parents identify the readiness signs in their child (see Guidelines box).*

Bowel training is usually accomplished before bladder training because of its greater regularity and predictability. There is a stronger sensation for defecation than for urination, and the sensation of defecation can be brought to the child's attention. In fact, nighttime bladder training may not be completed until 4 or 5 years of age, and even later training is normal.

A number of techniques can be helpful when initiating

*A helpful brochure is *Toilet Training: A Parent's Guide,* available from the **American Academy of Pediatrics,** 141 Northwest Point Blvd., P.O. Box 927, Elk Grove Village, IL 60009-0927; (800) 433-9016.

TABLE 12-1. Growth and development during toddler years

AGE (MONTHS)	PHYSICAL	GROSS MOTOR	FINE MOTOR
15	Steady growth in height and weight Head circumference 48 cm (19 inches) Weight 11 kg (24 pounds) Height 78.7 cm (31 inches)	Walks without help (usually since age 13 months) Creeps up stairs Kneels without support Cannot walk around corners or stop suddenly without losing balance Assumes standing position without support Cannot throw ball without falling	Constantly casting objects to floor Builds tower of two cubes Holds two cubes in one hand Releases a pellet into a narrow-necked bottle Scribbles spontaneously Uses cup well but rotates spoon
18	Physiologic anorexia from decreased growth needs Anterior fontanel closed Physiologically able to control sphincters	Runs clumsily, falls often Walks up stairs with one hand held Pulls and pushes toys Jumps in place with both feet Seats self on chair Throws ball overhand without falling	Builds tower of three to four cubes Release, prehension, and reach well developed Turns pages in a book two or three at a time In drawing, makes stroke imitatively Manages spoon without rotation
24	Head circumference 49 to 50 cm (19.5 to 20 inches) Chest circumference exceeds head circumference Lateral diameter of chest exceeds anteroposterior diameter Usual weight gain of 1.8 to 2.7 kg (4 to 6 pounds) Usual gain in height of 10 to 12.5 cm (4 to 5 inches) Adult height approximately double height at 2 years of age May have achieved readiness for beginning daytime control of bowel and bladder Primary dentition of 16 teeth	Goes up and down stairs alone with two feet on each step Runs fairly well, with wide stance Picks up object without falling Kicks ball forward without overbalancing	Builds tower of six to seven cubes Aligns two or more cubes like a train Turns pages of book one at a time In drawing, imitates vertical and circular strokes Turns doorknob, unscrews lid
30	Birth weight quadrupled Primary dentition (20 teeth) completed May have daytime bowel and bladder control	Jumps with both feet Jumps from chair or step Stands on one foot momentarily Takes a few steps on tiptoe	Builds tower of eight cubes Adds chimney to train of cubes Good hand-finger coordination; holds crayon with fingers rather than fist Moves fingers independently In drawing, imitates vertical and horizontal strokes, makes two or more strokes for cross

training. One is the selection of a potty-chair and/or use of the toilet. A freestanding potty-chair allows children a feeling of security. Planting the feet firmly on the floor also facilitates defecation (Stark, 1994). Another option is a portable seat attached to the regular toilet, which may ease the transition from potty-chair to regular toilet. Placing a small bench under the feet helps to stabilize the child's position. It is probably best to keep the potty in the bathroom and to let the child observe the excreta being flushed down the toilet to associate these activities with usual practices. If a potty-seat is not available, having the child sit *facing* the toilet tank provides added support. Boys may begin toilet training in the stand-up position or by sitting on a potty-chair or toilet. Imitating father during the preschool years is a powerful motivating force (Fig. 12-5).

Practice sessions should be limited to 5 or 10 minutes, a parent should stay with the child, and sanitary habits should be employed after every session. Children should be praised for cooperative behavior and/or successful evacuation. Dressing children in easily removed clothing; using training pants,

SENSORY	LANGUAGE	SOCIALIZATION
Able to identify geometric forms; places round object into appropriate hole Binocular vision well developed Displays an intense and prolonged interest in pictures	Uses expressive jargon Says four to six words, including names "Asks" for objects by pointing Understands simple commands May use head-shaking gesture to denote "no" Uses "no" even while agreeing to the request	Tolerates some separation from parent Less likely to fear strangers Beginning to imitate parents, such as cleaning house (sweeping, dusting), folding clothes May discard bottle Manages spoon but rotates it near mouth Kisses and hugs parents, may kiss pictures in a book Expresses emotions, has temper tantrums
	Says 10 or more words Points to a common object, such as a shoe or ball, and to two or three body parts	Great imitator (domestic mimicry) Takes off gloves, socks, and shoes and unzips Temper tantrums may be more evident Beginning awareness of ownership ("my toy") May develop dependency on transitional objects, such as "security blanket"
Accommodation well developed In geometric discrimination, able to insert square block into oblong space	Has vocabulary of approximately 300 words Uses two- to three-word phrases Uses pronouns "I," "me," "you" Understands directional commands Gives first name; refers to self by name Verbalizes need for toileting, food, or drink Talks incessantly	Stage of parallel play Has sustained attention span Temper tantrums decreasing Pulls people to show them something Increased independence from parent Dresses self in simple clothing
	Gives first and last name Refers to self by appropriate pronoun Uses plurals Names one color	Separates more easily from parent In play, helps put things away, can carry breakable objects, pushes with good steering Begins to notice sex differences; knows own sex May attend to toilet needs without help except for wiping

"pull-on" diapers, or panties; and encouraging imitation by watching others are other helpful suggestions. Forcing children to sit on the potty-chair or toilet for long periods, spanking them for having accidents, and other methods of negative control are avoided. Daytime accidents are common, particularly during periods of intense activity. Young children become so engrossed in play activity that if they are not reminded, they will wait until it is too late to reach the bathroom. Therefore frequent reminders and trips to the toilet are necessary.

Sibling Rivalry

The natural jealousy and resentment of children to a new child in the family is referred to as *sibling rivalry*. The arrival of a new infant represents a crisis for even the best-prepared toddlers. It is not the infant that toddlers hate or resent but the changes that this additional sibling produces, especially the separation from mother during the birth. The parents now share their love and attention with someone else, the usual routine is disrupted, and toddlers may lose their crib and/or room—all at a time when they thought they

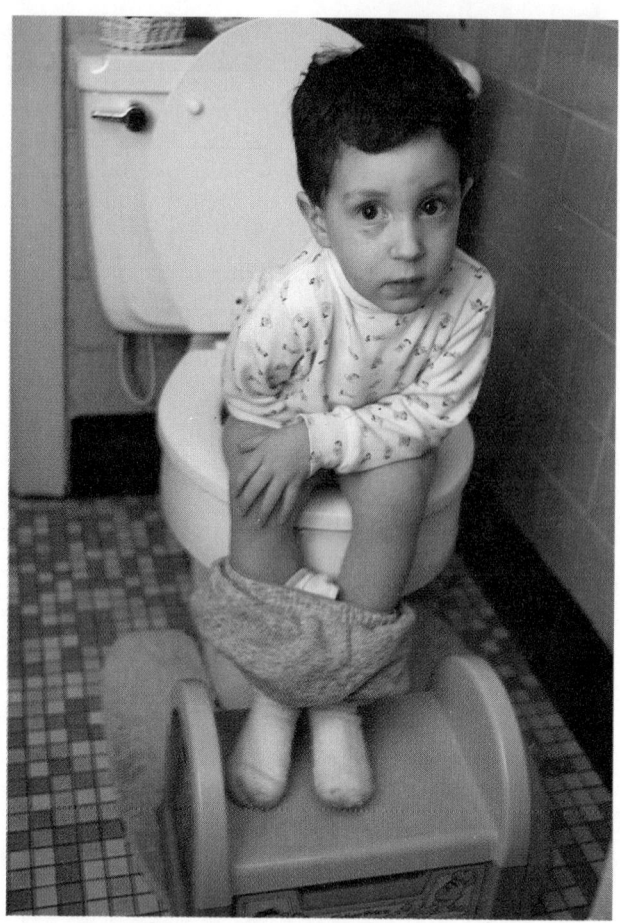

FIG. 12-5. Boys may begin toilet training sitting on a toilet. Note feet on small bench.

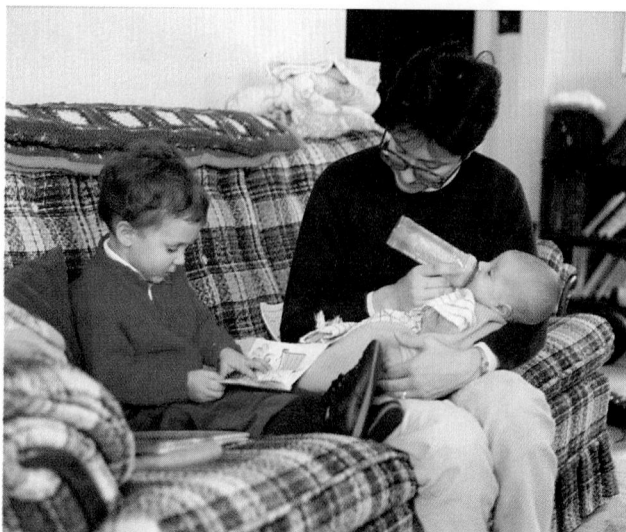

FIG. 12-6. To minimize sibling rivalry, parents should include the toddler in caregiving activities.

were in control of their world. Sibling rivalry tends to be most pronounced in the first-born, who experiences ***dethronement,*** (loss of sole parental attention). It also seems to be most difficult for young children, particularly in terms of mother-child interaction.

Preparation of children for the birth of a sibling is quite individual, but age dictates some important considerations. Time for toddlers is a vague concept. Tomorrow could be yesterday or next week, and a month from now could be never. Preparing children too soon for the birth may lessen their interest by the time the event occurs. A good time to start talking about the new baby is when toddlers become aware of the pregnancy and the changes taking place in the home in anticipation of the new member.

Toddlers need to have a realistic idea of what the newborn will be like. Telling them that a new playmate will come home soon sets up unrealistic expectations. Rather, parents should stress the activities that will take place when the baby arrives home, such as diapering, bottle- or breast-feeding, bathing, and dressing. At the same time, parents should emphasize which routines will stay the same, such as reading stories or going to the park. If toddlers have had no contact with an infant, it is a good idea to introduce them to one, if feasible. Providing a doll on which toddlers can imitate parental

behaviors is another excellent strategy. They can tend to the doll's needs (diapering, feeding) at the same time the parent is performing similar activities for the infant (Fig. 12-6).

A new sibling in the home is stressful, so any additional stresses for the toddler should be avoided or minimized. For example, moving the toddler to a regular bed or to a different room should be done well in advance of the infant's arrival.

Pregnancy is an abstraction for toddlers. They need concrete illustrations of how the baby is growing inside the mother. It is an excellent opportunity for introducing aspects of reproduction and sexuality. Seeing simple pictures of the uterus and fetus and feeling the fetus move help the child feel involved in the experience. Children also benefit from "siblings" classes that may be part of prenatal sessions.

When the new baby arrives, toddlers keenly feel the changed focus of attention. Visitors may initiate problems when they inadvertently shower the infant with attention and presents while neglecting the older child. Parents can minimize this by alerting visitors to the toddler's needs, having small presents on hand for the toddler, and including the child in the visit as much as possible.

How children exhibit jealousy is complex. Some will overtly hit the infant, push the child off mother's lap, or pull the bottle or breast from the infant's mouth. More often the expressions of hostility and resentment are more subtle and covert. Toddlers may verbally express a wish that the infant "go back inside mommy," or they will revert to more infantile forms of behavior, such as demanding a bottle, soiling their underpants, clinging for attention, using baby talk, or aggressively acting out toward others. For this reason, infants must be protected by parental supervision of the interaction between the siblings.

Temper Tantrums

Toddlers may assert their independence by violently objecting to discipline. They may lie down on the floor, kick their feet, and scream at the top of their lungs. Some have learned the effectiveness of holding their breath until the parent relents. Although holding one's breath may cause fainting from the lack of oxygen, the accumulation of carbon dioxide will stimulate the respiratory control center, resulting in no physical harm.

The best approach toward extinguishing such attention-seeking behavior is to ignore it, provided the behavior is not injuring the child, such as violently banging the head on the floor. However, the parent should remain close by. When the tantrum has subsided, the child needs to feel some control and security. At this time a toy or a favorite activity can be substituted for the ungranted request. (See also Limit setting and discipline, Chapter 4.)

Frequently temper tantrums can be avoided by giving the child advance warning of a request. For example, a popular time for tantrums is before bed. Active toddlers often have trouble slowing down and when placed in bed, resist staying there. One approach is to establish limited rituals that signal readiness for bed, such as a bath or story. Parents can reinforce the pattern by stating, "After this story it is bedtime," and consistently carrying out the routine.

Negativism

One of the more difficult aspects of rearing children in this age-group is their persistent "no" response to every request. The negativism is not an expression of being fresh or insolent, but a necessary assertion of self-control. One method of dealing with the negativism is reducing the opportunities for a "no" answer. Asking the child, "Do you want to go to sleep now?" is an almost certain example of a question that will be answered with an emphatic "no." Instead, tell the child that it is time to go to sleep and proceed accordingly.

In their attempt to exert control, children like to make choices. When confronted with appropriate choices, such as "You may have a peanut butter and jelly sandwich or chicken noodle soup for lunch," they are more likely to choose one rather than automatically say no. However, if their response is negative, parents should make the choice for the child.

Regression

The retreat from one's present pattern of functioning to past levels of behavior is referred to as *regression.* It usually occurs in instances of discomfort or stress when one attempts to conserve psychic energy by reverting to patterns of behavior that were successful in earlier stages of development. Regression is common in toddlers, because almost any additional stress hinders their ability to master present developmental tasks. Any threat to their autonomy, such as illness, hospitalization, separation, or adjustment to a sibling, represents a need to revert to earlier forms of behavior, such as increased dependency; refusal to use the potty-chair; temper tantrums; demand for the bottle, stroller, or crib; and loss of newly learned motor, language, social, and cognitive skills.

At first such regression appears acceptable and comfortable for children. The loss of newly acquired achievements is frightening and threatening, because children are aware of their helplessness. Parents become frightened of regressive behavior and frequently, in their efforts to deal with it, force the child to cope with an additional source of stress—the pressure to live up to expected standards.

When regression does occur, the best approach is to ig-

nore it while praising existing patterns of appropriate behavior. Regression is a child's way of saying, "I can't cope with this present stress and perfect this skill as well, but I will if given patience and understanding." For this reason it is advisable not to attempt new areas of learning when an additional crisis is present or expected, such as beginning toilet training shortly before a sibling is born or attempting new areas of learning during a brief period of hospitalization.

PROMOTING OPTIMUM HEALTH DURING TODDLERHOOD

NUTRITION

During the period from 12 to 18 months of age, the growth rate slows, decreasing the child's need for calories, protein, and fluid. However, the protein (1.2 g/kg) and caloric (102 kcal/kg) requirements are still relatively high to meet the demands for muscle tissue growth and high activity level (Forgac, 1995). The need for minerals such as iron, calcium, and phosphorus is still high, particularly when one considers the poor food habits of children in this age-group and the increased mineralization within bones.

At approximately 18 months of age, most toddlers manifest this decreased nutritional need with a decreased appetite, a phenomenon known as *physiologic anorexia.* They become picky, fussy eaters with strong taste preferences. They may eat large amounts one day and almost nothing the next. They are increasingly aware of the nonnutritive function of food: the pleasure of eating, the social aspect of mealtime, and the control of refusing food. They are influenced by factors other than taste when choosing food. If a family member refuses to eat something, toddlers are likely to imitate that response. If the plate is overfilled, they are likely to push it away, overwhelmed by its size. If food does not appear or smell appetizing, they will probably not agree to try it. In essence, mealtime is more closely associated with psychologic components than with nutritional ones.

Developmentally, by 12 months of age most children are eating the same food prepared for the rest of the family. Some may have mastered using a cup with occasional spilling, although most cannot adeptly use a spoon until 18 months of age or later and generally prefer using their fingers.

Nutritional Counseling

Eating habits established in the first 2 or 3 years of life tend to have lasting effects on subsequent years. If food is used as a reward or sign of approval, a child may overeat for nonnutritive reasons. If food is forced and mealtime is consistently unpleasant, the usual pleasure associated with eating may not develop. Mealtimes should be enjoyable rather than times for discipline or family arguments. The social aspect of mealtime may be distracting for young children; therefore an earlier feeding hour may be appropriate. Young children are unable to sit through a long meal and become fidgety and disruptive. This is particularly common when children are brought to the table just after active play. Calling them in from play 15 minutes before mealtime allows them ample opportunity to get ready for eating while settling down their active minds and bodies.

SAMPLE MENU FOR TODDLERS BASED ON FOOD GUIDE PYRAMID*	
Breakfast	½ cup dry, unsweetened cereal ½ cup orange juice 4 oz low-fat milk
Snack	½-1 whole banana
Lunch	1 tbsp peanut butter 2 tsp all-fruit preserves 1 slice whole-wheat bread 2 tbsp peas 4 oz low-fat milk
Snack	2 graham crackers 4 oz low-fat milk
Dinner	1 chicken leg, roasted without skin ¼-½ cup macaroni and cheese 2 tbsp green beans, cooked 2 tbsp carrots, cooked 4-6 oz low-fat milk
Snack	½ cup frozen yogurt
Total Servings	
Bread, cereal, rice, pasta	6-7
Vegetable	3
Fruit	3-4
Milk, yogurt, cheese	2-3
Meat, poultry, fish, dried beans, eggs, nuts	2

*Use fats, oils, and sweets sparingly. Increase fluids with servings of water. Serving sizes are minimums for nutritional adequacy. Many children eat more.

The method of serving food also takes on more importance during this period. Toddlers need to feel control and achievement in their abilities. Giving them large, adult-size portions can overwhelm them. In general, what is eaten is much more significant than how much is consumed. Small amounts of meat and vegetables supply greater food value than a large consumption of bread or potato. Serving sizes need to be appropriate for age (see box). Young children tend to like less spicy, bland food, although this is a culturally determined preference. Substitutions can be provided for foods that they do not enjoy, although this practice should not cater to all their desires. Frequent nutritious snacks can replace a meal. "Grazing"—nibbling and snacking—is a good way to ensure proper nutrition, provided appropriate foods are offered.

NURSING TIPS *Serving Size for Young Children*
A general guide to the serving size of food is 1 tablespoon of solid food per year of age or one fourth to one third the adult portion size.
Use the tablespoon guide for easily measured food such as vegetables or rice.
Use the fraction guide for bread or milk.

The ritualism of this age also dictates certain principles in feeding practices. Toddlers like the same dish, cup, or spoon every time they eat. They may reject a favorite food simply because it is served in a different utensil. If one food touches another, they often refuse to eat it. Mixed foods, such as stews or casseroles, are rarely favorites. Since toddlers are unpredictable in their table manners, it is best to use plastic dishes and cups, for both economy and safety. For some children a regular mealtime schedule also helps satisfy their desire and need for predictability and ritualism.

Most children by 12 months of age are eating the same food prepared for the rest of the family. However, appetite and food preferences are sporadic. Often the interest in food parallels a growth spurt, so that periods of good eating are interspersed with phases of poor eating. "Food jags" are common.

Such food fads do not ensure a well-balanced diet, but attempts to alter them are usually unsuccessful. It is preferable to accept such extremes and offer other foods in small portions. Introducing at least three items from the different food groups at each meal helps develop a variety of taste preferences and well-balanced eating habits.

SLEEP AND ACTIVITY
Total sleep decreases only slightly during the second year and averages about 12 hours a day. Most children take one nap a day, and by the end of the second or third year many relinquish this habit. The activity level is high, and there is rarely a problem with too little physical exercise, provided inappropriate restrictions are not instituted. With increasing numbers of young children being cared for outside the home, attention to the kinds of activity provided is important. For example, children with high activity levels may benefit from an environment in which outdoor play is encouraged.

Sleep problems are common, especially going to bed and falling asleep, and are probably related to fears of separation. Bedtime rituals (same hour of sleep, snack, quiet activity) are helpful, and transitional objects, such as a favorite stuffed animal or blanket, can help ease the child's insecurity at bedtime (see Fig. 12-3).

DENTAL HEALTH

Regular Dental Examinations
Ideally the child should see a dentist (or *pedodontist,* a pediatric dentist) soon after the first teeth erupt and no later than age 2½ years, when primary dentition is completed. Initial visits to the dentist should be nontraumatizing. Since toddlers react negatively to new and potentially frightening experiences, the initial visit can center around meeting the dentist, seeing the equipment, and sitting in the chair. If the child is cooperative, the dentist may just look at the teeth but reserve a more thorough examination for another visit. Modeling, in which the child observes procedures performed on the parent or a cooperative sibling, can also be effective.

Removal of Plaque
The objective of oral hygiene is removal of *plaque,* soft bacterial deposits that adhere to the teeth and cause *dental caries (decay* or *cavities)* and *periodontal (gum) disease.* The most effective methods for plaque removal are brushing and flossing. Several brushing techniques exist, although there is no universal agreement regarding the best method. One that is suitable for cleaning the primary teeth is the scrub method.

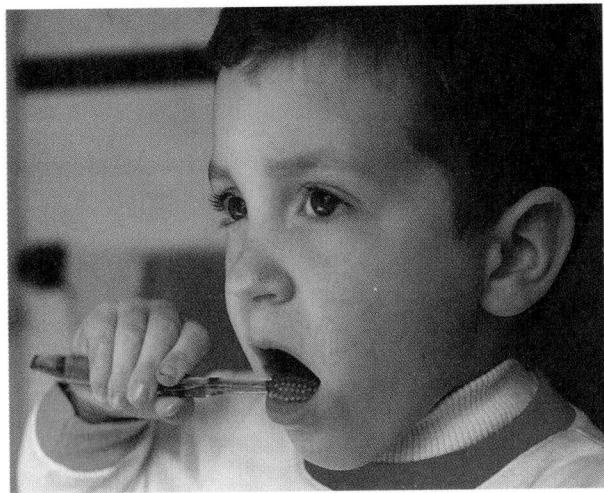

FIG. 12-7. Young children can participate in toothbrushing, but parents need to brush all the child's teeth thoroughly.

TABLE 12-2. Fluoride supplementation*

AGE	WATER FLUORIDE CONTENT (IN PPM)†		
	<0.3	0.3-0.6	>0.6
Birth-6 months	0	0	0
6 months-3 years	0.25	0	0
3-6 years	0.50	0.25	0
6-16 years	1.00	0.50	0

*Fluoride daily doses are given in milligrams
†Parts per million (ppm)
From American Academy of Pediatrics, Committee on Nutrition: Fluoride supplementation for children, *Pediatrics* 95(5):777, 1995.

The tips of the bristles are placed firmly at a 45-degree angle against the teeth and gums and moved back and forth in a vibratory motion. The ends of the bristles should be wiggling but not moving forcefully back and forth, which can damage the gums and enamel. All the surfaces of the teeth are cleaned in this manner except the lingual (inner) surfaces of the anterior teeth. To clean these surfaces, the toothbrush is placed vertical to the teeth and moved up and down. Only a few teeth are brushed at one time, using six to eight strokes for each section. A systematic approach is used so that all surfaces are thoroughly cleaned (Fig. 12-7).

For young children the most effective cleaning is done by parents. Several positions can be used that facilitate access to the mouth and help stabilize the head for comfort:

* Stand with child's back toward adult. (When done in front of a bathroom mirror, both child and adult can see what is being done in the mirror.)
* Sit on a couch or bed with child's head resting in adult's lap.
* Sit on the floor or a stool with child's head resting between adult's thighs.

With all positions, use one hand to cup the chin and one to brush the teeth. For easier access to back teeth, hold the mouth partially open.

NURSING TIPS
To encourage children to open their mouth, ask them to "tweet like a bird" to brush the front teeth and to "roar like a lion" to brush the back teeth.
Sing, tell stories, or talk to children during teeth cleaning to prevent boredom.

For effective cleaning, a small toothbrush with soft, rounded, multitufted nylon bristles that are short and uniform in length is recommended. Nylon bristles dry more rapidly after use and retain their shape better than natural bristles. Toothbrushes are replaced as soon as the bristles are frayed or bent. With young children, brushing may be more easily accomplished using only water, since many children dis-

like the foam from toothpaste and the foam interferes with visibility. There is also the danger of swallowing fluoridated toothpaste (see following discussion under Fluoride). When using toothpaste, children should select the flavor they like to encourage the brushing habit.

After the teeth have been cleaned, flossing with dental floss is done to remove plaque and debris from between the teeth and below the gum margin, where brushing is ineffective. Since young children do not have the dexterity to manipulate the floss, parents are taught the procedure.

A disclosing agent is helpful in identifying those areas of the teeth where plaque accumulates. It also helps motivate children to clean their teeth because plaque is difficult to see. After cleaning, the mouth is inspected to ensure that all traces of plaque have been removed. Where plaque remains, the teeth are rebrushed.

Ideally the teeth should be cleaned after each meal and especially before bedtime, and the child should be given nothing to eat or drink after the night brushing except water. At those times when brushing is impractical, the "swish-and-swallow" method of cleaning the mouth is taught: with a mouthful of water the child rinses the mouth and swallows, repeating the procedure three or four times.

Fluoride

Fluoride, a mineral, is found in water, foods, or drinks in which fluoridated water was used as part of the processing system. Because the water fluoridation process and manufacturing of fluoride toothpaste are almost impossible to unify in the United States, the dosage of fluoride supplements has been lowered to reduce the incidence of fluorosis. Increased fluoride ingestion leads to enamel protein retention, hypomineralization of the enamel and dentin, and disturbance of crystal formation. The effects caused by this change range from barely discernible white fiberlike lines or spots to gray-brown stains or pitted areas.

It is now recommended that fluoride supplementation be withheld from birth to 6 months, and decreased in dosage from 6 months to 6 years of age. When supplements are not needed, the level of fluoride in water has been decreased from 0.7 to 0.6 ppm (parts per million) (Table 12-2) (American Academy of Pediatrics, 1995).

Nurses have a responsibility to ensure an optimal fluoride regimen for children and to counsel families regarding correct use of supplements. The nurse should have a knowledge of the fluoride content of the community water supply and provide instruction to parents regarding correct administration of fluoride drops or tablets. Supplements should remain in the mouth for 30 seconds before swallowing and be taken on an empty stomach. Afterward the child should not drink or eat for 30 minutes. All fluoride products (toothpaste, supplements, and rinse) need to be stored away from young children to prevent poisoning. If the water supply is fluoridated, parents are encouraged to use water to prepare drinks and foods.

Low-Cariogenic Diet

Diet is critical to developing good teeth because the carious process depends primarily on fermentable sugars, especially sucrose. Refined table sugar, honey, molasses, corn syrup, and dried fruits such as raisins are highly cariogenic.

Ideally such foods should be eliminated. However, since this is impractical, some suggestions can be helpful. First, *the frequency with which sugar is consumed is more important than the total amount eaten*. Therefore, when sweets are eaten, they are less damaging if consumed immediately after a meal rather than as a snack between meals. When sweets are served as the dessert, the teeth can be cleaned afterward, decreasing the amount of time the sugar is in the mouth.

Second, the form of sugar is important. The more cariogenic foods are those that are sticky or hard, since they remain in the mouth longer. Consequently, sucking on lollipops is more cariogenic than eating a chocolate bar. Sometimes the source of the sugar is "hidden," such as in numerous prescription and nonprescription drugs and in many popular cereals, including the "all-natural" variety. Reading food labels is essential in eliminating sources of sucrose.

 Some snacks do not contribute to tooth decay. Aged cheeses, such as cheddar, may alter the pH and retard bacterial growth. Sugarless gum chewed after eating may actually protect against cavities by stimulating saliva that neutralizes acid. The artificial sweeteners saccharin and aspartame are noncariogenic; sorbitol has low cariogenic potential.

A special form of tooth decay in children between 18 months and 3 years of age is *nursing caries* (also called *nursing bottle caries* or *bottle-mouth caries*), which occurs when the child is routinely given a bottle of milk or juice at nap or bedtime or uses the bottle as a pacifier while awake. Frequent nocturnal breast-feeding for prolonged periods also leads to extensive destruction of the teeth. The practice of coating pacifiers in honey can also contribute to caries and may be a potential source of botulism poisoning. As the sweet liquid pools in the mouth, the teeth are bathed for several hours in this cariogenic environment. The maxillary (upper) incisors and molars are affected most, since the mandibular (lower) incisors are protected by the lower lip, tongue, and saliva (Fig. 12-8). Severely decayed teeth may require the application of stainless steel bands to preserve the spacing until the permanent teeth erupt.

Prevention involves eliminating the bedtime bottle completely, feeding the last bottle before bedtime, substituting a

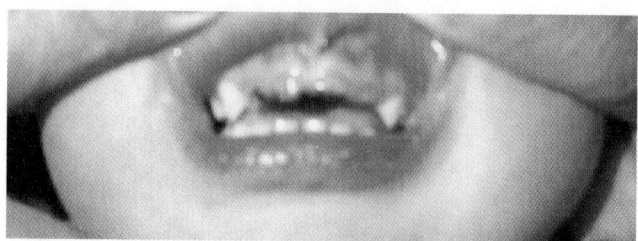

FIG. 12-8. Nursing caries. Note extensive carious involvement of maxillary primary incisors.

bottle of water for milk or juice, not using the bottle as a pacifier, and never coating pacifiers in sweet substances. Juice in bottles, especially commercially available ready-to-use bottles, is discouraged, since the beverage is especially damaging because the sugar is more readily converted to acid. Juice should always be offered in a cup in order to avoid prolonging the bottle-feeding habit. Nurses are in an excellent position to counsel parents regarding the dangers of this habit and other aspects of dental care.*

INJURY PREVENTION

Injuries cause more deaths in children between the ages of 1 to 4 years than in any other childhood age-group except adolescence. The injury death rate has remained relatively unchanged during the past decade; however, the corresponding rates from all other causes of death combined have declined significantly. Injury's prominence as the leading cause of death among toddlers and preschoolers underscores the need to emphasize safety awareness among parents. Child protection and parent education are key determinants in injury prevention.

A major factor in the critical increase of injuries during early childhood is the unrestricted freedom achieved through locomotion combined with an unawareness of danger within the environment. Specific categories of injuries and appropriate prevention are best understood by associating them with the major developmental achievements of young children (Table 12-3). The discussions of injuries in Chapters 1 and 10 are also relevant to safety concerns at this age.

---

*Sources of information about nursing bottle caries and other aspects of child dental health include **National Institute of Dental Research,** NIH, Building 31, Room 2C35, 31 Center Drive MSC 2290, Bethesda , MD 20892-2290, (301) 496-4261; **American Society of Dentistry for Children,** 211 E. Chicago Ave., Suite 1036, Chicago, IL 60611, (312) 337-2169 or 800-544-2174 (outside Illinois); **American Dental Association,** 211 E. Chicago Ave., Chicago, IL 60611, (312) 440-2500 or 800-621-8099 (outside Illinois); and **Canadian Dental Association,** 1815 Alta Vista Dr., Ottawa, Ontario K1G 3Y6, (613) 523-1770. Guidelines for children's dental care are available in Wong DL: *Wong and Whaley's Clinical manual of pediatric nursing,* ed 4, St Louis, 1996, Mosby.

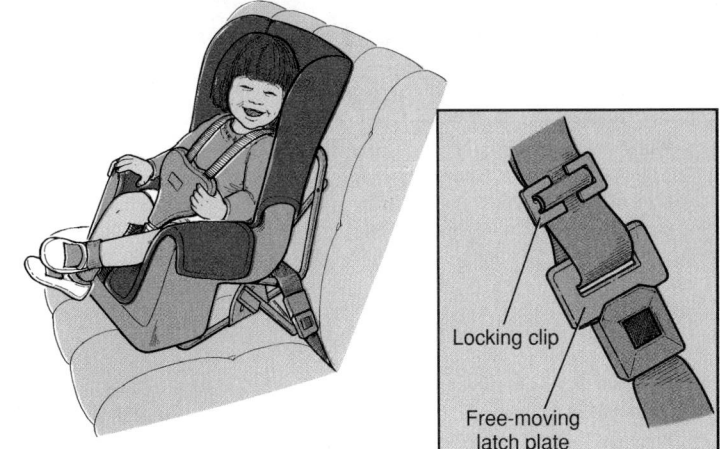

FIG. 12-9. Convertible seat in forward-facing position for older infants and children. *Inset:* Use of locking clip.

Motor Vehicle Injuries

Motor vehicle injuries cause more accidental deaths in all pediatric age-groups after age 1 year than any other type of injury or disease and are responsible for almost one half of all accidental deaths among children ages 1 to 4 years. Many of the deaths are caused by injuries within the car when restraints have not been used or have been used improperly. Approved restraints properly installed and applied can reduce the majority of fatalities and injuries (Osberg and DiScala, 1992).

Nurses have a responsibility for educating parents regarding the importance of car restraints and their proper use. Five types of restraints are available: (1) infant-only devices, (2) convertible models for both infants and toddlers, (3) boosters, (4) safety belts, and (5) devices for children with special needs (see Chapter 18). The infant-type restraints are discussed in Chapter 10; the convertible restraints and boosters are included here.

The ***convertible restraint*** is suitable for infants in the rearward-facing position and for toddlers in the forward-facing position (Fig. 12-9). The transition point for switching to the forward-facing position is defined by the manufacturer but is generally at a body weight of at least 9 kg (20 pounds) and 1 year of age (American Academy of Pediatrics, 1996). Convertible safety seats should be used until the child weighs at least 40 pounds. The restraint consists of a molded hard plastic or metal frame with energy-absorbing padding and a special harness system designed to hold the child firmly in the seat and distribute the forces to body areas that can withstand the impact.

Boosters are not restraint systems like the convertible devices, because they depend on the vehicle belts to hold the child and booster in place. Boosters are of two types: a ***low-shield model*** that primarily uses a lap belt (Fig. 12-10) and a ***belt-positioning model*** that uses a lap/shoulder belt. The combination lap/shoulder belt is preferred to the shield (lap belt) model (American Academy of Pediatrics, 1996).

Some older model restraints require the use of a top anchor (tether) strap to prevent the child from pitching forward

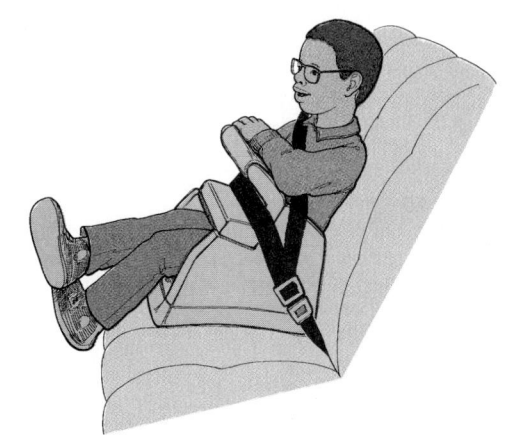

FIG. 12-10. Automobile booster seat. Note placement of shoulder strap (away from neck or face).

in a crash. If the tether strap is not used, up to 90% of the restraint's protection is lost. Instructions for proper installation of the tether strap and permanent bracket are included with the car restraint. Cars with free-sliding latchplates on the lap/shoulder belt require the use of a metal locking clip to keep the belt in a tight-holding position. The locking clip is threaded onto the belt above the latchplate (see inset, Fig. 12-9). If parents have newer cars with automatic lap/shoulder belts, they need to have additional lap belts installed to properly secure the restraint.

Children should use specially designed car restraints until they weigh at least 60 pounds or are 8 years old (American Academy of Pediatrics, 1996). Children who outgrow the convertible restraint may still be able to ride safely in a booster seat until the midpoint of the head is higher than the vehicle seat back. If a car safety seat is not available, the lap belt provides more protection than no restraint (except for infants, where there is no safe alternative to approved restraint devices). Shoulder-only automatic belts are designed to protect adults. Children should use the manual shoulder belts in the rear seat. Air bags do not take the place of child safety seats or seat belts. The safest area of the

TABLE 12-3. Injury prevention during early childhood

DEVELOPMENTAL ABILITIES RELATED TO RISK OF INJURY	INJURY PREVENTION

Walks, runs, and climbs
Able to open doors and gates
Can ride tricycle
Can throw ball and other objects
	Motor Vehicles
	Use federally approved car restraint; if restraint is not available, use lap belt
	Supervise child while playing outside
	Do not allow child to play on curb or behind a parked car
	Do not permit child to play in pile of leaves, snow, or large cardboard container in trafficked area
	Supervise tricycle riding
	Lock fences and doors if not directly supervising children
	Teach child to obey pedestrian safety rules
	    Obey traffic regulations; cross only at crosswalks and only when traffic signal indicates it is safe
	    Stand back a step from the curb until it's time to cross
	    Look left, right, and left again and check for turning cars before crossing street
	    Use sidewalks; when there is no sidewalk, walk on the left, facing traffic
	    Wear light colors at night, and attach fluorescent material to clothing

Able to explore if left unsupervised Has great curiosity Helpless in water; unaware of its danger; depth of water has no significance	**Drowning** Supervise closely when near any source of water Keep bathroom doors closed Have fence around swimming pool and lock gate Teach swimming and water safety
Able to reach heights by climbing, stretching, and standing on toes Pulls objects Explores any holes or opening Can open drawers and closets Unaware of potential sources of heat or fire Plays with mechanical objects	**Burns** Turn pot handles toward back of stove Place electric appliances, such as coffee maker and popcorn machine, toward back of counter Place guardrails in front of radiators, fireplaces, or other heating elements Store matches and cigarette lighters in locked or inaccessible area; discard carefully Place burning candles, incense, hot foods, and cigarettes out of reach Do not let tablecloth hang within child's reach Do not let electric cord from iron or other appliance hang within child's reach Cover electrical outlets with protective plastic caps Keep electrical wires hidden or out of reach Do not allow child to play with electrical appliance, wires, or lighters Stress danger of open flames; teach what "hot" means Always check bathwater temperature; adjust water heater temperature to 120° F or lower; do not allow children to play with faucets Apply a sunscreen when child is exposed to sunlight
Explores by putting objects in mouth Can open drawers, closets, and most containers Climbs Cannot read labels Does not know safe dose or amount	**Poisoning** Place all potentially toxic agents out of reach or in a locked cabinet Caution against eating nonedible items, such as plants Replace medications or poisons immediately; replace child-guard caps properly Administer medications as a drug, not as a candy Do not store large surplus of toxic agents Promptly discard empty poison containers; never reuse to store a food item or other poison Teach child not to play in trash containers Never remove labels from containers of toxic substances Have syrup of ipecac in home; use only if advised Know number and location of nearest poison control center (usually listed in front of telephone directory)
Able to open doors and some windows Goes up and down stairs Depth perception unrefined	**Falls** Keep screen in window, nail securely, and use guardrail Place gates at top and bottom of stairs Keep doors locked or use child-proof doorknob covers at entry to stairs, high porch, or other elevated area, including laundry chute Remove unsecured or scatter rugs Apply nonskid decals in bathtub or shower Keep crib rails fully raised and mattress at lowest level

TABLE 12-3. Injury prevention during early childhood—cont'd

DEVELOPMENTAL ABILITIES RELATED TO RISK OF INJURY	INJURY PREVENTION
	Falls, cont'd
	Place carpeting under crib and in bathroom
	Keep large toys and bumper pads out of crib or playpen (child can use these as "stairs" to climb out), then move to youth bed when child is able to climb out of crib
	Avoid using walkers, especially near stairs
	Dress in safe clothing (soles that do not "catch" on floor, tied shoelaces, pant legs that do not touch floor)
	Keep child restrained in vehicles; never leave unattended in shopping cart
	Supervise at playgrounds; select play areas with soft ground cover and safe equipment
Puts things in mouth May swallow hard or nonedible pieces of food	**Choking and Suffocation** Avoid large, round chunks of meat, such as whole hot dogs (slice lengthwise into short pieces) Avoid fruit with pits, fish with bones, dried beans, hard candy, chewing gum, nuts, popcorn, grapes, marshmallows Choose large sturdy toys without sharp edges or small removable parts Discard old refrigerators, ovens, and so on; if storing an old appliance, remove the door Keep automatic garage door transmitter in inaccessible place Select safe toy boxes or chests without heavy, hinged lids

Still clumsy in many skills
Easily distracted from tasks
Unaware of potential danger from strangers or other people
	Bodily Damage
	Avoid giving sharp or pointed objects—such as knives, scissors, or toothpicks—especially when walking or running
	Do not allow lollipops or similar objects in mouth when walking or running
	Teach safety precautions (e.g., to carry knife or scissors with pointed end away from face)
	Store all dangerous tools, garden equipment, and firearms in locked cabinet
	Be alert to danger of supervised animals and household pets
	Use safety glass and decals on large glassed areas, such as sliding glass doors
	Teach child name, address, and phone number and to ask for help from appropriate people (cashier, security guard, policeman) if lost; have identification on child (shown in clothes, inside shoe)
	Teach stranger safety
	   Avoid personalized clothing in public places
	   Never go with a stranger
	   Tell parents if anyone makes child feel uncomfortable in any way
	   Always listen to child's concerns regarding others' behavior
	   Teach child to say "no" when confronted with uncomfortable situations

car for children is the back seat. Children who must ride in the front passenger-side with an air bag should be positioned as far back as possible.

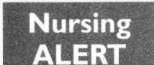 **Nursing ALERT** Safety belts should be worn low on the hips, snug, and not on the abdominal area. Children should be taught to sit up straight to allow for proper fit. The shoulder belt is used *only* if it does not cross the child's neck or face.

For any restraint to be effective, it must be used consistently and properly. Examples of misuse include misrouting the vehicle seat belt through the restraint, failing to use the vehicle seat belt to secure the restraint, failing to use a tether strap, failing to use the restraint's harness system, and incor-

rectly positioning the child, especially facing infants forward instead of rearward (Graham, Kittredge, and Stuemky, 1992). To address these issues, nurses must stress correct use of car restraints and rules that ensure compliance (see Family Home Care box on p. 378). Children riding in car safety seats are generally much better behaved than children left unrestrained, which can be a major benefit to parents and should be emphasized as an additional advantage of restraints.*

Injuries may also occur during sudden stops when objects

*American Academy of Pediatrics, 141 Northwest Point Blvd., P.O. Box 927, Elk Grove Village, IL 60007, (800) 433-9016; and local division of traffic safety or Department of Transportation, National Highway Traffic Safety Administration, (800) 424-9393. Guidelines for car seat safety are available in Wong DL: *Wong and Whaley's Clinical manual of pediatric nursing,* ed 4, St Louis, 1996, Mosby.

FAMILY HOME CARE
Using Car Safety Seats

Read manufacturer's directions and follow them exactly.
Anchor safety seat securely to car's seat and apply harness snugly to child.
Do not start the car until *everyone* is properly restrained.
Always use the restraint, even for short trips.
If child begins to climb out or undo the harness, firmly say, "No." It may be necessary to stop the car to reinforce the expected behavior. Use rewards, such as stars or stickers to encourage cooperative behavior.
Encourage child to help attach buckles, straps, and shields, but always double-check fastenings.
Decrease boredom on long trips. Keep soft toys in the car for quiet play; talk to child; point out objects and teach child about them. Stop periodically. If child wishes to sleep, make sure child stays in the restraint.
Insist that others who transport children also follow these safety rules.

are left unrestrained. On sudden impact a loose ball becomes a projectile missile. Therefore all items should be secured or stored in the trunk.

Children over 3 years of age are often involved in pedestrian traffic injuries. Because of their gross motor skills of walking, running, and climbing and their fine motor skills of opening doors and fence gates, they are likely to be in hazardous areas when unsupervised. Unaware of danger and unable to approximate the speed of a car, they are hit by moving vehicles. Running after a ball, playing in a pile of leaves or snow or inside a cardboard box, riding a tricycle, and playing behind a parked car or near the curb are common activities that may result in a vehicular tragedy. A precaution when children are playing in driveways is attaching to the tricycle a pole with a bright flag that is high enough to be visible through an automobile's back window. Another safeguard is the use of a device that beeps when the vehicle is driven in reverse to alert children to the oncoming car, van, or truck.

Preventing vehicular injuries involves protecting and educating children about the danger of moving or parked vehicles. Although preschool children are too young to be trusted to always obey, the parent should emphasize looking for moving vehicles before crossing the street, recognizing the stop and go colors of traffic lights, and following traffic officers' signals. Most important, what is preached must be practiced. Children learn through imitation, and consistency reinforces learning.

Drowning

Drowning, not including drowning from water transportation, ranks second among boys and third among girls ages 1 to 4 years as a cause of accidental death. With well-developed skills of locomotion, toddlers are able to reach potentially dangerous areas, such as bathtubs, toilets, buckets, swimming pools, hot tubs, and lakes. Their intense drive for exploration and investigation, combined with an unawareness of the danger of water and their helplessness in water, makes drowning always a viable threat. It is also one category of injuries that results in death within minutes, diminishing the chance for rescue and survival. Supervising children when near any

source of water is essential; teaching swimming and water safety can be helpful but cannot be regarded as sufficient protection.

Burns

Burns rank second to motor vehicle injuries among girls and third among boys in this age-group as a cause of accidental death. Their ability to climb, stretch, and reach objects above their head makes any hot surface a potential source of danger. Scalds from children pulling pots on top of themselves are a major source of burns. As a precaution, pot handles should be turned toward the back of the stove. Ideally, the knobs for controlling the range burners should be out of reach, not on the front panel where nimble fingers can turn them on and accidentally touch the hot burner. Oven doors should be closed whenever the oven is turned on or when it is cooling. The outside of doors of automatic self-cleaning ovens may become hot and, if touched, could cause a burn. Other sources of heat, such as radiators, fireplaces, accessible furnaces, kerosene heaters, or wood-burning stoves, should have guards placed in front of them. The tops of some of these heaters are designed to become hot enough to boil water to provide humidity. They are hazardous if touched or if the pan of water is spilled. Portable electric heaters must be placed in a high area, well out of reach of climbing young children.

Hot objects such as candles, incense, cigarettes, pots of tea or coffee, or irons must be placed away from children. The flame of a candle and the smoke of a cigarette invite investigation. Ashtrays with a center well are preferred to prevent the cigarette from falling off the rim, and adults should try not to smoke, cook, or drink hot liquids when children are physically close. If tablecloths are used, the edges should be placed out of reach to prevent injuries from both burns and falling objects.

Flame burns represent one of the most fatal types of burns and commonly occur when children play with matches and accidentally set themselves (and the home) on fire. To prevent flame burns, matches and lighters must be stored safely away from children, and parents need to teach children the dangers of playing with such objects. In addition, all homes should have smoke detectors installed to alert the occupants of a fire. A safety plan for immediate escape is also essential.

Electrical burns also represent an immediate danger to children. With preschoolers' ability to manipulate small, thin objects, they are able to insert hairpins or other conductive articles into electrical sockets. Young toddlers may explore outlets and wires by mouthing them. Since water is an excellent conductor, the chance for a severe circumoral electrical burn is great. Electrical outlets should have protective guards plugged into them when not in use (Fig. 12-11) or be made inaccessible by having furniture placed in front of them when feasible. Children should not be allowed to play with electrical cords or appliances, which should be kept out of reach as much as possible.

An example of an appliance that interests children and can present a hazard is an electric popcorn popper. Children can become so excited by the popping that they may inadvertently pull the electric cord and popper off the table, resulting in a burn from contact with the hot oil, corn, or appliance.

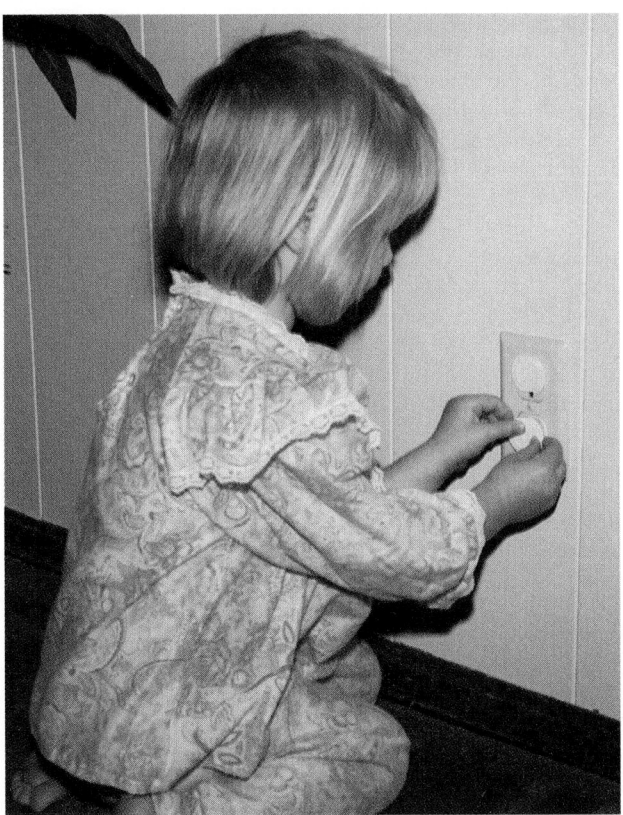

FIG. 12-11. Special plastic caps in electrical sockets prevent young fingers from exploring dangerous areas.

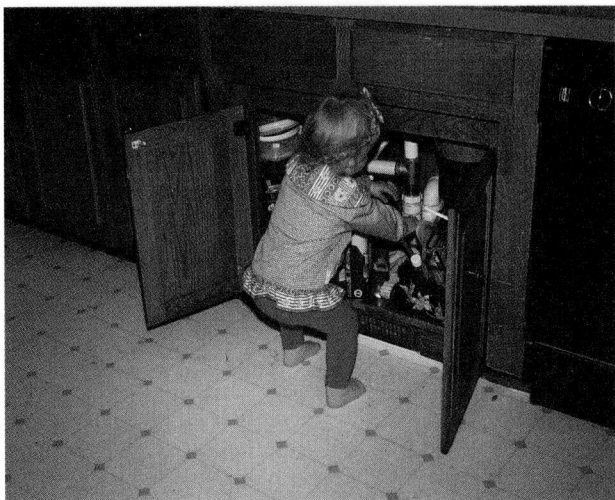

FIG. 12-12. Children are most likely to ingest substances that are on their level, such as cleaning agents stored under sinks, rat poison, or diaper pail deodorants.

Scald burns are the most common type of thermal injury in children. A scalding burn is often caused by high-temperature tap water, which children come in contact with either as a result of turning on the hot-water faucet, falling into a bathtub of hot water, or deliberate abuse. Always supervising youngsters when they are near tap water and checking bathwater temperatures are methods of prevention. Limiting household water temperatures to less than 49° C (120° F) is also recommended. At this temperature it takes 10 minutes of exposure to the water to cause a full-thickness burn. Conversely, water temperatures of 54° C (130° F), the usual setting of most water heaters, expose household members to the risk of full-thickness burns within 30 seconds. Nurses can help prevent such burns by advising parents of this common household danger and recommending that they readjust the water heater to a safe temperature. A meat or candy thermometer is a convenient way to measure water temperature. An easy-to-read hot-water gauge that changes color to show water temperatures between 120° and 150° is also available; it shows a "hot," "cool," or "OK" water temperature. A special device can also be added to the faucet that reduces the water flow once the set temperature is reached.

Poisoning

Ingestion of toxic agents is common during early childhood. The highest incidence occurs in children in the 2-year-old age-group. Although in many instances poisoning does not result in mortality, it may cause significant morbidity, such as

esophageal stricture from lye ingestion. Mouthing activity continues to be prevalent after 1 year of age, and exploring objects by tasting them is part of children's curious investigation. Almost every nonfood substance is potentially harmful, including many house plants, and by 2 years of age toddlers are able to climb most heights, open most drawers or closets, and unscrew most lids. By trial and error younger children also manage to undo tops of bottles, plastic containers, aerosol cans, and jars, including those with child-resistant lids. In addition, pharmacists often transfer drugs to regular containers for the elderly, who may have difficulty with child-resistant lids. Newer forms of drugs, such as transdermal patches and cough-suppressant lozenges, have created additional dangers, since they are not packaged with safety caps and the lozenges look like candy.

The major reason for poisoning is improper storage (Fig. 12-12). The guidelines suggested in Chapter 10 apply to children in this age-group as well. However, unlike the infant who was confined to certain heights and unable to unlatch inventive locks, young children manage to find access to many high-level, tight-security places. For this age-group only a locked cabinet is safe.

Parents should have two doses of ipecac syrup for each child in the home, know its proper use and administration in case of a poisoning, and have the phone number and location of the nearest poison control center. Emergency and preventive measures for accidental poisoning are discussed in Chapter 14.

Falls

Falls are still a hazard to children in this age-group, although by the later part of early childhood gross and fine motor skills are well developed, decreasing the incidence of falls down stairs or from chairs. However, playground injuries are common. Children need to be taught safety at play areas, such as no horseplay on high slides or jungle gyms, *sitting* on swings, and staying away from moving swings. Passive prevention includes placement of grass, sand, or wood chips under play equipment. Swing seats should be made of plastic, canvas, or rubber and have smooth or rounded edges. Slides should not exceed an incline of 30 degrees, have evenly spaced rungs for climbing, and have protective "tunnels."

The climbing and running of the typical toddler are complicated by the child's total neglect for and lack of appreciation of danger. Gates must be placed at both ends of stairs. Accessible windows that are left open during warm weather must be screened or guarded with a rail. Falling from open windows is a major cause of accidental death in urban, lower socioeconomic groups. Doors leading to stairwells or porches must be locked, since preschoolers can easily open them. Laundry chutes are another potential danger and typically are not locked because of their frequent use. A convenient type of lock is a sliding bar or hook that can be attached to the door and frame at a level higher than the child can reach.

Cribs and vehicles are other sources of falls. To avoid injury, crib rails should be fully raised, the mattress should be kept at the lowest position, and toys or bumper pads that may be used as steps to climb out should be removed. Ideally the floor should be carpeted. Once children reach a height of 89 cm (35 inches), they should sleep in a bed rather than a crib. If a bunk bed is selected, parents should be aware of possible dangers: falls and head entrapment between the mattress and guardrail or between the supporting mattress slats. If the beds are constructed of tubular metal, parents should check for breaks or cracks in the metal and welds, which may lead to collapse and injury. Children who sleep on the top bunk should be 6 years or older.

Children who are unrestrained can fall from high chairs, shopping carts, carriages, and car seats. Therefore proper restraint and adequate supervision are essential.

Clothing can also increase the chance of falling. Slippery shoes or socks, rubber-soled shoes that "catch" on the floor and rug, and loose or cuffed pants can easily make a child fall. Simple safety measures, such as checking clothing and shoes, keeping shoelaces tied with double knots or using self-adhering closures, can prevent accidents.

Aspiration and Suffocation

Usually by 1 year of age children chew well, but they may have difficulty with large pieces of food, such as meat and whole hot dogs, and with hard foods, such as nuts or dried beans. Young children cannot discard pits from fruit or bones from fish. It takes practice to learn how to chew gum without swallowing it. Therefore, the same precautions as discussed for infants regarding food selection must be implemented (see Chapter 10).

Play objects for toddlers must still be chosen with an awareness of danger from small parts. Large, sturdy toys without sharp edges or removable parts are safest. Coins, paper clips, pins, bells, button batteries, pull-tabs on cans, thumbtacks, nails, screws, jewelry (especially pierced earrings), and all types of pins are common household objects that can cause significant harm if swallowed or aspirated. Because of the danger of aspiration, parents should be taught emergency procedures for choking (see Airway Obstruction, Chapter 23).*

---

*Home care instructions on caring for the choking child are available in Wong DL: *Wong and Whaley's Clinical manual of pediatric nursing,* ed 4, St Louis, 1996, Mosby.

Another cause of death by traumatic asphyxiation is from electrically operated garage doors. Young children playing in the garage may become trapped under the door. Although the automatic doors should reverse when striking an object, they may not do so when hitting a flexible object or one that is very close to the ground. Precautions include placing controls where they are inaccessible to children, such as high on a wall and in a locked car, and instructing children that the transmitter is not a toy. Periodically the door should be checked to determine if it returns after striking an object.

Suffocation from causes seen during infancy is less frequent, but old refrigerators, ovens, and other large appliances are an ever-present threat. Toddlers can climb inside these appliances and, if they close the door behind them, can be trapped inside. Discarding old appliances or removing all doors during storage prevents such tragic deaths. Toddlers may also suffocate when unsafe toy box lids accidentally close on their head or neck. Parents should be advised of this danger and encouraged to buy storage chests with lightweight, removable covers.

Bodily Damage

Toddlers are still clumsy in many of their skills and can seriously harm themselves when walking while holding a sharp or pointed object or having food or objects such as spoons in their mouths. Preventing such occurrences is the best approach with toddlers. With preschoolers teaching safety is most important. The child should be taught that when walking with a pointed object such as a knife or scissors, the pointed end is held away from the face. Dangerous garden or workshop equipment and all firearms should be stored in a locked cabinet. Power lawn mowers are especially dangerous, and young children should not be allowed in an area where a mower is being used; nor should they be taken for a ride on a mower or allowed to operate the device. Safety education should include respect for firearms and their proper and appropriate use, including nonpowder guns, such as air guns and rifles, which cause serious penetrating injuries (Lie and others, 1994). In addition, the child should be warned of and protected against potential danger from animals (see Bodily Damage, Chapter 10, and Animal Bites, Chapter 30).

Toys can be a source of danger, and safety must be a prime consideration when selecting toys (see Family Home Care: Toy Safety, Chapter 4). Most toys have age ranges written on them to designate their safety, but this information must be used with knowledge of the specific child's readiness.

Household safety should be practiced and includes the usual precautions recommended for any age-group (see Family Home Care: Child Safety Home Checklist, Chapter 10). An additional safeguard for young children is the use of safety glass in doors, windows, and tabletops and the application of decals on glassed areas to lessen the likelihood of running through glass. Also, children should not be allowed to run, jump, wrestle, or play ball near glass structures (Armstrong and Molyneux, 1992).

ANTICIPATORY GUIDANCE— CARE OF FAMILIES

Understanding toddlers is fundamental to successful childrearing. Nurses, particularly those in ambulatory or child

FAMILY HOME CARE
Guidance During Toddler Years

Ages 12 to 18 Months

Prepare parents for expected behavioral changes of toddler, especially negativism and ritualism.

Assess present feeding habits and encourage gradual weaning from bottle and increased intake of solid foods.

Stress expected feeding changes of physiologic anorexia, presence of food fads and strong taste preferences, need for scheduled routine at mealtimes, inability to sit through an entire meal, and lack of table manners.

Assess sleep patterns at night, particularly habit of a bedtime bottle, which is a major cause of dental caries, and procrastination behaviors that delay hour of sleep.

Prepare parents for potential dangers of the home, particularly motor vehicle, poisoning, and falling injuries; give appropriate suggestions for safeproofing the home.

Discuss need for firm but gentle discipline and ways in which to deal with negativism and temper tantrums; stress positive benefits of appropriate discipline.

Emphasize importance for both child and parents of brief, periodic separations.

Discuss new toys that use developing gross and fine motor, language, cognitive, and social skills.

Emphasize need for dental supervision, types of basic dental hygiene at home, and food habits that predispose to caries; stress importance of supplemental fluoride.

Ages 18 to 24 Months

Stress importance of peer companionship in play.

Explore need for preparation for additional sibling; stress importance of preparing child for new experiences.

Discuss present discipline methods, their effectiveness, and parents' feelings about child's negativism; stress that negativism is important aspect of developing self-assertion and independence and is not a sign of spoiling.

Discuss signs of readiness for toilet training; emphasize importance of waiting for physical and psychologic readiness.

Discuss development of fears, such as darkness or loud noises, and of habits, such as security blanket or thumbsucking; stress normalcy of these transient behaviors.

Prepare parents for signs of regression in time of stress.

Assess child's ability to separate easily from parents for brief periods of separation under familiar circumstances.

Allow parents opportunity to express their feelings of weariness, frustration, and exasperation; be aware that it is often difficult to love toddlers at times when they are not asleep!

Point out some of the expected changes of the next year, such as longer attention span, somewhat less negativism, and increased concern for pleasing others.

Ages 24 to 36 Months

Discuss importance of imitation and domestic mimicry and need to include child in activities.

Discuss approaches toward toilet training, particularly realistic expectations and attitude toward accidents.

Stress uniqueness of toddlers' thought processes, especially through their use of language, poor understanding of time, causal relationships in terms of proximity of events, and inability to see events from another's perspective.

Stress that discipline still must be quite structured and concrete and that relying solely on verbal reasoning and explanation leads to injuries, confusion, and misunderstanding.

Discuss investigation of preschool or daycare center toward completion of second year.

---

health centers, are in a favorable position to assist parents in meeting the tasks and needs of children in this age-group. Prevention yields better results than treatment. Anticipatory guidance is paramount if one wishes to prevent future problems (see Family Home Care box). Advice is sometimes not the sole answer. Actual assistance, such as being available for home visiting or telephone consulting, should be part of the nurse's flexible repertoire of interventions. Whether parents

are experiencing the rearing dilemmas of a first or a subsequent child, they benefit from sharing their feelings, frustrations, and satisfactions. They need adult companionship, freedom from childrearing responsibilities, and periodic separations from their children. Part of a nurse's responsibility is to provide opportunities for parents to express their feelings and to meet their physical, mental, and spiritual needs.

KEY POINTS

- The toddler stage, extending from 12 to 36 months, is a period of intense exploration of the environment.
- Biologic development during the toddler years is characterized by the acquisition of fine and gross motor skills that allow children to master a wide variety of activities.

- Although most of the physiologic systems are mature by the end of toddlerhood, development of certain areas of the brain is still occurring, allowing for greater intellectual capacity.

- Locomotion is the major gross motor skill acquired during toddlerhood, followed by increased eye-hand coordination.
- Specific tasks in the psychosocial development of a toddler include differentiating self from others, tolerating separation from parent, coping with delayed gratification, controlling bodily functions, acquiring socially acceptable behavior, communicating verbally, and interacting with others in a less egocentric manner.
- According to Erikson the major developmental task of toddlerhood is acquiring a sense of autonomy while overcoming a sense of doubt and shame.
- Language is the major cognitive achievement in toddlerhood.
- In Piaget's sensorimotor and preconceptual phases of development, the toddler experiments by incorporating the old learning of secondary circular reactions with new skills and applies this knowledge to new situations. There is the beginning of rational judgment, an understanding of causal relationships, and discovery of objects as objects. Preconceptual thought is characterized by egocentrism, centration, global organization of thought processes, animism, and irreversibility.

- Development of body image occurs with increasing motor ability, at which point toddlers recognize the importance and capacity of body parts.
- The two phases of differentiation of self from significant others are separation and individuation.
- The most striking characteristic of language development during early childhood is the increasing level of comprehension.
- Parental concerns during the toddler years include toilet training, coping with sibling rivalry, limit-setting and discipline, dealing with temper tantrums, negativism, and regression.
- Effective discipline techniques for toddlers include reward, ignoring or extinction, and time-out.
- Nutrition is important at this stage because eating habits established in toddlerhood tend to have lasting effects in subsequent years.
- Regular dental examinations, fluoride supplementation, removal of plaque, and provision of a low-cariogenic diet promote optimum dental health.
- Because of increased locomotion, toddlers are at high risk for sustaining injuries. Fatal injuries are primarily the result of motor vehicle accidents, drownings, and burns.

REFERENCES

American Academy of Pediatrics, Committee on Injury and Poison Prevention: Selecting and using the most appropriate car seat safety seats for growing children: guidelines for counseling parents, *Pediatrics* 97(5):761-763, 1996.

American Academy of Pediatrics, Committee on Nutrition: Fluoride supplementation for children, *Pediatrics* 95(5):777, 1995.

Armstrong AM, Molyneux E: Glass injuries to children, *Br Med J* 304(6823):360, 1992.

Forgac MT: Timely statement of the American Dietetic Association: dietary guidance for healthy children, *J Am Dietetic Assoc* 95(3):370, 1995.

Graham CJ, Kittredge O, Stuemky JH: Injuries associated with child safety seat misuse, *Pediatr Emerg Care* 8:351-353, 1992.

Lidster CA, Horsburgh ME: Masturbation—beyond myth and taboo, *Nurs Forum* 29(3):18-27, 1994.

Lie L and others: American Public Health Association/American Academy of Pediatrics Injury Prevention Standards, *Pediatrics* 94(6:2):1046-1048, 1994.

Osberg JS, Di Scala C: Morbidity among pediatric motor vehicle crash victims: the effectiveness of seat belts, *Am J Public Health* 82(3):422-425, 1992.

Serwint JR and others: Child-rearing practices and nursing caries, *Pediatrics* 92(2):233-237, 1993.

Stark M: Assessment and management of the care of children with nocturnal enuresis: guidelines for primary care, *Nurs Pract Forum* 5(3):170-176, 1994.

BIBLIOGRAPHY

Growth and Development

Dixon SD, Stein MT: *Encounters with children: a practical guide to pediatric behavior and development*, ed 2, St Louis 1992, Mosby.

Fina DK: The spiritual needs of pediatric patients and their families, *AORN J* 62(4):556-564, 1995.

Gross D, Tucker S: Parenting confidence during toddlerhood: a comparison of mothers and fathers, *Nurs Pract: Am J Primary Health Care* 19(10):25, 29-30, 33-34, 1994.

Howard BT: Growing together: the toddler years need not be turbulent, *Contemp Pediatr* 7(6):21-40, 1990.

King EH, Logsdon DA, Schroeder SR: Risk factors for developmental delay among infants and toddlers, *Child Health Care* 21(1):39-52, 1992.

Zuckerman BS, Frank DA: Infancy and toddler years. In Levine MD and others, editors *Developmental-behavioral pediatrics*, ed 2, Philadelphia, 1992, WB Saunders.

Toilet Training

Berk L, Friman P: Epidemiologic aspects of toilet training, *Clin Pediatr* 29(5):278-282, 1990.

Brooks JG: *I'm a big kid now: a book about toilet training,* Neenah, WI, 1992, Kimberly Clark Corporation.

Loening-Baucke V: Management of chronic constipation in infants and toddlers, *Am Fam Physician* 49(2):397-400, 411-413, 1994.

Stadtler AC: Preventing encopresis, *Pediatr Nurs* 15(3):282-284, 1989.

Sibling Rivalry

Castiglia PT: Sibling rivalry, *J Pediatr Health Care* 3(1):52-54, 1989.

Lansky V: *A new baby at Koko bear's house,* Deephaven, MN, 1990, The Book Peddlers.

Leung AK, Robson LM: Sibling rivalry, *Clin Pediatr* 30(5):314-317, 1991.

Pakula LC: Sibling rivalry, *Pediatr Rev* 13(2):72-73, 1992.

Schmitt BD: Sibling rivalry toward a new baby, *Contemp Pediatr* 7(3):111-112, 1990.

Negativism/Temper Tantrums

Blum NJ and others: Disciplining young children: the role of verbal instructions and reasoning, *Pediatrics* 96(2:1):336-341, 1995.

Brayden RM, Poole SR: Common behavioral problems in infants and children, *Prim Care* 22(1):81-97, 1995.

Gross D, Conrad B: Temperament in toddlerhood, *J Pediatr Nurs* 10(3):146-151, 1995.

Needlman R, Howard B, Zuckerman B: Temper tantrums: when to worry, *Contemp Pediatr* 6(8):12-34, 1989.

Schmitt BD: The stubborn toddler who just says "No," *Contemp Pediatr* 7(4):71-72, 1990.

Socolar RR, Stein RE: Spanking infants and toddlers: maternal belief and practice, *Pediatrics* 95(1):105-111, 1995.

Nutrition

American Academy of Pediatrics, Committee on Nutrition: *Pediatric nutrition handbook,* Elk Grove Village, IL, 1993, The Academy.

Feeney B: Teaching aid . . . child health, nutrition, *Nurs Times* 91(10):42-44, 1995.

Lucas B: Nutrition in childhood. In Mahan LK, Arlin MT: *Krause's food, nutrition, and diet therapy,* ed 8, Philadelphia, 1992, WB Saunders.

McGarr B, Dwyer J, Holland HM: Delivering nutrition services in early intervention in rural areas, *Infants & Young Child* 7(3):52-62, 1995.

Pipes P, Trahms CM: *Nutrition in infancy and childhood,* ed 5, St Louis, 1993, Mosby.

Satter E: Feeding dynamics: helping children to eat well, *J Pediatr Health Care* 9(4):178-184, 1995.

Schmitt BD: A commonsense approach to sweets, *Contemp Pediatr* 8(9):63-65, 1991.

Dental Health

American Academy of Pediatric Dentistry: *Recommendations for preventive pediatric dental care,* Chicago, The Academy, May 1992.

Johnsen DC: The role of the pediatrician in identifying and treating dental caries, *Pediatr Clin North Am* 38(5):1173-1181, 1991.

Jones KF, Berg JH, Coody D: Update in pediatric dentistry, *J Pediatr Health Care* 8(4):160-167, 1994.

Lloyd S: Developments in oral health: teaching parents to look after children's teeth, *Prof Care Mother Child* 4(2):34-36, 1994.

McDonald RE, Avery DR: *Dentistry for the child and adolescent,* ed. 6, 1994, St Louis, Mosby.

Nowak AJ: What pediatricians can do to promote oral health, *Contemp Pediatr* 10(4):90-106, 1993.

Ogasawara T, Watanabe T, Kasahara H: Readiness for toothbrushing of young children, *J Dent Child* 59(5):353-359, 1992.

Schulte JR, Druyan ME, Hagen JC: Early childhood tooth decay, *Clin Pediatr* 31(12):727-730, 1992.

Von Burg MM, Sanders BJ, Weddell JA: Baby bottle tooth decay: a concern for all mothers, *Pediatr Nurs* 21(6):515-519, 1995.

Injury Prevention

Accident Facts, Chicago, 1995, National Safety Council.

Agran P, Winn D, Castillo D: Unsupervised children in vehicles: a risk for pediatric trauma, *Pediatrics* 87(1):70-73, 1991.

American Academy of Pediatrics, Committee on Injury and Poison Prevention: Children in pickup trucks, *Pediatrics* 88(2):393-394, 1991.

American Academy of Pediatrics Committee on Injury and Poison Prevention: Injuries associated with infant walkers, *Pediatrics* 95(5):778-780, 1995.

Bull MJ, Stroup KB, Doll JP: A parent guide: selecting and using car safety seats, *Contemp Pediatr* 7(7):113-118, 1990.

Bull MJ and others: Establishing special needs car seat loan program, *Pediatrics* 85(4):540-547, 1990.

Christoffel KK, Naureckas SM: Firearm injuries in children and adolescents: epidemiology and preventive approaches, *Curr Opin Pediatr* 6(5):519-524, 1994.

Gielen AC and others: In-home injury prevention practices for infants and toddlers: the role of parental beliefs, barriers, and housing quality, *Health Educ Q* 22(1):85-95, 1995.

Johnston C, Rivara FP, Soderberg R: Children in car crashes: analysis of data for injury and use of restraints, *Pediatrics* 93(6:1):960-965, 1994.

McFadden EA: Equipment safety for infants and children: beyond clinical practice, *J Pediatr Nurs* 9(5):335-336, 1994.

Schubert W, Ahrenholz DH, Solem LD: Burns from hot oil and grease: a public health hazard, *J Burn Care Rehabil* 11(6):558-562, 1990.

Sewell KH, Gaines SK: A developmental approach to childhood safety education, *Pediatr Nurs* 19(5):464-466, 1993.

Stuy M, Green M, Doll J: Child care centers: a community resource for injury prevention, *J Dev Behav Pediatr* 14(4):224-229, 1993.

Stylianos S, Eichelberger MR, Pediatric trauma: prevention strategies, *Pediatr Clin North Am* 40(6):1359-1368, 1993.

Swartz MK: Playground safety, *J Pediatr Health Care* 6(3):161-162, 1992.

Chapter 13

HEALTH PROMOTION OF THE PRESCHOOLER AND FAMILY

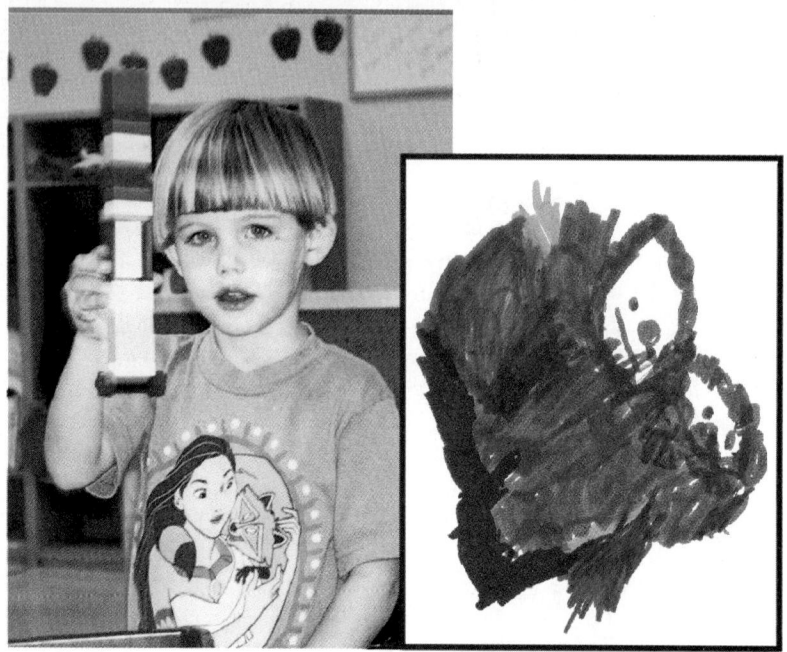

" *One day I played with my cousin Nicholas and I got these bumps. It's a virus.* " **Kaitlyn,** age 3 years

RELATED TOPICS *

LEARNING OBJECTIVES

On completion of this chapter the reader will be able to:

- Identify the major biologic, psychosocial, cognitive, moral, spiritual, and social developments that occur during the preschool years
- List the benefits of imaginary playmates
- Prepare preschoolers for preschool or daycare experience

- Provide parents with guidelines for sex education
- Provide parents with guidelines for dealing with a child's fears and sleep problems
- Recognize the causes of stuttering during the preschool years

- Offer parents suggestions for preventing speech problems
- Recognize feeding patterns of preschoolers
- Provide anticipatory guidance to parents regarding injury prevention based on the preschooler's developmental achievements

*See also Related Topics in Chapter 10.

PROMOTING OPTIMUM GROWTH AND DEVELOPMENT

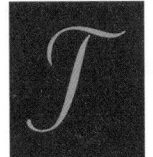

*T*he combined biologic, psychosocial, cognitive, spiritual, and social achievements during the *preschool period* (3 to 5 years of age) prepare preschoolers for their most significant change in life-style—entrance into school. Their control of bodily systems, experience of brief and prolonged periods of separation, ability to interact cooperatively with other children and adults, use of language for mental symbolization, and increased attention span and memory ready them for the next major period—the school years. Successful achievement of previous levels of growth and development is essential for preschoolers to refine many of the tasks that were mastered during the toddler years.

BIOLOGIC DEVELOPMENT

The rate of physical growth slows and stabilizes during the preschool years. The average *weight* at 3 years is 14.6 kg (32 pounds), at 4 years 16.7 kg (36¾ pounds), and at 5 years 18.7 kg (41¼ pounds). The average weight gain remains about 2.3 kg (5 pounds) per year.

Growth in *height* also remains steady at a yearly increase of 6.75 to 7.5 cm (2½ to 3 inches) and generally occurs in elongation of the legs rather than of the trunk. The average height at 3 years is 95 cm (37¼ inches), at 4 years 103 cm (40½ inches), and at 5 years 110 cm (43¼ inches).

Physical proportions no longer resemble those of the squat, potbellied toddler. The preschooler is slender but sturdy, graceful, agile, and posturally erect. There is little difference in physical characteristics according to sex, except as dictated by such factors as dress and hairstyle.

Most *bodily systems* are mature and stable and can adjust to moderate stress and change. During this period most children are toilet trained. Motor development consists for the most part of increases in strength and refinement of previously learned skills, such as walking, running, and jumping. However, muscle development and bone growth are still far from mature. Excessive activity and overexertion can injure delicate tissues. Good posture, appropriate exercise, and adequate nutrition and rest are essential for optimum development of the musculoskeletal system.

Gross and Fine Motor Behavior

Walking, running, climbing, and jumping are well established by age 36 months. Refinement in eye-hand and muscle coordination is evident in several areas. At age 3 the preschooler rides a tricycle, walks on tiptoe, balances on one foot for a few seconds, and broad jumps. By age 4 the child skips and hops proficiently on one foot (Fig. 13-1) and catches a ball reliably. By age 5 the child skips on alternate feet, jumps rope, and begins to skate and swim.

Fine motor development is evident in the child's increasingly skillful manipulation, such as in drawing and dressing. These skills provide readiness for learning and independence for entry into school.

Caryn Stoermer Hess, MS, RN, revised this chapter.

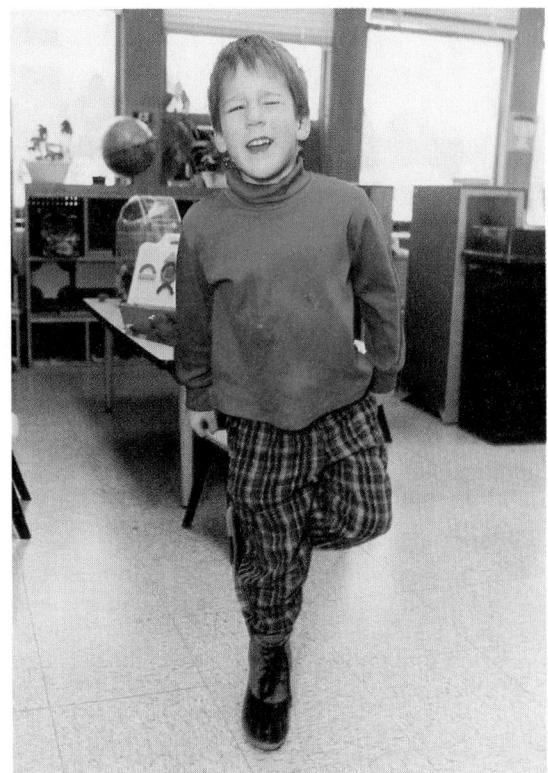

FIG. 13-1. A 4-year-old child has sufficient balance to walk or hop on one foot.

PSYCHOSOCIAL DEVELOPMENT

Developing a Sense of Initiative (Erikson)

If preschoolers have mastered the tasks of the toddler period, they are ready to face the developmental endeavors of this stage. The chief psychosocial task of the preschool period is acquiring a sense of *initiative.* Children are in a stage of energetic learning. They play, work, and live to the fullest and feel a real sense of accomplishment and satisfaction in their activities. Conflict arises when children overstep the limits of their ability and inquiry and experience a sense of *guilt* for not having behaved or acted appropriately. Feelings of guilt, anxiety, and fear may also result from thoughts that differ from expected behavior.

A particularly stressful thought is wishing one's parent dead. As a sense of rivalry or competition develops between the child and same-sex parent, the child may think of ways to get rid of the interfering parent. In most situations this rivalry is resolved by strongly identifying with the same-sex parent and peers during the school years. However, if that parent dies before the identification process is completed, the preschooler can be overwhelmed with feelings of guilt for having wished and therefore "caused" the death. Clarifying for children that wishes cannot and do not make events occur is essential in helping them overcome their guilt and anxiety.

Development of the *superego,* or *conscience,* has its beginnings toward the end of the toddler years and is a major task for preschoolers (see Cultural Awareness box). Learning right

CULTURAL AWARENESS
Learning Sociocultural Mores

Developing a conscience implies learning the sociocultural mores of the family's heritage. Depending on the type of attitudes conveyed, children will learn not only appropriate behaviors, but also tolerant, biased, or prejudicial values concerning their ethnic, religious, and social background and those of other groups. Much of this influence may remain dormant until they associate with children or adults of a different heritage. Then, depending on the particular group, they may be accepted or ostracized for their attitudes.

from wrong and good from bad is the beginning of morality (see Moral Development).

COGNITIVE DEVELOPMENT

One of the tasks related to the preschool period is readiness for school and scholastic learning. Many of the thought processes of this period are crucial for achieving such readiness, and it is intentional that the child begins school between ages 5 and 6 rather than at an earlier age.

Preoperational Phase (Piaget)

Piaget's cognitive theory actually does not include a period specifically for children 3 to 5 years old. The *preoperational phase* comprises the age span from 2 to 7 years and is divided into two stages: the *preconceptual phase,* ages 2 to 4, and the phase of *intuitive thought,* ages 4 to 7. One of the main transitions during these two phases is the shift from totally egocentric thought to social awareness and the ability to consider other viewpoints. However, egocentricity is still evident. (For a review of the characteristics of preoperational thought, see Chapter 12.)

Language continues to develop during the preschool period. Speech remains primarily a vehicle of egocentric communication. Preschoolers assume that everyone thinks as they do and that a brief explanation of their thinking makes the entire thought understood by others. Because of this self-referenced, egocentric verbal communication, it is frequently necessary to explore and understand the young child's thinking through other nonverbal approaches. For children in this age-group, the most enlightening and effective method is *play,* which becomes the child's way of understanding, adjusting to, and working out life's experiences.

Preschoolers increasingly use language without comprehending the meaning of words, particularly concepts of right and left, causality, and time. Children may use the concepts correctly but only in the circumstances in which they have learned them. For example, they may know how to put on shoes by remembering that the buckle is always on the outside of the foot. However, if different shoes have no buckles, they cannot reason which shoe fits which foot. In other words, they do not understand the concept of *right and left.*

Superficially, *causality* resembles logical thought. Preschoolers explain a concept as they heard it described by others, but their understanding is limited. An example is the concept of time. Since *time* is still incompletely understood, the child interprets it according to his or her own frame of ref-

erence, such as "A long time means until Christmas." Consequently, time is best explained in relationship to an event, such as "Your mother will visit you after you finish your lunch." Avoiding words such as "yesterday," "tomorrow," "next week," or "Tuesday" to express when an event is expected to occur and associating time with usual expected daily occurrences help children learn about temporal relationships while increasing their trust in others' predictions.

Preschoolers' thinking is often described as *magical thinking.* Because of their egocentrism and transductive reasoning, they believe that thoughts are all-powerful. Such thinking places them in the vulnerable position of feeling guilty and responsible for bad thoughts, which may coincide with the occurrence of a wished event. Their inability to logically reason the cause and effect of illness or an injury makes it especially difficult for them to understand such events.

MORAL DEVELOPMENT

Preconventional or Premoral Level (Kohlberg)

Young children's development of moral judgment is at the most basic level. There is little, if any, concern for why something is wrong. They behave because of the freedom or restriction that is placed on actions. In the *punishment and obedience orientation,* children (ages about 2 to 4 years) judge whether an action is good or bad depending on whether it results in reward or punishment. If children are punished for it, the action is bad. If they are not punished, the action is good, regardless of the meaning of the act. For example, if parents allow hitting, the child will perceive that hitting is good because it is not associated with punishment.

From approximately 4 to 7 years of age children are in the stage of *naive instrumental orientation,* in which actions are directed toward satisfying their needs and less frequently the needs of others. They have a very concrete sense of justice. Reciprocity or fairness involves the philosophy of "You scratch my back and I'll scratch yours," with no thought of loyalty or gratitude (Thomas, 1996).

SPIRITUAL DEVELOPMENT

Children's knowledge of faith and religion is learned from significant others in their environment, usually from the parents and their religious practices. However, young children's understanding of spirituality is influenced by their cognitive level. Preschoolers have a concrete conception of a God with physical characteristics, who is often like an imaginary friend. They understand simple Bible stories and memorize short prayers, but their understanding of the meaning of these rituals is limited. They benefit from concrete representations of religious practices, such as picture Bible books, and small statues, such as those of the Nativity scene.

Development of the conscience is strongly linked to spiritual development. At this age children are learning right from wrong and behave correctly to avoid punishment. Wrongdoing provokes feelings of guilt, and preschoolers often misinterpret illness as a punishment for real or imagined transgressions. It is important that children view God as one who bestows unconditional love, rather than as a judge of good or bad behavior. Praying to God and observing religious traditions, (e.g., prayers before meals or bedtime) can help children through stressful periods, such as hospitalization (Clutter, 1991).

DEVELOPMENT OF BODY IMAGE

The preschool years play a significant role in the development of body image. With increasing comprehension of language, preschoolers recognize that individuals have undesirable and desirable appearances. They recognize differences in skin color and racial identity and are vulnerable to learning prejudices and biases. They are aware of the meaning of words such as *pretty* or *ugly*, and they reflect the opinions of others regarding their own appearance. By 5 years of age children compare their size with their peers' and can become conscious of being large or short, especially if others refer to them as "so big" or "so little" for their age.

Despite the advances in body image development, preschoolers have poorly defined body boundaries and little knowledge of their internal anatomy. Intrusive experiences are frightening, especially those that disrupt the integrity of the skin, such as injections and surgery. There is a fear that if the skin is "broken," all their blood and "insides" can leak out. Therefore bandages are critical to "keeping everything from coming out."

DEVELOPMENT OF SEXUALITY

Sexual development during these years is a very important phase to a person's overall sexual identity and beliefs. Preschoolers are forming strong attachments to the opposite-sex parent while identifying with the same-sex parent.

As sexual identity is developing beyond gender recognition, modesty may become a concern, as well as fears of mutilation. There is sex-role imitation, and "dressing up" like Mommy or Daddy is an important activity. Attitudes and responses of others to role playing can condition the child to views of self or others. For example, comments such as "Boys shouldn't play with dolls" can influence a boy's self-concept of masculinity.

Sexual exploration may be more pronounced now than ever before, particularly in terms of exploring and manipulating the genitals. Questions about sexual reproduction may come to the forefront in the preschooler's search for understanding (see Sex Education, p. 392; also in Chapters 15 and 16).

SOCIAL DEVELOPMENT

During the preschool period the *individuation-separation process* is completed. Preschoolers have overcome much of the anxiety associated with strangers and the fear of separation of earlier years. They relate to unfamiliar people easily and tolerate brief separations from parents with little or no protest. However, they still need parental security, reassurance, guidance, and approval, especially when entering preschool or elementary school. Prolonged separation, such as that imposed by illness and hospitalization, is difficult, but preschoolers respond very well to anticipatory preparation and concrete explanation. They can cope with changes in daily routine much better than toddlers; however, they may develop more imaginary fears. They gain security and comfort from familiar objects, such as toys, dolls, or photographs of family members. They are able to work through many of their unresolved fears, fantasies, and anxieties through play,

especially if guided with appropriate play objects (e.g., dolls or puppets) that represent family members, medical and nursing staff, and other children.

Language

Compared with that of toddlerhood, language during the preschool years is more sophisticated and complex. Both cognitive ability and environment, particularly consistent role models, influence vocabulary, speech, and comprehension. Language becomes a major mode of communication and social interaction. Vocabulary increases dramatically, from 300 words at age 2 to more than 2100 words at the end of 5 years. Sentence structure, grammatical usage, and intelligibility also advance to a more adult level.

Children between the ages of 3 and 4 form sentences of about three to four words and include only the most essential words to convey a meaning. Such speech is often termed *telegraphic* for its brevity in length. Three-year-old children ask many questions and use plurals, correct pronouns, and the past tense of verbs. They name familiar objects, such as animals, parts of the body, relatives, and friends. They can give and follow simple commands. They talk incessantly, regardless of whether anyone is listening or answering them. They enjoy musical or talking toys or dolls and imitate new words proficiently.

From ages 4 to 5 preschoolers use longer sentences of four to five words and use more words to convey a message, such as prepositions, adjectives, and a variety of verbs. They follow simple directional commands, such as "Put the ball on the chair," but can carry out only one request at a time. They answer questions, such as "What do you do when you are hungry?" by describing the appropriate action. The pattern of asking questions is at its peak, and children usually repeat the question until they receive an answer.

By the end of age 5 children can use all parts of speech correctly, except for deviations from the rule. They can define simple things by describing their use, shape, or general category of classification, rather than simply describing their outward appearance. For example, they define a ball as "round, something you bounce, or a toy," rather than by its color. They can give some opposites, such as "If Mommy is a woman, Daddy is a man." By the time they are 6 years old, they can describe an object according to its composition, such as "A spoon is made of metal."

Personal-Social Behavior

The pervasive ritualism and negativism of toddlerhood gradually diminish during the preschool years. Although self-assertion is still a major theme, preschoolers demonstrate their sense of autonomy differently. They are able to verbalize their request for independence and perform independently because of their much-refined physical and cognitive development. By 4 or 5 years of age they need little if any assistance with dressing, eating, or toileting (Fig. 13-2). They can also be trusted to obey warnings of danger, although 3- or 4-year-old children may exceed their boundaries at times.

They are also much more sociable and willing to please. They have internalized many of the standards and values of the family and culture. However, by the end of early childhood they begin to question parental values and compare them with those of their peer group and other authority fig-

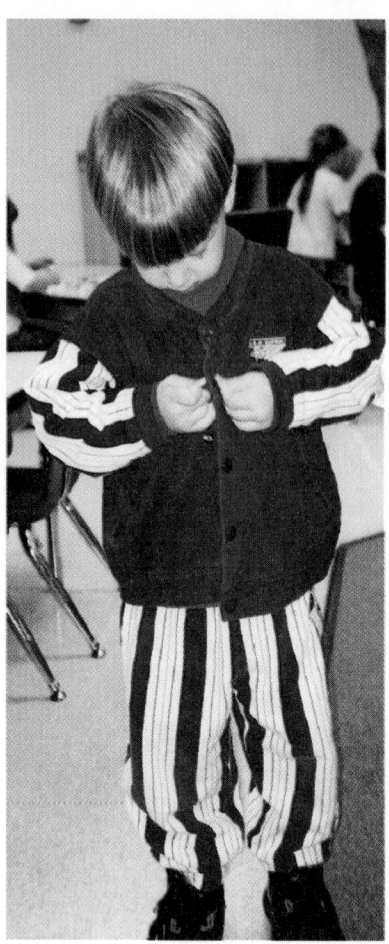

FIG. 13-2. Most preschoolers are able to dress themselves but need help with more difficult items of clothing.

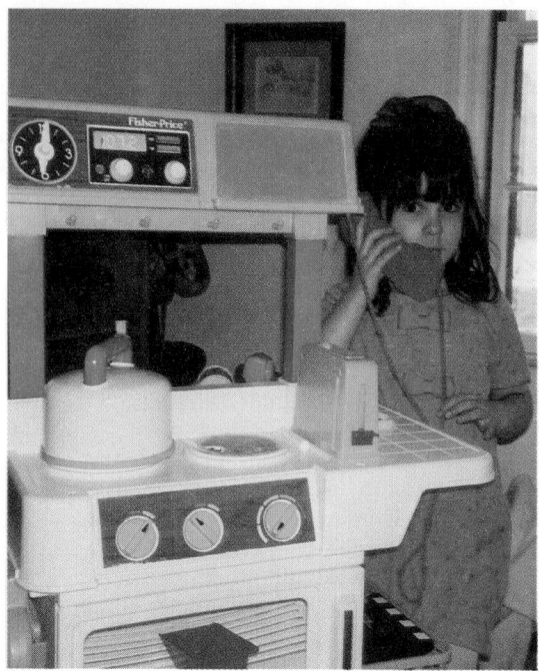

FIG. 13-3. Imaginative and dramatic play is typical of preschoolers, who enjoy using fantasy.

ures; as a result, they may be less willing to abide by the family's code of conduct. Preschoolers become increasingly aware of their position and role within the family. Although this is a more secure age for experiencing the addition of another sibling, relinquishing the position of first or youngest is still difficult and requires appropriate preparation (see Sibling Rivalry, Chapter 12).

Play

Various types of play are typical of this period, but preschoolers especially enjoy *associative play*—group play in similar or identical activities but without rigid organization or rules. Play should provide for physical, social, and mental development.

Play activities for physical growth and refinement of motor skills include jumping, running, and climbing. Tricycles, scooter trucks, wagons, gym and sports equipment, sandboxes, wading pools, and winter sleds can help develop muscles and coordination. Activities such as swimming, skating, and skiing teach safety, as well as muscle development and coordination.

Manipulative, constructive, creative, and educational toys provide for quiet activities, fine motor development, and self-expression. Easy construction sets, large blocks of various sizes and shapes, a counting frame, alphabet or number flash cards, paints, crayons, simple carpentry tools, musical toys, illustrated books, simple sewing or handicraft sets, large puzzles, and clay are suitable toys. Electronic games and educational computer programs are especially valuable in helping children learn basic skills, such as letters and simple words.

Probably the most characteristic and pervasive preschool activity is *imitative, imaginative, and dramatic play.* Dress-up clothes, dolls, housekeeping toys, dollhouses, play-store toys, telephones, farm animals and equipment, village sets, trains, trucks, cars, planes, hand puppets, and doctor and nurse kits provide hours of self-expression (Fig. 13-3). Probably at no other time is the reproduction of adult behavior so faithful and absorbing as in 4- and 5-year-old children (see Critical Thinking Exercise at the top left of p. 389). Toward the end of the preschool period, children are less satisfied with make-believe or pretend objects and enjoy actually doing the activity, such as cooking and carpentry.

Television and videotapes also have their places in children's play, although each should only be one part of children's total repertoire of social and recreational activities. Parents and other caregivers should supervise selection of programs, preview programs for appropriateness, and schedule hours for television viewing. (See the discussion on television, including the Parent Guidelines, in Chapter 5.)

Play is so much a part of the young child's life that reality and fantasy become blurred. The make-believe is reality during play and only becomes fantasy when the toys are put away or the dress-up clothes are removed. It is no wonder that *imaginary playmates* are so much a part of this age period.

The appearance of imaginary companions usually occurs between the ages of 2½ to 3 years, and for the most part

Imitative Play

In her bedroom 4-year-old Juanita is playing with her dolls. She pretends one doll is "Mommy" and is talking on the telephone: "Be quiet! Can't you see that I am busy? This is an important call. Go away." She hangs up the phone and chooses another doll, pokes it, and cries, "You're bad. Mommy doesn't like you."

Juanita's mother, Mrs. Ortiz, hears this play conversation and realizes she says similar things to Juanita when she is on the telephone. What advice would you give Mrs. Ortiz?

1. Reassure her that imitation is a normal and healthy activity in 4-year-olds.
2. Suggest that she use a telephone recorder to return calls at more convenient times.
3. Inquire about her reactions to the play conversation and discuss possible ways to avoid the situation.
4. Refer the child to a psychologist for further assessment of the apparent child-mother conflict.

The best answer is three. You want to capitalize on the mother's awareness of the possible messages the child's play has revealed. Your goal is also to empower the parent to find reasonable options that accommodate her life-style.

Although a telephone recorder is one option, it may not be the best one. Although this play behavior is typical of preschoolers, premature reassurance will not address the issue or solutions. More assessment is needed before suggesting a referral.

Imaginary Playmates

Mrs. Petner tells you, the nurse, that her 2½-year-old daughter, Kimberly, has an imaginary playmate named Alison. She was not very concerned about this until Kimberly started putting a plate on the table for Alison at mealtimes. Your best reply is which of the following?

1. "This is highly unusual behavior for children this age and indicates giftedness."
2. "This is normal for children this age, and it is fine to allow her to set a place for her imaginary playmate."
3. "It is best not to allow Kimberly to include her imaginary playmate in activities such as mealtimes."
4. "It is important that Kimberly separate reality from fantasy, and a referral to a mental health professional is indicated."

The best answer is two. Imaginary playmates are normal at this age and serve many purposes. Parents can acknowledge the presence of an imaginary companion as long as the child does not use the playmate to avoid punishment or responsibility. A referral is not necessary. Although the child may be gifted, this one behavior does not indicate that this is true.

COPING WITH CONCERNS RELATED TO NORMAL GROWTH AND DEVELOPMENT

Preschool and Kindergarten Experience

such playmates are relinquished when the child enters school. There seems to be a relationship between the level of intelligence and the presence of the imaginary companion. The more intelligent children tend to have the more vivid and complex pretend playmates.

Imaginary companions serve many purposes: they become friends in times of loneliness, they accomplish what the child is still attempting, and they experience what the child wants to forget or remember. It is not unusual for the "friend" to have a myriad of vices and to be blamed for wrongdoing. Sometimes the child hopes to escape punishment by saying, "My friend George broke the glass." At other times the child may fantasize that the companion misbehaved and play the role of parent. This becomes a way of assuming control and authority in a safe situation.

Parents often worry about the imaginary playmates, not realizing how normal and useful they are. They need to be reassured that children's fantasy is a sign of health that helps them differentiate between pretend and reality. Parents can acknowledge the presence of the imaginary companion by calling him or her by name and even agreeing to simple requests such as setting an extra place at the table, but they should not allow the child to use the playmate to avoid punishment or responsibility. For example, if the child blames the companion for messing a room, parents need to state clearly that the child is the only one they see and therefore the child is responsible for cleaning up (see Critical Thinking Exercise).

• • •

Table 13-1 summarizes the major developmental achievements for children 3, 4, and 5 years old.

During the preschool years many children attend some type of early childhood program, usually preschool or a daycare center. Group care has become commonplace with the large number of mothers presently employed outside the home (see Alternate Child Care Arrangements, Chapter 10). The effects of early education and stimulation on children have increasingly gained recognition and importance (for a discussion of the effects of daycare on young children, see Working Mothers, Chapter 4). Since social development widens to include age-mates and other significant adults, preschool provides an excellent vehicle for expanding children's experiences with others. It also is an excellent preparation for entrance into elementary school.

In preschool or daycare centers children are exposed to opportunities for learning group cooperation, adjusting to various sociocultural differences, and coping with frustration, dissatisfaction, and anger. If activities are tailored to provide mastery and achievement, children increasingly have feelings of success, self-confidence, and personal competence. Whether or not structured learning is imposed is less important than the social climate, type of guidance, and attitude toward the children that is fostered by the teacher or leader. With a teacher who is aware of preschoolers' developmental abilities and needs, children will learn from the activity that is provided. Most programs incorporate a daily schedule of quiet play, active outdoor activity, group activities such as games and projects, creative or free play, and snack and rest

TABLE 13-1. Growth and development during preschool years

AGE (YEARS)	PHYSICAL	GROSS MOTOR	FINE MOTOR	LANGUAGE
3	Usual weight gain of 1.8 to 2.7 kg (4 to 6 pounds) per year Average weight of 14.6 kg (32 pounds) Usual gain in height of 7.5 cm (3 inches) per year Average height of 95 cm (37¼ inches) May have achieved nighttime control of bowel and bladder	Rides tricycle Jumps off bottom step Stands on one foot for a few seconds Goes up stairs using alternate feet, may still come down using both feet on step Broad jumps May try to dance, but balance may not be adequate	Builds tower of nine or ten cubes Builds bridge with three cubes Adeptly places small pellets in narrow-necked bottle In drawing, copies a circle, imitates a cross, names what has been drawn, cannot draw stick figure but may make circle with facial features	Has vocabulary of about 900 words Uses primarily "telegraphic" speech Uses complete sentences of three to four words Talks incessantly regardless of whether anyone is paying attention Repeats sentence of six syllables Asks many questions
4	Pulse and respiration rates decrease slightly Growth rate is similar to that of previous year Average weight of 16.7 kg (36¾ pounds) Average height of 103 cm (40½ inches) Length at birth is doubled Maximum potential for development of amblyopia	Skips and hops on one foot Catches ball reliably Throws ball overhand Walks downstairs using alternate footing	Uses scissors successfully to cut out picture following outline Can lace shoes, but may not be able to tie bow In drawing, copies a square, traces a cross and diamond, adds three parts to stick figure	Has vocabulary of 1500 words or more Uses sentences of four to five words Questioning is at peak Tells exaggerated stories Knows simple songs May be mildly profane if associates with older children Obeys four prepositional phrases, such as "under," "on top of," "beside," "in back of," or "in front of" Names one or more colors Comprehends analogies, such as, "If ice is cold, fire is _____"
5	Pulse and respiration rates decrease slightly Average weight of 18.7 kg (41¼ pounds) Average height of 110 cm (43¼ inches) Eruption of permanent dentition may begin Handedness is established (about 90% are right-handed)	Skips and hops on alternate feet Throws and catches ball well Jumps rope Skates with good balance Walks backward with heel to toe Jumps from height of 12 inches and lands on toes Balances on alternate feet with eyes closed	Ties shoelaces Uses scissors, simple tools, or pencil very well In drawing, copies a diamond and triangle; adds seven to nine parts to stick figure; prints a few letters, numbers, or words, such as first name	Has vocabulary of about 2100 words Uses sentences of six to eight words, with all parts of speech Names coins (e.g., nickel, dime) Names four or more colors Describes drawing or pictures with much comment and enumeration Knows names of days of week, months, and other time-associated words Knows composition of articles, such as "A shoe is made of _____" Can follow three commands in succession

SOCIALIZATION	COGNITION	FAMILY RELATIONSHIPS
Dresses self almost completely if helped with back buttons and told which shoe is right or left Pulls on shoes Has increased attention span Feeds self completely Can prepare simple meals, such as cold cereal and milk Can help to set table; can dry dishes without breaking any May have fears, especially of dark and going to bed Knows own sex and sex of others Play is parallel and associative; begins to learn simple games but often follows own rules; begins to share	Is in preconceptual phase Is egocentric in thought and behavior Has beginning understanding of time; uses many time-oriented expressions, talks about past and future as much as about present, pretends to tell time Has improved concept of space, as demonstrated by understanding of prepositions and ability to follow directional command Has beginning ability to view concepts from another perspective	Attempts to please parents and conform to their expectations Is less jealous of younger sibling; may be opportune time for birth of additional sibling Is aware of family relationships and sex-role functions Boys tend to identify more with father or other male figure Has increased ability to separate easily and comfortably from parents for short periods

Very independent
Tends to be selfish and impatient
Aggressive physically as well as verbally
Takes pride in accomplishments
Has mood swings
Shows off dramatically, enjoys entertaining others
Tells family tales to others with no restraint
Still has many fears
Play is associative
    Imaginary playmates are common
    Uses dramatic, imaginative, and imitative devices
    Sexual exploration and curiosity demonstrated through play, such as being "doctor" or "nurse"
	Is in phase of intuitive thought
	Causality is still related to proximity of events
	Understands time better, especially in terms of sequence of daily events
	Unable to conserve matter
	Judges everything according to one dimension, such as height, width, or order
	Immediate perceptual clues dominate judgment
	Is beginning to develop less egocentrism and more social awareness
	May count correctly but has poor mathematic concept of numbers
	Obeys because parents have set limits, not because of understanding of right or wrong
		Rebels if parents expect too much, such as impeccable table manners
		Takes aggression and frustration out on parents or siblings
		Do's and don'ts become important
		May have rivalry with older or younger siblings; may resent older sibling's privileges and younger sibling's invasion of privacy and possessions
		May "run away" from home
		Identifies strongly with parent of opposite sex
		Is able to run simple errands outside the home

Less rebellious and quarrelsome than at age 4 years More settled and eager to get down to business Not as open and accessible in thoughts and behavior as in earlier years Independent but trustworthy; not foolhardy; more responsible Has fewer fears; relies on outer authority to control world Eager to do things right and to please; tries to "live by the rules" Has better manners Cares for self totally, occasionally needing supervision in dress or hygiene Not ready for concentrated close work or small print because of slight farsightedness and still unrefined eye-hand coordination Play is associative; tries to follow rules but may cheat to avoid losing	Begins to question what parents think by comparing them with age-mates and other adults May notice prejudice and bias in outside world Is more able to view other's perspective, but tolerates differences rather than understanding them May begin to show understanding of conservation of numbers through counting objects regardless of arrangement Uses time-oriented words with increased understanding Very curious about factual information regarding world	Gets along well with parents May seek out parent more often than at age 4 years for reassurance and security, especially when entering school Begins to question parents' thinking and principles Strongly identifies with parent of same sex, especially boys with their fathers Enjoys activities such as sports, cooking, and shopping with parent of same sex

periods. Preschool is particularly beneficial for children who lack a peer-group experience, such as an only child, and for children from impoverished homes. It also is an excellent preparation for kindergarten.

One of the issues that parents face is the child's readiness for preschool or kindergarten. There are no absolute indicators for school readiness, but children's social maturation, especially attention span, is as important as their academic readiness. Using a developmental screening tool that addresses cognitive (especially language), social, and physical milestones can identify children who may benefit from diagnostic testing.

Nurses can be helpful in guiding parents in locating suitable facilities with a well-qualified staff. State licensing agencies can help parents identify daycare centers that accept children of specific age-groups and are conveniently located. State-licensed programs are supposed to abide by established standards, which represent the *minimum* requirements and safeguards. However, enforcement of the standards is sometimes inadequate. Early childhood programs may also belong to a voluntary accreditation system, the National Academy of Early Childhood Programs, which serves as a model for *optimum* care.* References from other parents are also helpful, provided they have investigated the center carefully.

Other areas for parents to evaluate are the center's daily program, teacher qualifications, student/staff ratio, discipline policy, environmental safety precautions, provision of meals, sanitary conditions, adequate indoor/outdoor space per child, and fee schedule. In terms of an overall evaluation, there *is no substitute for a personal observation of the facility.* Parents should arrange to meet the director and some of the employees, especially those who would be caring for the child. Developing a checklist may be helpful to evaluate the center systematically and make comparisons with other facilities.

One of the areas that is increasingly important in selecting child care centers is the agency's health practices. Sub-

stantial evidence shows that children in daycare centers, especially those under 3 years of age, have more illnesses, especially diarrhea, hepatitis A, meningitis, otitis media, respiratory tract infections, and cytomegalovirus, than children not in daycare centers.

Nurses play an important role in infection control. Not only can they advise parents regarding the evaluation of a center's sanitary practices, but they can also take an active part in educating staff in measures to minimize transmission of infection. For example, in centers caring for children who are not toilet trained, reducing environmental contamination with urine and feces is an important infection control issue (Fig. 13-4).

Children need preparation for the preschool or kindergarten experience.* For young children it represents a change from their usual home environment and prolonged separation from parents.

Before the child begins the school experience, the parents should present the idea as exciting and pleasurable. Talking to the child about activities such as painting, building with blocks, or enjoying swings and other outdoor equipment allows the child to fantasize about the forthcoming event in a positive manner. When the first day of school arrives, the parents should behave confidently. Such behavior requires parents to have resolved their own feelings regarding the experience.

Parents should introduce their child to the teacher and the facility. In some instances it is helpful to remain for at least some part of the first day until the child is comfortable and at ease. Other specific actions that can help lessen separation anxiety include providing the school with detailed information about the child's home environment, such as familiar routines, favorite activities, food preferences, names of siblings or pets, and personal habits. Such information helps the child feel familiar in the strange surroundings. When schools automatically request this information, the parent has a valuable clue to evaluating the quality of the program, since the request represents the staff's awareness of each child's needs. Transitional objects, such as a favorite toy, may also help the child bridge the gap from home to school.

Sex Education

Preschoolers have experienced a tremendous amount of information during their short lifetimes. Although their thinking may not be mature, they search constantly for explanations and reasons that are logical and reasonable to them. The word "why" seems to supplant the word "no," which was common in toddlerhood. It is only natural that as they learn about "me," they will also want to know "why me" and "how me." Questions such as "Where do babies come from?" are as casual as "What makes it rain?" or "Who is that?" It is the *way* in which questions about procreation are answered that conditions children, even the youngest, to separate these questions from others about their world.

Two rules govern answering sensitive questions about topics such as sex. The first is to *find out what children know and think.* By investigating the theories children have pro-

---

*Information about the accreditation criteria and procedures of the National Academy of Early Childhood Programs is available from the **National Association for the Education of Young Children,** 1834 Connecticut Ave., N.W., Washington, DC 20009; (202) 232-8777 or (800) 424-2460. These criteria are excellent guidelines for evaluating preschools or daycare centers.

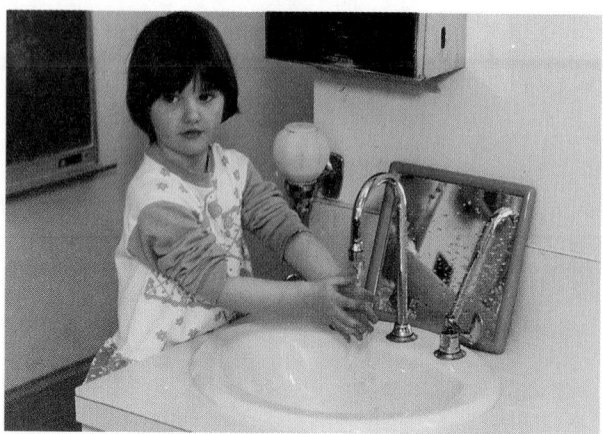

FIG. 13-4. Thorough handwashing is the single most effective method of preventing infection.

---

*Recommended books for preparing young children for daycare or school include *Going to Day Care* and *When Your Child Goes to School* by Fred Rogers (GP Putnam's Sons).

duced as a reasonable explanation, parents can not only give correct information but also help children understand why their explanation is inaccurate. Another reason for ascertaining what the child thinks before offering any information is that the "unasked for" answer may be given. For example, 4-year-old Sally asked her father, "Where did I come from?" Both parents quickly took this inquiry as a clue for offering sex education. After the explanation, Sally exclaimed, "I don't know about all that! All I know is Mary came from New York and I want to know where I was born."

The second rule for giving information is to *be honest.* It is true that much of the correct information will be forgotten or misunderstood by the preschooler, but what is more important is that the correct information can be restated until the child absorbs and comprehends the facts. Even though the correct anatomic words may be hard to pronounce or even more difficult to remember, they become foundational content for explaining other concepts later on.

Honesty does not imply imparting to children every fact of life or allowing excessive permissiveness in sexual curiosity. When children ask one question, they are looking for one answer. When they are ready, they will ask about the other "unfinished" parts of the story. Sooner or later they will wonder how the "sperm meets the egg" and "how the baby gets out," but it is best to wait until they ask.

Regardless of whether children are given sex education, they will engage in games of sexual curiosity and exploration. At about 3 years of age children are aware of the anatomic differences between the sexes and are very concerned with how the other "works." This is not really "sexual" curiosity, because many children are still unaware of the reproductive function of the genitals. Their curiosity is for the eliminative function of the anatomy. Little boys wonder how girls can urinate without a penis, so they watch girls go to the bathroom. Since they cannot see anything but the stream of water coming out, they want to observe further for what makes it come out. "Doctor play" is often a game invented for just such investigation. Little girls are no less curious about boys' anatomy. It is very intriguing to have a closer inspection of this "thing" that girls do not have.

One question that parents often have is how to handle such sexual curiosity. A positive approach is to neither condone nor condemn the sexual curiosity but to express that if children have questions, they should ask the parents; then the parents should encourage them to engage in some other activity. In this way children can be helped to understand that there are ways that their sexual curiosity can be satisfied other than through playing investigative games. This in no way condemns the act but stresses alternate methods to seek solutions and answers. Allowing children unrestricted permissiveness only intensifies their anxiety and concern, since exploring and searching usually yield little evidence to satisfy their curiosity.

Another concern for some parents is *masturbation,* or self-stimulation of the genitals. This occurs at any age for a variety of reasons and, if not excessive, is normal and healthy. It is most common at 4 years of age and during adolescence (Leung and Robson, 1993). For preschoolers it is a part of sexual curiosity and exploration. If parents are concerned about masturbation in their children, it is essential for nurses to investigate the circumstances associated with the activity,

because it may be an expression of anxiety, boredom, or unresolved conflicts. For example, a boy who repeatedly touches his penis is not masturbating for pleasure but may be reassuring himself that it is intact. Also, children who openly and publicly masturbate are inviting a reaction, such as discipline, punishment, or criticism. They may be overwhelmed by their sexual feelings and asking others to help them channel them into more constructive outlets. Since masturbation, like other forms of sex play, is a private act, parents should emphasize this to children as part of teaching them socially acceptable behavior.

Fears

The greatest number and variety of real and imagined fears are present during the preschool years and include fear of the dark, being left alone (especially at bedtime), animals (particularly large dogs and snakes), ghosts, sexual matters (castration), and objects or persons associated with pain. Parents often become perplexed about handling the fears because no amount of logical persuasion, coercion, or ridicule will send away the ghosts, boogeymen, monsters, and devils.

The best way to help children overcome their fears is by actively involving them in finding practical methods to deal with the frightening experience. This may be as simple as keeping a night light on in the child's bedroom for assurance that no monsters lurk in the dark. Exposing children to the feared object in a safe situation also provides a type of conditioning or *desensitization.* For instance, children who are afraid of dogs should never be forced to approach or touch one, but they may be gradually introduced to the experience by watching other children play with the animal. This type of modeling, demonstrating fearlessness in others, can be very effective if the child is allowed to progress at his or her own rate.

Usually by 5 or 6 years of age children relinquish these old fears. Explaining the developmental sequence of fears and their gradual disappearance may help parents feel more secure in handling preschoolers' fears. Sometimes fears do not subside with simple measures or developmental maturation. When children experience severe fears that disrupt family life, professional help is required.

Speech Problems

The most critical period for speech development occurs between 2 and 4 years of age. During this period children are using their rapidly growing vocabulary faster than they can produce the words. This failure to master sensorimotor integrations results in *stuttering* or *stammering* as children try to say the word they are already thinking about. This dysfluency in speech pattern is a *normal* characteristic of language development.

However, when parents or other significant persons place undue emphasis or stress on this pattern of dysfluency, an abnormal speech pattern may result. Chances for reversal of stuttering are good until about 5 years of age. Therefore prevention must begin early.

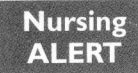 **Nursing ALERT** Dysfluency must be arrested before children develop an awareness or anticipation of the difficulty and begin to mistrust their speech skills.

FAMILY HOME CARE
Dealing with Stuttering in Children

To Be Encouraged

Viewing hesitancy and dysfluency as a normal part of speech development

Giving child plenty of time and the impression of not being rushed or in a hurry

Looking directly at child while he or she is talking; being patient and never ridiculing or criticizing

Setting a good example by speaking clearly and articulating well

Identifying situations when stuttering increases and avoiding them or ignoring the hesitancy

Capitalizing on periods of fluent speech with positive reinforcement, such as singing songs or repeating nursery rhymes

To Be Avoided

Giving in to the natural tendency to "help" by supplying word when child is having a block

Telling child to stop or start over, to think before speaking, or to take it easy and go slowly

Showing great concern, embarrassment, or disapproval for hesitancy

Doing *anything* that emphasizes stuttering and calls child's attention to speech skills

Promising reward for proper speech

The nurse should discuss with parents the normal dysfluencies in children's speech. When stuttering does occur, parents are advised to use the suggestions listed in the Family Home Care box to avoid inadvertently reinforcing this pattern. If excessive concern on the part of the parent or frustration and struggling by the child are noted, the child is referred for language and speech evaluation.

Children who are pressured into producing sounds ahead of their developmental level may develop *dyslalia* (articulation problems) or revert to using infantile speech. Prevention involves discussing with parents the usual achievement of speech production during childhood. The *Denver Articulation Screening Examination (DASE)* is an excellent tool to assess articulation skills in the child and to explain to parents the expected progression of sounds (Appendix C).

The DASE employs the word-imitative procedure. The child repeats 22 words but pronounces 30 different sound elements. The raw score, or the number of correctly pronounced sounds, is then compared with the percentile rank for children in that age-group. The examiner must be careful to evaluate the specific sound, rather than the quality of the entire word. For beginning examiners it is helpful to validate the final score by comparing the results with a different examiner, ideally a speech therapist. The child is also scored on intelligibility, by selection of one of four possible categories: (1) easy to understand, (2) understandable half the time, (3) not understandable, or (4) cannot evaluate. The DASE is a reliable, effective screening tool because it requires only 10 minutes to perform and is designed to discriminate between significant delay and normal variations in the acquisition of speech sounds.

PROMOTING OPTIMUM HEALTH DURING THE PRESCHOOL YEARS*

NUTRITION

Nutritional requirements for preschoolers are fairly similar to those for toddlers. The requirement for calories per unit of body weight continues to decrease slightly to 90 kcal/kg for an average daily intake of 1800 calories. Fluid requirements may also decrease slightly to about 100 ml/kg daily but depend on the activity level, climatic conditions, and state of health. The protein requirements are 1.2 g/kg for an average daily consumption of 24 g (Food and Nutrition Board, 1989). A moderately reduced fat diet may be recommended for healthy preschool children. However, it is important that the diet not be deficient in nutrients such as calcium (Shea and others, 1993).

Some preschoolers still have food habits that are typical of toddlers, such as food fads and strong taste preferences. When children reach 4 years of age, they seem to enter another period of finicky eating, which is generally characteristic of the more rebellious and rowdy behavior of children in this age-group. By age 5 years children are more agreeable to trying new foods, especially if encouraged by an adult who allows the child to help with food preparation or experiments with a new taste or different dish (Fig. 13-5). Mealtimes can become battlegrounds if parents expect perfect table manners. Usually the 5-year-old child is ready for the "social" side of eating, but the 3- or 4-year-old child still has difficulty sitting quietly through a long family meal.

The amount and variety of foods consumed by young children vary greatly from day to day. Consequently, parents sometimes worry about the quantity of food preschoolers consume. In general the quality is much more important than the quantity, a fact that should be stressed during nutritional counseling. Some evidence suggests that children self-regulate their caloric intake. If they eat less at one meal, they will compensate at another meal or will snack (Birch and others, 1991; Shea and others, 1992). Also, children's likes and dislikes may be related to genetic sensitivity to tastes (Anliker and others, 1991).

One approach toward lessening this parental concern is advising parents to keep a weekly record of everything the child eats. In particular, the need for measuring the amount of food, such as setting aside ½ cup of vegetables, and serving the child from this premeasured amount is stressed to provide a more accurate estimate of food intake at each meal. Usually by the end of the week, when they look at the food chart, parents are amazed at how much the child has consumed. In general, preschoolers consume only slightly more than toddlers, or about half an adult's portion.

SLEEP AND ACTIVITY

Sleep patterns vary widely, but the average preschooler sleeps about 12 hours a night and infrequently takes daytime naps. Activity levels continue to be high, although quiet activities,

---

*For a more comprehensive understanding the reader is urged also to review the material presented in Chapter 12 under Promoting Optimum Health During Toddlerhood.

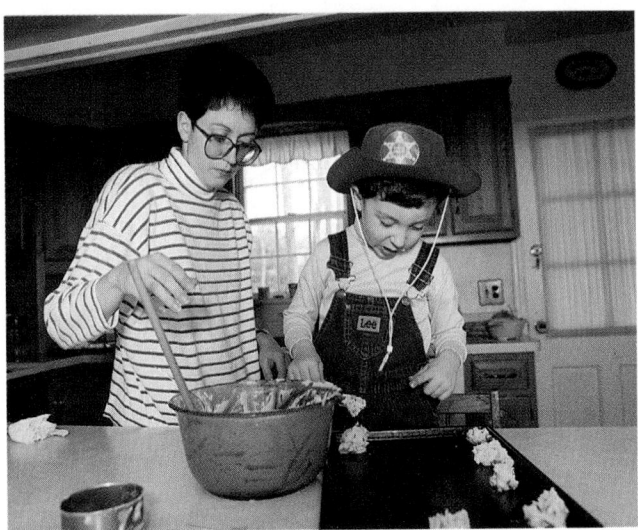

FIG. 13-5. Preschool-age children enjoy helping adults and are more likely to try new foods if they can assist in the preparation.

CULTURAL AWARENESS
Co-Sleeping

Although many experts recommend that infants and children be trained to sleep always in their own crib or bed, co-sleeping, or the "family bed" (in which parents allow the children to sleep with them or the siblings to sleep together in one bed), is a relatively common and accepted cultural practice, especially among black, Hispanic, and Asian families, such as the Japanese. Other groups that are adopting co-sleeping include (1) single parents, whose need for company may encourage this practice; (2) working parents, who desire the closeness at night that was lost during the day; and (3) parents who have had an issue about sleep or separation in their own past (Brazelton, 1992).

such as television, are increasingly appealing and can become an unhealthy substitute for active play. Preschoolers' increased gross motor abilities and coordination provide them with the opportunity to engage in many sports, if only at a novice level. Whether young children should begin formalized training in an activity at this early age is controversial. The American Academy of Pediatrics (1992) recommends that children's readiness to participate in organized sports should be determined individually. The decision should be based on the child's (not the parent's) motivation and enjoyment. The American Academy of Pediatrics encourages free play, a variety of physical activities, a noncompetitive atmosphere, and emphasis on fun and safety.

Sleep Problems*

The preschool years are a prime time for sleep problems. Young children sometimes have trouble going to sleep, especially after so much activity and stimulation during the day. Others may develop bedtime fears, wake during the night, or have nightmares or sleep terrors. Still others may prolong the inevitable through elaborate rituals. Children with reported sleep problems may be more likely to have a difficult temperament than those without sleep disturbances (Atkinson and others, 1995).

Recommendations for sleep disturbance are offered only *after* a thorough assessment of the problem has been completed. Cultural traditions may dictate sleep practices that are contrary to certain well-accepted professional recommendations. Therefore parents' perceptions of a sleep habit may not be considered a problem (see Cultural Awareness box).

Interventions can differ greatly; for example, **nightmares** (scary dreams that are followed by full waking) and **sleep terrors** (partial arousal from deep, nondreaming sleep) require very different approaches. Although sleep terrors require no

---

*Guidelines for helping parents deal with sleep problems are available in Wong DL: *Wong and Whaley's Clinical manual of pediatric nursing,* ed 4, St Louis, 1996, Mosby.

intervention (the best approach is to remain uninvolved so that the child remains asleep), nightmares respond best to the following interventions:

- Accept dream as real fear.
- Sit with child; offer comfort, assurance, and sense of protection.
- Lie down with child or take to own bed *only* if child is not calmed by other measures and understands this is special occasion.
- Consider professional counseling for recurrent nightmares unresponsive to above approaches.

For children who delay going to bed, a recommended approach involves counseling parents about the importance of a consistent bedtime ritual. Attention-seeking behavior is ignored, and the child is not taken into the parents' bed or allowed to stay up past a reasonable hour. Other measures that may be helpful include keeping a light on in the room, providing transitional objects such as a favorite toy, or leaving a drink of water by the bed.

Helping children slow down *before* bedtime also contributes to less resistance to going to bed. One approach is to establish limited rituals that signal readiness for bed, such as a bath or story. Parents can reinforce the pattern by stating, "After this story it is bedtime," and consistently carrying out the routine. If extra stimulation such as having visitors arrive at bedtime is disruptive to children's routine, it is advisable to settle children in bed beforehand.

DENTAL HEALTH

By the beginning of the preschool period the eruption of the deciduous teeth is complete. Dental care is essential to preserve these temporary teeth and to teach good dental habits (see Chapter 12). Although preschoolers' fine motor control is improved, they still require assistance and supervision with brushing, and flossing should be done by parents. Professional care and prophylaxis, especially fluoride supplements, should be continued. For children cared for away from home, parents are encouraged to monitor the dental care provided by others, including the diet to keep cariogenic foods to a minimum.

INJURY PREVENTION

Because of improved gross and fine motor skills, coordination, and balance, preschoolers are less prone to falls than are toddlers. They tend to be less reckless, listen more to paren-

Age 3 Years

Prepare parents for child's increasing interest in widening relationships.

Encourage enrollment in preschool.

Emphasize importance of setting limits.

Prepare parents to expect exaggerated tension-reduction behaviors, such as need for "security blanket."

Encourage parents to offer child choices when child vacillates.

Prepare parents to expect marked changes at 3½ years, when child becomes less coordinated (motor and emotional), becomes insecure, and exhibits emotional extremes.

Prepare parents for normal dysfluency in speech and advise them to avoid focusing on the pattern.

Prepare parents to expect extra demands on their attention as a reflection of child's emotional insecurity and fear of loss of love.

Warn parents that equilibrium of 3-year-old will change to aggressive, out-of-bounds behavior of 4-year-old.

Inform parents to anticipate more stable appetite with more food selections.

Stress need for protection and education of child to prevent injury (see Injury Prevention, Chapter 14).

Age 4 Years

Prepare parents for more aggressive behavior, including motor activity and offensive language.

Prepare parents to expect resistance to parental authority.

Explore parental feelings regarding child's behavior.

Suggest some kind of respite for primary caregivers, such as placing child in preschool for part of the day.

Prepare parents for child's increasing sexual curiosity.

Emphasize importance of realistic limit-setting on behavior and appropriate discipline techniques.

Prepare parents for highly imaginative 4-year-old, who indulges in "tall tales" (to be differentiated from lies) and for child's imaginary playmates.

Prepare parents to expect nightmares or an increase in them and suggest parents make sure child is fully awakened from a frightening dream.

Provide reassurance that a period of calm begins at 5 years of age.

Age 5 Years

Inform parents to expect tranquil period at 5 years.

Help parents to prepare child for entrance into school environment.

Make sure immunizations are up to date before entering school.

Suggest that nonemployed mothers (or fathers if appropriate) consider own activities when child begins school.

Suggest swimming lessons for child.

tal rules, and are aware of potential dangers, such as hot objects, sharp instruments, and dangerous heights. Putting objects in the mouth as part of exploration has all but ceased, although poisoning is still a danger. Pedestrian motor vehicle injuries increase from activities such as playing in the street, riding tricycles, running after balls, or forgetting safety regulations when crossing streets.

In general the guidelines suggested for injury prevention in Table 12-3 apply to children in this age-group as well. However, emphasis is now on *education* for safety and potential hazards, in addition to appropriate protection. Since preschoolers are great imitators, it is especially essential that parents set a good example by "practicing what they preach." Children quickly observe discrepancies in what they are told to do and what they see others do. Establishing habits at this time, such as wearing bicycle helmets, can create long-term safety behaviors.

ANTICIPATORY GUIDANCE— CARE OF FAMILIES

The preschool years present fewer childrearing difficulties than earlier years, and this stage of development is facilitated by appropriate anticipatory guidance in the areas already discussed (see Family Home Care box). There is a shift in childrearing practices from protection to education. Whereas injury prevention previously focused on safeguarding the immediate environment with less emphasis on reasoning, now the protective guardrails or electrical outlet caps may be substituted with verbal explanations of why danger exists and how to avoid it with appropriate judgment and understanding.

During this period an emotional transition between parent and child is also occurring. Although children are still attached to their parents and accepting of all parental values and beliefs, they are nearing the period of life when they will question previous teachings and prefer the companionship of peers. Entry into school marks a separation from home for parents, as well as for children. Parents need help in adjusting to this change, particularly if the mother has focused her daily activity primarily on home responsibilities. As preschoolers begin preschool or elementary school, mothers may need to seek activities beyond the family, such as community involvement or pursuing a career. In this way all family members are adjusting to change, which is part of the process of growth and development.

KEY POINTS

- The preschool years comprise the period from 3 to 5 years of age, a time that is considered critical for emotional and psychologic development.

- Biologic development in the preschool period is characterized by mature body systems and refinement in gross and fine motor behavior, as evidenced by participation in activities such as running, riding a bicycle, and drawing.

- According to Erikson, acquiring a sense of initiative is the chief psychosocial task of the preschooler. Development of the superego occurs during this period, and conscience begins to emerge.

- According to Piaget, the preschool age is characterized by intuitive or prelogical thinking and a move toward logical thought processes through advanced, complex learning, language, and understanding of causality.

- The seeds of moral development are planted during the preschool period. According to Kohlberg, children are in the stage of naive instrumental orientation, in which they are concerned with satisfying their own needs and less frequently the needs of others.

- Social development includes further individuation-separation, more sophisticated language, greater independence, and more complex, imaginative forms of play.

- Areas of special concern to parents during the preschool period are preschool and kindergarten experience, sex education, fears, and speech problems.

- In selecting a school, parents should inquire about daily programs, teacher qualifications, accreditation, student/staff ratio, safety, meals, fees, and health practices.

- Two rules that govern answering questions about sex and other sensitive issues are to find out what the child thinks and to be honest.

- Fears constitute a great part of the preschool period; objects, potential annihilation, and parent-induced fears are common sources.

- Hesitancy or dysfluency in speech patterns is a normal characteristic of language development. Speech problems can occur when parents express excessive concern over this pattern.

- Health promotion continues to be directed toward proper nutrition, adequate sleep, proper dental care, and injury prevention.

REFERENCES

American Academy of Pediatrics, Committee on Sports Medicine and Fitness: Fitness, activity, and sports participation in the preschool child, *Pediatrics* 90(6):1002-1004, 1992.

Anliker JA and others: Children's food preferences and genetic sensitivity to the bitter taste of 6-*n*propylthiouracil (PROP), *Am J Clin Nutr* 54(2):316-320, 1991.

Atkinson E and others: Sleep disruption in young children, *Child Care Health Dev* 21(4):233-246, 1995.

Birch LL and others: The variability of young children's energy intake, *N Engl J Med* 324(4):232-235, 1991.

Brazelton TB: *Touchpoints*, Reading, MA, 1992, Addison-Wesley.

Clutter L: Fostering spiritual care for the child and family. In Smith D and others, editors: *Comprehensive child and family nursing skills*, St Louis, 1991, Mosby.

Food and Nutrition Board, National Research Council: *Recommended dietary allowances*, ed 10, Washington, DC, 1989, National Academy Press.

Leung A, Robson W: Childhood masturbation, *Clin Pediatr* 32(4):238-241, 1993.

Shea S and others: Is there a relationship between dietary fat and stature or growth in children three to five years of age? *Pediatrics* 92:579-586, 1993.

Shea S and others: Variability and self-regulation of energy intake in young children in their everyday environment, *Pediatrics* 90:542-546, 1992.

Thomas RM: *Comparing theories of child development*, ed 4, Pacific Grove, CA, 1996, Brooks-Cole.

BIBLIOGRAPHY

Growth and Development

Ames LB, Ilg FI: *Your three-year-old: friend or enemy*, New York, 1980, Delacorte.

Ames LB, Ilg FI: *Your four-year-old: wild and wonderful*, New York, 1981, Delacorte.

Ames LB, Ilg FI: *Your five-year-old: sunny and serene*, New York, 1981, Delacorte.

Blum NJ and others: Disciplining young children: the role of verbal instructions and reasoning, *Pediatrics* 96(2):336-341, 1995.

Dixon SD, Stein MT: *Encounters with children: pediatric behavior and development*, ed 2, St Louis, 1992, Mosby.

Hauck MR: Cognitive abilities of preschool children: implications for nurses working with young children, *J Pediatr Nurs* 6(4):230-235, 1991.

Howard BJ: Growing together; learning independence in the preschool years, *Contemp Pediatr* 7(7):11-26, 1990.

Lavigne JB and others: Behavioral and emotional problems among preschool children in pediatric primary care: prevalence and pediatricians' recognition, *Pediatrics* 91(3):649-655, 1993.

Lowrey G: *Growth and development of children,* ed 8, St Louis, 1986, Mosby.

Lyytinen P: Developmental trends in children's pretend play, *Child Care Health Dev* 17(1):25, 1991.

Morrison CD, Bundy AC, Fisher AG: The contribution of motor skills and playfulness to the play performance of preschoolers, *Am J Occup Ther* 45(8):687-694, 1991.

Prior M and others: Sex differences in psychological adjustment from infancy to 8 years, *J Am Acad Child Adolesc Psychiatry* 32(2):291-304, 1993.

Rugg HA, Saltarelli LM: Exploratory play with objects: basic cognitive processes and individual differences, *New Dir Child Dev* (59):5-16, 1993.

Shonkoff JP: Preschool. In Levine MD and others, editors: *Developmental-behavioral pediatrics,* Philadelphia, 1992, Saunders.

Preschool and Kindergarten Experience

Byrd RS, Weitzman ML: Predictors of early grade retention among children in the United States, *Pediatrics* 93(3):481-487, 1994.

Casey PH, Evans LD: School readiness: an overview for pediatricians, *Pediatr Rev* 14(1):4-10, 1993.

Karp R and others: Growth and academic achievement in inner-city kindergarten children, *Clin Pediatr* 31(6):336-340, 1992.

Martin S, Ramey C, Ramey S: The prevention of intellectual impairment in children of impoverished families: findings of a randomized trial of educational day care, *Am J Public Health* 80:844-847, 1990.

Oberklaid F and others: Predicting preschool behavior problems from temperament and other variables in infancy, *Pediatrics* 91(1):113-120, 1993.

Palmer DJ and others: An exploratory study of the structure and validity of pediatric examination of educational readiness, *Dev Behav Pediatr* 11(6):317-321, 1990.

Robinson J: *Is your child ready for school?* New York, 1990, Simon & Schuster.

Wilson DA, Knudtson MD: Assessing school readiness through the school-entry screening exam, *Nurs Pract* 17(9):24-26, 29-30, 33, 1992.

Sex Education

Aquilino ML, Ely J: Parents and the sexuality of preschool children, *Pediatr Nurs* 11(1):41-46, 1985.

Calderone MS: Sexual health and the child, *Compr Ther* 6(12):3-7, 1980.

Castiglia PT: Masturbation, *J Pediatr Health Care* 2(2):111-112, 1988.

Masters WH, Johnson VE, Kolodny RC: *Human sexuality,* ed 3, Glenview, IL, 1988, Scott, Foresman.

Speech Problems

Biro P, Thompson M: Screening young children for communication disorders, *Matern Child Nurse J* 9(6):410-413, 1984.

Goldberg R: Identifying speech and language delays in children, *Pediatr Nurs* 15(4):252-259, 1984.

Pastore DR: Stuttering. In Hoekelman R and others, editors: *Primary pediatric care,* ed 2, St Louis, 1992, Mosby.

Schmitt BD: Does your child have a stuttering problem? *Contemp Pediatr* 8(3):83-84, 1991.

Sleep Problems

Beltramini A, Hertzig M: Sleep and bedtime behavior in preschool-aged children, *Pediatrics* 71(2):153-158, 1983.

Clore ER, Hibel J: The parasomnias of childhood, *J Pediatr Health Care* 7(1):12-16, 1993.

Crawford W, Bennet R, Hewitt K: Sleep problems in pre-school children, *Health Visit* 62(3):79-81, 1989.

DiMario F, Enery ES III: The natural history of night terrors, *Clin Pediatr* 26(10):505-511, 1987.

Edgil A and others: Sleep problems of older infants and preschool children, *Pediatr Nurs* 11(2):87-89, 1985.

Gates D, Morwessel N: Night terrors: strategies for family coping, *J Pediatr Nurs* 4(1):48-53, 1989.

Jimmerson KR: Maternal, environmental, and temperamental characteristics of toddlers with and toddlers without sleep problems, *J Pediatr Health Care* 5(2):71-77, 1991.

Leung AK, Robson WL: Nightmares, *J Natl Med Assoc* 85(3):233-235, 1993.

McMenamy C, Katz RC: Brief parent-assisted treatment for children's nighttime fears, *J Dev Behav Pediatr* 10(3):145-148, 1989.

Pagel J: Nightmares, *Am Fam Physician* 39(3):145-148, 1989.

Stores G: Sleep problems, *Arch Dis Child* 67(12):1420-1421, 1992.

HEALTH PROBLEMS OF TODDLERS AND PRESCHOOLERS

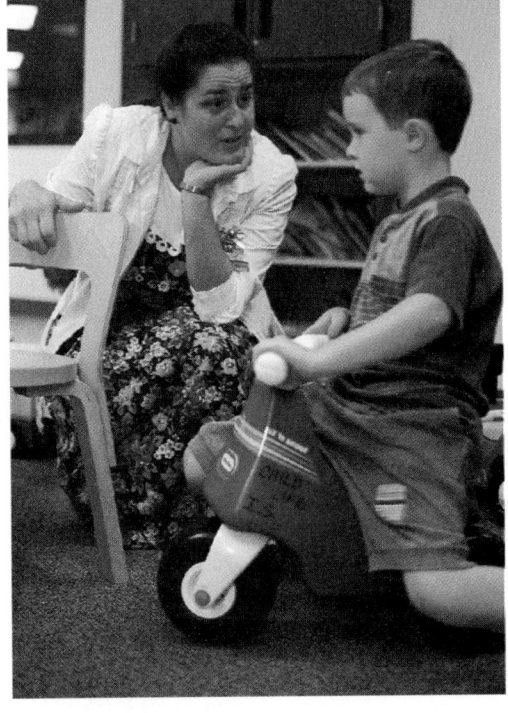

" *If I take medicine and it goes down to my stomach, how will it help my head?*"

Andrew, age 5 years, vehicle injury

RELATED TOPICS

399

INFECTIOUS DISORDERS

COMMUNICABLE DISEASES*

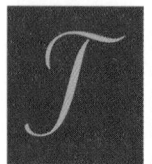he incidence of childhood communicable diseases has declined greatly since the advent of immunizations. Serious complications resulting from such infections have been further reduced with the use of antibiotics and antitoxins. However, infectious diseases do occur, and nurses must be familiar with the infectious agent in order to recognize the disease and institute appropriate preventive and supportive interventions (Table 14-1). See also Chapter 30 for a discussion of nursing care for dermatologic conditions.

Nursing Considerations

❖ Assessment

Identification of the infectious agent is of primary importance to prevent exposure to susceptible individuals. Nurses in ambulatory care settings, child care centers, and schools are often the first persons to see signs of a communicable disease, such as a rash or sore throat. The nurse must operate under a high index of suspicion for common childhood diseases in order to identify potentially infectious cases and to recognize diseases that require medical intervention. An example is the common complaint of sore throat. Although most often a symptom of a minor viral infection, it can signal diphtheria or a streptococcal infection, such as scarlet fever. Each of these bacterial conditions requires appropriate medical treatment to prevent serious sequelae.

Assessment of the following is helpful in identifying potentially communicable diseases: (1) recent exposure to a known case; (2) *prodromal symptoms* (symptoms that occur between early manifestations of the disease and its overt clinical syndrome) or evidence of constitutional symptoms, such as a fever or rash (see Table 14-1); (3) immunization history; and (4) history of having the disease. Because immunizations are available for several of the diseases, and since in almost each case an attack confers lifelong immunity, the possibility

*Renee Covey Harrison, MS, RN, revised this section.

of many infectious agents can be eliminated based on these two criteria.

❖ Nursing Diagnoses

A number of nursing diagnoses are prominent in the nursing care of the child with a communicable disease, and others specific to individual cases become evident. The most common nursing diagnoses are presented in the Nursing Care Plan on pp. 412-413.

❖ Planning

The principal nursing goals in addition to identification of the communicable disease (see Assessment) are as follows:

1. Child will not spread the infection to others.
2. Child will not experience complications.
3. Child will have minimal discomfort.
4. Child and family will receive adequate emotional support.

❖ Implementation

Prevent Spread. Prevention consists of two components: prevention of the disease and control of its spread to others. Primary prevention rests almost exclusively on immunization. (The nurse's role in immunization of children is discussed in Chapter 10.)

Control measures to prevent spread of the disease include appropriate techniques to reduce risk of cross-transmission of infectious organisms between patients and to protect health care workers from organisms harbored by patients. If the child is hospitalized, the facility's policies for infection control are followed (see Chapter 22). The most important procedure to stress is handwashing. Persons directly caring for the child or handling contaminated articles must wash their hands before beginning care of another patient. The child is instructed to practice good handwashing technique after toileting and before eating. For those diseases spread by droplets, the nurse instructs parents in measures aimed at reducing airborne transmission. The child who is old enough should use a tissue to cover the face during coughing or sneezing; otherwise the parent should cover the child's mouth with a tissue and then discard it. The usual hygiene measures of not sharing eating and drinking utensils are stressed to the family.

Nursing ALERT If a child is admitted to the hospital with an undiagnosed exanthema, strict isolation is instituted until a diagnosis is confirmed. Childhood communicable diseases requiring strict isolation are diphtheria and chickenpox.

Prevent Complications. Although most youngsters recover without any difficulty, certain groups of children are at risk for serious, even fatal, complications from communicable diseases, especially the viral diseases of chickenpox and erythema infectiosum (EI). Children with an immunodeficiency—those receiving steroid or other immunosuppressive therapy, those with a generalized malignancy such as leukemia or lymphoma, or those with an immunologic disorder—are at risk for viremia from replication of the *varicella-zoster virus (VZV)** in the blood. VZV is so named because it causes two distinct diseases: *varicella (chickenpox)* and *zoster (herpes zoster* or *shingles).* Varicella occurs primarily in children under 15 years of age. However, it leaves the threat of herpes zoster, an intensely painful varicella that is localized to a single dermatome (body area innervated by a particular segment of the spinal cord) (Straus, 1993). Patients who are immunocompromised and healthy infants under 1 year of age (who also have reduced immunity) are at a higher risk for reactivation of VZV, causing herpes zoster, probably as a result of a deficiency in cellular immunity (Terada and others, 1994).

Children with hemolytic disease, such as sickle cell disease, are at risk for aplastic anemia from EI. The *human parvovirus (HPV)* infects and lyses red blood cell precursors, thus interrupting the production of red blood cells. Therefore, in patients who need increased red blood cell production to maintain normal cell volumes, the virus may precipitate a severe aplastic crisis. Because the fetus depends on a high rate of red blood cell production and has an immature immune system, the fetus may develop severe anemia as a result of HPV infection in the mother.

Nursing ALERT High-risk children who have signs of these communicable diseases are referred to the practitioner immediately. School nurses are responsible for warning parents about recent outbreaks of these communicable diseases in order to prevent susceptible children's exposure to known cases. In most instances high-risk children are kept out of school until the outbreak is over.

Prevention of complications from diseases such as diphtheria and scarlet fever necessitates compliance with antibiotic therapy. With oral preparations the need to complete the entire course of therapy is stressed (see Compliance, Chapter 22). Varicella-zoster immune globulin (VZIG) may be given to high-risk children after exposure to chickenpox to prevent the development of varicella. The antiviral agent acyclovir (Zovirax) may be used to treat varicella infections; it is effective in decreasing the number of lesions, shortening the duration of fever, and decreasing itching, lethargy, and anorexia

*Educational materials for health care providers and families may be obtained from the **Varicella Zoster Virus Research Foundation,** 40 East 72nd St., New York, NY 10021; or Burroughs Wellcome Co., (800) 843-8889.

(Dunkle and others, 1991). Recent evidence suggests that vitamin A supplementation reduces both morbidity and mortality in measles and that all children with severe measles should be given vitamin A supplements (Glasziou and MacKerras, 1993). A single oral dose of 200,000 IU for children at least 1 year old (half that dose for children 6 to 12 months of age) is recommended. The higher dose may be associated with vomiting and headache for a few hours. The dose should be repeated the next day and at 4 weeks for children with ophthalmologic evidence of vitamin A deficiency (American Academy of Pediatrics, 1993).

Nursing ALERT Although the risk of vitamin A toxicity from these doses (they are 100 to 200 times the recommended dietary allowance) is very low, nurses should instruct parents on safe storage of the drug. Ideally, vitamin A should be dispensed in the age-appropriate unit dose to prevent excessive administration and possible toxicity.

Provide Comfort. Many of the communicable diseases cause skin manifestations that are bothersome to the child. The chief discomfort from most of the rashes is itching, and measures such as cool baths (usually without soap) and lotions (e.g., calamine) are helpful.

Nursing ALERT When lotions with active ingredients such as diphenhydramine in Caladryl are used, they are applied sparingly, especially over open lesions, where excessive absorption can lead to drug toxicity, and in children simultaneously receiving oral diphenhydramine.

To avoid overheating, which increases itching, children should wear lightweight, loose, nonirritating clothing and keep out of the sun. If the child persists in scratching, the nails are kept short and smooth; mittens and clothes with long sleeves or legs may be needed. For severe itching, antipruritic medication, such as diphenhydramine (Benadryl) or hydroxyzine (Atarax), may be required, especially when the child desires to sleep.

An elevated temperature is common, and both antipyretic medicine (acetaminophen or Children's Motrin) and environmental manipulation are implemented (see Controlling Elevated Temperature, Chapter 22). The acetaminophen is effective in lowering the fever, but evidence suggests that in chickenpox the medication does not significantly reduce the symptoms of itching, anorexia, abdominal pain, fussiness, or vomiting and that it may delay scabbing of the lesions (Doran and others, 1989).

A sore throat, another frequent symptom, is managed with lozenges, saline rinses (if the child is old enough to cooperate), and analgesics. Since most children are anorectic during an illness, bland foods and increased liquids are usually preferred. During the early stages of the disease, children voluntarily curtail their activity, and although bed rest is beneficial, it should not be imposed unless specifically indicated (e.g., with pertussis). During periods of irritability, quiet activity (e.g., reading, music, television, puzzles, coloring) helps distract children from the discomfort.

Text continued on p. 410.

TABLE 14-1. Communicable diseases of childhood

DISEASE

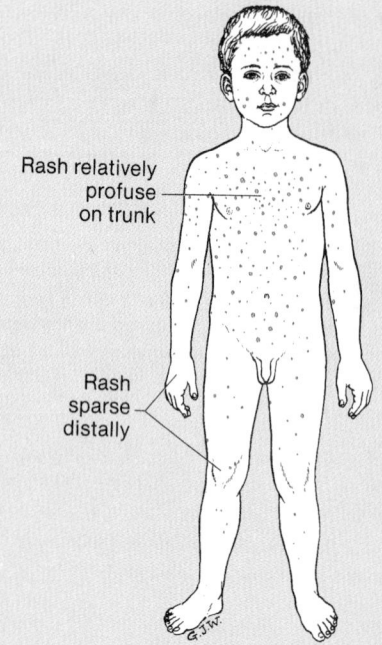

Rash relatively profuse on trunk

Rash sparse distally

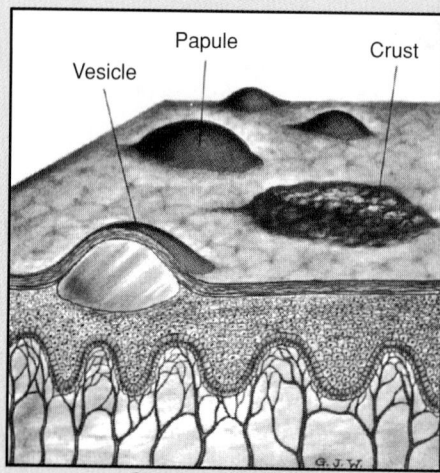

Vesicle Papule Crust

Simultaneous stages of lesions in chickenpox

Chickenpox (Varicella) (Fig. 14-1)

Agent: Varicella-zoster virus (VZV)

Source: Primary secretions of respiratory tract of infected persons; to a lesser degree, skin lesions (scabs not infectious)

Transmission: Direct contact, droplet (airborne) spread, and contaminated objects

Incubation period: 2 to 3 weeks, usually 13 to 17 days

Period of communicability: Probably 1 day before eruption of lesions (prodromal period) to 6 days after first crop of vesicles when crusts have formed

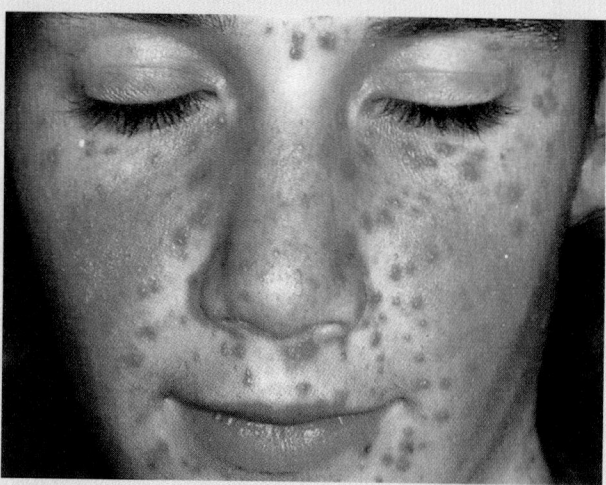

FIG. 14-1. Chickenpox (varicella). (Clinical view from Habif TP: *Clinical dermatology: a color guide to diagnosis and therapy,* ed 2, St Louis, 1990, Mosby.)

Diphtheria

Agent: Corynebacterium diphtheriae

Source: Discharges from mucous membranes of nose and nasopharynx, skin, and other lesions of infected person

Transmission: Direct contact with infected person, a carrier, or contaminated articles

Incubation period: Usually 2 to 5 days, possibly longer

Period of communicability: Variable; until virulent bacilli are no longer present (identified by three negative cultures); usually 2 weeks but as long as 4 weeks

CLINICAL MANIFESTATIONS	THERAPEUTIC MANAGEMENT/ COMPLICATIONS	NURSING CONSIDERATIONS
Prodromal stage: Slight fever, malaise, and anorexia for first 24 hours; rash highly pruritic; begins as macule, rapidly progresses to papule and then vesicle (surrounded by erythematous base, becomes umbilicated and cloudy, breaks easily and forms crusts); all three stages (papule, vesicle, crust) present in varying degrees at one time **Distribution:** Centripetal, spreading to face and proximal extremities but sparse on distal limbs and less on areas not exposed to heat (i.e., from clothing or sun) **Constitutional signs and symptoms:** Elevated temperature from lymphadenopathy, irritability from pruritus	**Specific:** Antiviral agent acyclovir (Zovirax); varicella-zoster immune globulin (VZIG) after exposure in high-risk children **Supportive:** Diphenhydramine hydrochloride or antihistamines to relieve itching; skin care to prevent secondary bacterial infection **Complications:** Secondary bacterial infections (abscesses, cellulitis, pneumonia, sepsis) Encephalitis Varicella pneumonia Hemorrhagic varicella (tiny hemorrhages in vesicles and numerous petechiae in skin) Chronic or transient thrombocytopenia	Maintain strict isolation in hospital Isolate child in home until vesicles have dried (usually 1 week after onset of disease), and isolate high-risk children from infected children Administer skin care: give bath and change clothes and linens daily; administer topical calamine lotion; keep child's fingernails short and clean; apply mittens if child scratches Keep child cool (may decrease number of lesions) Lessen pruritus; keep child occupied Remove loose crusts that rub and irritate skin Teach child to apply pressure to pruritic area rather than scratching it If older child, reason with child regarding danger of scar formation from scratching Avoid use of aspirin; use of acetaminophen controversial
Vary according to anatomic location of pseudomembrane **Nasal:** Resembles common cold, serosanguineous mucopurulent nasal discharge without constitutional symptoms; may be frank epistaxis **Tonsillar/pharyngeal:** Malaise; anorexia; sore throat; low-grade fever; pulse increased above expected for temperature within 24 hours; smooth, adherent, white or gray membrane; lymphadenitis possibly pronounced (bull's neck); in severe cases, toxemia, septic shock, and death within 6 to 10 days **Laryngeal:** Fever, hoarseness, cough, with or without previous signs listed; potential airway obstruction, apprehensive, dyspneic retractions, cyanosis	Antitoxin (usually intravenously); preceded by skin or conjunctival test to rule out sensitivity to horse serum Antibiotics (penicillin or erythromycin) Complete bed rest (prevention of myocarditis) Tracheostomy for airway obstruction Treatment of infected contacts and carriers **Complications:** Myocarditis (second week) Neuritis	Maintain strict isolation in hospital Participate in sensitivity testing; have epinephrine available Administer antibiotics; observe for signs of sensitivity to penicillin Administer complete care to maintain bed rest Use suctioning as needed Observe respirations for signs of obstruction Administer humidified oxygen if prescribed

Continued.

TABLE 14-1. Communicable diseases of childhood—cont'd

DISEASE

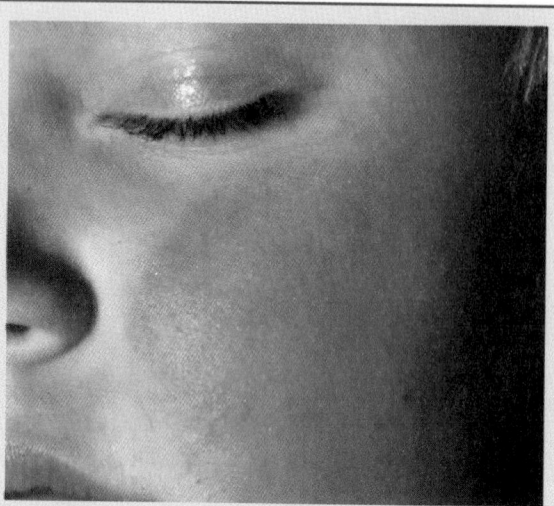

FIG. 14-2. Erythema infectiosum. (From Habif TP: *Clinical dermatology: a color guide to diagnosis and therapy*, ed 2, St Louis, 1990, Mosby.)

Erythema Infectiosum (Fifth Disease) (Fig. 14-2)
Agent: Human parvovirus B19 (HPV)

Source: Infected persons

Transmission: Unknown; possibly respiratory secretions and blood

Incubation period: 4 to 14 days, may be as long as 20 days

Period of communicability: Uncertain but before onset of symptoms in most children; also for about 1 week after onset of symptoms in children with aplastic crisis

Exanthema Subitum (Roseola) (Fig. 14-3)
Agent: Human herpes virus type 6 (HHV-6)

Source: Unknown

Transmission: Unknown (virtually limited to children between 6 months and 2 years of age)

Incubation period: Unknown

Period of communicability: Unknown

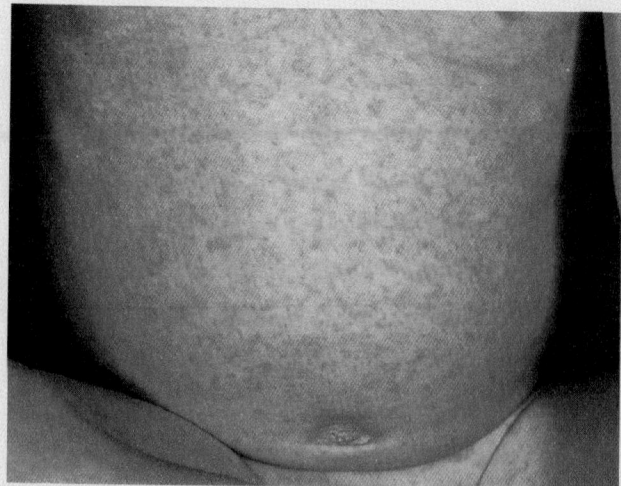

FIG. 14-3. Roseola infantum. (From Habif TP: *Clinical dermatology: a color guide to diagnosis and therapy*, ed 2, St Louis, 1990, Mosby.)

CLINICAL MANIFESTATIONS	THERAPEUTIC MANAGEMENT/ COMPLICATIONS	NURSING CONSIDERATIONS
Rash appears in three stages: I—Erythema on face, chiefly on cheeks, "slapped face" appearance; disappears by 1 to 4 days II—About 1 day after rash appears on face, maculopapular red spots appear, symmetrically distributed on upper and lower extremities; rash progresses from proximal to distal surfaces and may last a week or more III—Rash subsides but reappears if skin is irritated or traumatized (sun, heat, cold, friction) In children with aplastic crisis, rash is usually absent and prodromal illness includes fever, myalgia, lethargy, nausea, vomiting, and abdominal pain	*Symptomatic and supportive:* Antipyretics, analgesics, antiinflammatory drugs Possible blood transfusion for transient aplastic anemia *Complications:* Self-limited arthritis and arthralgia (arthritis may become chronic) (Nocton and others, 1993) May result in fetal death if mother infected during pregnancy, but no evidence of congenital anomalies Aplastic crisis in children with hemolytic disease or immunodeficiency Myocarditis (rare)	Isolation of child not **necessary, except** hospitalized child (immunosuppressed or with aplastic crises) suspected of HPV infection is placed on respiratory isolation and universal precautions Pregnant women: need not be excluded from workplace where HPV infection is present; should not care for patients with aplastic crises; explain low risk of fetal death to those in contact with affected children
Persistent high fever for 3 to 4 days in child who appears well Precipitous drop in fever to normal with appearance of rash *Rash:* Discrete rose-pink macules or maculopapules appearing first on trunk, then spreading to neck, face, and extremities; nonpruritic, fades on pressure, lasts 1 to 2 days *Associated signs and symptoms:* Cervical/postauricular lymphadenopathy, inflamed pharynx, cough, coryza	Nonspecific Antipyretics to control fever *Complications:* Recurrent febrile seizures (possibly from latent infection of central nervous system that is reactivated by fever) Encephalitis (rare)	Teach parents measures for lowering temperature (antipyretic drugs) If child is prone to seizures, discuss appropriate precautions, possibility of recurrent febrile seizures (Kondo and others, 1993)

Continued.

TABLE 14-1. Communicable diseases of childhood—cont'd

DISEASE

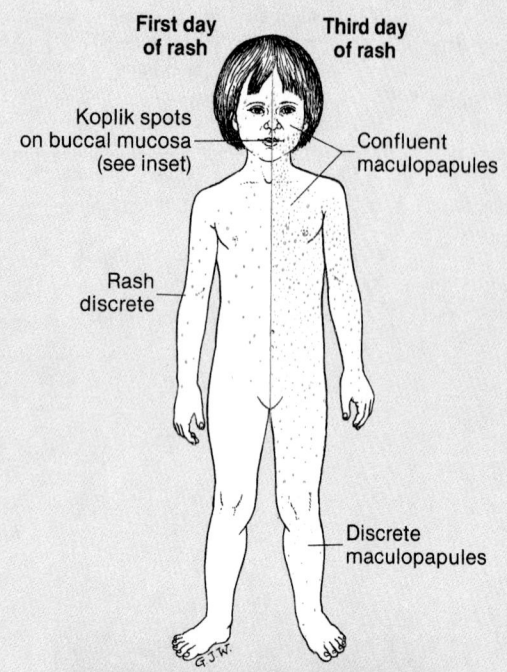

First day of rash / Third day of rash

Koplik spots on buccal mucosa (see inset)

Confluent maculopapules

Rash discrete

Discrete maculopapules

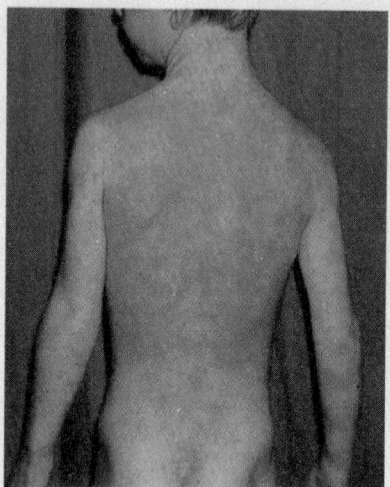

FIG. 14-4. Measles (rubeola). (Clinical view from Seidel HM and others: *Mosby's guide to physical examination,* St Louis, 1991, Mosby.)

Measles (Rubeola) (Fig. 14-4)
Agent: Virus

Source: Respiratory tract secretions, blood, and urine of infected person

Transmission: Usually by direct contact with droplets of infected person

Incubation period: 10 to 20 days

Period of communicability: From 4 days before to 5 days after rash appears but mainly during prodromal (catarrhal) stage

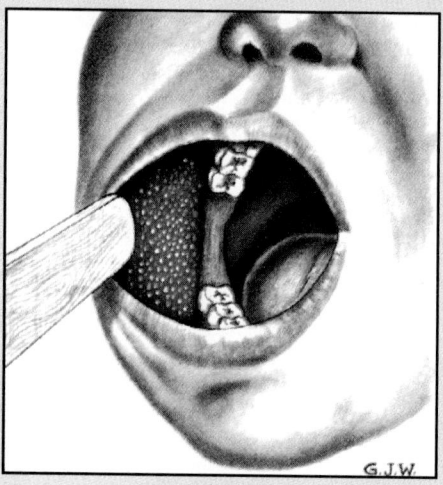

Koplik spots

Mumps
Agent: Paramyxovirus

Source: Saliva of infected persons

Transmission: Direct contact with or droplet spread from an infected person

Incubation period: 14 to 21 days

Period of communicability: Most communicable immediately before and after swelling begins

Pertussis (Whooping Cough)
Agent: Bordetella pertussis

Source: Discharge from respiratory tract of infected persons

Transmission: Direct contact or droplet spread from infected person; indirect contact with freshly contaminated articles

Incubation period: 5 to 21 days, usually 10

CLINICAL MANIFESTATIONS	THERAPEUTIC MANAGEMENT/ COMPLICATIONS	NURSING CONSIDERATIONS
Prodromal (catarrhal) stage: Fever and malaise, followed in 24 hours by coryza, cough, conjunctivitis, Koplik spots (small, irregular red spots with a minute, bluish white center first seen on buccal mucosa opposite molars 2 days before rash); symptoms gradually increase in severity until second day after rash appears, when they begin to subside *Rash:* Appears 3 to 4 days after onset of prodromal stage; begins as erythematous maculopapular eruption on face and gradually spreads downward; more severe in earlier sites (appears confluent) and less intense in later sites (appears discrete); after 3 to 4 days assumes brownish appearance, and fine desquamation occurs over areas of extensive involvement *Constitutional signs and symptoms:* Anorexia, malaise, generalized lymphadenopathy	Vitamin A supplementation (see p. 401) *Supportive:* Bed rest during febrile period; antipyretics Antibiotics to prevent secondary bacterial infection in high-risk children *Complications:* Otitis media Pneumonia Bronchiolitis Obstructive laryngitis and laryngotracheitis Encephalitis	Isolation until fifth day of rash; if hospitalized, institute respiratory precautions Maintain bed rest during prodromal stage; provide quiet activity *Fever:* Instruct parents to administer antipyretics; avoid chilling; if child is prone to seizures, institute appropriate precautions (fever spikes to 40° C [104° F] between fourth and fifth days) *Eye care:* Dim lights if photophobia present; clean eyelids with warm saline solution to remove secretions or crusts; keep child from rubbing eyes; examine cornea for signs of ulceration *Coryza/cough:* Use cool-mist vaporizer; protect skin around nares with layer of petrolatum; encourage fluids and soft, bland foods *Skin care:* Keep skin clean; use tepid baths as necessary
Prodromal stage: Fever, headache, malaise, and anorexia for 24 hours, followed by "earache" that is aggravated by chewing *Parotitis:* By third day, parotid gland(s) (either unilateral or bilateral) enlarges and reaches maximum size in 1 to 3 days; accompanied by pain and tenderness *Other manifestations:* Submaxillary and sublingual infection, orchitis, and meningoencephalitis	*Symptomatic and supportive:* Analgesics for pain and antipyretics for fever Intravenous fluid may be necessary for child who refuses to drink or vomits because of meningoencephalitis *Complications:* Sensorineural deafness Postinfectious encephalitis Myocarditis Arthritis Hepatitis Epididymo-orchitis Sterility (extremely rare in adult males)	Isolation during period of communicability; institute respiratory precautions during hospitalization Maintain bed rest during prodromal phase until swelling subsides Give analgesics for pain; if child is unwilling to chew medication, use elixir form Encourage fluids and soft, bland foods; avoid foods requiring chewing Apply hot or cold compresses to neck, whichever is more comforting To relieve orchitis, provide warmth and local support with tight-fitting underpants (stretch bathing suit works well)
Catarrhal stage: Begins with symptoms of upper respiratory tract infection, such as coryza, sneezing, lacrimation, cough, and low-grade fever; symptoms continue for 1 to 2 weeks, when dry, hacking cough becomes more severe	Antimicrobial therapy (e.g., erythromycin) Administration of pertussis immune globulin	Isolation during catarrhal stage; if hospitalized, institute respiratory precautions Maintain bed rest as long as fever present Keep child occupied during day (interest in play associated with fewer paroxysms) Reassure parents during frightening episodes of whooping cough

Continued.

TABLE 14-1. Communicable diseases of childhood—cont'd

DISEASE

Pertussis (Whooping Cough)—cont'd

Period of communicability: Greatest during catarrhal stage before onset of paroxysms and may extend to fourth week after onset of paroxysms

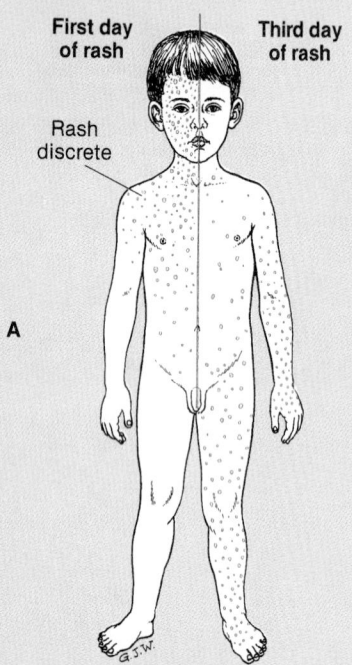

First day
of rash

Third day
of rash

Rash
discrete

A

Poliomyelitis

Agent: Enteroviruses, three types: type 1—most frequent cause of paralysis, both epidemic and endemic; type 2—least frequently associated with paralysis; type 3—second most frequently associated with paralysis

Source: Feces and oropharyngeal secretions of infected persons, especially young children

Transmission: Direct contact with persons with apparent or inapparent active infection; spread is via fecal-oral and pharyngeal-oropharyngeal routes

Incubation period: Usually 7 to 14 days, with range of 5 to 35 days

Period of communicability: Not exactly known; virus is present in throat and feces shortly after infection and persists for about 1 week in throat and 4 to 6 weeks in feces

B

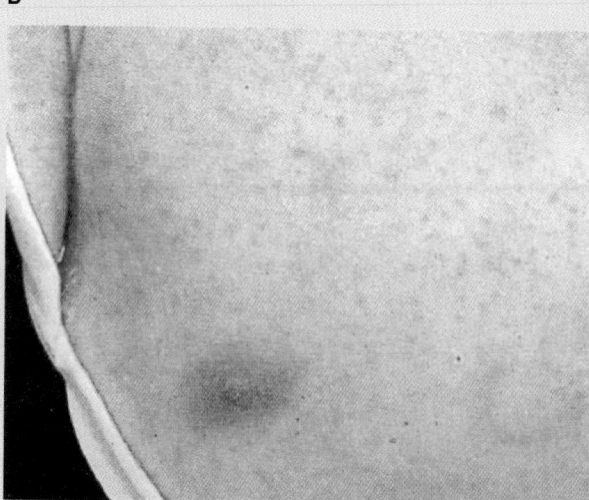

Rubella (German Measles) (Fig. 14-5)
Agent: Rubella virus

Source: Primarily nasopharyngeal secretions of person with apparent or inapparent infection; virus also present in blood, stool, and urine

Transmission: Direct contact and spread via infected person; indirectly via articles freshly contaminated with nasopharyngeal secretions, feces, or urine

Incubation period: 14 to 21 days

Period of communicability: 7 days before to about 5 days after appearance of rash

FIG. 14-5. Rubella (German measles). **A,** Progression of rash. **B,** Clinical view (From Habif TP: *Clinical dermatology: a color guide to diagnosis and therapy,* ed 2, St Louis, 1990, Mosby).

CLINICAL MANIFESTATIONS	THERAPEUTIC MANAGEMENT/ COMPLICATIONS	NURSING CONSIDERATIONS
Paroxysmal stage: Cough most often occurs at night and consists of short, rapid coughs followed by sudden inspiration associated with a high-pitched crowing sound or "whoop"; during paroxysms, cheeks become flushed or cyanotic, eyes bulge, and tongue protrudes; paroxysm may continue until thick mucous plug is dislodged; vomiting frequently follows attack; stage generally lasts 4 to 6 weeks, followed by convalescent stage	*Supportive treatment:* Hospitalization required for infants, children who are dehydrated, or those who have complications Bed rest Increased oxygen intake and humidity Adequate fluids Intubation possibly necessary *Complications:* Pneumonia (usual cause of death) Atelectasis Otitis media Convulsions Hemorrhage (subarachnoid, subconjunctival, epistaxis) Weight loss and dehydration Hernia Prolapsed rectum	Provide restful environment and reduce factors that promote paroxysms (dust, smoke, sudden change in temperature, chilling, activity, excitement); keep room well ventilated Encourage fluids; offer small amount of fluids frequently; refeed child after vomiting Provide high humidity (humidifier or tent); suction gently but often to prevent choking on secretions Observe for signs of airway obstruction (increased restlessness, apprehension, retractions, cyanosis) Involve public health nurse if child cared for at home
May be manifested in three different forms: *Abortive or inapparent*—Fever, uneasiness, sore throat, headache, anorexia, vomiting, abdominal pain; lasts a few hours to a few days *Nonparalytic*—Same manifestations as abortive but more severe, with pain and stiffness in neck, back, and legs *Paralytic*—Initial course similar to nonparalytic type, followed by recovery and then signs of central nervous system paralysis	No specific treatment, including antimicrobials or gamma globulin Complete bed rest during acute phase Assisted respiratory ventilation in case of respiratory paralysis Physical therapy for muscles following acute stage *Complications:* Permanent paralysis Respiratory arrest Hypertension Kidney stones from demineralization of bone during prolonged immobility	Maintain complete bed rest Administer mild sedatives as necessary to relieve anxiety and promote rest Participate in physiotherapy procedures (use of moist hot packs and range-of-motion exercises) Position child to maintain body alignment and prevent contractures or decubiti; use footboard Encourage child to move; administer analgesics for maximum comfort during physical activity Observe for respiratory paralysis (difficulty in talking, ineffective cough, inability to hold breath, shallow and rapid respirations); report such signs and symptoms to practitioner; have tracheostomy tray at bedside
Prodromal stage: Absent in children, present in adults and adolescents; consists of low-grade fever, headache, malaise, anorexia, mild conjunctivitis, coryza, sore throat, cough, and lymphadenopathy; lasts for 1 to 5 days, subsides 1 day after appearance of rash *Rash:* First appears on face and rapidly spreads downward to neck, arms, trunk, and legs; by end of first day, body is covered with a discrete, pinkish red maculopapular exanthema; disappears in same order as it began and is usually gone by third day *Constitutional signs and symptoms:* Occasionally low-grade fever, headache, malaise, and lymphadenopathy	No treatment necessary other than antipyretics for low-grade fever and analgesics for discomfort *Complications:* Rare (arthritis, encephalitis, or purpura); most benign of all childhood communicable diseases; greatest danger is teratogenic effect on fetus	Reassure parents of benign nature of illness in affected child Employ comfort measures as necessary Isolate child from pregnant women

Continued.

TABLE 14-1. Communicable diseases of childhood—cont'd

	DISEASE
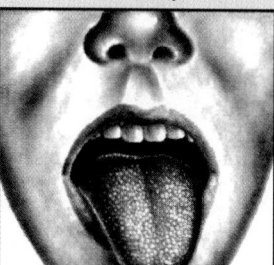 **First day of rash**: Flushed cheeks, White strawberry tongue (see inset), Increased density on neck, Transverse lines (Pastia sign), Increased density in groin. **Third day of rash**: Circumoral pallor, Red strawberry tongue (see inset), Increased density in axilla, Positive blanching test (Schultz-Charlton). **FIG. 14-6.** Scarlet fever.	**Scarlet Fever** (Fig. 14-6) *Agent:* Group A β-hemolytic streptococci *Source:* Usually from nasopharyngeal secretions of infected persons and carriers *Transmission:* Direct contact with infected person or droplet spread; indirectly by contact with contaminated articles or ingestion of contaminated milk or other food *Incubation period:* 2 to 4 days, with range of 1 to 7 days *Period of communicability:* During incubation period and clinical illness, approximately 10 days; during first 2 weeks of carrier phase, although may persist for months First day — White strawberry tongue / Third day — Red strawberry tongue

Support Child and Family. Most communicable diseases are benign, but they produce considerable concern and anxiety for some parents. Often the occurrence of a disease such as chickenpox is the first time the child is acutely uncomfortable. Parents need assistance to cope effectively with manifestations of the illness, such as intense itching. Sometimes a visiting nurse may be beneficial to help the family develop a plan of care and encourage compliance with any treatments.

The family and child need reassurance that recovery from the disease is generally rapid. However, visible signs of the dermatosis may be present for some time after the child is well enough to resume usual activities. When the disease involves noticeable signs, such as the crusts of chickenpox, the child may benefit from preparation before returning to school. For example, the parent can discuss the child's physical appearance with the teacher and/or school nurse and request that they explain the child's condition to classmates.

Nursing ALERT The occurrence of a communicable disease provides the opportunity to ask parents about the child's immunization status and reinforce the benefits of vaccines for children.

❖ Evaluation
The effectiveness of nursing interventions is determined by continual reassessment and evaluation of care based on the following observational guidelines and expected outcomes:

1. Observe or inquire about family members' use of control measures; observe for signs of disease in household contacts.
2. Monitor vital signs, especially temperature; inquire about the identification of high-risk contacts and appropriate isolation of the contact; observe or inquire about compliance with antibiotic or antiviral therapy.
3. Inquire about effectiveness of comfort measures.
4. Interview family and child regarding their feelings and concerns, especially when child returns to school.

Expected outcomes:
See Nursing Care Plan, pp. 412-413.

CONJUNCTIVITIS
Acute conjunctivitis, inflammation of the conjunctiva, occurs from a variety of causes that are typically age related. In newborns conjunctivitis can occur from infection during birth, most often from *Chlamydia trachomatis* (inclusion conjunctivitis). In infants recurrent conjunctivitis may be a sign of nasolacrimal duct obstruction. In children the usual causes

CLINICAL MANIFESTATIONS	THERAPEUTIC MANAGEMENT/ COMPLICATIONS	NURSING CONSIDERATIONS
Prodromal stage: Abrupt high fever, pulse increased out of proportion to fever, vomiting, headache, chills, malaise, abdominal pain	Treatment of choice is a full course of penicillin (or erythromycin in penicllin-sensitive children); fever should subside 24 hours after beginning therapy	Institute respiratory precautions until 24 hours after initiation of treatment
Enanthema: Tonsils enlarged, edematous, reddened, and covered with patches of exudate; in severe cases appearance resembles membrane seen in diphtheria; pharynx is edematous and beefy red; during first 1 to 2 days tongue is coated and papillae become red and swollen (white strawberry tongue); by fourth or fifth day white coat sloughs off, leaving prominent papillae (red strawberry tongue); palate is covered with erythematous punctate lesions	Antibiotic therapy for newly diagnosed carriers (nose or throat cultures positive for streptococci) *Supportive measures:* Bed rest during febrile phase, analgesics for sore throat *Complications:* Otitis media Peritonsillar abscess Sinusitis Glomerulonephritis Carditis, polyarthritis (uncommon)	Ensure compliance with oral antibiotic therapy (intramuscular benzathine penicillin G [Bicillin] may be given if parents' reliability in giving oral drugs is questionable) Maintain bed rest during febrile phase; provide quiet activity during convalescent period Relieve discomfort of sore throat with analgesics, gargles, lozenges, antiseptic throat sprays (Chloraseptic), and inhalation of cool mist Encourage fluids during febrile phase; avoid irritating liquids (citrus juices) or rough foods; when child is able to eat, begin with soft diet Advise parents to consult practitioner if fever persists after beginning therapy Discuss procedures for preventing spread of infection
Exanthema: Rash appears within 12 hours after prodromal signs; red pinhead-sized punctate lesions rapidly become generalized but are absent on face, which becomes flushed with striking circumoral pallor; rash is more intense in folds of joints; by end of first week desquamation begins (fine, sandpaper-like on torso; sheetlike sloughing on palms and soles), which may be complete by 3 weeks or longer		

are viral, bacterial, allergic, or related to a foreign body. Bacterial infection accounts for most instances of acute conjunctivitis in children. Diagnosis is made primarily from the clinical manifestations (see box), although cultures of purulent drainage may be needed to identify the specific cause.

Therapeutic Management

Treatment of conjunctivitis depends on the cause. Viral conjunctivitis is self-limiting, and treatment is limited to removal of the accumulated secretions. Bacterial conjunctivitis is usually treated with topical antibacterial agents. Drops may be used during the day and an ointment at bedtime because the ointment preparation remains in the eye longer. Ointments are usually not used in the daytime because they blur vision.

Nursing Considerations

Nursing goals include keeping the eye clean and properly administering ophthalmic medication. Accumulated secretions are always removed by wiping from the inner canthus downward and outward, away from the opposite eye. Warm, moist compresses, such as a clean washcloth wrung out with hot tap water, are helpful in removing the crusts. Compresses are *not* kept on the eye, because an occlusive covering promotes bacterial growth. Medication is instilled immediately after the

---

CLINICAL MANIFESTATIONS OF CONJUNCTIVITIS

Bacterial Conjunctivitis ("Pink Eye")
Purulent drainage
Crusting of eyelids, especially on awakening
Inflamed conjunctiva
Swollen lids
Usually both eyes infected

Viral Conjunctivitis
Usually occurs with upper respiratory tract infection
Serous (watery) drainage
Inflamed conjunctiva
Swollen lids
Usually both eyes infected

Allergic Conjunctivitis
Itching
Watery to thick, stringy discharge
Inflamed conjunctiva
Swollen lids
Usually both eyes affected

Conjunctivitis Caused by Foreign Body
Tearing
Pain
Inflamed conjunctiva
Usually only one eye affected

NURSING CARE PLAN
The Child with a Communicable Disease

NURSING DIAGNOSIS: High risk for infection related to susceptible host and infectious agents

PATIENT GOAL 1: Will not become infected

- **NURSING INTERVENTIONS/*RATIONALES***

Be highly suspicious of infectious diseases, especially in susceptible children

Identify high-risk children (e.g., those with an immunodeficiency or hemolytic disease) to whom communicable disease may be fatal; in case of an outbreak, advise parents to confine child to the home *to avoid exposure*

Participate in public education and service programs regarding prophylactic immunizations, method of spread of communicable diseases, proper preparation and handling of food and water supplies, control of animal vectors in regard to reservoirs of disease (not a factor in childhood communicable disease but in other infectious illness such as malaria), or screening programs to identify streptococcal infections

- **EXPECTED OUTCOME**

Susceptible children do not contract the disease

PATIENT GOAL 2: Will not spread disease

- **NURSING INTERVENTIONS/*RATIONALES***

Institute appropriate infection control practices (see Chapter 22)

Make referral to public health nurse when necessary *to ensure appropriate procedures in the home*

Work with families *to ensure compliance with therapeutic regimens*

Identify close contacts who may require prophylactic treatment (e.g., specific immune globulin or antibiotics)

Report disease to local health department if appropriate

- **EXPECTED OUTCOME**

Infection remains confined to original source

PATIENT GOAL 3: Will exhibit no evidence of complications

- **NURSING INTERVENTIONS/*RATIONALES***

Ensure compliance with therapeutic regimen (e.g., bed rest, antiviral therapy, antibiotics, adequate hydration)

Avoid giving aspirin to children with varicella *because of the possible risk of Reye syndrome*

Institute seizure precautions if febrile convulsions are a possibility

Monitor temperature; *unexpected elevations may signal an infection*

Maintain good body hygiene *to reduce risk of secondary infection of lesions*

Offer small, frequent sips of water or favorite drinks *to ensure adequate hydration* and soft, bland foods (gelatin, pudding, ice cream, soups), *since many children are anorectic during an illness;* feed again after vomiting; observe for signs of dehydration

- **EXPECTED OUTCOME**

Child exhibits no evidence of complications such as infection or dehydration

NURSING DIAGNOSIS: Pain related to skin lesions, malaise

PATIENT GOAL 1: Will experience minimal discomfort

- **NURSING INTERVENTIONS/*RATIONALES***

Use cool-mist vaporizer, gargles, and lozenges *to keep mucous membranes moist*

Apply petrolatum to chapped lips or nares

Cleanse eyes with physiologic saline solution *to remove secretions or crusts*

Keep skin clean; change bedclothes and linens at least daily

Administer oral hygiene

Keep child cool *because overheating increases itching*

Give cool baths and apply lotion such as calamine *to decrease itching*

Assess need for pain medication (see Chapter 22)

Employ nonpharmacologic pain reduction techniques (see Chapter 21)

*Administer analgesics, antipyretics, and antipruritics as needed

- **EXPECTED OUTCOMES**

Skin and mucous membranes are clean and free of irritants

Child exhibits minimal evidence of discomfort (specify)

NURSING DIAGNOSIS: Impaired social interaction related to isolation from peers

PATIENT GOAL 1: Will have some understanding of reason for isolation

- **NURSING INTERVENTIONS/*RATIONALES***

Explain reason for confinement and use of any special precautions *to increase child's understanding of restrictions*

Allow child to play with gloves, mask, and gown (if used) *to facilitate positive coping*

- **EXPECTED OUTCOME**

Child demonstrates understanding of restrictions

PATIENT GOAL 2: Will have opportunity to participate in suitable activities

- **NURSING INTERVENTIONS/*RATIONALES***

Always introduce self to child; allow to see face before donning protective clothing, if required

Provide diversionary activity

Encourage parents to remain with child during hospitalization *to decrease separation and provide companionship*

Encourage contact with friends via telephone (in hospital can use intercom between room and nurse's station)

Prepare child's peers for altered physical appearance, such as with chickenpox, *to encourage peer acceptance*

*Dependent nursing action.

NURSING CARE PLAN
The Child with a Communicable Disease—cont'd

- **EXPECTED OUTCOMES**

Child engages in suitable activities and interactions
Peers accept child

> **NURSING DIAGNOSIS:** High risk for impaired skin integrity related to scratching from pruritus

PATIENT GOAL 1: Will maintain skin integrity

- **NURSING INTERVENTIONS/RATIONALES**

Keep nails short and clean *to minimize trauma and secondary infection*
Apply mittens or elbow restraints *to prevent scratching*
Dress in lightweight, loose, and nonirritating clothing *because overheating increases itching*
Cover affected areas (long sleeves, pants, one-piece outfit) *to prevent scratching*
Bathe in cool water with no soap or apply cool compresses
Apply soothing lotions (sparingly on open lesions *because absorption of drug is increased*) *to decrease pruritus*
Avoid exposure to heat or sun, *which can aggravate rash* (e.g., chickenpox)

- **EXPECTED OUTCOME**

Skin remains intact

> **NURSING DIAGNOSIS:** Altered family processes related to child with an acute illness

PATIENT (FAMILY) GOAL 1: Will receive adequate emotional support

- **NURSING INTERVENTIONS/RATIONALES**

Inform parents of treatment options, especially acyclovir for varicella
Reinforce family's effort to carry out plan of care
Provide assistance when necessary, such as visiting nurse *to help with home care*
Keep family aware of child's progress *to encourage optimistic attitude*
Stress rapidity of recovery in most cases *to decrease anxiety*

- **EXPECTED OUTCOMES**

Family continues to comply with expectations
Family seeks needed support

---

eyes have been cleaned and according to correct procedure (see Chapter 22).

Prevention of infection in other family members is an important consideration with bacterial conjunctivitis. The child's washcloth and towel are kept separate from those used by others. Tissues used to clean the eye are discarded. The child should refrain from rubbing the eye and is instructed in good handwashing.

STOMATITIS

Stomatitis is inflammation of the oral mucosa, which may include the buccal (cheek) and labial (lip) mucosa, tongue, gingiva, palate, and floor of the mouth. It may be infectious or noninfectious and may be caused by local or systemic factors. In children aphthous stomatitis and herpetic stomatitis are typically seen.

Aphthous stomatitis (aphthous ulcer, canker sore) is a benign but painful condition whose cause is unknown. Its onset is usually associated with mild traumatic injury (biting the cheek, hitting the mucosa with a toothbrush, or a mouth appliance rubbing on the mucosa), allergy, and emotional stress. The lesions are painful, small, whitish ulcerations surrounded by a red border. They are distinguished from other types of stomatitis by healthy adjacent tissues, absence of vesicles, and no systemic illness. The ulcers persist for 4 to 12 days and heal uneventfully.

Herpetic gingivostomatitis (HGS) is caused by the her-

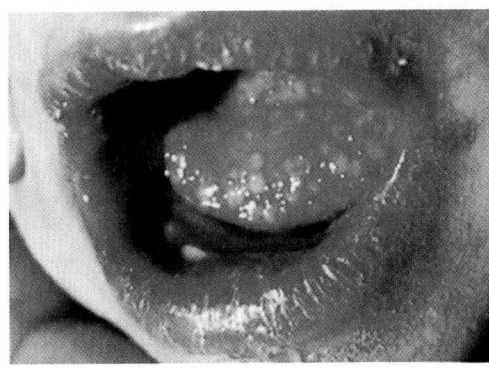

FIG. 14-7. Primary gingivostomatitis. (From Thompson JM and others: *Clinical nursing,* St Louis, 1986, Mosby.)

pes simplex virus (HSV), most often type 1, and may occur as a primary infection or recur in a less severe form known as recurrent herpes labialis (commonly called "cold sores" or "fever blisters"). The primary infection usually begins with a fever; the pharynx becomes edematous and erythematous; and vesicles erupt on the mucosa, causing severe pain (Fig. 14-7). Cervical lymphadenitis often occurs, and the breath has a distinctly foul odor. The disease can last 5 to 14 days with varying degrees of severity.

Therapeutic Management

Treatment for both types of stomatitis is aimed at relief of symptoms, primarily pain. Acetaminophen is usually sufficient for mild cases, but with more severe HGS, stronger analgesics such as codeine may be needed. Topical anesthetics are helpful and include over-the-counter preparations, such as Orabase, Anbesol, and Kanka, or prescription formulas, such as viscous xylocaine. Specific treatment for children with severe cases of HGS is the use of acyclovir (Zovirax).

Nursing Considerations

The chief nursing goals for children with stomatitis are relief of pain and prevention of spread of the herpes virus. Analgesics and topical anesthetics are used as needed to provide relief, especially before meals to encourage food and fluid intake. Drinking bland fluids through a straw is helpful in avoiding the painful lesions. An oral dressing (Orahesive)* that adheres to the mucosa can provide a barrier over the lesions. Mouth care is encouraged; the use of a very soft bristle toothbrush or disposable foam-tipped toothbrush provides gentle cleaning near ulcerated areas.

Careful handwashing is essential when caring for children with HGS. Since the infection is autoinoculable, children should keep their fingers out of the mouth; contaminated hands also can infect other body parts. Very young children may need elbow restraints to ensure compliance. All articles placed in the mouth are cleaned thoroughly. Newborns and individuals with immunosuppression should not be exposed to infected children.

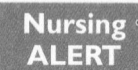 **Nursing ALERT** When examining herpetic lesions, wear gloves. The virus easily enters breaks in the skin and can cause herpetic whitlow of the fingers.

Because herpes infection is often associated with sexual transmission, the nurse should explain to parents and older children that HGS is usually caused by type 1 HSV, the type not associated with sexual activity.

INTESTINAL PARASITIC DISEASES†

Intestinal parasitic diseases, including helminths (worms) and protozoa, constitute the most frequent infections in the world. In the United States the incidence of intestinal parasitic disease, especially giardiasis, has increased among young children who are attending daycare centers.

Intestinal parasitic diseases in humans are caused by various infecting organisms. This discussion is limited to the two most common parasitic infections among children in the United States: giardiasis and pinworms. Table 14-2 describes the outstanding features of selected helminths that belong to the family of nematodes.

*Manufactured by Convatec, Princeton, NJ.
†Pamela DiVito-Thomas, MS, RN, revised this section.

GENERAL NURSING CONSIDERATIONS

Nursing responsibilities related to intestinal parasitic infections involve assistance with identification of the parasite, treatment of the infection, and prevention of initial infection or reinfection. Identification of the organism is accomplished by laboratory examination of substances containing the worm, its larvae, or ova. Most are identified by examining fecal smears from the stools of persons suspected of harboring the parasite. Fresh specimens are best for revealing parasites or larvae; therefore collected specimens should be taken directly to the laboratory for examination. If this is not feasible, the specimen is placed in a container with a preservative (see Stool Specimens, Chapter 22).

In most parasitic infections, examination of other family members, especially children, may be carried out to identify those who are similarly affected. Nurses frequently assume the responsibility for directing and instructing families in the collection and disposition of specimens. Parents need clear written instructions on obtaining an adequate sample and the number of samples required.

Once the diagnosis is confirmed and an appropriate treatment regimen is planned, parents need further explanation and reinforcement. Compliance in terms of drug therapy and any other measures, such as thorough handwashing, are essential for eradication of the parasite. The family needs to understand the nature of transmission and that in some cases the medication must be repeated in 2 weeks to 1 month to kill organisms hatched since initial treatment.

The nurse's most important function in relation to these parasites is preventive education of children and families regarding good hygiene and health habits. Thorough handwashing before eating or handling food and after using the toilet is the most important precautionary method. Other preventive practices are listed in the Family Home Care box.

 FAMILY HOME CARE
Preventing Intestinal Parasitic Disease

Always wash hands and fingernails with soap and water before eating and handling food and after toileting.
Avoid placing fingers in mouth and biting nails.
Discourage children from scratching bare anal area.
Use superabsorbent disposable diapers to prevent leakage.
Change diapers as soon as soiled and dispose of diapers in closed receptable out of children's reach.
Do not rinse diapers in toilet.
Disinfect toilet seats and diaper changing areas; use dilute household bleach (10% solution) or Lysol and wipe clean with paper towels.
Drink water that is specially treated, especially if camping.
Wash all raw fruits and vegetables and food that has fallen on the floor.
Avoid growing foods in soil fertilized with human excreta.
Teach children to defecate only in a toilet, not on the ground.
Keep dogs and cats away from playgrounds or sandboxes.
Avoid swimming in pools frequented by diapered children.
Wear shoes outside.

TABLE 14-2. Selected intestinal parasites

CLINICAL MANIFESTATIONS	COMMENTS
Ascariasis—*Ascaris lumbricoides* (Common Roundworm) Light infections: asymptomatic Heavy infections: anorexia, irritability, nervousness, enlarged abdomen, weight loss, fever, intestinal colic Severe infections: intestinal obstruction, appendicitis, perforation of intestine with peritonitis, obstructive jaundice, lung involvement—pneumonitis	Transferred to mouth by way of contaminated food, fingers, or toys Largest of the intestinal helminths Affects principally young children 1-4 years of age Prevalent in warm climates
Hookworm Disease—*Necator americanus* Light infections in well-nourished individuals: no problems Heavier infections: mild to severe anemia, malnutrition May be itching and burning ("ground itch") followed by erythema and a papular eruption in areas to which the organism migrates	Transmitted by discharging eggs on the soil, which are picked up, causing infection from direct skin contact with contaminated soil Wearing shoes is recommended, although children playing in contaminated soil expose many skin surfaces
Strongyloidiasis—*Strongyloides stercoralis* (Threadworm) Light infection: asymptomatic Heavy infection: respiratory signs and symptoms; abdominal pain, distention; nausea and vomiting; diarrhea—large, pale stools, often with mucus Threat to life in children with weakened immunologic defenses	Transmission is same as for hookworm except autoinfection common Older children and adults affected more often than young children Severe infections may lead to severe nutritional deficiency
Visceral Larva Migrans—*Toxocara canis* (Dogs); Intestinal Toxocariasis—*Toxocara cati* (Cats) Depends on reactivity of infected individual May be asymptomatic except for eosinophilia Specific diagnosis difficult	Transmitted by direct contamination of hands from contact with dog, cat, or objects or by ingestion of soil Dogs and cats should be kept away from areas where children play; sandboxes are especially important transmission areas Periodic deworming of diagnosed dogs and cats Control of dog and cat population Continued education and laws to prevent indiscriminate canine and feline defecation
Trichuriasis—*Trichuris trichiura* (Whipworm) Light infections: asymptomatic Heavy infections: abdominal pain and distention, diarrhea	Transmitted from contaminated soil, vegetables, toys, and other objects Most frequent in warm, moist climates Occurs most often in undernourished children living in unsanitary conditions

GIARDIASIS

Giardiasis is caused by the protozoan *Giardia lamblia* (also called *G. intestinalis,* *G. duodenalis,* and *Lamblia intestinalis*). It is the most common intestinal parasitic pathogen in the United States, and its prevalence among children in day-care centers may range from 17% to more than 50% during outbreaks (Bartlett and others, 1991). Breast-fed infants exposed to *Giardia* develop much less diarrhea but are not protected from becoming infected (Walterspiel and others, 1994).

The potential for transmission is great, since the cysts, the nonmotile stage of the protozoa, can survive in the environment for months. Chief modes of transmission are person to person; water, especially mountain lakes, streams, and pools frequented by diapered infants; food; and animals, especially puppies. In children, person-to-person transmission is the most likely cause.

Diagnostic Evaluation

Although individuals infected with giardiasis may be asymptomatic, young children, especially infants, usually manifest symptoms at any early stage (see box on p. 416). Unlike most other intestinal parasites, *G. lamblia* is not easily diagnosed from stool specimens. Since *Giardia* organisms are excreted in a highly variable pattern, six or more stool specimens collected over several weeks may be necessary to identify the trophozoites (active parasites) or cysts.

Since the organism lives in the upper intestine, aspiration or biopsy of the duodenum or upper jejunum may be performed. The *string test* may be used to aspirate duodenal fluid directly. A nylon string is attached to a gelatin capsule, which is swallowed; several hours later the string is withdrawn and the contents are examined microscopically for trophozoites. However, the string test is being used less often because other tests that detect *Giardia* antigen in the stool, such as

CLINICAL MANIFESTATIONS OF GIARDIASIS

Infants and young children:
Diarrhea
Vomiting
Anorexia
Failure to thrive
Children over 5 years of age:
Abdominal cramps
Intermittent loose stools
Constipation
Stools may be malodorous, watery, pale, and greasy
Most infections resolve spontaneously in 4 to 6 weeks
Rarely, chronic form occurs:
Intermittent loose, foul-smelling stools
Possibility of abdominal bloating, flatulence, sulfur-tasting belches, epigastric pain, vomiting, headache, and weight loss

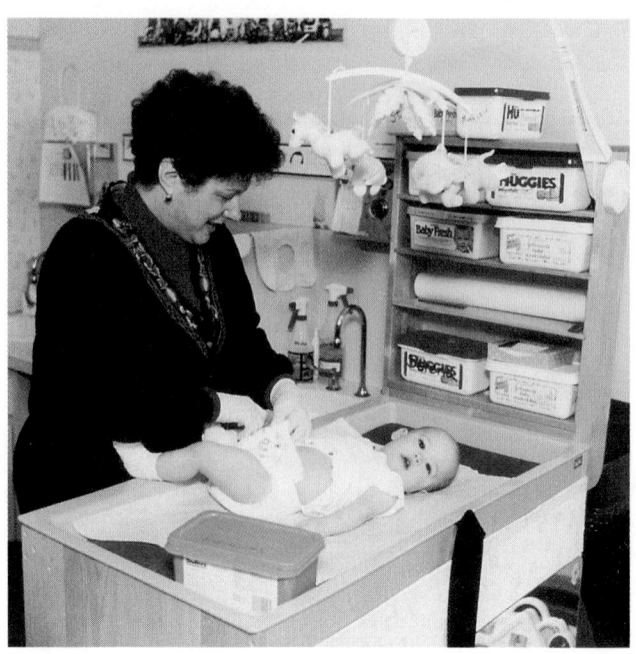

FIG. 14-8. Prevention of giardiasis, especially in daycare centers, requires sanitary practices during diaper changes, such as discarding paper diapers in a covered receptacle, changing paper covers on the diaper-changing surface, and having facilities for handwashing nearby. NOTE: Soiled cloth diapers and clothing should be stored in a plastic bag for transport home.

counterimmunoelectrophoresis (CIE) and enzyme-linked immunosorbent assay (ELISA), are available.

Therapeutic Management

The drugs available for treatment of giardiasis are quinacrine (Atabrine), furazolidone (Furoxone), and metronidazole (Flagyl). The drug of choice is furazolidone, unless cost is a factor, in which case quinacrine is substituted. Quinacrine is less than one-tenth the cost of furazolidone, and its long-term safety is established over the use of metronidazole. For pregnant women who need treatment, paromomycin may be used first, followed by metronidazole if the initial treatment is unsuccessful (Hill, 1993). Unfortunately, quinacrine has the highest frequency of side effects, especially nausea and vomiting; causes temporary yellow staining of the skin, sclera, and urine; and has a very bitter taste.

Nursing Considerations

The most important nursing consideration is prevention of giardiasis, especially among children and staff of daycare centers. Attention to meticulous sanitary practices, especially during diaper changes, is essential (see Family Home Care box on p. 414 and Fig. 14-8). Nurses can play an important role in educating daycare staff regarding appropriate sanitation practices (see Preschool or Daycare Experience, Chapter 13).

Once children are infected, family education regarding drug administration is essential. Parents often need suggestions for encouraging the child to take quinacrine. If other household members are infected, the nurse should inquire about their understanding and management of the disease.

NURSING TIPS To decrease the side effects of quinacrine and increase its palatability:
• Administer the drug with or after meals.
• Crush tablets and mix with a strong flavoring, such as jam or syrup.

ENTEROBIASIS (PINWORMS)

Enterobiasis, or pinworms, caused by the nematode *Enterobius vermicularis,* is the most common helminthic infection in the United States. It is universally present in temperate climatic zones and may infect more than 30% of all children at any one time. Crowded conditions, such as in classrooms and daycare centers, favor transmission.

Infection begins when the eggs are ingested. Since the eggs float in the air, they are also easily inhaled. The movement of the worms on skin and mucous membrane surfaces causes intense itching. As the child scratches, eggs are deposited on the hands and under the fingernails. The typical hand-to-mouth activity of youngsters makes them especially prone to continual reinfection. Pinworm eggs also persist in the home to contaminate anything they contact, such as toilet seats, doorknobs, bed linen, underwear, and food.

Diagnostic Evaluation

Except for the intense rectal itching associated with pinworms, the clinical manifestations (see box) are nonspecific. Diagnosis is most commonly made from the tape test (see Nursing Considerations). Repeated tests to collect eggs may be necessary, and if there is a possibility that other family members may be infected, a tape test should be performed on them.

<table>
<tr><td colspan="1">CLINICAL MANIFESTATIONS OF PINWORMS</td></tr>
<tr><td>

Intense perianal itching (principal symptom); evidence of itching in young children includes the following:
  General irritability
  Restlessness
  Poor sleep
  Bed-wetting
  Distractibility
  Short attention span
Perianal dermatitis and excoriation secondary to itching
If worms migrate, possible vaginal and urethral infection

</td></tr>
</table>

Therapeutic Management

The drugs available for treatment of pinworms include mebendazole (Vermox), pyrantel pamoate (Antiminth), piperazine phosphate, and pyrvinium pamoate (Povan). The drug of choice is mebendazole, which is safe, effective, and convenient, with few side effects. However, it is not recommended for children under 2 years of age. If pyrvinium pamoate is prescribed, parents are advised that the drug stains stool and vomitus bright red, as well as clothing or skin that comes in contact with the drug. Since pinworms are easily transmitted, all household members are treated. The drugs may be repeated in 2 weeks to prevent reinfection.

Nursing Considerations

Nursing care is directed at identifying the parasite, eradicating the organism, and preventing reinfection. Parents need clear, detailed instructions for the *tape test.* A loop of transparent (not "frosted" or "magic") tape, sticky side out, is placed around the end of a tongue depressor, which is then firmly pressed against the child's perianal area. A convenient, commercially prepared tape is also available for this purpose. Pinworm specimens are collected in the morning as soon as the child awakens and *before* the child has a bowel movement or bathes. The procedure may need to be repeated more than once before eggs are collected. Parents are instructed to place the tongue blade in a glass jar or loosely in a plastic bag so that it can be brought in for microscopic examination. For specimens collected in the hospital, practitioner's office, or clinic, the tape is placed smoothly on a glass slide, sticky side down, for examination.

Compliance with the drug regimen is usually excellent, because the duration of treatment is typically only one dose. However, the family is reminded of the need to take a second dose in 2 weeks. Posting a reminder on the refrigerator door or bathroom mirror is helpful.

To prevent reinfection, certain cleaning practices, such as washing all clothes and bed linen in hot water and vacuuming the house, may be recommended. However, there is little documentation on their effectiveness, since pinworms survive on so many surfaces. Suggestions that are helpful include handwashing after toileting and before eating, keeping the child's fingernails short to minimize the chance of ova collecting under the nails, dressing children in one-piece sleeping outfits, and daily showering rather than tub bathing.

INGESTION OF INJURIOUS AGENTS*

Since the passage of the Poison Prevention Packaging Act of 1970, which provides that certain potentially hazardous drugs and household products be sold in child-resistant containers, the incidence of poisonings in children has decreased dramatically. However, despite these advances, poisoning remains a significant health concern, with most cases occurring in children under 6 years of age. Children are poisoned by a variety of substances. Although the reported incidence of ingested substances varies, the most frequently ingested poisons are the following (Litovitz and others, 1993):

- Cosmetics and personal care products (perfume, cologne, aftershave)†
- Cleaning products (hypochlorite ["household"] bleach, pine oil disinfectants)
- Plants (nontoxic gastrointestinal irritants, oxalates; see box)
- Foreign bodies, toys, and miscellaneous substances (dessicants, thermometers, bubble-blowing solutions)
- Hydrocarbons (gasoline)

---

*Krena Hunter White, MS, MA, RN, revised this section.
†Most common substances in each category are in parentheses. Substances ingested are not necessarily most toxic but often represent ready availability.

<table>
<tr><td colspan="3">POISONOUS AND NONPOISONOUS PLANTS</td></tr>
<tr><td>Poisonous Plants</td><td>Toxic Parts</td><td>Nonpoisonous Plants</td></tr>
<tr><td>Apple</td><td>Leaves, seeds</td><td>African violet</td></tr>
<tr><td>Apricot</td><td>Leaves, stem, seed pits</td><td>Aluminum plant</td></tr>
<tr><td></td><td></td><td>Asparagus fern</td></tr>
<tr><td>Azalea</td><td>Foliage and flowers</td><td>Begonia</td></tr>
<tr><td>Buttercup</td><td>All parts</td><td>Boston fern</td></tr>
<tr><td>Cherry (wild or cultivated)</td><td>Twigs, seeds, foliage</td><td>Christmas cactus</td></tr>
<tr><td></td><td></td><td>Coleus</td></tr>
<tr><td>Daffodil</td><td>Bulbs</td><td>Gardenia</td></tr>
<tr><td>Dumb cane, dieffenbachia</td><td>All parts</td><td>Grape ivy</td></tr>
<tr><td></td><td></td><td>Jade plant</td></tr>
<tr><td>Elephant ear</td><td>All parts</td><td>Marigolds</td></tr>
<tr><td>English ivy</td><td>All parts</td><td>Piggyback</td></tr>
<tr><td>Foxglove</td><td>Leaves, seeds, flowers</td><td>begonia</td></tr>
<tr><td></td><td></td><td>Piggyback plant</td></tr>
<tr><td>Holly</td><td>Berries</td><td>Poinsettia†</td></tr>
<tr><td>Hyacinth</td><td>Bulbs</td><td>Prayer plant</td></tr>
<tr><td>Ivy</td><td>Leaves</td><td>Rubber tree</td></tr>
<tr><td>Mistletoe*</td><td>Berries, leaves</td><td>Snake plant</td></tr>
<tr><td>Oak tree</td><td>Acorn, foliage</td><td>Spider plant</td></tr>
<tr><td>Philodendron</td><td>All parts</td><td>Swedish ivy</td></tr>
<tr><td>Plum</td><td>Pit</td><td>Wax plant</td></tr>
<tr><td>Poison ivy, poison oak</td><td>Leaves, fruit, stems, smoke from burning plants</td><td>Weeping fig</td></tr>
<tr><td></td><td></td><td>Zebra plant</td></tr>
<tr><td>Pothos</td><td>All parts</td><td></td></tr>
<tr><td>Rhubarb</td><td>Leaves</td><td></td></tr>
<tr><td>Tulip</td><td>Bulbs</td><td></td></tr>
<tr><td>Water hemlock</td><td>All parts</td><td></td></tr>
<tr><td>Wisteria</td><td>Seeds, pods</td><td></td></tr>
<tr><td>Yew</td><td>All parts</td><td></td></tr>
</table>

*Eating one or two berries or leaves is probably nontoxic.
†Mildly toxic if ingested in massive quantities.

SELECTED POISONINGS IN CHILDREN

Corrosives (Strong Acids or Alkali)

Drain, toilet, or oven cleaners
Electric dishwasher detergent (liquid, because of higher pH, is more hazardous than granular)
Mildew remover
Batteries
Clinitest tablets
Denture cleaners

Clinical Manifestations

Severe burning pain in mouth, throat, and stomach
White, swollen mucous membranes, edema of lips, tongue, and pharynx (respiratory obstruction)
Violent vomiting (hemoptysis)
Drooling and inability to clear secretions
Signs of shock
Anxiety and agitation

Comments

Household bleach is a frequently ingested corrosive but rarely causes serious damage
Liquid preparations cause more damage than granular preparations

Treatment

Inducing emesis is contraindicated (vomiting redamages the mucosa)
Dilute corrosive with water (usually no more than 120 ml [4 oz]), not milk (coats membranes, making assessment difficult) unless vomiting occurs
Provide patent airway if needed
Administer analgesics
Do not allow oral intake
Esophageal stricture may require repeated dilations and/or surgery

Hydrocarbons

Gasoline
Kerosene
Lamp oil
Mineral seal oil (found in furniture polish)
Lighter fluid
Turpentine
Paint thinner and remover (some types)

Clinical Manifestations

Gagging, choking, and coughing
Nausea
Vomiting
Alterations in sensorium, such as lethargy
Weakness
Respiratory symptoms of pulmonary involvement
    Tachypnea
    Cyanosis
    Retractions
    Grunting

Comments

Immediate danger is aspiration (even small amounts can cause bronchitis and chemical pneumonia)
Gasoline, kerosene, lighter fluid, mineral seal oil, and turpentine cause severe pneumonia

Treatment (Controversial)

Inducing emesis is generally contraindicated
Gastric lavage may be used
Symptomatic treatment of chemical pneumonia includes high humidity, oxygen, hydration, and antibiotics for secondary infection

Acetaminophen
Clinical Manifestations

Occurs in four stages:
1. Initial period (2 to 4 hours after ingestion)
    Nausea
    Vomiting
    Sweating
    Pallor
2. Latent period (24 to 36 hours)
    Patient improves
3. Hepatic involvement (may last up to 7 days and be permanent)
    Pain in right upper quadrant
    Jaundice
    Confusion
    Stupor
    Coagulation abnormalities
4. Patients who do not die in hepatic stage gradually recover

Comments

Most common drug poisoning in children
Occurs from acute ingestion
Toxic dose is 150 mg/kg or greater in children
Toxicity from chronic therapeutic use is rare but may occur with ingestion of approximately 150 mg/kg/day, or about double the recommended maximum therapeutic dose (90 mg/kg/day) of acetaminophen, for several days (Douidar, Al-Khalil, and Habersang, 1994); toxicity is more likely in children with hepatic dysfunction (Cheung, Potts, and Meyer, 1994)

Treatment

Emesis, lavage, activated charcoal
Antidote N-acetylcysteine (NAC) is given, usually by nasogastric tube because of the antidote's offensive odor (smells like rotten eggs)
Given as one loading dose and usually 17 maintenance doses in different dosages
May be given intravenously, but use is investigational

Aspirin (ASA)
Clinical Manifestations

Acute poisoning
    Nausea
    Disorientation
    Vomiting
    Dehydration
    Diaphoresis
    Hyperpnea
    Hyperpyrexia
    Oliguria
    Tinnitus
    Coma
    Convulsions
Chronic poisoning
    Same as above but subtle onset (often confused with illness being treated)
Dehydration, coma, and seizures may be more severe
Bleeding tendencies

Comments

May be caused by acute ingestion (severe toxicity occurs with 300 to 500 mg/kg [4 to 7 gr/kg])
May be caused by chronic ingestion (i.e., more than 100 mg/kg/day for 2 or more days); can be more serious than acute ingestion
Time to peak serum salicylate level can vary with enteric aspirin or the presence of concretions (bezoars)

SELECTED POISONINGS IN CHILDREN—cont'd

Treatment
Home use of ipecac for moderate toxicity
Hospitalization for severe toxicity
Emesis, lavage, activated charcoal, and/or cathartic
Lavage will not remove concretions of ASA
Activated charcoal is important early in ASA toxicity
Sodium bicarbonate transfusions to correct metabolic acidosis and
 urinary alkalinization is effective in enhancing elimination
External cooling for hyperpyrexia
Diazepam for seizures
Oxygen and ventilation for respiratory depression
Vitamin K for bleeding
In extreme cases, hemodialysis (not peritoneal dialysis) may be used

Iron
Mineral supplement or vitamin containing iron

Clinical Manifestations
Occurs in five stages:
1. Initial period (½ to 6 hours after ingestion) (if child does not de-
 velop gastrointestinal symptoms in 6 hours, toxicity is unlikely)
 Vomiting
 Hematemesis
 Diarrhea
 Hematochezia (bloody stools)
 Gastric pain
2. Latency (2 to 12 hours)
 Patient improves
3. Systemic toxicity (4 to 24 hours after ingestion)
 Metabolic acidosis
 Fever
 Hyperglycemia
 Bleeding
 Shock
 Death (may occur)
4. Hepatic injury (48 to 96 hours)
 Seizures
 Coma
5. Rarely, pyloric stenosis develops at 2 to 5 weeks

Comments
Factors related to frequency of iron poisoning include:
 Widespread availability
 Packaging of large quantities in individual containers
 Lack of parental awareness of iron toxicity
 Resemblance of iron tablets to candy (e.g., M & Ms)
 Toxic dose is based on the amount of elemental iron in various
 salts (sulfate, gluconate, fumarate), which ranges from 20% to
 33%; ingestions of 60 mg/kg are considered dangerous

Treatment
Emesis or lavage
Lavage for all chewable tablets or liquids if spontaneous vomiting has
 not occurred
Chelation therapy with deferoxamine in severe intoxication (turns
 urine a red to orange color)
If intravenous deferoxamine is given too rapidly, hypotension, facial
 flushing, rash, urticaria, tachycardia, and shock may occur; stop the
 infusion, maintain the intravenous line with normal saline, and notify the practitioner immediately

Plants
See box on p. 417

Clinical Manifestations
Depends on type of plant ingested
May cause local irritation of oropharynx and entire gastrointestinal
 tract
May cause respiratory, renal, and central nervous system symptoms
Topical contact with plants can cause dermatitis

Comments
Some of most frequently ingested substances
Rarely cause serious problems, although some plant ingestions can be
 fatal
Can also cause choking and allergic reactions

Treatment
Remove plant parts (emesis)
Wash from skin or eyes
Supportive care as needed

More than 90% of poisonings occur in the home, although a significant number take place elsewhere, such as in a grandparent's or friend's home, in a school, or in a health care facility.

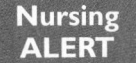 **Nursing ALERT** The following five commonly used and easily available drugs (first four are over-the-counter) can cause serious or fatal consequences if as little as ¼ teaspoon or ½ tablet is ingested: methyl salicylate, camphor, topical imidazolines (sympathomimetics such as those contained in Visine, Afrin, Otrivin, and Clear Eyes), benzocaine, and diphenoxylate-atropine (Lomotil and others). Stress to parents the importance of keeping such drugs away from children. If these agents are ingested, advise parents to seek medical treatment immediately. Emesis is not induced for significant camphor, topical imidazolines, or Lomotil ingestions (Liebelt and Shannon, 1993).

The developmental characteristics of young children predispose them to poisoning by ingestion. Infants and toddlers explore their environment through oral experimentation. Be-
cause the sense of taste is less discriminatory at this age, many unpalatable substances are ingested. In addition, toddlers and preschoolers are developing autonomy and initiative, which increase their curiosity and noncompliant behavior. Imitation is also a powerful motivator, especially when combined with lack of awareness of danger.

This section is primarily concerned with the immediate emergency treatment of ingestion of injurious agents. Specific management of corrosive, hydrocarbon, acetaminophen, salicylate, plant, and iron poisoning is summarized in the box that begins on p. 418. Because of the importance of lead poisoning among young children, ingestion of lead is discussed separately. Appropriate suggestions for poison prevention are discussed on p. 422 and in Chapter 12.

PRINCIPLES OF EMERGENCY TREATMENT

A poisoning may or may not require emergency intervention, but in every instance medical evaluation is necessary to ini-

Mrs. Berry, a neighbor, calls you. She is very upset because her 2-year-old son has eaten several chewable multivitamins with iron. She asks you if she should give syrup of ipecac. You advise her to:

1. First call the Poison Control Center.
2. Give the antiemetic.
3. Dilute the poison with several glasses of water.
4. Wait to see if the child develops symptoms.

The correct action for the mother is one, to first call the Poison Control Center, where they will advise her of home treatment, such as using ipecac. The goal is to remove the poison, not dilute it, making option three inappropriate. The most toxic ingredient in the drug is iron, which produces symptoms after several hours. Treatment, if needed, should begin long before symptoms appear.

tiate appropriate action. Parents are advised to call the **Poison Control Center (PCC)** *before* initiating any intervention. The local PCC telephone number (usually listed in the front of the telephone directory) should be posted near each phone in the house.* Some evidence indicates that the information given by PCCs is more accurate than instructions given by hospital emergency departments (see Critical Thinking Exercise).

Based on the initial telephone assessment, the PCC counsels the parents to begin treatment at home and/or to take the child to an emergency facility. When a call is taken, the name and telephone number of the caller are recorded to reestablish contact if the connection is interrupted. Since most poisonings are managed in the home, expert advice is essential in minimizing adverse effects. When the exact quantity or type of ingested toxin is not known, admission to a hospital for laboratory evaluation and surveillance is critical during the postingestion period.

General guidelines for emergency treatment of poisoning are listed on p. 421. Selected interventions, especially those that require professional intervention, are discussed next.

Assessment

The first and most important principle in dealing with a poisoning is to treat the child first, not the poison. This necessitates an immediate concern for life support; vital signs are taken and respiratory and/or circulatory support instituted as needed. The victim's condition is routinely reevaluated. Since shock is a complication of several types of household poisons, particularly corrosives, measures to reduce the effects of shock, such as elevation of the legs and head to the level of the heart to promote venous drainage and provision of warmth and rest, are important. Maintenance of respiratory function may require insertion of an airway and/or mechanical ventilation.

The emergency room nurse's responsibility is to be prepared for immediate intervention with any of the necessary

---

*Also available by calling (800) 555-1212 for any state in the United States.

equipment. Since time and speed are critical factors in recovery from serious poisonings, anticipation of potential problems and complications may mean the difference between life and death.

Gastric Decontamination

In general the immediate treatment is to remove the ingested poison by inducing vomiting. The preferred method for use at home is to administer *ipecac syrup*, an emetic that exerts its action by direct stimulation of the vomiting center and through an irritant effect on the gastric mucosa.

> **Nursing ALERT**
>
> The use of an emetic is generally contraindicated in conditions that increase the risk of aspiration and when emesis of the poison, such as a corrosive, redamages the mucosa of the esophagus and pharynx. Emesis is also contraindicated when there is existing or potential for rapid onset of central nervous system depression, dystonias (unusual muscle tone or movements), or seizures.

Proper administration of ipecac is essential (see Emergency Treatment box). Ipecac is available in 1-ounce (30 ml) vials. However, the label information does not include directions for a second dose if the child fails to vomit after the first dose. Therefore parents need clear instructions for proper use and dose. As a precaution, parents are advised to have full doses of ipecac for *each child* in the home, to carry the emetic when traveling, and to be certain that other caregivers (baby-sitters or relatives) have the emetic available. Because children share activities, more than one child may ingest the toxic substance. In an emergency, ipecac can be obtained from an all-night pharmacy, convenience store, emergency squad, or emergency department. Ipecac is also inexpensive.

Although out-of-date ipecac may be used in a dire emergency, the family is encouraged to replace the expired bottle. Since milk, fluid volume, food, and activity level do not alter ipecac's effectiveness, the common suggestions of forcing fluids and encouraging movement are unnecessary. If given, clear liquids are preferred for better visualization of white pill fragments. For maximum benefit in removing the poison, ipecac should be administered within 1 hour of a toxic ingestion.

If the child is admitted to an emergency facility, *gastric lavage* may also be done to empty the stomach of the toxic agent. Lavage is indicated for young infants in whom ipecac is contraindicated; if the patient is comatose or convulsing, or requires a protected airway; or if the ingested poison is rapidly absorbed (strychnine or cyanide). The use of lavage in petroleum distillate poisoning remains controversial because of the danger of aspiration. When lavage is performed, the largest-diameter tube that can be inserted is used to facilitate passage of gastric contents.

Another method of decontaminating the stomach is the use of *activated charcoal,* an odorless, tasteless, fine black powder that adsorbs many compounds, creating a stable complex. It is used within 1 hour of the poisoning but *after* giving an emetic, to avoid the charcoal also adsorbing the emetic and preventing its pharmacologic effect. It is mixed with water or a saline cathartic to form a slurry. Slurries are neither gritty nor distasteful but resemble black mud. Sorbitol, an ar-

FAMILY FOCUS
Poisoning

A poisoning is more than a physical emergency for the child. It usually represents an emotional crisis for the parents, particularly in terms of guilt, self-reproach, and insecurity in the parenting role. The emergency room is no place to admonish the family for negligence, lack of appropriate supervision, or failure to safe-proof the home. Rather, it is a time to calm and support the child and parents while unaccusingly exploring the circumstances of the injury. If the nurse prematurely attempts to discuss ways of preventing such an incident from recurring, the parents' anxiety will block out any suggestions or offered guidance. Therefore it is preferable for the nurse to delay the discussion until the child's condition is stabilized or, if the child is discharged immediately after emergency treatment, to make a public health referral or send a packet of information (Woolf, Saperstein, and Forjuoh, 1992).

EMERGENCY TREATMENT
Poisoning

1. Assess the victim:
   a. Take vital signs; reevaluate routinely.
   b. Initiate cardiorespiratory support if needed.
   c. Treat other symptoms, such as seizures.
2. Terminate exposure:
   a. Empty mouth of pills, plant parts, or other material.
   b. Flush eyes continuously with normal saline (room-temperature tap water at home) for 15 to 20 minutes.
   c. Flush skin and wash with soap and a soft cloth; remove contaminated clothes, especially if a pesticide, acid, alkali, or hydrocarbon is involved.
   d. Bring victim of an inhalation poisoning into fresh air.
   e. Give one sip of water to dilute ingested poison.
3. Identify the poison:
   a. Question the victim and witnesses.
   b. Look for environmental cues (empty container, nearby spill, odor on breath) and save all evidence of poison (container, vomitus, urine).
   c. Be alert to signs and symptoms of potential poisoning in absence of other evidence, including symptoms of ocular or dermal exposure
   d. Call Poison Control Center or other competent emergency facility for immediate advice regarding treatment.
4. Remove poison and prevent absorption:
   a. Induce vomiting; administer ipecac if ordered:
      (1) 6 to 12 months: 10 ml; do not repeat.*
      (2) 1 to 12 years: 15 ml; repeat dosage *once* if vomiting has not occurred within 20 minutes.
      (3) Over 12 years: 30 ml; repeat dosage *once* if vomiting has not occurred within 20 minutes.
      (4) Give 10 to 20 ml/kg of clear fluids after ipecac.
   b. Do not induce vomiting if:
      (1) Victim is comatose, in severe shock, or convulsing, or has lost the gag reflex.
      (2) Poison is a low-viscosity hydrocarbon (unless it contains a more toxic substance [e.g., pesticide or heavy metal] or a strong acid or alkali).
   c. Place child in side-lying, sitting, or kneeling position with head below chest to prevent aspiration.
   d. Administer activated charcoal with cathartic (unless used repeatedly; usual dose 1 g/kg unless amount of toxin is known) 30 to 60 minutes *after* vomiting from ipecac, if ordered.

*Emesis of children at home is generally contraindicated between ages 6 and 10 months. Ipecac can only be administered safely in a health care facility because of the high risk of aspiration.

tificial sweetener, is added to many commercial preparations (Actidose) as a flavoring and a cathartic. However, concentrated amounts of sorbitol have been known to cause severe dehydration in infants. Cathartics, such as sodium or magnesium, may be administered to stimulate evacuation of the bowel, thus decreasing systemic absorption of the poison and aiding in removal of the charcoal. However, the use of cathartics is controversial.

NURSING TIP To increase the child's acceptance of activated charcoal, mix it with flavoring or a sweetener and serve through a straw and in an opaque container with a cover, such as a disposable coffee cup and lid or an ordinary cup covered with aluminum foil or placed inside a small paper bag.

In a minority of poisonings, specific *antidotes* are available to counteract the poison. They are highly effective and should be available in all emergency facilities. The supply of antidotes should be checked routinely and replaced as used or according to expiration dates. Among the more frequently employed antidotes are *N*-acetylcysteine for acetaminophen poisoning, oxygen for carbon monoxide inhalation, naloxone for opioid overdose, flumazenil (Mazicon) for benzodiazepine (Valium, Versed) overdose, Digibind for digoxin toxicity, and antivenin for certain poisonous bites.

Prevention of Recurrence

The ultimate objective is to prevent poisonings from occurring or recurring. One effective counseling method is first to discuss the difficulties of constantly watching and safeguarding young children (see Family Focus box). In this way the challenging task of raising children can lead to a discussion of injury prevention as one part of the parental role. This approach also incorporates other contributory causes for the incident, such as inadequate support systems, marital discord, discipline techniques (especially use of physical punishment), and maternal distress. A visit to the home, especially after a repeat poisoning situation, is recommended as part of the follow-up care to assess hazards, including family factors, and to evaluate appropriate safe-proofing measures. One method of identifying risk areas is to ask specific questions or to have

the parent complete a questionnaire designed to isolate factors that predispose children to poisoning.

NURSING TIP Encourage parents to bend down to the child's eye level and survey the home environment for potential hazards. Have the parents try to open cabinets and reach shelves to access poisons.

Passive measures (those that do not require active participation) have been the most successful in preventing poisoning and include child-resistant closures and limiting the number of tablets in one container. However, these measures

GUIDELINES
Poison Prevention

Assess possible contributing factors in occurrence of injury, such as discipline, parent-child relationship, developmental ability, environmental factors, and behavior problems.

Institute anticipatory guidance for possible future injuries based on child's age and maturational level.

Refer to visiting nurse agency to evaluate home environment and need for safe-proofing measures.

Provide assistance with environmental manipulation when necessary, such as lead removal.

Educate parents regarding safe storage of toxic substances.

Advise parents to take drugs out of sight of children.

Advise parents to return all toxic substances *immediately* to safe storage.

Teach children the hazards of ingesting nonfood items without supervision.

Advise parents against using plants for teas or medicine.

Discuss problems of discipline and children's noncompliance and offer strategies for effective discipline (see Limit-Setting and Discipline, Chapter 3).

Instruct parents regarding correct administration of drugs for therapeutic purposes and to discontinue drug if there is evidence of mild toxicity.

Have syrup of ipecac available—two doses for each child in the family—but to use only if advised to do so by Poison Control Center (PCC) or practitioner.

Encourage grandparents or other frequent caregivers to keep syrup of ipecac in home.

Post number of local PCC with emergency phone list by telephone.

Include by the telephone the home address with nearest cross street in case an ambulance is needed. (In an emergency, family members may not remember the house address, and baby-sitters may not be aware of the information.)

alone are not sufficient to prevent poisoning, since most toxic agents in the home do not have safety closures. Therefore *active measures* (those that require participation) are essential. Guidelines for preventing the occurrence or recurrence of a poisoning are listed in the box.

See also Nursing Care Plan: The Child with Poisoning.*

HEAVY METAL POISONING

Heavy metal poisoning can occur from the ingestion of a variety of substances, the most common being lead. Other sources that are important in terms of children are iron (see box on p. 419) and mercury. *Mercury toxicity,* a rare form of heavy metal poisoning, has occurred in children from a variety of sources, such as broken thermometers or thermostats, broken fluorescent lights, and use of interior latex house paint. Elemental mercury (also called metallic mercury or quicksilver) is nontoxic if ingested and if the gastrointestinal tract is healthy (e.g., has no fistulas). However, mercury is volatile at room temperature and enters the bloodstream after it is inhaled, causing toxicity (tremors, memory loss, insomnia, gingivitis, diarrhea, anorexia, weight loss). The clas-

*In Wong DL: *Wong and Whaley's Clinical manual of pediatric nursing,* ed 4, St Louis, 1996, Mosby.

sic form of mercury poisoning is called *acrodynia* (or "painful extremities").

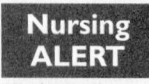 To prevent inhalation, spilled mercury must be cleaned up quickly, using disposable towels and rubber gloves and washing the hands well after removing the spill.

Heavy metals have an affinity for certain essential tissue chemicals, which must remain free for adequate cell functioning. When metals are bound to these substances, cellular enzyme systems are inactivated. Treatment involves *chelation,* use of a chemical compound that combines with the metal for rapid and safe excretion.

LEAD POISONING

Lead poisoning (sometimes termed *plumbism*) is a prevalent, significant, and preventable pediatric problem. Although lead poisoning associated with life-threatening encephalopathy is rarely seen today, many young children have lead levels sufficiently elevated to cause neurologic and intellectual damage. As the detrimental effects of low levels of lead on the developing central nervous system have been identified, blood lead levels indicating toxicity have decreased. For example, in 1991 the lower level of blood lead concentration was set at less than 10 μg/dl, a reduction from the 1985 level of less than 25 μg/dl (Centers for Disease Control and Prevention, 1991).

Factors Related to Lead Ingestion

The most important contributing factor to lead poisoning is the availability of lead in the environment. Lead enters the system either by ingestion or inhalation. In an unborn fetus, lead can enter the body transplacentally if the mother is exposed. The major environmental sources of lead are deteriorating lead-based paint, which contaminates household dust and soil; drinking water contaminated by exposed lead solder or old lead pipes; occupations and hobbies associated with parents or others in the house bringing home lead on clothes, shoes, and skin; and for some children, folk remedies or cosmetics, as well as the use of lead-containing pottery or leaded dishes for food storage. Lead-based paint from old housing remains the most frequent source of lead poisoning in children.

Most lead poisoning results from ingestion of lead dust during normal hand-to-mouth activity. A number of children have been known to eat loose lead paint chips. Some children are poisoned during renovation of their home. As mentioned earlier, sanding, scraping, and burning can release large amounts of lead into the air. In 1978 the *U.S. Consumer Product Safety Commission* banned the addition of lead to paints for residential use, but substantial amounts of lead remain on the painted interior and exterior surfaces of older homes. Although the child's home environment is usually the source of lead, other buildings, such as preschools or daycare centers, as well as a friend or relative's home, can contribute to lead exposure.

Other significant sources of lead in the child's environment are dust, soil, and air that become contaminated by emissions from lead smelters. Fortunately, the use of deleaded

POTENTIAL SOURCES OF LEAD

Ingested	Inhaled
Lead-based paint	Sanding and scraping of
Interior: walls, window	lead-based painted sur-
sills, floors, furniture	faces
Exterior: door frames,	Burning of leaded objects
fences, porches, siding	Automobile batteries
Plaster, caulking	Newspaper logs of col-
Unglazed pottery	ored paper
Cigarette butts and ashes	Leaded gasoline (automo-
Water from leaded pipes	bile exhaust)
Foods or liquids from cans	Sniffing leaded gasoline
soldered with lead	Dust
Household dust	Poorly cleaned urban
Soil, especially along	housing
heavily trafficked road-	Contaminated clothing and
ways	skin of household mem-
Food grown in contami-	bers working in smelting
nated soil	factories, in lead abate-
Urban playgrounds	ment projects, or as ur-
Folk remedies	ban policemen
Hobby materials (e.g.,	Lead-based insecticides
leaded paint or solder for	
stained-glass windows)	
Lead-containing dishware:	
pottery, ceramics, lead	
crystal	
Some antique pewterware	
Some dyes used in items	
such as papers, maga-	
zines, and wrappers	
Leaded objects: curtain	
weights, fishing sinkers,	
bullets	

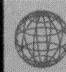

CULTURAL AWARENESS
Sources of Lead

In some cultures the use of traditional ethnic remedies may contain lead and increase children's risk of lead poisoning. These remedies include the following:

Azarcon (Mexico)—for digestive problems; a bright-orange powder; usual dose is ¼-1 teaspoon, often mixed with oil, milk, or sugar, or sometimes given as a tea; sometimes a pinch is added to a baby bottle or tortilla dough for preventive purposes

Greta (Mexico)—a yellow-orange powder, used in the same way as azarcon

Paylooah (Southeast Asia)—used for rash or fever; an orange-red powder given as ½ teaspoon straight or in a tea

Surma (India)—black powder applied to the inner lower eyelid that is used as a cosmetic to improve eyesight

Unknown ayurvedic (Tibet)—small, gray-brown balls used to improve slow development; two balls are given orally three times a day

Modified from Lead poisoning associated with use of traditional ethnic remedies—California, 1991-1992, *MMWR* 42(27):521-524, 1993.

gasoline has significantly reduced the level of lead in the air and the incidence of severe lead poisoning in children (Piomelli, 1994). Lead-soldered cans for food products, which have been outlawed in the United States, may still be found with imported products. Leaded containers, such as some water fountains and liquids stored in lead crystal, can also contribute to ingested sources of the heavy metal. Use of lead-contaminated water to prepare formula is a major source of poisoning in infants (Shannon and Graef, 1992).*

Potential sources of lead are listed in the box. Some ethnic groups, especially Hispanic, use improperly fired ceramic pottery and ethnic remedies that include lead (see Cultural Awareness box).

Developmentally, young children are at risk for lead poisoning because of their high level of oral activity. Particularly during late infancy and toddlerhood, children explore their environment by putting objects in their mouth. This normal hand-to-mouth activity contributes to the amount of lead they ingest in dust and dirt. Because of their size, young children inhale air that is closer to the ground, which is more heavily contaminated with lead. In addition, the child who ingests lead often practices *pica*, the habitual, purposeful, and compulsive ingestion of nonfood substances. Children under

the age of 6 are also most at risk for lead poisoning because of their developing nervous systems. In addition, three to five times more lead is absorbed in children than in adults. Diets deficient in iron and calcium and diets high in fats, such as those containing many fried foods, also increase the exposure risk for children living in leaded environments. These conditions make it possible for lead to be more quickly and readily absorbed. The greatest risk appears to be from iron deficiency, even in the absence of anemia (Wasserman and others, 1992).

Pathophysiology and Clinical Manifestations

Normally, ingested lead is very slowly excreted via the kidneys, alimentary tract, and to a small extent, sweat. Retained lead is stored chiefly in the bone and teeth, where it is inert. However, with chronic ingestion the rate of absorption exceeds the rate of excretion, and excess lead is deposited in the tissues and circulatory system, with about 90% attached to the erythrocytes. Even when the chronic ingestion stops, it takes the body twice as long to excrete the stored lead as it did to accumulate it. As a result, several body systems continue to be affected after the environmental removal of the poison (Fig. 14-9).

Central Nervous System. The most serious and irreversible side effects of lead intoxication are on the nervous system. Initially, membrane permeability increases, with a shift of fluid into the interstitial spaces of the brain. As a result, increased intracranial pressure causes cortical atrophy and *lead encephalopathy* (convulsions, mental retardation, paralysis, blindness, and ultimately coma and death), which is almost always associated with a blood lead concentration greater than 100 µg/dl.

However, before lead encephalopathy occurs, low-dose exposure to lead causes neurologic and intellectual deficits that may or may not be reversible. Hyperactivity, aggression, impulsiveness, decreased interest in play, lethargy, irritability,

*A suggested resource for families is *Lead in Your Drinking Water,* available from the U.S. Environmental Protection Agency, P.O. Box 42419, Cincinnati, OH 45242.

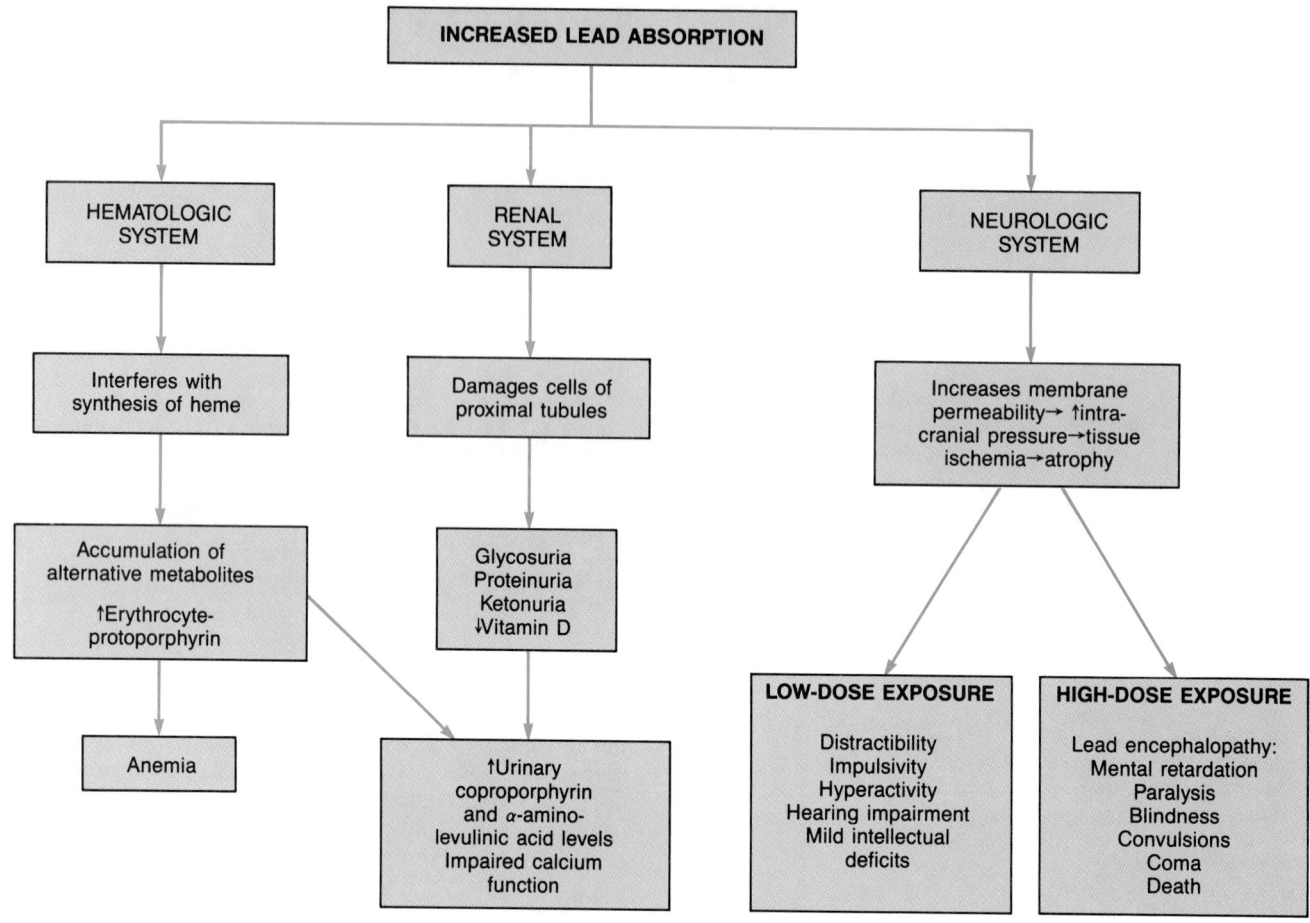

FIG. 14-9. Main effects of lead on body systems.

hearing impairment, learning difficulties, short attention span, and distractibility are common signs of low levels of lead poisoning. Studies demonstrate that as prenatal and postnatal lead levels increase, the child's intelligence quotient decreases (Bellinger, Stiles, and Needleman, 1992). Such manifestations of behavioral disturbance are important clues to the identification of children with early poisoning.

Hematologic System. Lead is extremely toxic to the biosynthesis of heme, preventing the formation of hemoglobin and causing its precursors, especially erythrocyte protoporphyrin, coproporphyrin, and delta-aminolevulinic acid (ALA), to increase in the body. *Erythrocyte protoporphyrin (EP)* is elevated in the blood when the blood lead concentration is moderately increased but is not a sensitive indicator for low lead exposure. Reduction of the heme molecule in the red blood cell results in anemia. However, with low levels of lead toxicity, anemia may not be present.

Renal System. Lead damages the cells of the proximal tubules, resulting in abnormal excretion of glucose, protein, amino acids, and phosphate and interference with the synthesis of vitamin D. With adequate treatment, kidney damage is usually reversible. Severe irreversible lead nephropathy is probably limited to prolonged childhood plumbism.

Other Manifestations. Other vague symptoms of plumbism are acute crampy abdominal pain, vomiting, con-

stipation, anorexia, headache, and fever. Some evidence suggests that in young children lead impairs growth, especially in infants with elevated prenatal and postnatal blood lead levels.

Diagnostic Evaluation

Diagnosis is made on measurement of blood lead levels. Since virtually all children are at risk for lead poisoning, universal screening is recommended. Priority for screening is given to children ages 6 to 72 months who are at highest risk: (1) those who live in or frequent deteriorated housing or such housing during remodeling, (2) those whose siblings or other close peers have lead poisoning, and (3) those whose household members have lead-related occupations or hobbies or those who live near lead-related industries (Centers for Disease Control and Prevention, 1991).

Screening tests are usually done on blood collected by finger or heel puncture. However, blood collected by venipuncture is needed to confirm the diagnosis. Other tests that are helpful in determining the presence of lead in the body are (1) radiographs of the long bones for "lead lines," caused by deposition of lead, and of the abdomen for the presence of recently ingested lead; (2) blood studies for evidence of anemia; and (3) a lead mobilization test to help predict the amount of lead that may be removed by chelation.

Therapeutic Management

The child's blood lead level determines the degree of risk and the type of intervention (Table 14-3). The objective of treatment is to remove lead in the body and prevent further accumulation of the metal. Therapeutic modalities include removing the source of lead, improving nutrition, and using chelation therapy. With emphasis on early detection of low blood lead levels, removing sources of lead in the environment is the major goal (see Family Home Care box on p. 426).

Chelation therapy is reserved for children with high blood lead levels. Drugs that may be used are calcium disodium edetate (CaNa$_2$EDTA), dimercaprol (also called BAL [British antilewisite]), D-penicillamine (Cuprimine, Depen), or succimer (Chemet).

The exact course of therapy depends on the severity of the child's condition and the practitioner's preference. CaNa$_2$EDTA is given preferably intravenously; intramuscular injections are very painful. BAL (prepared in peanut oil) is given only intramuscularly and is also a very painful injection. D-penicillamine and succimer are administered orally.

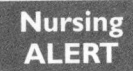 **Nursing ALERT** Children with allergy to peanuts or penicillin cannot receive BAL or D-penicillamine, respectively.

Symptomatic treatment during chelation therapy involves observing for and controlling seizures for which the child is at risk and taking measures to reduce the side effects of some of the medications, such as the nausea that can occur with BAL. Depending on the drug being used, serum electrolyte levels should be taken at prescribed intervals, urine specimens analyzed, and fluid intake and output measured. If numerous paint chips are visible in the gastrointestinal tract on radiologic examination, cleansing enemas or a cathartic may be ordered. Every effort is made to prevent infection and maintain adequate hydration. When succimer is given, adequate fluid intake is especially important, as is close monitoring of the absolute neutrophil l count. Neutropenia can occur during drug therapy. If nutritional deficiencies coexist, they are treated appropriately, such as with administration of supplemental iron for iron deficiency anemia. Iron should not be given during chelation, however, especially with BAL because of possible interactive effects.

Prognosis. Although most of the pathophysiologic effects of lead are reversible, the most serious consequences of both high and low lead exposure are the effects on the central nervous system. In children with lead encephalopathy, permanent brain damage results in mental retardation, behavior changes, possible paralysis, and seizures. However, low-dose exposure may also cause permanent neurologic deficits.

Nursing Considerations

The primary nursing goal in lead poisoning is to prevent the child's initial or further exposure to lead. For children with low-level exposure, this often requires identifying the sources of lead in the environment. Careful history taking is one of the most useful and valuable tools and should concentrate on the areas listed in the Guidelines box, especially those related to the home environment (Nordin, Rolnick, and Griffin,

TABLE 14-3. Classification of risk and treatment for lead poisoning	
BLOOD LEAD CONCENTRATION (mg/dl)	**INTERVENTION**
≤9	Child is not considered to be lead poisoned.
10-14	Many children with blood lead levels in this range should trigger community-wide childhood lead poisoning prevention activities. Children may need to be rescreened more frequently.
15-19	Child should receive nutritional and educational interventions and more frequent screening. If blood lead level persists in this range, environmental investigation and intervention should be done.
20-44	Child should receive environmental evaluation and remediation and a medical evaluation; may need pharmacologic treatment of lead poisoning.
45-69	Child will need both medical and environmental interventions, including chelation therapy.
≥70	Child is a medical emergency; medical and environmental management must begin immediately.

Modified from Centers for Disease Control and Prevention: *Preventing lead poisoning in young children,* Atlanta, 1991, CDC.

 GUIDELINES
Assessing Potential for Lead Poisoning

Does your child:
1. Live in a house or regularly visit a daycare center, preschool, the home of a baby-sitter or relative, or other house built before 1960 that has peeling or chipping paint?
2. Live in or regularly visit a house built before 1960 with recent, ongoing, or planned renovation or remodeling?
3. Have a brother or sister, housemate, or playmate being followed up or treated for lead poisoning (i.e., blood level ≥15 mg/dl)?
4. Live with an adult whose job, hobby, or use of ethnic remedies involves exposure to lead?
5. Live near an active lead smelter, battery-recycling plant, or other industry likely to release lead?

Modified from Centers for Disease Control and Prevention: *Preventing lead poisoning in young children,* Atlanta, 1991, CDC.

FAMILY HOME CARE
Reducing Blood Lead Levels

Make sure child does not have access to peeling paint or chewable surfaces painted with lead-based paint, especially window sills and wells.

If a house was built before 1960 (possibly before 1980) and has hard-surface floors, wet mop them at least once a week with a high-phosphate solution (e.g., trisodium phosphate [available in hardware stores]). Wipe other hard surfaces (e.g., window sills, baseboards) with the same kind of solution. If there are loose paint chips in an area, such as a window well, use a disposable cloth soaked with the high-phosphate (5% to 8%) solution to pick up and discard them. Do not vacuum hard-surfaced floors or window sills or wells, since this spreads dust. Use vacuum cleaners with agitators to remove dust from rugs rather than vacuum cleaners with suction only. If a rug is known to contain lead dust and cannot be washed, it should be discarded.

Wash and dry child's hands and face frequently, especially before eating.

Wash toys and pacifiers frequently.

If soil around home is or is likely to be contaminated with lead (e.g., if home was built before 1960 or is near a major highway), plant grass or other ground cover; plant bushes around outside of house so that child cannot play there.

During remodeling of older homes, be sure to follow correct procedures. Be certain children and pregnant women are not in the home, day or night, until process is completed. After deleading, thoroughly clean house using high-phosphate cleaning solution to damp mop and dust before inhabitants return.

In areas where lead content of water exceeds the drinking water standard, run cold water until it is as cold as possible before using it for drinking, cooking, and making formula; may use first-flush water for other purposes.

Do not store food in open cans, particularly if cans are imported.

Do not use pottery or ceramic ware that was inadequately fired or is meant for decorative use for food storage or service. Do not store drinks or food in lead crystal.

Avoid folk remedies or cosmetics that contain lead.

Make sure that home exposure is not occurring from parental occupations or hobbies. Household members employed in occupations such as lead smelting should shower and change into clean clothing before leaving work. Construction and lead abatement workers may also bring home lead contaminants.

Make sure child eats regular meals, since more lead is absorbed on an empty stomach.

Make sure child's diet contains sufficient iron and calcium and not excessive fat.

Modified from Centers for Disease Control and Prevention: *Preventing lead poisoning in young children*, Atlanta, 1991, CDC.

1994) (see Critical Thinking Exercise). Suggestions for reducing lead in the child's environment are listed in the Family Home Care box.

Children who must undergo chelation therapy are prepared for the injections and allowed to express their pain and anger. Playing with syringes and aggressive play, such as pounding clay or throwing beanbags, provides an excellent outlet for their frustrations. Children also deserve an explanation of the need for the treatment, particularly that it is not a punishment for eating lead or paint. During home oral chelation therapy, parents need to understand the importance of giving the drug as prescribed.

Chelating agents are administered deeply into a large muscle mass (see Atraumatic Care box). To lessen the pain from CaNa$_2$EDTA, the local anesthetic procaine is injected with the drug. Rotation of sites is essential to prevent the formation of painful areas of fibrotic tissue. Since CaNa$_2$EDTA and lead are toxic to the kidneys, records are kept of intake and output, and the results of urinalysis are assessed to monitor renal functioning. Because of the risk of seizures, appropriate precautions are instituted at the bedside of children with high blood lead levels.

CRITICAL THINKING EXERCISE
Lead Poisoning

The clinic in which you practice has received funds to begin a program to reduce lead poisoning in children. As a member of the planning committee, which of the following initial projects is effective and easy to implement?

1. Screening for blood lead levels by heel or finger puncture in all children under age 6 years
2. Questioning parents about the age and condition of their home(s) since the child's birth, including recent renovations
3. Screening for blood lead levels by venipuncture in all children under age 6 years who are at risk for lead exposure
4. Questioning parents about hobbies, occupations, and ethnic remedies that may expose the child to lead

The correct answer is two. Asking about the family's dwelling to identify instances where lead, especially on painted surfaces, could be present is the single most important screening procedure. Although asking about hobbies, occupations, and ethnic remedies should be considered, option four is not the priority question. Screening for blood lead levels is expensive and time consuming. Option three is incorrect because collection of blood by venipuncture is not a recommended screening procedure, and all children, regardless of risk, should be screened.

ATRAUMATIC CARE
Lead Chelation Therapy

To lessen the pain from CaNa$_2$EDTA, the local anesthetic procaine is injected with the drug. Apply EMLA cream over the puncture site 2½ hours before the injection.

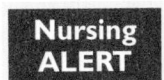 CaNa$_2$EDTA is never given in the absence of an adequate urine output. Children receiving the drug intramuscularly must be able to maintain adequate oral intake of fluids.

As in any situational crisis, parents need support and understanding if their child is treated for lead poisoning. Many of the families at highest risk for lead poisoning have the fewest resources to comply with measures such as relocation or deleading the home. Appropriate referrals are essential in locating assistance for parents. (See also Nursing Care Plan: The Child with Lead Poisoning.*)

CHILD MALTREATMENT†

The broad term *child maltreatment* includes intentional physical abuse or neglect, emotional abuse or neglect, and sexual abuse of children, usually by adults. It is one of the most significant social problems affecting children. In 1993 about 2.9 million children were reported as victims of child abuse and neglect to child protective services in the United States. However, this does not represent the number of children actually maltreated. Of these reported cases, about 35% were found to be substantiated or indicated (*In fact . . .*, undated). It is also likely that many other abuse cases are never brought to the attention of the authorities. Consequently, the best available statistics only partially reflect the true incidence of child maltreatment. According to the *National Center on Child Abuse and Neglect (NCCAAN)* (1993), the following statistics represent the incidence of child maltreatment in the United States‡: emotional neglect, 3.2 per 1000; emotional abuse, 3.0 per 1000; educational abuse, 4.5 per 1000; physical neglect, 8.1 per 1000; physical abuse, 4.9 per 1000; and sexual abuse, 2.1 per 1000. About 2000 children die from abuse or neglect each year, most of whom are under 4 years of age (*A nation's shame*, 1995).

CHILD NEGLECT

Child neglect is the most common form of maltreatment. About one half of all reported cases are associated with deprivation of necessities, and more than one third of deaths from maltreatment are in this group. Neglect is generally defined as the failure of a parent or other person legally responsible for the child's welfare to provide for the child's basic needs and an adequate level of care (Council on Scientific Affairs, 1985).

Little is known about the etiology of neglect, although it appears that many of the risk factors identified in physical abuse apply to neglect as well (see following discussion). Ignorance of the child's needs and a lack of resources are important contributing factors. For example, neglectful parents often demonstrate poor parenting skills. They may be unaware that an infant needs to be fed every 3 to 4 hours, may not know what to feed the child, and may have insufficient funds to buy food. The most serious lack of knowledge is failure to recognize emotional nurturing as an essential need of children. (See also Failure to Thrive, Chapter 11.)

Types of Neglect

Neglect takes many forms and can be classified broadly as physical or emotional maltreatment. *Physical neglect* involves the deprivation of necessities, such as food, clothing, shelter, supervision, medical care, and education. *Emotional neglect* generally refers to failure to meet the child's needs for affection, attention, and emotional nurturance. It may also include lack of intervention for or fostering of maladaptive behavior, such as delinquency or substance abuse. *Emotional abuse,* an even more difficult aspect of maltreatment to define, refers to the deliberate attempt to destroy or significantly impair a child's self-esteem or competence. Emotional abuse may take the following forms: rejecting, isolating, terrorizing, ignoring, or corrupting the child.

PHYSICAL ABUSE

The deliberate infliction of physical injury on a child, usually by the child's caregiver, is termed *physical abuse.* Minor physical injury is responsible for more reported cases of maltreatment than major physical injury, but major physical abuse causes more deaths. Despite the importance of the problem, a universally accepted definition of what constitutes minor and major physical abuse does not exist. Rather, each state in the United States defines abuse according to its individual reporting laws.

Munchausen Syndrome by Proxy (MSP)

One of the more unusual and perplexing types of abuse, usually physical, is MSP, which refers to illness that one person fabricates or induces in another person. In children, it is usually the mother who fabricates signs and symptoms of illness in her child, the proxy, to gain attention from the medical staff. Rarely, the father may be the perpetrator (Jones and others, 1993). MSP can take many forms, such as adding maternal blood to the child's urine to simulate hematuria, presenting a fictitious medical history, chronic poisoning of the child, or suffocating the child to cause apnea and seizures. Another form of MSP is alleging that the child has been sexually abused by someone else to gain recognition as the child's protector.

Such cases are often very difficult to confirm and require a high index of suspicion to protect the children. Warning signs of MSP include the following:

- Unexplained, prolonged, recurrent, or extremely rare illness
- Discrepancies between clinical findings and history
- Illness unresponsive to treatment
- Signs and symptoms occurring only in parent's presence
- Parent knowledgeable about illness, procedures, and treatments
- Parent very interested in interacting with health team members
- Parent very attentive toward child (refuses to leave hospital)
- Family members with similar symptoms

Consequences for children with MSP can be serious. They often undergo needless and painful medical procedures and treatments. The parent's actions may induce a serious illness in children; one that is fatal in almost 10% of the cases (Wilde

---

*In Wong DL: *Wong and Whaley's Clinical manual of pediatric nursing,* ed 4, St Louis, 1996, Mosby.
†Natalie Cloutman Arnold, MSN, RN, PNP, revised this section.
‡Additional information is available from the **Clearinghouse on Child Abuse and Neglect Information,** P.O. Box 1182, Washington, DC 20013-1182; (703) 385-7565 or (800) FYI-3366.

and Pedroni, 1993). Children may develop chronic invalidism, accepting the illness story and believing themselves to be ill. Finally, they may develop MSP as an adult. Even when some of these children are removed from the home, they continue to suffer severe psychologic trauma. Other siblings remaining in the home may become substitute victims.

Factors Predisposing to Physical Abuse

The exact cause of child abuse is not known, although three factors—parental characteristics, characteristics of the child, and environmental characteristics—influence the potential for abuse. However, no one factor or group of factors is predictive of abuse. Rather, the interaction of these factors is thought to increase the risk of abuse occurring in a particular family.

Parental Characteristics. Extensive research has focused on parental characteristics that distinguish abusive parents from nonabusive parents. Unfortunately, the findings from most of these studies provide conflicting evidence. For example, it is commonly believed that abusive parents were abused as children. However, few studies support this relationship. Although physical punishment tends to occur in abusive parents' childhood, most of the parents were not physically abused as children. However, abusive parents who report that they were severely punished as children are much more likely to injure their own children (Kotelchuck, 1982). If the abuse was not overt physical violence, abusive parents typically recall their punishment as unfair and severe, and they characterize their relationship with their parents as negative. Abusive parents tend to have difficulty controlling aggressive impulses, and the free expression of violence is one of the most consistent qualities of these families (Altemeier and others, 1982).

Another finding is that abusive families are often more socially isolated and have fewer supportive relationships than nonabusive parents. Children of teenage mothers are more at risk of abuse than those of older mothers (Stier and others, 1993). With little or no available support system and the presence of concurrent stresses imposed by the child or environment, these parents are extremely vulnerable to additional crises of any nature and literally strike out at the child as a method of releasing their increasing frustration and anxiety.

Other factors identified in abusive parents include low self-esteem and less adequate maternal functioning. Although inadequate knowledge of childrearing is often cited as a characteristic of abusive parents, research findings do not consistently support this belief. However, this does not mean that these parents cannot benefit from learning more constructive ways of rearing their children, especially nonviolent discipline methods.

Characteristics of the Child. The child also unintentionally contributes to the abusive situation. In families of two or more children, usually only one child is the victim of abuse. This child's temperament, position in the family, additional physical needs if ill or disabled, activity level, or degree of sensitivity to parental needs all contribute to the potential for physical abuse. For example, one child may not be abused if he or she fits into the "easy-child pattern," whereas another sibling with a difficult temperament may add to the parent's stress sufficiently to precipitate an abusive act. How-

ever, temperament alone is not the critical factor; rather, it is the "fit" or compatibility between the child's temperament and the parent's ability to deal with that behavioral style.

Occasionally the abused child is illegitimate, unwanted, brain damaged (especially in situations where the parents cannot accept the retardation), hyperactive, or physically disabled. Sometimes children are abused because they remind the parent of someone the parent dislikes, such as a younger brother or sister who received all the attention from their own parents. Premature infants may be at risk for maltreatment because of the failure of parent-child bonding during early infancy. Often a difficult pregnancy, labor, or delivery is a predisposing factor in abuse, especially when the infant is born prematurely or with congenital anomalies.

Although one child is usually the victim in an abusive family, removing that child from the home often places the other siblings at risk for abuse. Child maltreatment usually is not confined to one child because of a disturbed parent-child relationship but is a result of a family in distress. Therefore no child is safe if left in the abusive environment unless the parents can be helped to learn new parenting skills and to meet their needs and release their frustration through alternatives other than attacking their children.

Environmental Characteristics. The environment is a significant part of the potential abusive situation. Typically the environment is one of chronic stress, including problems of divorce, poverty, unemployment, poor housing, frequent relocation, alcoholism, and drug addiction. Increased exposure between children and parents, such as that which occurs in crowded living conditions, also increases the likelihood of abuse.

Although most reporting of abuse has been from lower socioeconomic populations, child abuse is by no means a problem of any one societal group. It spans all educational, social, and economic levels. Certainly, stresses imposed by poverty predispose lower socioeconomic families to abusive situations, and abuse in these groups is more apt to be reported. However, concealed crises can also be present in upper-class families. For example, a wealthy family experiencing major life changes, such as rehousing, the birth of an additional child, or marital discord, may have sufficient environmental stressors imposed on them to produce a potentially abusive situation. Wealthy families may be so overinvolved with commitments outside the home that abuse may be inflicted by substitute caregivers. Nurses need to be aware of such factors to identify the less obvious examples of child abuse and neglect.

SEXUAL ABUSE

Sexual abuse is one of the most devastating types of child maltreatment, and current estimates indicate that it has increased significantly during the past decade. However, the increased rate of reporting may not reflect a true increase in prevalence of sexual abuse and rather may be a result of changes in legislation and in society's attitudes toward women and children (Feldman and others, 1991). The number of reported occurrences was approximately 14% of all child maltreatment cases in 1993 (*In fact . . . ,* undated), but many authorities believe that this figure represents only a small percentage of the actual incidence.

As with all forms of child maltreatment, no universal definition for sexual abuse exists. The Child Abuse and Prevention Act (Public Law 100-294) defines *sexual abuse* as "the use, persuasion, or coercion of any child to engage in sexually explicit conduct (or any simulation of such conduct) for producing any visual depiction of such conduct, or rape, molestation, prostitution, or incest with children."

Sexual abuse includes several types of sexual maltreatment, including the following (see also Rape, Chapter 17):

Incest—any physical sexual activity between family members; blood relationship is not required (abusers can include stepparents, nonrelated siblings, grandparents, uncles, and aunts); does not include sexual relations between legally sanctional partners, such as spouses

Molestation—a vague term that includes "indecent liberties," such as touching, fondling, kissing, single or mutual masturbation, or oral-genital contact

Exhibitionism—indecent exposure, usually exposure of the genitals by an adult male to children or female adults

Child pornography—arranging and photographing in any media sexual acts involving children, alone or with adults or animals, regardless of consent by the child's legal guardian; also may denote distribution of such material in any form with or without profit

Child prostitution—involving children in sex acts for profit and usually with changing partners

Pedophilia—literally means "love of child" and does not denote a type of sexual activity but the preference of an adult for prepubertal children as the means of achieving sexual excitement

Characteristics of Abusers and Victims

Anyone, including siblings and mothers, can be sexual abusers, but a typical abuser is a male that the victim knows. Offenders come from all levels of society. Some are prominent persons in the community, and some, especially in the case of pedophiliacs (also called "child molesters"), are in positions, such as teaching and coaching, where they work closely with children.

Pornography and prostitution may involve strangers, as well as the children's own parents. There are no typical characteristics of these offenders, although the abused children tend to be runaways—young adolescents who engage in these activities to obtain money for food, shelter, drugs, and alcohol. Incestuous relationships between father or stepfather and daughter are generally prolonged, and the victims are usually reluctant to report the situation because of fear of retaliation and fear that they will not be believed. Typically, incestuous relationships begin later than other forms of child abuse, and the average age of the victim is 9 years (*Highlights*, 1988). The eldest daughter is usually abused, but in her absence, another sister is substituted. Sibling incest may also occur (Gilbert, 1992). Sexual abuse by relatives with a strong emotional bond with the victim is the most devastating to the child.

Boys are also victims of both intrafamilial and extrafamilial abuse. Males are much less likely to report abuse, and they may suffer much greater emotional harm from incestuous relationships, especially between mother and son, than female victims. Boys are likely to be subjected to anal penetration and oral-genital contact, to have subtle physical findings, and to be abused by a father, stepfather, or mother's boyfriend.

Initiation and Perpetuation of Sexual Abuse

The cycle of sexual abuse often starts innocently, unless it involves an isolated attack, such as rape. Often offenders spend

---

METHODS USED TO PRESSURE CHILDREN INTO SEXUAL ACTIVITY

The child is offered gifts or privileges.

The adult misrepresents moral standards by telling the child that it is "okay to do."

Isolated and emotionally and socially impoverished children are enticed by adults who meet their needs for warmth and human contact.

The successful sex offender pressures the victim into secrecy regarding the activity by describing it as a "secret between us" that other people may take away if they find out.

The offender plays on the child's fears, including fear of punishment by the offender, fear of repercussions if the child tells, and fear of abandonment or rejection by the family.

---

time with the victims to gain their trust before initiating any sexual contact. Most victims are then pressured into being an accessory to the sexual activity through various means (see box) and may be unaware that sexual activity is part of the offer. Children may not reveal the truth for fear that their parents would not believe them if they told, especially if the offender is a trusted member of the family. Some fear they will be blamed for the situation, and many young children with limited vocabulary have difficulty describing the activity when they do have the courage or opportunity to reveal the abuse.

Seductiveness by the child does not initiate incest. Most young girls experiment in seduction, especially during the preschool years, but the father's response normally differentiates this playfulness from overt sexual invitation. Although the reasons for incest are complicated and can occur in various family types, it does not occur in healthy families. Most incestuous relationships are directly tied to sexual maladjustment and estrangement between husband and wife. Most begin following the cessation of sexual relationships with the usual partner. Most fathers experience little guilt, and many wives at some level are aware of the incestuous affair. The wife may react by tolerating the situation or may resort to use of denial; some remain unaware of the activity. Consequently, the home offers little protection to young victims, since abusers have easy access to their victims and the children feel they cannot reveal their secret to other family members. However, not all incestuous relationships follow this pattern of silence. Currently, reports of father-daughter incest during child custody conflicts have become more common and have raised serious concerns regarding the possibility of false accusation. Rather than tolerating or denying the child's sexual abuse, the other parent (usually the mother) is typically the chief accuser.

NURSING CARE OF THE MALTREATED CHILD

❖ Assessment

One of the most critical responsibilities of all health professionals is identifying abusive situations as early as possible. The characteristics that may predispose members of some families to commit abuse can serve as a framework for assess-

GUIDELINES
Talking with Children Who Reveal Abuse

Provide a private time and place to talk.
Do not promise not to tell; tell them that you are required by law to report the abuse.
Do not express shock or criticize their family.
Use their vocabulary to discuss body parts.
Avoid using any leading statements that can distort their report.
Reassure them that they have done the right thing by telling.
Tell them that the abuse is not their fault, that they are not bad or to blame.
Determine their immediate need for safety.
Let the child know what will happen when you report.

WARNING SIGNS OF ABUSE

Physical evidence of abuse and/or neglect, including previous injuries
Conflicting stories about the "accident" or injury from the parents or others
Cause of injury blamed on sibling or other party
An injury inconsistent with the history, such as a concussion and broken arm from falling off a bed
History inconsistent with child's developmental level, such as a 6-month-old turning on the hot water
A complaint other than the one associated with signs of abuse (e.g., a chief complaint of a cold when there is evidence of first- and second-degree burns)
Inappropriate response of caregiver, such as an exaggerated or absent emotional response; refusal to sign for additional tests or agree to necessary treatment; excessive delay in seeking treatment; absence of the parents for questioning
Inappropriate response of child, such as little or no response to pain; fear of being touched; excessive or lack of separation anxiety; indiscriminate friendliness to strangers
Child's report of physical or sexual abuse
Previous reports of abuse in the family
Repeated visits to emergency facilities with injuries

ing vulnerability but are never predictive of actual abuse. Rather, a thorough physical examination and a careful, detailed history are the diagnostic tools needed to identify abuse. Nurses have a very special role because they may be the first person to see the child and parent and are the consistent caregivers if the child is hospitalized (see Guidelines box).

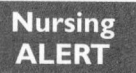

Nursing ALERT Nurses must be aware of their biases regarding child abuse. Studies show that nurses are less likely to report abuse when the child is female and from a middle-income, as opposed to lower-income, family (Pillitteri and others, 1992); are significantly less comfortable dealing with sexual abuse, abuse of infants, and fathers as the abusers (Seidl and others, 1993); and experience greater discomfort when dealing with abusers of children with disabilities than abusers of children without disabilities (Stanton and others, 1994).

Evidence of Maltreatment. Recognition of abuse or neglect necessitates a familiarity with both physical and behavioral signs that suggest maltreatment (see box on p. 431). No one indicator can diagnose maltreatment; rather, it is a pattern or combination of indicators that should arouse suspicion and further investigation. In addition, signs of possible abuse must be coupled with an understanding of diseases, such as bleeding disorders, osteogenesis imperfecta, or sudden infant death syndrome (SIDS), and cultural practices, such as cupping or coin rubbing (see Health Practices, Chapter 3), that may mimic physical abuse. Unintentional injuries may also be wrongly diagnosed as abuse, such as burns from metal buckles on car seats, lacerations from seat belts, or retinal hemorrhage after cardiopulmonary resuscitation. Normal variants, such as mongolian spots and congenital anomalies of genitalia, can be mistaken for abuse.

Not all forms of physical abuse demonstrate obvious signs. Violent shaking of children *(shaken baby syndrome [SBS])* can cause fatal intracranial trauma without signs of external head injury (American Academy of Pediatrics, 1993a). Nurses should suspect SBS in infants less than 1 year of age who present with subdural and/or retinal hemorrhages in the absence of external signs of trauma (Chiocca, 1995).

Nursing ALERT Stress to parents the dangers of shaking infants (can cause SBS). Advise against shaking as a method of burping or waking infant, tossing infant in air, and shaking infant when feeling angry or tense.

If MSP is suspected, nurses play an important role in monitoring the parent's activities to identify instances of causing the children's symptoms. Using a hidden video camera to document the parent's behavior is becoming a more common diagnostic procedure, but the parent's right of privacy must be considered (Wilde and Pedroni, 1993).

Neglect and Emotional Abuse. Neglect from deprivation of necessities is easier to identify than emotional neglect or abuse because physical signs are usually evident. Emotional maltreatment may be readily suspected, but it is very difficult to substantiate. Physical signs are often nonspecific, and nurses must rely on behavioral indicators, which range from depression to acting-out behavior, to help identify a possibly abusive situation. Any persistent and unexplained change in the child's behavior is an important clue to possible emotional abuse.

Sexual Abuse. Identifying instances of sexual abuse is particularly difficult because frequently few if any obvious physical indications of the activity may exist. Also, many individuals are hesitant to believe children and unwilling to report incidents. Even health professionals are sometimes at fault when they perform cursory physical examinations of the genitalia and ignore behavior or verbal comments that suggest abuse. When sexual abuse is suspected, other children in the family should also be evaluated, since multiple victims are not uncommon.

Unfortunately, there is no typical profile of the victim, and there must be a high index of suspicion to identify these children. Physical signs vary and may include any of those listed for sexual abuse in the box above. The victim may exhibit

CLINICAL MANIFESTATIONS OF POTENTIAL CHILD MALTREATMENT

Physical Neglect
Suggestive Physical Findings

Failure to thrive
Signs of malnutrition, such as thin extremities, abdominal distention, lack of subcutaneous fat
Poor personal hygiene, especially of teeth
Unclean and/or inappropriate dress
Evidence of poor health care, such as nonimmunized status, untreated infections, frequent colds
Frequent injuries from lack of supervision

Suggestive Behaviors

Dull and inactive; excessively passive or sleepy
Self-stimulatory behaviors, such as finger-sucking or rocking
Begging or stealing food ⎫
Absenteeism from school ⎬ in older child
Drug or alcohol addiction ⎪
Vandalism or shoplifting ⎭

Emotional Abuse and Neglect
Suggestive Physical Findings

Failure to thrive
Feeding disorders, such as rumination
Enuresis
Sleep disorders

Suggestive Behaviors

Self-stimulatory behaviors, such as biting, rocking, sucking
During infancy, lack of social smile and stranger anxiety
Withdrawal
Unusual fearfulness
Antisocial behavior, such as destructiveness, stealing, cruelty
Extremes of behavior, such as overcompliant and passive or aggressive and demanding
Lags in emotional and intellectual development, especially language
Suicide attempts

Physical Abuse
Suggestive Physical Findings

Bruises and welts
    On face, lips, mouth, back, buttocks, thighs, or areas of torso
    Regular patterns descriptive of object used, such as belt buckle, hand, wire hanger, chain, wooden spoon, squeeze or pinch marks
    May be present in various stages of healing
Burns
    On soles of feet, palms of hands, back, or buttocks
    Patterns descriptive of object used, such as round cigar or cigarette burns, "glovelike" sharply demarcated areas from immersion in scalding water, rope burns on wrists or ankles from being bound, burns in the shape of an iron, radiator, or electric stove burner
    Absence of "splash" marks and presence of symmetric burns
    Stun gun injury: lesions circular, fairly uniform (up to 0.5 cm), and paired about 5 cm (2 inches) apart (Frechette and Rimsza, 1992)
Fractures and dislocations
    Skull, nose, or facial structures
    Injury may denote type of abuse, such as spiral fracture or dislocation from twisting of an extremity or whiplash from shaking the child
    Multiple new or old fractures in various stages of healing

Lacerations and abrasions
    On backs of arms, legs, torso, face, or external genitalia
    Unusual symptoms, such as abdominal swelling, pain, and vomiting from punching
    Descriptive marks such as from human bites or pulling hair out
Chemical
    Unexplained repeated poisoning, especially drug overdose
    Unexplained sudden illness, such as hypoglycemia from insulin administration

Suggestive Behaviors

Wary of physical contact with adults
Apparent fear of parents or going home
Lying very still while surveying environment
Inappropriate reaction to injury, such as failure to cry from pain
Lack of reaction to frightening events
Apprehensive when hearing other children cry
Indiscriminate friendliness and displays of affection
Superficial relationships
Acting-out behavior, such as aggression, to seek attention
Withdrawal behavior

Sexual Abuse
Suggestive Physical Findings

Bruises, bleeding, lacerations or irritation of external genitalia, anus, mouth, or throat
Torn, stained, or bloody underclothing
Pain on urination or pain, swelling, and itching of genital area
Penile discharge
Sexually transmitted disease, nonspecific vaginitis, or venereal warts
Difficulty in walking or sitting
Unusual odor in the genital area
Recurrent urinary tract infections
Presence of sperm
Pregnancy in young adolescent

Suggestive Behaviors

Sudden emergence of sexually related problems, including excessive or public masturbation, age-inappropriate sexual play, promiscuity, or overtly seductive behavior
Withdrawn, excessive daydreaming
Preoccupied with fantasies, especially in play
Poor relationships with peers
Sudden changes, such as anxiety, loss or gain of weight, clinging behavior
In incestuous relationships, excessive anger at mother for not protecting daughter
Regressive behavior, such as bed-wetting or thumb-sucking
Sudden onset of phobias or fears, particularly fears of the dark, men, strangers, or particular settings or situations (e.g., undue fear of leaving the house or staying at the daycare center or the babysitter's house)
Running away from home
Substance abuse, particularly of alcohol or mood-elevating drugs
Profound and rapid personality changes, especially extreme depression, hostility, and aggression (often accompanied by social withdrawal)
Rapidly declining school performance
Suicidal attempts or ideation

various behavioral manifestations. Unfortunately, none of these behaviors is diagnostic of sexual abuse. When abused children exhibit these behaviors, the signs may be incorrectly attributed to the normal stresses of childhood, especially in older school-age children or adolescents. Even those signs considered most predictive of sexual abuse, such as certain genital findings, sexually inappropriate behavior for age, enactment of adult sexual activity, and intense focus on sexual activity (e.g., masturbation), do not always indicate that sexual abuse has occurred. Conversely, abused children may not demonstrate more knowledge of sexual activity than nonabused children. However, one difference in the abused children's explanation of sexual activity may be unusual affective responses. For example, abused children may relate stories that include fear of going to sleep or of being with a parent (Gordon, Schroeder, and Abrams, 1990).

 Many genital findings that have been reported as conclusive or highly suspect for sexual abuse, such as vaginal opening greater than 4 mm, hymenal tears and synechiae (tissue bands) inside the vagina, reflex anal dilatation, and condylomata acuminata (anogenital or venereal warts), may be found in unabused prepubertal children (Wong, 1991).

History Pertaining to the Incident. In addition to observable evidence of abuse, the type of history revealed by the parents or other caregiver, such as the baby-sitter or mother's boyfriend, is a significant factor. Areas of the history that should arouse suspicion of abuse are summarized in the box on p. 434.

Nursing ALERT Incompatibility between the history and the injury is probably the most important criterion on which to base the decision to report suspected abuse.

An important point to remember when taking a history is that maltreated children rarely betray their parents by admitting to the abuse they received. If questioned, they will repeat the same story as the parents and try to defend their parents' actions. If the interviewer directly accuses the parents of abuse, the child may accept responsibility for the act in an attempt to vindicate the parents. Whether children respond in this way out of fear is uncertain. However, children do fear losing whatever security and love they have. Between abusive acts, children may receive some measure of attention and love from the parents. If they betray the parents, they may lose this and be uncertain or fearful of the consequences, such as foster care. Preserving the present situation may be less frightening than the unknown future.

The *disclosure of sexual abuse* can occur in a variety of ways: the act is observed by others, resulting in a direct confrontation; the child tells someone, such as a parent of a friend; visible clues of the relationship are observed, such as an accumulation of coins, gifts, or candy; more obvious clues are seen, such as a child coming home disheveled or becoming pregnant; and physical or behavioral signs and symptoms are observed. Children usually describe the experience in terms of whether it was unpleasant or hurt or was pleasurable (usually a response to hand-genital contact); some indicate no reaction. Young children often feel no guilt or shame

because the act is pleasurable and they are unaware of its inappropriateness.

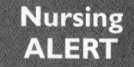 **Nursing ALERT** When children report potentially sexually abusive experiences, their reports need to be taken seriously, but also cautiously to avoid alarming the child or falsely accusing a person.

Children's reports of sexual abuse may vary from contradictory stories to unwavering versions of the experience. While their stories may sound contradictory, this may reflect the child's experiences in several instances of abuse. Also, children who repeatedly tell identical facts may have been prompted to do so. Increasing evidence suggests that the types of interrogation children are exposed to following reports of sexual abuse shape their thinking. Through the use of leading questions, closed questions (those requiring yes or no answers), intimidation, prodding, and selective reinforcement for certain answers, children begin to tell stories that never occurred. Eventually they may come to experience the tale as reality (Wakefield and Underwager, 1989). The Family Focus box discusses false allegations of abuse.

 FAMILY FOCUS
False Allegations of Abuse

Although most concern among health professionals is to detect child abuse early and to protect the child from further abuse, prevention of abuse must also include prevention of false allegations of abuse. Although some degree of overreporting is expected because the law requires the reporting of suspected maltreatment, the degree of overreporting is considered unreasonably high. Under the present child abuse laws, child protective services have the authority to remove a child from the home solely on the basis of allegations made to an abuse hotline (Radko, 1993).

Despite more than half of all reports being unfounded, little attention has been directed to the problem of false accusations and its devastating consequences, such as removal of the child from the home, termination of parental rights, public ridicule of the family, loss of employment, and excessive legal fees to regain custody of the child. Nurses play a critical role in carefully documenting all evidence of abuse, giving alleged offenders the opportunity to present their account of the incident, and recognizing diseases or cultural practices that may be confused with abuse (Wong, 1987). In the unfortunate event that a family is wrongly accused of abuse, they may benefit from the services of the **National Association of State VOCAL (Victims of Child Abuse Legislation) Organizations,*** a support group for persons who have experienced false accusations. Another organization that may be helpful to family members who have been accused of sexual abuse by their adult children is the **False Memory Syndrome (FMS) Foundation.†** The research and educational institution is dedicated to understanding and preventing allegations of abuse based on "false" memories. In recent years adult children, primarily women, claim to suddenly remember childhood sexual abuse, usually by fathers. The abuse is said to have been repressed for many years, but the memory is recovered with the help of a therapist (Loftus, 1995).

*1030 G. St., Suite 200, Sacramento, CA 95814
†3508 Market St., Suite 128, Philadelphia, PA 19104, (215) 387-1865.

Parental Behaviors. Certain behavioral responses of the parents to their child and to the interviewer should alert the nurse to the possibility of maltreatment. Although no one pattern of behaviors is characteristic of these parents, some responses include the following. Abusive parents have difficulty in showing concern toward their child. They are unable to comfort the child and give no indication of realizing how the child may feel, physically or emotionally. Instead, they are critical of and angry with the child for being injured. They maintain that the child is responsible for the injury, and, if asked any question regarding their responsibility of protecting or supervising the child, they become hostile and aggressive. They act as if the child's injury is an assault on them. Their entire perception of the incident is in terms of how it affects them, not the child, which is an indication of their preoccupation with their own needs and of their inability to give any support to others.

During the child's hospitalization they may not become involved in the child's care and may show little concern for his or her progress, eventual discharge, or need for follow-up care. However, if they are pressured during interrogation, they immediately demand to take the child home, regardless of the child's readiness for discharge.

Families respond to sexual abuse with a wide variety of emotional reactions, which range from not believing the child to being very supportive. Parents and other family members may display the same type of emotional responses as the victim, such as inability to eat or sleep, and somatic complaints, such as headache. In the acute emotional phase, parents have a need to blame someone. The three common targets are the offender, the child, and themselves. The parents frequently express anger at the child for "stupid" behavior and may even restrict the child's privileges as punishment. When the victim is a girl, the parents may question her sexual provocation of the event. Self-blaming parents assume full responsibility, believing that they have been inadequate parents or should not have allowed the child to go out. When a baby-sitter or trusted relative is involved in the assault and the child's complaint has not been believed until gross evidence is presented, the parents are often devastated by guilt.

Child Behaviors. Abused children's responses to their parents or the injury may also support the suspicion of abuse. Although no one pattern is typical, extremes of behavior may be observed. Children may be very unresponsive to the parent or excessively clinging and intolerant of separation. They may be overattached to the abusive parent, possibly in the hope of preventing any upset that may precipitate anger and another attack. During care of the injury, children may be passive and accepting of the discomfort or uncooperative and fearful of any physical contact. Some children maintain a wary watchfulness of all strangers; some shy away from strangers as if frightened; others are unusually affectionate and outgoing.

❖ Nursing Diagnoses

A number of nursing diagnoses are prominent in the nursing care of the maltreated child and family, and others specific to individual cases become evident. The most common nursing diagnoses are outlined in the Nursing Care Plan on pp. 436-437.

❖ Planning

The main nursing goals related to child maltreatment are as follows:

1. Child will be protected from further abuse.
2. Child and family will receive adequate support.
3. Hospitalized child and family, including foster parents if appropriate, will be prepared for discharge.
4. Child will not experience any maltreatment.

❖ Implementation

Protect Child From Further Abuse. Initially, identification of instances of suspected abuse or neglect is essential. The nurse may come in contact with abused children in an emergency room, practitioner's office, home, daycare center, or school.

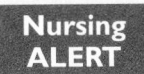 **Nursing ALERT** The priority is to remove the child from the abusive situation to prevent further injury.

All states and provinces in North America have laws for mandatory reporting of child maltreatment. Suspected child abuse is reported to the local authorities.* Referrals usually come to the state child welfare department and are assigned to a caseworker in an agency such as **Child Protective Services (CPS)**. Once a referral has been made, a caseworker is assigned to investigate the report. Based on the findings, the child is left in the home or temporarily removed.

A court proceeding may be necessary before the child can be placed outside the home or when parental rights are to be terminated. When the courts are involved, they usually require firsthand testimony by the referring parties. Nurses may be subpoenaed to appear in court, or their notes may be introduced as evidence in court hearings. Accurate and factual documentation is essential. A suggested outline for recording pertinent assessment data is presented in the Guidelines box on p. 434. Behaviors are described, not interpreted, and are recorded daily to establish a progress record. Conversations among the nurse, child, and parent are recorded verbatim as much as possible.

Support Child. Frequently, children suspected of abuse are hospitalized for medical management of their injuries. When the sexually abused child has been physically harmed, the care is consistent with that provided a rape victim (see Chapter 17). Regardless of the type of abuse, their needs are the same as those of any hospitalized child. The child should be treated as a child with the usual physical needs, developmental tasks, and play interests, not as a dramatic victim of abuse. The nurse is the child's advocate in this goal. The nurse also encourages the child's relationship with the parents. *The nurse does not become a substitute parent to the exclusion of the child's natural parents.* Such an intent only intensifies the parents' feelings of inadequacy, worthlessness, and isolation. It does not help them understand their child or promote their trust in health profession-

---

*Telephone numbers are usually listed under "Child Abuse" in the business white pages of the local directory, or call the emergency child abuse hotline: (800) 422-4453 ([800] 4-A-CHILD).

GUIDELINES
Recording Assessment Data
in Suspected Abuse

History of Injury
1. Date, time, and place of occurrence
2. Sequence of events with recorded times
3. Presence of witnesses, especially person caring for child at time of incident
4. Time lapse between occurrence of injury and initiation of treatment
5. Interview with child when appropriate, including verbal quotations and information from drawing or other play activities
6. Interview with parent, witnesses, or other significant persons, including verbal quotations
7. Description of parent-child interactions (verbal interactions, eye contact, touching, parental concern)
8. Name, age, and condition of other children in home (if possible)

Physical Examination
1. Location, size, shape, and color of bruises; approximate location, size, and shape on drawing of body outline
2. Distinguishing characteristics, such as a bruise in the shape of a hand; round burn (possibly caused by cigarette)
3. Symmetry or asymmetry of injury; presence of other injuries
4. Degree of pain; any bone tenderness
5. Evidence of past injuries; general state of health and hygiene
6. Developmental level of child; perform screening test (see Developmental Assessment, Chapter 7)

als. The goal of the *consistent* nurse-child relationship is to provide a role model for the parents in helping them to relate positively and constructively to their child and to foster a therapeutic environment for the child in his or her reprieve from the abusing situation.

Sexual Abuse.   The type of care needed by the child depends on the circumstances of the sexual abuse. It varies from reassurance and support when the act involves exhibitionism to long-term counseling in incestuous situations. In *interviewing* these children, nurses must be very careful to avoid biasing the child's retelling of the events. Some experts suggest that health professionals limit the interview to the child's physical and mental health concerns and leave the topics of the family's social, legal, or other problems to the police or CPS personnel (Koop, 1988).

In preparation for an interview, every effort is made to make the child feel comfortable with appropriate introductions and to avoid duplicating the behaviors typically used by offenders, such as touching the child without permission. The interview is conducted in a quiet and private location, preferably a neutral place, such as a school playroom or office, and not where the abuse occurred. Neutral questions are asked first, such as the child's reaction to the hospital (if appropriate). Then the incident is discussed in general terms. The interview should include such nonleading questions as "Do you know why you were brought to the hospital?" "Do you know what will happen here?" or "How do you feel about being here?" Later the question "Can you tell me what happened?" and other questions may then elicit an account of the incident. Sometimes the parents are able to help the

child describe the incident, and questions can then be directed to the circumstances of the assault. Questions should progress chronologically and proceed from the nonsexual to the more sexual content. If the child shows evidence of becoming too upset, the focus is redirected toward more neutral and less emotionally laden areas.

Children are given the opportunity to ask questions, but if they are hesitant, they are never pressured into talking. Young children in particular lack the verbal skills to describe body parts adequately. These children may benefit from play situations that provide opportunities for disclosure, such as drawing or playing with puppets or anatomically correct dolls or with dollhouses.

Considerable controversy exists regarding the use of children's *drawings* and *anatomically correct dolls* as *diagnostic* tests for sexual abuse. The presence of genitalia on a human figure drawing or sexual play with the dolls does not prove sexual abuse; the children's description and explanation of the drawing or play are more relevant than the content. Genitalia on drawings and sexual doll play may raise suspicion of abuse but are not diagnostic (Wakefield and Underwager, 1989).

Support Family.   One of the most difficult, yet essential, components of success with abusive parents is the quality of the *therapeutic relationship*. It must be one of genuine concern and treatment, not one of accusation and punishment. Nurses must examine their personal feelings toward these parents, particularly when sexual abuse is present. A therapeutic approach is to view the parent as the patient and the child as the victim of abuse. Unless the nurse's attitude is positive, abusive parents will not be motivated to change, since they will not be working with a trusting person who demonstrates the kind of behavior that is being asked of them.

When parental ignorance of childrearing practices has played a part in the abuse, the nurse can educate the parent regarding *children's physical and emotional needs*. Because of the parents' own childrearing, they may not be aware of nonviolent methods of discipline, such as time-out or consequences. They may also need help in dealing with their frustration so that they do not vent anger on the child. Since these parents may be sensitive to criticism or domination and already possess a very low self-esteem, teaching is implemented through demonstration and example rather than through lecturing. Any *competent parenting abilities* they demonstrate are praised to promote their sense of parental adequacy.

Sexual Abuse.   Care of the family also depends on the circumstances of the sexual abuse. With a nonparent offender the family may be more able to support the child than if incest were involved. Family members are encouraged to express their feelings of anger, guilt, shame, and/or embarrassment but are also cautioned to avoid displacing such feelings on the child. For example, it is easy for parents to admonish the child with a statement such as "We told you never to go with strangers," which makes the child feel responsible.

Family members are advised to encourage the child to resume normal activities and observe the child for signs of distress (see Posttraumatic Stress Disorder, Chapter 17). Children express their feelings primarily through behavior. Parents should be alert for changes in behavior that indicate distress resulting from the incident, such as remaining in the house, refusing to go to school, changes in sleeping patterns, and frequency of dreams and nightmares. Children are encouraged to talk about these feelings and nightmares, since the more they can talk about the experience, the more they are able to gain control over it.

Referral.   Referral to appropriate agencies is also essential. Most abusive parents tend to live in poverty, and the daily stresses imposed by their life-style are overwhelming. Resources for financial aid, improved housing, and child care should be sought. Self-help groups also provide important services. Such groups as **Parents Anonymous*** (a group for parents who have abused or fear that they may abuse their child, but only in terms of physical abuse, not sexual abuse) and **Parents United International, Inc.†** (a group devoted to helping sexually abused families) are very accepting and nonjudgmental, because everyone has been in the same position.

There is no way to predict which families will be successfully rehabilitated. With father-daughter incest, however, the best results occur when the father accepts full responsibility for the act, the mother acknowledges her role in failing to protect the child, and the child is able to understand and forgive the parents and develop a positive self-image despite the traumatic experience.

Plan for Discharge.   Discharge planning should begin as soon as the legal disposition for placement has been decided, which may be temporary foster home placement, return to the parents, or permanent termination of parental rights. The latter is the most drastic solution, but it is necessary in situations of repeated, life-threatening abuse. Whenever children are sent to a foster home or juvenile institution, they must be allowed an opportunity to express their feelings. No matter how severe the abuse, they usually mourn the loss of their parents. They need help to understand why they must not return home and that this new home is in no way a punishment. Whenever possible, foster parents are encouraged to visit in the hospital, and the nurse should take an active role in helping these new parents understand the child. It is unfortunate that some abused children live in torment as they are sent from one foster home to another, sometimes enduring worse circumstances than those that existed in their original home. Only through constant evaluation of the placement residence and the child's adjustment to a new environment can the vicious circle of abuse, abandonment, and neglect be stopped.

Prevent Abuse.   Prevention of child maltreatment has been an extremely difficult goal. Programs aimed at identifying potential abusers and instituting supportive intervention before the occurrence of an abusive act have met with variable success. However, nurses have played an important role in such programs. For example, prenatal and infancy home visiting by nurses to primiparas who were either teenagers, unmarried, or of low socioeconomic status resulted in significantly less reports of child abuse during the first 2 years (Olds and others, 1986). The nurses provided information on normal child growth and development and routine health care needs, served as informal support persons, and referred families to appropriate services when a need for assistance was identified.

Such programs provide models that can be used to reduce factors known to increase the risk of abuse. However, nurses in a variety of settings can implement similar activities. Nurses in prenatal clinics can prepare expectant families for the adjustment of parenthood. Nursery and postpartum nurses can foster the attachment process by encouraging parents to hold and look at their infant. In neonatal intensive care units, nurses can minimize the effects of separation by encouraging parents to visit and can help them become comfortable in the child's care. Those in ambulatory settings can teach parents appropriate methods of bathing, feeding, toileting, disciplining, and preventing injuries, while stressing the normal needs and developmental characteristics of children. Nurses need to

---

> ⌂ **FAMILY HOME CARE**
> **Preventing or Dealing with Sexual Abuse of Children**
>
> Sexual assault of children is much more common than most people realize. It may be preventable if children have good preparation. *To provide protection and preparation:*
> Pay careful attention to who is around children. (Unwanted touch *may* come from someone liked and trusted.)
> Back up a child's right to say "no."
> Encourage communication by taking seriously what children *say.*
> Take a second look at signals of potential danger.
> Refuse to leave children in the company of those not trusted.
> Include information about sexual assault when teaching about safety.
> Provide specific definitions and examples of sexual assault.
> Remind children that even "nice" people sometimes do mean things.
> Urge children to tell about *anybody* who causes them to be uncomfortable.
> Prepare children to deal with bribes and threats, as well as possible physical force.
> Virtually eliminate secrets between children and parents.
> Teach children how to say "no," ask for help, and control who touches them and how.
> Model self-protective and limit-setting behavior for children.
> Should it ever become necessary *to help a child recover from a sexual assault:*
> Listen carefully to understand children.
> Support the child for telling by praise, belief, sympathy, and lack of blame.
> Know local resources and choose help carefully.
> Provide opportunities to talk about the assault.
> Provide opportunities for the entire family to go through a recovery process.
> Sexual assault affects everyone. *To help deal with this social problem:*
> Provide sympathetic care and support to those who have been victimized.
> Recognize that offenders do not change without intervention.
> Organize neighborhood programs to support each other's efforts to protect children.
> Encourage schools to provide information about sexual assault as a problem of health and safety.
> Organize community groups to support educational treatment and law enforcement programs.

Modified from Adams C, Fay J: *No more secrets: protecting your child from sexual assault,* San Luis Obispo, CA, 1981, Impact.

---

*520 S. Lafayette, Park Plaza, Suite 316, Los Angeles, CA 90057.
†P.O. Box 952, San Jose, CA 95108; (408) 453-7616.

NURSING CARE PLAN
The Child Who Is Maltreated

NURSING DIAGNOSIS: High risk for trauma related to characteristics of child, caregiver(s), environment

PATIENT GOAL 1: Will experience no further abuse or neglect

- **NURSING INTERVENTIONS/*RATIONALES***

Implement measures *to prevent abuse:*
  Report suspicions to appropriate authorities
  Assist in removing child from unsafe environment and establishing in a safe environment
  Establish protective measures for the hospitalized child as indicated *to prevent continued abuse in hospital*
Refer family to social agencies for assistance with finances, food, clothing, housing, and health care *to help prevent neglect*
Keep factual, objective records *for documentation,* including:
  Child's physical condition
  Child's behavioral response to parents, others, and environment
  Interviews with family members
Collaborate efforts of multidisciplinary team *to continually evaluate progress of child in foster home or in return to own family*
Be alert for signs of continued abuse or neglect
Help parents identify those circumstances that precipitate an abusive act and alternative ways to deal with the release of anger other than attacking child
Refer for alternative placement when indicated *to prevent further injury or neglect*

- **EXPECTED OUTCOME**

Child experiences no further injury or neglect

NURSING DIAGNOSIS: Fear/anxiety related to negative interpersonal interaction, repeated maltreatment, powerlessness, potential loss of parents

PATIENT GOAL 1: Will experience reduction or relief of anxiety and stress

- **NURSING INTERVENTIONS/*RATIONALES***

Provide consistent caregiver and therapeutic environment during hospitalization *to relieve child's stress and to be a role model for family*
Demonstrate acceptance of child while not expecting same in return
Show attention while not reinforcing inappropriate behavior, *since all children have this need*
Plan appropriate activities for attention with nurse, other adults, and other children; use play *to work through relationships*
Praise child's abilities *in order to promote self-esteem*
Treat child as one who has a specific physical problem for hospitalization, not as "abused" victim

Avoid asking too many questions, *since this can upset child and interfere with other professionals' interrogations*
  Use play, especially family or dollhouse activity, *to investigate type of relationships perceived by child*
  Provide one consistent person to whom child relates regarding events of abuse *so that child is not overwhelmed*
  Help child grieve for loss of parents if their rights are terminated *because child may be very attached to parents despite abuse*
Encourage child to talk about feelings toward parents and future placement *to facilitate coping*
Encourage introduction to foster parents before placement if possible *to give child time to adjust*

- **EXPECTED OUTCOMES**

Child exhibits minimal or no evidence of distress
Child engages in positive relationships with caregivers
Child grieves for loss of parent

NURSING DIAGNOSIS: Altered parenting related to child, caregiver, or situational characteristics that precipitate abusive behavior

PATIENT (FAMILY) GOAL 1: Will exhibit evidence of positive interaction with children

- **NURSING INTERVENTIONS/*RATIONALES***

Identify families at risk for potential abuse *so that appropriate intervention is instituted*
Promote parental attachment to child, *since all children have this need*
Emphasize childrearing practices, especially effective methods of discipline, *since parents may lack knowledge about nonviolent discipline methods*
Increase parents' feeling of adequacy and self-esteem
Encourage support systems *that lessen stress and total responsibility of child care on one or both parents*
Teach children to recognize situations that place them at risk for sexual abuse and teach assertive responses *to discourage abuse*

- **EXPECTED OUTCOME**

Families exhibit evidence of positive interaction with children

PATIENT (FAMILY) GOAL 2: Will receive adequate support

- **NURSING INTERVENTIONS/*RATIONALES***

Provide "mothering" by directing attention to parent, taking over child care responsibilities until parent feels ready to participate, and focusing on parent's needs *so that parents can eventually meet child's needs*
Convey an attitude of genuine concern, not one of accusation and punishment, *since this only serves to further alienate family*
Refer parents to special support groups and/or counseling *for long-term support*
Help identify a support group for parents, such as extended family or nearby neighbors; help these significant others understand their important role in also preventing further abuse

NURSING CARE PLAN
The Child Who Is Maltreated—cont'd

Refer to social agencies that can provide assistance in areas such as financial support, adequate housing, and employment

• **EXPECTED OUTCOMES**

Parents demonstrate appropriate parenting activities
Parents seek group and individual support
Parents receive assistance with problems

PATIENT (FAMILY) GOAL 3: Will exhibit knowledge of normal growth and development

• **NURSING INTERVENTIONS/*RATIONALES***

Teach realistic expectations of child's behavior and capabilities

Emphasize alternate methods of discipline, such as reward, time-out, consequences, and verbal disapproval, *so that parents learn nonviolent discipline methods*
Suggest methods of handling developmental problems or goals, such as toddler negativism, toilet training, and independence, *since these situations may precipitate abuse*
Teach through demonstration and role modeling, rather than lecture; avoid authoritarian approach, *since family may be sensitive to criticism or domination and lack self-esteem*

• **EXPECTED OUTCOME**

Parents demonstrate an understanding of normal expectations for their child

---

be sensitive to the parents' needs for attention, reassurance, and reinforcement. Nurses need to know what kinds of community services are available, including self-help groups, and make timely referrals.

Sexual Abuse. Unlike preventive efforts for neglect and physical abuse, which have been aimed at the potential offender, *prevention of child sexual abuse* has centered on education of children to protect themselves. Currently, much controversy surrounds the effectiveness of these programs. The main issue is whether young children should be expected to participate in their own protection. Some experts suggest that in the struggle between sexual offender and potential child victim, most factors favor the adult, who has superior knowledge, strength, and skill to overcome most children's efforts at self-protection (Conte, Wolf, and Smith, 1989). Clearly, sexual abuse prevention is more than teaching children to say "no" or to recognize their right not to be touched in "private places." It is equally important to teach children safety in terms of potential risk situations. Several suggestions for parents regarding protecting and educating children against possible molestation are presented in the Family Home Care box on p. 435.

The nurse is frequently in a position to discuss this topic with parents as part of health maintenance and to provide guidelines. Books are available for parents that describe sexual abuse and its prevention.* Helpful games such as "What if the baby-sitter wants to wrestle and hug but tells you to keep it a secret?" can be used to explore dangerous situations in advance and help children learn the importance of saying

"no." They need reassurance that no matter what the other person says or does, the parents want to know about it and will not punish them. Even if children do participate in the activity before telling the parents, they must be reassured that it was not their fault.

In addition, parents need to be made aware that "nice" people, including friends and relatives, can be offenders; parents should carefully observe how others act toward the child. A sudden change in the child's behavior and a response such as "I don't like Uncle anymore" are clues to investigate the relationship. In the event of any doubt, further solitary encounters with this person and the child should be prevented. It is sometimes to the child's great misfortune that parents do not take certain comments seriously, such as "He hugs me too tight" or "I don't want to go with him." Casual parental statements such as "He just loves you" or "You do whatever adults tell you to do" can place children in jeopardy. Health professionals can alert parents to such dangers and guide them toward an appreciation of the problem, providing concrete guidelines toward child education and protection.

❖ Evaluation

The effectiveness of nursing interventions is determined by continual reassessment and evaluation of care based on the following observational guidelines and expected outcomes:

1. Observe child for additional physical and behavioral evidence of abuse; observe child's reactions to health professionals; if child is hospitalized, check staffing patterns for schedule of consistent group of nurses caring for child.
2. Interview parents regarding their knowledge of children's physical and development needs.
3. Interview child regarding feelings about returning home or placement outside the home.
4. Investigate community programs aimed at preventing child maltreatment.

Expected outcomes:
See Nursing Care Plan, pp. 436-437.

---

*Sources of information are the **National Committee for Prevention of Child Abuse**, Publishing Department, 332 S. Michigan Ave., Suite 1600, Chicago, IL 60604-4357, (312) 663-3520; **C. Henry Kempe National Center for the Prevention and Treatment of Child Abuse and Neglect**, 1205 Oneida St., Denver, CO 80220, (303) 321-3963; **American Association for Protecting Children, American Humane Association**, 63 Inverness Dr. E., Englewood, CO 80112, (800) 227-4645 (outside Colorado) or (303) 792-9900; and **National Resource Center on Child Sexual Abuse**, 107 Lincoln St., Huntsville, AL 35801, (800) 543-7006.

KEY POINTS

- Common infectious disorders during early childhood include communicable diseases, intestinal parasitic infections, conjunctivitis, and stomatitis.
- Nursing goals in the treatment of a communicable disease are identification, prevention of transmission, provision of comfort, and prevention of complications.
- Intestinal parasitic diseases constitute the most common infections in the world; giardiasis and enterobiasis are the most widespread parasitic infections among children in the United States.
- Although the incidence of poisoning has decreased in the last 30 years as a result of more stringent packaging regulations, childhood poisoning remains a serious health concern.
- The major principles of emergency treatment for poisoning are assessment, supportive measures, gastric decontamination, family support, and prevention of recurrence.
- Ipecac is an effective and safe emetic for home use in poisonings but is contraindicated in situations that increase the risk of aspiration and that involve ingestion of corrosives, in which vomiting redamages the mucosa.
- Three simple measures that can reduce the severity of a poisoning are knowing the telephone number of the Poison Control Center, having ipecac in the home (two doses per child), and administering it correctly.
- Acetaminophen poisoning is the most common drug poisoning among children and occurs primarily from acute overdose.
- The most important factor contributing to lead poisoning is its availability in the child's environment. Lead-based paint is the most toxic source of lead.
- With increasing awareness of the detrimental effects of low levels of lead on the developing nervous system, acceptable blood lead levels have been decreasing and now are at less than 10 μg/dl.
- Child maltreatment may take the form of physical abuse or neglect, emotional abuse or neglect, or sexual abuse.
- Parental, child, and environmental characteristics are criteria that may predispose children to maltreatment.
- Identification of abuse entails securing evidence of maltreatment, taking a history pertaining to the incident, and assessing parental and child behaviors.
- The reported incidence of sexual abuse has increased in the last decade; common forms are incest, molestation, rape, exhibitionism, child pornography, child prostitution, and pedophilia.

REFERENCES

Altemeier WA III and others: Antecedents of child abuse, *J Pediatr* 100(5):823-829, 1982.

American Academy of Pediatrics, Committee on Child Abuse and Neglect: Shaken baby syndrome—inflicted cerebral trauma, *Pediatrics* 92(2):872-873, 1993a.

American Academy of Pediatrics, Committee on Infectious Diseases: The use of oral acyclovir in otherwise healthy children with varicella, *Pediatrics* 91(3):674-676, 1993b.

Bartlett AV and others: Controlled trial of *Giardia lamblia*: control strategies in day care centers, *Am J Public Health* 81(6):1001-1006, 1991.

Bellinger DC, Stiles KM, Needleman HL: Low-level lead exposure, intelligence and academic achievement: a long-term follow-up study, *Pediatrics* 90(6):855-861, 1992.

Centers for Disease Control and Prevention: *Preventing lead poisoning in young children*, Atlanta, 1991, CDC.

Cheung L, Potts R, Meyer K: Acetaminophen treatment nomogram, *N Engl J Med* 330(26):1907-1908, 1994.

Chiocca EM: Shaken baby syndrome: a nursing perspective, *Pediatr Nurs* 21(1):33-38, 1995.

Conte J, Wolf S, Smith T: What sexual offenders tell us about prevention strategies, *Child Abuse Negl* 13:293-301, 1989.

Council on Scientific Affairs: AMA diagnostic and treatment guidelines concerning child abuse and neglect, *JAMA* 254(6):796-800, 1985.

Doran T and others: Acetaminophen: more harm than good for chickenpox? *J Pediatr* 114(6):1045-1048, 1989.

Douidar SM, Al-Khalil I, Habersang RW: Severe hepatotoxicity, acute renal failure, and pancytopenia in a young child after repeated acetaminophen overdosing, *Clin Pediatr* 33(1):42-45, 1994.

Dunkle LM and others: A controlled trial of acyclovir for chickenpox in normal children, *N Engl J Med* (325):1539-1544, 1991.

Feldman W and others: Is childhood sexual abuse really increasing in prevalence? An analysis of the evidence, *Pediatrics* 88(1):29-33, 1991.

Frechette A, Rimsza ME: Stun gun injury: a new presentation of the battered child syndrome, *Pediatrics* 89(5):898-901, 1992.

Gilbert CM: Sibling incest: a descriptive study of family dynamics, *J Child Adolesc Psychiatr Ment Health Nurs* 5(1):5-9, 1992.

Glasziou PP, MacKerras DEM: Vitamin A supplementation in infectious diseases: a meta-analysis, *Br Med J* 306(6874):366-370, 1993.

Gordon B, Schroeder C, Abrams M: Children's knowledge of sexuality: a comparison of sexually abused and nonabused children, *Am J Orthopsychiatry* 60(2):250-257, 1990.

Highlights of official child neglect and abuse reporting 1986, Denver, 1988, The American Humane Association.

Hill DR: Giardiasis: issues in diagnosis and management, *Infect Dis Clin North Am* 7(3):503-525, 1993.

In fact . . . answers to frequently asked questions on child abuse and neglect, Washington, DC, undated, National Clearinghouse on Child Abuse and Neglect Information.

Jones VF and others: The role of the male caretaker in Munchausen syndrome by proxy, *Clin Pediatr* 32:245-247, 1993.

Koop CE: *The surgeon general's letter on child sexual abuse,* Rockville, MD, 1988, US Department of Health and Human Services, Public Health Service, Health Resources and Services Administration, Bureau of Maternal and Child Health and Resources Development, Office of Maternal and Child Health.

Kotelchuck M: Child abuse and neglect: prediction and misclassification. In Starr RH, editor: *Child abuse prediction policy implications,* Cambridge, MA, 1982, Ballinger.

Liebelt EL, Shannon MW: Small doses, big problems: a selected review of highly toxic common medications, *Pediatr Emerg Care* 9(5):292-297, 1993.

Litovitz T and others: 1992 annual report of the American Association of Poison Control Centers Toxic Exposure Surveillance System, *Am J Emerg Med* 11(5):494-555, 1993.

Loftus E: Remembering dangerously, *Skeptical Inquirer* 19(2):20-29, 1995.

A nation's shame: fatal child abuse and neglect in the United States, Washington, DC, 1995, US Advisory Board on Child Abuse and Neglect.

National Center on Child Abuse and Neglect: *A coordinated response to child abuse and neglect: a basic manual,* Washington, DC, 1993, National Center.

Nocton JJ and others: Human parvovirus-associated arthritis in children, *J Pediatr* 122(2):186-190, 1993.

Nordin JD, Rolnick SJ, Griffin JM: Prevalence of excess lead absorption and associated risk factors in children enrolled in a midwestern health maintenance organization, *Pediatrics* 93:172-177, 1994.

Olds DL and others: Preventing child abuse and neglect: a randomized trial of nurse home visitation, *Pediatrics* 78(1):65-78, 1986.

Pillitteri A and others: Parent gender, victim gender, and family socioeconomic level influences on the potential reporting by nurses of physical child abuse, *Issues Compr Pediatr Nurs* 15:239-247, 1992.

Piomelli S: Childhood lead poisoning in the '90s, *Pediatrics* 93(4):508-510, 1994.

Radko K: Child abuse: guilty until proven innocent or legalized governmental child abuse, *Issues Child Abuse Accus* 5(2):96-101, 1993.

Seidl AH and others: Nurses' attitudes toward the child victims and the perpetrators of emotional, physical, and sexual abuse, *Issues Child Abuse Accus* 5(1):28-38, 1993.

Shannon M, Graef J: Lead intoxication in infancy, *Pediatrics* 89(1):87-90, 1992.

Stanton, M, and others: Nurses' attitudes toward emotional, sexual, and physical abusers of children with disabilities, *Rehabil Nurs* 19(4):214-218, 1994.

Stier DM and others: Are children born to young mothers at increased risk of maltreatment? *Pediatrics* 91(3):642-648, 1993.

Straus SE: Shingles: sorrows, salves, and solutions, *JAMA* 269(14):1836-1839, 1993.

Terada K and others: Varicella-zoster virus (VZV) reactivation is related to the low response of VZV-specific immunity after chickenpox in infancy, *J Infect Dis* 169:650-652, 1994.

Wakefield H, Underwager R: Interrogation of children, *Issues Child Abuse Accus* 1(1):14-28, 1989.

Walterspiel JN and others: Secretory anti-*Giardia lamblia* antibodies in human milk: protective effect against diarrhea, *Pediatrics* 93(1):28-31, 1994.

Wasserman G and others: Independent effects of lead exposure and iron deficiency anemia on developmental outcome at age 2 years, *J Pediatr* 121(5):695-703, 1992.

Wilde JA, Pedroni AT Jr: Privacy rights in Munchausen syndrome, *Contemp Pediatr* 10(1):83-91, 1993.

Wong DL: False allegations of child abuse: the other side of the tragedy, *Pediatr Nurs* 13(5):329-333, 1987.

Wong DL: The "evidence" is shaky at best, *Am J Nurs* 9(2):18, 1991.

Woolf AD, Saperstein A, Forjuoh S: Poisoning prevention knowledge and practices of parents after a childhood poisoning incident, *Pediatrics* 90(6):867-870, 1992.

BIBLIOGRAPHY

Communicable Diseases/Intestinal Parasitic Diseases

Addiss DG, Juranek DD, Spencer HC: Treatment of children with asymptomatic and nondiarrheal *Giardia* infection, *Pediatr Infect Dis J* 10(11):843-846, 1991.

American Academy of Pediatrics, Committee on Infectious Diseases: *1994 Red Book: Report of the Committee on Infectious Diseases,* ed 23, Elk Grove Village, IL, 1994, The Academy.

American Academy of Pediatrics, Committee on Infectious Diseases: Parvovirus, erythema infectiosum, and pregnancy, *Pediatrics* 85(1):131-133, 1990.

Cromer BA and others: Unrecognized pertussis infection in adolescents, *Am J Dis Child* 147:575-577, 1993.

Feder HM: Fifth disease, *N Engl J Med* 331(16):1062, 1994.

Glickman LT, Magnaval JF: Zoonotic roundworm infections, *Infect Dis Clin North Am* 7(3):717-732, 1993.

Gratz RR, Boulton P: Health considerations for pregnant child care staff, *J Pediatr Health Care* 8:18-26, 1994.

Gurevich I: Fifth disease and other parvovirus B 19 infections, *Heart Lung* 20(4):342-344, 1991.

Hall CB and others: Human herpesvirus-6 infection in children: a prospective study of complications and reactivation, *N Engl J Med* 331(7):432-438, 1994.

Kerfoot F: The perils of pertussis, *J Pediatr Nurs* 4(4):277, 1989.

Korman S: The duodenal string test, *Am J Dis Child* 144(7):803-805, 1990.

Kubiak M and others: Comparison of stool containment in cloth and single-use diapers using a simulated infant feces, *Pediatrics* 91(3):632-636, 1993.

Kuhls TL: Protozoal infections of the intestinal tract in children, *Adv Pediatr Infect Dis* 8:177-202, 1993.

Stevenson L, Brooke DS: Roseola (human herpesvirus 6), *J Pediatr Health Care* 8(6):283, 1994.

Conjunctivitis/Stomatitis

Bringing pinkeye under control, *Patient Care* 27:47-48, 1993.

Dunlap C, Barker B, Lowe J: 10 oral lesions you should know, *Contemp Pediatr* 8(12):16-28, 1991.

Lewis L, Glauser T, Joffie M: Gonococcal conjunctivitis in prepubertal children, *Am J Dis Child* 144(5):546-548, 1990.

Schmitt BD: When your child has an eye infection with pus, *Contemp Pediatr* 10(3):117-118, 1993.

Scully C, Porter S: Recurrent aphthous stomatitis: current concepts of etiology, pathogenesis and management, *J Oral Pathol Med* 18(1):21-27, 1989.

Sheahan SL, Seabolt JP: *Chlamydia trachomatis* infections: a health problem of infants, *J Pediatr Health Care* 3(3):144-149, 1989.

Stanker P and others: Protocol—conjunctivitis, *Sch Nurse* 5(2):34-36, 1989.

Trobe JD: *The physician's guide to eye care,* San Francisco, 1993, American Academy of Ophthalmology.

Weiss A, Brinser JH, Nazar-Stewart V: Acute conjunctivitis in childhood, *J Pediatr* 122(1):10-14, 1993.

Ingestion of Injurious Agents

Beware the hazards of activated charcoal, *Am J Nurs* 94(12):10, 1994.

Birkland P: International update: alternative treatment for common but dangerous acetaminophen overdoses, *J Emerg Nurs* 19(2):32A-33A, 1993.

Fine JS, Goldfrank LR: Update in medical toxicology, *Pediatr Emerg Med* 39(5):1031-1051, 1992.

Henretig F and others: Repeated acetaminophen overdosing causing hepatotoxicity in children, *Clin Pediatr* 28(11):525-528, 1989.

Kulig K: Initial management of ingestions of toxic substances, *N Engl J Med* 326(25):1677-1681, 1992.

Lewis RK, Paloucek FP: Assessment and treatment of acetaminophen overdose, *Clin Pharm* 10:765-774, 1991.

Lovejoy FH Jr: Diagnosis of the unknown poison, *Pediatr Rev* 13(7):273-274, 1992.

Mack R: Hydrocarbon ingestion—to Eyre is human, *Contemp Pediatr* 8(12):47-64, 1991.

Mack RB: Dishwasher detergent toxicity—here's looking at you, kid, *Contemp Pediatr* 10(11):49-58, 1993.

Manoguerra AS: Pediatric poisoning, *Emergency* 24(10):19-24, 1992.

Preventing strictures after caustic ingestion, *Emerg Med* 25(6):48, 1993.

Rogers GC, Matyunas NJ: *Handbook of common poisonings in children,* ed 3, Elk Grove Village, IL, 1994, American Academy of Pediatrics.

Vertrees J, McWilliams B, Kelly H: Repeated oral administration of activated charcoal for treating aspirin overdose in young children, *Pediatrics* 85(4):594-598, 1990.

Wigder HN and others: Emergency department poison advice telephone calls, *Ann Emerg Med* 25(3):349-352, 1995.

Wong D: Dispelling some myths about ipecac, *Am J Nurs* 88(7):952, 1988.

Heavy Metal Poisoning

Binder S: Childhood lead poisoning: the impact of prevention, *JAMA* 269(13):1679-1681, 1993.

Brown M, Bellinger D, Matthews J: In utero lead exposure, *MCN Am J Matern Child Nurs* 15(2):94-96, 1990.

Castiglia PT: Pica, *J Pediatr Health Care* 7(4):174-176, 1993.

Cummins SK, Goldman LR: Even advantaged children show cognitive deficits from low-level lead toxicity, *Pediatrics* 90(6):995-997, 1992.

DeRienzo-DeVivio S: Childhood lead poisoning: shifting to primary prevention, *Pediatr Nurs* 18(6):565-567, 1992.

Goldman LR: Childhood lead poisoning in 1994, *JAMA* 272(4):315-316, 1994 (editorial).

Kimbrough RD, LeVois M, Webb DR: Management of children with slightly elevated blood lead levels, *Pediatrics* 93(2):188-191, 1994.

Mahaffey KR: Exposure to lead in childhood: the importance of prevention, *N Engl J Med* 327(18):1308-1309, 1992.

Matte TD and others: Acute high-dose lead exposure from beverage contaminated by traditional Mexican pottery, *Lancet* 344(8928):1064-1065, 1994.

Needham DD: Diagnosis and management of lead-poisoned children: the pediatric nurse practitioner in a specialty program, *J Pediatr Health Care* 8(6):268-273, 1994.

Pirkle JL and others: The decline in blood lead levels in the United States, *JAMA* 272(4):284-291, 1994.

Swindell SL and others: Home abatement and blood lead changes in children with class III lead poisoning, *Clin Pediatr* 33(9):536-541, 1994.

Update: iron poisonings—so tragic, so preventable, *Contemp Pediatr* 10(4):123, 1993.

Weitzman M, Glotzer D: Lead poisoning, *Pediatr Rev* 13(12):461-468, 1992.

Weitzman M and others: Lead-contaminated soil abatement and urban children's blood lead levels, *JAMA* 269(13):1647-1654, 1993.

Zelman M and others: Toxicity from vacuumed mercury: a household hazard, *Clin Pediatr* 30(2):121-123, 1991.

Child Maltreatment

Alexander R and others: Incidence of impact trauma with cranial injuries ascribed to shaking, *Am J Dis Child* 144:724-726, 1990.

Alexander R and others: Serial abuse in children who are shaken, *Am J Dis Child* 144(1):58-60, 1990.

American Academy of Pediatrics, Committee on Bioethics: Religious exemptions from child abuse statutes, *Pediatrics* 81(1):169-171, 1988.

American Academy of Pediatrics, Committee on Child Abuse and Neglect and Committee on Community Health Services: Investigation and review of unexpected infant and child deaths, *Pediatrics* 92(5):734-735, 1993.

American Academy of Pediatrics, Committee on Early Childhood, Adoption, and Dependent Care: Developmental issues in foster care for children, *Pediatrics* 91(5):1007-1009, 1993.

American Academy of Pediatrics, Task Force on Child Abuse and Neglect: Public disclosure of private information about victims of abuse, *Pediatrics* 82(3):387, 1988.

Anderson CL: The parenting profile assessment: screening for child abuse, *Appl Nurs Res* 6(1):31-3, 1993.

Andrews AB: Developing community systems for the primary prevention of family violence, *Fam Community Health* 16(4):1-9, 1994.

Baldwin MA: Munchausen syndrome by proxy: neurological manifestations, *J Neurosci Nurs* 26(1):18-23, 1994.

Berenson AB: Appearance of the hymen at birth and one year of age: a longitudinal study, *Pediatrics* 91(4):820-825, 1993.

Berkowitz CD: Child sexual abuse, *Pediatr Rev* 13(12):443-452, 1992.

Besharov DJ: *Recognizing child abuse: a guide for the concerned,* New York, 1990, MacMillan.

Brucker JM: Battered child syndrome: educating the pediatric nurse, *J Pediatr Nurs* 6(6):428-429, 1991.

Burgess A, Hartman C, Kelley S: Assessing child abuse: the triads checklist, *J Psychosoc Nurs* 28(4):6-14, 1990.

Coleman L: Medical examination for sexual abuse: have we been misled? *Issues Child Abuse Accus* 1(3):1-9, 1989.

Dubowitz H, Black M, Harrington D: The diagnosis of child sexual abuse, *Am J Dis Child* 146(6):688-693, 1992.

Goldson E: The affective and cognitive sequelae of child maltreatment, *Pediatr Clin North Am* 38(6):1481-1496, 1991.

Hochhauser KG, Richardson, RA: Munchausen syndrome by proxy: an exploratory study of pediatric nurses' knowledge and involvement, *J Pediatr Nurs* 9(5):313-320, 1994.

Horsham P: Child sexual abuse: what parents need to know, *Can Nurse* 88(8):32-35, 1992.

Hyden PW, Gallagher TA: Child abuse intervention in the emergency room, *Pediatr Emerg Med* 39(5):1053-1081, 1992.

Kelley SJ: Methodological issues in child sexual abuse research, *J Pediatr Nurs* 6(1):21-29, 1991.

Kelley SJ: Parental stress response to sexual abuse and ritualistic abuse of children in day-care centers, *Nurs Res* 39(1):25-29, 1990.

Kempe RS, Kempe CH: *The common secret: sexual abuse of children and adolescents,* New York, 1984, Freeman.

Kemper KJ and others: Screening for maternal experiences of physical abuse during childhood, *Clin Pediatr* 33(6):333-339, 1994.

Krivacska JJ: Primary prevention of child sexual abuse: alternative, non-child directed approaches, *Issues Child Abuse Accus* 1(4):1-9, 1989.

Krowchuk H: Child abuser stereotypes: consensus among clinicians, *Appl Nurs Res* 2(1):35-39, 1989.

Legrand R, Wakefield H, Underwager R: Alleged behavioral indicators of sexual abuse, *Issues Child Abuse Accus* 1(2):1-5, 1989.

Lesniak LP: Penetrating the conspiracy of silence: identifying the family at risk for incest, *Fam Community Health* 16(2):66-76, 1993.

Lewin L: Establishing a therapeutic relationship with an abused child, *Pediatr Nurs* 16(3):263-264, 1990.

McCann J and others: Comparison of genital examination techniques in prepubertal girls, *Pediatrics* 85(2):182-187, 1990.

McCann J and others: Genital findings in prepubertal girls selected for nonabuse: a descriptive study, *Pediatrics* 86(3):428-439, 1990.

McCann J and others: Perianal findings in prepubertal children selected for nonabuse: a descriptive study, *Child Abuse Negl* 13:179-193, 1989.

Middleton C: Controversy . . . in best interests of the child!!! . . . , *Child Care Health Dev* 21(4):271-285, 1995.

Old D and others: Effects of prenatal and infancy nurse home visitation on surveillance of child maltreatment, *Pediatrics* 95(3):365-372, 1995.

Osborn M, Bryan S: Patient care guidelines: evidentiary examination in sexual assault, *J Emerg Nurs* 15(3):284-290, 1989.

Paradise JE: Predictive accuracy and the diagnosis of sexual abuse: a big issue about a little tissue, *Child Abuse Negl* 13:169-176, 1989.

Post CA: Play therapy with an abused child: a case study, *J Child Adolesc Psychiatr Ment Health Nurs* 3(1):34-36, 1990.

Saucier BL: The effects of play therapy on developmental achievement levels of abused children, *Pediatr Nurs* 15(1):27-30, 1989.

Schwab NC: Child abuse and neglect: legal and clinical implications for school nursing practice, *Sch Nurse* 5(4):17-28, 1989.

Senner A, Ott M: Munchausen syndrome by proxy, *Issues Compr Pediatr Nurs* 12(5):345-357, 1989.

Underwager R, Wakefield H: *The real world of child interrogations,* Springfield, IL, 1990, Thomas.

Wakefield H, Underwager R: *Accusations of child sexual abuse,* Springfield, IL, 1988, Thomas.

Widom CS: Does violence beget violence: a critical examination of the literature, *Psychol Bull* 106(1):3-28, 1989.

HEALTH PROMOTION OF THE SCHOOL-AGE CHILD AND FAMILY

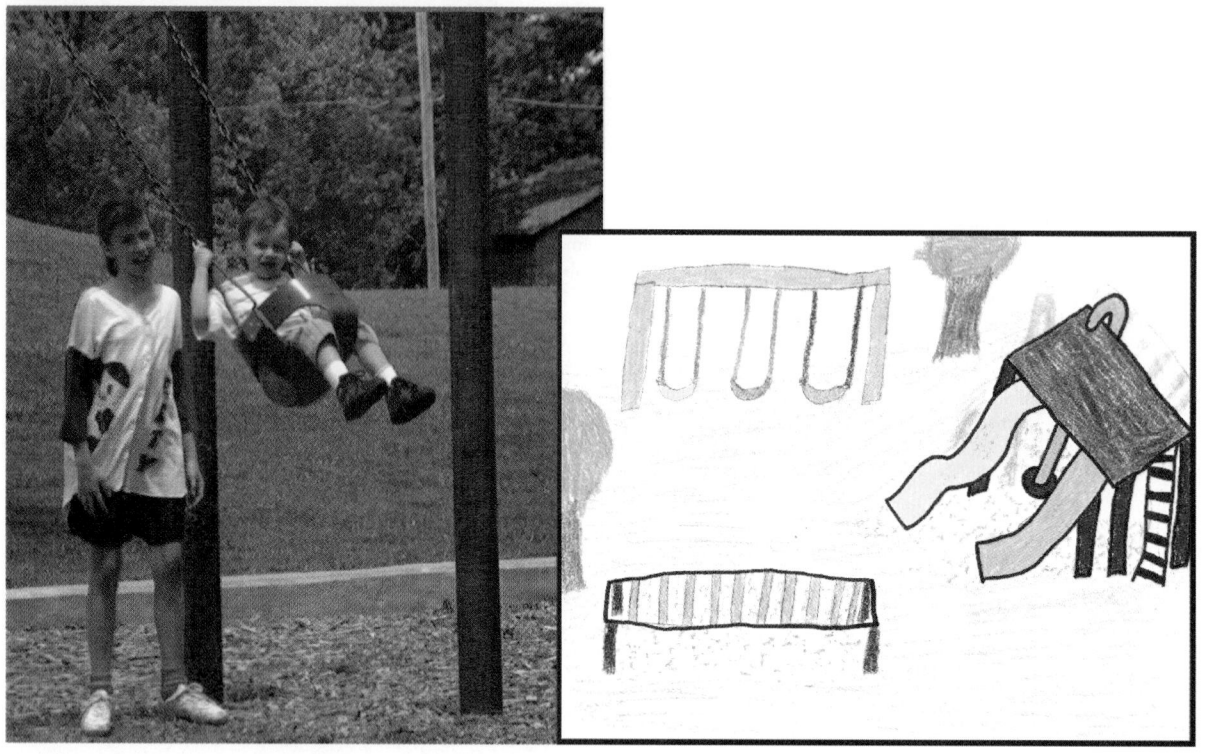

" To stay healthy, you need lots of fruit and water — and exercise, like running around or riding a bike. "

Anna, age 12 years

RELATED TOPICS

PROMOTING OPTIMUM GROWTH AND DEVELOPMENT

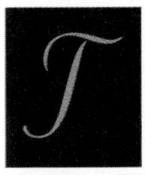

The segment of the life span that extends from age 6 years to approximately age 12 years has a variety of labels, each of which describes an important characteristic of the period. These middle years are most often referred to as *school-age* or the *school years.* This period begins with entrance into the wider sphere of influence represented by the school environment, which has a significant impact on development and relationships. This is the time that the child affiliates with age-mates and learns the culture of childhood. With peer groups children establish the first close relationships outside the family group.

Physiologically the middle years begin with the shedding of the first deciduous tooth and end at puberty with the acquisition of the final permanent teeth (with the exception of the wisdom teeth). During the preceding 5 to 6 years the child has progressed from a helpless infant to a sturdy, complicated individual with the capacity to communicate, conceptualize in a limited way, and become involved in complex social and motor behavior. Physical growth has been equally rapid. In contrast, the period of middle childhood, between the rapid growth of early childhood and the prepubescent growth spurt, is a time of gradual growth and development with steadier and more even progress in both physical and emotional aspects.

BIOLOGIC DEVELOPMENT

During middle childhood, growth in height and weight assumes a slower but steady pace as compared with the earlier years. Between ages 6 and 12 years, children will grow an average of 5 cm (2 inches) per year to gain 30 to 60 cm (1 to 2 feet) in height and will almost double their weight, increasing 2 to 3 kg (4½ to 6½ pounds) per year. The average 6-year-old child is about 116 cm (45 inches) tall and weighs about 21 kg (46 pounds); the average 12-year-old child stands about 150 cm (59 inches) tall and weighs approxi-

mately 40 kg (88 pounds). During this age period, girls and boys differ very little in size, although boys tend to be slightly taller and somewhat heavier than girls. Toward the end of the school-age years, both boys and girls begin to increase in size. Because many girls begin puberty midway through this school-age period, most girls surpass boys in both height and weight by the end of the school-age years (to the acute discomfort of both girls and boys).

Proportional Changes

School-age children are more graceful than they were as preschoolers, and they are steadier on their feet. Their body proportions take on a slimmer look, with longer legs, varying body proportion, and a lower center of gravity. Posture improves over that of the preschool period to facilitate locomotion and efficiency in using the arms and trunk. These proportions make climbing, bicycle riding, and other activities much easier. Fat gradually diminishes, and its distribution patterns change, contributing to the thinner appearance of the child during the middle years.

Accompanying the skeletal lengthening and fat diminution is an increase in the percentage of body weight represented by muscle tissue. By the end of this age period, both boys and girls will double their strength and physical capabilities, and their steady and relatively consistent acquisition of refined coordination will increase their poise and skill. However, this increased strength can be misleading. Although strength increases, muscles are still functionally immature when compared with those of the adolescent, and they are more readily damaged by muscular injury caused by overuse.

The most pronounced changes, and those that seem best to indicate increasing maturity in children, are a decrease in head circumference in relation to standing height, a decrease in waist circumference in relation to height, and an increase in leg length related to height. These observations often provide a clue to a child's degree of physical maturity that has proved useful in predicting readiness for meeting the demands of school. There appears to be a correlation between physical indications of maturity and success in school.

Facial Changes. Certain physiologic and anatomic characteristics are typical of children in the years of middle childhood. Facial proportions change as the face grows faster in relation to the remainder of the cranium. The skull and brain grow very slowly during this period and increase little in size thereafter. Since all the primary (deciduous) teeth are

---

Marilyn Winkelstein, PhD, RN, revised this chapter.

 For additional information, please view "Growth and Development" in *Whaley and Wong's Pediatric Nursing Video Series,* St Louis, 1996, Mosby; (800)426-4545.

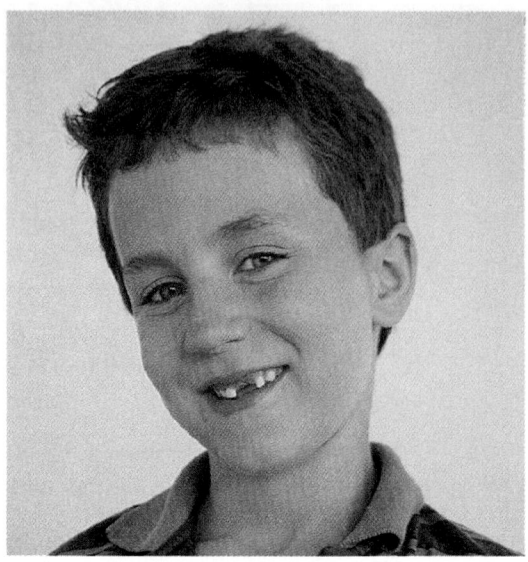

FIG. 15-1. Middle childhood is the stage of development when deciduous teeth are shed.

lost during this age span, middle childhood is sometimes known as the *age of the loose tooth* (Fig. 15-1) and the early years of middle childhood as the *ugly duckling stage,* when the new secondary (permanent) teeth appear to be much too large for the face.

Maturation of Systems

Maturity of the gastrointestinal system is reflected in fewer stomach upsets, better maintenance of blood glucose levels, and an increased stomach capacity, which permits retention of food for longer periods. The school-age child does not need to be fed as carefully, as promptly, or as frequently as before. Caloric needs are less than they were in the preschool years.

Physical maturation is evidenced in other body tissues and organs. *Bladder capacity,* although differing widely among individual children, is generally greater in girls than in boys. The *heart* grows more slowly during the middle years and is smaller in relation to the rest of the body than at any other period of life. Heart and respiratory rates steadily decrease and blood pressure increases during the ages from 6 to 12 years (see inside back cover).

The *immune system* becomes more competent in its ability to localize infections and produce an antibody-antigen response (Miller, 1989).

Bones continue to ossify throughout childhood but yield to pressure and muscle pull more than mature bones. Children should have ample opportunity to move around, and they should observe appropriate caution in carrying heavy loads. For example, they should shift books from one arm to the other, and those who carry tote bags slung from the shoulders should alternate the load from one shoulder to the other to avoid developing a low shoulder or spinal curvature.

There are wider differences between children at the end of middle childhood than at the beginning; such differences are sometimes striking. These differences become increasingly apparent and, if extreme or unique, may create emo-

tional problems unless the associated characteristics of height and weight relationships, rapid or slow growth, and other important features of development are recognized and explained to children and their families. Physical maturity is not necessarily correlated with emotional and social maturity. Seven-year-old children who look like 10-year-old children will, in fact, think and act like 7-year-old children. To expect behavior appropriate for 10-year-old children from them is unrealistic and can be detrimental to their development of competence and self-esteem. Conversely, to treat 10-year-old children as though they were 7 years old is an equal disservice to them.

Prepubescence

Preadolescence is the period that begins toward the end of middle childhood and ends with the thirteenth birthday. Since puberty signals the beginning of the development of secondary sex characteristics, *prepubescence,* the 2-year period that precedes puberty, typically occurs during preadolescence.

Toward the end of middle childhood the discrepancies in growth and maturation between boys and girls begin to be apparent. On the average, there is a difference of approximately 2 years between girls and boys in the age of onset of pubescence. This is a period of rapid growth in height and weight, especially for girls.

There is no universal age at which children assume the characteristics of prepubescence. The first physiologic signs begin to appear at about 9 years of age (particularly in girls) and are usually clearly evident in 11- to 12-year-old children. Although the preadolescent child does not want to be different, at this age the variability in physical growth and physiologic changes between children of the same sex and between the two sexes is often striking. This variability, especially in relation to the onset of secondary sexual characteristics, is of utmost concern to the preadolescent. Either early or late appearance of these characteristics can be a source of embarrassment and uneasiness to both sexes.

Preadolescence is a time when considerable overlapping of developmental characteristics occurs, with elements of both middle childhood and early adolescence. However, there are sufficient unique characteristics to set this period apart as an age category. Generally the earliest age at which puberty begins is 10 years in girls and 12 years in boys, although there has been an increase in the number of girls reaching puberty at age 9. The average age of puberty in girls is 12 years; for boys it is 14 years. Boys experience little visible sexual maturation during preadolescence.

PSYCHOSOCIAL DEVELOPMENT

Middle childhood is the period of psychosexual development that Freud described as the *latency period,* a time of tranquility between the Oedipal phase of early childhood and the eroticism of adolescence. During this time children experience relationships with same-sex peers following the indifference of earlier years and preceding the heterosexual fascination that accompanies puberty.

Developing a Sense of Industry (Erikson)

Successful mastery of Erikson's first three stages of psychosocial development is probably the most important accomplishment in terms of development of a healthy personality (Erikson, 1963). Successful completion of these stages requires a loving environment within a stable family unit that has prepared the child to engage in experiences and relationships beyond this intimate group.

It has been suggested that the individual's fundamental attitude toward work is established during middle childhood. A *sense of industry,* for which a more descriptive term is the *stage of accomplishment,* is achieved somewhere between age 6 and adolescence. School-age children are eager to develop skills and participate in meaningful and socially useful work. Children acquire a sense of industry through both formal and self-directed education.

Interests expand in the middle years, and with a growing sense of independence, the child wants to engage in tasks that can be carried through to completion (Fig. 15-2). During this time children receive the systematic instruction prescribed by their individual cultures and develop the skills needed to become useful, contributing members of their social communities. They gain great satisfaction from independent behavior in exploring and manipulating their environment and from interaction with peers. Often the acquisition of skills is a means for achieving success in social activities. Reinforcement in the form of grades, material rewards, additional privileges, and recognition provides encouragement and stimulation.

A sense of accomplishment also involves the ability to cooperate and to compete with others—to cope more effectively with people. Middle childhood is the time when children learn the value of doing things with others and the benefits derived from division of labor in the accomplishment of goals. Peer approval is a strong motivating power.

The danger inherent in this period of personality development is the occurrence of situations that might result in a sense of *inferiority.* This may happen if the previous stages have not been successfully achieved or if the child is incapable of or unprepared to assume the responsibilities associated with developing a sense of accomplishment. Feelings of inferiority or lack of worth can be derived from children themselves or from the social environment. Children with chronic

disabilities may be at a disadvantage for acquisition of certain skills and at risk for feeling inferior. However, no child is able to do well in everything, and children must learn that they will not be able to master each skill that they attempt. All children, even children who usually have positive attitudes toward work and their own capabilities, will feel some degree of inferiority in regard to a specific skill that they cannot master.

Children need and want real achievement. When they have access to tasks that need to be done, that they are able to do well despite individual differences in their innate capacities and emotional development, and for which they are suitably rewarded, children will be able to achieve a sense of industry and accomplishment.

COGNITIVE DEVELOPMENT (PIAGET)

When children enter the school years, they begin to acquire the ability to relate a series of happenings to mental representations that can be expressed both verbally and symbolically. This is the stage in development that Piaget describes as *concrete operations,* during which children are able to use thought processes to experience events and actions. The rigid, egocentric outlook of the preschool years is replaced by thought processes that allow children to see things from another's point of view.

During this stage children develop an understanding of relationships between things and ideas. They progress from making judgments based on what they see (*perceptual thinking*) to making judgments based on what they reason (*conceptual thinking*). They are increasingly able to master symbols and to use their memory store of past experiences in evaluating and interpreting the present.

One of the major cognitive tasks of school-age children is mastering the concept of *conservation* (Fig. 15-3). At an early age (about 5 to 7 years) they grasp the concept of reversibility of numbers as a basis for simple mathematic problems (e.g., $2 + 4 = 6$ and $6 - 4 = 2$). They learn that certain properties of the environment are not changed simply by altering their arrangement in space, and they become able to resist perceptual cues that suggest such alterations in the physical state of an object. For example, they recognize that changing the shape of a substance such as a lump of clay does not alter its total mass. They no longer perceive a tall, thin glass of water as containing a greater volume than a short, wide glass; they can distinguish between the weight of items regardless of their size. They recognize that size is not necessarily related to weight or volume. There appears to be a developmental sequence in children's capacity to conserve matter. Conservation of mass usually is accomplished earliest, weight some time later, and volume last.

School-age children also develop *classification* skills. They can group and sort objects according to the attributes that they share, place things in a sensible and logical order, and, in doing so, hold a concept in mind while making decisions based on that concept. It is characteristic of middle childhood that children derive great enjoyment from classifying and ordering their environment. They become occupied with numerous and varied collections of objects, such as stickers, stamps, shells, dolls, cars, stones, and anything that is classi-

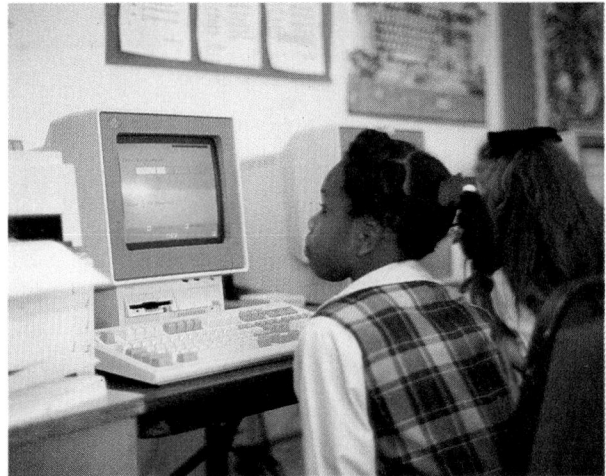

FIG. 15-2. School-age children are motivated to complete tasks working alone.

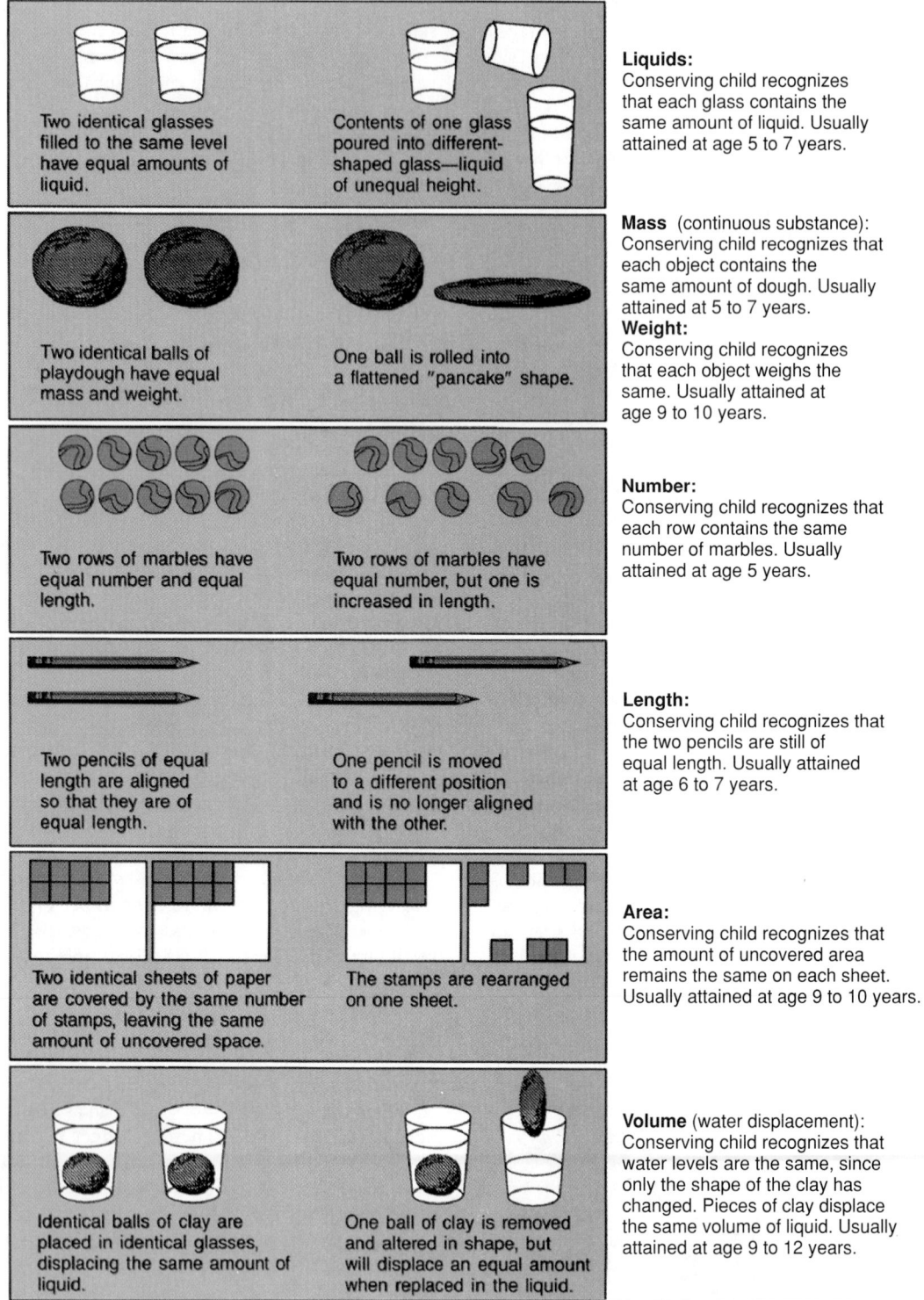

Liquids:
Conserving child recognizes that each glass contains the same amount of liquid. Usually attained at age 5 to 7 years.

Two identical glasses filled to the same level have equal amounts of liquid.

Contents of one glass poured into different-shaped glass—liquid of unequal height.

Mass (continuous substance): Conserving child recognizes that each object contains the same amount of dough. Usually attained at 5 to 7 years.
Weight: Conserving child recognizes that each object weighs the same. Usually attained at age 9 to 10 years.

Two identical balls of playdough have equal mass and weight.

One ball is rolled into a flattened "pancake" shape.

Number: Conserving child recognizes that each row contains the same number of marbles. Usually attained at age 5 years.

Two rows of marbles have equal number and equal length.

Two rows of marbles have equal number, but one is increased in length.

Length: Conserving child recognizes that the two pencils are still of equal length. Usually attained at age 6 to 7 years.

Two pencils of equal length are aligned so that they are of equal length.

One pencil is moved to a different position and is no longer aligned with the other.

Area: Conserving child recognizes that the amount of uncovered area remains the same on each sheet. Usually attained at age 9 to 10 years.

Two identical sheets of paper are covered by the same number of stamps, leaving the same amount of uncovered space.

The stamps are rearranged on one sheet.

Volume (water displacement): Conserving child recognizes that water levels are the same, since only the shape of the clay has changed. Pieces of clay displace the same volume of liquid. Usually attained at age 9 to 12 years.

Identical balls of clay are placed in identical glasses, displacing the same amount of liquid.

One ball of clay is removed and altered in shape, but will displace an equal amount when replaced in the liquid.

FIG. 15-3. Common examples that demonstrate the child's ability to conserve (ages are only approximate).

fiable. They even begin to order friends and relationships (e.g., first best friend, second best friend).

They develop the ability to understand relational terms and concepts, such as bigger and smaller; darker and paler; heavier and lighter; to the right of and to the left of; first, last, and intermediate relationships (fourth, second, and so on); and more than and less than. They can see family relationships in terms of reciprocal roles (e.g., in order to be a brother, one must have a sibling).

School-age children learn the alphabet and the ever-widening world of symbols called words that can be arranged in terms of structure and their relationship to the alphabet.

They learn to tell time, to see the relationship of events in time (history) and places in space (geography), and to combine time and space relationships (geology and astronomy).

The most significant skill, the *ability to read,* is acquired during the school years and becomes the most valuable tool for independent inquiry. Children's capacity for exploration, imagination, and expansion of knowledge is enhanced by the ability to read as they progress from the repetition and confusion of early efforts to increasing facility and comprehension.

MORAL DEVELOPMENT (KOHLBERG)

As children move from egocentrism to the more logical patterns of thought, they also move through stages in development of conscience and moral standards. Young children do not believe that standards of behavior come from within themselves but rather that rules are established and set down by others. During the preschool years children, to some extent, adopt and internalize the moral values of their parents. They learn the standards for acceptable behavior, act according to these standards, and feel guilty when they violate the standards. Although children of 6 or 7 years of age know the rules and behaviors expected of them, they do not understand the reasons behind them. Rewards and punishments guide their judgment; a "bad act" is one that breaks a rule or does harm. Young children may believe that what other people tell them to do is right and that what they think of to do themselves is wrong. Consequently, children 6 or 7 years old are more likely to interpret accidents and misfortunes as punishment for misdeeds or "bad" acts.

Older school-age children are able to judge an act by the intentions that prompted it rather than just by the consequences. Rules and judgments become less absolute and authoritarian and begin to be founded more on the needs and desires of others. For older children a rule violation is apt to be viewed in relation to the total context in which it appears; reactions are influenced by the situation as well as by the morality of the rule itself. Whereas a younger child can judge an act only according to whether it is right or wrong, older children will take into account a different point of view to make a judgment. They are able to understand and accept the concept of treating others as they would like to be treated.

SPIRITUAL DEVELOPMENT

Children at this age think in very concrete terms but are avid learners and have a great desire to learn about their God. They picture God as human and tend to describe him in terms of character traits such as loving and helping. He is a very important person in the lives of many children. They are fascinated by the concepts of hell and heaven, and with a developing conscience and concern about rules, they fear going to hell for misbehavior. School-age children want and expect to be punished for misbehavior and, if given the option, tend to choose a punishment that "fits the crime." Often they view illness or injury as a punishment for a real or imagined misdeed. The beliefs and ideals of family and religious personages are more influential than those of their peers in matters of faith.

School-age children begin to learn the difference between

the natural and the supernatural but have difficulty understanding abstractions. Consequently, religious concepts must be presented to them in concrete terms. They are comforted by prayer or other religious rituals, and if they are a part of their daily lives, these activities can help them cope with threatening situations. Their petitions to their God in prayers tend to be for very tangible rewards. Although younger children expect their prayers to be answered, as they get older, they begin to recognize that this does not always occur and become less concerned when prayers are not answered. They are able to discuss their feelings about their faith and how it relates to their lives (see Cultural Awareness box).

SOCIAL DEVELOPMENT

One of the most important socializing agents in the life of the school-age child is the peer group. Together, members explore ideas and the physical environment around them. In addition to parents and the schools, the peer group manages to convey a substantial amount of material to its members. Children have a culture all their own, with secrets, mores, and codes of ethics with which they promote feelings of group solidarity and detachment from adults. Through peer relationships children learn ways in which to deal with dominance and hostility and relate to persons in positions of leadership and authority.

Identification with peers appears to be a strong influence in the child's gaining independence from parents. The aid and support of the group provide the child with enough security to risk the moderate parental rejection brought about by each small victory in the development of independence.

Much of the child's concept of the appropriate sex role is acquired through relationships with peers. During the early school years there is little difference relative to sex in play experiences of children. Games and many other activities are shared by both girls and boys. However, in the later school years the differences become marked.

Social Relationships and Cooperation

Daily relationships with age-mates provide the most important social interactions in the life of school-age children. For the first time children are able to join in group activities with unrestrained enthusiasm and steady participation. Previous interactions had been limited to short periods under considerable adult supervision. With increased skills and wider opportunities, children are able to become involved with one or several peer groups in which they can gain status as respected members.

Valuable lessons are learned from daily interaction with age-mates. First, children learn to appreciate the numerous

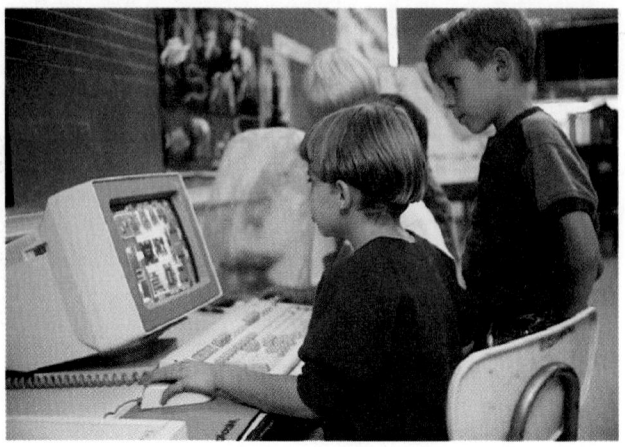

FIG. 15-4. School-age children enjoy engaging in activities with a "best friend."

and varied points of view that are represented in the peer group. As children interact with peers who see the world in ways that are somewhat different from the way they see it, they become aware of the limits of their own point of view. Because age-mates are peers and are not forced to accept each other's ideas as they are expected to accept those of adults, other children have a significant influence on decreasing the egocentric outlook of the child. Consequently, children learn to argue, persuade, bargain, cooperate, and compromise in order to maintain friendships.

Second, children become increasingly sensitive to the social norms and pressures of the peer group. The peer group establishes standards for acceptance and rejection, and children may be willing to modify their behavior to be accepted by the group. The need for peer approval becomes a powerful influence toward conformity. Children learn to dress, talk, and behave in a manner acceptable to the group. A variety of roles, such as class joker or class hero, may be assumed by individual children to gain approval from the group.

Third, the interaction among peers leads to the formation of intimate friendship between same-sex peers. School-age is the time when children have "best friends" with whom they share secrets, private jokes, and adventures; they come to one another's aid in times of trouble. In the course of these friendships children also fight, threaten, break up, and reunite. These dyadic relationships, in which the child experiences love and closeness for a peer, seem to be important as a foundation for heterosexual relationships in adulthood (Fig. 15-4).

Clubs and Peer Groups. One of the outstanding characteristics of middle childhood is the formation of formalized groups, or clubs. A prominent feature of many of these groups is the rigid rules imposed on the members. There is an exclusiveness in the selection of persons who have the privilege of joining. Acceptance in the group is often determined on a pass-fail basis according to social or behavioral criteria. Conformity is the core of the group structure. There are often secret codes, shared interests, and special modes of dress, and each child must abide by a standard of behavior established by the members. Understanding of and conformity to the rules provide children with feelings of security and relieve them of the responsibility of making decisions. By merging their identities with those of their peers, children are able to move from the family group to an outside group as a

step toward seeking further independence. They substitute conformity to a peer-group pattern for conformity to a family pattern while they are still too shaky and insecure to function independently.

During the early school years, groups are rather small and loosely organized, with changing membership and little formal structure. The more prolonged cohesiveness characteristic of groups or cliques in later school years is not obvious. As a rule, girls' groups are less formalized than boys', and although there may be a mixture of both sexes in the earlier school years, the groups of later school years are composed predominantly of children of the same sex. Common interests are a frequent basis around which a group is structured.

This is also a time for overnight or day camp, during which children learn that there may be different rules in different settings. Camp counselors may be the only other adults besides parents (and occasionally teachers) who require children to take responsibility for their physical cleanliness and personal belongings, but they also expect the children to cooperate with fellow campers and function as a unit.

Although peer-group identification and association are essential to a child's socialization, strong peer-group attachment can have inherent dangers. Peer pressures may force children into taking risks, even against their better judgment. Peer-group activities that result in unacceptable, unlawful, or criminal *gang violence* are increasing in the United States and represent a significant challenge for health professionals and teachers who work with children (Rollins, 1993).

Relationships with Families

Although the peer group is highly influential and necessary to normal child development, parents are still the primary influence in shaping the child's personality, setting standards for behavior, and establishing value systems. The family values usually predominate when parental and peer value systems come into conflict. Although children may appear to reject parental values while testing the new values of the peer group, ultimately they will retain and incorporate into their own value systems the parental values they have found to be of worth.

Peer associations seem to remain within the social class systems. Not infrequently, there may be discrimination in membership on the basis of ethnic or racial origin.

Children want to spend more time in the company of peers and may seem eager to leave the house; they often prefer activities of the peer group to family activities. This can be very disturbing to parents. Children become intolerant and critical of parents and their ways when they deviate from those of the group. They discover that parents can be wrong, and they begin to question the knowledge and authority of parents, who previously were considered to be all-knowing and all-powerful.

Although increased independence is the goal of middle childhood, children are not ready to abandon parental control. They need and want restrictions placed on their behavior; they are not yet prepared to cope with all the problems of their expanding environment. They feel more secure knowing that there is an authority greater than themselves to implement controls and restrictions. Children may complain loudly about the restrictions and try their best to break down parental barriers, but they are uneasy if they succeed in doing so. They respect the adults on whom they can rely to prevent them from acting on each and every urge. Children sense in this behavior an expression of love and concern for their welfare.

Children also need their parents as adults, not as pals. Sometimes parents, hurt at their children's rejection, attempt to maintain their love and gratitude by assuming the role of "pals." Children need the stable, secure strength provided by mature adults to whom they can turn during troubled relationships with peers or stressful changes in their world. During a disruption in their lives, such as times of failure, periods of illness, or a move that separates them from the security of friends, children need the firm, secure anchor of parental interest and concern. With a secure base in a loving family, children are able to develop the self-confidence and maturity needed to break loose from the group and stand independently.

Play

As children enter the school years, their play takes on new dimensions that reflect a new stage of development. Not only does play involve increased physical skill, intellectual skill, and fantasy, but as children form groups and cliques, they begin to develop a sense of belonging to a team or club. To belong to a group is of vital importance; clubs, secret societies, and organizations, such as Scouts, are part of the culture of childhood.

Rules and Ritual. The need for conformity in middle childhood is strongly manifested in the activities and games that are so important in the life of school-age children. Up to this point, they have played games they have invented themselves, or they have played in the company of a friend or an adult, when rules more or less evolved with the game. Now they begin to see the need for rules, and the games they begin to play have fixed and unvarying rules that may be bizarre and extraordinarily rigid (especially those made up by the group).

Conformity and ritual permeate the play of school-age children. Not only are they present in games, but they are also evident in much of the children's behavior and language. Childhood is full of chants and taunts, such as "Eeeny, meeny, miney, mo," "Last one is a rotten egg," and "Step on a crack, break your mother's back." Children derive great pleasure and power from such sayings, which have been handed down with few changes through generations.

Team Play. A more complex form of play that evolves from the need for peer interaction is the team game and sports that are part of the early school years. The rules of a team game may require the presence of a referee, umpire, or person of authority so that the rules can be followed more accurately. Through team play children learn to modify or exchange personal goals for goals of the group and learn that the concept of division of labor is an effective strategy for attaining a goal. They learn about the nature of competition and the importance of winning—an attribute highly valued in the United States.

Team play can also contribute to children's social, intellectual, and skill growth. Children will work hard to develop the skills needed to become team members, to improve their contribution to the group effort, and to anticipate the consequences of their behavior for the group. Team play helps stimulate cognitive growth as children are called on to learn many complex rules, make judgments about those rules, plan

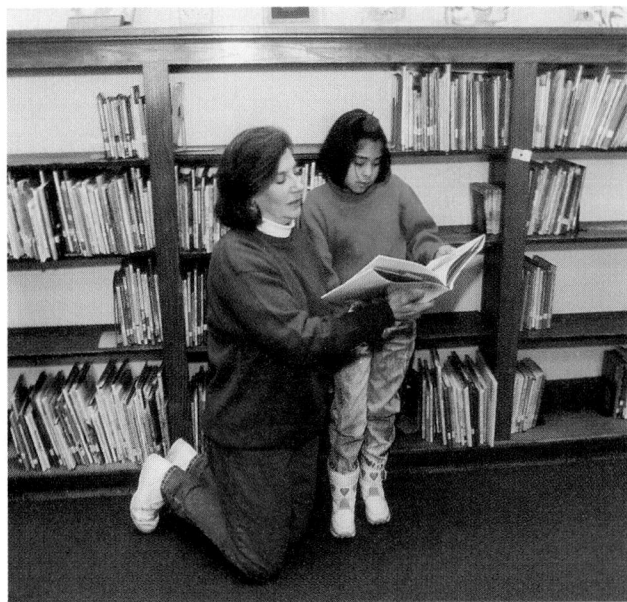

FIG. 15-5. Selecting a book with the assistance of an adult.

strategies, and assess the strengths and weaknesses of members of their own team and members of the opposing team.

Quiet Games and Activities. Although the play of school-age children is highly active, they also enjoy many quiet and solitary activities. The middle years are the time for collections, which constitute another ritual. The early school-age child's collections are an odd assortment of unrelated objects in messy, disorganized piles. Collections of later years are more orderly and selective, and they are organized neatly in scrapbooks, on shelves, or in boxes.

School-age children become fascinated with increasingly complex board or card games, such as Monopoly and rummy, that they can play with a best friend, family members, or a group. As in all games, their adherence to rules is fanatic. There is usually much discussion and argument, but the disagreement is easily resolved through reading the appropriate rule of the game.

The newly acquired skill of reading becomes increasingly satisfying as school-age children are able to expand their knowledge of the world through books (Fig. 15-5). School-age children never tire of stories, and just like preschool children, they love to have stories read aloud. Sewing, cooking, carpentry, gardening, and creative activities such as painting are other activities enjoyed. Many creative skills, such as music and art, as well as athletic skills, such as swimming, horseback riding, dancing, and skating, are learned and delighted in during childhood and continue to be enjoyed into adolescence and adulthood.

Ego Mastery. Play also affords children the means to acquire representational mastery over themselves, their environment, and others. Through play they can feel as big, as powerful, and as skillful as their imaginations will allow, and they can attain vicarious mastery and power over whomever and whatever they choose. They need to feel in control in their play. Schoolchildren still need the opportunity to use large muscles in exuberant outdoor play and the freedom to exert their newfound autonomy and initiative. They need space in which to exercise large muscles and to work off tensions, frustrations, and hostility. Physical skills practiced and mastered in play help them develop a feeling of personal competence, which contributes to a sense of accomplishment and helps provide a place of status in the peer group.

DEVELOPING A SELF-CONCEPT

The term *self-concept* refers to a conscious awareness of a variety of self-perceptions, such as one's physical characteristics, abilities (as determined by the sense of industry), values, self-ideals and expectancy, and idea of self in relation to others. It also includes one's body image, sexuality, and self-esteem. Although primary caregivers continue to impart the greatest influence on children's self-evaluation, the opinions of peers and teachers provide further input during middle childhood. With the emphasis on skill building and broadened social relationships, children are continually occupied in the process of self-evaluation.

The significant adults in children's lives can often manage, unobtrusively, to manipulate children's environments so that they meet with success. Each small success increases children's self-images. The more positive they feel about themselves, the more confident they feel in trying again for success. All children profit from feeling that they are in some way special to a significant adult. A positive self-concept makes children feel likable, worthwhile, and able to make a valuable contribution to their world. Such feelings lead to self-respect, self-confidence, and a general feeling of happiness. Negative feelings about one's self-concept lead to self-doubt.

Developing a Body Image

School-age children have a relatively accurate and positive perception of their physical selves, but in general they like their physical selves less as they grow older. The head appears to be the most important part of the school-age child's perceived image of self, with hair and eye color the characteristics used most frequently to describe the physical self.

Body image is influenced, but not solely determined, by significant others. The number of significant others influencing perception of physical self increases with age. Children are acutely aware of bodies—their own, those of their peers, and those of adults—and are acutely aware of deviations from the norm. It is important that children know body functions and that adults correct misinformation children may have about the body (e.g., what is fat).

At this time, physical impairments, such as hearing or visual defects, ears that "stick out," or birthmarks, assume greater importance. Increasing awareness of these differences, especially when accompanied by unkind comments and taunts from other children, may cause a child to feel inferior and less desirable. This is especially true if the defect interferes with the child's ability to participate in childhood games and activities. When children are teased or criticized about being different, the effect can be lasting.

COPING WITH CONCERNS RELATED TO NORMAL GROWTH AND DEVELOPMENT

School Experience

The school serves as the agent for transmitting the values of the society to each succeeding generation of children and as the setting for most of their relationships with peers. As a socializing agent second only to the family, schools exert a profound influence on the social development of children.

School entrance causes a sharp break in the structure of the child's world. For many children it is their first experience in conforming to a group pattern imposed by an adult who is not a parent and who has responsibility for too many children to be constantly aware of each child as an individual. Children want to go to school and usually adapt to the new conditions with little difficulty. Successful adjustment is directly related to the physical and emotional maturity of the child and to the parent's readiness to accept the separation associated with school entrance. Unfortunately, some parents express their subconscious attempts to delay the child's maturity by clinging behavior, particularly with their youngest child.

By the time they enter school, the majority of children have a fairly realistic concept of what school involves. The child receives information regarding the role of pupil from parents, siblings, playmates, and the media. In addition, most children have had experience with kindergarten, and some with preschool as well. However, the extent to which they are prepared differs. Middle-class children have fewer adjustments to make and less to learn about expected behavior, since the school tends to reflect dominant middle-class customs and values. If the child has attended a preschool program, the emphasis of the program significantly affects the child's adjustment. Some provide custodial care only, whereas others emphasize emotional, social, and intellectual development as well.

Classmates have a significant impact on the socialization of individual children. School is usually the first time that most children become members of a large group of individuals their own age. Peer relationships become increasingly important and influential as children proceed through school. The kind of influence exerted by the peer group depends on the background, interests, and abilities of the individual child.

Teachers.   To facilitate the transition from home to school, teachers should have personality characteristics that allow them to deal with the needs of young children. Children respond best to teachers with attributes that they would desire in a warm, loving parent. As a parent surrogate, the teacher in the early grades performs many of the activities formerly assumed by the parent, such as recognizing children's personal needs (e.g., a need to go to the bathroom or for help with clothing) and helping to develop their social behavior (e.g., manners).

Teachers, like parents, are concerned about the psychologic and emotional welfare of the child. Although the functions of teachers and parents differ, both place constraints on behavior and both are in a position to enforce standards of conduct. However, the teacher's primary responsibility is to stimulate and guide children's intellectual development, as opposed to providing for their physical welfare beyond the school setting. The teacher shares the parental influence in determining the child's attitudes and values.

Teachers serve as models with whom children identify and whom they try to emulate. Teacher approval is sought; teacher disapproval is avoided. The teacher is a very significant person in the life of the early schoolchild, and hero worship of a teacher may extend into late childhood and preadolescence (Fig. 15-6). Learner-centered behaviors of teachers,

FAMILY HOME CARE
Helping Children in School

General Guidelines

Be supportive—through companionship, share ideas and thoughts.

Be positive—every child should experience some success each day.

Share an interest in reading—use the library, discuss books they are reading.

Support and encourage activity rather than passivity.

Encourage originality—help children make their own projects from discarded articles or other available materials.

Foster the development of hobbies and collections.

Encourage children to wonder and reflect during free time.

Encourage family experiences and trips to places of interest.

Encourage questions—help children discover sources for information or places to explore and investigate.

Stimulate creative thinking and problem solving—help children try out new solutions to problems without fear of making mistakes.

Use rewards rather than punishment.

Specific Guidelines

Meet the teacher at the beginning of school and plan to visit the school to see what is taught and expected.

Send the child to school every day—teachers are concerned when parents make other plans for their children; it conveys the impression that school is unimportant.

Demonstrate an interest in what the child is learning.

Demonstrate an interest in content and growth more than in grades.

Make it clear to the child that schoolwork is between the child and the teacher; teacher and child should set goals for better school performance to allow the child to feel responsible for school successes and failures.

Take advantage of situations that support and reinforce school learning.

Share information with teachers that will help them understand the child better.

Communicate with the teacher if there appears to be a problem—avoid waiting for a scheduled conference.

Provide a quiet, well-lighted area for study that is safe from interruption; do not allow television or radio.

Avoid dictating a study time, but do enforce rules, such as no television until homework is done; accept the child's word that work is complete.

Help with homework should focus on explaining the question, not giving the answer.

Teach the child to break large tasks (e.g., a report) into smaller, manageable tasks spread over the allotted time rather than attempt the entire project the night before it is to be completed.

Limit home tutoring to special circumstances, such as when the teacher requests parental assistance after a child's prolonged absence.

Request special help for children with learning problems.

Support the school staff by showing respect for both the school system and the teacher, at least in the child's presence.

such as making supportive statements that reassure or commend children, making accepting and clarifying statements that help children refine ideas and feelings to provide a sense of being understood, and providing constructive assistance that aids children with their own problem solving, all contribute to the expansion and development of a positive self-concept.

Parents.   Parents share responsibility with the schools for helping children achieve their maximum potential. There are numerous ways in which parents can supplement the school (see Family Home Care box).

Cultivating responsibility is the goal of parental assistance. Being responsible for schoolwork helps children learn to keep promises, meet deadlines, and succeed at their jobs as adults. Responsible children may occasionally ask for help (e.g., with a spelling list), but usually they prefer to think through their work by themselves. Excessive pressure or lack of encouragement from parents may inhibit the development of these desirable traits (Schmitt, 1990).

Latchkey Children

The term *latchkey children* is used to describe children in elementary school who spend some amount of time, before or after school, without supervision of an adult or an older adolescent. The increasing numbers of single-parent families and working mothers, together with the lack of available child care, have created a stress-provoking situation for many

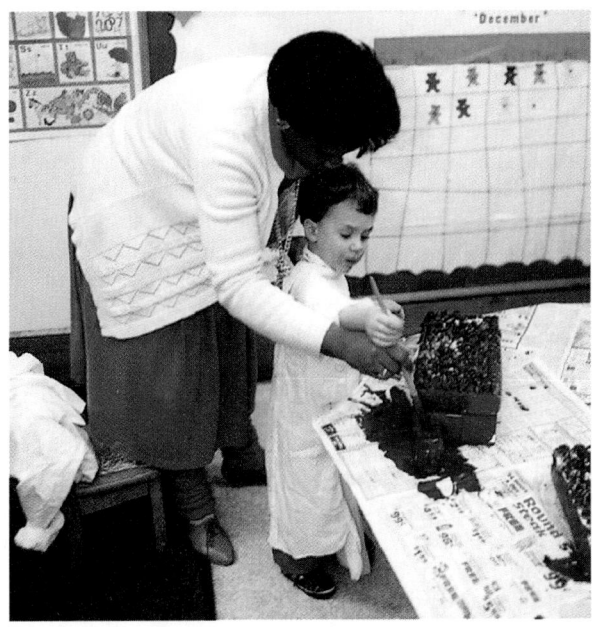

FIG. 15-6. Children can develop close relationships with their teachers.

schoolchildren. Some of these children may have a chronic illness as well (Holaday, Turner-Henson, and Swan, 1994).

The effect on these children is variable. Inadequate adult supervision after school leaves children at greater risk for injury and delinquent behavior. In some instances outside activities are curtailed and relationships with peers may be significantly diminished. Many latchkey children feel more lonely, isolated, and fearful than children who have someone to care for them. To cope with their fears and anxieties while alone, these children may devise strategies such as hiding, playing the television at loud volume, or using pets as a comfort.

Many communities and persons concerned about their welfare are trying to help children and their parents deal with this potentially serious problem. School-age care programs have been implemented by some communities and employers. It is important to teach self-help skills to these children and provide telephone check-in and reassurance programs.

Limit-Setting and Discipline

Numerous factors influence the amount and manner of discipline and limit-setting imposed on school-age children: the psychosocial maturity of the parents, the childhood and child-rearing experiences of the parents, the temperament of the children, the context of the children's misconduct, and the response of the children to rewards and punishments. As children are increasingly able to see a situation from the point of view of another, they are able to understand the effects of their reactions on others and themselves.

Disciplinary techniques should help children control their own behavior. Reasoning is an effective technique for this age-group. With advancing cognitive skills they are able to benefit from more complex types of disciplinary strategies. For example, withholding privileges, requiring compensation, imposing penalties, and contracting can be used with great success. Problem solving is the best approach to limit-setting, and children themselves can be included in the process of determining appropriate disciplinary measures.

Dishonest Behavior

During middle childhood children may engage in what is considered to be antisocial behavior. Lying, stealing, and cheating may become manifest in previously well-behaved children. It is especially disturbing to parents, who may have difficulty coping with this behavior.

Lying can occur for a number of reasons. Preschool children often have difficulty distinguishing between fact and fantasy. By the time they reach school age, they still "tell stories" but can distinguish between what is real and what is make-believe. If not, they need to be taught to distinguish between fantasy and reality. Often children will exaggerate a story or situation as a means to impress their family or friends.

Young children will lie to escape punishment or get out of some difficulty even when the evidence of their misbehavior is before their eyes. Older children may lie to meet expectations set by others to which they have been unable to measure up. However, most children are very concerned with the wrongness of lying and cheating—especially in their friends. They are quick to tell on others when they detect cheating.

Parents need to be reassured that all children lie sometimes and that they often have difficulty separating fantasy from reality. Parents should be helped to understand the importance of their own behavior as role models and of being truthful in their relationships with children.

Cheating is most common in young children ages 5 to 6. They find it difficult to lose at a game or contest, and so they cheat to win. They have not yet acquired the full realization of the wrongness of this behavior and do it almost automatically. It usually disappears as they mature. However, because children model observed behaviors, parents need to be aware of their own behavior. When parents set examples of honesty, children are more likely to conform to these standards.

As with other ethically related behavior, *stealing* is not an unexpected event in the younger child. Between 5 and 8 years of age, children's sense of property rights is limited, and they tend to take something simply because they are attracted to it or to take money for what it will buy. They are equally likely to give away something valuable that belongs to them. When young children are caught and punished, they are penitent—they "didn't mean to" and "promise never to do it again"—but it is quite likely that they will repeat the performance the following day. Often they not only steal but will lie about it as well or attempt to justify the act with excuses. It is seldom helpful to trap children into admission by asking directly if they committed the offense. Children do not take on such responsibility until nearer the end of middle childhood.

There are several reasons why children steal: a lack of a sense of property rights, an attempt to acquire the means with which to bribe favors from other children, a strong desire to own the coveted item, or a means for revenge to "get back at someone" (usually a parent) for what they consider to be unfair treatment. Older children may steal to supplement an inadequate income from other sources. Sometimes stealing is an indication that something is seriously wrong or lacking in the child's life. For example, children may steal to make up for love or another satisfaction that they feel is lacking.

In most situations it is best not to attempt to find a hidden or deep meaning to the stealing. An admonition, together with an appropriate and reasonable punishment, such as having the older child pay back the money or return the stolen items, will ordinarily take care of most cases. Most children can be taught to respect the property rights of others with little difficulty despite the temptations and opportunities presented to them. If children's personal rights are respected, they are more likely to respect the rights of others. Some children simply need more time to learn the importance of the culture's rules regarding private property.

Stress and Fear

Children today face more stresses than children in previous generations. Many children are stressed by conflict within the home and have constant anxiety regarding the separation that these disruptions can cause. The school environment is another stressful experience for some children. Competing with classmates for grades and teacher recognition and being labeled as "stupid" or "learning disabled" can result in emotional discomfort. Increasing violence within the family, the school, and the community also serves as a major stressor for children.

To help children cope with the stresses in their lives, the parent, teacher, or health worker must be able to recognize signs that indicate a child is undergoing stress and identify the source promptly.

The nurse who observes the following signs of stress in a child should explore the situation further:

> Stomach pains or headache
> Sleep problems
> Bed-wetting
> Changes in eating habits
> Aggressive or stubborn behavior
> Reluctance to participate
> Regression to earlier behaviors (e.g., thumbsucking)

Children need to be taught how to recognize signs of stress in themselves, such as a pounding heart, rapid breathing, or "butterflies" in the stomach. Once they are able to recognize that they are stressed, they can employ techniques for managing their stress. Probably the most useful technique is to help them plan a means for dealing with any stress through problem solving.

A wide variety and degree of anxiety symptoms, including fear of the dark, excessive worry about past behavior, self-consciousness, social withdrawal, and an excessive need for reassurance, are considered normal developmental events for children (Bell-Dolan, Last, and Strauss, 1990). School-age children are less fearful of body safety than they were as preschoolers, although they still fear being hurt, being kidnapped, or having to undergo surgery. They also fear death and are fascinated by all the aspects of death and dying. The fears of noises, darkness, storms, and dogs lessen. Most of the new fears that trouble school-age children are related to school and family.

• • •

Each child has a unique developmental pattern; therefore any attempt to describe the typical child can only represent an average and should not be considered an absolute criterion for any given child. Table 15-1 summarizes growth and development in middle childhood.

PROMOTING OPTIMUM HEALTH DURING THE SCHOOL YEARS

When school-age children enter school, they leave the relatively protected environment of home and neighborhood and experience interpersonal contacts with a larger number of children. Many childhood illnesses can be prevented or lessened by careful health supervision. The body's natural defenses against illness can be supported through careful attention to diet, rest, and exercise and protection from extreme mental and physical stress.

NUTRITION

Although caloric needs are diminished in relation to body size during middle childhood, resources are being laid down for the increased growth needs of the adolescent period. It is important to impress on children and their parents the value of a balanced diet to promote growth. Because children usually eat as their families do, the quality of their diet depends to a large extent on their families pattern of eating.

Likes and dislikes established at an early age continue in middle childhood, although the propensity for single food preferences begins to end and children acquire a taste for an increasing variety of foods. However, with the easy availability of fast-food restaurants, the influence of the mass media, and the temptation of an immense variety of "junk food," it is all too easy for children to fill up on empty calories—foods that do not promote growth, such as sugars, starches, and excess fats. The easy availability of high-calorie foods, combined with the tendency toward more sedentary activities, is contributing to an increasing prevalence of childhood obesity. This problem is discussed further in Chapter 17.

Parents do not know what their children eat when they are away from home. A parent may pack a lunch to be eaten at school but be unaware of how much is eaten, traded, sold, or thrown away. Nutrition education can and should be integrated with other classroom learning throughout the child's school years. In school the Food Guide Pyramid and the elements of a wholesome diet are learned, as well as how food products are grown, processed, and prepared. The school nurse can take an active role in nutrition education by working with teachers to plan and implement units on nutrition instruction and with parents and children to give nutritional guidance.

SLEEP AND REST

The amount of sleep and rest required during middle childhood is highly individualized. There is no specific amount needed by a child at any given age. Rather, the amount depends on the child's age, the activity level, and other factors, such as state of health. The growth rate has slowed; therefore less energy is expended in growth than was expended during the preceding periods.

During the school years children usually do not require a nap, but they spend 8 to 9½ hours in bed and sleep approximately 95% of that time (Coble and others, 1987). Although fewer bedtime problems occur during these years, occasional difficulties are still associated with the necessary bedtime ritual. Usually there is little problem for children 6 and 7 years old, and the task of going to bed can be facilitated by encouraging quiet activity before bedtime, such as coloring and reading. However, most children in middle childhood must be reminded frequently to go to bed; 8- to 9-year-old children and 11-year-old children are particularly resistant. Often children are unaware that they are tired; if they are allowed to remain up later than usual, they are fatigued the following day. Sometimes the bedtime resistance can be resolved by allowing a later bedtime in deference to the child's advancing age. Twelve-year-old children usually offer no difficulty in relation to bedtime. Some even retire early in order to enjoy slow preparations for bed, to read, or to listen to music.

EXERCISE AND ACTIVITY

The improved capabilities and adaptability of the school-age child permit greater speed and effort in motor activities; larger, stronger muscles permit longer and increasingly strenuous play without exhaustion. During middle child-

TABLE 15-1. Growth and development during school-age years

AGE (YEARS)	PHYSICAL AND MOTOR	MENTAL	ADAPTIVE	PERSONAL-SOCIAL
6	Growth and weight gain continues slowly Weight: 16-23.6 kg (35½-58 pounds); height: 106.6-123.5 cm (42-48 inches) Central mandibular incisors erupt Loses first tooth Gradual increase in dexterity Active age; constant activity Often returns to finger feeding More aware of hand as a tool Likes to draw, print, color Vision reaches maturity	Develops concept of numbers Counts 13 pennies Knows whether it is morning or afternoon Defines common objects such as fork and chair in terms of their use Obeys triple commands in succession Knows right and left hands Says which is pretty and which is ugly of a series of drawings of faces Describes the objects in a picture rather than simply enumerating them Attends first grade	At table, uses knife to spread butter or jam on bread At play, cuts, folds, pastes paper toys, sews crudely if needle is threaded Takes bath without supervision; performs bedtime activities alone Reads from memory; enjoys oral spelling game Likes table games, checkers, simple card games Giggles a lot Sometimes steals money or attractive items Has difficulty owning up to misdeeds Tries out own abilities	Can share and cooperate better Has great need for children of own age Will cheat to win Often engages in rough play Often jealous of younger brother or sister Does what adults are seen doing May have occasional temper tantrums Is a boaster Is more independent, probably influence of school Has own way of doing things Increases socialization
7	Begins to grow at least 5 cm (2 inches) a year Weight: 17.7-30 kg (39-66½ pounds); height: 111.8-129.7 cm (44-51 inches) Maxillary central incisors and lateral mandibular incisors erupt More cautious in approaches to new performances Repeats performances to master them Jaw begins to expand to accommodate permanent teeth	Notices that certain parts are missing from pictures Can copy a diamond Repeats three numbers backward Develops concept of time; reads ordinary clock or watch correctly to nearest quarter hour; uses clock for practical purposes Attends second grade More mechanical in reading; often does not stop at the end of a sentence, skips words such as *it*, *the*, and *he*	Uses table knife for cutting meat; may need help with tough or difficult pieces Brushes and combs hair acceptably without help May steal Likes to help and have a choice Is less resistant and stubborn	Is becoming a real member of the family group Takes part in group play Boys prefer playing with boys; girls prefer playing with girls Spends a lot of time alone; does not require a lot of companionship
8-9	Continues to grow at 5 cm (2 inches) a year Weight: 19.6-39.6 kg (43-87 pounds); height: 117-141.8 cm (46-56 inches) Lateral incisors (maxillary) and mandibular cuspids erupt Movement fluid; often graceful and poised Always on the go; jumps, chases, skips Increased smoothness and speed in fine motor control; uses cursive writing Dresses self completely Likely to overdo; hard to quiet down after recess More limber; bones grow faster than ligaments	Gives similarities and differences between two things from memory Counts backward from 20 to 1; understands concept of reversibility Repeats days of the week and months in order; knows the date Describes common objects in detail, not merely their use Makes change out of a quarter Attends third and fourth grades Reads more; may plan to wake up early just to read Reads classic books, but also enjoys comics	Makes use of common tools such as hammer, saw, screwdriver Uses household and sewing utensils Helps with routine household tasks such as dusting, sweeping Assumes responsibility for share of household chores Looks after all of own needs at table Buys useful articles; exercises some choice in making purchases Runs useful errands Likes pictorial magazines Likes school; wants to answer all the questions	Is easy to get along with at home Likes the reward system Dramatizes Is more sociable Is better behaved Is interested in boy-girl relationships but will not admit it Goes about home and community freely, alone or with friends Likes to compete and play games Shows preference in friends and groups Plays mostly with groups of own sex but is beginning to mix Develops modesty Compares self with others

TABLE 15-1. Growth and development during school-age years—cont'd

AGE (YEARS)	PHYSICAL AND MOTOR	MENTAL	ADAPTIVE	PERSONAL-SOCIAL
8-9— cont'd		More aware of time; can be relied on to get to school on time Can grasp concepts of parts and whole (fractions) Understands concepts of space, cause and effect, nesting (puzzles), conservation (permanence of mass and volume) Classifies objects by more than one quality; has collections Produces simple paintings or drawings	Is afraid of failing a grade; is ashamed of bad grades Is more critical of self Takes music and sport lessons	Enjoys Scouts, group sports
10-12	*Boys:* Slow growth in height and rapid weight gain; may become obese in this period Weight: 24.3-58 kg (54-128 pounds); height: 127.5-162.3 cm (50-64 inches) Posture is more similar to an adult's; will overcome lordosis *Girls:* pubescent changes may begin to appear; body lines soften and round out Remainder of teeth will erupt and tend toward full development (except wisdom teeth)	Writes brief stories Attends fifth to seventh grades Writes occasional short letters to friends or relatives on own initiative Uses telephone for practical purposes Responds to magazine, radio, or other advertising Reads for practical information or own enjoyment—stories or library books of adventure or romance, animal stories	Makes useful articles or does easy repair work Cooks or sews in small way Raises pets Washes and dries own hair Is responsible for a thorough job of cleaning hair, but may need reminding to do so Is sometimes left alone at home for an hour or so Is successful in looking after own needs or those of other children left in his or her care	Loves friends; talks about them constantly Chooses friends more selectively; may have a "best friend" Enjoys conversation Develops beginning interest in opposite sex Is more diplomatic Likes family; family really has meaning Likes mother and wants to please her in many ways Demonstrates affection Likes father, who is admired and may be idolized Respects parents

hood, youngsters acquire the coordination, timing, and concentration that are required to participate in adult-type activities, even though they may lack the strength, stamina, and control of the adolescent and adult. Consequently, a greater amount of physical activity should be expected and encouraged during the school years. However, it must be kept in mind that although school-age children are large and appear to be strong, they may not be ready for strenuous competitive athletics.

All growing children need some regular exercise and should be afforded opportunities of various kinds that provide satisfying experiences to meet individual likes and dislikes. Appropriate activities that promote coordination and development during the school-age years include running, jumping rope, swimming, roller skating, in-line skating, ice skating, and bicycle riding. Positive reinforcement achieved by experiencing increasingly smooth, rhythmic, and efficient use of the body conditions the child toward regular physical activity.

Exercise is essential for developmental progress in a number of areas, including muscle development and tone, refinement of balance and coordination, increased strength and endurance, and stimulation of body functions and metabolic processes. Children need ample space in which to run, jump, skip, and climb and safe facilities and equipment to use both indoors and outdoors. Most children need little encouragement to engage in physical activity. They have so much energy that they seldom know when to stop.

Children with disabling conditions or those who hesitate to become involved in active play, such as obese children, require special assessment and help so that activities that appeal to them, are compatible with their limitations, and meet their developmental needs can be determined.

Sports

Much controversy has surrounded the trend toward earlier participation in competitive athletics and the amount and type of competitive sports that are appropriate for children in the elementary grades. The current view is that virtually every child is suited for some type of sport, and authorities do not discourage participation if children are matched to the type of sport appropriate to their abilities and to their physical and emotional constitution. School-age children enjoy competition, and when those involved with children in this age-group understand children's physical limitations and teach them the proper techniques and safety measures necessary to avoid injury to developing bones and muscles, a safe and appropriate sport can be found for even the most unskilled and noncompetitive child (Fig. 15-7).

Various acceptable sports activities available to school-age children include baseball, soccer, gymnastics, and swimming. Equipment should be maintained in safe condition, and protective apparatus should be worn to prevent serious injury (see Traumatic Injury, Chapter 31).

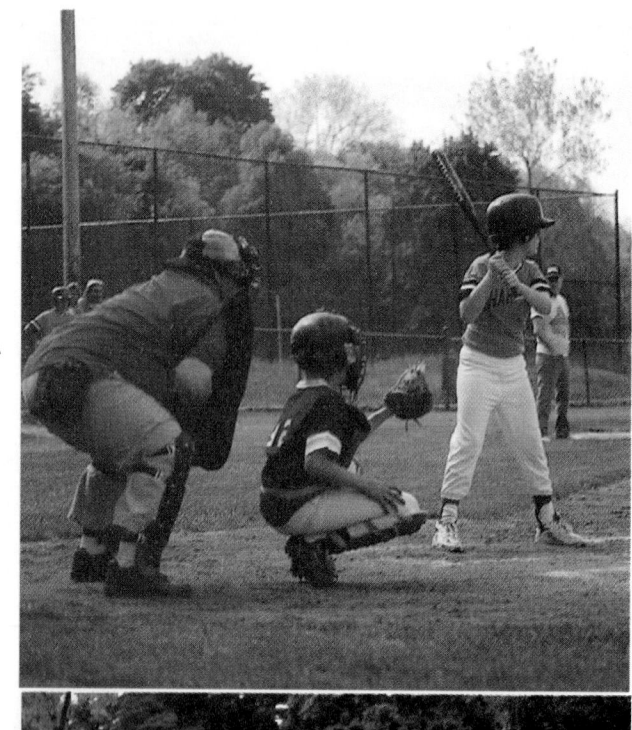

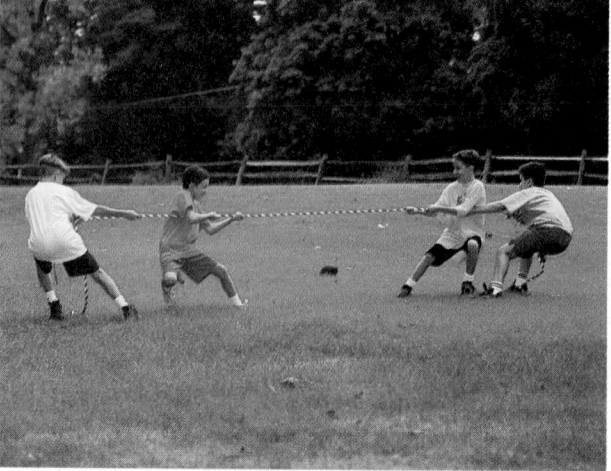

FIG. 15-7. The activities engaged in by school-age children vary according to interest and opportunity. **A,** Little League competitors. **B,** Playing tug-of-war.

During the school-age years girls have the same basic body structure as boys and thus have a similar response to systematic exercise training. At puberty, when boys become larger and have more muscle mass, it is usually recommended that girls compete only against other girls. Before puberty there is no essential difference in strength and size between girls and boys, making these precautions unnecessary (Metcalf and Roberts, 1993).

The American Academy of Pediatrics Committee on Sports Medicine and Committee on School Health (1989) recommend that preadolescence is a time to teach fundamental motor skills, develop fitness in a practical, safe, and gradual manner, and promote desired attitudes and values. Activities should include both practice sessions and unstructured play; the actual game or event should be managed in a manner that stresses mastery of the sport and enhancement of self-image rather than winning or pleasing others. All children should have an opportunity to participate, and special ceremonies should recognize all participants rather than individuals.

Acquisition of Skills

School-age children also demonstrate increasing capacities in fine muscle facility and complex artistic skills. Handedness is well established by the beginning of the school years, and children make great strides in writing and drawing during this age period. It is a time of energetic and vibrant creative productivity. With the tools of language and reading, children can create poems, stories, and plays. With more advanced fine motor skills, they are able to master an unlimited variety of handicrafts, such as ceramics, needlework, wood carving, and beadwork. They avidly pursue these skills in solitude, with a friend, or in programs offered through organized groups such as boys' or girls' clubs, Scouting, or special interest groups, which use crafts or other activities as a means to occupy, entertain, and educate children.

School-age children are capable of assuming responsibility for their own needs, although their distaste for soap and water and "dress" clothes is legendary. School-age children can and want to assume their share of household tasks, which usually are related to the male and female roles that have been defined by their culture. Many also assume responsibility for tasks outside the home, such as baby-sitting, mowing lawns, or paper routes.

DENTAL HEALTH

The first permanent (secondary) teeth erupt at about 6 years of age, beginning with the 6-year molar, which erupts posterior to the deciduous molars. The others appear in approximately the same order as eruption of the primary teeth (see Teething, Chapter 10) and follow shedding of the deciduous teeth (Fig. 15-8). With the appearance of the second permanent (12-year) molar, most of the permanent teeth are present. Permanent dentition, is somewhat more advanced in girls than it is in boys.

Because it is during the school-age years that the permanent teeth erupt, good dental hygiene and regular attention to dental caries are vital parts of health supervision during this period (see Dental Health, Chapter 12). Correct brushing techniques should be taught or reinforced, and the role that fermentable carbohydrates play in production of dental caries should be emphasized. It is also important to be alert

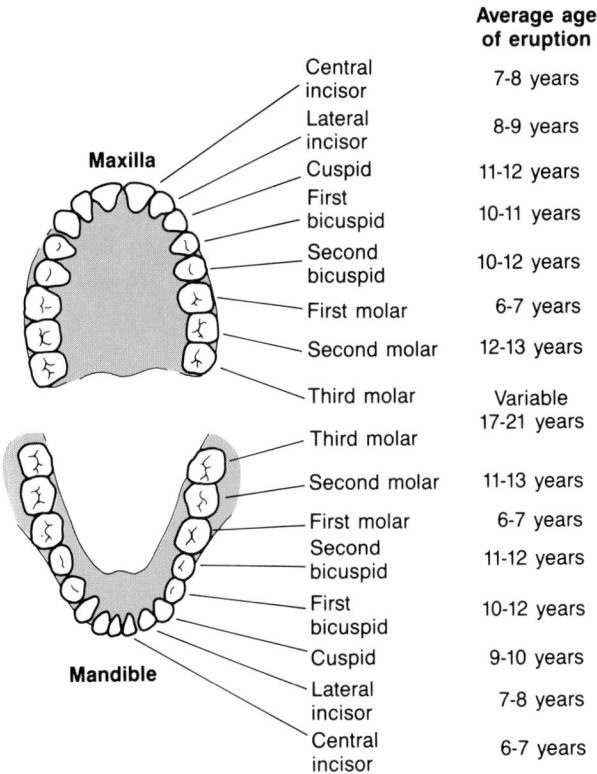

	Average age of eruption
Central incisor	7-8 years
Lateral incisor	8-9 years
Cuspid	11-12 years
First bicuspid	10-11 years
Second bicuspid	10-12 years
First molar	6-7 years
Second molar	12-13 years
Third molar	Variable 17-21 years
Third molar	
Second molar	11-13 years
First molar	6-7 years
Second bicuspid	11-12 years
First bicuspid	10-12 years
Cuspid	9-10 years
Lateral incisor	7-8 years
Central incisor	6-7 years

FIG. 15-8. Sequence of eruption of secondary teeth. (Data from McDonald RE, Avery DR: *Dentistry for the child and adolescent,* ed 6, St Louis, 1994, Mosby.)

to possible malocclusion problems that may result from irregular eruption of permanent teeth and that may impair function. Regular dental supervision and continued fluoride supplementation are as essential as regular medical supervision and should be an integral part of the health maintenance program.

The most effective means of preventing dental caries is proper oral hygiene. Children should be taught to carry out their own dental care with the supervision and guidance of the parents. Parents should learn the brushing technique along with their children, and they should inspect their children's efforts until the children can assume full responsibility.

Teeth should be brushed after meals, after snacks, and at bedtime. Children who brush their teeth frequently and become accustomed to the feel of a clean mouth at an early age usually maintain the habit throughout life. For the school-age child with mixed and permanent dentition, the best toothbrush is one of soft nylon bristles with an overall length of about 21 cm (6 inches). Numerous methods of brushing the teeth have been described and recommended for children, but no conclusive evidence indicates that one method is superior over another. The thoroughness of the cleaning is more important than the specific technique used. The dentist will assess all factors, such as manipulative skills and any special needs of the child, and suggest the most appropriate brushing technique and regimen. Flossing follows brushing. Parents do the flossing until children acquire the manual dexterity needed. Most children are not able to floss properly until about 8 or 9 years of age.

EMERGENCY TREATMENT
Evulsed Tooth

Recover tooth.
Hold tooth by crown; avoid touching root area.
If tooth is dirty, rinse it gently under running water or saline; be sure to insert stopper in sink or basin (to avoid tooth loss).
Insert tooth into socket.
Have child maintain tooth in place.
Transport child to dentist immediately.
Avoid sudden stops or sharp turns to prevent dislodging tooth.

If Reluctant to Reimplant Tooth:
Place evulsed tooth in suitable medium for transport:
 a. Cold milk
 b. Saliva—under child's or parent's tongue
If child is holding tooth in the mouth, avoid sudden stops to prevent swallowing tooth.
DON'T FORGET TO TAKE TOOTH.

Dental Problems

Limited or inadequate dental care results in the most prevalent of all childhood health problems: dental caries, malocclusion, and periodontal disease. Trauma, especially tooth evulsion, is also an important problem. All these conditions benefit from early intervention to prevent tooth loss.

Dental caries (cavities) is one of the most common chronic diseases that afflict humans at all ages; it is the principal oral problem in children and adolescents. Reducing the incidence and consequences of the disorder is of great importance in childhood because dental caries, if untreated, results in total destruction of involved teeth. The ages of greatest vulnerability are 4 to 8 years for the primary dentition and 12 to 18 years for the secondary or permanent dentition.

Dental caries is a multifactorial disease; it involves susceptible teeth, cariogenic microflora, and an appropriate oral environment. The incidence of lesions and the likelihood of progressive invasion vary considerably and depend on a number of factors being present in the right combination. Oral inspection is an integral part of the nursing assessment of the child. If there is any evidence of dental caries or other unhealthy state, the child is referred for dental services. An alarming number of children do not receive regular dental supervision, and a significant number reach adulthood without having been examined or treated by a dentist.

Periodontal disease, inflammatory and degenerative conditions involving the gums and tissues supporting the teeth, often begins in childhood and accounts for a significant amount of tooth loss in adulthood. The more common periodontal problems are *gingivitis* (simple inflammation of the gums) and *periodontitis* (inflammation of the gums and loss of connective tissue and bone in the supporting structures of the teeth).

The most prevalent periodontal disease, gingivitis, is a reversible inflammatory disease that begins very early in many children and is most often associated with the buildup of plaque on the teeth. Changes take place in the plaque bacteria, in both type and number of organisms, causing them to release a variety of destructive exotoxins, enzymes, and other noxious agents. They act to produce an inflammatory reaction in the gingival tissues, causing the gums to become red, edematous, tender, and subject to bleeding at the slightest irritation. Management is directed toward prevention by conscientious brushing and flossing, including the use of fluoride. The child should see the dentist at any signs of inflammation or irritation.

Malocclusion occurs when teeth of the upper and lower dental arches do not approximate in the proper relationships; the physiologic function of chewing is less effective and the cosmetic effect is less pleasing. Teeth that are uneven, crowded, or overlapping or are otherwise unable to meet their counterparts in the opposite jaw in the appropriate relationships may be predisposed to disease in later years.

Orthodontic treatment is usually most successful when it is started in the later school-age years or the early teenage years, after the last primary teeth have been shed and before growth ceases. However, referral should be made as soon as malocclusion is evident, since some deformities can be corrected at an earlier age.

Dental injury may occur in childhood and includes fractures of varying degrees of severity, chipping, dislocation, or evulsion. All tooth injuries require prompt treatment by a competent dentist to prevent permanent displacement or loss. Delayed examination and diagnosis of tooth damage can result in infection or pulp involvement. Also, because it can affect the remaining teeth, replacement of the lost tooth is needed to maintain normal alignment and position of the other teeth.

A tooth that is *evulsed* (avulsed, exarticulated, or "knocked out") should be replanted by the child, parent, or nurse and stabilized as soon as possible so that the blood supply to the tooth can be reestablished and the tooth kept alive (see Emergency Treatment box on p. 457). If the tooth is replaced within 30 minutes, there is a 70% chance that it will become reattached and roots will not resorb or the crown exfoliate. Evulsed primary teeth are usually not reimplanted.

As with all mouth trauma, an evulsed tooth causes a large amount of bleeding, which is most distressing to the child. Bleeding is frightening to children and their families; therefore the nurse or anyone faced with dental trauma should be prepared to cope with the emotionality that accompanies tooth evulsion. Using a calm approach and providing gentle reassurance to the child requires only a moment and does much to reduce anxiety.

SEX EDUCATION

Evidence indicates that many children experience some form of sex play during or before preadolescence as a response to normal curiosity, not as a result of love or sexual urge. Children are experimentalists by nature, and this play is incidental and transitory. Any adverse emotional consequences or guilt feelings depend on how the behavior is managed by the parents, if it is discovered, or whether children view their actions as wrong in the eyes of significant persons, particularly the parents (Levine, 1992).

The child's attitude toward sex is acquired indirectly at a very early age. Initial curiosity about differences in body structure between boys and girls and between children and adults arises in the preschool years. Middle childhood is an ideal time for formal sex education, and many authorities believe that the topic is best presented from a life-span approach. Information about sexual maturation and the process of reproduction helps to minimize the child's uncertainty, embarrassment, and feelings of isolation that often accompany puberty.

An important component of ongoing sex education is effective communication with parents. If parents either repress the child's sexual curiosity or avoid dealing with it, the sexual information that the child receives may be acquired almost entirely from peers. When peers are the primary source of sexual information, it is transmitted and exchanged in secret conversation and contains a large amount of misinformation.

Nurse's Role in Sex Education

No matter where nurses practice, they can provide information on human sexuality to both parents and children. To discuss the topic adequately, nurses must have not only an understanding of the physiologic aspects of sexuality and a knowledge of cultural and societal values, but also an awareness of their own attitudes, feelings, and biases about sexuality.

When sexual information is presented to school-age children, sex and sexuality should be treated as a normal part of growth and development. Questions should be answered honestly, matter-of-factly, and to the same extent as questions about other topics. Answers should be at the child's level of understanding. There may be times when boys and girls should be taught content separately.

Children need help to differentiate sex and sexuality. Exercises on clarifying values, identifying role models, engaging in problem-solving skills, and practicing responsibility are important prerequisites to the sexual information needed in early adolescence. In addition, children need to have much of the sexual information that is provided to them via the media or jokes explained and defused. Information concerning the acquired immunodeficiency syndrome (AIDS) should be presented in simple, accurate terms and should focus on how the AIDS virus is transmitted (Schonfeld and others, 1993).

Preadolescents need more precise information. They are interested in concrete information, such as "What if I start my period in the middle of class?" or "How can I keep people from telling I have an erection?" It is important to tell them what they want to know and what they can expect to happen as they become mature sexually.

During encounters with parents, nurses can be open and available for questions and discussion. They can set an example by the language they use in discussing body parts and their function and by the way in which they deal with problems that have emotional overtones, such as exploratory sex play and masturbation. Parents need to be helped to understand normal behaviors and to view sexual curiosity in their children as a part of the developmental process. Assessing the parents' level of knowledge and understanding of sexuality provides cues to their need for supplemental information that will better prepare them for the increasingly complex explanations that will be needed as their children grow older.

SCHOOL HEALTH

Child health maintenance is ultimately the responsibility of the parents; however, the public schools and health departments in the United States have contributed to the improvement of child health by providing a healthful school environment, health services, and health education that emphasizes sound health practices. Most of these functions constitute major components of community health services and involve large amounts of public funds and large numbers of health professionals, including nurses.

A school health program is involved in ongoing health maintenance through assessment, screening, and referral activities. Routine health services provided by most schools include health appraisal, emergency care, safety education, communicable disease control, counseling, and follow-up care. Health education of schoolchildren is primarily directed toward providing knowledge of health and influencing habits, attitudes, and conduct in relation to health and injury prevention.

Traditionally, school nurses have been viewed from a limited perspective that placed them in the role of disease detector, applier of bandages, and official caregiver in cases of illness and injury. Although these are still important functions, this traditional role is acquiring much broader dimensions. School nurses are being prepared to provide primary health care on a broader scale that includes assessment of physical, psychomedical, psychoeducational, behavioral, and learning disorder problems and to provide comprehensive well-child care. Many health care reformers are also proposing that school health services be enlarged to meet the needs of not only schoolchildren but also their families and the community (Igoe, 1993). School nurse practitioners will play an essential role in these school-based centers.

Since the passage of Public Laws 94-142 and 99-457, which require the integration of children with chronic illness or disability into regular classrooms, school health services are also responsible for the medical and nursing needs of these children. School nurse practitioners are vital to the development, implementation, and evaluation of health care plans and programs for these children. Unfortunately, not all schools have a school nurse, and the use of unlicensed assistive personnel (UAP) is increasing. School nurses are faced with the delegation to and supervision of UAP (Delegation of School Health Services to Unlicensed Assistive Personnel, 1995).

INJURY PREVENTION

Because school-age children have developed more refined muscular coordination and control and can apply their cognitive capacities to a more judicious course of action, the incidence of injury is diminished in children in this age-group when compared with the incidence in early childhood.

The most common cause of severe injury and death in school-age children is motor vehicle accidents—either as pedestrian or passenger. It is imperative that nurses continue to emphasize the importance of the three automobile safety measures that have been found to reduce the severity of injuries: effective restraint systems, door-lock mechanisms, and appropriate passenger seating locations in the motor vehicle.

The school-age child's desire for riding bicycles increases the risk of injury on streets and byways. Other serious injuries include accidents on skateboards, roller skates, in-line skates, skis, and other sports equipment. All-terrain vehicles (ATVs), popular with children under 16 years of age, are unstable, difficult to handle, and responsible for an increasing

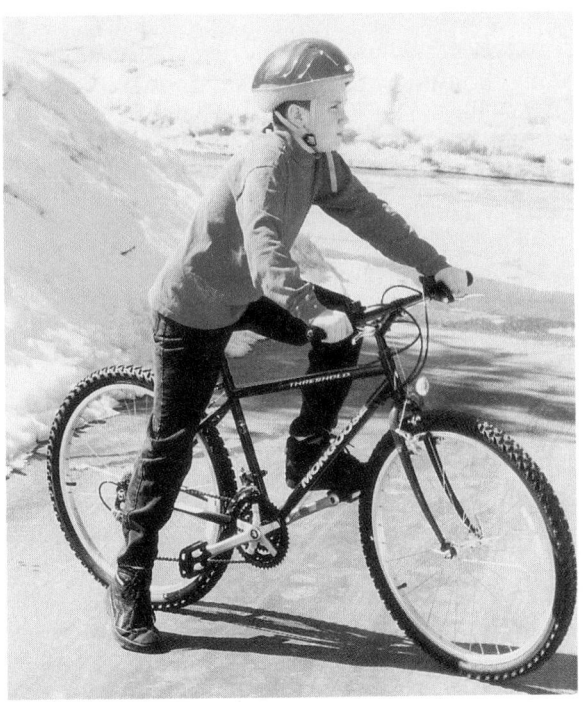

FIG. 15-9. The right-size bike is important; child should be able to sit on the bike and place balls of both feet on ground. Foot should comfortably reach and manipulate the pedal in the down position. Wearing a protective helmet is mandatory. Helmet should sit on top of head in a level position and should not rock back and forth or from side to side. Strap should always be fastened *securely* under the chin.

number of childhood injuries (Dolan, Knapp, and Andres, 1989). The two- and four-wheeled motorized vehicles are unlicensed and require no advanced training.

Most injuries occur in or near the home or school. The most effective means of prevention is education of the child and family regarding the hazards of risk taking and improper use of the equipment. Safety helmets, protective eye and mouth shields, and protective padding are strongly recommended for children engaged in active sports, even though they may not be required equipment. For example, falls from bicycles, ATVs, and skating devices are the cause of a significant number of head injuries in school-age children. Because head injury is the major cause of bicycle-related fatalities, probably the most important aspect of bicycle safety is to encourage the rider to wear a protective helmet (Fig. 15-9) (American Academy of Pediatrics, 1995). Physically active school-age children are highly susceptible to cuts and abrasions, and the incidence of childhood fractures, strains, and sprains is noteworthy. The incidence is significantly higher in school-age boys than in school-age girls. Injuries of a serious nature are discussed as appropriate elsewhere in the book—burns (Chapter 30), eye trauma (Chapter 19), near-drowning (Chapter 28), and head injuries (Chapter 28). The prevalence of injuries depends on the dangers present in the environment, the protection offered by adults, and the behavior patterns of the children. Table 15-2 lists the major developmental accomplishments and suggestions for injury prevention, and the Family Home Care boxes on p. 461 provide guidelines for bicycle, skateboard, and in-line skate safety.

TABLE 15-2. Injury prevention during school-age years

DEVELOPMENTAL ABILITIES RELATED TO RISK OF INJURY	INJURY PREVENTION
Is increasingly involved in activities away from home Is excited by speed and motion Is easily distracted by environment Can be reasoned with	**Motor Vehicle Accidents** Educate child regarding proper use of seat belts while a passenger in a vehicle. Maintain discipline while a passenger in a vehicle (e.g., keep arms inside, do not lean against doors or interfere with driver). Emphasize safe pedestrian behavior. Insist on wearing safety apparel (e.g., helmet) when applicable, such as riding bicycle, motorcycle, moped, or all-terrain vehicle (see Family Home Care boxes).
Is apt to overdo May work hard to perfect a skill Has cautious, but not fearful, gross motor actions Likes swimming	**Drowning** Teach child to swim. Teach basic rules of water safety. Select safe and supervised places to swim. Check sufficient water depth for diving. Swim with a companion. Use an approved flotation device in water or boat. Advocate for legislation requiring fencing around pools. Learn cardiopulmonary resuscitation (CPR).
Has increasing independence Is adventuresome Enjoys trying new things	**Burns** Instruct child in behavior in areas involving contact with potential burn hazards (e.g., gasoline, matches, bonfires or barbecues, lighter fluid, firecrackers, cigarette lighters, cooking utensils, chemistry sets); avoid climbing or flying kite around high-tension wires. Instruct child in proper behavior in the event of fire (e.g., fire drills at home and school). Teach child safe cooking (use low heat; avoid any frying; be careful of steam burns, scalds, or exploding foods, especially from microwaving).
Adheres to group rules May be easily influenced by peers Has strong allegiance to friends	**Poisoning** Educate child regarding hazards of taking nonprescription drugs and chemicals, including aspirin and alcohol. Teach child to say "no" if offered illegal or dangerous drugs or alcohol. Keep potentially dangerous products in properly labeled receptacles, preferably out of reach.
Has increased physical skills Needs strenuous physical activity Is interested in acquiring new skills and perfecting attained skills Is daring and adventurous, especially with peers Frequently plays in hazardous places Confidence often exceeds physical capacity Desires group loyalty and has strong need for friends' approval Attempts hazardous feats Accompanies friends to potentially hazardous facilities Delights in physical activity Is likely to overdo Growth in height exceeds muscular growth and coordination	**Bodily Damage** Help provide facilities for supervised activities. Encourage playing in safe places. Keep firearms safely locked up except during adult supervision. Teach proper care of, use of, and respect for devices with potential danger (e.g., power tools, firecrackers). Teach children not to tease or surprise dogs, invade their territory, take dogs' toys, or interfere with dogs' feeding. Stress eye, ear, or mouth protection when using potentially hazardous objects or devices or when engaged in potentially hazardous sports. Teach safety regarding use of corrective devices (glasses); if child wears contact lenses, monitor duration of wear to prevent corneal damage. Stress careful selection, use, and maintenance of sports and recreation equipment, such as skateboards and in-line skates (see Family Home Care box).

TABLE 15-2. Injury prevention during school-age years—cont'd

DEVELOPMENTAL ABILITIES RELATED TO RISK OF INJURY	INJURY PREVENTION
	Emphasize proper conditioning, safe practices, and use of safety equipment for sports or recreational activities.
	Caution against engaging in hazardous sports, such as those involving trampolines.
	Use safety glass and decals on large glassed areas, such as sliding glass doors.
	Teach name, address, and phone number and emphasize that child should ask for help from appropriate people (e.g., cashier, security guard, police) if lost; have identification on child (e.g., sewn in clothes, inside shoe).
	Teach personal safety:
	Avoid personalized clothing in public places.
	Never go with a stranger.
	Tell parents if anyone makes child feel uncomfortable in any way.
	Always listen to child's concerns regarding others' behavior.
	Stress for child to say "no" when confronted with uncomfortable situations.

FAMILY HOME CARE
Bicycle Safety

Always wear properly fitted bicycle helmet that is approved by Snell or the **American National Standards Institute (ANSI)**; replace damaged helmet.

Ride bicycles with traffic and away from parked cars.

Ride single file.

Walk bicycles through busy intersections only at crosswalks.

Give hand signals well in advance of turning or stopping.

Keep as close to the curb as practical.

Watch for drain grates, potholes, soft shoulders, and loose dirt or gravel.

Keep both hands on handlebars, except with signaling.

Never ride double on a bicycle.

Do not carry packages that interfere with vision or control; do not drag objects behind bike.

Watch for and yield to pedestrians.

Watch for cars backing up or pulling out of driveways; be especially careful at intersections.

Look left, right, then left before turning into traffic or roadway.

Never hitch a ride on a truck or other vehicle.

Learn rules of the road and respect for traffic officers.

Obey all local ordinances.

Wear shoes that fit securely while riding.

Wear light colors at night and attach fluorescent material to clothing and bicycle.

Be certain the bicycle is the correct size for rider.

Equip bicycle with proper lights and reflectors.

Have the bicycle inspected to ensure good mechanical condition.

Children riding as passengers must wear appropriate-size helmets in specially designed protective seats.

From American Academy of Pediatrics, Committee on Injury and Poison Prevention: Bicycle helmets, *Pediatrics* 95(4):609-610, 1995.

FAMILY HOME CARE
Skateboard and In-Line Skate Safety

Children younger than 5 years of age should not use skateboards or in-line skates. They are not developmentally prepared to protect themselves from injury.

Children who ride skateboards or in-line skates should wear helmets and other protective equipment, especially on knees, wrists, and elbows, to prevent injury.

Skateboards and in-line skates should never be ridden near traffic. Their use should be prohibited on streets and highways. Activities that bring skateboards together (e.g., "catching a ride") are especially dangerous.

Some types of use, such as riding homemade ramps on hard surfaces, may be particularly hazardous.

Modified from American Academy of Pediatrics, Committee on Injury and Poison Prevention: Skateboard injuries, *Pediatrics* 95(4):611-612, 1995.

ANTICIPATORY GUIDANCE— CARE OF FAMILIES

Parents of the school-age child find themselves in the position of sharing their child's time with the increasingly important peer group. It is through early peer relationships that children begin to prepare for moving from narrow, sheltered family relationships to a broader world of relationships and increased independence. Parents must learn to provide support as unobtrusively as possible without feeling rejected, hurt, or angry. The nurse can help parents of the school-age child by providing anticipatory guidance and reassurance throughout this period of child development and maturation (see Family Home Care box on p. 462).

FAMILY HOME CARE
Guidance During School Years

Age 6 Years

Prepare parents to expect strong food preferences and frequent refusal of specific food items.

Prepare parents to expect increasingly ravenous appetite.

Prepare parents for emotionality as child experiences erratic mood changes.

Help parents anticipate continued susceptibility to illness.

Teach injury prevention and safety, especially bicycle safety.

Encourage parents to respect child's need for privacy and to provide a separate bedroom for child, if possible.

Prepare parents for child's increasing interests outside the home.

Help parents understand the need to encourage child's interactions with peers.

Ages 7 to 10 Years

Prepare parents to expect improvement in health with fewer illnesses, but warn them that allergies may increase or become apparent.

Prepare parents to expect an increase in minor injuries.

Emphasize caution in selecting and maintaining sports equipment and reemphasize safety.

Prepare parents to expect increased involvement with peers and interest in activities outside the home.

Emphasize the need to encourage independence while maintaining limit-setting and discipline.

Prepare mothers to expect more demands at 8 years.

Prepare fathers to expect increasing admiration at 10 years; encourage father-child activities.

Prepare parents for prepubescent changes in girls.

Ages 11 to 12 Years

Help parents prepare child for body changes of pubescence.

Prepare parents to expect a growth spurt in girls.

Make certain child's sex education is adequate with accurate information.

Prepare parents to expect energetic but stormy behavior at 11 to become more even-tempered at 12.

Encourage parents to support child's desire to "grow up" but to allow regressive behavior when needed.

Prepare parents to expect an increase in masturbation.

Instruct parents that the amount of rest the child needs may increase.

Help parents educate child regarding experimentation with potentially harmful activities.

Health Guidance

Help parents understand the importance of regular health and dental care for the child.

Encourage parents to teach and model sound health practices, including diet, rest, activity, and exercise.

Stress the need to encourage children to engage in appropriate physical activities.

Emphasize providing a safe physical and emotional environment.

Encourage parents to teach and model safety practices.

KEY POINTS

- Middle childhood, also known as the school years, is a comfortable period of life that extends from 6 to 12 years of age.
- Although slower than previous years, there is a steady gain in height and weight with maturation of body systems; primary teeth are lost and replaced by permanent teeth.
- School-age children develop what Erikson terms a sense of industry or accomplishment.
- School-age children, although having a limited capacity for abstract thought, are able to use their thought processes in solving more complex problems, to make judgments based on reasoning, and to see a situation from the point of view of another.
- The child develops a conscience and is able to understand and adhere to rules and standards set by others.
- Entertaining different points of view, becoming sensitive to social norms, and forming peer friendships are the most important features of social development during the school years.
- Cooperative play, team activities, and acquisition of skills are prime elements of play during the school years; rules and rituals assume greater importance.

- School-age children become proficient at many types of activities.
- Typical parental concerns during middle childhood are beginning separation from the family unit, dishonest behavior, and scholastic achievement.
- Optimum nutrition is often hampered by an affinity for and availability of junk foods, irregular family meals, and schedules of working parents.
- Dental care continues to be important; dental problems include caries, periodontal disease, malocclusion, and dental injury.
- Increased socialization, earlier pubertal development, and constant media exposure make the school years an ideal time for sex education.
- School health ideally offers programs that include health appraisal, emergency care, safety education, communicable disease control, counseling, guidance, and health education with adjustment to individual student needs.
- Injury prevention is directed toward safety education, provision of safe play areas and equipment, and well-supervised sports activities.

REFERENCES

American Academy of Pediatrics, Committee on Injury and Poison Prevention: Bicycle helmets, *Pediatrics* 95(4):609-610, 1995.

American Academy of Pediatrics, Committee on Sports Medicine and Committee on School Health: Organized athletics for preadolescent children, *Pediatrics* 84:583-584, 1989.

Bell-Dolan D, Last C, Strauss C: Symptoms of anxiety disorders in normal children, *J Am Acad Child Adolesc Psychiatry* 29:759-765, 1990.

Coble PA and others: EEG sleep of healthy children 6 to 12 years of age. In Guilleminault C, editor: *Sleep and its disorders in children*, New York, 1987, Raven.

Delegation of school health services to unlicensed assisstive personnel: A position paper of the National Association of State School Nurse Consultants, *J School Nurs* 11(4):13-16, 1995.

Erikson EH: *Childhood and society*, ed 2, New York, 1963, Norton.

Holaday B, Turner-Henson A, Swan JH: Chronically-ill latchkey children, *Clin Pediatr* 33(5):303-306, 1994.

Igoe JB: School-linked family health centers in health care reform, *Pediatr Nurs* 19:67-68, 1993.

Levine MD: Middle childhood. In Levine MD and others: *Developmental-behavioral pediatrics*, ed 2, Philadelphia, 1992, Saunders.

Metcalf JH, Roberts SO: Strength training and the immature athlete: an overview, *Pediatr Nurs* 19:325-332, 1993.

Miller ME: Immunodeficiency of immaturity. In Stiehm R: *Immunologic disorders in infants and children*, Philadelphia, 1989, Saunders.

Rollins JA: Nurses as gangbusters: a response to gang violence in America, *Pediatr Nurs* 19:559-567, 1993.

Schmitt B: Preventing problems with schoolwork, *Contemp Pediatr* 7(9):31-32, 1990.

Schonfeld DJ and others: Understanding of acquired immunodeficiency syndrome by elementary school children—a developmental survey, *Pediatrics* 92:389-395, 1993.

BIBLIOGRAPHY

General

Adger H, DeAngelis C: Sexuality education: our schools can do better, *Contemp Pediatr* 6(10):56-67, 1989.

Carey WB: Temperament issues in the school-aged child, *Pediatr Clin North Am* 39:537-549, 1992.

Dixon SD, Stein MT: *Encounters with children: pediatric behavior and development*, ed 2, St Louis, 1992, Mosby.

Dworkin PH: Behavior during middle childhood: developmental themes and clinical issues, *Pediatr Ann* 18:347-355, 1989.

Eiden H, Thomas M, Fosarelli P: A teaching tool for children in self-care, *J Pediatr Health Care* 1:292-297, 1987.

Feldman H: The development of thinking skills in school-age children, *Pediatr Ann* 18:356-362, 1989.

Guilleminault C: Disorders of arousal in children: somnambulism and night terrors. In Guilleminault C, editor: *Sleep and its disorders in children*, New York, 1987, Raven.

Landman GB: Language development from six to twelve, *Pediatr Ann* 18:373-379, 1989.

Sandler A: Social development in middle childhood, *Pediatr Ann* 18:380-387, 1989.

Vessey JA, Braithwaite KB, Wiedmann M: Teaching children about their internal bodies, *Pediatr Nurs* 16:29-33, 1990.

Winkelstein ML: Fostering positive self-concept in the school-age child, *Pediatr Nurs* 15:229-233, 1989.

Wynn D, Schmidt CK, Aluin RM: Test-retest reliability of a body knowledge instrument in school-age children, *Matern Child Nurs J* 22:56-64, 1994.

Health Promotion

American Academy of Pediatrics, Committee on School Health: *School health: a guide for health professionals*, Elk Grove Village, IL, 1987, American Academy of Pediatrics.

American Academy of Pediatrics, Committee on Sports Medicine and Committee on School Health: Physical fitness and the schools, *Pediatrics* 80:449-450, 1987.

Bailey-Britton AM: The relationship between health and academic performance in school-age children, *Issues Compr Pediatr Nurs* 10:273-289, 1987.

Bausell RB: A national survey assessing pediatric preventive behaviors, *Pediatr Nurs* 11:438-444, 1985.

Cowell JM and others: School health services: a hub of services to children and their families, *Pediatr Nurs* 17:86-88, 1991.

Ferber R: Sleep schedule–dependent causes of insomnia and sleepiness in middle childhood and adolescence, *Pediatrician* 17:13-20, 1990.

Giordana BP, Igoe JB: Health promotion: the new frontier, *Pediatr Nurs* 17:490-492, 1991.

Hester ND: Health concerns of school-age children, *Issues Compr Pediatr Nurs* 10:251-262, 1987.

Pidgeon V, Olson S: A comparison of illness concepts of school-age children and adolescents, *Issues Compr Pediatr Nurs* 9:209-221, 1986.

Pipes PL, Trahms CM: *Nutrition in infancy and childhood*, ed 5, St Louis, 1993, Mosby.

Scanlon BJ: An holistic approach to school dental health, *J Sch Nurs* 7:12-15, 1991.

School Health

American Academy of Pediatrics, Committee on School Health: Guidelines for the administration of medication in school, *Pediatrics* 92:499-500, 1993.

Farren M, McKevitt RK: Nursing roles in school health. In Hoekelman RA and others, editors: *Primary pediatric care*, ed 2, St Louis, 1992, Mosby.

Fryer GE, Igoe JB: A relationship between availability of school nurses and child well-being, *J Sch Nurs* 11(3):12-16, 18, 1995.

Garbarino J and others: *Children in danger: coping with the consequences of community violence*, Jossey-Bass, San Francisco, 1992.

Groves BM and others: Silent victims: children who witness violence, *JAMA* 269:261-264, 1993.

Igoe JB: Healthy long-term attitudes on personal health can be developed in school-age children, *Pediatrician* 15:127-136, 1988.

Kornguth ML: School illnesses: who's absent and why? *Pediatr Nurs* 16:95-99, 1990.

Lear JG: Building a health/education partnership: the role of school-based health centers, *Pediatr Nurs* 18(2):172-173, 1992.

MacBriar BR and others: Development of a health concerns inventory for school-age children, *J Sch Nurs* 11(3):25-29, 1995.

Meeker R and others: A comprehensive school health initiative, *Image J Nurs Sch* 18:86-91, 1986.

Mudd KE, Noone SA: Management of severe food allergy in the school setting, *J Sch Nurs* 11(3):30-32, 1995.

Velsor-Friedrich B: Schools and health. Part II. School-based clinics, *J Pediatr Nurs* 10(1):62-63, 1995.

Injury Prevention

American Academy of Pediatrics, Committee on Accident and Poison Prevention: All-terrain vehicles: two-, three-, and four-wheeled unlicensed motorized vehicles, *Pediatrics* 79:306-308, 1987.

American Academy of Pediatrics, Committee on Accident and Poison Prevention: Injuries related to "toy" firearms, *Pediatrics* 79:473-474, 1987.

American Academy of Pediatrics, Committee on Accident and Poison Prevention: Bicycle helmets, *Pediatrics* 85:229-230, 1990.

American Academy of Pediatrics, Committee on Injury and Poison Prevention: Skateboard injuries, *Pediatrics* 95(4):611-612, 1995.

American Medical Association, Council on Scientific Affairs: Council report: Helmets and preventing motorcycle- and bicycle-related injuries, *JAMA* 272(19):1535-1538, 1994.

Boyce WT, Sobolewski S: Recurrent injuries in school children, *Am J Dis Child* 143:338-342, 1989.

Christoffel KK: Child passenger safety, *Am J Dis Child* 143:1271-1272, 1989.

Cushman R and others: Helmet promotion in the emergency room following a bicycle injury: a randomized trial, *Pediatrics* 88:43-47, 1991.

Dolan MA, Knapp JF, Andres J: Three-wheel and four-wheel all-terrain vehicle injuries in children, *Pediatrics* 84:694-698, 1989.

Jones NE: Childhood injuries: an epidemiologic approach, *Pediatr Nurs* 18:235-239, 1992.

Jones NE: Prevention of childhood injuries. I. Motor vehicle injuries, *Pediatr Nurs* 18:380-382, 1992.

Jones NE: Prevention of childhood injuries. II. Recreational injuries, *Pediatr Nurs* 18:619-621, 1992.

Lee EJ: Accident reports: survey of high school injuries, *Pediatr Nurs* 13:151-154, 1987.

Rivara FP and others: Attitudes and practices toward children as pedestrians, *Pediatrics* 84:1017-1021, 1989.

Schor EL: Unintentional injuries: patterns within families, *Am J Dis Child* 141:1280-1284, 1987.

Selbst SM, Alexander D, Ruddy R: Bicycle-related injuries, *Am J Dis Child* 141:140-144, 1987.

Senturia YD, Christoffel KK, Donovan AA: Children's household exposure to guns: a pediatric practice-based survey, *Pediatrics* 93(3):469-475, 1994.

Wilson MH: Preventing injury in the "middle years," *Contemp Pediatr* 6(6):20-54, 1989.

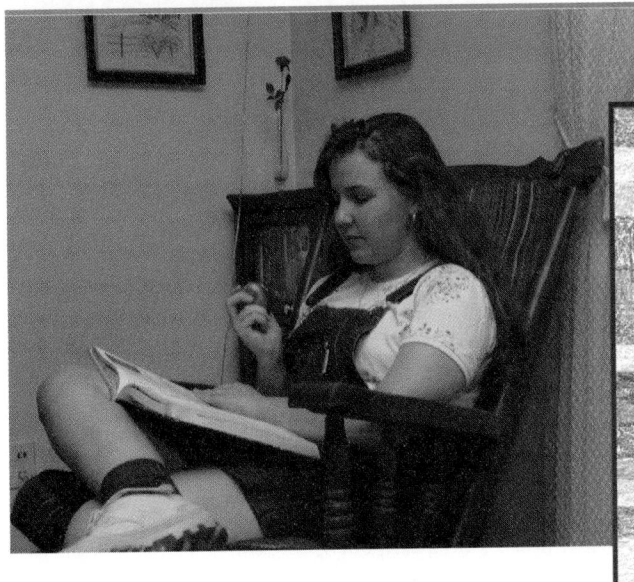

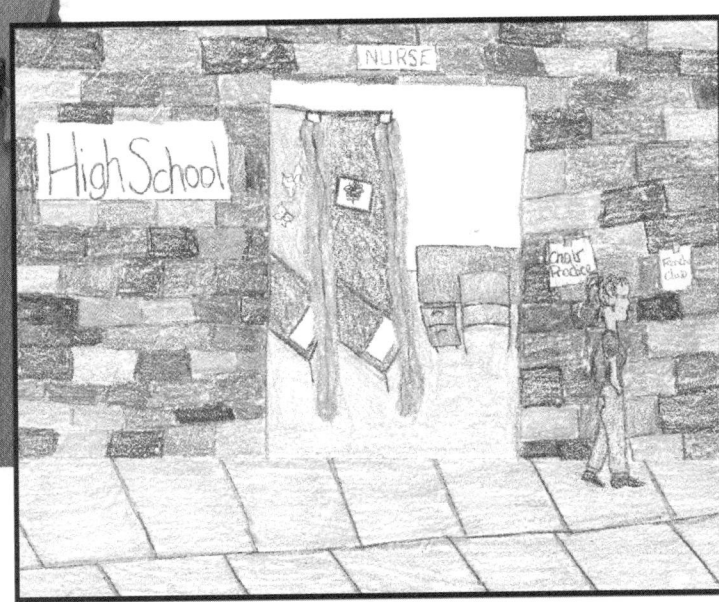

"Teenagers' moods switch a lot. Sometimes I work to be courteous all day, and then at home I'm worn out and find myself snapping at my family."

Amy, age 15 years

RELATED TOPICS

PROMOTING OPTIMUM GROWTH AND DEVELOPMENT

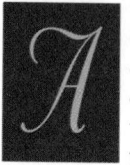

dolescence is a period of transition between childhood and adulthood—a time of rapid physical, cognitive, social, and emotional maturing as the boy prepares for manhood and the girl prepares for womanhood (see Cultural Awareness box). The precise boundaries of adolescence are difficult to define, but this period is customarily viewed as beginning with the gradual appearance of secondary sex characteristics at about 11 or 12 years of age and ending with cessation of body growth at 18 to 20 years.

Several terms are commonly used in reference to this particular stage of growth and development. *Puberty* primarily refers to the maturational, hormonal, and growth process that occurs when the reproductive organs begin to function and the secondary sex characteristics develop. This process is sometimes divided into three stages: *prepubescence,* the period of about 2 years immediately before puberty when the child is developing preliminary physical changes that herald sexual maturity; *puberty,* the point at which sexual maturity is achieved, marked by the first menstrual flow in girls but by less obvious indications in boys; and *postpubescence,* a 1- to 2-year period following puberty during which skeletal growth is completed and reproductive functions become fairly well established. *Adolescence,* which literally means "to grow into maturity," is generally regarded as the psychologic, social, and maturational process initiated by the pubertal changes. It involves three distinct subphases: *early adolescence* (ages 11 to 14), *middle adolescence* (ages 15 to 17), and *late adolescence* (ages 18 to 20). Adolescence tends to begin and end earlier in girls than in boys. The term *teenage years* is used synonymously with *adolescence* to describe ages 13 through 19.

BIOLOGIC DEVELOPMENT

The physical changes of puberty are primarily the result of hormonal activity under the influence of the central nervous

system, although all aspects of physiologic functioning are mutually interacting. The very obvious physical changes are noted in increased physical growth and in the appearance and development of secondary sex characteristics; less obvious are physiologic alterations and neurogonadal maturity, accompanied by the ability to procreate. Physical distinction between the sexes is determined on the basis of distinguishing characteristics: *primary sex characteristics* are the external and internal organs that carry out the reproductive functions (e.g., ovaries, uterus, breasts, penis); *secondary sex characteristics* are the changes that occur throughout the body as a result of the hormonal change (e.g., voice alterations, development of facial and pubertal hair, fat deposits) but play no direct part in reproduction.

Hormonal Changes of Puberty

It is generally accepted that the events of puberty are caused by hormonal influences and controlled by the anterior pituitary (adenohypophysis) in response to a stimulus from the hypothalamus. Stimulation of the gonads has a dual function: (1) production and release of gametes—production of sperm in the male and maturation and release of ova in the female—and (2) secretion of sex-appropriate hormones—estrogen and progesterone from the ovaries (female) and testosterone from the testes (male).

Sex Hormones. Sex hormones are secreted by the ovaries, testes, and adrenals; they are produced in varying amounts by both sexes throughout the life span. The adrenal cortex is responsible for the small amounts secreted before the pubescent years, but the sex hormone production that accompanies maturation of the gonads is responsible for the variety of biologic changes observed during puberty.

Estrogen, the feminizing hormone, is found in low quantities during childhood; it is secreted in slowly increasing amounts until about age 11 years. In males this gradual increase continues through maturation. In females the onset of estrogen production in the ovary causes a pronounced increase that continues until about 3 years after the onset of menstruation, at which time it reaches a maximum level that continues throughout the reproductive life of the female.

Androgens, the masculinizing hormones, are also secreted in small and gradually increasing amounts up to about 7 or 9 years of age, at which time there is a more rapid increase in both sexes, especially boys, until about age 15 years. These hormones appear to be responsible for most of the rapid

Judy Rollins, MS, RN, revised this chapter.

 For additional information, please view "Growth and Development" in *Whaley and Wong's Pediatric Nursing Video Series,* St Louis, 1996, Mosby; (800) 426-4545.

CULTURAL AWARENESS
The Adolescent Years

Other societies in which adolescence is seen as part of the life cycle may have ideas very different from American culture about how the adolescent years are to be spent. For example, some societies discourage contact between adolescent males and females. Sexual experimentation is outlawed, and all grown children, males and females, remain in the home of their parents until they wed. In America we tend to believe that the way our culture is organized is the way all cultures are or should be organized, but of course this is not so. Each society is unique. The way we describe adolescence, the way we experience it, and the predisposition of our adolescents toward violence are peculiar to our American culture.

Modified from Prothrow-Stith D: *Deadly consequences: how violence is destroying our teenage population and a plan to begin solving the problem,* New York, 1993, HarperCollins.

USUAL SEQUENCE OF MATURATIONAL CHANGES

Girls	Boys
Breast changes	Enlargement of testicles
Rapid increase in height and weight	Growth of pubic hair, axillary hair, hair on upper lip, hair on face and elsewhere on body (facial hair usually appears about 2 years after appearance of pubic hair)
Growth of pubic hair	
Appearance of axillary hair	
Menstruation (usually begins 2 years after first signs)	Rapid increase in height
Abrupt deceleration of linear growth	Changes in the larynx and consequently the voice (usually take place along with growth of penis)
	Nocturnal emissions
	Abrupt deceleration of linear growth

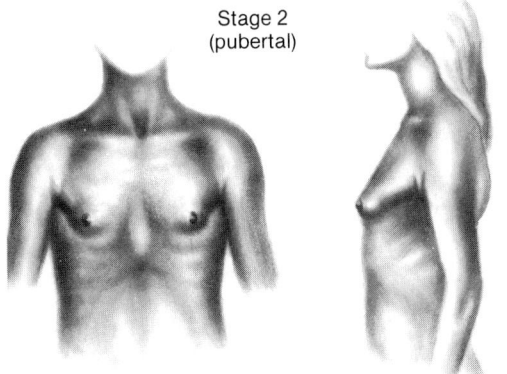

Stage 2
(pubertal)

Breast bud stage—small area of elevation around papilla; enlargement of areolar diameter

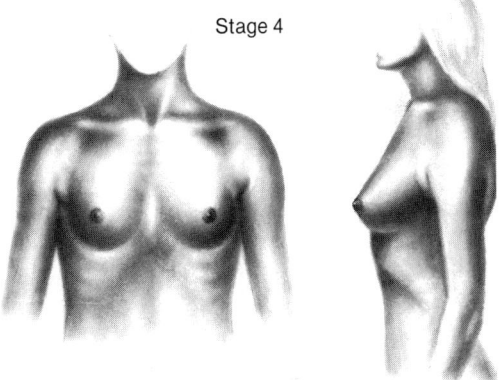

Stage 4

Projection of areola and papilla to form a secondary mound (may not occur in all girls)

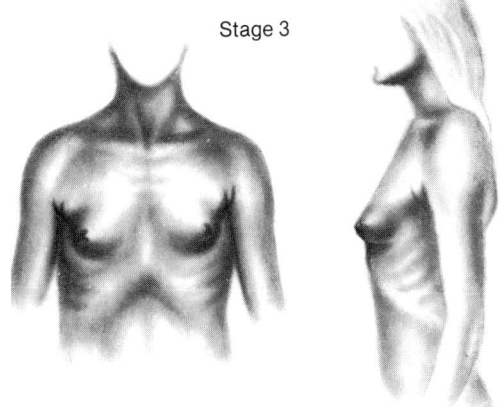

Stage 3

Further enlargement of breast and areola with no separation of their contours

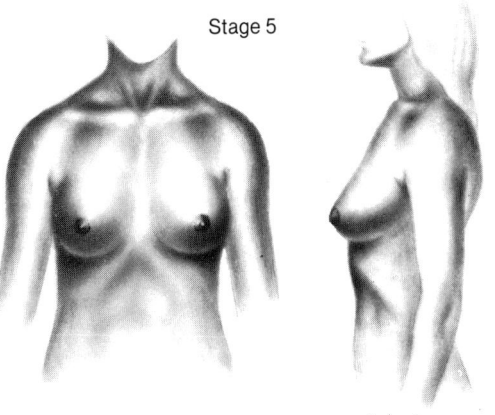

Stage 5

Mature configuration; projection of papilla only caused by recession of areola into general contour

FIG. 16-1. Development of the breast in girls—average age span, 11 to 13 years. Stage 1 (prepubertal—elevation of papilla only) is not shown. (Modified from Marshall WA, Tanner JM: *Arch Dis Child* 44:291, 1969; and Daniel WA, Paulshock BZ: *Patient Care,* May 13, 1979, pp 122-124.)

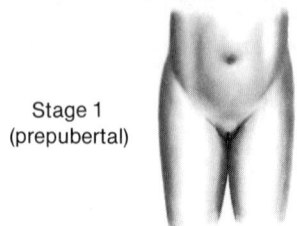

Stage 1
(prepubertal)

No pubic hair; essentially the same as
during childhood; no distinction between hair
on pubis and over the abdomen

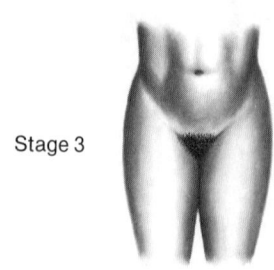

Stage 3

Hair darker, coarser, and curly and spread sparsely
over entire pubis in the typical female triangle

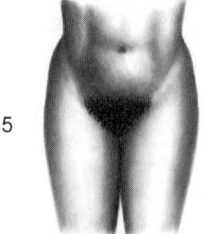

Stage 5

Hair adult in quantity, type, and pattern
with spread to inner aspect of thighs

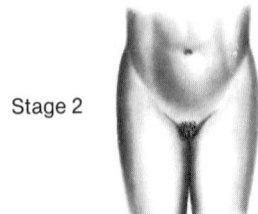

Stage 2

Sparse growth of long, straight, downy, and
slightly pigmented hair extending along labia;
between stages 2 and 3 begins to appear on pubis

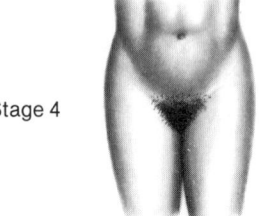

Stage 4

Pubic hair denser, curled, and adult in distribution
but less abundant and restricted to the pubic area

FIG. 16-2. Growth in pubic hair in girls—average age span for stages 2 through 5, 11 to 14 years. (Modified from Marshall WA, Tanner JM: *Arch Dis Child* 44:291, 1969; and Daniel WA, Paulshock BZ: *Patient Care*, May 13, 1979, pp 122-124.)

growth changes of early adolescence. With the onset of testicular function, the level of androgens (principally **testosterone**) in males increases over that in females and continues to increase until a maximum is attained at maturity.

Sexual Maturation

The visible evidence of sexual maturation is achieved in orderly sequence, and the state of maturity can be estimated on the basis of the appearance of these external manifestations. The age at which these changes are observed and the time required to progress from one stage to another may vary considerably among children. The time from the appearance of breast buds to full maturity may be 1½ to 6 years for adolescent girls; it may take 2 to 5 years for male genitalia to reach adult size. The stages of the development of secondary sex characteristics and genital development have been defined as a guide for estimating sexual maturity and are frequently referred to as the *Tanner stages*. The usual sequence of appearance of maturational changes is presented in the box on p. 467.

Sexual Maturation in Girls.   In most girls the initial indication of puberty is the appearance of breast buds, an event known as *thelarche,* which occurs between 9 and 13½ years (Fig. 16-1). This is followed in approximately 2 to 6 months by growth of pubic hair on the mons pubis, known as *adrenarche* (Fig. 16-2). In a minority of normally developing girls, however, pubic hair may precede breast development.

The initial appearance of menstruation, or *menarche,* occurs about 2 years after the appearance of the first pubescent changes, approximately 9 months after attainment of peak

height velocity and 3 months after attainment of peak weight velocity. Menarche has been related to a critical gain in body fat content (more fat content, earlier menarche), although this is controversial. The normal age range of menarche is usually 10½ to 15 years, with the average age being 12 years, 9½ months for North American girls. Initial menstrual periods are usually scanty, irregular, and anovulatory. Ovulation and regular menstrual periods usually occur 6 to 14 months after menarche. Girls may be considered to have *pubertal delay* if breast development has not occurred by age 13 or if menarche has not occurred within 4 years of the onset of breast development.

Sexual Maturation in Boys.   The first pubescent changes in boys are testicular enlargement accompanied by thinning, reddening, and increased looseness of the scrotum (Fig. 16-3). These events usually occur between 9½ and 14 years of age. Early puberty is also characterized by the initial appearance of pubic hair. Penile enlargement begins, and testicular enlargement and pubic hair growth continue throughout midpuberty. During this period there is also increasing muscularity, early voice changes, and development of early facial hair. Temporary breast enlargement and tenderness, *gynecomastia,* are common during midpuberty, occurring in up to one third of boys (see Critical Thinking Exercise on p. 470). The spurts in height and weight occur concurrently toward the end of midpuberty. For most boys, breast enlargement disappears within 2 years. By late puberty, there is a definite increase in the length and width of the penis, testicular enlargement continues, and first ejaculation occurs. Axillary hair develops, and facial hair extends to cover the anterior neck. Final voice changes occur secondary to the growth of

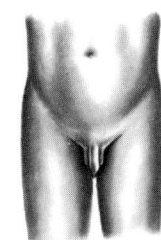

Stage 1 (prepubertal)

No pubic hair; essentially the same as
during childhood; no distinction between hair
on pubis and over the abdomen

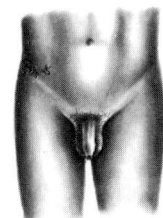

Stage 2 (pubertal)

Initial enlargement of scrotum and testes; reddening
and textural changes of scrotal skin; sparse growth of long,
straight, downy, and slightly pigmented hair at base of penis

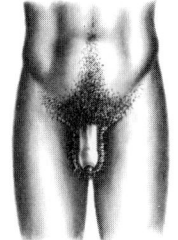

Stage 5

Testes, scrotum, and penis adult in size and shape;
hair adult in quantity and type with spread to inner
surface of thighs

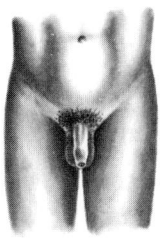

Stage 3

Initial enlargement of penis, mainly in length; testes
and scrotum further enlarged; hair darker, coarser,
and curly and spread sparsely over entire pubis

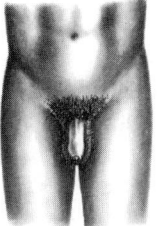

Stage 4

Increased size of penis with growth in diameter and
development of glans; glans larger and broader; scrotum
darker; pubic hair more abundant with curling but
restricted to pubic area

FIG. 16-3. Developmental stages of secondary sex characteristics and genital development in boys—average age span, 12 to 16 years. (Modified from Marshall WA, Tanner JM: *Arch Dis Child* 44:291, 1969; and Daniel WA, Paulshock BZ: *Patient Care*, May 13, 1979, pp 122-124.)

the larynx. Concerns about *pubertal delay* should be considered for boys who exhibit no enlargement of the testes or scrotal changes by ages 13½ to 14, or if genital growth is not complete 4 years after the testicles begin to enlarge.

Physical Growth

A constant phenomenon associated with sexual maturation is a dramatic increase in growth. The final 20% to 25% of height is achieved during puberty, and most of this growth occurs during a 24- to 36-month period—the adolescent *growth spurt.* This accelerated growth occurs in all children but, as in other areas of development, is highly variable in age of onset, duration, and extent. The growth spurt begins earlier in girls, usually between ages 9½ and 14½ years; on the average it begins between ages 10½ and 16 years in boys. During this period the average boy will gain 10 to 30 cm (4 to 12 inches) in height and 7 to 30 kg (15 to 65 pounds) in weight; the average girl, in whom the growth spurt is slower and less extensive, will gain 5 to 20 cm (2 to 8 inches) in height and 7 to 25 kg (15 to 55 pounds) in weight. Growth in height typically ceases 2 to 2½ years after menarche in girls and at age 18 to 20 years in boys.

This increase in size is acquired in a characteristic sequence of changes. Growth in length of the extremities and neck precedes growth in other areas, and since these parts are first to reach adult length, the hands and feet appear larger than normal during adolescence. Increases in hip and chest breadth take place in a few months, followed several months later by an increase in shoulder width. These changes are followed by increases in length of the trunk and depth of the chest. This sequence of changes is responsible for the characteristic long-legged, gawky appearance of the early adolescent child.

Sex Differences in General Growth Patterns. Sex differences in general growth and distribution patterns are apparent in skeletal growth, muscle mass, adipose tissue, and skin. Skeletal growth differences between boys and girls are apparently a function of hormonal effects at puberty and are evident primarily in limb length. The earlier cessation of growth in girls is caused by epiphyseal unity under the potent effect of estrogen secretion, and the hormonal effect on female bone growth is much stronger than the similar effect of testosterone in males. In boys the prolonged growth period before puberty and the less rapid epiphyseal closure are reflected in their greater overall height and longer arms and

CRITICAL THINKING EXERCISE
Embarrassing Body Changes

Twelve-year-old Sam and his mother arrive at the clinic for Sam's checkup for a health clearance to attend summer camp. "What are you looking forward to most about going to camp, Sam?" you ask. "Nothing," Sam replies. "I don't even want to go."

"Sam's just getting lazy," says his mother. "His physical education teacher called the other night and said that Sam has used every excuse in the world to get out of participating in class." She continues: "He even wants to quit the swim team. All he wants to do is sit around and watch TV and eat. Look at him. His laziness and all the food he eats are beginning to show." You glance over at Sam and see a slight pouch and enlarged breasts through his T-shirt. Which of the following would be your most appropriate response?

1. "Sam, you are at a time in your life when you want and really need to eat, but if you don't stay active, you will become overweight."
2. "Sam, I see that you have something in common with many boys your age. On the way to becoming a man, some boys get enlarged and tender breasts for a short time."
3. "Sam, I see why you don't want to go to camp; you're afraid the other kids will make fun of you."
4. "Sam, you should go to camp. It will be lots of fun and you will be able to work off some of the extra pounds you've gained."

Answer two is the most appropriate response. Sam has gynecomastia. You surmise that he is embarrassed or perhaps is even being teased about the condition. He needs to remove his shirt—further exposing his "problem"—during swim team practice or meets and during showers after physical education classes. This is likely why he has avoided both activities and is not looking forward to attending summer camp. The other three answers deny Sam the information he needs to adapt to this troublesome but temporary change in his body.

lows a less orderly pattern. There may be a transient increase in subcutaneous fat just before the skeletal growth spurt, especially in boys. This is followed 1 to 2 years later by a modest to marked decrease, again more marked in boys. Later, variable amounts of fat are deposited to fill out and contour the mature physique in patterns characteristic of the adolescent's sex, particularly in the regions over the thighs, hips, and buttocks and around the breast tissue.

Hormonal influences during puberty cause an acceleration in growth and maturation of the skin and its structural appendages. Sebaceous glands become extremely active at this time, especially those on the genitals and in the "flush areas" of the body (i.e., face, neck, shoulders, upper back, and chest). This increased activity and the structural nature of the glands are extremely important in the pathogenesis of a common problem of puberty: acne (see Chapter 30). The eccrine sweat glands, present almost everywhere on the human skin, become fully functional and respond to emotional as well as thermal stimulation. Heavy sweating appears to be more pronounced in boys than in girls. The apocrine sweat glands, nonfunctional in childhood, reach secretory capacity during puberty. Unlike the eccrine sweat glands, the apocrine glands are limited in distribution and grow in conjunction with hair follicles in the axillae, around the areola of the breast, around the umbilicus, on the external auditory canal, and in the genital and anal regions. Apocrine glands secrete a thick substance as a result of emotional stimulation that, when acted on by surface bacteria, becomes highly odoriferous.

Body hair assumes very characteristic distribution patterns and changes texture during puberty. Under the influence of gonadal and adrenal androgens, hair coarsens, darkens, and lengthens at sites related to secondary sex characteristics. Pubic and axillary hair appears in both sexes, although pubic hair is more extensive in males than in females. Beard, mustache, and body hair on the chest, upward along the linea alba, and sometimes on other areas (e.g., back and shoulders) appears in males and is androgen dependent. Extremity hair appears in varying amounts in both males and females but is also more prolific in the male.

Physiologic Changes

A number of physiologic functions are altered in response to some of the pubertal changes. The size and strength of the heart, blood volume, and systolic blood pressure increase, whereas the pulse rate and basal heat production decrease (see inside back cover). Blood volume, which has increased steadily during childhood, reaches a higher value in boys than in girls, a fact that may be related to the increased muscle mass in pubertal boys. Adult values are reached for all formed elements of the blood. Respiratory rate and basal metabolic rate, decreasing steadily throughout childhood, reach the adult rate in adolescence. Respiratory volume and vital capacity are increased, and to a far greater extent in males than in females. During this period, physiologic responses to exercise change drastically: performance improves, especially in boys, and the body is able to make the physiologic adjustments needed for normal functioning after exercise is completed. These capabilities are a result of the increased size and strength of muscles and the increased level of cardiac, respiratory, and metabolic functioning.

legs. Other skeletal differences are increased shoulder width in boys and broader hip development in girls.

Hypertrophy of the laryngeal mucosa and enlargement of the larynx and vocal cords occur in both boys and girls to produce voice changes. Girls' voices become slightly deeper and considerably fuller, but the effect in boys is striking. The "change of voice" in adolescent boys is one of the most noticeable traits of puberty, with the voice often shifting uncontrollably from deep to high tones in the middle of a sentence.

Growth of lean body mass, principally muscle, which tends to occur after the bone growth spurt, takes place steadily during adolescence. Lean body mass is both quantitatively and qualitatively greater in males than in females at comparable stages of pubertal development. Muscle development, under the influence of androgenic hormones, increases steadily. Muscles become remarkably well developed in boys, whereas in girls, muscle mass increase is proportionate to general tissue growth.

Nonlean body mass, primarily fat, is also increased but fol-

PSYCHOSOCIAL DEVELOPMENT

Developing a Sense of Identity (Erikson)

Traditional psychosocial theory holds that the developmental crisis of adolescence leads to the formation of a sense of identity (Erikson, 1963). Throughout childhood, individuals have been going through the process of identification as they concentrate on various parts of the body at specific times. During infancy children identify themselves as being separate from the mother; during early childhood they establish a gender-role identification with the appropriate-sex parent; and in later childhood they establish who they are in relation to others. In adolescence they come to see themselves as distinct individuals, somehow unique and separate from every other individual.

The early period of adolescence begins with the onset of puberty and extends to relative physical and emotional stability at or near graduation from high school. During this time the adolescent is faced with the crisis of *group identity vs alienation.* In the period that follows, the individual hopes to attain autonomy from the family and develop a sense of *personal identity* as opposed to *role diffusion.* A sense of group identity appears to be essential as a prelude to a sense of personal identity. Young adolescents must resolve questions concerning relationships with a peer group before they are able to resolve questions about who they are in relation to family and society.

Group Identity. During the early stage of adolescence the pressure to belong to a group is intensified. Teenagers find it essential to have a group to which they feel they can belong and that provides them with status. Belonging to a crowd helps adolescents to define the differences between themselves and their parents. They dress as the group dresses and wear makeup and hairstyles according to group criteria, all of which are different from those of the parental generation. Language, music, and dancing reflect a culture that is exclusive to the adolescent. When adults begin to emulate these fashions and interests, the style changes immediately. The evidence of adolescent conformity to the peer group and nonconformity to the adult group provides teenagers with a frame of reference in which they can display their own self-assertion while they reject the identity of their parents' generation. To be different is to be unaccepted and alienated from the group.

Individual Identity. The quest for personal identity is part of the ongoing identification process. As youngsters establish identity within a group, they are also attempting to incorporate multiple body changes into a concept of the self. Body awareness is part of self-awareness, and for some time the adolescent will engage in assimilating the self represented by this dimension. In this search for identity, adolescents consider the relationships that have developed between themselves and others in the past, as well as the directions they hope to be able to take in the future.

Significant others hold certain expectations for the behavior of the adolescent. Often these expectations or demands are persistent enough to result in certain decisions that might be made differently or not at all if the individual could be solely responsible for identity formation. It is all too easy to slip into the roles that are expected by these external influences without incorporating personal goals or questioning these decisions in relation to the developing personality. Thus individuals may become what parents or others wish them to be based on these premature decisions. Also, young persons might form a negative identity when society or their culture provides them with a self-image that is contrary to the values of the community. Labels such as "juvenile delinquent," "hood," or "failure" are applied to certain adolescents, who then accept and live up to these labels with behaviors that validate and strengthen them.

The process of evolving a personal identity is time-consuming and fraught with periods of confusion, depression, and discouragement. Determining an identity and a place in the world is a critical and perilous feature of adolescence (see Critical Thinking Exercise). However, as the pieces are gradually shifted and settled into place, a positive identity eventually emerges from the confusion. Role diffusion results when the individual is unable to formulate a satisfactory identity from the multiplicity of aspirations, roles, and identifications.

Sex-role Identity. Adolescence is the time for consolidation of a sex-role identity. During early adolescence the peer group begins to communicate some expectations regarding heterosexual relationships, and as development

---

CRITICAL **THINKING** **EXERCISE**

Discussing the Future

Jeremy, age 17, will be graduating from high school in the spring. His mother, a single parent, tells you that she is concerned because graduation is quickly approaching and Jeremy has made no plans for what he will do with his life after graduation. Whenever Jeremy mentions the topic, his mother tells him, "This is what you must do," and begins to outline the steps he must take. Jeremy just walks away. She asks, "What should I do?" Which of the following would be your most appropriate advice to Jeremy's mother?

1. "Think about Jeremy's interests and what he has been successful doing in the past. Arrange for him to speak to someone whose career builds on those interests."
2. "Continue to tell him what he must do. Eventually you will get through to him, and he will listen."
3. "Be open and available to him. Tell him what you think, but not what to do."
4. "You are wise to be concerned. We need to arrange some counseling for Jeremy."

The correct answer at this stage is three. Most adolescents want adult guidance and help, and messages are more likely to be heard if presented in an open-ended, nonjudgmental, nondictatorial fashion. Teenagers are unlikely to discuss their concerns on a timetable. Parents create the time and space and then wait. Parents who are available and willing to listen generally find that their adolescents are eager to talk. Answer one could be a good second step if Jeremy and his mother explore his interests together. Answer two is disrespectful to Jeremy, has not worked in the past, and likely will not work in the future. Answer four may be necessary at a later time if other strategies fail.

progresses, adolescents encounter expectations for mature sex-role behavior from both peers and adults. Expectations such as these vary from culture to culture, among geographic areas, and among socioeconomic groups.

Emotionality.   Adolescents vacillate in their emotional states and between considerable maturity and childlike behavior. One minute they are exuberant and enthusiastic; the next minute they are depressed and withdrawn. Unpredictable, but essentially normal, outbursts of primitive behavior appear as the teenager loses control over instinctual drives. As the tension is relieved, emotion is brought under control and individuals retreat in order to review what has happened, to attempt to master their anger, and in the overall process to grow in their ability to control their emotions and gain from the new experience. Because of these "tantrums" and mood swings, adolescents are frequently labeled as unstable, inconsistent, and unpredictable. Little things can cause an emotional upheaval and, depending on the teenager's interpretation, can mean a great deal.

Teenagers are better able to control their emotions in later adolescence. They can approach problems more calmly and rationally, and although they are still subject to periods of depression, their feelings are less vulnerable and they begin to demonstrate the more mature emotions of later adolescence. Whereas early adolescents react immediately and emotionally, older adolescents can control their emotions until socially acceptable times and places for expression present themselves. They are still subject to heightened emotion, and when it is expressed, their behavior reflects feelings of insecurity, tension, and indecision.

COGNITIVE DEVELOPMENT (PIAGET)

Cognitive thinking culminates with the capacity for *abstract thinking.* This stage, the period of *formal operations,* is Piaget's fourth and last stage. Adolescents are no longer restricted to the real and actual, which was typical of the period of concrete thought; they are also concerned with the possible. They now think beyond the present. Without having to center attention on the immediate situation, they can imagine a sequence of events that might occur, such as college and occupational possibilities; how things might change in the future, such as relationships with parents; and the consequences of their actions, such as dropping out of school. At this time their thoughts can be influenced by logical principles rather than just their own perceptions and experiences. They now become increasingly capable of scientific reasoning and formal logic.

Adolescents are capable of mentally manipulating more than two categories of variables at the same time. For example, they can consider the relationship between speed, distance, and time in planning a trip. They can detect logical consistency or inconsistency in a set of statements and evaluate a system or set of values in a more analytic manner. For instance, they question the parent who insists on honesty in the youngster but at the same time cheats on an income tax report or expense account.

Young people are now able to think about both their own thinking and the thinking of others. They wonder what opinion others have of them, and they are increasingly able to imagine the thoughts of others. With this capacity comes the ability to differentiate between others' thoughts and their own and to interpret thoughts of others more accurately. Thus they are able to understand that few concepts are absolute or independent of other influencing factors. As they come to know that other cultures and communities have different norms and standards from their own, it becomes easier to accept members of these other cultures, and the decision to behave in their own culture in an accepted manner becomes a more conscious commitment to that culture.

MORAL DEVELOPMENT (KOHLBERG)

Whereas younger children merely accept the decisions or point of view of adults, adolescents, to gain autonomy from adults, must substitute their own set of morals and values. When old principles are challenged but new and independent values have not yet emerged to take their place, young people search for a moral code that preserves their personal integrity and guides their behavior, especially in the face of strong pressure to violate the old beliefs. Their decisions involving moral dilemmas must be based on an *internalized set of moral principles* that provides them with the resources to evaluate the demands of the situation and to plan a course of action that is consistent with their ideals.

Late adolescence is characterized by a serious questioning of existing moral values and their relevance to society and the individual. Adolescents can easily take the role of another. They understand duty and obligation based on reciprocal rights of others, as well as the concept of justice that is founded on making amends for misdeeds and repairing or replacing what has been spoiled by wrongdoing. However, they seriously question established moral codes, often as a result of observing that adults verbally ascribe to a code but do not adhere to it.

SPIRITUAL DEVELOPMENT

As youngsters move toward independence from parents and other authorities, some begin to question the values and ideals of their families. Others cling to these values as a stable element in their lives as they struggle with the conflicts of this turbulent period. Adolescents need to work out these conflicts for themselves, but they also need support from authority figures and/or peers for their resolution. Often the peer group is more influential than parents, although values acquired during the formative years are usually maintained.

Adolescents are capable of understanding abstract concepts and of interpreting analogies and symbols. They are able to empathize, philosophize, and think logically. Most are searching for ideals and speculate about illogical statements and conflicting ideologies. Their tendency toward introspection and emotional intensity at this age often makes it difficult for others to know what they are thinking. They tend to keep their thoughts private, fearing that no one will understand these feelings that they perceive to be unique and special. However, they may reveal deep spiritual concerns. They need support and encouragement in their struggle for understanding and the freedom to question without censure.

Young people may reject formal worship services but engage in individual worship in the privacy of their room. They may need to explore the concept of the existence of God. Comparing their religion with that of others may result in their questioning their own beliefs but ultimately results in formulating and solidifying their spirituality.

SOCIAL DEVELOPMENT

To achieve full maturity, adolescents must free themselves from family domination and define an identity independent of parental authority. However, this process is fraught with ambivalence on the part of both teenagers and their parents. Adolescents want to grow up and to be free of parental restraints, but they are fearful as they try to comprehend the responsibilities that are linked with independence. Feelings of immortality and exemption from the consequences of risk-taking behavior, although viewed as negative, can serve an important developmental function at this time. These feelings can give adolescents the courage to separate from their parents and become independent (Prothrow-Stith, 1993). Part of this emancipation involves developing social relationships outside the family that help teenagers identify their role in society. Adolescence is a time of intense sociability and often a time of equally intense loneliness. Acceptance by peers, a few close friends, and the secure love of a supportive family are requisites for the interpersonal maturation process.

Relationships with Parents

During adolescence the parent-child relationship changes from one of protection-dependency to one of *mutual affection and equality.* The process of achieving independence often involves turmoil and ambiguity as both parent and adolescent learn to play new roles and work toward this end while, at the same time, resolving the often painful series of rifts essential to establishing the ultimate relationships.

Most of the behavior observed in the adolescent is related to the struggle for independence and the external restrictions and checks that are placed on this spontaneous maturation process. On the one hand, adolescents are accepted as maturing preadults. They are allowed privileges heretofore denied, and they are provided with increasing responsibilities. On the other hand, because of their unpredictability and insecurity in evaluating situations and making sound judgments, they must conform to regulations and restrictions set by adults. This state of affairs is particularly exemplified by the struggle between parents and adolescents concerning the nightly curfew.

As teenagers assert their rights for grown-up privileges, they frequently create tensions within the home. They resist parental control, and conflicts can arise from almost any situation or any subject. Some of the favorite topics of dispute include use of the telephone, manners, dress, chores and duties, homework, disrespectful behavior, friendships, dating, money, automobiles, drinking and/or drugs, and time schedules. Present in these areas of conflict are the overriding argument that "Everyone else has one" or is allowed the desired item or privilege and the ever-present assertions that "You don't understand me or trust me" and "You always treat me like a baby." Spoken or unspoken, parents' reactions consist of "Is this all the thanks I get for what I have done, or am doing, for you?"

The teenager's earliest attempts to achieve emancipation from parental controls are manifested in a period of rejection

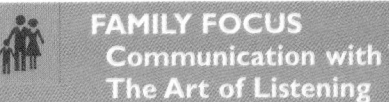

FAMILY FOCUS
Communication with Teens:
The Art of Listening

Conflicts between parents and their adolescents are often a result of a very natural characteristic of parenthood: the desire to protect one's offspring—from harm or from simply doing something "stupid" or embarrassing or something they may later regret. Teens sometimes "bounce" their thoughts and ideas off adults. At times they really want some feedback; at other times they simply want to elicit a reaction.

I found it easy to listen openly, thoughtfully, and without interrupting when my teenagers' friends discussed troublesome topics. However, one day, when one of my own teenagers had a similar conversation with me, the parent part kicked in. I felt responsible and spoke my piece on the spot. This brought communication to a halt and resulted in defensiveness. It was a long time before my child tried to talk to me about anything controversial again.

The next time one of my teenagers started a similar conversation, I decided to try to trick myself. Throughout the entire conversation, I told myself over and over again to act as if this were not my teenager, but rather someone else's child. I found this actually worked quite well and I was able to listen without interrupting. I continued to use the system, sometimes with more success than at other times.

Mother of four

of the parents. Adolescents are critical, argumentative, and generally remote with both parents. They absent themselves from home and family activities and spend an increasing amount of time with the peer group. They confide less in their parents. This rejection is not consistent, however, and varies with mood changes.

With advancing adolescence, teenagers become more competent, and with this competence comes a need for more autonomy. However, although they are psychologically better prepared for independence, they are often thwarted in their efforts by lack of money or by other parental barriers. Much conflict arises in relation to the teenager's outside activities and the elements of privacy and trust. Too many parents believe that they must know all their adolescent's activities and feelings; they may go through the teenager's belongings in an attempt to find out what the youngster is doing. However, to gain the respect and trust of adolescents, parents must respect their youngster's privacy, as well as show an honest and sincere interest in what the adolescent believes and feels (see Family Focus box).

The recent trends in society in terms of equality and relaxation of previous moral standards have made the adjustments of teenagers and parents increasingly difficult. The so-called generation gap is widening in relation to a number of attitudes, values, and beliefs. Parents can no longer find guidance from their own experiences in understanding the needs of today's teenagers.

Relationships with Peers

Although parents remain the primary influence in their lives, for the majority of teenagers, peers assume a more significant role in adolescence than they did during childhood. The peer group serves as a strong support to teenagers, individually and collectively, providing them with a sense of belonging and a feeling of strength and power. It forms that transitional world between dependence and autonomy.

Peer Group. Adolescents are usually social, gregarious, and group minded. Thus the peer group has an intense influence on adolescents' self-evaluation and behavior. To gain acceptance by a group, younger teenagers tend to conform completely in such things as mode of dress, hairstyle, taste in music, and vocabulary, often at the expense of individuality and self-assertion. The teenagers' entire being is measured by the reactions of their peers.

The school is psychologically important to adolescents as a focus of social life. Teenagers usually distribute themselves into a relatively predictable social hierarchy. They know to which groups they and others belong.

Within the larger groups are smaller, distinct, and rather exclusive crowds or cliques of selected close friends who are emotionally attached to each other. The selection is based on common tastes, interests, and background. Although cliques may become formalized, most remain informal and small. However, each has an identifying feature that proclaims its difference from others and its solidarity within itself, in much the same manner as the adolescent generation as a whole sets itself apart from the adult generation. Cliques are usually made up of one sex, and girls tend to be more cliquish than boys and to have a greater need for close friendships (Fig. 16-4). Within the intimacy of the group, adolescents gain support in learning about themselves, consideration for the feelings of others, and increased ego development and self-reliance.

To belong is of utmost importance; thus adolescents behave in a way that will ensure their establishment in a group. Adolescents are highly susceptible to social approval, acceptance, and demands. To be ignored or criticized by peers creates feelings of inferiority, inadequacy, and incompetence.

Best Friends. Personal friendships of the one-on-one variety usually develop between same-sex adolescents. This relationship is closer and more stable than it is in middle childhood, and it is important in the quest for identity. A best friend is the best audience on whom to try out possible roles and identities that an adolescent wants to test. Best friends may try a role together, each providing support for the other. Each cares about what the other thinks and feels. Since a sense of intimacy grows within a permanent relationship, the stability of this same-sex friendship is an important link in the progress toward an intimate heterosexual relationship in young adulthood.

Heterosexual Relationships

During adolescence, relationships with members of the opposite sex take on new importance (see Family Focus box). Although there seems to be a trend toward earlier dating, on the *average,* dating activities begin in the seventh and eighth grades and are usually "crowd" dates at organized school functions. For example, a group of girls just happens to be around a certain group of boys at most activities. During high school, crowd dates are still popular, but now there is more pairing off of couples. Double-dating and then single-pair dating follow group dating. Most adolescents are dating to some degree by the time they leave high school.

The type and degree of seriousness of heterosexual relationships vary. The initial stage is usually noncommittal, extremely mobile, and seldom characterized by any deep romantic attachments. Crushes, those strong feelings of attachment to an important or well-liked adult in the youngster's life who embodies the qualities considered most valuable by the adolescent, are common in early adolescence; they constitute one of the earliest "love" attachments.

During early midadolescence, as their sexual capacity is evolving, young boys may feel the need to test the power of their sexuality by numerous exploits and conquests. It may

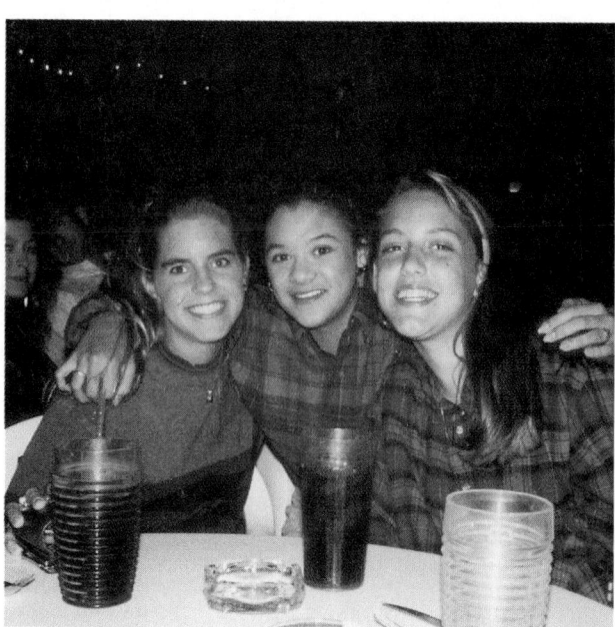

FIG. 16-4. Teenagers like to gather in small groups.

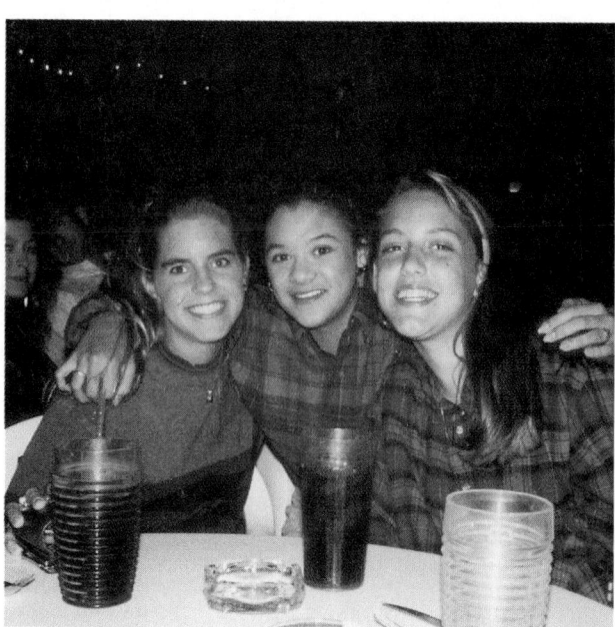

FAMILY FOCUS
Reflecting on What Teenage Boys Want in Girls

Jimmy, 17 years old: "Someone who's nice."

Kurt, 17 years old: "It's how they act, how they treat you."

Jamil, 18 years old: "Sometimes looks get you talking to the girl. But you wouldn't talk to a good-looking girl if she was really rude to you. And you probably would talk to a girl who isn't that good-looking but was nice to you."

Matt, 16 years old: "You wouldn't usually go talk to an ugly girl."

Kurt: "I met my girlfriend when I was in seventh grade, but I wasn't attracted to her at all. Then, as we became friends, I got really attracted to her—the way she acted, her personality, her sense of humor. And then I thought she started to look really pretty."

Matt: "I just like pretty girls. I can't do anything about it. I would always go and talk to the pretty girl first."

Jamil: "The girls do the same thing, though. They want the perfect guy. They can be standing there talking to me, and then when someone more popular walks down the hall—oh, well, let's forget me and go talk to the more popular guy."

From Minton L: Fresh voices, *Parade Magazine,* p 15, Feb 4, 1996.

be a response to inner sexual pressures or a need to conform to group expectations. With advancing adolescence and a more firm sexual identity, steady dating and boy-girl love relationships with deeper commitment become more numerous. The relationship continues until misunderstanding or boredom ends the association, and the process is often repeated with another partner.

Authorities disagree regarding the value of early opposite-sex relationships in the development of a sexual identity. Some believe that longer same-sex relationships are necessary to develop fully the characteristics of one's own sex, whereas others believe that dating provides adolescents with experience in human relationships, promotes social skills, and enhances their ability to choose a mate wisely (Fig. 16-5).

Sexual Activity. Because puberty occurs at earlier ages than it did a half-century ago, and since the line between sexuality and sex is blurred, sexual activity among adolescents is an area that must be addressed. Masturbatory activity usually begins at puberty. Although both genders engage in this behavior, it is more frequently reported by boys. Masturbation provides an opportunity for sexual self-exploration before development of regular social-sexual interaction with another individual. Participation in this behavior is greatly influenced by learned cultural attitudes, religion, and sex-role expectations (see also p. 477).

During adolescence, most youngsters indulge in kissing and petting, the traditional first steps in the sequence of heterosexual activity. In addition, a greater proportion of teenagers are sexually experienced with each successive year of adolescence. About one third of males and one fourth of females have had sexual intercourse by age 15; by the age of 18 or 19, three quarters of American youth have had sexual relations with another person (Seidman and Rieder, 1994).

Adolescents engage in sexual relationships for pleasurable sensations, to satisfy sexual drives, to satisfy curiosity, as a conquest, as an expression of some degree of affection, or from inability to withstand pressures to conform. Often the urge to belong to and gain reassurance from a group and the wish to really belong to someone provoke a series of increasingly

intimate physical contacts with a favored boyfriend or girl-friend, with each contact being more sexually provocative than the last. Eventually, sexual intercourse becomes established as a behavior pattern and a method for ensuring social participation—or even as an end in itself. Early dating can involve an adolescent pair in a close sexual relationship before they are ready for intimacy.

The current trend toward greater permissiveness regarding adolescent sexual behavior will undoubtedly have an effect on the adolescent developmental experience. However, the recent concern with transmission of human immuno-deficiency virus (HIV) may influence these sexually permissive attitudes. It has been predicted that attitudes toward sex will shift from a moral context to a predominantly health context within a few years. Unfortunately, many adolescents cling to the fallacy that heterosexual behaviors are "AIDS free."

Homosexuality in Adolescents

The development of homosexuality during childhood or adolescence has been greatly ignored and thought to be either a transient experience or a pathologic event. The pediatric community has recognized the special needs of these adolescents in order to foster a healthy transition during this period.

Confusion about sexual orientation is common in adolescence. However, most adolescents who participate in homosexual activity or have homosexual feelings do not become gay or lesbian adults (Friedman and Downey, 1994). Nurses need to recognize the potential for same-gender attraction and to be sensitive to the fact that not all youths will be involved in heterosexual relationships. Nurses need to evaluate their own attitudes and beliefs about homosexuality to determine their own comfort level in providing health care to gay or lesbian youths.

 In one study, 0.4% of junior and senior high-school students reported a homosexual identity. However, a greater percentage reported homosexual fantasies, attractions, and behaviors. These findings illustrate the complexities in assigning sexual orientation labels to adolescents (Remafedi and others, 1992).

In addition to all the normal tasks of adolescence, gay males and females have their own unique issues of identity formation. This process, which can begin as early as preadolescence, has been called *coming out* and does not refer to any particular event or time, but to a series of events that lead adolescents to establish an integrated sense of who they are.

Interests and Activities

During early adolescence the interests and activities of girls and boys are in rather sharp contrast. Boys spend much time in active outdoor sports or "just going out with the guys." They enjoy hobbies and clubs, and television and video or computer games take up much of their time. Girls and mixed-sex activities are of interest to boys but do not become prominent concerns until their development more nearly approaches that of the more rapidly maturing girls. As their bodies gain strength and size, "making the team" is a major concern for many youths, and a boy may spend an excessive amount of time in attempting to perfect athletic skills. The essential bicycle of middle childhood is replaced by the auto-

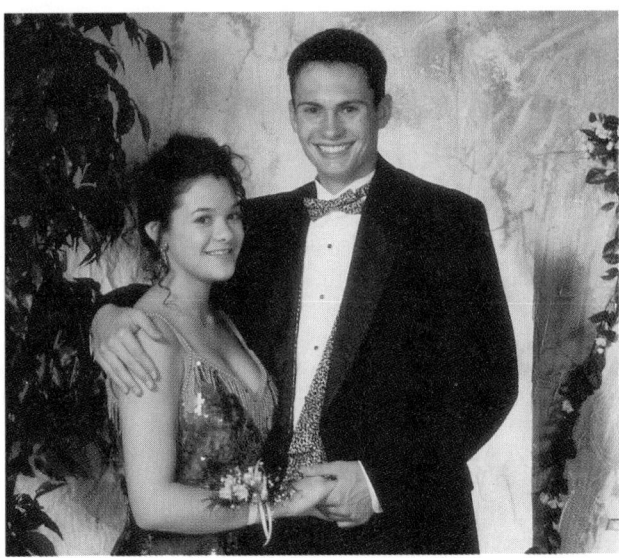

FIG. 16-5. Heterosexual friendships are characteristics of adolescence.

mobile, the symbol of status to the adolescent. If a car cannot be acquired, a motorcycle or motorbike is preferable to walking, riding the bus, or the humiliation of being chauffeured by a parent or sibling. Many boys avidly seek part-time employment, some because of economic necessity.

Although girls' leisure interests may involve outdoor activities, an increased interest in parties and social activities is evident. They may be interested in hobbies and volunteer activities, and many seek part-time jobs through necessity or to purchase more clothes and other teenage "necessities." They are avid conversationalists and spend much of their time in the company of other girls, talking, listening to music, and experimenting with makeup, hairstyles, and clothes. They enjoy shopping for clothes. Many of their thoughts and feelings are confessed in a diary.

Members of both sexes enjoy movies, rock concerts, dancing, and other communal activities and entertainment, including "cruising" favorite streets in automobiles and gathering in shopping malls. Teenage horror films attract teenagers in large numbers, and X-rated movie theaters are crowded with adolescents. With the availability of movies on videotape, adolescents congregate in small groups to watch films on home video players.

Dancing has always occupied a central place in the customs of many cultures. There is delight in physical movement and a feeling of relief that comes from release of tension in activity. Dancing can also serve as a means of expressing specific sexual and aggressive urges in symbolic form and action. Many of the popular dances have sexual overtones and erotic movements. At the same time, the structure of today's teen dances is such that the dancers seldom touch one another. In this way the urges can be expressed without the danger of close physical contact. Conversely, slow dancing provides a socially acceptable mode of close physical contact.

Reading is still a favorite occupation of many teenagers and may serve to satisfy some of their needs for vicarious experiences. Reading is more purposeful at this stage than at earlier ages, and adolescents read magazines, books, and comics.

Traditional television viewing may decline in adolescence, and many teenagers have a decided preference for music. Teenagers often are avidly addicted to the portable radios and cassette tape or compact disc (CD) players that accompany many of their other activities (e.g., studying, walking, working). Closely associated with the radio is the stereo, which assumes an important role in teenagers' lives. Much of their money may be spent on recorded media, which are collected in much the same way as books.

When they are not engaged in other activities, teenagers enjoy participating in "rap sessions" or in endless telephone conversations. The telephone provides that essential link between peers when they are physically removed from one another. It fulfills the need for flight from parents to peers without leaving the home. For boy-girl conversations, the telephone provides a way to experience closeness without the fear of complications that physical proximity may engender (Fig. 16-6).

Teenage interests and activities are subject to rapid change. Each succeeding "generation" of teenagers has its own peculiar characteristics, which are evidenced in behavior, vocabulary, dress, and other external manifestations that reflect

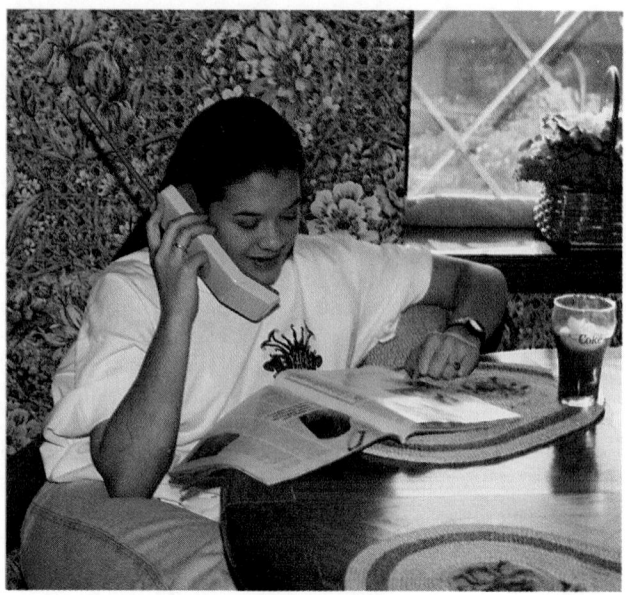

FIG. 16-6. The telephone, especially the portable phone, provides teenagers with hours of conversation with same-sex and opposite-sex friends.

and establish a clear line of separateness, although superficial, between the peer and the adult cultures. The rapidity with which these external trappings change is often astonishing.

DEVELOPMENT OF SELF-CONCEPT AND BODY IMAGE

The sudden growth that takes place in early adolescence creates feelings of confusion for adolescents. They have lost the security of a familiar body and feel a strangeness about their altered bodies. Consequently, they may try either to hide them or to advertise them, or they may alternate between the two extremes. Teenagers are acutely aware of their appearance as they begin to acquire images of themselves as adults, but they see discrepancies between their ideal and actual skills and abilities.

Adolescents are continually comparing themselves with their peers and making judgments about their own normality based on these observations. Pubertal children feel most comfortable when they are just like their friends and age-mates. Perceived defects or deviations from the group average are threatening to their idealized image. Any blemish is likely to be magnified out of proportion, and any delay of the visible evidence of maturity is cause for worry. Unfortunately, this is also the time when the hormonal effect of the sebaceous glands produces acne that creates problems for many youngsters. To the adolescent, even the most insignificant pimple may be viewed as a gross disfigurement; every blemish is a major catastrophe. The advent of chronic disease or a permanent physical disability has very special significance during adolescence and creates additional stresses for both the youngster with the condition and health workers.

It has been determined that the body image established during adolescence is the one that individuals retain throughout life. Much of adolescents' search for identity takes place before a mirror as they try to read from the reflected features just who they are and what they look like to other people. Adolescents practice facial expressions and postures, try out hair arrangements, worry about a pimple, and in other ways attempt to assess the best means to achieve a maximum effect—to reveal the "true self."

The self-concept becomes more differentiated as adolescents acquire a more complex picture of themselves, one that takes situational factors into account. The self-concept becomes more individuated, more distinct from the concepts of others. Whereas younger teens describe themselves in terms of similarities with peers, as adolescence advances, young people describe themselves more in terms of their special characteristics.

Boys' Responses to Puberty

The early adolescent increases in height and muscle mass are welcomed by the adolescent boy, whose growth, for several months, has lagged significantly behind that of his female age-mates. Although his more mature physique brings a highly valued increase in strength and more mature athletic skills, this rapid growth is uneven. When bones grow faster than muscles, muscles are taut and respond with quick, jerky movements; when muscles grow faster than bones, they become somewhat loose and sluggish. For a time he is awkward and uncoordinated.

The development of secondary sex characteristics, especially the growth of facial and body hair, has psychologic and social meaning for the adolescent boy. This, more than any other secondary characteristic, is associated with the masculine sex role, and the ritual act of shaving at the slightest evidence of growth is a way for the young boy to validate his identification with this role. Shaving also provides a legitimate excuse to gaze at and admire the broadening shoulders and altered features of his changing body image (Fig. 16-7).

The growth of the penis and testes creates some important problems for the adolescent male. Unlike the reproductive organs in the female, the male reproductive organs are readily visible and provide the boy with concrete evidence of his masculine character. He knows by the sensations localized within these organs that he is maturing. His reproductive organs become sensitive to sexual stimulation. Sexual feelings are directly related to the genitals, desire is urgent, and he

seeks rapid relief from pressure and tension through ejaculation.

The maturation of male genital function allows the male to produce seminal fluid. This may be released spontaneously as a nocturnal emission, or "wet dream." Spontaneous ejaculations are frequently puzzling, troublesome, and embarrassing events. Unless he has been prepared in advance for this eventuality, the boy often finds it difficult to seek an explanation from his parents. Therefore he turns to friends or reading material to gain information, or he may puzzle about the meaning in his own mind.

The frequency of erections is increased in response to a variety of stimuli, as is the frequency of sexual outlet through masturbation or intercourse. The opportunity for gratification of these genital urges through heterosexual expression is often limited by Western cultural standards; early premarital sexual involvement is fraught with many problems and conflicts. In addition, homosexual activities are not universally accepted by society. As a consequence, the teenage boy resorts to masturbation, manipulating the genitals for the purpose of ejaculation, to relieve himself of the accumulated pressures in his genital organs. Almost every boy masturbates alone or in relation to sexual experimentation with others of the same sex. However, this, too, is often associated with guilt and anxiety. Misconceptions still dominate the feelings of many people who believe masturbation to be evil, unmanly, or "not nice" and who attribute a wide assortment of ills to the practice. Adolescent males need to be reassured that engaging in the practice from time to time is normal and that it temporarily helps provide the young man with important information about how his body works and how adult physical sexuality and reproduction are accomplished.

Girls' Responses to Puberty

As girls begin the pubertal changes, they, too, become very body conscious. Because in girls the onset of puberty is almost 2 years in advance of that in boys, their initial reaction to increased height may be embarrassment as they find themselves towering above their male classmates. They worry about becoming too tall. Adolescent girls often slouch or adopt a hunched posture in an attempt to minimize this increased height, especially early-maturing girls, who are normally of above-average height. The increase in weight and the normal plumping of features with fat deposition are predominant concerns of the pubescent girl. They perceive these changes to be evidence of a tendency toward obesity; many attempt to avoid them by strict and rather faddish dieting. This poorly timed strategy can deprive their bodies of essential nutrients during a period of rapid body development.

The young girl is interested in her changing form and feminine curves. The average girl looks on her budding breasts with pleasure as a sign of approaching maturity and evidence of her femininity. She observes and may even measure the progress of her developing breasts and continually compares her own progress with that of her friends and classmates. She begins to wear a bra. Some girls are sensitive about their breast development and attempt to hide it, whereas others are delighted with their new figures and wear tight sweaters and clothes that accentuate their curves.

Development of some of the secondary sex characteristics may be less pleasing to girls than they are to boys, particu-

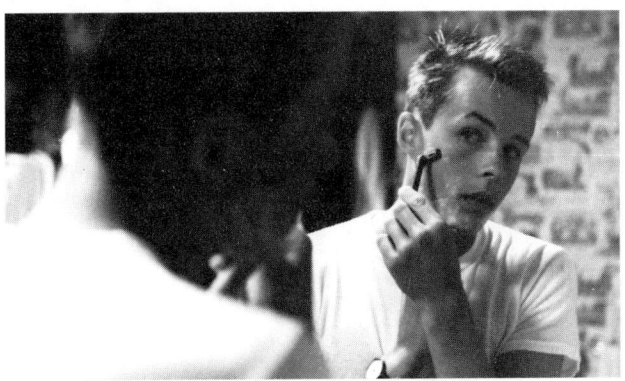

FIG. 16-7. The act of shaving offers the adolescent male the opportunity to study his changing appearance.

TABLE 16-1. Growth and development during adolescence

EARLY ADOLESCENCE (11-14 YEARS)	MIDDLE ADOLESCENCE (15-17 YEARS)	LATE ADOLESCENCE (18-20 YEARS)
Growth Rapidly accelerating growth Reaches peak velocity Secondary sex characteristics appear	Growth decelerating in girls Stature reaches 95% of adult height Secondary sex characteristics well advanced	Physically mature Structure and reproductive growth almost complete
Cognition Explores newfound ability for limited abstract thought Clumsy groping for new values and energies Comparison of "normality" with peers of same sex	Developing capacity for abstract thinking Enjoys intellectual powers, often in idealistic terms Concern with philosophic, political, and social problems	Established abstract thought Can perceive and act on long-range options Able to view problems comprehensively Intellectual and functional identity established
Identity Preoccupied with rapid body changes Trying out of various roles Measurement of attractiveness by acceptance or rejection of peers Conformity to group norms	Modifies body image Very self-centered; increased narcissism Tendency toward inner experience and self-discovery Has a rich fantasy life Idealistic Able to perceive future implications of current behavior and decisions; variable application	Body image and gender-role definition nearly secured Mature sexual identity Phase of consolidation of identity Stability of self-esteem Comfortable with physical growth Social roles defined and articulated
Relationships with Parents Defining independence-dependence boundaries Strong desire to remain dependent on parents while trying to detach No major conflicts over parental control	Major conflicts over independence and control Low point in parent-child relationship Greatest push for emancipation; disengagement Final and irreversible emotional detachment from parents; mourning	Emotional and physical separation from parents completed Independence from family with less conflict Emancipation nearly secured
Relationships with Peers Seeks peer affiliations to counter instability generated by rapid change Upsurge of close, idealized friendships with members of the same sex Struggle for mastery takes place within peer group	Strong need for identity to affirm self-image Behavioral standards set by peer group Acceptance by peers extremely important—fear of rejection Exploration of ability to attract the opposite sex	Peer group recedes in importance in favor of individual friendship Testing of male-female relationships against possibility of permanent alliance Relationships characterized by giving and sharing
Sexuality Self-exploration and evaluation Limited dating, usually group Limited intimacy	Multiple plural relationships Decisive turn toward heterosexuality (if homosexual, knows by this time) Exploration of "sex appeal" Feeling of "being in love" Tentative establishment of relationships	Forms stable relationships and attachment to another Growing capacity for mutuality and reciprocity Dating as a male-female pair Intimacy involves commitment rather than exploration and romanticism
Psychologic Health Wide mood swings Intense daydreaming Anger outwardly expressed with moodiness, temper outbursts, and verbal insults and name-calling	Tendency toward inner experiences; more introspective Tendency to withdraw when upset or feelings are hurt Vacillation of emotions in time and range Feelings of inadequacy common; difficulty in asking for help	More constancy of emotion Anger more apt to be concealed

larly the growth of body hair. The dominant culture in which smooth-skinned females are preferred makes it necessary for the girl to shave her underarms and legs regularly to meet the standards for feminine appearance. The girl becomes increasingly conscious of the feminine ideal and, in an effort to approach this standard, experiments with a variety of cosmetics and hairstyles. Alone and together, she and her friends spend endless hours before the mirror posing, applying cosmetics, and combing their hair.

The advent of menstruation, that exclusive feature of female puberty, provides the greatest impetus toward full realization and acceptance of female sexuality. Menstruation is positive evidence of womanhood and the potential for pregnancy and childbearing. Most girls are adequately prepared for the event and take this new function in stride, looking forward to menstruation, feeling satisfaction at its onset, and seeing it as the symbol of their passage from childhood to womanhood. Others find it distressing, frightening, and difficult to accept. Because of its sudden onset, the first menstruation can be a traumatic experience for the girl who has not been taught what to expect.

Unlike the adolescent boy, strong sexual feelings in the adolescent girl are not usually centered in the genital region but are more generalized. Girls' first sexual experiences are likely to be different from and have different meanings than those of boys. Masturbation is less regularly practiced. Adolescent girls are more likely than boys to experience sex for the first time in a perceived close relationship than through masturbation.

• • •

The changes that occur during the early, middle, and late phases of adolescence are summarized in Table 16-1.

PROMOTING OPTIMUM HEALTH DURING ADOLESCENCE

Adolescents are, on the whole, healthy individuals. The disease level is low during this age period, but there is heightened concern about the body (McKay and Diem, 1995). Most of the health problems and the more common illnesses are in some way related to the body changes of puberty or to engaging in high-risk behaviors.

Health promotion in persons in this age-group is primarily one of health teaching and guidance. There is a growing consensus that the most effective adolescent health promotion efforts involve multiple systems and address multiple issues (Willard and Schoenborn, 1995). Research suggests that interventions integrating programs and expertise from health care, school, and community-based settings can effectively increase adolescents' prevention skills, improve their access to health care services, build adult motivation and support for adolescent prevention practices, and change physical environments and social norms to support healthy behavior (Pentz, 1993).

Adolescents are able to assume the major responsibility for their own health, including maintaining health practices (e.g., toothbrushing, caring for appliances), taking prescribed medications, keeping appointments, and performing proce-

GUIDELINES
Interviewing Adolescents

Ensure confidentiality and privacy; interview adolescent without parents.

Show concern for adolescent's perspective: "First, I'd like to talk about your main concerns" and "I'd like to know what you think is happening."

Offer a nonthreatening explanation for the questions you ask: "I'm going to ask a number of questions to help me better understand your health."

Maintain objectivity; avoid assumptions, judgments, and lectures.

Ask open-ended questions when possible; move to more directive questions if necessary.

Begin with less sensitive issues and proceed to more sensitive ones.

Use language that both the adolescent and you understand.

Restate: reflect back to adolescents what they have said, along with feelings that may be associated with their descriptions.

dures when necessary. Interview approaches should consider the adolescent's increasing independence and responsibility (see Guidelines box above and Critical Thinking Exercise on p. 480).

IMMUNIZATIONS

An immunization update is an important part of adolescent preventive care. Obtaining a record of the teen's prior immunizations is important. Adolescents should receive a tetanus-diphtheria (Td) vaccine 10 years after their most recent childhood diphtheria-pertussis-tetanus (DPT) vaccination, which is typically given at 4 to 5 years of age. With the exception of pregnant teens, all adolescents should receive a second measles-mumps-rubella (MMR) vaccine unless they have documentation of two MMR vaccinations during childhood but not before 12 months of age. All adolescents who have not previously received three doses of hepatitis B vaccine should be vaccinated against hepatitis B virus (Recommended childhood immunization schedule, 1996), (see also Immunizations, Chapter 10).

NUTRITION

The rapid and extensive increase in height, weight, muscle mass, and sexual maturity of adolescence is accompanied by greater nutritional requirements. Since nutritional needs are closely related to the increase in body mass, the peak requirements occur in the years of maximum growth, during which the body mass almost doubles. The caloric and protein requirements during this time are higher than at almost any other time of life. As a result of this increased anabolic need, the adolescent is highly sensitive to caloric restrictions.

Adolescents' appetites soar. A fast-growing boy's stomach may be too small to accommodate the amount of food he requires to meet his growth needs unless he eats at very frequent intervals.

The nutritional needs of adolescents are difficult to determine because of meager nutritional information on members of this age-group. This difficulty is further complicated by the influence of emotional and other stress factors affecting nutrient utilization and the psychologic factors that influence

CRITICAL **THINKING EXERCISE**
Respecting Privacy

Jamie S., a 17-year-old female, arrives with her mother for a routine history and physical examination for college entrance. As you are taking Jamie to an examination room, her mother whispers to you, "I need to speak with you in private." What would be your most appropriate response?

1. Ask Jamie to undress to prepare for the examination while you take her mother to another room to find out what's on her mind.
2. Say to Jamie's mother in Jamie's presence, "Mrs. S., whatever you have to say to me, you need to say in front of Jamie."
3. Say to Jamie and her mother, "I would like to begin by speaking with both of you together, then spend some time just with you, Mrs. S., then just with you, Jamie."
4. Say to Jamie and her mother, "I would like to begin by speaking with both of you together, then spend some time just with you, Jamie, then just with you, Mrs. S."

The most appropriate response is four. Jamie and her mother need to know ahead of time that they will each have an opportunity to express their concerns in private. Since Jamie is your patient, she should be first. Knowing that her mother will also have an opportunity to express concerns, Jamie will likely be more open and may even say, "I know what my mother will tell you," and address the issue herself. Option one is disrespectful of Jamie, and option two is disrespectful of Jamie's mother and her concerns. Number one is poor for two additional reasons. First, an explanation of what will occur and the interview should precede getting undressed for an examination. Second, Jamie likely will be aware that you are speaking with her mother, feel that her privacy is being violated, and become defensive and distrustful of both you and her mother. Although response three gives both mother and daughter an opportunity to express concerns, if Mrs. S. goes first, Jamie is likely to spend time trying to draw from you what her mother said and/or become defensive.

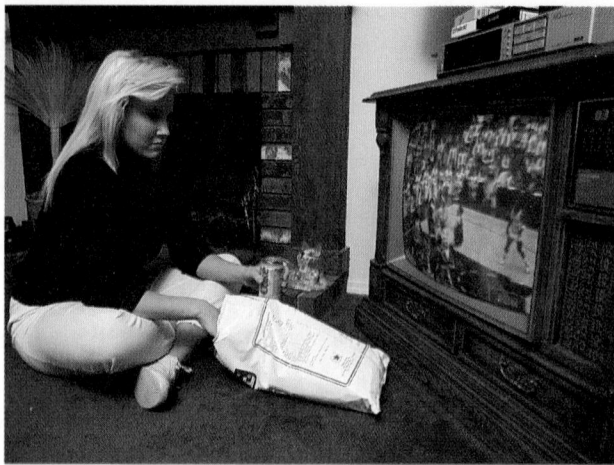

FIG. 16-8. Snacking on empty calories is common among adolescents, especially during inactivity.

Eating Habits and Behavior

Eating and attitudes toward food are primarily family centered during early and middle childhood, and food habits are largely related to cultural and individual family preferences and patterns. With adolescence and the move toward independence, family influences on the child change. Children's interests, attitudes, and routines are altered as an increasing number of meals are eaten away from home. These changes are largely a result of the high value that teenagers place on peer acceptability and sociability; therefore their eating habits are easily influenced by their associates.

Pressure for time and commitments to activities adversely affect the teenager's eating habits. Omitting breakfast or eating a breakfast that is nutritionally poor in quality is also frequently a problem. Snacks, usually selected on the basis of accessibility rather than nutritional merit, become more and more a part of the habitual eating pattern during adolescence (Fig. 16-8). Adolescents characteristically reject or only infrequently eat a sufficient amount of fresh fruits and vegetables, especially those that are rich in ascorbic acid. Milk is usually passed over in favor of soft drinks.

Overeating or undereating during adolescence presents special problems. As they experience the normal increase in weight and fat deposition of the growth spurt, teenage girls often resort to dieting. The desire for the admired slim figure and a fear of becoming "fat" prompt teenage girls to embark on nutritionally inadequate reducing regimens that drain their energy and deprive their growing bodies of essential nutrients. They resort to diets on their own or with peers in an effort to conform. Many adopt the current fad diets and are victims of food misinformation. Boys are less inclined to undereat. They are more concerned about gaining size and strength. However, they tend to eat foods high in calories but low in other essential nutrients.

The number of overweight adolescents is increasing (Troiano and others, 1995). Along with increased availability of energy-dense foods, the U.S. population has moved toward a sedentary life-style. Although some overweight adolescents will lose their excess weight as they mature and develop, many will go on to become overweight adults. Because treatment

eating habits. In addition, the wide variations in growth rates during adolescence and the equally wide variations in ages at which these changes take place complicate any attempt to set minimum dietary standards for any given age.

Adolescents usually have sufficient intake of protein to meet their needs, except those who limit their food intake because of economic problems or in an attempt to lose weight. There is a substantial increase in the need for the minerals calcium, iron, and zinc during periods of rapid growth: calcium for skeletal growth, iron for expansion of muscle mass and blood volume, and zinc for the generation of both skeletal and bone tissue. Girls may be especially susceptible to iron deficiency at menarche. Maximum bone mass is acquired during adolescence; therefore the calcium deposited during these years determines the risk of osteoporosis (Key and Key, 1994). A balanced intake of protein, fats, and carbohydrates is recommended to prevent the chronic degenerative disorders of adulthood (Agostoni and others, 1994). Dietary intervention should promote the regular consumption of breakfast, a balanced intake of animal and vegetable foods, and an increased calcium supply to maximize bone density.

of obesity for adults is largely ineffective and dietary treatment of adolescents is complicated by possible interference with growth, preventing obesity by encouraging increased physical activity may provide the greatest promise.

Nursing Considerations

Healthy dietary habits should be discussed with all adolescents. Adolescents need to learn about the Food Guide Pyramid (see Chapter 11); the relationships among dietary fat, weight status, and health; and food sources of fat, salt, and fiber (Murphy and others, 1994). Their food habits must be considered when planning nutritional education and guidance because they reflect many influences and conditions.

In helping teenagers select a nutritious diet, it is best to begin with their present diet and actively involve them in the process. Teenagers do not respond well to judgmental attitudes and dislike being preached to, but they do respond when their independence is respected and they are given the opportunity to make their own decisions regarding food choices.

In general, adolescents are body conscious and concerned about their appearance. When diet is associated with clear skin, firm flesh, and glossy hair, the teenager is more likely to be receptive to nutritional education. However, helping young persons arrive at a decision for change is more difficult than providing information. They respond best when the counselor provides straightforward information, uses instructional methods that actively involve them, talks *with* them and not at them, and listens to what they have to say.

SLEEP AND REST

Teenagers vary in their need for sleep and rest. Rapid physical growth, the tendency toward overexertion, and the overall increased activity of this age contribute to fatigue in adolescents. During growth spurts the need for sleep is increased. Their propensity for staying up late makes it very difficult to arise in the morning, and they may sleep late at every opportunity. Adequate sleep and rest at this time are important to a total health regimen.

EXERCISE AND ACTIVITY

Although today's youth are less fit than children 20 years ago, adolescents probably spend more time and energy practicing and participating in sports activities than do members of any other age-group. The number of girls and boys participating in youth sports within and outside school settings has increased dramatically in recent years (Ostrum, 1993) (Fig. 16-9).

School-based, health-oriented physical education may provide both immediate effects of the activity and sustained effects through encouragement of lifelong activity patterns. Unfortunately, games and competitive sports are the mainstays of existing programs, instead of moderate-intensity activities that contribute to the public health goal of lifelong activity (Troiano and others, 1995).

The practice of sports, games, and even dancing contributes significantly to growth and development, the education process, and better health. It provides exercise for growing muscles, interactions with peers, and a socially acceptable means of enjoying stimulation and conflict. In addition, competitive activities help the teenager in the process of self-

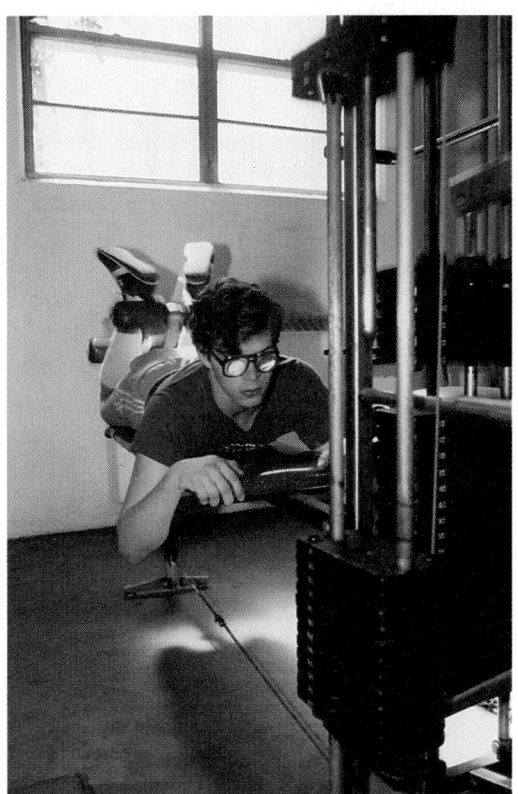

FIG. 16-9. Adolescents should be encouraged to participate in activities that contribute to lifelong physical fitness.

appraisal, development of self-respect, and concern for others. Because physical fitness appears to be a major influence on one's lifelong health status, children should be encouraged to participate in activities that contribute to lifelong physical fitness. Nurses can encourage participation as an excellent means for health promotion and building of self-esteem. However, youngsters should not be encouraged to engage in physical activity that is beyond their physical or emotional capacity (see also Health Problems Related to Sports Participation, Chapter 17).

DENTAL HEALTH

Dental health should not be neglected during adolescence, although the rate of caries formation is not as great as in childhood. Early adolescence is usually when corrective orthodontic appliances are worn, and these are frequently a source of embarrassment and concern to the youngster. Reassurance regarding the temporary nature of the annoyance and anticipation of an improved appearance help to make the inconvenience tolerable. It is also important to reinforce the orthodontist's directions regarding use and care of the appliances and to emphasize careful attention to toothbrushing during this time (see also Chapters 12 and 15).

PERSONAL CARE

The body-conscious teenager is highly amenable to discussion and counseling about personal care and hygiene. Body changes associated with puberty bring with them special needs for cleanliness. The hyperactive sebaceous glands and newly functioning apocrine glands make frequent bathing or showering a necessity, and underarm deodorants assume an important place in personal care. The adolescent will find that hair requires more frequent shampooing, and girls will have questions about hair removal, use of cosmetics, and menstrual hygiene. Many group discussions center around the virtues of particular products or methods. Adolescents are continually bombarded with messages from the media regarding the best means of enhancing their popularity and appeal to the opposite sex. Nurses are in a position to help them evaluate the relative merits of commercial products.

Vision

Regular vision testing is a vital part of health care and supervision during adolescence. At this time the incidence of visual refractive difficulties reaches a peak that is not exceeded until the fifth decade of life. The increased demands of schoolwork make good vision important for academic success. Consequently, teenagers are more likely to be referred for visual evaluation. The need for corrective lenses can create psychologic problems for teenagers if they believe that glasses spoil their appearance or do not fit their body image. For those who can afford them, contact lenses are a preferred solution. For some the impact of a visual defect, no matter how slight, may prove to be a great personal concern.

Hearing

Considerable concern has surrounded current teenage practices causing possible damage to the hearing. Cochlear damage from relatively continuous exposure to the loud sound levels of rock music, has been documented. The popularity of portable radios and stereo cassette and compact disc (CD) players with lightweight earphones, which enable the listener to adjust the volume, are of particular concern to health care professionals. When these units are used for extended periods, permanent hearing loss can occur. Appealing to individual youngsters for more judicious use is not always successful, although they should be informed of the risk. Efforts directed toward legislating legal limits to the noise exposure that can be achieved through the sets along with widespread education may be possible solutions. (See Chapter 19 for a discussion of noise-related hearing loss.)

Posture

The process of normal development during adolescence may result in altered posture. The rapid skeletal growth that is usually associated with a significant lag in muscular growth leads to weakness, easy fatigability, and awkwardness. This situation predisposes teens to slumping and makes them less inclined to stand or sit erect. A reduction in physical activity, which often accompanies the rapid skeletal growth, aggravates the situation, especially in teenage girls. (The adolescent who is routinely engaged in vigorous physical activity appears to have fewer problems with posture.) Most postural problems resolve as the adolescent matures, and most do not require special attention.

The best approach to counseling teenagers about posture is to show, not tell, them and to serve as a proper model. Good posture can be demonstrated best by having the adolescent stand before a full-length mirror or by taking a photograph of the adolescent's body profile. Postural defects and desired alterations can be pointed out in full view of both the young person and the nurse. A sunken chest, winged scapulas, swayback, protuberant abdomen, and drooping head and shoulders are clearly visible, and the nurse is able to demonstrate the simple corrections that can transform the youngster into a more attractive and ultimately healthier person. Adolescents will need reassurance that the fatigue they feel when attempting to maintain correct posture is a transient effect caused by weak muscles, especially those of the back, and that they will soon acquire the strength and endurance to maintain the desired posture. If they concentrate on assuming correct positioning several times each day, with regular practice it will eventually become a permanent aspect of their person.

Serious postural defects detected in the process of a physical assessment require early medical intervention. Scoliosis is usually intensified during adolescence, and tight muscles often produce postural problems that need special attention. Nurses can refer a youngster to the appropriate source, such as the family physician, pediatrician, or health clinic, for evaluation and implementation of corrective therapy. (See Scoliosis, Chapter 31.)

Body Piercing

The popular trend of ear or, less often, nose, nipple, navel, penis, or tongue piercing may sometimes create a health problem in the uninformed teenager. It is a nursing responsibility to caution girls or boys against the practice of having piercing performed by friends, mothers, or themselves. Although in most cases there are few if any serious side effects, there is always a danger of complications such as infection, cyst or keloid formation, bleeding, dermatitis, or metal allergy. Therefore the procedure should be performed by a qualified operator using proper sterile technique. This is especially important if a youngster has a history of diabetes, allergies, or skin disorders.

 Using the same unsterilized needle to pierce body parts of multiple teens presents the same risk of human immunodeficiency virus (HIV) transmission as occurs with other needle-sharing activities.

Suntanning

The continuous quest for an attractive appearance leads many teenagers to excessive sunbathing and artificial means for acquiring a tan skin. However, the practice has serious long-term risks, and the adolescent should be educated regarding the detrimental effects of sunlight on the skin (see Sunburn, Chapter 30). Some long-term effects include premature aging of the skin, increased risk of skin cancer, and in susceptible individuals, phototoxic reactions.

The increasing popularity of artificial suntanning has prompted concern from health professionals regarding the use of sunlamps and suntanning machines. The long-term effects of tanning machines are similar to those of the sun; dermatologists do not recommend suntanning by this means. Those who insist on using suntanning equipment should be warned that goggles must be worn in tanning booths to prevent serious corneal burning. Education on the use of sunscreens, including hypoallergenic products,

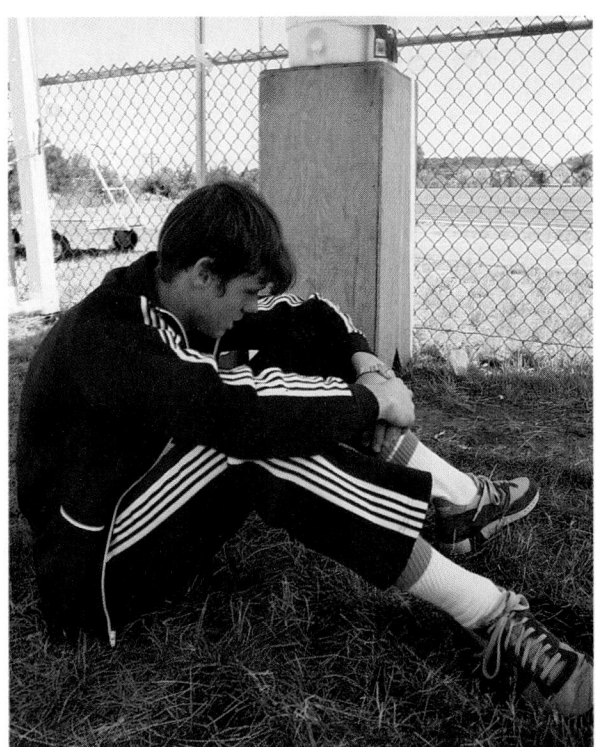

FIG. 16-10. Adolescents use being alone as a method of coping with stress.

AREAS OF STRESS IN ADOLESCENCE
Body image
Sexuality conflicts
Scholastic pressures
Competitive pressures
Relationships with parents
Relationships with siblings
Relationships with peers
Finances
Decisions about present and future roles
Career planning
Ideologic conflicts

with a sun protective factor (SPF) of at least 15 is important health teaching.

STRESS REDUCTION

The multiple changes occurring in adolescence potentially result in great stress (see Fig. 16-10 and box). The adolescent is faced with pressures from peers to conform, which often involve flaunting adult authority and even serious health risks. Health risks include pressures for sexual experimentation and use of drugs, alcohol, and cigarettes, as well as potentially dangerous physical activities.

Early-maturing girls and late-maturing children are especially sensitive to the stresses of being different from their peers. Many feel intense anxiety over their identity. Both early- and late-maturing children feel out of place among their classmates, but slow-maturing children appear to suffer the most pronounced inner turmoil and may be hesitant to voice their concerns. Slow-maturing youngsters need support and reassurance that they are not abnormal and need only be patient until the time comes when they, too, will develop the characteristics for which they yearn.

SEXUALITY EDUCATION AND GUIDANCE

Contemporary adolescents are constantly exposed to sexual symbolism and erotic stimulation from the mass media. At the same time, the development of primary and secondary sex characteristics and the increased sensitivity of the genitals produce thoughts and fantasies about sexual relationships. Young people are at the stage of life when the sexual aspects of interpersonal relationships become particularly important.

Societal expectations push them toward dating, and their own inner sex drive urges them toward exploration. Although many adolescents have received sexuality education from parents and school throughout childhood, they are not always adequately prepared for the impact of puberty. A large portion of their knowledge is acquired from peers, television, movies, and magazines. Even information acquired from parents may be inaccurate (McGrory, 1995). Consequently, much of the sex information they accumulate is incomplete, inaccurate, riddled with cultural and moral values, and not very helpful.

The responsibility for providing sexuality education has been assumed by parents, schools, churches, community agencies such as **Planned Parenthood Federation of America, Inc.,*** and health professionals, especially nurses. The public perceives nurses as having authoritative information and as willing to take time with patients (Croft and Asmussen, 1993). To be able to discuss the topic with teenagers adequately, nurses must have not only an understanding of the physiologic aspects of sexuality and a knowledge of cultural and societal values, but also an awareness of their own attitudes, feelings, and biases about sexuality.

The most comprehensive approach to sexuality education is offered by the **Sexuality Information and Education Council of the United States (SIECUS)†** and the **Sex Information and Education Council of Canada (SIECCAN),‡** interdisciplinary organizations founded to establish sexuality as a health entity and to dignify it through an open approach, study, and scientific research. SIECUS maintains that every sexuality education program should present the topic from six aspects: biologic, social, health, personal adjustments and attitudes, interpersonal associations, and the establishment of values.

Whether nurses counsel young people on an individual basis, in mixed groups, or in groups segregated by gender makes little difference. Ideally, boys and girls should be able to discuss sexuality objectively with one another and in groups, but this is not always possible. The difference in the rate of maturation between boys and girls and between different members of the same sex often makes it desirable to discuss certain aspects of sexuality in segregated groups. As a general

---

*810 Seventh Ave., New York, NY 10019; (212) 541-7800 or (800) 829-7732.
†130 W. 42nd St., Suite 350, New York, NY 10036; (212) 819-9770.
‡850 Coxwell Ave., E. York, Ontario M4C 5R1; (416) 466-5304.

rule, the need for separate discussion groups diminishes as young people progress toward maturity.

Sexuality education should consist of instruction concerning normal body functions and should be presented in a straightforward manner using correct terminology. When discussing sex and sexual activities, nurses should use simple but correct language, not street language, highly scientific terminology, or evasive jargon. Once the meanings of biologic terms such as uterus, testicles, and vagina are understood, most teenagers prefer to use them in their discussions.

Many girls arrive at menarche with conflictive attitudes, myths, and illogical beliefs. Even girls adequately prepared for menstruation do not always understand its relationship to the total process of reproduction. Many are under the incorrect impression that the "safe" time for sexual intercourse is midway between menstrual periods.

Teenagers' curiosity and desire for information extend beyond the need for anatomic and physiologic knowledge. They need to know more than the mechanics of conception, pregnancy, and birth. Adolescents, girls in particular, want answers to questions such as "What is it like?" "Does it hurt?" "What happens when . . .?" and "Is it all right if you . . .?" Boys are often concerned about the fallacy that a relationship exists between penis size and sexual function. They need reassurance that masturbation is a normal and common practice, that some degree of homosexuality is not unusual in early adolescence, and that oral-genital relations can be normal substitutes for intercourse.

However, sexuality education cannot end there. Teens need to discuss intercourse, alternative methods of sexual satisfaction, and how to resist peer pressure. With the increased incidence of sexually transmitted diseases, especially AIDS, the topic of "safe sex," especially abstinence or the use of condoms and abstinence, is essential. Role playing can help them learn effective approaches to dealing with difficult situations. Sex and sexuality cannot be taught without discussions on mature decision making, sexual responsibility, and values clarification.

Adolescents need role models and life experiences with delayed gratification. Most important, they need problem-solving experience and decision-making skills so that they can anticipate the positive and negative outcomes of a decision. With these types of assistance, teenagers can become sexually responsible young adults.

INJURY PREVENTION

Physical injuries are the greatest single cause of death in the adolescent age-group and claim more lives than all other causes combined. The most vulnerable ages are the years 15 to 24, when accidental injuries account for about 60% of deaths in boys and 40% of deaths in girls. The tragedy of this is that these figures remain fairly constant from year to year and that almost all fatal injuries are preventable.

During adolescence, peak physical, sensory, and psychomotor function gives teenagers a feeling of strength and confidence that they have never experienced before, and the physiologic changes of puberty give impetus to many basic instinctual forces. One manifestation of this is an increase in energy that simply must be discharged through action, often at the expense of logical thinking and other control mechanisms. Their propensity for risk-taking behavior plus feelings of indestructibility make adolescents especially prone to inju-

ries. Some of the developmental characteristics of teenagers and the common injuries associated with this age-group are outlined in Table 16-2.

Vehicle-Related Injuries

The adolescent's newly acquired ability to drive and the normal developmental need for independence and freedom make the automobile an attractive part of an adolescents' life. Motor vehicle crashes are the single greatest cause of death, accounting for nearly two thirds of fatal injuries among young people (Bearinger and Blum, 1994). The majority of fatal and nonfatal motor vehicle crashes involve alcohol. Adolescents practice other behaviors that may increase their likelihood of death in a motor vehicle. In a survey of high-school students, 19.1% reported rarely or never using a seat belt, and 35.3% had ridden within the previous month with a driver who had been drinking alcohol (Kann and others, 1995).

Nonautomotive Vehicle Injuries. The increasing use of other motorized vehicles, such as motorized bicycles, all terrain vehicles (ATVs), jet skis, and snowmobiles, has caused an increase in injuries, especially among youngsters below the legal age for driving automobiles. Many adolescents ride bicycles without helmets and without lights at night, and the overwhelming majority of deaths from bicycle injuries (primarily head injuries) involve teenagers. Most injuries involve the motorcycle and another vehicle, but burn injuries have been reported from contact with the hot muffler, especially when youngsters are riding double.

Firearms

Improper use of firearms continues to be one of the leading causes of accidental death in the adolescent age-group. Most of these deaths occur in or on home premises. Almost half the victims of firearm fatalities are between the ages of 15 and 24 years. Most accidental injuries can be prevented when proper safety precautions are taken in the use and storage of firearms. For example, loaded guns should never be permitted in or around the home, and guns and ammunition must be stored where only appropriate adults have access to them. Asking families about the presence of a gun in the home and offering these preventive actions if one is present may be the most effective action health professionals can take (American Academy of Pediatrics, 1992). Firearms are increasingly a factor in intentional as well as unintentional death for adolescents. The murder rate for teenage boys ages 15 to 19 more than doubled between 1985 and 1991; for black males in this age-group, the rate nearly tripled (Children's Defense Fund, 1995). Virtually all this increase (97%) was attributed to the use of guns.

Nonpowder Firearms. Nonpowder guns (air rifles, BB guns), although viewed as toys by many, account for almost as many injuries as powder guns. The regulations regarding nonpowder guns are relaxed; they can be purchased legally by youngsters and are labeled as suitable for children as young as 8 years. Few states regulate their use. As child advocates, nurses can press for legislation to regulate the sale of these potentially dangerous "toys."

Sports Injuries

Because the degree of physical maturation, size, coordination, and endurance varies greatly among adolescents of the same

TABLE 16-2. Injury prevention during adolescence

DEVELOPMENTAL ABILITIES RELATED TO RISK OF INJURY	INJURY PREVENTION

Need for independence and freedom
Testing independence
Age permitted to drive a motor vehicle (varies)
Inclination for risk taking
Feeling of indestructibility
Need for discharging energy, often at expense of logical thinking and other control mechanisms
Strong need for peer approval
May attempt hazardous feats
Peak incidence for practice and participation in sports
Access to more complex tools, objects, and locations
Can assume responsibility for own actions
	Motor/Nonmotor Vehicles
	Pedestrian—emphasize and encourage safe pedestrian behavior
	Passenger—promote appropriate behavior while riding in a motor vehicle
	Driver—provide competent driver education; encourage judicious use of vehicle, discourage drag racing, "playing chicken"; maintain vehicle in proper condition (brakes, tires, etc.)
	Teach and promote safety and maintenance of two-wheeled vehicles
	Promote and encourage wearing of safety apparel such as helmet, long trousers, sturdy shoes
	Reinforce the dangers of drugs, including alcohol, when operating a motor vehicle
	
	Drowning
	Teach nonswimmer to swim
	Teach basic rules of water safety
	    Judicious selection of place to swim
	    Sufficient water depth for diving
	    Swimming with companion
	
	Burns
	Reinforce proper behavior in areas involving contact with burn hazards (gasoline, electric wires, fires)
	Advise regarding excessive exposure to natural or artificial sunlight (ultraviolet burn)
	Discourage smoking
	Encourage use of sunscreen
	
	Poisoning
	Educate in hazards of drug use, including alcohol
	
	Falls
	Teach and encourage general safety measures in all activities
	
	Bodily Damage
	Promote acquisition of proper instruction in sports and use of sports equipment
	Instruct in safe use of and respect for firearms and other devices with potential danger (e.g., power tools, firecrackers)
	Provide and encourage use of protective equipment when using potentially hazardous devices
	Promote access to and/or provision of safe sports and recreational facilities
	Discourage use of and/or availability of hazardous sports equipment (e.g., trampoline, surfboards)
	Instruct regarding proper use of corrective devices (e.g., glasses, contact lenses, hearing aids)
	Encourage and foster judicious application of safety principles and prevention
	Be alert for signs of depression (potential suicide)

age, sports competition between young people who differ greatly in strength and agility is unfair and hazardous. Matching candidates for sports should be done relative to physical maturity, height, weight, and physical fitness and skills, particularly in a sport involving rigorous body contact. Age is a less important consideration.

Every sport has some potential for injury, whether one par-

ticipates in serious competition or is actively engaged in the activity for pure enjoyment. A large number of severe or fatal injuries occur to persons who are not physically prepared for the activity. The increase in strength and vigor in adolescence may tempt youngsters to overextend themselves, especially boys who are egged on by teammates or are stimulated by the admiration of female observers. The range of injuries

FAMILY HOME CARE
Guidance During Adolescence

Encourage Parents to:
Accept adolescent as a unique individual.
Respect adolescent's ideas, likes and dislikes, and wishes.
Be involved with school functions and attend adolescent's performances, whether it be a sporting event or a school play.
Listen and try to be open to teen's views, even when they disagree with parental views.
Avoid criticism about no-win topics.
Provide opportunity for choosing options and accept natural consequences of these choices.
Allow young person to learn by doing, even when choices and methods differ from those of adults.
Provide adolescent with clear, reasonable limits.
Clarify house rules and consequences for breaking them.
Let society's rules and consequences teach responsibility outside the home.
Allow increasing independence within limitations of safety and well-being.
Be available but avoid pressing teen too far.
Respect adolescent's privacy.
Try to share adolescent's feelings of joy or sorrow.

Respond to feelings as well as words.
Be available to answer questions, give information, and provide companionship.
Try to make communication clear.
Avoid comparisons with siblings.
Assist adolescent in selecting appropriate career goals and preparing for adult role.
Welcome adolescent's friends into the home and treat them with respect.
Provide unconditional love
Be willing to apologize when mistaken.

Be Aware that Adolescents:
Are subject to turbulent, unpredictable behavior.
Are struggling for independence.
Are extremely sensitive to feelings and behavior that affect them.
May receive a different message than what was sent.
Consider friends extremely important.
Have a strong need "to belong."

---

sustained in sports or recreational activities can involve any part of the body and extend from relatively minor cuts, bruises, and abrasions to totally incapacitating central nervous system injuries or death.

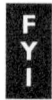 The leading cause of serious sports injuries among boys is participation in football, whereas most girls are injured while participating in gymnastics.

Nursing Considerations

Injury prevention is an ongoing part of nursing responsibility throughout the childhood years. Anticipatory guidance to parents and children regarding the expected problems and hazards related to growth and development does not end as children approach maturity. They need the same education in basic safety precautions, as well as instruction in skills required in performance of activities such as sports, instruction in handling motor vehicles and firearms, and instruction in proper maintenance of equipment. During adolescence, however, health and safety education and guidance are more effective when the young people are involved directly; parents and health professionals can emphasize the importance of safety during performance of activities and the proper conditioning and preparation for sports.

Prevention can occur on a variety of levels. Safety advocacy, changing public policy, and legislation can curtail injuries. Examples of such approaches are laws that mandate wearing seat belts, mandatory helmet use while driving moving vehicles other than automobiles, keeping the legal drinking age at 21 years, and instituting curfews for teen drivers. In addition to improving the environment, health education for teenagers and significant adults is essential. Helping adolescents understand their need for engaging in risky behavior, exploring possible negative outcomes, and weighing possible alternatives are critical components of injury prevention.

ANTICIPATORY GUIDANCE—CARE OF FAMILIES

The parents of the adolescent are usually as confused and perplexed about the changes and behavior of this stage of development as the youngster is. Parents also need support and guidance to help them through this trying time. They need to understand the changes taking place and to understand and accept the expected behaviors that accompany the process of detachment, to be prepared to "let go," and to promote the changed relationship from one of dependence to one of mutuality (see Family Focus box). The Family Home Care box lists suggestions for anticipatory guidance of parents with an adolescent.

FAMILY FOCUS
Family Rules for Adolescents

U.S. society does little to help adolescents mature and separate. Americans have remarkably few rites of passage that mark the stages of life. Few ceremonies and tests are practiced to determine eligibility for specific adult privileges. Obtaining a driver's license, graduating from high school, and reaching the 21-year-old legal age for drinking are among the few that exist. U.S. society also does not have many generally agreed-on social dictums. When is the right age to begin dating? What is a reasonable curfew? Should an 18-year-old be allowed to stay out all night? There are few areas of general agreement. Every family makes up its own rules, influenced, but uninstructed, by the society at large. Many families have great difficulty with this process.

Modified from Prothrow-Stith D: *Deadly consequences: how violence is destroying our teenage population and a plan to begin solving the problem,* New York, 1993, HarperCollins.

KEY POINTS

- The pubescent growth spurt that begins around age 10 in girls and age 12 in boys signals the beginning of adolescence.
- Biologic development during puberty is characterized by increased activity of the pituitary gland, which results in sexual maturity and the appearance of secondary sex characteristics.
- According to Erikson, the major developmental crisis of adolescence is establishing a sense of identity.
- Cognitive development in adolescence includes abstract thought, thinking beyond the present, logical reasoning, and a sense of idealism.
- Development of body image is closely tied to body changes and social interactions.
- According to Kohlberg's theory of moral development, adolescents begin to question existing moral values and learn to make choices.

- Spiritual development is characterized by the questioning of family values and ideals, a move to more philosophic thinking, and emphasis on personal religion.
- Adolescent relationships with parents may be strained, whereas the influence of the peer group increases and heterosexual relationships assume importance.
- Teenagers demonstrate a wide variety of interests, and their increased physical and cognitive skills allow them to engage in increasingly difficult and complex activities.
- Adolescents' emotions fluctuate.
- Nutritional needs, especially for calcium, zinc, and iron, may not be met by teenagers' eating habits, such as snacking and irregular mealtimes.
- Motor vehicle injuries are the primary cause of death from injury in the adolescent years.

REFERENCES

Agostoni C and others: Dairy products and adolescent nutrition, *J Int Med Res* 22(2):67-76, 1994.

American Academy of Pediatrics, Committee on Adolescence: Firearms and adolescents, *Pediatrics* 89(4):784-787, 1992.

Bearinger L, Blum R: Adolescent health care. In Wallace H, Nelson R, Sweeney P, editors: *Maternal and child health practices,* ed 4, Oakland, CA, 1994, Third Party.

Children's Defense Fund: *The state of America's children yearbook,* Washington, DC, 1995, The Fund.

Croft C, Asmussen L: A developmental approach to sexuality education: implications for medical practice, *J Adolesc Health* 24(2):109-114, 1993.

Erikson EH: *Childhood and society,* ed 2, New York, 1963, Norton.

Friedman R, Downey J: Homosexuality, *N Engl J Med* 331(14):923-930, 1994.

Kann L and others: Youth risk behavior surveillance—United States, 1993, *MMWR CDC Surveill Summ* 44(1):1-56, 1995.

Key JD, Key LL Jr: Calcium needs of adolescents, *Curr Opin Pediatr* 6(4):379-382, 1994.

McGrory A: Education for the menarche, *Pediatr Nurs* 21(5):439-443, 1995.

McKay L, Diem E: Health concerns of adolescent girls, *J Pediatr Nurs* 10(1):19-27, 1995.

Murphy AS and others: Nutrition education needs and learning preferences of Michigan students in grades 5, 8, and 11, *J Sch Health* 64(7):273-278, 1994.

Ostrum G: Sports-related injuries in youths: prevention is the key—and nurses can help! *Pediatr Nurs* 19(4):333-342, 1993.

Pentz M: Benefits of integrating strategies in different settings. In Elster A, Panzarine S, Holt K, editors: *American Medical Association State of the Art Conference on Adolescent Health Promotion: proceedings,* Arlington, VA, 1993, National Center for Education in Maternal and Child Health.

Prothrow-Stith D: *Deadly consequences: how violence is destroying our teenage population and a plan to begin solving the problem,* New York, 1993, HarperCollins.

Recommended childhood immunization schedule—United States, January-June 1996, *MMWR* 44(51/52):940-941, 1996.

Remafedi G and others: Demography of sexual orientation in adolescents, *Pediatrics* 89(4):714-721, 1992.

Seidman S, Rieder R: A review of sexual behavior in the United States, *Am J Psychiatry* 151(3):330-341, 1994.

Troiano R and others: Overweight prevalence and trends for children and adolescents, *Arch Pediatr Adolesc Med* 149:1085-1091, 1995.

Willard JC, Schoenborn CA: Relationship between cigarette smoking and other unhealthy behaviors among our Nation's youth: United States, 1992, *Advance Data for Vital and Health Statistics,* No 263, Hyattsville, MD, 1995, National Center for Health Statistics.

BIBLIOGRAPHY

General

American Medical Association: *Guidelines for adolescent preventive services,* Chicago, 1992, The Association.

Andersen LB: Changes in physical activity are reflected in changes in fitness during late adolescence: a 2-year follow-up study, *J Sports Med Phys Fitness* 34(4):390-397, 1994.

Bearinger L, Gephart J: Interdisciplinary education in adolescent health, *J Pediatr Child Health* 29(suppl 1):S10-S15, 1993.

Bearinger L and others: Nursing competence in adolescent health: anticipating the future needs of youth, *J Prof Nurs* 8(2):80-86, 1992.

Blum RW and others: American Indian–Alaska Native youth health, *JAMA* 267(12):1637-1644, 1992.

Braun BL, Wagenaar AC, Flack JM: Alcohol consumption and physical fitness among young adults, *Alcohol Clin Exp Res* 19(4):1048-1054, 1995.

Fulton RAB, Moore CM: Spiritual care of the school-age child with a chronic condition, *J Pediatr Nurs* 10(4):224-231, 1995.

Groer MW and others: Adolescent stress and coping: a longitudinal study, *Res Nurs Health* 15(3):209-217, 1992.

Grubbs S and others: Self-efficacy in normal adolescents, *Issues Ment Health Nurs* 13:121-128, 1992.

Haggerty R: Care of the poor and underserved in America: older adolescents: a group at special risk, *Am J Dis Child* 145:569-571, 1991.

Hendee W and others: *The health of adolescents*, San Francisco, 1991, Jossey-Bass.

Kollar M et al: Adolescent anger: a developmental study, *J Child Adolesc Psychiatr Ment Health Nurs* 4(1):9-15, 1991.

Millstein S: A view of health from the adolescent's perspective. In Millstein S, Petersen A, Nightingale E, editors: *Promoting the health of adolescents: new directions for the twenty-first century*, New York, 1993, Oxford University Press.

Moffit TE and others: Childhood experience and the onset of menarche: a test of a sociobiological model, *Child Dev* 63(1):59-67, 1992.

Piaget J: *The theory of stages in cognitive development*, New York, 1969, McGraw-Hill.

Rosella JD, Albrecht SA: Anticipatory guidance: alcohol, adolescents, and recognizing abuse and dependence, *Issues Compr Pediatr Nurs* 16(4):207-218, 1993.

Schmitt B: Dealing with normal adolescent rebellion, *Contemp Pediatr* 7(7):55-60, 1990.

Slusher IL and others: State of the art of nursing research and theory development in adolescent health, *Issues Compr Pediatr Nurs* 16:1-11, 1993.

Steinberg L and others: Impact of parenting practices on adolescent achievement: authorative parenting, school involvement, and encouragement to succeed, *Child Dev* 63(5):1266-1281, 1992.

Vaughn VC, Litt IF: *Child and adolescent development: clinical implications*, Philadelphia, 1990, Saunders.

Health Promotion

Alderman EM, Fleischman AR: Should adolescents make their own health-care choices? *Contemp Pediatr* 10(1):65-82, 1993.

Availability of comprehensive adolescent health services, *MMWR* 42(26):507-515, 1993.

Blum RW: Global trends in adolescent health, *JAMA* 265(20):2711-2719, 1991.

Council on Scientific Affairs, American Medical Association: Confidential health services for adolescents, *JAMA* 269(11):1420-1424, 1993.

Crockett L, Petersen A: Adolescent development: health risks and opportunities for health promotion. In Millstein, S, Petersen, A, Nightingale, E, editors: *Promoting the health of adolescents: new directions for the twenty-first century*, New York, 1993, Oxford University Press.

Cromer BA and others: Compliance with breast self-examination instruction in high school students, *Clin Pediatr* 31(4):215-220, 1992.

Ell K, Northern H: *Families and health care: psychosocial practice*, New York, 1990, Adline de Gruyter.

Glenmark B, Hedberg G, Jansson E: Prediction of physical activity level in adulthood by physical characteristics, physical performance and physical activity in adolescence: an 11-year follow-up study, *Eur J Appl Physiol* 69(6):530-538, 1994.

Isaacs M: Developing culturally competent strategies for adolescents of color. In Elster A, Panzarine S, Holt K, editors: *American Medical Association State of the Art Conference on Adolescent Health Promotion: proceedings*, Arlington, VA, 1993, National Center for Education in Maternal and Child Health.

Ranade B: Nutritional recommendations for children and adolescents, *Int J Clin Pharmacol Ther Toxicol* 31(6):285-290, 1993.

Schreiner B, Brondum LA: Nutrition in pediatric primary care: assessment and common problems, *Nurse Pract Forum* 5(1):13-23, 1994.

Sobczk W and others: Health promotion schools of excellence: a model program for Kentucky and the nation, *J Ky Med Assoc* 93(4):142-147, 1995.

VandenBergh MF and others: Physical activity, calcium intake, and bone mineral content in children in The Netherlands, *J Epidemiol Community Health* 49(3):299-304, 1995.

Yarcheski A, Scoloveno A, Mahon N: Social support and well-being in adolescents: the mediating role of hopefulness, *Nurs Res* 43(5):288-292, 1994.

Sexuality and Sexuality Education

American Academy of Pediatrics, Committee on Adolescence: Homosexuality and adolescence, *Pediatrics* 92(4):6341-634, 1993.

Crooks R, Baur K: *Our sexuality*, ed 4, Redwood City, CA, 1990, Benjamin/Cummings.

Flaming D, Morse J: Minimizing embarrassment: boys' experiences of pubertal changes, *Issues Compr Pediatr Nurs* 14(4):211-230, 1991.

Laumann D and others: *The social organization of sexuality*, Chicago, 1995, University of Chicago Press.

Meeropool E: One of the gang: sexual development of adolescents with physical disabilities, *J Pediatr Nurs* 6(4):243-249, 1991.

Mellanby A, Phelps F, Tripp JH: Teenagers, sex, and risk taking, *Br Med J* 307(6895):25, 1993.

Roth B: Fertility awareness as a component of sexuality education: preliminary research findings with adolescents, *Nurse Pract* 18(3):40, 43, 47-48, 1993.

Taylor BA, Remafedi G: Youth coping with sexual orientation issues, *J Sch Nurs* 9(2):26-39, 1993.

Tucker S: Adolescent patterns of communication about the menstrual cycle, sex, and contraception, *J Pediatr Nurs* 5(6):393-400, 1990.

Woodcock A, Stenner K, Ingham R: "All these contraceptives, videos and that. . . ": young people talking about school sex education, *Health Educ Res* 7(4):517-531, 1992.

Yarber W, Parrillo A: Adolescents and sexually transmitted diseases, *J Sch Health* 62(7):331-338, 1992.

Injury Prevention

Dexheimer Pharris M, editor: *The community responds to youth violence: what works? What doesn't?* Monograph, Minneapolis, MN: 1994, Division of General, Pediatric, and Adolescent Health, University of Minnesota Medical School.

Dryfoos J: Preventing high-risk behavior, *Am J Public Health* 81(2):157-158, 1991.

Fingerhut L and others: *Firearm mortality among children, youth, and young adults, 1-34 years of age: trends and current status—United States, 1979-1990*, Washington, DC, 1991, US Government Printing Office.

Garmezy N: Resilience in children's adaptation to negative life events and stressed environments, *Pediatr Ann* 20(9):459-466, 1991.

Lawrence HS: Fatal nonpowder firearm wounds: case report and review of the literature, *Pediatrics* 85:177-181, 1990.

Lipp E, Trimble N: Health behaviors of adolescent male football athletes, *Pediatr Nurs* 19(4):395-397, 399, 1993.

Meehan PJ, O'Carroll PW: Gangs, drugs, and homicide in Los Angeles, *Am J Dis Child* 146(6):683-687, 1992.

Metcalf J, Roberts S: Strength training and the immature athlete: an overview, *Pediatr Nurs* 19(4):325-332, 1993.

Sheley JF, McGee ZT, Wright JD: Gun-related violence in and around inner-city schools, *Am J Dis Child* 146(6):677-682, 1992.

Wilson P, Testani-Dufour L: Bicycle safety programs: targeting injury prevention through education, *Pediatr Nurs* 19(4):343-346, 1993.

HEALTH PROBLEMS OF SCHOOL-AGE CHILDREN AND ADOLESCENTS

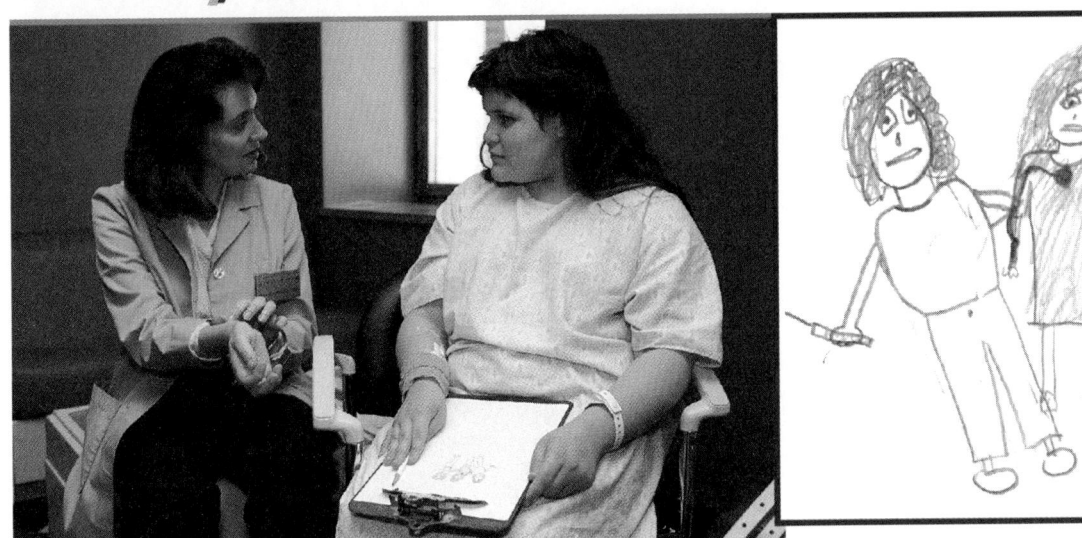

" *Putting in PICC line was freaky, not fun. They said it wouldn't hurt, but it did.* "

Melissa, age 13 years, infected fracture

RELATED TOPICS

COMMON HEALTH PROBLEMS

INFECTIOUS MONONUCLEOSIS

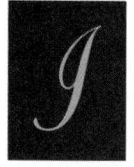 nfectious mononucleosis is an acute, self-limiting infectious disease that is common among young persons up to 25 years of age. The disease is characterized by an increase in the mononuclear elements of the blood and by general symptoms of an infectious process. The course is usually mild but occasionally can be severe or, rarely, accompanied by serious complications.

Etiology/Pathophysiology

The herpeslike Epstein-Barr virus is the principal cause of infectious mononucleosis. It appears in both sporadic and epidemic forms, the sporadic cases being more common. The mechanism of spread has not been proved, although it is believed to be transmitted by direct intimate contact with oral secretions. It also appears to be only mildly contagious, and the period of communicability is unknown. The incubation period following exposure is 4 to 6 weeks.

Diagnostic Tests

The onset of symptoms may be acute or insidious. The common presenting symptoms vary greatly in type, severity, and duration (see box). The leukocyte count may be normal or low, but usually lymphocytic leukocytosis develops. There is also an increase in atypical leukocytes in the peripheral blood smear. The heterophil antibody test determines the extent to which the patient's serum will agglutinate sheep red blood cells. In infectious mononucleosis, a titer of 1:160 is considered diagnostic, although a rising titer during the earlier stages is the best indicator.

The *"spot test" (Monospot),* a slide test of high specificity, is rapid, sensitive, inexpensive, and easy to perform, and has the advantage that it can detect significant agglutinins at lower levels, thus permitting earlier diagnosis. Blood is usually obtained for the test by finger puncture.

Marilyn Winkelstein, PhD, RN, revised this chapter.

Therapeutic Management

There is no specific treatment for infectious mononucleosis. Common symptoms are ordinarily relieved by simple remedies. A mild analgesic is usually sufficient to relieve the bothersome symptoms of headache, fever, and malaise. Bed rest is encouraged for fatigue but is not imposed for any specified period of time. Affected youngsters are instructed to regulate activities according to their own tolerance unless complicating factors are present. If the spleen is enlarged, activities in which children might receive a blow to the abdomen or chest are avoided.

A short course of oral penicillin is sometimes prescribed for sore throat, especially if β-hemolytic streptococci are present. Administration of ampicillin frequently precipitates a maculopapular rash in affected persons; therefore its use is contraindicated. Sore throat, which can be severe, can be relieved by gargles, hot drinks, analgesic troches, or analgesics,

---

CLINICAL MANIFESTATIONS OF INFECTIOUS MONONUCLEOSIS

Early Signs
Headache
Malaise
Fatigue
Chilliness
Low-grade fever
Loss of appetite
Puffy eyes

Full-Blown Disease
Cardinal Features
Fever
Sore throat
Cervical adenopathy

Common Features
Splenomegaly (may persist for several months)
Palatine petechiae
Macular eruption (especially on trunk)
Exudative pharyngitis/tonsillitis
Hepatic involvement to some degree, often associated with jaundice

including opioids. The use of corticosteroids has demonstrated effectiveness in reducing respiratory distress from tonsillar hypertrophy, hemolytic anemia, thrombocytopenia, and neurologic complications. Although steroids can shorten the course of the illness, their use is reserved for complicated cases.

Prognosis. The course of infectious mononucleosis is self-limiting and usually uncomplicated. Acute symptoms usually disappear within 7 to 10 days, and the persistent fatigue subsides within 2 to 4 weeks. A number of affected youngsters may need to restrict activities for 2 to 3 months; the disease rarely extends for longer periods. Complications are uncommon but can be serious and require appropriate management.

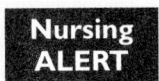

| Nursing ALERT | Advise family to seek medical evaluation of the youngster if: Breathing becomes difficult. Abdominal pain develops. Sore throat pain is so severe that the child is unable to eat or drink. |

Nursing Considerations

Nursing responsibilities are directed toward providing comfort measures to relieve the symptoms and helping affected youngsters and their families determine appropriate activities according to the stage of the disease and their interests. They may need diet counseling to select foods that contain sufficient calories to meet growth and energy needs but are easy to swallow. Every effort should be made to prevent a secondary infection; therefore, the adolescent is counseled to limit exposure to persons outside the family, especially during the acute phase of illness.

The illness and its associated weakness and fatigue can cause depression and resentment on the part of usually vigorous, active teenagers. It is important to spend time with youngsters to listen to their concerns and to allow them to express their feelings and vent their anger. Adolescents need reassurance that the limitations are only temporary, that social activities—so essential at this stage of development—can be resumed after the acute phase, and that they will have sufficient autonomy to determine the extent of their capabilities and the rate of resumption of activities.

SMOKING

Seventy percent of children experiment with cigarettes during the course of their childhood, many while in elementary school. Some youngsters then progress to occasional use (on weekends, at parties, on dates). By the end of high school about 20% to 30% of senior high school boys and 25% to 35% of senior high school girls report having smoked in the past 30 days (Johnston, Bachman, and O'Malley, 1992).

The hazards of smoking at any age are undisputed; however, a preventive approach to teenage smoking is especially important. Smoking almost immediately brings about reduced lung function, "smoker's" cough, and other respiratory difficulties. Most harmful of all is the likelihood of lifelong addiction, since the earlier a person starts smoking, the more difficult it is to quit later in life. Furthermore, research findings indicate a clear association between the use of to-bacco and the use of alcohol and other drugs (Torabi, Bailey and Majd-Jabbari, 1993).

Etiology

There are a variety of reasons why teenagers begin smoking, such as imitation of adult behavior, peer pressure, and emulation of traits popularly attributed to smokers. Teenagers least likely to smoke are those whose families and friends do not smoke, those who are interested in academics or athletics (particularly high-performance sports, such as basketball, swimming, and track), and those who plan to go on to college (see Family Focus box).

Smokeless Tobacco

Tobacco products that are placed in the mouth but not ignited (e.g., snuff and chewing tobacco) are referred to as smokeless tobacco. This increasingly popular substitute for cigarettes is now posing a serious hazard to children and adolescents, as well as young adults. These products have been shown to be carcinogenic, and regular use has been reported to cause foul-smelling breath, periodontal disease, and tooth erosion or loss. A 1994 report of the Surgeon General (U.S. Department of Health and Human Services, 1994) concluded that smokeless tobacco is also associated with lesions in oral soft tissue and can lead to cigarette smoking.

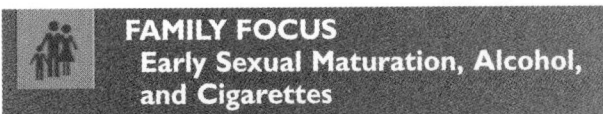

FAMILY FOCUS
Early Sexual Maturation, Alcohol, and Cigarettes

Cigarette smoking and the drinking of alcohol among adolescents are complex behaviors that cannot be explained by any single causative factor. However, theorists and investigators have looked at the relationship between biologic maturation and these behaviors. In particular, early sexual maturation in girls is related to the earlier onset of cigarette smoking and alcohol use (Wilson and others, 1994). One explanation for this association focuses on the rationale that girls who enter puberty early have a decreased self-image because their bodies are out of synchrony with those of other girls in their age group. Consequently a young girl who is sexually mature at the age of 12 years may be attracted to a group of 14–16-year-old girls and boys who smoke and drink. If these teens have not been in any motor vehicle injuries while drinking, the young girl reasons that she, too, will be safe if she smokes, drinks, or is in an automobile with friends who are drinking.

Although parents and nurses cannot influence the time of biologic maturation, they can identify young girls who are at risk for the initiation of smoking and drinking because of early puberty. Parents need to understand that an early maturing daughter might be uncomfortable with her body, and take advantage of all opportunities to build her self-esteem. Parental sensitivity to the importance of peer group acceptance is crucial. Parents need to be very supportive of a teenage daughter who feels left out or different. School nurses are in an excellent position to provide anticipatory guidance to girls who enter puberty early and to help them role play responses they can use to cope with situations that involve offers to smoke and drink. In addition, school nurses can provide information on the bodily changes that accompany puberty and emphasize the fact that not all teens enter puberty at the same time.

Nursing Considerations

Prevention of regular smoking in teenagers appears to be the most effective way to reduce the overall incidence of smoking. A variety of methods have been employed to deal with the problem. For the most part, smoking-prevention programs that focus on negative long-term effects of smoking on health have been ineffective. Those emphasizing immediate effects and youth-to-youth programs have been somewhat more effective, but primarily in improving teenagers' attitudes toward smoking. Because smoking and smoking-related behavior function as a key social symbol, antismoking campaigns must be addressed to the norms of the potential smokers without ridicule or threat to the social norms of the group.

Two areas of focus are gaining interest among health advocates: (1) peer-led programming emphasizing social consequences of smoking and (2) use of media, such as videotapes and films, in smoking prevention. If a significant number of influential peers can "sell" their classmates on the idea that the habit is not popular, the followers will imitate their behavior. Short-term rather than long-term consequences are emphasized (e.g., the effects of smoking on personal appearance, such as the unattractive stains on teeth and hands and the unpleasant odor that smoking gives to the breath and clothing). Several strategies are recommended for health professionals (see box).

Schools are ideal settings for tobacco use prevention programs. The majority of states have mandated that schools in-

corporate education that relays the adverse effects of smoking to students (Clubb, 1991). Smoking bans in schools also accomplish several goals: (1) they discourage students from starting to smoke; (2) they reinforce knowledge of the health hazards of cigarette smoking and exposure to environmental tobacco smoke; and (3) they promote a smoke-free environment as the norm. There is also pressure from the United States federal government for states to enforce the legal age for buying cigarettes.

HEALTH PROBLEMS RELATED TO SPORTS PARTICIPATION

Every sport has some potential for injury to the participant—whether the youngster engages in serious competition or participates for enjoyment. Serious injury can occur during rough contact sports or to persons who are not physically prepared for the activity. The risk of injury is greater if the youngster's body build is not suited to the sport, if the muscles and support systems (respiratory and cardiovascular) are insufficiently conditioned to withstand the rigors of the physical stress, or if the youngster lacks the insight and judgment to recognize when an activity is beyond his or her capabilities. More injuries occur during recreational sports participation than during organized athletic competition.

Not only does the activity itself pose a hazard of greater or lesser degree (Fig. 17-1), but the environment and the sports or recreational equipment present additional risks. Children participate in physical activity in a variety of environments, both indoors and outdoors, on floors, on the ground, on snow, on or beneath water surfaces, and sometimes in free air space. These activities frequently involve equipment that intensifies the risk factor.

Acute overload injuries are those that occur suddenly during an activity and produce immediate symptoms. They can be caused by a blow or overstretching, twisting, or sudden stress to tissues. For descriptions and management of traumatic injuries see Chapter 31.

OVERUSE SYNDROMES

To excel in sports, the young athlete is forced to train longer, harder, and earlier in life than previously. The rewards are an increased level of fitness, better performances, faster times, and the satisfaction of attaining a personal goal. However, the risk of overuse injury is always present and can be related to several factors: training errors, muscle-tendon imbalance, anatomic malalignment, incorrect footwear or playing surface, an associated disease state, and growth.

The common feature in overuse injuries is the repetitive microtrauma that occurs to a particular anatomic structure when the same movements are performed over a long period of time; the end result is inflammation of the involved structure with complaints of pain, tenderness, swelling, and disability. Examples of overuse syndromes include "Little League elbow" (tendinitis and osteochondritis from repetitive throwing), "tennis elbow" (lateral epicondylitis from repetitive elbow strain), and Osgood-Schlatter disease (traction apophysitis of tibial tubercle).

RECOMMENDED NONSMOKING STRATEGIES

Provide only a cursory mention of long-term health consequences (e.g., cardiovascular and cancer risks)

Discuss immediate physiologic consequences in some detail (e.g., changes in heart rate and blood pressure, minor respiratory symptoms, and blood carbon monoxide concentrations)

Mention alternatives to smoking for establishing a self-image that appears tough, independent, mature, or sophisticated (e.g., establishing a weight-lifting regimen, jogging and dancing, joining a Boys' Club or a Girls' Club, engaging in volunteer work for a hospital or political or religious group)

Mention the negative effects of smoking (e.g., earlier wrinkling of skin, yellow stains on teeth and fingers, tobacco odor on breath and clothing)

Mention the increasing ostracism of smokers by nonsmokers, both legal and informal, in places of work and public places

Mention the increasing evidence that second-hand smoke is injurious to the health of nonsmokers who are regularly exposed, especially small children

Acknowledge that many adults once believed that important social benefits were associated with smoking, but point out that the vast majority of adult smokers would now quit smoking if they could

Arm the cooperative adolescent with arguments for dealing with peer pressure (e.g., by not smoking, a teenager demonstrates independence and nonconformity, traits normally prized by youth)

Request posters and pamphlets from local voluntary agencies (e.g., American Cancer Society, American Heart Association, and American Lung Association) to display prominently

Modified from Wong-McCarthy WJ, Gritz ER: Preventing regular teenage cigarette smoking, *Pediatr Ann* 11:683-689, 1982.

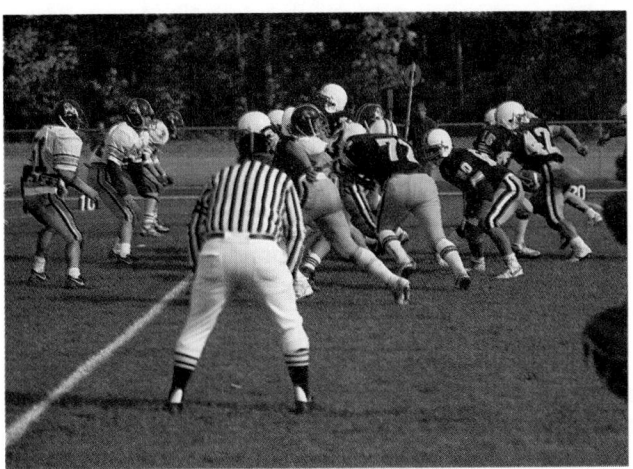

FIG. 17-1. Football is an example of a strenuous collision sport.

Stress Fractures

Stress fractures occur as a result of repeated muscle contraction and are seen most often in repetitive weightbearing sports such as running, gymnastics, and basketball. They occur less often in swimmers. The most common symptoms are a sharp, persistent, progressive pain or a deep, persistent, dull ache located over the bone. Sometimes there is pain on impact (heel strike), but the most important clinical sign is pain over the involved bony surface. Diagnosis is established on the basis of clinical observation; occasionally a bone scan may be needed.

Therapeutic Management

Development of inflammation is common to all overuse syndromes; therefore the management is directed toward rest or alteration of activities, physical therapy, and medication. Rest is the primary therapy and is usually interpreted as reduced activity and the use of alternative exercise—*not* bed rest or immobilization with casting. The primary purpose is to alleviate the repetitive stress that initiated the symptoms. It is important to keep the youngster mobile. Training can be continued with alternative exercise that maintains conditioning without aggravating the injury. For example, pool running (treading water in the deep end of a pool) can use the same movements as running but without the weight bearing.

Other modalities include cryotherapy and cold whirlpools. Sometimes taping, bracing, splinting, and other orthotics are employed (treatment is very specific to the injury). Medications such as nonsteroidal antiinflammatory drugs are prescribed for discomfort. Topical medications are of questionable value.

NURSE'S ROLE IN SPORTS FOR CHILDREN AND ADOLESCENTS

Nurses may become involved in sports activities in the areas of preparation and evaluation for activities, prevention of injury, treatment of injuries, and rehabilitation after injury. Selecting an appropriate sport for both recreation and competition is a joint effort of youngster, parents, and health professionals. The best approach to counseling children and parents regarding sports participation is to encourage activities that are most likely to provide pleasure and physical benefits throughout childhood and into adulthood. Exposure to a variety of sports activities is probably better for young children than limiting them to one sport. Parents should be cautioned against overprogramming children in order that the children have ample time for other activities and associations.

When children sustain athletic injuries, nurses are often responsible for instructing the children and their parents regarding care. Instructions (e.g., schedule for appointments, application of ice, and any restrictions in activity) should be made clear and preferably be accompanied by written directions. The importance of taking medications as prescribed is emphasized, because they may be needed for an extended period of time and compliance may be difficult.

Prevention of sports injuries is probably the most important aspect of any athletic program. Children should be suited to the activity, and the environment and equipment should be safe for physical activity. Children should be adequately prepared for the sport, especially if it requires strenuous and/or continuous physical exertion. Nurses collaborate with coaches and athletic trainers to ensure that safety measures are carried out. Stretching exercises, warming up and cooling down activities, and an appropriate training program are only some of the requisites for safe participation. Protective measures, such as pads, taping, wrapping, or other devices, are employed for areas at risk. Nurses are also on the alert for environmental safety risks.

ALTERED GROWTH AND MATURATION

The absence of physical and/or sexual maturation at a time when other children are experiencing positive evidence of sexual development and its associated spurt in growth and physical strength is a matter of concern to both the parents and their affected child. Fortunately, in most instances the delay in development is a simple physiologic or *constitutional delay* that merely represents one end of the normal genetically influenced variation of pubertal growth. These children will go through a delayed but normal puberty to finally catch up, in their late teens, with their more rapidly developing agemates. Less benign causes of delayed development may be of endocrine origin or chromosomal aberrations. In other situations delayed development may be a result of chronic diseases (such as malabsorption or chronic asthma) that are serious enough to retard the developmental process or environmental factors (such as stress or poor nutrition).

The rate of maturation is important during the school years, but at puberty it assumes gigantic proportions to youngsters and their parents as well. Girls or boys who lag behind their peers in physical maturation are painfully aware of their shortcomings. Adolescent girls feel out of place among companions whose hips and breasts are developing, feel cheated if they have not yet menstruated, and are not a part of the giggling and boy-talk of friends. Adolescent boys feel weak and small compared with more muscular companions with whom they can no longer compete. Slow-maturing youngsters need support and reassurance that they are not abnormal and that they too will develop the characteristics for which they yearn.

Serial measurements of growth are plotted periodically on standard growth charts to determine the pattern of growth and to compare the individual child with the norm for that particular age-group. When assessing children in the extremes of height ranges, it is important to compare their height with the height of their parents and siblings.

TALL OR SHORT STATURE

Tall Stature

Despite the fact that the average height of both boys and girls is steadily increasing, there is still a small group of children who, because of some organic disorder or a familial tendency, are excessively tall when compared with their contemporaries. To some, especially boys, it may be a source of pride; to others, especially girls, it may be a source of intense anxiety and a severe social handicap.

When the rate of height change before puberty suggests the probability of excessive adult height, treatment with hormones may be considered, although there is a great deal of controversy regarding their use for this purpose. The use of estrogens has proved effective in controlling height when therapy is initiated prior to menarche and before the end of the adolescent growth spurt that normally precedes menarche. The selection of children for hormonal therapy is made on the basis of a careful evaluation of physical, psychologic, and social factors.

Short Stature

Short stature is a nonspecific finding that may be the first manifestation of a serious disorder, or it may be of no consequence medically. From a worldwide point of view, the most common cause of short stature and/or delayed development is probably inadequate nutrition; however, the major disorders that produce delayed development are chronic diseases, endocrine dysfunction, and syndromes of primary gonadal failure.

Chronic diseases can interfere with growth, but unless the illness is unduly prolonged, catch-up growth will occur. Diseases and disorders that usually cause some degree of growth delay include asthma, cystic fibrosis, gastrointestinal diseases (such as parasitic infections), malabsorption syndromes, cardiac anomalies, and chronic renal disturbances. The duration of the illness is more significant than the intensity in terms of the effect on growth, although the precise length of time necessary to affect growth permanently has not been determined.

Skeletal disorders that affect growth in stature are principally those described as dwarfism. Most are caused by a variety of congenital defects and disorders, such as achondroplasia, and by some of the inborn errors of metabolism, such as Hurler or Hunter syndrome.

Psychosocial or *deprivation dwarfism* is a stress-induced growth failure that appears to be more common than previously thought. It is defined as growth retardation in children over 2 years of age caused by environmental (emotional) stress and is associated with a marked delay in physical growth, delayed developmental skills, and immature behavior. When these children are removed from the deprived en-

vironment, their growth proceeds at a normal or increased rate. (See also Failure to Thrive, Chapter 11, and Child Maltreatment, Chapter 14.)

Management consists of continued medical observation, attention to general health and nutrition, and psychologic support. Where growth delay is accompanied by poor self-esteem, many authorities recommend hormonal therapy. Testosterone in carefully regulated doses has proved effective in some cases. Growth hormone is capable of increasing height and is used to treat growth hormone deficiency. Its use with children who have constitutional delay is highly controversial (see Hypopituitarism, Chapter 29).

Nursing Considerations

Deviation from the normal course of puberty is always of concern to the affected adolescent, and to some it assumes monumental proportions. Most of the problems of delayed development are those caused by simple constitutional delay of puberty, and in this situation the child can be assured that the normal course of events will eventually take place.

One of the difficulties related to a size that is incongruent with chronologic and mental age is the manner in which others, especially adults, relate to the child. People quite naturally respond to children with short stature as though they are younger than their age. Consequently, these children often react with babyish or juvenile behavior, thus setting in motion a circular pattern of behavior and response. Conversely, children who are tall or physically advanced for their age are frequently treated as though they are more advanced than their years. They are often considered to be retarded or behaviorally immature when they actually perform according to the normal behavioral expectations for their age.

Listening to distressed adolescents and conveying to them interest and concern are prerequisite to any successful intervention. Counseling and therapy are individualized to meet the needs of each youngster. Encouraging these children to accentuate the positive aspects of their bodies and personalities with sound health practices and good grooming helps foster a more positive self-image.

SEX CHROMOSOME ABNORMALITIES

Compared with most hereditary disorders, sex chromosome abnormalities are encountered with relatively high frequency. Most are caused by an alteration in sex chromosome number, some of which are listed in Table 17-1. The more common of these are Turner and Klinefelter syndromes. Some general characteristics of sex chromosome abnormalities are the following:

1. There is a direct relationship between the male or female body type and the presence or absence of a Y chromosome. It appears that the Y chromosome is essential for development of male characteristics.
2. The severity of defects is not related to the number of extra X chromosomes, except for mental retardation, which increases proportionately with each X chromosome.
3. The presence of more than one Y chromosome appears to have variable but as yet not well defined effects on an individual.
4. The majority of these conditions are due to nondisjunction.

TABLE 17-1. Common sex chromosome abnormalities

SYNDROME	CHROMOSOMAL NOMENCLATURE	PHENOTYPE	INCIDENCE (LIVE BIRTHS)	CLINICAL MANIFESTATIONS
Turner	45,X or 45XO	Female	1:2500 female births*	Short stature; webbed neck; low posterior hairline; shield-shaped chest with widely spaced nipples; sterile; no development of secondary sex characteristics
Triple X, or superfemale	47,XXX (can also be 48,XXXX or 49,XXXXX)	Female	1:850-1250 female births	Normal female characteristics; usually tall; variable mental capacity and behavior; at risk for impaired learning; fertile
XYY male	47,XYY (can also be 48,XYYY or mosaic)	Male	1:900 male births*	Usually normal sexual development; tendency to be tall with long head; poor coordination; may demonstrate aberrant behavior
Klinefelter	47,XXY (48,XXYY, 48,XXXY, 49,XXXXY, and so on, mosaics)	Male	1:850 male births*	Tall with long legs; hypogenitalism; sterile; male secondary sex characteristics may be deficient; may demonstrate aberrant behavior; learning disabled; possible gynecomastia
Fragile X (see also Chapter 19)	46,XY or 46,XX	Predominantly male	Not established	Normocephaly or macrocephaly; prominent mandible; large ears; macroorchidism; mental retardation

*Data from Nora JJ, Fraser FC: *Medical genetics: principles and practice,* ed 3, Philadelphia, 1989, Lea & Febiger.

Turner Syndrome

Turner syndrome is caused by absence of one of the X chromosomes; as a result, the number of chromosomes in these girls is 45—44 pairs of autosomes and 1 X chromosome (45,X). The incidence of the condition in the population has been estimated at 1 in 2500 female births. Although this disorder is often recognized at birth with the signs of a webbed neck, low posterior hairline, widely spaced nipples, and edema of the hands and feet, it is diagnosed most frequently at puberty because of three outstanding features: short stature, sexual infantilism, and amenorrhea.

Girls with Turner syndrome will always be sterile. They have been found to have difficulty with peer relationships and understanding social cues. They exhibit more behavioral problems, especially in relation to immature, socially isolated behavior. Definitive diagnosis is confirmed on the basis of a negative sex chromatin test; chromosomal analysis is rarely necessary.

Therapy is always individualized for these girls and consists primarily of hormone treatment and psychologic counseling for both child and parents. Linear growth often can be increased by the administration of growth hormone, provided therapy is begun early. Estrogen therapy is initiated during the usual time for puberty to promote the development of secondary sex characteristics. Responses to estrogen therapy vary from girl to girl, but gradual feminization is accomplished to some degree in most individuals.

Klinefelter Syndrome

The most common of all chromosomal abnormalities, Klinefelter syndrome, is caused by the presence of one or more additional X chromosomes. The majority of males with this syndrome have a chromosomal complement of 47,XXY. In young boys this disorder is seldom seen before puberty, at which time varying degrees of failure of adolescent virilization occur. Some males are not detected until they appear for evaluation for infertility. All have absence of sperm in the semen (azoospermia), small testes, and defective development of secondary sex characteristics. The incidence of Klinefelter syndrome is estimated to be approximately 1 in 850 live male births. In 80% of these boys there is a chromatin-positive buccal smear, and the extra chromosome is apparent on chromosomal analysis.

Cognitive impairment of varying degrees is a frequent finding and appears to have a direct relationship to the number of X chromosomes in the cells. Boys with Klinefelter syndrome may also have gross motor skill difficulties, developmental language delay, poor verbal skills, and reduced auditory memory. Shyness, passivity, behavioral problems, and school difficulties are often associated with the disorder, but this may be related to the difference in body build and delayed development.

The major effort in medical treatment is directed toward enhancing the masculine characteristics through the administration of male hormones, principally testosterone. Cosmetic surgery will eliminate embarrassment for the boy with gynecomastia.

Nursing Considerations

The nursing care of children with Turner or Klinefelter syndrome is primarily supportive. Nurses assist in diagnosis, explain tests and therapies to children and families, and provide support and encouragement. Because both disorders render the individual unable to reproduce, psychologic counseling, as well as modification of sex education, will be an important aspect of care. Marriage and sexual relationships are still possible, and alternative reproductive options, such as artificial insemination and adoption, should be discussed.

DISORDERS RELATED TO THE REPRODUCTIVE SYSTEM

AMENORRHEA

It is not unusual for an adolescent girl to skip a menstrual period or two when establishing normal menstrual and ovulatory cycles. Delay in initiation of menstruation is ordinarily a temporary problem resulting from late onset of puberty and requires no intervention. This is of little concern unless it creates undue anxiety on the part of the girl and her parents, which can ordinarily be allayed by explanation and reassurance. Careful examination will reveal any congenital defects of the genital tract (a rare cause).

Primary amenorrhea is defined as no menses by age 16 in the presence of normal secondary sex characteristics, no menses 1 to 2 years after reaching Tanner stage V, or no menses 3 to 5 years after the onset of breast development (see Fig. 16-1). Primary amenorrhea may result from absence or malformation of the female genital structures, the inability of normal structures to respond to hormonal stimulation, or strenuous physical activity. The most common cause of *secondary amenorrhea* (prolonged absence of menstruation for 6 months or more in the first 2 years following menarche or when more than three periods have been missed after menses have become established) is pregnancy. Other factors include immaturity, extreme physical stress, severe emotional stress, sudden environmental change, hyperthyroidism or hypothyroidism, chronic systemic illness, extreme weight loss or gain, anorexia nervosa (even before marked weight loss), ovarian disturbance, and pharmacologic agents (e.g., some prescribed medications, abused substances, hormones).

Exercise-Related Menstrual Dysfunction

Delayed menarche has been associated with girls who engage in strenuous exercise. It is not clear whether exercise delays menarche, or menarcheal delay promotes athletic success. Some attribute delayed menarche and maintenance of regular ovulation to lack of development of body fat. Alterations have also been noted in menstrual bleeding patterns of girls who engage in strenuous exercise. The activities that appear to be associated with delayed or altered menstruation are ballet dancing, running, gymnastics, and swimming. This condition may cause embarrassment and concern to the youngster and her parents, which can be minimized by explanation and reassurance regarding its benign and temporary nature.

DYSMENORRHEA

A certain amount of discomfort during the first day or two of the menstrual flow is extremely common. Most girls experience cramping, abdominal pain, backache, and leg ache,

but in a few the pain is intolerable and incapacitating. *Primary dysmenorrhea* is painful menses not related to any pelvic disease. When the discomfort can be attributed to endometriosis, infection, adhesions from peritonitis, or other pelvic disease, the complaint is termed *secondary dysmenorrhea.*

Primary dysmenorrhea is directly related to the occurrence of prior ovulation. There is also a relationship between uterine contractility and the secretion of prostaglandins. Psychogenic factors such as sexual abuse, familial conditioning, sexrole confusion, and school avoidance may also contribute to dysmenorrhea.

A thorough gynecologic examination is carried out to exclude any pelvic abnormalities, and a careful history is taken regarding the type and duration of pain, its relationship to menstrual flow, and any associated symptoms. These questions not only provide information to the examiner, but also serve to provide the girl with evidence that her problem is being taken seriously. An explanation of the physiology of menstruation is reassuring.

Therapeutic Management

The treatment of choice for adolescents is the administration of nonsteroidal antiinflammatory drugs that block the formation of prostaglandins for 2 to 3 days of the menstrual cycle. Cyclic estrogen therapy and oral contraceptives are also effective. Simple exercises such as pelvic rocking, assuming the knee-chest position, and breathing exercises, may be beneficial. Encourage good hygiene and participation in regular activities.

Nursing Considerations

All young teens need reassurance that menstruation is a normal function. The nurse who is sought out for advice regarding menstrual problems has an opportunity to engage in health teaching concerning menstrual physiology and hygiene, as well as the importance of a well-balanced diet, exercise, and general health maintenance. Health teaching can also dispel any myths in relation to menstruation and femininity. When assessment indicates a potential problem and the need for evaluation, referral to an appropriate practitioner, health service, or clinic may be necessary.

One of the most difficult experiences facing the adolescent girl is the gynecologic examination. Whether it is her first experience or not, she is most likely filled with apprehension. Almost all adolescents are extremely self-conscious about their bodies and the changes taking place. They need continuing support in the form of anticipatory guidance regarding what to expect and suggestions of what to do to help relax during the procedure. Usually the stressful experience of being placed in stirrups for the pelvic examination can be avoided. The young female who is relaxed may be examined in the supine position with hips and knees flexed and legs abducted. If a female nurse is not the examiner, it is essential for her to remain with the patient during the examination to offer support and guidance.

VAGINITIS

Vaginitis can be caused by physical, chemical, or infectious agents. Physical causes may include a forgotten tampon or contraceptive sponge. Chemical irritants include bubble bath, douching, and deodorant pads. Removal of the offending material or discontinuing use of the irritating substance is usually all that is necessary to treat physical or chemical vaginitis. Infectious vaginitis can be caused by the *Candida* fungi (yeast), *Trichomonas* protozoa parasites, or bacteria. Diagnosis is confirmed with microscopic evaluation of vaginal secretions. Treatment varies depending on the infectious agent.

Health teaching is important in the prevention and management of all types of vaginitis. Adolescent females need to be reassured that increased vaginal mucus can occur at the time of ovulation, before menstruation, or with sexual excitement. Many teens mistake these variations as signs of infection. Young females should be taught to wipe front to back after toileting and to realize that vaginitis can result from irritation, foreign objects, and sexual activity. Nurses need to stress the importance of an evaluation to determine the exact cause.

DISORDERS OF THE MALE REPRODUCTIVE SYSTEM

Most obvious anomalies, such as hypospadias, hydrocele, phimosis, and cryptorchidism, have been identified, and corrective measures have been instituted during early childhood. The most frequent problems related to the reproductive organs in later childhood are (1) infections, such as urethritis (see Urinary Tract Infection, Chapter 27); (2) hematuria; (3) penile problems, such as nonretractable foreskin in uncircumcised males, carcinoma, and trauma; (4) scrotal conditions, such as varicocele (elongation, dilation, and tortuosity of the veins superior to the testicle); and (5) testicular torsion (a condition in which the testicle hangs free from its vascular structures, which can result in partial or complete venous occlusion with rotation). Tumors of the testes are not a common condition, but when manifested in adolescence, they are generally malignant and demand immediate evaluation.

The usual presenting symptom for testicular cancer is a heavy, hard painless mass (either smooth or nodular) that is palpated on the testis. Treatment involves surgical removal of the affected testicle (orchiectomy) and possibly chemotherapy and radiation if metastasis has occurred.

Nursing Considerations

The adolescent male is extremely self-conscious about his changing body and needs preparation for a genital examination. The most successful approach is to assume a matter-of-fact attitude toward the examination, explain precisely what will take place, and maintain a continuous commentary about what is being done and the findings at each phase of the examination. The adolescent male is approached as someone important as a person, with the nurse interested in his concerns. To supplement routine health assessment, every adolescent male should be taught frequent testicular self-examination (TSE) to familiarize himself with his own anatomy and to ensure early detection of any abnormality.

The normal testicle is a firm organ with a smooth, egg-shaped contour; the epididymis is palpated as a raised swelling on the superior aspect of the testicle and should not be confused as an abnormality. (See Critical Thinking Exercise above.)

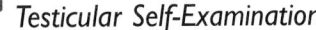

CRITICAL THINKING EXERCISE
Testicular Self-Examination

At a recent faculty meeting the school nurse presented plans for a class on testicular self-examination (TSE) to be delivered to the sophomore boys. Several faculty members questioned the value of providing such a class when there is limited time to deliver content relating to "routine academic subjects." Which of the following responses could the nurse use to justify including the TSE class in the curriculum?

1. TSE provides an opportunity for adolescent males to pick up early cases of epididymitis, a common infection in this age group.
2. TSE allows adolescent boys to determine if they have an asymptomatic sexually transmitted disease.
3. TSE permits detection of any tumors of the testes, which are not common in adolescence, but which are often malignant and demand immediate attention when they occur.
4. TSE allows easy identification of malignant testicular tumors that occur in 5% of adolescent males.

The correct response is three. TSE is an easily learned technique that allows the adolescent male to become familiar with his own anatomy and to determine any abnormalities. Although testicular cancer is not common in adolescence, when it does occur the tumors are often malignant and early detection is essential. Although TSE is easily learned by adolescents, the method does not allow the adolescent male to determine if he has a sexually transmitted disease or epididymitis.

GYNECOMASTIA

The male breast, although not strictly part of the male reproductive system, responds to hormonal changes. Some degree of bilateral or unilateral breast enlargement occurs frequently in boys during puberty. It is estimated that approximately half of adolescent boys have transient gynecomastia, usually lasting less than 1 year (Biro and others, 1990), that subsides spontaneously with achievement of male development. Occasionally, however, it is associated with abnormalities such as Klinefelter syndrome or endocrine dysfunction; therefore appropriate diagnostic examination rules out these possibilities.

If the condition persists or is extensive enough to cause embarrassment or to produce doubts about gender identity in the young boy, plastic surgery is indicated for cosmetic and psychologic considerations. Administration of testosterone has no effect on breast development or regression and may even aggravate the condition.

Nursing Considerations

Treatment usually consists of assurance to the adolescent and his parents that this is a benign and temporary situation. Adolescents who are distressed about physical integrity and masculinity may benefit from the knowledge that it occurs in more than 50% of all adolescent males.

HEALTH PROBLEMS RELATED TO SEXUALITY

More than half of all young people in grades 9 to 12 have had sexual intercourse; male students and black students are more likely to engage in sexual intercourse than white or Hispanic students (Sexual behavior, 1992). Adolescents express various reasons for wanting to be sexually active, such as (1) the need to be loved, (2) the desire for conquest, (3) the need to feel grown up, (4) the need to conform and be accepted by peers, and (5) rebellion against parents. The increasing incidence of adolescent pregnancy, sexually transmitted disease (STD), and sexual trauma make it imperative that health professionals understand these problems as well as the psychosocial dynamics that may have led to them.

ADOLESCENT PREGNANCY

Each year 1 in 10 adolescent girls in the United States becomes pregnant—approximately 1 million females under the age of 20 years. About 554,000 of these pregnancies result in a birth; more than 400,000 are terminated by abortion (McAnarney and Hendee, 1989). Today most teenage mothers choose to keep their babies; consequently, there are 1.3 million infants living with teenage mothers, about half of whom are not married. Today in most cases teenage pregnancy is no longer considered to be biologically disadvantageous to the unborn child, but it is still regarded as socially, educationally, psychologically, and economically disadvantageous to the mother.

With better facilities available for care, the mortality for teenage pregnancies is decreasing, but the morbidity remains high. Teenage girls and their unborn infants are at greater risk for complications of both pregnancy and delivery. The most frequent complications are premature labor and infants of low birth weight, high neonatal mortality, pregnancy-induced hypertension (PIH), iron deficiency anemia, fetopelvic disproportion, and prolonged labor. It now appears that the major obstetric difficulties are related to the smaller maternal size rather than the younger age or developmental immaturity.

Although teenagers have special needs, the obstetric risk should be no greater than for any pregnant patient. When quality prenatal care is available early in the pregnancy, the progress and outcome of teenage pregnancies compare favorably with those of older women.

Nursing Considerations

The most important goal in nursing care of the pregnant teenager is to help her obtain prenatal care. The importance of early prenatal care, especially adequate nutrition, is well known for the welfare of both mother and infant when the adolescent chooses to continue the pregnancy and to facilitate a safe abortion if this option is selected. For guidelines, teaching, and general support measures during pregnancy, the reader is directed to the excellent textbooks available on nursing care throughout the maternity cycle.*

---

*For example, see Bobak IM, Jensen MD: *Maternity and gynecologic care: the nurse and the family,* ed 5, St Louis, 1997, Mosby.

CONTRACEPTION

Family planning services have developed and expanded during recent years, and with the increase in sexual activity among the teenage population the need for contraceptive services as part of the health care of adolescents is great.

Teenagers want contraceptive information, but many do not use birth control methods consistently. For example, condom use among adolescent females who engage in high-risk behaviors, such as substance or alcohol abuse and minor delinquency, is much lower than among adolescents who do not engage in high-risk behaviors (Orr and others, 1992). Therefore contraceptive counseling may need to be broader than just providing birth control information and devices; it should be part of a comprehensive health education program.

The choice of a safe and effective contraceptive method must be suited to the individual (Table 17-2). The choice is based on preference after the adolescent is informed of the benefits and disadvantages. Motivation is necessary for most methods. For example, the pill is very effective if used correctly, but the adolescent must remember to take the pill every day. For many young women the use of a levonorgestrel implant (Norplant) is an ideal choice, because it is extremely effective and eliminates the need for compliance. However, sexually active adolescents need to remember that contraceptive devices other than condoms do not prevent STDs. Condom use is still important and must be discussed with all adolescents who seek contraceptive advice.

SEXUALLY TRANSMITTED DISEASES (STDs)

STDs are among the most prevalent of the communicable diseases with a disproportionate number occurring in adolescents and young adults. Sexually active adolescents are particularly at risk because they are often late in seeking medical attention, they are at higher risk for developing ectopic pregnancies due to scarring from the infection, and the mortality and morbidity associated with human immunodeficiency virus (HIV) infection is positively correlated to the number of sexual partners. When a patient has one STD, it is important to check for others in the history and examination.

The most prevalent STDs in the adolescent and adult populations are gonorrhea and chlamydial infections. These and other STDs are outlined in Table 17-3.

Although few adolescents have acquired immunodeficiency syndrome (AIDS), adolescents are at high risk for HIV infection because of the trend toward sexual intercourse at earlier ages, the high prevalence of STDs in adolescence, and increasing heterosexual transmission of the HIV virus. Most people diagnosed with AIDS in their early 20s were infected during adolescence. The risk of HIV infection in teenagers must not be underestimated (Hoffman, Kelly, and Futterman, 1996).

Therapeutic Management

Effective treatment of both males and females with an STD involves administration of the appropriate therapeutic agent. It is also suggested that all patients with gonorrhea receive a course of tetracycline therapy because of the high rate of mixed gonococcal and chlamydial infections. Treatment of sexual partners is also an essential part of therapy.

TABLE 17-2. Advantages and disadvantages of contraceptive methods in the adolescent

METHOD	ADVANTAGES	DISADVANTAGES
Abstinence	100% effective in preventing STDs and pregnancy	Peer pressure to conform Relatively high failure rate from noncompliance
Withdrawal Withdrawal of penis before ejaculation	Reduced risk of pregnancy No medical visit necessary	High failure rate Some seminal fluid often released before ejaculation Ejaculate at vaginal orifice may enter vagina No STD protection
Rhythm Refrain from intercourse during fertile period (time of ovulation)	Teaches women about their menstrual cycle Encourages couple participation	High failure rate Requires a regular, predictable menstrual cycle (unusual in early and middle adolescence) No STD protection
Barrier Methods Condom	No medical complications Easy to use Available without prescription	Requires consistent use Requires premeditated intent for sexual union May decrease sensation
Male: penile covering to trap sperm Spermicidal condoms increase effectiveness for pregnancy and STD prevention	Provides protection against STDs No side effects Female participation	High failure rate (unless used properly)
Female: inserted into vagina with base covering part of perineum	Girl can carry with her for unexpected sexual encounter Male participation	Interrupts sex
Diaphragm Cervical covering to prevent sperm from reaching egg Must be used in conjunction with spermicidal jelly	Virgins can be fitted May be inserted 4 to 6 hours before intercourse Low failure rate when used correctly Few contraindications May be reused	High failure rate in adolescents because of inconvenience of use Requires consistent use Requires fitting and instruction by medical personnel If inserted early, should be checked for placement before coitus Requires premeditated intent for sexual union Requires body awareness and comfort with touching oneself for insertion Little STD protection May increase incidence of urinary tract infection
Sponge Cervical covering Releases a spermicide	Can be obtained without a prescription May be inserted up to 6 hours before sex	Similar to diaphragm, but less effective Minimal STD protection Difficult to remove Requires body awareness and comfort with touching self Decreased effectiveness in parous women
Chemicals—spermicidal foam, jelly, cream, and suppositories Substance injected into vagina to kill sperm	Available without prescription Inexpensive Easy to use Provides some protection against STDs No major health concerns	High failure rate unless combined with condom Possible for sperm to be ejaculated directly into uterine os, bypassing spermicide in vagina Must be used shortly before coitus; therefore requires interruption of sexual experience Repeated sexual union requires repeated application Requires premeditated intent for sexual union Messy

Continued.

TABLE 17-2. Advantages and disadvantages of contraceptive methods in the adolescent—cont'd

METHOD	ADVANTAGES	DISADVANTAGES
Oral Contraceptives Estrogen and progesterone-like compounds Inhibit ovulation by blocking release of gonadotropins from anterior pituitary gland	99% effective if used correctly Exceedingly safe for adolescents Method of choice for most youngsters Administered by mouth Becomes a ritual not associated with sexual activity Regulates menses, decreases dysmenorrhea and acne	Higher failure rate in adolescents than in older women Need to follow precise instructions; requires continued motivation, consistent use Requires prescription Price substantial for teenager No STD protection Side effects: numerous; of special concern to teenagers: weight gain, tiredness, depression, breast tenderness, breakthrough bleeding, spotting, and heavy bleeding with clots
Implanted Contraceptives Levonorgestrel implants (Norplant) Synthetic and biologically active progestin Inhibits ovulation in the majority of menstrual cycles Increases thickness of cervical mucus, preventing sperm penetration into cervical canal	Theoretically 100% effective Eliminates need for compliance (convenient) Long-term continuous protection (up to 5 years if desired) Safe for adolescents Very low dose of hormones and no estrogen Reversible No interruption of sex	Invasive at time of insertion into inner aspect of upper arm; some discomfort from local anesthetic; removal may be difficult Requires prescription Price substantial for teenagers (may be paid by Medicaid) No STD protection Side effects: irregular and possibly heavy menstrual bleeding that persists for many women during first few months' use; amenorrhea, headache, nervousness, nausea, dizziness, significant weight gain
Depo Provera Progestin that suppresses hormonal cycle and prevents ovulation Injection given every 3 months	No interruption of sex Invisible method	No STD protection Significant weight gain Irregular menses or amenorrhea Decreased libido Fertility may be delayed Must return to care provider every 3 months for injection
Postcoital Contraception Combined estrogen-progestin pill containing ethinyl estradiol; given within 72 hours of unprotected sex and repeated 12 hours later; prevents implantation	Useful in unplanned sexual intercourse	No STD protection May cause nausea Effectiveness dependent on phase of menstrual cycle Not intended for repeated use

A totally effective prophylaxis against infection is not yet available; therefore preventive efforts must be directed toward finding and treating affected persons, locating and examining contacts of affected persons, educating young people regarding the facts of the disease and its spread, and encouraging the use of condoms in sexually active young people.

Nursing Considerations

Nursing responsibilities encompass all aspects of sexually transmissible disease education, confidentiality, prevention, and treatment. Part of the sex education of young people should include providing information about these diseases, their symptoms and treatment, and dispelling the myths associated with their mode of transmission. Many vulnerable adolescents are uninformed or misinformed about these.

The major efforts of counseling should be directed toward prevention, with emphasis on avoiding sex or, when this does not seem feasible, avoiding casual sex with multiple partners and promoting the use of condoms. The school nurse may be involved in the controversial issue of whether or not to distribute condoms to sexually active high school students as a possible measure to control the spread of STDs, especially HIV infection, in this population.

PELVIC INFLAMMATORY DISEASE (PID)

PID is an infection of the upper female genital tract (endometrium and fallopian tubes), most commonly caused by STDs. Teenagers account for 16% to 20% of all cases of PID,

TABLE 17-3. Selected sexually transmitted diseases

MANIFESTATIONS	THERAPY	NURSING CONSIDERATIONS
Gonorrhea *(Neisseria Gonorrhoeae)*		
Male: Urethritis—dysuria with profuse yellow discharge, frequency, urgency, nocturia	Single dose IM ceftriaxone	Find and treat sexual contacts Educate young people regarding facts of the disease and its spread Encourage use of condoms in sexually active young people
Female: Cervicitis (postpubertal)—may be associated with discharge, dysuria, dyspareunia; vulvovaginitis (prepubertal)	Single oral dose of cefixime, ciproflaxin or ciprofloxacin	High rate of mixed disease; therefore treatment for chlamydia is recommended
Chlamydia *(Chlamydia Trachomatis)*		
Male: Meatal erythema, tenderness, itching, dysuria, urethral discharge	Doxycycline Azithromycin	Same as above
Female: Mucopurulent cervical exudate with erythema, edema, congestion	If pregnant: erythromycin	
Syphilis *(Treponema Pallidum)*		
Primary stage: Chancre—a hard, painless, red, sharply defined lesion with indurated base, raised border, eroded surface, and scanty yellow discharge; usually located on penis, vulva, or cervix	Penicillin or doxycycline	Viability of organism outside body is short Rapidly killed by oxygen, soap, common bacterial agents, and drying About 95% transmitted sexually; affected person most infectious during first year of disease
Secondary stage: Systemic influenza-like symptoms and lymphadenopathy, rash; usually appears 1 to 3 weeks after healing of chancre		May be transmitted to fetus Increased risk for HIV when open lesions are present
Herpes Progenitalis *(Herpesvirus Hominis*—Type II)		
Small (usually painful) vesicles on genital area, buttocks, and thighs; itching usually initial symptom; when vesicles break, shallow, circular, extremely painful lesions remain	No known cure Acyclovir orally or IV	Use of condoms to avoid spread or infection with other organisms. Pregnancy should be avoided in sexually active girls Infection can be transmitted to infant during birth
Trichomoniasis *(Trichomonas Vaginalis)*		
Pruritus and edema of external genitalia; foul-smelling, greenish vaginal discharge; sometimes postcoital bleeding May be asymptomatic, especially in males	Oral metronidazole	Patient should not consume alcohol while taking medication and for at least 48 hours following last dose Can be sexually transmitted, therefore sexual partners should be treated.
Candidiasis, or Moniliasis *(Candida Albicans)*		
Edema and erythema of vulva and thick white, cheesy vaginal discharge May be satellite lesions on groin, thighs, and buttocks Cutaneous lesions on penis May be asymptomatic	Nystatin vaginal suppositories Miconazole vaginal cream or suppository Butoconazole cream Clotrimazole vaginal tablets	Possibility of predisposing factors such as oral contraceptives (which alter vaginal environment), antibiotics, diabetes, pregnancy, depressed cellular immunity Increased risk of neonatal oral candidiasis
Human Papillomavirus (HPV)		
Warts may be found on any part of male or female genitalia	Topical application of chemical agents (podophyllin or trichloroacetic acid [TCA]) Freezing with liquid nitrogen Intravaginal and external application of 5-fluorouracil Laser therapy	All external lesions are treated because of concern regarding relationship of HPV to cancer
Acquired Immunodeficiency Syndrome (Human Immunodeficiency Virus [HIV])		
See Chapter 26	Primarily supportive	See Chapter 26

which often result from untreated gonorrheal or chlamydial infections.

Presenting symptoms in the adolescent may be generalized, with fever, abdominal pain, urinary tract symptoms, and vague influenza-like manifestations, such as malaise, nausea, diarrhea, or constipation. A pelvic examination is indicated for every sexually active female who complains of lower abdominal pain to evaluate the possibility of PID.

PID is of major concern to nurses because of the devastating effects on the reproductive tract of affected adolescents. Approximately 25% of females experiencing PID may have short-term complications, such as acute abscess formation in the fallopian tubes (tubo-ovarian abscess), or long-term complications, such as chronic pelvic pain, dyspareunia (painful coitus), or adhesion formation. Most significant, however, is the increased risk for ectopic pregnancy and/or infertility, which results from tubal scarring.

Prevention is the primary concern of health care professionals. Barrier contraceptive methods, such as condoms with the addition of spermicide, seem to offer the best protection for preventing STDs and this serious complication. Sexually active teenage females should be screened routinely to detect asymptomatic STDs, and treatment should be initiated to prevent PID and all associated complications.

RAPE

The adolescent girl is particularly vulnerable to sexual assault, and it is estimated that more than 50% of rape victims are between 15 and 19 years of age. In each instance the victim is potentially subject to serious physical or emotional harm, or both. Males may also be assaulted (usually homosexually) and experience a range of symptoms similar to that observed in female victims.

Rape is broadly defined as sexual intercourse or attempted intercourse without the victim's consent. Most of the current definitions of rape are expanded to include all forms of sexual victimization, including anal, oral, and genital penetration. Rape also includes intrusion of any object or body part into the genital or anal area of another person's body. Fitting the penis between the labia without disruption of the hymen or evidence of ejaculation is also considered sufficient penetration to constitute rape. *Statutory rape* may be charged when the victim is unable to give consent legally by virtue of age (age varies from state to state from 12 to 18 years of age), mental deficiency, psychosis, or an altered state of consciousness caused by sleep, drugs (including alcohol), or illness.

Three relationships are identified for adolescent assault: stranger (person unknown to the victim), nonstranger (person known to the victim; sometimes referred to as *acquaintance* or *date rape*), and incest (see Sexual Abuse, Chapter 14). Although all can have serious and long-lasting effects, they are presumed to be different in a number of important ways: in the nature of the dominant, psychologic, and cognitive behavior they provoke; in the issues they raise for service providers and other potential helpers; and in the techniques that may be helpful for treating existing and new cases.

Diagnostic Evaluation

The rape victim may exhibit any of a variety of reactions (see box), and the circumstances of the initial medical evaluation may also be frightening and stressful. The initial contact with

CLINICAL MANIFESTATIONS OF RAPE VICTIMS

May Display a Variety of Behaviors:
Hysterical crying
Giggling
Agitation
Feelings of degradation
Anger and rage
Helplessness
Nervousness
Rapid mood swings
Appear calm and controlled (masking inner turmoil)
Confused
Self-blame
Fear—of the rape and of injury

Evidence of Physical Force from:
Roughness
Nonbrutal beating (slapping)
Brutal beating (slugging, kicking, beating repeatedly with fists)
Choking or gagging

Medical Examination Provides Evidence of:
Penetration
Ejaculation
Use of force

the rape victim must be supportive because the interrogation and associated activities have the potential to add to the trauma of the sexual assault. First of all the victim needs to know that she (or he) is (1) all right and (2) not being blamed for the situation.

It is important to obtain a clear account of the circumstances of an alleged rape without forcing the victim to relive a very painful experience. Information includes date, time, location, and an accurate description of any type of sexual contact. The physical examination is carried out as soon as possible, since physical evidence deteriorates rapidly. The victim should not bathe or shower before the examination.

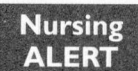 **Nursing ALERT** It is not uncommon for rape victims to delay seeking help, especially in cases of acquaintance or date rape. Nurses can be most supportive by acknowledging the painful and sometimes confusing feelings that surround such experiences and focusing on the fact that the victim is seeking assistance now.

The young person is always told in advance in understandable terms exactly what to expect in the way of tests and procedures, and the explanation is accompanied by strong emotional support. The victim is examined thoroughly, including nongenital areas, for evidence of injury that might substantiate the use of force.

Specimens are obtained for examination, including vaginal secretions for evidence of sperm and blood for serology, and a gonococcal culture is obtained to prove that the victim did not have any preexisting infection. The child is reexamined at appropriate intervals (4 to 6 weeks for syphilis; 2 to 3 days for gonorrhea) to determine if the child acquired disease from the assailant. If testing for HIV is performed, it is carried out at the initial examination and again after a 2-month period.

Therapeutic Management

Adolescents who have been raped arrive at the emergency room or practitioner's office under a variety of circumstances. They are usually brought in by parents, friends, or police officers, but some may seek medical help on their own. It is advisable to obtain parental consent for examination, but the examination may be performed without consent if the adolescent is mature and the parents are unavailable. A female observer should be present during the history and examination of female victims who are examined by a male practitioner. Whether a parent should be present during the examination is determined on an individual basis. The parent's presence is usually encouraged if the parent is supportive and the young person agrees.

Any injuries sustained by the victim that require surgical treatment are repaired. Lacerations of the vagina are not uncommon. Most practitioners prescribe, and many victims and/or their parents prefer the youngster to receive, prophylactic administration of penicillin at the time of initial examination. Pregnancy prophylaxis with high-dose estrogen is offered to the victim who is not using oral contraceptives or who is not pregnant or menstruating. Follow-up care is needed to observe for possible development of PID or other sexually transmitted disease.

Rape Trauma Syndrome

The term *rape trauma syndrome* refers to the reaction to a sexual assault. The syndrome involves two phases: (1) the acute phase of disorganization of life-style, and (2) a long-term process of reorganization. These phases encompass behavioral, somatic, and psychologic reactions to the stressful event. Rape crisis organizations have excellent resources to help victims through these phases.*

Acute Phase of Disorganization. During the acute phase victims exhibit either an expressed style or a controlled style of demonstrating emotional reactions in coping with the stress of the experience. Those with the expressed style are able to express their feelings of fear, anger, and/or anxiety. Those with the controlled style hide or mask their feelings and display a calm, subdued affect. However, the controlled victim is as upset as the victim who expresses feelings. Other acute reactions include physical reactions such as body soreness, disturbances in sleep patterns, and alterations in eating patterns. Many youngsters feel very embarrassed and focus on how the event will affect them at school.

Long-Term Reorganization Process. Changes in life-style are often observed during the reorganization phase. Victims may continue previous activities such as attending school but achieve only a minimal level of functioning. Teenagers may attend school but be apprehensive that other students know about the incident and are talking about them. Most children experience nightmares, phobias about being left alone, and panic reactions on seeing the assailant, the scene of the crime, or a symbolic reminder of the assault. Sexual fears are prominent and difficult for the victim to discuss.

Feelings of helplessness and powerlessness are experienced

---

*For information about local organizations contact the **National Organization for Victim Assistance,** 1757 Park Rd., N.W., Washington, DC 20010; (202) 232-6682.

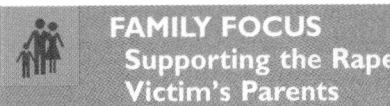

FAMILY FOCUS
Supporting the Rape Victim's Parents

In addition to the needs of the adolescent rape victim, the nurse is also sensitive to the needs and reactions of the youngster's parents. Some will be angry and blame the adolescent; others will feel guilty and embarrassed. Many reactions can be expected at the time of the incident, ranging from despair to extreme agitation. Frequently the parents require as much support and reassurance as the victim. Agitated, angry, or incapacitated parents are unable to provide support for their youngster. Meeting their needs can facilitate their ability to support the teenager during the crisis.

as victims feel that events are totally beyond their control. Victims are concerned about the potential effects that the assault will have on their relationships with others, particularly regarding the extent to which persons close to them will blame them for the assault. There are concerns about whom to tell about the event and how to tell them.

Nursing Considerations

Many of the approaches that have been described for the sexually abused child (see Chapter 14) apply to the adolescent. Sexual assault is a devastating experience with long-lasting effects. The primary goal of nursing care is to avoid inflicting further stress on the youngster who is often angry, confused, frightened, embarrassed, and filled with self-blame. The nurse must do everything possible to reduce the stress of the interrogation and examination. Although most health professionals and law enforcement officers are sensitive to the needs of the youngster and attempt to make the process as nonstressful as possible, the nurse should be alert to cues that indicate the victim is being overstressed.

Follow-up care of the rape victim is essential and extends over a long period of time. Aside from the universal need for emotional support, the needs of rape victims vary widely and depend on the nature of the incident, when it took place, the physical and emotional injuries sustained by the victim, the actions being considered as a result, the resources available for informal support, and the anticipated reactions of persons in the informal support network (see Family Focus box).

EATING DISORDERS

OBESITY

Few health problems related to childhood and adolescence are so obvious to others, so difficult to treat, and have such long-term effects on psychologic and physical health status as obesity. It is the most common nutritional disturbance of children and one of the most challenging contemporary health problems at all ages.

There is no generally accepted definition for obesity or being overweight. Some authorities consider obesity to occur if the child's actual body weight is greater than 120% of ideal body weight for height and age. However, this definition does not take into account the proportion of lean body mass (muscle) to fat. It is possible for two children to be of the same height and weight and for one to be obese and the other not. Regardless of the criteria used to define obesity, the number of overweight children in the United States is increasing. The increase parallels the findings of a large increase in the prevalence of overweight adults (Troiano and others, 1995).

Etiology/Pathophysiology

Obesity results from a caloric intake that consistently exceeds caloric requirements and expenditure. The causes that produce this disequilibrium are complex and may involve a variety of influences, including metabolic, hypothalamic, hereditary, social, cultural, and psychologic factors (Fig. 17-2). Less than 5% of cases of childhood obesity can be attributed to an underlying disease such as hypothyroidism, adrenal hypercorticoidism, hyperinsulinism, and dysfunction of or damage to the central nervous system.

The metabolism of glucose plays an important role in the regulation of fat deposition because excess calories from carbohydrates are stored as fat and a lack of glucose prompts the release of fat as a source of energy. Apparently people who are obese are able to store fat easily but are unable to release this fat or burn it for energy. People who are obese may be more efficient in fat storage and have less heat-producing brown fat than people who are not obese.

Heredity is an important factor in the development of obesity. For example, identical twins reared apart tend to resemble their natural parents to a greater extent than they do their adoptive parents. Obesity can develop in infancy, during childhood, at the onset of puberty, or at any time during adolescence. It is almost impossible to distinguish between hereditary and environmental factors, since both may be operating in any situation when other family members are obese.

Children who are obese are less active than lean children, although it is uncertain whether the inactivity creates the obesity or whether the obesity is responsible for the inactivity. Many people who are obese also demonstrate an overwhelming appetite and often overeat when they are not hungry or have no appetite. They eat more rapidly and tend to ingest more calories at one meal rather than over a period of time. Adolescents who are obese are characteristically night eaters and often skip meals, particularly breakfast.

Theories that attempt to explain the development of obesity are:

Adipose cell theory. The number of cells in adipose tissue is increased, the size of the fat cells is increased, or a combination of these. It is believed that there are sensitive periods in development when cell numbers increase. Children who are obese have larger cells that stay the same size once they reach a maximum, and their fat cells appear to increase in number during childhood.

Set point theory. Individuals have a predetermined level for body weight that remains relatively stable during adulthood. With increased caloric intake the metabolic rate increases to burn the excess; when intake is reduced, metabolism decreases to conserve energy.

Sociocultural factors also play an important role in weight gain. Patterns of eating are culturally and socially based in most instances, and in some the food preferences of the culture contribute to the development of obesity. Many cultures consider plump children to be a sign of health, and some look on obesity as evidence of well-being and foster weight gain as a desirable feature.

Psychologic factors may provide a basis for eating patterns in childhood. In infancy the child first experiences relief from discomfort through feeding and learns to associate eating with feelings of well-being, security, and the comforting presence of the nurturing person. Soon eating is deeply associated with the feeling of being loved. Many parents use food, such as candy and other "treats," as a positive reinforcer for desired behavior. This practice soon acquires symbolic significance to the extent that the child continues to use food as a reward, a comfort, and a means by which to deal with feelings of depression, hostility, boredom, or loneliness.

Obesity is a serious handicap to the social life of a child and, to an even greater extent, to the social life of a teenager. The common emotional sequelae of obesity in adolescence are defective body image, low self-esteem, social isolation, and feelings of rejection and depression.

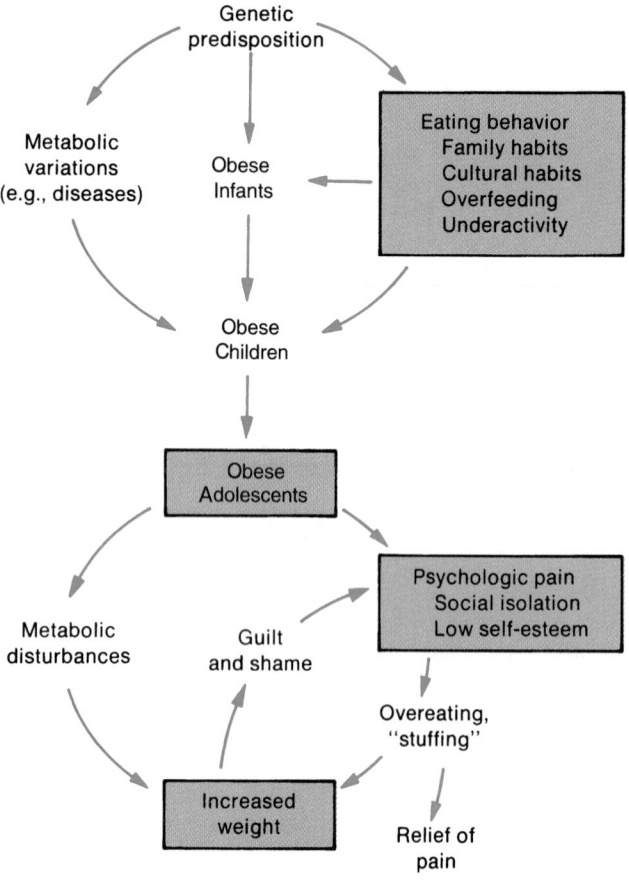

FIG. 17-2. Complex relationships in adolescent obesity.

CLINICAL MANIFESTATIONS OF OBESITY
Child appears overweight
Weight over established standards
Skinfold thickness greater than established standards
Body fat increased above established standards

NURSING DIAGNOSES: THE CHILD WHO IS OBESE
Altered nutrition: more than body requirements related to dysfunctional eating patterns, hereditary factors Activity intolerance related to sedentary life-style, physical bulk Ineffective individual coping related to little or no exercise, poor nutrition, personal vulnerability Self-esteem disturbance related to perception of physical appearance, internalization of negative feedback Altered family processes related to management of child who is obese

ESSENTIALS OF A WEIGHT REDUCTION DIETARY REGIMEN FOR CHILDREN AND ADOLESCENTS

The diet should provide for the following:
  Steady slow weight loss
  Lack of metabolic complications
  Lack of hunger
  Preservation of lean body mass
  Absence of psychiatric reactions
  Normal activity
  Growth

Diagnostic Evaluation

An obese child looks "too fat." Several tests can be employed to assess obesity (see box on p. 504). Skinfold measurements, as well as body fat measurements as determined by bioelectric impedance, computed tomography, or magnetic resonance imaging measurements, may be used for additional data. Appropriate diagnostic tests rule out suspected metabolic and endocrine disorders.

Nursing Considerations

❖ Assessment

The presence of obesity is obvious from appearance alone, and a gross determination can be made by a rough comparison of height and weight with standard growth charts. Children who are 20% over the normal for their height and weight should be evaluated further. Evaluation includes height and weight history of the child, parents, and siblings, as well as eating habits, appetite and hunger patterns, and physical activities in which the child is engaged. It is useful to have an estimation of the degree of fatness in order to have some idea of the component of body weight that can be modified. In addition to the above, a psychosocial history is helpful to understand the impact this condition has on the child's life.

❖ Nursing Diagnoses

Based on a thorough assessment of the child or adolescent who is obese, nursing diagnoses become apparent. Although the diagnoses vary according to the needs of the individual child, some of the more prominent ones are outlined in the box above.

❖ Planning

The goals of a weight-loss program include the following:

1. Child will follow a diet that provides loss of fat content without interfering with growth, normal activity, and psychologic well-being.
2. Child will engage in a regular exercise program.
3. Child will modify eating behavior.
4. Child and family will receive psychologic support.

❖ Implementation

Motivation to lose weight is the key to success. The reasons behind youngsters' desire to lose weight need to be explored with them, but success is rarely achieved unless youngsters are motivated to lose weight and take personal responsibility for their dietary habits and exercise program. Children who are forced by parents to seek help are seldom sufficiently motivated, become rebellious of parental nagging, and are unwilling to control dietary intake. An approach that focuses on healthy eating habits and enjoyable exercise for all members of the family is more likely to be successful.

Diet. Planning caloric restriction for the adolescent during the rapid growth period requires a careful design (see box). Because obesity is usually a lifelong problem, it is best to provide the individual with a diet that can be maintained throughout life with the emphasis on restricting calories. The most successful diets are those that use ordinary foods in controlled portions rather than diets that require the avoidance of any specific food. The youngster is taught how to incorporate favorite foods into the diet and how to select satisfying substitutes. The dieting youngster should eat what the rest of the family eats, but less of it, and should be allowed favorite foods in small amounts. There are a multitude of restricted calorie diets available from a number of sources, such as the American Dietetic Association. The caloric values for a wide variety of commercial foods are also available to facilitate meal planning.

For children, especially teenagers, snacking is an integral part of the daily routine, which makes dieting particularly difficult for children who are obese. They have little concept of the caloric content of even the most commonplace snack foods. Vending machines are usually stocked with high-calorie, low-nutrient temptations; they are readily accessible; and children often have pocket money with which to purchase these items. Following pressures from concerned parents and nutritionists, many schools are providing more wholesome "treats," such as fruit, juices, and raw vegetables, in vending machines in school cafeterias. However, the favorite gathering places for children and teens are the fast-food establishments, which are often located near large schools.*

No child or adolescent should be encouraged to initiate a reduction diet without a health assessment and counseling. It is also important to emphasize the undesirable nature of the fad diets and crash programs that continually appear in various publications. Exotic diets have not been successful, and their unbalanced nature makes them potentially dangerous for growing children or adolescents. To be successful from all aspects, a dietary program should be nutritionally sound with sufficient satiety value, produce the desired

---

*Information on the nutrient value of name brand foods, including several fast-food restaurants, is available from the **Nutrition Coordinating Center,** 2221 University Ave., S.E., Suite 310, Minneapolis, MN 55414; (612) 627-4862.

weight loss, and be accompanied by nutrition education and continued support.

Exercise. Because weight loss will occur only when caloric expenditure is greater than caloric intake, physical activity in the form of regularly scheduled exercise, progressively increased over the child's usual activity, is an integral part of a weight-reduction program. Activities should be those that stress self-improvement rather than competition, and teenagers need continued psychologic support and encouragement to prevent the beginning of the destructive cycle of passivity, withdrawal, and rejection.

Behavioral Therapy. Probably the most successful method for treating obesity is diet and exercise combined with behavior modification, which emphasizes identification and elimination of inappropriate eating habits as well as problem-solving techniques to identify solutions to use in situations that encourage overeating. Attention is focused not on food but on the social and behavioral aspects surrounding food consumption.

Group Involvement. Some persons on weight-reduction programs find that support and mutual reinforcement provided by a group of persons with a similar problem help them to adjust to the changes needed for successful accomplishment of their goals, including weight loss. Commercial groups, such as Weight Watchers, TOPS, or diet workshops, composed primarily of adults, may be helpful to a few teenagers; however, a group composed of persons their own age is more effective. Some types of groups for youngsters who are obese include summer camps designed and conducted by health professionals, school groups organized and led by the school nurse, and groups associated with special clinics.

The group is concerned not only with weight loss but also with the development of a positive self-image. Nutrition education and diet planning are essential elements of the group function, but equally important are discussions centered around better grooming and improvement of social skills. Improvement is measured by positive changes in all aspects of endeavor.

Medical Therapies. There is little evidence that drugs are more effective than diet and exercise in maintaining weight loss. There is also some concern that the use of appetite-suppressing drugs may become a habit for some adolescents. Surgical techniques are available that bypass a substantial portion of the intestine or occlude a large segment of the stomach to produce a marked diet restriction and resultant weight loss. These shunting techniques are hazardous surgical procedures with many metabolic complications. The complex metabolic effects need clarification and this procedure should be restricted to those instances when obesity is life-threatening or when disease states demand weight loss for effective management.

Prevention. Unfortunately, weight loss programs do not enjoy the success rate that therapeutic interventions for most other disorders do; the failure rate is dismally high. The most successful treatment of preadolescent obesity (which often leads to adult obesity) is to treat preschool obesity with programs that include frequent visits (Davis and Christoffel, 1994). The ultimate goal is to prevent obesity in children.

❖ **Evaluation**

The effectiveness of nursing interventions is determined by continual reassessment based on the following observational guidelines and expected outcomes:

1. Assess weight at regular intervals (usually weekly); discuss with child his or her feelings, reactions, concerns; analyze daily recordings (log) of activities (eating, behavior, exercise) and feelings.
2. Review exercise program with child or teen.
3. Review log of eating behaviors; discuss observations with child or teen.
4. Interview child or teen about the plan of care and progress toward short-term and long-term goals.

Expected outcomes:

1. Eating patterns lead to weight loss; child or teen expresses feelings and concerns regarding problems.
2. Child or teen engages in preferred exercise and activities regularly.
3. Child or teen demonstrates an understanding of eating patterns.
4. Child or teen evidences a steady weight loss (or weight maintenance in a growing child).

See also Nursing Care Plan: The Child Who Is Obese.*

ANOREXIA NERVOSA (AN)

AN is an eating disorder characterized by a refusal to maintain a minimally normal body weight and by severe weight loss in the absence of obvious physical causes. It occurs predominantly in adolescent or young adult females, and the incidence is increasing.

The onset of AN generally takes place at or near menarche, but it may begin in preadolescence or in adulthood. The disease has two peaks: between ages 12 and 14 years and between ages 16 and 17 years. Young people who have this disorder are most frequently from the upper or middle socioeconomic groups; are often described as "good children"; are academically high achievers, conforming, and conscientious; and have a high energy level, even with marked emaciation. These adolescents are usually strongly dependent on their parents, and frequently an ambivalent mother-daughter relationship is present for females. Sexual abuse may be a factor in some cases of AN and/or bulimia.

Etiology/Pathophysiology

The etiology of the disorder remains unclear. There is a distinct psychologic component, and the diagnosis is based primarily on psychologic and behavioral criteria. Nevertheless, the physical manifestations of anorexia lend support to possible organic factors in the etiology.

Dominating the psychologic aspects of anorexia nervosa are a relentless pursuit of thinness and a fear of fatness, usually preceded by a period of a year or two of mood disturbances and behavior changes. The weight loss is usually triggered by a typical adolescent crisis such as the onset of menstruation or traumatic interpersonal incidents that precipitate serious dieting that continues out of control.

Frequently there is an exaggerated misinterpretation of the normal fat deposition characteristic of the early adolescent period, or someone may comment that the adolescent girl is

*In Wong DL: *Wong and Whaley's Clinical manual of pediatric nursing,* ed 4, St Louis, 1996, Mosby.

putting on weight. The weight loss may be a response to teasing or to changing schools or going to college. Youngsters entering the growth phase of puberty, when biologic fat accumulation is normal, are particularly vulnerable. The current emphasis on slimness is a very significant factor. The standard for beauty is one exemplified by tall, thin, small-breasted models in all forms of media.

In some situations the adolescent is experiencing severe family stress, such as parental separation or divorce. In these and other circumstances in which the youngster perceives having no personal control, the decision to eat or not eat becomes one area where individual control can be exercised.

Diagnostic Evaluation

Diagnosis is made on the basis of clinical manifestations (see box) and conformity to the criteria established by the American Psychiatric Association (1994) (see box).

Therapeutic Management

The initial goal is to treat the life-threatening malnutrition with strict adherence to dietary requirements, which sometimes necessitates intravenous and tube feedings (these methods are usually reserved for severe situations). Rapid weight gain should be avoided as it can be medically unsafe, and often overwhelms the patient. Many deaths associated with AN occur during rehabilitation as a result of cardiovascular overload. A safe and reasonable target weight is calculated by the physician and dietitian—usually 18% fat.

One treatment approach that has met with varied degrees of success is behavior modification. This requires team involvement with the following essential aspects:

1. The health team determines an approach with the patient and adheres to it consistently.
2. All team members are involved.
3. There is continuity of caregivers (team members).
4. There is clear communication among team members and with the patient so that the patient understands precisely what is expected.
5. The patient is supported in his or her efforts, (e.g., positive feedback for accomplishments).

Individuals whose disorder can be clearly related to a dysfunctional family situation will need intensive family therapy. Many of those whose therapy plan is implemented in the hospital need a continued behavior modification program after discharge to maintain the desired weight.

Family therapy seems to be effective when begun soon after the onset of illness, but it is less successful when the condition has existed for some time. Therapy is directed toward disengagement and redirection of malfunctioning processes in the family. Individual psychotherapy is aimed at helping the young person resolve the adolescent identity crisis, particularly as it relates to a distorted body image.

Nursing Considerations

The management of AN is directed toward correction of the severe state of malnutrition and resolution of the psychologic dynamics. Because of the psychogenic nature of the disorder, treatment is difficult and lengthy. All of those involved in therapy must keep in mind the adolescent's distorted sense of body image and self-awareness, as well as feelings of self-doubt, ineffectiveness, and helplessness that prompt such self-damaging behavior in order to feel in control.

Nurses need to adopt and maintain a kind, supportive, yet firm manner in managing the care of a teen with AN. The child requires sustained support and reassurance to cope with ambivalent feelings related to the body concept and the desire to see oneself as a cooperative and reliable person worthy of receiving kindness. Encouraging the child with education and activities that strengthen self-esteem facilitates the resocialization process and promotes social acceptance among peers.

It is important for nurses to be aware of some of the physical side effects of AN. Patients with AN often limit their fluid intake, leading to urinary tract problems: ketones and protein may be detected in the urine as a result of breakdown of fat and protein. Vital sign instability can be severe (including orthostatic hypotension). The pulse becomes irregular, and the rate decreases markedly. Bradycardia and hypothermia can result in cardiac arrest (see Critical Thinking Exercise on p. 508).

Health professionals, patients, and families can find assistance and information from any of the following organizations: The *National Eating Disorders Organization**, the *National Association of Anorexia Nervosa and Associated*

---

*445 E. Granville Rd., Worthington, OH 43085 (614) 436-1112.

CLINICAL MANIFESTATIONS OF ANOREXIA NERVOSA

Severe and profound weight loss
Signs of altered metabolic activity:
   Secondary amenorrhea (if menarche attained)
   Primary amenorrhea (if menarche not attained)
   Bradycardia
   Lowered body temperature
   Decreased blood pressure
   Cold intolerance
   Dry skin and brittle nails
   Appearance of lanugo hair

DIAGNOSTIC CRITERIA FOR ANOREXIA NERVOSA

A. Refusal to maintain body weight over a minimal normal weight for age and height, e.g., weight loss leading to maintenance of body weight less than 85% of that expected; or failure to make expected weight gain during period of growth, leading to body weight less than 85% of that expected.
B. Intense fear of gaining weight or becoming fat, even though underweight
C. Disturbance in the way in which one's body weight, size, or shape is experienced, e.g., the person claims to "feel fat" even when emaciated, believes that one area of the body is "too fat" even when obviously underweight
D. In females, absence of at least three consecutive menstrual cycles when otherwise expected to occur (primary or secondary amenorrhea) (A woman is considered to have amenorrhea if her periods occur only following hormone, e.g., estrogen, administration.)

From American Psychiatric Association: *Diagnostic and statistical manual of mental disorders,* ed 4 (DSM-IV), Washington, DC, 1994, The Association.

Anorexia Nervosa

Jane is a 13-year-old whose grades have been excellent and whom the teachers describe as a "model student." Recently some of Jane's friends have expressed concern to the school nurse practitioner that Jane has begun to "jog" at lunch time and seldom eats with them. Jane has told her friends that she gained weight over the winter months and that she is "jogging" because she wants to qualify for the track team this spring. In addition to severe weight loss, which of the following symptoms of anorexia nervosa is the school nurse practitioner likely to observe when she interviews Jane and performs a sports physical?

1. Decreased body temperature
2. History of dysmenorrhea
3. Tachycardia
4. Heat intolerance

The correct answer is one. Anorexia nervosa is a condition in which several alterations in metabolic activity can occur following excessive weight loss. These alterations include lowered body temperature, bradycardia, secondary amenorrhea, decreased blood pressure, and cold intolerance. When the nutritional status improves and normal body weight has been restored, these metabolic changes are usually reversed.

DIAGNOSTIC CRITERIA FOR BULIMIA

A. Recurrent episodes of binge eating (rapid consumption of a large amount of food in a discrete period of time)
B. A feeling of lack of control over eating behavior during the eating binges
C. The person regularly engages in either self-induced vomiting, use of laxatives or diuretics, strict dieting or fasting, or vigorous exercise in order to prevent weight gain
D. A minimum average of two binge eating episodes a week for at least 3 months
E. Persistent overconcern with body shape and weight

From American Psychiatric Association: *Diagnostic and statistical manual of mental disorders,* ed 4-revised (DSM-IV) Washington, DC, 1994, The Association.

Disorders, Inc., * and the *American Anorexia/Bulimia Association, Inc.*†

See also Nursing Care Plan: The Adolescent with Anorexia Nervosa.‡

BULIMIA

Bulimia is an eating disorder characterized by binge eating. The binge behavior consists of secretive, frenzied consumption of large amounts of high-calorie (or "forbidden") foods during a brief period of time (usually less than 2 hours). The binge is counteracted by a variety of weight-control methods (purging), including self-induced vomiting, diuretic and laxative abuse, and rigorous exercise. The frequency of bingeing can be anywhere from once a week to seven or eight times a day. These binge/purge cycles are followed by self-deprecating thoughts, a depressed mood, and an awareness that the eating pattern is abnormal.

The disorder is observed more frequently in older adolescent girls and young women. Characteristically, affected persons have been unsuccessful dieters, have low impulse control, and may have been self-conscious about being overweight in childhood. They fall into two categories: (1) those who consume vast quantities of food followed by purging but who, if unable to purge, still consume large amounts, and (2) those who restrict their caloric intake, especially when unable to purge. Some are of normal weight or (more often) are slightly above normal weight; others become as underweight as anorectic individuals—*bulimarexia.*

Diagnostic Evaluation

The diagnosis may be first suspected from the presence of complications, including fluid and electrolyte disturbances from gastrointestinal losses, abdominal complaints from laxative abuse, erosion of tooth enamel and increased dental caries from vomited gastric acid, and throat complaints. The diagnosis is established on the basis of criteria established by the American Psychiatric Association (1994) (see box).

Therapeutic Management

Therapy is similar to management of anorexia nervosa. Hospitalization may be required, especially for complications such as potassium depletion and esophageal damage. Intravenous fluids and potassium replacement are essential elements of care, and cardiac monitoring is indicated; behavior therapy may also be used.

Nursing Considerations

Nursing care is similar to care of the patient with AN. Acute care also involves careful monitoring of fluid and electrolyte alterations and observation for signs of cardiac complications.

DISORDERS WITH BEHAVIORIAL COMPONENTS

ATTENTION DEFICIT HYPERACTIVITY DISORDER (ADHD) AND LEARNING DISABILITY (LD)

ADHD refers to developmentally inappropriate degrees of inattention, impulsiveness, and hyperactivity. The symptoms of ADHD must have been present before the age of 7 years, and must be present in at least two settings. In addition the persistence of developmentally inappropriate and marked inattention must not be a symptom of another disorder (American Psychiatric Association, 1994). An *LD* refers to a heterogeneous group of disorders manifested by significant difficulties in acquisition and use of listening, speaking, reading, writing, reasoning, mathematic abilities, or social skills.

ADHD and LD conditions affect every aspect of the child's life but are most obvious in the classroom. Early iden-

*Box 7, Highland Park, IL 60035; (708) 831-3438.
†Regents Hospital, 425 E. 61st St., New York, NY 10021; (212) 891-8686.
‡In Wong DL: *Wong and Whaley's Clinical manual of pediatric nursing,* ed 4, St Louis, 1996, Mosby.

tification of affected children is needed, since the characteristics of the disorder significantly interfere with the normal course of emotional and psychologic development. Many children develop maladaptive behavior patterns that impede psychosocial adjustment while they try to cope with cognitive dysfunction. Their behavior evokes negative responses from others, and repeated exposure to negative feedback adversely affects their self-concept. Constant failure despite honest effort can also affect their self-esteem.

Diagnostic Evaluation

The behaviors exhibited by the child with ADHD are not unusual aspects of child behavior. The difference lies in the quality of motor activity and developmentally inappropriate inattention, impulsivity, and hyperactivity the child displays. The manifestations may be numerous or few, mild or severe, and will vary with the developmental level of the child. Any given child will not have every manifestation that is characteristic of the syndrome. The diagnostic criteria established by the **American Psychiatric Association** (1994) for identifying the child with ADHD are outlined in the box.

A comprehensive battery of tests is needed to confirm a learning disability. These include intelligence tests (these children tend to have normal or above-average IQs), hand-eye coordination tests, and measurements of auditory and visual perception, comprehension, and memory. Often there is a wide gap between verbal and performance scores on IQ tests.

Therapeutic Management

Management of the child with ADHD or LD usually involves multiple approaches that include family education and coun-seling, medication, proper classroom placement, environmental manipulation, and sometimes psychotherapy for the child.

Medication. Many drugs have been advocated for management of symptoms of ADHD. The most frequently prescribed medications are dextroamphetamine (Dexedrine) or methylphenidate (Ritalin). However, not all children benefit from medications. Children taking stimulant medication may have symptoms that include nervousness, insomnia, and decreased appetite with subsequent weight loss. Long-term use of dextroamphetamine may result in suppression of growth. (See Critical Thinking Exercise on p. 510.)

Environmental Manipulation. The child's environment is simplified by decreasing external stimuli and distractions, reducing alternatives, and encouraging desired patterns of behavior. Parents need to develop firm but reasonable limits and provide a stable and predictable environment with regular routines of sleeping, eating, working, and playing.

Classroom Education. Special activities in the schools are designed to offer a direct attack on such areas of deficit as visual perception, auditory perception, and other areas involving integration and coordination. The purpose of programs for children with special learning disabilities is to assist them toward more successful achievement, personal adjustment, and eventual retention in the regular classroom. However, according to Public Law 94-142, The Education for All Handicapped Children's Act, children with ADHD or LD must receive free public education in the least restrictive environment (see Chapters 1 and 18).

Course of ADHD. In the majority of affected children the disorder is relatively stable through early adolescence. In

---

DIAGNOSTIC CRITERIA FOR ATTENTION DEFICIT HYPERACTIVITY DISORDER

A. Either (1) or (2):
 (1) six (or more) of the following symptoms of **_inattention_** have persisted for at least 6 months to a degree that is maladaptive and inconsistent with developmental level:
   Inattention
   (a) often fails to give close attention to details or makes mistakes in schoolwork, work, or other activities
   (b) often has difficulty sustaining attention in tasks or play activities
   (c) Often does not seem to listen when spoken to directly
   (d) often does not follow through on instructions and fails to finish schoolwork, chores, or duties in the workplace (not because of oppositional behavior or failure to understand instructions)
   (e) often has difficulty organizing tasks and activities
   (f) often avoids, dislikes, or is reluctant to engage in tasks that require sustained mental effort (such as schoolwork or homework)
   (g) often loses things necessary for tasks or activities (e.g., toys, school assignments, pencils, books, or tools)
   (h) is often easily distracted by extraneous stimuli
   (i) is often forgetful in daily activities
 (2) six (or more) of the following symptoms of **_hyperactivity-impulsivity_** have persisted for at least 6 months to a degree that is maladaptive and inconsistent with developmental level:
   Hyperactivity
   (a) often fidgets with hands or feet or squirms in seat

   (b) often leaves seat in classroom or in other situations in which remaining seated is expected
   (c) often runs about or climbs excessively in situations in which it is inappropriate (in adolescents or adults, may be limited to subjective feelings of restlessness)
   (d) often has difficulty playing or engaging in leisure activities quietly
   (e) is often "on the go" or often acts as if "driven by a motor"
   (f) often talks excessively
   Impulsivity
   (g) often blurts out answers before questions have been completed
   (h) often has difficulty awaiting turn
   (i) often interrupts or intrudes on others (e.g., butts into conversations or games)
B. Some hyperactive-impulsive or inattentive symptoms that caused impairment were present before age 7 years.
C. Some impairment from the symptoms is present in two or more settings (e.g., at school, work, and at home).
D. There must be clear evidence of clinically significant impairment in social, academic, or occupational functioning.
E. The symptoms do not occur exclusively during the course of or are not accounted for by another mental disorder.

From American Psychiatric Association: *Diagnostic and statistical manual of mental disorders,* ed 4-revised (DSM-IV), Washington, DC, 1994, The Association.

CRITICAL THINKING EXERCISE
Attention Deficit Hyperactivity Disorder

Johnnie, age 8 years, is a third grader who was diagnosed with attention deficit hyperactivity disorder (ADHD) 1 year ago. Johnnie has been taking the drug methylphenidate (Ritalin) for the past year. Which of the following behaviors indicates that Johnnie may need to have the administration times of his medications changed?

1. For the past week, Johnnie has not eaten his lunch. He states that he is not hungry.
2. During this school year Johnnie's math grade has increased from a letter grade of D to a grade of B.
3. Johnnie's mother told the school nurse that Johnnie has been sleeping very well at night.
4. During the past year, Johnnie's teacher has noted that Johnnie has been socializing more with his classmates and that he now has a "best friend."

The correct answer is one. Children taking stimulant medications often experience positive effects such as improvement in school work and increasing self-confidence in social skills. However, there are also negative side effects for some of the drugs used to treat ADHD. For example, side effects for methylphenidate include nervousness, decreased appetite, and insomnia. The absorption rate of methylphenidate is increased when this drug is taken with meals; therefore, side effects such as decreased appetite may become more pronounced when the medication is taken with meals. Side effects can be alleviated by changing the times that the drug is administered or by switching to a sustained time-release form of the drug that can be given once a day in the morning. When evaluating a child's response to the medication, it is important to obtain reports from the child's teacher, the school nurse, and the parents. Information concerning the child's behavior in at least two settings should be obtained before adjustments are made in the medication dosage or scheduling.

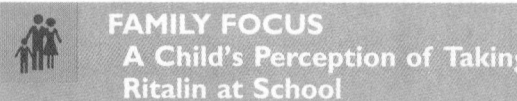
FAMILY FOCUS
A Child's Perception of Taking Ritalin at School

I feel embarrassed by having to leave class early to go take my medication. The other kids always ask where I'm going and why. It would be better if we could leave class at the same time as everyone else, go take the medication and then just be a little late to the next class. Students don't ask why people are late for class, only why they leave early. It also bothers me when kids tell other kids, "Go take a pill," and other mean things just because someone is acting up.

What could nurses and teachers do to help? Most kids do not understand why other kids have to take medication. I think it would help if a nurse or teacher talked with the other kids and explained why some children take the medication and how ADHD affects people. That way there would be more understanding among all the kids.

Marissa White, age 16

most individuals, symptoms diminish during late adolescence and adulthood, although a minority experience the full complement of symptoms of ADHD into middle adulthood. Other adults may no longer have the full disorder but still retain some symptoms that cause functional impairment (American Psychiatric Association, 1994).

Children with LD grow up to be adults with LD. The goal is to help them identify their area of weakness and to compensate for it.

Nursing Considerations

Nurses are active participants in all aspects of management of the child with ADHD or LD. Nurses in the community setting work with families in the home and with school personnel on a long-term basis to help plan and implement therapeutic regimens and to evaluate the effectiveness of therapy. They should explain that children taking stimulant medication need to have it administered in the morning to maximize its effectiveness in the classroom and to decrease its insomnia-producing potential. Parents benefit from practical, specific strategies for helping children with ADHD, such as the need for structure and consistency in dressing,

meals, sleep, and discipline (Comfort, 1992) (see Family Focus box).

Nurses must understand which type of LD a child has in order to best provide direction for the child, parents, and teachers. Children with an auditory perceptual deficit appear unable to follow directions or to comprehend large amounts of verbal teaching. These children need to be taught with diagrams, pictures, demonstration, and written lists. Children with a visual perceptual deficit may have difficulty reading, lining up numbers for mathematic operations, or judging distance. These children may have dyslexia (letter reversals) and do better with demonstration and a verbal approach. Children with an integrative deficit may have difficulty sequencing data or storing and retrieving sensory data. Multisensory techniques should be used, and comprehension should be checked frequently throughout instruction. Children with motor deficits may need to use typewriters in the classroom, since their handwriting will *not* improve. They may need to find alternatives to physical competition that requires coordination of movement (Selekman and Snyder, 1996).

ENURESIS

Enuresis (bed-wetting) is a common and troublesome disorder that is difficult to define because of the variable ages at which children achieve bladder control. In a broad sense the disorder can be defined as repeated involuntary urination (usually nocturnal) in children who are beyond the age when voluntary bladder control should normally have been acquired. The chronologic or developmental age of the child must be at least 5 years; the voiding of urine must occur at least twice a week for at least 3 months. The predominant symptom is urgency that is immediate and accompanied by acute discomfort, restlessness, and sometimes urinary frequency.

Enuresis affects 5 million children in the United States and is more common in boys than in girls (Houts, 1991). It is primarily an alteration of neuromuscular bladder functioning and is often benign and self-limiting. Nocturnal bed-wetting usually ceases between 6 and 8 years of age, although it some-

CULTURAL AWARENESS
Enuresis

The age at which children attain urinary continence varies widely. For example, white children in the United States tend to achieve continence earlier than African-American children. In addition, children in Great Britain and Sweden appear to attain continence slightly earlier than children in the United States, and in the extreme, the East African Digos often achieve bladder control by the age of 12 months. Therefore practitioners must be sensitive to the differences among groups before labeling a child enuretic (Rappaport, 1992).

FAMILY FOCUS
Helping Families Understand
Encopresis

The prevailing attitude of nurses toward the family of a child with encopresis should be one of no-fault, thus relieving the guilt of both parents and child. Since parents and children are often reluctant to volunteer information, direct questioning about the soiling is more successful. Parents are usually relieved to know that other parents share this problem and are surprised to know that functional changes that take place as the condition develops make control of seepage impossible. Many parents complain that their children soil because they do not take time from play for a bowel movement. Actually, the children may be unaware of a prior sensation and unable to control the urge once it begins. They may be so accustomed to bowel accidents that they are unable to smell or feel it and even deny soiling when it occurs.

times continues into adolescence. (See Cultural Awareness box.)

Organic causes that may be related to enuresis should be ruled out before psychogenic factors are considered. These include structural disorders of the urinary tract, urinary tract infection, neurologic deficits, disorders that increase the normal output of urine, such as diabetes, and disorders such as chronic renal failure or sickle cell disease that impair the concentrating ability of the kidneys. A bladder volume of 300 to 350 ml is sufficient to hold a night's urine. In other cases the enuresis is influenced by emotional factors, although it is doubtful that they are causative factors. Parents report that these children sleep more soundly than other children; however, the depth of sleep has not been identified as the cause of nocturnal enuresis (Rappaport, 1993). Enuresis has a strong familial tendency.

NURSING TIP Have child void in a measuring cup after holding urine for as long as possible. Normal bladder capacity (in ounces) is the child's age plus 2 (e.g., a 6-year-old's normal capacity is 8 ounces) (Schmitt, 1990).

Various therapeutic techniques are employed in the management of enuresis. These include drugs, bladder training, restriction or elimination of fluids after the evening meal, interruption of sleep to void, and some type of electrical device designed to establish a conditioned reflex response to waken the child at the initiation of voiding.

Anticholinergic drugs, especially oxybutynin, reduce uninhibited bladder contractions and may be helpful for children with daytime urinary frequency. Desmopressin (DDAVP) nasal spray, an analog of vasopressin, reduces nighttime urine output to a volume less than functional bladder capacity.

Nursing Considerations

No matter what techniques are employed, the nurse can help both children and parents to understand the problem of enuresis, the treatment plan, and the probable difficulties they may encounter in the process. More importantly the nurse can provide consistent support and encouragement to help sustain them through the inconsistent and unpredictable treatment process. Children need to believe that they are helping themselves and to sustain feelings of confidence and hope.

ENCOPRESIS

Encopresis is the repeated voluntary or involuntary passage of feces of normal or near-normal consistency into places not appropriate for that purpose according to the individual's own sociocultural setting. The fecal incontinence must not be caused by any physiologic effect, such as a laxative, or a general medical condition. The fecal incontinence may be related to emotional problems. The disorder is less common than enuresis, but the two may coexist.

Primary encopresis is identified by age 4 when the child has not achieved fecal continence. Secondary encopresis is fecal incontinence occurring in a child over 4 years of age after a period of established fecal continence. Predisposing factors seem to be inconsistent toilet training and psychosocial stress, such as entering school or the birth of a sibling. The disorder is more common in boys than in girls. Incontinence frequently occurs secondary to constipation, painful impaction, or retention of feces with subsequent overflow. It is not unusual for soiling to take place after bathing because of reflex stimulation.

School performance and attendance is affected as the child's offensive odor becomes a target for scorn and derision from classmates. This causes further withdrawal and other behavioral manifestations. Therapeutic management consists of determining the cause of the soiling and application of appropriate interventions to correct the problem. It may involve dietary changes, relief of a fecal impaction, and/or behavioral therapy. Frequently psychotherapeutic intervention with the child and the family becomes necessary.

Nursing Considerations

The nursing care of the child with encopresis involves primarily education and support of the family, as well as treatment of existing constipation. Families are taught the physiology of normal defecation, toilet training as a developmental process, and the treatment outlined for the particular family. Family counseling is directed toward reassurance that most problems resolve successfully, although relapses during periods of stress are possible (see Family Focus box).

POSTTRAUMATIC STRESS DISORDER (PTSD)

PTSD is frequently observed following an overwhelming stimulus (e.g., physical abuse or experiencing a sibling dying while in the child's care). Disasters initiate similar psychologic effects, and PTSD has been diagnosed in many children who have experienced such events. Children with PTSD tend to relive or visualize traumatic experiences for years and retain some fear specific to the event. They continue to function as always but have a feeling of foreboding regarding the future. The way in which children react depends on what resources the individual child brings to the situation—coping strategies used, defense mechanisms summoned, and the child's social environment. Although studies indicate that children do not outgrow the trauma, they can be helped to overcome their sense of hopelessness.

The response to the event takes place in three stages. The *initial response* to the stressor is intense arousal, which usually lasts for a few minutes to 1 or 2 hours. The stress hormones are at the maximum as the individual prepares for "fight" or "flight." A prolonged arousal phase may indicate psychosis.

The *second phase,* which lasts approximately 2 weeks, is one in which defense mechanisms are mobilized. It is a period of quiescence in which the event appears to have produced no impression. The victims feel numb, and stress hormone secretion is absent. The reaction is outside their awareness, not well controlled, and involves some type of behavioral pattern. Defense mechanisms are less adaptive to specific situations and may not be what the situation demands. Denial that anything is wrong is a frequently observed defense mechanism.

The *third phase* is one of coping, which normally extends over 2 to 3 months. It is one of consciously directed inquiry. The victims want to know what happened and appear to be getting worse, when actually they are getting better. Numerous psychologic symptoms may be apparent, such as depression, repetitive phenomenon, phobic symptoms, anxiety symptoms, and conversion reactions. Children frequently display repetitive actions. They play out the situation over and over again in an attempt to come to terms with their fear. Flashbacks are common. This phase can be self-perpetuating, and a prolonged reaction can develop into an obsession with the traumatic event. Some traumatic effects remain indefinitely (Terr, 1989).

Nursing Considerations

Children need to deal with any traumatic event; much depends on the intensity of the event and their reaction to it. They usually react in much the same manner as their caregivers (contagious pathology); therefore it is important to be aware of these reactions also. In the second, or defense, phase of the PTSD the appropriateness of the defense mechanism must be assessed, and children must be assisted in application of their defense. If children do not engage in some catharsis, or if their defense phase is prolonged, they may need referral for special psychologic help.

Coping is a learned response, and children in the third phase can be helped to use their coping strategies to deal with their fear. Children usually are willing to accept reasoning. Those who are assisted in their catharsis and allowed expression will survive without serious lasting effects. It is impor-

tant for children to be reassured regarding the randomness of an event such as a playground shooting, rape, attack, or natural disaster (e.g., hurricane, earthquake). They should be encouraged to play out the stress and/or discuss their feelings about the event. If they are unable to do this, they may become obsessed with the traumatic event and need professional help. Conversion reactions are common obsessive behaviors in children.

Children need professional help if any of the phases of PTSD are prolonged. Boys tend to have a prolonged defense phase more often than girls. Occasionally the event will be unrecognized, and the affected child will engage in what is considered to be unusual behavior. Children exhibiting any sudden change in behavior need to be assessed for a traumatic event—"Did something happen?" When the change in behavior is traced to a traumatic event, treatment can be implemented.

SCHOOL PHOBIA

Children, other than beginning students, who resist going to school because of dread of the school situation, concerns with leaving home, or both, are said to have school phobia. Anxiety—especially anxiety over separation from the parent, usually the mother—that frequently verges on panic is a constant manifestation. Some children are afraid the parent will not be home when they get there. Simple reassurance is often sufficient for these children.

Physical symptoms are prominent and may affect any part of the body (e.g., anorexia, nausea, vomiting, diarrhea, dizziness, headache, leg pains, abdominal pains, or even a low-grade fever). A striking feature of school phobia is the prompt subsiding of symptoms when it is evident that the child can remain at home. Another significant observation is absence of symptoms on weekends and holidays unless they are related to other places such as Sunday school or parties. Occasional mild reluctance is not uncommon among schoolchildren, but if the fear continues for longer than a few days it must be considered a serious problem—a warning of an important personality problem.

Nursing Considerations

The interventions for school phobia depend on the cause. The primary goal is to return the child to school. The longer a child is permitted to stay out of school, the more difficult it is to reenter. Parents must be convinced gently but firmly that *immediate* return is essential and that it is their responsibility to insist on school attendance.

The child with severe symptoms may require modified school attendance, such as part-time class attendance and spending time in the counselor's or nurse's office, then getting homework from the teacher after class. It may be necessary for a parent to attend class with the child. If the problem persists, professional help is recommended.

RECURRENT ABDOMINAL PAIN (RAP)

RAP is one of the somatic complaints of childhood that is almost always attributed to a psychogenic etiology, although it can be a symptom of either psychosomatic or organic disease. Children with RAP have real pain that the child usually locates in the periumbilical area. However, on palpation the pain is more likely to be experienced in the epigastric area or in the lower right or left quadrant and is accompanied by vague tenderness without muscle guarding. The pain is irregular in time, duration, and intensity and is associated with either loose or pellet-formed stools. Other symptoms that may accompany the abdominal pain are headache, pallor, dizziness, and dysuria.

Support for the psychologic aspects of this disorder is based on observations of aggravation of symptoms during times of tension or stress. Children with RAP tend to be highly sensitive, have a poor self-image, and are uncomfortable with expressions of anger or argument, especially in those persons who are significant in their life. School attendance is adversely affected, and these children generally exhibit poor learning performance. It is not uncommon for symptoms to be aggravated during school days.

Treatment is difficult. Hospitalization may be necessary, and the child frequently shows improvement in the hospital environment. Initial efforts are directed toward ruling out organic causes of the pain, relieving discomfort, and attempting to determine the situations that precipitate attacks. A high-fiber diet and bowel training are emphasized. When simple measures are ineffective, an antispasmodic drug such as propantheline bromide may be prescribed to relieve the muscle spasm.

Nursing Considerations

Once the diagnosis has been established, the parents and the child need an explanation of the pain, which can be compared to a skeletal muscle cramp or "charley horse" for easier comprehension. Reassurance that the symptoms are not unique to their child and that the pain can be expected to subside is helpful in relieving parental fears and anxieties. When parents are reassured that there is no organic cause of the pain, they will need some guidance regarding what they can do during a painful episode. All too often they feel helpless and anxious, which tends to compound the child's distress.

The simple expedient of having the child rest in a peaceful, quiet environment and providing comfort will often relieve the symptoms in a short time. A heating pad may also help ease the discomfort. Teaching children relaxation exercises and guided imagery may also be helpful (see Pain Management, Chapter 21). If pain is not relieved by these simple measures, the parents are taught how to administer antispasmodics, if prescribed. For example, if pain is precipitated by meals, having the child take the medication 20 to 30 minutes before mealtime may prevent an episode.

The most valuable measures that the nurse can provide are support and reassurance to the family. When open communication is established and families are able to see a relationship between stress-provoking situations and the child's symptoms, the chance for remedial action is enhanced. Follow-up care and continued support are essential, because the symptoms tend to remit and exacerbate; therefore the availability of a supportive health professional can be a source of comfort to the child and family.

CONVERSION REACTION

Conversion reaction, also known as hysteria, hysterical conversion reaction, and childhood hysteria, is a psychophysiologic disorder with a sudden onset that can usually be traced to a precipitating environmental event. Once considered rare in childhood, the diagnosis of conversion reaction occurs more frequently than has generally been acknowledged. In childhood the disorder is observed with equal frequency in both sexes, but girls outnumber boys during adolescence.

The manifestations involve primarily the voluntary musculature and special senses and include abdominal pain, fainting, pseudoseizures, paralysis, headaches, and visual field restriction. The most commonly observed symptom is seizure activity, which can be differentiated from symptoms of neurogenic origin by formal tests, the most useful of which is the finding of a normal electroencephalogram.

It has been observed that nearly all children with conversion reaction have experienced a major family crisis before the onset of symptoms, such as loss of a parent or other significant person through death, divorce, or moving.

Nursing Considerations

Nursing care is similar to that for the child with recurrent abdominal pain.

CHILDHOOD DEPRESSION

Depression in childhood is often difficult to detect. Children may be unable to express their feelings and tend to act out their problems and concerns. Some states of depression are of a temporary nature (e.g., acute depression precipitated by a traumatic event). This might include a period of hospitalization, loss of a parent through death or separation, or loss of a significant relationship with something (a pet), someone (a friend or family member), or a place (move from a familiar home, neighborhood, or city). The characteristics of children with depression are outlined in the accompanying box. The child tends to spend more time in solitary activities, especially television viewing, and schoolwork is impaired. Some

---

CHARACTERISTICS OF CHILDREN WITH DEPRESSION

Behavior
Predominantly sad facial expression with absence or diminished range of affective response
Solitary play or work; tendency to be alone; disinterest in play
Lowered grades in school; lack of interest in doing homework or achieving in school
Diminished motor activity; tiredness
Change in appetite resulting in weight loss or gain
Alterations in sleeping pattern
Tearfulness or crying

Internal States
Utterance of statements reflecting lowered self-esteem, sense of hopelessness, or guilt
Suicidal ideations

Physiology
Constipation
Nonspecific complaints of not feeling well
Lowered urinary excretion of 30 methoxy-4-hydroxyphenylglycol (MHPG)
Abnormal dexylmethazone suppression test (DST)
Hypersecretion of growth hormone during sleep
Blunting of growth hormone to insulin-induced hypoglycemia, suggestive of endogenous depression

Modified from Brantly DK, Takacs DJ: Anxiety and depression in preschool and school-aged children. In Clunn PA, editor: *Child psychiatric nursing,* St Louis, 1991, Mosby.

children become more dependent and clinging; others become more aggressive and disruptive. The manifestations may last a few days or weeks, usually resolving spontaneously.

More serious and less common are depressive responses to more chronic stress and loss; these are frequently observed in children with chronic illness or disability. There is usually no apparent precipitating event, but there is often a history of frequent disruptions in important relationships. Manifestations are as varied as those observed in acute depression but occur more frequently and extend over a longer period of time.

Nursing Considerations

The management of childhood depression is usually psychotherapeutic and highly individualized. Nurses should be aware that depression is a problem that can easily be overlooked in the child and one that can interrupt normal growth and development. Recognizing depression and making appropriate referrals is an important nursing function. Identification of the depressed child requires a careful history (health, growth and development, social, and family health), interviews with the child, and observations by the nurse, parents, and teachers. (See also Suicide, p. 517.)

CHILDHOOD SCHIZOPHRENIA

Childhood schizophrenia refers to severe deviations in ego functioning and is generally reserved for psychotic disorders that appear after the first 4 or 5 years of life. Schizophrenia in adults occurs with relative frequency, and although childhood psychosis is not as common, it is by no means rare.

Childhood schizophrenia is characterized by a gradual onset of neurotic symptoms that show wide variation according to each affected child's developmental level, the age of onset, the nature of early childhood experiences, and the type of defense mechanisms used. However, the basic core disturbance is a lack of contact with reality and the subsequent development of a world of the child's own. Secondary characteristics represent impairment in a wide number of areas of development, including cognition, perception, emotion, language, and physical motor control. The most common manifestations involve language disturbances, impaired interpersonal relationships, and inappropriate affect (outward expression of emotion).

Nursing Considerations

Nursing of psychotic children is a highly specialized area, but since these problems are being recognized with increasing frequency, nurses should be alert to the possibility. A child who consistently demonstrates abnormal behavior should be referred for evaluation.

SERIOUS HEALTH PROBLEMS OF LATER CHILDHOOD AND ADOLESCENCE

SUBSTANCE ABUSE

The use of other substances, primarily drugs, by children and adolescents to produce an altered state of consciousness is believed to reflect the variety of changes taking place in their lives and the stresses engendered by these changes. Experimenting with drugs is widespread during adolescence, but most teens do not become high-risk users. Today's youth are much less likely to use illicit drugs (e.g., hallucinogens, heroin, and nonmedical use of psychotherapeutic drugs) than were youths of the 1970s. However, alcohol, tobacco, and marijuana consumption among adolescents remains high, and cocaine use—particularly "crack"—appears to be increasing (National Institute on Drug Abuse, 1991).

Drug abuse is the regular use of drugs for other than the accepted medical purposes and to the extent that it results in physical or psychologic harm to the user and/or is detrimental to society. *Drug abuse, misuse,* and *addiction* are culturally defined and are voluntary behaviors. *Drug tolerance* and *physical dependence* are involuntary behaviors based on physiologic changes. Consequently an individual can be addicted to a narcotic with or without being physically dependent, whereas a person may be physically dependent on a narcotic without being addicted, such as patients who are experiencing pain. (See discussion on fear of addiction under Pain Assessment, Chapter 21.)

Most drugs to which young people turn induce changes in perception, a feeling of well-being, and a sense of closeness. To most, they provide a feeling of happiness. In the majority of cases drug use begins with experimentation. The individual may try a drug only once, may use it occasionally, or may make it an integral part of a drug-centered life-style.

Motivation

There are several common motives for drug use. Children and adolescents try drugs out of curiosity, for "kicks." Drugs produce for some persons a dreamy state of altered consciousness and a feeling of power, excitement, heightened acuity, or confidence. Others seek visual hallucinatory experiences and sexual sensation. Many youngsters use drugs not only for the perceptual and sensory experiences, but also for the social aspects. They use drugs because others use them, and because they want to "belong." Teenagers are highly influenced by society's fads and fashions, and they are, developmentally, sensation-hungry risk takers. Adolescents are also trying to find a means to cope with the stress of the adult world, its social and technologic concerns, and their powerlessness to change it. Adolescents seek escape from reality and want to achieve a sense of closeness and intimacy with other people, to escape from distress or decision making, and to feel a sense of insight into the mysteries of life and death.

Types of Drugs Abused

Any drug can be abused, and most are potentially harmful to youngsters still going through formative life experiences. Although rarely conceived of as drugs by society, the chemically active substances most frequently abused are caffeine and theobromines contained in chocolate and in common beverages such as tea, coffee, and colas. Common analgesics (e.g., Darvon Compound, Fiorinal), ethyl alcohol (ethanol), and nicotine are others that, although recognized as drugs, are sanctioned by society. These drugs can produce mild to moderate euphoric and/or stimulant effects and can lead to physical and psychic dependence. Many of the hazards associated with drug use are also related to adolescents driving a car while under the influence of drugs.

Drugs with mind-altering capacity that are available on the

black market and that are of medical and legal concern are the hallucinogenic, narcotic, hypnotic, and stimulant drugs. In addition, those of concern to health professionals are alcohol and various volatile substances, such as antifreeze, plastic model airplane cement, typewriter correction fluid, and organic solvents, which are inhaled to achieve altered sensation in the user. Drugs available on the street are often mixed with other compounds and fillers so that the purity of the drug, its strength, and the nature of additives are highly variable.

Alcohol. Acute or chronic abuse of ethanol, a socially accepted depressant, is responsible for many acts of violence, suicide, accidental injury, and death. It is the most widely accepted drug, can be purchased legally by adults, is relatively inexpensive, is often used as part of a meal (wine and beer), and is approved by adults throughout the world when used in moderation. Youngsters may be afraid of hard drugs but feel comfortable with alcohol, which is increasingly being used by children of elementary school age.

The most noticeable effects of alcohol are on the central nervous system—incoordination, emotional lability, and impaired judgment, memory, and perception. Young alcoholics enjoy the effect of the alcohol and look forward to becoming intoxicated. They drink rapidly to obtain a "high" emotional state, often drink alone, and cannot predictably control their use of alcohol. Not all of these characteristics are observed in the alcoholic but if several signs are evident, the youngsters should be considered at risk and detoxification therapy initiated to ensure safe and complete withdrawal from the drug. Information about alcohol and answers to questions can be obtained by calling the *Alcohol Hotline.**

Cocaine. The use of cocaine by adolescents is increasing more rapidly than any other form of substance abuse. Cocaine is available in two forms: water-soluble cocaine hydrochloride administered by "snorting" and a nonsoluble alkaloid (freebase) used primarily for smoking. "Crack" is a purer and more menacing form of the drug; it can be produced cheaply and smoked in either water pipes or mentholated cigarettes. The increased use of cocaine is related to its availability and affordability, the false perception of safety in its use, its association with persons in glamorous occupations, its snob appeal, its reputation as a sexually enhancing drug, and peer pressure.

Cocaine creates a sense of euphoria, or an indefinable high. Withdrawal does not produce the dramatic symptoms observed in withdrawal from other substances. The effects are those more commonly seen in depression, including lack of energy and motivation, irritability, appetite changes, psychomotor retardation, and irregular sleep patterns. More serious symptoms include cardiovascular manifestations and seizures. Withdrawal is not to be confused with the so-called crash after a cocaine high, which consists of a long period of sleep. Answers to questions about the health risks of cocaine can be obtained by calling the *National Cocaine Hotline.†* It also provides referrals to support groups and treatment centers.

Narcotics. Narcotic drugs include opiates such as heroin, morphine, meperidine hydrochloride (Demerol), fentanyl, hydromorphone (Dilaudid) and codeine. They produce a state of euphoria by removing painful feelings and creating a pleasurable experience and a sense of success accompanied by clouding of consciousness and a dreamlike state. Physical signs of narcotic abuse include constricted pupils, respiratory depression, and, often, cyanosis. Needle marks may be visible on the arms or legs in chronic users. Withdrawal from opiates is extremely unpleasant unless controlled with supervised substitution of methadone.

Perhaps more important are the indirect consequences related to the illegal status of narcotic use and the problems associated with securing the drug—time-consuming searches and often illegal methods used to meet the high cost. Health problems result from self-neglect of physical needs (nutrition, cleanliness, dental care), overdose, contamination, and infection, including HIV infection and hepatitis.

Central Nervous System Depressants. A variety of hypnotic drugs that produce physical dependence and withdrawal symptoms on abrupt discontinuation may be used by adolescents. They create a feeling of relaxation and sleepiness but impair general functioning. Drugs in this category include both barbiturates and nonbarbiturates (such as methaqualone [Quaalude]), as well as alcohol. Barbiturates combined with alcohol produce a profound depressant effect.

Central Nervous System Stimulants. Amphetamines and cocaine do not produce strong physical dependence and can be withdrawn without much danger. However, psychologic dependence is strong, and acute intoxication can lead to violent aggressive behavior or psychotic episodes characterized by paranoia, uncontrollable agitation, and restlessness. When combined with barbiturates, the euphoric effects are particularly addictive.

Methamphetamine is gradually assuming an important place in drug abuse. The drug can be snorted, injected, swallowed, or smoked and produces a burst of energy in its users, along with intense, alternating attacks of boldness and paranoia. It provokes excitement far more intense than that caused by crack and cocaine. The drug, with the street names "crank," "meth," and "crystal," is inexpensive and has a longer period of action than cocaine. Instead of a short (few minutes) high, as achieved with crack, a user can remain "up" for hours on a similar dose of crank.

Mind-Altering Drugs. Hallucinogens (psychedelic, psychotomimetic, psychotropic, or illusionogenic) are drugs that produce vivid hallucinations and euphoria. These drugs do not produce physical dependence, since they can be abruptly withdrawn without ill effect. However, acute and long-term effects are variable, and in some individuals the dissociative behavior may be unduly prolonged. This category includes cannabis (marijuana, hashish) and lysergic acid diethylamide (LSD).

Inhalants. Glue "sniffing," the inhalation of plastic cement, and inhalation of other volatile substances that youngsters breathe and rebreathe in paper or plastic bags produce euphoria and altered consciousness. These substances are extremely hazardous to the individual, causing rapid loss of consciousness and respiratory arrest. Many persons taking these drugs do not have time to remove the bag from their heads and quickly become asphyxiated.

 An important addition to the list of "sniffing" substances is air dusters, cans of pressurized gas used to blow dust from such surfaces as computers and camera lenses. The dusters contain chemical solvents and usually a form of freon, which can cause fatal cardiac dysrhythmias.

---

*(800) ALCOHOL.

†(800) COCAINE.

Nursing Considerations Related to Therapeutic Management

Nurses in almost every setting are increasingly likely to have contact with young drug abusers or to be in a position to serve as educator and patient advocate. The nurse most often encounters young drug abusers when they are (1) experiencing overdose symptoms, (2) experiencing withdrawal symptoms, (3) manifesting bizarre behavior or confusion secondary to drug ingestion, (4) worried that they are becoming or will become addicted, or (5) worried about a friend or family member who is addicted.

Drug use may be encountered in relation to other health problems; therefore, nurses caring for adolescents who are in the hospital or under treatment for other illnesses need to know if the youngsters use drugs compulsively, since withdrawal phenomena can seriously complicate the illness. Nurses should be able to recognize physical or behavioral clues that indicate the onset of withdrawal or the effects of drugs that might have been brought to the youngster secretly by well-meaning relatives or friends.

Acute Care. Adolescents experiencing toxic drug effects or withdrawal symptoms are frequently seen as emergencies. Experienced emergency room personnel are familiar with the management of acute drug toxicosis; the signs, symptoms, and behavioral characteristics of a variety of substances; and differences and similarities among them. Observation of or description of the behavior is often of more value than a report by patients or their friends as to the chemical agent taken.

The treatment for drug toxicity or withdrawal varies according to the drug and the method used. Every effort is made to determine the type and amount of drug taken, the time it was taken, the mode of administration, and factors related to the onset of presenting symptoms. It is helpful to know the individual's pattern of use. For example, if two types of drugs are involved, they may require different treatments. Gastric lavage may be employed when the drug has been ingested recently and the cough reflex is intact, but it would be of little value when the drug has been administered by the intravenous ("mainlined") or intranasal ("sniffed") route. Since the actual content of most street drugs is highly questionable, other pharmaceutical agents are administered with caution, except perhaps naloxone (Narcan) or flumazenil (Mazicon) in cases of suspected opiate or benzodiazepine overdose, respectively. It is also necessary to assess for possible trauma sustained while the patient was under the influence of the drug.

Long-Term Management. A major factor in the treatment and rehabilitation of young drug users is careful assessment, in the nonacute stage, to determine the function that the drug plays in the youngster's life. Adolescents need help to identify the problem that motivated them to use drugs and to recognize their own role in self-destructive, inappropriate drug abuse behavior before they can embark on a rehabilitation program.

Rehabilitation begins when youngsters decide, with the help of concerned and supportive adults, that they can and are willing to change. The family is an integral part of the rehabilitation process. Rehabilitation implies not only environmental manipulation and involvement in therapy, but also commitment on the part of the youth to substitute dependency on people for dependency on drugs and to explore alternative mechanisms for problem solving and coping with stress. Persons working with troubled youth must be prepared for recidivism, or the tendency to relapse, and maintain a plan for reentry into the treatment process.

Family Support. Organizations that have achieved success in helping others cope with problems of drug abuse are excellent sources for both youngsters and their families. The *Tough Love** philosophy first employed by Alcoholics Anonymous and Al-Anon is based on the conviction that parents have the right and responsibility to be the policymakers in the family, set limits on the behavior of their children, and take control of the household from out-of-control youngsters. The premise is that allowing teenagers to experience the negative consequences of their behavior will bring them closer to accepting help and/or changing their behavior.

Another group that provides support and counseling for families experiencing crises with their children is *Parents Anonymous†*, which maintains crisis counseling on a 24-hour basis. *Al-Anon, Ala-Teen,* and *Ala-Tot* are support groups for children and families who have an alcoholic family member. Information can be obtained from *Alcoholics Anonymous* listings in local telephone directories.

Prevention. Substance abuse in adolescence is both an individual and a community problem, and nurses play an important role in education and legislation, as well as in individual observation, assessment, and therapy. In this drug-oriented society, patterns of drug use may be established through parental models and the influence of the media as an effective means to make the user "feel better." Impressionable youth need to be educated regarding appropriate use of chemicals. More important, those associated with adolescents should listen to what they are saying, determine what is bothering them, and try to help them meet these needs through alternative methods before they resort to drugs.

Peer pressure is a powerful tool and can be used effectively in prevention. A group that has had some success in reducing injury from drunk driving is *Students Against Driving Drunk (SADD),‡* an organization designed to help eliminate teenage drunk driving. Some of the techniques used by the group include peer counseling, parental guidelines for teenage parties, and community awareness. Nurses can encourage the formation of chapters of SADD in the high schools in their communities.

Researchers have identified specific individual and environmental factors believed to make some children more vulnerable than others to substance abuse. An important predictor is age of initial use. Drug use initiated before the age of 15 is a major risk factor for serious drug abuse problems (National Institute on Drug Abuse, 1991). Therefore prevention efforts must begin well before children reach adolescence.

---

*Tough Love International, P.O. Box 1069, Doylestown, PA, 18901; (215) 348-7090.

†2230 Hawthorne Blvd., No. 208, Torrance, CA 90505; (800) 352-0386 in California and (800) 421-0353 elsewhere. Other sources of information include the *National Clearinghouse for Alcohol and Drug Information,* P.O. Box 2345, Rockville, MD 20847-2345, (800) 729-6686; *National Federation of Parents for Drug-Free Youth,* (800) 554-KIDS or (301) 585-5437 (Maryland); and *Center for Substance Abuse Prevention,* 5600 Fishers Lane, Rockville, MD 20857, (301) 443-0365.

‡P.O. Box 800, Malboro, MA 01752; (508) 481-3568.

The most effective substance abuse prevention strategies are part of a broader, generic prevention effort to promote health and success. Health-compromising behaviors tend to be interconnected and to have common antecedents. Prevention efforts that focus on changing only one behavior (e.g., alcohol and other drug use) are less likely to be successful.

SUICIDE

Suicide is the third leading cause of death during the teenage years, surpassed only by death from injury and homicide (see Chapter 1). A striking feature is the rise among persons in the younger age-groups. During the years 1950 to 1988 the suicide rate quadrupled in adolescents between the ages of 15 and 19 (Attempted suicide, 1991).

Most authorities distinguish between suicidal ideation, gesture, and attempt, and all three must be acknowledged. *Suicidal ideation* involves thoughts about or plans for suicide. A *gesture* is made without any real attempt to cause either serious injury or death but rather to send out a signal that something is wrong. An *attempt*, unlike a gesture, is intended to cause injury or death but is unsuccessful. Teenagers sometimes make a number of gestures to draw attention to the fact that they are unable to cope. If the signals are not detected and responded to promptly, they may escalate in seriousness until they become serious attempts or completed acts. Another category, an *impulsive act*, describes a rage response designed to punish or manipulate a loved person perceived as withdrawing that love. Moreover, many experts believe that numerous "accidental" deaths are actually suicides.

Etiology

Adolescence has always been characterized by turmoil, heightened emotionality, and wide variations in mood. With limited capacities for problem solving and with fewer and less sophisticated resources for resolving difficulties, some teenagers have difficulty coping with critical events, especially a situation that is forced on them, such as the death of a friend, parent, or sibling. Impulsive behavior, characteristic of younger children, places children and adolescents at high risk for unintentional suicide.

Biologic, sociologic, and psychologic factors may be involved. Suicidal youngsters almost invariably come from a disturbed family situation, with economic stresses, family disintegration, medical problems, or psychiatric illness. Divorce, separation, abandonment, alcoholism, and death are highly significant factors that are frequently noted in the histories of suicidal youth. During a family crisis youngsters may become suicidal when they feel overwhelmed by the crisis and unable to help the family recover equilibrium. A history of suicide by another family member is a common finding. Suicide risk is greater among youngsters with depression, chemical dependency, or psychosis. Gay and lesbian adolescents are at high risk for suicide especially if they lack a support system (see Family Focus Box). The availability of firearms in the United States has also been identified as a risk factor for adolescent suicide.

Suicidal Methods

The outcome of suicidal behavior is influenced to some extent by the method used. Violent methods of destruction used by adults, such as jumping from heights or in front of

FAMILY FOCUS
Suicide and Homosexuality

Thirty percent of all teen suicides each year occur among homosexual youths. Gay or lesbian adolescents who live in families or communities that do not accept homosexuality are very likely to suffer from low self-esteem and may even internalize homophobic feelings of their family or community. Such internalization can lead to self-loathing, despair, hopelessness, and eventually suicide. Supportive parents, friends, or relationships serve as protective factors against suicide.

However, many gay or lesbian adolescents have no friends and are not supported by their parents or families. Nurses who interact with adolescents must be aware of the association between adolescent homosexuality and suicide. School nurses may be the first individuals to identify and discuss issues of homosexuality with an adolescent. In their professional capacity, nurses can also serve as support persons for adolescents who are homosexual and provide the supportive relationship that will help to prevent suicide. Nurses must also capitalize on those opportunities or experiences that promote the healthy development of self-esteem in gay, lesbian, and bisexual youths. One experience might include providing educational programs in the school to raise the level of consciousness about the risk factors for suicide and its warning signs. Another experience could be programs conducted in or outside of school that are designed to foster peer relationships and competency in social skills among high-risk adolescents and young adults.

trains, are less frequently employed by youths. Overdose of drugs is the method of choice for most adolescents who attempt suicide. Drugs used by adolescents include medications prescribed for parents (such as barbiturates and antidepressants), those intended for household use (aspirin or acetaminophen), or solvents. Ingestion of medications and wrist lacerations are the methods favored by females; males use more lethal methods involving knives, guns, and automobiles. Younger children (under 13½) are more likely to resort to hanging.

Motivation

Many youngsters cannot identify a cause for their suicidal ideas. Ambivalence about life and death and hopelessness are common feelings. Most suicidal gestures are impulsive acts committed to force parents or other significant persons to pay attention to the youngster's need for help. The attempt usually is the culmination of a behavioral pattern. These youngsters often have a history of attention-getting behaviors that range from minor acts to increasingly dramatic ones. With the ultimate act of attempted suicide, youngsters finally make themselves heard. They seldom actually plan a suicidal act because they really want to die; successful suicides are committed either impulsively or accidentally.

Suicidal ideation is not uncommon in adolescents. It represents numerous fantasies, such as relief from suffering, a means to gain comfort and sympathy, or a means of revenge against those who have hurt them. Adolescents have the erroneous perception that the act of suicide will evoke remorse and pity and that they will be able to return and witness the grief. Some children and younger adolescents desire to punish others who will be grieved by their death. Angry children who are unable to punish directly those who have injured or insulted them will take revenge on those who love them through self-destruction ("They'll be sorry when they find me dead"; "They'll be sorry they were mean to me").

Occasionally there are adolescents who are so severely depressed that suicide seems to be the only means of release from their despair. These youngsters rarely give evidence of their intent, concealing their suicidal thoughts for fear of outside intervention. Most adolescents tell their peers of their suicidal thoughts or plans but avoid telling adults. Sometimes this self-destructive behavior on the part of adolescents is a desire to punish themselves for guilt-filled actions or thoughts. Peer pressure also has convinced many young persons that there is something wrong with them if they feel lonely or depressed; therefore they direct these feelings inward to avoid the risk of rejection. Social isolation is the most significant factor in distinguishing adolescents who will kill themselves from those who will not. It is also more characteristic of those who complete suicide than of those who make attempts or threats.

A cluster phenomenon, known as "contagion," has also been observed. Sometimes referred to as a teenage "epidemic," this situation occurs when one suicide appears to trigger several other suicides in a group such as a school or community. Suicide of a public figure sometimes prompts a number of suicides.

Diagnostic Evaluation

Depression is a symptom common to adolescents who attempt suicide. Depression is characterized by both subjective symptoms and objective signs that reflect the adolescent's grief. Adolescents describe feelings of sadness, despair, helplessness, hopelessness, boredom, loss of interest, and isolation. They may also feel self-reproach, self-deprecation, and guilt. Subjective symptoms of depression or specific changes in behavior may place an adolescent at risk for suicide (see box).

Therapeutic Management

Suicidal threats must be taken very seriously. There has been a general tendency to dismiss a suicide attempt as an impulsive act resulting from a temporary crisis or depression. If this drastic move to gain attention fails to draw attention to their problems or makes them worse, adolescents may conclude that suicide is the only answer to their escalating, unsolvable, and unbearable problems.

Children need to know that someone cares and must be provided with swift and efficient crisis intervention. Although an acute depressive reaction can be managed without difficulty by ordinary practitioners, the youngster who has made a serious attempt or has made a plan for suicide should receive immediate attention and competent psychiatric care.

Nursing Considerations

Care of the suicidal youngster includes early recognition, management, and prevention. Probably the most important aspect of management is the recognition of warning signs that indicate a youngster is troubled and might attempt suicide. Health professionals need to be alert to the signs of depression, and anyone who exhibits such behavior, subtle or overt, should be referred for thorough psychologic assessment. De-

---

CLINICAL MANIFESTATIONS ASSOCIATED WITH SUICIDE RISK

Mood/Affect
Marked persistent depression
Feelings of hopelessness, helplessness, isolation
Deteriorating schoolwork
Remains distant, sad, remote
Flat affect—has "frozen" facial expression
Persistently looks or sounds sad and unhappy
Describes self as worthless
Feelings of self-hatred or excessive guilt
Feelings of humiliation, often brought on by inadequate performance at school
Sudden cheerfulness following deep depression*
Wish to be punished

Behavior
Changes in physical appearance—a child previously neat and well-groomed who stops bathing and begins to look slovenly
Loss of function due to illness or trauma
Loss of energy—loss of interest, listlessness, exhaustion without obvious cause
Sleep disturbances—difficulty going to sleep or sleeping excessively, taking voluntary naps during afternoon or evening
Increased irritability, argumentativeness, or stubbornness
Physical complaints—recurrent stomachaches, headaches
Repeated visits to doctor's office or emergency room for treatment of injuries
Antisocial behavior—engages in drinking, uses drugs, fights, commits acts of vandalism, runs away from home, becomes sexually promiscuous
Preoccupation with death—focuses on morbid thoughts; speaks repeatedly about people getting killed*
May begin referring to own death

School and Interpersonal Relationships
Resists or refuses to go to school
May become truant, cuts classes, does not complete assignments
Social withdrawal from friends, activities, interests that were previously enjoyed
Wants to give away cherished possessions*
Lacks an effective social support system

Coping Skills
Loses reality boundaries
Withdraws and isolates self
No use of support systems
Sees self as totally helpless, a victim of fate

*Absolute "red flags" or danger signals.

---

pression can be manifested in two different ways: young people who feel depressed may talk about suicide and feelings of worthlessness, or they may build themselves a solid defense against such intolerable feelings of depression with behavioral or psychosomatic disturbances.

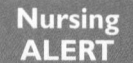 **Nursing ALERT**   No threat of suicide should be ignored or challenged in any way. It is a symptom that must be taken seriously. Too often, suicidal threats or minor attempts are confused with bids for attention. It is also a mistake to be lulled into a false sense of security when the adolescent's depression is apparently relieved. The improvement in attitude may very well mean that the youngster has made the decision to carry out the threat.

Peers or other confidants are excellent sources of information and valuable observers. They may not be able to diagnose depression, but they are able to sense when a friend has undergone a marked personality change. It is important to emphasize that the peer who detects any changes in a friend is a potential rescuer and should not remain quiet about the observations. Friendship does not imply collusion. A peer who believes that a friend may be suicidal should alert someone who is in a position to help—a parent, teacher, guidance counselor, school nurse, or other person.

As soon as the youngster who attempts suicide is out of danger from medical problems resulting from the attempt, the data-gathering process should begin. It should include information from several sources to help evaluate the extent to which the child is suffering, the direction for therapy, and the probability of a repeated attempt. The youngster is questioned directly about the depression or suicidal behavior. Clues to a youngster's feelings may be elicited by questions such as the following (Greydanus and Pratt, 1995):

- Do you consider yourself more a happy person, an unhappy person, or somewhere in the middle?
- Have you ever been so unhappy or upset that you felt like being dead?
- Have you ever thought about hurting yourself?
- Have you ever developed a plan to hurt yourself or kill yourself?
- Have you ever attempted to kill yourself?

NURSING TIP Ask youngsters to give their written word that they will not attempt suicide during an agreed-on period of time (a week, a day, maybe even just 5 minutes) and that they will contact help immediately if they feel that they cannot keep their contract. The length of time a youngster suggests provides valuable information regarding the seriousness of the threat. Furthermore, most teenagers attach significance to signing their name to a document, and if they sign a no-suicide contract, will usually honor it. Contracts can be extended when the time limit expires.

Since the suicide attempt is frequently an outgrowth of family distress, it is essential to deal with the family as well. Ideally the most effective approach is recognition of susceptible youngsters during the early stages of intrafamily distress so that family counseling can be started. This emphasizes again the importance of parent-child relationships and the role of the nurse in assessing family interactions and recognizing disturbed relationships. Prevention efforts must be directed toward improving childrearing practices through support and education of parents and changing societal conditions that generate defeat, despair, and maladaptive behavior.

Follow-up care is of utmost importance. Although confidentiality is the usual approach with adolescent counseling, in the case of self-destructive behaviors this cannot be honored. The suicidal behavior is reported to the family and other professionals, and youngsters are informed that this will be done. Such action conveys an important message to an attempter—that the professionals understand and care.

Some schools have instituted suicide-prevention programs. Most are designed for high school–age youth, but many are attempting to reach elementary school–age children as well. Schools with programs in operation offer services such as drop-in counseling and a peer-counseling telephone line. Information can be obtained from the **American Association of Suicidology.***

See also Nursing Care Plan: The Child Who Is Suicidal.†

---

*2459 S. Ash, Denver, CO 80222.
†In Wong DL: *Wong and Whaley's Clinical manual of pediatric nursing,* ed 4, St Louis, 1996, Mosby.

KEY POINTS

- The rapid changes, growth, and stress accompanying the transition to adulthood may predispose youngsters to faulty problem solving.
- Smoking is a widespread problem among teenagers; reasons for smoking include social pressures and mass media influence, and a need to develop a self-concept.
- Participation in sports predisposes children and adolescents to both acute injuries and overuse syndromes.
- Alterations in growth and maturation may be manifest in short or tall stature, precocious puberty, and delayed sexual development.
- Tools for assessment of growth include a family history, previous growth patterns, physical examination, bone age determination, and endocrine studies.
- The most frequent health problems related to the female reproductive system involve menstrual dysfunction.
- Health problems related to sexuality include pregnancy, rape, and sexually transmitted diseases; prevention includes sex education and contraceptive counseling.

- Eating disorders observed in middle and late childhood are obesity, anorexia nervosa, and bulimia.
- Effective therapies for attention deficit hyperactivity disorder and learning disabilities usually involve a multiple approach: family education and counseling, medication, remedial education, environmental manipulation, and psychotherapy.
- Behavior problems in middle childhood can result from attention deficit hyperactivity disorder, enuresis, encopresis, school phobia, recurrent abdominal pain, childhood depression, conversion reaction, and childhood schizophrenia.
- The substances abused by children and adolescents are alcohol, marijuana, narcotics, central nervous system depressants, central nervous system stimulants, hydrocarbons and fluorocarbons, and mind-altering drugs.
- Suicide, the deliberate act of self-injury with the intent to kill, may occur because of difficulties coping with stress, disturbed family environment, chemical dependency, or psychoses.

REFERENCES

American Psychiatric Association: *Diagnostic and statistical manual of mental disorders,* ed 4 (DSM-IV), Washington, DC, 1994, The Association.

Attempted suicide among high school students—United States, 1990, *MMWR* 40(37):633-635, 1991.

Biro FM and others: Hormonal studies and physical maturation in adolescent gynecomastia, *J Pediatr* 116:450-455, 1990.

Clubb R: Promoting non-tobacco use in childhood, *Pediatr Nurs* 17(6):566-570, 1991.

Comfort RL: Living with an unconventional child, *J Pediatr Health Care* 6(3):114-120, 1992.

Davis K, Christoffel KK: Obesity in preschool and school-age children: treatment early and often may be best, *Arch Pediatr Adolesc Med* 148(12):1257-1261, 1994.

Greydanus DE, Pratt HD: *Adolescent health update: emotional and behavioral disorders of adolescence;* part 2, vol 8, no 1, Elk Grove Village, IL, 1995, American Academy of Pediatrics.

Hoffmen N, Kelly C, Futterman D: Tuberculosis infection in human immunodeficiency virus-positive adolescents and young adults: a New York City cohort, *Pediatrics* 97(2):198-203, 1996.

Houts AC: Nocturnal enuresis as a biobehavioral problem, *Behav Ther* 22:133-151, 1991.

Johnston LD, Bachman JG, O'Malley PM: *Monitoring the future questionnaire responses from the nation's high school seniors 1989,* Ann Arbor, MI, 1992, Institute for Social Research, University of Michigan.

McAnarney ER, Hendee R: Adolescent pregnancy and its consequences, *JAMA* 262:74-77, 1989.

National Institute on Drug Abuse: *Drug abuse and drug abuse research,* Rockville, MD, 1991, The Institute.

Orr DP and others: Factors associated with condom use among sexually active female adolescents, *J Pediatr* 120(2):311-317, 1992.

Rappaport LA: Enuresis. In Levine M and others: *Developmental-behavioral pediatrics,* ed 2, Philadelphia, 1992, Saunders.

Rappaport LA: The treatment of nocturnal enuresis—where are we now, *Pediatrics* 92:465-466, 1993.

Schmitt B: Nocturnal enuresis: finding the treatment that fits the child, *Contemp Pediatr* 7(9):70-97, 1990.

Selekman J, Snyder M: Primary care of the child with a learning disability. In Jackson P, Vessey J: *Primary care of children with chronic conditions,* ed 2, St Louis, 1996, Mosby.

Sexual behavior among high school students—United States, 1990, *MMWR* 40(51, 52):885-888, 1992.

Terr L: Traumatic events in childhood have lasting effects, *AAP News* 5(5):1, 1989.

Torabi MR, Bailey WJ, Majd-Jabbari, M: Cigarette smoking as a predictor of alcohol and other drug use by children and adolescents: evidence of the "gateway drug effect", *J Sch Health* 63:302-306, 1993.

Troiano R and others: Overweight prevalence and trends for children and adolescents, *Arch Pediatr Adolesc Med* 149(10):1085-1091, 1995.

US Department of Health and Human Services: Preventing tobacco use among young people: a report of the surgeon general, Atlanta, 1994, US Department of Health and Human Services, Public Health Service, Centers for Disease Control and Prevention, National Center for Chronic Disease Prevention and Health Promotion, Office on Smoking and Health.

Wilson DM and others: Timing and rate of sexual maturation and the onset of cigarette and alcohol use among teenage girls, *Arch Pediatr Adolesc Med* 148:789-795, 1994.

BIBLIOGRAPHY

General

American Academy of Pediatrics, Committee on Infectious Disease: *Red book: Report of the Committee on Infectious Disease,* ed 23, Evanston, IL, 1994, American Academy of Pediatrics.

Levine MD, Carey WB, Crocker AC, editors: *Developmental-behavioral pediatrics,* ed 2, Philadelphia, 1992, WB Saunders.

Panzarine S and others: Adolescent health care: a challenge for nursing educators, *J Nurs Educ* 27:278-280, 1988.

Pipes PL, Trahms CM: *Nutrition in infancy and childhood,* ed 5, St Louis, 1993, Mosby.

Sumaya CV: Infectious mononucleosis and Epstein-Barr virus. In Hoekelman RA and others, editors: *Primary pediatric care,* ed 2, St Louis, 1992, Mosby.

Smoking

American Academy of Pediatrics, Committee on Substance Abuse: "Smokeless cigarettes" and other nicotine delivery devices, *Pediatrics* 87:410-411, 1991.

American Academy of Pediatrics, Committee on Substance Abuse: Tobacco-free environment: an imperative for the health of children and adolescents, *AAP News* 10(4):25-27, 1994.

Cigarette smoking among youth—United States, 1989, *MMWR* 40(41):712-715, 1991.

Davis R, Tollestrup K, Milham S: Trends in teenage smoking during pregnancy, *Am J Dis Child* 144(12):1297-1301, 1990.

Winkelstein M: Adolescent smoking: influential factors, past preventive efforts and future nursing implications, *J Pediatr Nurs* 7:120-127, 1992.

Disorders Related to Sports

American Academy of Pediatrics, Committee on Sports Medicine: Amenorrhea in adolescent athletes, *Pediatrics* 84:394-395, 1989.

American Academy of Pediatrics, Committee on Sports Medicine: Knee brace use by athletes, *Pediatrics* 85:228, 1990.

Backous DD and others: Soccer injuries and their relation to physical maturity, *Am J Dis Child* 142:839-842, 1988.

Council on Scientific Affairs: Drug abuse in athletes, *JAMA* 259:1703-1705, 1988.

Goldberg B and others: Injuries in youth football, *Pediatrics* 81:255-261, 1988.

Hergenroeder AC: Diagnosis and treatment of ankle sprains, *Am J Dis Child* 144:809-814, 1990.

Kris-Etherton PM: Nutrition and athletic performance, *Contemp Nutr* 14(8), 1989.

Mansfield MJ, Emans SJ: Growth in female gymnasts: should training decrease during puberty, *J Pediatr* 122:237-240, 1993.

McLain LG, Reynolds S: Sports injuries in a high school, *Pediatrics* 84:446-450, 1989.

Ostrum G: Sports-related injuries in youth: prevention is the key and nurses can help, *Pediatr Nurs* 19:333-342, 1993.

Pratt M: Strength, flexibility, and maturity in adolescent athletes, *Am J Dis Child* 143:560-563, 1989.

Rowland TW, Kelleher JF: Iron deficiency in athletes, *Am J Dis Child* 143:197-200, 1989.

Runyan CW, Gerkin EA: Epidemiology and prevention of adolescent injury: a review and research agenda, *JAMA* 262:2273-2279, 1989.

Terney R, McLain LG: The use of anabolic steroids in high school students, *Am J Dis Child* 144:99-103, 1990.

Yelverton GA: Anabolic steroids, *Pediatr Nurs* 15:63, 1989.

Altered Growth and/or Maturation

Bercu B: Growth hormone treatment and the short child: to treat or not to treat, *J Pediatr Health Care* 110:991-995, 1987.

Henry JJ: Routine growth monitoring and assessment of growth disorders, *J Pediatr Health Care* 6:291-301, 1992.

Mandoki M, Sumner G: Klinefelter syndrome: the need for early identification and treatment, *Clin Pediatr* 30(3):161-164, 1991.

Moore KC and others: Clinical diagnoses of children with extremely short stature and their response to growth hormone, *J Pediatr* 122:687-692, 1992.

Rapaport R and others: Immune functions during treatment of growth hormone-deficient children with biosynthetic human growth hormone, *Clin Pediatr* 30(1):22-27, 1991.

Rohn R: Comparative heights of mothers and fathers whose children are short, *Am J Dis Child* 144(9):995-997, 1990.

Schwartz ID, Root AW: Puberty in girls: early, incomplete, or precocious? *Contemp Pediatr* 7(1):147-156, 1990.

Stabler B: Psychosocial outcomes of short stature, *Pediatr Rounds* 2:5-7, 1993.

Walker J and others: Treatment of short normal children with growth hormone—a cautionary tale? *Lancet* 336:1331-1334, 1990.

Disorders of the Reproductive System

Coupey SM, Ahlstrom P: Common menstrual disorders, *Pediatr Clin North Am* 36:551-571, 1989.

Cumming DC, Cumming CE, Kieren DK: Menstrual mythology and sources of information about menstruation, *Am J Obstet Gynecol* 164:472-476, 1991.

Elvik S: Vaginal discharge in the prepubertal girl, *J Pediatr Health Care* 4(4):181-185, 1990.

Greydanus DE, Shearin RB: *Adolescent sexuality and gynecology,* Philadelphia, 1990, Lea & Febiger.

Higgs D: The patient with testicular cancer: nursing management of chemotherapy, *Clin Rev* 17(2):243-249, 1990.

Klein TF, Berry CC, Felice M: The development of a testicular self-examination instructional booklet, *J Adolesc Health Care* 11:235-239, 1990.

Tuttle J: Menstrual disorders during adolescence, *J Pediatr Health Care* 5(4):197-203, 1991.

Adolescent Pregnancy

American Academy of Pediatrics, Committee on Adolescence: Adolescent pregnancy, *Pediatrics* 83:132-133, 1989.

Association of Maternal and Child Health Programs: *Adolescent fathers: directory of services,* Washington, DC, 1991, National Center for Education in Maternal and Child Health.

Castiglia P: Adolescent fathers, *J Pediatr Health Care* 4(6):311-313, 1990.

Davis S: Pregnancy in adolescents, *Pediatr Clin North Am* 36:665-680, 1989.

East PL, Matthews KL, Felice ME: Qualities of adolescent mothers' parenting, *J Adolesc Health* 15:163-168, 1994.

Fielding JE, Williams CA: Adolescent pregnancy in the United States: a review and recommendation for clinicians and research needs, *Am J Prev Med* 7:47-52, 1991.

Jones M, Bonte C: Conceptualizing community interventions in social service needs of pregnant adolescents, *J Pediatr Health Care* 4(4):193-201, 1990.

Klerman LV: Adolescent pregnancy and parenting: controversies of the past and lessons for the future, *J Adolesc Health* 14:553-561, 1993.

McAnarney ER, Hendee R: The prevention of adolescent pregnancy, *JAMA* 262:78-82, 1989.

Palmore S, Millar K: An intervention program for pregnant teens and teen parents, *School Nurse* 6(4):14-17, 1990.

Palmore S, Millar K, Millar M: An interview for pregnant teens—identifying special needs in a school setting, *School Nurse* 6(4):18-20, 1990.

Porter C: Clinical and research issues related to teen mothers' childrearing practices, *Issues Compr Pediatr Nurs* 13(1):41-58, 1990.

Rhodes AM: Parental notification, *MCN* 17(3):155, 1992.

Winter L, Brackenmaker L: Tailoring family planning services to the special needs of adolescents, *Fam Plann Perspect* 23(1):24-30, 1991.

Contraception

Bullough B and others: Contraceptives for teenagers, *J Pediatr Health Care* 5(5):237-244, 1991.

Demetriou E, Kaplan DW: Adolescent contraceptive use and parental notification, *Am J Dis Child* 143:1166-1172, 1989.

Harbin R: Female adolescent contraception, *Pediatr Nurs* 21(3):221-226, 1995.

Hatcher RA and others: *Contraceptive technology,* ed 16, New York, 1994, Irvington.

Jay MS, DuRant RH, Litt IF: Female adolescents' compliance with contraceptive regimens, *Pediatr Clin North Am* 36:731-746, 1989.

Kulig JW: Adolescent contraception: nonhormonal methods, *Pediatr Clin North Am* 36:717-730, 1989.

Mashburn M: Levonorgestrel implant use among adolescents, *J Pediatr Health Care* 8(6):255-260, 1994.

Rhodes AM: Norplant and the "coerced conception" controversy, *MCN* 16(5):277, 1991.

Sharts-Engel NC: Levonorgestrel subdermal implants (Norplant) for long-term contraception, *MCN* 16(4):232, 1991.

Shearin RB, Boehlke JR: Hormonal contraception, *Pediatr Clin North Am* 36:697-715, 1989.

Sexually Transmitted Diseases

Cates W, Rolfs RT, Aral SO: Sexually transmitted diseases, pelvic inflammatory disease and infertility: an epidemiological report, *Epidemiol Rev* 12:199-220, 1990.

English A: Treating adolescents: legal and ethical considerations, *Med Clin North Am* 74:1097-1112, 1990.

Holmes KK and others, editors: *Sexually transmitted diseases,* ed 2, New York, 1990, McGraw-Hill.

Khoiny FL: Pelvic inflammatory disease in the adolescent, *J Pediatr Health Care* 3:230-236, 1989.

Nettina SM, Kauffman FH: Diagnosis and management of sexually transmitted genital lesions, *Nurse Pract* 15(1):20-39, 1990.

Rice RJ and others: Sociodemographic distribution of gonorrhea incidence: implications for prevention and behavioral research, *Am J Public Health* 81(10):1252-1258, 1991.

Steiner JD and others: Are adolescents getting smarter about acquired immunodeficiency syndrome? *Am J Dis Child* 144:302-306, 1990.

US Department of Health and Human Services: Recommendations for the prevention and management of *Chlamydia trachomatis* infections, *MMWR* 42(RR-12):1-39, 1993.

Wendell D and others: Youth at risk: sex, drugs, and human immunodeficiency virus, *Am J Dis Child* 146:76-81, 1992.

Wilk S: Pediatric management problems, *Pediatr Nurs* 17(2):186-197, 1991.

Rape

Beckman C and others: Treating sexual assault victims: a protocol for health professionals, *Physician Assist* 14(2):123-126, 1990.

Browne A: Violence against women by male partners: prevalence and outcomes and policy implications, *Am Psychol* 48:1077-1087, 1993.

Goodman LA and others: Male violence against women, *Am Psychol* 48:1054-1058, 1993.

Lenehan GP: Sexual assault nurse examiners: a SANE way to care for rape victims, *J Emerg Nurs* 17(1):1-2, 1991.

Mayer RA, Boggio NT: The adolescent rape victim, *Emerg Med* 24(3):98-115, 1992.

Obesity

Alexander MA: Obesity in school children, *School Nurse* 7(4):6-10, 1991.

Castiglia PT: Obesity in adolescence, *J Pediatr Health Care* 3:221-223, 1989.

Dietz WH Jr: The overweight child: psychosocial effects and treatment, *Feelings Med Signif* 31(1):1-4, 1989.

Epstein L and others: Growth in obese children treated for obesity, *Am J Dis Child* 14(12):1360-1364, 1990.

Feldman W, Feldman E, Goodman JT: Culture versus biology: children's attitudes toward thinness and fatness, *Pediatrics* 81:190-194, 1988.

Moore DC: Body image and eating behavior in adolescent boys, *Am J Dis Child* 144:475-479, 1990.

Schmitt BD: A weight reduction program for overweight older children and adolescents, *Contemp Pediatr* 8(8):85-91, 1991.

Stunkard A, Berkowitz R: Treatment of obesity in children, *JAMA* 264(19):2550-2551, 1990.

Anorexia Nervosa/Bulimia

Castiglia PT: Anorexia nervosa, *J Pediatr Health Care* 3:105-107, 1989.

Castiglia PT: Bulimia, *J Pediatr Health Care* 3:167-169, 1989.

Comerci GD: Eating disorders in adolescents, *Pediatr Rev* 10:1-6, 1988.

Ferraro AR: Bulimia: a look from within, *Pediatr Nurs* 16:187-191, 1990.

Flood M: Addictive eating disorders, *Nurs Clin North Am* 24:65-69, 1989.

Garner D: Pathogenesis of anorexia nervosa, *Lancet* 431:1631-1634, 1993.

Muscari ME: Effective nursing strategies for adolescents with anorexia nervosa and bulimia nervosa, *Pediatr Nurs* 14:475-482, 1988.

Stewart DE and others: Infertility and eating disorders, *Am J Obstet Gynecol* 163:1196-1199, 1990.

Attention Deficit Hyperactivity Disorder/Learning Disabilities

Adesman AR, Wender EH: Improving the outcome for children with ADHD, *Contemp Pediatr* 8(3):122-139, 1991.

Amaya-Jackson L, Cantwell D: Controversies in psychopharmacological management of attention deficit and related disorders, *Int Pediatr* 6(2):176-183, 1991.

American Academy of Pediatrics: Learning disabilities, dyslexia, and vision, *Pediatrics* 90:124-126, 1992.

Castiglia P: Dyslexia, *J Pediatr Health Care* 4(4):206-208, 1990.

Murphy MA, Hagerman RJ: Attention deficit hyperactivity disorder in children: diagnosis, treatment, and follow-up, *J Pediatr Health Care* 6(1):2-11, 1992.

Smitherman CH: A drug to ease attention deficit-hyperactivity disorder, *MCN* 15(6):362-365, 1990.

Vatz RE, Weinberg LS: Treatment of attention-deficit hyperactivity disorder, *JAMA* 269:2368, 1993.

Voeller K: The neurological basis of attention deficit hyperactivity disorder, *Int Pediatr* 5(2):171-176, 1990.

Enuresis/Encopresis

Castiglia PT: Encopresis, *J Pediatr Health Care* 1:335-337, 1987.

Castiglia PT: Nocturnal enuresis, *J Pediatr Health Care* 1:280-282, 1987.

Corkery J: Nintendo power, *Am J Dis Child* 144(9):959, 1990.

Friman PC, Warzak WJ: Nocturnal enuresis: a prevalent, yet curable parasomnia, *Pediatrician* 17:38-45, 1990.

Gibson LY: Bedwetting: a family's recurrent nightmare, *MCN* 14:270-272, 1989.

Miller K: Concomitant nonpharmacologic therapy in the treatment of primary nocturnal enuresis, *Clin Pediatr* 32:32-37, 1993.

Piazza C and others: Reinforcement of incontinent stools in the treatment of encopresis, *Clin Pediatr* 30(1):28-32, 1991.

Rushton H: Nocturnal enuresis: epidemiology, evaluation, and current available treatment options, *J Pediatr* 114:691-696, 1989.

Stroh SE, Stern HP, McCarthy SG: Fecal incontinence in children: a clinical update, *MCN* 14:252-254, 1989.

Terho P: Desmospressin in nocturnal enuresis, *J Urol* 145:818-820, 1991.

Behavior Disorders

Carpenter WT, Buchanan RW: Medical progress: schizophrenia, *N Engl J Med* 330:681-690, 1994.

Castiglia P: School phobias/school avoidance, *J Pediatr Health Care* 7:229-232, 1993.

Conway A, Bernardo L, Tontala K: The effects of disasters on children: implications for emergency nurses, *J Emerg Nurs* 16(6):393-397, 1990.

Davis B: Loneliness in children and adolescents, *Issues Compr Pediatr Nurs* 13(1):59-69, 1990.

Hodgman C and others: Managing depression in children, *Patient Care* 27:51-60, 1993.

Jacobson J: The relationship between social support and depression in adolescents, *J Child Adolesc Psychiatr Ment Health Nurs* 4(1):20-24, 1991.

Lipovsky JA: Posttraumatic stress disorder in children, *Fam Commun Health* 14(3):42-51, 1991.

Puskar K, Dvorsak K: Relocation stress in adolescents: helping teenagers cope with a moving dilemma, *Pediatr Nurs* 17(3):295-297, 1991.

Weller EB, Weller RA: Pediatric management of depression, *Pediatr Ann* 18:104-113, 1989.

Wyllie R, Kay M: Causes of recurrent abdominal pain, *Clin Pediatr* 32:369-371, 1993.

Substance Abuse

Alexander DE, Gwyther RE: Alcoholism in adolescents and their families: family-focused assessment and management, *Pediatr Clin North Am* 42(1):217-234, 1995.

American Academy of Pediatrics, Committee on Adolescence, Committee on Bioethics, and Provisional Committee on Substance Abuse: Screening for drugs of abuse in children and adolescents, *Pediatrics* 84:396-398, 1989.

Bateman DA, Heagarty MC: Passive freebase cocaine ("crack") inhalation by infants and toddlers, *Am J Dis Child* 143:25-27, 1989.

Brown BS and others: Kids and cocaine—a treatment dilemma, *J Subst Abuse Treat* 6:3-8, 1989.

Casswell S and others: What children know about alcohol and how they know it, *Br J Addict* 3:223-227, 1988.

Castiglia PT and others: Influences on children's attitudes toward alcohol consumption, *Pediatr Nurs* 15:263-266, 1989.

Clouet D, Asghar K, Brown R, editors: *Mechanisms of cocaine abuse and toxicity,* NIDA Research Monograph 88, Washington, DC, 1988, US Government Printing Office.

Estroff TW, Schwartz RH, Hoffmann NG: Adolescent cocaine abuse, *Clin Pediatr* 28:550-555, 1989.

Heagarty MC: Crack cocaine: a new danger for children, *Am J Dis Child* 14:756-757, 1990.

Rich J: Action stat! Acute alcohol intoxication, *Nursing 89* 19(9):33, 1989.

Robinson DP, Green JW: The adolescent alcohol and drug problem: a practical approach, *Pediatr Nurs* 14:305-310, 1988.

Schubiner H: Treatment: validating toughlove, *Child Teens Today* 11(4):1-3, 1991.

Washburn P: Identification, assessment, and referral of adolescent drug abusers, *Pediatr Nurs* 17(2):137-40, 1991.

Suicide

American Academy of Pediatrics, Committee on Adolescence: Suicide and suicide attempts in adolescents and young adults, *Pediatrics* 81:322-324, 1988.

Bakkala CF: The role of the school nurse in suicide prevention, *School Nurse* 6(1):13-15, 1990.

Berman AL, Jobes DA: *Adolescent suicide: assessment and intervention,* Washington, DC, 1991, American Psychological Association.

Brent DA and others: Risk factors for adolescent suicide, *Arch Gen Psychiatry* 45:581-588, 1988.

Gemma PB: Coping with suicidal behavior, *MCN* 14:101-103, 1989.

Gyulay JE: What suicide leaves behind, *Issues Compr Pediatr Nurs* 12:103-118, 1989.

Lamb JM: The suicidal adolescent: how you can help, *Nursing 90* 20(5):72-76, 1990.

Pfeffer CR: Spotting the red flags for adolescent suicide, *Contemp Pediatr* 6(2):59-70, 1989.

Reinherz H, Frost A, Pakiz B: Changing faces: correlates of depressive symptoms in late adolescence, *Fam Commun Health* 14(3):53-63, 1991.

Reynolds WM: A school-based procedure for the identification of adolescents at risk for suicidal behaviors, *Fam Commun Health* 14(3):64-75, 1991.

Chapter 18

IMPACT OF CHRONIC ILLNESS, DISABILITY, OR DEATH ON THE CHILD AND FAMILY

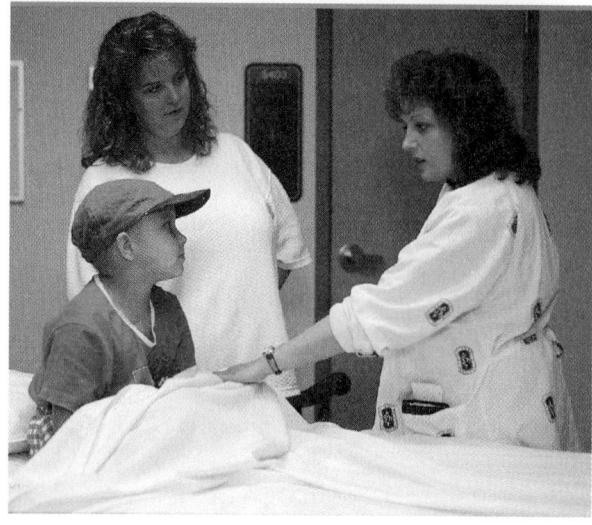

Connie, age 8 years, cancer

RELATED TOPICS

PERSPECTIVES IN THE CARE OF CHILDREN WITH SPECIAL NEEDS

SCOPE OF THE PROBLEM

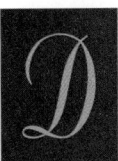espite the interest and concern for these children, exact definitions and prevalence rates of chronic illness, disability, and terminal illness do not exist. For the purposes of this chapter, see the definitions listed in the accompanying box.

Statistics regarding chronic illness and disability are at best only estimates of the actual prevalence of the problem. In the United States an estimated 20% of children under 18 years of age experienced mild chronic conditions, 9% experienced chronic conditions of moderate severity, and 2% experienced severe chronic conditions (Newacheck, Stoddard, and Mc-Manus, 1993). Cancer and mental health problems without physical manifestations are not included in these figures. Asthma and congenital heart defects account for two thirds of all cases of chronic illness in children.

Although there has been little change in the survival patterns for asthma and acquired immunodeficiency syndrome (AIDS), there have been improvements in other diseases, such as cancer, cystic fibrosis, and spina bifida. In addition, technologic advances have increased survival rates of extremely and very low–birth-weight infants. The resulting progress for these children at risk contributes to the growing number of children who have chronic and/or disabling conditions, many of whom remain dependent on technology.

Broadly expanding chronic conditions that include speech, learning, emotional, sensory, and cognitive disorders yields an even greater number of children who have a significant long-term condition. Terminal illness also significantly adds to the number of children with special needs. Cancer is the leading cause of death from disease in children ages 1 through 15 years (*Cancer facts*, 1994). However, many children survive for long periods and experience problems typically associated with chronic illness or physical disability. Considering also those who care deeply about the child, the number of individuals intimately affected by these children's illnesses and disabilities is staggering.

Elizabeth Ahmann, ScD, RN, revised this chapter.

CHANGING TRENDS IN CARE

Developmental Focus

One change is in the focus on the child's *developmental age* rather than chronologic age or diagnosis. Using the developmental approach emphasizes the child's abilities and strengths rather than disabilities. Attention focuses on normalizing experiences, environmental adaptations, and promoting coping skills. Nurses often are in vital positions to redirect attention from the pathologic model with its focus on weaknesses and

COMMON TERMS REGARDING CHILDREN WITH SPECIAL NEEDS

Chronic illness—a condition that interferes with daily functioning for more than 3 months in a year, causes hospitalization of more than 1 month in a year, or (at time of diagnosis) is likely to do either of these

Congenital disability—a disability that has existed since birth but is not necessarily hereditary

Developmental delay—a maturational lag; an abnormal, slower rate of development in which a child demonstrates a functioning level below that observed in normal children of the same age

Developmental disability—any mental and/or physical disability that is manifested before age 22 years and is likely to continue indefinitely

Disability—a functional limitation that interferes with a person's ability, for example, to walk, lift, hear, or learn

Handicap—a condition or barrier imposed by society, the environment, or one's own self; not a synonym for disability

Impairment—a loss or abnormality of structure or function

Technology-dependent child—a child between the ages of birth to 21 years with a chronic disability that requires the routine use of a medical device to compensate for the loss of a life-sustaining body function; daily ongoing care and/or monitoring is required by trained personnel

Data from Research and Training Center on Independent Living (RTC/IL): *Guidelines for reporting and writing about people with disabilities*, ed 3, Lawrence, KS, 1990, The Center; Hobbs N, Perrin J, editors: *Issues in the care of children with chronic illness*, San Francisco, 1985, Jossey-Bass; *Report to Congress and the Secretary by the Task Force on Technology-Dependent Children: Fostering home and community-based care for technology-dependent children*, vol 2, Health Care Financing Administration, HCFA Pub No 88-02171, Washington, DC, 1988, US Department of Health and Human Services; and Childhood-disability definition created, *AAP News* 11(7):4, 1995.

problems to the developmental model to meet the unique needs of the child and family.

A developmental focus also considers family development. The life cycle of the family unit reflects changing ages and needs of family members as well as changing external demands. A family member's serious illness or disability can cause significant stress or crisis at any stage of the family life cycle. Just as with individual development, family development may be interrupted or even regress to an earlier level of functioning. Nurses can use the concept of family development to plan meaningful interventions and evaluate care (see Developmental Theory, Chapter 4).

Family-Centered Care

The importance of family-centered care—a philosophy that considers the family as the constant in the child's life—is especially evident in the care of children with special needs (see also Family-Centered Care, Chapter 1). As parents learn about the youngster's health care needs, they often become experts in delivering care. Health care providers, including nurses, are adjuncts to the child's care and need to form partnerships with parents. Collaboration is essential to forming trusting and effective partnerships. Collaborative relationships are characterized by communication, dialogue, active listening, awareness, and acceptance of differences (Bishop, Woll, and Arango, 1993).

Communicating with Families. Families whose child is ill react along what health care providers may view as a continuum from the "good" to the "difficult" family stereotype. Nurses readily form relationships with the "good" family, who perceives staff as having power or control and accepts this hierarchy (Satariano and Briggs, 1989). However, this is often not the case with the "difficult" family, who is characterized as being underinvolved or overinvolved in the child's care. Dixon (1993; personal communication, 1996) describes four patterns of involvement in parents' relationships with nurses. *Silent in care parents* choose to have limited involvement with the hospitalized child and nursing staff. These parents do not initiate relationships with nurses and are difficult to engage in decision making. *Recipients of care* believe nurses both know what is best for the child and should be in control. Their level of trust in professionals is very high, whereas their level of need for information is low. Parents who are *monitors of care* keep track of the performance of all hospital staff, seek care from nurses, and request detailed information. Finally, *managers of care* are in control of health-related decisions and use nurses for direct care and consultation. They are frequently involved in providing technologically complex care to their chronically ill child.

Nurses should respect families' varying styles of interacting with health care providers and can base strategies for working with families on understanding a family's style (Table 18-1). Care conferences, especially multidisciplinary meetings that include the family and key health professionals, provide an opportunity for joint sharing of ideas and expression of feelings or concerns. Individual discussions, especially with the case manager, primary nurse, or clinical nurse specialist (advanced nurse practitioner), help establish a consistent and flexible plan of care that can prevent conflicts or deal with them before they become major issues. In family-centered

TABLE 18-1. Strategies for facilitating parent-nurse interaction	
PARENT CHARACTERISTICS	**STRATEGIES**
Silent in Care	
Have trust and mistrust	Do not force participation
May not accompany child; prefer to wait outside	Avoid authoritarian stance
Are very uncertain, quiet	Use simple terms and demystify surroundings
Use little verbal communication	Explain what will happen
Visit on limited or irregular basis	Point out how their presence helps child
Recipient of Care	
Have total trust	Offer/provide information; elicit feedback to ensure their understanding
Want nurse to make decisions	
Offer numerous positive comments	Allow unlimited contact with child
Are easily impressed with information	Engage them in gaining child's cooperation
Are prone to misunderstandings	
Comply with rules	
Focus on child while visiting	
Monitor of Care	
Have high levels of mistrust	Believe that you can build trust
Have attitude that "mistakes can happen"	Negotiate, negotiate, negotiate!
Monitor everyone's performance	Be flexible regarding rules
Involved in all decisions	Avoid issues of control
Want high levels of information	Ask their opinion and use their suggestions
Know agency's hierarchy	
Seek care from nurses	
Ask for rule changes	
Manager of Care	
Are similar to monitors, but less angry	Recognize them as experts about their child
Achieve complex coordination of child's chronic care	Recognize need for respite

Developed by Donna M. Dixon, Memorial Medical Center, Springfield, IL, 1993. Used with permission. Modified from Knafl KA, Cavallari KA, Dixon DM: *Pediatric hospitalization: family and nurse perspectives,* Glenview, IL, 1988, Scott, Foresman.

care the goal is to maintain the integrity of the family, empower family members to assume a leadership role, and support the family during stressful times (Baker, 1994).

Issues of culture, ethnicity, and race affect access to services, utilization, and follow-through with referrals and recommendations (Huber, Holditch-Davis, and Brandon, 1993; Newacheck, Stoddard, and McManus, 1993). For some ethnic and minority populations, cultural understandings of illness and disability, the structure of family life, social roles for individuals who are disabled, and other factors related to the perception of children may differ from "mainstream" American culture (Groce and Zola, 1993). These factors may affect family needs and family choices regarding the care of their child with special needs. Nurses play an important role in explaining the health care system to the family. Nurses should also listen to the family's understanding, needs, and concerns and should assist the family in incorporating their cultural preferences and priorities into the plan of care.

Normalization

Another principle that is increasingly employed is that of *normalization*, which refers to establishing a normal pattern of living (see also box on p. 544). By applying the principles of normalization, the environment for the child is "normalized" and "humanized." Normalization principles can be applied to service delivery and patterns of daily care for the child.

Another trend is the earlier discharge of children from acute or chronic care facilities to the family and community. *Home care* represents the return to a system and set of priorities in which family values are as important to the care of a child with a chronic health problem as they are in the care of other children. Home care seeks to achieve goals that are consistent with the developmental model (Stein, 1985):

1. Normalize the life of a child with special needs, including those with technologically complex care, in a family and community context and setting.
2. Minimize the disruptive impact of the child's condition on the family.
3. Foster the child's maximum growth and development.

With appropriate training and support, families provide complex procedures and treatments in the home. Parents are challenged to retain a homelike setting among monitors, ventilators, and other sophisticated equipment. Throughout the text, home care is discussed as appropriate for specific conditions. The process of transition from hospital to home is elaborated in Chapters 20 and 21.

Paralleling normalization and home care is a trend toward *mainstreaming*, or integrating children with special needs into regular classrooms. Just as the home is the natural environment for children, so school must also be included as an essential component of the children's overall physical, intellectual, and social development. Children who attend school have the advantages of learning and socializing with a wide group of peers. There is an increased focus on individualization as the academic needs of these children are planned along with those of the rest of the students. A variety of supplemental programs have been designed in the school system to accommodate special needs, both at school age and younger, through early intervention programs, thus providing these children with an equal educational opportunity. This change and increasing opportunities for normalization for children with special needs in large part have resulted from the passage of Public Law 94-142 (the Education of All Handicapped Children Act of 1975) and its 1990 amendments (Public Law 101-47b), which changed the name of the act to the Individuals with Disabilities Education Act (IDEA); Public Law 99-457 (the Education of the Handicapped Act Amendments of 1986); and the Americans with Disabilities

Act (ADA) of 1990 (see also Chapter 1). Nurses can provide parents with information about these laws* and in some cases may participate in the development of individualized educational programs (IEPs) or individualized family service plans (IFSPs) for children with special needs.†

THE FAMILY OF THE CHILD WITH SPECIAL NEEDS

REACTIONS OF FAMILIES TO A CHRONIC ILLNESS OR DISABILITY

When the diagnosis of a disability or chronic illness is made, the family progresses through a fairly predictable sequence of stages, regardless of the actual nature of the condition. Although a number of "stages" have been described, no one set of phases is universally accepted. Not all families experience this process, and each family member varies widely in the time needed to progress through any of the stages and the need to use earlier stages. The nurse explores family reactions for all possible interpretations, not just negative ones. Too often a parent's angry reaction is attributed to a stage of adjustment or a maladaptive reaction rather than an appropriate response to, for instance, an insulting remark.

Shock and Denial

The initial stage, or impact, is intensely emotional and is characterized by *shock, disbelief,* and sometimes *denial,* especially if the disorder is not obvious, such as in chronic illness. Denial is probably the least understood and most poorly dealt with reaction. Health professionals tend to label denial as "maladaptive" and may actively attempt to remove it by repeated and sometimes blunt explanations of prognosis. However, denial is often an adaptive approach.

Denial is a necessary cushion to prevent disintegration and is a normal response to any type of loss. Probably all family members experience various degrees of adaptive denial as they learn of the impact that the diagnosis has on their lives. Denial becomes maladaptive when it prevents recognition of treatment or rehabilitative goals necessary for the child's optimum survival or development.

Shock and denial can last from days to months, sometimes even longer. Examples of denial that may be exhibited at the time of diagnosis include (1) shopping for physicians, (2) attributing the symptoms of the actual illness to a minor condition, (3) refusing to believe the diagnostic tests, (4) delaying agreement to treatment, (5) acting very happy and optimistic despite the revealed diagnosis, (6) refusing to tell or talk to anyone about the condition, (7) insisting that no one is telling the truth, regardless of others' attempts to do so, (8) denying the reason for admission, and (9) asking no questions about the diagnosis, treatment, or prognosis. Each of

---

*The *NICHCY New Digest,* vol 1, no 1, 1991, was entirely devoted to the topic "The Education of Children and Youth with Special Needs: What do the Laws Say?" (NICHCY, P.O. Box 1492, Washington, DC 20013.)
†The following resource is recommended for developing an IFSP: *Guidelines and Recommended Practices for the Individualized Family Service Plan* by B. Johnson, M. McGonigel, and R. Kaufmann, available from the **Association for the Care of Children's Health,** 7910 Woodmont Ave., Suite 300, Bethesda, MD 20814; (301) 654-6549.

these mechanisms allows individuals to distance themselves from the onslaught of a tremendous emotional impact and to collect and mobilize their energies toward goal-directed, problem-solving behaviors.

In some instances, various indicators of denial can be viewed as adaptive. Searching for another professional opinion may mean that parents cannot obtain answers to their questions or that they are looking for a different approach to treatment that better meets the needs of their child and family. When parents discuss their strengths and the benefits they derive from caring for their child with special needs, it does not necessarily reflect refusal to accept their difficult circumstances. Sometimes delay in making decisions or failure to ask questions simply reflects a lack of information.

Partial denial, such as seeking additional professional consultations or occasionally acting as if nothing were wrong, is common for families with children who have life-threatening conditions. Without such a temporary protective mechanism, few people could survive the constant emotional drain of anticipating their own death or the death of a family member. Partial denial allows the child and family to absorb stressful information, or "dose" themselves, in amounts they can personally manage at the time.

The importance of children's denial has repeatedly been demonstrated as a factor in their positive coping with the diagnosis. Denial allows an individual to maintain hope in the face of overwhelming odds. As with hope, denial may be an adaptive mechanism for dealing with loss that persists until a family or patient is ready for or needs other responses.

Adjustment

Adjustment gradually follows shock and is usually characterized by an open admission that the condition exists. This stage is manifested by several responses, probably the most universal of which are guilt and anger. *Guilt* arises from a human need to find rational causes for events. The concept of cause and effect implies an ability to change future events. It is often greatest when the cause of the disorder is directly traceable to the parent, such as in genetic diseases or from an injury. However, it occurs even without any scientific or realistic basis for parental responsibility. Frequently the guilt stems from a false assumption that the disability is a result of personal failing or wrongdoing, such as drinking alcohol, taking drugs, smoking, not eating correctly, having sex or an affair, or not doing something correctly during pregnancy or the birth. Guilt may also be related to thoughts of wishing the child dead, especially when the demands of care seem overwhelming and unrelenting, and may be associated with religious beliefs, either as a punishment or as a test of faith. Children, too, may interpret their serious illness as retribution for past misbehavior.

> **Nursing ALERT**
>
> Be particularly sensitive to the child who passively accepts all painful procedures. This child may believe that such acts are inflicted as deserved punishment. It is always vital to assure children that what happens to them during diagnosis or treatment is to make them well.

Another common reaction in family members is *anger.* Anger directed inwardly may be evident as self-reproaching

or punitive behavior, such as neglecting one's health and verbally degrading oneself. Anger directed outwardly may be manifest in open arguments or withdrawal from communication and may be evident in the person's relationship with any number of individuals, such as the spouse, the child, and siblings. Passive anger toward the ill child may be evident in decreased visiting, refusal to believe how sick the child is, or inability to provide comfort. One of the most common targets for parental anger is a staff member.

The child who is sick or disabled and the well siblings are also apt to respond with anger. Affected children are aware of the loss engendered by the illness or disability and may react angrily to the imposed restrictions or the feelings of being different. Siblings also feel anger and resentment toward the ill child and parents for the loss of routine and for decreased parental attention. It is difficult for older children and almost impossible for younger children to comprehend the plight of the affected child. Their perception is of a brother or sister who has the undivided attention of their parents, receives cards and gifts, and is the focus of everyone's concern.

A number of other reactions among family members, especially parents, are typical and include:

Lowered self-esteem, in which parents perceive a defect in their child as a defect in themselves; their life goals may be abruptly and dramatically altered, and they lose the fantasy of immortality through their child

Shame, in which family members anticipate social rejection, pity, or ridicule and related loss of social prestige and may experience social withdrawal

Ambivalence, in which the simultaneous experience of love and hatred normally experienced by parents toward their children is likely to be greatly intensified

Depression, in which parents experience chronic feelings of sorrow; for example, to some parents, mental retardation symbolizes the child's death and therefore precipitates a grief reaction.

During the period of adjustment, four types of parental reactions to the child may occur that influence the child's eventual response to the disorder (see box; see also p. 529). The most common initial response, especially among mothers, is *benevolent overreaction.* This is usually a consequence of unresolved guilt or fear, such as ambivalent feelings or not wanting the child during pregnancy, feeling responsible for the disorder, believing that the child would die at the time of birth or diagnosis, or reactivated feelings about a previous death of a loved one. The benevolent overreaction results in a vicious cycle of overprotective, permissive parent and de-

---

PARENTAL RESPONSES THAT INFLUENCE CHILD'S RESPONSE TO THE DISORDER

Overprotection, in which the parents fear letting the child achieve any new skill, avoid all discipline, and cater to the child's every desire so as to prevent frustration

Rejection, in which the parents detach themselves emotionally from the child but usually provide adequate physical care or constantly nag and scold the child

Denial, in which parents act as if the disorder does not exist or attempt to have the child overcompensate for it

Gradual acceptance, in which parents place necessary and realistic restrictions on the child, encourage self-care activities, and promote reasonable physical and social abilities

pendent, demanding child. Early intervention and anticipatory guidance can intervene in this pattern, which otherwise might prevent the child from developing self-control, independence, initiative, and self-esteem.

Reintegration and Acknowledgment

For many families a final stage in adjustment is characterized by realistic expectations for the child and reintegration of family life with the illness or disability in proper perspective. Since a large portion of the adjustment phase is one of grief for a loss, total resolution is not possible until the child dies or leaves home as an independent adult.

This adjustment phase also involves social reintegration, in which the family broadens its activities to include relationships outside of the home, with the child as an acceptable and participating member of the group. This last criterion often differentiates gradual acceptance during the adjustment period from total acceptance or acknowledgment.

Many parents of children with special needs experience *chronic sorrow,* an emotional response that is manifested through the life span of the parent-child interaction (Clubb, 1991). Acceptance is interspersed with periods of intensified sorrow for the loss, especially at certain landmarks of the child's development (e.g., entry into school, onset of puberty), since each new age traditionally brings new expectations and a reminder of what could have been. Situational stress, such as inability to pay the child's medical bills, may also cause grief to resurface. Consequently, even families who have achieved a high level of adjustment and acceptance are, at predictable times (see box), in need of support from professionals or other families who have coped successfully with similar experiences.

IMPACT OF CHILD'S CHRONIC ILLNESS OR DISABILITY ON FAMILY MEMBERS

Parents

Besides grieving for the loss of a perfect child, parents may or may not receive positive feedback from transactions with their child. Many parents feel satisfaction and fulfillment from

the parenting role. For others, parenting may be a series of unrewarding experiences, which contribute to parental feelings of inadequacy and failure. These responses may be most evident in parents who are responsible for the child's care. For example, parents may become preoccupied with their ability to carry out certain procedures, overlooking the child's personal comfort and satisfaction or failing to offer praise for anything less than perfect cooperation or performance. They may pursue a frustrating activity until they achieve "success"—long after the child has become irritable and uncooperative. As a result, parents can become caught in a pattern of interaction that is mutually unrewarding and minimally productive. For these parents, several strategies may be helpful: education regarding what can reasonably be expected of their child, assistance in identifying the child's strengths, praise for a parental job well done, and finding respite care so that parents can renew their energies.

Parental Roles. Excessive demands may be placed on parental time, energy, and financial resources. Depending on the roles assumed by each spouse, these responsibilities may be shared or shifted more heavily to one member. In a shared approach, parents often divide tasks in a very specific way, according to their skills or level of comfort. For example, the parent with patience for waiting may be the logical person to take the child for tests, examinations, and procedures. The parent who deals best with the sickness and side effects of treatment can ready the environment for the child's return home. It is important for nurses to realize that the absence of one parent from the hospital or clinic does not necessarily indicate that the shared parent pattern is not in effect (Clements, Copeland, and Loftus, 1990). On the other hand, making efforts to involve both parents in decision making and in learning how to care for the child's special needs can reduce some of the burden of care often placed on mothers.

In other families, changing sex roles mean added responsibilities for one parent. For example, the working mother may feel the need to continue employment to help defray the expenses, but she also incurs the added burden of additional child/home responsibilities. The result can eventually be marital conflicts as one partner views his or her share as unequal.

In addition, the partner who is not included in the caregiving activities may feel neglected, since all the attention is directed toward the child, and resentful that he or she is not sufficiently informed to be competent in the care. Without active participation in the child's care, the parent has little appreciation of the time and energy involved in performing those activities. When the less prepared partner does attempt to participate, the other parent frequently criticizes the less skillful efforts. As a result, communication and support for each other may be adversely affected.

Although marital stress often increases, divorce rates in these families are not substantially higher than those for the general population. Research suggests that families of children with chronic conditions who adjust poorly are those who had problems before the illness. A couple's marital functioning before the birth or diagnosis of a child with special needs may well be the best predictor of long-term marital adjustment.

The nurse can assist the family in avoiding conflicts by providing anticipatory guidance early on. Guidance can address

---

ANTICIPATED PARENTAL STRESS POINTS

Diagnosis of the condition—requires considerable learning, as well as dealing with emotional response

Developmental milestones—times that children normally achieve walking, talking, and self-care are delayed or impossible for the child

Start of schooling—particularly stressful are situations in which appropriate schooling will not be in a regular class placement

Reaching the ultimate attainment—situations, such as realizing that ambulation will be impossible or that the child will not learn to read, must be handled

Adolescence—issues such as sexuality and independence become prominent

Future placement—decisions about placement must be made when the child becomes an adult or when the parents can no longer care for the child

Death of the child

the stressors often cited as having an impact on the marriage: (1) the home care program with the burden of care assumed by primarily one parent, (2) the financial burden, (3) the fear of the child dying, (4) pressure from relatives, (5) the hereditary nature of the disease (if applicable), and (6) fear of pregnancy. Other causes of tension may center on the inconveniences associated with care, such as long waiting for appointments, lack of parking near care facilities, or lack of overnight accommodations. Certainly, these last stressors are within health professionals' domain to minimize, if not eliminate.

Mother/Father Differences.   Mothers and fathers in the same family often adjust and cope as parents of a child with special needs. Some mothers experience a peaks-and-valleys periodic crisis pattern, whereas most fathers tend to experience a steady, gradual recovery. Some research suggests that mothers of children with certain conditions may be more susceptible to psychologic distress than fathers. Furthermore, mothers are more likely to have to deal with delaying or forfeiting personal goals (Fisman and Wolf, 1991).

The father of a child with special needs struggles with issues that may be quite distinct from those of the mother. He may feel that his role of protector is challenged because he does not know how to help and cannot protect the family from the seemingly overwhelming recurring problems. Dreams of lineage, ego fulfillment, and athletic and vocational achievement are threatened and in turn may threaten the father's self-esteem. Because the traditional paternal role, particularly with sons, emphasizes joint recreation over caregiving, fathers seem to have more difficulty adjusting to a son with special needs than to a daughter with special needs. With today's increased emphasis on fathers' involvement in the lives of their children, this loss is felt more profoundly than in the past. The extensive stresses in the family can leave the father feeling depressed, weak, guilty, powerless, isolated, embarrassed, and very angry. Fearful that he will lose control or be viewed as weak or ineffectual, however, the father will often hide his feelings and display an outward confidence that may lead others to believe that everything is fine. Feelings are further exacerbated by a health care system that frequently excludes and disregards men. Too often the father feels like an afterthought in the care of his child (May, 1990).

Fathers worry about what the future holds for their children, as well as about their ability to manage the increasing financial burden. Some fathers escape in their work as a means for dulling the pain. Others view all the difficulties of having a child with special needs as challenges to overcome and are not afraid to push limits and be assertive to acquire the needed services for their children (May, 1990).

Single-Parent Families.   Single-parent families are of special concern. The absence of a parent may result from divorce or death, or the parents may never have married. As the only parent of a child who may require extensive, sophisticated, and lifelong care, the single parent may feel an enormous burden. Available financial and emotional resources may already be stretched to the limit. Nurses must recognize that external sources of support and personal inner strength are particularly crucial for single parents to enable them to care for their child (Clements, Copeland, and Loftus, 1990). A special effort should be made to assist the single parent in finding financial and support services that can ease the bur-

den of care. Nurses can also assist the single parent in identifying helping roles that may be acceptable to relatives and friends.

Siblings

Results of studies on how siblings are affected by having a brother or sister with special needs are inconsistent. Some confirm that brothers and sisters of children with chronic or disabling conditions are at high risk for maladjustment; others report no significant differences between siblings of children with special needs and siblings of children without chronic or disabling conditions; and still others note the absence of effects (Gallo and others, 1992). However, most investigators do agree that brothers and sisters of children with special needs are no more at risk for *severe* psychiatric problems than are siblings of children without chronic or disabling conditions.

Some difficulties for siblings arise from the demands of the child's condition. For example, at diagnosis the child with special needs by necessity becomes the focus of parental attention and concern. Frequent hospitalizations or trips to the physician or clinic disrupt the family routine. Siblings are pushed to the background, often staying at the homes of family and friends. The child's condition may interfere with holiday celebrations, vacations, and other special events. Siblings may resent these intrusions, which frequently demand self-sacrifice. Their parents may be unable to attend their school functions, ball games, or other activities and at times may be physically and emotionally unavailable for them. The family's financial and emotional resources may be directed toward the child with special needs. When this occurs, there is often not only a decrease in normal family activities, but a decrease in personal items for the other children as well.

Many of the difficulties siblings encounter are a result of the nature of the sibling relationship itself (see Chapter 4). It is within the sibling relationship that children learn to share, compete, and compromise with others close to them in status. The equality of this relationship is often lost when a brother or sister has special needs. The child with special needs is suddenly "out of tune," unable to contribute to the family or the sibling relationship in his or her usual way. Because identification is another characteristic of sibling relationships, some siblings believe that they, too, will "catch" the condition, a reasonable assumption considering experiences with contagious diseases, such as chickenpox. Identification, combined with a young child's egocentric thinking, may lead a sibling to feel responsible for a brother or sister's condition. For example, siblings may believe that playing

 FAMILY FOCUS
Reflection of an Older Brother

My youngest sister Kerry was on an apnea monitor 3 years ago, when I was 15. I was never embarrassed about Kerry being on the monitor, except for the time it went off in church and everyone turned around to look at us.

Joey Bellino
Oldest sibling of an infant on an apnea monitor
Washington, DC

rough with their brother or sister or even thinking bad thoughts about the sibling caused the condition.

Most brothers and sisters experience mixed and sometimes contradictory feelings. They may feel left out of new family developments and changing roles, guilty that they escaped getting the condition, or sad when their brother or sister is unable to participate in a particular activity or event. Some siblings feel embarrassed and ashamed; having a child in the family who is ill, disfigured, or disabled marks the family as "different" (see Family Focus box). Siblings may actually experience a *courtesy stigma*—a spoiled identity because of a close relationship with someone who is devalued and avoided because he or she is different. These painful feelings may lead to isolation and loneliness.

When parents give the child with special needs preferential treatment, siblings may feel resentful and jealous—feelings that are often distorted by their own sense of loss and concern. Older siblings in particular may resent stepping in as surrogate parents for their younger brothers and sisters. Siblings may be angry at parents for being unable to protect their brother or sister from getting the condition or angry at insensitive friends and classmates. Some siblings must also deal with anger from the child with special needs who resents them for escaping the experience.

Some siblings develop adjustment or behavior problems, especially younger male or older female siblings. Younger children having difficulty tend to become withdrawn and irritable, whereas older siblings tend to act out. Some typical problems include bed-wetting, headaches and other physical complaints, changes in school performance, school phobia, sleep problems, proneness to injury, depression, and severe separation anxiety.

Often overlooked is the positive caring between children with special needs and their brothers and sisters. Siblings can experience pride and satisfaction in their own contributions to the family, joy and excitement in their brother or sister's accomplishments, and genuine love. Parents may report an increased closeness among the siblings or an increase in their home responsibilities (Ferrell and others, 1994). Ultimately, most brothers and sisters seem to adapt well, and many demonstrate high levels of self-confidence, independence, maturity, altruism, and tolerance.

Certain factors (e.g., family size, age between children) seem to influence sibling adjustment. However, the most im-

portant factors appear to be parental feelings, perceptions, and reactions. Siblings are more at risk for adjustment problems when parents are unaccepting of the child with special needs. Also, certain times seem to be more difficult for siblings (see box).

How siblings react will have an important impact on the child's overall adjustment. When siblings act in a normal fashion, a secure, stable training ground is provided for social relationships for the child with special needs.

Extended Family Members and Society

Two other groups of people may experience the effects of a child's chronic illness or disability: (1) significant nonnuclear family members or friends and (2) society as a whole. Although extended family relationships are often helpful to parents in rearing a child with special needs, they may also be sources of stress. For example, grandparents or other well-meaning relatives may have more difficulty accepting the diagnosis than the parents themselves do. They may attempt to reassure the parents that the child "will grow out of" his or her slowness at a time when parents are struggling to accept reality.

Most grandparents experience some ambivalence: they love their grandchild and yet feel personal disappointment. They often experience a double grief, both for their grandchild and for their child, the parent. The future is now unpredictable not only for the grandchild, but for the child's parents as well. Grandparents do not often acknowledge these emotions and are left to adapt on their own. Support groups for grandparents, although uncommon, can be beneficial (Burns and Madian, 1992).

Although society's views of individuals with chronic illness or disability are changing toward a more accepting, nonjudgmental, and open attitude, parents, siblings, and the child with special needs frequently are victims of prejudice, ostracism, or criticism. Much of this stems from public ignorance and fear, and this remains a crucial area for intervention by health professionals. Other areas in which society could better meet the needs of families of children with chronic illness or disability include the development of support services such as respite care, financing care, and insurance practices that do not discriminate against individuals with chronic illness.

FACTORS AFFECTING THE FAMILY'S ADJUSTMENT

Although it is easy to assume that families of children with the most severe illnesses or disabilities would have the poorest adjustment, the severity of the condition reflects only one part of the overall picture. The family's ability to adjust to having a child with special needs is influenced by factors such as their available support system, perception of the event, coping mechanisms, reactions to the child, available resources, and concurrent stresses within the family (see Table 18-3).

A family's level of adjustment is significantly influenced by the *functional burden* on the individual family (Stein, 1985). This concept considers the issues related to caring for and living with the child in relation to the family's resources and ability to cope. Thus the family of a child with multiple disabilities demanding complex care—yet having many re-

---

ANTICIPATED SIBLING STRESS POINTS

Birth of another child—may be the sibling with special needs or the subsequent birth of another child

Diagnosis of condition—in certain illnesses, times of remission and exacerbations are difficult

When the child is hospitalized—parental time and attention are focused on the child with special needs

Start of schooling—particularly stressful if friends reject the child with special needs

Adolescence—when dating begins, may be embarrassed to bring dates home

Future placement—may worry about responsibility for the sibling with special needs, especially if the parents are ill or die

Death of the child

sources and coping skills—may adjust more successfully to their situation than the family of a child with a less serious condition and few resources to counter the balance.

The significant others who are available to individuals for emotional strength during periods of crisis comprise their *support system.* Support systems may be available through a variety of relationships and may consist of one significant other, such as a spouse, or a group of significant others, such as the extended family or the health team.

The source of support is a determining factor in the effectiveness of certain forms of support. For example, *expressive support* is best provided by individuals with whom one has strong ties and who are similar to oneself. On the other hand, *instrumental support* can often be provided by those to whom the family has weaker ties and who can link the family to a broader, more diverse social network. Therefore the most appropriate sources of informational support might include both professionals who have theoretic and practical knowledge and nonprofessionals—parents—whose experience equips them as experts. Parent-to-parent support is unique and unobtainable from any other source.* When professionals develop a strong therapeutic relationship with the family, they, too, can be appropriate sources of emotional support (see discussion on therapeutic relationships in Chapter 1).

Although a support system exists, it may not be effective unless the individual is able to use the system through mutual channels of communication. Providing parents with written information they can share with extended family can often help them in reaching out to others during a difficult time.

When necessary, nurses can assist family members to recognize their strengths and employ their adaptive *coping mechanisms,* which may include information seeking, utilizing social support networks, drawing on personal strengths, or relying on their faith life, in adjusting to and managing chronic illness, disability, or life-threatening illness in a child. At times nurses can assist family members in developing new coping mechanisms.

REACTIONS OF FAMILIES TO CHILDHOOD DEATH: THE GRIEF PROCESS

No event is more devastating for families than the threatened or actual loss of a child. Families, especially parents, are deprived of the joy and fulfillment of watching a child grow. All family members are affected by the loss, and their needs must be recognized to resolve their grief. Nurses require a basic understanding of the grief process before (if the death is anticipated), at the time of, and after the death to provide guidance and emotional support to the survivors.

---

*The *Parent Resource Directory* lists more than 400 parents of children with chronic illness or disabilities in the United States and Canada, including addresses, phone numbers, the child's condition, and the health facility where the child receives care. It is available from the **Association for the Care of Children's Health,** 7910 Woodmont Ave., Suite 300, Bethesda, MD 20814; (301) 654-6549. Information about self-help groups and books and pamphlets are available from the **National Self-Help Clearinghouse,** CUNY Graduate Center, 25 W. 43rd St., New York, NY 10036; (212) 642-2944.

In response to any loss there is a grief reaction. Anticipatory grief may precede an anticipated death. *Acute grief* develops within hours to days after a death and is characterized by somatic symptoms and intense subjective distress. *Grief work,* or *mourning,* refers to the lengthy process that begins with acute grief and extends into a period of reorganization of psychologic life, with attachment to new people and interests. *Bereavement* often refers to the period of mourning, although grief, mourning, and bereavement are used interchangeably.

In expected death the child and family are generally involved in the plan for intervention both before and after the death. In unexpected death the survivors face the tremendous task of integrating the loss into their lives, with no opportunity for anticipatory grief. In either situation nurses can facilitate the grief process by being aware of expected psychologic and somatic reactions and by dialoguing with family members, ascertaining their needs, and supporting their efforts to cope, adapt, and grieve. The application of principles of family-centered care is as important at this time as any other.

Anticipatory Grief

When death is the expected or possible outcome of a disorder, the child and family members experience behavioral reactions of anticipatory grief. Anticipatory grief may be manifest in varying behaviors and intensities and may include denial, anger, depression, and other psychologic and somatic symptoms. The "stages" of dying described by Kübler-Ross (1969) are not included here because they were not based on work with children. The importance of the work of Kübler-Ross to the care of children and families lies in its emphasis on recognizing the dying person as being alive and dying itself as a process in which the dying person is engaged. Care providers are most effective when actively engaging those coping with death and empowering them to address their remaining needs (Corr, 1993).

Acute Grief

When death occurs, whether it is expected or unexpected, acute grief develops within hours to days. Acute grief is a definite syndrome with psychologic and somatic symptoms that cause intense distress (see box). Reactions such as hearing the dead person's voice, feeling distant from others who want to help, or feeling overwhelming guilt for failing to prevent the death may make grieving persons fear that they are approaching a mental breakdown. On the contrary, these symptoms are normal, necessary, and expected responses. They signify that survivors are working through the acute grief and will probably satisfactorily resolve the loss and resume or restructure a meaningful role in their social environment.

Although grief symptoms should appear immediately after a crisis, they may be delayed, exaggerated, or apparently absent. In the place of normal grief responses, *distorted reactions,* such as excessive hostility, depression with signs of suicide, or overactivity without a sense of loss, may occur. Such distorted reactions can be transformed into normal grief with appropriate intervention, such as by a grief counselor. Nurses working with grieving families should be aware of the symptomatology of normal grief (see box) to recognize the rare occurrence of morbid grief reactions.

CHARACTERISTICS OF NORMAL GRIEF REACTION

Sensations of Somatic Distress

Feeling of tightness in the throat
Choking, with shortness of breath
Marked tendency toward sighing
Empty feeling in abdomen
Lack of muscular power
Intense subjective distress described as tension or mental pain

Preoccupation with Image of the Deceased

Hears, sees, or imagines that the dead person is present
Slight sense of unreality
Feeling of emotional distance from others
Feeling of approaching a mental breakdown

Feelings of Guilt

Searches for evidence of failure in preventing the death
Accuses self of negligence or exaggerates minor omissions

Feelings of Hostility

Loss of warmth toward others
Tendency toward irritability and anger
Does not want to be bothered by friends or relatives

Loss of Usual Pattern of Conduct

Restlessness, inability to sit still, aimless moving about
Continual searching for something to do or thinking about
    what should be done
Lack of capacity to initiate and maintain organized patterns of
    activity

Modified from the landmark publication by Lindemann E: Symptomatology and management of acute grief, *Am J Psychiatry* 101:141-143, 1944.

Mourning

After the death the lengthy process of grief work or mourning begins and extends into a period of adjustment to the loss, with attachment to new people and the development of new interests. Contrary to the common belief that mourning is completed in a year, research indicates that resolution of grief may take years and that there may be an *intensification* of grief during the early years.

Shock and Disbelief.   Shock, numbness, and disbelief are seen during the immediate phase of grief. As one parent described, "We were as prepared for our son's death as anyone could be, but it was a shock when in a moment his life was finished. I just can't get over the rapidity with which life ends." This temporary numbness protects the survivors from the overwhelming pain associated with grief. Often decisions are made automatically and only certain details are remembered.

Expression of Grief.   When the numbness fades, a period of intense grief begins and is characterized by a yearning and loneliness for the deceased. During this stage many of the signs of acute grief are evident, and physical complaints such as inability to sleep and appetite changes are common. There is a tendency to review the events of the deceased's life and to evaluate the relationship with the loved one. At this time feelings of guilt and anger are common.

Disorganization and Despair.   During this stage the pain of the loss is replaced primarily by emptiness, apathy, and deep depression. There is a feeling that life has no meaning and that the pain will never end. This is particularly relevant for parents. For example, mothers often comment that they feel they have suffered a double loss—loss of their child and loss of the mothering role. Feelings of estrangement from other loved ones are common, and social isolation may foster the depression.

Reorganization.   Reorganization refers to recovery from the loss. During this very gradual process the survivors again find meaning in living, readjust to life without the deceased, develop new or renewed relationships, and learn to live with the memory of the deceased with much less pain. It never means that the loved one is forgotten and the pain is gone. There always remains a deep ache that is never totally replaced with happiness and one that returns more intensely, for example, on holidays or anniversaries (see Postdeath, p. 559).

THE CHILD WITH SPECIAL NEEDS

IMPACT OF CHRONIC ILLNESS OR DISABILITY ON THE CHILD

The child's reaction to chronic illness or disability depends to a great extent on his or her developmental level, temperament, and available coping mechanisms; on the reactions of family members or significant others; and to a lesser extent on the condition itself. A child's conceptual understanding of his or her own illness is based not only on age and developmental level but also on the duration and type of experience accumulated with the disease (Yoos, 1994). Knowledge of these variables is essential in providing the kind of information and support needed by these children to cope with a sometimes overwhelming situation.

Developmental Aspects

The impact of a chronic illness or disability is influenced by the age at onset. Chronic illness affects children of all ages, but the developmental aspects of each age-group dictate particular stresses and risks for the child. The nurse must also recognize that children need to redefine their condition and its implications as they develop and grow. Children's developmental concepts of illness are discussed in Chapter 21. An understanding of these developmental factors facilitates planning care to support the child and minimize the risks.

Infancy.   During infancy the child is engaged in the task of developing trust, which necessitates a reciprocal satisfying relationship between child and parent. When illness or disability occurs, this relationship is potentially affected. For example, a visible defect can retard parent bonding as the parent mourns the loss of the perfect child. In addition, prolonged illness may impose separations that prevent the child and parent from normal attachment and deprive the infant of the nurturing relationship.

The illness itself affects the infant, especially since sensorimotor experiences are critical at this age. Illness and/or disability often impairs the child's motor abilities by confining the child to a crib and lessening contact with the environment. The messages transmitted to infants about their bodies are influenced by the amount of pain and discomfort they experience. Associating touch with pain can compromise the infant's ability to give and receive affection. Lack of pleasurable sensations can lead to an irritable and unhappy child. Consequently, parents may interpret the behaviors as evidence that they are not adequately meeting the child's physical and emotional needs, which further affects the parent-child relationship and the acquisition of trust. Nursing intervention can be important in helping parents work with the irritable child in a way that encourages understanding and caring.

Nurses should advocate for policies and practices that will best meet the needs of the infant and family. Twenty-four-hour visitation in the neonatal intensive care unit and other infant units is of primary importance. Showing parents how to touch and hold the infant will promote their confidence and competence. "Kangaroo care" has been shown to be both safe and beneficial to the infant. Mothers who choose to breast-feed can be encouraged, with a private space provided for them to nurse or pump and storage facilities made available for breast milk. Sibling visitation can be facilitated.

Toddler. The toddler is in the stage of autonomy; the need for mastery of locomotor and language skills is paramount. The child learning to walk and talk progresses toward becoming a separate person, both physically and psychologically. However, illness or disability can hinder mobility and deprive the child of mastery. In addition, overprotective parents can magnify the problem by setting limits on the child's exploration and experimentation for fear of injury or exertion. Even the most basic self-help skills, such as feeding and dressing, may be done for the child. Age-appropriate tasks such as toilet training may be delayed. With such limited opportunities for testing mastery, children soon fear to venture on their own and develop little confidence in their abilities. Over time they may feel defeated and become apathetic, passive, and clinging.

Illness can impose separations that are detrimental to the toddler. As with the infant, separation is the most anxiety-producing event. A chronic illness or disability can necessitate repeated hospitalizations and painful procedures. If the need to preserve the parent-child relationship is not appreciated, the child may become depressed and eventually detach from the parent. Children seem to have a tremendous capacity to withstand stress, provided their attachment to the parent is preserved.

Preschooler. The preschooler is in the stage of initiative; numerous tasks are achieved during this age that can be severely hampered by chronic illness and disability. Impairment can limit the preschooler's learning about the environment, especially in terms of social development. Rather than being encouraged to play with peers and participate in nursery school activities, the preschooler may be confined to the home, where socialization is limited to the secure and tolerant family. Immature behavior may be tolerated because age-appropriate standards and discipline are not enforced. Consequently, when paired with children the same age or placed in school, the child may not know how to act and can easily be criticized by peers and viewed as a "baby." The illness or disability may provoke much less criticism than his or her inappropriate behavior. Faced with such reactions from others, in contrast to the security of the home, the child may gradually choose a life of social isolation and loneliness, especially during the school-age years.

One of the major tasks of this period is establishing sexual identity, and one of the principal methods is through imitation of sex-related activities. However, the sick child may have fewer opportunities to engage in such activity and may view the parent predominantly in the caregiving role, since this may be the focus of their relationship. Some families expect the mother to assume the care of the child while the father provides the financial base by working outside the home. This can limit the child's identification with the male role.

In addition to sexual identity, the child's body image is forming. Children's knowledge of their bodies is limited to what they see, feel, and use. If the child is chronically ill, body awareness is focused on the personal pain and anxiety it causes. The young child may lose control over newly acquired bowel and bladder function and feel embarrassed and inferior. The child with a disability may have difficulty forming a mental image of impaired body parts, such as paralyzed extremities. This poorly developed sense of body integrity makes children especially fearful of intrusive or mutilating experiences, which can be frequent during prolonged illness.

One of the more critical influences of chronic illness or disability on preschoolers is the feeling of guilt that they "caused" the condition by a real or imagined misdeed. This is probably less a factor if the child is born with the disorder than if it occurs during the preschool years. Such guilt can greatly affect the child's developing but fragile self-esteem. Unlike the child with a temporary physical impairment who has additional opportunities for achieving mastery and thus overcoming feelings of guilt and inferiority, the child with a chronic illness or disability experiences continual insults. Unless situations are structured for success, life can become a series of failures—of never being strong enough or good enough to compete with peers.

School-Age Child. The child of school age is striving to achieve a sense of accomplishment while overcoming a sense of inferiority. Successful mastery of this task depends on the child's ability to cooperate and compete with others. Consequently, physical impairments can greatly affect the ability to achieve and compete. For example, physical disability may hinder participation in sports, and repeated absences from school caused by illness can place the child at an academic disadvantage. To repeat a grade can saddle the child with feelings of shame, inadequacy, and inferiority. However, the decision to remain in the same grade can also enhance feelings of success because the work requirements may be easier and new classmates provide a second chance for forming friendships.

During this age there is a transition from relationships with family members to strong identification with peers. Peers increasingly influence school-age children's views of themselves and their self-esteem. Anything that labels children as "different" can affect their sense of belonging to the group. Many children cope with their "differentness" by retreating from socialization. As they withdraw farther from the group, their sense of belonging diminishes and intense loneliness and isolation dominate. However, if they are helped to deal with their feelings of being different and to recognize their unique abilities, these children can cope very well. Nurses can help families promote social competence in their children by addressing feelings of inadequacy and assisting children to recognize their unique abilities (Breitmayer and others, 1992). Specific training in social skills may be useful (Hills and Lutkenoff, 1993; Turner-Henson and others, 1994). Naturally, all children will be unable to master some tasks and will feel some degree of inferiority. If this is stressed to children with physical impairment, the burden to achieve is lessened.

As school-age children identify more with the peer group and authority figures outside the home, there is a concurrent striving for independence from the family. However, the ill child may be forced into an extended period of dependency either from the disorder or from parental overprotectiveness. Attempts to demonstrate independence may be manifested as resentment toward the parents, refusal to comply with treatment, or risk-taking behavior, such as cheating on the special diet. If parents can understand that these behaviors represent a normal phase of development, they may be more tolerant and able to find appropriate outlets for independence (e.g., increasing the child's responsibility for home care or increasing the child's control in non-disease-related activities).

Adolescence.   The impact of illness or disability can be most detrimental during adolescence. The major task of the adolescent is to establish a personal identity. Pubertal changes must be integrated into the self-image while the teenager is gaining control and mastery over increased physical capabilities and sexuality. During early adolescence this takes place primarily within the peer group. Illness or injury at this time interferes with teenagers' sense of mastery and control over a changing body. They are different at a stage of development when being different is unacceptable to the peer group, who may view a disability in one member as a threat to the established uniformity by which all are measured. At no time of life is an individual so vulnerable to the emotional stress of biologic impairment. In fact, adolescents with physical differences tend to blame most of their problems on the fact that they have something wrong with them. Appearance, skills, and abilities are highly valued by peers (Fig. 18-1); a teenager who is limited in any of these qualities is subject to rejection. This is especially marked when a physical disability interferes with sexual attractiveness.

Teenagers with special needs are faced with the task of incorporating their disabilities into the changing self-concept. The youngster who develops the illness or acquires the disability during the crucial adolescent years has more difficulty

accomplishing this task than has the teenager who has been affected since childhood. It appears that the earlier the onset of a limiting condition, the better the individual is able to adapt to it. The youngster with a newly acquired disorder will have the additional task of grieving for a lost "perfection" while adjusting to the changes taking place as a natural course of events. He or she often feels rejected because of personal appearance or an inability to engage in activities expected of a healthy adolescent. The threat is greatest during middle adolescence, when the teenager has less available energy to cope with illness, since emotional resources are being used to meet the normal demands of this developmental phase.

Adolescence is a time for achieving independence from the family and planning for future goals and responsibilities. Adolescents with long-term chronic illness may be less future directed and less independent than well peers. Enforced dependency caused by physical impairment can exacerbate the parent-child conflicts surrounding independence. Lack of understanding from both parties can result in bitter feelings and intrafamilial turmoil. The tendency toward rebellion may be directed at the disorder and reflected in decreased compliance with treatment, denial of the disorder to preserve a sense of normalcy with peers, and risk-taking behavior that can place the teenager in jeopardy, such as driving a car despite a disorder that increases the chance of an injury. Such behaviors can further strain an already tense parent-child relationship. On the other hand, parents can promote independence by giving the adolescent a greater role in his or her own treatment regimen, encouraging the adolescent to develop a relationship with the health care team that is not mediated by parents, and promoting normalization principles.

Coping Mechanisms

Children's innate and learned coping mechanisms are very important in their ability to deal with their disorder. Individual characteristics and the social support afforded the child are critically important influences on the child's ability to cope with stress. The better the family copes, the better the child is able to deal with the stressors imposed by the illness or disability. Individual characteristics associated with positive coping are female sex, early infancy and older than 4 years, active or easy temperament, high self-esteem, above-average intelligence, and strong social skills (Garmezy, 1991).

Children with chronic conditions tend to use five distinct patterns of coping (see box on p. 536). Children with more positive and accepting attitudes about their chronic illness use a more adaptive coping style characterized by optimism, competence, and compliance. They show fewer behavior problems at home and at school. The two maladaptive coping patterns—"Feels different and withdraws" and "Is irritable, moody and acts out"—are associated with poorer adaptation; children using these strategies have poorer self-concepts, more negative attitudes about their conditions, and more behavior problems at home and at school (Austin, Patterson, and Huberty, 1991).

Well-adapted children gradually learn to accept their physical limitations but find achievement in a variety of compensatory motor and intellectual pursuits. They function well at home, at school, and with peers. They have an understanding of their disorder that allows them to accept their limitations, assume responsibility for care, and assist in treatment and rehabilitation regimens. They express appropriate emo-

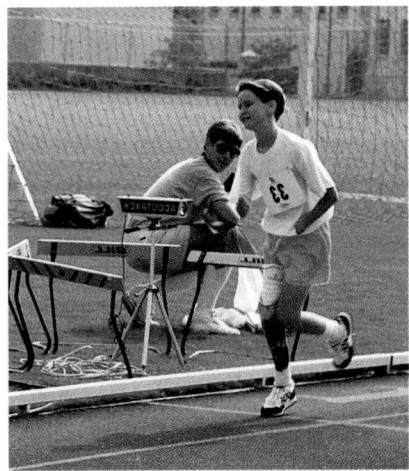

FIG. 18-1. Children with any type of impairment should have the opportunity to develop their skills. (Courtesy Poyo/Hinton Photography.)

COPING PATTERNS USED BY CHILDREN WITH SPECIAL NEEDS

Develops competence and optimism. Accentuates the positive aspects of the situation and concentrates more on what has or can do rather than on what is missing or cannot do; is as independent as possible.

Feels different and withdraws. Sees self as being different from other children because of the chronic health condition; views being different as negative; sees self as less worthy than others; focuses on things cannot do, and sometimes over-restricts activities needlessly.

Is irritable, moody, and acts out. Uses proactive and self-initiated coping behaviors, although usually counterproductive in that the behaviors are not ego enhancing or socially responsible and do not result in desired outcomes; acts out irritability, which may or may not be associated with condition's symptoms.

Complies with treatment. Takes necessary medications, treatments; adheres to activity restrictions; also uses behaviors that indicate developing independence (e.g., assumes responsibility for taking medication).

Seeks support. Talks with adults, children, physicians, and nurses; develops plans to handle problems as they occur; uses downward comparison (i.e., realizes that others have it worse).

Modified from Austin J, Patterson J, Huberty T: Development of the Coping Health Inventory for Children, *J Pediatr Nurs* 6(3):166-174, 1991.

---

tions, such as sadness, anxiety, and anger, at times of exacerbations but confidence and guarded optimism during periods of clinical stability (Fig. 18-2). They are able to identify with other similarly affected individuals, promoting positive self-images and displaying pride and self-confidence in their ability to master a productive, successful life despite the disability.

Responses to Parental Behavior

The parents' behavior toward the child, especially in terms of childrearing, is one of the most important influencing factors in the child's adjustment. For example, children whose parents are overprotective tend to have marked dependency (especially on the mother), fearfulness, inactivity, and lack of outside interests. Children who are raised by overly solicitous and guilt-ridden parents are often overly independent, defiant, and risk takers. Children who are reared by parents who emphasize their deficits and tend to "hide" or isolate them appear as shy and lonely individuals who harbor resentful and hostile attitudes toward unaffected persons. In contrast, children who are reared by parents who establish reasonable limits tend to develop age-appropriate independence and achievement commensurate with their limitations. In addition, family organization and illness-related support and involvement of parents influence the child's adjustment to chronic illness (Savinetti-Rose, 1994). They often display pride and confidence in their ability to cope successfully with the challenges imposed by their disorder. Anticipatory guidance by the nurse and encouragement of normalizing practices may assist parents in facilitating positive adjustment in their children.

Type of Illness or Disability

The type of illness or disability also influences the child's emotional response. Interestingly, children with *more severe* disorders often cope better than those with milder conditions. However, the presence of multiple conditions may place a child at risk for more behavioral problems (Newacheck, McManus, and Fox, 1991). Considering children's cognitive ability and their delay in achieving abstract thinking until adolescence, it is likely that an obvious condition is easier to accept because its limitations are concrete. For example, children who are blind or crippled are constantly reminded of their inability to run. However, children with cardiac defects not only live by rules they do not understand, but also only vaguely and occasionally sense their illness, such as when they try to run and experience dyspnea and fatigue. Therefore some chronic illnesses pose special threats to children.

The onset of a disabling condition may generate a state of confusion for children, who may have trouble differentiating between actual body functions and their image of their bodies. They may also experience problems in identifying themselves and those extensions of self (e.g., wheelchairs, braces, crutches, or other mechanical or prosthetic devices) and may have difficulty in accepting functional aids.

IMPACT OF IMPENDING DEATH ON THE CHILD

Children with life-threatening conditions must face the possibility of death, a realization that can have a profound effect

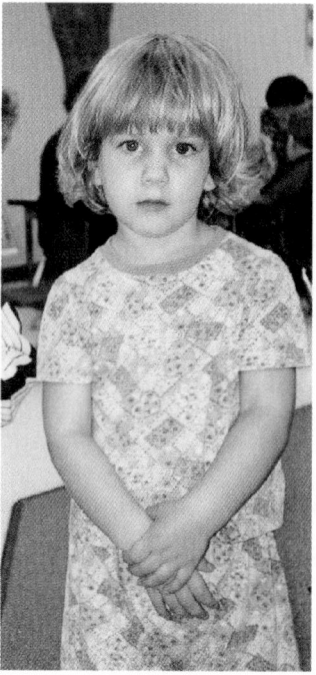

FIG. 18-2. Periods of sadness and anger are appropriate in the child's adjustment to a chronic illness or disability, especially during exacerbations of the disorder.

on their lives. However, the impact of impending death is greatly influenced by a number of factors, including the child's developmental age, the child's experience with the diagnosis, and the role and reaction of the child's parents.

Developmental Concepts of Death

Children's understanding of death parallels their cognitive and psychosocial development. Exactly how preverbal children view death is a mystery, because there is no way of reliably assessing their views of death. It is quite likely, on the basis of their cognitive abilities, that they have no concept of death. Toddler's egocentricity and vague separation of fact and fantasy make it impossible for them to comprehend absence of life.

Children between 3 and 5 years of age usually have heard the word *death,* and they have some idea of its meaning. They see death as a departure, possibly as a kind of sleep. They may recognize the fact of physical death, but they do not see that it involves the loss of the abilities a person has in life. The dead person in the coffin still breathes, eats, and sleeps. Death is temporary and gradual; life and death can change places with one another. Because of their immature concept of time, they have no real understanding of the universality and inevitability of death. Words such as *forever* and *everyone* have meaning only in the child's egocentric thinking.

Much of what pertains to the preschool period regarding the understanding of death also relates to school-age children, particularly those near 6 or 7 years of age. However, these children have a deeper understanding of death in the concrete sense. They may attempt to ascribe a more comprehensible meaning to the event by personifying death as a devil, God, a ghost, or a bogeyman. As some of these names imply, children attach a destructive connotation to death that is often associated with fear of mutilation and punishment. Naturalistic and physiologic explanations of death, such as "When you die, your body decays in the ground," are also common.

By 9 or 10 years of age most children have an adult concept of death. They realize that it is inevitable, universal, and irreversible. Their attitudes toward death are greatly influenced by the reactions and attitudes of others, particularly their parents.

Table 18-2 summarizes children's concepts of and reactions to death and outlines supportive interventions for each developmental stage.

Influence of Experience

Although children's concept of death is limited by their cognitive abilities, children develop an appreciation for what is happening to them through their experience with life-threatening illness. As these children acquire information about their situation, they develop different conceptions of themselves, a process that occurs in five stages (Bluebond-Langner, 1989):

Stage 1. Disease is a serious illness. New identity of "sick" child.
Stage 2. Discovery of the relationship of medication and recovery. Learns the taboos of disease and death.
Stage 3. Marked by an understanding of the purposes and implications of special procedures. Sense of well-being begins to fade, and perceives self as different from other children.
Stage 4. Illness is viewed as a permanent condition. Sense of always being sick and never getting better.

Stage 5. Realization that there is only a finite number of medications. Awareness (directly or indirectly) of the fatal prognosis.

The time lapse between stages tends to be the same for all children regardless of age. Passage from the first stage to the second stage occurs rapidly on relapse. Passage through the second, third, and fourth stages takes somewhat longer, but passage to the fifth stage may take place as soon as the child learns of the death of another, and all knowledge from previous stages is quickly synthesized into a new self-awareness. Since experience, not age or intellectual ability, is the critical factor in passing through these stages, young children who have undergone treatment for several months may know more about their prognosis than adolescents whose disease is newly diagnosed.

NURSING CARE OF THE FAMILY AND CHILD WITH SPECIAL NEEDS

❖ Assessment

Since the nurse may meet a family during any phase of the adjustment process, several assessment areas are important. Knowledge of the family's available support system is essential and may include the marital relationship, nonmarital partners, extended family, colleagues and co-workers, friends, and professionals. The family's perception of the illness or disability is also an area that influences family adjustment. Assessment questions should focus on members' general knowledge of the condition even before the child's diagnosis was made, the influence of religion on their thinking, imagined causes of the condition, and the effects of the child's disorder on the family.

Since the family's ability to cope with previous stresses influences the current situation, answers to questions about their usual coping skills are enlightening. Knowledge of concurrent stresses, such as financial, marital or nonmarital, career, or unemployment, helps identify families who may have fewer resources to cope with the child's needs.

Nursing ALERT Be aware that many families do not have a telephone, a service most practitioners consider essential for families of children with special needs. Other families may have telephones but are reluctant to reveal the telephone number. To overcome these difficulties, use the following strategies:

Help family identify telephone access close to home (e.g., neighbor's home, nearby store).

Explore methods to obtain telephone service for the family (e.g., social service agencies, charitable organizations).

Be sensitive to family's concern for privacy when asking for a telephone number; explain reason for needing number and to whom it will be given.

Finally, awareness of the family members' reactions to the child and the illness or disability is important. Sample questions that the nurse and family can use to evaluate the support system, perception of the illness, coping mechanisms, resources, and concurrent stresses are listed in Table 18-3. Because factors affecting the family's response may change at

TABLE 18-2. Children's understanding of and reactions to death

CONCEPTS OF DEATH	REACTIONS TO DEATH	INTERVENTIONS
Infants and Toddlers Death has least significance to children under 6 months After parent-child attachment and the development of trust is established, the loss, even temporary, of the significant person is profound Prolonged separation during the first several years is thought to be more significant in terms of future physical, social, and emotional growth than at any subsequent age Toddlers are egocentric and can only think about events in terms of their own frame of reference—living Their egocentricity and vague separation of fact and fantasy make it impossible for them to comprehend absence of life Instead of understanding death, this age-group is affected more by any change in life-style	With the death of someone else, they may continue to act as though the person is alive As children grow older, they will be increasingly able and willing to let go of the dead person Ritualism is important; a change in life-style could be anxiety producing This age-group reacts more to the pain and discomfort of a serious illness than to the probable fatal prognosis This age-group also reacts to parental anxiety and sadness	Help parents deal with their feelings, allowing them more emotional reserve to meet the needs of their children Encourage parents to remain as near to child as possible, yet be sensitive to parents' needs Maintain as normal an environment as possible to retain ritualism If a parent has died, encourage having consistent caregiver for child Promote primary nursing
Preschool Children Believe their thoughts are sufficient to cause death; the consequence is the burden of guilt, shame, and punishment Their egocentricity implies a tremendous sense of self-power and omnipotence Usually have some connotation of its meaning Seen as a departure, a kind of sleep May recognize the fact of physical death but do not separate it from living abilities Seen as temporary and gradual; life and death can change places with one another No understanding of the universality and inevitability of death	If they become seriously ill, they conceive of the illness as a punishment for their thoughts or actions May feel guilty and responsible for the death of a sibling Greatest fear concerning death is separation from parents May engage in activities that seem strange or abnormal to adults Because of their fewer defense mechanisms to deal with loss, young children may react to a less significant loss with more outward grief than to the loss of a very significant person The loss is so deep, painful, and threatening that the child must deny it for the present in order to survive its overwhelming impact Behavior reactions such as giggling, joking, attracting attention, or regressing to earlier developmental skills indicate children's need to distance themselves from tremendous loss	Help parents deal with their feelings, allowing them more emotional reserve to meet the needs of their children Help parents to understand behavioral reactions of their children Encourage parents to remain near the child as much as possible, to minimize the child's great fear of separation from parents If a parent has died, encourage having a consistent caregiver for child Promote primary nursing
School-Age Children Still associate misdeeds or bad thoughts with causing death and feel intense guilt and responsibility for the event Because of their higher cognitive abilities, they respond well to logical explanations and comprehend the figurative meaning of words Have a deeper understanding of death in a concrete sense Particularly fear the mutilation and punishment they associate with death Personify death as devil, monster, or bogeyman May have naturalistic/physiologic explanations of death	Because of their increased ability to comprehend, they may have more fears, for example: The reason for the illness Communicability of the disease to themselves or others Consequences of the disease The process of dying and death itself Their fear of the unknown is greater than the known The realization of impending death is a tremendous threat to their sense of security and ego strength Likely to exhibit fear through verbal uncooperativeness rather than actual physical aggression	Help parents deal with their feelings, allowing them more emotional reserve to meet the needs of their children Encourage parents to remain near child as much as possible, yet be sensitive to parents' needs Because of children's fear of the unknown, anticipatory preparation is very important Since the developmental task of this age is industry, helping children maintain control over their bodies and increasing their understanding allow them to achieve independence, self-worth, and self-esteem and avoid a sense of inferiority

TABLE 18-2. Children's understanding of and reactions to death—cont'd		
CONCEPTS OF DEATH	REACTIONS TO DEATH	INTERVENTIONS
School-Age Children—cont'd By 9 or 10, children have an adult concept of death, realizing that it is inevitable, universal, and irreversible	Very interested in postdeath services May be inquisitive about what happens to the body	Encourage children to talk about their feelings and provide aggressive outlets Encourage parents to honestly answer questions about dying rather than avoiding or fabricating euphemisms Encourage parents to share their moments of sorrow with their children Provide preparation for postdeath services
Adolescents Have a mature understanding of death Still very much influenced by "remnants" of magical thinking and are subject to guilt and shame Likely to see deviations from accepted behavior as reasons for their illness	Straddle transition from childhood to adulthood Have the most difficulty in coping with death Least likely to accept cessation of life, particularly if it is their own Concern is for the present much more than for the past or the future May consider themselves alienated from their peers and unable to communicate with their parents for emotional support, feeling alone in their struggle Adolescents' orientation to the present compels them to worry about physical changes even more than the prognosis Because of their idealistic view of the world, they may criticize funeral rites as barbaric, money making, and unnecessary	Help parents deal with their feelings, allowing them more emotional reserve to meet the needs of their children Avoid alliances with either parent or child Structure hospital admission to allow for maximum self-control and independence Answer adolescents' questions honestly, treating them as mature individuals and respecting their needs for privacy, solitude, and personal expressions of emotions Help parents understand their child's reactions to death/dying, especially that concern for present crises, such as loss of hair, may be much greater than for future ones, including possible death

any point during the illness, assessment must be a continuous process.

Special challenges exist in assessing the child's feelings about having a disability. Chapter 6 presents several approaches to encourage a child to discuss feelings about the condition. The nurse should use a variety of communication techniques, such as drawing and play, as assessment tools rather than rely solely on parental reports. Often children are neglected partners in their care, and their unique needs are not identified.

The needs of working parents and siblings also should be assessed, a goal that requires flexibility in scheduling appointments to include these important family members. When working parents know that their input is valuable, they will often change their work schedule to meet with a health professional. Since siblings can be of any age, the use of appropriate communication strategies for assessment must be considered. Nonverbal techniques such as those discussed in Chapter 6 should be considered for these children. Several instruments can be used to assist the family in assessing their overall functioning and support system (see Chapter 6).

❖ Nursing Diagnoses

A number of nursing diagnoses are prominent in the nursing care of the family and child with special needs. Others specific to individual cases become evident, especially when the child's actual disorder is considered. The most common nursing diagnoses are outlined in the Nursing Care Plan on pp. 551-555.

❖ Planning

The nursing plan depends to a large extent on the child's actual illness or disability. However, the following are basic goals for all families and children with special needs:

1. Child and family receive support at time of diagnosis.
2. Family's emotional reactions are accepted.
3. Child and family cope with stresses of situation.
4. Child and family receive appropriate information about the condition.
5. Family establishes an environment of normalization for the child.

FAMILY FOCUS
Identifying Family Needs

To ensure an effective plan of care, attention to *family-identified needs and priorities* is essential. For example, a family may have difficulty focusing on treatment issues if their current priority is obtaining enough food to feed their children.

TABLE 18-3. Assessment of factors affecting family adjustment

FACTORS AFFECTING ADJUSTMENT	ASSESSMENT QUESTIONS
Available Support System	
Status of marital relationship	Whom do you talk to when you have something on your mind? (If answer is not the spouse, ask for the reason.)
Alternate support systems	When something is worrying you, what do you do?
	What helps you most when you are upset?
Ability to communicate	Does talking seem to help when you feel upset?
Perception of the Illness/Disability	
Previous knowledge of disorder	Have you ever heard the word (name of diagnosis) before? Tell me about it (if answer is yes).
Influence of religion	Has your religion or faith been of help to you? Tell me how (if answer is yes).
Imagined cause of disorder	What are your thoughts about the causes of the disorder?
Effects of illness or disability on family	How has your child's illness or disability affected you and your family?
	How has your life-style changed?
Coping Mechanisms	
Reactions to previous crises	Tell me one time you've had another crisis (problem, bad time) in your family. How did you solve that problem?
Reactions to the child	Do you find yourself being a little more cautious with this child than with your other children?
Childrearing practices	Do you feel as comfortable disciplining this child compared with your other children?
Attitudes	How is this child different from the siblings or other children of similar age?
	Describe your child's personality. Is it easy, difficult, or in-between?
	When you think of your child's future, what thoughts come to mind?
Available Resources	What parts of your child's care are causing the most difficulty for you and/or your family?
	What services are available to help?
	What services do you need that presently are not available?
Concurrent Stresses	What other problems are you facing now? (Be specific; ask about financial, marital, sibling, and extended family/friends concerns.)

❖ Implementation

The main objective in working with the family is to assist them to cope effectively with those stresses imposed by the child's special needs. To achieve this goal, the entire family should be considered in every aspect of the implementation process (see Family Focus box on p. 539).

Provide Support at Time of Diagnosis

The time of diagnosis may be experienced as a crisis by some families. The impact of the crisis may occur at the time of birth, following a long period of physical and/or psychologic testing, or immediately after a tragic injury. The impact may begin before the diagnosis is made, when parents are aware that something is wrong with their child but before medical confirmation (Clements, Copeland, and Loftus, 1990). It is a critical time for parents. Although they may not hear or remember all that is said to them, they frequently sense a certain attitude of acceptance, rejection, hope, or despair that may influence their ability to absorb the shock and begin adapting to the family's altered future.

Parents should be encouraged to be together when they are informed of their child's condition, thus avoiding the problem of one parent having to interpret complex findings and deal with the initial emotional reaction of the other. The informing session should take place in a private, comfortable setting free of distractions and interruptions, in an atmosphere in which the parents feel free to express their emo-

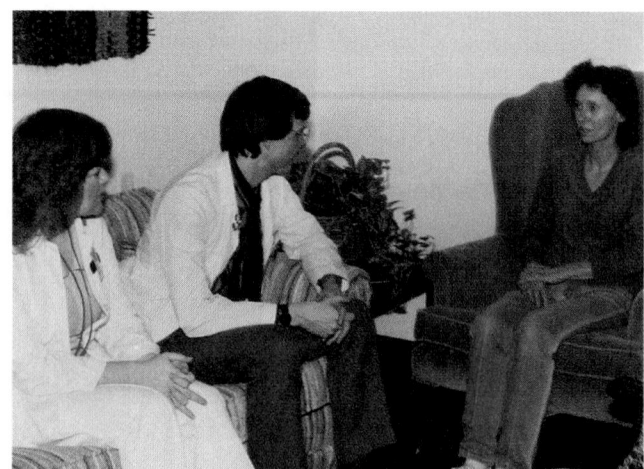

FIG. 18-3. Informing session should take place in a private, comfortable setting free of distractions and interruptions.

tions (Fig. 18-3). If their feelings can be expressed and acknowledged, the parents can be helped to deal openly with them. Their emotional needs are acknowledged by showing acceptance of such expressions as crying, sadness, anger, and disappointment. Emotional support is offered by having tissues available if a family member cries and demonstrating through facial and bodily language that indeed this is a difficult and painful period. Although touching is a powerful expression of empathy, it must be used wisely. For example, it can prematurely terminate free expression of feelings, especially when combined with statements such as "Everything will be all right." Nurses should also be aware of cultural issues regarding touching (see Chapter 3).

Parents should receive the kind of information they desire. Most parents want a clear, simple explanation of the diagnosis, a prediction of possible futures for the child, advice on what to do next, an opportunity to ask questions, a warm and sympathetic listener, and most important, time. Clarification of explanations is elicited with such questions as "Do you see what I mean?" or "Is this clear to you?" Technical terms are used with simple definitions. If the parents are unaware of the term, they are given written literature or at least a written summary of the diagnosis.

NURSING TIP Develop a glossary of commonly used terms, acronyms, and "initials" to distribute to parents. The list can stand alone or become a part of patient or parent handbooks.

Finally, the informing conference should not end with the presentation of devastating news. Instead, the child's strengths, appealing behaviors, and potential for development

---

GUIDELINES
Situations Requiring Special Consideration

CONGENITAL ANOMALY. Tension in delivery room conveys the sense that something is seriously wrong. Communication is often delayed while physician is involved with mother's care. The manner in which the infant is presented may well set the tone for the early parent-child relationship.

Clarify role with physician in regard to revealing information, to enable immediate parental support.

Explain to parents briefly in simple language what the defect is and something concerning the immediate prognosis before showing them the infant, when they are more apt to "hear" what is said.

Be aware of nonverbal communication. Parents watch the facial expressions of others for signs of revulsion or rejection.

Present the infant as something precious.

Emphasize the well-formed aspects of the infant's body.

Allow time and opportunity for parents to express their initial response.

Encourage parents to ask questions and provide honest, straightforward answers without undue optimism or pessimism.

COGNITIVE IMPAIRMENT. Unless cognitive impairment (mental retardation) is associated with other physical problems, it is often easy for parents to miss clues to its presence or to make defensive excuses regarding diagnosis.

Plan situations that help parents become aware of the problem.

Encourage parents to discuss their observations of the child, but withhold diagnostic opinions.

Focus on what the child can do and appropriate interventions to promote progress (e.g., infant stimulation programs) to involve parents in their child's care while helping them gain an awareness of the child's disability.

PHYSICAL DISABILITY. If loss of motor or sensory ability occurs during childhood, diagnosis is readily apparent. The challenge lies in helping the child and parents over the period of shock and grief and toward the phase of acceptance and reintegration.

Institute early rehabilitation (e.g., using a prosthetic limb, learning to read braille, learning to read lips).

Be aware that physical rehabilitation usually precedes psychologic adjustment.

When the cause of the disability is accidental, avoid implying that parents or child was responsible for the injury, yet allow them the opportunity to discuss feelings of blame.

Encourage expression of feelings (see Communication Techniques, Chapter 6).

CHRONIC ILLNESS. Realization of the true impact may take months or years. Conflict over parent's vs child's concerns may result in serious problems. When condition is inherited, parents may blame themselves and/or child may blame parents.

Help each family member gain an appreciation of the other's concerns.

Discuss hereditary aspect of condition with parents at time of diagnosis to lessen guilt and accusatory feelings.

Encourage child to express feelings by using third-person technique (e.g., "Sometimes when a person has an illness that was passed on by the parents, that person feels angry or bitter toward them").

MULTIPLE DISABILITIES. The child or parent may require additional time for the shock phase and may only be able to attend to one diagnosis before hearing significant information regarding other disorders.

Acknowledge parents' understanding and acceptance of all diagnoses, especially when an obvious and more hidden disability coexists.

Appreciate the devastating consequences of more than one disability to a child, especially if they interfere with expressive-receptive abilities.

TERMINAL ILLNESS. Parents require much support to deal with their own feelings and guidance in how to tell the child the diagnosis. They may want to conceal the diagnosis from the child. They may believe that the child is too young to know, will not be able to cope with the information, or will lose hope and the will to live.

Approach the subject of disclosure in a positive way by asking, "How will you tell your child about the diagnosis?"

Help parents understand the disadvantages of not telling children (e.g., deprives them of the opportunity to discuss their feelings openly and ask questions, incurs the risk of them learning the truth from outside and sometimes less tactful sources, may lessen children's trust and confidence in their parents once they learn the truth).

Guide parents to see the potential problems involved in fostering a conspiracy.

Offer parents guidelines for how and what to tell children about their disease or the possibility of death. Explanations should be tailored to the child's cognitive ability, be based on knowledge child already has, and be honest. Honesty must be tempered with concern for the child's feelings.

Assure parents that telling a child the name of the illness and the reason for treatment instills hope, provides support from others, and serves as a foundation for explaining and understanding subsequent events.

Acknowledge that being honest is not always easy because the truth may prompt children to ask other distressing questions, such as "Am I going to die?" However, even this difficult question must be answered.

are stressed, as well as available rehabilitation efforts or treatment. Parents can be encouraged to view their experiences as a series of challenges that they are capable of handling, particularly with available professional feedback. The parents are assured that the nurse will be available to answer questions and to provide further assistance as needed.

The preceding discussion relates primarily to the initial informing interview. However, because of the need for long-term follow-up, it is only one in a series of continuing discussions. In all interactions the family's input is solicited and incorporated into the plan of care. Some situations require consideration of special problems (see Guidelines box on p. 541).

Accept Family's Emotional Reactions

One of the most supportive interventions is to accept the family's emotional reactions to the child's condition in as nonjudgmental a manner as possible. Although all families respond differently and in varying degrees of intensity, three responses are so common and often so poorly handled that they deserve special consideration.

Denial.   The nurse's response to denial is a critical component of the individual's continuing need for this defense mechanism. The most effective method of support is active listening. Silence neither reinforces nor rejects denial (or any other emotional reaction) but implies a willingness and acceptance of the person's need for this behavior. However, silence alone can be misinterpreted. For example, if the person demonstrates denial, such as by saying, "I am sure the doctors made a mistake," and the nurse responds silently and leaves, the person may infer disapproval, agreement, avoidance, or rejection from this behavior.

To be effective, silence and listening must be accompanied by physical and mental concentration and use of body language to communicate interest and concern. Direct eye contact, touch, physical closeness, and body posture, such as sitting and leaning slightly forward, demonstrate silent but effective communication. (See also Communication Techniques, Chapter 6.)

Guilt.   Since guilt is such a common response and can cause family members tremendous anxiety, they should be told directly that there is no known cause of the disorder (when appropriate) and that they are not to be blamed. Using the third-person technique is valuable in eliciting thoughts of guilt. For example, with children an appropriate statement may be, "When people get sick, they often wonder if they did anything to make themselves sick." This allows children an opportunity to explore any feelings of responsibility they harbor.

If family members are expressing feelings of guilt, it is important to allow them to talk about their feelings rather than quickly trying to dispel them with long "scientific" explanations. Statements such as "If you believe you are responsible for Johnny's condition, then no wonder you feel so bad" acknowledge the family member's feelings. This step is frequently appreciated and necessary before the facts can be presented and absorbed. An effective method in lessening guilt is to *encourage the irrationality of thought.* For example, one mother stated that her son probably developed cancer by sitting too close to the television, which she could have prevented by being more strict. By following her reasoning and

GUIDELINES
Encouraging Expression of Emotion

Describe the behavior: "You seem angry at everyone."
Give evidence of understanding: "Being angry is only natural."
Give evidence of caring: "It must be difficult to endure so many painful procedures."
Help focus on feelings: "Maybe you wonder why this happened to your child."

talking about how *many* children sit close to the television and how *few* of them ever have cancer, the nurse was able to help the mother realize that this activity was not a cause.

Anger.   Anger is one of the more difficult reactions to accept and deal with therapeutically. The responses to anger may be reciprocal anger, fear, acceptance, and/or encouragement. The first two reactions impede communication and express disapproval and rejection of the person. They most frequently occur when the listener views the anger as a personal assault. The last two responses allow the individual to express his or her feelings in an atmosphere of nonjudgmental acceptance. Two basic rules for dealing with the angry person are to avoid losing one's temper and to encourage the person to talk (see Guidelines box). One essential element to the successful implementation of this process is to wait for the person to respond to a statement before proceeding to the next step. Since the objective of each statement is for the person to speak freely, the responses should avoid "yes" or "no" types of answers.

Help Family Cope

For the family to meet the stresses of optimally adjusting to the child's condition, each member must be individually supported so that the family system is strong. Although the family can indefinitely support a member who is in need of assistance, its greatest strength lies in every member supporting each other. The nurse should bear in mind that the family member in greatest need is not necessarily the affected child but may be a parent or sibling who is dealing with stresses that require intervention.

Parents.   The nurse can provide support by being attentive to families' responses to their children. Mothers and fathers need to experience success, joy, and pride in their children to give the support they need. Children, too, require support for their interactions, adjustments, and efforts. They must be reinforced for attempts to get to know their care providers and to communicate their needs to them.

Nurses must examine their attitudes to determine their ability to engage in parent-professional partnerships. An essential characteristic is the belief that parents are equal to professionals and that parents are experts regarding their child. (See Guidelines box for developing successful partnerships with parents.)

Since most mothers and fathers of children with special needs have little or no experience with children who have chronic or disabling conditions, the nurse can role model appropriate interactions with the child. Above all, the nurse should ensure that the parents and siblings learn to perceive the child as a child first, with unique and individual needs.

GUIDELINES
Developing Successful
Parent-Professional Partnerships

Promote primary nursing; in nonhospital settings designate a case manager.

Acknowledge parents' overall competence and their unique expertise with their child.

Respect parents' time as having equal value to that of other members of child's health care team.

Explain or define any medical, technical, or disciplinary-specific terms.

Tell families, "I am not sure" or "I don't know," when appropriate.

Facilitate family's effectiveness in team meetings (e.g., provide parents with same information as other participants).

The nurse needs to convey a humanistic, accepting approach to the child to enable the parents to observe this acceptance. This attitude of liking, concern for, and acceptance of the child should begin in early infancy and continue throughout the child's life.

Communication among all family members is encouraged. Parent group sessions are helpful in assisting parents to verbalize thoughts and feelings to each other but often do not take into account siblings' or the child's viewpoint. Therefore the nurse may need to set up a family session, such as during a home or clinic visit. Although the ideal situation is to have all the members present at once, this is often not possible. However, inviting members to participate at various visits is an appropriate alternative.

Parents can be encouraged to discuss their feelings toward the child, the impact of this event on their marriage, and associated stresses, such as financial burdens. For most families, regardless of their income or insurance coverage, financial concerns exist. The costs of caring for a child with special needs can be overwhelming. In addition, the family wage earner may have to sacrifice job opportunities to remain close to a medical facility or to avoid losing insurance benefits.*

The nurse should regard fathers as able, effective parents, competent and capable of coping with the challenges they face. Every effort is made to include the father in visits, such as to the nursery, clinic, special school, and stimulation programs. The father should be included in the assessment process, with specific emphasis on having him describe the child's strengths and difficulties. It is not unusual to find two parents who have differing views of the child's abilities, especially in the area of developmental disabilities.†

Numerous volunteer and community resources are available that provide assistance, rehabilitation, equipment, and funding for a variety of health problems.* National and local disease-oriented organizations may provide needed assistance and support to families that qualify. Many of these are discussed elsewhere in the text under the diagnosis. State and federal departments of health, mental health, social service, and labor may be able to help locate appropriate regional resources. For example, state **Programs for Children with Special Health Needs** (formerly Crippled Children's Services) provide financial assistance for children with many disabling conditions. Local and national sources of respite care and medical daycare may be useful to families. Nurses should become acquainted with those in their communities and with vocational programs for special groups.

Although community resources may exist, it is often very difficult for parents to locate suitable services, and coordination among several agencies may be lacking. Fragmented care is one of the chief complaints from families. Consequently, community networking for improved services is essential. Although this topic is beyond the scope of the present discussion, nurses can become key figures in coordinating services.

Parent-to-Parent Support. The support a parent receives from another parent is unique and unobtainable from any other source. A growing number of hospitals and clinics now have a parent on staff. The services these parents provide are particularly valuable for parents of children with special needs who are likely to experience frequent and lengthy hospitalizations, as well as numerous routine clinic visits.

Just being with another parent who has shared similar experiences is helpful. A parent of a child with the same diagnosis is not always necessary, since parents in the process of adjusting to a child with special needs—or finding respite services, educational or rehabilitative services, special equipment vendors, and financial counseling—tread a common path. If the agency does not have a parent staff position, the nurse can contact parent groups, who will often send a representative. Another strategy is ask another parent to talk to the parents.† The nurse should seek out a parent who is a good listener, has a nonjudgmental approach to differences in families, and possesses good advocacy and problem-solving skills.

---

*Information regarding financial issues is available from the **Federation for Children with Special Needs**, 95 Berkeley St., Suite 104, Boston, MA 02116; (617) 482-2915. A helpful book for families is Rosenfeld L: *Your Child and Health Care: a "Dollars and Sense" Guide for Families with Special Needs,* Baltimore, 1994, Brookes, available from the **Association for the Care of Children's Health**, 7910 Woodmont Ave., Suite 300, Bethesda, MD 20814; (301) 654-6549.

†Excellent resources on fathers' issues are presented in a training film, *Special Kids, Special Dads: Fathers of Children with Disabilities,* and a monograph, *Fathers of Children with Special Needs: New Horizons,* which are available from the **Association for the Care of Children's Health,** 7910 Woodmont Ave., Suite 300, Bethesda, MD 20814; (301) 654-6549.

---

*General sources of information are **Clearinghouse for Disability Information**, Room 3132, Switzer Building, C St., S.W., Washington, DC 20202-2524; **National Information Center for Children and Youth with Disabilities,** P.O. Box 1492, Washington, DC 20013, (202) 884-8200 or (800) 695-0285; **National Information Clearinghouse for Infants with Disabilities and Life-Threatening Conditions,** Center for Developmental Disabilities, The University of South Carolina, Benson Building, Columbia, SC 29208, or (800) 922-9234, ext 201; and **National Center for Children with Chronic Illness and Disability,** Box 721-UMHC, Harvard St. at E. River Rd., Minneapolis, MN 55455, (612) 626-4032. A comprehensive list of books and pamphlets for parents and teachers is available from the **National Easter Seal Society,** 230 West Monroe St., Suite 1800, Chicago, IL 60606; (312) 726-6200. In Canada: **Coalition of Provincial Organizations of the Handicapped,** Suite 926, 294 Portage Ave., Winnipeg, Manitoba R3C 0B9, (204) 947-0303; and **Canadian Rehabilitation Council for Disabled,** 45 Sheppard Ave., E., Suite 801, Toronto, Ontario M2N 5W9, (416) 250-7490. †The *Parent Resource Directory* lists more than 400 parents of children with chronic illness or disabilities in the United States and Canada, including addresses, phone numbers, the child's condition, and the health facility where the child receives care. It is available from the **Association for the Care of Children's Health,** 7910 Woodmont Ave., Suite 300, Bethesda, MD 20814; (301) 654-6549.

The parent self-help group is another way to promote parent-to-parent support.* Group members feel less alone and have the opportunity to observe both coping and mastery role modeling from other members. Parents' groups are rich resources for information. Even if parents are unable to attend meetings, they can still benefit from group newsletters and other literature that often accompany membership. The nurse can foster parent participation in self-help groups by serving as a referral agent, a group advisory board member, a resource person, a group member, or an assistant in founding a group. Sometimes all that is required in starting a group is identifying one or two parents as leaders; sharing with them the names, telephone numbers, and addresses of other families who have expressed both an interest and a willingness to release their phone number and address; and guiding them in how to initiate a first meeting.†

Advocate for Empowerment. Nurses can advocate for methods that foster opportunities for parent empowerment. For example, nurses can suggest reimbursement for travel and child care, plus stipends to enable parents' voices to be heard at meetings and conferences. They can encourage parent membership on staff, committees, and boards. They can keep parents informed of pending legislation on child health issues or take action when parents inform them.

The Child. Through ongoing contacts with the child, the nurse (1) observes the child's responses to the disorder, ability to function, and adaptive behaviors within the environment and with significant others; (2) explores the child's own understanding of the nature of his or her illness or condition; and (3) provides support while the child learns to cope with his or her feelings. Children are encouraged to express their concerns rather than allowing others to express them for them, since open discussions may reduce anxiety.

Parents sometimes convey concern because children cannot express their anxieties. If children cannot or will not talk, they may have to play out their feelings. They can be provided with toys to express threatening or stressful emotions. The nurse may find that children respond best to drawing pictures or telling stories (see Chapter 6). Puppets can also be used. By demonstrating to parents how useful these techniques are, the nurse also helps them learn new ways of communicating with their child. For youngsters with extremely serious handicaps and/or persistent maladjustment, psychiatric evaluation and management may be needed.

One of the most important interventions is alleviating the child's feeling of being different and normalizing his or her life as much as possible. The guidelines in the accompanying box are fundamental in implementing the normalizing process. Whenever possible, the nurse should assist the family to assess the child's daily routine for indications of normalizing

GUIDELINES
Promoting Normalization

Preparation. Prepare child in advance for changes that may occur from the illness or disability; for example, the child is told in advance of the possible side effects of drug therapy.

Participation. Include child in as many decisions as possible, especially those relating to his or her care regimen; for example, the child is responsible for taking medications or scheduling home treatments.

Sharing. Allow both family members and child's peers to be a part of the care regimen whenever possible; for example, the child is given his or her medication when the other siblings receive their vitamins; the parent cooks the same menu for the whole family; and if the child is invited to another's home, the parent advises the family of the child's dietary restrictions.

Control. Identify areas where child can be in control so that feelings of uncertainty, passivity, and helplessness are decreased; for example, the child identifies activities that are appropriate to his or her energy level and chooses to rest when fatigued.

Expectation. Apply the same family rules to the child with a chronic illness or disability as to the well siblings or peers; for example, the child is disciplined, expected to fulfill household responsibilities, and attends school in accordance with abilities.

practices. For example, the child who remains in a bedroom all day is in need of a restructured daily routine to provide activities in different parts of the house, such as eating in the kitchen or dining room with the family. Such children may also be deprived of social, recreational, and academic activities that can be recognized by applying normalization practices. For example, home and out-of-home health-related treatments should be planned at times that least interfere with normal daily activities.

Children who are concerned that their condition detracts from their physical attractiveness need attention focused on the normal aspects of appearance and capabilities. Health professionals must help strengthen and consolidate the self-image by emphasizing the normal, while at the same time allowing children to express anger, isolation, fear of rejection, feelings of sadness, and loneliness. They need positive reinforcement for compliance and any evidence of improvement. Anything that might improve attractiveness and contribute to a positive self-image is employed, such as makeup for a teenager with a scar, clothing that disguises a prosthesis, or a hairstyle or wig to cover a deformity or lost hair.

Siblings. The presence of a child with special needs in a family may result in parents paying less attention to the other children. Siblings may respond by developing negative attitudes toward the child or by expressing anger in different forms. The nurse can help by using "anticipatory guidance," questioning the parents about what they believe is the best way to have siblings respond to the child and guiding them through ways to meet their other children's needs for attention. This questioning should take place before serious negative effects occur.

Siblings may also experience embarrassment associated with courtesy stigma. Parents are then faced with the diffi-

---

*Information about self-help groups and books and pamphlets are available from the **National Self-Help Clearinghouse,** 25 W. 43rd St., Room 620, New York, NY 10036; (212) 642-2944.

†The following resources are recommended: *Organizing and Maintaining Support Groups for Parents of Children with Chronic Illness and Handicapping Conditions* by Minna Newman Nathanson, available from the **Association for the Care of Children's Health,** 7910 Woodmont Ave., Suite 300, Bethesda, MD 20814; and *The Self-Help Sourcebook: Finding and Forming Mutual Aid Self-Help Groups* by E.J. Madara and A. Meese, available from the **New Jersey Self-Help Clearinghouse,** Saint Clares–Riverside Medical Center, Denville, NJ 07834, (201) 625-9565.

culty of responding to this embarrassment in an understanding and appropriate manner without punishing the siblings for how they feel. Parents should talk with the siblings about how they view their affected sibling. For example, siblings of a child who is retarded may express fears about their ability to bear normal children. Adolescents in particular may not be able to discuss these vital issues with their parents and may prefer to consult with the nurse. Many siblings benefit from sharing their concerns with other young people who are experiencing a similar situation.* Support groups for siblings can help decrease isolation, promote expression of feelings, and provide examples of effective coping skills.

Many parents express concern about when and how to inform the other children in the family about a sibling's disability. The answer depends on each child's level of sophistication and understanding. However, it is usually best to inform the siblings before a neighbor or other nonfamily member does so. Uninformed siblings may fantasize or develop apprehensions that are out of proportion to the child's actual condition. Furthermore, if parents choose to be silent or deceptive about the issue, they are setting a negative precedent for the siblings to follow, rather than encouraging the siblings to cope with the experience in a healthy and nurturing way.

---

*For information on the **Sibling Information Network,** contact the Information Network, CUAP, 991 Main St., Suite 3A, East Hartford, CT 06108.

The nurse must be sensitive to the reactions of siblings and whenever possible intervene to promote more positive adjustments. For example, siblings often mention that they are expected to take on additional responsibilities to help the parents care for the child. It is not unusual for them to express a positive reaction to assuming the extra duties but a negative response to feeling unappreciated for doing so. Such feelings can often be minimized by encouraging siblings to discuss this with the parents and by suggesting to parents ways of showing gratitude, such as an increase in allowance, special privileges, and most significantly, verbal praise (see Family Focus box).

Extended Family Members and Community.   The nurse must also be sensitive to family's cues regarding sources of stress from extended members, such as grandparents. For example, the nurse may encourage the parents to invite the grandparents to be present during one of the child's visits to a clinic, during the diagnostic workup, or to a parent conference or to provide appropriate literature. Including grandparents in a discussion in which they can share their concerns may help them deal with their feelings, thus reducing stress on the entire family. Grandparents' feelings of blame and anger as well as any "cure fantasies" they harbor can be brought out in the open and discussed if necessary. Grandparents can be helped to understand the effects of their behavior on the family with an appropriate statement, such as "Your daughter is currently experiencing a great deal of pain and anguish.

FAMILY FOCUS
Supporting Siblings

Promote Healthy Sibling Relationships

Value each child individually, and avoid comparisons. Remind each child of his or her positive qualities and contribution to other family members.

Help siblings see the differences and similarities between themselves and a child with special needs. Create a climate in which children can achieve successes without feeling guilty.

Teach siblings ways to interact with the child.

Seek to be fair in terms of discipline, attention, and resources; require the affected child to do as much for himself or herself as possible.

Let siblings settle their own differences; intervene only to prevent siblings from hurting one another.

Legitimize reasonable anger. Even children with special needs behave badly sometimes.

Respect a sibling's reluctance to be with or to include the child with special needs in activities.

Help Siblings Cope

Listen to siblings to let them know that their thoughts and suggestions are valued.

Praise siblings when they have been patient, have sacrificed, or have been particularly helpful. Do not expect siblings to always act in this manner.

Acknowledge the personal strengths of siblings and their ability to cope with stress successfully.

Provide age-appropriate information about the child's condition, and update when appropriate.

Let teachers know what is happening so they can be understanding and helpful.

Recognize special stress times for siblings and plan to minimize negative effects.

Schedule special time with siblings; have a friend or family member substitute when parent is unavailable.

Encourage sibling to join or help establish a sibling support group.

Use the services of professionals when needed. If parent feels that such a service is necessary, it should be provided in as vigorous a manner as a service for the child with special needs.

Involve Siblings

Seek out ways to include siblings realistically in the care and treatment of the child with special needs.

Limit caregiving responsibilities, and give recognition when siblings perform them.

Develop a library of children's books on special needs.

Invite siblings to attend meetings to develop plans for the child with special needs.

Discuss future plans with them.

Solicit their ideas on treatment and service needs.

Have them visit professionals who work with the child.

Help them develop competencies to teach the child new skills.

Provide opportunities for siblings to advocate for the child.

Allow siblings to set their own pace for learning and involvement.

Modified from Powell T, Ogle P: *Brothers and sisters—a special part of exceptional families,* Baltimore, 1985, Brookes; Spokane Washington Deaconess Medical Center Pediatric Oncology Unit: Tips for dealing with siblings, *Candlelighters Childhood Cancer Foundation Quarterly Newsletter* 11(3, 4):7, 1987; and Carlson J, Leviton A, Mueller M: Services to siblings: an important component of family-centered practice, *ACCH Advocate* 1(1):53-56, 1993.

We realize that this is difficult for you as well as your daughter; however, you can be of tremendous help by being supportive toward her."

Considerable stress can also arise from nonfamilial sources, such as friends, neighbors, or strangers. Inability to cope with comments about the disorder or curious stares by others may foster the tendency to isolate and protect the child within the home. The family needs guidance in preparing for these inevitable experiences. One approach is encouraging parents to dress the child as much as possible like other children. Good grooming is very important in minimizing differences in appearance. Through role playing, parents can practice responses to comments such as "Is your child retarded?" or "Has he always been crippled?" Through parent groups, family members can share experiences and learn from each other how they successfully deal with probing questions or unkind remarks. Interventions should include the siblings and the affected child, who also must face and deal with these events. Nurses can teach young children about disabilities to familiarize them with the special needs and abilities of these individuals. For example, school nurses can simulate experiences such as having only one leg through role playing, can use books or films, or can invite community guests with physical limitations to visit the class.

Educate About the Disorder and General Health Care

Educating the family about the disorder is actually an extension of revealing the diagnosis.* Education involves not only supplying technical information, but also discussing how the condition will affect the child. Parents may be able to digest only so much information at a time. It may be helpful to provide essential information followed by asking, "What else would you like to know about your child's condition?" Responding to parents' questions and concerns ensures that their information needs are met.

Activities of Daily Living. Parents also need guidance in how the condition may interfere with or alter activities of daily living, such as eating, dressing, sleeping, and toileting. Guidance in normalizing these activities for the child and family and in promoting age-appropriate self-care should be provided (Ahmann and Bond, 1992). One area frequently affected is nutrition. Common problems are undernutrition, resulting from food being inappropriately restricted, loss of appetite, vomiting, or motor deficits that interfere with feeding, and overnutrition, usually caused by a caloric intake in excess of energy expenditure or boredom and lack of stimulation in other areas. Although the child requires the same basic nutrients as other children, the daily requirements may differ. Special nutritional considerations are discussed as appropriate throughout the text.

Safe Transportation. Modifications may also be needed regarding car safety. Children with conditions such as low birth weight (see Discharge Planning and Home Care, Chapter 9) or orthopedic, neuromuscular, or respiratory problems often cannot safely use conventional car restraints. For example, children with hip spica casts cannot sit properly in child safety seats (see Congenital Hip Dysplasia, Chapter 31). Modifications can be made to some commercial models, and for older children a special vest is available that secures the child to the back seat in a lying-down position.*

If a child requires a wheelchair, the family should consult the wheelchair manufacturer for specific instructions regarding safe car transportation. Considerations for wheelchairs used for vehicle transportation must address securing both the wheelchair and the occupant in the wheelchair. Wheelchairs should be secured facing forward with tie downs at four points. The tie-down system should be dynamically crash tested, as should the occupant securement system that secures the child in the wheelchair. For example, use of trays would not be recommended for transportation. With children who must travel with additional medical equipment, this equipment (i.e., oxygen, monitors, ventilators) should be anchored to the floor or underneath the vehicle seat or wheelchair. Soft padding should be added around the equipment to reduce movement. A second adult should be present to monitor the condition of a medically fragile child while traveling.

Primary Health Care. Children with special needs require all the usual health care recommended for any child. Attention to injury prevention, immunizations, dental health, and regular physical examinations is essential. Nurses can play an important role in reminding parents of these aspects of care that are so often neglected when the concern is focused on the child's specific illness or disability. Specific discussions of nutrition, sleep and activity, dental health, and injury prevention are presented in the chapters on health promotion for specific age-groups. Immunizations are discussed in Chapter 10.

Parents also need to be aware of the importance of communicating the child's condition in the event of a medical emergency. Young children are unable to give information about their disorder, and although older children may be reliable sources, after an accident they may be physically unable to speak. Therefore all children with any type of chronic condition that may affect medical care should wear some type of identification, such as Medic-Alert bracelet,† or carry a card in their wallet, which lists the medical condition and a phone number for emergency medical records and other personal information.

Children need information about their condition, the therapeutic plan, and how the disease or the therapy might affect their particular situation. Children nearing puberty also need to understand the maturation process and how their disability may alter this event. Information should not be given all at once but be timed appropriately to meet the changing needs of the youngsters, and it should be described and repeated as often as the situation demands. The subject of sexuality related to the effects of the disorder is a prominent concern of adolescents, but they rarely initiate a discussion of this sensitive topic. Any probable interference in sexual function because of the disability should be discussed openly and candidly with the teenager.

---

*See Wong DL: *Wong and Whaley's Clinical manual of pediatric nursing,* ed 4, St Louis, 1996, Mosby, for home care instruction sheets, which may be copied and given to families.

*Information on car safety restraints for children with special needs is available from **Automotive Safety for Children Program,** Riley Hospital for Children, 702 Barnhill Dr., S-139, Indianapolis, IN 46223; (317) 274-2977 or (800) KID-N-CAR (in Indiana).
†P.O. Box 1009, Turlock, CA 95381-1009, (800) ID-ALERT.

Promote Normal Development

Aside from knowledge of the condition and its effect on the child's abilities, the family must be guided toward fostering appropriate development in their child. Although each stage may take longer to achieve, parents are guided to helping the child fully realize potential in preparation for the next developmental stage. Table 18-4 outlines developmental aspects of chronic illness or disability and supportive interventions. With appropriate planning and knowledge of strategies to improve the child's functional abilities, most children can live fulfilling and productive lives.

One important aspect of promoting normal development is to encourage the child's self-care abilities in both activities of daily living and the medical regimen. An assessment of the child's age and physical, emotional, and mental capacities, as well as the support and structure provided by the family, should be considered in determining the appropriate level of self-care in the medical regimen (Savinetti-Rose, 1994). Even toddlers can be involved in their own care by holding supplies for the parent during a procedure. Over time children should be encouraged toward greater autonomy in the self-care arena.

Early Childhood. During infancy the child is achieving basic *trust* through a satisfying, intimate, consistent relationship with his or her parents. However, the affected child's early existence may be stressful, chaotic, and unsatisfying. Consequently, he or she may need more parental support and expressions of affection to achieve trust. Likewise, the parents require assistance in finding ways to meet the infant's needs, such as how to hold a rigid or flaccid infant, how to feed a child with tongue thrust or episodes of dyspnea, and how to stimulate a child who seems incapable of achieving any skills. If hospitalizations are frequent or prolonged, every effort is made to preserve the parent-child relationship (see also Chapter 21). Hospital policies should promote visitation by and involvement of families.

During early childhood the goal is to achieve separation from parents, autonomy, and initiative. However, the natural parental response to having a sick child is overprotection. Parents need help in realizing the importance of brief separations from the child and from others involved in the child's care and of providing social experiences outside the home whenever possible. Respite care, which provides temporary relief for family members, can be essential in allowing caregivers time away from the daily burdens.

Young children also need the opportunity to develop independence. Frequently the child is able to learn self-help skills, such as holding the bottle, finger feeding, and removing simple articles of clothing, but the parent continues to perform the act. The nurse can guide parents to the usual milestones expected from the child.

When the young child has a disability that interferes with motor development, intervention must be based on providing activities that allow maximum motor development. Also, the activity must take into account the child's need for social interaction, sense of control over the body, feeling of competence and achievement, and an outlet for aggression.

When a child is unable to perform a skill independently, functional aids should be used. With innovation, many adaptations can be implemented in children's environments to increase their mobility and independence and allow them to

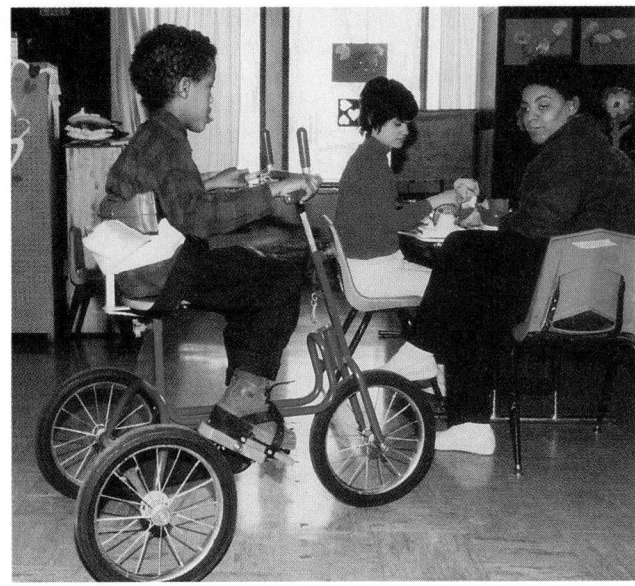

FIG. 18-4. A modified tricycle with block pedals, self-adhesive straps for support, and modified seat and handle bars can help a child with disabilities gain mobility.

play like other children their age. For example, with slight modifications, a child with physical limitations may be able to ride a tricycle (Fig. 18-4).

Another critical component for normal child development is discipline. Discipline and guidance serve several purposes, such as providing children with boundaries on which to test out their behavior and teaching them socially acceptable behavior. Resentment and hostility can arise among siblings if different standards are applied to each child. The nurse's responsibility is to help parents learn successful methods of managing a child's behaviors before they become problems (see Chapter 4).

School Age. For school-age children the major tasks are entry into school and achieving a sense of *industry*. Although the importance of school in the life of all children is well known, school absences are significantly higher among children with chronic illness than among their healthy peers. The more school absences the child experiences, the more difficult it is to resume attendance, and "school phobia" may result. The child should return to school as soon as possible after diagnosis or treatments.

Preparation for entry into or resumption of school is best accomplished through a team approach with the parents, child, schoolteacher, school nurse, and primary nurse in the hospital. Ideally this planning should begin before hospital discharge, provided the child is well enough to resume usual activities. A structured plan should be developed, with attention to those aspects of care that must be continued during school hours, such as administration of medication or other treatments.

Children also need preparation before entering or resuming school. Having a tutor in the hospital or home as soon as children are physically able helps them realize that school will continue and gives them time to consider this prospect

TABLE 18-4. Developmental aspects of chronic illness or disability on children		
AGE/DEVELOPMENTAL TASKS	**POTENTIAL EFFECTS OF CHRONIC ILLNESS OR DISABILITY**	**SUPPORTIVE INTERVENTIONS**
Infancy		
Develop a sense of trust	Multiple caregivers and frequent separations, especially if hospitalized	Encourage consistent caregivers in hospital or other care settings
	Deprived of consistent nurturing	Encourage parental presence, "rooming in" during hospitalization, and participation in care
Bond/attach to parent	Delayed because of separation, parental grief for loss of "dream" child, parental inability to accept the condition, especially a visible defect	Emphasize healthy, perfect qualities of infant
Learn through sensorimotor experiences	Increased exposure to painful experiences over pleasurable ones	Help parents learn special care needs of infant for them to feel competent
	Limited contact with environment from restricted movement or confinement	Expose infant to pleasurable experiences through all senses (touch, hearing, sight, taste, movement)
Begin to develop a sense of separateness from parent	Increased dependency on parent for care	Encourage age-appropriate developmental skills (e.g., holding bottle, finger feeding, crawling)
	Overinvolvement of parent in care	Encourage all family members to participate in care to prevent overinvolvement of one member
		Encourage periodic respite from demands of care responsibilities
Toddlerhood		
Develop autonomy	Increased dependency on parent	Encourage independence in as many areas as possible (e.g., toileting, dressing, feeding)
Master locomotor and language skills	Limited opportunity to test own abilities and limits	Provide gross motor skill activity and modification of toys or equipment, such as modified swing or rocking horse
Learn through sensorimotor experience, beginning preoperational thought	Increased exposure to painful experiences	Give choices to allow simple feeling of control, (e.g., choice of what book to look at or what kind of sandwich to eat)
		Institute age-appropriate discipline and limit-setting
		Recognize that negative and ritualistic behavior are normal
		Provide sensory experiences (e.g., water play, sandbox, finger paint)
Preschool		
Develop initiative and purpose Master self-care skills	Limited opportunities for success in accomplishing simple tasks or mastering self-care skills	Encourage mastery of self-help skills
		Provide devices that make task easier (e.g., self-dressing)
Begin to develop peer relationships	Limited opportunities for socialization with peers; may appear "like a baby" to age-mates	Encourage socialization (e.g., inviting friends to play, daycare experience, trips to park)
	Protection within tolerant and secure family may cause child to fear criticism and withdraw	Provide age-appropriate play, especially associative play opportunities
		Emphasize child's abilities; dress appropriately to enhance desirable appearance
Develop sense of body image and sexual identification	Awareness of body may center on pain, anxiety, and failure	Encourage relationships with same-sex and opposite-sex peers and adults
	Sex role identification focused primarily on mothering skills	Help child deal with criticisms; realize that too much protection prevents child from realities of world
Learn through preoperational thought (magical thinking)	Guilt (thinking he or she caused the illness/disability or is being punished for wrongdoing)	Clarify that cause of child's illness or disability is not his or her fault or a punishment
School Age		
Develop a sense of accomplishment	Limited opportunities to achieve and compete (e.g., many school absences or inability to join regular athletic activities)	Encourage school attendance; schedule medical visits at times other than school; encourage child to make up missed work
Form peer relationships	Limited opportunities for socialization	Educate teachers and classmates about child's condition, abilities, and special needs

TABLE 18-4. Developmental aspects of chronic illness or disability on children—cont'd

AGE/DEVELOPMENTAL TASKS	POTENTIAL EFFECTS OF CHRONIC ILLNESS OR DISABILITY	SUPPORTIVE INTERVENTIONS
School Age—cont'd Learn through concrete operations	Incomplete comprehension of the imposed physical limitations or treatment of the disorder	Encourage sports activities (e.g., Special Olympics) Encourage socialization (e.g., Girl Scouts, Campfire, Boy Scouts, 4-H Clubs, having a best friend or club membership) Provide child with knowledge about his or her condition Encourage creative activities (e.g., Very Special Arts)
Adolescence Develop personal and sexual identity Achieve independence from family Form heterosexual relationships Learn through abstract thinking	Increased sense of feeling different from peers and less able to compete with peers in appearance, abilities, special skills Increased dependency on family; limited job/career opportunities Limited opportunities for heterosexual friendships; less opportunity to discuss sexual concerns with peers Increased concern with issues such as why did he or she get the disorder, can he or she marry and have a family Decreased opportunity for earlier stages of cognition may impede achieving level of abstract thinking	Realize that many of the difficulties the teenager is experiencing are part of normal adolescence (rebelliousness, risk taking, lack of cooperation, hostility toward authority) Provide instruction on interpersonal and coping skills Encourage socialization with peers, including peers with special needs and those without special needs Provide instruction on decision making, assertiveness, and other skills necessary to manage personal plans Encourage increased responsibility for care and management of the disease or condition (e.g., assuming responsibility for making and keeping appointment [ideally alone], sharing assessment and planning stages of health care delivery, contacting resources) Encourage activities appropriate for age (e.g., attending mixed-sex parties, sports activities, driving a car) Be alert to cues that signal readiness for information regarding implications of condition on sexuality and reproduction Emphasize good appearance and wearing stylish clothes, use of makeup Understand that adolescent has same sexual needs and concerns as any other teenager Discuss planning for future and how condition can affect choices

(Fig. 18-5). They need to investigate possible answers to the many questions others will ask. One method of anticipatory preparation is to role play, with the child as the "returned pupil" and the nurse or parent as "other schoolmates." If the child returns to school with some obvious physical change, such as hair loss, amputation, or visible scar, the nurse might also ask questions about these alterations to prompt preparatory responses from the child.

Classroom peers also need preparation, and a joint plan of the schoolteacher, nurse, and child is best. At a minimum the classmates should be given a description of the child's condition, prepared for any visible changes in the child, and allowed an opportunity to ask questions. The child should have the option of attending this session. As the child's condition changes, particularly if the illness is potentially fatal,

school personnel, including the students, need periodic appraisal of the child's status and preparation for what to expect.

Children with special needs are encouraged to maintain or reestablish relationships with peers and to participate according to their capabilities in any age-appropriate activities. Alternative activities may be substituted for those that are impossible or that place a strain on the child's condition. Programs such as the **Special Olympics*** offer children an op-

*1350 New York Ave., N.W., Suite 500, Washington, DC 20005-1581; (202) 628-3630. Several pamphlets on sports and recreation for children with disabilities are available from the **National Easter Seal Society**, 70 E. Lake St., Chicago, IL 60601, (312) 726-6200; and the **American Alliance for Health, Physical Education, Recreation and Dance (AAHPERD)**, 1900 Association Dr., Reston, VA 22091, (703) 476-3400.

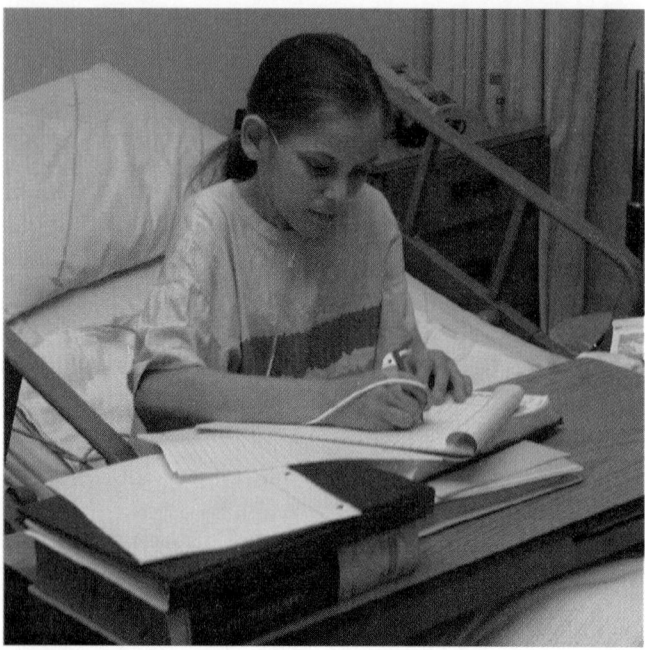

FIG. 18-5. Children with special needs should continue their schooling as soon as their condition permits.

portunity to compete with their peers and to achieve athletic skill. Summer camps* allow children to associate with peers and develop a wide variety of skills. Children with special needs can derive enormous benefits from expressive activities, such as art, music, poetry, dance, and drama. With adaptive equipment and imagination, children can participate in a variety of activities. Organizations such as **Very Special Arts** offer children an opportunity to celebrate and share their accomplishments.† Children need the opportunity to interact with healthy peers, as well as to engage in activities with groups or clubs composed of similarly affected age-mates. Such organizations as ostomy clubs, diabetes clubs, and cerebral palsy groups share information and provide support related to the special problems the members face.

Adolescence.   Adolescence can be a particularly difficult period for the teenager and family. All the needs discussed before apply to this age-group as well. Developing *independence* or *autonomy,* however, is a major task for the adolescent as planning for the future becomes a prominent concern. Although the emphasis in the past has been on achieving independence from physical assistance, recent developments in the fields of special education, adolescent development, and family systems suggest redefining autonomy in terms of individuals' capacities to take responsibility for their own behavior, to make decisions regarding their own

lives, and to maintain supportive social relationships. Given this understanding, even individuals with severe impairment can be viewed as autonomous if they perceive their own needs and take responsibility for meeting them, either directly or by engaging the assistance of others. As adolescents become more autonomous, the nurse can help them articulate needs, participate in developing their own plan of care, and discover and express how others can be of greatest assistance.

Physical symptoms are high on the teenager's list of health-related concerns. Because adolescence is a time of enormous physical and emotional changes, it is important for the nurse to make a distinction between body changes that are related to disability and those that are a result of normal body development. It can be a great comfort for teenagers with disabling conditions to know that many of the changes they experience are normal developmental outcomes.

A sense of feeling different from peers can lead to loneliness, isolation, and depression. Participation in groups of teenagers with chronic conditions or disabilities can alleviate feelings of isolation and smooth the transition to a meaningful relationship with one person in adulthood.

Establish Realistic Future Goals

One of the most difficult adjustments is setting realistic future goals for the child and for those involved in his or her continued care. Sometimes the impact of this decision does not surface until the child finishes school or the parents near retirement, when a crisis can arise because all the family roles and relationships that maintained stability are now disrupted.

Planning for the future should be a gradual process. All along, the parents should cultivate realistic vocations for the child. For example, if children have physical disabilities, they are directed to intellectual, artistic, or musical pursuits. Children with developmental disabilities are taught manual skills. In this way the child's development proceeds in the direction of self-support through gainful employment.

With prolonged survival young people with chronic illnesses must deal with new decisions and problems, such as marriage, employment, and insurance coverage. With appropriate guidance, gainful employment, marriage, and a family are attainable goals. For those whose conditions are genetic, counseling is needed regarding future offspring. Prospective spouses often benefit from an opportunity to discuss their feelings regarding marriage to an individual with continued health needs and possibly a limited life span. Health insurance coverage is a critical issue because some private carriers may no longer insure a young person who leaves home or may be unwilling to reinsure the person who is independent. Life insurance is another dilemma, especially when children have serious defects, such as congenital heart anomalies.

Unfortunately, vocational pursuits and completely independent living are not realistic goals for all persons. Persons with multiple or severe disabilities may require lifelong care and assistance. In these situations parents must look to the time when they will no longer be able to care for their child. Residential placement may be very difficult unless the family mutually participates in the decision-making and planning process. Placement outside the home should not be viewed as abandonment. Not infrequently it is the only way to preserve the family unit. The nurse should help the family investigate suitable placements, discuss their feelings regarding

*A directory of camps for children with a variety of chronic illnesses or general physical disabilities is available for a fee from **American Camping Association,** Publications Service, 5000 State Rd., 67 N., Martinsville, IN 46151; (800) 428-CAMP.
†Very Special Arts has affiliate chapters in all 50 states and in selected sites internationally; yearly festivals are held throughout the world. Information is available from **Very Special Arts,** Education Office, John F. Kennedy Center for the Performing Arts, Washington, DC 20566; (202) 628-2800.

Text continued on p. 556.

NURSING CARE PLAN
The Child with Chronic Illness or Disability

NURSING DIAGNOSIS: Altered growth and development related to chronic illness or disability, parental reactions (overbenevolence), repeated hospitalization

PATIENT GOAL 1: Will attain maximum expected growth and developmental potential

- **NURSING INTERVENTIONS/RATIONALES**

See Table 18-4

- **EXPECTED OUTCOME**

Child achieves appropriate physical, psychosocial, and cognitive development for age and abilities

NURSING DIAGNOSIS: Altered family processes related to situational crisis (child with a chronic disease or disability)

PATIENT (FAMILY) GOAL 1: Will exhibit positive adjustment behaviors to the diagnosis

- **NURSING INTERVENTIONS/RATIONALES**

Provide opportunity for family to adjust to discovery of diagnosis

Anticipate grief reaction to loss of the "perfect" child *because this usually occurs in the adjustment process*

Explore family's feelings regarding child and their ability to cope with the disorder

Encourage family to express their concerns

Repeat information as often as necessary *to reinforce family's understanding*

Serve as a role model regarding attitudes and behavior toward child

- **EXPECTED OUTCOMES**

Parents verbalize feelings and concerns regarding implications of the disease

Family demonstrates an attitude of acceptance and adjustment

PATIENT (FAMILY) GOAL 2: Will demonstrate understanding of disorder

- **NURSING INTERVENTIONS/RATIONALES**

Help family to understand the disorder, its therapies, and implications

Reinforce information given by others *to promote better understanding*

Clarify misconceptions

Provide accurate information at a rate family can absorb *because information given too rapidly will not be learned*

Discuss advantages and limitations of therapeutic plan

Encourage family to ask questions and express concerns

- **EXPECTED OUTCOME**

Family demonstrates an understanding of the disease (specify)

PATIENT (FAMILY) GOAL 3: Will experience reduction of fear and anxiety

- **NURSING INTERVENTIONS**

Explore family's concerns and feelings of irritation, guilt, anger, disappointment, inadequacy, and other feelings

Help family distinguish between realistic fears and unfounded fears; eliminate unfounded fears

Discuss with parents their fears regarding:
  Dealing with child's anxiety about condition
  Fear of dreadful developments
  Fear of death
  Fear of tests and procedures
  Child's ability to compete with peers

Explore their feelings regarding prescribed therapies

- **EXPECTED OUTCOME**

Family members discuss their fears and concerns

PATIENT (FAMILY) GOAL 4: Will exhibit positive adaptation behaviors to child

- **NURSING INTERVENTIONS/RATIONALES**

Explore family's reaction to child and the disorder

Assess family's coping skills, abilities, and resources *so that these can be reinforced*

Help family to achieve a realistic view of child and capabilities and limitations

Foster positive family relationships *so that their ability to cope is maximized*

Assess interpersonal relationships within family, especially behaviors that reflect family's attitudes toward affected child

Intervene appropriately if there is evidence of maladaptation; refer for counseling if appropriate

Encourage parents in their attempts to promote child's development

Emphasize positive aspects of child's abilities or attributes

Help family gain confidence in their ability to cope with child, the disorder, and its impact on other family members

- **EXPECTED OUTCOMES**

Family verbalizes feelings and concerns regarding special needs of child and their effect on the family process

Family members demonstrate an attitude of confidence in their ability to cope

PATIENT (FAMILY) GOAL 5: Will exhibit ability to care for child

- **NURSING INTERVENTIONS/RATIONALES**

Help family develop a thorough plan of care

Teach skills needed *to provide optimum care*

Interpret child's behavior to parents (e.g., anger, depression, regression, physical modifications as a result of disorder) *to prevent any unwarranted negative reaction (e.g., punishment) toward child*

Help family plan for the future

- **EXPECTED OUTCOME**

Family sets realistic goals for selves, child, and others

Continued.

Nursing Care Plan
The Child with Chronic Illness or Disability—cont'd

PATIENT (FAMILY) GOAL 6: Will exhibit positive family relationship

- **NURSING INTERVENTIONS/RATIONALES**

Identify family support systems (immediate family, extended family, friends, health service providers)

Assess systematically the number, affiliation, and interrelationships (if any) of persons the family sees as important

Help family to assign specific tasks to specific people *so that family receives support they need*

Reinforce positive coping mechanisms

Encourage family members to discuss their feelings about each other

Impress on parents the importance of providing as normal a life as possible for the affected child

Emphasize the growth and developmental progress of their child *to help family feel adequate in their maternal/ paternal roles*

Help family foster child's development by stimulating child to age-appropriate goals consistent with activity tolerance

- **EXPECTED OUTCOMES**

Family demonstrates positive, growth-promoting behaviors

Family avails itself of support

PATIENT (FAMILY) GOAL 7: Will receive adequate support

- **NURSING INTERVENTIONS/RATIONALES**

Be available to family *to provide support*

Listen to family members, singly or collectively

Allow for expression of feelings, including feelings of guilt, helplessness, and their perception of the impact that the condition may have (or does have) on family

Refer to community agencies or special organizations providing assistance: financial, social, and support

Refer to genetic counseling if appropriate

Help family learn to expect feelings of frustration and anger toward child; reassure them that it is not a reflection on their parenting

Assist family in problem solving

Encourage interaction with other families who have a similarly affected child

Introduce to families

Provide information regarding support groups

Help families learn when to accept and when to "fight" for the care and services they believe are needed

- **EXPECTED OUTCOMES**

Family maintains contact with health providers

Family demonstrates an understanding of child's needs and the impact the condition will have on them

Problems are dealt with early

Family becomes involved with local agencies and support groups as needed

PATIENT (FAMILY) GOAL 8: Will be prepared for home care

- **NURSING INTERVENTIONS/RATIONALES**

Teach skills needed *to ensure optimum home care*

Assess home situation, including family's strengths, weaknesses, and support systems

Help devise an individualized plan of care based on assessment of family's needs and resources

Encourage family involvement in care while still in the hospital *so that they are better prepared to assume child's care*

Encourage family to ask questions regarding posthospital care

Explore family's attitudes toward child's entry (or reentry) into the home

Help family acquire needed drugs, supplies, and equipment

Refer to special agencies, based on need assessment, *for ongoing support and assistance*

Arrange for regular follow-up care *to assess effectiveness of home management*

- **EXPECTED OUTCOMES**

Family demonstrates an understanding of needed skills (specify skills and method of demonstration)

Family members avail themselves of resources within their community (specify)

Family complies with home care program

PATIENT (FAMILY) GOAL 9: Will participate in ongoing care

- **NURSING INTERVENTIONS/RATIONALES**

Participate in follow-up care *to ensure continuity of care*

Coordinate team management of child and family

Be alert to comments by child or family members that indicate possible problems *so that problems are identified early*

Assess interpersonal relationships within family, especially behaviors that reflect family's attitudes toward child

Be alert for cues that signal undue anxiety and guilt: preoccupation with causative factors, constant analysis of effects of therapies, experimentation with diets and folk remedies, and seeking magical cures

Be alert for overprotective behaviors, such as assuming self-care activities for child and restricting child's activities or interaction with peers

Allow family to express discouragement at interference with activities and what appears to be slow progress

- **EXPECTED OUTCOMES**

Family participates in follow-up care

Family expresses both positive and negative reactions to child's progress

*Signs that may indicate family's difficulty in adjusting to child's condition are identified early

---

*Nursing outcome.

NURSING CARE PLAN

The Child with Chronic Illness or Disability—cont'd

PATIENT (SIBLINGS) GOAL 10: Will exhibit positive attachment behaviors with child

- **NURSING INTERVENTIONS/*RATIONALES***

Assess siblings *to identify areas of concern*

Communicate honestly with siblings about child's disease or disability

Provide opportunity for siblings to ask questions and express feelings, but avoid lengthy explanations before they ask *so that they are not overwhelmed*

Help parents talk to siblings about child's condition and interpret siblings' needs and questions

Encourage parents to spend special time with their children who are not ill or disabled

Help siblings and family understand that it is normal for them to sometimes have negative feelings about child

Prepare siblings in advance for any household changes, *since preparation encourages coping*

Allow sibling(s) to participate in child's care and therapy as appropriate

Help siblings learn how to explain child's condition to their peers and others

Acknowledge siblings' strengths and abilities to cope

Refer to sibling groups and networks composed of siblings of children with the same or similar conditions *for ongoing support*

Assess siblings periodically *to determine their adjustment to the family situation*

- **EXPECTED OUTCOMES**

Siblings verbalize or otherwise demonstrate their feelings and concerns

Parents include siblings in discussions about disabled child

Parents make an effort to spend time with other children

Siblings exhibit an understanding of household changes

Siblings assist with affected child's care (specify)

Siblings become involved in support groups (specify)

NURSING DIAGNOSIS: Anxiety/fear related to tests, procedures, hospitalization, etc. (specify)

PATIENT GOAL 1: Will demonstrate understanding of hospitalization, procedures, etc. (specify)

- **NURSING INTERVENTIONS/*RATIONALES***

See Preparation for Procedures, Chapter 22

See Nursing Care Plan: The Child in the Hospital, Chapter 21

- **EXPECTED OUTCOME**

Child copes with stresses of procedures, tests, etc. (specify)

NURSING DIAGNOSIS: High risk for injury (specify)

PATIENT GOAL 1: Will experience no injury

- **NURSING INTERVENTIONS/*RATIONALES***

Assess environment for hazards if indicated

Teach safety precautions *to decrease risk of injury*

Encourage activities that are compatible with the disease or disability

- **EXPECTED OUTCOME**

Child remains free of injury and complications

PATIENT GOAL 2: Will cope with limitations positively

- **NURSING INTERVENTIONS/*RATIONALES***

Help devise alternatives for restricted activities and help child cope with physical limitations *so that child's ability to cope is maximized*

- **EXPECTED OUTCOME**

Child demonstrates appropriate adaptation to limitations (specify)

PATIENT GOAL 3: Will experience no complications

- **NURSING INTERVENTIONS/*RATIONALES***

Stress importance of sound health practices and frequent health supervision *so that complications are less likely to develop*

Make certain child and family understand the therapeutic measures prescribed *to promote optimum health*

Encourage older child to choose activities but take responsibility for own safety

Plan appropriate activities with allied personnel (e.g., teachers, coaches, counselors)

Confer with school nurse (or other person) regarding any special needs of child

Discuss with parents any indicated limit-setting

- **EXPECTED OUTCOME**

Child maintains optimum health

NURSING DIAGNOSIS: Diversional activity deficit related to environmental lack of diversion, physical limitations (specify), hospitalization

---

PATIENT GOAL 1: Will have opportunity to participate in diversionary activities

- **NURSING INTERVENTIONS/*RATIONALES***

Provide appropriate stimulation

Encourage activities appropriate to age, interest, and capabilities of child

Encourage physical exercise that does not overtax child (if indicated)

Continued.

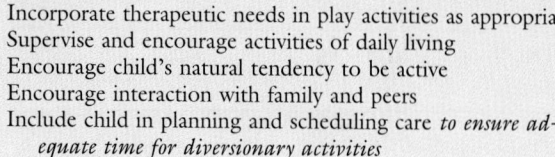

Incorporate therapeutic needs in play activities as appropriate

Supervise and encourage activities of daily living

Encourage child's natural tendency to be active

Encourage interaction with family and peers

Include child in planning and scheduling care *to ensure adequate time for diversionary activities*

• **EXPECTED OUTCOMES**

Child engages in age-appropriate activities within limits of capabilities

Child accepts efforts of family and caregivers

PATIENT GOAL 2: Will engage in appropriate exercise

• **NURSING INTERVENTIONS/RATIONALES**

Encourage child to participate in normal childhood activities commensurate with interests and capabilities

Encourage and reinforce age-appropriate behaviors, experiences, and socialization with peers

Discourage physical inactivity *so that child receives needed exercise*

• **EXPECTED OUTCOME**

Child engages in nonsedentary activities within limits of disability

---

NURSING DIAGNOSIS: Impaired social interaction related to hospitalization, confinement to home, frequent illness, activity intolerance, fatigue (specify)

PATIENT GOAL 1: Will experience positive interpersonal relationships

• **NURSING INTERVENTIONS/RATIONALES**

Encourage child to maintain usual activities

Arrange for continued interpersonal contacts while hospitalized or otherwise confined

Provide opportunities for interaction with others, especially peers *for optimum growth and development*

Encourage regular school attendance, including daycare, beginning school, and return to school

Arrange for rest periods at school if needed *so that child is better able to attend school*

Promote peer contact whenever possible *so that relationships can develop and be maintained*

Encourage recreational outlets and after-school activities appropriate to child's interests and capabilities

Discourage activities that increase isolation from others

• **EXPECTED OUTCOMES**

Child engages in appropriate activities

Child associates with peers and family

Child attends school with reasonable regularity

NURSING DIAGNOSIS: Self-care deficit (specify) related to specific impairment (specify)

PATIENT GOAL 1: Will engage in self-care activities

• **NURSING INTERVENTIONS/RATIONALES**

Teach child about the disease and therapies *to ensure optimum safety and results*

Encourage child to assist in own care as age and capabilities permit

Provide and/or help devise methods to facilitate maximum functioning

Incorporate play that promotes desired behavior *to encourage cooperation and compliance*

Select toys and activities that allow maximum participation by child

Modify environment if needed (specify) *so that child can assume self-care activities*

Assist with self-care activities when needed (specify)

Avoid undue persistence to accomplish a goal

Provide incentives *to achieve desired behavior*

Instruct when to seek assistance from family or health care providers

• **EXPECTED OUTCOME**

Child engages in self-help activities commensurate with capabilities (specify activities and extent of involvement)

PATIENT GOAL 2: Will achieve sense of competence and mastery

• **NURSING INTERVENTIONS/RATIONALES**

Capitalize on child's assets; help child compensate for liabilities

Praise child for accomplishments and "near" accomplishments, such as partial completion of a task, *to encourage sense of competency*

Ensure adequate rest before attempting energy-expending activities

Emphasize child's abilities and focus on realistic endeavors

Emphasize positive coping behaviors

Discourage activities that are beyond child's capabilities; promote and reinforce successful endeavors

Encourage participation in own care to the extent that child is able

Teach and encourage responsibility for use of equipment, appliances, testing, and medication (specify)

Help child become adept at self-management to maximum capabilities

• **EXPECTED OUTCOMES**

Child takes responsibility for self-care according to age and capabilities (specify)

Child engages in appropriate activities without undue fatigue

NURSING DIAGNOSIS: Body image disturbances related to perception of disability (self and others), feeling of differentness, inability to participate in specific activities (specify)

PATIENT GOAL 1: Will maintain positive attitude

• **NURSING INTERVENTIONS/*RATIONALES***

Convey an attitude of understanding, caring, and acceptance *to encourage positive body image*
Maintain open communications with child
Relate to child on appropriate cognitive level
Serve as role model for others *so that they are more accepting*

• **EXPECTED OUTCOME**

Child maintains a positive attitude (specify behaviors)

PATIENT GOAL 2: Will express feelings and concerns

• **NURSING INTERVENTIONS**

Encourage verbalization of feelings and perceptions, especially feelings of "differentness"
Explore feelings concerning disease or disability and its implications: stress of being "different," physical limitations, difficulty competing, relationships with peers, self-image
Encourage child to discuss feelings about how he or she thinks others feel about the disorder

• **EXPECTED OUTCOME**

Child openly discusses feelings and concerns about the condition, therapies, and perceived reactions of others

PATIENT GOAL 3: Will cope with actual or perceived changes caused by illness

• **NURSING INTERVENTIONS/*RATIONALES***

Acknowledge feelings and facilitate sharing feelings with family and other health professionals
Clarify misconceptions child may have acquired
Help child to identify positive aspects of situation *to facilitate coping*

• **EXPECTED OUTCOME**

Child discusses the disorder and feelings regarding limitations imposed by it

PATIENT GOAL 4: Will cope with disorder and its effects

• **NURSING INTERVENTIONS/*RATIONALES***

Help child assess own strengths and assets; emphasize strengths
Identify coping behaviors *so that they can be reinforced*
Support positive coping mechanisms and extinguish negative ones
Help child set realistic goals *to facilitate coping*
Encourage as much independence as condition allows
Introduce child to other children who have adjusted well to this or a similar disorder
Suggest involvement with special groups and facilities for children with similar problems

• **EXPECTED OUTCOMES**

Child identifies own assets and strengths realistically
Child verbalizes positive suggestions for adjusting to the disability
Child becomes involved with special group activities

PATIENT GOAL 5: Will exhibit improved self-esteem and self-concept

• **NURSING INTERVENTIONS/*RATIONALES***

Encourage an appealing physical appearance: good body hygiene, clean straight teeth, good grooming, stylish hair and clothing, makeup for teenage girls
Assist with improving appearance and grooming
Point out positive aspects of own coping, appearance, and other capabilities
Promote constructive thinking in child; encourage child to maximize strengths
Reinforce positive behaviors
Help child to determine and engage in activities that foster self-esteem
Promote independence, *since this is an important part of self-esteem*

• **EXPECTED OUTCOMES**

Child demonstrates a positive appearance and attitude (specify)
Child appears clean, well groomed, and attractively dressed
Child exhibits behaviors that indicate elevated self-esteem (specify)

PATIENT GOAL 6: Will exhibit appropriate sense of control

• **NURSING INTERVENTIONS/*RATIONALES***

Channel need for control and feeling of effectiveness in appropriate directions
Encourage child to monitor own care as appropriate
Provide opportunities for child to make choices and participate in care when appropriate *to ensure sense of control*
Assess child with vocational planning when appropriate

• **EXPECTED OUTCOME**

Child becomes actively involved in own care and management

PATIENT GOAL 7: Will be prepared for discharge

• **NURSING INTERVENTIONS/*RATIONALES***

Begin early in hospitalization to discuss "going home"
Help child develop independence and self-help capabilities
Encourage visits from friends *to help child assess the impact of any change in appearance or behavior that might interfere with returning to previous environments*

• **EXPECTED OUTCOME**

Child verbalizes and otherwise demonstrates interest in going home

See also:
Nursing Care Plan: The Child in the Hospital, Chapter 21
Nursing Care Plan: The Family of the Ill or Hospitalized Child, Chapter 21
Nursing Care Plan: The Child Who Is Terminally Ill or Dying, pp. 561-563

this decision, and help the family explore measures to maintain meaningful communication between family members.

❖ Evaluation

The effectiveness of nursing interventions is determined by continual reassessment and evaluation of care based on the following observational guidelines and expected outcomes:

1. Observe family members' responses to the diagnosis and the types of questions or concerns they have.
2. Interview family regarding their knowledge and understanding of the child's condition; observe if they have instituted suggestions, such as the use of identification devices for children with certain conditions.
3. Observe the response of professionals to reactions such as denial, guilt, and anger and whether supportive interventions are used with the family.
4. Observe family's communication patterns with each other and their ability to discuss feelings about issues such as the impact of the child's condition on the marriage or additional care responsibilities; investigate family's use of services, such as self-help groups or other community resources.
5. Perform a developmental screening test on young children and compare the results to expected milestones for the child's abilities; investigate the use of functional aids to assist children in developing to their potential; question family about the child's attendance at school and interaction with peers.
6. Interview family to determine whether their self-identified needs and concerns have been adequately addressed.

Expected outcomes:
See Nursing Care Plan, pp. 551-555.

NURSING CARE OF THE FAMILY AND CHILD WHO IS TERMINALLY ILL OR DYING

UNEXPECTED CHILDHOOD DEATH

With sudden, unexpected death the family is deprived of any of the advantages of anticipatory grief. There is no opportunity to prepare oneself or others for the death, no time exists to complete "unfinished business," and initial denial may be very strong. Because of this lack of time to prepare, many families feel great guilt and remorse for not having done something additional or different with the child. For example, they may berate themselves for depriving the child of some desired material object or privilege or, more painfully, for not having prevented the sudden death in some way. "If only I'd been a better parent" is a common feeling at this time.

Nursing intervention for families who experience the sudden death of a child must be sensitive to the special needs and concerns of these families. The box outlines four major areas for intervention with survivors of sudden death. Arriving at the hospital and awaiting news of the child's condition is a vulnerable time. The communication of the child's death must be done with great sensitivity, and the physician or nurse should be prepared to handle feelings of denial, guilt, and anger without judgment. Offering an opportunity to view the body, even if it is disfigured, can be important, since a parent's imagined view of the child is often worse than the reality. Informing the family of what to expect when they view the child can lessen the shock. The need for autopsy and the fact that it will not influence an open viewing at a funeral

---

STRATEGIES FOR INTERVENTION WITH SURVIVORS OF SUDDEN CHILDHOOD DEATH

Arrival of the Family

Meet the family immediately and escort to a private area.
A health care worker with bereavement training should remain with the family.
Provide information about the extent of illness or injury and treatment efforts.
If the health care worker must leave the family or the family requests privacy, return in 15 minutes so the family does not feel forgotten.
Provide tissues, telephone, coffee, and a Bible.

Pronouncement of Death

When available, the family's own physician should inform them of the child's death.
Alternatively, the physician or nurse should introduce themselves and establish calm, reassuring eye contact with the parents.
Honest, clear communication that avoids misinterpretation is essential.
Nonverbal communication such as hugging, touching or remaining with the family in silence may be most empathetic.
Acknowledge the family's guilt, attempt to alleviate it, and deal openly and nonjudgmentally with anger.
Provide information, answer questions, and offer reassurance that everything possible was done for the child.

Viewing the Body

Offer the parents the opportunity to see the body; repeat the offer later if they decline.
Before viewing, inform the parents of bodily changes they should expect (tubes, injuries, cold skin).
A single staff member should accompany the family but remain inconspicuous.
Offer the opportunity to hold the child.
Allow the family as much time as they need.
Offer parents the opportunity for siblings to view the body.

Formal Concluding Process

Discuss and answer questions concerning autopsy and funeral arrangements; obtain signatures on the body release and autopsy forms.
Provide anticipatory guidance regarding symptoms of grief response and their normalcy.
Provide written materials about grief symptoms.
Escort the family to the exit or to their car if necessary.
Provide a follow-up phone call in 24 to 48 hours to answer questions and provide support.
Provide referrals to local support and resource groups (e.g., bereavement groups, bereavement counselors, sudden infant death syndrome [SIDS] groups, Parents of Murdered Children, Mothers Against Drunk Driving [MADD]).

Modified from Back K: Sudden, unexpected pediatric death: caring for the parents, *Pediatr Nurs* 17(6):571-574, 1991.

should be explained. Finally, formal closure and follow-up with the family are important.

Families who experience a child's sudden death may experience recurrent memories of both the child and the death experience and may long grieve over missed opportunities (Kachoyeanos and Selder, 1993). Support and resource groups that may be useful to families include the **Sudden Infant Death Syndrome Alliance,*** **National Sudden Infant Death Syndrome Resource Center,†** **American Sudden Infant Death Syndrome Institute,‡** **Mothers Against Drunk Driving,§** and **National Organization of Parents of Murdered Children, Inc.‖**

ANTICIPATED DEATH

When death is anticipated, a *terminal phase,* the time of dying before the actual death, presents the opportunity for the family to make plans in advance, such as where the child should spend the last days or what type of funeral arrangements are desired. When death is unexpected, the shock is sufficient to render the survivors incapable of making even simple decisions. Those in attendance at the death and those caring for the dying child can be instrumental in initiating discussions that may facilitate the grief process.

Especially in the traditional hospital setting, many families are not given the option of terminating treatment when cure is unlikely, and staff may be reluctant to make decisions about "no code" or "do not resuscitate" (DNR) orders (withholding cardiopulmonary resuscitation in response to cardiac arrest). Some of these situations, such as the dying child's right to refuse additional treatment, often pose difficult ethical questions. Of even greater complexity is the cessation of life-sustaining measures, such as artificial ventilation or tube feeding, in patients who are in a persistent vegetative state.

As the group of health professionals who are most involved with families, nurses are in an excellent position to ensure that families are given the options available to them at the time of death. The nurse's first responsibility is to explore the family's wishes and empower them to be sure the wishes are met (see Family Focus box). Statements such as "Tell me about your thoughts for the kind of care you want your child to receive when he [or she] is dying" or "Have you considered the kinds of interventions you would like us to use when your child is near death?" can begin discussion of this sensitive but critical aspect of terminal care.

To make an informed decision, the family needs an honest appraisal of the child's prognosis, especially if the condition is a sudden illness or injury. Nurses can also assist the family in the decision-making process by minimizing environmental stressors, providing relevant information, discussing relief of pain the child may experience, and encouraging the family to use formal and informal sources of support (relatives, pastors, professionals) as they face difficult decisions (Rushton and Glover 1990). If parents choose "no code," they are assured that this does not mean "no care" and that

everything possible will be done to make the child comfortable. For example, the family may want oxygen given to the child for difficult breathing but not want active resuscitation.

 Nursing ALERT Once a decision not to resuscitate is made, it must be communicated to all members of the health team, including a *written* medical order that specifies the exact nature of the treatments that are to be withheld. DNR orders are reviewed on a regular basis.

Another important option for the family should be the choice of hospice* or hospital care for the terminal stage of illness. *Hospital care* refers to the traditional practices of caring for dying patients in an acute care facility; *hospice* is a concept, not necessarily a facility. Hospice services provide palliative care for the child with no reasonable expectation of

---

*Information on hospice services for children is available from the **National Hospice Organization,** 1901 N. Moore St., Arlington, VA 22209; (800) 658-8898. A recommended resource is *Home Care for Seriously Ill Children: A Manual for Parents* by D. Moldow and I. Martinson, available from **Children's Hospice International,** 901 N. Washington St., 7th Floor, Alexandria, VA 22314; (800) 24-CHILD.

FAMILY FOCUS
Family of the Dying Child

No matter whether you have a PhD or you have many children, when your child dies, it is a new experience and nothing can prepare you for it. Like so many things in life, experience is the best teacher.

Three of our children have died, and by the time the third was dying, we handled many things differently. We learned a lot about dignity and the rights of the child and family. For example, at first, we didn't know that we had a right to have our child die at home. We also didn't understand pain medications and that if children are taking these medicines and are still in agony, they have not overdosed on the medication.

We learned a lot about case management. With our first two children, lots of different people were making decisions and disagreeing about what was best and what should be done. No one had primary authority. With our third child, one doctor took a primary role. Any questions and problems were handled by one person. I could call him 24 hours a day. It made a lot of difference, and I felt our concerns and needs were better heard and respected.

The nurses caring for our third child at home enabled me to step back and just be his mommy. When I could do this, I realized that we were fighting so hard for his life that we weren't really letting him die. His nurses had worked with him for a long time and really loved him. It was hard for them when we decided to let him die. In his last several days we wanted a lot of family time with our son, and I think the nurses felt left out. Something about their reaction to our increased time with him in the last few days made us feel guilty. If we had all been able to communicate a little more openly, I would have understood that they needed more time with him at the end, too. Everyone's needs could have been met.

Jeni Stepanek
Mother
Upper Marlboro, MD

---

*10500 Little Patuxent Parkway, Suite 420, Columbia, MD 21044; (800) 221-7437.
†8201 Greensboro Dr., Suite 600, McLean, VA 22102; (703) 821-8955.
‡6065 Roswell Rd., Suite 876, Atlanta, GA 30328; (800) 232-SIDS (in Georgia: [800] 847-SIDS).
§P.O. Box 541688, Dallas, TX 75354-1688; (800) 438-6233.
‖100 E. 8th St., Rm. B41, Cincinnati, OH 45202; (513) 721-5683.

cure so that he or she can live life to the fullest without pain, with choices and dignity, and with family support (Sumner and Hurula, 1993). The three basic ways of providing hospice care are in a hospice, in a facility that employs the hospice concept, or in the child's home. If the home is chosen, the goal is to enable the child and family to have the best possible quality of life until the time of death. The child may or may not die in the home. Nurses working in hospice settings and with children dying at home are critical members of the health team. They often prepare the family for the home care experience, provide psychologic support for the family, and teach the physical care, especially comfort measures, such as pain control (see Chapter 21).

Regardless of where the child is cared for during the terminal stage, both the child and the family usually experience the following fears: (1) fear of what the actual death will be like, (2) fear of dying alone or not being present when the child dies, and (3) fear of pain. Nurses play a major role in managing care so that each of these fears is lessened. Although no one can predict exactly what the child's death will be like, the nurse can explore the family's expectations, clarify misconceptions, and supply information based on how the death is most likely to occur. Since the child and family have fears of isolation and loneliness, their wishes to be together must be respected (Fig. 18-6). If the family members temporarily leave the child's room, they need reassurance that they will be summoned if the child's condition worsens (see box for signs of approaching death).

All parents want their child's death to be comfortable, and no nursing intervention is more important than control of

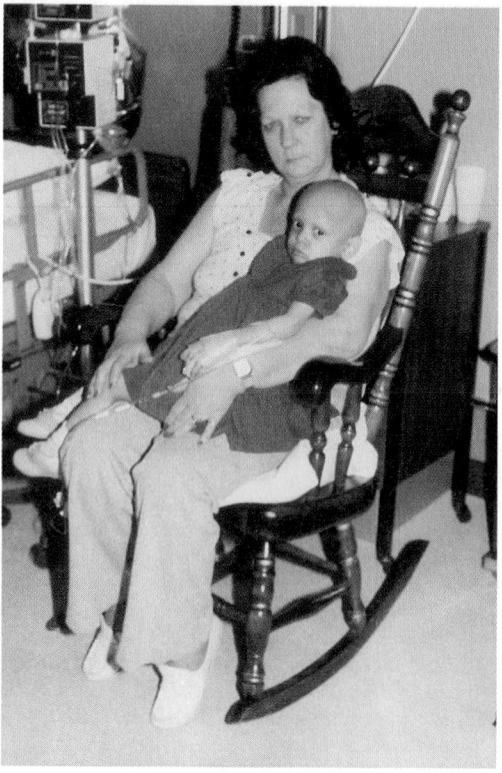

FIG. 18-6. For the dying child there is no greater comfort than the security and closeness of a parent.

pain. Pain is managed on a *preventive schedule,* with adjustments made as needed to provide maximum comfort. Optimum pain relief requires using opioid analgesics such as morphine, increasing doses of opioids as needed, decreasing the duration between doses, and changing routes of administration to comply with the child's needs and wishes. Whenever possible, the oral route is preferred, but when that is no longer possible, continuous intravenous or subcutaneous infusion may provide the greatest benefit. Any nonpharmacologic measures that may augment pain relief and promote relaxation are employed, such as cutaneous stimulation (e.g., rocking or stroking the skin) or diversion (e.g., reading to the child or playing music). (See also Chapter 21 for a discussion of pain assessment and management.)

The experience of a child with life-threatening illness and/or the child's death has profound effects on the family, including the siblings. Parents may turn to nurses for advice on how to inform siblings of a child's impending death and how to incorporate siblings into the child's final days. When a brother or sister dies, the sibling's reaction will depend on many factors, including the circumstances of the death, the quality of the prior sibling relationship, the age of the child, parental reactions, and family communication patterns (Gibbons, 1992).

Predominant feelings of children when a sibling's diagnosis is potentially fatal, such as serious trauma or a disease such as cancer, include isolation and displacement. The parents devote most their time to care for the ill or injured child, causing the siblings to feel left out of the parent/sick child partnership and regarded as unimportant family members.

Siblings may also express concern for their own health status, recognizing the possibility of death and at times manifesting physical symptoms similar to those of the child. Siblings' knowledge of the ill child's diagnosis is often inadequate, although many children perceive cancer to be the "scariest disease" (Martinson and others, 1990).

Sibling's responses to death arise in part from their cognitive understanding of death. Two common feelings are guilt and shame. Books and articles can be used to help children deal with death (see Bibliography, Terminal Illness/Death).

AT THE TIME OF DEATH

As death approaches, the nurse should both recognize and assist the family to recognize the physical signs (see box) and institute appropriate care to make the death as peaceful as possible (see Nursing Care Plan, pp. 561-563). The nurse should explain everything that is being done to make the child comfortable, even if the child does not appear to be coherent. The nurse can offer support to the family by visiting frequently, sitting quietly with them, and attending to their needs, such as bringing them some nourishment. Immediately after the death the family is encouraged to stay with the child as long as they wish. Many parents want to hold or rock the child one last time.

A topic that should be considered when a child dies is tissue donation. For some families this may be a meaningful act—one that benefits another human being despite the loss of their child. In centers where transplants are performed, a full-time transplant coordinator is usually available to inform the family about organ donation and to take care of details. If a transplant coordinator's services are not available, the

---

PHYSICAL SIGNS OF APPROACHING DEATH

Loss of sensation and movement in the lower extremities, progressing toward the upper body
Sensation of heat, although body feels cool
Loss of senses:
    Tactile sensation decreases
    Sensitive to light
    Hearing is last sense to fail
Confusion, loss of consciousness, slurred speech
Muscle weakness
Loss of bowel and bladder control
Decreased appetite/thirst
Difficulty swallowing
Change in respiratory pattern:
    Cheyne-Stokes respirations (waxing and waning of depth of breathing with regular periods of apnea)
    "Death rattle" (noisy chest sounds from accumulation of pulmonary and pharyngeal secretions)
Weak, slow pulse; decreased blood pressure

FAMILY FOCUS
Children Need to Say Good-Bye

As a nurse/grief counselor, I conduct grief workshops with children who have experienced the death of someone special. Children often communicate their feelings of being excluded through drawings. They may draw a picture of the dying person in a hospital bed that is raised too high for them to see the person's face clearly. Sometimes children reveal that they did not get to say good-bye because a family member told them, for example, "You don't want to see your grandma this way. She is too sick for you to visit." If the special person died at home, the children had to stay in their room when the funeral home staff took away the body.

I have learned never to underestimate the importance of allowing children to be involved with the dying person and the significance of a child's loss. Once, when I asked a 6-year old girl to draw a picture with the theme, "This is what I was doing when my _____ died," she drew a picture and completed the sentence with "when my *home* died." Her grandmother had been like her mother; to the child, her home was gone. We need to give children the choice of being included in the family's activities of saying good-bye.

    Barbara Bilderback, MS, MA, RN
    Bereavement Supervisor, Saint Francis Hospice
    Tulsa, OK

---

staff needs to decide which members should discuss this topic with the family. Ideally this should be the person who knows the family best, knows when the death is expected, or has the opportunity to spend time with the family when the death is unexpected. Often nurses are in an optimum position to suggest tissue donation after consultation with the attending physician. The request should be made in a private and quiet area of the hospital and should be simple and direct, with questions such as "Are you a donor family?" "Have you ever considered organ donation?" or "Did [the child's name] ever express such a wish?"* Words such as "options" or "choices" should be used to reiterate that the decision is theirs and that no pressure will be applied. Family members should also be reassured that everything possible has been done or is being done to save their child (Cerney, 1993). Finally, written consent is required. Any number of body tissues or organs can be donated (skin, eyes, bone, kidney, heart, liver, pancreas), and their removal does not mutilate or desecrate the body or cause any suffering. The family may have an open casket, and there is no delay in the funeral. There is no cost to the donor family.

In cases of unexplained death, violent death, or suspected suicide, autopsy is required by law. In other instances it may be optional, and parents should be informed of this choice. The procedure, as well as forms that require signing, should be explained. The family should know that the child can be in an open casket after an autopsy.

At some point the nurse should discuss if the family has made preparations for the burial service and if the staff can help in any way. Parents often have concerns about the funeral, such as siblings' involvement in the death rituals. Although no absolute answers exist regarding the question of siblings attending the funeral or burial services, the general consensus is that the surviving children benefit from being involved in these events. However, children need preparation for postdeath services. They should be told what to expect,

particularly how the deceased person will look if the coffin is open, allowed their private time to say good-bye, and permitted to stay as long as they wish. Ideally the parents should prepare the siblings. If the parents' grief prevents this communication, a significant family member or friend should substitute (see Family Focus box).

POSTDEATH

The crisis of loss does not end with the child's death. In many ways it only begins. Unfortunately, the child's death often marks the close of the family's contacts with health professionals involved in the care. Consequently, many of these families never receive the support and guidance that could assist them in resolving the loss. Fortunately, hospice programs recognize this need and provide regular follow-up after the death. In addition, self-help groups are present in many communities (e.g., **The Compassionate Friends,*** an international organization for bereaved parents and siblings, and specialty groups such as **Parents of Murdered Children†**).

Follow-up can help the family understand the process of mourning, particularly its duration and pain, and can provide assistance in making decisions that involve the loss. One especially difficult dilemma faced by many parents is the decision to have additional children. The advisability of having another child soon after the death is controversial. Consequently, the nurse's role is not to give answers but to assist parents in assessing their readiness for another pregnancy through knowledge of the parents' progress through grief and their motivations for conceiving.

---

*Information about being an organ donor is available from **The Living Bank**, P.O. Box 6725, Houston, TX 77265, (800) 528-2971; and **The United Network for Organ Sharing (UNOS)**, (800) 24-DONOR.

*P.O. Box 3696, Oak Brook, IL 60522-3696; (708) 990-0010.
†100 E. 8th St., Rm. B41, Cincinnati, OH 45202; (513) 721-5683.

At times family members may need assistance in their grieving (see Guidelines box). Mothers, in particular, often feel a great sense of loneliness and emptiness, and part of their resolving the grief is finding a substitute role that is fulfilling and rewarding. Nurses can be instrumental in this process by

GUIDELINES
Supporting Grieving Families*

General

Stay with the family; sit quietly if they prefer not to talk; cry with them if desired.

Accept the family's grief reactions; avoid judgmental statements (e.g., "You should be feeling better by now").

Avoid offering rationalizations for the child's death (e.g., "You should be glad your child isn't suffering anymore").

Avoid artificial consolation (e.g., "I know how you feel," or "You are still young enough to have another baby").

Deal openly with feelings such as guilt, anger, and loss of self-esteem.

Focus on feelings by using a feeling word in the statement (e.g., "You're still feeling all the pain of losing a child").

Refer the family to an appropriate self-help group or for professional help if needed.

At the Time of Death

Reassure the family that everything possible is being done for the child, if they want lifesaving interventions.

Do everything possible to ensure the child's comfort, especially relieving pain.

Provide the child and family with the opportunity to review special experiences or memories in their lives.

Express personal feelings of loss and/or frustrations (e.g., "We will miss him so much," "We tried everything; we feel so sorry that we couldn't save her").

Provide information that the family requests and be honest.

Respect the emotional needs of family members, such as siblings, who may need brief respites from the dying child.

Make every effort to arrange for family members, especially parents, to be with the child at the moment of death, if they want to be present.

Allow the family to stay with the dead child for as long as they wish and to rock, hold, or bathe the child.

Provide practical help when possible, such as collecting the child's belongings.

Arrange for spiritual support, such as clergy; pray with the family if no one else can stay with them.

Postdeath

Attend the funeral or visitation if there was a special closeness with the family.

Initiate and maintain contact (e.g., sending cards, telephoning, inviting them back to the unit, making a home visit).

Refer to the dead child by name; discuss shared memories with the family.

Discourage the use of drugs or alcohol as a method of escaping grief.

Encourage all family members to communicate their feelings rather than remaining silent to avoid upsetting another member.

Emphasize that grieving is a painful process that often takes years to resolve.

*"Family" refers to all significant persons involved in the child's life, such as the parents, siblings, grandparents, or other close relatives or friends.

(1) preparing the mother for anticipating the *normal* feelings of emptiness, loneliness, and sometimes even failure; (2) helping her reevaluate her role as parent and spouse, stressing that giving up the lost child must occur before she can reestablish emotional relationships; (3) encouraging her to explore fulfilling activities that utilize her special interests, talents, and qualifications; and (4) supporting her as her role changes, particularly assisting with communication between affected family members.

Nurses should also be aware of behaviors that indicate siblings' difficulty with resolving their grief, such as persistent blame and guilt, patterns of overactivity with aggressive and destructive outbursts, compulsive caregiving, persistent anxieties (e.g., fear of another family death or of their own), excessive clinging to the parent, difficulty with forming new relationships, problems at school, or delinquency (e.g., stealing). Providing anticipatory guidance to parents regarding behaviors to watch for may be helpful. Even siblings as young as 2 years of age can experience survivor guilt (Gibbons, 1992). In these situations, professional assistance may be required, and the nurse can provide appropriate referral.

 In a study of adolescent reactions to a sibling's death, fathers' perceptions of their teenagers' reactions were more accurate and reliable than mothers' perceptions (Hogan and Balk, 1990). This observation stresses the importance of including fathers in follow-up family assessments.

Communication with the bereaved family is essential, but often there is a feeling of not knowing what to say and of helplessness in offering words of comfort. The most supportive approach is to avoid judging the family's reactions or offering advice or rationalizations and to focus on feelings. Perhaps the most valuable supportive measure the nurse can perform for families is to listen (Parkman, 1992). Families understand that no words will relieve their pain; all they want is acceptance, understanding, and respect for their grief. A plan for regular follow-up with bereaved families can be beneficial.

It is important for families to understand that mourning takes a long time. Whereas acute grief may last only weeks or months, resolving the loss is measured in years. Holidays and anniversaries can be particularly difficult, and people who previously had been supportive may now expect the family to have "adjusted." Consequently, prolonged mourning is often silent and lonely.

Many families never receive the support and guidance that could help them resolve the loss. At a minimum, one follow-up phone call or meeting with the family should be arranged, possibly 1 month after the child's death, to give the family time to overcome the phase of shock and disbelief (Jankovic and others, 1989). Families can also be referred to self-help groups. When such groups are not available, nurses can be instrumental in networking families or facilitating parent and sibling groups. Formal bereavement programs or bereavement counseling can be helpful as well.*

*A manual that can be useful in the development of a family-centered bereavement program is *Whispers of Hope: A Hospital-Based Program for Bereaved Parents and Their Families* by T. Rose and E.S. Stewart (1993), available from Duke University Pediatric Brain Tumor Family Support Program, Durham, NC 27710; (919) 684-5301.

NURSING DIAGNOSIS: Altered growth and development related to terminal illness and/or impending death

PATIENT GOAL 1: Will receive adequate support during terminal phase

• **NURSING INTERVENTIONS/*RATIONALES***

Encourage family to remain near child as much as possible *to provide support through their presence*

Encourage child to talk about feelings; help family as they encourage child to express feelings

Provide safe, acceptable outlets for aggression

Answer questions as honestly as possible while maintaining a positive, hopeful approach

Explain all procedures and therapies, especially physical effects child will experience

Help child distinguish between consequences of therapies and manifestations of disease process

Structure hospital environment to allow for maximum self-control and independence within the limitations imposed by child's developmental level and physical condition

Respect child's need for privacy without neglecting child

Provide for presence of customary support systems

• **EXPECTED OUTCOMES**

Child expresses feelings freely

Child demonstrates an understanding of symptoms

PATIENT GOAL 2: Will exhibit minimal or no evidence of physical discomfort

• **NURSING INTERVENTIONS/*RATIONALES***

Appreciate that pain control is essential component of physical and emotional care during terminal stage

Provide pain relief around the clock *to prevent the recurrence of pain*

Encourage family to provide comfort measures child prefers (e.g., rocking, stroking)

Avoid excessive noise or light *that may irritate child*

Place all commodities within easy reach *to increase child's control and lessen need for excessive movement*

Use gentle, minimal physical manipulation

Avoid pressure (bedclothes, sheets) on painful areas

Experiment with using heat or cold on painful areas *(use cautiously because of easy skin breakdown)*

Whenever possible, make use of procedures (e.g., noninvasive temperature monitoring) *to minimize discomfort*

Change position frequently; if difficult for child, coordinate with pain relief from analgesics *to make moving easier and less distressing*

Avoid pressure on bony prominences or painful sites (water bed, flotation mattress); ensure good body alignment *to prevent skin breakdown*

Keep fresh air circulating in room (open window, use small fan)

Use pillows or other supports to prop child in comfortable position

Carry child (if possible) to other areas for diversion if desired

Place absorbent pads under hips *because child may be incontinent*

Help child to toilet if desired

Limit care to essentials

May need to forego usual hygienic measures such as bath or clothing change but provide comfort measures (e.g., mouth care, wiping forehead, gentle back rub)

*Administer anticholinergic drugs (atropine or scopolamine) *to reduce secretions (lessens "death rattle," which can be distressing to family)*

• **EXPECTED OUTCOME**

Child exhibits minimal or no evidence of physical discomfort

PATIENT GOAL 3: Will receive adequate emotional support at time of dying

• **NURSING INTERVENTIONS/*RATIONALES***

Preserve child's physical closeness with family members (e.g., parent may want to rock child in chair or lie next to child in bed)

Teach family about supportive interventions

Talk to child even though child may not appear to be awake

Position self and others where child can easily see face (e.g., sit at head of bed)

Speak to child in clear, distinct voice; avoid whispering

Avoid conversation about child in child's presence *to reduce anxiety/fear*

Offer calm reassurance and orient child to surroundings when awake

Phrase questions for "yes" or "no" answers *to conserve energy*

Avoid repeated measurements of vital signs, *which only disturb child*

Play favorite music *(may soothe child)*

• **EXPECTED OUTCOME**

Child appears calm and relaxed

NURSING DIAGNOSIS: Altered nutrition: less than body requirements related to loss of appetite, disinterest in food

PATIENT GOAL 1: Will receive optimum nutrition

• **NURSING INTERVENTIONS/*RATIONALES***

Offer any food and fluids child desires

Provide small meals and snacks several times a day

Avoid excessive encouragement to eat or drink

Avoid foods with strong odors *because they may cause nausea*

Provide pleasant environment for eating

Serve foods that require the least energy to eat (soups, shakes)

Feed slowly *to conserve energy*

*Administer antiemetic as prescribed if nausea/vomiting is a problem

Provide mouth care before and after eating; lubricate lips with petrolatum *to prevent cracking and promote comfort*

• **EXPECTED OUTCOME**

Child consumes some nutrients

*Dependent nursing action.

Continued.

NURSING CARE PLAN
The Child Who Is Terminally Ill or Dying—cont'd

NURSING DIAGNOSIS: Fear/anxiety related to diagnosis, tests, therapies and prognosis

PATIENT GOAL 1: Will experience reduction of anxiety

- **NURSING INTERVENTIONS/RATIONALES**

Limit interventions to palliation only; discuss need for non-palliative treatment with family and physician

Explain all procedures and other aspects of care to child *to reduce anxiety/fear*

Remain with child or provide for constant attendance

Determine what child has been told about prognosis *so this information can be reinforced*

Determine what family wants child to know about prognosis

Emphasize importance of honesty

Answer child's questions as openly and honestly as possible

Involve parents in child's care

Remain nonjudgmental regarding child's behavior

- **EXPECTED OUTCOME**

Child discusses fears without evidence of stress

NURSING DIAGNOSIS: Anticipatory grieving related to potential loss of a child

PATIENT (FAMILY) GOAL 1: Will receive adequate support

- **NURSING INTERVENTIONS/RATIONALES**

Discuss the grieving process with family *so that family better understands normalcy of feelings*

Provide opportunities for family to express emotions

Help parents deal with their feelings, *allowing them more emotional reserve to meet the needs of their children*

Encourage parents to remain as near to child as possible, yet be sensitive to parents' needs

Provide information regarding child's status and anticipated reactions *to decrease anxiety/fear*

Help parents to understand behavioral reactions of their children, especially that concern for present crisis, such as loss of hair, may be much greater than for future ones, including possible death

Facilitate family's assistance with child's care

Provide comfort measures for child and family

Encourage family to maintain own health care needs

Provide as much privacy as possible

Assist family in assessing their need for referral services (e.g., hospice services, specific organizations for grieving families)

Encourage parents to answer questions about dying honestly rather than avoiding questions or using euphemisms

Encourage parents to share their moments of sorrow with their children

---

Discuss with parents appropriate involvement of siblings

Identify religious and cultural beliefs related to death (e.g., prayer, rites, rituals)

Provide preparation for postdeath services

Discuss with family their preferences for care if death is imminent

Arrange for appropriate spiritual care in accordance with family's beliefs and/or affiliations

Maintain contact with family

Provide support for families who choose home care for their child

See Guidelines box on p. 541

- **EXPECTED OUTCOMES**

Family expresses fear, concerns, and any special desires for terminal child

Family demonstrates an understanding of child and his or her needs (specify)

Family members avail themselves of services as desired

See also:

Nursing Care Plan: The Child in the Hospital, Chapter 21

Nursing Care Plan: The Family of the Ill or Hospitalized Child, Chapter 21

PATIENT GOAL 2: Will exhibit no evidence of loneliness

- **NURSING INTERVENTIONS/RATIONALES**

Offer calm reassurance to child

Reassure child of the love of others

Continue to set some limits for child *to provide a sense of security*

Spend time with child when not directly involved in care

Reinforce to child that what is happening is not child's fault *to decrease feelings of guilt*

Involve child in routine activities as tolerated

Maintain a "normal" atmosphere

Play favorite music and read stories to child

Orient child to surroundings when child is awake

Phrase questions for "yes" or "no" answers when possible *to conserve child's energy*

- **EXPECTED OUTCOME**

Child exhibits no evidence of loneliness

NURSING DIAGNOSIS: Anticipatory grieving related to imminent death of a child

PATIENT (FAMILY) GOAL 1: Will receive adequate support

- **NURSING INTERVENTIONS/RATIONALES**

Be available to family

Inform family of what to expect at time of death

Convey an attitude of caring for both child and family

NURSING CARE PLAN

The Child Who Is Terminally Ill or Dying—cont'd

Encourage at least one family member to stay with child

Help family to provide care of child as they desire without forcing involvement

*Administer medications or other agents as prescribed *to reduce unpleasant manifestations*

Oxygen *for respiratory distress*

Anticonvulsants *for seizures*

Anticholinergic drugs *to reduce secretions ("death rattle")*

Analgesics *for pain*

Stool softeners/laxatives *for constipation*

Antiemetics *for nausea/vomiting*

Help and encourage family to express feelings appropriately

Encourage family to meet their own physical needs

Provide privacy

Provide for physical comfort of family

Provide emotional support and comfort to family

Encourage family to talk to child

Involve family and other children in decision making whenever possible, especially regarding alternatives for terminal care (hospital, home, hospice)

Support and assist family in giving explanations to other family members regarding child's status

*Dependent nursing action.

Maintain nonjudgmental attitude toward behavior of family members

• **EXPECTED OUTCOMES**

Family members discuss their feelings

Family members are actively involved in child's care

PATIENT (FAMILY) GOAL 2: Will receive adequate support for home care

• **NURSING INTERVENTIONS/RATIONALES**

Teach family physical care of child

Provide family with means for contacting health professionals at any time (e.g., phone numbers)

Maintain daily contact with family (e.g., telephone call, home visit)

Refer to community agencies as appropriate *for ongoing support*

Reassure family that they can readmit child to the hospital at any time

Help plan with family what to do when the child dies and what to expect

• **EXPECTED OUTCOMES**

Family demonstrates ability to provide care for child

Family is in contact with appropriate support groups

NURSES' REACTIONS TO CARING FOR DYING CHILDREN

The death of a patient is one of the most stressful aspects of critical care or oncology nursing (see Family Focus box). Nurses experience reactions to a fatal illness that are very similar to the responses of family members, including denial, anger, depression, guilt, and ambivalent feelings.

Strategies that can assist the nurse in maintaining the ability to work effectively in these settings include maintaining good general health, developing well-rounded interests, using distancing techniques such as taking time off when needed, developing and using professional and personal support systems, cultivating the capacity for empathy, focusing on the positive aspects of the caregiver role, and basing nursing interventions on sound theory and empiric observations. Attending shared-remembrance rituals assists some nurses in resolving grief (Zappa and Parks, 1993). Similarly, attending the funeral services can be a supportive act for both the family and the nurse and in no way detracts from the professionalism of care.

FAMILY FOCUS
A Dying Child: A Nurse's Perspective

Claire was unresponsive with slow, gasping breathing. Her mother asked me what I thought was happening. I replied honestly, "Your baby is dying because of her brain tumor." The mother put her arms around me and cried. We arranged for Claire to be baptized.

Honesty. Painful as the loss of a child is, my job is to assist the family through this experience. Although I usually wait until a private moment, such as driving home, I found tears streaming down my face as family and friends gathered for Claire's baptism. I went into the kitchen to compose myself, only to find several of my colleagues crying as well. Saying good-bye to a dying child will always be a difficult but shared experience.

Jeanne O'Connor Egan, RN, MSN
Pediatric clinical specialist, Children's Hospital
Washington, DC

KEY POINTS

- Trends in the treatment of children with chronic illness or disability have focused on developmental age, the child's strengths and uniqueness, family-centered care, establishment of normalization, early discharge, home care, mainstreaming, and early intervention.
- Families' reactions to disability or chronic illness are manifested in the following stages: shock and denial, adjustment, reintegration, and acknowledgment.
- Assessment of the family's adjustment to a child's chronic illness, disability, or death includes the availability of a support system, their perception of the event, their coping mechanisms, concurrent stressors, and their response to the child.
- To help parents cope with their child's chronic illness or disability, nurses must offer attentiveness, humanistic support, solicitation of suggestions for care, facilitation of communication, verbalization of feelings, and referral to volunteer and community agencies.
- Supporting the child involves encouraging self-expression, alleviating feelings of being different, and strengthening self-image.
- In response to the child with chronic illness or disability, parents may be affected by feelings of inadequacy and failure; excessive demands on time, energy, and financial resources; and strain on the marital relationship.
- Acute grief is a syndrome with intense and distressing psychologic and somatic symptoms that appear at the time of death.
- Mourning is a prolonged, painful process that consists of four phases: shock and disbelief, expression of grief, disorganization and despair, and reorganization.
- The child's reaction to illness or disability depends on developmental level, coping mechanisms, others' reactions, and the illness itself.
- Children's concept of death is determined by their cognitive ability and their experience with life-threatening illness.
- Young children see death as temporary and reversible and mainly fear separation.
- School-age children view death as irreversible but not necessarily inevitable and may fear mutilation.
- Children beyond 9 to 10 years of age realize death is irreversible, universal, and inevitable but may resist the thought of their own death.
- Siblings have special needs, including the need for information, reassurance about their own health status, assurance that they are not responsible for the illness or death, and support for their own grieving process.
- Special needs of the family facing the unexpected death of a child include support while awaiting news of the child's status; a sensitive pronouncement of death; acknowledgment of feelings of denial, guilt, and anger; an opportunity to view the body; closure; and referrals for support.
- Special decisions at the time of dying and death may involve hospital or hospice care, the child's right to die, visualization of the body, tissue donation and autopsy, and siblings' attendance at the funeral.
- In dealing with stress related to the dying patient, the nurse can cope successfully through self-awareness, consciousness raising, knowledge and practice, available support system, maintaining general good health, and focusing on the positive rewards of involvement with dying children and their families.

REFERENCES

Ahmann E, Bond NJ: Promoting normal development in school age children and adolescents who are technology dependent: a family centered model, *Pediatr Nurs* 18(4):399-405, 1992.

Austin J, Patterson J, Huberty T: Development of the Coping Health Inventory for Children, *J Pediatr Nurs* 6(3):166-174, 1991.

Baker NA: Avoiding collisions with challenging families, *MCN Am J Matern Child Nurs* 19:97-101, 1994.

Bishop KK, Woll J, Arango P: *Family/professional collaboration for children with special health care needs,* Burlington, 1993, Department of Social Work, University of Vermont.

Bluebond-Langner M: Worlds of dying children and their well siblings, *Death Stud* 13:1-16, 1989.

Breitmayer BJ and others: Social competence of school aged children with chronic illnesses, *J Pediatr Nurs* 7(3):181-188, 1992.

Burns CE, Madian N: Experiences with a support group for grandparents of children with disabilities, *Pediatr Nurs* 18(1):17, 1992.

Cancer facts and figures—1994, Atlanta, 1994, American Cancer Society.

Cerney MS: Solving the organ donor shortage by meeting the bereaved family's needs, *Crit Care Nurs* 13(1):32-36, 1993.

Clements D, Copeland L, Loftus M: Critical times for families with a chronically ill child, *Pediatr Nurs* 16(2):157-161, 224, 1990.

Clubb R: Chronic sorrow: adaptation patterns of parents with chronically ill children, *Pediatr Nurs* 17(5):461-466, 1991.

Corr CA: Coping with dying: lessons that we should and should not learn from the work of Elisabeth Kübler-Ross, *Death Stud* 17(1):69-83, 1993.

Dixon DM: *Parent participation during hospitalization: understanding differences,* Unpublished manuscript, Springfield, IL, 1993, Memorial Medical Center.

Ferrell BR and others: The experience of pediatric cancer pain. Part I. Impact of pain on the family, *J Pediatr Nurs* 9(6):368-379, 1994.

Fisman S, Wolf L: The handicapped child: psychological effects of parental, marital, and sibling relationships, *Psychiatr Clin North Am* 14(1):199-217, 1991.

Gallo AM and others: Well siblings of children with chronic illness: parent's reports of their psychologic adjustment, *Pediatr Nurs* 18(1):23-29, 1992.

Garmezy N: Resilience in children's adaptation to negative life events and stressed environments, *Pediatr Ann* 20(9):459-466, 1991.

Gibbons MB: A child dies, a child survives: the impact of sibling loss, *J Pediatr Health Care* 6(2):65-72, 1992.

Groce NE, Zola IK: Multiculturalism, chronic illness, and disability, *Pediatrics* 91(5):1048-1055, 1993.

Hills RG, Lutkenhoff ML: Social skills group for physically challenged school-age children, *Pediatr Nurs* 19(6):573-577, 1993.

Hogan NS, Balk DE: Adolescent reactions to sibling death: perceptions of mothers, fathers, and teenagers, *Nurs Res* 39(2):103-106, 1990.

Huber C, Holditch-Davis D, Brandon D: High risk preterm infants at 3 years of age: parental response to the presence of developmental problems, *Child Health Care* 22(2):107, 124, 1993.

Jankovic M and others: Meetings with parents after the death of their child from leukemia, *Pediatr Hematol Oncol* 6:155-160, 1989.

Kachoyeanos MK, Selder FE: Life transitions of parents at the unexpected death of a school-age and older child, *J Pediatr Nurs* 8(1):41-49, 1993.

Kübler-Ross E: *On death and dying*, New York, 1969, Macmillan.

Martinson IM and others: Impact of childhood cancer on healthy school-age siblings, *Cancer Nurs* 13(3):183-190, 1990.

May J: *Fathers of children with special needs: new horizons*, Washington, DC, 1990, Association for the Care of Children's Health.

Newacheck PW, McManus MA, Fox HB: Prevalence and impact of chronic illness among adolescents, *Am J Dis Child* 145(12):1367-1373, 1991.

Newacheck PW, Stoddard JJ, McManus M: Ethnocultural variations in the prevalence and impact of childhood chronic conditions, *Pediatrics* 91(5):1031-1039, 1993.

Parkman S: Helping families say good-bye, *MCN Am J Matern Child Nurs* 17(1):14-17, 1992.

Rushton CH, Glover JJ: Involving parents in decisions to forego life-sustaining treatment for critically ill infants and children, *AACN Clin Issues Crit Care Nurs* 1(1):206-214, 1990.

Satariano HJ, Briggs NJ: The good family syndrome, *Pediatr Nurs* 15(3):285-286, 1989.

Savinetti-Rose B: Developmental issues in managing children with diabetes, *Pediatr Nurs* 20(1):11-15, 1994.

Stein REK: Home care: a challenging opportunity, *Child Health Care* 14(2):90-95, 1985.

Sumner L, Hurula J: Pediatric hospice nursing: making the most of each moment, *Nursing '93*, Aug 1993, pp 50-55.

Turner-Henson A and others: The experiences of discrimination: challenges for chronically ill children, *Pediatr Nurs* 20(6):571-577, 1994.

Yoos HL: Children's illness concepts: old and new paradigms, *Pediatr Nurs* 20(2):134-140, 1994.

Zappa S, Parks G: A remembrance ceremony to help families and staff work through the grieving process, *J Pediatr Oncol Nurs* 10(2):65-66, 1993 (abstract).

BIBLIOGRAPHY

Chronic Illness/Disability

Ahmann E, Lierman C: Promoting normal development in technology dependent children: an introduction to the issues, *Pediatr Nurs* 18(2):143-148, 1992.

Ahmann E, Lipsi K: Developmental assessment of the technology dependent infant and young child, *Pediatr Nurs* 18(3):299-305, 1992.

American Academy of Pediatrics, Committee on Children with Disabilities: Pediatric services for infants and children with special health care needs, *Pediatrics* 92(1):163-165, 1993.

Baker NA: Avoiding collisions with challenging families, *MCN Am J Matern Child Nurs* 19:97-101, 1994.

Bluebond-Langner M and others: Children's knowledge of cancer and its treatment: impact of an oncology camp experience, *J Pediatr* 116(2):207-213, 1990.

Bossert E, Martinson I: Kinetic family drawings—revised: a method of determining the impact of cancer on the family as perceived by the child with cancer, *J Pediatr Nurs* 5(3):204-213, 1990.

Bossert E and others: Strategies of normalization used by parents of chronically ill school-age children, *Child Adolesc Psychiatr Ment Health Nurs* 3(2):57-61, 1990.

Brookins GK: Culture, ethnicity, and bicultural competence: implications for children with chronic illness and disability, *Pediatrics* 91(5, Pt 2):1056-1062, 1993.

Burke S, Roberts C: Nursing research and the care of chronically ill and disabled children, *J Pediatr Nurs* 5(5):316-327, 1990.

Cardoso P: Family-centered care, *Child Health Care* 20(4):258-260, 1991.

Chambas K: Sexual concerns of adolescents with cancer, *J Pediatr Oncol Nurs* 8(4):165-172, 1991.

Clark HB and others: A social skills development model: coping strategies for children with chronic illness, *Child Health Care* 18(1):19-29, 1989.

Cooper E: Helping parents cope with the reality of parenting a child with a disabling condition, *Child Health Care* 20(3):189-190, 1991.

Crowley A: Integrating handicapped and chronically ill children into day care centers, *Pediatr Nurs* 16(1):39-44, 1990.

Davis B, Steele S: Case management for young children with special health care needs, *Pediatr Nurs* 17(1):15-19, 1991.

Davis P, May J: Involving fathers in early intervention and family support programs: issues and strategies, *Child Health Care* 20(2):87-92, 1991.

Deatrick JA, Knafl KA: Management behaviors: day-to-day adjustments to childhood chronic conditions, *J Pediatr Nurs* 5(1):15-22, 1990.

Diehl S, Moffitt K, Wade S: Focus group interview with parents of children with medically complex needs: an intimate look at their perceptions and feelings, *Child Health Care* 20(3):170-178, 1991.

Faux S: Sibling relationships in families with congenitally impaired children, *J Pediatr Nurs* 6(3):175-184, 1991.

Fraley A: Chronic sorrow: a parental response, *J Pediatr Nurs* 5(4):268-273, 1990.

Gallo AM and others: Stigma in childhood chronic illness: a well sibling perspective, *Pediatr Nurs* 17(1):21-25, 1991.

Heiney SP and others: Lasting impressions: a psychosocial support program for adolescents with cancer and their parents, *Cancer Nurs* 13(1):13-20, 1990.

Hewson M and others: Comprehensive team care, *MCN Am J Matern Child Nurs* 18(4):198-205, 1993.

Hixson D, Stoff E, White P: Parents of children with chronic health impairments: a new approach to advocacy training, *Child Health Care* 21(2):111-115, 1992.

Hockenberry-Eaton M, Minick P: Living with cancer: children with extraordinary courage, *Oncol Nurs Forum* 21(6):1025-1031, 1994.

Jackson B, Finkler D, Robinson C: A case management system for infants with chronic illnesses and developmental disabilities, *Child Health Care* 21(4):224-232, 1992.

Jackson P, Vessey J: *Primary care of the child with a chronic condition,* ed 2, St Louis, 1996, Mosby.

Jellinek MS and others: Coping with the truly difficult parent, *Contemp Pediatr* 8(2):19-49, 1991.

Knafl KA and others: Learning from stories: parents' accounts of the pathway to diagnosis, *Pediatr Nurs* 21(5):411-415, 1995.

Knafl KA and others: Parent's views of health care providers: an exploration of the components of a positive working relationship, *Child Health Care* 21(2):90-95, 1992.

Krahn GL, Hallum A, Kime C: Are there good ways to give bad news? *Pediatrics* 91(3):578-582, 1993.

Liptak GS, Weitzman M: Children with chronic conditions need your help at school, *Contemp Pediatr* 12(9):64-80, 1995.

Meeropol E: One of the gang: sexual development of adolescents with physical disabilities, *J Pediatr Nurs* 6(4):243-250, 1991.

Patterson JM and others: Caring for medically fragile children at home: the parent-professional relationship, *J Pediatr Nurs* 9(2):98-106, 1994.

Selekman J, McIlvain-Simpson G: Sex and sexuality for the adolescent with a chronic condition, *Pediatr Nurs* 17(6):535-538, 1991.

Wells PW and others: Growing up in the hospital. I. Let's focus on the child, *J Pediatr Nurs* 9(2):66-73, 1994.

Whyte DA: A family nursing approach to the care of a child with a chronic illness, *J Adv Nurs* 17(3):317-327, 1992.

Zagorsky ES: Caring for families who follow alternative health practices, *Pediatr Nurs* 19(1):71-75, 1993.

Terminal Illness/Death

American Academy of Pediatrics, Committee on Pediatric Emergency Medicine: Death of a child in the emergency department, *Pediatrics* 93(5):861-862, 1994.

Antonacci M: Sudden death: helping bereaved parents in the PICU, *Crit Care Nurse* 10(4):65-70, 1990.

Black KJ: Sudden, unexpected pediatric death: caring for the parents, *Pediatr Nurs* 17(6):571-575, 1991.

Bosworth T: Leukemia through a teenager's eyes, *MCN Am J Matern Child Nurs* 14(2):93-94, 1989.

Brahams D: Medicine and the law: a life-sustaining treatment for brain-damaged child, *Lancet* 339(8807):1472-1473, 1992.

Brett AS: Limitations of listing specific medical interventions in advance directives, *JAMA* 266(6):825-828, 1991.

Carlson JAS: The psychologic effects of sudden infant death syndrome on parents, *J Pediatr Health Care* 7(2):77-81, 1993.

Cassidy M: Supportive care and the dying child, *J Home Health Care Pract* 3(1):34-38, 1990.

Davies B, Eng B: Factors influencing nursing care of children who are terminally ill, *Pediatr Nurs* 19(1):9-14, 1993.

Davis FD: Organ procurement and transplantation, *Nurs Clin North Am* 24(4):823-836, 1989.

Dufour DF: Home or hospital care for the child with end-stage cancer: effects on the family, *Issues Compr Pediatr Nurs* 12(5):371-383, 1989.

Dychkowski LB: Caring for the terminally ill child in the school setting, *Sch Nurse* 6(2):8-10, 12, 1990.

Gary GA: Facing terminal illness in children with AIDS: developing a philosophy of care for patients, families, and caregivers, *Home Healthc Nurse* 10(2):40-43, 1992.

Grogan LB: Grief of an adolescent when a sibling dies, *MCN Am J Matern Child Nurs* 15(1):21-24, 1990.

Hall MD: The way it is . . . caring for dying children, *Am J Nurs* 90(7):86, 1990.

Hammer M and others: A ritual of remembrance . . . grief suffered by nurses themselves, *MCN Am J Matern Child Nurs* 17(6):310-313, 1992.

Hoekstra-Weebers JEH and others: A comparison of parental coping styles following the death of adolescent and preadolescent children, *Death Stud* 15(6):565-575, 1991.

Hogan NS, Balk DE: Adolescent reactions to sibling death: perceptions of mothers, fathers, and teenagers, *Nurs Res* 39(2):103-106, 1990.

Jefidoff A, Gasner R: Helping the parents of the dying child: an Israeli experience, *J Pediatr Nurs* 8(6):413-415, 1993.

Jezewski MA: Obtaining consent for do-not-resuscitate status: advice from experienced nurses, *Nurs Outlook* 44(3):114-119, 1996.

Jezewski MA and others: Consenting to DNR: critical care nurses' interactions with patients and family members, *Am J Crit Care* 2(4):302-309, 1993.

Kahn EC: A comparison of family needs based on the presence or absence of DNR orders, *Dimens Crit Care Nurs* 11(5):286-292, 1992.

Mahon MM: Death of a sibling: primary care interventions, *Pediatr Nurs* 20(3):293-295, 1994.

McCown DE: When children face death in a family, *J Pediatr Health Care* 2(1):14-19, 1988.

Miles A: Caring for families when a child dies, *Pediatr Nurs* 16(4):346-347, 1990.

Pazola KJ, Gerberg AK: Privileged communication—talking with a dying adolescent, *MCN Am J Matern Child Nurs* 15(1):16-21, 1990.

Pengra H, Morgan D, Warren L: Nursing implementation of do not resuscitate policy into home healthcare, *Home Healthc Nurse* 10(2):32-39, 1992.

Perrone J: Adolescents with cancer: are they at risk for suicide? *Pediatr Nurs* 19(1):22-25, 1993.

Redding B: Facilitating grieving. In Smith D and others, editors: *Comprehensive child and family nursing skills*, St Louis, 1991, Mosby.

IMPACT OF COGNITIVE OR SENSORY IMPAIRMENT ON THE CHILD AND FAMILY

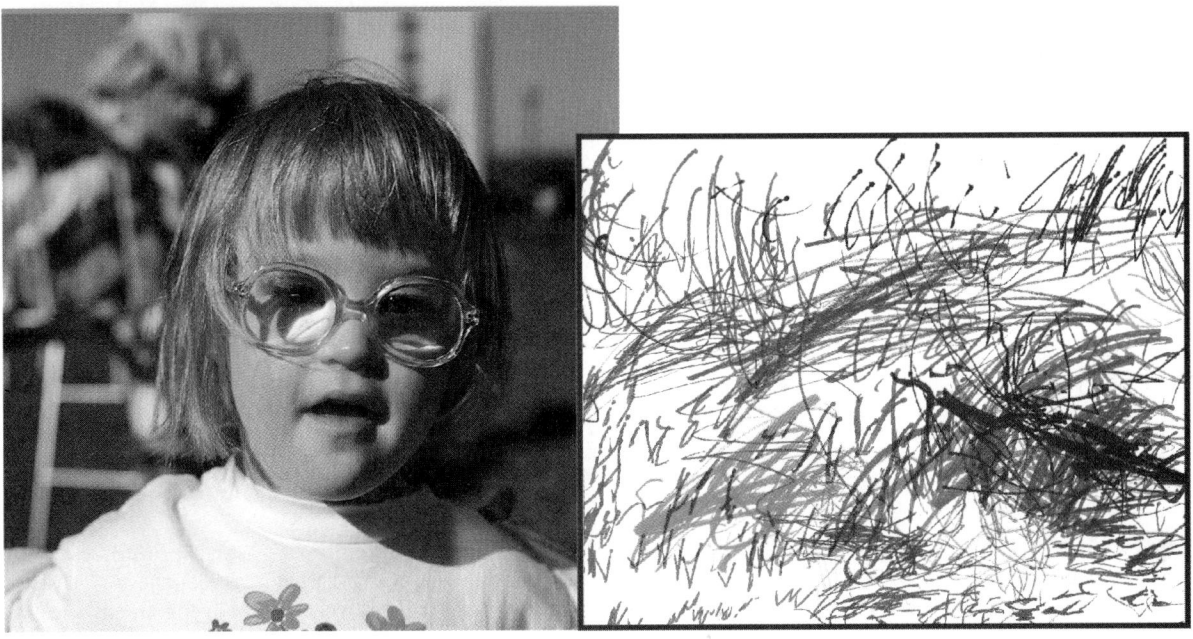

Emily, age 3 years, Down syndrome

RELATED TOPICS

COGNITIVE IMPAIRMENT

GENERAL CONCEPTS

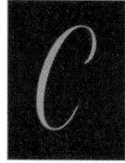*ognitive impairment* is a general term that encompasses any type of mental difficulty or deficiency. In this chapter the term is used synonymously with *mental retardation (MR)*. Although the needs and concerns of the family are a primary focus throughout the chapter, the reader is encouraged to review Chapter 18, which details the family's adjustment to disabilities in general.

The classic definition of MR has three components: subaverage intellectual functioning, deficits in adaptive behavior, and onset before 18 years of age (Batshaw, 1993). Recently the **American Association on Mental Retardation (AAMR)** significantly changed this definition by raising the upper limit of subaverage intellectual functioning from an intellectual quotient (IQ) of 70 to 75 and defining more clearly the deficit in adaptive behaviors. Adaptive limitations must occur in two or more of the following ten areas: communication, self-care, home living, social skills, leisure, health and safety, self-direction, functional academics, community use, and work (Luckasson, 1992).

It is critical to note that a low IQ is not the sole criterion for MR. For example, individuals with IQ scores near 75 may not be classified as retarded if they are able to adapt to the environment. Also, if cognitive impairment accompanied by adaptive limitations occurs from injury and disease after age 18, the person is not considered retarded.

The new definition also does not include a classification based on IQ scores as it did previously (Table 19-1). Rather, it emphasizes abilities, environments, supports, and empowerment. The intensity of needed support is classified as intermittent, limited, extensive, or pervasive. The underlying assumption is that with appropriate supports over a prolonged period, the ability of the person with MR to function each day will generally improve.

Renee Harrison, MS, RN, revised this chapter.

Diagnosis and Classification

The diagnosis of MR is usually made after a period of suspicion, by professionals and/or the family, that the child's developmental progress is delayed. In some cases it is confirmed at birth because of recognition of distinct syndromes, such as Down syndrome. At the other extreme, the diagnosis is made after the child begins school, when problems such as speech delays arouse concern. In all cases a high index of suspicion for developmental delay and behavioral signs (see box) is necessary for early diagnosis, and routine developmental screening (see Chapter 7) can assist in early identification. Delays are typically seen in gross and fine motor and speech development, although the latter is most predictive.

Results of standardized tests are used in making the diagnosis of MR. The most frequently used IQ tests include the Stanford-Binet Test and Wechsler Intelligence Scale for Children–Revised (WISC-R). Tests for assessing adaptive behaviors include the Vineland Social Maturity Scale and the AAMR Adaptive Behavior Scale. Informal appraisal of adaptive behavior may be made by those fully acquainted with the child (e.g., teachers, parents, other care providers). Frequently these observations lead parents to seek evaluation of the child's development.

A more useful approach for clinical application is classification based on educational potential or symptom severity. For educational purposes the terms *educable mentally retarded (EMR)* or *trainable mentally retarded (TMR)* may

EARLY BEHAVIORAL SIGNS SUGGESTIVE OF COGNITIVE IMPAIRMENT

Nonresponsiveness to contact
Poor eye contact during feeding
Diminished spontaneous activity
Decreased alertness to voice or movement
Irritability
Slow feeding

From Crocker A, Nelson R: Mental retardation. In Levine M and others: *Developmental-behavioral pediatrics*, Philadelphia, 1983, Saunders.

TABLE 19-1. Classification of mental retardation

LEVEL (IQ)*	PRESCHOOL (BIRTH-5 YEARS)—MATURATION AND DEVELOPMENT	SCHOOL-AGE (6-21 YEARS)—TRAINING AND EDUCATION	ADULT (21 YEARS AND OLDER)—SOCIAL AND VOCATIONAL ADEQUACY
Mild—50-55 to approximately 70	Often not noticed as retarded by casual observer but is slower to walk, feed self, and talk than most children; follows same sequence in development as normal children	Can acquire practical skills and useful reading and arithmetic to a third- to sixth-grade level with special education; can be guided toward social conformity; achieves mental age of 8 to 12 years	Can usually achieve social and vocational skills adequate to self-maintenance; may need occasional guidance and support when under unusual social or economic stress; can adjust to marriage but not childrearing
Moderate—35-40 to 50-55	Noticeable delays in motor development, especially in speech; responds to training in various self-help activities	Can learn simple communication, elementary health and safety habits, and simple manual skills; does not progress in functional reading or arithmetic; achieves mental age of 3 to 7 years	Can perform simple tasks under sheltered conditions: participates in simple recreation; travels alone in familiar places; usually incapable of self-maintenance
Severe—20-25 to 35-40	Marked delay in motor development; little or no communication skills; may respond to training in elementary self-care (e.g., self-feeding)	Usually walks, barring specific disability; has some understanding of speech and some response; can profit from systematic habit training; achieves mental age of toddler	Can conform to daily routines and repetitive activities; needs continuing direction and supervision in protective environment
Profound—below 20-25	Gross retardation; minimum capacity for functioning in sensorimotor areas; needs total care	Obvious delays in all areas of development; shows basic emotional responses; may respond to skillful training in use of legs, hands, and jaws; needs close supervision; achieves mental age of young infant	May walk; needs complete custodial care; has primitive speech; usually benefits from regular physical activity

*Data from American Psychiatric Association: *Diagnostic and statistical manual of mental disorders* ed 4, *(DSM-IV),* Washington, DC, 1994, The Association.

be used. EMR corresponds to the mildly retarded group, which constitutes about 85% of all people with MR. TMR is generally equivalent to children with moderate levels of cognitive impairment and accounts for about 10% of the MR population (American Psychiatric Association, 1994). Although nurses may be familiar with the approximate range of IQ for classifying severity, they should refrain from using numbers as the criterion for assessing or evaluating the child's abilities, since numbers are of little value in counseling parents or training these children.

Etiology

The causes of severe MR are primarily genetic, biochemical, and infectious. Although the etiology is unknown in the majority of cases, general categories of events that may lead to retardation include the following (Grossman, 1983):

1. Infection and intoxication, such as congenital rubella, syphilis, maternal drug consumption (e.g., excessive alcohol), chronic lead ingestion, or kernicterus
2. Trauma or physical agent, that is, injury to the brain suffered during the prenatal, perinatal, or postnatal period
3. Inadequate nutrition and metabolic disorders, such as phenylketonuria

4. Gross postnatal brain disease, such as neurofibromatosis and tuberous sclerosis
5. Unknown prenatal influence, including cerebral and cranial malformations, such as microcephaly and hydrocephalus
6. Gestational disorders, including prematurity, low birth weight, and postmaturity
7. Psychiatric disorders that have their onset during the child's developmental period up to age 18 years, such as autism
8. Environmental influences, including evidence of a deprived environment associated with a history of MR among parents and siblings
9. Chromosomal abnormalities, such as Down syndrome and fragile X syndrome

NURSING CARE OF CHILDREN WITH COGNITIVE IMPAIRMENT

❖ Assessment

Nurses play a major role in identifying children with cognitive impairment. In the newborn and early infancy period, few signs are present, with the exception of Down syndrome (see p. 575). After this age, however, delayed developmental milestones are the major clues to MR. In addition, nurses must have a high index of suspicion for early behavior patterns that may suggest cognitive impairment (see box on p. 568) and be aware of stereotypes that may delay diagnosis, such as "retarded children have to look dumb." Parental concerns, such as delayed development compared with siblings, need to be taken seriously. All children should receive regular developmental assessment, and the nurse is often the person responsible for performing such assessments (see Chapter 7). When delays are found, the nurse must use sensitivity and discretion in revealing this finding to parents.

❖ Nursing Diagnoses

A number of nursing diagnoses are prominent in the nursing care of the child with cognitive impairment and the child's family; other diagnoses specific to individual cases become evident. The most common nursing diagnoses are outlined in the Nursing Care Plan on p. 574.

❖ Planning

The goals of nursing care for the child with MR and family are as follows:

1. Child will be educated using effective teaching strategies.
2. Child's optimum development will be promoted.
3. Child will learn self-care skills.
4. Family will plan for future care.
5. Child will be cared for appropriately during hospitalization.

❖ Implementation

Educate Child and Family. To teach children with cognitive impairment, it is necessary to investigate their learning abilities and deficits. This is important for the nurse who may be involved in a home care type of program or who may be caring for the child in a health care setting. The nurse who understands how these children learn can effectively teach them basic skills or prepare them for various health-related procedures.

Children with cognitive impairment have a marked deficit in their ability to discriminate between two or more stimuli because of difficulty in recognizing the relevance of specific cues. However, these children can learn to discriminate if the cues are presented in an exaggerated, concrete form and if all extraneous stimuli are eliminated. For example, the use of colors to emphasize visual cues or the use of singing or rhymes to stress auditory cues can help them learn. Their deficit in discrimination also implies that concrete ideas are learned much more effectively than abstract ideas. Therefore demonstration is preferable to verbal explanation, and learning should be directed toward mastering a skill rather than understanding the scientific principles underlying a procedure.

Another cognitive deficit is in short-term memory. Whereas children of average intelligence can remember several words, numbers, or directions at one time, these children are less able to do so. Therefore they need simple one-step directions. Learning through a step-by-step process requires a *task analysis,* in which each task is separated into its necessary components and each step is taught completely before proceeding to the next activity.

One critical area of learning that has had a tremendous impact on education for cognitively impaired individuals is

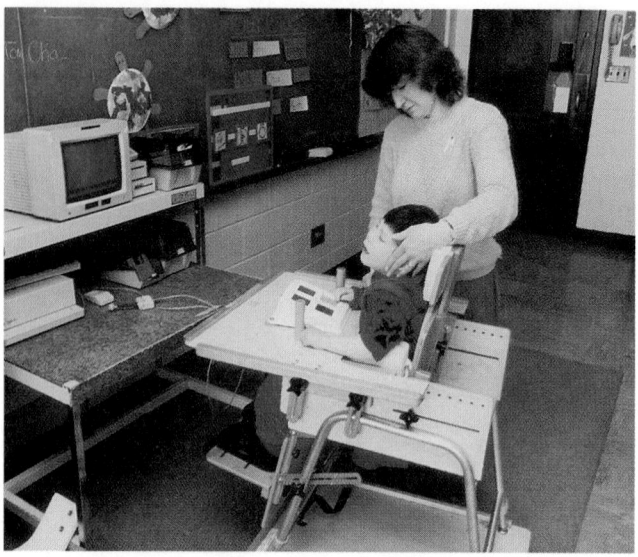

FIG. 19-1. A push panel allows a child with cognitive impairment to turn a computer on and off.

motivation. Programs based on the motivational principles of behavior modification, employing positive reinforcement for specific tasks or behaviors, have demonstrated marked improvement in children's ability to learn. Advances in technology have greatly aided in providing reinforcement, especially in children who are severely retarded and who may have physical disabilities that limit their range of capabilities. For example, with the use of specially designed switches, children are given control of some event in the environment, such as turning on the television (Fig. 19-1). The television picture becomes reinforcement for activating the switch. Repetitive use of these switches provides an early, simplistic association with a technical device that may progress to increasingly more complex aids.

Early intervention programs have been widely promoted for children with developmental disabilities, and there is considerable evidence that these programs are valuable for cognitively impaired children. Nurses working with these families need to be aware of the types of programs in their community. Under Public Law 101-476, the Individuals with Disabilities Education Act of 1990, states are encouraged to provide full early intervention services and are required to provide educational opportunities for all children with disabilities from birth to 21 years of age. Services may be provided under state **Programs for Children with Special Health Needs** (formerly **Crippled Children's Program**) or by private organizations such as the **National Easter Seal Society***** and the **Association of Retarded Citizens of the United States.†** Parents should inquire about these programs by contacting the appropriate agencies. The child's education should begin as soon as possible, not at 5 or 6 years

---

*70 E. Lake St., Chicago, IL 60601; (312) 726-6200 or (800) 221-6827.
†500 East Border, Suite 300, Arlington, TX 76010; (817) 261-6003.
Information on early intervention programs in each state is available from the **National Down Syndrome Society,** 666 Broadway, New York, NY 10012; (212) 460-9330 or (800) 221-4602.

of age. As children grow older, their education should be directed toward vocational training that prepares them for as independent a life-style as possible within their scope of abilities.

Teach Child Self-Care Skills. When a child with cognitive impairment is born, parents need assistance in promoting normal developmental skills that are almost automatically learned by other children. These include self-care skills such as feeding, toileting, dressing, and grooming. Teaching these skills requires a basic knowledge of the developmental sequence in learning the skills demonstrated by children of average intelligence. For example, children with subaverage intelligence would not be expected to dress themselves as early as unaffected youngsters.

Teaching self-care skills also necessitates a working knowledge of the individual steps needed to master a skill. For example, before beginning a self-feeding program, a task analysis is performed. After a task analysis, the child is observed in a particular situation, such as eating, to determine what skills are possessed and the child's developmental readiness to learn the task. Family members are included in this process because their "readiness" is as important as the child's. Numerous self-help aids are available to facilitate independence and can be most helpful in eliminating some of the difficulties of learning, such as using a plate with suction cups to prevent accidental spills (Fig. 19-2).

Promote Child's Optimum Development. Optimum development involves more than achieving independence. It requires appropriate guidance for establishing acceptable social behavior and personal feelings of self-esteem, worth, and security. These attributes are not simply learned through a stimulation program. Rather, they must arise from the genuine love and caring that exist among family members. However, families need guidance in providing an environment that fosters optimum development. Often it is the nurse who can provide assistance in these areas of childrearing.

Another important area for promoting optimum development and self-esteem is ensuring the child's physical well-being. Any congenital defects should be repaired, such as cardiac, gastrointestinal, or orthopedic anomalies. Plastic surgery may be considered when the child's appearance may be substantially improved. Dental health is very significant, and orthodontic and restorative procedures can immensely improve facial appearance.

Play/Exercise. Children who are cognitively impaired have the same needs for recreation and exercise as other children. However, because of the child's slower development, parents may be less aware of the need to provide such activities. Therefore the nurse guides parents toward selection of suitable play and exercise activities. Since play has been discussed for children in each age-group in earlier chapters, only the exceptions are presented here.

The type of play is based on the child's developmental age, although the need for sensorimotor play may be prolonged for several years. Parents should use every opportunity to expose the child to as many different sounds, sights, and sensations as possible. Appropriate play includes musical mobiles, stuffed toys, water play, floating toys, rocking chair or horse, swing, bells, and rattles. The child should be taken on outings, such as trips to the grocery store or shopping center; other people should be encouraged to visit in the home; and the child should be related to directly, such as by cuddling, holding, rocking, talking to the child in the *en face* (face to face) position, and giving "rides" on the parents' shoulders.

Toys are selected for their recreational and educational value. For example, a large inflatable beach ball is a good water toy; it encourages interactive play and can be used to learn motor skills, such as balance, rocking, kicking, and throwing. A doll with removable clothes and different types of closures can help the child learn dressing skills. Musical toys that mimic animal sounds or respond with social phrases are excellent ways of encouraging speech. Toys should be simple in design so that the child can learn to manipulate them without help. For children with severe cognitive and physical impairment, electronic switches can be used to allow them to operate toys (Fig. 19-3).

Suitable activities for physical activity are based on the child's size, coordination, physical fitness and maturity, motivation, and health (Fig. 19-4). Some children may have physical problems that prevent certain sports, such as atlantoaxial instability in children with Down syndrome (see p. 576). These children often have greater success in individual and dual sports than in team sports and enjoy themselves

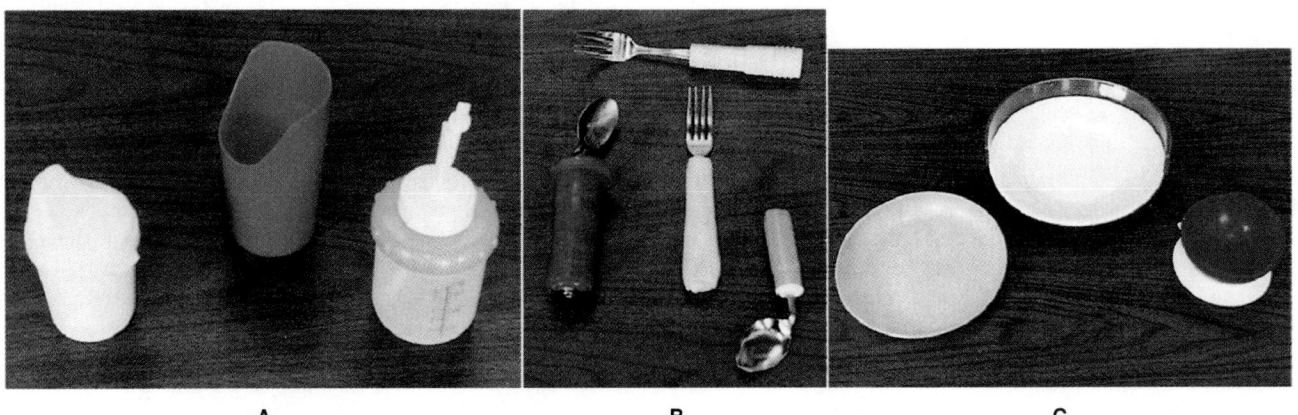

FIG. 19-2. Self-help aids for feeding. **A,** Modified drinking cups. **B,** Modified utensils. **C,** Modified dishes.

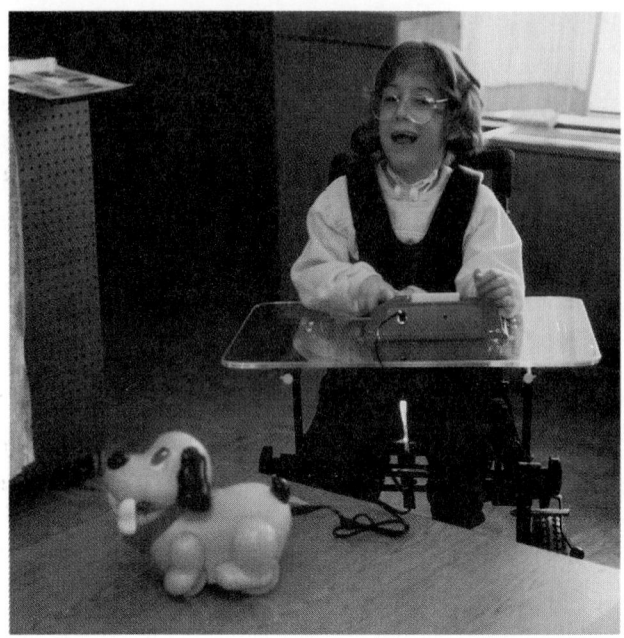

FIG. 19-3. A manual switch allows a child with cognitive impairment to play with a battery-operated toy.

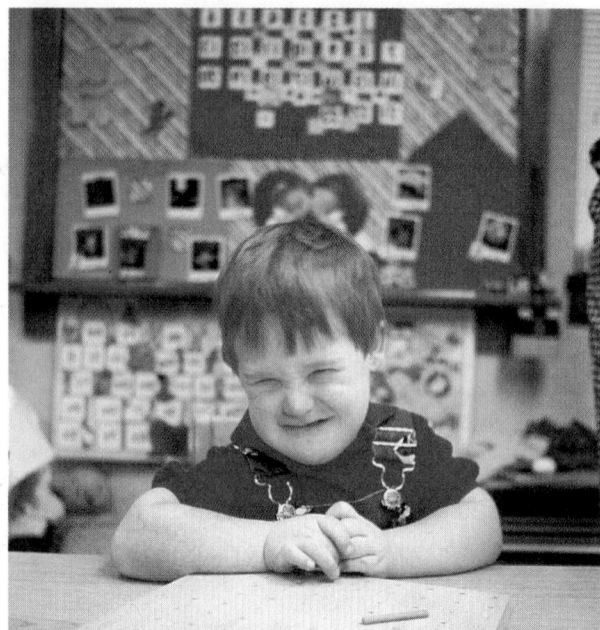

FIG. 19-4. Play activities for children with cognitive impairments need to be appropriate for their abilities.

most with children of the same developmental level. The **Special Olympics*** provide these children with a unique competitive opportunity.

Safety is a major consideration in selecting recreational and exercise activities. For example, toys that may be appropriate developmentally may present dangers to a child who is strong enough to break them or use them incorrectly.

Communication.   Verbal skills are typically delayed more than other physical skills. Speech requires hearing and interpretation *(receptive skills)* and facial muscle coordination *(expressive skills)*. Since both types of skills may be impaired, these children need frequent audiometric testing and should be fitted with hearing aids if this is indicated. In addition, they may need help in learning to control their facial muscles. For example, some children may need tongue exercises to correct the tongue thrust or gentle reminders to keep the lips closed.

Nonverbal communication may be appropriate for some of these children, and various devices are available. For the child without associated physical disabilities, a talking picture board is helpful. For children with physical limitations, several adaptations or types of communication devices are available to facilitate selection of the appropriate picture or word (Fig. 19-5). Some children may be taught sign language or *Blissymbols*—a highly stylized system of graphic symbols that represent words, ideas, and concepts. Although they require education to learn their meaning, no reading skill is needed. The symbols are usually arranged on a board, and the person points or uses some type of selector to convey a message.

Discipline.   Discipline must begin early. Limit-setting

*1350 New York Ave., N.W., Suite 500, Washington, DC 20005-4709; (202) 628-3630. In Canada: **Canadian Special Olympics, Inc.,** 40 St. Clair Ave., W., Suite 209, Toronto, Ontario M4V 1M6.

measures need to be simple, consistently applied, and appropriate for the child's mental age. Control measures are based primarily on teaching a specific behavior rather than on understanding the reasons behind it. Stressing moral lessons is of little value to a child who lacks the cognitive skills to learn from self-criticism or from a lesson based on previous wrongdoing. Behavior modification, especially reinforcement of desired actions, and time-out are appropriate forms of behavior control.

Socialization.   Acquiring social skills is a complex task, as is learning self-care procedures. Active rehearsal with role playing and practice sessions and positive reinforcement for desired behavior have been the most successful approaches. Parents should be encouraged early to teach their child socially acceptable behavior: waving goodbye, saying hello and thank you, responding to his or her name, greeting visitors but not being overly affectionate, and sitting modestly. The teaching of socially acceptable sexual behavior is especially important to minimize sexual exploitation. Parents also need to expose the child to strangers so he or she can practice manners, since there is no automatic transfer of learning from one situation to another.

Dressing and grooming are also important aspects of socialization. A child who is dressed in age-appropriate clothing and is well groomed is much more likely to be accepted and to develop good self-esteem. Clothes should be clean, up-to-date, and well fitted. Many attractive outfits can be adapted with self-adhering fasteners and elastic openings to facilitate self-dressing.

Children of all ages need peer relationships, and these children are no exception. As soon as possible, parents should enroll the child in appropriate preschool programs. Not only do these programs provide education and training, but they also offer an opportunity for social experiences among the

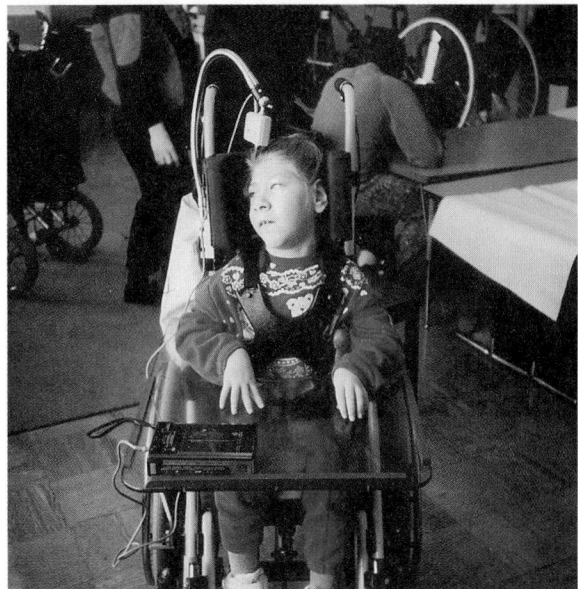

FIG. 19-5. A child with cognitive and physical impairments can play a tape recorder by moving a device near her head.

children. As children grow older, they should have peer experiences similar to those of other children, including group outings, sports, and organized activities, such as Boy Scouts, Girl Scouts, or Special Olympics. They are encouraged to form a close relationship with a best friend.

Sexuality. Adolescence may be a particularly difficult time for the family, especially in terms of the child's sexual behavior, possibility of pregnancy, future plans to marry, and ability to be independent. Frequently, little anticipatory guidance has been offered parents to prepare the child for physical and sexual maturation. The nurse can help in this area by providing parents with information about sexuality education that is geared to the child's developmental level. For example, the adolescent female needs a *simple* explanation of menstruation and instructions on personal hygiene during the menstrual cycle.

These adolescents also need practical sexual information regarding anatomy, physical development, and conception.* Because of their easy persuasion and lack of judgment, they need a well-defined, concrete code of conduct. The subtleties of social sexual behavior are less beneficial than specific instructions for handling certain situations. For example, a girl should be firmly told never to go alone anywhere with any person she does not know well. A boy should be warned about intimate advances from other males. To protect him or her from abusive sexual activities, parents must closely observe their teenager's activities and associates.

The question of contraceptive protection for female retarded adolescents is often a parental concern. Permanent contraception through sterilization is a special dilemma because of moral and ethical questions, as well as psychologic

---

*Sources of information on sexuality and conception are the **Association for Retarded Citizens of the United States,** 500 East Border, Suite 300, Arlinton, TX 76010, (817) 261-6003; and **Planned Parenthood Federation of America,** 810 7th Ave., New York, NY 10019, (212) 541-7800.

effects on the adolescent. State laws vary; some allow no sterilization, and others permit review of sterilization requests.

Parents of these adolescents are often very concerned about the advisability of marriage between two individuals with significant cognitive impairment. There is no conclusive answer; each situation must be judged individually. In some instances marriage is possible, but parenthood is usually not desirable because of the complexity of childrearing and the potential problem of perpetuating mental deficiency. The nurse should discuss this topic with parents and with the prospective couple, stressing suitable living accommodations and contraceptive methods to prevent pregnancy. If children are conceived, these parents require specialized assistance in learning to meet the needs of their offspring (Keltner and Tymchuk, 1992).

Help Family Adjust to Future Care. Not all families are able to cope with home care of their affected child, especially one who is severely or profoundly retarded and/or multidisabled. Older parents may not be able to assume care responsibilities once they reach retirement or old age. For these parents, the decision regarding residential placement is a difficult one, and the availability of such facilities varies widely. The nurse working with a family should help them investigate and evaluate various programs, in addition to assisting them in their adjustment to the decision for placement.

Care for Child During Hospitalization. Caring for the child during hospitalization can be a special challenge. Frequently, nurses are unfamiliar with children who are cognitively impaired, and they may cope with their feelings of insecurity and fear by ignoring or isolating the child. Not only is this approach nonsupportive, but it may also be destructive for the child's sense of self-esteem and optimum development, and it may hamper the parents' ability to cope with the stress of the experience. One method that successfully avoids this nontherapeutic approach is the use of the mutual participation model in planning the child's care. Parents are encouraged to room with their child but should not be made to feel as if the responsibility is totally theirs.

When the child is admitted, a detailed history is taken (see Chapter 21), especially in terms of all self-care activity. During the interview the child's developmental age is assessed. It is best to avoid directly asking about IQ levels, because this may make the parents uncomfortable and often tells little about the child's actual abilities. Questions are approached positively. For example, rather than asking, "Is your child toilet trained yet?" the nurse may state, "Tell me about your child's toileting habits." The assessment should also focus on any special devices the child uses, effective measures of limit-setting, unusual or favorite routines, and any behaviors that may require intervention. For example, if the parent states that the child engages in self-stimulatory activities, the nurse inquires about events that precipitate them and techniques that the parents use to manage them.

The child's functional level of eating and playing, ability to express needs verbally, progress in toilet training, and relationship with objects, toys, and other children are also assessed. The child is encouraged to be as independent as possible in the hospital.

Realizing that the child may be lonely in the hospital, the nurse makes certain that toys and other activities are

NURSING CARE PLAN
The Child with Mental Retardation

NURSING DIAGNOSIS: Altered growth and development related to impaired cognitive functioning

---

PATIENT GOAL 1: Will achieve optimum growth and development potential

• NURSING INTERVENTIONS/*RATIONALES*

Involve child and family in an early infant stimulation program *to help maximize child's development*

Assess child's developmental progress at regular intervals; keep detailed records to distinguish subtle changes in functioning *so that plan of care can be revised as needed*

Help family determine child's readiness to learn specific tasks, *since readiness may not be easily recognized*

Help family set realistic goals for child *to encourage successful attainment of goals and self-esteem*

Employ positive reinforcement for specific tasks or behaviors *because this improves motivation and learning*

Encourage learning of self-care skills as soon as child is ready

Reinforce self-care activities *to facilitate optimum development*

Encourage family to investigate special daycare programs and educational classes as soon as possible

Emphasize that child has same needs as other children (e.g., play, discipline, social interaction)

Before adolescence, counsel child and parents regarding physical maturation, sexual behavior, marriage, and childrearing

Encourage optimum vocational training

• EXPECTED OUTCOMES

Child and family are actively involved in infant stimulation program

Family applies concepts and continues activities in home care of child

Child performs activities of daily living at optimum capacity

Family investigates educational programs

Appropriate limit-setting, recreation, and social opportunities are provided

Adolescent issues are explored as appropriate

PATIENT GOAL 2: Will achieve optimum socialization

• NURSING INTERVENTIONS/*RATIONALES*

Emphasize that child has same need for socialization as other children

Encourage family to teach child socially acceptable behavior (e.g., saying "hello" and "thank you," manners, appropriate touch)

Encourage grooming and age-appropriate dress *to encourage acceptance by others and self-esteem*

Recommend programs that provide peer relationships and experiences (e.g., mainstreaming, Boy Scouts, Girl Scouts, Special Olympics) *to promote optimum socialization*

Provide adolescent with practical sexual information and a well-defined, concrete code of conduct *because child's easy persuasion and lack of judgment may place child at risk*

• EXPECTED OUTCOMES

Child behaves in socially acceptable manner

Child has peer relationships and experiences

Child does not experience social isolation

NURSING DIAGNOSIS: Altered family processes related to having a child with MR

PATIENT (FAMILY) GOAL 1: Will receive adequate support

• NURSING INTERVENTIONS/*RATIONALES*

Inform family as soon as possible at or after birth, *since family may suspect a problem and need immediate support*

Have both parents present at informing conference *to avoid problem of one parent having to relay complex information to the other parent and deal with the initial emotional reaction of the other*

Give family written information about the condition, when possible (e.g., a specific syndrome or disease), *for family to refer to later*

Discuss with family members benefits of home care; allow them opportunities to investigate all residential alternatives before making a decision

Encourage family to meet other families with a similarly affected child *so that they can receive additional support*

Refrain from giving definitive answers about the degree of retardation; stress the potential learning abilities of these children, especially with early intervention, *to encourage hope*

Demonstrate acceptance of child through own behavior *because parents are sensitive to the affective attitude of the professional*

Emphasize normal characteristics of child *to help family see child as an individual with strengths, as well as weaknesses*

Encourage family members to express their feelings and concerns *because this is part of the adaptation process*

• EXPECTED OUTCOMES

Family expresses feelings and concerns regarding the birth of a child with MR and its implications

Family members make realistic decisions based on their needs and capabilities

Family members demonstrate acceptance of child

PATIENT (FAMILY) GOAL 2: Will be prepared for long-term care of child

• NURSING INTERVENTIONS/*RATIONALES*

As child grows older, discuss with parents alternatives to home care, especially as parents near retirement or old age, *so that appropriate long-term care can be provided*

Encourage family to consider respite care as needed *to facilitate family's ability to cope with child's long-term care*

Help family investigate residential settings, *since this may be needed for child's optimum care*

Encourage family to include affected member in planning and to continue meaningful relationships after placement

Refer to agencies that provide support and assistance

• EXPECTED OUTCOMES

Family identifies realistic goals for future care of child

Family avails themselves of supportive services

See also Nursing Care Plan: The Child with Chronic Illness or Disability, Chapter 18

provided. The child is placed in a room with other children of approximate developmental age, preferably a room with two beds, to avoid overstimulation. The nurse discusses with the other parents the child's abilities and introduces the parents and children to each other. By the nurse's example of treating the child with dignity and respect, others who may be fearful of what they do not understand are encouraged to accept the child.

Procedures are explained to the child through methods of communication that are at the appropriate cognitive level. Generally, explanations should be simple, short, and concrete, emphasizing what the child will experience *physically*. Demonstration either through actual practice or with visual aids is always preferable to verbal explanation. The nurse repeats instructions often and evaluates the child's understanding by asking questions such as "What will it feel like?" "What will the doctor look like?" "Show me how you must lie," or "Where will the dressing be?" Parents are included in preprocedural teaching for their own learning and to help the nurse learn effective methods of communicating with the child.

During hospitalization the nurse should also focus on growth-promoting experiences for the child. For example, hospitalization may be an excellent opportunity to emphasize to parents abilities that the child does have but has not had the opportunity to practice, such as self-dressing. It may also be an opportunity for social experiences with peers, group play, or new educational and recreational activities. For example, one child who had the habit of screaming and kicking demonstrated a definite decrease in those behaviors after he learned to pound pegs and use a punching bag. Through social services the parents may become aware of specialized programs for the child. Hospitalization may also offer parents a respite from everyday care responsibilities and an opportunity to discuss their feelings with a concerned professional.

Assist in Measures to Prevent Retardation. Besides having a responsibility to families with a child with MR, nurses also need to be involved in programs aimed at preventing MR. Many of the familial, social, and environmental factors known to cause mild retardation are preventable. Counseling and education can reduce or eliminate such factors (e.g., poor nutrition, cigarette smoking, and chemical abuse, which increase the risk of prematurity and intrauterine growth retardation). Consequently, the major interventions are directed at improving maternal health and educating women regarding the dangers of chemicals, including alcohol, during pregnancy. Other preventive strategies that play an important role include optimum medical care for high-risk newborns; rubella immunization; genetic counseling and prenatal screening, especially in terms of Down or fragile X syndrome; newborn screening for treatable inborn errors of metabolism, such as congenital hypothyroidism, phenylketonuria, and galactosemia; and early appropriate therapies and rehabilitation services for children with developmental disabilities.

❖ Evaluation

The effectiveness of nursing interventions is determined by continual reassessment and evaluation of care based on the following observational guidelines and expected outcomes:

1. Observe techniques used to teach child and child's success in ability to learn; inquire if child is enrolled in early stimulation program.
2. Interview family regarding provision of appropriate socialization, discipline, and play for child; observe child's ability to communicate with others; if possible, interview child regarding feelings of self-worth.
3. Observe those activities of daily living that child can completely or partially perform.
4. Interview family regarding any plans for future care and their awareness of community services.
5. Check patient record for evidence of nursing admission history, especially for self-help activities; observe parent's involvement in child's care; observe social interaction of child and family with other patients.
6. Investigate community programs aimed at preventing retardation and inquire as to nursing involvement in these efforts.

Expected outcomes:
See Nursing Care Plan, p. 574.

DOWN SYNDROME

Down syndrome is the most common chromosomal abnormality of a generalized syndrome, occurring in 1 in 800 to 1000 live births. It owes its once common but unacceptable name, *mongolism*, to the particular facial characteristics, which resemble those of the Mongol race.

Etiology

The cause of Down syndrome is not known, but evidence from cytogenetic and epidemiologic studies supports the concept of multiple causality. Approximately 95% of all cases of Down syndrome are attributable to an extra chromosome 21 (group G), thus the name *trisomy 21*. Although children with trisomy 21 are born to parents of all ages, there is a statistically greater risk in older women, particularly those over 35 years of age. For example, in women 30 years of age the incidence of Down syndrome is about 1 in 1500 live births, but in women age 40 it is about 1 in 100. However, the majority (about 80%) of infants with Down syndrome are born to women under age 35. In less than 5% of cases, paternal age is a factor, especially in men 55 years of age or older (Cooley and Graham, 1991).

About 3% to 4% of the cases may be caused by *translocation* of chromosomes 15 and 21 or 22. This type of genetic aberration is usually hereditary and is not associated with advanced parental age. From 1% to 2% of affected persons demonstrate *mosaicism*, which refers to cells with both normal and abnormal chromosomes. The degree of physical and cognitive impairment is related to the percentage of cells with the abnormal chromosome makeup.

Diagnostic Evaluation

Down syndrome can usually be diagnosed by the clinical manifestations alone (see box on p. 576 and Fig. 19-6), but a chromosomal analysis should be done to confirm the genetic abnormality.

Several physical problems are associated with Down syndrome. Many of these children have congenital heart malformations, the most common being septal defects. Respiratory tract infections are very prevalent and, when combined with cardiac anomalies, are the chief cause of death, particularly during the first year of life. Hypotonicity of chest and

CLINICAL MANIFESTATIONS OF DOWN SYNDROME

Head
*Separated sagittal suture
Brachycephaly
Skull rounded and small
Flat occiput
Enlarged anterior fontanel
Sparse hair (variable)

Face
Flat profile

Eyes
*Oblique palpebral fissures (upward, outward slant)
Inner epicanthal folds
Speckling of iris (Brushfield spots)
Short, sparse eyelashes
Blepharitis

Nose
*Small
*Depressed nasal bridge (saddle nose)

Ears
Small
Short pinna (vertical ear length)
Overlapping upper helices
Narrow canals

Mouth
*High, arched, narrow palate
Small, osseous orbit
Protruding tongue; may be fissured at lip and furrowed on surface
Hypoplastic mandible
Downward curve (especially noted when crying)
Mouth kept open

Teeth
Delayed eruption
Alignment abnormalities common
Microdontia
Periodontal disease

Chest
Shortened rib cage
Twelfth rib anomalies
Pectus excavatum/carinatum

Neck
*Skin excess and lax
Short and broad

Abdomen
Protruding
Muscles lax and flabby
Diastasis recti
Umbilical hernia

Genitalia
Small penis
Cryptorchidism
Bulbous vulva

Hands
Broad, short
Stubby fingers
Incurved little finger (clinodactyly)
Transverse palmar crease
Characteristic dermal ridge patterns
Distally located axial triradius
Increased ulnar loops on fingers

Feet
*Wide space between big and second toes
*Plantar crease between big and second toes
Broad, stubby, short

Musculoskeleton
*Hyperflexibility
*Muscle weakness
Hypotonia
Atlantoaxial instability

Skin
Dry, cracked, and frequent fissuring
Cutis marmorata (mottling)

Other
Reduced birth weight

*Most common findings (Pueschel, 1992).

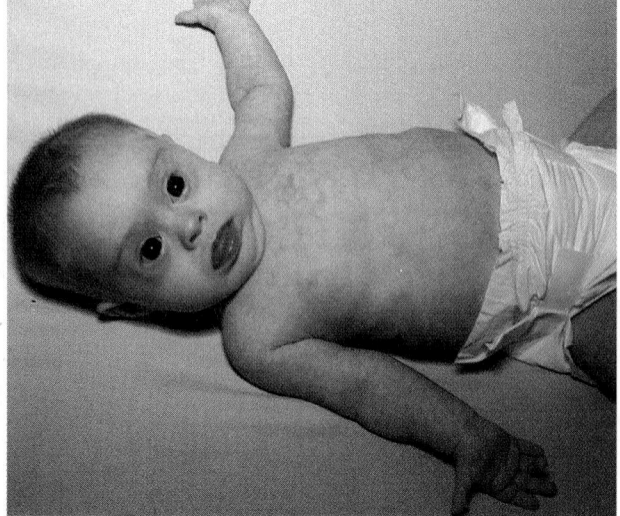

FIG. 19-6. Down syndrome in infant. Note small, square head with upward slant to the eyes, flat nasal bridge, protruding tongue, mottled skin, and hypotonia.

abdominal muscles and dysfunction of the immune system probably predispose to the development of respiratory tract infection. Other physical problems include thyroid dysfunction, especially congenital hypothyroidism, and an increased incidence of leukemia.

Therapeutic Management

Although no cure exists for Down syndrome, a number of therapies are advocated, such as surgery to correct serious congenital anomalies and possibly the physical stigmata, although the latter is controversial. These children also benefit from regular medical care. Evaluation of sight and hearing is essential, and treatment of otitis media is required to prevent auditory loss, which can influence cognitive function. Periodic testing of thyroid function is recommended, especially if growth is severely delayed. Children participating in sports that may involve stress on the head and neck, such as gymnastics, diving, butterfly stroke in swimming, high jump, and soccer, should be evaluated radiologically for *atlantoaxial instability*. Symptoms of the disorder include neck pain, weakness, and torticollis. Affected children are at risk for spinal cord compression.

Nursing ALERT	Report immediately any child with the following signs of spinal cord compression: Persistent neck pain Loss of established motor skills and bladder or bowel control Changes in sensation

Prognosis. Life expectancy has improved in recent years but remains lower than that for the general population. More than 80% survive to age 30 years and beyond. Down syndrome is associated with earlier aging, and virtually all deceased individuals have neurologic changes associated with Alzheimer disease (Cooley and Graham, 1991).

Nursing Considerations

Support Family at Time of Diagnosis. Because of the unique physical characteristics, the infant with Down syndrome is usually diagnosed at birth, and parents should be informed of the diagnosis at this time. Parents usually prefer that both of them be present during the informing interview so that they can support one another emotionally. They appreciate receiving reading material about the syndrome* and being referred to others for help or advice, such as parent groups or professional counseling.

Once parents are aware of the diagnosis, they are confronted with the crisis of losing their perfect or dream child and grieving for and accepting their reality child. Consequently, the parents' responses to the child may greatly influence decisions regarding future care. Whereas some families willingly want to take the child home, others consider immediate residential placement. The nurse must carefully answer questions regarding developmental potential. Institutionalization is no longer an option. For families unable or unready to choose taking the newborn home, specialized foster care or adoption are other options (see Critical Thinking Exercise).

Assist Family in Preventing Physical Problems. Many of the physical characteristics of Down syndrome present nursing problems. The hypotonicity of muscles and hyperextensibility of joints complicate positioning. The limp, flaccid extremities resemble the posture of a rag doll; as a result, holding the infant is difficult and cumbersome. Sometimes parents perceive this lack of molding to their bodies as evidence of inadequate parenting. The extended body position promotes heat loss because more surface area is exposed to the environment. Parents are encouraged to swaddle or wrap the infant tightly in a blanket before picking up the child to provide security and warmth. The nurse also discusses with parents their feelings concerning attachment to the child, emphasizing that the child's lack of clinging or molding is a physical characteristic, not a sign of detachment or rejection.

Decreased muscle tone compromises respiratory expansion. In addition, the underdeveloped nasal bone causes a

---

*Sources of information include the **Association for Retarded Citizens of the United States,** 500 East Border Suite 300, Arlinton, TX 76010, (817) 261-6003; **American Association on Mental Retardation,** 1719 Kalorama Rd., N.W., Washington, DC 20009, (202) 387-1968 or (800) 424-3688; the **National Down Syndrome Society,** 141 5th Ave., New York, NY 10011, (800) 221-4602; and the **National Down Syndrome Congress,** 1605 Chantilly Dr., Suite 250, Atlanta, GA 30324, (404) 633-1555 or (800) 232-6372.

CRITICAL THINKING EXERCISE
Diagnosis of Down Syndrome

The parents of Melissa, a newborn diagnosed as having Down syndrome, ask you, "What are we supposed to do with her?" They further state that they already have three other children at home. How should you respond?

1. Encourage the parents to consider placement arrangements.
2. Actively listen to the parents' concerns.
3. Refer the parents to their pediatrician.
4. Ask the social worker to see the parents.

The correct answer is two. The parents of a newborn child who has Down syndrome need time to process information given to them. The best choice for the nurse is to listen and then be able to guide them to appropriate resources, not to give them suggestions that would affect their family's future. Options three and four are appropriate interventions but should not replace the nurse's role with the family.

chronic problem of inadequate drainage of mucus. The constant stuffy nose forces the child to breathe by mouth, which dries the oropharyngeal membranes, increasing the susceptibility to upper respiratory tract infections. Measures to lessen these problems include clearing the nose with a bulb-type syringe,* rinsing the mouth with water after feedings, using a cool-mist vaporizer to keep the mucous membranes moist and the secretions liquefied, changing the child's position frequently and performing postural drainage and percussion if necessary, practicing good handwashing, and properly disposing of soiled articles, such as tissues. If antibiotics are ordered, the importance of completing the full course of therapy for successful eradication of the infection and prevention of growth of resistant organisms is stressed.

Inadequate drainage and pooling of mucus in the nose also interfere with feeding. Because the child breathes by mouth, sucking for any length of time is difficult. When eating solids, the child may gag on the food because of mucus in the oropharynx. Parents are advised to clear the nose before each feeding, give small, frequent feedings, and allow opportunities for rest at mealtime.

The protruding tongue also interferes with feeding, especially solid foods. Parents need to know that the tongue thrust is not an indication of refusal to feed, but a physiologic response. Parents are advised to use a small but long, straight-handled spoon to push the food toward the back and side of the mouth. If food is thrust out, it is refed.

Dietary intake needs supervision. Decreased muscle tone affects gastric motility, predisposing the child to constipation. Dietary measures such as increased fiber and fluid promote evacuation. The child's eating habits may need careful scrutiny to prevent obesity. Height and weight measurements should be obtained on a serial basis, especially during infancy. Since these children's growth is slower than the general pe-

---

*Home care instructions on using a bulb syringe are available in Wong DL: *Wong and Whaley's Clinical manual of pediatric nursing,* ed 4, St Louis, 1996, Mosby.

diatric population's trends, special growth charts developed for these children should be used (Cronk and others, 1988).

During infancy the child's skin is pliable and soft. However, it gradually becomes rough and dry and is prone to cracking and infection. Skin care involves the use of minimum soap and application of lubricants. Lip balm is applied to the lips, especially when the child is outdoors, to prevent excessive chapping.

Assist in Prenatal Diagnosis and Genetic Counseling. Prenatal diagnosis of Down syndrome is possible through chorionic villus sampling and amniocentesis, since chromosomal analysis of fetal cells can detect the presence of trisomy or translocation. However, analysis will not identify sporadic cases in young women when there is no indication for prenatal testing. Testing for low maternal serum α-fetoprotein, high chorionic gonadotropin, and low unconjugated estriol levels may identify affected young women, who can then undergo amniocentesis (American Academy of Pediatrics, 1989; Haddow and others, 1992).

The nurse has a role in genetic counseling of women who are of advanced maternal age or who have a family history of the disorder to discuss the possibility of amniocentesis. If the fetus is affected, the nurse must allow the parents to express their feelings concerning elective abortion and support their decision to terminate or proceed with the pregnancy.

See also Nursing Care Plan: The Child with Down Syndrome.*

FRAGILE X SYNDROME†

Fragile X syndrome is the most common inherited cause of MR and the second most common genetic cause of MR after Down syndrome. It has been described in all ethnic groups and races; the incidence of affected males is 1 in 1250; 1 in 2500 females are affected, and 1 in 259 females are carriers. Because its identification as a disorder is relatively new, many health professionals and educators lack the necessary familiarity with the manifestations for appropriate referral and management once fragile X syndrome is diagnosed (Hagerman and Cronister, 1996).

The syndrome is caused by an abnormal gene on the lower end of the long arm of the X chromosome. Chromosome analysis may demonstrate a *fragile site* (a region that fails to condense during mitosis and is characterized by a nonstaining gap or narrowing) in the cells of affected males and females and in carrier females. This fragile site has been determined to be caused by a gene mutation that results in excessive repeats of nucleotide in a specific deoxyribonucleic acid (DNA) segment of the X chromosome. The number of repeats in a normal individual is between 6 and 50. An individual with 50 to 200 base-pair repeats is said to have a *premutation* and is therefore a carrier. When passed from a parent to a child, these base-pair repeats can expand from 200 or more, which is termed a *full mutation.* This expansion only occurs when a carrier mother passes the mutation to her offspring; it does not occur when a carrier father passes the mutation to his daughters.

The inheritance pattern has been termed *X-linked domi-*

nant with reduced penetrance. It is in distinct contrast to the classic X-linked recessive pattern in which all carrier females are normal, all affected males have symptoms of the disorder, and no males are carriers. Consequently, genetic counseling of affected families is more complex than that for families with a classic X-linked disorder, such as hemophilia. Prenatal diagnosis of the fragile X gene mutation is now possible with direct DNA testing in a family with an established history, using amniocentesis or chorionic villus sampling (Brown and others, 1993). Both affected sexes are fertile and therefore capable of transmitting the fragile X disorder.

Clinical Manifestations

The classic trend of physical findings in adult males with fragile X syndrome consists of a long face with a prominent jaw (prognathism); large, protruding ears; and large testes (macro-orchidism). In prepubertal children, however, these features may be less obvious, and behavioral manifestations may initially suggest the diagnosis (see box). In carrier females the clinical manifestations are extremely varied.

Therapeutic Management

No cure exists for fragile X syndrome. Medical treatment may include the use of serotonin agents such as carbamazepine (Tegretol) or fluoxetine (Prozac) to control violent temper outbursts and the use of central nervous system (CNS) stimulants or clonidine (Catapres) to improve attention span and decrease hyperactivity. The use of folic acid, which affects the metabolism of CNS transmitters, is controversial.

All affected children require early speech and language therapy, occupational therapy, and special education assistance. Without appropriate intervention, a progressive decline in IQ can occur.

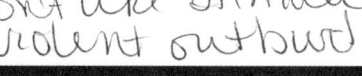

CLINICAL MANIFESTATIONS OF FRAGILE X SYNDROME

Physical Features
Long, wide, and/or protruding ears
Long, narrow face, with prominent jaw
In postpubertal males, enlarged testicles
Long palpebral fissures
High, arched palate
Strabismus
Increased head circumference
Mitral valve prolapse/aortic root dilatation
Hypotonia
Hyperextensible finger joints
Transpalmar crease
Pes planus (flat feet)

Behavioral Features
Mild to severe MR (occasional normal IQ with learning disabilities)
Speech delay; speech may be rapid, with stuttering and repetition of words
Short attention span, hyperactivity
Mouthing beyond expected age for behavior
Hypersensitivity to taste, sounds, touch
Intolerance to change in routine
Autistic-like behaviors
May exhibit aggressive behavior

---

*In Wong DL: *Wong and Whaley's Clinical manual of pediatric nursing,* ed 4, St Louis, 1996, Mosby.
†Donna Phillips Smith, MS, RN, revised this section.

Prognosis.   Individuals with fragile X syndrome are expected to live a normal life span. Their cognitive impairment may be improved by behavioral and educational interventions.

Nursing Considerations

Since cognitive impairment is a fairly consistent finding in individuals with fragile X syndrome, the care given to these families is the same as for any child with MR. Because the disorder is hereditary, genetic counseling is necessary to inform parents and siblings of the risks of transmission. In addition, any male or female with unexplained or nonspecific mental impairment should be referred for genetic testing and, if needed, counseling. Families with a member affected by the disorder should be referred to the **National Fragile X Foundation.***

meet educ. program level

SENSORY IMPAIRMENT

HEARING IMPAIRMENT

Hearing impairment is one of the most common disabilities in the United States. An estimated 1 in 1000 infants are born deaf. For infants admitted to the neonatal intensive care unit, the incidence rises sharply to approximately 1 to 3 per 100 neonates (National Institutes of Health, 1993). There are about 1 million children with hearing impairment ranging in age from birth to 21 years in the United States, and almost a third of these children have other disabilities, such as visual or cognitive deficits.

Definition and Classification

Hearing impairment is a general term indicating disability that may range in severity from mild to profound and includes the subsets of deaf and hard-of-hearing. *Deaf* refers to a person whose hearing disability precludes successful processing of linguistic information through audition, with or without a hearing aid. *Hard-of-hearing* refers to a person who, generally with the use of a hearing aid, has residual hearing sufficient to enable successful processing of linguistic information through audition. Other terms, such as *deaf and dumb, mute,* or *deaf-mute,* are unacceptable. Persons with hearing impairments are not dumb and, if mute, have no physical speech defect other than that caused by the inability to hear.

Hearing defects may be classified according to etiology, pathology, or symptom severity. Each is important in terms of treatment, possible prevention, and rehabilitation.

Etiology.   Hearing loss may be caused by a number of prenatal and postnatal conditions. These include a family history of childhood hearing impairment, anatomic malformations of the head or neck, low birth weight, severe perinatal asphyxia, perinatal infection (cytomegalovirus, rubella, herpes, syphilis, toxoplasmosis, bacterial meningitis), chronic ear infection, cerebral palsy, Down syndrome, or administration of ototoxic drugs.

In addition, high-risk neonates who are surviving formerly fatal prenatal or perinatal conditions may be susceptible to

hearing loss from the disorder or its treatment. For example, sensorineural hearing loss may be a result of continuous humming noises or high noise levels associated with incubators, oxygen hoods, or intensive care units, especially when combined with the use of potentially ototoxic antibiotics.

Environmental noise is a special concern. Sounds loud enough to damage sensitive hair cells of the inner ear can produce irreversible hearing loss. Very loud, brief noise, such as gunfire, can cause immediate, severe, and permanent loss of hearing. Longer exposure to less intense but still hazardous sounds, such as music, can also produce hearing loss (Consensus Conference, 1990). The exact sound level that produces hearing loss is unknown.

Pathology.   Disorders of hearing are divided according to location of the defect. *Conductive* or *middle-ear hearing loss* results from interference of transmission of sound to the middle ear. It is the most common of all types of hearing loss and most frequently is a result of recurrent serous otitis media. Conductive hearing impairment involves mainly interference with loudness of sound.

Sensorineural hearing loss, also called *perceptive* or *nerve deafness,* involves damage to the inner ear structures and/or the auditory nerve. The most common causes are congenital defects of inner ear structures or consequences of acquired conditions, such as kernicterus, infection, administration of ototoxic drugs, or exposure to excessive noise. Sensorineural hearing loss results in distortion of sound and problems in discrimination. Although the child hears some of everything going on around him or her, the sounds are distorted, severely affecting discrimination and comprehension.

Mixed conductive-sensorineural hearing loss results from interference with transmission of sound in the middle ear and along neural pathways. It frequently results from recurrent otitis media and its complications.

Central auditory imperception includes all hearing losses that do not demonstrate defects in the conductive or sensorineural structures. They are usually divided into organic or functional losses. In the *organic type* of central auditory imperception, the defect involves the reception of auditory stimuli along the central pathways and the expression of the message into meaningful communication. Examples are *aphasia,* an inability to express ideas in any form, either written or verbally; *agnosia,* the inability to interpret sound cor-

TABLE 19-2. Intensity of sounds expressed in decibels	
DECIBELS (dB)	REPRESENTATIVE SOUND
0	Softest sound normal ear can hear
10	Heartbeat, rustling of leaves
20	Whisper at 1.8 m (5 feet)
30-45	Normal conversation
60	Noise in average restaurant
70-80	Street noises
80	Loud radio in home
90-100	Train
120	Thunder, rock music
140	Jet airplane during departure
>140	Pain threshold

*1441 York St., Suite 303, Denver, CO 80206; (800) 688-8765 or (303) 333-6155 in Colorado.

rectly; and *dysacusis,* difficulty in processing details or discrimination among sounds.

In the *functional type* of hearing loss, no organic lesion exists to explain a central auditory loss. Examples of functional hearing loss are conversion hysteria (an unconscious withdrawal from hearing to block remembrance of a traumatic event), infantile autism, and childhood schizophrenia.

Symptom Severity. Hearing impairment is expressed in terms of a *decibel (dB),* a unit of loudness (Table 19-2); it is measured at various frequencies, such as 500, 1000, and 2000 cycles per second, the critical listening speech range. Hearing impairment can be classified according to *hearing-threshold level* (the measurement of an individual's hearing threshold by means of an audiometer) and the degree of symptom severity as it affects speech (Table 19-3). These classifications offer only general guidelines regarding the effect of the impairment on any individual child, since children differ greatly in their ability to use residual hearing.

Therapeutic Management

Treatment of hearing loss depends on the cause and type of hearing impairment. Many conductive hearing defects respond to medical or surgical treatment, such as antibiotic therapy for acute otitis media or insertion of tympanostomy tubes for chronic otitis media. When the conductive loss is permanent, hearing can be improved with the use of a hearing aid to amplify sound.

Treatment for sensorineural hearing loss is much less satisfactory. Since the defect is not one of intensity of sound, hearing aids are of less value in this type of defect. The use of *cochlear implants* (a surgically implanted prosthetic device) provides hope for some affected children. Cochlear implants convert sounds to electrical impulses and feed the impulses directly to the auditory nerve, providing information the brain can process to make speech sounds intelligible. Many experts doubt the devices can help children who are born deaf or become so before they learned to talk.

Disorders of central auditory imperception depend on the cause. Functional types, such as conversion hysteria, may re-

TABLE 19-3. Classification of hearing loss based on symptom severity	
HEARING LEVEL (dB)	**EFFECT**
Slight—<30 (hard of hearing)	Has difficulty hearing faint or distant speech Usually is unaware of hearing difficulty Likely to achieve in school but may have problems No speech defects
Mild to moderate— 30-55 (hard of hearing)	Understands conversational speech at 1 to 1.8 m (3 to 5) feet but has difficulty if speech is faint or if not facing speaker May have speech difficulties
Marked—55-70 (hard of hearing)	Unable to understand conversational speech unless loud Considerable difficulty with group or classroom discussion Requires special speech training
Severe—70-90 (deaf)	May hear a loud voice if nearby May be able to identify loud environmental noises Can distinguish vowels but not most consonants Requires speech training
Profound—>90 (deaf)	May hear only loud sounds Requires extensive speech training

RISK CRITERIA FOR SENSORINEURAL HEARING IMPAIRMENT IN YOUNG CHILDREN

Neonates (Birth to 28 Days)
1. Family history of congenital or delayed-onset childhood sensorineural impairment
2. Congenital infection known or suspected to be associated with sensorineural hearing impairment such as toxoplasmosis, syphilis, rubella, cytomegalovirus, and herpes
3. Craniofacial anomalies, including morphologic abnormalities of the pinna and ear canal, absent philtrum, and low hairline
4. Birth weight less than 1500 g (<3.3 pounds)
5. Hyperbilirubinemia at a level exceeding indication for exchange transfusion
6. Ototoxic medications, including but not limited to the aminoglycosides, used for more than 5 days (e.g., gentamicin, tobramycin, kanamycin, streptomycin), and loop diuretics used in combination with aminoglycosides
7. Bacterial meningitis
8. Severe depression at birth, which may include infants with Apgar scores of 0 to 3 at 5 minutes and those who fail to initiate spontaneous respiration by 10 minutes or those with hypotonia persisting to 2 hours of age
9. Prolonged mechanical ventilation for a duration equal to or greater than 10 days (e.g., persistent pulmonary hypertension)
10. Stigmata or other findings associated with syndromes known to include sensorineural hearing loss (e.g., Waardenburg or Usher syndrome)

Risk Criteria: Infants (29 Days to 2 Years)
1. Parent/caregiver concern regarding hearing, speech, language, and/or developmental delay
2. Bacterial meningitis
3. Neonatal risk factors that may be associated with progressive sensorineural hearing loss (e.g., cytomegalovirus, prolonged mechanical ventilation, inherited disorders)
4. Head trauma, especially with either longitudinal or transverse fracture of the temporal bone
5. Stigmata or other findings associated with syndromes known to include sensorineural hearing loss (e.g., Waardenburg or Usher syndrome)
6. Ototoxic medications, including but not limited to the aminoglycosides, used for more than 5 days (e.g., gentamicin, tobramycin, kanamycin, streptomycin), and loop diuretics used in combination with aminoglycosides
7. Children with neurodegenerative disorders such as neurofibromatosis, myoclonic epilepsy, Werdnig-Hoffmann disease, Tay-Sachs disease, Niemann-Pick disease, any metachromatic leukodystrophy, or any infantile demyelinating neuropathy
8. Childhood infectious diseases known to be associated with sensorineural hearing loss (e.g., mumps, measles)

From American Speech-Language Hearing Association: Joint Committee on Infant Hearing 1990 position statement, *ASHA* 33(suppl 5):3-6, 1991.

quire psychologic intervention, but others, such as autism, may not respond to any therapy.

Tactile devices are another option for persons with profound hearing impairment to improve their speech perception. A vibrotactile or electrotactile signal is used to transmit impulses to a point of stimulation, usually the fingers or hands. This information is then transmitted to the language-processing center in the brain (Sarant and others, 1993).

❖ Assessment

Assessment of children for hearing impairment is a critical nursing responsibility. Discovery of a hearing impairment within the first 6 to 12 months of life is essential to prevent social, physical, and psychologic damage to the child. Assessment involves (1) identifying those children who by virtue of their history are at risk (see box on p. 580), (2) observing for behaviors that indicate a hearing loss, and (3) screening all children for auditory function. This discussion focuses on developmental and behavioral indices associated with hearing impairment. Auditory testing is presented in Chapter 7.

Infancy.   At birth the nurse can observe the neonate's response to auditory stimuli, as evidenced by the startle reflex, head turning, eye blinking, and cessation of body movement. The infant may vary in the intensity of the response, depending on the state of alertness. However, a consistent absence of a reaction should lead to suspicion of hearing loss. The box summarizes other clinical manifestations of hearing impairment in the infant.

CLINICAL MANIFESTATIONS OF HEARING IMPAIRMENT

Infants

Lack of startle or blink reflex to a loud sound
Failure to be awakened by loud environmental noises
Failure to localize a source of sound by 6 months of age
Absence of babble or inflections in voice by age 7 months
General indifference to sound
Lack of response to the spoken word; failure to follow verbal directions
Response to loud noises as opposed to the voice

Children

Use of gestures rather than verbalization to express desires, especially after age 15 months
Failure to develop intelligible speech by age 24 months
Monotone quality, unintelligible speech, lessened laughter
Vocal play, head banging, or foot stamping for vibratory sensation
Yelling or screeching to express pleasure, annoyance (tantrums), or need
Asking to have statements repeated or answering them incorrectly
Responding more to facial expression and gestures than verbal explanation
Avoidance of social interaction; often puzzled and unhappy in such situations; prefer to play alone
Inquiring, sometimes confused facial expression
Suspicious alertness, sometimes interpreted as paranoia, alternating with cooperation
Frequently stubborn because of lack of comprehension
Irritable at not making themselves understood
Shy, timid, and withdrawn
Often appear "dreamy," "in a world of their own," or extremely inattentive

---

Childhood.   The child who is profoundly deaf is much more likely to be diagnosed during infancy than the less severely affected one. If the defect is not detected during early childhood, it likely will become evident during entry into school, when the child has difficulty in learning. Unfortunately, some of these children are mistakenly placed in special classes for students with learning disabilities or MR. Therefore it is essential that the nurse suspect a hearing impairment in any child who demonstrates the behaviors listed in the box.

Of primary importance is the effect of hearing impairment on speech development. A child with a mild conductive hearing loss may speak fairly clearly but in a loud, monotone voice. A child with a sensorineural defect usually has difficulty in articulation. For example, inability to hear higher frequencies may result in the word *spoon* being pronounced "poon." Children with articulation problems need to have their hearing tested.

Nursing ALERT   When parents express concern about their child's hearing and speech development, refer the child for a hearing evaluation. Absence of well-formed syllables ("da," "na," "yaya") by 11 months of age should result in immediate referral (Eilers and Oller, 1994).

❖ Nursing Diagnoses

A number of nursing diagnoses are prominent in the nursing care of the child with hearing impairment and the child's family; other diagnoses specific to individual cases become evident. The most common nursing diagnoses are outlined in the Nursing Care Plan on pp. 584-585.

❖ Planning

The goals of nursing care for the child with hearing impairment and family are as follows:

1. Child will achieve optimum development through enhancement of the communication process and socialization.
2. Child and family will receive support.
3. Child will receive appropriate care during hospitalization.

❖ Implementation

Promote Communication Process.   The nurse's initial role in rehabilitation is to encourage the family to participate in an auditory training program.* Rehabilitation training consists of using a hearing aid and learning lipreading (speech reading), sign language, and verbal communication.

Hearing Aids.   The nurse should be familiar with the types, basic care, and handling of hearing aids, especially when the child is hospitalized.† Types of aids include those

---

*Home training correspondence programs are sponsored by the **John T. Tracy Clinic,** 806 West Adams Blvd., Los Angeles, CA 90007; (213) 748-5481. Other sources of information on several aspects of hearing loss and on the International Parents' Organization are the **Alexander Graham Bell Association for the Deaf,** 3417 Volta Place, N.W., Washington, DC 20007, (202) 337-5220; and **Canadian Hearing Society,** 271 Spadina Rd., Toronto, Ontario M5R 2V3, (416) 964-9595.
†Information about hearing aids is available from the **National Hearing Aid Society,** 20361 Middlebelt Rd., Livonia, MI 48152; (800) 521-5247 or (313) 478-2610 (in Michigan).

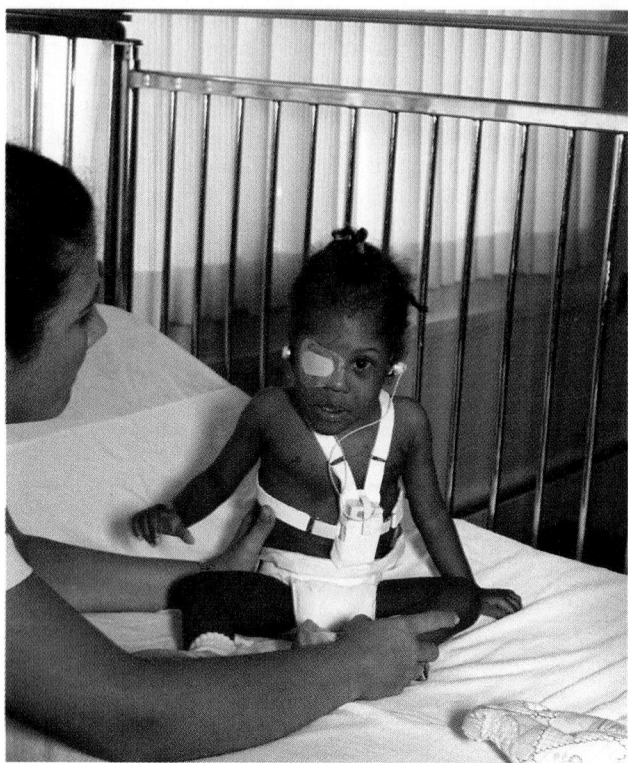

FIG. 19-7. On-the-body hearing aids are convenient for young children, such as this child with severe bilateral hearing loss. Note eye patching for strabismus.

worn in or behind the ear, models incorporated into an eyeglass frame, or types worn on the body with a wire connection to the ear (Fig. 19-7). One of the most common problems with a hearing aid is *acoustic feedback,* an annoying whistling sound usually caused by improper fit of the ear mold. Sometimes the whistling may be at a frequency that the child cannot hear but that is annoying to others. In this case, if children are old enough, they are told of the noise and asked to readjust the aid.

NURSING TIP To reduce or eliminate whistling from a hearing aid, try reinserting the aid, making certain that no hair is caught between the ear mold and canal, cleaning the ear mold or ear, or lowering the volume of the aid.

As children grow older, they may be self-conscious about the device. Every effort is made to make the aid inconspicuous, such as an appropriate hairstyle to cover behind-the-ear or in-the-ear models, attractive frames for glasses, and placement of the on-the-body type where it is not seen, such as under a blouse or sweater. Children are given responsibility for the care of the device as soon as they are able, since fostering independence is a primary goal of rehabilitation.

Nursing ALERT Stress to parents the importance of storing batteries for hearing aids in a safe location and to teach children or supervise young children not to remove the battery from the hearing aid. Ingestion of batteries is most often of those from hearing aids, including the child's own aid (Litovitz and Schmitz, 1992).

 GUIDELINES
Facilitating Lipreading

Attract child's attention before speaking; use light touch to signal speaker's presence.
Stand close to child.
Face child directly or move to a 45-degree angle.
Stand still; do not walk back and forth or turn away to point or look elsewhere.
Establish eye contact and show interest.
Speak at eye level and with good lighting on speaker's face.
Be certain nothing interferes with speech patterns, such as chewing food or gum.
Speak clearly and at a slow and even rate.
Use facial expression to assist in conveying messages.
Keep sentences short.
Rephrase message if child does not understand the words.

Lipreading. Even though the child may become an expert at lipreading, only about 40% of the spoken word is understood, and less if the speaker has an accent, mustache, or beard. Exaggerating pronunciation or speaking in an altered rhythm further lessens comprehension. Parents can help the child understand the spoken word by using the suggestions in the Guidelines box. The child learns to supplement the spoken word with sensitivity to visual cues, primarily body language and facial expression (e.g., tightening the lips, muscle tension, eye contact).

Cued Speech. This method of communication is an adjunct to straight lipreading. It uses hand signals to help the child with a hearing impairment distinguish between words that look alike when formed by the lips (e.g., "mat," "bat"). It is most often used by children with hearing impairments who are using speech rather than those who are nonverbal.

Sign Language. Sign language, such as the **American Sign Language (ASL)** or **British Sign Language (BSL),** is a visual-gestural language that uses hand signals that roughly correspond to specific words and concepts in the English language. Family members are encouraged to learn signing because using or watching hands requires much less concentration than lipreading or talking. Also, a symbol method enables some children to learn more and to learn faster.

Speech Therapy. The most formidable task in the education of a child who is profoundly hearing impaired is learning to speak. Speech is learned through a multisensory approach, using visual, tactile, kinesthetic, and auditory stimulation. Since the usual mechanism for learning language (imitation and reinforcement) is not available to the child, systematic formal education is required. Parents are encouraged to participate fully in the learning process.

Additional Aids. Everyday activities present problems for older children with hearing impairment. For example, they may not be able to hear the telephone, doorbell, or alarm clock. Several commercial devices are available to help them adjust to these dilemmas. Flashing lights can be attached to a telephone or doorbell to signal its ringing. Trained hearing ear dogs can provide great assistance because they alert the person to sounds, such as someone approaching, a moving car, a signal to wake up, or a child's cry. Special *teletypewriters* or *telecommunications devices for the deaf (TDD)* help people with impaired hearing communicate with each other over the telephone; the typed message is conveyed via the telephone lines and displayed on a small screen.*

Any audiovisual medium presents dilemmas for these children, who can see the picture but cannot hear the message. However, with *closed captioning* a special decoding device is attached to the television, and the audio portion of a program is translated into subtitles that appear on the screen.†

As children learn to compensate for their lack of hearing, they become extremely perceptive to visual and vibratory changes. They often know when another person wants to talk to them because the person will walk close by but not pass. They learn to be alert to other people approaching them by seeing their shadows or feeling the vibrations of their footsteps. They are acutely aware of facial expressions and may comprehend the unspoken word more quickly than the spoken word.

Socialization. Since socialization is extremely important to the child's development, the nurse discusses with the family methods of fostering social contact. If children attend a special school for the deaf, they are able to socialize with peers in that setting. Classmates become a potential source of close friendships because they communicate more easily among themselves. Parents are encouraged to promote these relationships whenever possible.

Children with a hearing impairment may need special help in school or social activities. For those children wearing hearing aids, background noise should be kept to a minimum. Since many of these children are able to attend regular classes, the teacher may need assistance in adapting methods of teaching for the child's benefit. The school nurse is often in an optimum position to emphasize methods of facilitated communication, such as lipreading (see Guidelines box). Since group projects and audiovisual teaching aids may hinder the child's learning, these educational methods should be carefully evaluated.

In a group setting it is helpful for the other members to sit in a semicircle in front of the child. Since one of the difficulties in following a group discussion is that the child is unaware of who will speak next, someone should point out each speaker. Speakers can also be given numbers, or their names can be written down as each person talks. If one person writes down the main topic of the discussion, the child is able to follow lipreading more closely. Such suggestions can increase the child's ability to participate in sports, clubs such as Boy Scouts or Girl Scouts, and group projects.

Support Child and Family. Once the diagnosis of hearing impairment is made, parents need extensive support to adjust to the shock of learning about their child's disability and an opportunity to realize the extent of the hearing loss. If the hearing loss occurs during childhood, the child also requires sensitive, supportive care during the long and often difficult adjustment to this sensory loss. Early rehabilitation is one of the best strategies for fostering adjustment. However, progress in learning communication may not always coincide with emotional adjustment. Depression or anger is common, and such feelings are a normal part of the grieving process. (See also Chapter 18 for an extensive discussion of the emotional support of the child and family.)

Care for Child During Hospitalization. The needs of the hospitalized child with impaired hearing are the same as those of any other child, but the disability presents special challenges to the nurse (see Critical Thinking Exercise). For example, verbal explanations must be supplemented with tactile and visual aids, such as books or actual demonstration and practice. Children's understanding of the explanation needs to be constantly reassessed. If their verbal skills are poorly developed, they can answer questions through drawing, writing, or gesturing. For example, if the nurse is attempting to clarify where a spinal tap is done, the child is asked to point to where the procedure will be done on the body. Since these children often need more time to grasp the full meaning of an explanation, the nurse needs to be patient, allowing ample time for understanding.

When communicating with the child, the nurse should use the same principles as those outlined for facilitating lipreading. Ideally, nurses without foreign accents should be assigned to the child. The child's hearing aid is checked to ensure that it is working properly. If it is necessary to awaken the child at night, the nurse gently shakes the child or turns on the hearing aid before arousing the child. The nurse always makes sure that the child can see him or her before any procedures, even routine ones such as changing a diaper or

---

CRITICAL THINKING EXERCISE
Hearing Impairment

Five-year-old Jason has a severe congenital hearing impairment. You have been assigned to care for him in the outpatient surgery postanesthesia care unit (PACU), where he has just been admitted following a herniorrhaphy. As he emerges from anesthesia, he becomes more and more agitated. The most likely cause for his behavior is which of the following?

1. This is a normal reaction to anesthesia.
2. He is experiencing separation anxiety.
3. He is unable to communicate properly.
4. He is in pain.

The correct answer is three. Because Jason became increasingly more agitated as he emerged from anesthesia, his behavior does not suggest the transitory confusion associated with the initial emergence from anesthesia. Rather, it suggests that as he became more aware of his surroundings and tried to communicate with the staff, Jason became increasingly frustrated. Reasons for this might include (a) not having his hearing aid in place; (b) having his arms restrained by intravenous lines, pulse oximetry monitors, and a blood pressure cuff, thus restricting his use of sign language; (c) being unable to read the nurse's lips from a prone position; or (d) not having a nurse who could understand his speech or know or recognize his attempts to use sign language. Although pain is a possibility and needs to be evaluated, regional blocks are typically given during the surgery to keep children comfortable until after they are discharged home. It is unlikely that Jason is having separation anxiety, since this usually occurs in younger children.

Nursing Care Plan
The Child with Hearing Impairment

NURSING DIAGNOSIS: Sensory/perceptual alterations (auditory) related to hearing impairment

PATIENT GOAL 1: Will experience maximum hearing potential

- **NURSING INTERVENTIONS/*RATIONALES***

Help family investigate hearing aid dealers *to locate a reliable dealer*

Discuss types of hearing aids and their proper care *to ensure maximum benefit*

Stress to family importance of storing hearing aid batteries safely and of teaching children (or supervising young children) not to remove the battery *to prevent ingestion or aspiration of batteries*

Teach child how to regulate hearing aid *for maximum benefit*

Help child focus on all sounds in the environment and talk about them *to maximize hearing*

For older child, discuss methods of camouflaging the aid *to make it less conspicuous*

- **EXPECTED OUTCOMES**

Child acquires and uses hearing aid properly

Child does not ingest or aspirate hearing aid battery

NURSING DIAGNOSIS: Impaired verbal communication related to inability to hear auditory cues

PATIENT GOAL 1: Will engage in communication process within limits of impairment

- **NURSING INTERVENTIONS/*RATIONALES***

Encourage family to attend the rehabilitation program *in order to continue learning in the home;* encourage them to learn sign language *as a method of communication*

Teach language that serves a useful purpose *for communication*

Encourage use of language and books in the home *to stimulate verbal communication and promote normal development*

Encourage spontaneous language and correct speech *to promote speech development*

- **EXPECTED OUTCOMES**

Family continues communication practices in home environment

Family provides stimulation to child

PATIENT GOAL 2: Will demonstrate ability to lipread.

- **NURSING INTERVENTIONS/*RATIONALES***

Test child for visual problems *that may interfere with learning to lipread or use sign language*

Teach family and others involved with child (e.g., teacher)

behaviors that facilitate lipreading (see box on p. 582) *to promote communication process*

- **EXPECTED OUTCOMES**

Child communicates with others in manner taught (specify)

Persons communicating with child use good communication techniques

NURSING DIAGNOSIS: Altered growth and development related to impaired communication

PATIENT GOAL 1: Will achieve optimum independence level for age

- **NURSING INTERVENTIONS/*RATIONALES***

Help family transfer normal childrearing practices to this child *to promote optimum development*

Emphasize importance of attaining independence in self-care

Provide child with devices that foster independence (e.g., hearing ear dog, special signaling aids for telephone or doorbell)

Discuss with family importance of discipline and limit-setting, *since all children have these needs*

- **EXPECTED OUTCOMES**

Child performs activities of daily living appropriate to level of development

Appropriate discipline and limit-setting are provided

PATIENT GOAL 2: Will have opportunity to participate in activities for play and socialization

- **NURSING INTERVENTIONS/*RATIONALES***

Guide family in selection of toys *to maximize visual and tactile senses, as well as residual hearing*

Encourage child to participate in group activities (e.g., scouting, sports) *to promote socialization*

Help child follow group discussion by pointing out the speaker and arranging the group in a semicircle *to facilitate hearing and/or lipreading*

Help child develop friendships among hearing and deaf peers *to promote socialization*

Recommend closed-captioned television *for child's enjoyment*

- **EXPECTED OUTCOMES**

Child engages in activities appropriate to developmental level

Child has peer relationships and experiences

PATIENT GOAL 3: Will be provided educational opportunities within a regular classroom

- **NURSING INTERVENTIONS/*RATIONALES***

Discuss with teacher and children ways of communicating effectively with child (e.g., through facilitating lipreading) *to facilitate child's education*

Promote socialization with classmates *to encourage enjoyment of education*

- **EXPECTED OUTCOMES**

Child attends school regularly

Child communicates with others in the classroom

NURSING CARE PLAN
The Child with Hearing Impairment—cont'd

NURSING DIAGNOSIS: Altered family processes related to diagnosis of deafness of a child

PATIENT (FAMILY) GOAL 1: Will adjust to child's hearing loss

- **NURSING INTERVENTIONS/*RATIONALES***

Anticipate grief reaction as part of adjustment to loss

Provide opportunities for family to express feelings and concerns *to promote adjustment*

Help family deal with feelings regarding previous responses to child when true nature of the problem was unknown *to minimize feelings of guilt*

Help family realize extent of child's disability and its tremendous influence on speech and language development

Discuss advantages and limitations of amplifying devices with different types of hearing loss *so that family can make informed decisions*

Encourage formal rehabilitation as soon as possible *to foster normal growth and development of child*

- **EXPECTED OUTCOMES**

Family expresses feelings and concerns regarding child's loss of hearing

Family demonstrates an understanding of the implications of hearing loss

Family becomes involved in appropriate programs

PATIENT (FAMILY) GOAL 2: Will receive emotional support

- **NURSING INTERVENTIONS/*RATIONALES***

Be available to family *for assistance and support*

Encourage family members to discuss their feelings regarding the disability *to enhance coping*

Stress child's abilities rather than disability *to promote child's optimum development*

Become familiar with techniques used for communication if following the family on a long-term basis

Refer family to appropriate community agencies for medical, psychiatric, educational, vocational, or financial assistance *to ensure that their overall needs are met*

Involve parents in local parent groups for deaf children *for continuing support*

- **EXPECTED OUTCOMES**

Family expresses feelings and concerns about the disability and its ramifications

Family members avail themselves of available resources

PATIENT (FAMILY) GOAL 3: Will demonstrate attachment to child

- **NURSING INTERVENTIONS/*RATIONALES***

Help family identify clues other than verbal ones that signify infant's communication with them, *since communication is an important part of attachment process*

Encourage family to stimulate child with visual and tactile cues, *since auditory cues are absent or diminished*

Stress importance of continuing to talk to child even though child may not hear their voices *to promote normalization*

- **EXPECTED OUTCOME**

Parents and child demonstrate a positive relationship

NURSING DIAGNOSIS: High risk for injury related to environmental hazards, infection

PATIENT (OTHERS) GOAL 1: Will not acquire or have greater hearing loss

- **NURSING INTERVENTIONS/*RATIONALES***

Infancy

Encourage immunization at appropriate age *to prevent acquired sensorineural hearing loss from childhood diseases*

Minimize noise levels in intensive care unit, *since this is associated with hearing loss*

Prevent ear infection; detect early *because this is the most common cause of impaired hearing*

Childhood

Assess hearing ability of infants and children receiving ototoxic antibiotics *for early detection*

Promote compliance with treatment regimens for otitis media, *since this is a common cause of impaired hearing*

Discuss with parents measures to prevent otitis media (see Chapter 23)

Evaluate auditory ability of children prone to chronic ear or respiratory problems *for early detection of impaired hearing*

Assess sources of excessive noise in child's environment; institute appropriate measures to decrease sound levels (e.g., turn music lower, use ear protection) *because exposure to excessive noise is a cause of sensorineural hearing loss*

Participate in immunization programs for children *to prevent childhood diseases that may result in hearing loss*

- **EXPECTED OUTCOMES**

Infant or child does not develop hearing loss

Child is not exposed to excessive noise levels

Child is properly immunized

See also Nursing Care Plan: The Child with Chronic Illness or Disability, Chapter 18

regulating an infusion, are performed. It is important to remember that the child may not be aware of one's presence until alerted through visual or tactile cues.

Ideally, parents are encouraged to room with the child. However, it must be conveyed to them that this is not to serve as a convenience to the nurse but as a benefit to the child. Although the parents' aid can be enlisted in familiarizing the child with the hospital and explaining procedures, the nurse also talks directly to the youngster, encouraging expression of feelings about the experience. If there is difficulty in understanding the child's speech, an effort is made to become familiar with his or her pronunciation of words. Parents often can be helpful by explaining the child's usual speech habits. Nonvocal communication devices that employ pictures or words that the child can point to are also available (see p. 572). Such boards can also be made by drawing pictures or writing the words of common needs on cardboard, such as *parent, food, water,* or *toilet.*

The nurse has a special role as child advocate with the child and is in a strategic position to alert other health team members and other patients to the child's special needs regarding communication. For example, the nurse should accompany other practitioners on visits to the child's room to ensure that they speak to the child and that the child understands what is said. Caregivers sometimes forget that the child has the abilities to perceive and learn despite a hearing loss, and consequently they communicate only with the parents. As a result, the child's needs and feelings remain unrecognized and unmet.

Because children with impaired hearing may have difficulty in forming social relationships with other children, the child is introduced to roommates and encouraged to engage in play activities. The hospital setting can provide growth-promoting opportunities for social relationships. With the assistance of a child-life specialist, the child can learn new recreational activities, experiment with group games, and engage in therapeutic play. The use of puppets, dollhouses, role playing with dress-up clothes, building with a hammer and nails, finger painting, playing with syringes, and water play can help the child express feelings that previously were suppressed.

Assist in Measures to Prevent Hearing Impairment. A primary nursing role is prevention of hearing loss. Since the most common cause of impaired hearing is chronic otitis media, it is essential that appropriate measures be instituted to treat existing infections and prevent recurrences (see Chapter 23). Children with histories of ear or respiratory infections or any other condition known to increase the risk of hearing impairment should receive periodic auditory testing.

To prevent the causes of hearing loss that begin prenatally and perinatally, pregnant women need counseling regarding the necessity of early prenatal care, including genetic counseling for known familial disorders; avoidance of all ototoxic drugs, especially during the first trimester; tests to rule out syphilis, rubella, or blood incompatibility; medical management of maternal diabetes; control of alcoholism; and adequate dietary intake. The necessity of routine immunization during childhood to eliminate the possibility of acquired sensorineural loss from rubella, mumps, or measles (encephalitis) is stressed.

Exposure to excessive noise pollution is a well-established cause of sensorineural hearing loss. The nurse should routinely assess the possibility of environmental noise pollution and advise children and parents of the potential danger. When individuals engage in activities associated with high-intensity noise, such as flying model airplanes, target shooting, or snowmobiling, they should wear ear protection such as earmuffs or earplugs (not ordinary dry cotton). However, any protection is better than none. Even common household equipment, such as lawn mowers, power vacuum cleaners, and cordless telephones, can be hazardous.

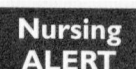 **Nursing ALERT** Suspect hazardous noise if the listener experiences (1) difficulty in communication while hearing the sound, (2) ringing in the ears (tinnitus) after exposure to the sound, or (3) muffled hearing after leaving the sound.

❖ Evaluation

The effectiveness of nursing interventions is determined by continual reassessment and evaluation of care based on the following observational guidelines and expected outcomes:

1. Observe the techniques used to communicate with the child; inquire if child is enrolled in auditory training program; inquire about socialization opportunities for the child (i.e., who are child's friends, what are his or her extracurricular activities).
2. Interview family regarding their adjustment to the sensory impairment; observe family members' relationship with the child; interview child regarding feelings about the sensory impairment and its effect on activities of daily living (especially important if impairment is recent).
3. Observe types of preparation and communication used to prepare child for hospitalization or procedures; observe parents' involvement in child's care; observe interaction of child and family with other patients.
4. Investigate community programs aimed at preventing or detecting hearing loss and inquire as to nursing involvement in these efforts.

Expected outcomes:
See Nursing Care Plan, pp. 584-585.

VISUAL IMPAIRMENT

Visual impairment is a common problem during childhood. In the United States the prevalence of blindness and serious visual impairment in the pediatric population is estimated at 30 to 64 children per 100,000 population. Another 100 children per 100,000 have less serious impairment (Davidson, 1992). The nurse's role is clearly one of assessment, prevention, referral, and in some instances rehabilitation.

Definition and Classification

Visual impairment is a general term that refers to visual loss that cannot be corrected with regular prescription lenses. However, more useful definitions for classifying visual impairments include the following. *School vision* (also known as *partially sighted*) refers to visual acuity between 20/70 and 20/200. The child should be able to obtain an education in the usual public school system with the use of normal-sized print. Near vision is almost always better than distance vision. *Legal blindness,* visual acuity of 20/200 or less and/or a visual field of 20 degrees or less in the better eye, is useful only as a legal definition, not as a medical diagnosis. It allows special considerations with regard to taxes, entrance into special schools, eligibility for aid, and other benefits.

Refractive Errors

Myopia

Nearsightedness—ability to see objects clearly at close range but not at a distance

PATHOPHYSIOLOGY

Results from eyeball that is too long, causing image to fall in front of retina

CLINICAL MANIFESTATIONS

Rubs eyes excessively

Tilts head or thrusts head forward

Has difficulty in reading or other close work

Holds books close to eyes

Writes or colors with head close to table

Clumsy; walks into objects

Blinks more than usual or is irritable when doing close work

Is unable to see objects clearly

Does poorly in school, especially in subjects that require demonstration, such as arithmetic

Dizziness

Headache

Nausea after close work

TREATMENT

Corrected with biconcave lenses that focus rays on retina

Hyperopia

Farsightedness—ability to see objects at a distance

PATHOPHYSIOLOGY

Results from eyeball that is too short, causing image to focus beyond retina

CLINICAL MANIFESTATIONS

Because of accommodative ability, child can usually see objects at all ranges

Most children normally hyperopic until about 7 years of age

TREATMENT

If correction is required, use convex lenses to focus rays on retina

Astigmatism

Unequal curvatures in refractive apparatus

PATHOPHYSIOLOGY

Results from unequal curvatures in cornea or lens that cause light rays to bend in different directions

CLINICAL MANIFESTATIONS

Depends on severity of refractive error in each eye

May have clinical manifestations of myopia

TREATMENT

Corrected with special lenses that compensate for refractive errors

Anisometropia

Different refractive strength in each eye

PATHOPHYSIOLOGY

May develop amblyopia as weaker eye is used less

CLINICAL MANIFESTATIONS

Depends on severity of refractive error in each eye

May have clinical manifestations of myopia

TREATMENT

Treated with corrective lenses, preferably contact lenses, to improve vision in each eye so they work as a unit

Amblyopia

Lazy eye—reduced visual acuity in one eye

PATHOPHYSIOLOGY

Results when one eye does not receive sufficient stimulation

Each retina receives different images, resulting in diplopia (double vision)

Brain accommodates by suppressing less intense image

Visual cortex eventually does not respond to visual stimulation, with loss of vision in that eye

CLINICAL MANIFESTATIONS

Poor vision in affected eye

TREATMENT

Preventable if treatment of primary visual defect, such as anisometropia or strabismus, begins before 6 years of age

Strabismus

"Squint" or *cross-eye*—malalignment of eyes (Fig. 19-8)

Estropia—inward deviation of eye

Exotropia—outward deviation of eye

PATHOPHYSIOLOGY

May result from muscle imbalance or paralysis, poor vision, or congenital defect

Since visual axes are not parallel, brain receives two images, and amblyopia can result

CLINICAL MANIFESTATIONS

Squints eyelids together or frowns

Has difficulty in focusing from one distance to another

Inaccurate judgment in picking up objects

Unable to see print or moving objects clearly

Closes one eye to see

Tilts head to one side

If combined with refractive errors, may see any of the manifestations listed for refractive errors

Diplopia

Photophobia

Dizziness

Headache

Cross-eye

TREATMENT

Treatment depends on cause of strabismus

May involve occlusion therapy (patching stronger eye) or surgery to increase visual stimulation to weaker eye

Early diagnosis is essential to prevent vision loss

Cataracts

Opacity of crystalline lens

PATHOPHYSIOLOGY

Prevents light rays from entering eye and refracting them on retina

CLINICAL MANIFESTATIONS

Gradually less able to see objects clearly

May lose peripheral vision

Nystagmus (with complete blindness)

Gray opacities of lens

Strabismus

Absence of red reflex

TREATMENT

Requires surgery to remove cloudy lens and replace lens (intraocular lens implant, removable contact lens, prescription glasses)

Must be treated early to prevent blindness from amblyopia

Glaucoma

Increased intraocular pressure

PATHOPHYSIOLOGY

Congenital type results from defective development of some component related to flow of aqueous humor

Increased pressure on optic nerve causes eventual atrophy and blindness

CLINICAL MANIFESTATIONS

Mostly seen in acquired types—loses peripheral vision

May bump into objects not directly in front

Sees halos around objects

May complain of mild pain or discomfort (severe pain, nausea, vomiting, if sudden rise in pressure)

Redness

Excessive tearing (epiphora)

Photophobia

Spasmodic winking (blepharospasm)

Corneal haziness

Enlargement of eyeball (buphthalmos)

TREATMENT

Requires surgical treatment (goniotomy) to open outflow tracts

May require more than one procedure

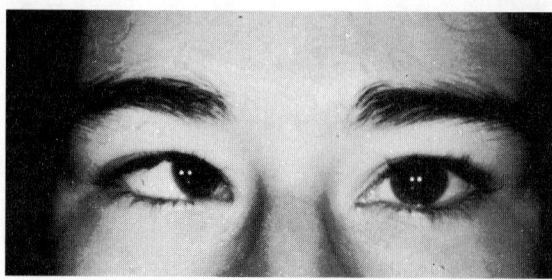

FIG. 19-8. Strabismus (esotropia). Note obvious malalignment of eyes. Light reflections are centered in the left cornea and to the side of the right cornea. (From Havener WH and others: *Nursing care in eye, ear, nose, and throat disorders,* ed 3, St Louis, 1974, Mosby.)

Etiology

Visual impairment can be caused by a number of genetic and prenatal or postnatal conditions. These include perinatal infections (herpes, chlamydia, gonococci, rubella, syphilis, toxoplasmosis), retinopathy of prematurity, trauma, postnatal infections (meningitis), and disorders such as sickle cell disease, juvenile rheumatoid arthritis, Tay-Sachs disease, albinism, and retinoblastoma. In many instances, such as with refractive errors, the cause of the defect is unknown.

Refractive errors are the most common types of visual disorders in children. The term *refraction* means bending and refers to the bending of light rays as they pass through the lens of the eye. Normally, light rays enter the lens and fall directly on the retina. However, in refractive disorders the light rays either fall in front of the retina *(myopia)* or beyond it *(hyperopia)*. Other eye problems, such as strabismus, may or may not include refractive errors, but they are very important because, if untreated, they result in blindness from amblyopia. These, along with other less frequent visual disorders, are summarized in the box on p. 587. In addition to these disorders, other visual problems can be the result of infection or trauma.

Trauma. Trauma is a common cause of blindness in children. Injuries to the eyeball and adnexa (supporting or accessory structures, e.g., eyelids, conjunctiva, lacrimal glands) can be classified as penetrating or nonpenetrating. *Penetrating wounds* are most often a result of sharp instruments, such as sticks, knives, or scissors; propulsive objects, such as firecrackers, guns, bows and arrows, or slingshots; or a powerful contusion by a blunt object, which may occur during a fight or from a serious car accident. *Nonpenetrating injuries* may be a result of foreign objects in the eyes, lacerations, a blow from a blunt object such as a ball (baseball, softball, basketball, racquet sports) or fist, or thermal or chemical burns.

Treatment is aimed at preventing further ocular damage and is primarily the responsibility of the ophthalmologist. It involves adequate examination of the injured eye (with the child sedated or anesthetized in severe injuries), appropriate immediate intervention such as removal of the foreign body or suturing of the laceration, and prevention of complications, such as administration of antibiotics or steroids and complete bed rest to allow the eye to heal and blood to reabsorb (see Emergency Treatment box on p. 589). The prog-

nosis varies according to the type of injury. It is usually guarded in all cases of penetrating wounds because of the high risk of serious complications.

Infections. Infections of the adnexa and the structures of the eyeball or globe may occur in children. The most common eye infection is *conjunctivitis* (see Chapter 14). Treatment is usually ophthalmic antibiotics. Severe infections may require systemic antibiotic therapy. Steroids are used cautiously because they exacerbate viral infections such as herpes simplex, increasing the risk of damage to the involved structures.

Nursing Considerations

❖ Assessment

Assessment of children for visual impairment is a critical nursing responsibility. Discovery of a visual impairment as early as possible is essential to prevent social, physical, and psychologic damage to the child. Assessment involves (1) identifying those children who by virtue of their history are at risk, (2) observing for behaviors that indicate a vision loss, and (3) screening all children for visual acuity and signs of other ocular disorders, such as strabismus. This discussion focuses on clinical manifestation of various types of visual problems (see box on p. 587). Vision testing is discussed in Chapter 7.

Infancy. At birth the nurse should observe the neonate's response to visual stimuli, such as following a light or object and cessation of body movement. The infant may vary in the intensity of the response, depending on the state of alertness.

Of special importance in detecting visual impairment during infancy are the parents' concerns regarding visual responsiveness in their child. Their concerns, such as lack of eye contact from the infant, must be taken seriously. During infancy the child should be tested for strabismus. Lack of binocularity after 4 months of age is considered abnormal and must be treated to prevent amblyopia.

Nursing ALERT	Suspect blindness if the infant does not react to light and in any-age child if parents express concern.

Childhood. Since the most common visual impairment during childhood is refractive errors, testing for visual acuity is essential. The school nurse usually assumes major responsibility for vision testing in schoolchildren. Besides refractive errors, the nurse should be aware of signs and symptoms that indicate other ocular problems. If a referral is made to the family requesting further eye testing, the nurse is responsible for follow-up concerning the recommendation.

❖ Nursing Diagnoses

A number of nursing diagnoses are prominent in the nursing care of the child with visual impairment and the child's family (see box on p. 588); other diagnoses specific to individual cases become evident.

❖ Planning

The goals of care for the child with visual impairment and family are as follows:

1. Child and family will receive support and education.
2. Parent-child attachment will develop.
3. Child will achieve optimum development.
4. Child will receive appropriate care during hospitalization.

❖ Implementation

Support Child and Family. The shock of learning that their child is blind or partially sighted is an immense crisis for families. Of all types of disabilities, many people fear loss of sight the most. Vision is involved in almost every activity of daily living. Parents need support during the initial phase of learning about the diagnosis and help to gain a realistic understanding of their child's abilities. The family is encouraged to investigate appropriate stimulation and educational programs for their child as soon as possible. Sources of information include state **Commissions for the Blind,** local schools for the blind, the **American Foundation for the Blind,*** **National Federation of the Blind,**† **National Association for Parents of the Visually Impaired, Inc.**‡ **National Association for Visually Handicapped,**§ and **American Council of the Blind.**‖

When blindness is not congenital but acquired, newly blind children need much support to help them adjust to the disability. They are usually frightened and confused by the sudden or progressive loss of sight and benefit from an environment that provides security and familiarity.

Promote Parent-Child Attachment. A crucial time in the life of blind infants is when they and their parents are getting acquainted with each other. Pleasurable patterns of interaction between the infant and parents may be lacking if there is not enough reciprocity. For example, if the parent gazes fondly at the infant's face and seeks eye contact but the infant fails to respond because he or she cannot see the parent, a troubled cycle of responses may occur. The nurse can help parents learn to look for other cues that indicate the infant is responding to them, such as whether the eyelids blink; whether the activity level accelerates or slows; whether respi-

---

*11 Penn Plaza, Suite 300, New York, NY 10001, (212) 502-7600.
†1800 Johnson St., Baltimore, MD 21230; (410) 659-9314.
‡2180 Linway Dr., Beloit, WI 53511; (800) 562-6265.
§22 W. 21st St., New York, NY 10010; (212) 889-3141.
‖1155 15th St., N.W., Washington, DC 20005; (202) 467-5081 or (800) 424-8666 (afternoons only).
Sources of information in Canada include the **Canadian National Institute for the Blind,** 1931 Bayview Ave., Toronto, Ontario M4G 4C8; **Low Vision Association of Canada,** 145 Adelaide St. West, Toronto, Ontario M5H 3H4; and **Blind Organization of Ontario,** 597 Parliament St., Suite B-3, Toronto, Ontario M4X 1W3.

EMERGENCY TREATMENT
Eye Injuries

Foreign Object
Examine eye for presence of a foreign body (evert upper lid to examine upper eye).
Remove a freely movable object with pointed corner of gauze pad lightly moistened with water.
Do not irrigate eye or attempt to remove a penetrating object (see below).
Caution child against rubbing eye.

Chemical Burns
Irrigate eye copiously with tap water for 20 minutes.
Evert upper lid to flush thoroughly.
Hold child's head with eye under tap of running luke-warm water.
Take to emergency room.
Have child rest with eyes closed.
Keep room darkened.

Ultraviolet Burns
If skin is burned, patch both eyes (make sure lids are completely closed); secure dressing with Kling bandages wrapped around head rather than tape.
Have child rest with eyes closed.
Refer to an ophthalmologist.

Hematoma ("Black Eye")
Use a flashlight to check for gross *hyphema* (hemorrhage into anterior chamber; visible fluid meniscus across iris; more easily seen in light-colored than in brown eyes).
Apply ice for first 24 hours to reduce swelling if no hyphema is present.
Refer to an ophthalmologist immediately if hyphema is present.
Have child rest with eyes closed.

Penetrating Injuries
Take child to emergency room.
Never remove an object that has penetrated eye.
Follow strict aseptic technique in examining eye.
Observe for:
    Aqueous or vitreous leaks (fluid leaking from point of penetration)
    Hyphema
    Shape and equality of pupils, reaction to light
    Prolapsed iris (not perfectly circular)
Apply a Fox shield if available (not a regular eye patch) and apply patch over unaffected eye to prevent bilateral movement.
Maintain bed rest with child in 30-degree Fowler position.
Caution child against rubbing eye.

ratory patterns change, such as faster or slower breathing, when the parents come near; and whether the infant makes throaty sounds when they speak to the infant. In time parents learn that the infant has unique ways of relating to them. They are encouraged to show affection using nonvisual methods, such as talking or reading, cuddling, and walking the child.

Promote Child's Optimum Development. Promoting the child's optimum development requires rehabilitation in a number of important areas. These include learning self-help skills and appropriate communication techniques to become independent. Although nurses may not be directly involved in such programs, they can provide direction and guidance to families regarding the availability of programs and the need to promote these activities in their child.

Development and Independence. Motor development depends on sight almost as much as verbal communication depends on hearing. From earliest infancy, parents are encouraged to expose the infant to as many visual-motor experiences as possible, such as sitting supported in an infant seat or swing and being given opportunities for holding up the head, sitting unsupported, reaching for objects, and crawling.

Despite visual impairment the child can become independent in all aspects of self-care. The same principles used for promoting independence in sighted children apply, with additional emphasis on nonvisual cues. For example, the child may need help in dressing, such as special arrangement of clothing for style coordination and braille tags to distinguish colors and prints.

The blind child also must learn to become independent in navigational skills. The two main techniques are the ***tapping method*** (use of a cane to survey the environment for direction and to avoid obstacles) and ***guides,*** such as a sighted human guide or a dog guide, such as a Seeing Eye dog. Children who are partially sighted may benefit from ocular aids, such as a monocular telescope.

Play and Socialization. Blind children do not learn to play automatically. Because they cannot imitate others or actively explore the environment as sighted children do, they depend much more on others to stimulate and teach them how to play. Parents need help in selecting appropriate play material, especially those that encourage fine and gross motor development and stimulate the senses of hearing, touch, and smell. Toys with educational value are especially useful, such as dolls with various clothing closures.

Blind children have the same needs for socialization as sighted children. Since they have little difficulty in learning verbal skills, they are able to communicate with age-mates and participate in suitable activities. The nurse discusses with parents opportunities for socialization outside the home, especially regular preschools. The trend is to include these children with sighted children to help them adjust to the outside world for eventual independence.

To compensate for inadequate stimulation, these children may develop ***blindisms*** (self-stimulatory activities, e.g., body rocking, finger flicking, arm twirling). Such habits restrict the child's social acceptance and are discouraged. Behavior modification is often successful in reducing or eliminating blindisms.

Education. The main obstacle to learning is the child's total dependence on nonvisual cues. Although the child can learn via verbal lecturing, he or she is unable to read the written word or to write without special education. Therefore the child must rely on ***braille,*** a system that uses raised dots to represent letters and numbers. The child can then read the braille with the fingers and can write a message using a braille writer. However, unless others read braille, this type of communication is not useful for communicating with others. A more portable system for written communication is the use of a braille slate and stylus (Fig. 19-9) or a microcassette tape recorder. A recorder is especially helpful for leaving messages

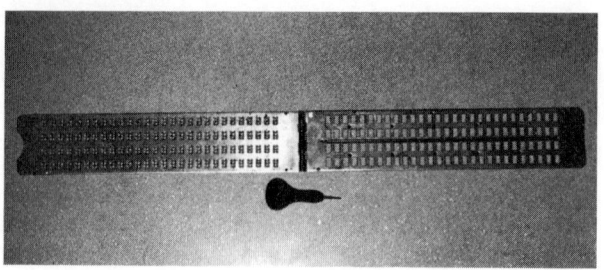

FIG. 19-9. Braille slate and stylus. The hinged slate consists of a series of open rectangles on one side and standard braille cells on the other. The paper is clamped or sandwiched between these two metal bars, and the appropriate dots are punched with the stylus.

for others and for note taking during classroom lecturing. For mathematic calculations, portable calculators with voice synthesizers are available.*

Records and tapes are significant sources of reading material other than braille books, which are large and cumbersome. The **Library of Congress†** has talking books, braille books, and a special records program, which are available at many local and state libraries and directly from the Library of Congress. The talking book machine and tape player are provided at no cost to families, and there is no postage fee for returning the materials. **Recording for the Blind, Inc.,‡** also provides texts and tapes of books, which are very helpful for secondary and college students who are blind.

Learning to use a regular typewriter is another form of writing but has the disadvantage of the blind person's being unable to check the accuracy of the typing. Computers eliminate this drawback; a home computer with a voice synthesizer can be adapted to speak each letter or word that has been typed.

The child with partial sight benefits from specialized visual aids, which produce a magnified retinal image. The basic devices are accommodation (e.g., bringing the object closer), special plus lenses, hand-held and stand magnifiers, telescopes, video projection systems, and large print. Special equipment is available to enlarge print. Information about services for the partially sighted is available from the **National Association for Visually Handicapped** and **American Foundation for the Blind** (see previous footnote for addresses). Children with diminished vision often prefer to do close work without their glasses and compensate by bringing the object very near to their eyes. This should be allowed. The exception is the child with vision in only one eye, who should always wear glasses for protection.

Care for Child During Hospitalization. Because nurses are more likely to care for children who are hospitalized for procedures that involve temporary loss of vision than for children who are blind, the following discussion concentrates primarily on the needs of such children. The nursing care objectives in either situation are to (1) reassure the child

---

*A catalog of numerous products for people with vision problems is available from the American Foundation for the Blind (see previous footnote).
†Division for the Blind and Visually Handicapped, 1291 Taylor St., N.W., Washington, DC 20542; (202) 707-5100 or (800) 424-8567.
‡20 Roszel Rd., Princeton, NJ 08540; (609) 452-0606.

and family throughout every phase of treatment, (2) orient the child to the surroundings, (3) provide a safe environment, and (4) encourage independence. Whenever possible, the same nurse should care for the child to ensure consistency in the approach. These same principles also apply to a blind child who requires hospitalization.

When sighted children temporarily lose their vision, almost every aspect of the environment becomes bewildering and frightening. They are forced to rely on nonvisual senses for help in adjusting to the blindness without the benefit of any special training. Nurses have a major role in minimizing the effects of temporary loss of vision. They need to talk to the child about everything that is occurring, emphasizing aspects of procedures that are felt or heard. They should approach the child by always identifying themselves as soon as they enter the room. Since unfamiliar sounds are especially frightening, these are explained. Parents are encouraged to room with their child and participate in the care. Familiar objects, such as a teddy bear or doll, should be brought from home to help lessen the strangeness of the hospital. As soon as the child is able to be out of bed, he or she is oriented to the immediate surroundings. If the child is able to see on admission, this opportunity is taken to point out significant aspects of the room. The child is encouraged to practice ambulating with the eyes closed to become accustomed to this experience.

The room is arranged with safety in mind. For example, a stool or chair is placed next to the bed to help the child climb in and out of bed. The furniture is always placed in the same position to prevent collisions. Cleaning personnel are reminded of the need to keep the room in order. If the child has difficulty navigating by feeling the walls, a rope can be attached from the bed to the point of destination, such as the bathroom. Attention to details such as well-fitting slippers or robes that do not hang on the floor is important in preventing tripping. Unlike the child who is blind, these children are not familiar with navigating with a cane.

The child is encouraged to be independent in self-care activities, especially if the visual loss may be prolonged or potentially permanent. For example, during bathing the nurse sets up all the equipment and encourages the child to participate. At mealtime the nurse explains where each food item is on the tray, opens any special containers, prepares cereal or toast, but encourages the child in self-feeding. Favorite finger foods, such as sandwiches, hamburgers, hot dogs, or pizza, may be good selections. The child is praised for efforts at being cooperative and independent. Any improvements made in self-care, no matter how small, are stressed.

Appropriate recreational activities are provided, and if a child-life specialist is available, such planning is done jointly. Since children with temporary blindness have a wide variety of play experiences to draw on, they are encouraged to select activities. For example, if they like to read, they may enjoy being read to. If they prefer manual activity, they may appreciate playing with clay or building blocks or feeling different textures and naming them. If they need an outlet for aggression, activities such as pounding or banging on a drum can be helpful. Simple board and card games can be played with a "seeing partner" or if the opponent helps with the game. They should have familiar toys from home to play with, since familiar items are more easily manipulated than new ones. If

parents want to bring presents, they should be objects that stimulate hearing and touch, such as a radio, music box, or stuffed animal.

Occasionally, children who are blind come to the hospital for procedures to restore their vision. Although this is an extremely happy time, it also requires intervention to help them adjust to sight. They need an opportunity to take in all that they see. They should not be bombarded with visual stimuli. They may need to concentrate on people's faces or their own to become accustomed to this experience. They often need to talk about what they see and to compare the visual images with their mental ones. The child may also go through a period of depression, which must be respected and supported. The nurse or parents should refrain from statements such as "How can you be so sad when you can see again?" Instead the child should be encouraged to discuss how it feels to see, especially in terms of seeing himself or herself.

Newly sighted children also need time to adjust to the ability to engage in activities that were impossible before. For example, they may prefer to use braille to read, rather than learning a new "visual approach," because of familiarity with the touch system. Eventually, as they learn to recognize letters and numbers, they will integrate these new skills into reading and writing. However, parents and teachers must be careful not to push them before they are ready. This applies to social relationships and physical activities as well as learning situations.

Assist in Measures to Prevent Visual Impairment. An essential nursing goal is to prevent visual impairment. This involves many of the same interventions discussed under hearing impairments, that is, (1) prenatal screening for pregnant women at risk, such as those with rubella or syphilis infection and family histories of genetic disorders associated with visual loss; (2) adequate prenatal and perinatal care to prevent prematurity and iatrogenic (result of medical treatment) damage from excessive administration of oxygen; (3) periodic screening of all children, especially newborns through preschoolers, for congenital blindness and visual impairments caused by refractive errors, strabismus, and other disorders; (4) rubella immunization of all children; and (5) safety counseling regarding the common causes of ocular trauma.

Safety counseling should include safe practices when working with, playing with, or carrying objects such as scissors, knives, and balls.

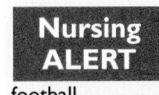 **Nursing ALERT** A helmet with a face guard should be required gear for *all* children playing baseball or softball (not only catcher, batter, umpire, and base runner), hockey, or football.

After detection of eye problems, the nurse has a responsibility to prevent further ocular damage by ensuring that corrective treatment is employed. For the child with strabismus, this often necessitates occlusion patching of the stronger eye. Compliance with the procedure is greatest during the early preschool years. It is more difficult to encourage school-age children to wear the occlusive patch because the poor visual acuity of the uncovered weaker eye interferes with schoolwork and the patch sets them apart from their peers. In school they benefit from being positioned favorably (closer to the chalkboard or other visual media) and allowed extra time to read or complete an assignment. If treatment of the eye disorder requires instillation of ophthalmic medication, the family is taught the correct procedure (see Chapter 22).*

For the child with refractive errors, the nurse helps the child adjust to wearing *glasses.* Young children who often pull glasses off benefit from temporal pieces that wrap around the ears or an elastic strap attached to the frames and around the back of the head to hold the glasses on securely. Once children appreciate the value of clear vision, they are more likely to wear the corrective lenses.

Glasses should not interfere with any activity. Special protective guards are available during contact sports to prevent accidental injury, and all corrective lenses should be made from safety glass, which is shatterproof. Often, corrective lenses improve visual acuity so dramatically that children are able to compete more effectively in sports. This in itself is a tremendous inducement to continue wearing glasses.

Contact lenses are a popular alternative, especially for adolescents. Several types are available, such as hard lenses, including gas permeable ones, and soft lenses, which may be designed for daily or extended wear. Contact lenses offer several advantages over glasses, such as greater visual acuity, total corrected field of vision, convenience (especially with the extended-wear type), and optimum cosmetic benefit. Unfortunately, they are usually more expensive and require much more care than glasses, including considerable practice to learn techniques for insertion and removal. If they are prescribed, the nurse can be very helpful in teaching parents or older children how to care for the lenses.

Since trauma is the leading cause of blindness, the nurse has the major responsibility of preventing further eye injury until the specific treatment is instituted. The major principles to follow when caring for an eye injury are outlined in the Emergency Treatment box on p. 589. Since patients with a serious eye injury fear blindness, the nurse should stay with the child and family to provide support and reassurance.

❖ Evaluation

The effectiveness of nursing interventions is determined by continual reassessment and evaluation of care based on the following observational guidelines and expected outcomes:

1. Interview family regarding their adjustment to the sensory impairment; observe family members' relationship with the child; interview child regarding feelings about the sensory impairment and its effect on activities of daily living (especially important if a visual loss).

2. Have parents identify those cues that indicate the infant is responding to them; observe nonvisual behaviors of parents as they respond to infant.

3. Observe the techniques the child uses to read and navigate; inquire if the child is enrolled in a visual training program; inquire about socialization opportunities for the child (i.e., who are the child's friends, what are the child's extracurricular activities).

4. Observe preparation of the room and self-care activities that provide for safety and independence during hospitalization.

Expected outcomes:

1. Parents express their feelings and concerns regarding loss of sight and demonstrate an understanding of child's disability and its implications.

2. Parents demonstrate attachment behaviors.

3. Infant or child engages in appropriate activities for level of development (specify); child demonstrates an attitude of security in the environment.

4. Child and family receive safe and supportive care during hospitalization.

See also Nursing Care Plan: The Child with Visual Impairment.*

DEAF-BLIND CHILDREN

The most traumatic sensory impairment is loss of sight and hearing. Obviously, auditory and visual disabilities have profound effects on the child's development. They interfere with the normal sequence of physical, intellectual, and psychosocial growth. Although such children often achieve the usual motor milestones, their rate of development is slower. These children learn communication only with specialized training. Some deaf-blind children, especially those with residual hearing or sight, can learn to speak. Whenever possible, speech is encouraged, since it allows communication with other individuals.

The future prospects for deaf-blind children are at best unpredictable. Congenital blindness and/or deafness may be accompanied by other physical or neurologic problems, which further lessen the child's learning potential. The most favorable prognosis is for children who have acquired deafness and blindness and have few, if any, associated disabilities. Their learning capacity is greatly potentiated by their developmental progress before the sensory impairments. Although total independence, including gainful vocational training, is the goal, some deaf-blind children are unable to develop to this level. They may require lifelong parental or residential care. The nurse working with such families helps them deal with future goals for the child, including possible alternatives to home care during the parents' advancing years.

RETINOBLASTOMA†

Retinoblastoma is a rare congenital malignant tumor arising from the retina. It may be present at birth or may arise in the retina during the first 2 years of life. Retinoblastoma may be hereditary or nonhereditary and unilateral or bilateral. Hereditary retinoblastomas are transmitted as an autosomal dominant trait with incomplete penetrance.

Diagnostic Evaluation

Retinoblastoma has few grossly obvious signs (see box). Typically it is the parent who first observes a whitish "glow" in the pupil. The white reflex or white pupil (*leukokoria*), known as the *cat's eye reflex,* represents visualization of the tumor as the light momentarily falls on the mass (Fig. 19-10).

---

*Home care instructions on giving eye medications are available in Wong DL: *Wong and Whaley's Clinical manual of pediatric nursing,* ed 4, St Louis, 1996, Mosby.

*In Wong DL: *Wong and Whaley's Clinical manual of pediatric nursing,* ed 4, St Louis, 1996, Mosby.
†Marilyn Hockenberry-Eaton, PhD, RN, C, PNP, and Nancy Kline, MS, RN, CPNP, revised this section.

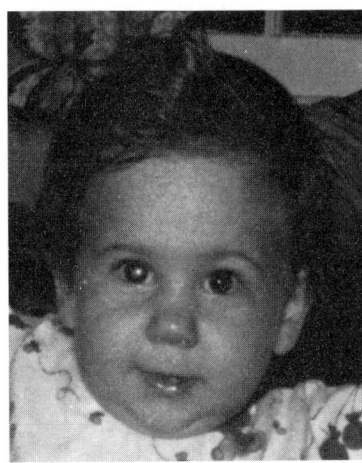

FIG. 19-10. Cat's eye reflex. Whitish appearance of lens is produced as light falls on tumor mass in right eye.

The first step in diagnosis is carefully listening to and recognizing the significance of reports from family members regarding suspected abnormalities within the eye. Since the cat's eye reflex is a momentary sign visualized only under specific conditions, the practitioner must attempt to duplicate those conditions necessary to observe the tumor. Children suspected of having this disorder are referred to an ophthalmologist. Definitive diagnosis is usually based on indirect ophthalmoscopy, which is performed with the patient under general anesthesia with maximum dilation of the pupils.

Therapeutic Management

Treatment of retinoblastoma depends chiefly on the stage of the tumor at the time of diagnosis. Staging includes five groups; group I refers to a small localized tumor(s), whereas group V is reserved for tumors involving more than half the retina and vitreous seeding. In general, early-stage unilateral retinoblastomas are treated with irradiation or other techniques, such as cryotherapy, which freezes the tumor. The aim of therapy is to preserve useful vision in the affected eye and eradicate the tumor.

With advanced tumor growth, especially optic nerve involvement, *enucleation* (removal) of the affected eye is the treatment of choice. The use of chemotherapy in advanced disease is controversial but, if employed, may include the drugs vincristine, cyclophosphamide, and adriamycin.

With bilateral disease, every attempt is made to preserve useful vision in the least affected eye with enucleation of the severely diseased eye. When bilateral tumors are found early, radiotherapy or other treatments to both eyes may prevent the need for enucleation.

Prognosis.   The overall prognosis for retinoblastoma is very favorable, with a survival rate of nearly 90% for both unilateral and bilateral tumors. Retinoblastoma is one of the tumors that may spontaneously regress.

Of major concern in long-term survivors is the development of secondary tumors, especially osteogenic sarcoma. Children with bilateral disease (hereditary form) are more likely to develop secondary cancers than are children with unilateral disease. It is thought that these individuals are predisposed to developing cancer, and radiation increases their risk.

Nursing Considerations

One of the most important nursing goals is to have a high index of suspicion for this rare malignancy. If parents report noticing a strange light in the eye or expression, these concerns must be taken seriously. Families with a history of retinoblastoma require follow-up, and the nurse can be instrumental in reminding parents of appointments.

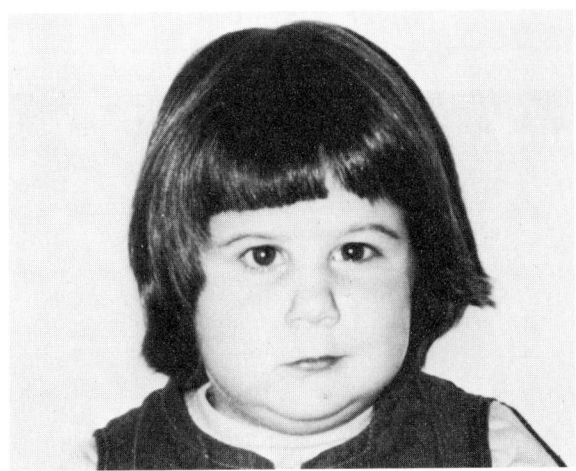

FIG. 19-11. Preschooler with right prosthetic eye.

Since the tumor is usually diagnosed in infants or very young children, most of the preparation for diagnostic tests and treatment involves parents. After indirect ophthalmoscopy, the child may not see very clearly, or the eyes may be sensitive to light because of pupillary dilation. Parents are made aware of these normal reactions before the procedure. They also are informed that a battery of screening tests, such as bone surveys and bone marrow aspiration, may be performed to detect metastasis.

Once the disease is staged, the physician confers with the parents regarding treatment. Unless the diagnosis is made very early, an enucleation is performed. Parents are told about the procedure, as well as about the positive benefits of a prosthesis. Showing them pictures of another child with an artificial eye may be very helpful in their adjusting to the thought of disfigurement (Fig. 19-11).

After surgery the parents are prepared for the child's facial appearance. An eye patch is in place, and the child's face may be edematous or ecchymotic. Parents often fear seeing the surgical site because they imagine a cavity in the skull. On the contrary, the lids are usually closed and the area does not appear sunken, because a surgically implanted sphere maintains the shape of the eyeball. The implant is covered with conjunctiva, and when the lids are open, the exposed area resembles the mucosal lining of the mouth. Once the child is fitted for a prosthesis, usually within 3 weeks, the facial appearance returns to normal. Initial instructions for care of the prosthesis are given by the ocularist, who fits and manufactures the device.

Care of the socket is minimal and easily accomplished. The wound itself is clean and has little or no drainage. If an antibiotic ointment is prescribed, it is applied in a thin line on the surface of the tissues of the socket. To cleanse the site, an irrigating solution may be ordered and is instilled daily or more frequently if necessary, *before* application of the antibiotic ointment. The dressing consists of an eye pad taped over the surgical site with nonirritating tape; it is changed daily. Once the socket has healed completely, a dressing is no longer

necessary, although it is a preventive measure against infection.

A long-term consideration is the survivor's ability to transmit the defective gene to his or her offspring. Parents are encouraged to seek genetic counseling for themselves and for the child during puberty.

Support Family.   Families with a history of the disorder may feel great guilt for transmitting the defect to their offspring. In families with no history of retinoblastoma, the discovery of the diagnosis is a shock, frequently complicated by guilt for not having found it sooner. Since parents frequently are the first to observe the cat's eye reflex, they may feel angry at themselves or others, especially health professionals, for delaying a more thorough examination. The nurse assesses each of these variables in planning care based on understanding the family's emotional reactions and adjustment (see Chapter 18).

See also Nursing Care Plan: The Child with Cancer, Chapter 26.

KEY POINTS

- Mental retardation (MR) is the most common developmental disability in the United States, affecting about 3% of the population.
- According to the American Association of Mental Deficiencies, MR is a "significantly subaverage general intellectual functioning existing concurrently with deficits in adaptive behavior and manifested during the developmental period."
- Causes of severe MR are primarily genetic, biochemical, viral, and developmental. Mild MR is associated primarily with familial, social, and environmental causes, whereas severe MR is more likely to be associated with specific syndromes.
- Education of children with cognitive impairment emphasizes sensory and verbal discrimination, improvement of short-term memory, motivation, and technologic support.
- Promoting optimum development may be achieved through family guidance regarding play, communication, discipline, socialization, and sexuality.
- Prevention efforts regarding MR focus on support for the premature neonate and other high-risk newborns, rubella immunization, genetic counseling, and maternal education regarding the risks of chemical use and the importance of adequate nutrition.
- Down syndrome, a chromosomal abnormality, is characterized by retarded intelligence of variable degree, slowed language development, congenital anomalies, sensory problems, and diminished growth and sexual development.
- Fragile X syndrome is characterized by MR and phenotypic findings in affected males. It is considered the

second leading chromosomal cause of MR after Down syndrome, and the most common hereditary cause.
- Hearing disorders may be classified according to the location of the defect: conductive, sensorineural, mixed conductive-sensorineural, and central auditory imperception.
- Rehabilitation for hearing loss involves parent education and support, hearing aids, lipreading, sign language, speech therapy, and promotion of socialization.
- Prevention of hearing loss includes treatment of infection, auditory testing, immunization, pregnancy and genetic counseling, and reduction of noise pollution.
- Visual impairments in childhood include refractive errors, amblyopia, strabismus, cataracts, glaucoma, trauma, and infections.
- Nursing goals in visual rehabilitation include helping the family and child adjust to the child's visual impairment, promoting parent-child attachment, fostering optimum development and independence, providing for play and socialization, and being aware of educational facilities.
- For the child undergoing ocular surgery, nursing care is aimed at reassuring the child and family throughout treatment, orienting the child to the surroundings, providing a safe environment, and encouraging independence.
- Prevention of visual impairment focuses on prenatal screening, prenatal and perinatal care, periodic vision screening, immunization, and safety counseling.
- Retinoblastoma is a rare congenital malignant tumor; its most common clinical manifestations are cat's eye reflex (white pupil) and strabismus.

REFERENCES

American Academy of Pediatrics, Committee on Genetics: Prenatal diagnosis for pediatricians, *Pediatrics* 84(4):741-744, 1989.

American Psychiatric Association: *Diagnostic and statistical manual of mental disorders,* ed 4 *(DSM-IV),* Washington, DC, 1994, The Association.

Batshaw, ML: Mental retardation, *Pediatr Clin North Am* 40(3):465-692, 1993.

Brown WT and others: Rapid fragile X carrier screening and prenatal diagnosis using a nonradioactive PCR test, *JAMA* 270(13):1569-1575, 1993.

Consensus Conference: Noise and hearing loss, *JAMA* 263(23): 3185-3190, 1990.

Cooley SC, Graham JM: Down syndrome—an update and review for the primary pediatrician, *Clin Pediatr* 30(4):233-253, 1991.

Cronk C and others: Growth charts for children with Down syndrome: 1 month to 18 years of age, *Pediatrics* 81(1):102-110, 1988.

Davidson PW: Visual impairment and blindness. In Levine MD, Carey WB, Crocker AC, editors: *Developmental-behavioral pediatrics,* ed 2, Philadelphia, 1992, Saunders.

Eilers RE, Oller DK: Infant vocalizations and the early diagnosis of severe hearing impairment, *J Pediatr* 124:199-203, 1994.

Grossman HJ, editor: *Classification in mental retardation,* Washington, DC, 1983, American Association on Mental Retardation.

Haddow JE and others: Prenatal screening for Down's syndrome with use of maternal serum markers, *N Engl J Med* 327:588-593, 1992.

Hagerman RJ, Cronister A: Fragile X syndrome. In Jackson PL, Vessey, JA: *Primary care of the child with a chronic condition,* ed 2, St Louis, 1996, Mosby.

Keltner BR, Tymchuk AJ: Reaching out to mothers with mental retardation, *MCN Am J Matern Child Nurs* 17(3):136-140, 1992.

Litovitz T, Schmitz BF: Ingestion of cylindrical and button batteries: an analysis of 2382 cases, *Pediatrics* 89:747-757, 1992.

Luckasson R, editor: *Mental retardation: definition, classification and systems of support,* ed 9, Washington, DC, 1992, American Association on Mental Retardation.

National Institutes of Health: *NIH consensus statement: early identification of hearing impairment in infants and young children,* vol 11, no 1, Washington, DC, 1993, NIH.

Pueschel SM: The child with Down syndrome. In Levine MD and others, editors: *Developmental-behavioral pediatrics,* ed 2, Philadelphia, 1992, Saunders.

Sarant JZ and others: The effect of handedness in tactile speech perception, *J Rehabil Res* 30:423-435, 1993.

Updates: Do deaf children benefit from cochlear implants? *Contemp Pediatr* 12(8):9-10, 1995.

BIBLIOGRAPHY

Cognitive Impairment

American Academy of Pediatrics, Committee on Bioethics: Sterilization of women who are mentally handicapped, *Pediatrics* 85(5):868-871, 1990.

American Academy of Pediatrics, Committee on Children With Disabilities: Screening infants and young children for developmental disabilities, *Pediatrics* 93(5):863-865, 1994.

Brizee L, Sophos C, McLaughlin J: Nutrition issues in developmental disabilities, *Inf Young Child* 2(3):10-21, 1990.

Brown FR and others: Intellectual and adaptive functioning in individuals with Down syndrome in relation to age and environmental placement, *Pediatrics* 85:450-452, 1990.

Chomicki S, Wilgosh L: Health care concerns among parents of children with mental retardation, *Child Health Care* 21(4):206-212, 1992.

Cronister AE, Hagerman RJ: Fragile X syndrome, *J Pediatr Health Care* 3(1):9-19, 1989.

Forness SR, Hecht B: Special education for handicapped and disabled children: classification, programs, and trends, *J Pediatr Nurs* 3(2):75-88, 1988.

Friedrich WN, Cohen DS, Wilturner LT: Specific beliefs as moderator variables in maternal coping with mental retardation, *Child Health Care* 17(1):40-44, 1988.

Hayes A, Batshaw ML: Down syndrome, *Pediatr Clin North Am* 40(3):523-535, 1993.

Krais WA: The incompetent developmentally disabled person's right of self-determination, right to die, sterilization and institutionalization, *Am J Law Med* 15(2-3):333-361, 1989.

Oehler JM and others: How to target infants at highest risk for developmental delay, *MCN Am J Matern Child Nurs* 18(1):20-23, 1993.

Steele S: Assessing developmental delays in preschool children, *J Pediatr Health Care* 2(3):141-145, 1988.

Steele S: Fostering potentiality in persons with mental retardation, *Issues Compr Pediatr Nurs* 11:283-290, 1988.

Steele S: Down syndrome: nursing interventions, newborn through preschool age years, *Issues Compr Pediatr Nurs* 13(2):111-126, 1990.

Steele S: Preschool children with developmental delays: nursing intervention, *J Pediatr Health Care* 2(5):245-252, 1988.

Steele S and others: Home management of URI in children with Down syndrome, *Pediatr Nurs* 15(5):484-488, 1989.

Taylor EH: Understanding and helping families with neurodevelopmental and neuropsychiatric special needs, *Pediatr Clin North Am* 42:143-152, 1995.

Taylor MO: Teaching parents about their impaired adolescent's sexuality, *MCN Am J Matern Child Nurs* 14:109-112, 1989.

Vessey JA: Care of the hospitalized child with a cognitive developmental delay, *Holistic Nurs Pract* 2:48-54, 1988.

Vessey JA: Down syndrome. In Jackson PL, Vessey JA: *Primary care of the child with a chronic condition,* ed 2, St Louis, 1996, Mosby.

Vessey JA, Swanson MN: Caring for the child with Down syndrome, *J School Nurs* 9(14):20-33, 1993.

Walden BJ: The newborn infant with Down syndrome: realities and possibilities, *J Perinat Neonat Nurs* 2(4):72-82, 1989.

Hearing Impairment

American Academy of Otolaryngology–Head and Neck Surgery Subcommittee on Cochlear Implants, Kveton J, Balkany TJ: Status of cochlear implantation in children, *J Pediatr* 118(25):1-7, 1991.

Badger T, Jones E: Deaf and hearing children's conceptions of the body interior, *Pediatr Nurs* 16(2):201-205, 1990.

Coplan J: Deafness: ever heard of it? Delayed recognition of permanent hearing loss, *Pediatrics* 79(2):206-213, 1987.

Epstein S, Reilly JS: Sensorineural hearing loss, *Pediatr Clin North Am* 36(6):1501-1520, 1989.

Harrison LL: Minimizing barriers when teaching hearing-impaired clients, *MCN Am J Matern Child Nurs* 15(2):113, 1990.

Jackson CB: Primary health care for deaf children. Part I, *J Pediatr Health Care* 3(6):316-318, 1989.

Jackson CB: Primary health care for deaf children. Part II, *J Pediatr Health Care* 4(1):39-41, 1990.

Kravitz L, Selekman J: Understanding hearing loss in children, *Pediatr Nurs* 18:591-594, 1992.

McGarr N: Research on the use of sensory aids for hearing-impaired people, *Volta Rev* 91(5):1-138, 1989.

Oberklaid F, Harris C, Keir E: Auditory dysfunction in children with school problems, *Clin Pediatr* 28(9):397-403, 1989.

Roush J: Acoustic amplification for hearing-impaired infants and young children, *Inf Young Child* 2(4):59-71, 1990.

Thomas KA: How the NICU environment sounds to a preterm infant, *MCN Am J Matern Child Nurs* 14:249-251, 1989.

Thompson M, Thompson G: Early identification of hearing loss: listen to parents, *Clin Pediatr* 30(2):77-80, 1991.

Weibley T: Inside the incubator, *MCN Am J Matern Child Nurs* 14(2):96-100, 1989.

Vision Impairment

Bailey C, Buckley R: Ocular prostheses and contact lenses. II. Contact lenses, *Br Med J* 302(6784):1066-1069, 1991.

DeRespinis PA: Cyanoacrylage nail glue mistaken for eye drops, *JAMA* 263(17):2301, 1990.

Donaldson SS, Smith LM: Retinoblastoma: biology, presentation, and current management, *Oncology* 3(4):45-51, 1989.

Dudley N: Aids for visual impairment, *Br Med J* 302(6761):1151-1153, 1990.

Friendly DS: Development of vision in infants and young children, *Pediatr Clin North Am* 40:693-704, 1993.

Gallie BL and others: The genetics of retinoblastoma, *Pediatr Clin North Am* 38:299-315, 1991.

Kodadek SM, Haylor MJ: Using interpretive methods to understand family caregiving when a child is blind, *J Pediatr Nurs* 5(1):42-49, 1990.

Kovalesky A: *Nurses guide to children's eyes,* New York, 1985, Grune & Stratton.

Nelson LB, Wilson TW, Jeffers, JB: Eye injuries in childhood: demography, etiology, and prevention, *Pediatrics* 84(3):438-441, 1989.

Phillips S, Hartley JT: Developmental differences and interventions for blind children, *Pediatr Nurs* 14(3):201-204, 1988.

Rollins JA: National Library Service for the Blind and Physically Handicapped, *Pediatr Nurs* 14(6):522, 1988.

Schraeder B, McEvoy-Shields K: Visual acuity, binocular vision, and ocular muscle balance in VLBW children, *Pediatr Nurs* 17(1):30-33, 1991.

Servodidio CA, Abramson DH, Romanella A: Retinoblastoma, *Cancer Nurs* 14(2):117-123, 1991.

Tongue AC: Refractive errors in children, *Pediatr Clin North Am* 34(6):1425-1437, 1987.

Multiple Impairments: Deaf-Blind

Luiselli JK: Training self-feeding skills in children who are deaf and blind, *Behav Mod* 17:457-473, 1993.

Programs for deaf-blind children and adults, *Am Ann Deaf* 138:205-209, 1993.

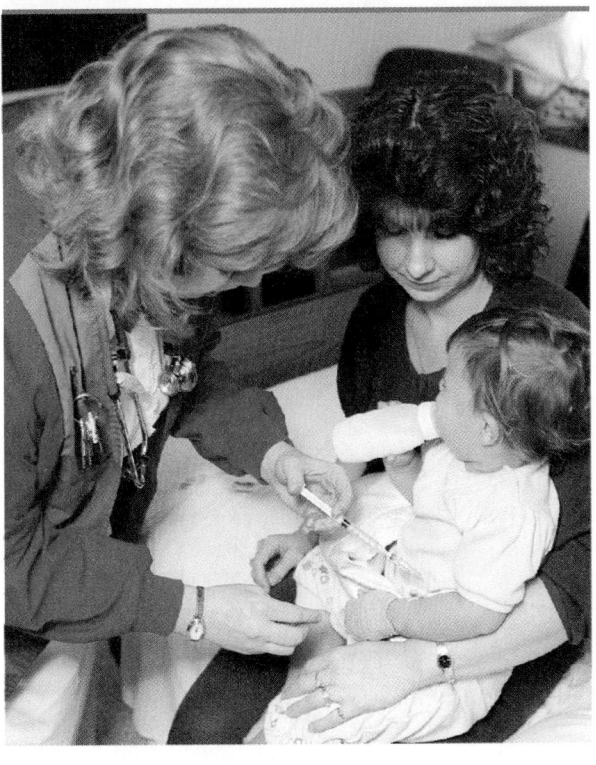

RELATED TOPICS

GENERAL CONCEPTS OF HOME CARE

DEFINITION

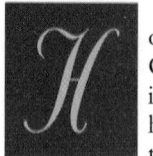 ome care is not a new concept in pediatrics. Over time the term has referred to parents caring for mildly ill children at home, to nursing home visits after children are discharged from the hospital, to hospice care, and more recently, to care at home for children with more serious chronic illness and dependence on medical technology. Also, with insurance companies encouraging earlier hospital discharge for healthy newborns, public and community health nurses may increasingly return to providing parenting education for postpartum women at home.

As discussed in this chapter, *home care* refers to care provided in the family's residence for children with complex health care needs and their families. The purpose of home care services is to promote, maintain, or restore health or to maximize the level of independence while minimizing the effects of disability and illness, including terminal illness. Home care differs from *hospice care,* which is a program of palliative and supportive care services providing physical, psychologic, social, and spiritual care for dying persons, their families, and other loved ones. Hospice services are available in both the home and inpatient settings.

IMPETUS FOR HOME CARE

The initial impetus for home care for children with complex medical conditions came from a parental desire to have these children at home and from professionals' willingness to work with families to achieve this goal. Improving the quality of life for both the child and the family was the driving force in the efforts to move technology-dependent children from the hospital to the home setting.

Other factors eventually influenced the shift toward an emphasis on home care for this population, including increasing numbers of children requiring long-term complex medical

and nursing care and lower costs for home care as compared with hospital care.

Dramatic advances in medical care over the past 2 decades have resulted in increased numbers of children requiring long-term complex medical care as a result of (1) improvements in trauma care and the survival of severe trauma victims; (2) increased survival rates for children with leukemia and other cancers, chronic kidney disorders, sickle cell anemia, cystic fibrosis, spina bifida, and cardiac or intestinal malformations; (3) more aggressive care for muscular dystrophy and degenerative neuromuscular disorders; and (4) more children with acquired immunodeficiency syndrome (AIDS).

The cost of care is another critical factor. For third-party payers and the government, the cost of home care is generally less than the cost of hospital care for children dependent on medical technology and requiring substantial and complex care. However, families may absorb many of the costs of home care, including medication, supplies, transportation, shelter, utilities, food, laundry, and housekeeping. Families generally provide at least some portion of the nursing care as well, and some may become unemployed or only partially employed to stay at home. These out-of-pocket expenses and the loss of income can become a financial burden for the family.

EFFECTIVENESS OF HOME CARE

Home care is effective for many children; however, it may not be possible in all circumstances. A number of factors must be present to make it effective. First, the child's condition must be medically stable so that care can be managed in the home setting and supported by available home care equipment. Second, the family must want the child at home and must have the motivation and ability to learn the child's care. Families must also be able to live with the intrusion of the child's equipment, care schedule, and nurses and other providers in their daily life. Third, professionals and the community must be prepared to provide the necessary support to make home care successful, including nursing and other therapeutic services, transportation, accessible emergency facilities, and case management. Fourth, financial support, both public and private, is essential.

Even if home care is initially successful for a child and family, changing factors may influence the plan. Alterations in the child's medical condition, the lack of adequate community resources, depletion of the family's financial resources, high levels of family stress and exhaustion, and disagreements be-

Elizabeth Ahmann, ScD, RN, authored this chapter.
Portions of this text are modified from Ahmann E: An overview of issues in pediatric high-tech home care. In Gorski L: *High tech home care manual,* Gaithersburg, MD, 1994, Aspen; and Ahmann E: Family-centered care: shifting our orientation, *Pediatr Nurs* 20(2):113-117, 1994.

tween the family members and the health care team can all affect the success of home care (Harris, 1988). Changes in the home care plan or short-term or long-term residential placement may be alternatives if any of these occur.

DISCHARGE PLANNING AND SELECTION OF A HOME CARE AGENCY

Much of the success of home care for the child who is dependent on medical technology depends on careful planning and preparation. Despite the rapid growth of home care for technology-dependent children, negotiation with the insurance company may be required. General principles of discharge planning and transition to home care are addressed in Chapter 21. *Discharge planning must begin early, be a multidisciplinary process, and involve the family.* Early involvement of the home care agency promotes continuity of care and a smooth transition from hospital to home. The home care plan for a child with complex care requirements should address the many health and community services that may need to be mobilized. Comprehensive written home care instructions facilitate continuity of care across settings and providers (see box).*

NURSING TIP An excellent method of providing home care instructions is with video recordings. Once the family masters the procedures, consider video recording their performance on tape. Visual learning is most helpful for people who cannot read or are not fluent in English (Curry and Cullen, 1990).

The plans for transition from hospital to home should include family members (at least two persons) both learning and demonstrating all aspects of the child's care in the hospital. An in-hospital trial period during which parents provide total care for the child is generally beneficial as well. After a successful trial, the family may benefit from taking the child home on a brief pass before making final discharge plans. (This may need to be negotiated with the insurance company.) The home care nurse will play an important role in assessing this experience with the family. Whether or not

---

*Numerous home care instructions are available in Wong DL: *Wong and Whaley's Clinical manual of pediatric nursing,* ed 4, St Louis, 1996, Mosby.

the child is taken home on a pass, a predischarge home visit offers the home care nurse the opportunity to meet the family, help them assess their preparedness and the preparedness of the home environment, discuss plans for arranging the child's equipment at home (Fig. 20-1), reinforce prior discharge teaching, and implement any additional teaching that may be necessary.

CASE MANAGEMENT

Parents of children with complex care requirements often experience frustration about the fragmentation of services and desire competent case management. Traditional definitions of *case management* generally focus on cost control, attainment of desired clinical outcomes, and monitoring and evaluation of care provided. However, for optimum home care of the child who is technology dependent, case management—or *care coordination*—should be viewed more broadly (see also Chapter 1).

Care coordination has several purposes. Its primary goal is ensuring continuity for the child and family across hospital, home, educational, therapeutic, and other settings. Care should be coordinated among multiple providers to reduce the complexity of care for the child, reduce fragmentation of care, and decrease the burden of care for the family. Care coordination should ensure that the medical, nursing, and health maintenance needs of the child are addressed, as well as the financial issues, psychosocial concerns, and educational issues of the child and family.

Although professionals must always see part of their role as ensuring that integrated, coordinated care is provided, care coordination should promote the family's role as primary decision maker and enhance the family's capability to meet the special needs of the child and the family unit (Johnson, Jeppson, and Redburn, 1992). Care coordination is most effective if a single person works with the family to accomplish the many tasks and responsibilities involved. These include assessing needs and resources, planning for comprehensive care, coordinating services and referrals, monitoring and evaluating services, and providing administrative support and

---

MINIMUM CONTENTS OF WRITTEN HOME CARE INSTRUCTIONS

A schedule of routine care needs
Correct settings for any equipment required
A list of signs, symptoms, and parameters (physical and behavioral) that are normal for the individual child
A list of signs, symptoms, and parameters (physical and behavioral) that indicate a problem for the individual child
Guidelines and a list for whom to contact about what problems
An explanation of pertinent emergency procedures

From Ahmann E: An overview of issues in pediatric high tech home care. In Gorski L: *High tech home care manual,* Gaithersburg, MD, 1994, Aspen.

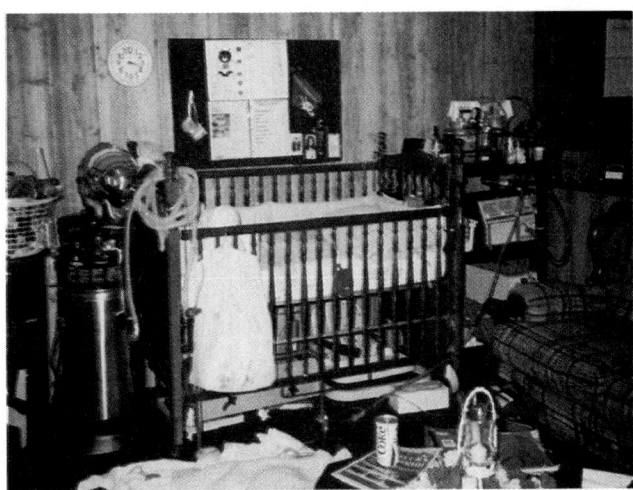

FIG. 20-1. An essential aspect of preparation for home care is arranging equipment and supplies.

advocacy. The American Nurses Association (ANA, 1988) recommends that the nurse case manager have a minimum of a baccalaureate degree in nursing and 3 years of experience.

ROLE OF THE NURSE, TRAINING, AND STANDARDS OF CARE

The home care nurse must share a level of technical expertise with the critical care nurse while being able to adapt equipment, procedures, and the nursing process to the home setting. (See Chapter 22 for specific technical skills that may be required in home care practice.) The need for technical expertise must be matched by a knowledge of child development and the ability to work creatively with the child challenged by chronic illness and technology dependence. When practicing in the home, the nurse must be comfortable making independent nursing judgments and problem solving with no immediate assistance. At the same time the nurse must have excellent interpersonal skills, an ability to work with other professionals and the family, and most important, an ability to respect family autonomy.

When working with a home care agency, nurses should expect to receive patient placements appropriate to their expertise. They should also expect orientation in the following areas: to the individual patient's care plan and equipment needs; to the agency's policies and procedures, including procedures for addressing any problems that may occur when care is provided in the home; to documentation procedures (reimbursement-driven documentation in home care differs from documentation practices in the hospital setting); and to legal liability issues. Supervision of practice, including occasional on-site visits by a nursing supervisor, should be provided.

Home care agencies, public or private, that participate in the Medicare or Medicaid programs must be certified by a federally designated, state-certifying body and abide by federal and state regulations. Private agencies that do not participate in the federal programs are not mandated to meet the federal standards. The trend is for large, national, private agencies to develop a certifying process that will ensure greater credibility and acceptable standards of practice (Klug, 1992). The ANA has developed standards of nursing practice for both community health and home care nurses that should guide practice in the home setting (ANA, 1986a, 1986b). Despite some important differences between pediatric and adult care in the home, as of this writing, no national standards specific to pediatric home care nursing practice have been developed.

FAMILY-CENTERED HOME CARE

Technology dependence, chronic illness, and complex care requirements cross social, cultural, spiritual, and economic boundaries. No matter what a family's background, family values must be respected in the provision of home care services. *The home is the family's domain,* and the child is at home because the family's central role is to nurture and raise their child. The nurse must respect the family's central role in the

care of the child and must work in collaboration with the family in efforts to care for the child. Family-centered nursing practice is essential in the home setting.

The first of the nine key components of family-centered care (see Chapter 1) provides the philosophic basis for family-centered practice: recognition that the family is the constant in the child's life, whereas the service systems and personnel within those systems fluctuate (Shelton and Stepanek, 1994). Nurses working with families of children with complex chronic problems must respect the family's central, caring role, their knowledge, and their particular and unique expertise. Families have the most intimate knowledge of the child's strengths and abilities, the challenges of providing care, and the abilities and needs of other family members (Bishop, Woll, and Arango, 1993). *Believing that no one knows the child better than the family is critical* to the success of any health care plan.

RESPECT FOR DIVERSITY

Respect for varied family structures and for racial, ethnic, cultural, spiritual, and socioeconomic diversity among families is essential in home care (see also Chapter 3). Nurses work in close relationship with family members and in the family's own domain. The family's background and their life-style choices are respected. Particular attention is given to communication. The meaning of words used and the way they are said may affect various cultural groups in different ways. For example, the words "family support" may be interpreted by some families as an implication that they are weak and in need of help (Patterson and Blum, 1993). Families may also differ in their cultural view of children, in childrearing practices, and in their views of illness, its causes, and its meaning. The views of illness may influence the type or level of investment a family will make in the child's care. Families may have beliefs about health care and healing practices that are for-

---

FAMILY FOCUS
Developing a Relationship with Culturally Diverse Families

I work in the inner city, and my home care patients come from a variety of racial and ethnic backgrounds. I am Caucasian, from Australia. Often, when I first visit a family, there is an initial coolness or apprehension toward me. This is understandable because I am a stranger, and perhaps families think I'll judge them in one way or another. By the end of the first visit, however, there is usually a smile as I leave; by the second visit they often greet me with a smile at the door; and by the third visit we usually have a friendship, a trust, and an ease of communication.

If I'm working on a case for an extended time, I use a holistic nursing approach. This involves being aware of how the illness of the child affects the entire family. As I listen over many weeks to their fears and questions, and often as I share faith perspectives, a bond begins to form. I find it a privilege to share in their joys and their pain, and I feel rewarded by the trust that they invest in me.

Julie Edgerton, RN
Home Care Nurse
Children's National Medical Center
Washington, DC

CRITICAL THINKING EXERCISE
Medical Neglect

The home care nurse notes that the family has failed to give a dose of the child's medication. The nurse is responsible for all the following actions *except:*

1. Educate and counsel the family about the child's medication requirements and schedule.
2. Report the family for medical neglect.
3. Assess the child's condition.
4. Document the missed dose and any corrective measures taken.

The correct answer is two. Some behaviors that might be considered medical neglect may result from the family feeling overwhelmed, not being fully educated about the child's care requirements, and/or experiencing denial. The nurse has a responsibility to address these issues with the family. At the same time the nurse should be cognizant that home care providers may have legal liability not only for their own actions but also for those of parents who are "noncompliant" with medical orders. The frequency and severity of "noncompliance" will affect the nurse's responsibility. For example, one missed medication dose may be appropriately handled by documentation and counseling. On the other hand, regularly missing doses or one instance of turning off a ventilator alarm requires a more vigorous response. The point at which these instances cross the line into reportable medical neglect depends in part on the definitions of abuse or neglect in the state in which services are provided.

Modified from Ahmann E: Thinking critically about family-centered home care nursing, *Pediatr Nurs* 20(6):588-590, 1994.

eign to the nurse's background and experience. The home care nurse, aware that value systems drive behavior, needs to learn about the family's culture, ask questions without implying judgment, interpret the mainstream medical culture, and help families design interventions that meet their preferences (Stone and Hoffman, 1993) (see Family Focus box).

Respect for family diversity and awareness of both family developmental stages (see Chapter 4) and the stages of a family's adjustment to illness in a child (see Chapter 18) will assist the home care nurse in recognizing and promoting family strengths and in respecting varied coping mechanisms. Labels such as "dysfunctional," "difficult," and "noncompliant" can reinforce negative expectations and shape behaviors of both parents and professionals (see Critical Thinking Exercise). On the other hand, emphasizing, identifying, and building on family strengths and coping mechanisms are strategies that promote a central goal in nursing care of the child and family: family empowerment (see Chapter 1). The nurse working with families should remain flexible and open-minded, since new family strengths may emerge over time and coping mechanisms may wax and wane with the stresses of caring for a child with serious or multiple problems.

PARENT-PROFESSIONAL COLLABORATION

Family-centered nursing practice is built on a foundation of parent-professional collaboration, which represents a shift

from the traditional unidirectional relationships between health care providers and families. *Collaborative relationships,* essential in the home care setting, are characterized by several features (Bishop, Woll, and Arango, 1993):

Communication—Including complete and unbiased sharing of information with parents about their child's care and prognosis

Dialogue—Exchanging of information and sharing of reactions and ideas

Active listening—Listening beyond the words to hear and understand concerns, including checking to be certain that interpretations are correct

Awareness and acceptance of difference—Willingness to examine one's own cultural biases and to accept that others may think and act out of different value systems

Negotiation—The process of examining different options, priorities, and preferences to best meet the needs of the child and family

Communication with the family should not be invasive. There is no need to collect information from the family that can be obtained from the child's records. The nurse should explain to the family the reason for questions, particularly those that the family may perceive as intrusive, and should inform families of who will have access to the information. The nurse must also assure families that they have a right to expect confidentiality in regard to the data collected. When working in the home, the nurse must respect the privacy of family members' communications with each other that may be overheard.

> **Nursing ALERT**
> Home care nurses should restrict their communications with other professionals to clinically relevant information about the family.

Communication with family members should include sharing with the family, in a supportive manner, complete and unbiased information about all aspects of the child's condition and care (Shelton and Stepanek, 1994). Parents can feel overwhelming frustration related to obtaining accurate information about their child's illness and its management. Nurses should answer a family's questions in a straightforward manner, including not knowing the answers. Information should be shared with families in a way that will have meaning in their cultural context (Huber, Holditch-Davis, and Brandon, 1993). Many parents report a preference for interactions with professionals who communicate empathy and concern. Although they want accurate information, many parents prefer that providers moderate the amount of information on possible complications and unfavorable prognoses (Knafl and others, 1992). A resource guide for families in which they can record pertinent medical information can assist parents in managing their child's care (Lobosco and others, 1991).

Disagreements may arise between parents and nurses over proper procedures for care of the child (see Thinking Critically About . . . box). In any situation that will not pose danger or risk for the child, nurses should respect parental preferences. If disagreements cannot be resolved, a home care supervisor or case manager should be contacted to assist with problem solving (Ahmann and Bond, 1992). If parents wish to alter a plan of treatment that is part of medical orders, the nurse should ask that they negotiate the change with the prac-

THINKING CRITICALLY ABOUT . . .
Respecting Parental Choices in Home Care

The nurse working in a home care setting has certain professional responsibilities. The nurse has medical orders to follow and professional training and perhaps agency standards to guide the provision of care. At times, however, parental decisions and choices may differ from those the nurse might make.

These disagreements between the parents and nurse can arise in the development of care plans (e.g., parents and nurse see different goals for the child), in implementation of procedures (e.g., parents and nurse have different methods for suctioning), and in styles of interacting with or disciplining a child. Ahmann and Bond (1992) outline a number of steps that the nurse can take in negotiating areas of disagreement with the family (see p. •••) but suggest that in general the nurse should respect the family's choices even when the nurse has different priorities or approaches than the family. Klug (1993) suggests that a parent's authority should be respected unless either risk or harm is posed to the child or the written medical orders are not followed. Issues of legal liability cannot be overlooked (Hogue, 1992). Honest, respectful communication and careful documentation are important when any disagreement arises. Agency policies will guide the nurse's practice. Case managers or nursing supervisors may be called on to help negotiate areas of disagreement.

Copyright Elizabeth Ahmann, 1994.

FAMILY FOCUS
What I Learned about Home Care

I learned many things as a result of having home care for four children over a period of 8 years. Two of the major areas I learned about were communication and families' rights. It took a long time to learn some of these things.

Initially, I tried very hard to be sensitive to the professionals and often put my own feelings and needs aside. It took a while to learn that I could stand up for myself and my family and that my child could continue to receive good care. One area that was important to me was to have nurses withhold judgment on our parenting style, even if they might have parented differently.

Communication needs to be open and two-way. Families and nurses ought to tell each other what is going well. For example, "Thanks for keeping the room so neat while you're here" can help a nurse see a family's appreciation. There was so little I could do as just "Mommy" that it really meant a lot to me when nurses would say, "That's such a cute outfit you picked out for him today." Communicating about little things, even inconsequential topics such as favorite TV shows, makes it easier to communicate about more important things and about problems. Communication has to be open about problems, too.

Jeni Stepanek
Mother
Upper Marlboro, MD

titioner, since the nurse must follow the written medical orders (Klug, 1993).

Other options to help resolve conflicts include the following (Ahmann and Bond, 1992):

Work with the family's priorities and reevaluate over time.
Provide the family with additional information that may affect their perception of priorities.
Share the nurse's perception of priorities and rationales without judgment.
Suggest an additional priority goal if the family agrees.

THE NURSING PROCESS

In the home the family is a partner in each step of the nursing process. The use of formal self-report assessment tools can help families identify needs they may have for information, training, services, and support. Assessment should also address family strengths and resources (see Family Assessment, Chapter 6). The principles of communication discussed previously guide data collection. The nurse's observations are shared neutrally, without value judgment, and in a way that preserves the family's own role in decision making (Bond, Phillips, and Rollins, 1994).

All the information gathered as part of the assessment process is shared with the family. The nurse should recognize that the family's perception of their most important need will generally guide their behavior and consume their attention and energy. For this reason, family priorities guide the planning process.

Both short-term and long-term goals should be outlined and agreed on by the child, family, and professionals involved. The plan of care should integrate various disciplines that may be involved with the child in order to minimize duplication

and consolidate care requirements. Cross-training of professionals and a transdisciplinary mode of treatment can also be useful when a child has multiple and complex care requirements. For example, certain physical or occupational therapy routines may be incorporated into the child's morning nursing procedures, or speech therapy interventions may be conducted by the parent or nurse around eating times so that the entire day is not occupied by procedures. A written schedule of daily routines should be developed and followed by all caregivers.

Goals of care are supported by intervention strategies that reflect normalization (see Chapter 18) and the interests and abilities of the child and family. Nurses can help families explore a range of alternative strategies, services, and resources so that the family can choose the best match for their situation.

Family participation in evaluating a home care plan can occur on several levels. Families and care providers should regularly review the goals of care and then update the care plan as required. The nurse can also ask the family open-ended questions at regular intervals to assess their opinions on the effectiveness of care (Bond, Phillips, and Rollins, 1994). As part of the evaluation process, families should be acknowledged for their successes and accomplishments. Finally, families should be given an opportunity to evaluate individual home care nurses, the home care agency, and other service providers on a periodic basis. The evaluation should address the nurse's knowledge, skills, and respect for the family's choices. It also should address the agency's handling of the schedule, provision of qualified nurses, and problem-solving abilities (Klug, 1992). The evaluations should be used by the agency to improve quality of care (see Family Focus box).

Home care nursing encourages a close and rewarding relationship with the family. One of the most important aspects

CRITICAL THINKING EXERCISE
Maintaining Therapeutic Boundaries

You are a home care nurse who has been working with a 3-year-old child who is ventilator dependent. You have been visiting the Jones family several days a week for the last 5 months. You notice that the parents are arguing increasingly. Some of the arguments are about whether Mr. Jones helps enough with the child's care. Mrs. Jones approaches you to complain about her husband. Depending on your relationship with the family, you might do any of the following except:

1. Mention that home care can be stressful for a family.
2. Indicate that you can provide referrals for counseling should the parents want them.
3. Agree with Mrs. Jones that her husband is not contributing enough to the child's care.
4. Listen and reflect with Mrs. Jones about her feelings.

The correct answer is three. Therapeutic boundaries are not rigid and fixed. They must be responsive to the relationship preferred by the family and the style with which the family operates. For this reason, depending on the family, options one, two, or four (or a combination) might be most appropriate. In any circumstance it would be inappropriate to agree with Mrs. Jones that her husband is not helping enough with the child's care. Such an action implies a judgment that is not within the nurse's role to make and undermines rather than supports the family system.

of this relationship is maintaining professional boundaries and a therapeutic role that is supportive but not intrusive. Some of these issues are discussed under Therapeutic Relationship, Chapter 1 (see also Critical Thinking Exercise).

PROMOTION OF OPTIMUM DEVELOPMENT, SELF-CARE, AND EDUCATION

There is little question that living at home offers most children with complex medical problems great social and emotional advantages over living in the hospital or other institutional setting. However, in infancy and throughout the developmental stages, a child's medical condition(s) and the dependence on medical technology can place constraints on and pose challenges to *normal development.* For example, the child may have lengthy and repeated hospitalizations; developmental regression can occur in response to stress; fatigue may be due to underlying pathology, the flare of an illness, or medication side effects; and equipment requirements may impede mobility, exploration, and independence. The challenge of providing support for normal development in a child who is chronically ill and technology dependent is to optimize opportunities for developmentally appropriate experiences within the constraints posed by the medical condition and the equipment requirements.

Home care plans are designed to promote optimum child development through initial and periodic assessment, planning, referrals for further assessment or therapeutic services, and by interventions that address normalization issues and self-care. (See Chapter 18 for a discussion of normalization.) General principles for a family-centered assessment and planning process have been addressed earlier in this chapter and are applied in developmental assessment and planning as well.

Some parents may not pursue early developmental intervention because they do not view their child as needing the services. In this case professionals need to explain the child's developmental needs to parents in ways that are meaningful from the parents' own cultural and socioeconomic perspectives (Huber, Holditch-Davis, and Brandon, 1993). Only then can parents make truly informed decisions. Once parents have been fully informed of the child's condition, likely developmental sequelae, and the expected benefits of intervention, developmental goals outlined by the child and family should guide planning and intervention.

Each family is entitled to an *individual family service plan (IFSP)* to help ensure early intervention. All states in the United States provide agencies that develop IFSPs (American Academy of Pediatrics, 1995).

Several principles underlie appropriate developmental intervention plans for children with complex medical problems (Ahmann and Lierman, 1992). First, understanding a child's medical condition ensures that the nurse and family can plan to maximize developmental opportunities at times when the child has the most energy and endurance and that stress signals that determine the child's tolerance for type, intensity, and duration of activity will be noted (Ahmann and Lipsi, 1991). Second, plans for developmental support must be flexible and tailored to the individual child's abilities, interests, and needs. Third, familiarity with the child's medical equipment will facilitate the planning of creative ways to meet the child's developmental needs. For example, the use of lengthy oxygen tubing allows the active toddler freedom of movement during the day (Fig. 20-2); portable equipment of any type facilitates family outings; and mounting a ventilator to a wheelchair allows the adolescent greater independence.

Many developmental aspects of chronic illness or disability in children are discussed in Chapter 18 (see Promote Normal Development). Some additional factors apply when children are or have been dependent on medical technology and should be considered in developing plans to promote normal development (Ahmann and Lierman, 1992). These special needs may include the following:

For infants, attention to promoting oral-motor development
For toddlers, efforts to encourage mobility and exploration, and extra assistance with language development
For preschoolers, assistance in self-care
For school-age children, provision of games and tasks for mastery, and socialization opportunities
For adolescents, increased independence in managing their own medical care

Promoting coping and capability can buffer stress and contribute to mental health and self-esteem in a child with chronic illness (Patterson and Geber, 1991). The extent to which a child is involved in his or her own care depends on many factors, including the child's developmental age, level of interest, and physical ability, as well as parental comfort and support. *Self-care,* both in activities of daily living and in regard to the medical condition, is important.

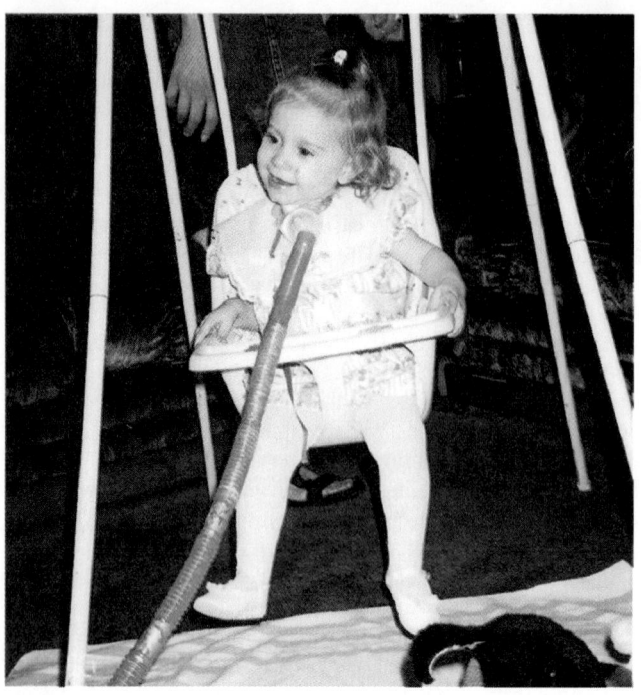

FIG. 20-2. Use of lengthy tubing facilitates a child's freedom of movement.

The frame of reference for self-care in activities of daily living should be the goal of attaining age-appropriate competence. Some modifications in the environment, in the medical equipment, and/or in the techniques for daily activities may be required to promote and support self-care. Effective teaching for self-care is focused at the child's own level of conceptual understanding and may be augmented by the use of dolls, other models and diagrams, simple explanations, and repetition.

For the school-age child or adolescent dependent on medical technology, *educational planning* is important. Despite laws that ensure a "free appropriate public education" to these children, conflict over payment for health care services in the school setting has often been an impediment to mainstreaming children with complex medical problems (Walker, 1991). When a child requiring special medical care is to be placed in an educational setting, the parents, child, school health coordinator, educational evaluation team, and education and administrative staff should meet to determine safe and appropriate placement, as well as necessary services and personnel to enable the child to attend school in the least restrictive environment. Training of educational staff and caregivers is essential to ensuring the child's safety in the educational setting* (Haynie, Porter, and Palfrey, 1989; Krier, 1993). Special assistance can also be beneficial in reintegrating previously schooled children, such as those with cancer, into the school setting. Parents may need assistance in developing the skills necessary to advocate effectively for their child in the educational system (DiGregorio-Hixson, Stoff, and White, 1992).

---

*A thorough discussion of training issues, content, and guidelines for care in the school are provided in Haynie, Porter, and Palfrey, 1989.

SAFETY ISSUES IN THE HOME

Safety is an important consideration in pediatric home care and should be addressed in the home care plan. First, before hospital discharge, emergency preparations must be made. The home should have a telephone.

NURSING TIP If the family does not have a telephone, arrangements may be made with the telephone company to supply service. Alternatively, one or two nearby neighbors may agree to let the family use their services. In rural areas a local pharmacy or police or ranger station may be willing to receive messages and relay them to the family.

The telephone and electric companies (if use of medical equipment requires electricity) are notified that the family needs to be placed on a priority service list so that the family will learn of any anticipated interruptions in service and receive priority in reinstatement of interrupted services. Prior contact with rescue squad and local emergency facility personnel can help ensure prompt and appropriate interventions if required.

Before hospital discharge, emergency protocols are developed and reviewed with both the parents and the professional caregivers. Cardiopulmonary resuscitation (CPR) guidelines, if appropriate, should be posted near the child's bedside or in another accessible location. A list of emergency telephone numbers can be placed near each home phone and should include those of the rescue squad, emergency room, managing physician(s), nursing agency, and equipment vendor(s).

Another aspect of safety relates to the provision of care by appropriately trained individuals. Family members should receive thorough training in the child's care requirements and have the opportunity to demonstrate knowledge and confidence before hospital discharge. Professional staff caring for the child should have the appropriate background and training for the child's particular care needs. Because of the child's body size, special skill and caution are required both in performing procedures (e.g., gastrostomy feedings, suctioning) and in monitoring the use of equipment (e.g., ventilator settings, intravenous flow rates, total fluid volumes) (see Chapter 22).

The activity level and curiosity of young children raise additional safety considerations in the provision of home care. All medications, needles, syringes, and any contaminated materials are securely stored well out of the reach of curious hands. Special attention is paid to childproofing the control panels for ventilators, pumps, monitors, and other equipment. Use of clear plastic tape, covers, or panels to cover control knobs or buttons reduces the risk of accidental changes in settings. Electrical cords are kept short and out of reach, and safety covers are used on any open outlets. When not in use, equipment is unplugged, and any wires (e.g., lead wires for an apnea monitor) are stored out of reach.

Care at night poses other safety concerns. Care must be taken to prevent accidental strangulation on apnea, oximeter, or cardiac monitor wires or lengthy intravenous tubing during sleep. Parents or other caregivers need to be able to clearly hear monitor, ventilator, or pump alarms at night; an inexpensive intercom system or baby monitor can be used.

NURSING TIP Coiling extra tubing and taping it at the exit site, as well as running wires or tubes out the bottoms of pajamas, is a precaution against strangulation.

Safe transportation is a vitally important concern. In many cases wheelchairs and other medical equipment must be properly secured to the vehicle, including vans and buses. Additional information on car safety and general health supervision is provided in Chapter 18 (see Educate About the Disorder and General Health Care).

FAMILY-TO-FAMILY SUPPORT

Family-to-family support networks can be an important source of emotional and instrumental support and empowerment for families of children with chronic health problems.

Family-to-family support does not replace professional sources of support but rather is a unique resource promoting family strengths through shared experience (Johnson, Jeppson, and Redburn, 1992). Existing parent support groups may not necessarily meet an individual family's needs; when nurses refer a family to a particular group, they should inform the family of the group's purposes (Betz and others, 1990). The value of informal support networks should not be overlooked. Similarly, the support needs of fathers, grandparents, and siblings may be different from those of mothers and should be acknowledged as part of the plan of care. (Some sources of information and support for families are listed at the end of this chapter.) Peer support for school-age children and adolescents with complex care may also be beneficial.

KEY POINTS

- Effective home care depends on many factors, including the child's relative medical stability; the family's willingness, training, and ability to accommodate the child's care requirements; and professional, financial, and community support.
- Comprehensive, multidisciplinary discharge planning should begin early and should include the family and a home care representative in addition to hospital personnel.
- Thorough training of the family, including a trial of care, a predischarge pass to home, and a predischarge home visit, can ease the transition to home.
- Care coordination ensures continuity of care and reduces fragmentation of services. The family may assume varying degrees of care coordination over time.
- The home care nurse must share a level of technical expertise with the critical care nurse while being able to adapt equipment, procedures, and the nursing process to the home setting.
- Federal standards apply to agencies that participate in Medicare or Medicaid; standards of practice by The American Nurses Association can guide nurses in the home setting.
- Family-centered nursing practice is applied in the

home setting; diversity in family structures, cultural backgrounds, strengths, and coping mechanisms is respected.
- Collaborative relationships are characterized by communication, dialogue, active listening, awareness and acceptance of difference, and negotiation.
- The nursing process is adapted to involve the family in each step and to preserve the family's central role in decision making.
- "House rules" agreed on by the nurse and family allow a family to maintain a feeling of control over their own environment when professionals are present.
- Home care plans are designed to promote optimum development of the child and focus on normalization, on the impact of the child's medical condition and technologic requirements on development, on self-care, and on educational needs.
- Safety in the provision of home care services involves emergency preparations and protocols, appropriate training of family and home care personnel, and safe use and childproofing of medical equipment.
- Family-to-family support networks can both provide emotional and instrumental support and encourage family em powerment.

REFERENCES

Ahmann E: An overview of issues in pediatric high-tech home care. In Gorski LA, editor: *High tech home care manual,* Gaithersburg, MD, 1994, Aspen.

Ahmann E, Bond NJ: Promoting normal development in school-age children and adolescents who are technology dependent: a family centered model, *Pediatr Nurs* 18:399-405, 1992.

Ahmann E, Lierman C: Promoting normal development in technology dependent children: an introduction to the issues, *Pediatr Nurs* 18:143-152, 1992.

Ahmann E, Lipsi KA: Early intervention for technology dependent infants and young children, *Infants Young Child* 3(4):67-77, 1991.

American Academy of Pediatrics: *The medical home and early intervention,* Elk Grove Village, IL, 1995, The Academy.

American Nurses Association: *Nursing case management,* Washington, DC, 1988, The Association.

American Nurses Association: *Standards of community health nursing practice,* Washington, DC, 1986a, The Association.

American Nurses Association: *Standards of home health nursing practice,* Washington, DC, 1986b, The Association.

Betz CL and others: A survey of self-help groups in California for parents of children with chronic conditions, *Pediatr Nurs* 16(3):293-296, 1990.

Bishop KK, Woll J, Arango P: *Family/professional collaboration,* Burlington, VT, 1993, Department of Social Work, University of Vermont.

Bond N, Phillips P, Rollins JA: Family-centered care at home for families with children who are technology-dependent, *Pediatr Nurs* 20(2):123-130, 1994.

Curry R, Cullen J: Using videorecordings in pediatric nursing practice, *Pediatr Nurs* 16(5):501-504, 1990.

DiGregorio-Hixson D, Stoff E, White PH: Parents of children with chronic health impairments: a new approach to advocacy training, *Child Health Care* 21(2):111-115, 1992.

Harris PJ: Sometimes pediatric home care doesn't work, *Am J Nurs* 88:851-854, 1988.

Haynie M, Porter SM, Palfrey JS: *Children assisted by medical technology in educational settings: guidelines for care,* Boston, 1989, The Children's Hospital (Project School Care).

Hogue E: Parental noncompliance in home care, *Pediatr Nurs* 18(6):603-606, 1992.

Huber C, Holditch-Davis D, Brandon D: High-risk preterm infants at 3 years of age: parental response to the presence of developmental problems, *Child Health Care* 22(2):107-124, 1993.

Johnson BH, Jeppson ES, Redburn L: *Caring for children and families: guidelines for hospitals,* Bethesda, MD, 1992, Association for the Care of Children's Health.

Klug RM: Clarifying roles and expectations in home care, *Pediatr Nurs* 19:374-376, 1993.

Klug RM: Selecting a home care agency, *Pediatr Nurs* 18:504-507, 1992.

Knafl K and others: Parents' view of health care providers: an exploration of the components of a positive working relationship, *Child Health Care* 21(2):90-95, 1992.

Krier JJ: Involvement of educational staff in the health care of medically fragile children, *Pediatr Nurs* 19(3):251-254, 1993.

Lobosco AF and others: Local coalitions for coordinating services to children dependent on technology and their families, *Child Health Care* 20(2):75-86, 1991.

Patterson JM, Blum RW: A conference on culture and chronic illness in childhood: conference summary, *Pediatrics* 91:1025-1030, 1993.

Patterson JM, Geber G: Preventing mental health problems in children with chronic illness or disability, *Child Health Care* 20(3):150-161, 1991.

Shelton TL, Stepanek JS: *Family-centered care for children needing specialized health and developmental services,* Bethesda, MD, 1994, Association for the Care of Children's Health.

Stone M, Hoffman R: *Cultural understanding: how far do you go?* Paper presented at the ACCH local conference on Incorporating Cultural Awareness into Pediatric Healthcare, Washington, DC, April 30, 1993.

Walker P: Where there is a way there is not always a will: technology, public policy, and the social integration of children who are technology-assisted, *Child Health Care* 20(2): 68-74, 1991.

BIBLIOGRAPHY

Aday LA, Aitken MJ, Wegener DH: *Pediatric home care: results of a national evaluation of programs for ventilator assisted children,* Chicago, 1988, Pluribus.

Ahmann E: "Chunky stew": appreciating cultural diversity while providing health care for children, *Pediatr Nurs* 20(3):320-324, 1994.

Ahmann E: Family-centered care: the time has come, *Pediatr Nurs* 20(1):52-53, 1994.

Ahmann E: *Home care for the high risk infant: a family-centered approach,* Gaithersburg, MD, 1996, Aspen.

Ahmann E: Thinking critically about family-centered home care nursing, *Pediatr Nurs* 20(6):588-590, 1994.

Ahmann E, Lipsi KA: Developmental assessment of the technology-dependent infant and young child, *Pediatr Nurs* 18:299-313, 1992.

American Academy of Pediatrics, Committee on Children with Disabilities: Pediatric services for infants and children with special health care needs, *Pediatrics* 92(1):163-165, 1993.

Barnsteiner J, Gillis-Donovan J: Being related and separate: a standard for therapeutic relationships, *MCN Am J Matern Child Nurs* 15:223-228, 1990.

Britton LJ, Johnston JD: Dependent on technology: a child grows up hospitalized, *Pediatr Nurs* 19(6):579-584, 1993.

Buehler JA, Lee HJ: Exploration of home care resources for rural families with cancer, *Cancer Nurs* 15(4):299-308, 1992.

Burns CE, Madian N: Experiences with a support group for grandparents of children with disabilities, *Pediatr Nurs* 18:17-22, 1992.

Cady C, Yoshioko RS: Using a learning contract to successfully discharge an infant on home total parenteral nutrition, *Pediatr Nurs* 17:67-74, 1991.

Davis BD, Steele S: Case management for young children with special care needs, *Pediatr Nurs* 17:15-19, 1991.

Diehl SF, Moffitt KA, Wade SM: Focus group interview with parents of children with medically complex needs: an intimate look at their perceptions and feelings, *Child Health Care* 20(3):170-178, 1991.

Dunst C, Trivette C, Deal A: *Enabling and empowering families,* Cambridge, MA, 1988, Brookline.

Dunst C and others: Enabling and empowering families of children with health impairments, *Child Health Care* 17(2):71-81, 1988.

Fields A and others: Home care cost-effectiveness for respiratory technology-dependent children, *Am J Dis Child* 145(7):729-733, 1991.

Fleming J and others: Impact on the family of children who are technology dependent and cared for in the home, *Pediatr Nurs* 20(4):379-388, 1994.

Gallo AM: Stigma in childhood chronic illness: a well sibling perspective, *Pediatr Nurs* 75:21-25, 1991.

Gallo AM and others: Well siblings of children with chronic illness: parents' reports of their psychological adjustment, *Pediatr Nurs* 18:23-27, 1992.

Grammatica G: Developing a quality home care program for children, *Pediatr Nurs* 15(1):33-35, 1989.

Groce NE, Zola IK: Multiculturalism, chronic illness and disability, *Pediatrics* 91:1048-1055, 1993.

Haas DL: Family-centered, community-based, coordinated care for children with special health care needs. Part II, *Issues Compr Pediatr Nurs* 15(2, entire issue), 1992.

Hamilton B, Vessey J: Pediatric discharge planning, *Pediatr Nurs* 18:475-480, 1992.

Hewson M and others: Comprehensive team care, *MCN Am J Matern Child Nurs* 18(4):198-205, 1993.

Hogue E: Liability for premature discharge: an update, *Pediatr Nurs* 17(1):76-78, 1991.

Jackson B, Finkler DE, Robinson C: A case management system for infants with chronic illnesses and developmental disabilities, *Child Health Care* 21(4):224-232, 1992.

Jones ML: *Home care for the chronically ill or disabled child,* New York, 1985, Harper & Row.

Kasprisin C: Home care instructions. In Wong DL: *Wong and Whaley's Clinical manual of pediatric nursing,* ed 4, St Louis, 1996, Mosby.

Kaufman J: An overview of public sector financing for pediatric home care. Part I, *Pediatr Nurs* 17:280-281, 1991.

Kaufman J: An overview of public sector financing for pediatric home care. Part II, *Pediatr Nurs* 17(4):380, 381, 422, 1991.

Klug RM: Understanding private insurance for funding pediatric home care, *Pediatr Nurs* 17:197-198, 1991.

Leff P, Walizer E: *Building the healing partnership,* Cambridge, MA, 1992, Brookline.

Leighton EM, Davis RH, Anderson LJW: An orientation program for high-technology home care nursing, *Pediatr Nurs* 16:182-185, 1990.

Marrelli TM: *Handbook of home health standards and documentation: guidelines for reimbursement,* ed 2, St Louis, 1994, Mosby.

McClowry S: Pediatric nursing psychosocial care: a vision beyond hospitalization, *Pediatr Nurs* 19(2):146-148, 1993.

McClung RL: Considerations for the use of a conceptual model in home health nursing, *Pediatr Nurs* 21(1):68-70, 1995.

Nissam LG, Sten MB: The ventilator assisted child: a case for empowerment, *Pediatr Nurs* 17:507-511, 1991.

Nugent K and others: A practice model for a parent support group, *Pediatr Nurs* 18:11-16, 1992.

Office of Technology Assessment (OTA), Congress of the United States: *Technology dependent children: hospital v. home care—a technical memorandum* (OTA-TM-H-38), Washington, DC, 1987, US Government Printing Office.

Parette HP, Bartlett CR, Holder-Brown L: The nurse's role in planning for inclusion of medically fragile and technology-dependent children in public school settings, *Issues Compr Pediatr Nurs* 17(2):61-72, 1994.

Steele S: Nurse and parent collaborative case management in a rural setting, *Pediatr Nurs* 19(6):612-615, 1993.

Stein R, Jessop DJ: Does pediatric home care make a difference for children with chronic illness? Findings from the Pediatric Ambulatory Care Treatment Study, *Pediatrics* 73(6):845-853, 1984.

Stutts AL: Selected outcomes of technology-dependent children receiving home care and prescribed child care services, *Pediatr Nurs* 20(5):501-507, 1994.

Wegener DH, Aday LA: Home care for ventilator assisted children: predicting family stress, *Pediatr Nurs* 15:371-376, 1989.

Wells PW and others: Growing up in the hospital. Part II. Nurturing the philosophy of family-centered care, *J Pediatr Nurs* 9(3):141-149, 1994.

Wheeler TW, Lewis CC: Home care for medically fragile children: urban versus rural settings, *Issues Compr Pediatr Nurs* 16:13-30, 1993.

Worthington RC: Effective transitions for families: life beyond the hospital, *Pediatr Nurs* 21(1):86-87, 1995.

Youngblut JM, Brennan PF, Swegart LA: Families with medically fragile children: an exploratory study, *Pediatr Nurs* 20(5):463-468, 1994.

Zagorsky ES: Caring for families who follow alternative health care practices, *Pediatr Nurs* 19(1):71-75, 1993.

Zanoa JS: Beyond the stack of bills: what home care of cancer patients really costs, *Cancer Nurs News* 10(3):13, 1992.

Selected Resources on Home Care

Association for the Care of Children's Health
7910 Woodmont Ave., Suite 300
Bethesda, MD 20814
(301) 654-6549

National Association for Home Care
519 C Street, N.E.
Washington, DC 20002-5809
(202) 547-7424

National Father's Network
The Kindering Center
16120 Northeast 8th St.
Bellevue, WA 98008
(206) 747-4004

National Information Center for Children and Youth with Disabilities
PO Box 1492
Washington, DC 20013
(202) 884-8200 or (800) 695-0285

National Information Clearinghouse for Infants with Disabilities and Life Threatening Conditions
NIS
CDD/USC
Benson Building
Columbia, SC 29208
(800) 922-9234, ext. 201 (voice or TDD)
In South Carolina: (800) 922-1107

Project Copernicus
(Family-Centered Care)
Kennedy-Krieger
Community Resources
2911 E. Biddle St.
Baltimore, MD 21213
(410) 550-9700
(410) 550-9758 (TDD)

Sibling Support Project
Children's Hospital and Medical Center
4800 Sand Point Way, N.E.
Seattle, WA 98105
(206) 368-4911

Skip (Sick Kids Need Involved People, Inc.)
545 Madison Ave., 13th Floor
New York, NY 10022
(212) 421-9160

FAMILY-CENTERED CARE OF THE CHILD DURING ILLNESS AND HOSPITALIZATION

Chapter 21

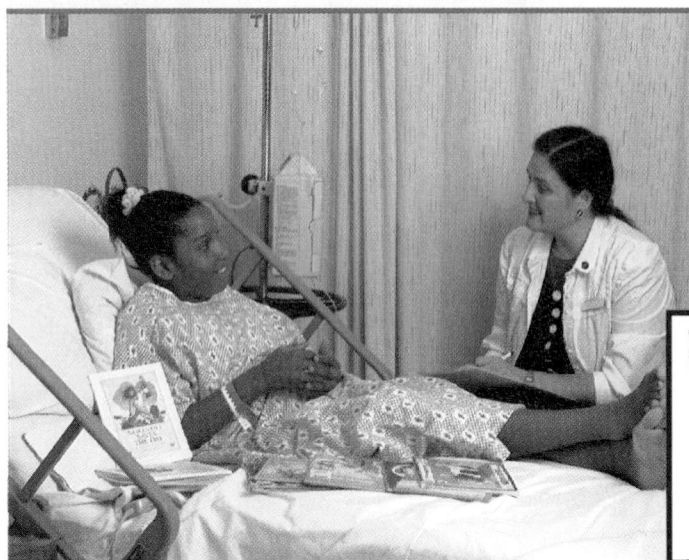

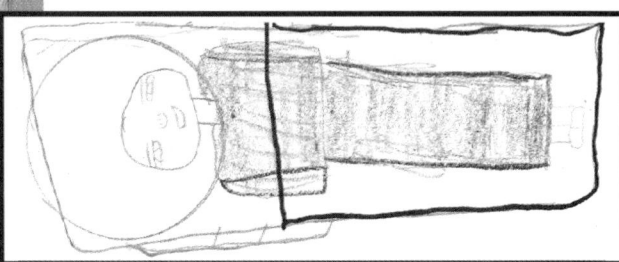

" I've had three surgeries — one across my stomach (where my spleen and gallbladder were taken out), but it doesn't hurt anymore. "

Evonne, age 10 years, sickle cell anemia

RELATED TOPICS

STRESSORS OF HOSPITALIZATION AND CHILDREN'S REACTIONS

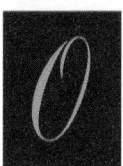 ften illness and hospitalization are the first crises children must face. Children, especially during the early years, are particularly vulnerable to the crises of illness and hospitalization because (1) stress represents a change from the usual state of health and environmental routine, and (2) children have a limited number of coping mechanisms to resolve *stressors* (those events that produce stress). Children's reactions to these crises are influenced by their developmental age; previous experience with illness, separation, or hospitalization; innate and acquired coping skills; the seriousness of the diagnosis; and the support system available.

SEPARATION ANXIETY

The major stress from middle infancy throughout the preschool years, especially for children ages 6 to 30 months, is separation anxiety. The principal behavioral responses to this stressor during early childhood are summarized in the box.

During the phase of *protest,* children react aggressively to the separation from the parent. They cry and scream for their parents, refuse the attention of anyone else, and are inconsolable in their grief (Fig. 21-1). During the phase of *despair,* the crying stops, and depression is evident. The child is much less active, is uninterested in play or food, and withdraws from others (Fig. 21-2).

The third stage is *detachment,* which is sometimes also called *denial.* Superficially it appears that the child has finally adjusted to the loss. The child becomes more interested in the surroundings, plays with others, and seems to form new relationships. However, this behavior is the result of resignation and is not a sign of contentment. The child detaches from the parent in an effort to escape the emotional pain of desiring the parent's presence and copes by forming shallow relationships with others, becoming increasingly self-centered, and attaching primary importance to material objects. This is the most serious stage in that reversal of the potential adverse effects is less likely to occur once detachment is established. However, in most situations the temporary

---

Judy Holt Rollins, MS, RN, revised this chapter.

MANIFESTATIONS OF SEPARATION ANXIETY IN YOUNG CHILDREN

Phase of Protest

Observed behaviors during later infancy:
  Cries
  Screams
  Searches for parent with eyes
  Clings to parent
  Avoids and rejects contact with strangers
Additional behaviors observed during toddlerhood:
  Verbally attacks strangers (e.g., "Go away")
  Physically attacks strangers (e.g., kicks, bites, hits, pinches)
  Attempts to escape to find parent
  Attempts to physically force parent to stay
Behaviors may last from hours to days
Protest, such as crying, may be continuous, ceasing only with physical exhaustion
Approach of stranger may precipitate increased protest

Phase of Despair

Observed behaviors:
  Inactive
  Withdraws from others
  Depressed, sad
  Uninterested in environment
  Uncommunicative
  Regresses to earlier behavior (e.g., thumb-sucking, bedwetting, use of pacifier, use of bottle)
Behaviors may last for variable length of time
Child's physical condition may deteriorate from refusal to eat, drink, or move

Phase of Detachment

Observed behaviors:
  Shows increased interest in surroundings
  Interacts with strangers or familiar caregivers
  Forms new but superficial relationships
  Appears happy
Detachment usually occurs after prolonged separation from parent; rarely seen in hospitalized children
Behaviors represent a superficial adjustment to loss

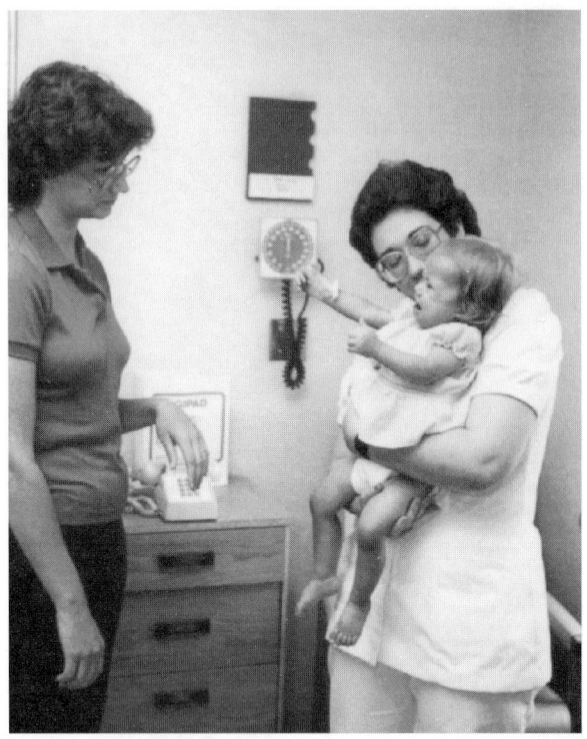

FIG. 21-1. In the protest phase of separation anxiety, children cry loudly and are inconsolable in their grief for the parent.

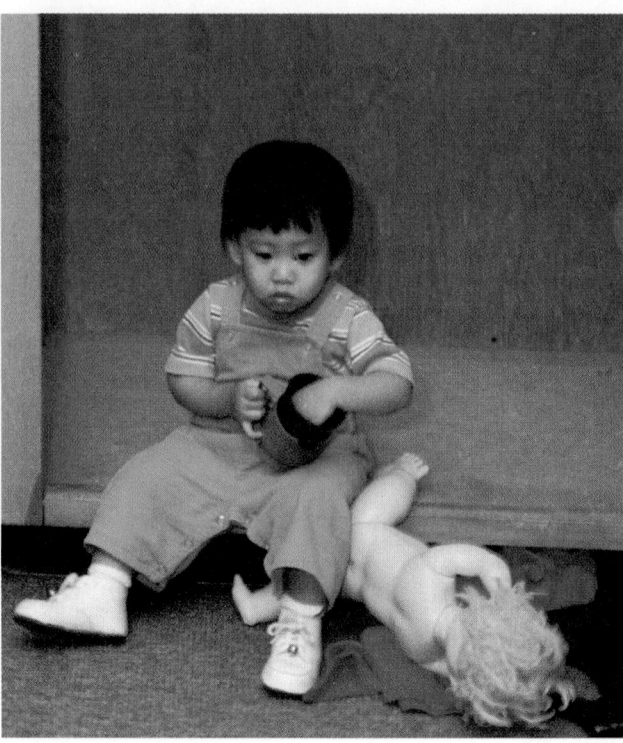

FIG. 21-2. During the despair phase of separation anxiety, children are sad, lonely, and uninterested in play or food.

separations imposed by hospitalization do not cause such prolonged parental absences that the child enters into detachment. In addition, considerable evidence suggests that even with stressors such as separation, children are remarkably adaptable and permanent ill effects are rare.

Although progression to the stage of detachment is uncommon, the initial stages are frequently observed even with very brief separations from either parent. Unless health team members understand the meaning of each stage of behavior, they may erroneously label the behaviors as positive or negative. For example, they may see the loud crying of the protest phase as "bad" behavior. Since the protesting increases when a stranger approaches the child, they may interpret that reaction as meaning they should stay away. During the quiet, withdrawn phase of despair, health team members may think the child is finally "settling in" to the new surroundings, and they may see the detachment behaviors as proof of a "good adjustment." The faster this stage is reached, the more likely that the child will be regarded as the "ideal patient."

Since children seem to react "negatively" to visits by their parents, uninformed observers feel justified in restricting parental visiting privileges. For example, during the protest stage, children outwardly do not appear happy to see their parents. In fact, they may even cry louder. If they are depressed, they may reject their parents or begin to protest once more. Often they cling to their parents in an effort to ensure their continued presence. Consequently, such reactions may be regarded as "disturbing" the child's adjustment to the new surroundings. If the separation has progressed to the phase of detachment, children will respond no differently to their parents than they would to any other strange or familiar person.

Such reactions are equally distressing to parents, who are unaware of their meaning. If parents are regarded as intruders, they will see their absence as "beneficial" to the child's adjustment and recovery. They may respond to the child's behavior by staying for only short periods, visiting less frequently, or deceiving the child when it is time to leave. The result is a destructive cycle of misunderstanding and unmet needs.

Early Childhood

Separation anxiety is the greatest stress imposed by hospitalization during early childhood. If separation is avoided, young children have a tremendous capacity to withstand any other stress. During this age period the typical reactions previously described are seen. However, children in the toddler stage demonstrate more goal-directed behaviors. For example, they may plead with the parents to stay and physically try to keep the parents with them or try to find parents who have left. They may demonstrate displeasure on the parents' return or departure by having temper tantrums; refusing to comply with the usual routines of mealtime, bedtime, or toileting; or regressing to more primitive levels of development. However, temper tantrums, bed-wetting, or other behaviors may also be expressions of anger or even a physiologic response to stress.

Since preschoolers are more secure interpersonally than toddlers, they can tolerate brief periods of separation from their parents and are more inclined to develop substitute trust in other significant adults. However, the stress of illness usually renders preschoolers less able to cope with separation; as a result, they manifest many of the stage behaviors of separation anxiety, although in general the protest behaviors are more subtle and passive than those seen in younger children. Preschoolers may demonstrate separation anxiety by refusing to eat, experiencing difficulty in sleeping, crying quietly for their parents, continually asking when the parents will visit, or withdrawing from others. They may express anger indirectly by breaking their toys, hitting other children, or refusing to cooperate during usual self-care activities. Nurses need to be sensitive to these less obvious signs of separation anxiety in order to intervene appropriately.

Later Childhood and Adolescence

Previous research, usually based on adult recollections, indicated that the family does not play as important a role for school-age children as it does during the toddler and preschool years. However, in a recent study that asked children about their fears when hospitalized, children ranked "being away from my family" higher than any other fear associated with hospitalization (Hart and Bossert, 1994). Although school-age children are better able to cope with separation in general, the stress and often accompanying regression imposed by illness or hospitalization may increase their need for parental security and guidance. This is particularly true for young school-age children who have only recently left the safety of the home and are struggling with the crisis of school adjustment. Middle and late school-age children may react more to the separation from their usual activities and peers than to the absence of their parents. These children have a high level of physical and mental activity that frequently finds no suitable outlets in the hospital environment, and even when they dislike school, they admit to missing its routine and worry that they will not be able to compete or "fit in" with their classmates when they return. Feelings of loneliness, boredom, isolation, and depression are common. Such reactions may occur more as a result of separation than from concern over the illness, treatment, or hospital setting.

School-age children may need and desire parental guidance or support from other adult figures but be unable or unwilling to ask for it. Because the goal of attaining independence is so important to them, they are reluctant to seek help directly for fear that they will appear weak, childish, or dependent. Cultural expectations to "act like a man" or to "be brave and strong" bear heavily on these children, especially boys, who tend to react to stress with stoicism, withdrawal, or passive acceptance. Often the need to express hostile, angry, or other negative feelings finds outlets in alternate ways, such as irritability and aggression toward parents, withdrawal from hospital personnel, inability to relate to peers, rejection of siblings, or subsequent behavioral problems in school.

For adolescents, separation from home and parents may be a welcomed and appreciated event. However, loss of peer-group contact may pose a severe emotional threat because of loss of group status, inability to exert group control or leadership, and loss of group acceptance. Deviations within peer groups are poorly tolerated, and, although group members may express concern for the adolescent's illness or need for hospitalization, they continue their group activities, quickly filling the gap of the absent member. During the temporary separation from their usual group, ill adolescents may benefit from group associations with other hospitalized age-mates.

LOSS OF CONTROL

One of the factors influencing the amount of stress imposed by hospitalization is the amount of control that persons perceive themselves as having. Lack of control increases the perception of threat and can affect children's coping skills. Many hospital situations decrease the amount of control a child feels. Although the usual sensory stimulations are lacking, the additional hospital stimuli of sight, sound, and smell may be overwhelming. Without an insight into the type of environment conducive to children's optimum growth, the hospital experience can at best temporarily slow development and at worst permanently restrict it. Because children's needs vary greatly depending on their age, the major areas of loss of control in terms of physical restriction, altered routine or rituals, and dependency are discussed for each age-group.

Infants

Infants are developing the most important attribute of a healthy personality—trust. Trust is established through consistent, loving care by a mothering person. Infants attempt to control their environment through emotional expressions, such as crying or smiling. In the hospital setting, cues may be missed or misinterpreted, and routines may be established to meet the hospital staff's needs instead of the infant's needs. Inconsistent care and deviations from the infant's daily routine may lead to mistrust and a decreased sense of control (Wells and others, 1994).

Toddlers

Toddlers are striving for autonomy, and this goal is evident in most of their behaviors—motor skills, play, interpersonal relationships, activities of daily living, and communication. When their egocentric pleasures meet with obstacles, toddlers react with negativism, especially temper tantrums. Any restriction or limitation of movement, such as the simple act of making toddlers lie down, can cause forceful resistance and noncompliance.

Loss of control also results from altered routines and rituals. Toddlers rely on the consistency and familiarity of daily rituals to provide a measure of stability and control in their complex world of growing and developing. The experience of hospitalization or illness severely limits their sense of expectation and predictability, since practically every detail of the hospital environment differs from that of the home.

Toddlers' main areas for rituals include eating, sleeping, bathing, toileting, and play. When the routines are disrupted, difficulties can occur in any or all of these areas. The principal reaction to such change is regression. For example, when mealtime and food choices differ from those at home, toddlers often refuse to eat, demand a bottle, or ask others to feed them. Although regression to earlier forms of behavior may seem to increase toddlers' security and comfort, in reality it is very threatening for them to relinquish their most recently acquired achievements.

Enforced dependency is a chief characteristic of the sick role and accounts for the numerous instances of toddler negativism. For example, rigid schedules, different clothes, altered caregiving activities, unfamiliar surroundings, separation from parents, and medical procedures usurp toddlers' control over their world. Although most toddlers initially react negatively and aggressively to such dependency, prolonged loss of autonomy may result in passive withdrawal from interpersonal relationships and regression in all areas of development. Therefore the effects of the sick role are most severe in instances of chronic, long-term illnesses or in those families who foster the sick role despite the child's improved state of health.

Preschoolers

Preschoolers also suffer from loss of control caused by physical restriction, altered routines, and enforced dependency. However, their specific cognitive abilities, which make them feel omnipotent and all-powerful, also make them feel out of control. This loss of control in the context of their sense of self-power is a critical influencing factor in their perception of and reaction to separation, pain, illness, and hospitalization.

Preschoolers' egocentric and magical thinking limits their ability to understand events because they view all experiences from their own self-referenced (egocentric) perspective. Without adequate preparation for unfamiliar settings or experiences, preschoolers' fantasy explanations for such events are usually more exaggerated, bizarre, and frightening than the actual facts. One typical fantasy to explain the reason for illness or hospitalization is that it represents punishment for real or imagined misdeeds (see Family Focus box). In response to such thinking the child usually feels shame, guilt, and fear.

Preschoolers' concrete thinking means that explanations are understood only in terms of real events. Purely verbal instructions are often inadequate for them because they are unable to abstract and synthesize beyond what their senses tell them. When combined with their egocentric and magical thinking, this characteristic may lead them to interpret messages according to their particular past experiences. Even with the best preparation for a procedure, they may misconstrue the details.

Transductive reasoning implies that preschoolers deduct from the particular to the particular, rather than from the specific to the general, or vice versa. For example, if preschoolers' concept of nurses is that they inflict pain, preschoolers will think that every nurse (or everyone wearing a similar uniform) will also inflict pain.

School-Age Children

Because of their striving for independence and productivity, school-age children are particularly vulnerable to events that may lessen their feeling of control and power. In particular, altered family roles; physical disability; fears of death, abandonment, or permanent injury; loss of peer acceptance; lack of productivity; and inability to cope with stress according to perceived cultural expectation may result in loss of control.

Because of the nature of the patient role, many routine hospital activities usurp individual power and identity. For school-age children, dependent activities such as enforced bed rest, use of a bedpan, inability to choose a menu, lack of privacy, help with a bed bath, or transport by a wheelchair or stretcher can be a direct threat to their security. Although all

FAMILY FOCUS
A Reflection on Hospitalization

Upon my initial hospitalization, determination of an appropriate insulin dosage meant approximately 7 to 10 injections a day for 10 days. While concrete memories of the hospitalization remain sketchy, remnants of my overwhelming feelings of fright persist. In my mind, hospitalization symbolizes the beginning of my diabetic life: daily injections, food restrictions, glucose monitoring, and blood tests administered by my parents, whom I idolized. As children less than age 7 often view illness as a result of human action, I blamed myself for my illness. I considered the daily injections, tests, doctors, and hospitalization punishment because I was bad or inferior, and thus, deserving of these regimens and limitations.

After all, I was "different." During early childhood, I could not eat candy, have birthday cake, choose what and when I wanted to eat, or sleep over at a friend's house without my parents coming to administer my insulin injection. None of my other friends, classmates, family members, nor siblings had to adhere to such regulations. In my mind, the adversity of these regulations implied wrongdoing and misbehavior on my part, and required punishment. Because I continually received the punishment, there was only one conclusion: I was different, I was bad—I was diabetic.

Modified from Levi R: Childhood illness through a child's eyes, *The ACCH Advocate* 2(1):43-44, 1995.

these usual hospital procedures seem routine and inconsequential, to children who want to "act grown-up" they allow no freedom of choice. However, when children are allowed to exert a measure of control, regardless of how limited, they generally respond very well to any procedure. For example, some of the most cooperative, satisfied, and contented patients are those school-age children who help make their beds, choose their schedule of activities, assist in procedures, and help the nurses care for the younger children. An increased sense of control is usually an outcome of feeling useful and productive.

Besides the hospital environment, illness also may cause a feeling of loss of control. One of the most significant problems of children in this age-group centers on boredom. When physical or enforced limitations curtail their usual abilities to care for themselves or to engage in favorite activities, school-age children generally respond with depression, hostility, or frustration. Keeping a normally active child on bed rest is no small challenge. However, by emphasizing areas of control for the child and capitalizing on quiet activities, particularly hobbies such as building models or collecting specific objects, nurses can promote school-age children's adjustment to physical restriction. Nursing judgment regarding selection of a roommate is one of the most important contributing factors to the overall adjustment of children in this age-group to illness and hospitalization.

Adolescents

Adolescents' struggle for independence, self-assertion, and liberation centers on the quest for personal identity. Anything that interferes with this poses a threat to their sense of identity and results in a loss of control. Illness, which limits their physical abilities, and hospitalization, which separates them from their usual support systems, constitute major situational crises.

The patient role fosters dependency and depersonalization. Adolescents may react to dependency with rejection, uncooperativeness, or withdrawal. They may respond to depersonalization with self-assertion, anger, or frustration. Regardless of response, hospital personnel often regard them as difficult, unmanageable patients. Parents may not be a source of help because these behaviors serve to isolate them further from understanding the adolescent. Although peers may visit, they may not be able to offer the kind of support and guidance needed. Sick adolescents often voluntarily isolate themselves from age-mates until they feel they can compete on an equal basis and meet group expectations. As a result, adolescents may be left with virtually no support system.

Loss of control also occurs for many of the reasons discussed for school-age children. However, adolescents are more sensitive to potential instances of loss of control and dependency than are younger children. For example, both groups seek information about their physical status and rely heavily on anticipatory preparation to decrease fear and anxiety. However, adolescents react not only to the kinds of information supplied them but also to the means by which it is conveyed. They may feel very threatened by others who relate facts in a condescending manner. Adolescents want to know that others can relate to them on their own level. This necessitates a careful assessment of their intellectual abilities, previous knowledge, and present needs.

BODILY INJURY AND PAIN

In caring for children, nurses must have an appreciation of a child's concerns about bodily harm and the reactions to pain at different developmental periods. Table 21-1 summarizes developmental considerations related to children's understanding of illness and pain. The box on p. 614 outlines developmental characteristics of children's reactions to pain.

Infants

Research exploring children's development of illness concepts and how their understanding of illness relates to fears of bodily injury includes no findings for preverbal children. Consequently, the following discussion is limited to infants' reactions to pain (see Infant Pain, Chapter 9).

Infants' response to pain after the neonatal period is quite similar to earlier reactions, although there is marked variability in measures of distress, especially initial cry and heart rate, which may decrease in some infants. The most consistent indicator of distress is a facial expression of discomfort (Fig. 21-3). Body movements include squirming, writhing, jerking, and flailing. Some infants may cry loudly after the procedure, whereas others are easily calmed by a gentle hug. It is important to recognize and respect such early signs of individuality and to realize that children who react less intensely may still be experiencing significant discomfort (Broome and others, 1990).

Children's response to pain is increasingly influenced by their prior painful experiences and the emotional reaction of parents during the procedure. Older infants react intensely with physical resistance and uncooperativeness. They may refuse to lie still, attempt to push the person away, or try to escape with whatever motor activity they have achieved. Distraction does little to lessen their immediate reaction to pain, and anticipatory preparation, such as showing them the equipment, can increase their fear and resistance.

TABLE 21-1. Children's developmental concepts of illness and pain

CONCEPT OF ILLNESS*	CONCEPT OF PAIN†
Preoperational Thought (2 to 7 Years) *Phenomenism:* Perceives an external, unrelated, concrete phenomenon as the cause of illness (e.g., "being sick because you don't feel well") *Contagion:* Perceives cause of illness as proximity between two events that occurs by "magic" (e.g., "getting a cold because you are near someone who has a cold")	Relates to pain primarily as physical, concrete experience Thinks in terms of magical disappearance of pain May view pain as punishment for wrongdoing Tends to hold someone accountable for own pain and may strike out at person
Concrete Operational Thought (7 to 10+ Years) *Contamination:* Perceives cause as a person, object, or action external to the child that is "bad" or "harmful" to the body (e.g., "getting a cold because you didn't wear a hat") *Internalization:* Perceives illness as having an external cause but as being located inside the body (e.g., "getting a cold by breathing in air and bacteria")	Relates to pain physically (e.g., headache, stomachache) Is able to perceive of psychologic pain (e.g., someone dying) Fears bodily harm and annihilation (body destruction and death) May view pain as punishment for wrongdoing
Formal Operational Thought (13 Years and Older) *Physiologic:* Perceives cause as malfunctioning or nonfunctioning organ or process; can explain illness in sequence of events *Psychophysiologic:* Realizes that psychologic actions and attitudes affect health and illness	Is able to give reason for pain (e.g., fell and hit nerve) Perceives several types of psychologic pain Has limited life experiences to cope with pain as adult might cope despite mature understanding of pain Fears losing control during painful experience

*From Bibace R, Walsh ME: Development of children's concepts of illness, *Pediatrics* 66(6):912-917, 1980.
†From Hurley A, Whelan EG: Cognitive development and children's perception of pain, *Pediatr Nurs* 14(1):21-24, 1988.

DEVELOPMENTAL CHARACTERISTICS OF CHILDREN'S RESPONSES TO PAIN

Young Infant

Generalized body response of rigidity or thrashing, possibly with local reflex withdrawal of stimulated area

Loud crying

Facial expression of pain (brows lowered and drawn together, eyes tightly closed, and mouth open and squarish) (Fig. 21-3)

Demonstrates no association between approaching stimulus and subsequent pain

Older Infant

Localized body response with deliberate withdrawal of stimulated area

Loud crying

Facial expression of pain and/or anger (same facial characteristics as pain but eyes are open)

Physical resistance, especially pushing the stimulus away *after* it is applied

Young Child

Loud crying, screaming

Verbal expressions of "Ow," "Ouch," "It hurts"

Thrashing of arms and legs

Attempts to push stimulus away *before* it is applied

Uncooperative; needs physical restraint

Requests termination of procedure

Clings to parent, nurse, or other significant person

Requests emotional support, such as hugs or other forms of physical comfort

May become restless and irritable with continuing pain

All these behaviors may be seen in anticipation of actual painful procedure

School-Age Child

May see all behaviors of young child, especially *during* actual painful procedure but less in anticipatory period

Stalling behavior, such as "Wait a minute" or "I'm not ready"

Muscular rigidity, such as clenched fists, white knuckles, gritted teeth, contracted limbs, body stiffness, closed eyes, wrinkled forehead

Adolescent

Less vocal protest

Less motor activity

More verbal expressions, such as "It hurts" or "You're hurting me"

Increased muscle tension and body control

Data from Craig KD and others: Developmental changes in infant pain expression during immunization injections, *Soc Sci Med* 19(12):1331-1337, 1984; and Katz ER, Kellerman J, Siegel SE: Behavioral distress in children with cancer undergoing medical procedures: developmental considerations, *J Consult Clin Psychol* 48(3):356-365, 1980.

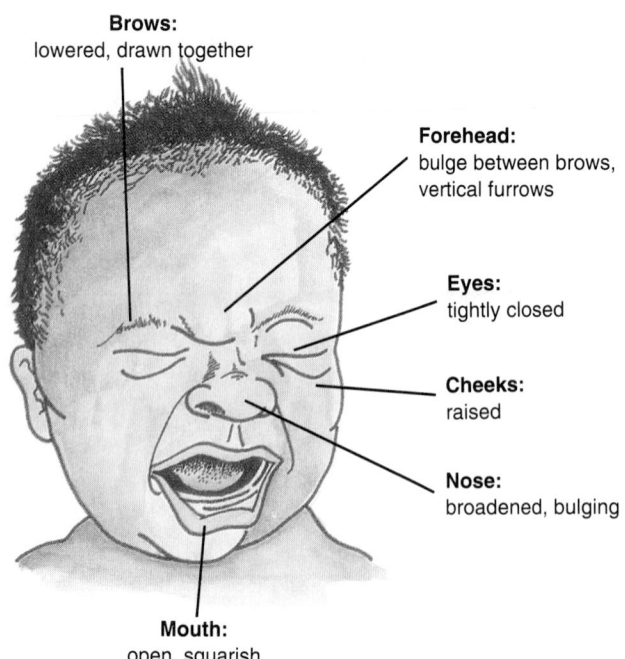

Brows:
lowered, drawn together

Forehead:
bulge between brows, vertical furrows

Eyes:
tightly closed

Cheeks:
raised

Nose:
broadened, bulging

Mouth:
open, squarish

FIG. 21-3. Facial expression of physical distress is the most consistent behavioral indicator of pain in infants.

Toddlers

Toddlers' concept of body image, particularly the definition of body boundaries, is very poorly developed. Intrusive experiences, such as examining the ears or mouth or checking a rectal temperature, are very anxiety producing. Toddlers may react to such painless procedures as intensely as they do to painful ones.

Toddlers' reactions to pain are similar to those seen during infancy, except that the number of variables influencing the individual response is highly complex and varied. Memory, physical restraint, separation from parents, emotional reactions of others, and lack of preparation partially determine the intensity of the behavioral response. In general, children in this age-group continue to react with intense emotional upset and physical resistance to any actual or perceived painful experience. Behaviors indicating pain include grimacing, clenching their teeth and/or lips, opening their eyes wide, rocking, rubbing, and acting aggressively, such as biting, kicking, hitting, or running away. Unlike adults, who usually decrease their activity when in pain, young children typically become restless and overly active; frequently this response is not recognized as a consequence of pain.

By the end of this age period, toddlers usually are able to communicate about their pain. Although they have not developed the ability to describe the type or intensity of the pain, they usually are able to localize it by pointing to a specific area.

Preschoolers

Concepts of illness begin during the preschool period and are influenced by the cognitive abilities of the preoperational stage. Preschoolers differentiate poorly between themselves and the external world. Their thinking is focused on externally perceived events, and causality is based on the proximity of two events. Consequently, children define illness according to what they are told or are given external evidence of, such as "You are sick because you have a fever." The cause of illness is seen as a concrete action the child does or fails to do, such as "Catching a cold because you go out into cold weather"; consequently, it implies a degree of responsibility and self-blame. Another explanation may be based on contagion, that the proximity of two objects or persons causes the illness; for example, "A person gets a cold when someone else with a cold gets near him."

The psychosexual conflicts of children in this age-group make them very vulnerable to threats of bodily injury. Intrusive procedures, whether painful or painless, are threatening to preschoolers, whose concept of body integrity is still poorly developed. Preschoolers may react to an injection with as much concern for withdrawal of the needle as for the actual pain. They fear that the intrusion or puncture will not re-close and that their "insides" will leak out.

Concerns of mutilation are paramount during this age period. Loss of any body part is threatening, but preschool boys' fears of castration complicate their understanding of surgical or medical procedures associated with the genital area, such as circumcision, repair of hypospadias or epispadias, cystoscopy, or catheterization. Their limited comprehension of body functioning also increases their difficulty in understanding how or why body parts are "fixed." For example, telling preschoolers that their tonsils are to be removed may be interpreted as "taking out their voice," or having the penis "fixed" may be understood as cutting it off. Words such as "dye," "cut off," "take out," or "draw" (e.g., "draw some blood") are understood literally and can lead to confusion and fear (see Communicating with Children, Chapter 6).

Reactions to pain tend to be similar to those seen during toddlerhood, although some differences become apparent. For example, preschoolers respond more favorably than younger children to preparatory interventions, such as explanation and distraction. Physical and verbal aggression are more specific and goal directed. Instead of showing total body resistance, preschoolers may push the offending person away, try to secure the equipment, or attempt to lock themselves in a safe place. Much more thought is evident in their plan of attack or escape.

Verbal expression in particular demonstrates their advanced development in response to stress. They may verbally abuse the nurse by stating, "Get out of here" or "I hate you." They may also use the more cunning approach of trying to persuade the person to give up the intended activity. A common plea is, "Please don't give me a shot; I'll be good." Some statements are not only attempts to avoid the event but also evidence of children's perceptions about the experience.

Preschoolers can locate their pain and can use appropriate pain scales. Children as young as 3 years can use assessment tools that employ facial expressions of pain (see Table 21-2).

School-Age Children

Fears concerning the physical nature of the illness surface at this time. School-age children may be less concerned with pain than with disability, uncertain recovery, or possible death. Children with chronic illness are more likely to identify intrusive procedures as stressful, whereas children who are acutely ill are more likely to indicate physical symptoms (Bossert, 1994). Girls tend to express more and stronger fears than boys, and previous hospitalizations may have no effect on the frequency or intensity of these fears. Because of their developing cognitive abilities, school-age children are aware of the significance of different illnesses, the indispensability of certain body parts, potential hazards of treatments, life-long consequences of permanent injury or loss of function, and the meaning of death. A major concern of school-age children when hospitalized is their fear of being told that something is "wrong" with them (Hart and Bossert, 1994). They generally take a very active interest in their health or illness. Even those children who rarely ask questions usually reveal detailed knowledge of their condition by attentively listening to all that is said around them. They request factual information and quickly perceive lies or half-truths. Seeking information tends to be one way of coping or maintaining a sense of control despite the stress and uncertainty of the condition.

The school-age child defines illness by a set of multiple concrete symptoms, such as signs of a cold, and views the cause as primarily germs or bacteria. The germs have a powerful, almost magical quality, so that in the child's mind, illness can be prevented by avoiding people with the germs. There is also the notion of contamination, which is similar to that seen in the younger age-group; for example, the illness occurs because of physical contact or because the child engaged in a harmful action and became contaminated. Consequently, feelings of self-blame and guilt may be associated with the reason for becoming ill.

School-age children begin to show concern for the potential beneficial and hazardous effects of procedures. Besides wanting to know if a procedure will hurt, they want to know what it is for, how it will make them better, and what injury or harm could result. For example, these children may fear the actual procedure of anesthesia. Unlike preschoolers, who fear the mask and the strange surroundings, school-age children fear what may happen while they are asleep, whether they will wake up, and that they may die. Preadolescents also worry about the procedure itself, particularly if it is one that will result in visible changes in body appearance.

Intrusive procedures of a nonsexual nature, such as routine physical examination of the ears, nose, mouth, and throat, are generally well tolerated. However, concerns for privacy become evident and increasingly significant. Although school-age children may cooperate during examination of, or procedures performed on, the genital area, it is usually very stressful for them, especially for preadolescents who are beginning pubertal changes. Nurses who respect children's need for privacy can provide them with much assurance and support.

By age 9 or 10, most school-age children show less fright or overt resistance to pain than younger children. They generally have learned coping methods of dealing with discomfort, such as holding rigidly still, clenching their fists or teeth, or trying to act brave by the "grin-and-bear-it" routine. If they do display signs of overt resistance, such as biting, kicking, pulling away, trying to escape, crying, or plea bargaining, they may deny such reactions later, especially to their peers for fear of embarrassment.

School-age children verbally communicate about their

pain in respect to its location, intensity, and description. Unlike younger children, who may have difficulty choosing words to describe pain, children 8 years and older use a wide variety of words and phrases, such as hurting, sore, burning, stinging, aching, and "like a sharp knife" (Tesler and others, 1991).

School-age children also use words as a means of controlling their reactions to pain. For example, these children may ask the nurse to talk to them during a procedure. Some prefer to participate in a procedure, whereas others choose to distance themselves by not looking at what is happening. Most appreciate an explanation of the procedure and seem less fearful when they know what to expect. Others try to gain control by attempting to postpone the event. A typical request is, "Give me the shot when I am finished with this." Although the ability to make decisions does increase their sense of control, unlimited procrastination results in heightened anxiety. When choices are allowed, such as selection of the injection site, it is best to structure the number of possible sites and to limit the number of "procrastination" techniques.

Similar to their more passive acceptance of pain is their nondirective request for support or help. School-age children will rarely initiate a conversation about their feelings or request someone to stay with them during a lonely or stressful period. Their visible composure, calmness, and acceptance often mask their inner longing for support. It is especially important to be aware of nonverbal clues, such as a serious facial expression, a half-hearted reply of "I am fine," silence, lack of activity, or social isolation, as signs of the need for help. Usually when someone identifies the unspoken messages and offers support, they readily accept it.

Adolescents

Although the development of body image begins at birth, its relevance is paramount during adolescence. Injury, pain, disability, and death are viewed primarily in terms of how each affects adolescents' views of themselves in the present. Any change that differentiates the adolescent from peers is regarded as a major tragedy. For example, diseases such as diabetes mellitus often present a more difficult adjustment period for children in this age-group than for younger children because of the necessary changes in the adolescent's lifestyle. Conversely, serious, even life-threatening illnesses that entail no visible body changes or physical restrictions may have less immediate significance for the adolescent. Therefore the nature of bodily injury may be more important in terms of adolescents' perception of the illness than its actual degree of severity.

Adolescents' rapidly changing body image during pubertal development often makes them feel insecure about their bodies. Illness, medical or surgical intervention, and hospitalization increase their existing concerns for normalcy. They may respond to such events by asking numerous questions, withdrawing, rejecting others, or questioning the adequacy of care. Frequently their fear for loss of control and body image change is demonstrated as overconfidence, conceit, or a "know-it-all" attitude.

Because of sexual changes, adolescents are very concerned about privacy. Lack of respect for this need can cause greater stress than physical pain. In addition, adolescents look for

signs that indicate that they are developing normally and according to acceptable standards. When illness occurs, they fear that growth may be retarded, leaving them behind their peers. Although they may not voice this concern, they may demonstrate it by carefully observing others' reactions to them.

Adolescents typically react to pain with much self-control. Physical resistance and aggression are less likely at this age, unless the adolescent is totally unprepared for a procedure. As with older school-age children, adolescents are very concerned with remaining composed and feel embarrassed and ashamed of losing control. They are able to describe their pain experience and to use any of the pain assessment tools developed for adults. However, they may be reluctant to disclose their pain, requiring the nurse to listen closely and observe physical indications, such as limited movement, excessive quiet, or irritability. They may also believe that the nurse knows how they feel; thus they may see no need to ask for analgesia (Favaloro and Touzel, 1990).

EFFECTS OF HOSPITALIZATION ON THE CHILD

Children may react to the stresses of hospitalization before admission, during hospitalization, and after discharge. A child's conception of illness is even more important than age and intellectual maturity in predicting the level of adjustment before hospitalization (Carson, Gravley, and Council, 1992). Although age and intellectual ability are strongly related to children's concepts of illness, research indicates that regardless of the duration of a child's medical condition, total hospitalization days, and more life-threatening medical condition, he or she may not have more sophisticated illness concepts (Kury and Rodrigue, 1995). Therefore nurses should avoid overestimating the illness concepts of children with prior medical experience.

POSTHOSPITAL BEHAVIORS IN CHILDREN

Young Children

Some initial aloofness toward parents; may last from a few minutes (most common) to a few days

Frequently followed by dependency behaviors:
  Tendency to cling to parents
  Demand parents' attention
  Vigorously oppose any separation (e.g., staying at preschool or with a baby-sitter)

Other negative behaviors include the following:
  New fears (e.g., nightmares)
  Resistance to going to bed, night waking
  Withdrawal and shyness
  Hyperactivity
  Temper tantrums
  Food finickiness
  Attachment to blanket or toy
  Regression in newly learned skills (e.g., self-toileting)

Older Children

Negative behaviors include the following:
  Emotional coldness, followed by intense, demanding dependence on parents
  Anger toward parents
  Jealousy toward others (e.g., siblings)

Many children, especially those under 4 years of age, demonstrate temporary behavioral changes after discharge (see box on p. 616). These changes are a result of (1) separation from significant people, (2) a lack of opportunity to form new attachments, and (3) a strange environment.

Individual Risk Factors

A number of risk factors make certain children more vulnerable than others to the stresses of hospitalization (see box below). It has also been noted that rural children exhibit significantly greater degrees of psychologic upset than urban children, possibly because urban children have opportunities to become familiar with a local hospital (Gillis, 1990). Perhaps because separation is such an important issue surrounding hospitalization for young children, children who are active and strong willed tend to fare better when hospitalized than youngsters who are passive. Consequently, nurses should be alert to children who passively accept all changes and requests; these children may need more support than the "oppositional" child.

The development of subsequent long-term emotional disturbance may be related to the *length* and *number* of hospital admissions and the type of hospital practices. A single hospitalization of 4 weeks or more and repeated hospital admissions have been associated with later disturbances. However, supportive practices, such as frequent family visiting, may lessen the detrimental effects of such admissions.

Changes in the Pediatric Population.   The pediatric population in hospitals today has changed dramatically over the last two decades. A greater percentage of the children hospitalized today have more serious and complex problems than those hospitalized in the past. Many of these children are fragile newborns and children with severe injuries or disabilities who survived because of incredible technologic advances, yet were left with chronic or disabling conditions that require frequent and lengthy hospital stays. Research suggests that prior experience and familiarity with medical events related to hospitalization do not reduce fears in children (Hart and Bossert, 1994). Rather, prior experience may simply replace fear of the unknown with fear of the known. The nature of their conditions increases the likelihood that they will experience more invasive and traumatic procedures while they are hospitalized. These factors make them more vulnerable to the emotional consequences of hospitalization and result in their needs being significantly different from those of the short-term patients of the past (see Chapter 18 for further discussion on children with special needs). The majority of these children are infants and toddlers, the age-group most vulnerable to the effects of hospitalization.

RISK FACTORS THAT INCREASE CHILDREN'S VULNERABILITY TO THE STRESSES OF HOSPITALIZATION

"Difficult" temperament
Lack of fit between child and parent
Age (especially between 6 months and 5 years)
Male gender
Below-average intelligence
Multiple and continuing stresses (e.g., frequent hospitalizations)

Concern in recent years has focused on the increasing numbers of these children "growing up in hospitals" (Britton and Johnston, 1993). Discharge is prolonged because of complex medical and nursing care, elusive diagnoses, complicated psychosocial issues, and inconsistent community resources (Wells and others, 1994). Without special attention devoted to meeting the child's psychosocial and developmental needs in the "artificial" hospital environment, the detrimental consequences of prolonged hospitalization may be severe.

Beneficial Effects of Hospitalization

Although hospitalization can be and usually is stressful for children, it can also be beneficial. The most obvious benefit is the recovery from illness, but hospitalization also can present an opportunity for children to master stress and feel competent in their coping abilities. The hospital environment can provide children with new socialization experiences that can broaden their interpersonal relationships. Sciarillo (1995) suggests that a simple paradigm shift—from "promoting adaptation" to "participating in growth"—can be strategic in changing how individuals view illness and hospitalization. By viewing these events as challenges rather than as problems, children, families, and health care professionals are presented with an opportunity for growing in new ways. The psychologic benefits need to be considered and maximized during hospitalization. Appropriate nursing strategies to achieve this goal are presented on p. 648.

NURSING CARE OF THE CHILD WHO IS HOSPITALIZED

❖ Assessment

A number of important areas must be assessed to identify nursing diagnoses and plan care for an individual child. In some instances, such as with elective admission, assessment begins even before the child is hospitalized so that appropriate preadmission preparation can be instituted. At other times, assessment occurs at the time of admission and should be integrated into other admission procedures so that the child's specific needs are recognized *early* in the hospitalization. Another critical area is assessment of pain for implementing appropriate relief of discomfort. Although assessment is discussed under nursing care of the child who is hospitalized, a comprehensive approach must involve the child's parents or other caregivers.

The nurse's primary intent is to provide *atraumatic care* (see Chapter 1). Therefore patient assessment should be individualized and include an evaluation of the child's growth and development, psychosocial needs, educational needs, and the effects of the illness on the child's family or guardian.

Admission Assessment

A nursing admission history should be taken to ensure a systematic collection of data about the child and family that allows the nurse to plan individualized care. The nursing admission history presented in the box on pp. 618-619 is organized according to the Functional Health Patterns outlined by Gordon (1994, 1995) (see Nursing Diagnosis, Chapter 2) to facilitate the formulation of nursing diagnoses.

NURSING ADMISSION HISTORY ACCORDING TO FUNCTIONAL HEALTH PATTERNS*

Health Perception–Health Management Pattern

Why has your child been admitted?

How has your child's general health been?

What does your child know about this hospitalization?

　Ask the child why he or she came to the hospital.

　If answer is "For an operation or for tests," ask the child to tell you about what will happen before, during, and after the operation or tests.

Has your child ever been in the hospital before?

　How was that hospital experience?

　What things were important to you and your child during that hospitalization? How can we be most helpful now?

What medications does your child take at home?

　Why are they given?

　When are they given?

　How are they given (if a liquid, with a spoon; if a tablet, swallowed with water; or other)?

　Does your child have any trouble taking medication? If so, what helps?

　Is your child allergic to any medications?

What, if any, forms of complementary medicine practices are being used?

Nutrition-Metabolic Pattern

What are the family's usual mealtimes?

Do family members eat together or at separate times?

What are your child's favorite foods, beverages, and snacks?

　Average amounts consumed or usual size of portions

　Special cultural practices, such as family eats only ethnic food

What foods and beverages does your child *dislike*?

What are your child's feeding habits (bottle, cup, spoon, eats by self, needs assistance, any special devices)?

How does your child like the food served (warmed, cold, one item at a time)?

How would you describe your child's usual appetite (hearty eater, picky eater)?

　Has being sick affected your child's appetite? In what ways?

Are there any known or suspected food allergies?

Is your child on a special diet?

Are there any feeding problems (excessive fussiness, spitting up, colic); any dental or gum problems that affect feeding?

What do you do for these problems?

Elimination Pattern

What are your child's toilet habits (diaper, toilet trained—day only or day and night, use of word to communicate urination or defecation, potty chair, regular toilet, other routines)?

What is your child's usual pattern of elimination (bowel movements)?

Do you have any concerns about elimination (bed-wetting, constipation, diarrhea)?

What do you do for these problems?

Have you ever noticed that your child sweats a lot?

Sleep-Rest Pattern

What is your child's usual hour of sleep and awakening?

What is your child's schedule for naps; length of naps?

Is there a special routine before sleeping (bottle, drink of water, bedtime story, nightlight, favorite blanket or toy, prayers)?

Is there a special routine during sleep time, such as waking to go to the bathroom?

What type of bed does your child sleep in?

Does your child have a separate room or share a room; if shares, with whom?

What are the home sleeping arrangements (alone or with others, e.g., sibling, parent, other person)?

What is your child's favorite sleeping position?

Are there any sleeping problems (falling asleep, waking during night, nightmares, sleep walking)?

Are there any problems in awakening and getting ready in the morning?

What do you do for these problems?

Activity-Exercise Pattern

What is your child's schedule during the day (preschool, daycare center, regular school, extracurricular activities)?

What are your child's favorite activities or toys (both active and quiet interests)?

What is your child's usual television-viewing schedule at home?

　What are your child's favorite programs?

　Are there any TV restrictions?

Does your child have any illness or disabilities that limit activity? If so, how?

What are your child's usual habits and schedule for bathing (bath in tub or shower, sponge bath, shampoo)?

What are your child's dental habits (brushing, flossing, fluoride supplements or rinses, favorite toothpaste); schedule of daily dental care?

Does your child need help with dressing or grooming, such as hair combing?

Are there any problems with the above (dislike of or refusal to bathe, shampoo hair, or brush teeth)?

What do you do for these problems?

Are there special devices that your child requires help in managing (eyeglasses, contact lenses, hearing aid, orthodontic appliances, artificial elimination appliances, orthopedic devices)?

NOTE: Use the following code to assess functional self-care level for feeding, bathing/hygiene, dressing/grooming, toileting:

　O: Full self-care

　I: Requires use of equipment or device

　II: Requires assistance or supervision from another person

　III: Requires assistance or supervision from another person and equipment or device

　IV: Is dependent and does not participate

Cognitive-Perceptual Pattern

Does your child have any hearing difficulty?

　Does the child use a hearing aid?

　Have "tubes" been placed in your child's ears?

Does your child have any vision problems?

　Does the child wear glasses or contact lenses?

Does your child have any learning difficulties?

　What is the child's grade in school?

For information on pain, see box on p. 623.

Self-Perception–Self-Concept Pattern

How would you describe your child (e.g., takes time to adjust, settles in easily, shy, friendly, quiet, talkative, serious, playful, stubborn, easygoing)?

What makes your child angry, annoyed, anxious, or sad? What, helps?

How does your child act when annoyed or upset?

What have been your child's experiences with and reactions to temporary separation from you (parent)?

Does your child have any fears (places, objects, animals, people, situations)? How do you handle them?

Do you think your child's illness has changed the way he or she thinks about self (e.g., more shy, embarrassed about appearance, less competitive with friends, stays at home more)?

Role-Relationship Pattern

Does your child have a favorite nickname?

What are the names of other family members or others who live in the home (relatives, friends, pets)?

*The focus of the admission history is the child's psychosocial environment. Most of the questions are worded in terms of parental responses. Depending on the child's age, they should be addressed directly to the child when appropriate.

NURSING ADMISSION HISTORY ACCORDING TO FUNCTIONAL HEALTH PATTERNS—cont'd

Who usually takes care of your child during the day/night (especially if other than parent, such as baby-sitter, relative)?

What are the parents' occupations and work schedules?

Are there any special family considerations (adoption, foster child, stepparent, divorce, single parent)?

Have any major changes in the family occurred lately (death, divorce, separation, birth of a sibling, loss of a job, financial strain, mother beginning a career, other)? Describe child's reaction.

Who are your child's play companions or social groups (peers, younger or older children, adults, prefers to be alone)?

Do things generally go well for your child in school or with friends?

Does your child have "security" objects at home (pacifier, bottle, blanket, stuffed animal or doll)? Did you bring any of these to the hospital?

How do you handle discipline problems at home? Are these methods always effective?

Does your child have any condition that interferes with communication? If so, what are your suggestions for communicating with your child?

Will your child's hospitalization affect the family's financial support or care of other family members (e.g., other children)?

What concerns do you have about your child's illness and hospitalization?

Who will be staying with your child while hospitalized?

How can we contact you or another close family member outside of the hospital?

Sexuality-Reproductive Pattern

(Answer questions that apply to your child's age-group.)

Has your child begun puberty (developing physical sexual characteristics, menstruation)? Have you or your child had any concerns?

Does your daughter know how to do breast self-examination?

Does your son know how to do testicular self-examination?

How have you approached topics of sexuality with your child?

Do you feel you might need some help with some topics?

Has your child's illness affected the way he or she feels about being a boy or a girl? If so, how?

Do you have any concerns with behaviors in your child, such as masturbation, asking many questions or talking about sex, not respecting others' privacy, or wanting too much privacy?

Initiate a conversation about an adolescent's sexual concerns with open-ended to more direct questions and using the terms "friends" or "partners" rather than "girlfriend" or "boyfriend":

Tell me about your social life.

Who are your closest friends? (If one friend is identified, could ask more about that relationship, such as how much time they spend together, how serious they are about each other, if the relationship is going the way the teenager hoped.)

Might ask about dating and sexual issues, such as the teenager's views on sexuality education, "going steady," "living together," or premarital sex.

Which friends would you like to have visit in the hospital?

Coping–Stress Tolerance Pattern

(Answer questions that apply to your child's age-group.)

What does your child do when tired or upset?

If upset, does your child want a special person or object?

If so, explain.

If your child has temper tantrums, what causes them and how do you handle them?

Whom does your child talk to when worried about something?

How does your child usually handle problems or disappointments?

Have there been any big changes or problems in your family recently? If so, how have you handled them?

Has your child ever had a problem with drugs or alcohol or tried suicide?

Do you think your child is "accident prone"? If so, explain.

Value-Belief Pattern

What is your religion?

How is religion or faith important in your child's life?

What religious practices would you like continued in the hospital (e.g., prayers before meals/bedtime; visit by minister, priest, or rabbi; prayer group)?

One of the main purposes of the history is to assess the child's usual health habits at home to promote a more normal environment in the hospital. Therefore questions related to activities of daily living in the nutritional-metabolic, elimination, sleep-rest, and activity-exercise patterns are a major part of the assessment.

The questions found under the health perception–health management pattern are directed toward evaluation of the child's preparation for hospitalization and are key factors in determining if additional preparation is needed. The questions included in the self-perception–self-concept and role-relationship patterns offer insight into the child's potential reaction to hospitalization, especially in terms of separation. The nurse should also inquire about the use of any complementary medicine practices (see box). In a national survey, more than a third of adults had used at least one unconventional therapy within the previous year, yet 72% did not inform their medical doctor that they had done so (Eisenberg and others, 1993). It is reasonable to expect that many of these adults have children who also use complementary medicine practices (see Critical Thinking Exercise on p. 620).

Once the data are collected, the information must be applied to the nursing process and communicated to other staff. It makes little sense to assess a child's home routine if none

COMPLEMENTARY MEDICINE PRACTICES AND EXAMPLES

Nutrition, diet, and life-style/behavioral health changes— Macrobiotics, megavitamins, diets, life-style modification, health risk reduction/health education, wellness

Mind/body control therapies— Biofeedback, relaxation, prayer therapy, guided imagery, hypnotherapy, music/sound therapy, aromatherapy, education therapy

Traditional and ethnomedicine therapies— Acupuncture, ayurvedic medicine, herbal medicine, homeopathic medicine, Native-American medicine, natural products, traditional Oriental medicine

Structural manipulation and energetic therapies— Acupressure, chiropractic medicine, massage, reflexology, rolfing, therapeutic touch, QI Gong

Pharmacologic and biologic therapies— Antioxidants, cell treatment, chelation therapy, metabolic therapy, oxidizing agents

Bioelectromagnetic therapies— Diagnostic and therapeutic application of electromagnetic fields (e.g., transcranial electrostimulation, neuromagnetic stimulation, electroacupuncture)

CRITICAL **THINKING EXERCISE**
Complementary Medicine Practices

Maria, a 10-year-old Hispanic female, has had severe nose-bleeds. She is admitted to the hospital for a complete workup in an attempt to determine the cause. Her parents and grandparents have gathered around her bed. When you enter her room to begin admitting procedures, you notice an unusual scent. Maria's mother is rubbing the contents from an unfamiliar bottle of liquid on Maria. Meanwhile, the grandmother is rubbing Maria's head. She is startled at your entry and drops something on the floor near your feet. You bend over to pick it up and discover that it is a penny. After introducing yourself and explaining the purpose of your visit, your most appropriate response would be which of the following?

1. "Here is your penny."
2. "I need to take this bottle and have the lab examine its contents."
3. "Many families tell me that they use certain medicine practices that are traditional in their families. Can you tell me about yours?"
4. "What is going on here?"

The correct answer is three. The third-person technique (see Chapter 6) gives families permission to share information. What you have probably observed is Santeria, the African-Caribbean religion that was brought to the New World by slaves from West Africa. Although it is common among immigrants from Cuba, Puerto Rico, Brazil, and Santo Domingo, it is believed that a majority of Latin immigrants will have contact with Santeria sometime in their lives. Answer one avoids the issue, which could be very important. Although at some point you may need to have the contents of the bottle examined (answer two), it is an inappropriate initial response. Answer four is confrontive and disrespectful.

---

of this knowledge is integrated into the plan of care. Most nursing units have provisions for care plans in which specific information about the child's habits and needs are recorded and incorporated in the hospital routine.

Besides taking the nursing admission history, nurses should also perform a physical assessment (see Chapter 7) or obtain the information from the medical examination before planning care. At the very least, the nurse's physical assessment of the child should include observation of the body for any bruises, rashes, signs of neglect, deformities, or physical limitations. The nurse should also listen to the heart and lungs to assess overall physical status. For example, it is impossible to evaluate improvement in respiratory function in a child admitted with pulmonary disease unless there are baseline data with which to compare subsequent findings.

Pain Assessment

Pain assessment is a critical component of the nursing process. Unfortunately, health professionals, including nurses, tend to underestimate pain in children (see Thinking Critically About . . . box). One of the reasons for inadequate management of pain is a lack of understanding of what pain

---

For additional information, please view "Pain Assessment and Management" in Whaley and Wong's Pediatric Nursing Video Series, St Louis, 1996, Mosby; (800) 426-4545.

---

is—a personal phenomenon that *cannot* be experienced by any other individual. Therefore defining pain in terms of another's perceptions is inappropriate and inaccurate. An operational definition that is useful in clinical practice follows: *pain is whatever the experiencing person says it is, existing whenever the person says it does* (McCaffery and Beebe, 1989). This definition implies a very important attitude toward patients—*that they are believed.* It includes both verbal and nonverbal expressions of pain.

Fallacies and Facts. Children are undertreated for pain for a number of complex and interrelated reasons, including professionals' misconceptions about pain; the complexities of pain assessment, particularly in nonverbal children; and the lack of information regarding currently available pain reduction techniques. A number of fallacies continue to flourish because of incorrect knowledge about pain in infants and children, despite these fallacies having been disproved by current research on pediatric pain (see box on p. 622).

Fear of Addiction. A major concern that prevents health professionals from adequately using opioids* to relieve pain is an unwarranted fear of addiction. Studies on addiction rates in patients treated with opioids have found an incidence of less than 1% (Friedman, 1990). The Acute Pain Management Guideline Panel (1992) has made the following statement regarding addiction from opioid use in pain management for children: *There is no known aspect of childhood development or physiology that indicates any increased risk of physiologic or psychologic dependence from the brief use of opioids for acute pain management.*

One of the reasons for the unfounded and prevalent fear regarding addiction is confusion among three terms: narcotic addiction, drug tolerance, and physical dependency. Health professionals erroneously equate all three terms with addiction, when in reality these terms reflect completely different behavioral and physiologic actions:

Narcotic addiction—*Behavioral, voluntary* pattern characterized by compulsive drug-seeking behavior leading to overwhelming involvement with use and procurement of drug for purposes other than such medical reasons as pain relief
Drug tolerance—*Physiologic, involuntary* need for larger dose of opioid to maintain original analgesic effect
Physical dependence—*Physiologic, involuntary* effect manifested by withdrawal symptoms when chronic use of opioid is abruptly discontinued or opioid antagonist, such as naloxone (Narcan), is administered

Fear of Respiratory Depression. Although respiratory depression is the most serious side effect of opioids, it is a rare occurrence in children receiving appropriate doses. Evidence suggests that in children over 3 to 6 months of age, opioids cause no greater respiratory depression than in adults. Respiratory depression is most likely to occur when the opioid is administered with other sedating drugs, such as hydroxyzine (Vistaril), promethazine (Phenergan), chlorpromazine (Thorazine), midazolam (Versed), or diazepam (Valium). Unlike many sedatives, opioids have the advantage of the antidote naloxone (Narcan), which rapidly reverses the

---

*The term *opioid* refers to natural or synthetic analgesics with morphine-like actions. It is preferred to the term *narcotic,* which in a legal context refers to any substance that causes psychologic dependence, such as cocaine, which is not an opioid. The word "narcotic" also engenders fears of addiction in older children and parents that are unwarranted when opioids are used for pain control.

THINKING CRITICALLY ABOUT . . .
Undermedication of Pain in Children

Several studies have examined the pattern of pain medication for children as compared with adults and have found remarkably consistent findings—that children have been undermedicated for pain. Eland and Anderson (1977) investigated the incidence of administration of analgesics to 25 hospitalized children for postoperative pain. Twelve of the children received a total of 24 doses of analgesics; the remaining 13 children were never given any medication for pain relief. In contrast, 18 adults with identical diagnoses received 372 opioid analgesic doses and 299 nonopioid analgesic doses for a total of 671 doses. One of the saddest findings was that more than twice as many children had pain medication ordered as received it. This lack of response to the need for pain medication directly relates to the nurses who failed to administer the analgesic.

Another study investigating analgesic prescriptions given to children and adults after open heart surgery found that all the adults received medication, for a total of 564 doses, but only three-fourths the children were given medication, for a total of 237 doses during the first 3 postoperative days. This difference was even greater on the fifth postoperative day, when 83% of the adults continued to receive analgesics (a total of 136 doses) but only 12% of the children were medicated (a total of 10 doses) (Beyer and others, 1983).

Another study on postoperative pain found that 75% of the children reported pain on the day of surgery, and if orders for opioid or nonopioid analgesics were written, the nonopioid was given exclusively. In addition, the doses ordered were usually too small and/or too infrequent to be maximally effective. Most orders were written "PRN," which was often interpreted by nursing staff to mean "as little as possible" (Mather and Mackie, 1983).

A review of analgesic use in the emergency department reported significantly low use in children with mild to moderate trauma, including children with painful fractures. Head injury was associated with especially low use of analgesics (Friedland and Kulick, 1994).

The situation is even more serious with infants. One analysis of anesthetic practices with newborns undergoing surgical ligation of patent ductus arteriosus found that 76% of the infants received only nitrous oxide and a paralyzing agent. These infants could not move during surgery but could feel all the pain of a thoracotomy.

(Anand and Aynsley-Green, 1985). In a survey of nurses working in neonatal intensive care units, 79% believed that infants were undermedicated for pain. The same study found that more than half the medications used for pain relief had no analgesic properties (Franck, 1987). A study comparing premedication for procedures, such as arterial line or chest tube placement, found that infants in neonatal intensive care units received no premedication much more often than children in pediatric intensive care units (Bauchner, May, and Coates, 1992).

Fortunately, professionals' response to recognizing and treating pediatric pain has been improving. Studies such as those described above have prompted the **American Academy of Pediatrics** (1987) and the **American Society of Anesthesiologists** to publish jointly a statement on neonatal anesthesia that encourages the use of local or systemic pharmacologic agents "according to the usual guidelines for the administration of anesthesia to high-risk, potentially unstable patients." If medication is withheld, the decision should be based on the same medical criteria used for older patients, not on the infant's age or perceived degree of cortical maturity.

Guidelines are also available that help practitioners to assess and manage pain using methods based on the published scientific literature. In the United States the **Agency for Health Care Policy and Research (AHCPR)** has published guidelines developed by pain experts that focus on the issues of postoperative, procedure-related or trauma, and cancer pain. Other national and international organizations have also contributed research-based recommendations that nurses can use to improve pain control (see box at the top of p. 622).

In your agency, see if these references are readily available to staff. If not, order them, especially the free AHCPR publications, and distribute them, stressing that they provide state-of-the-art information. As you practice, carry your copy of the guidelines; mark sections, such as those discussing addiction and listing drug dosages, for quick reference. Compare your pain assessment and management interventions with those in the published guidelines, and make a commitment to increase your knowledge. *Remember: to relieve pain effectively, its management must be based on scientific research, not personal opinion or belief.*

---

respiratory depressant effect. Fortunately, the benzodiazepines, such as diazepam and midazolam, have the drug flumazenil (Romazicon) to treat respiratory depression (see also p. 643).

In addition, as tolerance to the analgesic effect of opioids occurs, tolerance to the respiratory depressant effect also occurs. Pain acts as a natural antagonist to the respiratory depressant effect of opioids. With increased pain, a patient can receive increased doses of opioids without necessarily experiencing clinically significant respiratory depression. Respiratory depression is rare in children receiving long-term opioid therapy, since tolerance to the respiratory depression develops.

Principles of Pain Assessment in Children. Since pain is both a sensory and an emotional experience, several assessment strategies should be used to gather information about pain. One approach to pain assessment in children is QUESTT:

Question the child.
Use pain rating scales.

Evaluate behavior and physiologic changes.
Secure parents' involvement.
Take cause of pain into account.
Take action and evaluate results.

Question Child. Children's verbal statements and descriptions of pain are the *most* important factors in assessing pain. However, young children may not know what the word "pain" means and may need help in describing it using familiar language. Therefore using a variety of words to describe pain, such as "owie," "boo-boo," "feel funny," or "hurt," is necessary. The nurse also should use appropriate foreign language words; for example, in Spanish, pain is "duele," "dolor," or "ai ai." Older children benefit from using simple words to describe pain. Suggested questions for obtaining information about children's experiences with pain are presented in the box on p. 623. Asking children to locate the pain is also helpful, and play can provide other means for helping children to reveal discomfort.

Acute Pain Management: Operative or Medical Procedures and Trauma

Acute Pain Management in Infants, Children and Adolescents; Operative and Medical Procedures

Management of Cancer Pain

Quick Reference Guide for Clinicians: Management of Cancer Pain: Adults

Available at no charge from the Agency for Health Care Policy and Research Publications, P.O. Box 8527, Silver Spring, MD 20907; (800) 358-9295.

Principles of Analgesic Use in the Treatment of Acute Pain and Chronic Cancer Pain

Available from the American Pain Society, 4700 West Lake Ave., Glenview, IL 60025; (847) 375-4700.

Management of Acute Pain: A Practical Guide

Available from the International Association for the Study of Pain (IASP), 909 N.E. 43rd St., Suite 306, Seattle, WA 98105-6020; (206) 547-6409.

Handbook of Cancer Pain Management

Available from the Wisconsin Cancer Pain Initiative, 3675 Medical Sciences Center, University of Wisconsin Medical School, 1300 University Ave., Madison, WI 53706; (608) 262-0978.

Report of the Consensus Conference on the Management of Pain in Childhood Cancer

In *Pediatrics* 86(5, suppl):813-834, 1990; available from the American Academy of Pediatrics, P.O. Box 927, Elk Grove Village, IL 60009-0927; (800) 433-9016.

Guidelines for Standard of Care of Acute Painful Episodes in Patients with Sickle Cell Disease

Available from Samir K. Ballas, MD, Cardeza Foundation, 1015 Walnut St., Philadelphia, PA 19107.

Clinical Reference Guide for Health Care Providers

Sickle Cell Related Pain: Assessment and Management Conference Proceedings

Available from the New England Regional Genetics Group (NERGG), P.O. Box 670, Mt. Desert, ME 04660; (207) 288-2704; FAX (207) 288-2705.

ANA Position Statements on Promotion of Comfort and Relief of Pain in Dying Patients and on the Role of the Registered Nurse in the Management of Patients Receiving IV Conscious Sedation for Short-Term Therapeutic, Diagnostic, or Surgical Procedures

Published in *The American Nurse,* Feb 1992, pp 7-8. May be available from American Nurses' Association Publications Distribution Center, P.O. Box 4100, Kearneysville, WV 25430; (800) 637-0323.

Oncology Nursing Society position paper on cancer pain

By Spross JA, McGuire DB: *Oncol Nurs Forum* 17(5):753, 1990.

Mayday Pain Resource Center

From City of Hope National Medical Center, Nursing Research and Education/Mayday Pain Resource Center, 1500 East Duarte Rd., Duarte, CA 91010; (818) 359-8111, ext. 3829; FAX (818) 301-8941.

Whaley and Wong's Pediatric Pain Assessment and Management

Videotape available from Mosby, 11830 Westline Industrial Dr., St. Louis, MO 63146; (800) 426-4545.

ALSO AVAILABLE FOR FAMILIES:

Pain Control After Surgery: A Patient's Guide

Managing cancer pain: patient guide

Available at no charge from the Agency for Health Care Policy and Research Publications, P.O. Box 8527, Silver Spring, MD 20907; (800) 358-9295.

Children's Cancer Pain Can Be Relieved: A Guide for Parents and Families

Available from Wisconsin Cancer Pain Initiative, 3675 Medical Sciences Center, University of Wisconsin Medical School, 1300 University Ave., Madison, WI 53706; (608) 262-0978.

Pain Relief: How to Say No to Acute, Chronic, and Cancer Pain!

By Jane Cowles, 1993; available from MasterMedia Limited, 17 E. 89th St., New York, NY 10128; (212) 546-7650.

Questions and Answers About Pain Control: A Guide for People with Cancer and Their Families

Available at no charge from the Office of Cancer Communications, Bldg. 31, Rm. 10A24, Bethesda, MD 20892, (800) 4-CANCER; and from local branches of the American Cancer Society, or call (800) ACS-2345.

Sickle Cell Related Pain: Assessment and Management—A Guide for Patients and Parents

Available from the New England Regional Genetics Groups (NERGG), P.O. Box 670, Mt. Desert, ME 04660; (207) 288-2704; FAX (207) 288-2705.

Fallacy: Infants do not feel pain.

Fact: Infants demonstrate behavioral, especially facial, and physiologic, including hormonal, indicators of pain. Neonates have the neural mechanisms to transmit noxious stimuli by 20 weeks of gestation. (See also Neonatal Pain, Chapter 9.)

Fallacy: Children tolerate pain better than adults.

Fact: Children's tolerance for pain actually *increases* with age. Younger children tend to rate procedure-related pain higher than older children.

Fallacy: Children cannot tell you where they hurt.

Fact: By 4 years of age, children can accurately point to the body area or mark the painful site on a drawing; children as young as 3 years old can use pain scales, such as faces.

Fallacy: Children always tell the truth about pain.

Fact: Children may not admit having pain to avoid an injection; because of constant pain, they may not realize how much they are hurting; children may believe that others know how they are feeling and not ask for analgesia.

Fallacy: Children become accustomed to pain or painful procedures.

Fact: Children often demonstrate *increased* behavioral signs of discomfort with repeated painful procedures.

Fallacy: Behavioral manifestations reflect pain intensity.

Fact: Children's developmental level, coping abilities, and temperament, such as activity level and intensity of reaction to pain, influence pain behavior. Children with more active, resisting behaviors may rate pain lower than children with passive, accepting behaviors.

Fallacy: Parents do not want to be involved in their child's pain control.

Fact: Parents *do* want to be involved. They know their child best and can help in assessing pain and pain relief measures. Since they may not have seen their child in severe pain, they may need guidance in interpreting pain responses.

Fallacy: Narcotics are more dangerous for children than they are for adults.

Fact: Narcotics (opioids) are no more dangerous for children than they are for adults. Addiction to opioids used to treat pain is extremely rare in children. Reports of respiratory depression in children are also uncommon. By 3 to 6 months of age, healthy infants can metabolize opioids similarly to older children.

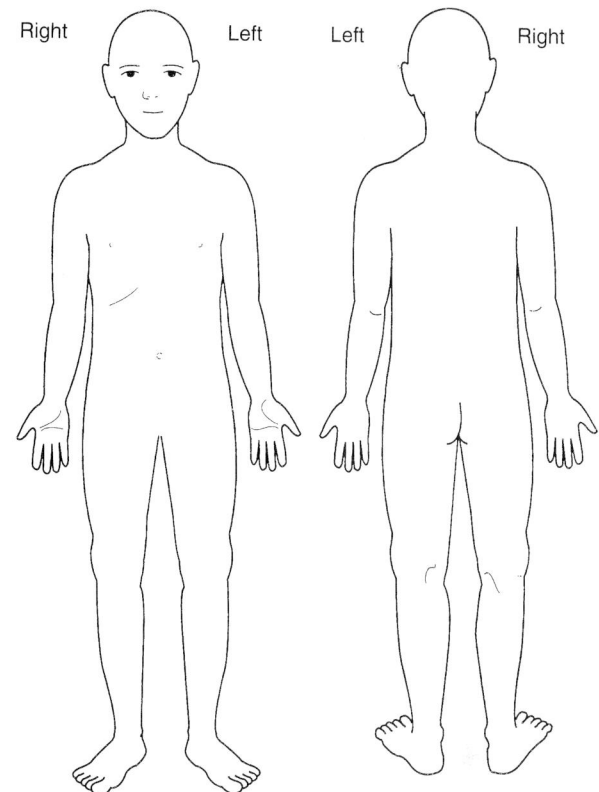

FIG. 21-4. Adolescent pediatric pain tool (APPT): body outlines for pain assessment. Instructions: "Color in the areas on these drawings to show where you have pain. Make the marks as big or as small as the place where the pain is." (From Savedra MC, Tesler MD, Holzemer WL, and Ward JA, School of Nursing, University of California–San Francisco, San Francisco, CA. Copyright ©1989, 1992.)

NURSING TIPS

Ask child to point to where it hurts or to "where Mommy or Daddy would put a Band-Aid."
Have child mark or color the painful area on a drawing of a human figure (Fig. 21-4).
Ask child to tell how a puppet, doll, or stuffed animal is feeling or to point out areas on these models that "hurt" or "don't feel good."

When asking children about pain, the nurse must remember that they may deny pain because they fear receiving an injectable analgesic or because they believe they deserve to suffer as punishment for some misdeed. They may also deny pain to a stranger but readily admit it to a parent. This behavior should not be interpreted as seeking attention from the parent, but as a valid indication of pain.

Use a Pain Rating Scale. Pain rating scales (tools) provide a quantitative self-reporting measure of pain. Although various pain scales exist (Table 21-2), not all of them are appropriate for young children. For the most valid and reliable pain intensity rating, a scale is selected that is suitable to the child's age, abilities, and preference. Scales using facial expressions are readily accepted by children and can be used by very young children. Some evidence indicates that children may prefer a faces scale to other tools (West and others, 1994; Wong and Baker, 1988).

It is best to use the same scale with children to avoid confusing them with different instructions and to use the pain assessment scale for pain only. Multiple uses of the scale (e.g., as a general measure of the child's feelings) can cause the child to lose interest in the scale. In introducing the pain scale, nurses should explain that this is one way for children to let nurses know how they are feeling. Ideally, children should be taught to use the scale before pain is expected, such as preoperatively. Familiarizing children with the scale facilitates its use when children are actually in pain.

Evaluate Behavioral and Physiologic Changes. Behavioral changes are common indicators of pain and are especially valuable in assessing pain in nonverbal children. Children's behavioral responses to pain change with age and follow a developmental trend (see box on p. 613). However, children vary widely in their responses and may exhibit behaviors at one age that are more typically seen at a different age. In addition, temperament affects coping style, and children with more positive moods may appear to be in less pain than they actually are. Children who use passive coping behaviors (offering no resistance, cooperating) may rate pain as more intense than children who use active coping behaviors (resisting, attacking) (Broome and others, 1990). Cultural background may also play a role in children's pain responses, although the influence appears slight (Pfefferbaum, Adams, and Aceves, 1990). Unfortunately, nurses often make judgments about pain based on behavior, which results in some children receiving inadequate pain medication (Wallace, 1989). (See also Critical Thinking Exercise on p. 626.)

TABLE 21-2. Pain rating scales for children

PAIN SCALE/ DESCRIPTION	INSTRUCTIONS	RECOMMENDED AGE/COMMENTS
FACES Pain Rating Scale* (Wong and Baker, 1988, Wong 1996): Consists of six cartoon faces ranging from smiling face for "no pain" to tearful face for "worst pain"	Explain to child that each face is for a person who feels happy because there is no pain (hurt) or sad because there is some or a lot of pain. FACE 0 is very happy because there is no hurt. FACE 1 hurts just a little bit. FACE 2 hurts a little more. FACE 3 hurts even more. FACE 4 hurts a whole lot, but FACE 5 hurts as much as you can imagine, although you don't have to be crying to feel this bad. Ask child to choose face that best describes own pain. Record the number under chosen face on pain assessment record.	Children as young as 3 years Using same instructions without affect words, such as *happy* or *sad*, results in same pain rating, probably reflecting child's rating of pain intensity.

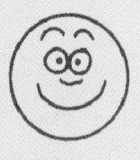 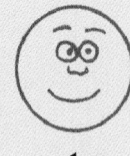 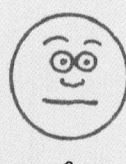 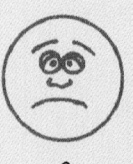 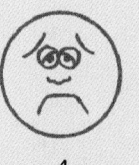 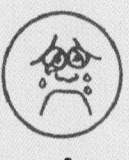

| 0 | 1 | 2 | 3 | 4 | 5 |

PAIN SCALE/ DESCRIPTION	INSTRUCTIONS	RECOMMENDED AGE/COMMENTS
Oucher† (Beyer and others, 1995): Consists of six photographs of child's face representing "no hurt" to "biggest hurt you could ever have"; also includes a vertical scale with numbers from 0 to 100; scales for black and Hispanic children have been developed (Villarruel and Denyes, 1991)	*Numeric scale* Point to each section of scale to explain variations in pain intensity: "0 means no hurt." "This means little hurts" (pointing to lower part of scale, 1 to 29). "This means middle hurts" (pointing to middle part of scale, 30 to 69). "This means big hurts" (pointing to upper part of scale, 70 to 99). "100 means the biggest hurt you could ever have." Score is actual number stated by child. *Photographic scale* Point to each photograph on Oucher and explain variations in pain intensity using following language: first picture from the bottom is "no hurt," second is "a little hurt," third is "a little more hurt," fourth is "even more hurt than that," fifth is "pretty much or a lot of hurt," and the sixth is the "biggest hurt you could ever have." Score pictures from 0 to 5, with the bottom picture scored as 0. *General* Practice using Oucher by recalling and rating previous pain experiences (e.g., falling off a bike). Child points to number or photograph that describes pain intensity associated with experience. Obtain current pain score from child by asking "How much hurt do you have right now?"	Children 3 to 13 years Use numeric scale if child can count to 100 by ones and identify larger of any two numbers, or by tens. Determine whether child has cognitive ability to use photographic scale; child should be able to seriate six geometric shapes from largest to smallest. Determine which ethnic version of Oucher to use. Allow the child to select a version of Oucher, or use version that most closely matches physical characteristics of child.
Numeric Scale Uses straight line with end points identified as "no pain" and "worst pain"; divisions along line are marked in units from 0 to 10 (high number may vary)	Explain to child that at one end of the line is a 0, which means that a person feels no pain (hurt). At the other end is a 10, which means the person feels the worst pain imaginable. The numbers 1 to 9 are for a very little pain to a whole lot of pain. Ask child to choose a number that best describes own pain.	Children as young as 5 years, as long as they can count and have some concept of numbers and their values in relation to other numbers

*Several variations of faces scales exist. Wong-Baker FACES Pain Rating Scale is available from Purdue Frederick Co., 100 Connecticut Ave., Norwalk CT 06856; (203) 853-0123, ext. 7236. For translations of FACES and brief instructions, see Appendix H. *Reference manual for the Wong-Baker FACES Pain Rating Scale* is also available from the City of Hope National Medical Center, Nursing Research and Education/Mayday Pain Resource Center, 1500 East Duarte Rd., Duarte, CA 91010; (818) 359-8111 ext. 3829; FAX (818) 301-8941.

†Oucher is available from Association for the Care of Children's Health, 7910 Woodmont Ave., Suite 300, Bethesda, MD 20814; (301) 654-6549 or (800) 808-ACCH.

TABLE 21-2. Pain rating scales for children—cont'd

PAIN SCALE/ DESCRIPTION	INSTRUCTIONS	RECOMMENDED AGE/COMMENTS

Numeric Scale—cont'd

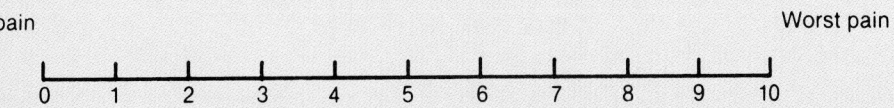

No pain   Worst pain

0 1 2 3 4 5 6 7 8 9 10

Poker Chip Tool*

Uses four red poker chips placed horizontally in front of child (Hester, Foster, and Kristensen, 1990)

Tell child, "These are pieces of hurt." Beginning at the chip nearest child's left side and ending at the one nearest child's right side, point to chips and say, "This [the first chip] is a little bit of hurt and this [the fourth chip] is the most hurt you could ever have." For a young child or for any child who does not comprehend the instructions, clarify by saying, "That means this [the first chip] is just a little hurt; this [the second chip] is a little more hurt; this [the third chip] is more hurt; and this [the fourth chip] is the most hurt you could ever have." Ask child, "How many pieces of hurt do you have right now?" Children without pain will say they don't have any. Clarify child's answer by words such as, "Oh, you have a little hurt? Tell me about the hurt." Elicit descriptors, location, and cause. Ask the child, "What would you like me to do for you?" Record number of chips selected.

Spanish instructions: Follow English instructions, substituting the following words. Tell parent, if present: "Estas fichas son una manera de medir dolor. Usamos cuatro fichas." Say to child: "Estas son pedazos de dolor: una es un poquito de dolor y cuatro son el dolor maximo que tu puedes sentir. Cuantos pedazos de dolor tienes?"

Children as young as 4 to 4½ years, provided they can count and have some concept of numbers

Word Graphic Rating Scale*†

(Tesler and others, 1991): Uses descriptive words (may vary in other scales) to denote varying intensities of pain

Explain to child, "This is a line with words to describe how much pain you may have. This side of the line means no pain and over here the line means worst possible pain." (Point with your finger where "no pain" is, and run your finger along the line to "worst possible pain," as you say it.) "If you have no pain, you would mark like this." (Show example.) "If you have some pain, you would mark somewhere along the line, depending on how much pain you have." (Show example.) "The more pain you have, the closer to worst pain you would mark. The worst pain possible is marked like this." (Show example.) "Show me how much pain you have right now by marking with a straight, up-and-down line anywhere along the line to show how much pain you have right now." With a millimeter rule, measure from the "no pain" end to the mark and record this measurement as the pain score.

Children 4 to 17 years

No
pain

Little
pain

Medium
pain

Large
pain

Worst
possible pain

*Instructions for Poker Chip Tool and Word Graphic Rating Scale from Acute Pain Management Guideline Panel: *Acute pain management in infants, children, and adolescents: operative and medical procedures; quick reference guide for clinicians,* ACHPR Pub No 92-0020, Rockville, MD, 1992, Agency for Health Care Policy and Research, Public Health Service, US Department of Health and Human Services. Poker Chip Tool developed in 1975 by Nancy O. Hester, University of Colorado Health Sciences Center, Denver, CO. Spanish instructions from Jordan-Marsh M and others: *The Harbor-UCLA Medical Center Humor Project for Children,* Los Angeles, 1990, Harbor-UCLA Medical Center.
†Word Graphic Rating Scale is part of the Adolescent Pediatric Pain Tool and is available from Pediatric Pain Study, University of California, School of Nursing, Department of Family Health Care Nursing, San Francisco, CA 94143-0606; (415) 476-4040.

Continued.

TABLE 21-2. Pain rating scales for children—cont'd

PAIN SCALE/ DESCRIPTION	INSTRUCTIONS	RECOMMENDED AGE/COMMENTS
Visual Analogue Scale Uses 10 cm horizontal line with end points marked "no pain" and "worst pain"	Ask child to place a mark on line that best describes amount of own pain. With a centimeter ruler, measure from the "no pain" end to the mark and record this measurement as the pain score.	Children as young as 4½ years Vertical or horizontal scale may be used.
Color Tool (Eland, 1993): Uses markers for child to construct own scale that is used with body outline	Present eight markers to child in a random order. Ask child, "Of these colors, which color is like . . .?" (the event identified by the child as having hurt the most). Place the marker (represents severe pain) away from the other markers. Ask child, "Which color is like a hurt, but not quite as much as . . .?" (the event identified by the child as having hurt the most). Place the marker with the marker chosen to represent severe pain. Ask child, "Which color is like something that hurts just a little?" Place the marker with the other colors. Ask child, "Which color is like no hurt at all?" Show the four marker choices to child in order from the worst to the no-hurt color. Ask child to show on the body outlines where they hurt, using the markers chosen. After child has colored the hurts, ask if they are current hurts or hurts from the past. Ask if child knows why the area hurts if it is not clear to you why it does.	Children as young as 4 years, provided they know their colors, are not color blind, and are able to construct the scale if in pain

> **Nursing ALERT** If children's behaviors appear to differ from their rating of pain, believe their pain rating.

CRITICAL THINKING EXERCISE
Pain Assessment

Stacy is 14 years old, and this is her second day after abdominal surgery. As you enter her room, she smiles at you and continues to talk and joke with her visitor. Stacy rates her pain a 4 on a scale of 0 to 5, no to worst pain, respectively. Her roommate, Jill, is 12 years old, and this is her third day after scoliosis surgery. She does not smile and is lying very still in bed. Jill rates her pain a 4 on the same scale. Based on your assessment, you write the following in their charts (choose two items):

1. Stacy: In no acute distress and appears comfortable, talking and joking with a visitor.
2. Jill: Rates her surgical pain a 4 on a 0 to 5 scale and is unable to move because of pain; she appears depressed.
3. Stacy: Rates her surgical pain a 4 on a 0 to 5 scale.
4. Jill: Rates her surgical pain a 4 on a 0 to 5 scale.

The correct answers are three and four. The best estimate of pain is the person's self-report. Responses one and two are based on subjective impressions. In response one the adolescent's report of pain is totally disregarded. In response two there is no assessment data to support that Jill's behavior indicates inability to move or depression.

Depending on the type and location of pain, children may display behaviors that indicate local body pain, such as pulling the ears for ear pain, rolling the head from side to side for head and ear pain, lying on the side with legs flexed for abdominal pain, limping for leg or foot pain, and refusing to move a body part. Children who experience chronic or repeated pain often develop effective behavioral coping strategies, such as squeezing a hand, talking, counting, relaxing, or thinking about pleasant events. Once these coping skills are identified, the child is encouraged to use them in future experiences with pain.

Physiologic responses indicating pain include flushing of the skin; increases in sweating, blood pressure, pulse, and respiration; restlessness; and dilation of the pupils. However, these signs vary considerably—for example, heart rate may actually decrease—and they may be produced by emotions such as fear, anger, or anxiety. They occur primarily in acute pain from stimulation of the sympathetic nervous system. If pain persists, the body begins to adapt and these responses decrease or stabilize. Consequently, if nurses rely primarily on observing these physiologic indications or expecting "pain" behaviors before believing that pain exists, many instances of pain will go unrecognized.

One of the most valuable clues to pain is a change in behavior and vital signs after administration of an analgesic. Behaviors such as less irritability or cessation of crying and decreased pulse, respirations, and blood pressure provide important evidence for pain existing before treatment. Often the

PAIN ASSESSMENT RECORD

Directions for each column:

1. Record date and time of administering analgesic; assess analgesic effect _____ minutes later and then _____ .

2. Use a pain rating scale if child understands its use. Name of scale _____ .

   Ratings: No pain = _____ . Worst pain = _____ . Acceptable pain rating _____ .

3. Record analgesic, dose, and route.

4. Record possible indications or effects of pain, such as shallow breathing due to incisional pain, parental request for pain relief; record indications or effects of pain relief, such as "moves easily, playing."

5. Record level of arousal using sedation scale in box. Also, record any other side effects (e.g., nausea, itching).

6. R = respiratory function. Record breaths per minute and/or other observations of respiratory status (e.g., depth of respiration, change in color of skin).

7. Signature or initials of person recording information.

SEDATION SCALE

S = Sleeping, easliy aroused.*

1 = Awake and alert.*

2 = Occasionally drowsy, easy to arouse.*

3 = Frequently drowsy, arousable, drifts off to sleep during conversation.†

4 = Somnolent, minimal or no response to stimuli.†

* Requires no action.

† Notify practitioner.

---

1 Date/ time	2 Pain rating	3 Analgesic	4 Possible effects/indications of pain or relief of pain	5 Arousal/ side-effects	6 R	7 Signature

FIG. 21-5. Pain assessment record.

change in vital signs is attributed to the depressant effect of opioids, when in reality the return to more normal physiologic functioning is due to pain relief.

Secure Parents' Involvement. Parents know their child, are sensitive to changes in their child's behavior, and typically want to be involved in their child's pain relief. Parents' ability to recognize pain in their children varies. Some parents may never have seen their child in severe pain and may equate certain responses, such as irritability or withdrawal, with discomfort. However, others are aware that certain behaviors signal pain because the child has acted similarly during previous painful events. In addition, parents usually know what comforts their child, such as rocking, stroking, or talking. They are the persons most consistently caring for the child and want to be involved in pain relief (Watt-Watson, Everden, and Lawson, 1990). Encouraging their participation gives them control and a sense of helping.

To better assess the child's pain, the nurse can interview the parents about their child's previous pain experiences (see box on p. 623). Ideally, this questioning should occur before the child is in pain, such as on admission to the hospital. Parents need to realize that their knowledge of their child is important in providing care. Parents sometimes leave the assessment of pain up to the nurse because "nurses are more experienced," and consequently parents do not report pain. Parents need to be taught nonverbal pain behaviors in children and encouraged to inform the staff when they occur.

Take Cause of Pain into Account. When children exhibit behaviors or other clues that suggest pain, reasons for discomfort should be investigated. Pathology may give clues to the expected intensity and type of pain. For example, pain associated with vaso-occlusive crises in sickle cell disease is severe. Pain caused by bone marrow puncture is typically greater than the discomfort associated with a venipuncture. However, it is a mistake to believe that certain conditions or procedures always produce a standard amount of pain. For example, sore throat pain may be mild or severe—only the child knows the intensity.

> **Nursing ALERT**
>
> A golden rule to follow in pain assessment is this: Whatever is painful to an adult is painful to an infant or child until proved otherwise.

Take Action and Evaluate Results. The reason for assessing pain is to relieve it (see p. 633). Total pain relief should be the goal, with the combined use of pharmacologic and nonpharmacologic interventions. However, complete relief may not be possible. When children are able, they can tell the nurse what level of pain is acceptable to them.

Regardless of the type of pain intervention, *evaluation of the results is essential.* No one pain reduction technique is effective for all children. Therefore a pain assessment record is used to monitor the effectiveness of the interventions (Fig. 21-5). With nonverbal children, behavioral and physiologic signs are evaluated for evidence of pain relief. With verbal children, their statements about pain relief and pain ratings are also recorded. Changes in the medication regimen are made as needed to provide the maximum pain relief with the minimum side effects. Family members are often excellent partners for keeping a pain assessment record for the nurse.

> **Nursing ALERT**
>
> Presenting practitioners with objective documentation of pain, rather than opinion, is more likely to lead to a favorable change in analgesic disorders (Walker and Wong, 1991).

❖ Nursing Diagnoses

A number of nursing diagnoses are prominent in the nursing care of children who are ill and/or hospitalized. Other nursing diagnoses specific to individual cases may become evident in addition to those outlined in the Nursing Care Plan on pp. 648-653.

❖ Planning

An effective plan of care for the child who is hospitalized is based on patient- and family-identified needs, as well as those identified by the nurse. Family members and the child should play active roles in developing the plan whenever possible.

The main goals for the child who is ill and/or hospitalized are as follows:

1. Child will be prepared for hospitalization.
2. Child will experience little or no separation.
3. Child will maintain a sense of control.
4. Child will exhibit decreased fear of bodily injury.
5. Child will experience a reduction of pain that is acceptable to child.
6. Child will have opportunities to participate in developmentally appropriate diversional activities.
7. Child will experience maximum benefits from hospitalization.

❖ Implementation

Prepare Child for Hospitalization

The rationale for preparing children for the hospital experience and related procedures is based on the principle that fear of the unknown (fantasy) exceeds fear of the known. Therefore decreasing the elements of the unknown results in less fear. When children do not have paralyzing fear to cope with, they are able to direct their energies toward dealing with the other, unavoidable stresses of hospitalization and to benefit optimally from the growth potential of the experience.

The preparation process may be elaborate, with tours, puppet shows, and playtime with miniature hospital equipment; it may involve the use of books (see p. 671) and/or films; or it may be limited to a brief description of the major aspects of any hospital stay. No firm consensus exists on the timing of the event. Some authorities recommend preparing children 4 to 7 years of age about 1 week in advance so they can assimilate the information and ask questions. For older children the time may be longer. However, for young children, who may begin to fantasize about what they observed, 1 or 2 days before admission is sufficient time for anticipatory preparation (Petrillo and Sanger, 1980). Children ages 5 to 12 years prefer to know about impending hospitalization from several weeks to a few minutes before the event. Because standardized programs cannot adequately meet the needs of the full age range of pediatric patients, some hospitals have developed preparation programs that target a specific age-group, such as toddlers or adolescents (Johnson, Jeppson, and Redburn, 1992). The length of the session should be suited to the children's attention span—the younger the child, the shorter the program. The optimum approach is one that is individualized for each child and family. Regardless of the specific type of program, all children, even those who have been hospitalized before, benefit from an introduction to the environment and routine of the unit.

> **FYI** In many hospitals, *child-life specialists,* health care professionals with extensive knowledge of child growth and development and of the special psychosocial needs of children who are hospitalized and their families, help prepare children for hospitalization, surgery, and procedures. A *collaborative effort* between the nurse, child-life specialist, and other members of the child's health care team helps ensure the best possible hospital experience for the child and family.

Hospital Admission.   The preparation that children require on the day of admission depends on the kind of prehospital counseling they have received. If they have been prepared in a formalized program, they will usually know what to expect in terms of initial medical procedures, inpatient facilities, and nursing staff. However, prehospital counseling does not preclude the need for support during procedures such as obtaining blood specimens, x-ray tests, or physical examination. For example, undressing young children before they feel comfortable in their new surroundings can be very upsetting. Causing needless anxiety and fear during admission may adversely affect the nurse's establishment of trust with these children. Therefore nursing assistance during the admission procedure is vital, regardless of how well prepared any child is for the experience of hospitalization. In addition, spending this time with the child gives the nurse an opportunity to evaluate the child's understanding of subsequent procedures (Fig. 21-6). Ideally, a primary nurse is assigned whenever possible to allow for individualized care and to provide a substitute support person for the child (see Chapter 1).

When a child is admitted, nurses follow several fairly universal admission procedures, which are outlined in the box. One particularly important decision is room assignment. The minimum considerations for room assignment are age, sex, and nature of the illness. Ideally, however, room selection should be based on a variety of developmental and psychobiologic needs. Determining compatible roommates, both for the children and for rooming-in parents, greatly influences the growth potential from the hospital experience.

No absolute rules govern room selection, but in general, placing children of the same age-group and with similar types of illness in the same room is both psychologically and medically advantageous. However, there are many exceptions. For example, a school-age child may thrive on the responsibility of caring for a younger child. A child in traction may be very therapeutic for another child confined to bed because of a serious illness. A child who is very independent despite physical disabilities may help another child with similar or different limitations, and the parents of the child with disabilities may achieve deeper insight and acceptance of their child's disorder.

Age-grouping is especially important for adolescents. Many hospitals make an effort to place teenagers on their own unit or in a separate designated section of the pediatric or general unit whenever possible.

Prevent or Minimize Separation

A primary nursing goal is to prevent separation, particularly in children under 5 years of age. Changes in hospitals' policies over recent years reflect a changed attitude toward parents; many hospitals no longer consider parents "visitors" and welcome their presence at all times throughout the child's hospitalization. Today most hospitals offer unrestricted visiting hours for parents on general pediatric units. Limitations

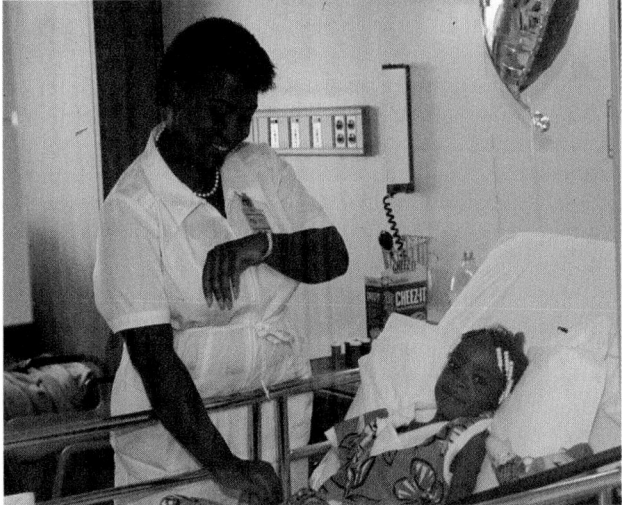

FIG. 21-6. The initial admission procedures give the nurse an opportunity to get to know the child and to assess the child's understanding of the hospital experience. (Courtesy St. Louis Children's Hospital.)

> **GUIDELINES FOR ADMISSION**
>
> **Preadmission**
>
> Assign a room based on developmental age, seriousness of diagnosis, communicability of illness, and projected length of stay.
>
> Prepare roommate(s) for the arrival of a new patient; when children are too young to benefit from this consideration, prepare parents.
>
> Prepare room for child and family, with admission forms and equipment nearby to eliminate need to leave child.
>
> **Admission**
>
> Introduce primary nurse to child and family.
>
> Orient child and family to inpatient facilities, especially to assigned room and unit; emphasize positive areas of pediatric unit.
>
> > Room: explain call light, bed controls, television, bathroom, telephone, etc.
> >
> > Unit: direct to playroom, desk, dining area, or other areas.
>
> Introduce family to roommate and his or her parents.
>
> Apply identification band to child's wrist, ankle, or both (if not done).
>
> Explain hospital regulations and schedules (e.g., visiting hours, mealtimes, bedtime, limitations [give written information if available]).
>
> Perform nursing admission history (see box on pp. 618-619).
>
> Take vital signs, blood pressure, height, and weight.
>
> Obtain specimens as needed and order needed laboratory work.
>
> Support child and assist practitioner with physical examination (for purposes of nursing assessment).

on visitation are primarily due to hospital policy or nursing judgment (Whitis, 1994). Many provide facilities such as a chair or bed for at least one person per child, unit kitchen privileges, and other amenities that create a welcoming atmosphere for parents. However, not all hospitals provide such an invitation, and parents' own schedules may prevent rooming-in. In such instances, strategies to minimize the effects of separation must be implemented.

As previously mentioned, ideally a primary nurse, along with associates, is assigned to meet the child's needs. A thorough, detailed nursing history (see box on pp. 618-619) specifically identifies the child's established daily routine. Usual daily activities such as food preparation and method of feeding help establish a complementary schedule of caregiving practices. Incorporating these normal activities also helps the parents feel that they are participating in the child's care, even if through another person. A consistent staff member can be designated to keep the family informed of the child's condition and to support the family's concerns and priorities without being judgmental (Stepanek and Ahmann, 1995).

Nurses must have an appreciation of the child's separation behaviors. As discussed earlier, the phases of protest and despair are normal. The child is allowed to cry. Even if the child rejects strangers, the nurse provides support through physical presence. *Presence* is defined as spending time being physically close to the child while using a quiet tone of voice, appropriate choice of words, eye contact, and touch in ways that establish rapport and communicate empathy (Pederson, 1993). If behaviors of detachment are evident, the nurse maintains the child's contact with the parents by frequently talking about them, encouraging the child to remember them, and stressing the significance of their visits, telephone calls, or letters.

Separation may be equally as difficult for parents, especially when they do not understand the behaviors of separation anxiety. To avoid the immediate protest, parents may sneak out or lie to the child about leaving. As a result, the child does not learn that absence is associated with a guaranteed return, but that absence means loss of parents. Helping parents recognize that separation behaviors are normal and expected can decrease the parents' anxiety and may ease their fears about leaving without telling the child. Explaining to parents how the child reacts after they leave may also be helpful. Many parents imagine that the child cries for hours after they leave, whereas in reality the child may cry for a few minutes but settle down when comforted by someone else.

Toddlers and preschoolers have a very limited concept of time. The young child's question, "Will my mommy come yesterday?" symbolizes a lack of understanding for usual measurements of time, such as days, hours, and weeks. Time is measured in associations, such as eating dinner "when daddy comes home." Therefore, when helping parents with their fears of separation, nurses need to suggest ways of explaining leaving and returning. For example, if parents must leave to go to work or to make meals for the other family members, they should tell the child the reason for leaving. They also need to convey the expected time of return in terms of anticipated events. For example, if the parents will return in the morning, they can say to the child, "We'll see you after the sun comes up" or "We'll come back when (a favorite program) is on television."

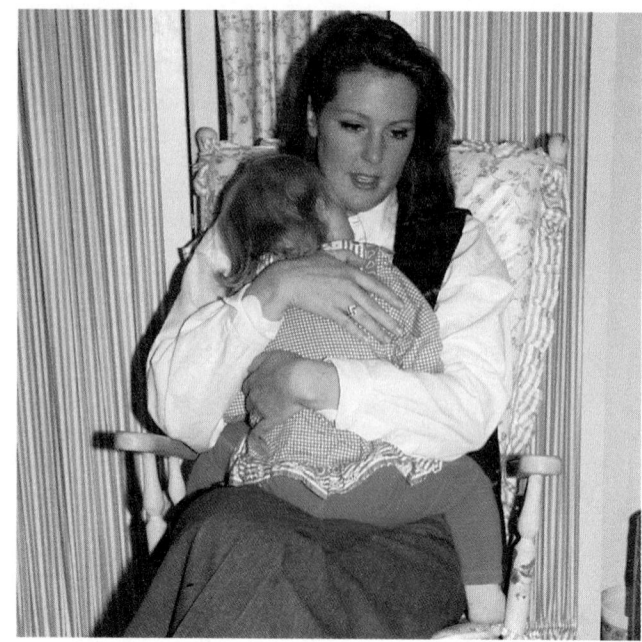

FIG. 21-7. When parents cannot visit, other significant persons can provide comfort to the hospitalized child.

The young child's ability to tolerate parental absence is very limited. Therefore parental visits should be frequent (e.g., visiting three times a day for short periods rather than once a day for an extended time). This may necessitate that each parent visit at different times to lessen the length of separation. When parents cannot visit, the presence of other significant people can be most comforting for the child (Fig. 21-7).

If parents leave after the child is asleep, they still need to communicate their absence. The parents of a 5-year-old boy solved this problem by devising a sign; on one side they drew a picture of a telephone, and on the other they drew a hamburger. Before they left, they turned the sign to the appropriate side to tell the child when he awoke that they were out using the telephone or eating.

Older children who know how to tell time may find it helpful to have a clock or watch. However, these children have the same need for honesty from their parents regarding visiting schedules. Because their peer groups are important, adolescents often appreciate planning visiting hours with their parents to ensure that the patient has some private time for friends.

Familiar surroundings also increase the child's adjustment to separation. If parents cannot room-in, they should leave favorite home articles with the child, such as a blanket, toy, bottle, feeding utensil, or article of clothing. Since young children associate such inanimate objects with significant people, they gain comfort and reassurance from these possessions. They make the association that if the parents left this, the parents will surely return. Placing an identification band on the toy lessens the chances of its being misplaced and provides a symbol that the toy is experiencing the same needs as the child. Other mementos of home include photographs and audiotape or videocassette recordings of family members reading a story, singing a song, saying prayers before bedtime, relating events at home, or taking a "talking walk" through the home. The tapes can be played at lonely times, such as on awakening or before sleeping. Some units allow pets to visit, which can have therapeutic benefits for a child. Animals should be carefully screened for medical or behavioral problems, and patients should be screened for allergies.

Older children also appreciate familiar articles from home, particularly photographs, a radio, a favorite toy or game, and the usual pajamas. Often the importance of treasured objects to school-age children is overlooked or criticized. However, many school-age children have a special object to which they formed an attachment in early childhood. Therefore such treasured or transitional objects can help even older children feel more comfortable in a strange environment.

The strange sights, smells, and sounds in the hospital that are commonplace for the nurse can be frightening and confusing for children. It is important for the nurse to try to evaluate stimuli in the environment from the child's point of view (considering also what the child may see or hear happening to other patients) and to make every effort to protect the child from frightening and unfamiliar sights, sounds, and equipment. The nurse should offer explanations or prepare the child for those experiences that are unavoidable. Combining familiar or comforting sights with the unfamiliar can relieve much of the harshness of medical equipment.

NURSING TIP "Soften" medical equipment (e.g., clip a bear or other animal to a stethoscope; use paper, fabric, or stickers to transform an IV pump into a friendly animal) to create a pleasant and more familiar environment for children (Rollins, 1991).

Helping children maintain their usual nonhome contacts also minimizes the effects of separation imposed by hospitalization. This includes continuing school lessons during the illness and confinement, visiting with friends either directly or through letter writing or telephone calls, and participating in stimulating projects whenever possible (Fig. 21-8). For extended hospitalizations, youngsters enjoy personalizing the hospital room to make it "home" by decorating the walls with

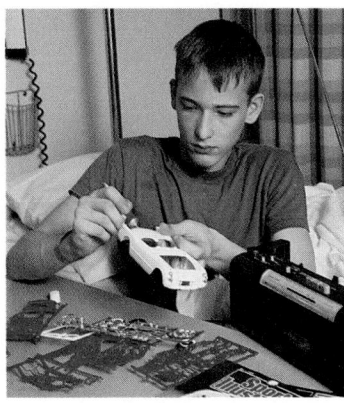

FIG. 21-8. For extended hospitalizations, children enjoy having projects to occupy time. (Courtesy St. Louis Children's Hospital.)

posters and cards, rearranging the furniture (when possible), and displaying a collection or hobby.

Minimize Loss of Control

Feelings of loss of control result from separation, physical restriction, changed routines, enforced dependency, and magical thinking. Although some of these cannot be prevented, most can be minimized through individualized planning of nursing care.

Promote Freedom of Movement. Younger children react most strenuously to any type of physical restriction or immobilization. Although some restraint, such as immobilizing an extremity for insertion of an intravenous line, is frequently necessary, most physical restriction can be prevented if the nurse gains the child's cooperation.

For young children, particularly infants and toddlers, preserving parent-child contact is the best means of decreasing the need for or stress of restraint. For example, almost the entire physical examination can be done in a parent's lap, with the parent hugging the child for procedures such as otoscopy. For painful procedures the parents' preferences for assisting, observing, or waiting outside the room are assessed (see also Parental Support, p. 678).

Environmental factors also influence the need for physical restraint. Keeping children in cribs or playpens may not represent immobilization in a concrete sense, but it certainly limits sensory stimulation. Increasing mobility by transporting children in carriages, wheelchairs, carts, wagons, or on stretchers or beds provides them with mechanical freedom.

Maintain Child's Routine. Altered daily schedules and loss of rituals are particularly stressful for toddlers and early preschoolers and may increase the stress of separation. The nursing admission history provides a baseline for planning care around the child's usual home activities.

A frequently neglected aspect of altered routines is the change in the child's daily activities. A nonhospitalized child's day, especially during the school years, is structured with specific times for eating, dressing, going to school, playing, and sleeping. However, this time structure vanishes when the child is hospitalized. Although the nurses have a set schedule, the child is frequently unaware of it; new schedules are imposed that may be rigid or flexible. For example, some units have uniform nap times and bedtimes for all children, whereas others allow children to stay up very late. Many children obtain significantly less sleep in the hospital than at home; the primary causes are delay in sleep onset and early termination of sleep because of hospital routines. Not only are hours of sleep disrupted, but waking hours are spent in passive activities. For example, few institutions impose any regulation on the amount of time the child spends watching television.

One technique that can minimize the disruption in the child's routine is *time structuring*. This approach is most suitable for the noncritically ill school-age and adolescent child who has mastered the concept of time. It involves scheduling the child's day to include all those activities that are important to the child and nurse, such as treatment procedures, schoolwork, exercise, television, playroom, and hobbies. Together, the nurse, parent, and child then plan a daily schedule with times and activities written down (Fig. 21-9). This is left in the child's room, and a clock or watch is avail-

ERIC'S DAILY SCHEDULE:

7:00 AM	Breakfast, Watch TV, Brush Teeth, Wash up	3:00 PM	Tutor (M,W,F) Study Time (T,Th)
9:00	Tub Room, Dressing Change	4:00	Physical Therapy
10:00	Rest, TV, Snack	5:00	Dinner
11:00	Physical Therapy	6:30	Dressing Change
12:00 PM	Lunch	7:00 to 9:00	TV, Reading, Snack, Friends Visit
1:00	Playroom, Quiet Play, Rest, Friends Visit	9:00	Brush Teeth, Wash up
		9:15	Bedtime

FIG. 21-9. Time structuring is an effective strategy for normalizing the hospital environment and increasing the child's sense of control.

BILL OF RIGHTS FOR CHILDREN AND TEENS

In this hospital you and your family have the right to:
Respect and personal dignity
Care that supports you and your family
Information you can understand
Quality health care
Emotional support
Care that respects your need to grow, play, and learn
Make choices and decisions

From Association for the Care of Children's Health: *A pediatric bill of rights*, Bethesda, MD, 1991, The Association. A detailed explanation of each right plus a separate "Bill of Rights for Parents" is available from the Association for the Care of Children's Health, 7910 Woodmont Ave., Suite 300, Bethesda, MD 20814; (301) 654-6549, (800) 808-ACCH.

able for the child's use. Whenever possible, a calendar is also constructed with special events marked, such as favorite television programs, visits by friends or relatives, events in the playroom, and holidays or birthdays. If specific changes in treatment are expected (e.g., "beginning physical therapy in 2 days"), these are added.

NURSING TIP Ask the young child to select or draw pictures or symbols to represent daily or weekly fun activities (e.g., favorite TV programs, family visits, playroom times). Draw a clock face with the hands of the clock depicting the time each event will occur next to the child's representation. Have the child compare the clock on the schedule with a clock or watch in the room. When the two match, the child knows that it is time for a favorite activity and exactly what that activity is.

Encourage Independence. The dependent role of the hospitalized patient imposes tremendous feelings of loss on older children. Principal interventions should focus on respect for individuality and the opportunity for decision making. Although these sound simple, their efficacy lies with nurses who are flexible, tolerant, and personally secure. The last is particularly important because when decision making is geared toward the patient, nurses can feel threatened by a sense of lessened control.

Promoting children's control involves maintaining independence, and the concept of self-care can be most beneficial. *Self-care* refers to the practice of activities that individuals personally initiate and perform on their own behalf in maintaining life, health, and well-being (Orem, 1995). Although self-care is limited by the child's age and physical condition, most children beyond infancy can perform some activities with little or no help. Whenever possible, these activities are encouraged in the hospital. Other approaches include jointly planning care; time structuring; wearing street clothes; making choices in food selections, bedtime, and so on; continuing school activities; and rooming with an appropriate age-mate.

Promote Understanding. Loss of control can occur from feelings of having too little influence on one's destiny,

as well as from sensing overwhelming control or power over fate. Although preschoolers' cognitive abilities predispose them most to magical thinking and self-power, all children are vulnerable to misinterpreting causes for stresses such as illness and hospitalization.

Most children feel more in control when they know what to expect, because the element of fear is reduced. Anticipatory preparation and providing information help greatly to lessen stress and prevent lack of understanding (see Preparation for Procedures, Chapter 22).

Informing children of their rights while hospitalized fosters greater understanding and may relieve some of the feelings of powerlessness they typically experience. Hospitals providing services to children should have a hospital-wide policy on the rights and responsibilities of these patients and of their parents and/or guardians. An increasing number of hospitals and organizations have developed a "Bill of Rights" that is prominently displayed throughout the hospital or is presented to children and their families on admission (see box for example).

Prevent or Minimize Bodily Injury

Beyond early infancy all children fear bodily injury either from mutilation, bodily intrusion, body image change, disability, or death. In general, preparation of children for painful procedures decreases their fears. Manipulating procedural techniques for children in each age-group also minimizes fear of bodily injury. For example, since toddlers and young preschoolers are traumatized by insertion of a rectal thermometer, axillary temperatures or temperatures taken with electronic or tympanic membrane devices can effectively be substituted. Whenever procedures are performed on young children, the most supportive intervention is to do the procedure as quickly as possible while maintaining parent-child contact.

Because of young children's poorly defined body boundaries, the use of bandages may be particularly helpful. For example, telling children that the bleeding will stop after the needle is removed does little to relieve their fears, whereas applying a small Band-Aid usually provides much reassurance. The size of bandages is also significant to children in this age-group; the larger the bandage, the more importance is attached to the wound. Watching their surgical dressings become successively smaller is one way young children can measure healing and improvement. Prematurely removing a dressing may cause these children considerable concern for their well-being.

For children who fear mutilation of body parts, it is essential that the nurse repeatedly stress the reason for a procedure and evaluate the child's understanding. For example, explaining cast removal to preschoolers may seem simple enough, but children's comprehension of the details may vary considerably from the explanation. Asking them to draw a picture of what they think will happen presents substantial evidence of the perceived events.

Children may fear bodily injury from a great variety of sources. X-ray machines, use of strange equipment for examination, unfamiliar rooms, or awkward positions can be perceived as potentially hazardous. In addition, thoughts and actions can be imagined sources of bodily damage. For older children, masturbation or sex play may be perceived as powerful weapons of potential destruction. Therefore it is important to investigate imagined reasons, particularly of a sexual nature, for illness. Since children may fear revealing such thoughts, using projective techniques such as drawing or doll play may elicit previously undisclosed misconceptions.

Older children fear bodily injury of both internal and external origins. For example, school-age children are aware of the significance of the heart and may fear the actual operation as much as the pain, the stitches, and the possible scar. Adolescents may express concern about the actual procedure but be much more anxious over the resulting scar. An appreciation of each child's special concerns helps nurses focus on critical areas during preparation for procedures or when giving explanations of the disease processes.

Children can grasp information only if it is presented on or close to their level of cognitive development. This necessitates an awareness of the words used to describe events or processes. For example, young children told that they are going to have a CAT scan may wonder, "Will there be cats? Or something that scratches?" It is clearer to describe the procedure in simple terms and explain what the letters of the common name stand for (Gaynard and others, 1990). When children are upset about their illness, their perception can be changed by (1) providing a somewhat different and less negative account of the disease or (2) offering an explanation that is characteristic of the next stage of cognitive development. An example of the first strategy is reassuring a preschooler who fears that after a tonsillectomy, another sore throat means a second operation. Explaining that once tonsils are "fixed" they do not need fixing again can help relieve the fear. An example of the latter strategy is to explain that germs made the tonsils sick and even though germs can cause another sore throat, they cannot cause the tonsils to ever be sick again. This higher-level explanation is based on the school-age child's concept of germs as a cause of disease.

Provide Pain Management

Relief of pain is a basic need and right of all children. Effective pain management requires that health professionals be willing to try a number of interventions to achieve optimum results. Basically, pain-reducing methods can be grouped into two categories: nonpharmacologic and pharmacologic. Whenever possible, both should be used; however, nonpharmacologic measures are not substitutes for analgesics.

Nonpharmacologic Management. A number of nonpharmacologic techniques exist for lessening the perception of pain or making the pain more tolerable, and, when used with analgesics, can enhance these drugs' effectiveness. However, nonpharmacologic strategies can also produce a cooperative child who continues to suffer "in silence." Therefore nurses must carefully evaluate the effectiveness of the intervention in truly reducing pain and avoid setting an expectation of passive acceptance. Aside from this risk, nonpharmacologic methods are extremely safe and most are independent nursing functions.

Nonpharmacologic interventions include *general strategies* that are effective with most children, especially those who can benefit from explanations. However, *specific nonpharmacologic strategies* are more effective with certain children than with others (see Guidelines box on p. 634). Experimentation with several strategies that are suitable to child's age, pain intensity, and abilities is often necessary to determine the most effective approach.

Nursing ALERT Most specific nonpharmacologic strategies require children's understanding and cooperation. Therefore try to match the strategy with the pain severity. Children in severe pain may not be able to expend the effort necessary to learn the technique, and those with very mild symptoms may not be motivated to learn. Therefore these strategies may be most useful with midrange pain.

In the selection of a pain reducer, it is best to use a strategy familiar to the child or to describe several strategies and let the child select the most appealing one. Parents should be involved in the selection process; they may be familiar with the child's usual coping skills and can help identify potentially successful strategies. Involving parents also encourages their participation in learning the skill with the child and acting as coach. If the parent cannot assist the child, other appropriate persons may include a grandparent, older sibling, nurse, or child-life specialist.

Children should learn a specific strategy *before* pain occurs or before it becomes severe. To reduce the child's effort, instructions for a strategy, such as distraction or relaxation, can be audiotaped and played during a period of discomfort.

Pharmacologic Management. Using pharmacologic methods to control pain requires attention to four "rights": right drug, right dose, right route, and right time. Although nurses may not prescribe the medication, knowledge of these essential principles assists in optimally implementing analgesic orders and discussing with other practitioners possible strategies to improve pain control.

Right Drug. Nonopioids, including acetaminophen (Tylenol, paracetamol) and nonsteroidal antiinflammatory drugs (NSAIDs), are suitable for mild to moderate pain; opioids are needed for moderate to severe pain. A combination of the two analgesics attacks pain on two levels: nonopioids at the peripheral nervous system (PNS) and opioids at the central nervous system (CNS). This approach provides increased analgesia without increased side effects. Several commercially available combinations, such as Tylenol with Codeine, may have increasing doses of the opioid but a constant dose of the nonopioid (see box on p. 635). Therefore, before increasing the opioid, it may be preferable to increase the nonopioid

General Strategies

Form a trusting relationship with child and family.

Express concern regarding their reports of pain.

Take an active role in seeking effective pain management strategies.

Use general guidelines to prepare child for procedure (see Chapter 22)

Prepare child before potentially painful procedures but avoid "planting" the idea of pain. For example, instead of saying, "This is going to (or may) hurt," say, "Sometimes this feels like pushing, sticking, or pinching, and sometimes it doesn't bother people. Tell me what it feels like to you."

Use "nonpain" descriptors when possible (e.g., "It feels like intense heat" rather than "It's a burning pain").

This allows for variation in sensory perception, avoids suggesting pain, and gives child control in describing reactions.

Avoid evaluative statements or descriptions (e.g., "This is a terrible procedure" or "It really will hurt a lot").

Stay with child during a painful procedure.

Encourage parents to stay with child if child and parent desire; encourage parent to talk softly to child and to remain near child's head.

Involve parents in learning specific nonpharmacologic strategies and assisting child in their use.

Educate child about the pain, especially when explanation may lessen anxiety (e.g., that child's pain is expected after surgery and does not indicate something is wrong; reassure that child is not responsible for the pain).

For long-term pain control, give child a doll, which becomes "the patient," and allow child to do everything to the doll that is done to the child; pain control can be emphasized through the doll by stating, "Dolly feels better after the medicine."

Teach procedures to child and family for later use.

Specific Strategies

Distraction

Involve parent and child in identifying strong distractors.

Involve child in play; use radio, tape recorder, record player; have child sing or use rhythmic breathing.

Have child take a deep breath and blow it out until told to stop (French, Painter, and Coury, 1994).

Have child blow bubbles to "blow the hurt away."

Have child concentrate on yelling or saying "ouch" by focusing on "yelling loud or soft as you feel it hurt: that way I know what's happening."

Have child look through kaleidoscope (type with glitter suspended in fluid-filled tube) and encourage to concentrate by asking, "Do you see the different designs? (Vessey, Carlson, and McGill, 1994).

Use humor, such as watching cartoons, telling jokes or funny stories, or acting silly with child.

Have child read, play games, or visit with friends.

Relaxation

With an infant or young child:

Hold in a comfortable, well-supported position, such as vertically against the chest and shoulder.

Rock in a wide, rhythmic arc in a rocking chair or sway back and forth, rather than bouncing child.

Repeat one or two words softly, such as "Mommy's here."

With a slightly older child:

Ask child to take a deep breath and "go limp as a rag doll" while exhaling slowly, then ask child to yawn (demonstrate if needed).

Help child assume a comfortable position (e.g., pillow under neck and knees).

Begin progressive relaxation: starting with the toes, systematically instruct child to let each body part "go limp" or "feel heavy"; if child has difficulty with relaxing, instruct child to tense or tighten each body part and then relax it.

Allow child to keep eyes open, since children may respond better if eyes are open rather than closed during relaxation.

Guided Imagery

Have child identify some highly pleasurable real or pretend experience.

Have child describe details of the event, including as many senses as possible (e.g., "feel the cool breezes," "see the beautiful colors," "hear the pleasant music").

Have child write down or record script.

Encourage child to concentrate only on the pleasurable event during the painful time; enhance the image by recalling specific details, such as reading the script or playing the record.

Combine with relaxation.

Positive Self-Talk

Teach child positive statements to say when in pain (e.g., "I will be feeling better soon," "When I go home, I will feel better, and we will eat ice cream.")

Thought Stopping

Identify positive facts about the painful event (e.g., "It does not last long").

Identify reassuring information (e.g., "If I think about something else, it does not hurt as much").

Condense positive and reassuring facts into a set of brief statements, and have child memorize them (e.g.: "Short procedure, good veins, little hurt, nice nurse, go home").

Have child repeat the memorized statements whenever thinking about or experiencing the painful event.

Cutaneous Stimulation

Includes simple rhythmic rubbing; use of pressure, electric vibrator; massage with hand lotion, powder, or menthol cream; application of heat or cold, such as an ice cube on the site before giving injection or application of ice to the site opposite the painful area (e.g., if right knee hurts, place ice on left knee).

A more sophisticated method is transcutaneous electrical nerve stimulation (TENS) (use of controlled low-voltage electricity to the body via electrodes placed on the skin).

Behavioral Contracting

Informal—May be used with children as young as 4 or 5 years of age:

Use stars or tokens as rewards.

Give uncooperative or procrastinating children (during a procedure) a limited time (measured by a visible timer) to complete the procedure.

Proceed as needed if child is unable to comply.

Reinforce cooperation with a reward if the procedure is accomplished within specified time.

Formal—Use written contract, which includes the following:

Realistic (seems possible) goal or desired behavior

Measurable behavior (e.g., agrees not to hit anyone during procedures)

Contract written, dated, and signed by all persons involved in any of the agreements

Identified rewards or consequences are reinforcing

Goals can be evaluated

Requires commitment and compromise from both parties, e.g., while timer is used, nurse will not nag or prod child to complete procedure.

SELECTED COMBINATION OPIOID AND NONOPIOID ORAL ANALGESICS

Nonaspirin Products

Darvocet-N 50	50 mg propoxyphene napsylate
	325 mg acetaminophen
Darvocet-N 100	100 mg propoxyphene napsylate
	650 mg acetaminophen
Lortab	2.5, 5, or 7.5 mg hydrocodone bitartrate
	500 mg acetaminophen
Lortab Liquid (each 5 ml)	2.5 mg hydrocodone bitartrate
	120 mg acetaminophen
Percocet-5*	5 mg oxycodone HCl
	325 mg acetaminophen
Tylenol with Codeine No. 1	7.5 mg codeine
	300 mg acetaminophen
Tylenol with Codeine No. 2	15 mg codeine
	300 mg acetaminophen
Tylenol with Codeine No. 3	30 mg codeine
	300 mg acetaminophen
Tylenol with Codeine No. 4	60 mg codeine
	300 mg acetaminophen
Tylenol and Codeine Elixir (each 5 ml)	12 mg codeine
	120 mg acetaminophen
	7% alcohol
Tylox*	5 mg oxycodone HCl
	500 mg acetaminophen
Vicodin	5 mg hydrocodone
	500 mg acetaminophen

Aspirin Products†

Darvon Compound	32 mg propoxyphene HCl
	389 mg aspirin
	32.4 mg caffeine
Darvon Compound-65	65 mg propoxyphene HCl
	389 mg aspirin
	32.4 mg caffeine
Darvon with A.S.A.	65 mg propoxyphene HCl
	325 mg aspirin
Darvon-N with A.S.A.	100 mg propoxyphene napsylate
	325 mg aspirin
Percodan*	4.5 mg oxycodone HCl
	0.38 mg oxycodone terephthalate
	325 mg aspirin
Percodan-Demi*	2.25 mg oxycodone HCl
	0.19 mg oxycodone terephthalate
	325 mg aspirin

*All medications require a prescription, but these are classified as schedule II drugs (like morphine), and each filling requires a written prescription that includes the patient's name and address, the practitioner's DEA (Drug Enforcement Agency) number, and the date. The prescription must be filled within 5 days.
†Aspirin is not recommended for children because of its possible association with Reye syndrome.

for postoperative pain control, because of the accumulation of its metabolite, *normeperidine*. Normeperidine is a CNS stimulant that can produce anxiety, tremors, myoclonus, and generalized seizures. Normeperidine's half-life is 15 to 20 hours, compared with 3 hours for meperidine, and the CNS excitation is not reversed with naloxone. According to the **Acute Pain Management Guideline Panel** (1992), "Meperidine should be reserved for very brief courses in otherwise healthy patients who have demonstrated an unusual reaction (e.g., local histamine release at the infusion site) or allergic response during treatment with other opioids such as morphine or hydromorphone."

Nursing ALERT Assess the child at least every 8 hours for early signs of normeperidine toxicity, such as tremors in the outstretched hand, episodes of twitching or jerking, or increased agitation or excitability (may be upset easily). If toxicity is suspected, discontinue the meperidine, maintain the IV, and notify the practitioner (Love, 1994). If symptoms worsen, a CNS depressant may be needed. The pharmacist should complete an adverse drug reaction report (Form 3500A) to MedWatch.*

Opioids are frequently combined with other drugs that are considered "potentiators." However, little evidence indicates that any drug potentiates the analgesic effect of opioids; rather, drugs that produce sedation are erroneously equated with producing analgesia. One common drug combination—*meperidine (pethidine [Demerol])*, *promethazine (Phenergan)*, and *chlorpromazine (Thorazine)*, known as *DPT* or *lytic cocktail*—is used for conscious sedation for procedures (see Preoperative Care, Chapter 22). Meperidine, a short-acting analgesic, provides pain relief for 2 to 3 hours but is irritating to the tissues when given intramuscularly. Promethazine has antianalgesic properties, produces excessive sedation, and can cause extrapyramidal reactions (spasms of neck, face, tongue, and back; fixed eyeballs). All these drugs cause respiratory depression and lower the seizure threshold, a particular risk to those with a convulsive disorder. In addition, the "cocktail" is usually administered intramuscularly, causing additional pain. For these reasons, DPT is not recommended for general use and should be used only in exceptional circumstances (Acute Pain Management Guideline Panel, 1992). Appropriate drugs for conscious sedation are listed in the box on p. 636.

Several drugs, known as *adjuvant analgesics* or *coanalgesics*, may be used alone or with opioids to control pain symptoms. Frequently used drugs to relieve anxiety, cause sedation, and provide amnesia are diazepam (Valium) and midazolam (Versed); however, they are not analgesics. Other adjuvants include tricyclic antidepressants (i.e., amitriptyline, imipramine) and antiepileptics for neuropathic pain (brief, lancinating pain); steroids for inflammation and bone pain; and dextroamphetamine and caffeine for increased analgesia and decreased sedation (McCaffery, 1996).

---

*The FDA Medical Products Reporting Program, Food and Drug Administration, 5600 Fishers Lane, Rockville, MD 20852-9787; (800) FDA-1088, FAX (800) FDA-0178.

component, for example, adding one plain Tylenol (300 mg) to Tylenol with Codeine No. 3 before advancing to Tylenol with Codeine No. 4. However, if this approach is not successful, the pain most likely requires a stronger opioid.

Actions of various opioids differ. Morphine is considered the drug of choice. When morphine is not a suitable opioid, drugs such as hydromorphone (Dilaudid) and fentanyl (Sublimaze) are effective substitutes. Although fentanyl is used as an anesthetic in the operating room, it is classified as an analgesic. It can be safely administered by nurses (Willens, 1994).

Meperidine (Demerol, pethidine) is not recommended for chronic use (or for more than 48 hours at a time), such as

EFFECTIVE MEDICATIONS FOR CONSCIOUS SEDATION

Opioids*

Morphine sulfate, 0.05 to 0.10 mg/kg IV over 1 to 2 minutes given 5 minutes before procedure

Fentanyl, 1 to 2 μg/kg (0.001 to 0.002 mg/kg) IV 3 minutes before procedure

Fentanyl Oralet, 5 to 15 μg/kg, maximum to 400 μg, orally 20 to 40 minutes before procedure†

Meperidine (if morphine sulfate or fentanyl is not available), 0.5 to 1.0 mg/kg IV over 1 to 2 minutes given 2 to 5 minutes before procedure or 1.5 mg/kg orally 45 to 60 minutes before procedure

Sedatives‡

Diazepam (Valium), 0.2 to 0.3 mg/kg, maximum to 10 mg, orally 45 to 60 minutes before procedure

Midazolam (Versed), 0.2 to 0.4 mg/kg, maximum to 15 mg (IV solution), orally 30 to 45 minutes, or 0.05 mg/kg IV 3 minutes before procedure

Pentobarbital (Nembutal), 1 to 3 mg/kg IV boluses to maximum of 100 mg until asleep

Chloral hydrate, 50 to 75 mg/kg, maximum to of 100 mg/kg or 2.0 g, orally or rectally 60 minutes before procedure

Modified from Zeltzer LK and others: Report of the subcommittee on the management of pain associated with procedures in children with cancer, *Pediatrics* 86(suppl):826-831, 1990; and Coté CJ: Sedation for the pediatric patient, *Pediatr Clin North Am* 41(1):31-58, 1994.
*Provide analgesia and sedation.
†Not recommended for children less than 15 kg. Lozenge should be sucked, not chewed and swallowed. If chewed, drug is less effective because part of it is metabolized by liver before entering bloodstream. Swallowing drug rapidly does not increase risk of respiratory depression during first 15 to 30 minutes, period of greatest risk for decreased respiration.
‡Provide sedation but no analgesia.

At times health professionals question whether pain really exists and administer *placebos* to "see if the pain is real." This practice is unjustified and unethical; a positive response to a placebo, such as a saline injection, is common in patients who have a documented organic basis for pain. Therefore the deceptive use of placebos does not provide useful information about the presence or severity of pain. In addition, the use of placebos can cause side effects similar to those of opioids, can destroy the client's trust in the health care staff, and raises serious ethical and legal questions (Hinnant, 1995). Therefore the use of placebos is avoided (American Pain Society, 1992).

Right Dosage. The optimum dosage is one that controls pain without causing severe side effects. This usually requires *titration,* the gradual adjustment of drug dosage (usually by increasing or decreasing the dose) until optimum pain relief without excessive sedation is achieved. Dosage recommendations, such as those in Tables 21-3 and 21-4, are only safe initial dosages, not optimum dosages. Children (except infants younger than about 3 to 6 months of age) metabolize drugs more rapidly than adults; younger children may require higher doses of opioids to achieve the same analgesic effect. Therefore the therapeutic effect and duration of analgesia vary. Children's dosages are usually calculated according to body weight, except in children who weigh 50 kg (110 pounds) or more, when the weight formula may exceed the average adult dose. In this case the adult dose is used.

A reasonable starting dose of opioid for the neonate who is *not* mechanically ventilated is one fourth to one third of the recommended starting dose for older children. The infant is monitored very closely for signs of pain relief and respiratory depression. The dose is titrated to effect. Since tolerance can develop rapidly, very large opioid doses may be needed for continued severe pain (American Pain Society, 1992).

If pain relief is inadequate, the initial dosage is increased (usually by 25% to 50% and sometimes more to provide greater analgesic effectiveness). Decreasing the interval between doses may also provide more continuous pain relief. A major difference between opioids and nonopioids is that nonopioids have a *ceiling effect,* which means that doses higher than the recommended dose will not produce greater pain relief. Opioids do not have a ceiling effect other than that imposed by side effects; therefore larger dosages can be given safely for increasing severity of pain. (See Critical Thinking Exercise on p. 639.)

Nursing ALERT A frequent error in attempts to improve pain control is to change to another analgesic. If an opioid, such as morphine, hydromorphone, or fentanyl, is used, rarely is the problem one of drug choice. Rather, the problem is usually one of inadequate dosage. If changing to another analgesic is warranted because of adverse side effects, the new drug should be at least equal in potency to the original analgesic.

Parenteral and oral dosages of opioids are not the same. Because of the *first-pass effect,* an oral opioid is rapidly absorbed from the gastrointestinal tract and enters the portal circulation, where it is partially metabolized before reaching the central circulation. Therefore oral dosages must be larger to compensate for the partial loss of analgesic potency to achieve *equianalgesia* (equal analgesic effect). Conversion factors for selected opioids, when a change is made from intramuscular (IM) or intravenous (IV) to oral, are listed in Tables 21-4 and 21-5. Immediate conversion from IM or IV to the suggested equianalgesic oral dose may result in a substantial error in the individual child. For example, the dose may be significantly more or less than what the child requires. Small changes ensure small errors.

Right Route. Several routes of administration exist (see box on pp. 640-641). Children should not have to endure pain, such as from IM injections, to achieve pain relief. Therefore the most effective and least traumatic route of administration should be selected.

A significant advance in the administration of IV or subcutaneous (SC) analgesics is the use of *patient-controlled analgesia (PCA).* As the name implies, the patient controls the amount and frequency of the analgesic, which is typically delivered through a special infusion device. Children who are physically able to "push a button" and who can understand the concept of "pushing a button" to obtain pain relief (usually during later preschool age) can use PCA (Gureno and Reisinger, 1991). Although it is controversial, parents and nurses have used the PCA system for the child (Ruble and Billet, 1993; Webb, Paarlberg, and Sussman, 1991). Nurses can efficiently use the infusion device on any-age child to administer analgesics without the need for signing for and pre-

TABLE 21-3. Nonopioid analgesic drugs approved for children*

DRUG (TRADE NAME)	DOSE	COMMENTS
Acetaminophen (paracetamol; Tylenol and other brands)	10-20 mg/kg/dose every 4-6 hours not to exceed 5 doses in 24 hours	Available in drops (80 mg/0.8 ml), elixir (160 mg/5 ml), tablets (80 mg), swallowable caplets (160 mg), and rectal suppositories (several dosages) Nonprescription Higher dosage range may provide increased analgesia
Choline magnesium trisalicylate (Trilisate)	Children 37 kg or less: 50 mg/kg/day divided into 2 doses Children over 37 kg: 2250 mg/day divided into 2 doses	Available in elixir 500 mg/5 ml Prescription
Ibuprofen Children's Motrin	Children 6 months to 12 years: 5-10 mg/kg/dose every 6-8 hours not to exceed 40 mg/kg/day for fever Children over 12 years: 200-400 mg/dose every 6-8 hours	Available in suspension (100 mg/5 ml) Nonprescription Recommended for fever reduction in children 6 months to 12 years, but also indicated for juvenile rheumatoid arthritis and mild to moderate pain in children over 12 years
Children's Advil	Children 6 months and older: 5-10 mg/kg/dose every 6-8 hours not to exceed 40 mg/kg/day for fever	Available in suspension (100 mg/5 ml) Prescription Dosage recommendation is for juvenile rheumatoid arthritis and fever
Naproxen (Naprosyn)	Children over 2 years: 10 mg/kg/day divided into 2 doses	Available in elixir (125 mg/5 ml) Prescription
Tolmetin (Tolectin)	Children over 2 years: 20 mg/kg/day divided into 3 or 4 doses	Available in scored 200 mg tablets Prescription

*All drugs except acetaminophen are nonsteroidal antiinflammatory drugs (NSAIDs).
Acetylsalicylic acid (aspirin) is also an NSAID but is not recommended for children because of its possible association with Reye syndrome. The NSAIDs in the table have no known association with Reye syndrome. However, caution should be exercised in prescribing any salicylate-containing drug (e.g., Trilisate) for children with known or suspected viral infection.
Ketorolac (Toradol) is the only NSAID that can be given intravenously. Although it is not approved for patients less than 16 years of age, it is used in children.
Side effects of ibuprofen, naproxen, and tolmetin include nausea, vomiting, diarrhea, constipation, gastric ulceration, bleeding nephritis, and fluid retention.
Acetaminophen and choline magnesium trisalicylate are well tolerated in the gastrointestinal tract and do not interfere with platelet function. NSAIDs except acetaminophen should not be given to patients with allergic reactions to salicylates. All the NSAIDs should be used cautiously in patients with renal impairment.

paring opioid injections every time one is needed. When used as "nurse"- or "parent"-controlled analgesia, the concept of patient control is negated and may lead to excessive dosing.

PCA infusion devices typically allow for the following three methods or modes of drug administration to be used alone or in combination:

1. **Patient-administered boluses** that can only be infused according to the preset amount and lockout interval (time between doses); more frequent "pushing of the button" means no drug is delivered, but the patient may need the dose and/or time adjusted for better pain control
2. **Nurse-administered boluses** that are typically used to give an initial loading dose to increase blood levels rapidly and to relieve *breakthrough pain* (pain not relieved with the usual programmed dose)
3. **Continuous basal** or **background infusion** that delivers a constant amount of analgesic and prevents pain from returning during those times, such as sleep, when the patient cannot control the infusion; may decrease safety of PCA

At present the optimum use of these three modes is under investigation. However, as with any type of analgesic management plan, continued assessment of the child's pain relief is essential for the greatest benefit from PCA (see Critical Thinking Exercise on p. 639). Typical uses of PCA are for controlling pain from surgery, sickle cell crisis, trauma, and cancer.

Morphine is the drug of choice for PCA and is usually prepared in a concentration of 1 mg/ml. Other options are hydromorphone and fentanyl. Because PCA is typically used for continuous and extended pain control, meperidine should not be administered (see p. 635). Another risk of using meperidine is confusion between its concentration (10 mg/ml) and that of morphine when the PCA pump is programmed, which can result in undermedication or overmedication.

Another advance is the use of the *epidural* or *intrathecal route,* primarily postoperatively or in selected cases of terminal care. A catheter is placed into the epidural or intrathecal

TABLE 21-4. Dosage of selected opioids for children

DRUG	APPROXIMATE EQUIANALGESIC ORAL DOSE	APPROXIMATE EQUIANALGESIC PARENTERAL DOSE	RECOMMENDED STARTING DOSE (CHILDREN LESS THAN 50 kg BODY WEIGHT)[a]	
			ORAL	PARENTERAL[b]
Morphine[c]	30 mg every 3-4 hours (around-the-clock dosing) 60 mg every 3-4 hours (single dose or inter-mittent dosing)	10 mg every 3-4 hours	0.2-0.4 mg/kg every 3-4 hours 0.3-0.6 mg/kg time released every 12 hours	0.1-0.2 mg/kg IM every 3-4 hours 0.02-0.1 mg/kg IV bolus every 2 hours 0.015 mg/kg every 8 minutes PCA 0.01-0.02 mg/kg/hr IV infusion (neo-nates) 0.01-0.06 mg/kg/hr IV infusion (child)
Fentanyl (Sublimaze) (oral mucosal form—**Fentanyl Oralet**)[d]	Not available	0.1 mg IV	5-15 μg/kg; maximum dose 400 μg	0.5-1.5 μg/kg IV bo-lus every ½ hour 1-2 μg/hr IV infusion
Codeine[e]	200 mg every 3-4 hours	130 mg every 3-4 hours	1 mg/kg every 3-4 hours	Not recommended
Hydromorphone[e] (**Dilaudid**)	7.5 mg every 3-4 hours	1.5 mg every 3-4 hours	0.04-0.1 mg/kg every 4-6 hours	0.02-0.1 mg/kg IM every 3-4 hours 0.005-0.2 mg/kg IV bolus every 2 hours
Hydrocodone (in **Lorcet, Lortab, Vi-codin**, others)	30 mg every 3-4 hours	Not available	0.2 mg/kg every 3-4 hours[g]	Not available
Levorphanol (**Levo-Dromoran**)	4 mg every 6-8 hours	2 mg every 6-8 hours	0.04 mg/kg every 6-8 hours	0.02 mg/kg every 6-8 hours
Meperidine (**Demer-ol**)[f]	300 mg every 2-3 hours	100 mg every 3 hours	Not recommended	0.75 mg/kg every 2-3 hours
Methadone (**Dolo-phine**, others)	20 mg every 6-8 hours	10 mg every 6-8 hours	0.2 mg/kg every 6-8 hours	0.1 mg/kg every 6-8 hours
Oxycodone (**Roxi-codone, Oxycontin**; also in **Percocet, Percodan, Tylox,** others)	30 mg every 3-4 hours	Not available	0.2 mg/kg every 3-4 hours[g]	Not available

Data from Acute Pain Management Guideline Panel: *Acute pain management: operative or medical procedures and trauma: clinical practice guideline,* AHCPR Pub No 92-0032, Rockville, MD, 1992, Agency for Health Care Policy and Research, Public Health Service, US Department of Health and Human Services; and Berde C and others: Report of the subcommittee on disease-related pain in childhood cancer, *Pediatrics* 86(5, pt 2):820, 1990. *IV*, Intravenous; *IM*, intramuscular; *PCA*, patient-controlled analgesia.

Note: Published tables vary in the suggested doses that are equianalgesic to morphine. Clinical response is the criterion that must be applied for each patient; titration to clinical response is necessary. Because there is not complete cross-tolerance among these drugs, it is usually necessary to use a lower than equianalgesic dose when changing drugs and to retitrate to response. **Caution:** Recommended doses do not apply to patients with renal or hepatic insufficiency or other conditions affecting drug metabolism and kinetics.

[a]**Caution:** Doses listed for patients with body weight less than 50 kg cannot be used as initial starting doses in infants less than 6 months of age. For nonventilated infants under 6 months of age, the initial opioid dose should be about one fourth to one third of the dose recommended for older infants and children. For example, morphine could be used at a dose of 0.03 mg/kg instead of the traditional 0.1 mg/kg.

[b]IM injections should not be used.

[c]For morphine, hydromorphone, and oxymorphone, rectal administration is an alternate route for patients unable to take oral medications, but equi-analgesic doses may differ from oral and parenteral doses because of pharmacokinetic differences.

[d]Fentanyl Oralet is indicated for use in a hospital setting only (1) as an anesthetic premedication in the operating room setting or (2) to induce conscious sedation before a diagnostic or therapeutic procedure in other monitored anesthesia care settings in hospital; is contraindicated in children who weigh less than 15 kg (33 lb).

[e]**Caution:** Codeine doses above 65 mg often are not appropriate because of diminishing incremental analgesia with increasing doses but continually increasing constipation and other side effects. Dosages are from McCaffery M, Beebe A: *Pain: Clinical manual for nursing practice,* St Louis, 1989, Mosby.

[f]Meperidine is not recommended for continuous pain control, i.e., postoperatively, because of risk of normeperidine toxicity (see p. 635).

[g]**Caution:** Doses of aspirin and acetaminophen in combination with opioid/NSAID preparations must also be adjusted to patient's body weight.

TABLE 21-5. Selected analgesics (equianalgesia)

GENERIC (TRADE) DRUG*	EQUAL TO ORAL MORPHINE (mg)	EQUAL TO IM/IV MORPHINE (mg)
Propoxyphene hydrochloride (Darvon) 65 mg	4.8	1.6
Propoxyphene napsylate + acetaminophen (Darvocet-N 50)	4.8	1.6
30 mg codeine + 300 mg acetaminophen (Tylenol No. 3)	7.2	2.4
Oxycodone 5 mg + 325 mg acetaminophen (Percocet)	7.2	2.4
Oxycodone 5 mg + 325 mg aspirin (Percodan)	7.2	2.4
Hydrocodone 5 mg + 500 mg acetaminophen (Vicodin)	9	3
Oxycodone 5 mg + 500 mg acetaminophen (Tylox)	9	3
Acetaminophen (Tylenol Extra Strength) 500 mg	4	1.3
Transdermal fentanyl patch (Duragesic) (based on 25 μg patch applied q 3 days = 50 mg oral morphine q 24 hr or divided into 6 doses = 8.3 mg)	8.3	2.77

Table by Betty R. Ferrell, PhD, FAAN, 1994.
*Oral medication with exception of fentanyl.

CRITICAL THINKING EXERCISE

Pain Management—Patient-Controlled Analgesia (PCA)

Juan, 9 years old, is hospitalized for a fractured pelvis and multiple other trauma as a result of a motor vehicle injury. Since admission he has been receiving PCA ordered as "morphine, 2.0 to 2.5 mg/hr, lockout 10 minutes; bolus dose 1.5 mg, not to exceed one dose per hour." In assessing his pain, you note that he rates the pain a 4 on a scale of 0 to 5, no pain to worst pain, respectively, and he has been pushing the PCA button an average of 15 times an hour. The first action you take is which of the following?

1. Tell Juan that he is pushing the button too often; he should wait 10 minutes before using the PCA machine.
2. Administer the bolus dose of morphine and reassess pain in 10 minutes.
3. Increase the hourly dose of morphine from 2.0 to 2.5 mg and reassess pain in 1 hour.
4. Contact the surgeon about Juan's inadequate pain management.

The correct answer is two. Juan's pain is inadequately treated, and your first intervention is to give the ordered bolus dose. If the bolus dose relieves the pain to an acceptable level for Juan, the next step is to increase the hourly dose to 2.0 mg. Since the PCA order allows titrating (adjusting) the dosage upward, this action precedes calling the surgeon. It is absolutely inappropriate to tell Juan to push the PCA button less often; this response disregards his need for improved pain control and eliminates a valuable assessment parameter, the number of PCA uses.

space of the spinal column. An opioid (usually fentanyl or preservative-free morphine), often with a long-acting local anesthetic (usually bupivacaine) is instilled via continuous-drip or intermittent administration. Analgesia results primarily from the drug's direct effect on opiate receptors in the spinal cord, rather than in the brain, which is responsible for undesirable effects (e.g., sedation and respiratory depression). Respiratory depression is rare, but if it occurs, it develops slowly and is evident several hours after the infusion.

Nursing ALERT When the epidural or intrathecal route is used, check the child's level of consciousness and respiratory rate and depth hourly for the first 24 hours to detect delayed-onset respiratory depression (American Pain Society, 1992).

Other routes that have benefited from new products for pain control are the *oral transmucosal* and *transdermal routes.* Oral transmucosal *fentanyl* (Fentanyl Oralet) provides atraumatic preoperative oral sedation and analgesia. Fentanyl is also available as a transdermal patch (Duragesic). It may be used for older children and adolescents who have chronic cancer pain.

One of the most significant improvements in the ability to provide atraumatic care to children is the anesthetic cream, *EMLA,** a eutectic mixture of local anesthetics (lidocaine 2.5% and prilocaine 2.5%). The eutectic mixture, whose melting point is lower than that of the two anesthetics alone, permits effective concentrations of the drug to penetrate *intact* skin. A thick layer of cream is applied under an occlusive transparent dressing for 1 hour or more before procedures, such as lumbar, venous, arterial, finger, heel, or earlobe punctures; implanted port access; insertion of peripherally inserted central catheters (PICC lines); superficial biopsy; skin graft; laser treatment of port wine stains; removal of epicardial (pacing) wires, chest tubes, or hair (electrolysis); bone marrow examination; allergy testing; and IM or SC injections. For deeper pain, such as IM injections, the application time should be extended up to 2 hours (see Guidelines box on p. 641). The duration of anesthesia is up to 4 hours.

EMLA is approved for children over 1 month of age but

---
*For additional information about EMLA, contact Astra Pharmaceuticals, (800) 228-EMLA.

ROUTES AND METHODS OF ANALGESIC DRUG ADMINISTRATION

Oral

Preferred because of convenience, cost, and relatively steady blood levels

Higher dosages of oral form of opioids required for equivalent parenteral analgesia

Peak drug effect occurs after 1½ to 2 hours for most analgesics
 Delay in onset is disadvantage when rapid control of severe pain or fluctuating pain is desired

Sublingual/Buccal/Transmucosal

Tablet or liquid placed between cheek and gum (buccal) or under tongue (sublingual)

Highly desirable because more rapid onset than oral
 Avoids first-pass effect through liver, which normally reduces analgesia from oral opioids (unless sublingual/buccal form swallowed, which occurs often in children)

Few drugs commercially available in this form
 Many drugs can be compounded into a sublingual troche or lozenge*

Fentanyl Oralet—Fentanyl in hard confection base on a plastic holder used for preoperative or preprocedural sedation/analgesia

Intravenous (IV) (Bolus)

Preferred for rapid control of severe pain

Provides most rapid onset of effect, usually in about 5 minutes
 Advantage for acute pain, procedural pain, and "breakthrough" pain

Initial bolus dose is controversial; one recommendation is one-half IM dose

Needs to be repeated hourly for continuous pain control
 Drugs with short half-life (morphine, fentanyl, hydromorphone) are preferred, to avoid toxic accumulation of drug

Intravenous (Continuous)

Preferred over bolus and IM for maintaining control of pain

Provides steady blood levels

Easy to titrate dosage

Suggested initial dose is controversial; one approach to calculating hourly infusion rate is to divide IM dose by drug's expected duration for IM route

Full peak effect is delayed; best if combined with initial IV bolus dose

Subcutaneous (SC) (Continuous)

Used when oral and IV routes not available

Provides equivalent blood levels to continuous IV infusion

Suggested initial bolus dose to equal 2-hour IV dose; total 24-hour dose usually equal to total IV or IM 24-hour dose

Patient-Controlled Analgesia (PCA)

Generally refers to self-administration of drugs, regardless of route

Typically uses programmable infusion pump (IV or SC) that permits self-administration of boluses of medication at preset dose and time interval (*lockout interval* is time between doses)

Best pain control may be achieved with initial bolus and continuous (basal or background) infusion of opioid

Optimum lockout interval not known, but must be at least as long as time needed for onset of drug
 Should effectively control pain during movement or procedures
 Longer lockout requires larger dose

May be used as a convenient analgesic delivery system for neonates; nurse pushes button for increased pain control

Intramuscular (IM)

Available in many opioid preparations

Painful administration (hated by children)

Some drugs (e.g., meperidine) can cause tissue damage

Wide fluctuation in absorption of drug from muscle

Faster absorption from deltoid than gluteal sites

Shorter duration and more expensive than oral drugs

Time consuming for staff

Intranasal

Midazolam (Versed) has been used as nasal spray
 Although effective, may be traumatic route for children

Available commercially as Stadol NS (butorphanol); approved for those over 18 years of age; should not be used in patient receiving morphine-like drugs because butorphanol is partial antagonist

Intradermal

Used primarily for skin anesthesia (e.g., for lumbar puncture, bone marrow aspiration, arterial puncture, skin biopsy)

Local anesthetics (lidocaine) cause stinging, burning sensation
 Duration of stinging may depend on type of "caine" used

To avoid stinging sensation associated with lidocaine:
 Buffer the solution by adding 1 part sodium bicarbonate (1 mEq/ml) to 10 parts 1% or 2% lidocaine (see Guidelines box on p. 642)

Topical/Transdermal

EMLA (eutectic mixture of local anesthetics [lidocaine/prilocaine]) cream
 Eliminates or reduces pain from most procedures involving skin puncture
 Must be placed over puncture site under occlusive dressing for 1 hour or more before procedure (see Guidelines box on p. 641)

TAC (tetracaine/adrenalin/cocaine) or *TC (without adrenalin)* or *LAT (lidocaine/adrenaline/tetracaine)*
 Provides skin anesthesia about 15 minutes after application
 Gel (preferably) or liquid placed on wounds for suturing (nonintact skin)
 Cocaine must not be used on mucous membranes and denuded areas because of the risk of systemic absorption and toxicity
 Adrenalin must not be used on end arterioles (fingers, toes, tip of nose, penis, earlobes) because of vasoconstriction
 LAT is safer and less expensive

Transdermal Fentanyl (Duragesic)

Available as "patch" for continuous cancer pain control

Safety and efficacy not established in children under 12 years

Not appropriate for initial relief of acute pain because of long interval to peak effect (from 12 to 24 hours)

Orders for "rescue doses" of an opioid should be available for pain that "breaks through"

Has duration of up to 72 hours for prolonged pain relief

If respiratory depression occurs, several doses of naloxone may be needed

Rectal

Alternative to oral or parenteral routes

Variable absorption rate

Generally disliked by children, but often preferred over IM injection

Many drugs can be compounded into rectal suppositories

Regional Nerve Block

Use of long-acting anesthetic (bupivacaine) injected into site, usually at end of surgery

---

Data primarily from American Pain Society: *Principles of analgesic use in the treatment of acute pain or chronic cancer pain,* ed 2, Skokie, IL, 1992, The Society; and McCaffery M, Beebe A: *Pain: clinical manual for nursing practice,* St Louis, 1989, Mosby.
*For further information about compounding drugs in troches or suppositories, contact Technical Staff, Professional Compounding Centers of America, P.O. Box 368, Sugarland, TX 77487; (800) 331-2498.

ROUTES AND METHODS OF ANALGESIC DRUG ADMINISTRATION—cont'd

Provides prolonged analgesia postoperatively, such as after inguinal herniorrhaphy

May be used to provide local anesthesia for surgery, such as dorsal penile nerve block for circumcision

Inhalation

Use of anesthetics, such as nitrous oxide or halothane, to produce partial or complete analgesia for painful procedures

Occupational exposure to high levels of nitrous oxide may cause side effects

Epidural/Intrathecal

Involves catheter placed into epidural or intrathecal space for continuous drip or intermittent administration of opioid (with or without a long-acting anesthetic, e.g., bupivacaine)

Analgesia primarily from drug's direct effect on opiate receptors in spinal canal

Provides steady drug levels and long-lasting analgesia

Respiratory depression is very rare but may have slow and delayed onset; can be prevented by checking level of consciousness and respiratory rate and depth hourly for initial 24 hours

Nausea, itching, and urinary retention are common dose-related side effects

---

GUIDELINES
Using EMLA *(Eutectic Mixture of Local Anesthetics—Lidocaine 2.5% and Prilocaine 2.5%)*

Explain to child that EMLA is like a "magic cream that takes hurt away." Tap or lightly scratch site of procedure to show child that "skin is now awake."

Apply thick layer (dollop) of EMLA over normal intact skin to anesthetize site (about ½ of 5 g tube; can use ⅓ of tube if puncture site is localized and superficial, e.g., intradermal injection or heel/finger puncture).

For venous access, apply to two sites; place enough cream on antecubital fossa to cover medial and lateral veins. Do not rub.

Place transparent adhesive dressing (e.g., Tegaderm) over EMLA. Make sure cream remains dollop. A piece of plastic film (e.g., food wrap) with tape to seal the edges can be used. Use only as much adhesive as needed to prevent leakage.

To make the dressing less accessible, cover it with a self-adhering Ace-type bandage, such as *Coban,* or an IV protector, such as *IV House.** Label the dressing with "EMLA applied," the date, and the time to distinguish it from other types of dressings. Instruct older children not to disturb the dressing. (Covering the dressing with an opaque material may reduce the attraction and discourage "fingering.") Supervise younger or cognitively compromised children throughout the application time.

Leave EMLA on skin for at least 60 minutes for superficial puncture and 120 minutes for deep penetration (e.g., IM injection, biopsy). EMLA may be applied at home and may need to be kept on longer in persons with dark and/or thicker skin. Anesthesia may last up to 3 hours after EMLA is removed.

Remove dressing before procedure and wipe cream from skin. With transparent adhesive, grasp opposite sides, and while holding dressing *parallel* to skin, pull sides away from each other to stretch and loosen dressing. An adhesive remover may be used.

Observe skin reaction, either blanched or reddened. If there is no obvious skin reaction, EMLA may not have penetrated adequately; test skin sensitivity and, if needed, reapply.

Repeat tapping or lightly scratching skin to show child that "skin is asleep" so that "it cannot feel a needle either."

After procedure, assess behavioral response. If child was upset, use pain scale (e.g., FACES) to help child distinguish between pain and fear.

In the United States, EMLA is not approved for use in infants under 1 month of age.† It should not be used in those rare patients with congenital or idiopathic methemoglobinemia and in infants under age 12 months who are receiving treatment with methemoglobin-inducing agents, e.g., sulfonamides, phenytoin (Dilantin), phenobarbital, and acetaminophen (Tylenol).

NOTE: EMLA is contraindicated in anyone with a known history of sensitivity or allergy to amide-type local anesthetics (lidocaine, prilocaine, mepivacaine, bupivacaine, etidocaine) or to any other component of the product.

EMLA cream maximum recommended application area to intact skin for infants and children

BODY WEIGHT (kg)	MAXIMUM APPLICATION AREA (cm^2)
up to 10 kg	100 (4″ × 4″)
10 to 20 kg	600 (10″ × 10″)
above 20 kg	2000 (18″ × 18″)

These are broad guidelines for avoiding systemic toxicity in applying EMLA to patients with normal, intact skin and with normal renal function and hepatic function.

For more individualized calculation of how much lidocaine and prilocaine may be absorbed, practitioners can use the following estimates of lidocaine and prilocaine absorption for children and adults:

The estimated mean (+SD) absorption of lidocaine is 0.045 (+0.016) mg/cm^2/hr.

The estimated mean (+SD) absorption of prilocaine is 0.077 (+0.036) mg/cm^2/hr.

Modified from Wong DL: Overcoming 'needle phobia' with EMLA, *Am J Nurs* 95(2):24, 1995.
*For more information, contact I.V. House, 7400 Foxmont Dr., Hazelwood, MO 63042-2198; 800-530-0400; FAX 314-831-3683.
†In Canada, EMLA is not approved for use in infants under 6 months of age.

has been used safely on newborns for circumcision and on preterm neonates for heel punctures (Benini and others, 1993; Taddio and others, 1995). It should be used cautiously on infants between ages 1 and 12 months who are receiving treatment with methemoglobin-inducing agents, such as sulfonamides, phenytoin (Dilantin), and acetaminophen (Tylenol). However, the use of these drugs is not a contraindication for applying EMLA, and there are no published reports of methemoglobinemia caused by EMLA when an infant received acetaminophen. Because of their diminished levels of erythrocyte-methemoglobin reductase, infants less than 3 months old are more susceptible to prilocaine-induced *methemoglobinemia,* a very rare and reversible side effect. *Methemoglobin* is a dysfunctional form of hemoglobin that reduces the oxygen-carrying capacity of the blood, causing cyanosis and hypoxemia. The use of IV methylene blue promptly eliminates the methemoglobinemia (Farrington, 1993). Other side effects are very mild and include pallor or erythema or edema at the application site.

The *intradermal route* is often used to inject a local anesthetic, typically lidocaine (Zylocaine), into the skin to reduce the pain from a lumbar puncture, bone marrow aspiration, or venous or arterial access. One problem with the use of lidocaine is the stinging and burning that initially occur. However, the use of *buffered lidocaine* reduces the stinging sensation (Orlinsky and others, 1992) (see Guidelines box). Warming the lidocaine to 37° C (98.6° F) may also accomplish the same effect (Davidson and Boom, 1992).

Right Time. The right timing for administering analgesics depends on the type of pain. For continuous pain control, such as for postoperative or cancer pain, a preventive schedule of medication *around the clock (ATC)* is effective. The ATC schedule avoids the low plasma concentrations that permit breakthrough pain. If analgesics are administered only when pain returns (a typical use of the PRN, or "as needed," order), pain relief may take several hours. This may require higher doses, leading to a cycle of undermedication of pain alternating with periods of overmedication and drug toxicity. This cycle of erratic pain control also promotes "clock watch-

ing," which may be erroneously equated with "addiction." Nurses can effectively use PRN orders by giving the drug at regular intervals, since "as needed" can be interpreted to mean "as needed to prevent return of pain."

Preventive pain control is best provided through continuous IV infusion rather than intermittent boluses. If intermittent boluses are given, the intervals between doses should not exceed the drug's expected duration of effectiveness. For extended pain control with fewer administration times, drugs that provide longer duration of action (e.g., some NSAIDs, time-released morphine or oxocodone, methadone, levorphanol) can be used.

> **Nursing ALERT**
>
> Since breakthrough pain can occur even with optimum ATC scheduling, there should be an order for PRN "rescue" doses of an analgesic.

Continuous analgesia is not always appropriate, because not all pain is continuous. Frequently, temporary pain control is needed to provide analgesia before a scheduled procedure. When pain can be predicted, the drug's peak effect should be timed to coincide with the painful event. For example, with opioids the peak effect is only a few minutes for the IV route; with nonopioids the peak effect occurs about 2 hours after oral administration. For rapid onset and peak of action, opioids that quickly penetrate the blood-brain barrier (e.g., IV fentanyl) provide excellent pain control.

Observe for Side Effects. Both NSAIDs and opioids have side effects, although the major concern is with those from opioids (see box below). Respiratory depression is the most serious complication and is most likely to occur in sedated patients. The respiratory rate may decrease gradually or may cease abruptly; lower limits of normal are not established for children, but any significant change from a previous rate calls for increased vigilance. A slower respiratory rate does not necessarily reflect decreased arterial oxygenation; an increased depth of ventilation may compensate for the altered

---

GUIDELINES
Using Buffered Lidocaine (BL)

Supplies: 8.4% sodium bicarbonate (1 mEq/ml), 1% or 2% lidocaine with or without epinephrine, syringe with removable needle, and a 30-gauge needle

Instructions:
Use 1 part sodium bicarbonate to 10 parts lidocaine (i.e., draw up 1 ml of lidocaine and 0.1 ml of sodium bicarbonate).
Change needle used to withdraw BL to 30-gauge needle for intradermal injection.
For venipuncture or port access, inject 0.1 ml or less BL intradermally directly over intended puncture site; anesthesia occurs almost immediately.
Suggested maximum dose of lidocaine for local anesthesia is 4.5 mg/kg.
If buffering lidocaine vial (e.g., 20 ml lidocaine with 2 ml sodium bicarbonate), use solution for 7 days or less and preferably when freshly prepared.

SIDE EFFECTS OF OPIOIDS

General
Constipation (possibly severe)
Respiratory depression
Sedation
Nausea and vomiting
Agitation, euphoria
Mental clouding
Hallucinations
Orthostatic hypotension
Pruritus
Urticaria
Sweating
Miosis (may be sign of toxicity)
Anaphylaxis (rare)

Signs of Tolerance
Decreasing pain relief
Decreasing duration of pain relief

Signs of Physical Dependence
Initial signs of withdrawal:
  Lacrimation
  Rhinorrhea
  Yawning
  Sweating
Later signs:
  Restlessness
  Irritability
  Tremors
  Anorexia
  Dilated pupils
  Gooseflesh

GUIDELINES
Managing Opioid-Induced
Respiratory Depression

If respirations are depressed:
Assess sedation level (see Fig. 21-5 for sedation scale)
Reduce infusion by 25% when possible.
Stimulate patient (shake gently, call by name, ask to breathe).
If patient cannot be aroused or is apneic (American Pain Society, 1992):
Administer naloxone (Narcan):
For children less than 40 kg: dilute 0.1 mg of naloxone in 10 ml of sterile saline to make 10 μg/ml solution and give 0.5 μg/kg.
For children over 40 kg: dilute 0.4 mg ampule in 10 ml of sterile saline and give 0.5 ml.
Administer bolus slow IV push every 2 minutes until effect is obtained.
Closely monitor patient. Naloxone's duration of antagonist action may be shorter than that of opioid, requiring repeated doses of naloxone
NOTE: Respiratory depression caused by benzodiazepines (e.g., diazepam [Valium] or midazolam [Versed]) can be reversed with flumazenil (Romazicon). Pediatric dosing experience suggests 0.01 mg/kg (0.1 ml/kg) as loading dose followed by 0.005 mg/kg/min (0.05 ml/kg/min) until awake or to a maximum of 1 mg (10 ml) (Deshpande and Tobias, 1996). The recommended initial dose for children 20 kg or more is 0.2 mg (2 ml) IV over 15 seconds; if no response after 45 seconds, administer same dose and repeat as needed at 60-second intervals for maximum dose of 1 mg (10 ml).

• Gradually reduce dose (similar to tapering of steroids):
Give one half of previous daily dose in q 6 hr doses for first 2 days.
Then reduce dose by 25% every 2 days.
• Continue this schedule until total daily dose of 0.6 mg/kg/day of morphine (or equivalent) is reached.
• After 2 days on this dose, discontinue opioid.
• May also switch to oral methadone, using one fourth of equianalgesic dose as initial weaning dose and proceeding as described above.

Use Supportive Statements When Administering Analgesics. The effectiveness of analgesics can be enhanced by a supportive attitude toward the child. By reinforcing the cause and effect of the medication and analgesia, the nurse can condition the child to expect pain relief, provided the regimen is likely to be effective. Although IM injections should *not* be given, when they are, children need to understand that the "little hurt from the needle will take away the bigger hurt for a long time."

Parents and older children may have concerns about the use of opioids because of fear of addiction. These concerns should be addressed with assurance that any such risk is extremely low. It may be helpful to ask the question, "If you did not have this pain, would you want to take this medicine?" The answer is invariably no, which reinforces the solely therapeutic nature of the drug. It is also important to avoid making statements to the family such as "We don't want you to get used to this medicine" or "By now you shouldn't need this medicine," which may reinforce the fear of becoming addicted.

Provide Developmentally Appropriate Activities

A primary goal of nursing care for the child who is hospitalized is to minimize threats to the child's development. Many strategies (e.g., minimizing separation) have been discussed and may be all that the short-term patient requires. However, children who experience prolonged or repeated hospitalization are at greater risk for developmental delays or regression. The nurse who provides opportunities for the child to participate in developmentally appropriate activities further normalizes the child's environment and helps reduce interference with the child's ongoing development (see Normalization, Chapter 18).

Play is the "work" of children of all ages and assumes a critical role in their development. Because of its other important purposes in the hospital setting, play is the focus of a separate discussion.

Perhaps at no other age is the concept of interference with normal development more crucial than when it is applied to the rapidly developing infant and toddler. The nurse plays a primary role in identifying children at risk and helping to plan, implement, and evaluate developmental intervention (see Chapters 10 and 12).

School is an integral part of the school-age child's and adolescent's development. Accreditation standards for hospitals serving children consider access to appropriate educational services a key factor in the accreditation decision process when a child's treatment requires a significant absence from school. The nurse can encourage children to resume schoolwork as quickly as their condition permits, help them sched-

rate (Rowbotham and others, 1989). If respiratory depression or arrest occurs, the nurse must be prepared to intervene quickly (Pasero and McCaffery, 1994) (see Guidelines box).

Although respiratory depression is the most feared side effect, constipation is a common side, and sometimes serious, effect of opioids, which decrease peristaltic activity and increase anal sphincter tone. Prevention with stool softeners and laxatives is more effective than treatment once constipation occurs. Dietary treatment, such as increased fiber, is usually not sufficient to promote regular bowel evacuation. However, dietary measures, such as increased fluid, fruit, and bran intake, and especially activity, are encouraged.

Pruritus from epidural or intrathecal infusion can be treated with low doses of naloxone infused slowly or with IV nalbuphine. Pruritus from IV infusion usually responds to oral antihistamines. Nausea, vomiting, and sedation usually subside after 2 days of opioid administration, although intravenous, oral, or rectal antiemetics may be necessary.

Both tolerance and physical dependence can occur with prolonged use of opioids. Treatment of tolerance involves increasing the dose or decreasing the duration between doses. Treatment of physical dependence involves gradually reducing the dose over several days to prevent occurrence of withdrawal symptoms (similar to tapering of steroid dosages after chronic steroid therapy). The following are suggested guidelines for treating physical dependence (American Pain Society, 1992):

ule and protect a selected time for studies, and help the family coordinate hospital educational services with their children's schools. Children should have the opportunity to "keep up" with art and music classes, as well as their academic subjects.

To meet the unique developmental needs of adolescents, special units have been developed that provide privacy, increased socialization, and appropriate activities for these young people. Typically these units are set apart from the general pediatric facility so that the teenagers do not share space with younger children, who are often perceived as a threat to their maturity.

NURSING TIP When adolescents must share a common activity room with younger patients, referring to the area as the "activity" room rather than the "playroom" may entice them to visit the room and participate in activities.

These units also provide more flexible routines and activities, such as more group activity, wearing of street clothes, provisions to leave the adolescent unit temporarily, and access to the items so critical to teenagers—telephones, compact disc and tape players, videocassette recorders (VCRs), computers, and televisions. Because adolescents' food habits are rarely limited to the three traditional meals a day, a ready supply of snacks should be available. However, the most important benefit of these units is increased socialization with peers. In addition, staff members usually enjoy working with this age-group and are well suited to establishing the trust so essential for communication.

Provide Opportunities for Play/Expressive Activities

Play is one of the most important aspects of a child's life and one of the most effective tools for managing stress. Since illness and hospitalization constitute crises in a child's life, and since these situations are often fraught with overwhelming stresses, children need to play out their fears and anxieties as a means of coping with these stresses.

Play is essential to children's mental, emotional, and social well-being, and as with their developmental needs, the need for play does not stop when children are ill or in the hospital. On the contrary, play in the hospital serves many functions (see box).

FUNCTIONS OF PLAY IN THE HOSPITAL

Provides diversion and brings about relaxation
Helps the child feel more secure in a strange environment
Helps to lessen the stress of separation and the feelings of homesickness
Provides a means for release of tension and expression of feelings
Encourages interaction and development of positive attitudes toward others
Provides an expressive outlet for creative ideas and interests
Provides a means for accomplishing therapeutic goals (see Use of Play in Procedures, Chapter 22)
Places child in active role and provides opportunity to make choices and be in control

---

Engaging in such activities puts children in charge, removing them for a time from the usual passive role of recipients of a constant stream of "things" being done to them. In the hospital environment, most decisions are made for the child; play and other expressive activities offer the child much-needed opportunities to make choices. Even if a child chooses not to participate in a particular activity, the nurse has offered the child a choice, perhaps one of but a few real choices the child has had that day (Rollins, 1993).

Of all hospital facilities, probably no room does more to alleviate the stressors of hospitalization than the playroom or activity room. In this room children temporarily distance themselves from the fears of separation, loss of control, and bodily injury. They can work through their feelings in a nonthreatening, comfortable atmosphere and in the manner that is most natural for them. They also know that the boundaries of this room are safe from intrusive or painful procedures and probing questions (see Critical Thinking Exercise).

Diversional Activities. Almost any form of play can be used for diversion and recreation, but the activity should be selected on the basis of the child's age, interests, and limitations (Fig. 21-10). Children do not necessarily need special direction for using play materials. All they require is the raw materials with which to work and adult approval and supervision to help keep their natural enthusiasm or expression of feelings from getting out of control. Small children enjoy a variety of small, colorful toys that they can play with in bed or in their room, or more elaborate play equipment, such as playhouses, sandboxes, rhythm instruments, or large boxes and blocks, that may be a part of the hospital playroom.

CRITICAL **THINKING EXERCISE**
The Playroom

You are watching 7-year-old Hannah playing Candyland with her brother, sister, and several other children in the playroom. A laboratory technician enters the playroom and says, "Hannah, I need to take some blood. I can see that you are playing a game, so I'll just do it while you play. It will just take a minute." Your most appropriate response would be which of the following?

1. "Go right ahead. It's silly to have to interrupt her game."
2. "Let me help you so that you can finish sooner."
3. "Hannah, is this okay with you?"
4. "We don't allow any procedures in the playroom."

Number four is the best response. The playroom should be considered a safe place—a sanctuary—and therefore off-limits for procedures. In many hospitals the child's bed is accorded the same status; children are taken to a treatment room. Even if it is "okay" with Hannah (number three), it is important to consider the possible impact on the other children in the room, who may be confused about even a simple procedure (e.g., checking blood pressure) or the sanctuary status of the playroom for themselves.

An exception is sometimes made when all the children present are older and the procedure is a quick, painless one (e.g., checking blood pressure or giving oral medication) that all the children present have experienced. In such cases the patient and the other children are asked if it is okay and give permission before the procedure is undertaken.

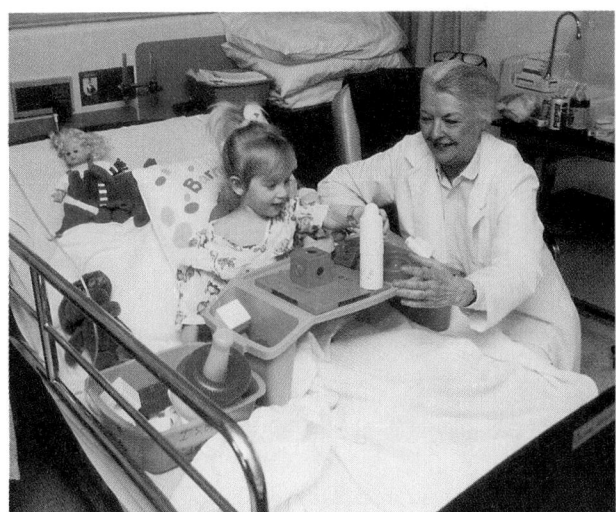

FIG. 21-10. Play materials for children in the hospital need to be appropriate for their age, interests, and limitations.

Games that can be played alone or with another child or an adult are popular with older children, as are puzzles; reading material; quiet, individual activities, such as sewing, stringing beads, and weaving; and Lego blocks and other building materials. Assembling models is an excellent pastime, but one should make certain that all pieces and necessary materials are included in the package. It is disappointing to the child to be ready to begin a project only to find that an essential item, such as glue, is missing from the set.

Well-selected books are of infinite value to the child. Children never tire of stories; having someone read aloud gives them endless hours of pleasure and is of special value to the child who has limited energy to expend in play. A radio, VCR, electronic games, and television, included among most hospital room equipment, are useful tools for entertaining a child, but parents and nurses should monitor program selection and the time spent using these devices to avoid their becoming a substitute for social interaction or therapeutic play.

When supervising play for ill or convalescent children, it is best to select activities that are simpler than would normally be chosen according to the specific developmental level of the child. These children usually do not have the energy to cope with more challenging activities. Other limitations also influence the type of activities. Special consideration must be given to the child who is confined in terms of movement, has a restricted extremity, or is isolated. Toys for isolated children may need to be disinfected before and/or after use.

Toys. Parents of hospitalized children often ask nurses about the types of toys that would be best to bring for their child. It is wise to assure the parents that although it is natural to want to provide new toys for their child, it is often better to wait awhile to bring new things, especially in the case of younger children. Small children need the comfort and reassurance of familiar things, such as the stuffed animal the child hugs for comfort and takes to bed at night. These familiar items are a link with home and the world outside the hospital.

Large numbers of toys often confuse and frustrate a small child. A few small, well-chosen toys are usually preferred to one large, expensive one. Children who are hospitalized for an extended time benefit from changes. Rather than a confusing accumulation of toys, older toys should be replaced periodically as interest wanes.

NURSING TIP Have parents provide the child with a shoe box, a child's small suitcase, or a knapsack to attach to the bed for an easy storage receptacle to prevent small items from becoming lost in the sheets or under the bed.

Children love putting things in and taking things out of a larger container. Many simple items, such as a small magnifying glass, a magnet, grooming aids, a small mirror, crayons and drawing paper, colorful paper with scissors and paste, a magic slate, small dolls or toy soldiers, small cars, and beads to string, afford endless hours of amusement. It is the nurse's responsibility to assess the safety of the toys brought to the child.

A highly successful diversion for a child who is hospitalized for a length of time and whose parents are unable to visit frequently is having the parents bring a box with seven small, inexpensive, brightly wrapped items with a different day of the week printed on the outside of each package. The child will eagerly anticipate the time for opening each one. When the parents know when their next visit will be, they can provide the number of packages that corresponds to the days between visits. In this way the child knows that the diminishing packages also represent the anticipated visit from the parent.

Expressive Activities. Play and other expressive activities provide one of the best opportunities for encouraging emotional expression, including the safe release of anger and hostility. Nondirective play that allows children freedom for expression can be tremendously therapeutic. Therapeutic play, however, should not be confused with *play therapy,* a psychologic technique reserved for use by trained and qualified therapists as an interpretative method with emotionally disturbed children. *Therapeutic play,* on the other hand, is a very effective, nondirective modality for helping children deal with their concerns and fears, and at the same time it often helps the nurse to gain insights into children's needs and feelings.

Tension release can be facilitated through almost any activity, and with younger ambulatory children, large-muscle activity such as use of tricycles and wagons is especially beneficial. Much aggression can be safely directed into pounding and throwing games and activities. Beanbags are often thrown at a target or open receptacle with surprising vigor and hostility. A pounding board is employed with enthusiasm by young children; clay and playdough are marvelous media for use at any age.

Creative Expression. Although all children derive physical, social, emotional, and cognitive benefits from engaging in art or other creative activities, children's need for such activities is intensified when they are hospitalized (Rollins, 1995). Children are more at ease expressing their thoughts and feelings through art, since humans think first in images and later learn to translate these images into words. A child's drawing before surgery, for example, will often re-

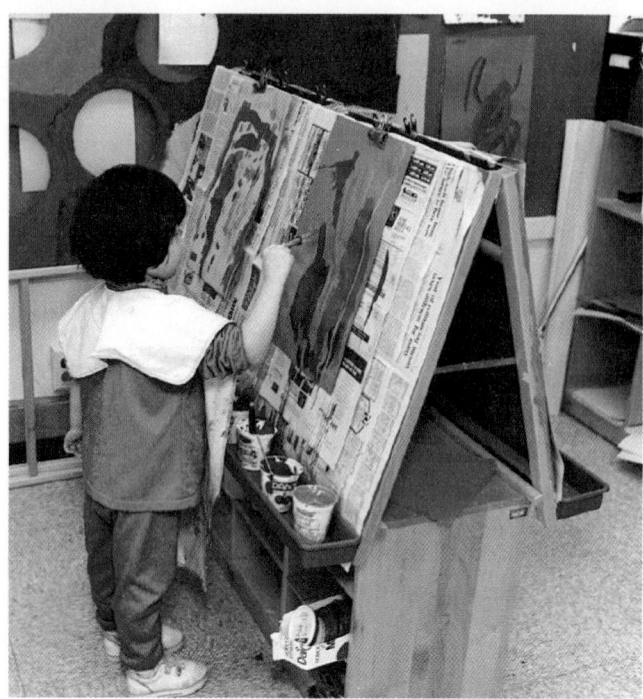

FIG. 21-11. Drawing and painting are excellent media for expression.

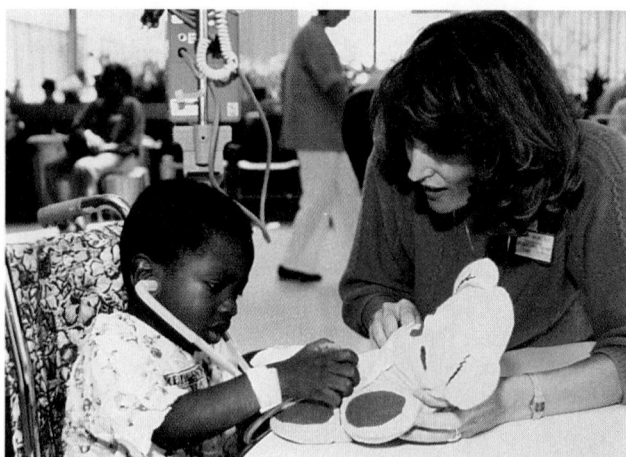

FIG. 21-12. Playing with stuffed animals allows children to safely explore feelings and concerns. (Courtesy St. Louis Children's Hospital.)

veal unvoiced concerns about mutilation, body changes, and loss of self-control (O'Malley and McNamara, 1993). Drawing and painting are excellent media for expression. The child needs only to be supplied with the raw materials, such as crayons and paper; pots of bright poster color, large brushes, and an ample supply of newsprint supported on easels; or materials for finger painting (Fig. 21-11). Children can work individually or collaborate on a group project, such as a mural painted on a long piece of paper. For children confined to bed, an old sheet (acquired from the laundry) spread over the bed and a large gown that extends down over the bedclothes to cover the child's own gown provide protection for clean linen.

Although interpretation of children's drawing requires special training, observing changes in a series of the child's drawings over time can be helpful in assessing psychosocial adjustment and coping (Rae, 1991). The nurse can use children's drawings, stories, poetry, and other products of creative expression as a springboard for discussion of thoughts, fears, and understanding of concepts or events (see Communication Techniques, Chapter 6).

Nurses can incorporate opportunities for musical expression into routine nursing care. For example, simple musical instruments, such as bracelets with bells, can be placed on infants' legs for them to shake to accompany mealtime music or dressing changes. Dance and movement suggestions may encourage a child to ambulate.

Holidays provide stimulus and direction for unlimited creative projects. Children can participate in decorating the pediatric unit, and making pictures and decorations for their rooms gives the children a sense of pride and accomplishment. This is especially beneficial for children who are im-

mobilized and isolated. Making gifts for someone at home helps to maintain interpersonal ties.

Dramatic Play.   Dramatic play is a well-recognized technique for emotional release, allowing children to reenact frightening or puzzling hospital experiences. Through use of puppets, replicas of hospital equipment, or some actual hospital equipment, children can play out the situations that are a part of their hospital experience. Dramatic play enables children to learn about procedures and events that will concern them and to assume the roles of the adults in the hospital environment.

Puppets are universally effective for communicating with children. Most children see them as peers and readily communicate with them. Children will relate to the puppet feelings that they hesitate to express to adults. Puppets can share children's own experiences and help them to find solutions to their problems. Puppets dressed to represent figures in the child's environment—for example, a physician, nurse, child patient, therapist, and members of the child's own family— are especially useful (Fig. 21-12). Small, appropriately attired dolls are equally effective in encouraging the child to play out situations, although puppets are usually best for direct conversation.

NURSING TIP Make a simple puppet using a large handkerchief. Place some cotton balls in the center of the cloth and wrap a rubberband over the handkerchief and cotton balls to form a "head." Place the head over the index finger so that the rubberband secures it to the finger. Let the cloth drape over the front and back of the hand. The cloth forms four parts of the puppet: the index finger is the head, the thumb and other fingers are the arms, and the draped cloth is the body. Decorate the head by drawing features on it.

Play must consider medical needs, but at times a procedure can be postponed for a short time to allow the child to complete a special activity (see Critical Thinking Exercise). Play must consider any limitations imposed by the child's condition. For example, small children may eat paste and other creative media; therefore a child who is allergic to wheat

Robert, 5 years old, is recovering from abdominal surgery. You enter his room to check his dressing. His mother is reading him a story. Your most appropriate response would be which of the following?

1. To Robert's mother: "I need to check Robert's dressing."
2. "Robert, I need to check your dressing, but I can see that you are in the middle of a story right now. I'll check back in about 5 minutes and do it then."
3. "It's time to check your dressing, Robert. Let's get started."
4. "Robert, I need to check your dressing. It should take about 5 minutes. Would you like me to check it now, or to come back in about 10 minutes when you have finished hearing the story?"

Your best response would be number four, although number two would also be acceptable. Number four not only indicates that you value and respect the activity Robert is engaged in, but also offers him an opportunity to make a choice: to interrupt the story and complete the procedure, or to finish the story and wait for your return. If, because of your own schedule, you are unable to offer such choices, express your desire come back later, but explain that this time it is impossible. Number one ignores Robert's presence; number three fosters a passive role.

should not be given finger paint made from wallpaper paste or playdough made with flour. A child on a restricted salt intake should not play with modeling dough, since salt is one of its major constituents. At home the play program can be planned around the therapy regimen. However, play can be satisfactorily incorporated into the child's care if the nurse and others involved allow some flexibility and use creativity in planning for play.

Maximize Potential Benefits of Hospitalization

Foster Parent-Child Relationships. The crisis of illness and/or hospitalization can mobilize parents into more acute awareness of the needs of their children. For example, one school-age child who was diagnosed with a serious physical condition commented to the nurse that he "enjoyed" the hospital because it was the first time that he had seen so much of his parents. He expressed concern over discharge because he anticipated the loss of the intensified love and attention. The nurse was able to discuss these feelings with the parents and to increase their awareness of their child's need for them.

Hospitalization provides opportunities for parents to learn more about their children's growth and development. When parents are helped to understand children's usual reactions to stress, such as regression or aggression, they are not only better able to support the child through the hospital experience, but also may extend their insights into childrearing practices after discharge.

Difficulties in parent-child relationships that may result in feeding problems, negative behavior, and sleep disturbances may decrease during hospitalization. The temporary cessation

of such problems sometimes alerts parents to the role they may be playing in propagating the negative behavior. With assistance from health professionals, parents can restructure ways of relating to their children to foster more positive behavior.

Hospitalization may also represent a temporary reprieve or refuge from a disturbed home. Typically, abused or neglected children's dramatic physical and social improvement during hospitalization is proof of the growth potential of this experience. Hospitalized children temporarily are able to seek support, reassurance, and security from new relationships, particularly with nurses and hospitalized peers.

Provide Educational Opportunities. Illness and hospitalization represent excellent opportunities for children and other family members to learn more about their bodies, each other, and the health professions. For example, during a hospital admission for a diabetic crisis, the child may learn about the disease; the parents may learn about the child's needs for independence, normalcy, and appropriate limits; and each of them may find a new support system in the hospital staff.

The special tutoring that children may receive during extended hospitalizations can help them advance their studies and concentrate on subjects that were difficult. The child's relationship with a tutor can foster a more positive attitude toward school and learning.

Illness or hospitalization can also help older children in choosing a vocation. Frequently children have impressions of physicians or nurses that are disproportionately glorified or horrified. Actual experience with different health professionals can influence their attitude about health professionals and even a decision regarding a health career.

Promote Self-Mastery. The experience of facing a crisis such as illness or hospitalization, coping successfully with it, and maturing as a result of it constitutes an opportunity for self-mastery. Younger children have the chance to test fantasy vs reality fears. They realize that they were not abandoned, mutilated, castrated, or punished. In fact, they were loved, cared for, and treated with respect for their individual concerns. It is not unusual for children who have undergone hospitalization or surgery to tell others that "it was nothing" or to display proudly their scars or bandages. For older children, hospitalization may represent an opportunity for decision making, independence, and self-reliance. They are proud of having survived the experience and may feel a genuine self-respect for their achievements. Nurses can facilitate such feelings of self-mastery by emphasizing aspects of personal competence in the child and not focusing on uncooperative or negative behavior.

Provide Socialization. Hospitalization may offer children a special opportunity for social acceptance. Lonely, asocial, sometimes delinquent children find a sympathetic environment in the hospital. Children who are physically deformed or in some other way "different" from their age-mates may find an accepting social peer group (Fig. 21-13). Although this does not always spontaneously occur, nurses can structure the environment to foster a supportive child group. For example, selection of a compatible roommate can help children gain a new friend and learn more about themselves. Forming relationships with significant members of the health care team, such as the physician, nurse, child-life spe-

Text continued on p. 654.

NURSING CARE PLAN
The Child in the Hospital

NURSING DIAGNOSIS: Anxiety/fear related to separation from accustomed routine and support system; unfamiliar surroundings

PATIENT GOAL 1: Will experience minimized separation

- **NURSING INTERVENTIONS/RATIONALES**

Assign same nursing personnel as much as possible and a primary nurse *to provide the consistency that builds trust*
Arrange workload and schedule to allow personal contact with child
Encourage parents to room-in whenever possible *to prevent separation*
Provide an atmosphere of warmth and acceptance for both child and parents
Encourage parents and others to cuddle, hug, and otherwise demonstrate affection for child
Recognize child's separation behaviors as normal
    Allow child to cry, *since this is a normal response to separation*
    Provide support through physical presence
Maintain child's contact with parents and siblings
    Talk about child's parents frequently
    Encourage child to talk about and remember family members, pets
    Stress significance of parents' and siblings' visits, telephone calls, or letters
Help parents understand the behaviors of separation anxiety and suggest ways of supporting the child
    Explain to child when parents leave and when they will return
    Tell hospitalized child the reason for leaving
    Convey the expected time of return in terms of anticipated events; for example, if the parents will return in the morning, they can say they will see the child "After the sun comes up" or "When (a favorite program) is on television"
    Use a clock or calendar for an older child *so child can anticipate next family visit*
    Visit for short but frequent times rather than one long time; encourage parents and relatives to take turns visiting
    Encourage siblings, grandparents, and other significant persons in child's life to visit
    Leave favorite articles from home, such as a blanket, toy, bottle, feeding utensil, or article of clothing, with child, *since this helps child tolerate separation*
    Respect treasured objects of older children, such as a stuffed animal
    Encourage family to provide photographs of family members and recordings of the parents' voices (e.g., reading a story, singing a song, saying prayers before bedtime, relating events at home) *to familiarize the unfamiliar environment and to provide comfort during times of separation*
Play family recordings at lonely times, such as before sleep

Suggest that the family leave small gifts for the child to open each day: if the parents know when their next visit will be, have them leave the number of packages that correspond to the days between visits
Assign a "foster grandparent" or consistent volunteer to be with child if available

- **EXPECTED OUTCOMES**

Child has consistent caregivers
Parents visit as much as possible
Parents cooperate in care (specify)
Child accepts and responds positively to comforting measures
Child discusses the family, including pets
Parents demonstrate an understanding of separation behaviors
Siblings, grandparents, and other significant persons visit as much as possible
Family provides child with familiar and/or cherished articles from home
Assigned person spends time with child (specify amount)

PATIENT GOAL 2: Will express feelings

- **NURSING INTERVENTIONS/RATIONALES**

Accept expression of feelings *so that child continues these expressions*
Provide an atmosphere that encourages free expression of feelings
Provide opportunities for the child to verbalize, "play out," or otherwise express feelings without fear of punishment
Encourage drawing and other expressive activities *because children often find it easier to express themselves in images instead of words*
Encourage keeping a journal or diary *to allow child to review progress and changes in feelings*

- **EXPECTED OUTCOME**

Child verbalizes or plays out feelings or concerns

PATIENT GOAL 3: Will remain calm

- **NURSING INTERVENTIONS/RATIONALES**

Do nothing to make child more anxious, remembering that what may not provoke anxiety in an adult may make a child very anxious
Maintain a calm, relaxed, and reassuring manner
Spend time with child and family *to establish rapport*
Give competent, consistent nursing care *to instill confidence in both parents and child*
Try to avoid intrusive procedures

- **EXPECTED OUTCOMES**

Child exhibits no signs of apprehension
Parents relate readily with personnel and calmly with child
Child rests quietly and calmly

PATIENT GOAL 4: Will exhibit trusting behaviors

- **NURSING INTERVENTIONS/RATIONALES**

Be positive in approach to child
Be honest with child *to encourage child to trust*
Convey to child the behaviors expected

NURSING CARE PLAN
The Child in the Hospital—cont'd

Be consistent in expectations and relationships with child *because consistency is an important component of the development of trust*

Treat child fairly and help child to feel this

Encourage parents to maintain a truthful relationship with the child

Make certain child has call light or other signal device within reach

• EXPECTED OUTCOMES

Child develops rapport with primary nurse

Child maintains trust of family

PATIENT GOAL 5: Will experience feelings of security

• NURSING INTERVENTIONS/*RATIONALES*

Maintain child's identity

    Address child by name or usual nickname

    Avoid assigning a nickname to child or converting a given name to its counterpart in another language (e.g., using Joe instead of José)

Avoid communicating any signals of rejection, distaste, or other negative feelings to child

Criticize or communicate disapproval of unacceptable *behavior,* not disapproval of the *child*

Communicate (verbally and nonverbally) that the child is a valued person

Discourage treatments or procedures in the child's room or playroom *to maintain these areas as "safe places"*

• EXPECTED OUTCOMES

Child interacts with staff

*Staff demonstrates respect for child

PATIENT GOAL 6: Will experience reduction of or no fear

• NURSING INTERVENTIONS/*RATIONALES*

Explain routines, items, procedures, and events in a language and method appropriate to the child's developmental level; use simple language, drawings, and play *to facilitate understanding and mastery*

Reassure child and repeat reassurance as necessary

Ask child to explain reason for hospitalization and correct if necessary *to help absolve child from any guilt about being hospitalized*

Encourage parent(s) to participate in child's care

Encourage child to handle items that may seem strange or threatening *to reduce fear of the unknown*

Give encouragement and positive feedback for cooperation in care

• EXPECTED OUTCOMES

Child exhibits understanding of information presented (specify information and means of demonstration)

Child discusses procedures and activities without evidence of anxiety

*Nursing outcome.

PATIENT GOAL 7: Will be allowed to regress

• NURSING INTERVENTIONS/*RATIONALES*

Recognize that regressive behavior is a feature of illness *so that it is not viewed as abnormal*

Accept regressive behavior and help child with dependency

Assist child in reconquering the negative counterpart of the psychosocial stage to which child has regressed (e.g., overcome mistrust; facilitate development of trust)

• EXPECTED OUTCOME

*Staff and parents exhibit an attitude of acceptance of regressive behaviors

PATIENT GOAL 8: Will experience adequate comfort level

• NURSING INTERVENTIONS/*RATIONALES*

Provide pacifier, if appropriate, *to meet oral needs and to provide comfort*

Hold infant or young child when this does not interfere with therapy

Touch, talk, and otherwise comfort child who cannot be held

Provide sensory stimulation and diversion appropriate to child's level of development

Encourage family members to visit and allow them to comfort and care for child to the extent possible

• EXPECTED OUTCOMES

Child engages in nonnutritive sucking

Child exhibits no signs of distress

Family is involved in care

> **NURSING DIAGNOSIS:** Anxiety/fear related to distressing procedures, events

PATIENT GOAL 1 Will be prepared for hospitalization

• NURSING INTERVENTIONS/*RATIONALES*

Prepare child as needed *to reduce fear of the unknown and to promote cooperation*

Select appropriate preparatory materials

Involve parents *to enable them to serve as effective resources for their child*

Modify preparation in special situations (e.g., ambulatory/outpatient setting, emergency admission, ICU) (see pp. 663-666)

• EXPECTED OUTCOME

Child is prepared for hospital experience

PATIENT GOAL 2: Will exhibit decreased fear of bodily injury

• NURSING INTERVENTIONS/*RATIONALES*

Recognize developmental fears associated with illness and procedures *to ensure appropriate intervention*

Provide age-appropriate explanations for procedures, especially those that are intrusive or involve the genitals, and include information about what body parts will not be affected, as well as those that will

Continued.

Provide age-appropriate explanations for procedures the child may see or hear performed on other patients *to decrease child's fears*

Reassure child that certain body parts can be removed without producing harm (e.g., blood, tonsils, appendix)

Provide privacy for any procedure that exposes the body

Protect child from seeing unclothed patients

Use interventions that preserve child's concept of body integrity (e.g., bandages over puncture sites)

• **EXPECTED OUTCOME**

Child displays minimum fear of bodily injury

PATIENT GOAL 3: Will receive support during tests and procedures

• **NURSING INTERVENTIONS/***RATIONALES*

Prepare child for procedures according to age and level of understanding, including strategies for coping

Remain with child *to provide support by physical presence*

Prepare child and family for surgery if appropriate

Answer questions and explain purposes of activities

Keep child (and family) informed of progress

• **EXPECTED OUTCOME**

Child remains calm and cooperative during procedures

NURSING DIAGNOSIS: Pain related to (specify)

PATIENT GOAL 1: Will perceive less pain by using appropriate strategies

• **NURSING INTERVENTIONS/***RATIONALES*

Employ nonpharmacologic strategies to help child manage pain *because techniques such as relaxation, rhythmic breathing, and distraction can make pain more tolerable*

Use strategy that is familiar to child or describe several strategies and let child select one (see Guidelines, p. 634) *to facilitate child's learning and use of strategy*

Involve parent in selection of strategy *because parent knows child best*

Select appropriate person(s), usually parent, to assist child with strategy

Teach child to use specific nonpharmacologic strategies before pain occurs or before it becomes severe, *since these approaches appear to be most effective for mild pain*

Assist or have parent assist child with using strategy during actual pain *because coaching may be needed to help child focus on required actions*

• **EXPECTED OUTCOMES**

Child exhibits acceptable pain level

Child learns and implements effective coping strategies

Parent learns coping skills and is effective in assisting child to cope

PATIENT GOAL 2: Will experience no pain or reduction of pain to level acceptable to child when receiving analgesics

• **NURSING INTERVENTIONS/***RATIONALES*

Plan to administer prescribed analgesic before procedure *so that its peak effect coincides with painful event*

Plan preventive schedule of medication around the clock (ATC) or "PRN as needed to prevent pain" when pain is continuous and predictable (e.g., postoperatively) *to maintain steady blood levels of analgesic*

Administer analgesia by least traumatic route whenever possible *to avoid causing additional pain;* avoid intramuscular or subcutaneous injections (see box, p. 640)

Prepare child for administration of analgesia by using supportive statements (e.g., "This medicine I am putting in the IV will make you feel better in a few minutes")

Reinforce effect of analgesic by saying that child will begin to feel better in (fill in appropriate amount of time, according to drug use); use clock or timer to measure onset of relief with child; reinforce cause and effect of pain and analgesic *so that child becomes conditioned to expecting relief*

If injection must be given, avoid saying, "I am going to give you an injection for pain," *since this is another pain in addition to the existing pain;* if child refuses injection, explain that the little hurt from the needle will take away the bigger hurt for a long time

Avoid statements such as "This is enough medicine to take away anyone's pain" or "By now you shouldn't need so much pain medicine," *because they convey a judgmental and belittling attitude*

Give child control whenever possible (e.g., using patient-controlled analgesia, choosing which arm for a venipuncture, taking bandages off, holding tape or other equipment)

*Administer prescribed analgesic; nonopioids, including acetaminophen (Tylenol, paracetamol) and nonsteroidal anti-inflammatory drugs (NSAIDs), are suitable for mild to moderate pain (Table 21-3); opioids are needed for moderate to severe pain (Table 21-4); combination of the two analgesics (see Table 21-5) attacks pain at peripheral nervous system and at central nervous system and provides increased analgesia without increased side effects

Titrate (adjust) dosage for maximum pain relief

Begin with recommended dosage for age and weight

Increase dosage and/or decrease dose interval between dosages if pain relief is inadequate

If using parenteral route, change to oral route as soon as possible using equianalgesic dosages (see Tables 21-4 and 21-5) *because of first-pass effect (oral opioid is rapidly absorbed from gastrointestinal tract and enters portal circulation, where it is partially metabolized before reaching central circulation; therefore oral dosages must be larger)*

*Avoid combining opioids with so-called "potentiators," *since combining drugs such as promethazine (Phenergan) and chlorpromazine (Thorazine) adds risk of sedation and respiratory depression without increasing analgesia (for alternative drugs to the Demerol, Phenergan, and Thorazine (DPT) mixture, see box, p. 636)*

---

*Dependent nursing action.

NURSING CARE PLAN
The Child in the Hospital—cont'd

Do not use placebos in the assessment or treatment of pain, *since deceptive use of placebos does not provide useful information about presence or severity of pain, can cause side effects similar to those of opioids, can destroy child's and family's trust in health care staff, and raises serious ethical and legal questions*

• **EXPECTED OUTCOMES**

Child exhibits absence or minimal evidence of pain
Child accepts administration of analgesia with minimal distress

---

NURSING DIAGNOSIS: High risk for poisoning or injury related to sensitivity, excessive dose, decreased gastrointestinal motility

---

PATIENT GOAL 1: Will exhibit normal respiratory function

• **NURSING INTERVENTIONS/*RATIONALES***

Monitor rate and depth of respirations and level of sedation *because depression of these functions can lead to apnea*
Have emergency drugs and equipment in case of respiratory depression from opioids (see box, p. 643) to begin therapy as soon as needed

• **EXPECTED OUTCOME**

Child's respirations and sedation level remain within acceptable limits (see inside back cover for normal variations)

PATIENT GOAL 2: Will not develop constipation and will receive treatment for other opioid-related side effects

• **NURSING INTERVENTIONS/*RATIONALES***

*Administer stool softener or laxative *to prevent constipation*
Stop or decrease medication if evidence of rash
*Administer antipruritic *for itching*
*Administer antiemetic for nausea and vomiting
Encourage child to lie quietly *because movement increases nausea and vomiting*
Recognize signs of tolerance: decreasing pain relief, decreasing duration of pain relief
Recognize signs of withdrawal after discontinuation of drug (physical dependence) (see box, p. 642)
†Help treat tolerance and physical dependence appropriately *because these are involuntary, physiologic responses that occur from prolonged use of opioids*
Never refer to child who is tolerant or physically dependent as "addicted"

• **EXPECTED OUTCOMES**

Child has regular bowel movements
Child exhibits no evidence of rash or itching
Child receives appropriate therapy for tolerance or dependency
See also Preparation for Procedures, Chapter 22
See also Administration of Medications, Chapter 22

---

*Dependent nursing action.
†Nursing outcome.

NURSING DIAGNOSIS: Powerlessness related to the health care environment

---

PATIENT GOAL 1: Will experience "homelike" atmosphere in the hospital environment

• **NURSING INTERVENTIONS/*RATIONALES***

Determine child's customary routine and usual manner of handling child from parents or other caregiver (see box, pp. 618-619)
Maintain a routine similar to one that child is accustomed to at home
Minimize a hospital-like environment as much as possible; allow child to sit at table to eat and wear own pajamas or street clothes
Use terms familiar to child, such as those for body functions
Encourage patients with extended hospitalizations to decorate room (e.g., pictures, bedspread from home) *to make it more "homelike"*
Encourage sibling visitation
Explore possibility of pet visitation for children with extended hospitalizations

• **EXPECTED OUTCOME**

Child's routines and environment are similar to those at home (specify)

PATIENT GOAL 2: Will experience opportunities to exert control

• **NURSING INTERVENTIONS/*RATIONALES***

Allow child choices whenever possible, such as food selection, clothing, options for time of basic care (bath, play, bedtime), selection of television channels, and choice of activities, *to give child some measure of control*
Use time structuring with an older child (a jointly planned and written schedule of daily activities)
Permit freedom on the unit within defined and enforced limitations
Explain reason for physically restraining a child to both child and parents
Encourage self-care according to child's abilities
Assign tasks to an older child, especially in extended hospitalization (e.g., making the bed, supervising younger children, distributing menus, collating charts)
Respect child's need for privacy

• **EXPECTED OUTCOMES**

Child participates in planning care (specify)
Child moves about the unit but respects limits
Child participates in care activities (specify activities)
Child assumes responsibility for tasks (specify)
*Child's need for privacy is maintained

NURSING DIAGNOSIS: Diversional activity deficit related to impaired mobility, musculoskeletal impairment, confinement to hospital or home, effects of illness

---

Continued.

NURSING CARE PLAN
The Child in the Hospital—cont'd

PATIENT GOAL 1: Will have opportunity to participate in activities

- **NURSING INTERVENTIONS/***RATIONALES*

Schedule therapies and periods of rest to allow for activities
Involve child in planning care to the extent of capabilities *to reduce feelings of passivity*
Arrange for and encourage interaction with others as feasible *to promote socialization*
Encourage visits from family and friends
Provide opportunity to socialize with noninfectious children

- **EXPECTED OUTCOMES**

Child helps plan care and schedule
Child interacts with family and other children

PATIENT GOAL 2: Will have opportunity to participate in diversional activities

- **NURSING INTERVENTIONS/***RATIONALES*

Spend time with child
Query child and parents regarding child's favorite diversional activities
Change position of bed in room periodically *to alter sensory stimuli* if child is confined to bed
Provide activities appropriate to child's condition, physical limitations, and developmental level
Encourage family to caress and hold infant or child
Maintain accustomed home routine of diversional activities, when possible
Consult with a child-life specialist *to provide diversional activities*
Encourage interaction with other children
Choose a roommate compatible in age, sex, and physical abilities
Monitor time spent watching television or playing electronic games vs interactive or creative activities
Allow ample time for play
Make play, art, music, and other expressive materials available to child
Encourage play activities and diversions appropriate to child's age, condition, and capabilities
Help facilitate an activity by acting under child's instructions to perform tasks child is unable to do
Use play as a teaching strategy and an anxiety-reducing technique
Promote the use of a separate activity room or area for adolescents

- **EXPECTED OUTCOMES**

Child engages in activities appropriate for age, interests, and physical limitations (specify activities)
Child receives attention and comfort
Child engages in age-appropriate play (specify)

NURSING DIAGNOSIS: Activity intolerance related to generalized weakness, fatigue, imbalance between oxygen supply and demand

PATIENT GOAL 1: Will maintain adequate energy levels

- **NURSING INTERVENTIONS/***RATIONALES*

Assess child's level of physical tolerance
Anticipate child's need for rest, as evidenced by irritability, short attention span, and fretfulness; assist child in those activities of daily living that may be beyond tolerance
Provide entertainment and quiet diversional activities appropriate to child's age and interest *to conserve energy*
Provide diversional play activities *that promote rest and quiet but prevent boredom and withdrawal*
Choose an appropriate roommate of similar age and interests and one who requires restricted activity *to decrease feelings of loneliness and sadness*
Instruct child to rest when feeling tired
Balance rest and activity when ambulatory

- **EXPECTED OUTCOMES**

Child plays and rests quietly and engages in activities appropriate to age and capabilities (specify)
Child exhibits no evidence of intolerance
Child tolerates increasingly more activity

PATIENT GOAL 2: Will receive optimum rest

- **NURSING INTERVENTIONS/***RATIONALES*

Provide quiet environment *to promote rest*
Organize activities for maximum sleep time
Schedule visiting to allow for sufficient rest
Keep visiting periods with friends and family short
Encourage parents to remain with child *to decrease separation and anxiety*
*Administer sedatives and analgesics as indicated, if ordered, *for restlessness and pain*
Encourage frequent rest periods
Enforce regular sleep times
Follow child's usual routine for bedtime, nap time
Implement measures to ensure sleep, such as quiet, darkened room
Be alert to signs that child is tired or overstimulated *to allow flexibility in scheduling or enforcing rest and sleep periods*

- **EXPECTED OUTCOMES**

Child remains calm, quiet, and relaxed
Child has sufficient amount of rest (specify)

NURSING DIAGNOSIS: High risk for injury/trauma related to unfamiliar environment, therapies, hazardous equipment

---

*Dependent nursing action.

Nursing Care Plan

The Child in the Hospital—cont'd

PATIENT GOAL 1: Will experience no injury

• NURSING INTERVENTIONS/*RATIONALES*

Employ environmental safety measures *to prevent injuries*

Report any potential hazards (e.g., slippery floors, poor illumination, electrical hazards, damaged or malfunctioning furniture or equipment, unprotected windows, stairwells)

Dispose of small breakable items appropriately (thermometers, bottles)

Keep potentially hazardous articles out of child's reach

Check bathwater for temperature before bathing infant or child *to prevent burns*

Maintain surveillance of children in bathtub/shower

Keep crib sides up and securely fastened; use siderails for children who may fall out of bed

Use safety restraints only when absolutely necessary
    Remove as often as possible
    Discontinue as soon as possible
    Check regularly for adequate circulation to restrained area and any pressure points and that restraint is applied properly

Maintain hand contact while caring for a child in a crib with siderails down *to prevent falls*

Transport infants and children appropriately
    Hold with proper support
    Fasten safety belt on gurney, wheelchair

Alert parents and ancillary hospital personnel regarding child's physical tolerance and need for assistance during activity

Fasten safety belts in high chairs, swings

• EXPECTED OUTCOME

Child remains free of injury

NURSING DIAGNOSIS: Bathing/hygiene and dressing/grooming self-care deficit related to physical or cognitive disability, mechanical restrictions

PATIENT GOAL 1: Will engage in self-help activities

• NURSING INTERVENTIONS/*RATIONALES*

Allow child to help plan own daily routine and choose from alternatives when appropriate *to promote sense of control*

Encourage participation in self-care activities according to developmental level and capabilities *to promote mastery and decrease regression*

Provide devices, equipment, and methods to assist child in self-care

Advocate for child-sized features *that foster independence* (e.g., bathroom door handles low enough for children to reach)

Assist with dressing, grooming, bathing as indicated

• EXPECTED OUTCOME

Child engages in self-help activities to maximum capabilities

NURSING DIAGNOSIS: Toileting self-care deficit related to physical or cognitive disability, mechanical restrictions

PATIENT GOAL 1: Will exhibit normal elimination patterns

• NURSING INTERVENTIONS/*RATIONALES*

Solicit information from child and parents regarding child's normal patterns and procedures of elimination

Sit child in upright position when possible *to encourage elimination*

Employ special devices when appropriate (e.g., fracture pan, commode, elevated toilet seat)

Carry out bowel-training program with hydration, high-fiber diet, stool softeners, and mild laxatives if needed

Provide privacy *to promote relaxation needed for elimination*

• EXPECTED OUTCOME

Child has daily bowel movement

NURSING DIAGNOSIS: Altered patterns of urinary elimination related to discomfort, positioning

PATIENT GOAL 1: Will exhibit normal voiding

• NURSING INTERVENTIONS/*RATIONALES*

Solicit information from child and parents regarding child's normal patterns and procedures of elimination

Position child as upright as possible to void

Hydrate child *to ensure adequate urine output for age*

Stimulate bladder emptying with warm water, running water, stroking suprapubic area

Catheterize as indicated

See also:
    Nursing Care Plan: The Child with Chronic Illness or Disability, Chapter 18
    Nursing Care Plan: The Child Undergoing Surgery, Chapter 22
    Nursing Care Plan: The Child Who Is Terminally Ill or Dying, Chapter 18
    Nursing Care Plan for specific health problem(s)

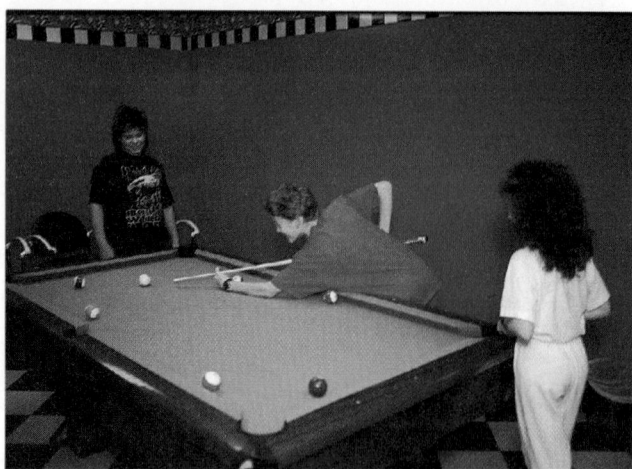

FIG. 21-13. The hospital environment can present an opportunity for forming new friendships and an accepting peer group for children.

cialist, or minister, can greatly enhance children's adjustment in many areas of life.

Parents may also encounter a new social group in other parents who have similar problems. The waiting room or hallway "self-help" groups are inherent to every institution. Nurses can capitalize on this informal gathering by encouraging parents to discuss collectively their concerns and feelings. Nurses can also refer parents to organized parent groups or can use the help and support of recovered hospitalized patients.

❖ Evaluation

The effectiveness of nursing interventions is determined by continual reassessment and evaluation of care based on the following observational guidelines and expected outcomes:

1. Interview child and parents regarding the type of preparation for hospitalization the child received.
2. Review the medical record for evidence of parental visitation; interview parents and child regarding strategies used to minimize separation.
3. Observe child's hospital schedule and compare it with the schedule the child typically follows at home; interview child and family for examples of when they were allowed choices in the child's care.
4. Review the medical record for evidence of pain assessment and administration of analgesics or nonpharmacologic pain reducers. Compare child's behavior and pain scores before and after administration of pain reducers for evidence of pain relief.
5. Interview child regarding the types of play and other activities that were introduced by the nurses or child-life specialist and the times the child visited the playroom. For preverbal child, observe child's use of play materials.
6. Interview child and parents regarding their perception of any beneficial aspects of the hospitalization. Observe behaviors that indicate benefits, such as the formation of new friendships.

Expected outcomes:
See Nursing Care Plan, pp. 648-653.

STRESSORS AND REACTIONS IN THE FAMILY OF THE CHILD WHO IS HOSPITALIZED

PARENTAL REACTIONS

Parents' reactions to illness in their child depend on a variety of influencing factors. Although which factors are most likely to influence their response cannot be predicted, a number of variables have been identified (see box). (See also Chapter 18.)

Almost all parents respond to their child's illness and hospitalization with remarkably consistent reactions. Initially, parents may react with *disbelief*, especially if the illness is sudden and serious. Following the realization of illness, parents react with *anger* or *guilt* or both. They may blame themselves for the child's illness or become angry at others for some wrongdoing. Even in the mildest of illnesses, parents question their adequacy as caregivers and review any actions or omissions that could have prevented or caused the illness. When hospitalization is indicated, parental guilt is intensified because the parents feel helpless in alleviating the child's physical and emotional pain.

Fear, anxiety, and *frustration* are common feelings expressed by parents. Fear and anxiety may be related to the seriousness of the illness and the type of medical procedures involved. Often great anxiety is related to the trauma and pain inflicted on the child. Feelings of frustration are often related to lack of information about procedures and treatments, unfamiliarity with hospital rules and regulations, a sense of unwelcomeness from the staff, or fear of asking questions. Much frustration can be alleviated in a pediatric unit when parents are aware of what to expect and what is expected of them, are encouraged to participate in their child's care, and are regarded as the most significant contributors to the child's total health.

Parents eventually may react with some degree of *depression*. The depression usually occurs when the acute crisis is over, such as after hospital discharge or complete recovery. Mothers often comment on their feeling of physical and mental exhaustion after all the other family members have adapted to the crisis. Parents may also worry about and miss their other children, who may be left in the care of family, friends, or neighbors. Other reasons for anxiety and depression are related to concerns for the child's future well-being, including negative effects produced by the hospitalization and any financial burden incurred from the hospitalization.

FACTORS AFFECTING PARENTS' REACTIONS TO THEIR CHILD'S ILLNESS

Seriousness of the threat to the child
Previous experience with illness or hospitalization
Medical procedures involved in diagnosis and treatment
Available support systems
Personal ego strengths
Previous coping abilities
Additional stresses on the family system
Cultural and religious beliefs
Communication patterns among family members

SIBLING REACTIONS

Siblings' reactions to a sister's or brother's illness or hospitalization are discussed in Chapter 18 and differ little when a child becomes temporarily ill. They experience loneliness, fear, and worry, as well as anger, resentment, jealousy, and guilt. Various factors have been identified that influence the effects of the child's hospitalization on siblings. Although these factors are similar to those seen when a child has a chronic illness, Craft (1993) reported that the following factors regarding siblings are related specifically to the hospital experience and have been found to increase the effects on the sibling:

- Younger and experiencing many changes
- Cared for outside the home by care providers who are not relatives
- Received little information about their ill brother or sister
- Perceived their parents to be treating them differently compared with before their sibling's hospitalization

Simon (1993) asked 45 siblings of children who were hospitalized their perceptions of the stress of the hospitalization of a brother or sister. The siblings' perceptions of the stress they experienced were equal to the level of stress of hospitalized children.

Parents are often unaware of the number of effects that siblings experience during the sick child's hospitalization and of the benefit of simple interventions to minimize such effects, such as explicit explanations about the illness and provisions for the siblings to remain at home. Sibling visitation seems to increase the parent's awareness of the changes older siblings are experiencing, but not those of younger siblings. This may be due to the tendency of parents and health professionals to include older siblings in discussions about the child, whereas younger siblings are sent to the playroom or given some toys to occupy their time (Craft and Craft, 1989).

ALTERED FAMILY ROLES

In addition to the effects of separation on family roles, loss of parenting, sibling, and offspring roles may affect each family member differently. One of the most common reactions of parents is specialized and intensified attention toward the sick child. The other children usually regard this as unfair and interpret the parents' attitude toward them as rejection. Although such responses are usually unconscious and unintended, they place unique burdens on ill children. For example, the ill child may feel obligated to play the sick role in order to meet parents' expectations, especially children who have had limited physical ability and regain normal health status, such as after corrective heart surgery. Parents may be unable to perceive the child's recovery and therefore need to continue the pattern of overprotection and indulgent attention.

Ill children may also feel jealousy and resentment from other siblings. Because of their singular position in the family, they may be denied the companionship of their brothers and sisters. Rivalry between siblings tends to be greatest in the sibling who is nearest in age to the ill child. Without an understanding of the interpersonal dynamics between siblings, parents are likely to blame the well children for antisocial behavior. Illness may also result in children's loss of status within either their family or social group. For example, illness in the oldest child may temporarily terminate special privileges as "big" brother or sister.

NURSING CARE OF THE FAMILY

❖ Assessment

Assessment involves those factors that are most likely to influence the family's responses to the child's illness and/or hospitalization. Although it is not possible to predict exactly which factors are most likely to have an effect on the family's reactions, the areas discussed in Table 18-2 should be included in the assessment process. Other important variables are (1) the seriousness of the child's illness, (2) the family's previous experience with hospitalization, and (3) the medical procedures involved in the diagnosis and treatment. Important information is also obtained in the nursing admission history (see box on pp. 618-619).

Discharge Assessment

Throughout the hospitalization the nurse should be aware of the need for discharge planning and those assessment factors that affect the family's ability to provide home care. Discharge planning must begin early in the hospital admission to permit sufficient time to assess the family's ability to perform care at home and to institute needed teaching. With the current concern for cost containment and recognition of children's emotional needs, home care for children with technologically complex care, such as youngsters on ventilators, has become increasingly common.

In terms of home care for children with complex care, a thorough assessment of the family and home environment should be performed to ensure that the family's emotional and physical resources are sufficient to manage the tasks of home care. (For a discussion of family and home assessment strategies, see Chapter 6. See also Chapter 20 on home care.) In addition to adequate family resources, an investigation of community services, including respite care, is needed to ensure that appropriate support agencies are available, such as emergency facilities, home health agencies, and equipment vendors. Financial resources may also be a consideration. To coordinate the immense task of assessment and to plan implementation, a care coordinator or manager should be appointed early in the discharge program.

Discharge planning is also concerned with those skills that parents or children are expected to continue at home. Assessment for planning appropriate teaching includes knowledge of (1) the actual and perceived complexity of the skill, (2) the parents' or child's ability to learn the skill, and (3) the parents' or child's previous or present experience with such procedures.

❖ Nursing Diagnoses

A number of nursing diagnoses are prominent in the nursing care of the family of the hospitalized child, and others specific to individual cases become evident. The most common nursing diagnoses are outlined in the Nursing Care Plan on pp. 659-662.

❖ Planning

The main goals for the family are as follows:

1. Family will participate in child's care to the extent they desire.
2. Family will receive support.
3. Family will be informed of child's care.
4. Family will be prepared for discharge and home care.

❖ Implementation
Encourage Parent Participation

Preventing or minimizing separation is a key nursing goal with the child who is hospitalized, but maintaining parent-child contact is also beneficial for the family. One of the best approaches is encouraging parents to stay with their child and to participate in the care whenever possible. Although some health facilities provide special accommodations for parents, the concept of "rooming-in" can be instituted anywhere. The first requirement is the staff's positive attitude toward parents. When hospital staff genuinely appreciate the importance of continued parent-child attachment, they foster an environment that encourages parents to stay. When parents are included in the care planning and understand that they are a contributing factor to the child's recovery, they are more inclined to remain with their child and have more emotional reserves to support themselves and the child through the crisis. An empowerment model of helping allows the nurse to focus on parents' strengths and seek ways to promote growth and family functioning so that the parents become empowered in caring for their child (Fig. 21-14).

Since the mother tends to be the usual family caregiver, she usually spends more time in the hospital than the father. However, not all mothers (or fathers) feel equally comfortable in assuming responsibility for their child's care. Some may be under such great emotional stress that they need a temporary reprieve from total participation in caregiving activities. Others may feel insecure in participating in specialized areas of care, such as bathing the child after surgery. On the other hand, some mothers may feel a great need to have control of their child's care. This seems particularly true of young mothers who have more recently established their role as a parent, mothers of children too young to verbalize their needs, and ethnic minority mothers when the hospital setting is predominantly staffed by nonminority personnel (Schepp, 1992). Individual assessment of each parent's preferred involvement is necessary to prevent the effects of separation while supporting parents in their needs as well. Both

underinvolvement and overinvolvement of parents in the child's care can be detrimental; therefore every effort is extended to help parents identify moderate amounts of visiting and participation.

With life-styles and sex roles changing, fathers may assume all or some of the usual "mothering" roles in the household. In this case it may be the father-child relationship that requires preservation. Fathers need to be included in the plan of care and respected for their parental role. For some fathers the child's hospitalization may represent an opportunity to alter their usual caregiving role and increase their involvement. In single-parent families the caregiver may not be a parent but an extended family member, such as a grandparent or aunt.

One of the potential problems with continuous parent rooming-in is neglect of the parent's need for sleep, nutrition, and relaxation (see Family Focus box). Often the sleeping accommodations are limited to a chair, and sleep is disrupted by nursing procedures. Encouraging the parents to leave for brief periods, arranging for sleeping quarters on the unit but outside the child's room, and planning a schedule of alternating visiting with another family member can minimize the stresses for the parent.

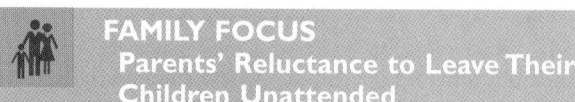

NURSING TIP If parents are reluctant to leave the hospital (usually for fear of not being there when the child awakens or the practitioner visits), arrange for them to have a remote "beeper" that can provide immediate communication regardless of their location (Ashenberg and others, 1996).

All too often, nurses respond to parent participation by abandoning their patient responsibilities. Nurses need to restructure their roles to complement and augment the caregiv-

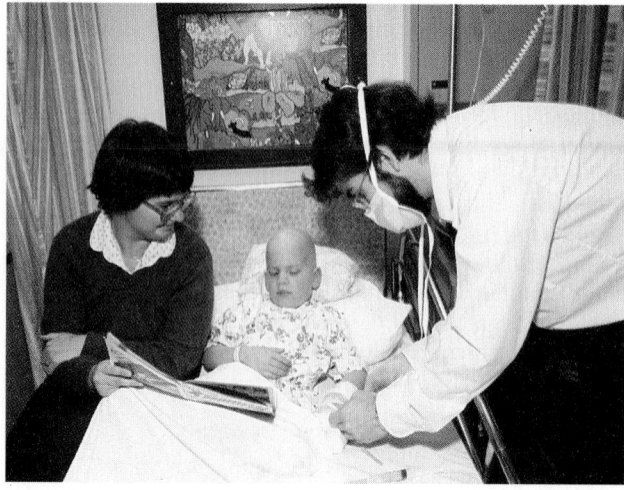

FIG. 21-14. Parental presence during hospitalization, including during procedures, provides emotional support for the child and increases the parent's sense of empowerment in the caregiver role. (Courtesy St. Louis Children's Hospital.)

FAMILY FOCUS
Parents' Reluctance to Leave Their Children Unattended

Parents are often very reluctant to leave their children or to ask the nurse to watch their children while they take a break. In his research on the experiences of nurses and parents when parents room-in, Darbyshire (1994) found that many parents did not eat properly, or in some cases, at all. The following are two mothers' experiences:

I just about starved to death the first couple of days . . . just . . . I mean, it was my own fault really, 'cos I wouldn't leave the wee one. There was always going to be something else happening and I thought . . . if he gets upset I'd better be there when it finishes.

There was one day I couldn't get any of the visitors to look after the wee chap so I could go for something to eat and it was about six o'clock at night and nurse said, "You look awful, are you OK?" and I said, "No, actually I feel awful and I think I'm going to pass out," and she said, "Oh, you've just gone a funny colour," and I said, "What time is it?" and I said, "It's OK, it's just because I haven't eaten all day"—because none of my family had come to take the child from me, and I didn't think to say to a nurse, "Could you watch him till I go for something to eat?"

From Darbyshire P: *Living with a sick child in hospital*, London, 1994, Chapman & Hall.

ing functions of parents. Even in units structured to provide care by parents, parents frequently feel anxiety in their caregiving responsibilities; those more involved in direct care may feel more anxiety than those less involved in direct care. Therefore 24-hour responsibility may be too much for some parents. Assistance and relief by nursing personnel should always be available to these families, and nurses must often work diligently to establish the strong bond of trust some parents need to take advantage of these opportunities.

Support Family Members

Support involves the willingness to stay and listen to parents' verbal and nonverbal messages. Sometimes the nurse does not give this support directly. For example, the nurse may offer to stay with the child to allow the parents time alone or may discuss with other family members the parents' need for extra relief. Often relatives and friends want to help but do not know how. Suggesting ways, such as baby-sitting, preparing meals, tending the garden or home, doing laundry, or transporting the siblings to school, can prompt others to help lessen the responsibilities that burden parents. An ongoing parent support group held on the pediatric unit during the children's traditional nap time has also proved effective in helping parents share emotions and concerns related to hospitalization (Nugent and others, 1992).

Support may also be provided through the clergy. Parents with deep religious beliefs may appreciate the counsel of a clergy member, but because of their stress they may not have sufficient energy to initiate the contact. Nurses can be supportive by arranging for clergy to visit, upholding parents' religious beliefs, and respecting the individual meaning and significance of those beliefs.

Support involves an acceptance of cultural, socioeconomic, and ethnic values. For example, health and illness are defined differently by various ethnic groups. For some, a disorder that has few outward manifestations of illness, such as diabetes, hypertension, or cardiac problems, is not a sickness. Consequently, following a prescribed treatment may be seen as unnecessary. Nurses who appreciate the influences of culture are more likely to intervene therapeutically. (See also Chapter 3 for an extensive discussion of cultural and religious influences on health care.)

Parents need help in accepting their own feelings toward the ill child. If given the opportunity, parents often disclose their feelings of loss of control, anger, and guilt. They often resist admitting to such feelings because they expect others to disapprove of behavior that is less than perfect. Unfortunately, health personnel, including nurses, sometimes do exercise little tolerance for deviation from the expected norm. This only increases the psychologic impact of a child's illness on family members. Helping parents identify the specific reason for such feelings and emphasizing that each is a normal, expected, and healthy response to stress provides the parents with an opportunity to lessen their emotional burden.

Support may also involve preparing siblings for hospital visits, assessing their adjustment, and providing appropriate interventions or referrals when needed. The nurse can invite visiting siblings to participate in playroom activities or other unit events. Siblings' needs are often neglected as parents and health personnel focus attention on the child who is hospitalized.

Provide Information

One of the most important nursing interventions is providing information about (1) the disease, its treatment, prognosis, and home care; (2) the child's emotional, as well as physical, reaction to illness and hospitalization; and (3) the probable emotional reactions of family members to the crisis.

For many families the child's illness is the first contact they have with the hospital experience. Often parents are not prepared for the child's behavioral reactions to hospitalization, such as separation behaviors, regression, aggression, and hostility. Providing the parents with information about these normal and expected behavioral responses can lessen the parents' anxiety during the hospital admission. The family is equally unfamiliar with hospital rules, which often adds to feelings of confusion and anxiety. Therefore the family needs clear explanations about what to expect and what is expected of them.

Parents also need to be aware of the effects of illness on the family and strategies that prevent negative changes. Specifically, parents should keep the family well informed and communicating as much as possible. They should treat all the children as equally and as normally as before the illness occurred. Discipline, which initially may be lessened for the ill child, should be continued to provide a measure of security and predictability. When ill children know that their parents expect certain standards of conduct from them, they feel certain that they will recover. Conversely, when all limits are removed, they fear that something catastrophic will happen.

Nurses should help parents understand and accept the meaning of posthospitalization behaviors so that the parents can tolerate and support such behaviors. Consequently, parents should be forewarned of the usual continuance of such reactions after discharge (see box on p. 616). Parents who do not expect such reactions may misinterpret them as evidence of the child's "being spoiled" and demand perfect behavior at a time when the child is still reacting to the stress of illness and hospitalization. If the behaviors, especially the demand for attention, are dealt with in a supportive manner, most children are able to relinquish them and assume precrisis levels of functioning.

Nurses should also forewarn parents of the reactions of siblings, particularly anger, jealousy, and resentment. Older siblings may deny such reactions because they provoke feelings of guilt. However, everyone needs outlets for emotions, and the repressed feelings may surface as problems in school, with age-mates, as psychosomatic illnesses, or in delinquent behavior.

Probably one of the most neglected areas involves giving information to siblings. Frequently age becomes the only factor that leads to an awareness of this problem, because older children may begin to ask questions or request explanations. Even in this situation, however, the information may be seriously inadequate. Children in every age-group deserve some explanation of the sibling's illness or hospitalization. Although the exact wording may differ, the explanation should focus on the following concerns: (1) "Will I get sick and have to go to the hospital?" (2) "Did I cause the illness?" (for actual or imagined reasons), and (3) "Will my parents abandon me if my brother or sister doesn't recover?" If parents or nurses address the explanations to these three questions, the siblings' own fears of illness, guilt, and abandonment are

FAMILY HOME CARE
Supporting Siblings During Hospitalization

Trade off staying at the hospital with spouse or have a parent surrogate who knows the siblings well stay in the home.

Offer information about the child's condition to young siblings as well as older siblings; respect the sibling who avoids information as a means of coping with the situation.

Arrange for children to visit their brother or sister in the hospital if possible.

Encourage phone visits and mail between brothers and sisters; provide children with phone numbers, writing supplies, and stamps.

Help each sibling identify an extended family member or friend to be their support person, and provide extra attention during parental absence.

Make or buy inexpensive toys or trinkets for siblings, one gift for each day the child will be hospitalized.

    Wrap each gift separately and place in a basket, box, or other container at each child's bedside.

    Instruct siblings to open one gift each night at bedtime and to remember that he or she is in the parent's thoughts.

If the child's condition is stable and distance is not prohibitive, plan a special time at home with the siblings or have spouse or another relative or friend bring the children to meet parent(s) at a restaurant or other location near the hospital.

    Have extended family members or friends schedule a visit to the child in the hospital during parental absence.

    Arrange a pass for the child to leave the hospital to join the family if the child's condition permits.

Modified from Craft M, Craft J: Perceived changes in siblings of hospitalized children: a comparison of sibling and parent reports, *Child Health Care* 18(1):42-48, 1989; and Rollins J: *Brothers and sisters: a discussion guide for families,* Landover, MD, 1992, Epilepsy Foundation of America.

minimized. See Family Home Care box for ways parents can support siblings during hospitalization.

Prepare for Discharge and Home Care

Most hospitalizations necessitate some type of discharge preparation. Often this involves education of the family for continued care and follow-up in the home. Depending on the diagnosis, this may be relatively simple or highly complex. Preparing the family for home care demands a high degree of competence in planning and implementing discharge instructions. Although this is usually a team effort, nurses are often key individuals in initiating the process and collaborating with others in the planning and implementing stages.

Nurses frequently are responsible for all or some of the teaching as well. The teaching plan incorporates levels of learning, such as observing, participating with assistance, and finally, acting without help or guidance. The skill is divided into discrete steps, and each step is taught to the family member until it is learned. Return demonstration of the skill is requested before new skills are introduced. A record of teaching and performance provides an efficient checklist for evaluation. All families need to receive detailed *written* instructions

CRITICAL THINKING EXERCISE
Discharge Planning and Home Care

Two-year-old Rhonda comes from a rural home 150 miles from the medical center. Last month she suffered a severe case of meningitis that left her profoundly cognitively impaired. During her hospitalization her parents have called infrequently and have never visited because they do not have a telephone or car as a result of their low income. Rhonda is now ready to be discharged from the tertiary care center. As the primary nurse who is responsible for Rhonda's discharge planning, which of the following activities would you initiate?

1. Arrange for Rhonda to be institutionalized because her family will be unable to care for her.
2. Give a list of local services with an encouraging note about the importance of arranging follow-up care to the transport team to give to her parents.
3. Call and arrange for the public health nurse from Rhonda's district to make a home visit shortly after her return.
4. Arrange for a multidisciplinary care conference to discuss Rhonda's discharge.

The correct answer is four. A multidisciplinary care conference, including the parents, can be arranged with some planning. The public health department can be asked to either escort Rhonda's parents to the medical center or arrange for them to participate over a speaker phone. The public health nurse from Rhonda's district also will be able to advise the team of the services available in Rhonda's community. Since Rhonda will need care from a variety of professionals, this conference will help ensure that there are no gaps or overlaps in services.

Providing Rhonda's parents with a list of agencies is inappropriate. First, they do not own their own phone. Second, the parents are not in the position of knowing what services they will need. Third, dealing with professional agencies is often an arduous task and one that parents should not be expected to do while adjusting to the child's disability. Although contacting the local public health nurse is a good idea, this should be done well in advance of discharge. This way the nurse could perform a home assessment to help arrange for appropriate services. Institutionalization of children with mental retardation is considered a last resort. All other options should be explored first.

about home care,* with telephone numbers for assistance, before they leave the hospital (see Critical Thinking Exercise).

Videocassette recordings offer another excellent vehicle for home teaching. The actual teaching session in the hospital can be recorded and played for the family as often as needed. If the family has a VCR at home, the filmed instructions serve as a refresher when parents have questions about the procedure.

Once the family is competent in performing the skill, they are given responsibility for the care. Whenever possible, the

*Home care instructions for a wide variety of technical skills are available in Wong DL: *Wong and Whaley's Clinical manual of pediatric nursing,* ed 4, St Louis, 1996, Mosby. Home modifications for numerous technical skills are available in Smith DP and others, editors: *Comprehensive child and family nursing skills,* St Louis, 1991, Mosby.

NURSING CARE PLAN
The Family of the Ill or Hospitalized Child

NURSING DIAGNOSIS: Anxiety/fear related to situational crisis, threat to role functioning, change in environment

FAMILY GOAL 1: Will adjust to hospital environment

- **NURSING INTERVENTIONS/RATIONALES**

Introduce family to significant staff members

Describe hospital routine that affects child

Acclimate family to the new and strange surroundings (e.g., physical layout of unit, including playroom, unit kitchen, toilet, telephone, where they can stay, where they can store their belongings)

Direct family to areas they may need to use outside the unit (e.g., dining room, chapel)

Direct family to "destinations" (places within the hospital that are interesting to look at or talk about)

Provide an atmosphere that promotes questioning, expression of doubts and feelings

Be available to family *to facilitate their adjustment*

Be alert to signs of tension in family members

Provide for privacy

- **EXPECTED OUTCOMES**

Family demonstrates familiarity with hospital environment

Family members ask questions

FAMILY GOAL 2: Will feel a part of the health care team

- **NURSING INTERVENTIONS/RATIONALES**

Employ a polite approach and demeanor

Greet family by name when they arrive on the unit

Encourage family's presence

Include family in planning patient care

Encourage family to select and assume specific roles in child's care

Offer encouragement for their efforts

Ask family to share with staff what they know about child's care and needs

Convey an attitude of collegiality with family, not competition

- **EXPECTED OUTCOME**

Family becomes involved in planning and carrying out care for the child

FAMILY GOAL 3: Will experience reduced apprehension

- **NURSING INTERVENTIONS/RATIONALES**

Allow for expression of feelings about child's hospitalization and illness

Provide needed information *to alleviate fear of the unknown*

Prepare family for what to expect (e.g., procedures, behaviors)

Explore family's expectations

Explore family's concerns and feelings of irritation, guilt, anger, disappointment, inadequacy

Explore family's fears and anxieties regarding child's status and expectations of results of procedures or therapy

Introduce parents to other families who have a child in the hospital, especially a child who is similarly affected, *to facilitate family-to-family support*

Provide something constructive and meaningful for family to focus on (e.g., keeping record of intake and output, pain relief record, ensuring a specified amount of fluid intake, collecting a specimen)

- **EXPECTED OUTCOMES**

Family members verbalize feelings and concerns

Family demonstrates an understanding of procedures and behaviors (specify manner of demonstration and learning)

Family interacts with other families

Family complies with directions (specify)

FAMILY GOAL 4: Will be prepared for special procedures (e.g., radiology, diagnostic tests, surgery)

- **NURSING INTERVENTIONS**

Assess family's understanding of the procedure and its purpose

Provide needed information; clarify misconceptions

Explain special preparation needed (e.g., nothing by mouth [NPO], shaving, preprocedural medication or equipment)

Describe

   Where child will be during the procedure

   Whether family can be with child

   Where family can wait

   Approximate length of time procedure requires

Reassure family that they will be notified regarding progress of the procedure

- **EXPECTED OUTCOME**

Family demonstrates an understanding of procedures and tests (specify)

FAMILY GOAL 5: Will receive support during child's absence

- **NURSING INTERVENTIONS/RATIONALES**

Provide a comfortable place for family to wait

Suggest activities to help reduce anxiety (e.g., go to the coffee shop or dining room, take a short walk [specify activity])

Be available to family *for support*

Make contact with family at frequent intervals *to relay information, provide comfort*

- **EXPECTED OUTCOME**

Family takes advantage of suggestions (specify)

Continued.

NURSING CARE PLAN

The Family of the Ill or Hospitalized Child—cont'd

FAMILY GOAL 6: Will adjust to child's appearance and behavior after procedure(s) or in special care unit

- **NURSING INTERVENTIONS/*RATIONALES***

Remain calm *to decrease family's anxiety*
Describe the environment, if appropriate (e.g., ICU)
Apply principles of learning to explanations
    Begin with small amounts of information
    Begin with very general information
    Allow ample time for family to absorb information and to
        ask questions
    Use age-appropriate explanations and techniques for sib-
        lings
Explain how child will look and the reasons for the child's
    appearance and equipment
Explain what child is experiencing
Prepare child and surroundings *to lessen impact of the first
    impression*
    Tidy the bed
    Personalize the bed and bedside with a toy or other
        item(s)
    Provide chairs for family
    Be prepared for possible adverse reaction (e.g., fainting)
Convey an attitude of caring *about*, as well as *for*, the child
Accompany the family to the child's bedside
Allow time for follow-up discussion of questions and con-
    cerns

- **EXPECTED OUTCOME**

Family comes to child's bedside without evidence of distress

FAMILY GOAL 7: Will experience reduction of or no fear

- **NURSING INTERVENTIONS**

Help family distinguish between realistic and unfounded fears
Help eliminate unfounded fears
Discuss with family their fears regarding
    Child's signs and symptoms
    Child's anxiety
    Consequences of disease or therapy
    Deterioration of child's condition
    Tests and procedures
    Death
Answer questions honestly and compassionately

- **EXPECTED OUTCOME**

Family members verbalize fears and explore nature and rami-
    fications of these fears

NURSING DIAGNOSIS: Powerlessness related
to health care environment

FAMILY GOAL 1: Will experience a sense of control

- **NURSING INTERVENTIONS/*RATIONALES***

Encourage family's presence at times convenient for them;
    consider variations (e.g., cultural, occupational) in visiting
Encourage expression of concerns regarding child's care and
    progress
Explore family's feelings regarding prescribed therapies
Encourage family to assume as much control as possible in
    child's management
    Encourage participation in child's care
    Include family in setting goals for care
    Involve family in scheduling and other aspects of care
    Explain what family can do for child and how to handle
        child to maintain therapy (e.g., how to pick up the child
        who has an intravenous line)
    Employ family's suggestions regarding child's care when-
        ever possible

- **EXPECTED OUTCOMES**

Family schedules time to be with child
Family readily discusses feelings and concerns
Family contributes to care and management of child
*Family's suggestions are incorporated into plan of care

NURSING DIAGNOSIS: Altered family processes related to situational crisis (threat to role
functioning, hospitalization of a child)

FAMILY GOAL 1: Will demonstrate knowledge of child's illness

- **NURSING INTERVENTIONS/*RATIONALES***

Recognize family's concern and need for information, sup-
    port
Assess family's understanding of diagnosis and plan of care
Reinforce and clarify health professional's explanation of
    child's condition, suggested procedures and therapies, and
    the prognosis
Use every opportunity to increase family's understanding of
    the disease and its therapies
Repeat information as often as necessary *to facilitate under-
    standing*
Interpret technical information, *since family may not under-
    stand*
Help family interpret infant's or child's behaviors and re-
    sponses
Do not appear rushed; if time is inappropriate, set a time for
    discussion as soon as feasible
    Keep appointment faithfully

- **EXPECTED OUTCOME**

Family demonstrates an understanding of the disease and its
    therapies (specify knowledge)

---

*Nursing outcome.

NURSING CARE PLAN
The Family of the Ill or Hospitalized Child—cont'd

FAMILY GOAL 2: Will experience reduction of or no guilt feelings

- **NURSING INTERVENTIONS**

Acknowledge feelings of guilt
Provide accurate and specific information regarding the cause of the illness
Clarify misconceptions and false assumptions

- **EXPECTED OUTCOME**

Family verbalizes their understanding of the cause of the illness (specify)

FAMILY GOAL 3: Will receive adequate support

- **NURSING INTERVENTIONS/***RATIONALES*

Respect parental rights
Convey an attitude of respectful caring for both child and family
Support and emphasize family's strengths and abilities
Provide feedback and praise
Refer to other professionals *for additional interpersonal and concrete support* (e.g., social service, clergy)

- **EXPECTED OUTCOMES**

Family exhibits behaviors that indicate a feeling of self-respect
Family uses supportive services

FAMILY GOAL 4: Will demonstrate positive coping behaviors toward child

- **NURSING INTERVENTIONS**

Determine family's understanding of the normal childhood responses to the stress of illness and hospitalization
Explain child's regression, magical thinking, egocentricity, separation anxiety, fears
Explain behavioral reactions generally expected of child (specify according to age and developmental level)
Explain what child is (family are) permitted to do in coping with child's behavior
Reinforce family's endeavors

- **EXPECTED OUTCOME**

Family demonstrates an understanding of child's unfamiliar behaviors (specify manner of demonstration: verbalization, physical attitude, behaviors with child)

FAMILY GOAL 5: Will assist child in coping effectively with hospitalization

- **NURSING INTERVENTIONS**

Help parents determine the best way to prepare child for hospitalization, procedures
Provide family with precise information about what will take place so they know what child is likely to experience
Encourage family to trust child's capacity to cope
Impress on family the need for honesty in relating to child
Encourage family to use play as a coping strategy

Suggest appropriate items to bring to child (e.g., pajamas, favorite toys)
See also Nursing Care Plan: The Child in the Hospital, pp. 648-653

- **EXPECTED OUTCOMES**

Family helps in planning strategies
Family is honest with child and staff
Family uses play as a tool for relating with child

FAMILY GOAL 6: Will experience positive relationships

- **NURSING INTERVENTIONS/***RATIONALES*

Recognize that family members know child best and are "cued in" to child's needs
Welcome unlimited family presence *to promote family relationships*
Encourage family to bring other significant family members to visit (e.g., siblings, grandparents, and [where permitted] pets)
Encourage family to provide child with significant, but manageable, items from home *to provide security*
Arrange for family members to have a meal together

- **EXPECTED OUTCOMES**

Child and family exhibit behaviors that indicate positive coping
Family is with child at appropriate times and in appropriate numbers
Child demonstrates an attitude of security with familiar persons and things

FAMILY GOAL 7: Will exhibit evidence of optimum health

- **NURSING INTERVENTIONS/***RATIONALES*

Stress importance of maintaining family members' health during child's illness and hospitalization
Encourage adequate rest *to promote health of family*
    Provide sleeping facilities where possible
    Encourage members to alternate visiting with child *to allow some time at home*
    Explore means for respite care of dependent family members
Assure family that child will receive optimum care in their absence
Provide relief for family from direct care of child as needed
Promote adequate nutrition
Provide meals for parents if possible
Direct family to nutritious resources for meals
Encourage regular mealtimes away from unit
Provide access to unit kitchen to store and prepare snacks

- **EXPECTED OUTCOMES**

Family shows no evidence of illness
Family members appear well rested
Family members eat regularly

Continued.

NURSING CARE PLAN
The Family of the Ill or Hospitalized Child—cont'd

FAMILY GOAL 8: Will experience smooth transition from hospital to home

- **NURSING INTERVENTIONS**

Assess family's learning needs
Outline and carry out a teaching plan
Determine services needed and make necessary referrals
Include family in planning and problem solving
Maintain open communication between family and health care providers

- **EXPECTED OUTCOME**

Child and family demonstrate ability to provide needed care in the home

FAMILY GOAL 9: Will demonstrate knowledge of home care

- **NURSING INTERVENTIONS/*RATIONALES***

Assess family's knowledge *to facilitate planning*
Teach family the skills needed to carry out the therapeutic program (specify)
   Allow ample time for preparation
   Teach necessary techniques and observations
   Help family by demonstration
   Distribute appropriate home care instructions and/or other educational materials
   Encourage questions and expression of feelings and concerns
   Allow sufficient time for family to perform procedures under supervision
Inform parents of
   Signs of progress to observe for
   Any unfavorable signs to be alert for
   Problems that can be anticipated (e.g., care of equipment or devices)

   Behaviors that indicate special needs (e.g., pain medication, imminent seizures)
   A course of action to follow (e.g., seizure care)
   Make certain family knows how to contact appropriate persons if or when needed
Prepare family for possible posthospital behaviors of the child (see box on p. 616)
Ensure family's comprehension of child's needs before discharge

- **EXPECTED OUTCOMES**

Family demonstrates procedures needed to care for child in the home (specify learning and method of demonstration)
Family is aware of how to seek help

FAMILY GOAL 10: Will demonstrate understanding of continuity of care

- **NURSING INTERVENTIONS**

Inform family of community resources available
Refer to agencies as appropriate (specify)
Help identify support group(s) for family
Be available to family by telephone or other means
Schedule follow-up appointments as needed

- **EXPECTED OUTCOMES**

Family seeks appropriate assistance
Family keeps appointments

See also:
   Nursing Care Plan: The Child in the Hospital, p. 648
   Nursing Care Plan: The Child with Chronic Illness or Disability, Chapter 18
   Nursing Care Plan: The Child Who Is Terminally Ill or Dying, Chapter 18

---

family should have a transition or trial period to assume care with minimum supervision. This may be arranged on the unit, during a home pass, or in a facility, such as a motel, near the hospital. Such transitions provide a safe practice period for the family, with assistance readily available when needed, and are especially valuable when the family lives at a distance from the treating center.

In many instances parents need only simple instructions and understanding of follow-up care. However, the often overwhelming care assumed by some families, coupled with other stressors they may be experiencing, necessitates continued professional support after discharge. A follow-up home visit or telephone call gives the nurse a better opportunity to individualize care and provide information in perhaps a less stressful learning environment than the hospital (Snowdon and Kane, 1995). Appropriate referrals and resources may in-

clude visiting nurse or home health agencies, private nurse services, the school system, physical therapist, mental health counselor, social worker, or any number of community agencies, including special organizations, such as **SKIP.*** Sharing the important issues surrounding the child's and family's needs is essential. Referral summaries should be concise, specific, and factual. When numerous support services are involved, periodic collaboration among the professionals involved and the family is an excellent strategy to ensure efficient usage and comprehensive delivery of services.

---

*SKIP (Sick Kids need Involved People) serves as an educational, support, and resource agency that provides assistance to families who have chosen home care for their child with complex medical needs. The address of the national headquarters is 545 Madison Ave., 13th Floor, New York, NY 10022, (212) 421-9160.

❖ Evaluation

The effectiveness of nursing interventions is determined by continual reassessment and evaluation of care based on the following observational guidelines and expected outcomes:

1. Observe schedule of parental presence and amount of participation in child's care; observe parents' willingness and ability to take care of their own needs, such as regular breaks to eat, sleep, and care for the family's needs at home.
2. Interview family regarding their concerns; observe support offered by others, such as relatives, friends, and clergy; observe if special cultural practices (if applicable) are respected in the hospital.
3. Interview family regarding their knowledge of the child's illness, the child's expected reactions to the hospitalization experience, and the emotional needs of the other family members, especially siblings. Observe frequency of siblings' visits and interview siblings regarding their understanding of the ill child's condition.
4. Observe family's performance of skills and determine their understanding of other aspects of home care before discharge; interview family and/or resource persons regarding the family's use of appropriate referral services.

Expected outcomes:
See Nursing Care Plan, pp. 659-662.

CARE OF THE CHILD AND FAMILY IN SPECIAL HOSPITAL SITUATIONS

AMBULATORY/OUTPATIENT SETTING

The ambulatory or outpatient setting provides needed medical services for the child while eliminating the necessity of overnight admission. Among the benefits of ambulatory care are (1) minimization of the stressors of hospitalization, especially separation from the family; (2) reduced chance of infection; and (3) cost savings. Admission to the ambulatory or outpatient hospital setting usually is for surgical or diagnostic procedures, such as insertion of tympanostomy tubes, hernia repair, adenoidectomy, tonsillectomy, cystoscopy, or bronchoscopy.

Because of the limited contact with the child, nursing admission procedures are extremely important. Ideally, each child and family should receive preadmission counseling, including a tour of the facility and a review of the expected day's procedures. When this is not possible, surgery should be scheduled to allow time for children to become acquainted with their surroundings and for nurses to assess, plan, and implement appropriate teaching. Waiting is usually inevitable in ambulatory settings, a factor families often report as the most stressful part of the hospitalization experience. Providing a pager allows the family (and in many instances, the child) to leave the area and then be paged to return when needed (Ashenberg and others, 1996).

Discharge instructions must also be explicit (see Prepare for Discharge and Home Care, p. 658). Parents need guidelines on when to call their practitioner regarding a change in the child's condition. It is helpful for the nurse to make a follow-up telephone call or to specify a time for the family to report on the child's progress. Even hints for taking the child home in the car are appreciated.

NURSING TIPS Help the family prepare for the transportation home by offering these suggestions:
- Have a blanket and pillow in the car. (Always use the car safety system.)
- Take a basin or plastic bag in case of vomiting.
- Use a cup with a cap and straw for the child to drink fluids.
- Give any prescribed pain medication before leaving facility.

ISOLATION

Admission to an isolation room increases all the stressors typically associated with hospitalization. There is further separation from familiar persons, additional loss of control, and added environmental changes, such as sensory deprivation and the strange appearance of visitors. Children may feel depersonalized from reduced interaction with the environment and the people in it (Hart and others, 1992). Their orientation to time and place is affected. These stressors are compounded by children's limited understanding of isolation. Preschool children have difficulty understanding the rationale for isolation because they cannot comprehend the cause-and-effect relationship between germs and illness. They are likely to view isolation as punishment. Older children understand the causality better but still require information to decrease fantasizing or misinterpretation.

When a child is placed in isolation, preparation is essential for the child to feel in control. With young children the best approach is a simple explanation, such as "You need to be in this room to help you get better. This is a special place to make all the germs go away. The germs made you sick, and you could not help that."

All children, but especially younger ones, need preparation in terms of what they will see, hear, or feel in isolation. Therefore they are shown the mask, gloves, and gown and are encouraged to "dress up" in them. Playing with the strange apparel lessens the fear of seeing "ghostlike" people walk into the room. Before entering the room, nurses and other health personnel should introduce themselves and let the child see their face before donning a mask. In this way the child associates them with significant experiences and gains a sense of familiarity in an otherwise strange and lonely environment.

When the child's condition improves, appropriate play activities are provided to minimize boredom, stimulate the senses, provide a real or perceived sense of movement, orient the child to time and place, provide social interaction, and reduce depersonalization.* For example, the environment can be manipulated to increase sensory freedom by moving the bed toward the door or window. Opening window shades; providing musical, visual, or tactile toys; and increasing interpersonal contact can substitute mental mobility for the limitations of physical movement. Rather than dwelling on the negative aspects of isolation, the child can be encouraged to view this experience as challenging and positive. For example, the nurse can help the child look at isolation as a method of keeping others out and letting only special people in. Children often think of intriguing signs for their doors, such as "Enter at your own risk" or "Many have entered but few have left." These signs also encourage people "on the outside" to talk with the child about the ominous greetings.

---

*An excellent resource for activities for children in isolation is *Therapeutic Play Activities for Hospitalized Children* by R.H. Hart and others (1992, Mosby).

NURSING TIP Have the child select a place he or she would like to visit. Help the child decorate the bed and equipment to suit the theme (e.g., truck, circus tent, spaceship, sky). At a set time each day pretend to go with the child to the special place. Consider including props such as a suitcase or picnic basket (Hart and others, 1992).

EMERGENCY ADMISSION

One of the most traumatic hospital experiences for the child and parents is an emergency admission. The sudden onset of an illness or the occurrence of an injury leaves little time for preparation and explanation. Sometimes the emergency admission is compounded by admission to an intensive care unit or the need for immediate surgery. However, even in those instances requiring only outpatient treatment, the child is exposed to a strange, frightening environment and to people who often inflict pain. Thus every medical emergency requires psychologic intervention to reduce the fear and anxiety frequently associated with the experience.

Lengthy preparatory admission procedures are often inappropriate for emergency situations. In such instances, nurses must focus their nursing interventions on the essential components of admission counseling (see box) and complete the process as soon as the child's condition is stabilized.

Unless an emergency is life-threatening, children need to participate in their care to maintain a sense of control. Because emergency rooms are frequently hectic, there is a tendency to rush through procedures to save time. However, the extra few minutes needed to allow children to participate may save many more minutes of useless resistance and uncooperativeness during subsequent procedures. Other supportive measures include ensuring privacy, accepting various emotional responses to fear or pain, preserving parent-child contact, explaining all events before or as they occur, and personally remaining calm.

At times, because of the child's physical condition, little or no preparatory counseling for emergency hospitalization can be done. In such situations the implementation of *postvention*, or counseling subsequent to the event, has therapeutic value. The process of postvention involves evaluating children's thoughts regarding admission and related procedures. It is similar to precounseling techniques; however, instead of supplying information, the nurse listens to the explanations offered by the child. Projective techniques such as drawing, doll play, or storytelling are especially effective. The

---

NEONATAL/PEDIATRIC ICU STRESSORS FOR THE CHILD AND FAMILY

Physical Stressors

Pain and discomfort (e.g., injections, intubation, suctioning, dressing changes, other invasive procedures)
Immobility (e.g., use of restraints, bed rest)
Sleep deprivation
Inability to eat or drink
Changes in elimination habits

Environmental Stressors

Unfamiliar surroundings (e.g., crowding)
Unfamiliar sounds
    Equipment noise (e.g., monitors, telephone, suctioning, computer printout)
    Human sounds (e.g., talking, laughing, crying, coughing, moaning, retching, walking)
Unfamiliar people (e.g., health care professionals, patients, visitors)
Unfamiliar and unpleasant smells (e.g., alcohol, adhesive remover, body odors)
Constant lights (disturb day/night rhythms)
Activity related to other patients
Sense of urgency among staff
Unkind or thoughtless comments from staff

Psychologic Stressors

Lack of privacy
Inability to communicate (if intubated)
Inadequate knowledge and understanding of situation
Severity of illness
Parental behavior (expression of concern)

Social Stressors

Disrupted relationships (especially with family and friends)
Concern with missing school or work
Play deprivation

Data primarily from Tichy AM and others: Stressors in pediatric intensive care units, *Pediatr Nurs* 14(1):40-42, 1988.

ESSENTIAL COMPONENTS OF EMERGENCY ADMISSIONS COUNSELING

Appropriate introduction to family
Use of child's name, not terms such as "honey" or "dear"
Determination of child's age and some judgment made about developmental age (if the child is of school age, asking about the grade level will offer some evidence for concurrent intellectual ability)
Information about the chief complaint from both parents and child
Information about child's general state of health, any problems that may interfere with medical treatment, such as sensitivity to medication, and previous experience with hospital facilities

---

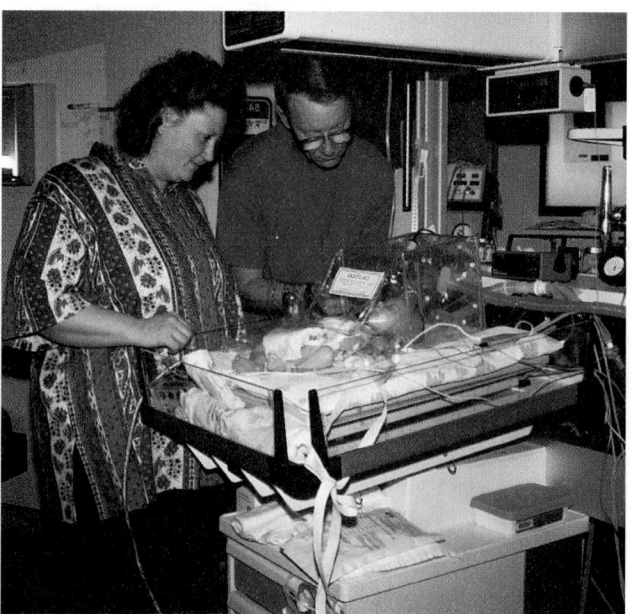

FIG. 21-15. Parents can be overwhelmed when their child is critically ill and requires care in an ICU.

nurse then bases additional information on what has already been revealed.

Intensive Care Unit (ICU)

Admission to an ICU can be a particularly traumatic event for both the child and the parents (Fig. 21-15). The nature and severity of the illness and the circumstances surrounding the admission are major factors, especially for parents. Parents experience significantly more stress when the admission is unexpected rather than expected. Stressors for the child and parent are described in the box on p. 664. Although several studies have described what parents perceive as most stressful, the most effective strategy may be to simply ask parents what is stressful and what they are doing to cope with the stressors they identify (Hughes and others, 1994). Assessment should be repeated periodically to account for changes in perceptions over time.

The emotional needs of the family are paramount when a child is admitted to an ICU. Although the same interventions discussed earlier for the stressors of separation, loss of control, and bodily injury and pain apply here, additional interventions may also benefit the family and child (see Guidelines and Family Focus boxes).

Critically ill children become the focus of the parents' lives, and parents' most pressing need is for information (Fisher, 1994). They want to know if their child will live, and if so,

FAMILY FOCUS
Artists as Partners in Care

A teenaged boy with a rare genetic disorder, having made steady progress after awakening from a coma, relapsed and seemed very depressed. When told that a musician was visiting the pediatric intensive care unit (PICU), he immediately perked up and asked to have his room lights turned on. He whispered endless song requests to the musician. Family members and staff were treated to some of his first smiles in days; his biggest came when the musician held his hand and guided it across the guitar stings while they sang "Born to Be Wild" together at the boy's request. His dad was misty-eyed as he thanked the musician for the visit.

A few weeks later the boy's condition worsened and he again lapsed into a coma. There was nothing more to be done. His parents began the necessary preparations to take their son home to die.

We continued to visit our friend and his family, offering a song, a story, or just simply to say hello. I hold a vivid picture of our final visit. We stood around the boy's bed with his parents singing together songs they remembered from their youth, from more carefree times. Song and laughter filled the boy's room.

Perhaps the boy heard his parents' laughter and knew then that they would be okay. He died a few days later on the morning he was to have been discharged.

Judy Rollins, MS, RN
Washington, DC

Modified from Rollins J: *Placed in our keeping*, 1995, unpublished.

GUIDELINES
Providing Support During ICU Admission

Prepare child and parents for elective ICU admission, such as for postoperative care after cardiac surgery.

Prepare child and parents for unanticipated ICU admission by focusing primarily on the sensory aspects of the experience and on usual family concerns (e.g., persons in charge of child's care, schedule for visiting, area where family can stay).

Prepare parents regarding child's appearance and behavior when they first visit child in ICU.

Accompany family to bedside to provide emotional support and answer questions.

Prepare siblings for their visit; plan length of time for sibling visitation; monitor siblings' reactions during visit to prevent them from becoming overwhelmed.

Encourage parents to stay with their child:
 If visiting hours are limited, allow flexibility in schedule to accommodate parental needs.
 Give family members a written schedule of visiting times.
 If visiting hours are liberal, be aware of family members' needs and suggest periodic respites.
 Assure family they can call the unit at any time.

Prepare parents for expected role changes and identify ways for parents to participate in child's care without overwhelming them with responsiblities:
 Help with bath or feeding.
 Touch and talk to child.
 Help with procedures.

Provide information about child's condition in understandable language:
 Repeat information often.
 Seek clarification of understanding.

During bedside conferences, interpret information for family members and child or, if appropriate, conduct report outside room.

Prepare child for procedures, even if this involves explanation while procedure is performed.

Assess and manage pain; recognize that a child who cannot talk, such as an infant or child in a coma or on a ventilator, can be in pain.

Establish a routine that maintains some similarity to daily events in child's life whenever possible:
 Organize care during normal waking hours.
 Keep regular bedtime schedules, including quiet times when television or radio is lowered or turned off.
 Provide uninterrupted sleep cycles (60 minutes for infant, 90 minutes for older child).
 Close and open drapes and dim lights to allow for day/night.
 Place curtain around bed for privacy.
 Orient child to day and time; have clocks or calendars in easy view for older children.

Schedule a time when child is left undisturbed (e.g., during naps, visit with family, playtime, or favorite program).

Reduce stimulation in environment:
 Refrain from loud talking or laughing.
 Keep equipment noise to a minimum:
  Turn alarms as low as safely possible.
  Perform treatments requiring equipment at one time.
  Turn off bedside equipment that is not in use, such as suction and oxygen.
  Avoid loud, abrupt noises, such as clattering bedpans or toilets flushing.

whether the child will be the same as before. They need to know why various interventions are being done for the child, that the child is being treated for pain and/or is comfortable, and that the child may be able to hear them even though not awake.

Despite the stresses normally associated with ICU admission, a special security develops from being carefully monitored and receiving individualized care. Therefore planning for transition to the regular unit is essential and should include (1) assignment of a primary nurse on the regular unit who visits before the transfer, (2) continued visits by the ICU staff to assess the child's and parents' adjustment and to act as a temporary liaison with the nursing staff, (3) explanation of the differences between the two units and the rationale for the change to less intense monitoring of the child's physical condition, and (4) selection of an appropriate room, such as one that is close to the nursing station, and a compatible roommate.

KEY POINTS

- Children are particularly vulnerable to the stresses of illness and hospitalization because stress represents a change from the usual state of health and routine and because they possess limited coping mechanisms.
- The three phases of separation anxiety are protest, despair, and detachment.
- Feelings of loss of control are caused by unfamiliar environmental stimuli, physical restriction, altered routine, and dependency.
- Fear of bodily pain may be manifested in the following ways: infants—facial expressions, body movements; toddlers—intense emotional upset, physical resistance; preschoolers—aggression, verbal expression, dependency; school-age children—precise verbalization of pain, passive requests for support or help, procrastination technique; adolescents—self-control, limited movement.
- Because of their separation from significant people, children who are hospitalized may lack the opportunity to form new attachments in the strange environment of the hospital and exhibit negative behaviors after discharge.
- Nursing care of the child in the hospital is aimed at preventing or minimizing separation, decreasing loss of control, minimizing bodily injury and pain, promoting normal development, using play/expressive activities to lessen stress, and maximizing the potential benefits of hospitalization.
- Pain assessment includes questioning the child, using pain rating scales, evaluating behavior, securing parents' involvement, taking the cause of the pain into account, and taking action. Pain management should incorporate both pharmacologic and nonpharmacologic methods.
- The nurse can maximize potential benefits of hospitalization by fostering parent-child relations, providing educational opportunities, promoting self-mastery, and encouraging socialization.
- Family reactions are influenced by the seriousness of the illness; experience with illness or hospitalization and diagnostic or therapeutic procedures; available support systems; personal ego strengths; coping abilities; presence of additional stresses; cultural and religious beliefs; and family communication patterns.
- Fear of contracting illness, their younger age, a close relationship with the ill sibling, substitute child care, minimum explanation of the illness, and perceived changes in parenting all increase the deleterious effects of a brother's or sister's illness and hospitalization on siblings.
- Nursing care of the family involves listening to parents' verbal and nonverbal messages; providing clergy support; accepting cultural, socioeconomic, and ethnic values; giving information to families and siblings; and preparing for discharge and home care.
- Admission to an outpatient setting, emergency department, isolation room, or intensive care unit requires additional intervention strategies to meet the child's and family's needs.

REFERENCES

Acute Pain Management Guideline Panel: *Acute pain management in infants, children, and adolescents: operative and medical procedures: quick reference guide for clinicians,* AHCPR Pub No 92-0020, Rockville, MD, 1992, Agency for Health Care Policy and Research, Public Health Service, US Department of Health and Human Services.

American Academy of Pediatrics: Neonatal anesthesia, *Pediatrics* 80(3):446, 1987.

American Pain Society: *Principles of analgesic use in the treatment of acute pain and chronic cancer pain,* ed 3, Skokie, IL, 1992, The Society.

Anand K, Aynsley-Green A: Metabolic and endocrine effects of surgical ligation of patent ductus arteriosus in the human preterm neonate: are there implications for further improvement of postoperative outcome? *Mod Probl Paediatr* 23:143-157, 1985.

Ashenburg MD and others: Easing the wait: development of a pager program for families, *Pediatr Nurs* 22(2):103-107, 1996.

Bauchner H, May A, Coates E: Use of analgesic agents for invasive medical procedures in pediatric and neonatal intensive care units, *J Pediatr* 121(4):647-649, 1992.

Benini F and others: Topical anesthesia during circumcision in new-born infants, *JAMA* 270(7):850-853, 1993.

Beyer JE and others: Patterns of postoperative analgesic use with adults and children following cardiac surgery, *Pain* 17:71-81, 1983.

Beyer JE and others: *The Oucher: a user's manual and technical report,* Bethesda, MD, 1995, Association for the Care of Children's Health.

Bossert E: Stress appraisals of hospitalized school-age children, *Child Health Care* 23(1):33-49, 1994.

Britton LJ, Johnston JD: Dependent on technology: a child grows up hospitalized, *Pediatr Nurs* 19(6):579, 1993.

Broome M and others: Children's medical fears, coping behaviors, and pain perceptions during a lumbar puncture, *Oncol Nurs Forum* 17(3):361-367, 1990.

Carson D, Gravley J, Council J: Children's prehospitalization conceptions of illness, cognitive development, and personal adjustment, *Child Health Care* 21(2):103-110, 1992.

Craft M: Siblings of hospitalized children: assessment and intervention, *J Pediatr Nurs* 8(5):289-297, 1993.

Craft M, Craft J: Perceived changes in siblings of hospitalized children: a comparison of sibling and parent reports, *Child Health Care* 18(1):42-48, 1989.

Darbyshire P: *Living with a sick child in hospital,* London, 1994, Chapman & Hall.

Davidson JAH, Boom SJ: Warming lignocaine to reduce pain associated with injection, *Br Med J* 305:617-618, 1992.

Eisenberg DM and others: Unconventional medicine in the United States: prevalence, costs, and patterns of use, *N Engl J Med* 328(4):246-252, 1993.

Eland J: Children with pain. In Jackson OB, Saunders RB: *Child health nursing,* Philadelphia, 1993, Lippincott.

Eland J, Anderson JE: The experience of pain in children. In Jacox A, editor: *Pain: a source book for nurses and other health professionals,* Boston, 1977, Little, Brown.

Farrington E: Lidocaine 2.5%/prilocaine 2.5% EMLA Cream, *Pediatr Nurs* 19(5):484-486, 488, 1993.

Favaloro R, Touzel B: A comparison of adolescents' and nurses' postoperative pain ratings and perceptions, *Pediatr Nurs* 16(4):414-417, 424, 1990.

Fisher M: Identified needs of parents in a pediatric intensive care unit, *Crit Care Nurse* 14(3):82-90, 1994.

Franck L: A national survey of the assessment and treatment of pain and agitation in the neonatal intensive care unit, *J Obstet Gynecol Neonatal Nurs* 16:387-393, 1987.

French GM, Painter EC, Courty DL: Blowing away shot pain: a technique for pain management during immunization, *Pediatrics* 93(3):384-388, 1994.

Friedland LR, Kulick RM: Emergency department analgesic use in pediatric trauma victims with fractures, *Ann Emerg Med* 23(2):203-207, 1994.

Friedman DP: Perspectives on the medical use of drugs of abuse, *J Pain Symptom Manage* 5(1):52-55, 1990.

Gaynard L and others: *Psychosocial care of children in hospitals,* Bethesda, MD, 1990, Association for the Care of Children's Health.

Gillis A: Hospital preparation: the children's story, *Child Health Care* 19(1):19-27, 1990.

Gordon M: *Manual of nursing diagnosis: 1995-1996,* St Louis, 1995, Mosby.

Gordon M: *Nursing diagnosis: process and application,* ed 3, St Louis, 1994, Mosby.

Gureno MA, Reisinger CL: Patient-controlled analgesia for the young pediatric patient, *Pediatr Nurs* 1991.

Hart D, Bossert E: Self-reported fears of hospitalized school-age children, *J Pediatr Nurs* 9(2):83-90, 1994.

Hart RH and others: *Therapeutic play activities for hospitalized children,* St Louis, 1992, Mosby.

Hester NO, Foster RL, Kristensen K: Measurement of pain in children: generalizability and validity of the pain ladder and poker chip tool. In Tyler D, Krane E, editors: *Advances in pain research and therapy: pediatric pain 15,* New York, 1990, Raven.

Hinnant DC: Reality check on placebos *Am J Nurs* 95(8):20, 1995.

Hughes M and others: How parents cope with the experience of neonatal intensive care, *Child Health Care* 23(1):1-14, 1994.

Johnson BH, Jeppson ES, Redburn L: *Caring for children and families: guidelines for hospitals,* Bethesda, MD, 1992, Association for the Care of Children's Health.

Kury S, Rodrigue J: Concepts of illness causality in a pediatric sample: relationship to illness duration, frequency of hospitalization, and degree of life-threat, *Clin Pediatr* 34(4):178-184, 1995.

Levi R: Childhood illness through a child's eyes, *ACCH Advocate* 2(1):43-45, 1995.

Love G: The dangers of normepederine toxicity, *Am J Nurs* 94(6):14, 1994.

Mather L, Mackie J: The incidence of postoperative pain in children, *Pain* 15:271-282, 1983.

McCaffery M: Analgesics: mapping out pain relief, *Nurs '96* 26(1):41-16, 1996.

McCaffery M, Beebe A: *Pain: clinical manual for nursing practice,* St Louis, 1989, Mosby.

Nugent K and others: A practice model for a parent support group, *Pediatr Nurs* 18(1):11-16, 1992.

O'Malley M, McNamara S: Children's drawings: a preoperative assessment tool, *AORN J* 57(5):1074-1089, 1993.

Orem D: *Nursing: concepts of practice,* ed 5, New York, 1995, Mosby.

Orlinsky M and others: Pain comparison of unbuffered versus buffered lidocaine in local wound infiltration, *J Emerg Med* 10:411-415, 1992.

Pasero CL, McCaffery M: Avoiding opiod-induced respiratory depression, *Am J Nurs* 94(4):25-31, 1994.

Pederson C: Presence as a nursing intervention with hospitalized children, *Matern Child Nurs J* 21(3):75-81, 1993.

Petrillo M, Sanger S: *Emotional care of hospitalized children,* ed 2, Philadelphia, 1980, Lippincott.

Pfefferbaum B, Adams J, Aceves, J: The influence of culture on pain in Anglo and Hispanic children with cancer, *J Am Acad Child Adolesc Psychiatry* 29(4):642-647, 1990.

Rae W: Analyzing drawings of children who are physically ill or hospitalized using the Ipsative method, *Child Health Care* 20(4):198-207, 1991.

Rollins J: Art: helping children meet the challenges of hospitalisation, *Interacta* 15(3):36-41, 1995.

Rollins J: Medical students as facilitators of the arts for children in hospitals, *Int J Arts Med* 2(1):7-13, 1993.

Rollins J: Supporting the child. In Smith DP and others, editors: *Comprehensive child and family nursing skills,* St Louis, 1991, Mosby.

Rowbotham D and others: Transdermal fentanyl for the relief of pain after upper abdominal surgery, *Br J Anaesth* 63:56-59, 1989.

Ruble K, Billett C: Innovative pain management for toddlers: parent-controlled analgesia, *Oncol Nurse Forum* 20(2):321, 1993.

Schepp K: Correlates of mothers who prefer control over their hospitalized child's care, *J Pediatr Nurs* 7(2):83-89, 1992.

Sciarillo W: Humanizing health care for children and families: revitalizing the spirit of our work, *ACCH Advocate* 2(11):4-8, 1995.

Simon K: Perceived stress of nonhospitalized children during the hospitalization of a sibling, *J Pediatr Nurs* 8(5):298-304, 1993.

Snodgrass WR, Dodge WF: Lytic/"DPT" cocktail: time for rationale and safe alternatives, *Pediatr Clin North Am* 36(5):1285-1291, 1985.

Snowdon A, Kane D: Parental needs following the discharge of a hospitalized child, *Pediatr Nurs* 21(5):425-428, 1995.

Stepanek JS, Ahmann E: Parent-professional collaboration when hospital visits are infrequent, *Pediatr Nurs* 21(5):466-468, 1995.

Taddio A and others: Safety of lidocaine-prilocaine cream in the treatment of preterm neonates, *J Pediatr* 127(6):1002-1005, 1995.

Tesler M and others: The word-graphic rating scale as a measure of children's and adolescents' pain intensity, *Res Nurs Health* 14:361-371, 1991.

Vessey JA, Carlson KL, McGill J: Use of distraction with children during an acute pain experience, *Nurs Res* 43(6):369, 1994.

Villarruel AM, Denyes MJ: Pain assessment in children: theoretical and empirical validity, *Adv Nurs Sci* 14(2):32-41, 1991.

Walker M, Wong DL: A battle plan for patients in pain, *Am J Nurs* 91(6):32-36, 1991.

Wallace M: Temperament: a variable in children's pain management, *Pediatr Nurs* 15(2):118-121, 1989.

Watt-Watson JH, Evernden C, Lawson C: Parents' perceptions of their child's acute pain experience, *J Pediatr Nurs* 5(5):344-349, 1990.

Webb C, Paarlberg J, Sussman M: The use of a PCA device by parents or nurses for postoperative pain in children with cerebral palsy, *J Pain Symptom Manage* 6(3):160, 1991.

Wells P and others: Growing up in the hospital. Part 1. Let's focus on the child, *J Pediatr Nurs* 9(2):66-73, 1994.

West N and others: Measuring pain in pediatric patients in the ICU, *J Pediatr Oncol Nurs* 11(2):64-68, 1994.

Whitis G: Visiting hospitalized patients, *J Adv Nurs* 19(1):85-88, 1994.

Willens JS: Giving fentanyl for pain outside the OR, *Am J Nurs* 94(2):24-28, 1994.

Wong D, Baker C: Pain in children: comparison of assessment scales, *Pediatr Nurs* 14(1):9-17, 1988.

Wong D, Baker C: *Reference manual for the Wong-Baker FACES Pain Rating Scale,* Tulsa, OK, 1996, Wong & Baker.

BIBLIOGRAPHY

Hospitalization: The Child and Family

Adams H: Humor: strong medicine . . . in a children's burn unit in a hospital in Tallinn, Estonia, *IJAM* 2(2):22-23, 1993.

American Academy of Pediatrics, Committee on Hospital Care: Staffing patterns for patient care and support personnel in a general pediatric unit, *Pediatrics* 93(5):850-854, 1994.

Baker N: Avoiding collisions with challenging families, *MCN Am J Matern Child Nurs* 19(2):97-101, 1994.

Banks E: Concepts of health and sickness of preschool- and school-aged children, *Child Health Care* 19(1):43-48, 1990.

Balayewich C, Gasson A: Oh, Suzanna! A nursing challenge, *Axone* 15(1):9-12, 1993.

Biddinger L: Bruner's theory of instruction and preprocedural anxiety in the pediatric population, *Issues Compr Pediatr Nurs* 16(3):147-154, 1993.

Biehler B: Impact of role-sets on implementing self-care theory with children, *Pediatr Nurs* 18(1):30-34, 1992.

Bolig R, Brown R, Kuo J: A comparison of never-hospitalized and previously hospitalized adolescents: self-esteem and locus of control, *Adolescence* 27(105):227-234, 1992.

Bossert E: Factors influencing the coping of hospitalized school-age children, *J Pediatr Nurs* 9(5):299-306, 1994.

Brown J, Ritchie JA: Nurses' perceptions of parent and nurse roles in caring for hospitalized children, *Child Health Care* 19(1):28-36, 1990.

Burke SO and others: Hazardous secrets and reluctantly taking charge: parenting a child with repeated hospitalizations, *Image J Nurs Sch* 23(1):39-45, 1991.

Chambers M: Play as therapy for the hospitalized child, *J Clin Nurs* 2(6):349-353, 1993.

Coffman S, Levitt MJ, Guacci-Franco N: Mothers' stress and close relationships: correlates with infant health status, *Pediatr Nurs* 19(2):135-140, 1993.

Coyne I: Partnership in care: parents' views of participation in their hospitalized child's care, *J Clin Nurs* 4(2):71-79, 1995.

Curley MA, Wallace J: Effects of the nursing Mutual Participation Model of Care on parental stress in the pediatric intensive care unit: a replication, *J Pediatr Nurs* 7(6):377-385, 1992.

Curtin L: There's no place like home, *Nurs Manage* 26(1):26-29, 1995.

Darbyshire P: Parents, nurses and paediatric nursing: a critical review, *J Adv Nurs* 18(11):1670-1680, 1993.

Darbyshire P: Parents in paediatrics, *Paediatr Nurs* 7(1):8-9, 1995.

Denholm CJ: Memories of adolescent hospitalization: results from a 4-year follow-up study, *Child Health Care* 19(2):101-105, 1990.

Dixon DM: Parent and nurse interaction during acute care, pediatric hospitalization, *Capsules Comments Pediatr Nurs* 2(2):91-99, 1995.

Evans M: An investigation into the feasibility of parental participation in the nursing care of their children, *J Adv Nurs* 20(3):477-482, 1994.

Gaynard L, Goldberger J, Laidley L: The use of stuffed body-outline dolls with hospitalized children and adolescents, *Child Health Care* 20(4):216-224, 1991.

Glendon K and others: Using a personal storybook and Mr Potato Head toy as a creative approach to individualized teaching, *ACCH Advocate* 1(12):49-51, 1993.

Goodill S and others: The role of dance/movement therapy with medically involved children, *IJAM* 2(2):24-27, 1993.

Graves JK, Ware ME: Parents' and health professionals' perceptions concerning parental stress during a child's hospitalization, *Child Health Care* 19(10):37-42, 1990.

Greenberg LA: Teaching children who are learning disabled about illness and hospitalization, *MCN Am J Matern Child Nurs* 16(5):260-263, 1991.

Grey M: Stressors and children's health, *J Pediatr Nurs* 8(2):85-91, 1993.

Grimm DL, Pefley PT: Opening doors for the child "inside," *Pediatr Nurs* 16(4):368-369, 1990.

Johnson A, Lindschau A: Staff attitudes toward parent participation in the care of children who are hopitalized, *Pediatr Nurs* 22(2):99-102, 1996.

Jones D: Effect of parental participation on hospitalized child behavior, *Issues Compr Pediatr Nurs* 17(2):81-92, 1994.

Kennedy C, Gyr P, Garst K: A nursing tool to assess children upon hospital admission, *MCN Am J Matern Child Nurs* 16(2):78-82, 1991.

Kristjansdottir G: A study of the needs of parents of hospitalized 2- to 6-year-old children, *Issues Compr Pediatr Nurs* 14(1):49-64, 1991.

Lau C: Parents in partnership: a family centered care program, *Paediatr Nurs* 6(2):11-15, 1993.

LeVieux-Anglin L and others: Incorporating play interventions into nursing care, *Pediatr Nurs* 19(5):459-463, 1993.

Lipsi K, Clements-Shafer K, Rushton C: Developmental rounds: an intervention strategy for hospitalized infants, *Pediatr Nurs* 17(5):433-437, 468, 1991.

Lloyd J and others: Screening for psychosocial dysfunction in pediatric inpatients, *Clin Pediatr* 34(1):18-24, 1995.

Logsdon DA: Conceptions of health and health behaviors of preschool children, *J Pediatr Nurs* 6(6):396-406, 1991.

Mabe P, Treiber F, Riley W: Examining emotional distress during pediatric hospitalization for school-aged children, *Child Health Care* 20(3):162-169, 1991.

McBurney BH, Schultz C: Defining quality services in a general pediatric unit, *J Nurs Care Qual* 7(3):51-60, 1993.

McClowry SG: Behavioral disturbances among medically hospitalized school-age children, *J Child Adolesc Psychiatr Ment Health Nurs* 4(2):62-67, 1991.

McClowry SG: The relationship of temperament to pre- and posthospitalization behavioral responses of school-age children, *Nurs Res* 39(1):30-35, 1990.

McClowry SG, McLeod SM: The psychosocial responses of school-age children to hospitalization, *Child Health Care* 19(3):155-161, 1990.

McLeod SM, McClowry SG: Using temperament theory to individualize the psychosocial care of hospitalized children, *Child Health Care* 19(2):79-85, 1990.

Merkens MJ: A pediatric chronic illness transition unit, *Child Health Care* 19(1):4-9, 1990.

Miron J: What children think about hospitals, *Can Nurs* 86(3):23-25, 1990.

Nelson-Smith J: Programs for play . . . real benefits of computers for children in hospital, *Nurs Times* 87(42):55-57, 1991.

Nix KS: Children and the health care system. In Smith DP and others, editors: *Comprehensive child and family nursing skills*, St Louis, 1991, Mosby.

Palmer S: Care of sick children by parents: a meaningful role, *J Adv Nurs* 18(2):185-191, 1993.

Porter CP, Villarruel AM: Socialization and caring for hospitalized African- and Mexican-American children, *Issues Compr Pediatr Nurs* 14(1):1-16, 1991.

Price S: The special needs of children, *J Adv Nurs* 20(2):227-232, 1994.

Rape R, Bush J: Psychological preparation for pediatric oncology patients undergoing painful procedures: a methodological critique of the research, *Child Health Care* 23(1):51-67, 1994.

Rikard-Bell C: The impact of critical incidents in paediatric hospitals: a review, *Aust J Adv Nurs* 12(1):29-35, 1994.

Schepp KG: Factors influencing the coping effort of mothers of hospitalized children, *Nurs Res* 40(1):42-46, 1991.

Slusher IL, McClure MJ: Infant stimulation during hospitalization, *J Pediatr Nurs* 7(4):276-279, 1992.

Strachan R: Emotional responses to paediatric hospitalisation, *Nurs Times* 89(46):45-49, 1993.

Thomas S: Child's play? . . . physical and emotional needs of sick children, *Nurs Times* 90(3):42-44, 1994.

Tiedman M, Clatworthy S: Anxiety responses of 5- and 11-year-old children during and after hospitalization, *J Pediatr Nurs* 5(5):334-343, 1990.

Tye V and others: Children's distress during magnetic resonance imaging procedures, *Child Health Care* 24(1):5-19, 1995.

Vessey J, Mahon M: Therapeutic play and the hospitalized child, *J Pediatr Nurs* 5(5):328-333, 1990.

Wells P and others: Growing up in the hospital: nurturing the philosophy of family-centered care. Part 2, *J Pediatr Nurs* 9(3):141-149, 1994.

While A: The contribution of nurses to children's well-being in hospital: a selective review of the literature, *J Clin Nurs* 1(3):117-121, 1992.

White MA and others: Sleep onset latency and distress in hospitalized children, *Nurs Res* 39(3):134-139, 1990.

Wilson C: Use of children's artwork to evaluate the effectiveness of a hospital preparation program, *Child Health Care* 20(2):120-121, 1991.

Wright MC: Behavioral effects of hospitalization in children, *J Paediatr Child Health* 31:165-167, 1995.

Yoos HL: Children's illness concepts: old and new paradigms, *Pediatr Nurs* 20(2):134-140, 145, 1994.

Young J: Changing attitudes towards families of hospitalized children from 1935 to 1975: a case study, *J Adv Nurs* 17(12):1422-1429, 1992.

Ziegler D and others: Preparation for surgery and adjustment to hospitalization, *Nurs Clin North Am* 29(4):655-669, 1994.

Special Hospital Situations

Bernardo LM, Conway K, Bove M: The ABC method of emotional assessment and intervention: a new approach in pediatric emergency care, *J Emerg Nurs* 16(2):70-76, 1990.

Braun R and others: Transitional family care: PICU to pediatrics, *Crit Care Nurse* 14(4):65-68, 1994.

Brunnquell D, Kohen D: Emotions in pediatric emergencies: what we know, what we can do, *Child Health Care* 20(4):240-247, 1991.

Curley MAQ: Caring for parents of critically ill children, *Crit Care Med* 21(9, suppl):S386-S387, 1993.

Doll-Speck L, Miller B, Rohrs K: Sibling education: implementing a program for the NICU, *Neonatal Network* 12(4)P:49-52, 1993.

Gillis AJ: Hospital preparation: the children's story, *Child Health Care* 19(1):19-27, 1990.

Heuer L: Parental stressors in a pediatric intensive care unit, *Pediatr Nurs* 19(2):128-131, 1993.

LaMontagne L, Pawlak R: Stress and coping of parents of children in a pediatric intensive care unit, *Heart Lung* 19(4):416-421, 1990.

LaMontagne L and others: Psychophysiological responses of parents to pediatric critical care stress, *Clin Nurs Res* 3(2):104-118, 1994.

Lynch M: Preparing children for day surgery, *Child Health Care* 23(3):78-85, 1994.

Melnyk B: Coping with unplanned childhood hospitalization: effects of informational interventions on mothers and children, *Nurs Res* 43(1):50-55, 1994.

Miles M, Funk S, Carelson J: Parental stressor scale: neonatal intensive care unit, *Nurs Res* 42(3):148-152, 1993.

Miles M, Mathes M: Preparation of parents for the ICU experience: what are we missing? *Child Health Care* 20(3):132-137, 1991.

Page N and others: Visitation in the pediatric intensive care unit: controversy and compromise, *AACN Clin Issues Crit Care Nurs* 5(3):289-295, 1994.

Pawlak R, Chiafery M: Parental coping and activities during pediatric critical care, *Am J Crit Care* 1(2):76-80, 1992.

Prudhoe C, Peters D: Social support of parents and grandparents in the neonatal intensive care unit, *Pediatr Nurs* 21(2):140-146, 1995.

Rushton CH: Child/family advocacy: ethical issues, practical strategies, *Crit Care Med* 21(9, suppl):S387, 1993.

Rushton CH: Family-centered care in the critical care setting: myth or reality? *Child Health Care* 19(2):68-78, 1990.

Rushton CH: Strategies for family-centered care in the critical care setting, *Pediatr Nurs* 16(2):195-199, 1990.

Saunders A: Changing nurses' attitudes toward parenting in the NICU, *Pediatr Nurs* 20(4):392-394, 1994.

Small M, Engler A, Rushton C: Saying goodbye in the intensive care unit: helping caregivers grieve, *Pediatr Nurs* 17(1):103-105, 1991.

Stern HP and others: Communication, decision making, and perception of nursing roles in a pediatric intensive care unit, *Crit Care Nurs Q* 14(3):56-68, 1991.

Thomas DO: How to deal with children in the emergency department, *J Emerg Nurs* 17(1):49-50, 1991.

Todres ID: Communication between physician, patient, and family in the pediatric intensive care unit, *Crit Care Med* 21(9, suppl):S383-S385, 1993.

Tughan L: Visiting in the PICU: a study of the perceptions of patients, parents, and staff members, *Crit Care Nurs Q* 15(1):57-68, 1992.

Vessey J, Farley J, Risom L: Iatrogenic developmental effects of pediatric intensive care, *Pediatr Nurs* 17(3):229-232, 1991.

Voepel-Lewis T, Andrea CM, Magee SS: Parent perceptions of pediatric ambulatory surgery: using family feedback for program evaluation, *J Post Anesth Nurs* 7(2):106-114, 1992.

While A, Wilcox V: Paediatric day surgery: day-case unit admission compared with general paediatric ward admission, *J Adv Nurs* 19(1):52-57, 1994.

Youngblut JM, Shiao SP: Child and family reactions during and after pediatric ICU hospitalization: a pilot study, *Heart Lung* 22:46-53, 1993.

Pain Assessment

Beard J: Pain control: when your patient can't speak, *Am J Nurs* 94(4):22-23, 1994.

Beyer JE, Denyes MJ, Villarruel AM: The creation, validation and continuing development of the Oucher: a measure of pain intensity in children, *J Pediatr Nurs* 7(5):335-346, 1992.

Beyer JE, Knapp TR: Methodologic issues in the measurement of children's pain, *Child Health Care* 14(4):233-241, 1986.

Beyer JE, McGrath PJ, Berde CB: Discordance between self-report and behavioral pain measures in children aged 3-7 years after surgery, *J Pain Symptom Manage* 5(6):350-356, 1990.

Beyer JE, Wells N: The assessment of pain in children, *Pediatr Clin North Am* 36(4):837-854, 1989.

Bieri D and others: The Faces Pain Scale for the self-assessment of the severity of pain experienced by children: development, initial validation, and preliminary investigation for ratio scale properties, *Pain* 41(2):139-150, 1990.

Broome M: Measurement of pain: self-report strategies, *J Pediatr Oncol Nurs* 8(3):131-133, 1991.

Eland JM, Banner W: Assessment and management of pain in children. In Hazinski MF: *Nursing care of the critically ill child*, ed 2, St Louis, 1992, Mosby.

Ernst AA and others: Lidocaine adrenaline tetracaine gel versus tetracaine adrenaline cocaine gel for topical anesthesia in linear scalp and facial lacerations in children aged 5 to 17 years, *Pediatrics* 95(2):255-258, 1995.

Franck LS: Pain in the nonverbal patient: advocating for the critically ill neonate, *Pediatr Nurs* 15(1):65, 1989.

Gujol MC: A survey of pain assessment and management practices among critical care nurses, *Am J Crit Care* 3(2):123-128, 1994.

Harbeck C, Peterson L: Elephants dancing in my head: a developmental approach to children's concepts of specific pains, *Child Dev* 63:138-149, 1992.

Hester NO: Pain in children. In Fitzpatrick JJ, Stevenson JS, editors: *Annual review of nursing research*, vol 11, New York, 1993, Springer.

Jordan-Marsh M and others: Alternate Oucher form testing gender ethnicity and age variations, *Res Nurs Health* 17:111-118, 1994.

Knott C and others: Using the Oucher: developmental approach to pain assessment in children, *MCN* 19(6):314-320, 1994.

Kuttner L, LePage T: Face scales for the assessment of pediatric pain: a critical review, *Can J Behav Sci* 21(2)198-209, 1989.

LaMontagne LL and others: Children's ratings of postoperative pain compared to ratings by nurses and physicians, *Issues Compr Pediatr Nurs* 14(4):241-247, 1991.

Lincoln LM: Children's response to acute pain: a developmental approach, *J Am Acad Nurse Practitioners* 4(4):139-141, 1992.

Mackey D, Jordan-Marsh M: Innovative assessment of children's pain, *J Emerg Nurs* 17(4):250-215, 1991.

McCaffery M: How reliable is your patient's pain assessment? *Nursing '94* 24(1):19, 1994.

McCaffery M, Ferrel B: Opioid analgesics: nurses' knowledge of doses and psychological dependence, *J Nurs Staff Dev* 8(2):77-84, 1992.

McGrath PA: Evaluating a child's pain, *J Pain Symptom Manage* 4(4):198-214, 1989.

McGrath PJ, Craig KD: Developmental and psychological factors in children's pain, *Pediatr Clin North Am* 36(4):823-836, 1989.

McGrath PJ, Unruh A: *Pain in children and adolescents,* New York, 1988, Elsevier Science.

Miller D: Comparisons of pain ratings from postoperative children, their mothers, and their nurses, *Pediatr Nurs* 22(2):145-149, 1996.

Pasero CL: The right tool for the job, *Am J Nurs* 94(2):22, 1994.

Ross DM, Ross SA: *Childhood pain: current issues, research, and management,* Baltimore, 1988, Urban & Schwarzenberg.

Savedra MC and others: Assessment of postoperative pain in children and adolescents using the adolescent pediatric pain tool, *Nurs Res* 42(1):5-9, 1993.

Schechter NL: The undertreatment of pain in children: an overview, *Pediatr Clin North Am* 36(4):781-794, 1989.

Schmidt K, Eland J, Weiler K: Pediatric cancer pain management: a survey of nurses' knowledge, *J Pediatr Oncol Nurs* 11(1):4-12, 1994.

Smith GA and others: Comparison of topical anesthetics without cocaine to tetracaine-adrenaline-cocaine and lidocaine infiltration during repair of lacerations: Bupivacaine-norepinephrine is an effective new topical anesthetic agent, *Pediatrics* 97(3):301-307, 1996.

Stevens B: Development and testing of a pediatric pain management sheet, *Pediatr Nurs* 16(6):543-548, 1990.

Van Cleve L, Savedra M: Pain location: validity and reliability of body outline markings for 4- to 7-year-old children who are hospitalized, *Pediatr Nurs* 19(3):217-220, 1993.

Wilkie DJ and others: Measuring pain quality: validity and reliability of children's and adolescents' pain language, *Pain* 41:151-159, 1990.

Wong DL: Pediatric pain assessment scales: where do we go from here? *J Pediatr Oncol Nurs* 11(2):69-70, 1994.

Wong DL: The FACES pain rating scale, *Home Health Focus* 2(8):63, 1996.

Wong DL, Baker C: The school nurse and the child in pain, *Sch Nurs* 5(2):14-28, 1989.

Pain Management

Bonadio W, Wagner V: Adrenaline-cocaine gel topical anesthetic for dermal laceration repair in children, *Ann Emerg Med* 21(12):1435-1438, 1992.

Bostrom B, McCormick P, Hooke C: Painless procedures with propofol, *J Pediatr Oncol Nurs* 10(2):64-65, 1993.

Broome M, Lillis P, Smith MC: Pain management with children: a meta-analysis of the research, *Nurs Res* 2:154-158, 1989.

Engebo D: Safe and effective use of tetracaine, adrenaline, and cocaine (TAC) solution anesthetic for anesthetizing of lacerations, *J Emerg Nurs* 16(2):100-101, 1990.

French JP, Nocera M: Drug withdrawal symptoms in children after continuous infusions of fentanyl, *J Pediatr Nurs* 9(2):107-113, 1994.

Fox AE: Confronting the use of placebos for pain, *Am J Nurs* 9(9):42-46, 1994.

Goode IA, Betcher DL: EMLA, *J Pediatr Oncol Nurs* 11(1):38-41, 1994.

Gordon D: Hydroxyzine doesn't 'help' opioids, *Am J Nurs* 95(8):20, 1995.

Heiney S: Helping children through painful procedures, *Am J Nurs* 1(11):20-24, 1991.

Howe CJ: A new standard of care for pediatric pain management, *MCN Am J Matern Child Nurs* 18(6):325-329, 1993.

Leahy S, Hockenberry-Eaton M, Sigler-Price K: Clinical management of pain in children with cancer: selected approaches and innovative strategies, *Cancer Pract* 2(1):37-45, 1994.

Pederson C: Ways to feel comfortable: teaching aids to promote children's comfort, *Issues Compr Pediatr Nurs* 17(1):37-46, 1994.

Position statement in the role of the RN in the management of patients receiving IV conscious sedation for short-term therapeutic, diagnostic, or surgical procedures, *AORN J* 55:207-208, 1992.

Proudfoot J: Analgesia, anesthesia, and conscious sedation, *Emerg Med Clin North Am* 13(2):357-379, 1995.

Sacchetti A and others: Pediatric analgesia and sedation, *Ann Emerg Med* 23:237-250, 1994.

Schechter NL, Altman A, Weisman S: Report of the Consensus Conference on the Management of Pain in Childhood Cancer, *Pediatrics* 86(5, suppl):813-834, 1990.

Schechter NL and others: The use of oral transmucosal fentanyl citrate for painful procedures in children, *Pediatrics* 95(3):335-339, 1995.

Selbst SM, Clark M: Analgesic use in the emergency department, *Ann Emerg Med* 19:1010-1013, 1990.

Steward DJ: Management of childhood pain: new approaches to procedure-related pain, *J Pediatr* 122(5, pt 2):entire issue, 1993.

Taddio A and others: Use of lidocaine-prilocaine cream for vaccination pain in infants, *J Pediatr* 124(4):643-648, 1994.

Terndrup TE: Pediatric pain control, *Ann Emerg Med* 27(4):466-470, 1996.

Tobias JD: Indications and applications of epidural anesthesia in a pediatric population outside the perioperative period, *Clin Pediatr* 32(2):81-85, 1993.

Tobias JD, Rasmussen GE: Pain management and sedation in the pediatric intensive care unit, *Pediatr Clin North Am* 41(6):1269-1292, 1994.

Tobias JD and others: Oral ketamine premedication to alleviate the distress of invasive procedures in pediatric oncology patients, *Pediatrics* 90(4):537-541, 1992.

Tyler DC: Pharmacology of pain management, *Pediatr Clin North Am* 41(1):59, 1994.

Valente S: Using hypnosis with children for pain management, *Oncol Nurs Forum* 18(4):699-704, 1991.

Weisman SJ, Schechter NL: The management of pain in children, *Pediatr Rev* 12(8):237-243, 1991.

Wong DL: DPT pedi-cocktail: not a good mix, *Am J Nurs* 94(6):14-15, 1994.

Wong DL: Managing pain. In Smith DP and others, editors: *Comprehensive child and family nursing skills,* St Louis, 1991, Mosby.

Wong DL: Overcoming 'needle phobia' with EMLA, *Am J Nurs* 65(2):24, 1995.

Yaster M: Pain relief, *Pediatrics* 95(3):427-428, 1995.

Yaster M and others: Local anesthetics in the management of acute pain in children, *J Pediatr* 124(2)165-176, 1994.

Zajac J: Pediatric pain management, *Crit Care Nurse Q* 15(2):35-51, 1992.

Discharge Planning and Home Care

Cady C, Yoshioka R: Using a learning contract to successfully discharge an infant on home total parenteral nutrition, *Pediatr Nurs* 17(1):67-71, 74, 1991.

Crummette B, Boatwright D: Case management in inpatient pediatric nursing, *Pediatr Nurs* 17(5):469-473, 1991.

Curry R, Cullen J: Using videorecordings in pediatric nursing practice, *Pediatr Nurs* 16(5):501-504, 1990.

DeWitt P and others: Obstacles to discharge of ventilator-assisted children from the hospital to home, *Chest* 103(5):1560-1565, 1993.

Hill DS: Coordinating a multidisciplinary discharge for the technology-dependent child based on parental needs, *Issues Compr Pediatr Nurs* 16(4):229-237, 1993.

Hogue E: Liability for premature discharge: an update, *Pediatr Nurs* 17(1):76, 78, 1991.

Isaacman DJ and others: Standardized instructions: do they improve communication of discharge information from the emergency department? *Pediatrics* 89(6):1204-1208, 1992.

Kasprisin C: Home care instructions. In Wong DL: *Wong and Whaley's clinical manual of pediatric nursing,* ed 4, St Louis, 1996, Mosby.

McClowry SG: Pediatric nursing psychosocial care: a vision beyond hospitalization, *Pediatr Nurs* 19(2):146-148, 1993.

Nuttall P, Nicholes P: Cystic fibrosis: adolescent and maternal concerns about hospital and home care, *Issues Compr Pediatr Nurs* 15(3):199-213, 1992.

Scharer K and others: Evaluating written discharge instructions in a pediatric setting, *J Nurs Qual Assur* 4(4):63-71, 1990.

Sheikh L, O'Brien M, McCluskey-Fawcett K: Parent preparation for the NICU-to-home transition: staff and parent perceptions, *Child Health Care* 22(3):227-239, 1993.

Siarkowski-Amer K, Piegeon V: Documentation of discharge teaching before and after use of a discharge teaching tool, *J Pediatr Nurs* 6(5):296-301, 1991.

While AE: Consumer views of health care: a comparison of hospital and home care, *Child Care Health Dev* 18(2):107-116, 1992.

Wong DL: Transition from hospital to home for children with complex medical care, *J Pediatr Oncol Nurs* 8(1):3-9, 1991.

Worthington R: Family matters. Effective transitions for families: life beyond the hospital, *Pediatr Nurs* 21(1):86-87, 1995.

Selected Books for Children

Banks A: *Hospital journal: a kid's guide to a strange place,* New York, 1989, Viking Penguin.

Chase F, Coleman L: *A visit to the hospital,* New York, 1974, Grosset & Dunlap.

Clark B: *Going to the hospital,* New York, 1970, Random House (pop-up book).

Collier J: *Danny goes to the hospital,* New York, 1970, Norton.

Drescher J: *The moon balloon,* Bethesda, MD, 1996, Association for Care of Children's Health.

Howe J: *The hospital book,* New York, 1981, Crown.

Moore A: *Broken Arrow boy,* Kansas City, MO, 1990, Landmark Editions.

Rey M, Rey H: *Curious George goes to the hospital,* New York, 1966, Houghton Mifflin.

Stein S: *A hospital story,* New York, 1974, Walker.

Weber A: *Elizabeth gets well,* New York, 1970, Crowell.

Other Resources

Association for Care of Children's Health, 7910 Woodmont Ave., Suite 300, Bethesda, MD 20814; (301) 654-6549; (800) 808-ACCH.

Centering Corporation, 1531 N. Saddle Creek Rd., Omaha, NE 68104; (402) 555-1200.

Talks About the Hospital, a series written by Fred Rogers, is available from Family Communications, Inc., 4802 Fifth Ave., Pittsburgh, PA 15213; (412) 687-2990.

Chapter 22

PEDIATRIC VARIATIONS OF NURSING INTERVENTIONS

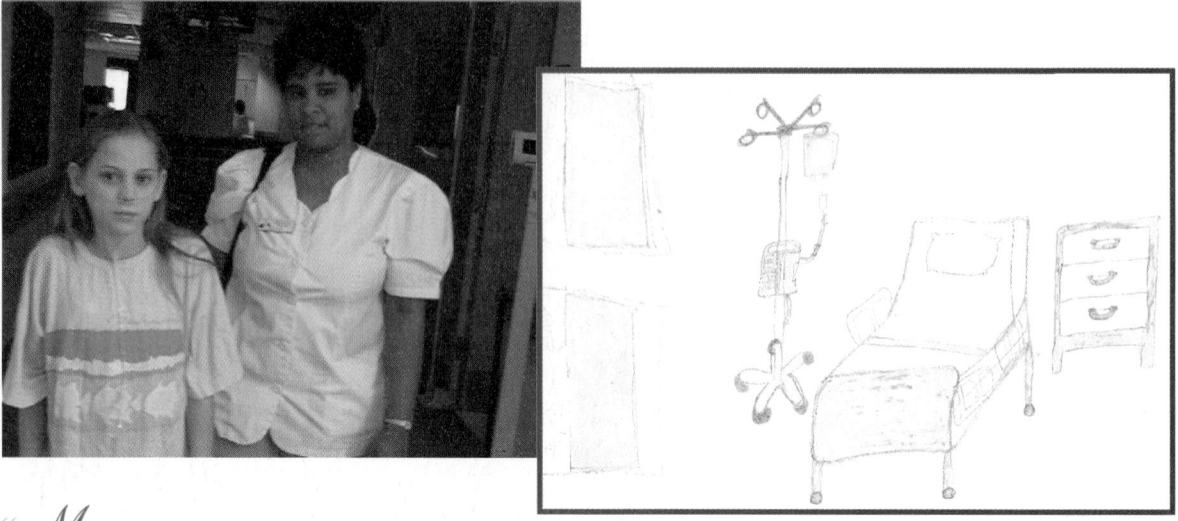

" *My nurse stayed with me through the whole thing when I had a chest tube put in. It really helped.* "

Tefawna, age 16 years, cystic fibrosis

LEARNING OBJECTIVES
On completion of this chapter the reader will be able to:

- Identify those instances in which informed consent is required and in which minors may be considered emancipated
- Formulate general guidelines for preparing children for procedures, including surgery
- Implement play in therapeutic procedures
- List general strategies for enhancing compliance in children and families
- Outline general hygiene and care procedures for hospitalized children

- Implement feeding techniques that encourage food and fluid intake
- Describe methods of reducing temperature in a child with fever or hyperthermia
- Describe systems that can be used for infection control
- Describe safe methods of administering oral, parenteral, rectal, optic, otic, and nasal medications to children

- Identify nursing responsibilities in maintaining fluid balance
- Demonstrate correct procedures for postural drainage and tracheostomy care
- Describe the procedures involved in providing nutrition via gavage, gastrostomy, and parenteral routes
- Describe the procedures involved in administering an enema and ostomy care to children

GENERAL CONCEPTS RELATED TO PEDIATRIC PROCEDURES

INFORMED CONSENT

Informed consent refers to the legal and ethical requirement that the patient clearly, fully, and completely understand the proposed medical treatment to be performed, including significant risks associated with the treatment. The patient must also be informed of alternative treatments that could be offered, including their benefits and risks and the risks of nontreatment, before giving informed consent. To obtain valid informed consent, the following three conditions must be met (Hogue, 1988):

1. The person must be capable of giving consent; he or she must be over the age of majority (usually age 18) and must be considered competent (i.e., possess the mental capacity to make choices and understand their consequences).
2. The person must receive the information needed to make an intelligent decision.
3. The person must act voluntarily when exercising freedom of choice without force, fraud, deceit, duress, or other forms of constraint or coercion.

Kathryn A. Perry, MSN, APRN, RN,C, CNS revised this chapter.

Because of the numerous variations of the laws and institutional policies within the United States, the following discussion of informed consent is presented in general terms and is not to be interpreted as legal advice. Although informing patients of the risks, benefits, and alternatives of a procedure is the physician's responsibility, nurses frequently are responsible for securing the person's signature on a written consent form. In caring for children, special dilemmas may arise regarding who may sign the consent for treatment when parental consent is not available. The *age of majority* is especially important when caring for adolescents, and *competence* is a key issue in decisions involving minors who are retarded. Also, the judicial system may intervene in cases where the parents' views and the child's best interests conflict (Nix, 1991). Consequently, nurses need to be familiar with the issues involved in this highly significant and complex subject and must keep current on legal aspects of practice within their community.

Requirements for Obtaining Informed Consent

Written informed consent of the parent or legal guardian is usually required for medical or surgical treatment, including many diagnostic procedures. One blanket consent is not sufficient. Separate informed permissions must be obtained for each surgical or diagnostic procedure, including the following:

1. Major surgery
2. Minor surgery (e.g., cutdown, biopsy, dental extraction, suturing a laceration [especially one that may have a cosmetic effect], removal of a cyst, closed reduction of a fracture)
3. Diagnostic tests with an element of risk (e.g., bronchoscopy, needle biopsy, angiography, electroencephalogram, lumbar puncture, cardiac catheterization, ventriculography, bone marrow aspiration)
4. Medical treatments with an element of risk (e.g., blood transfusion, thoracentesis or paracentesis, radiation therapy, shock therapies)

In addition, certain situations are not directly related to medical treatment but require parental consent, such as the following:

1. Taking photographs for medical, educational, or other public use
2. Removal of the child from the health care institution against the advice of the physician
3. Postmortem examinations, except in unexplained deaths, such as sudden infant death, violent death, or suspected suicide
4. Examination of medical records by unauthorized persons, such as attorneys or insurance representatives (family members have legal right to medical records) (see Thinking Critically About . . . box)

The need for informed consent is also an issue with proposed treatments or research involving children with a mental age of 7 years or older. *Assent* (usually verbal agreement) requires that the child be informed about the proposed treatment or research and agree or concur with the decisions made by the person(s) who can give informed consent. By including children in the decision-making process and gaining their acceptance, children are treated with respect. Assent is not a legal requirement but an ethical one to protect the rights of children.

Eligibility for Giving Informed Consent

In most situations the parent or legal guardian gives informed consent. However, problems may arise when parents are not available to give informed consent, the child is a borderline or emancipated minor, or the parents neglect or refuse care for their minor children.

THINKING CRITICALLY ABOUT . . .
Informed Consent and Parental
Right to the Child's Medical Chart

Does the right to certain types of information before giving valid informed consent include the right to review medical records? Since the process of consent continues throughout the patient's treatment, is there an ongoing right of parents to see their children's medical charts?

The answer to these questions varies depending on state law. Some state statutes give parents the unrestricted right to a copy of children's medical records. Other states have no statutes that address this point. In these states the best practice is to allow parents to review or have a copy of minors' charts under reasonable circumstances. That is, records should be available in a reasonable time. In addition, practitioners should avoid restrictive requirements such as review permitted only in the presence of a clinician. Rather, an appropriate practitioner should be available to answer any questions that parents may have during their review.

Informed Consent of Parents or Legal Guardians. Parents have full responsibility for the care and rearing of their minor children, including legal control over them. Therefore, as long as children are minors, their parents or legal guardians are required to give informed consent before medical treatment is rendered or any procedure is performed on them. Parents also have a right to withdraw consent later.

Evidence of Consent.   A signed consent form is only evidence that the process of informed consent has occurred; it is not legally required, although it may be an institutional policy. Verbal consent is also evidence of the process (Cushing, 1991). For example, when parents are unavailable to sign consent forms, verbal consent may be obtained via telephone. Verbal consent may also be obtained from parents who are unable to sign (e.g., because of injury). It is good risk management to have a witness to a parent's or guardian's verbal consent. Another nurse may be present or listening on a telephone extension. Both nurses record that informed consent was given and the name, address, and relationship of the person giving consent, together with their signatures indicating that they witnessed the consent.

Informed Consent of Mature and Emancipated Minors.   State laws differ with regard to the so-called age of majority. Although some variation still exists, children become adults on their eighteenth birthday in most states. Competent adults can give informed consent on their own behalf. Nonetheless, some courts have permitted minors to consent to their treatment based on the *mature minors' doctrine,* which permits minors to give consent even though they are not technically adults as long as they understand the consequences of their decisions (Brent, 1991). For example, statutes in many states permit minors to give consent on their own behalf to certain treatments, such as for sexually transmitted diseases, contraceptive services, pregnancy, or drug or alcohol abuse.

An *emancipated minor* is one who is legally under the age of majority but is recognized as having the legal capacity of an adult under circumstances prescribed by state law, such as pregnancy, marriage, high school graduation, living independently, or military service.

Consent to abortion is more complex. The issue of parental notification before or after an abortion is still undecided, although several states have enacted laws that state minors seeking abortions must involve their parents or obtain court permission (Johannsen, 1995). A woman's right to abortion is an extremely controversial legal and moral issue in the United States.

Treatment Without Parental Consent.   Exceptions to requiring parental consent before treating minor children occur in situations in which children need prompt medical or surgical treatment and a parent is not readily available to give consent or refuses to give consent. In the absence of parents or legal guardians, some providers permit persons in charge of the child to give informed consent for treatment. In emergencies, consent is not needed; it is implied according to the law (Hogue, 1988). Emergencies include danger to life or possibility of permanent injury.

Refusal to give consent can occur when the treatment, such as blood transfusions, conflicts with the parents' religious beliefs. All states recognize such exceptions and have statutory procedures to permit treatment if the life or health of such a minor is in jeopardy or if delayed treatment would create a risk to the minor's health. The state is also able to intervene in situations that jeopardize the health and welfare of children, as in cases in which parents neglect or impose excessive or improper punishment on a child. Most communities have procedures by which custody of the child can be transferred to a governmental or a private agency when parental neglect or abuse can be proved.

PREPARATION FOR PROCEDURES

For most procedures, no special physical preparation is needed, and the focus of care is psychologic preparation of the child and family (see next section). However, some procedures require physical preparation before the procedure, such as cleansing and shaving of the skin before surgery. One area of special concern is the administration of appropriate sedation and/or analgesia before stressful procedures (see p. 685). The drug is given before the procedure to allow time for the medication to reach its peak effect. Whenever possible, the intravenous (through an existing infusion), oral, or rectal route is used rather than the intramuscular route be-

cause children dislike injections. Some institutions are using short-acting anesthetics, such as ketamine, or potent analgesics, such as fentanyl, to eliminate the pain and trauma associated with treatments, such as bone marrow tests, lumbar punctures, burn débridement, and suturing. (See also Pain Management, Chapter 21.)

Psychologic Preparation

Preparing children for procedures decreases their anxiety, promotes their cooperation, supports their coping skills and may teach them new ones, and facilitates a feeling of mastery in experiencing a potentially stressful event. Preparatory methods may be formal, such as group preparation for hospitalization. Most preparation strategies used by nurses are informal, focus on providing information about the experience, and are directed at stressful and/or painful procedures. In general, young children respond better to play materials, and older youngsters benefit more from viewing peer-modeling films (Bates and Broome, 1986). Especially for painful procedures, the most effective preparation includes the provision of sensory-procedural information and helping the child develop coping skills, such as imagery or relaxation (Broome, 1990).

General guidelines for preparing children for procedures are described in the box, and age-specific guidelines that consider children's developmental needs and cognitive abilities are presented in the box on pp. 676-677. In addition to these suggestions, nurses should consider the child's temperament, existing coping strategies, and previous experiences in individualizing the preparatory process. Children who are distractible and highly active, as well as those who are "slow to warm up," may need individualized sessions that are shorter for the active child but more slowly paced for the shy child. Youngsters who tend to cope well may need more emphasis on using their present skills, whereas those who appear to cope less adequately can benefit from more time devoted to simple coping strategies, such as relaxing, breathing, counting, squeezing a hand, or singing.

NURSING TIPS Prepare a basket (toy or treasure chest or cart) to keep near the treatment area. Items ideal for the basket are a Slinky; a sparkling "magic" wand (clear, acrylic tube sealed on both ends and partially filled with liquid in which is suspended metallic confetti); a soft foam ball; bubble solution; party blowers; pop-up books with foldout, three-dimensional scenes; real medical equipment, such as a syringe, adhesive bandages, and alcohol packets; toy medical supplies or a toy medical kit; marking pens; a note pad; and stickers. Have the child choose an item to use during a procedure, such as a party blower to help distract and relax the youngster. After the procedure, allow the child to choose a small gift, such as a sticker, or to play with items, such as medical equipment (Heiney, 1991).

Children also are different in their "information-seeking dimension"; some want and actively solicit information about the intended procedure, whereas others characteristically avoid information.

The exact timing of the preparation for a procedure varies with the child's age and the type of procedure. There are no exact guidelines to govern timing, but in general the younger

---

GENERAL GUIDELINES FOR PREPARING CHILDREN FOR PROCEDURES

Determine details of exact procedure to be performed.

Review parents' and child's present level of understanding.

Plan actual teaching based on child's developmental age and existing level of knowledge.

Incorporate parents in the teaching if they desire, especially if they plan to participate in care.

Inform parents of their role during procedure, such as stand near child's head or in line of vision and talk softly to child.

While preparing child and family, allow for ample discussion to prevent information overload and ensure adequate feedback.

Use concrete, not abstract, terms and visual aids to describe procedure. For example, use a simple line drawing of a boy or girl (Fig. 22-1), and mark the body part that will be involved in the procedure.

Emphasize that no other body part will be involved.

If the body part is associated with a specific function, stress the change or noninvolvement of that ability (e.g., following tonsillectomy, child can still speak).

Use words appropriate to child's level of understanding (a rule of thumb for number of words is age in years plus 1).

Avoid words and phrases with dual meanings (see Guidelines box on p. 678) unless child understands such words.

Clarify all unfamiliar words (e.g., "Anesthesia is a *special* sleep").

Emphasize sensory aspects of procedure—what child will feel, see, smell, and touch and what child can do during procedure (e.g., lie still, count out loud, squeeze a hand, hug a doll).

Allow child to practice those procedures that will require cooperation (e.g., turning, deep breathing, using an incentive spirometer or mask).

Introduce anxiety-laden information last (e.g., the preoperative injection).

Be honest with child about unpleasant aspects of a procedure but avoid creating undue concern. When discussing that a procedure may be uncomfortable, state that it feels differently to different people and have child describe how it felt.

Emphasize end of procedure and any pleasurable events afterward (e.g., going home, seeing the parent).

Stress positive benefits of procedure (e.g., "After your tonsils are fixed, you won't have as many sore throats").

AGE-SPECIFIC GUIDELINES FOR PREPARING CHILDREN FOR PROCEDURES BASED ON DEVELOPMENTAL CHARACTERISTICS

Infant: Developing a Sense of Trust and Sensorimotor Thought
Attachment to Parent

*Involve parent in procedure if desired.

Keep parent in infant's line of vision.

If parent is unable to be with infant, place familiar object with infant (e.g., stuffed toy).

Stranger Anxiety

*Have usual caregivers perform or assist with procedure.

Make advances slowly and in nonthreatening manner.

*Limit number of strangers entering room during procedure.

Sensorimotor Phase of Learning

During procedure use sensory soothing measures (e.g., stroking skin, talking softly, giving pacifier).

*Use analgesics (e.g., local anesthetic, intravenous opioid) to control discomfort.

Cuddle and hug child after stressful procedure; encourage parent to comfort child.

Increased Muscle Control

Expect older infants to resist.

Restrain adequately.

Keep harmful objects out of reach.

Memory for Past Experiences

Realize that older infants may associate objects, places, or persons with prior painful experiences and will cry and resist at the sight of them.

*Keep frightening objects out of view.

*Perform painful procedures in a separate room, not in crib (or bed).

*Use nonintrusive procedures whenever possible (e.g., axillary or tympanic temperatures, oral medications).

Imitation of Gestures

Model desired behavior (e.g., opening mouth).

Toddler: Developing a Sense of Autonomy and Sensorimotor to Preoperational Thought

Use same approaches as for infant in addition to the following:

Egocentric Thought

Explain procedure in relation to what child will see, hear, taste, smell, and feel.

Emphasize those aspects of procedure that require cooperation (e.g., lying still).

Tell child it's okay to cry, yell, or use other means to express discomfort verbally.

Negative Behavior

Expect treatments to be resisted; child may try to run away.

Use firm, direct approach.

Ignore temper tantrums.

Use distraction techniques (e.g., singing a song *with* a child).

Restrain adequately.

Animism

Keep frightening objects out of view (young children believe objects have lifelike qualities and can harm them).

Limited Language Skills

Communicate using behaviors.

Use a few, simple terms familiar to child.

Give one direction at a time (e.g., "Lie down," then "Hold my hand").

Use small replicas of equipment; allow child to handle equipment.

Use play; demonstrate on doll but avoid child's favorite doll, since child may think doll is really "feeling" procedure.

Prepare parents separately to avoid child's misinterpreting words.

Limited Concept of Time

Prepare child shortly or immediately before procedure.

Keeping teaching sessions short (about 5 to 10 minutes).

Have preparations completed before involving child in procedure.

Have extra equipment nearby (e.g., alcohol swabs, new needle, adhesive bandages) to avoid delays.

Tell child when procedure is completed.

Striving for Independence

Allow choices whenever possible but realize that child may still be resistant and negative.

Allow child to participate in care and to help whenever possible (e.g., drink medicine from a cup, hold a dressing).

Preschooler: Developing a Sense of Initiative and Preoperational Thought
Egocentric

Explain procedure in simple terms and in relation to how it affects child (as with toddler, stress sensory aspects).

Demonstrate use of equipment.

Allow child to play with miniature or actual equipment.

Encourage "playing out" experience on a doll both before and after procedure to clarify misconceptions.

Use neutral words to describe the procedure (see box on p. 678).

Increased Language Skills

Use verbal explanation but avoid overestimating child's comprehension of words.

Encourage child to verbalize ideas and feelings.

Concept of Time and Frustration Tolerance Still Limited

Implement same approaches as for toddler but may plan longer teaching session (10 to 15 minutes); may divide information into more than one session.

Illness and Hospitalization May Be Viewed as Punishment

Clarify why each procedure is performed; a child will find it difficult to understand how medicine can make him or her feel better and can taste bad at the same time.

Ask child thoughts regarding why a procedure is performed.

State directly that procedures are never a form of punishment.

Animism

Keep equipment out of sight, except when shown to or used on child.

Fears of Bodily Harm, Intrusion, and Castration

Point out on drawing, doll, or child where procedure is performed.

Emphasize that no other body part will be involved.

Use nonintrusive procedures whenever possible (e.g., axillary temperatures, oral medication).

Apply an adhesive bandage over puncture site.

Encourage parental presence.

Realize that procedures involving genitals provoke anxiety.

Allow child to wear underpants with gown.

Explain unfamiliar situations, especially noises or lights.

Striving for Initiative

Involve child in care whenever possible (e.g., hold equipment, remove dressing).

Give choices whenever possible but avoid excessive delays.

Praise child for helping and attempting to cooperate; never shame child for lack of cooperation.

*Applies to any age.

AGE-SPECIFIC GUIDELINES FOR PREPARING CHILDREN FOR PROCEDURES BASED ON DEVELOPMENTAL CHARACTERISTICS—cont'd

School-Age Child: Developing a Sense of Industry and Concrete Thought

Increased Language Skills; Interest in Acquiring Knowledge

Explain procedures using correct scientific/medical terminology.

Explain reason for procedure using simple diagrams of anatomy and physiology.

Explain function and operation of equipment in concrete terms.

Allow child to manipulate equipment; use doll or another person as model to practice using equipment whenever possible (doll play may be considered "childish" by older school-age child).

Allow time before and after procedure for questions and discussion.

Improved Concept of Time

Plan for longer teaching sessions (about 20 minutes).

Prepare in advance of procedure.

Increased Self-Control

Gain child's cooperation.

Tell child what is expected.

Suggest ways of maintaining control (e.g., deep breathing, relaxation, counting).

Striving for Industry

Allow responsibility for simple tasks (e.g., collecting specimens).

Include in decision making (e.g., time of day to perform procedure, preferred site).

Encourage active participation (e.g., removing dressings, handling equipment, opening packages).

Developing Relationships with Peers

May prepare two or more children for same procedure or encourage one to help prepare another peer.

Provide privacy from peers during procedure to maintain self-esteem.

Adolescent: Developing a Sense of Identity and Abstract Thought

Increasingly Capable of Abstract Thought and Reasoning

Supplement explanations with reasons why procedure is necessary or beneficial.

Explain long-term consequences of procedures.

Realize that adolescent may fear death, disability, or other potential risks.

Encourage questioning regarding fears, options, and alternatives.

Conscious of Appearance

Provide privacy.

Discuss how procedure may affect appearance (e.g., scar) and what can be done to minimize it.

Emphasize any physical benefits of procedure.

Concerned More with Present Than with Future

Realize that immediate effects of procedure are more significant than future benefits.

Striving for Independence

Involve in decision making and planning (e.g., choice of time; place; individuals present during procedure, such as parents; clothing to wear).

Impose as few restrictions as possible.

Suggest methods of maintaining control.

Accept regression to more childish methods of coping.

Realize that adolescent may have difficulty in accepting new authority figures and may resist complying with procedures.

Developing Peer Relationships and Group Identity

Same as for school-age child but assumes even greater significance.

Allow adolescents to talk with other adolescents who have had the same procedure.

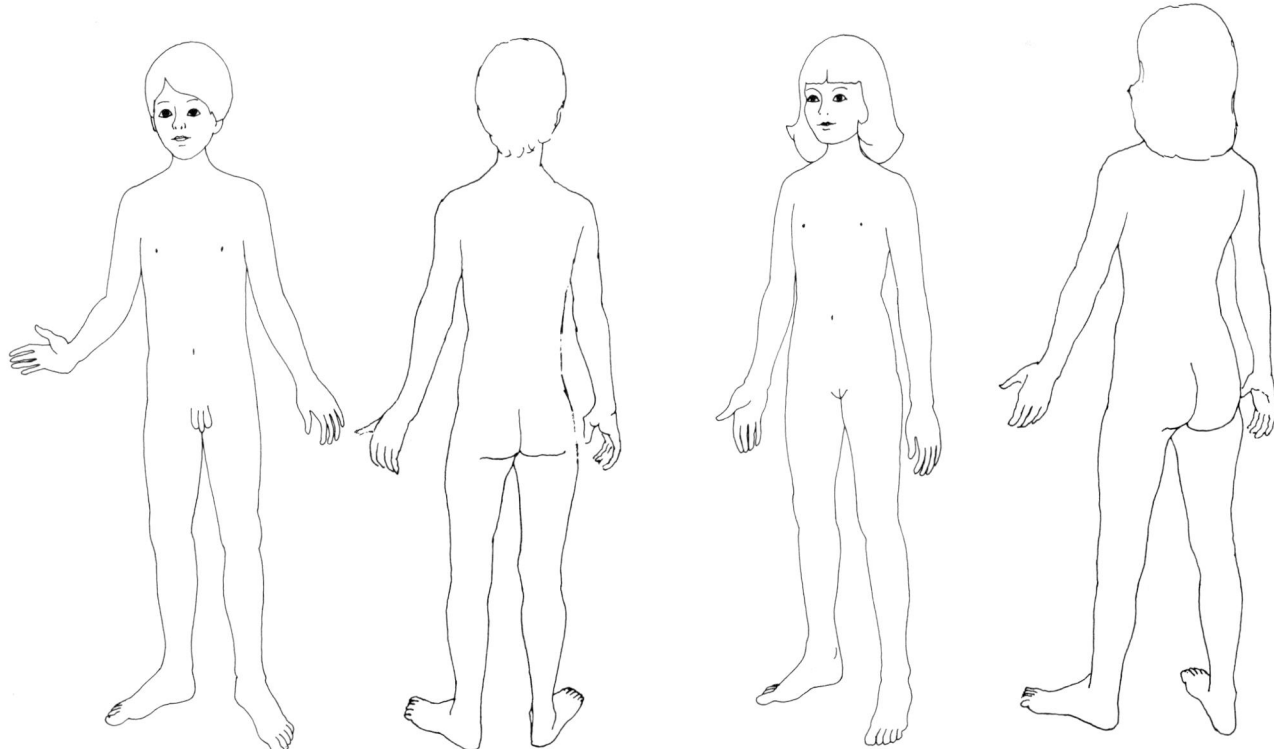

FIG. 22-1. Examples of line drawings to be used in preparing child for procedures.

the child, the closer the explanation should be to the actual procedure to prevent undue fantasizing and worrying. With complex procedures, more time may be needed for assimilation of information, especially with older children. For example, the explanation for an injection can immediately precede the procedure for all ages, but preparation for surgery may begin the day before for young children and a few days before for older children, although older children's preferences should be elicited (see Prepare Child for Hospitalization, Chapter 21).

Establish Trust and Provide Support. The nurse who has spent time with and who has established a positive relationship with a child will usually find it easier to gain the child's cooperation. If the relationship is based on trust, the child will associate the nurse with caregiving activities that give comfort and pleasure most of the time and not regard the nurse as someone who brings discomfort and stress. If the nurse does not know the child, it is best that the nurse be introduced by another staff person whom the child trusts. The first visit with the child should not include any painful procedure and ideally should focus on the child first, then on the explanation of the procedure. When talking with the child, the nurse uses the same guidelines for communicating with children that are discussed in Chapter 6.

Parental Support. Children need support during procedures, and for young children the greatest source of comfort is the parents. However, controversy exists regarding the role parents should assume during the procedure, especially if discomfort is involved. Nurses need to consider the issues in deciding whether parental presence is beneficial. The parents' preferences for assisting, observing, or waiting outside the room should be assessed, as well as the child's preference for parental presence. The child's choice should be respected. Parents who want to stay should be educated, since they do not automatically know what to do, where to be, and what to say to help their child through the procedure (Acute Pain Management Guideline Panel, 1992). Simple instructions

such as clarifying where parents can stay in the room and positioning them where they have eye contact with the child provide support and lessen anxiety. Parents who do not want to be present or participate are supported in their decision and encouraged to remain close by so that they can be available to console the child immediately after the procedure (see Thinking Critically About . . . box). Parents should also know that someone will be with their child to provide support. Ideally this person should inform the parents after the procedure about how the child performed.

Provide an Explanation. Children need an explanation for anything that involves them directly. Before performing a procedure, the nurse explains to children what is to be done and what is expected of them. The explanation should be short, simple, and appropriate to the child's level of comprehension. Long explanations are not necessary and may only increase anxiety in a small child. This is especially true regarding painful procedures. When explaining the procedure to parents with the child present, the nurse uses language appropriate to the child because unfamiliar words can be misunderstood (see Guidelines box). If the parents need additional preparation, this is done in an area away from the child. Teaching sessions are planned at times most conducive to the child's learning (e.g., after a rest period) and for the usual span of attention.

Special equipment is not necessary for preparing a child, but for young children who cannot yet think in concepts, using objects to supplement verbal explanation is important. Allowing children to handle actual items that will be used in their care, such as a stethoscope, sphygmomanometer, or oxygen mask, helps them to develop familiarity with these items and to reduce the threat often associated with their use. Miniature versions of hospital items such as gurneys and x-ray and intravenous equipment can be used to explain what the chil-

---

THINKING CRITICALLY ABOUT . . .
Parental Presence During Their Child's Stressful Procedure

Many institutions permit parents and children to be together during painful or stressful situations. However, allowing parents to stay with the child during induction of anesthesia, recovery from anesthesia, and cardiopulmonary resuscitation during an arrest tends to remain restricted. When parents and children are asked their preference regarding visiting during these times, however, the results favor offering the family a choice. For example, more than 80% of children ages 5 to 11 years wanted parents at the time of anesthesia induction, and more than 90% wanted them to be in the postanesthesia care unit (Hanna and Sherlock, 1983). (See also discussion above). When parents were offered the choice of staying during an arrest, 100% stated they would choose this option again (Villarreal, 1992). When one hospital considered a policy of allowing parents in the operating room if the child was dying, the parent advisory committee simply asked, "What right has Children's Hospital to dictate to families how they should experience the death of a child or how they should grieve?" (Fina, 1994). Shouldn't this question apply to all "visiting" policies?

GUIDELINES
Selecting Nonthreatening Words or Phrases

Words/Phrases to Avoid	Suggested Substitutions
Shot, bee sting, stick	Medicine under the skin
Organ	Special place in body
Test	See how [specify body part] is working
Incision	Special opening
Edema	Puffiness
Stretcher, gurney	Rolling bed
Stool	Child's usual term
Dye	Special medicine
Pain	Hurt, discomfort, "owie," "boo-boo"
Deaden	Numb, make sleepy
Cut, fix	Make better
Take (as in "take your temperature" and "take your blood pressure")	See how warm you are Check your pressure; hug your arm
Put to sleep, anesthesia	Special sleep
Catheter	Tube
Monitor	TV screen
Electrodes	Stickers, ticklers
Specimen	Sample

dren can expect and permit them to safely experience situations that are unfamiliar and potentially frightening. Written and illustrated materials are also valuable aids to preparation.*

NURSING TIP *Use photographs of children in different areas of the hospital (e.g., radiology department, operating room) to give children a more realistic idea of equipment they may encounter.*

Performance of the Procedure

Supportive care continues during the procedure and can be a major factor in a child's ability to cooperate and achieve mastery. Before the procedure is begun, all equipment is assembled and the room is readied to prevent unnecessary delays and interruptions that only serve to increase the child's anxiety.

NURSING TIP *To avoid a delay during a procedure, have extra supplies handy. For example, have tape, bandages, alcohol swabs, and an extra needle in your pocket when giving an injection or performing a venipuncture.*

If at all possible, procedures are performed in a special treatment room rather than the child's hospital room. Traumatic procedures should never be performed in "safe" areas, such as the playroom. If the procedure is lengthy, conversation that could be misinterpreted by the child is avoided. As the procedure is nearing completion, the nurse should inform the child that it is almost over in language that the child understands.

Expect Success. Nurses who approach children with confidence and who convey the impression that they expect to be successful are less likely to encounter difficulty. It is best to approach children as though cooperation is expected. Children sense anxiety in another and may respond to a perceived threat by striking out or with active resistance. Although some children will still exhibit such behavior, a firm approach with a positive attitude on the part of the nurse tends to convey a feeling of security to most children.

Involve Child. As in any other aspect of care, involving children helps to gain their cooperation. Permitting them to make choices gives them some measure of control. However, a choice is given only in situations in which one is available. Asking children, "Do you want to take your medicine now?" or "I'm going to give you an injection now, okay?" leads them to believe that there is an option and provides them with the opportunity to legitimately refuse or delay the medication. This places the nurse in an awkward, if not impossible, position. It is much better to state firmly, "It's time to drink your medicine now." Children usually like to make choices, but the choice must be one that they may have (e.g., "It's time for your medicine. Do you want to drink it plain or with a little water?").

*Sources of preparatory materials are the *You're Gonna Do What?* series of diagnosis and treatment procedures, available from Arkansas Children's Hospital, Attn: Barbara Widell, 800 Marshall St., Little Rock, AR 72202, (501) 320-1199; *Talks About the Hospital Series* by Fred Rogers, available from Family Communications, Inc., Attn: Marketing Department, 4802 Fifth Ave., Pittsburgh, PA 15213, (412) 687-2990; and *Hospital Friends,* available from the Centering Corp., 1531 N. Saddle Creek Rd., Omaha, NE 68104, (402) 553-1200.

Many children respond to tactics that appeal to their maturity or courage. This approach also gives them a sense of participation and achievement. For example, preschool children will be proud that they can hold the dressing during the procedure or remove the tape. The same is true for the school-age child, who often cooperates with minimal resistance.

Provide Distraction. When children are occupied with some activity that interests them, they are less likely to focus on the procedure. For example, when an injection is given, it is helpful to give the child something to do or something on which to focus attention. For example, asking the child to point the toes inward and wiggle them not only helps relax the gluteal muscles but provides a diversion. Other strategies for diverting attention are to have the child tightly squeeze the hands of a parent or an assistant, count aloud, sing a familiar song such as a nursery rhyme, or verbally express discomfort.

NURSING TIP *Help the child to select and practice a coping technique before the procedure. Consider having the parent or some other supportive person, such as a child-life specialist, "coach" the child in learning and using the coping skill.*

(For other interventions that may lessen discomfort, see Pain Management, Chapter 21.)

Allow Expression of Feelings. The child is allowed to express feelings of anger, anxiety, fear, frustration, or any other emotion. It is natural for children to strike out in frustration or to try to avoid stress-provoking situations. The child needs to know that it is all right to cry. Behavior is children's primary means of communication and coping and should be permitted unless it inflicts harm on them or those caring for them.

Postprocedural Support

After the procedure the child continues to need reassurance that he or she performed well and is accepted and loved. If the parents did not participate, the child is united with them as soon as possible so that they can provide comfort.

Encourage Expression of Feelings. Planned activity after the procedure is helpful in encouraging constructive expression of feelings. For verbal children, reviewing the details of the procedure can help clarify misconceptions and provide feedback for improving the nurse's preparatory strategies. Play is an excellent activity for all children. Infants and young children are given the opportunity for gross motor movement. Older children can vent their anger and frustration in acceptable pounding or throwing activities. Play dough is a remarkably versatile medium for pounding and shaping. Dramatic play provides an outlet for anger and places the child in a position of control, in contrast to the position of helplessness in the real situation. Puppets may also be used to allow the child to communicate in a nonthreatening way. One of the most effective interventions is *therapeutic play,* which includes activities such as permitting the child to give an injection to a doll or stuffed toy to reduce the stress of injections (Fig. 22-2).

Praise Child. Children need to hear from adults that they know the youngsters did the best they could in the situation, no matter how they behaved. It is important for children to know that their worth is not being judged on the basis of their behavior in a stressful situation. Reward systems, such as earning stars or tokens or saving the empty medicine cup as evidence of achievement, are often helpful. Children who require distasteful medications or injections over time can look with pride on a series of stars or stickers on a calendar, especially if an accumulated number represents a special privilege or reward.

Returning to the child a short while after the procedure helps the nurse to strengthen a supportive relationship. Re-

lating with the child in a relaxed and nonstressful period allows him or her to see the nurse not only as someone associated with stressful situations but also as someone with whom to share pleasurable experiences as well.

Use of Play in Procedures

The use of play is an integral part of relationships with children. As such, its value in specific situations is discussed throughout this book, such as in Chapter 21 in relation to hospitalization. Nurses can easily include play activities as part of nursing care. Play can be used in teaching, for expression

---

PLAY ACTIVITIES FOR SPECIFIC PROCEDURES

Fluid Intake

Make freezer pops using child's favorite juice.
Cut gelatin into fun shapes.
Make game of taking sip when turning page of book or in games such as "Simon Says."
Use small medicine cups; decorate the cups.
Color water with food coloring or powdered drink mix.
Have tea party; pour at small table.
Let child fill a syringe and squirt it into mouth or use it to fill small decorated cups.
Cut straws in half and place in small container (much easier for child to suck liquid).
Decorate straw: cut out small design with two holes and pass straw through; place small sticker on straw.
Use a "crazy" straw.
Make a "progress poster"; give rewards for drinking a predetermined quantity.

Deep Breathing

Blow bubbles with bubble blower.
Blow bubbles with straw (no soap).
Blow on pinwheel, feathers, whistle, harmonica, balloons, toy horns, party blowers.
Practice band instruments.
Have blowing contest using balloons,* boats, cotton balls, feathers, marbles, Ping-Pong balls, pieces of paper; blow such objects on a table top over a goal line, over water, through an obstacle course, up in the air, against an opponent, or up and down a string.
Suck paper or cloth from one container to another using a straw.
Use blow bottles with colored water to transfer water from one side to the other.
Dramatize stories, such as "I'll huff and puff and blow your house down" from the Three Little Pigs.
Do straw-blowing painting.
Take a deep breath and "blow out the candles" on a birthday cake.
Use a little paint brush to "paint" nails with water and blow nails dry.

Range of Motion and Use of Extremities

Throw beanbags at fixed or movable target or wadded paper into wastebasket.
Touch or kick Mylar balloons held or hung in different positions (if child is in traction, hang balloon from trapeze).
Play "tickle toes"; wiggle them on request.
Play Twister game or "Simon Says."
Play pretend and guess games (e.g., imitate a bird, butterfly, or horse).
Have tricycle or wheelchair races in safe area.
Play kickball or throw ball with soft foam ball in safe area.
Position bed so that child must turn to view television or doorway.
Climb wall like a "spider."

Pretend to teach "aerobic" dancing or exercises; encourage parents to participate.
Encourage swimming if feasible.
Play video games or pinball (fine motor movement).
Play "hide and seek" game: hide toy somewhere in bed (or room if ambulatory) and have child find it using specified hand or foot.
Provide clay to mold with fingers.
Paint or draw on large sheets of paper placed on floor or wall.
Encourage combing own hair; play "beauty shop" with "customer" in different positions.

Soaks

Play with small toys or objects (cups, syringes, soap dishes) in water.
Wash dolls or toys.
Bubbles may be added to bath water if permissible; move bubbles to create shapes or "monsters."
Pick up marbles or pennies* from bottom of bath container.
Make designs with coins on bottom of container.
Pretend a boat is a submarine by keeping it immersed.
Read to child during soaks, sing with child, or play game, such as cards, checkers, or other board game (if both hands are immersed, move the board pieces for the child).
Sitz bath: give child something to listen to (music, stories) or look at (Viewmaster, book).
Punch holes in bottom of plastic cup, fill with water, and let it "rain" on child.

Injections

Let child handle syringe, vial, and alcohol swab, and give an injection to doll or stuffed animal.
Use syringes to decorate cookies with frosting, squirt paint, or target shoot into a container.
Draw a "magic circle" on area before injection; draw smiling face in circle after injection, but avoid drawing on puncture site.
Allow child to have a "collection" of syringes (without needles); make "wild" creative objects with syringes.
If multiple injections or venipunctures, make a "progress poster"; give rewards for predetermined number of injections.
Have child count to 10 or 15 during injection.

Ambulation

Give child something to push.
  Toddler: push-pull toy
  School-age child: wagon or decorated IV stand
  Adolescent: a baby in a stroller or wheelchair
Have a parade; make hats, drums, etc.

Extending Environment (Patients in Traction, etc.)

Make bed into a pirate ship or airplane with decorations.
Put up mirrors so patient can see around room.
Move patient's bed frequently, especially to playroom, hallway, or outside.

*Small objects such as marbles or coins, as well as gloves or balloons, are unsafe for young children because of possible aspiration.

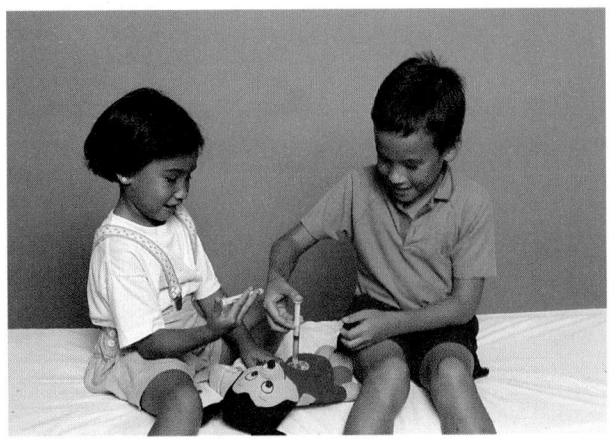

FIG. 22-2. Playing with syringes provides children with the opportunity to play out fears and concerns.

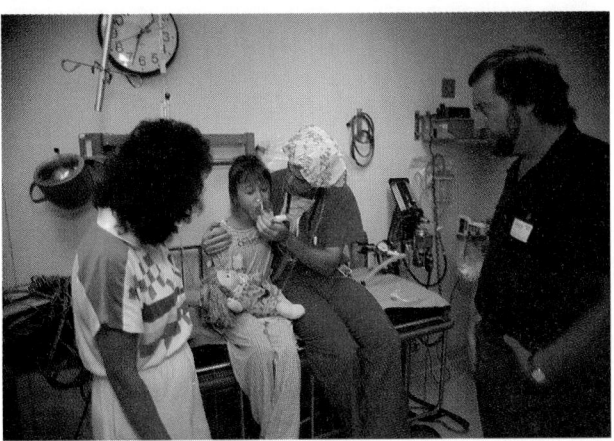

FIG. 22-3. Parental presence during induction of anesthesia can minimize the child's and parents' anxiety during the preoperative period.

of feelings, or as a method to achieve a therapeutic goal. Consequently, it should be included in preparing children for and encouraging their cooperation during procedures. Play sessions after procedures can be structured, such as directed toward playing with syringes, or general, with a wide variety of equipment available for children to play with. Suggestions for incorporating play into nursing procedures and activities for the hospitalized child that facilitate learning and adjustment to a new situation are described in the box on p. 680.

NURSING TIP Play can also be spontaneous at the bedside and does not always require many supplies or much nursing time. Small items, such as finger puppets or a small bottle of bubbles, can be kept in the nurse's pocket for immediate use.

SURGICAL PROCEDURES

Preoperative Care

Children experiencing surgical procedures require both psychologic and physical preparation. In general, psychologic preparation is similar to that discussed for any procedure and may employ many of the same techniques used in preparing a child for hospitalization, such as films, books, play, and tours. However, some important differences exist. Even though children are asleep for the actual surgical intervention, they are subjected to numerous preoperative and postoperative procedures, which require a series of preparatory sessions to prevent overstressing the child with too much information.

Psychologic intervention consisting of systematic preparation, rehearsal of the forthcoming events, and supportive care during times of stress (e.g., admission) has been shown to be more effective than a single-session preparation or consistent supportive care without systematic preparation and rehearsal. Play is always an effective strategy in preparing children, and increased familiarity with medical procedures decreases anxiety.

Although fear of anesthesia is thought to be a major concern among children, little evidence for this exists. One study

of school-age children found that the most feared events were the injection and the mask on the face.

Parental presence during induction is becoming a more common practice, although few institutions endorse the policy (Fig. 22-3). Reports from parents who attend the induction are very favorable. Even though some may become anxious, most parents can control their anxiety, do not disrupt the induction, and support the child (Hall and others, 1995; LaRosa-Nash and others, 1995). Some concern surrounds the appropriateness of this practice for all parents. A few parents are visibly upset by the rapid succession of induction events, observing their child becoming limp, and leaving the child in the care of strangers (Vessey, Caserza, and Bogetz, 1990).

However, based on the parents' favorable response to the practice and most children's desire to have parents with them during any stressful procedure, a policy of offering parents the option of attending the induction, combined with a program that prepares them for what to expect and what is expected of them, is recommended. When parents choose not to or are not allowed to attend this induction, leaving a favorite possession with the child and uniting the child and parents as soon as possible after surgery (preferably in the postanesthesia care unit [PACU]) are important interventions. During surgery the family should have a designated place to wait and needs to be kept informed of the child's progress. Family members also should know where and when they can visit the child after surgery.

Aside from possibly being separated from the parents before and after surgery, children may be cared for by a number of unfamiliar practitioners. Although the same supportive nurse should remain with the child through as many of the procedures as possible, the child may have other nurses, especially if the patient returns to a special care unit postoperatively. Many hospitals have surgical tours for children and parents to familiarize them with the strange environment and to introduce them to other individuals who will be involved in their care.

In addition to psychologic preparation, children usually require various types of physical care before surgery, such as

Nursing Care Plan
The Child Undergoing Surgery

Preoperative Care

> **NURSING DIAGNOSIS:** High risk for injury related to surgical procedure, anesthesia

NURSE GOAL 1: Will receive fully informed consent and sign appropriate documents

- **NURSING INTERVENTIONS/*RATIONALES***

Inquire whether parents have any questions about procedure *to determine their level of understanding and to provide for additional information (from nurse or other professional)*
Check chart for signed informed consent form or obtain informed consent
  Contact physician to determine if parents have been informed of procedure *because informed consent is physician's responsibility*
Obtain and/or witness signature if not obtained earlier

- **EXPECTED OUTCOMES**

Family receives fully informed consent
Family signs appropriate documents

PATIENT GOAL 1: Will receive proper hygiene measures

- **NURSING INTERVENTIONS/*RATIONALES***

Bathe child, groom hair
Provide mouth care *to promote comfort while NPO*
Cleanse operative site according to prescribed method, if ordered, *to minimize risk of infection*

- **EXPECTED OUTCOME**

Child is cleansed and prepared appropriately (specify)

PATIENT GOAL 2: Will receive proper preparation

- **NURSING INTERVENTIONS/*RATIONALES***

Carry out special procedure as prescribed (e.g., colonic enemas)
*Administer antibiotics as ordered, observing for known side effects
Order and/or assist with special tests, such as x-ray films
Consult with practitioner for appropriate change in schedule or route of administration of any medication child ordinarily receives
Attire child appropriately (e.g., special operating room gown)
  Allow child to wear underwear or pajama bottoms, if possible, *to provide privacy*
  Label personal articles and clothing
Remove any makeup and/or nail polish *to observe for cyanosis*
Remove jewelry and/or prosthetic devices (e.g., mouth retainers) *because they may be lost or interfere with anesthesia and surgery*
Check for loose teeth
  Inform anesthesiologist, if detected, *to prevent aspiration of teeth during anesthesia*

- **EXPECTED OUTCOME**

Child is prepared appropriately (specify)

---

*Dependent nursing action.

PATIENT GOAL 3: Will experience no complications

- **NURSING INTERVENTIONS/*RATIONALES***

Maintain child NPO (nothing by mouth) as ordered *to prevent aspiration during anesthesia* (clear liquids up to 2 hours before surgery for children at any age pose no additional risk for pulmonary aspiration during elective surgery)
Be sure child is well hydrated before NPO begins, especially infants *who are more at risk for dehydration*
Take and record vital signs
  Report any deviations from admission readings, especially elevated temperature, *which may indicate infection*
Have child void before preoperative medication is administered *to prevent bladder distention or incontinence during anesthesia*
  Record time of last voiding if unable to void
Be certain allergies are clearly indicated on chart *to decrease risk of adverse reaction*
Check laboratory values for any sign of systemic abnormality, such as infection (increased white blood cells), anemia (decreased hemoglobin and/or hematocrit), or bleeding tendencies (reduced platelets or prolonged bleeding or clotting time)
Keep small infants warm during transport and waiting time

- **EXPECTED OUTCOMES**

Child is NPO for designated time preoperatively
Child voids
Pertinent information about child is visible

PATIENT GOAL 4: Will experience no injury

- **NURSING INTERVENTIONS/*RATIONALES***

Check that identification band is securely fastened
Check identification band with surgical personnel *to ensure correct identification*
Fasten siderails of bed or crib *to prevent falls*
Use restraints during transport by stretcher (or other conveyance) *to prevent falls*
Do not leave child unattended

- **EXPECTED OUTCOMES**

Child is safe from immediate harm
Child is clearly and correctly identified

> **NURSING DIAGNOSIS:** Anxiety/fear related to separation from support system, unfamiliar environment, knowledge deficit

PATIENT GOAL 1: Will demonstrate optimum sense of security

- **NURSING INTERVENTIONS/*RATIONALES***

Institute preoperative teaching *to reduce anxiety/fear*
Orient child to strange surroundings
Explain where parents will be while child is in operating room
Have someone stay with child *to provide increased sense of security*

- **EXPECTED OUTCOME**

Child demonstrates minimum insecurity or anxiety

PATIENT/FAMILY GOAL 2: Will demonstrate understanding of surgery and postoperative care

- **NURSING INTERVENTIONS/RATIONALES**

Prepare for postoperative procedures, as indicated (e.g., nasogastric tube, intravenous (IV) fluids, nothing by mouth, dressing changes, wound drains if necessary)

Explain reason for surgery; if special operative procedure is to be performed, explain basic principles and briefly outline care if needed *to reinforce information given by practitioner*

Explain all preoperative procedures (e.g., blood work, other laboratory tests)

In emergency situation, explain most essential components of surgery (e.g., where child will be before and after surgery, anesthesia, dressing)

Accept behavioral reactions of parents and child *because these can vary greatly*

- **EXPECTED OUTCOMES**

Child and family demonstrate an understanding of forthcoming events (specify methods of learning and evaluation)
*Family's behavioral reactions are accepted and supported

PATIENT GOAL 3: Will exhibit signs of optimum relaxation, sedation, and support before arriving in operating room

- **NURSING INTERVENTIONS/RATIONALES**

†Administer preoperative sedation (preferably oral), if ordered, *to promote relaxation and sleep*

Place unfamiliar equipment out of child's view *to decrease anxiety/fear*

Place child in quiet room with minimum distraction *to promote relaxation and encourage sleep*

Do not leave child unattended

Explain what is happening, unless child is asleep

Encourage parents to stay with child as long as permitted and according to their wishes

Permit parent to hold child until child falls asleep, if desired

Encourage parents to accompany child as far as possible, preferably through induction of anesthesia

Allow significant objects to accompany child (e.g., a favorite toy) *to provide comfort and sense of security*

- **EXPECTED OUTCOMES**

Child falls asleep or lies quietly
Child is not left alone

NURSING DIAGNOSIS: Altered family processes related to a surgical procedure

---

PATIENT (FAMILY) GOAL 1: Will receive adequate support and reassurance

- **NURSING INTERVENTIONS/RATIONALES**

Reinforce and clarify information given by practitioner

Explain associated diagnostic tests and procedures (e.g., x-ray examinations)

Explain child's schedule
   When child will receive premedication
   Time child will leave for surgery
   Where parents can wait for child to return
   Room to which child will return
   Postprocedural care and routines

Explore family's feelings regarding the procedure and its implications *to assess need for further intervention*

Include parents in preparation of child

Be available to family *to provide support and reassurance as needed*

See also Nursing Care Plan: The Family of the Ill or Hospitalized Child, Chapter 21

- **EXPECTED OUTCOMES**

Family demonstrates an understanding of procedure (specify demonstration) and related information (specify)
Family complies with directives (specify)

Postoperative Care

NURSING DIAGNOSIS: High risk for injury related to surgical procedure, anesthesia

---

NURSE GOAL 1: Receive child on return from surgery

- **NURSING INTERVENTIONS/RATIONALES**

Place child in bed (unless transported in own bed or crib) using techniques appropriate to type of surgery *to prevent injury*

Hang IV apparatus and connect any needed equipment (e.g., suction apparatus, traction)

Place child in position of comfort and safety in accordance with surgeon's orders

Perform stat (immediate) activities

- **EXPECTED OUTCOME**

Child is transferred to bed without injury and with minimum stress

PATIENT GOAL 1: Will exhibit signs of wound healing without evidence of wound infection

- **NURSING INTERVENTIONS/RATIONALES**

Use proper handwashing techniques and other universal precautions, especially if wound drainage is present

Employ careful wound care *to minimize risk of infection*
   Keep wound clean and dressings intact
   Apply dressings *that promote moist wound healing* (i.e., hydrocolloid dressings [e.g., Duoderm])
   Change dressings if indicated, whenever soiled; carefully dispose of soiled dressings
   Carry out special wound care as prescribed (e.g., irrigation, drain care)

---

*Nursing outcome.
†Dependent nursing action.

Continued.

NURSING CARE PLAN
The Child Undergoing Surgery—cont'd

Cleanse with prescribed preparation (if ordered)

*Apply antibacterial solutions and/or ointments as ordered *to prevent infection*

Report any unusual appearance or drainage *for early detection of infection*

Place diapers below abdominal dressing, if appropriate, *to prevent contamination*

When child begins oral feedings, provide nutritious diet as ordered *to promote wound healing*

• **EXPECTED OUTCOME**

Child exhibits no evidence of wound infection

PATIENT GOAL 2: Will exhibit no evidence of complications

• **NURSING INTERVENTIONS/RATIONALES**

Ambulate as prescribed *to decrease complications associated with immobility*

Maintain child NPO until fully awake *to prevent aspiration*

Encourage to void when awake

    Offer bedpan

    Boys may be allowed to stand at bedside

Notify practitioner if unable to void *to ensure appropriate intervention*

Maintain abdominal decompression, chest tubes, or other equipment, if prescribed

Provide diet as prescribed; advance as appropriate

• **EXPECTED OUTCOME**

Child exhibits no evidence of complications

NURSING DIAGNOSIS: Anxiety/fear related to surgery, unfamiliar environment, separation from support systems, discomfort

PATIENT GOAL 1: Will experience reduced anxiety

• **NURSING INTERVENTIONS/RATIONALES**

Maintain calm, reassuring manner

Encourage expression of feelings *to facilitate coping*

Explain procedures and other activities before initiating

Answer questions and explain purposes of activities

Keep informed of progress

Remain with child as much as possible

Give encouragement and positive feedback for cooperation in care

Encourage parental presence as soon as permitted *to decrease stress of separation*

If emergency procedure, review child's memory of previous events *so that misconceptions can be clarified*

• **EXPECTED OUTCOMES**

Child rests quietly and calmly

Child discusses procedures and activities without evidence of anxiety

---

NURSING DIAGNOSIS: Pain related to surgical incision

PATIENT GOAL 1: Will experience no pain or reduction of pain to level acceptable to child

• **NURSING INTERVENTIONS/RATIONALES**

Do not wait until child experiences severe pain to intervene *in order to prevent pain from occurring*

Avoid palpating operative area unless necessary

Insert rectal tube, if indicated, *to relieve gas*

Encourage to void, if appropriate, *to prevent bladder distention*

Administer mouth care *to provide comfort*

Lubricate nostril *to decrease irritation* from nasogastric tube, if present

Allow child position of comfort if not contraindicated

Perform nursing activities and procedures (e.g., dressing change, deep breathing, ambulation) after analgesia

†Administer analgesics prescribed *for pain*

†Administer antiemetics as ordered *for nausea and vomiting*

Monitor effectiveness of analgesics

• **EXPECTED OUTCOME**

Child rests quietly and exhibits minimal or no evidence of pain (specify)

NURSING DIAGNOSIS: High risk for fluid volume deficit related to NPO status before and/or after surgery, loss of appetite, vomiting

PATIENT GOAL 1: Will receive adequate hydration

• **NURSING INTERVENTIONS/RATIONALES**

Monitor IV infusion at prescribed rate *to ensure adequate hydration*

    Attach pediatric IV apparatus if not done in operating room

Offer fluids as soon as ordered or child tolerates

    Start with small sips of water and advance as tolerated

Encourage to drink

    Tempt with favorite fluids, ice chips, or flavored ice pops

• **EXPECTED OUTCOMES**

Child exhibits no evidence of dehydration

Child takes and retains fluid when allowed (specify)

NURSING DIAGNOSIS: High risk for infection related to weakened condition, presence of infective organisms

PATIENT GOAL 1: Will maintain normal respiratory function

---

*Nursing outcome.

†Dependent nursing action.

NURSING CARE PLAN
The Child Undergoing Surgery—cont'd

• **NURSING INTERVENTIONS/***RATIONALES*

Assess need for pain medication before respiratory therapy
Help to turn and deep breathe
> Splint operative site with hand or pillow if possible before coughing (if coughing prescribed) *to minimize pain*

Assist with use of incentive spirometer or blow bottle
Perform percussion and vibration if indicated
Suction secretions if needed
Assess respirations, including breath sounds

• **EXPECTED OUTCOME**

Lungs remain clear

> **NURSING DIAGNOSIS:** Altered family processes related to situational crisis (emergency hospitalization of child), knowledge deficit

PATIENT/FAMILY GOAL I: Will receive adequate support and reassurance

• **NURSING INTERVENTIONS/***RATIONALES*

Explain all procedures *to reduce anxiety/fear*
Keep family informed of child's progress
Encourage expression of feelings *to facilitate coping*
Refer to public health nurse, if indicated, *for follow-up care*
Refer to appropriate agency or persons for specific help (e.g., social service, clergy)

See also Nursing Care Plan: The Child in the Hospital, Chapter 21
See also Nursing Care Plan: The Family of the Ill or Hospitalized Child, Chapter 21

• **EXPECTED OUTCOMES**

Family discusses child's condition and therapies comfortably
Family demonstrates an awareness of child's progress (specify method of evaluation)
Family members avail themselves of appropriate assistance

PATIENT (FAMILY) GOAL 2: Will demonstrate understanding of home care

• **NURSING INTERVENTIONS/***RATIONALES*

If dressing changes are required at home, teach parents sterile or aseptic procedures; provide written list of necessary equipment and instructions *for referral at home*
Instruct parents regarding administration of medications, if ordered, including possible side effects and untoward reactions, *to ensure adequate home care*
Instruct parents in care and management of special procedures (e.g., ostomy care, irrigations) *to ensure adequate home care*

• **EXPECTED OUTCOME**

Family demonstrates an understanding of instructions (specify methods of learning and evaluation)

---

those listed in the Nursing Care Plan on pp. 682-685 and in the preoperative checklist (see Guidelines box on p. 686 [left]). An important concern is restriction of food and fluids before surgery to avoid aspiration during anesthesia. Before fluids are restricted, children are encouraged to drink to promote hydration and minimize the dryness and thirst they experience. Infants require special attention to fluid needs. They should not be without oral fluids for an extended period preoperatively to avoid glycogen depletion and dehydration. Typical recommendations for food or fluids before anesthesia induction are no milk or solids after midnight before scheduled procedures and no clear liquids from 4 to 8 hours before the procedure. However, research indicates that clear liquids up to 2 hours before surgery for children at any age pose no additional risk for pulmonary aspiration during elective surgery (Schreiner, 1994) (see Guidelines box on p. 686 [right]).

Although most preoperative care procedures are routine, nurses should keep in mind that they can be anxiety provoking for children and parents. For example, for young children, having to wear a loose-fitting hospital gown without the security of underpants or pajama bottoms can be traumatic. Therefore these articles of clothing should be allowed.

The most upsetting event for children is generally the preoperative injection. Unfortunately, little research has been done on the value of this practice. If children have no preoperative pain, are well prepared psychologically for surgery, and have their parents nearby, preanesthetic medication may be unnecessary. When drugs are used, they should be "atraumatic" by using oral, existing intravenous, or rectal routes.

Numerous preanesthetic drug regimens are used with children, and no consensus exists on the optimum method. Drugs used should achieve five goals (American Academy of Pediatrics, 1992): (1) to guard the patient's safety and welfare; (2) to minimize physical discomfort or pain; (3) to minimize negative psychologic responses to treatment by providing analgesia, and to maximize the potential for amnesia; (4) to control behavior; and (5) to return the patient to a state in which safe discharge, as determined by recognized criteria, is possible.

The use of sedating drugs for procedures has serious associated risks, such as hypoventilation, apnea, airway obstruction, and cardiopulmonary impairment. They produce ***conscious sedation***—a medically controlled state of depressed consciousness that (1) allows protective reflexes to be maintained, (2) retains the patient's ability to maintain a patent airway independently and continuously, and (3) permits appropriate response by the patient to physical stimulation or verbal command (e.g., "Open your eyes").

GUIDELINES
Preoperative Checklist

☐ Signed informed consent on chart and properly witnessed.
☐ Child NPO (nothing by mouth) for appropriate length of time.
☐ Child's medication orders changed as needed because of NPO status.
☐ Results of laboratory tests and vital signs reviewed for abnormal findings, such as elevated temperature, and reported to practitioner.
☐ Any specific physical preparation of surgical area, such as shaving or administration of enemas, performed.
☐ Child appropriately attired and any personal items (e.g., underwear, favorite toy) labeled.
☐ Dental appliances (e.g., retainers) contact lenses, prosthesis, hearing aid, nail polish, and makeup removed.
☐ Loose teeth and appliances remaining with child noted on chart.
☐ Child voided before preoperative sedation administered.
☐ Child wearing correct patient identification.
☐ Child's identification charge care on chart.
☐ Child and family adequately prepared for surgery experience (i.e., where family can wait for surgeon's report; whether parents can accompany the child to perioperative suite, induction area, or PACU).
☐ Any special circumstances, such as allergies,* skin problems, respiratory or cardiac conditions, paralysis, or family history of malignant hyperthermia, clearly displayed on front of chart.
☐ History and physical examination, including child's weight and laboratory test results, indicated on chart.

*For a discussion of latex allergy, see Spina Bifida, Chapter 32.

GUIDELINES
Recommended Preoperative Feeding

At 8 PM or midnight the evening before surgery, **stop all food,** including the following:
  Solid food, candy,* and chewing gum*
  Milk, milk products, and formulas†
  Orange juice and juice containing pulp
Breast-feeding may continue until **3 hours** before surgery.
Clear fluids may be continued until **2 hours** before surgery.
Clear fluids include water, apple juice, clear juice drinks, plain gelatin, clear broth, Pedialyte, and ice pops.

Modified from Schreiner MS: Preoperative and postoperative fasting in children, *Pediatr Clin North Am* 41(1):111-120, 1994.
*Hard sucking candy is probably of little concern, and a variety of opinions exist regarding the significance of gum chewing.
†The duration for fasting after formulas is uncertain at present, and shorter intervals may be appropriate.

Guidelines box on p. 687). Although most of these interventions are prescribed by physicians, it is the nurse's responsibility to exercise judgment in their implementation. For example, vital signs are taken as frequently as necessary until they are stable. Simply recording temperature, pulse, respiration, and blood pressure without comparing the present readings with previous ones is a useless technical function. Each vital sign is evaluated in terms of side effects from anesthesia and signs of impending shock, respiratory compromise, or pain. The nurse should also be alert for the development of malignant hyperthermia, a potentially lethal genetic myopathy. In susceptible children, certain anesthetic agents trigger the disorder, producing elevated temperature, muscle rigidity, hypermetabolism, and muscle cell destruction. The symptoms may or may not occur during surgery; therefore alert observation in the PACU and regular care unit is essential (Wlody, 1991). Early signs of the disorder include tachycardia, rising blood pressure, tachypnea, mottled skin, and muscle rigidity.

Nursing ALERT   When taking the preoperative history, ask the family if any relatives have had anesthetic difficulties suggesting malignant hyperthermia; report findings immediately.

The American Academy of Pediatrics (1992) has developed policies that provide guidelines for conscious sedation. These guidelines include provision of emergency equipment, such as a positive-pressure oxygen delivery system, airway management and breathing equipment, and an emergency cart. The patient's level of consciousness and responsiveness, heart rate, blood pressure, respiratory rate, and oxygen saturation (via pulse oximetry) must be monitored during the procedure by an individual present for this purpose. In all cases the patient's condition after the procedure is also documented.

Children may also fear induction of anesthesia by mask. Practices that can minimize anxiety related to inhalation anesthesia are (1) disguising the unpleasant odor of anesthetic gases by applying a pleasant-smelling substance on the mask; (2) using a transparent plastic mask rather than an opaque black mask and gradually bringing it toward the face; (3) directing a stream of gas toward the child's face from the bare tube until the child becomes drowsy, then using the mask; and (4) allowing the child to sit up rather than lie down for anesthesia induction.

Postoperative Care

After surgical procedures, various psychologic and physical interventions and observations are required to prevent or minimize possible untoward effects from anesthesia and the surgical procedure (see Nursing Care Plan, pp. 683-685, and

Providing comfort is a major nursing responsibility after surgery. Pain is assessed and analgesics are administered to provide comfort and to facilitate the child's cooperation with postoperative procedures, such as ambulating and deep breathing. Routinely scheduled intravenous analgesics and the use of patient-controlled analgesia (PCA), rather than PRN (as necessary) orders, afford more satisfactory pain control (see Pain Management, Chapter 21). Mouth care is another important aspect of care, because most children are allowed nothing orally until bowel sounds return (see p. 693).

Since respiratory infections are a potential complication, every effort is taken to aerate the lungs and remove secretions. The lungs are auscultated regularly to identify abnormal sounds or any areas of diminished or absent breath sounds. To prevent hypostatic pneumonia, respiratory movement can be encouraged with incentive spirometers or other

GUIDELINES
Postoperative Care

Ensure that preparations are made to receive child.
Bed or crib is ready.
Intravenous equipment, such as pumps, and any other relevant equipment, such as suction apparatus, oxygen flow meter, or Gomco suction, is at bedside.
Obtain baseline information:
Take vital signs, including blood pressure (BP); keep BP cuff in place and deflated to lessen amount of disturbance to child.
Take and record vital signs more frequently if any value fluctuates.
Inspect operative area.
Check dressing if present.
Outline any bleeding area on dressing or cast with pen.
Reinforce, but do not remove, loose dressing.
Observe areas below surgical site for blood that may have drained toward bed.
Assess for bleeding and other symptoms in areas not covered with a dressing, such as throat after tonsillectomy.
Assess skin color and characteristics.
Assess level of consciousness and activity.
Notify physician of any irregularities in child's condition.
Assess for evidence of pain (see Pain Assessment, Chapter 21).
Review surgeon's orders after completing initial assessment, and check that any preoperative orders, such as seizure or cardiac medications, have been reordered and can be given by available routes (oral preparations may be contraindicated).
Monitor vital signs as ordered and more often if indicated.
Check dressings for bleeding or other abnormalities.
Check bowel sounds.
Observe for signs of shock, abdominal distention, and bleeding.
Assess for bladder distention.
Observe for signs of dehydration.
Detect presence of infection:
Take vital signs every 2 to 4 hours, as ordered.
Collect or request needed specimens.
Inspect wound for signs of infection—redness, swelling, heat, pain, and purulent drainage.

FACTORS THAT POSITIVELY INFLUENCE COMPLIANCE

Individual/Family Factors

High self-esteem
Positive body image
High degree of autonomy (increased locus of control)
Supportive and well-adjusted family
Effective family communication
Family expectation for successful completion of therapy

Care Setting Factors

Perceived satisfaction with care
Positive interactions with practitioners
Continuity of care
Individualized care
Minimum waiting time for appointments
Convenient care setting

Treatment Factors

Simple regimen
Minimum disruption in usual life-style
Short duration
Inexpensive
Visible benefits
Tolerable side effects

or correct their perceptions and assist children in feeling a sense of mastery for having gone through a stressful procedure.

COMPLIANCE

The extent to which the patient's behavior in terms of taking medication, following diets, or executing other life-style changes coincides with the prescribed regimen is known as *compliance* (or *adherence*). Reviews of compliance rates in children and adolescents with chronic diseases estimate that the rate of noncompliance ranges from 36% to more than 80% (Pidgeon, 1989). Since nurses are frequently responsible for teaching families about treatment protocols, they must have knowledge of factors that influence compliance, methods to measure compliance, and strategies to enhance adherence to prescribed treatment.

Assessment of Compliance

In developing strategies to provide compliance, the nurse must first assess factors that influence compliance in the patient. Since many children are too young to assume partial or total responsibility for their care, parents are usually the primary caregivers in terms of home management. Consequently, the nurse needs to assess their ability to carry out instructions. The first approach to assessment is knowledge of those factors that influence compliance, and the second is to apply methods to assess compliance more objectively.

Several factors influence compliance (see box), although no typical characteristics of noncompliers exist, and even education is not correlated with compliance (Rosenstock, 1988). Basically, any aspect of the health care environment that increases the family's satisfaction with the care they are receiving positively influences adherence to the treatment regimen. However, the more complex, expensive, inconvenient, and disruptive the treatment protocol, the less likely the family is

motivating activities (see p. 680). If these measures are presented as games, the child is more likely to comply. The child's position is changed every 2 hours, and deep breathing is encouraged.

NURSING TIP Because deep breathing is usually painful after surgery, premedicate the child for pain and have the child splint the operative site (depending on its location) by hugging a small pillow or a favorite stuffed animal.

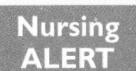

Nursing ALERT Early signs of respiratory involvement are abnormal rate, shallow depth, and cough. These findings are reported immediately.

During the recovery period, some time should be spent with children to assess their perception of surgery. Play, drawing, and storytelling are excellent methods of discovering their thoughts. With such information the nurse can support

to comply. During long-term conditions that involve multiple treatments and considerable rearrangement of life-style, compliance is severely affected.

Although it is helpful to know those factors that influence compliance, assessment must include more direct measurement techniques. A number of methods exist, but no one method is totally reliable. The most successful approach combines at least two of the following methods:

Clinical judgment. The nurse judges family compliance. This is a very poor method that is subject to bias and inaccuracy unless the nurse carefully evaluates the criteria used in evaluation.

Self-reporting. The family is asked about their ability to carry out the prescribed treatments, although most people overestimate their compliance by about 20% even when they admit to lapses in treatment.

Direct observation. The nurse directly observes the patient or family performing the treatment. This method is difficult to employ outside the health care setting, and the family's awareness of being observed frequently affects their performance.

Monitoring appointments. The family's attendance at scheduled appointments is recorded, although this method only indirectly indicates compliance with the prescribed care.

Monitoring therapeutic response. The child's response in terms of benefit from treatment is monitored and preferably recorded on a graph or chart. Unfortunately, few treatments yield directly measurable results.

Pill counts. The nurse counts the number of pills remaining in the original container and compares the amount missing with the number of days the medication should have been taken. Although this is a simple method, families may forget to bring the container or deliberately alter the number of pills to avoid detection. This method is also poorly suited to liquid medication, which is so often prescribed in pediatrics. Another strategy is to call the pharmacy and check on the number of refills for long-term prescriptions.

Chemical assay. For certain drugs, such as digoxin and phenytoin, measurement of plasma drug levels provides information on the amount of drug recently ingested. However, this method is expensive, indicates only short-term compliance, and requires precise timing of the assay for accurate results.

Strategies to Enhance Compliance

Organizational strategies refer to those interventions that involve the care setting and the therapeutic plan. They include employing the factors listed in the box that are known to positively affect compliance. Depending on the individual situation, this may involve increasing the frequency of appointments, designating a primary practitioner, reducing the cost of medication by purchasing generic brands, reducing the treatment's disruption of the family's life-style, and using "cues" to minimize forgetting. Numerous devices are available commercially or can be improvised for cueing, such as pill dispensers; watches with alarms; charts to record completed therapy; reminders, such as messages on the refrigerator or morning coffee pot; and treatment schedules that incorporate the treatment plan into the daily routine, such as physical therapy after the evening bath.

Educational strategies are concerned with instructing the family about the treatment plan. Although education is an important component in enhancing compliance and patients who are more knowledgeable about their condition are more likely to comply, education alone does not ensure compliant behavior. Also, for education to be effective, it must incorporate teaching principles known to enhance understanding

GUIDELINES
Effective Teaching of Family Members

Establish rapport; reduce anxiety and fear.

Assess what family knows and expects to learn, especially if they have concerns, and address their concerns before beginning teaching.

Assess family's learning style; ask if they prefer to have everything explained in detail or if they prefer knowing only the major facts.

Use a variety of teaching materials (lecture, demonstration, video or slide presentation, written material).

Speak family's language, avoid jargon, and clarify all terms.

Be specific when giving information.

Divide the information into small steps.

Keep information short, simple, and concrete.

Introduce most important information first.

Use "verbal" headings to organize information, such as "There are two things you need to learn: how to give the medicine and what side effects to look for. First, how to give. . . . Second, what side effects. . . ."

Stress how important the instructions are and the expected benefits; explain the detrimental effects of inadequate treatment but avoid fear tactics.

Evaluate the teaching by eliciting feedback to ensure that the family understands the information.

Repeat information as needed.

Reward the family for learning through verbal praise.

Use "teachable moments"—times when family is most likely to accept new information (e.g., when member asks a question or when symptoms are present).

Use "hands on" demonstration and return demonstration to encourage mastery of skills and retention of information.

and retention of material (see Guidelines box). Written materials are essential, especially in any regimen requiring multiple or complex treatments, and need to be understandable to the average individual, who reads at about the fourth-grade level. Including the culturally significant decision maker (e.g., maternal grandmother) in teaching sessions will help improve compliance (Faber, 1986).

One study found that 30% to 50% (depending on the educational level) of mothers failed to understand basic medical terms that residents presumed the mother would understand, such as *asthma, vitamin, fever, development,* and *virus* (Gablehouse and Gitterman, 1990).

Treatment strategies are related to the child's refusal or inability to take the prescribed medication. The family may also have difficulty following a prescribed treatment regimen. They may remember and understand the instructions but may not be able to give the medicine as prescribed. It is essential to assess the reason for refusal. For example, the child may not be able to swallow pills. In this case, perhaps they can be crushed or a liquid medication substituted. The opposite also may occur; the child may have difficulty drinking a liquid medication but is able to swallow pills.

Also assess the treatment and medication schedule to determine if it is reasonable for a home situation. Although an every-6-hour or every-8-hour schedule is reasonable for hospitals, a parent would have difficulty awakening one or two

ing privileges for older children may be needed to reduce noncompliance.

CRITICAL THINKING EXERCISE

Discharge Instructions

Ms. Jordan is preparing to take 2-month-old Brittany home from the hospital after a 4-day admission for a severe ear infection and eye infection. Brittany will be going home taking an antibiotic that you have been giving every 8 hours and eye drops that you have been giving every 6 hours. The infant is fed about every 4 hours. Choose the appropriate home schedule.

1. 12 AM—Feed and give antibiotic and eye drops
    4 AM—Feed
    6 AM—Give eye drops
    8 AM—Feed and give antibiotic
   12 PM—Feed and give eye drops
    4 PM—Feed and give antibiotic
    6 PM—Give eye drops
    8 PM—Feed
2. 12 AM—Feed and give antibiotic
    4 AM—Feed
    8 AM—Feed and give eye antibiotic and eye drops
   12 PM—Feed and give eye drops
    4 PM—Feed and give antibiotic and eye drops
    8 PM—Feed and give eye drops
3. 12 AM—Feed and give antibiotic and eye drops
    6 AM—Feed and give antibiotic and eye drops
  10 AM—Feed and give eye drops
    2 PM—Feed and give antibiotic
    6 PM—Feed and give eye drops
    9 PM—Feed

The best answer is two. Even though you followed the every-6-hour schedule for the eye drops in the hospital, it is unlikely that the parent could manage this at home. It is sometimes difficult getting eye drops into an infant's eyes, and giving the parent a schedule in which they must be given twice during the night would be difficult. Reducing the number of times the parent and infant must awaken during the night decreases the likelihood of a missed dose because the parent forgot to awaken.

If this were an older child, the antibiotic schedule could also be altered to waking hours only so the child and parent would not have to awaken at night for medication.

Although not every medication can be given on a more flexible schedule, most can. Ask the practitioner if the medication can be given three times a day instead of every 8 hours or four times a day instead of every 6 hours, etc. Medications or treatments given at unusual times are more likely to be missed. Discharge instructions should always be given keeping in mind the parent's ability to be compliant with them.

NURSING TIP To encourage a child to perform a treatment for a certain time frame (e.g., soaking a foot), ask the child to soak during a favorite TV show, including commercials. This technique also helps evaluate compliance by asking the child what show was watched (Woolverton, 1991).

GENERAL HYGIENE AND CARE

MAINTAINING HEALTHY SKIN

Skin, the largest organ of the body, is not merely a covering but also a complex structure that serves many functions, the most important of which is to protect the tissues that it encloses and to protect itself. Many routine nursing activities—maintaining an intravenous line, removing a dressing, positioning a child in bed, changing a diaper, using electrode patches, or maintaining restraints—have the potential to contribute to skin injury. Skin care must go beyond the daily bath and become a part of each nursing intervention. General guidelines for skin care are listed in the Guidelines box on p. 691. Specific guidelines for skin care of neonates are provided in Chapter 9 under Skin Care.

Assessment of the skin is most easily accomplished during the bath, but often the nurse is not the one who bathes the child. In this case the nurse needs to plan a time to observe the child's skin and to request feedback from the caregiver. The skin is examined for any early signs of injury, especially for the child who is at risk. Risk factors include impaired mobility, protein malnutrition, edema, incontinence, sensory loss, anemia, and infection. Identification of risk factors helps to determine those children who need a more thorough skin assessment.

When capillary blood flow is interrupted by pressure, the blood flows back into the tissue when the pressure is relieved. As the body attempts to reoxygenate the area, a bright-red flush appears. This *reactive hyperemia,* or flush, may be present for one-half to three-fourths as long as the time the pressure occluded the blood flow to the area.

Nursing ALERT If the redness persists, this may be the first sign of skin breakdown, including the possibility of more extensive damage below the skin.

Staging of pressure ulcers is used to classify the amount of tissue damage that has occurred. The tissue in the wound must be visible to be staged; it is difficult to assess a wound that is covered with necrotic tissue or a scab (see box on p. 690). Accurate documentation of redness or obvious skin breakdown is essential. Color, size (diameter and depth), location, presence of sinus tracts, odor, exudate, and response to treatment are observed and recorded at least daily. (For treatment of wounds, see Chapter 30; see also Critical Thinking Exercise on p. 691).

The nurse must also have an understanding of the types of mechanical damage that can occur, such as pressure, friction, shearing, and epidermal stripping. When a combination

times at night when a medication could be given during the day at times that would be easy to remember (see Critical Thinking Exercise).

Behavioral strategies encompass those interventions designed to modify behavior directly. Several strategies exist that are effective in encouraging the desired behavior and are very useful with children. Also, positive reinforcement may be employed to strengthen the behavior; this may consist of earning stars or tokens, which gains the child a special privilege or gift. A more formal method is the use of contracting (see Limit-setting and Discipline, Chapter 4). However, at times techniques such as time-out for young children or withhold-

Stage I

Nonblanchable erythema of intact skin; the heralding lesion of skin ulceration.* NOTE: Reactive hyperemia can normally be expected to be present for one-half to three-fourths as long as the pressure occluded blood flow to the area. This should not be confused with a stage I pressure ulcer.

Stage II

Partial-thickness skin loss involving epidermis and/or dermis. The ulcer is superficial and presents clinically as an abrasion, blister, or shallow crater.

Stage III

Full-thickness skin loss involving damage or necrosis of subcutaneous tissue that may extend down to, but not through, underlying fascia. The ulcer presents clinically as a deep crater with or without undermining of adjacent tissue.†

Stage IV

Full-thickness skin loss with extensive destruction, tissue necrosis or damage to muscle, bone, or supporting structures (e.g., tendon or joint capsule). NOTE: Undermining and sinus tracts may also be associated with stage IV pressure ulcers.

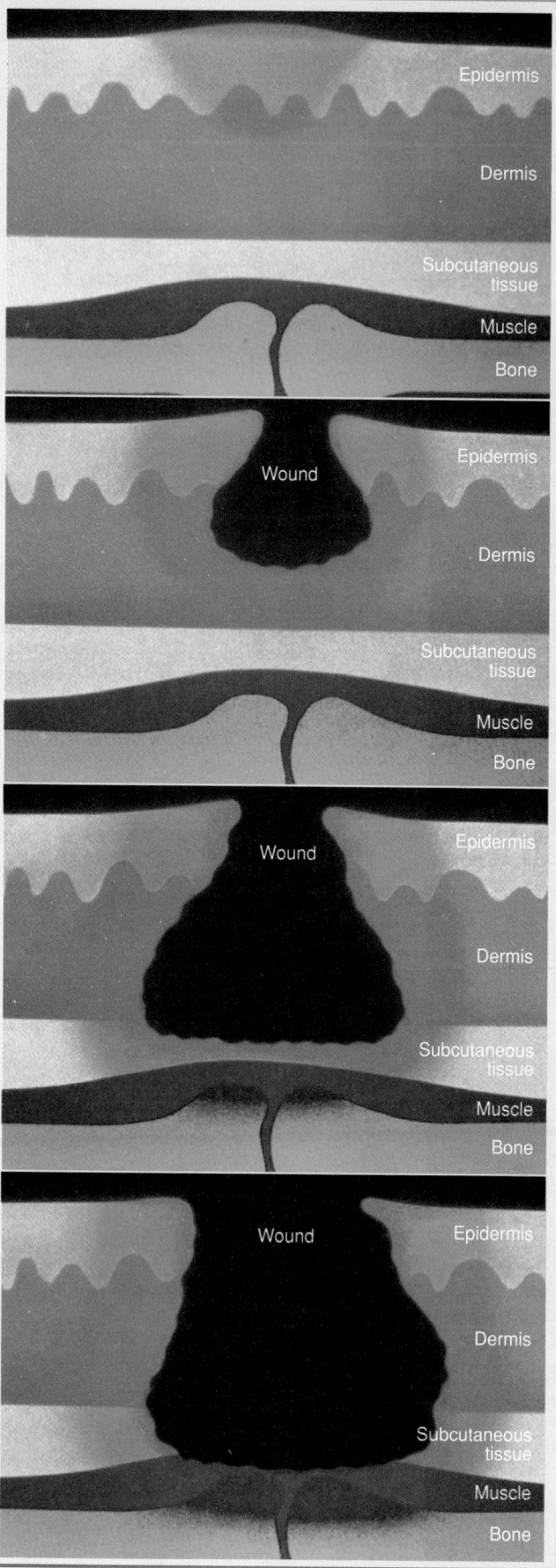

From Panel for the Prediction and Prevention of Pressure Ulcers in Adults: *Pressure ulcers in adults: prediction and prevention*, Clinical Practice Guideline Number 3, AHCPR Pub No 92-0047, Rockville, MD, 1992, Agency for Health Care Policy and Research, Public Health Service, US Department of Health and Human Services. Illustrations courtesy ConvaTec, Princeton, NJ.
*Identification of stage I pressure ulcers may be difficult in patients with darkly pigmented skin.
†When eschar is present, accurate staging of the pressure ulcer is not possible until the eschar has sloughed or the wound has been débrided.

GUIDELINES
Skin Care

Cleanse skin with gentle soap (e.g., Dove) or cleanser (e.g., Cetaphil). Rinse well with plain warm water.

Provide daily cleansing of eyes, oral and diaper or perianal areas, and any areas of skin breakdown.

Apply moisturizing agents after cleansing to retain moisture and rehydrate skin; however, cleanse skin of any old cream before adding a new layer.

Use minimum tape or adhesive. On very sensitive skin, use a protective, pectin-based or hydrocolloid skin barrier between skin and tape or adhesives.

Use water or possibly adhesive remover (if skin is not fragile) when removing tape or adhesives.

Place pectin-based or hydrocolloid skin barriers directly over excoriated skin. Leave barrier undisturbed until it begins to peel off. With wet, oozing excoriations, place a small amount of stoma powder (as used in ostomy care) on site, remove excess powder, and apply skin barrier. Hold barrier in place for several minutes to allow barrier to soften and mold to skin surface.

Alternate electrode placement and thoroughly assess skin underneath electrodes at least every 24 hours.

Be certain fingers or toes are visible whenever extremity is used for intravenous or arterial line.

Reduce friction by keeping skin dry (may apply absorbent powder, e.g., cornstarch) and using soft, smooth bed linen and clothes.

Use a draw sheet to move a child in bed or onto a gurney to reduce friction and shearing injuries; do not drag the child from under the arms.

Identify children who are risk for skin breakdown before it occurs. Employ measures, such as pressure-reducing or pressure-relieving devices, to prevent breakdown.

Do not massage reddened bony prominences because it can cause deep tissue damage; provide pressure relief to those areas instead.

Keep skin free of excess moisture (i.e., urine or fecal incontinence, wound drainage, excessive perspiration).

Routinely assess the child's nutritional status. A child who is NPO (nothing by mouth) for several days and is only receiving intravenous fluid is nutritionally at risk, which can also affect the skin's ability to maintain its integrity. Hyperalimentation should be considered for these children before they are at risk.

---

of risk factors and mechanical injury is present, skin breakdown can occur (Hagelgans, 1993).

When a child is identified as at risk for skin breakdown, nursing interventions are directed toward prevention of mechanical injury. Wounds caused by pressure can be prevented by using current technology and resources (Bryant, 1992). *Pressure ulcers* can develop when the pressure on the skin and underlying tissues is greater than the capillary closing pressure, causing capillary occlusion. If the pressure remains unrelieved, vessels can collapse, resulting in tissue anoxia and cellular death. Pressure ulcers most often occur over bony prominences. These lesions are usually very deep (stage IV), extending into subcutaneous tissue or even deeper into muscle, tendon, or bone. Prevention of pressure ulcers includes measures that reduce or relieve pressure.

A *pressure-reduction device* reduces pressure more than

would usually occur on a regular hospital bed or chair. These products do not prevent pressure from causing capillary closing; therefore turning and repositioning are always included when using these devices. Most of these items are overlays that are placed on top of the regular mattress. A *pressure-relief device* maintains pressure below that which would cause capillary closing. These devices are usually high-technology beds that are used for patients who have multiple problems and cannot be turned effectively.

Nursing ALERT

Convoluted foam mattress pads with a base of 5 cm (2 inches) (measured from where the convolutions begin, not the peak of the convolution) and soft padding, such as sheepskin, do not significantly reduce pressure when compared with a regular hospital mattress (Krouskop and others, 1985).

Friction and shear both contribute to pressure ulcers. *Friction* occurs when the surface of the skin rubs against another surface, such as the sheets on the bed. The skin may have the appearance of an abrasion. The skin damage is usually limited to the epidermal and upper layers. It most often occurs over the elbows or heels. Prevention of friction injury includes the use of protective sheepskin over the elbows or heels, moisturizing agents, transparent dressings over susceptible areas, and soft, smooth bed linen and clothing. Friction alone does not cause tissue necrosis, but when it acts with gravity, it results in shear injury.

Shear is the result of the force of gravity pushing down on the body and friction of the body against a surface, such

CRITICAL THINKING EXERCISE
Risk of Skin Breakdown

You work on a pediatric surgical unit. In a recent continuous quality improvement report, it was noted that 10% of the patients developed some type of skin breakdown, most often stage II wounds. Which of the following variables identified about this patient population should be investigated further?

1. Average age of the child is 6 years and sex is more often male.
2. Major reason for surgery is orthopedic repair, especially as a result of trauma.
3. Average length of surgery is 4 hours, and average duration until appearance of wound is 24 to 48 hours.
4. All children received adequate pain medication.

The correct answer is three. During prolonged surgery, patients are often placed on an inadequately padded surface. The excessive pressure on bony prominences causes redness and deeper tissue damage that may not be apparent until hours or days later. The fact that these children are most likely to need orthopedic surgery (this age-group and sex are at risk for injuries) may also be a risk factor if mobility is impaired. However, with good pain control, these children should be able to move quite easily. If pressure ulcers develop postoperatively from immobility, they are most likely to develop later than during the first 2 days.

as the bed or chair. For example, when a patient is in the semi-Fowler position and begins to slide to the foot of the bed, the skin over the sacral area remains in the same place because of the resistance of the bed surface. The blood vessels in the area are stretched and may cause small-vessel thrombosis and tissue death (Bryant, 1992). The same type of damage can occur when a patient is pulled up in the bed if the skin does not move with the patient. Prevention of shear injury includes using "lift sheets" when repositioning a patient, elevating the bed no more than 30 degrees for short periods, and using the knee gatch to interrupt the pull of gravity on the body toward the foot of the bed.

Epidermal stripping results when the epidermis is unintentionally removed with tape removal. These lesions are usually shallow and irregularly shaped. Prevention of epidermal stripping includes recognizing fragile skin, such as in neonates; using minimum tape; using solid-wafer skin barriers, transparent dressings, or laced binders to secure dressings (Montgomery straps) on areas where tape must be changed frequently; using skin sealants under adhesives unless skin is fragile; and using porous tapes. Tape is placed so there is no tension, traction, or wrinkles on the skin. To remove tape, the nurse slowly peels the tape away while stabilizing the underlying skin. Adhesive remover may be used to break the adhesive bond but may be drying to the skin (Bryant, 1992). Wetting the tape with water may facilitate removal.

Chemical factors can also lead to skin damage. Fecal incontinence, especially when mixed with urine; wound drain-age; or gastric drainage around gastrostomy tubes can erode epidermis. The skin can very quickly progress from redness to denudement if exposure continues. Moisture barriers, gentle cleansing as soon after exposure as possible, and skin barriers can be used to prevent damage caused by chemical factors (see also Diaper Dermatitis, Chapter 30).

BATHING

Unless contraindicated, most infants and children can be bathed in a tub at the bedside, on the bed, or in a standard bathtub or shower located on the unit, which is often conveniently adapted for pediatric use. For infants and young children confined to bed, the towel method can be used. Two towels are immersed in a dilute soap solution and wrung damp. With the child lying supine on a dry towel, one damp towel is placed on top of the child and used to gently clean the body. This towel is discarded, and the child is dried and turned prone. The procedure is repeated using the second damp towel.

Infants and small children are *never* left unattended in a bathtub, and infants who are unable to sit alone are securely held with one hand during the bath. The infant's head is supported securely with one hand, or the farther arm is firmly grasped in the nurse's hand while the head rests comfortably on the nurse's wrist or arm. This hold provides secure control of the infant while the other hand is free to wash the infant's body (Fig. 22-4). Infants or children who are able to sit without assistance need only close supervision and a pad

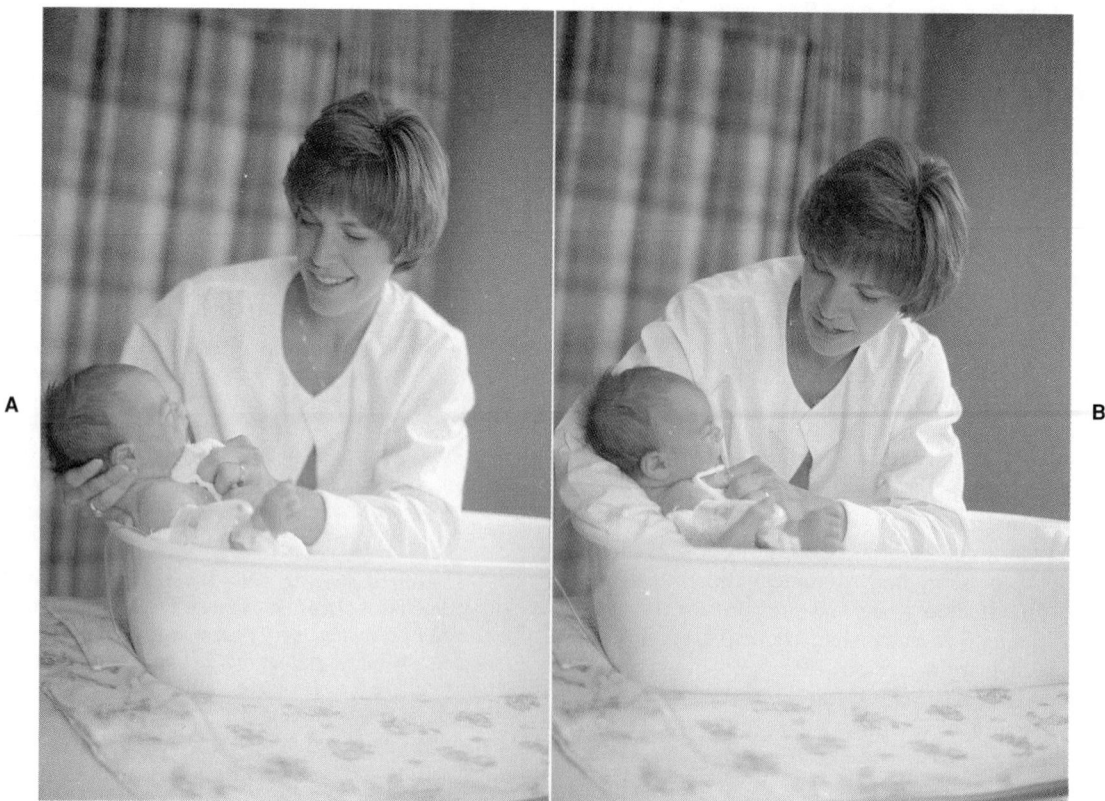

FIG. 22-4. Two methods of supporting infant during tub bath. **A,** Using hand to support neck and head. **B,** Using arm to support neck and head.

placed in the bottom of the tub to prevent slipping and loss of balance, which could result in a bumped head or submersion of the face.

Older children may enjoy a shower if it is available. School-age children may be reluctant to bathe, and many are not accustomed to a daily bath. However, most children who feel well require little encouragement to participate in their daily care. Nurses need to use judgment regarding the amount of supervision the child requires. Some can be trusted to assume this responsibility unaided, whereas others will need someone in constant attendance. Children with mental or physical limitations and suicidal or psychotic children (who may commit bodily harm) require close supervision.

Areas that require special attention during bed baths and for children performing their own care are the ears, between skinfolds, the neck, the back, and the genital area. The genital area should be carefully cleansed and dried with particular care to skinfolds, and in uncircumcised boys, usually those over 3 years of age, the foreskin should be gently retracted and the exposed surfaces cleansed and then the foreskin replaced. Do not attempt to retract the foreskin in newborns. If the condition of the glans indicates inadequate cleaning, such as accumulated smegma, inflammation, phimosis, or foreskin adhesions, teaching proper hygiene is indicated. In the Vietnamese and Cambodian cultures the foreskin is traditionally not retracted until adulthood (Krueger and Osborn, 1986). Older children have the tendency to avoid these areas; therefore they may need a gentle reminder.

Children who are ill or debilitated need more extensive assistance with bathing and other aspects of hygienic care, but they should be encouraged to perform as much as they can without overtaxing their energies. Increasing involvement can be expected with improved strength and endurance. Children with limited capacity for self-care but no other contraindications benefit greatly from tub baths. They can be transported to the tub and, with the aid of lifting devices and/or an appropriate number of persons to assist, gain the advantages of a tub bath.

ORAL HYGIENE

Mouth care is an integral part of daily hygiene and should be continued in the hospital. Infants and debilitated children require the nurse to perform mouth care. Although young children can manage a toothbrush and should be encouraged to use it, most will need assistance to perform a satisfactory job. Older children, although capable of brushing and flossing without assistance, sometimes need to be reminded that this is a part of their hygienic care. Most hospitals have equipment available for those children who do not have a toothbrush or toothpaste of their own. (See Dental Health, Chapters 10 and 12, for specific oral hygiene techniques; mouth care of children with mucosal ulcers is discussed under nursing care of the child with leukemia in Chapter 26.)

HAIR CARE

Brushing and combing hair are a part of the daily care for all persons in the hospital, including infants and children. If the child does not have a brush or comb, many hospitals provide one as part of the usual admission kit. If not, the parents should be asked to bring hair care equipment for the child's use. Both boys and girls should be helped to comb or brush their hair, or it should be done for them, at least once daily. The hair is styled for comfort and in a manner pleasing to the child and parents. A satisfactory style for girls with longer hair is French braiding, which is done by starting with three equal portions of hair from the top of the scalp; as the hair is braided, segments of hair are added at successive intervals until all the hair has been incorporated into one or more neat, head-hugging braids. The ends are firmly anchored with a coated elastic band or barrette. The hair should not be cut without parental permission, although shaving hair to provide access to a scalp vein for intravenous needle insertion may be necessary.

If children are hospitalized for more than a few days, the hair may need shampooing. With infants the hair may be washed during the daily bath or less frequently. For most children washing the hair and scalp once or twice weekly is sufficient, unless there is an indication to wash it more frequently, such as following a high fever and profuse sweating. Some hospitals have shampoo basins, but almost any child can be conveniently transported by a gurney to an accessible sink or washbasin for shampooing. Those who are unable to be transported can receive a shampoo in their beds with adequate protection and/or specially adapted equipment or positioning. A convenient method involves positioning the child near the edge of the bed, placing towels under the shoulders, and draping a large plastic garbage bag at the edge of the bed with one open side under the shoulders and the other side opened away from the head so that the hair is inside the opening. Water can be transported in a basin or placed in a clean enema bag. The nurse should fill a clean enema bag with warm water, hang the bag from an intravenous pole, and use the clamp on the bag's tubing to adjust the flow of water.

Teenagers, with their normally increased oily sebaceous secretions, are particularly in need of frequent hair care and usually require more frequent shampoos. Commercial no-rinse products also may prove useful on a short-term basis.

Black children require special hair care, and this need is frequently neglected or inadequately managed. For the black child with kinky hair, most standard combs are inadequate and may cause hair breakage and discomfort to the child. If a special comb with widely spaced teeth is not available on the unit, the parent can be reminded to bring a comb, if possible, for the child's use. It is also much easier to comb the hair after shampooing when it is wet. This type of hair also requires a special hair dressing or pomade, which usually has a coconut oil base. The preparation is rubbed on the hands and then transferred to the hair to make it more pliable and manageable. The child's parents should be consulted regarding the preparation they want to be used on their child's hair, and they should be asked if they can provide some for use during the child's hospitalization. Petroleum jelly should *not* be used. If braiding or plaiting the hair is desired, the hair should be damp and loosely woven. The hair tightens as it dries, which could result in tension folliculitis (Joyner, 1988).

FEEDING THE SICK CHILD

Loss of appetite is a symptom common to most childhood illnesses and is frequently the initial evidence of illness, preceding fever and other overt signs of infection. In most cases children can be permitted to determine their own need for food. Since an acute illness is usually short, the nutritional state is seldom compromised. In fact, urging foods on the sick child may precipitate nausea and vomiting and in some cases even cause an aversion to the feeding situation that can extend into the convalescent period and beyond.

Refusing to eat may also be one way children can exert power and control in an otherwise helpless situation. For young children, loss of appetite may be related to the depression of separation from their parents and their natural tendency toward negativism. Parents' concern with eating can intensify the problem. Forcing a child to eat only meets with rebellion and reinforces the behavior as a control mechanism. Parents are encouraged to relax any pressure during the period of acute illness. Although it is best to encourage high-quality nutritious foods, the child may desire foods and liquids that contain mostly empty or nonnutritional calories. Some well-tolerated foods include gelatin, clear soups, carbonated drinks, flavored ice pops, dry toast, crackers, and hard candy. Even though these substances are not nutritious, they can provide necessary fluid and calories.

Dehydration is always a hazard when children are febrile or anorexic, especially when this is accompanied by vomiting or diarrhea. An adequate fluid intake is encouraged by offering small amounts of favored fluids at frequent intervals and by offering salty foods (that increase thirst) if allowed. If di-

arrhea is present, high-carbohydrate liquids (e.g., carbonated beverages, gelatin, flavored ice pops) are avoided because they may aggravate the diarrhea by an osmotic effect. Also, replacing abnormal losses with plain water or undiluted broth, which may worsen the electrolyte imbalance, is not advocated. Fluids should not be forced, and the child should not be wakened from rest to take fluids. Forcing fluids may create the same difficulties as urging unwanted food. Gentle persuasion with preferred beverages will usually meet with success. Using play techniques can also be very effective (see Guidelines box).

When children are placed on special diets, such as clear liquids after surgery or during episodes of diarrhea, assessment of their intake and readiness to advance to more complex foods is essential.

Nursing ALERT	Evidence of lack of readiness to advance the diet includes the following:

Vomiting or diarrhea
Decrease in appetite
Abdominal cramping or distention
Absence of bowel sounds
Dehydration or weight loss

GUIDELINES
Feeding the Sick Child

Take a dietary history (see Chapter 6) and use information to make eating time as much like home as possible.

Encourage parents or other family members to feed child or to be present at mealtimes.

Have children eat at tables in groups; bring nonambulatory children to eating area in wheelchairs, beds, strollers, gurneys, or wagons.

Use familiar eating utensils, such as a favorite plate, cup, or bottle for small children.

Make mealtimes pleasant; avoid any procedures immediately before or after eating; make sure child is rested and pain free.

Have a nurse present at mealtimes to offer assistance, prevent disruptions, and praise children for their eating.

Serve small, frequent meals rather than three large meals or serve three meals and nutritious between-meal snacks.

Bring in foods from home, especially if food preparation is very different from hospital's; consider cultural differences.

Provide finger foods for young children.

Involve children in food selection and preparation whenever possible.

Serve small portions, and serve each course separately, such as soup first, followed by meat, potatoes, and vegetables, and ending with dessert; with young children, camouflage size of food by cutting meat thicker so less appears on plate or by folding a cheese slice in half; offer second helpings; ensure a variety of foods, textures, and colors.

Provide food selections that are favorites of most children, such as peanut butter and jelly sandwiches, hot dogs, hamburgers, macaroni and cheese, pizza, spaghetti, tacos, fried chicken, corn on the cob, and fruit yogurt.

Avoid foods that are highly seasoned, have strong odors, are served hot, or are all mixed together, unless typical of cultural practices.

Provide fluid selections that are favorites of most children, such as fruit punch, cola, ginger ale, sweetened tea, ice pops, sherbet, ice cream, milk and milkshakes, eggnog, pudding, gelatin, clear broth, or creamed soups (see also box on p. 680).

Offer nutritious snacks, such as frozen yogurt or pudding, ice cream, oatmeal or peanut butter cookies, hot cocoa, cheese slices or "kisses," pieces of raw vegetable or fruit, and dried fruit or cereal.

Make food attractive and different, for example:
Serve a "picnic lunch" in a paper bag.
Pack food in a Chinese-food container; decorate container.
Put a "face" or a "flower" on a hamburger or sandwich with pieces of vegetable.
Use a cookie cutter to shape a sandwich.
Serve pudding, yogurt, or juice frozen as an ice pop.
Make slurpies or snow cones by pouring flavored syrup on crushed ice.
Add vegetable coloring to water or milk.
Serve fluids through brightly colored or unusually shaped straws.
Make "bowtie" sandwiches by cutting them in triangles and placing two points together.
Slice sandwiches into "fingers."
Grate mounds of cheese.
Cut apples horizontally to make circles.
Put a banana on a hot dog bun and spread with peanut butter.
Break uncooked spaghetti into toothpick lengths and skewer cheese, cold meat, vegetables, or fruit chunks.

Praise children for what they do eat.

Do *not* punish children for not eating by removing their dessert or putting them to bed.

Once the child is feeling better, the appetite usually begins to improve. It is best to take advantage of any hungry period by serving high-quality foods and snacks. If the child still refuses to eat, nutritious fluids, such as prepared breakfast drinks, should be encouraged. Parents can be very helpful by bringing in favorite food items from home, especially if the family's cultural eating habits differ from the hospital's food services.

In general, hot dogs, hamburgers, peanut butter and jelly sandwiches, fruit yogurt, milkshakes, spaghetti, tacos, macaroni and cheese, and pizza are favorite foods of most children. Although alone they may not typify well-balanced diets, they can be adjusted to include sufficient amounts from the different food groups. It is better to work with preferred food choices than with selections that children rarely eat. A number of creative approaches to food preparation can increase the child's interest in eating (see Guidelines box).

Regardless of the type of diet, charting of the amount consumed is an important nursing responsibility. Descriptions need to be detailed and accurate, such as "4 ounces of orange juice, one pancake, no bacon, and 8 ounces of milk." Comments such as "ate well" or "ate poorly" are inadequate. Charting the percentage of the meal eaten is also inadequate unless food is measured before serving.

> **Nursing ALERT**
> Ask the parent if the child ate all the food from the tray. Occasionally a parent may eat something from the tray because the child did not eat or want it. If a family member has eaten some of the food, this makes a marked difference in the report of how much the child ate.

If parents are involved in the child's care, they are encouraged to keep a list of everything eaten. Using a premeasured cup for fluids ensures a more accurate estimate of intake. A comparison of the intake at each meal can isolate food deficiencies, such as insufficient intake of meat or vegetables. Behaviors associated with mealtime also identify possible factors influencing appetite. For example, the observation that "Child eats well when with other children but plays with food if left alone in room" helps the nurse plan mealtime activities that stimulate the appetite.

CONTROLLING ELEVATED TEMPERATURES

An elevated temperature, most frequently from fever but occasionally caused by hyperthermia, is one of the most common symptoms of illness in children. This manifestation is frequently misunderstood and of great, but often unnecessary, concern to parents. To facilitate an understanding of fever, the following terms are defined:

Set point—the temperature around which body temperature is regulated by a thermostat-like mechanism in the hypothalamus

Fever—an elevation in set point such that body temperature is regulated at a higher level; may be arbitrarily defined as temperature above 38° C (100° F)

Hyperthermia—a situation in which body temperature exceeds the set point, which usually results from the body or external conditions creating more heat than the body can eliminate, such as in heatstroke, aspirin toxicity, seizures, or hyperthyroidism

Body temperature is regulated by a thermostat-like mechanism in the hypothalamus. This mechanism receives input from centrally and peripherally located receptors. When temperature changes occur, these receptors relay the information to the thermostat, which either increases or decreases heat production to maintain a constant set point temperature. During an infection, however, pyrogenic substances cause an increase in the body's normal set point, a process that is mediated by prostaglandins. Consequently the hypothalamus increases heat production until the core (internal) temperature reaches the new set point.

Most fevers in children are of viral origin, are of relatively brief duration, and have limited consequences. In addition, fever probably plays a role in enhancing the development of both specific and nonspecific immunity and in aiding recovery and survival from infection. Contrary to popular belief, neither the rise in temperature nor its response to antipyretics indicates the severity or etiology of infection, which casts doubt on the value of using fever as a diagnostic or prognostic indicator.

Measures to Reduce Elevated Temperature

Treatment of elevated temperature depends on whether it is caused by a fever or hyperthermia. Because the set point is normal in hyperthermia but increased in fever, different approaches must be used to lower body temperature successfully.

Fever. The principal reason for treating fever is the relief of discomfort; there is no specific degree of fever that requires treatment. Relief measures include pharmacologic and/or environmental intervention. The most effective intervention is the use of antipyretics to lower the set point.

Antipyretic drugs include acetaminophen, aspirin, and nonsteroidal antiinflammatory drugs (NSAIDs). Acetaminophen is the preferred drug; aspirin should *not* be given to children because of the association between aspirin use in children with influenza virus or chickenpox and Reye syndrome. One nonprescription NSAID, ibuprofen (Children's Motrin or Children's Advil), is approved for fever reduction in children as young as 6 months of age. Dosage is based on the initial temperature level: 5 mg/kg of body weight for temperatures less than 39.1° C (102.5° F) or 10 mg/kg for temperatures greater than 39.1° C. The duration of fever reduction is generally 6 to 8 hours and is longer with the higher dose (Simon, 1996). Table 22-1 lists the recommended dosages of acetaminophen. It may be given every 4 hours but no more than five times in 24 hours. Since body temperature normally decreases at night, three to four doses in 24 hours are usually sufficient to control most fevers. The temperature is usually retaken 30 minutes after the antipyretic is given to assess its effect but should not be repeatedly measured; the child's level of discomfort is the best indication for continued treatment.

Environmental measures to reduce fever may be used if tolerated by the child and if they do not induce shivering. Shivering is the body's way of maintaining the elevated set point by producing heat. Compensatory shivering greatly increases metabolic requirements above those already caused by the fever.

TABLE 22-1. Dosage recommendations for acetaminophen (Tylenol)*

AGE	WEIGHT (POUNDS)	DOSE (MG)	FORM†
Under 3 months	6-11	40	½ dropper
4-11 months	12-17	80	1 dropper or ½ tsp elixir
12-23 months	18-23	120	1½ dropper or ¾ tsp elixir or 1½ chewable tablet (80 mg)
2-3 years	24-35	160	2 droppers or 1 tsp elixir or 2 chewable tablets (80 mg)
4-5 years	36-47	240	1½ tsp elixir or 3 chewable tablets (80 mg)
6-8 years	48-59	320	2 tsp elixir or 4 chewable tablets (80 mg) or 2 swallowable tablets
9-10 years	60-71	400	2½ tsp elixir or 5 chewable tablets (80 mg) or 2½ swallowable tablets
11 years	72-95	480	3 tsp elixir or 6 chewable tablets (80 mg) or 3 swallowable tablets
12 years and above	96+	640	4 swallowable tablets

*Doses should be administered four or five times daily but should not exceed five doses in 24 hours.
†1 dropper = 80 mg/0.8 ml; elixir = 160 mg/5 ml; chewable tablet = 80 mg each; junior-strength chewable tablets = 160 mg each; junior-strength swallowable tablets = 160 mg each. Rectal suppositories and sprinkle caps acetaminophen (Feverall) are also available from Upsher-Smith Laboratories, Inc, 14905 23rd Ave. N., Minneapolis, MN 55447; (800) 328-3344.

Nursing ALERT   Treatment of shivering is directed at modifying or interfering with the rate of heat loss by warming the body with increased clothing (especially on the extremities), higher environmental temperature, and warm baths (Holtzclaw, 1990).

Traditional cooling measures, such as wearing minimum clothing, exposing the skin to the air, reducing room temperature, increasing air circulation, and applying cool, moist compresses to the skin (e.g., the forehead), are effective if employed approximately 1 hour *after* an antipyretic is given so that the set point is lowered. Cooling procedures such as sponging or tepid baths are ineffective in treating febrile children either when used alone or in combination with antipyretics, and they cause considerable discomfort (Newman, 1985).

Seizures associated with a fever occur in 3% to 4% of all children, usually those 3 months to 5 years of age. Although most children never have febrile seizures after the first occurrence, a younger age at onset and a family history of febrile seizures are associated with recurring episodes. For children who have febrile seizures, administration of antipyretics does not prevent recurrences.

Hyperthermia.   Unlike with fever, antipyretics are of no value in hyperthermia, because the set point is already normal. Consequently, cooling measures are used. Cool applications to the skin help to reduce the core temperature. Cooled blood from the skin surface is conducted to inner organs and tissues, and warm blood is circulated to the surface, where it is cooled and recirculated. The surface blood vessels dilate as the body attempts to dissipate heat to the environment and facilitate this cooling process.

Commercial cooling devices, such as cooling blankets or mattresses, are available to reduce body temperature. They are placed on the bed and covered with a sheet or lightweight blanket. Frequent temperature monitoring is essential to prevent excessive cooling of the body.

Traditionally, cool compresses have been used to decrease high temperature. However, no particular temperature of water is agreed on as optimum. For tepid tub baths it is usually best to start with warm water and gradually add cool water until the desired water temperature of 37° C (98.6° F) is reached to accustom the child to the lower water temperature. Generally the temperature of the water only has to be 1° to 2° (usually a warm temperature) less than the child's temperature to be effective (Kinmonth, Fulton, and Campbell, 1992). The child is placed directly in the tub of tepid water for 20 to 30 minutes while water is gently squeezed from a washcloth over the back and chest or gently sprayed over the body from a sprayer. In the bed or crib, cool washcloths or towels are used, exposing only one area of the body at a time. The sponging is continued for approximately 30 minutes.

Nursing ALERT   Isopropyl alcohol should never be used for sponging; neurotoxic effects such as stupor, coma, and even death have been reported (Arditi and Killner, 1987).

After the tub or sponge bath, the child is dried and dressed in lightweight pajamas, nightgown, or diaper and placed in a dry bed. The temperature is retaken 30 minutes after the tub bath or sponge bath. The child is dried by gently rubbing the skin surface with a towel to stimulate circulation. The tub or sponge bath should not be continued or restarted until the skin surface is warm or if the child feels chilled. Chilling causes vasoconstriction, which defeats the purpose of the cool applications. In this condition, little blood is carried to the skin surface; the blood remains primarily in the viscera to become heated.

Whether a temperature elevation in the critically ill child is caused by fever or hyperthermia, it should be treated more aggressively. The metabolic rate increases 10% for every 1° C increase in temperature and three to five times during shivering, increasing oxygen, fluid, and caloric requirements. If the child's cardiovascular or neurologic system is already compromised, these increased needs are especially hazardous (Bruce and Grove, 1992). In all children with elevated temperature, attention to adequate hydration is essential. Most children's needs can be met through additional oral fluids.

FAMILY TEACHING AND HOME CARE

Nurses have a unique opportunity for teaching the family about health care practices while the child is hospitalized. Although most children have learned self-care and hygiene in the home or at school, many have not. For some young children, this is their first introduction to the use of a toothbrush. Much health teaching can be accomplished even when the child is hospitalized for only a short time. The daily bath, handwashing before meals and after bowel and bladder evacuation, and conscientious dental hygiene are taught by example during routine care. Clean hair, nails, and clothing, as well as good grooming, are emphasized as essential to a pleasing appearance. Positive reinforcement of good hygiene practices helps to create a positive body image, promote the development of self-esteem, and prevent health problems (e.g., teaching girls to wipe the genital area from front to back after toileting).

Although sick children's appetites may be poor and not characteristic of their home eating habits, the hospital stay provides numerous opportunities for nurses to assess the family's knowledge of good nutrition and to implement teaching as needed to improve nutritional intake.

Parental education about elevated temperatures is essential, since many parents are unaware of what constitutes a fever, have unrealistic fears about the dangers of fever, and are apt to overmedicate or undermedicate the febrile child. Parents also need to know that sponging is indicated for elevated temperatures from hyperthermia rather than fever and that ice water and alcohol are inappropriate, potentially dangerous, solutions. Parents should know how to take the child's temperature, read the thermometer accurately, and have guidelines for seeking professional care (see Family Home Care Box).* Some of the newer temperature-measuring devices, such as tympanic membrane sensors, plastic strips, or digital thermometers, may be better suited for home use, since many parents are unable to read a mercury thermometer or calculate the correct decimal point (see Temperature, Chapter 7).

If the use of acetaminophen is indicated, the parents need instruction in administering the drug.* It is important to emphasize accuracy in both the amount of drug given and the time intervals at which the drug is administered. Since many forms of acetaminophen are available, the nurse must be certain of the type being used in the home when discussing dosage. For example, the chewable tablets come in *two* strengths (80 and 160 mg), and the specially coated, swallowable tablets for older children are 160 mg. The nurse should alert the parents to this because the tablets for older children may contain *twice* the amount of drug as the lower-dose chewable ones. If parents switch from the infant drops to the elixir, they are cautioned against using the dropper to measure the elixir, which is much less concentrated than the drops. Also, as children grow, the dosage needs to be recalculated. To ensure the correct dose, it is recommended that a dose for a small child be calculated on the basis of 15 mg/kg/dose rather than 10 mg/kg/dose (Gribetz and Cronley, 1987).

FAMILY HOME CARE
The Child with Fever

Call Immediately If:
Child is <2 months of age.
Fever is >40.5° C (105° F).
Child is crying inconsolably.
Child is difficult to awaken.
Child is confused or delirious.
Child has had a seizure.
Child has a stiff neck.
Child has purple spots on the skin.
Breathing is difficult, and child does not feel better after nose is cleared.
Child is acting very sick.
Child has an underlying risk factor for serious infection (e.g., sickle cell disease).

Call During Office Hours If:
Child is 2 to 4 months old (unless fever is caused by a diphtheria-pertussis-tetanus [DPT] vaccination).
Fever is 40° to 40.5° C (104° to 105° F), especially if child is <2 years old.
Burning or pain occurs with urination.
Fever has been present for >72 hours.
Fever has been present for >24 hours without an obvious cause or location of infection.
Fever disappeared for >24 hours and then returned.
Child has a history of febrile seizures.
Parents have other questions.

Modified from Schmitt BD: Fever in childhood, *Pediatrics* 74(5, suppl):934, 1984.

SAFETY

Safety is an essential component of any patient's care, but children have special characteristics that require an even greater concern for safety. Since small children are separated from their usual environment and do not possess the capacity for abstract thinking and reasoning, it is the responsibility of everyone who comes in contact with them to maintain protective measures throughout their hospital stay. Nurses need to understand the age level at which each child is operating and plan for safety accordingly.

Name bands, a part of hospital safety practices, are particularly important for children in the pediatric age-group. Infants and unconscious patients are unable to tell or respond to their names. Toddlers may answer to any name or to a nickname only. Older children may exchange places, give an erroneous name, or choose not to respond to their own names as a form of joke, unaware of the hazards of such practices.

INFECTION CONTROL

The use of medical asepsis and appropriate barrier precautions to reduce the risk of *nosocomial* (hospital-acquired) infections is essential in caring for children. Children are infected frequently with organisms, such as varicella (chickenpox), that are transmissible and may be dangerous to others, especially immunocompromised patients. In addition, children

---

*Home care instructions on measuring temperature and giving medications are available in Wong DL: *Wong and Whaley's Clinical manual of pediatric nursing,* ed 4, St Louis, 1996, Mosby.

may not have developed good hygiene habits, such as hand-washing after toileting. Young children are especially at risk for infection because of their high oral activity. Children in diapers present infection risks if caregivers do not practice meticulous cleaning and disposal techniques.

To assist hospitals in maintaining up-to-date isolation practices, the **Centers for Disease Control and Prevention (CDC)** and the **Hospital Infection Control Practices Advisory Committee (HICPAC)** have revised the "CDC Guideline for Isolation Precautions in Hospitals," which was published in 1983. The guideline was revised to meet the following objectives: (1) to be epidemiologically sound; (2) to recognize the importance of all body fluids, secretions, and excretions in the transmission of nosocomial pathogens; (3) to contain adequate precautions for infections transmitted by the airborne, droplet, and contact routes of transmission; (4) to be as simple and user friendly as possible; and, (5) to use new terms to avoid confusion with existing infection control and isolation systems.*

The revised guideline contains two levels of precautions. In the first, and most important, level are those precautions designed for the care of all patients in hospitals regardless of their diagnosis or presumed infection status. Implementation of these "Standard Precautions" is the primary strategy for successful nosocomial infection control. In the second level are precautions designed only for the care of specified patients. These additional "Transmission-Based Precautions" are used for patients known or suspected to be infected or colonized with epidemiologically important pathogens that can be transmitted by airborne or droplet transmission or by contact with dry skin or contaminated surfaces.

Standard Precautions synthesize the major features of Universal (Blood and Body Fluid) Precautions (UP) (designed to reduce the risk of transmission of bloodborne pathogens) and Body Substance Isolation (BSI) (designed to reduce the risk of transmission of pathogens from moist body substances). Standard Precautions involve the use of *barrier protection*, such as gloves, goggles, gown, and/or mask, to prevent contamination from (1) blood; (2) all body fluids, secretions, and excretions *except sweat*, regardless of whether or not they contain visible blood; (3) nonintact skin; and (4) mucous membranes. Standard Precautions are designed to reduce the risk of transmission of microorganisms from both recognized and unrecognized sources of infection in hospitals.

Transmission-Based Precautions are designed for patients documented or suspected to be infected or colonized with highly transmissible or epidemiologically important pathogens for which additional precautions beyond Standard Precautions are needed to interrupt transmission in hospitals. There are three types of Transmission-Based Precautions: Air-

---

*This section is modified from Garner JS: Guideline for isolation precautions in hospitals, *Infection Control Hosp Epidemiol* 17(1):54-80, 1996.

SUMMARY OF TYPES OF PRECAUTIONS AND PATIENTS REQUIRING THEM

Standard Precautions

Use Standard Precautions for the care of all patients

Airborne Precautions

In addition to Standard Precautions, use Airborne Precautions for patients known or suspected to have serious illnesses transmitted by airborne droplet nuclei. Examples of such illnesses include measles, varicella (including disseminated zoster), tuberculosis

Droplet Precautions

In addition to Standard Precautions, use Droplet Precautions for patients known or suspected to have serious illnesses transmitted by large particle droplets. Examples of such illnesses include the following:
Invasive *Haemophilus influenzae* type b disease, including meningitis, pneumonia, epiglottitis, and sepsis
Invasive *Neisseria meningitidis* disease, including meningitis, pneumonia, and sepsis
Other serious bacterial respiratory infections spread by droplet transmission, including diphtheria (pharyngeal), Mycoplasma pneumonia, pertussis, pneumonic plague, streptococcal pharyngitis, pneumonia, or scarlet fever in infants and young children
Serious viral infections spread by droplet transmission, including Adenovirus, influenza, mumps, parvovirus B19, rubella

Contact Precautions

In addition to Standard Precautions, use Contact Precautions for patients known or suspected to have serious illnesses easily transmitted by direct patient contact or by contact with items in the patient's environment. Examples of such illnesses include the following:
Gastrointestinal, respiratory, skin, or wound infections or colonization with multidrug-resistant bacteria judged by the infection control program, based on current state, regional, or national recommendations, to be of special clinical and epidemiologic significance
Enteric infections with a low infectious dose or prolonged environmental survival, including *Clostridium difficile*. For diapered or incontinent patients: enterohemorrhagic *Escherichia coli* O157:H7, *Shigella*, hepatitis A, or rotavirus
Respiratory syncytial virus, parainfluenza virus, or enteroviral infections in infants and young children
Skin infections that are highly contagious or that may occur on dry skin, including diphtheria (cutaneous), herpes simplex virus (neonatal or mucocutaneous), impetigo, major (noncontained) abscesses, cellulitis, or decubiti, pediculosis, scabies, staphylococcal furunculosis in infants and young children, zoster (disseminated or in the immunocompromised host)
Viral/hemorrhagic conjunctivitis
Viral hemorrhagic infections (Ebola, Lassa, or Marburg)

From Garner JS: Guideline for isolation precautions in hospitals, *Infection Control Hosp Epidemiol* 17(1):66, 1996.

borne Precautions, Droplet Precautions, and Contact Precautions. They may be combined for diseases that have multiple routes of transmission (see box on p. 698). When used either singularly or in combination, they are to be used in addition to Standard Precautions.

Airborne Precautions are designed to reduce the risk of airborne transmission of infectious agents. Airborne transmission occurs by dissemination of either airborne droplet nuclei (small-particle residue [5 μm or smaller in size] of evaporated droplets that may remain suspended in the air for long periods of time) or dust particles containing the infectious agent. Microorganisms carried in this manner can be dispersed widely by air currents and may become inhaled by or deposited on a susceptible host within the same room or over a longer distance from the source patient, depending on environmental factors; therefore, *special air handling* and *ventilation* are required to prevent airborne transmission. Airborne Precautions apply to patients known or suspected to be infected with epidemiologically important pathogens that can be transmitted by the airborne route. Examples of such illnesses include measles, varicella (chickenpox), and tuberculosis.

Droplet Precautions are designed to reduce the risk of droplet transmission of infectious agents. Droplet transmission involves contact of the conjunctivae or the mucous membranes of the nose or mouth of a susceptible person with large-particle droplets (larger than 5 μm in size) containing microorganisms generated from a person who has a clinical disease or who is a carrier of the microorganism. Droplets are generated from the source person primarily during coughing, sneezing, or talking and during the performance of certain procedures such as suctioning and bronchoscopy. Transmission via large-particle droplets requires close contact between source and recipient persons, because droplets do not remain suspended in the air and generally travel only short distances, usually 3 ft or less, through the air. Because droplets do not remain suspended in the air, special air handling and ventilation are not required to prevent droplet transmission. Droplet Precautions apply to any patient known or suspected to be infected with epidemiologically important pathogens that can be transmitted by infectious droplets (see box on p. 698).

Contact Precautions are designed to reduce the risk of transmission of epidemiologically important microorganisms by direct or indirect contact. *Direct-contact transmission* involves skin-to-skin contact and physical transfer of microorganisms to a susceptible host from an infected or colonized person, such as occurs when personnel turn patients, bathe patients, or perform other patient-care activities that require physical contact. Direct-contact transmission also can occur between two patients (e.g., by hand contact), with one serving as the source of infectious microorganisms and the other as a susceptible host. *Indirect-contact transmission* involves contact of a susceptible host with a contaminated intermediate object, usually inanimate, in the patient's environment. Contact Precautions apply to specified patients known or suspected to be infected or colonized (presence of microorganism in or on patient but without clinical signs and symptoms of infection) with epidemiologically important microorganisms that can be transmitted by direct or indirect contact.

Nurses caring for young children are frequently in contact with body substances, especially urine, feces, and vomitus. Nurses need to exercise judgment for those situations when gloves, gowns, or masks are necessary. For example, gloves and possibly gowns should be worn for changing diapers when there are loose or explosive stools. Otherwise, the plastic lining of disposable diapers provides a sufficient barrier between the hands and body substances. The type of diaper may be an important aspect of infection control. Superabsorbent disposable diapers with elastic legs contain urine and feces better than cloth diapering systems, and their use can reduce fecal contamination in the environment (Van and others, 1991).

Nursing ALERT   Handwashing is the most critical infection control practice.

During feedings, gowns should be worn if the child is likely to vomit or spit up, which often occurs during burping. If aprons with minimal shoulder protection are worn, the child should be sitting on the nurse's lap, not upright against the shoulder, when the child is bubbled. When gloves are worn, the hands are washed thoroughly after removing the gloves, because both latex and vinyl gloves fail to provide complete protection. The absence of visible leaks does not indicate that gloves are intact. In addition, glove leaks occur more frequently with vinyl than with latex gloves (Olsen and others, 1993). An additional consideration is that some people are allergic to latex (see Spina Bifida, Chapter 32).

Nursing ALERT   Patients and staff may be sensitive to latex and demonstrate allergic reactions ranging from hives, wheezing, and localized swelling to anaphylaxis. Latex is present in numerous health care products, including gloves, tourniquets, airway equipment, catheters, IV supplies, and dressings.

Another essential practice of infection control is that all needles (uncapped and unbroken) are disposed of in a rigid, puncture-resistant container located near the site of use. Consequently, these containers are installed in patients' rooms. Since children are naturally curious, extra attention is needed in selecting a suitable type of container and a location that discourages access to the disposed needles (Fig. 22-5). The use of needleless systems allow secure syringe or IV tubing attachment to vascular access devices without the risk of needle stick injury to the child or nurse. These devices also help maintain IV line integrity.

ENVIRONMENTAL FACTORS

All the environmental safety measures in operation for the protection of adults apply to children as well, such as good illumination; floors clear of fluid or objects that might contribute to falls; nonskid surfaces in showers and tubs; electrical equipment that is maintained in good working order, is operated only by personnel familiar with its use, and is not in contact with moisture or near tubs, where it could prove to be a shock hazard; beds of ambulatory patients locked in place and at a height that allows easy access to the floor (a special hazard for children is the danger of entrapment un-

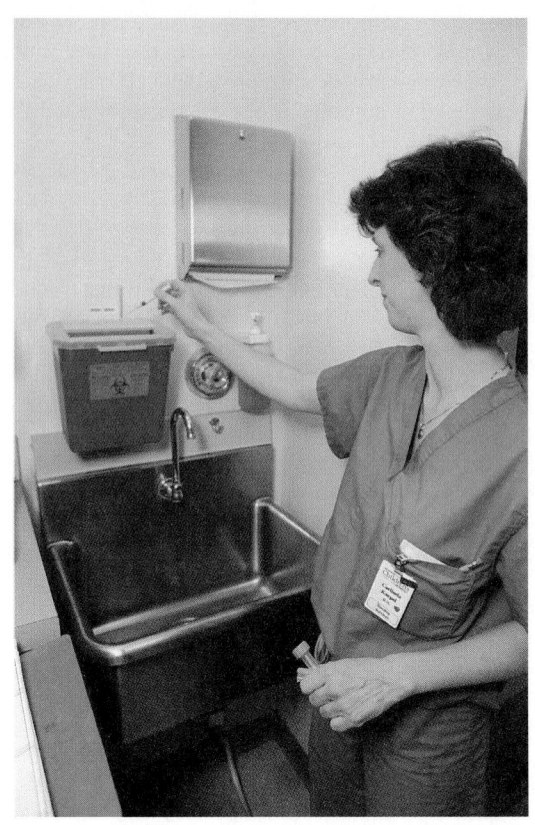

FIG. 22-5. To prevent needle stick injuries, used needles (and other sharp instruments) are not capped or broken and are disposed of in a rigid, puncture-resistant container located near the site of use. Note placement of the container to prevent children's access to the contents.

der an electronically controlled bed when it is activated to descend); proper care and disposal of small breakable items such as thermometers and bottles; and a well-organized fire plan known to all staff members.

All windows should be securely screened and elevators and stairways made safe. Ideally, electrical outlets should be provided with covers to prevent burns in small children whose exploratory activities may extend to inserting objects into the small openings. Bathwater is carefully checked before placing the child in it, and children must never be left alone in a bathtub. Infants are helpless in water, and small children (and some older ones) may turn on the hot water faucet and be severely burned.

Furniture is safest when it is scaled to the child's proportions, is sturdy, and is well balanced to prevent its being easily tipped over. Infants and small children must be securely strapped into infant seats, feeding chairs, and strollers. Baby walkers should be discouraged because they provide access to hazards, resulting in burns, falls, and poisonings. Infants, young children, and those who are weak, paralyzed, agitated, confused, sedated, or cognitively impaired are never left unattended on treatment tables, on scales, or in treatment areas. Even premature infants are capable of surprising mobility; therefore portholes in incubators must be securely fastened when not in use. Beds of ambulatory patients should remain locked in place and at a height that allows easy access to the floor.

Crib sides should be elevated and fastened securely unless an adult is at the bedside. It is safer to leave crib sides up, regardless of the child's ability to get out and even when the crib is unoccupied, to remove the child's temptation to climb

in. Anyone attending an infant or small child in a crib with the sides down should never turn away without maintaining hand contact with the child; that is, one hand should be kept on the child's back or abdomen to prevent the child from rolling, crawling, or jumping from the open crib (Fig. 22-6). A child who is apt to or has demonstrated the inclination to climb over the sides of the crib is safest when placed in a specially constructed crib with a cover or one that has a safety net placed over the top. If the net is used, it must be tied to the frame in such a manner that there is ready access to the child in case of emergency. Nets are never tied to the movable crib sides, and the knots should be tied in a manner that

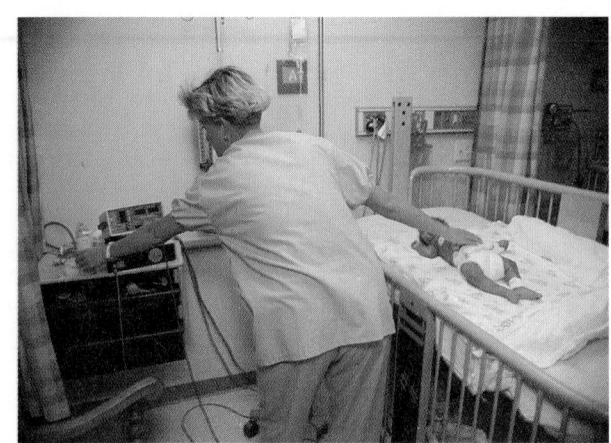

FIG. 22-6. Nurse maintains hand contact when back is turned.

permits quick release. Cribs are not placed within reach of heating units, appliances, dangling cords, or other objects that can be grabbed by curious hands, and toys are not tied to or across crib rails once children are old enough to reach them.

Toys. Toys play a vital role in the everyday life of children, and they are no less important in the hospital setting. However, nurses are responsible for assessing the safety of toys brought to the hospital by well-meaning parents and friends. Toys and gifts should be appropriate to the child's age, condition, and treatment. For example, if the child is in an oxygen tent, electrical or friction toys cannot be placed in the tent. Toys are inspected to make certain that they are non-allergenic, washable, and unbreakable and that they have no small, removable parts that can be aspirated or swallowed or that can in other ways inflict injury to a child.

> **Nursing ALERT** Plants and flowers harbor gram-negative bacteria and molds that may be a risk to the immunocompromised child. These items may also pose the danger of poisoning to curious toddlers.

LIMIT-SETTING

Setting limits is essential to a child's safety. Children must understand where they are permitted to go and what they are permitted to do in the hospital. These limitations should be made clear to them, consistently enforced, and repeated as frequently as necessary to make certain that they are understood. The nurse is responsible for a child's whereabouts at all times. Children can easily wander off unnoticed, and their access to tubs, laundry chutes, medication rooms and carts, and elevators must be prevented. Normally active older children often become restless when their activity is restricted and may resort to pillow fights, water fights, and other rough play that might endanger the safety of the involved children or other children, staff, or visitors. Children in the hospital require supervision, and appropriate tension-reducing activities can be planned and supervised by nurses and/or by the play therapist. A useful discipline technique is time-out (see Limit-setting and Discipline, Chapter 4).

TRANSPORTING INFANTS AND CHILDREN

In the course of a hospital stay, infants and children usually need to be transported within the unit and to areas outside the pediatric unit. Infants and small children can be carried for short distances within the unit, but for more extended trips the child should be securely transported in a suitable conveyance.

Small infants can be held or carried in the horizontal position with the back supported and the thigh grasped firmly by the carrying arm (Fig. 22-7, *A*). In the football hold the infant is carried on the nurse's arm with the head supported by the hand and the body held securely between the nurse's body and elbow (Fig. 22-7, *B*). Both these holds leave the nurse's other arm free for activity. The infant can be held in the upright position with the buttocks on the nurse's forearm and the front of the body resting against the nurse's chest. The infant's head and shoulders are supported by the nurse's other arm to allow for any sudden movement by the infant (Fig. 22-7, *C*). Older infants are able to hold their heads erect but can still make sudden movements.

Infants can be transported to other areas, such as the radiography department, in their bassinets or cribs. Baby carriages are sometimes used for infants who are not likely to

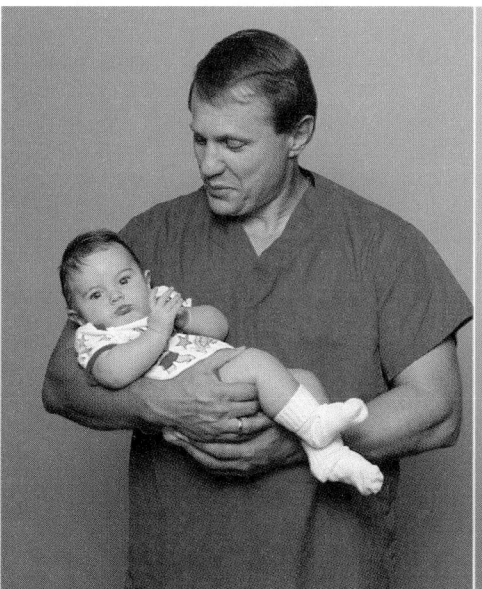 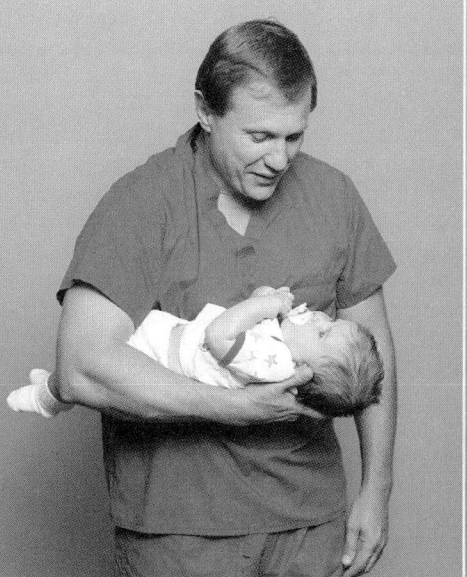 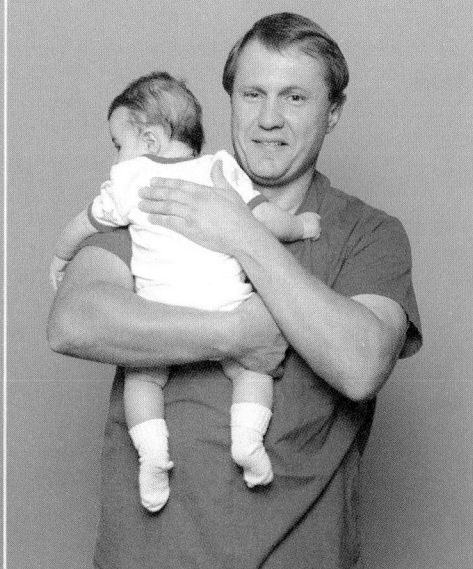

| A | B | C |

FIG. 22-7. Transporting infants. **A,** Infant's thigh firmly grasped in nurse's hand. **B,** Football hold. **C,** Back supported.

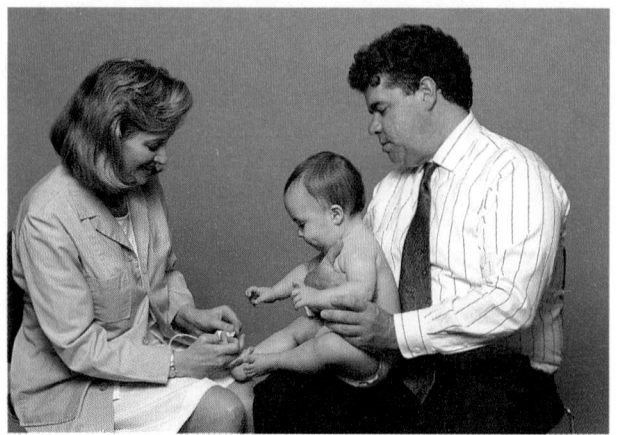

FIG. 22-8. Parent provides comfort and security to infant while nurse carries out procedure.

stand up. Strollers and wheeled feeding chairs or tables are also convenient transporters in some situations, such as trips to the playroom or nurse's station.

The method of transporting children is determined by their age, condition, and destination. Most older children are safe in wheelchairs or on gurneys. A younger child can be transported in a crib, on a gurney, in a wagon with raised sides, or in a wheelchair with a safety belt. Gurneys should be equipped with high sides and a safety belt, both of which are secured during transport.

RESTRAINTS

Frequently some method of restraint is needed to ensure a child's safety or comfort, to facilitate examination, or to carry out procedures. Restraint can be accomplished manually or with physical devices. Restraining the child manually provides an element of human contact that is lacking in restraint by mechanical means (Fig. 22-8). A physician's order and parental consent are required for restraints used for reasons other than procedures. These requirements are controversial, and nurses should be aware of their agencies' policies. These requirements originated from some concerns in elderly persons. Restraints can often be avoided with adequate preparation of the child, parental or staff supervision of the child, and adequate protection of a vulnerable site, such as an infusion device.

Mechanical restraints are never used as a punishment or as a substitute for observation. When a child must be restrained, the child and parents need a simple explanation, and if the restraint is applied for an extended time, the explanation must be repeated often to gain cooperation and to help the child understand that it is not a punishment. Restraining devices are not without risk and must be checked and documented every 1 to 2 hours to ensure that they are accomplishing their purpose, that they are applied correctly, and that they do not impair circulation, sensation, or skin integrity.

Parents need to know the purpose of restraints, how to remove and reapply them, and the signs of complications from their use. Parents are sometimes upset when their child must be restrained and need to understand how they can help

to ensure the maximum benefit and to minimize the stress related to the use of restraints. Children, too, should be prepared for the procedure or the circumstance for which the restraint is required.

Removing restraints whenever possible (at least every 2 hours when children are awake) is an essential part of nursing care of children who are restrained for treatments or other purposes. Alternate methods may be devised to replace the need for passive restraints. Holding children for periods is a pleasant alternative, as is restraining them in a high chair, where they can observe the surrounding activities. If feasible, distraction techniques such as play and reading to the child should be employed to gain cooperation without resorting to restraints. Parental participation is always encouraged.

Jacket Restraint

A jacket restraint is sometimes used as an alternative to the crib net to prevent the child from climbing out of the crib or to keep the child safe in various chairs. The jacket is put on the child with the ties in back so that the child is unable to manipulate them, and the long tapes, secured to the understructure of the crib, keep the child inside the crib. The jacket restraint is also useful as a means to maintain the child in a desired horizontal position. A Posey belt scaled to fit the child is an alternative device. The jacket-type restraint has been associated with accidental strangulation deaths in elderly persons.

Mummy Restraint

When an infant or small child requires short-term restraint for examination or treatment that involves the head and neck, such as venipuncture, throat examination, and gavage feeding, the mummy device effectively controls the child's movements. A blanket or sheet is opened on the bed or crib with one corner folded to the center. The infant is placed on the blanket with shoulders at the fold and feet toward the opposite corner (Fig. 22-9, *A*). With the infant's right arm straight down against the body, the right side of the blanket is pulled firmly across the infant's right shoulder and chest and secured beneath the left side of the body (Fig. 22-9, *B*). The left arm is placed straight against the child's side, and the left side of the blanket is brought across the shoulder and chest and locked beneath the child's body on the right side. The lower corner is folded and brought over the body and tucked or fastened securely with safety pins (Fig. 22-9, *C*). Safety pins can be used to fasten the blanket in place at any step in the process.

To modify the mummy restraint for chest examination, the folded edge of the blanket is brought over each arm and under the back, after which the loose edge is folded over and secured at a point below the chest to allow visualization and access to the chest (Fig. 22-9, *D*).

Arm and Leg Restraints

Occasionally, one or more extremities must be restrained or limited in motion. Several commercial restraining devices are available, or a restraint can be fashioned from gauze tape, muslin strips, or a length of narrow stockinette. When this type of restraint is used, it must be appropriate to the size of the child; it must be padded to prevent undue pressure, constriction, or tissue injury; and the extremity must be observed

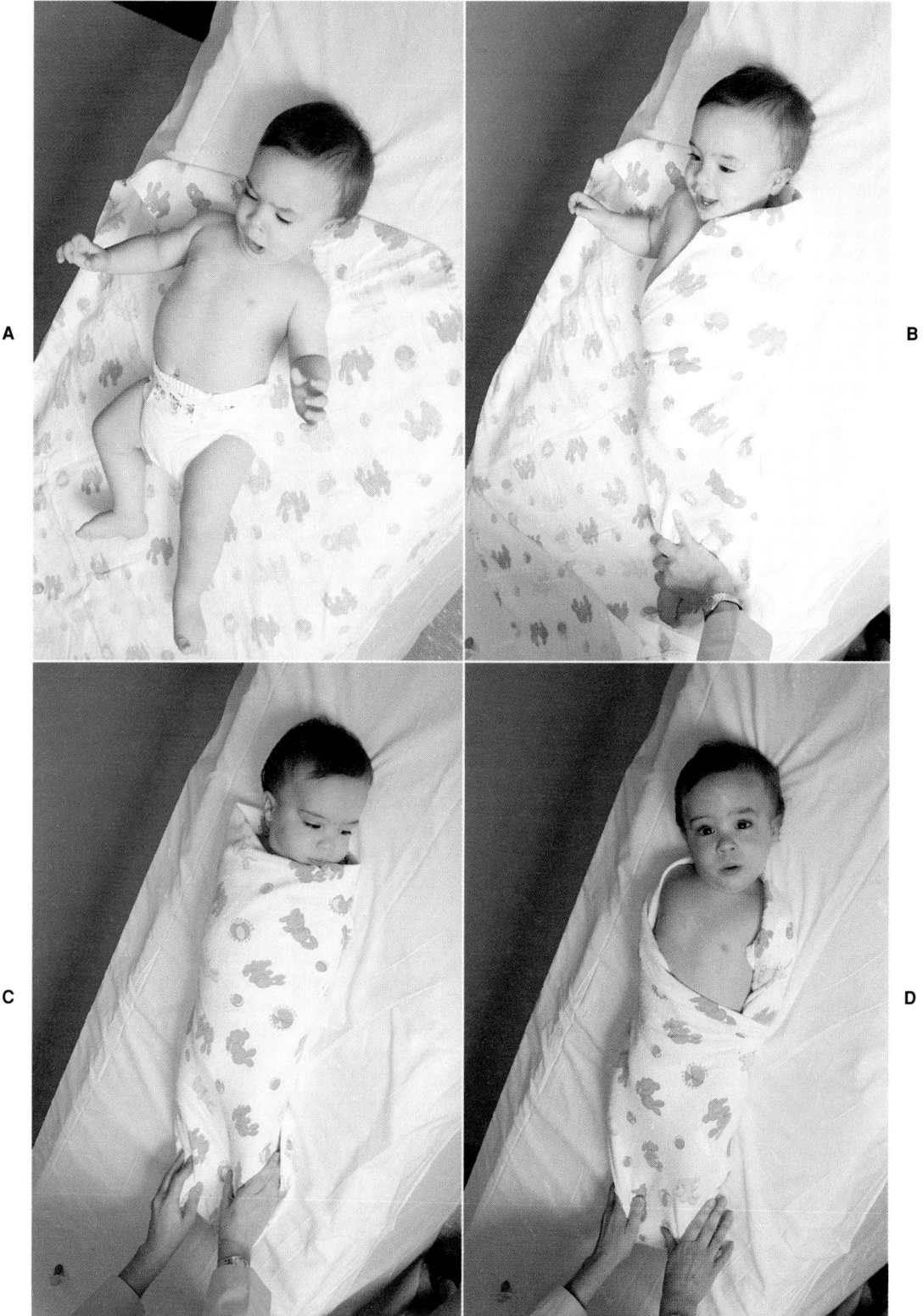

FIG. 22-9. Application of mummy restraint. **A,** Infant placed on folded corner of blanket. **B,** One corner of blanket brought across body and secured beneath body. **C,** Second corner brought across body and secured, and lower corner folded and tucked or pinned in place. **D,** Modified mummy restraint with chest uncovered.

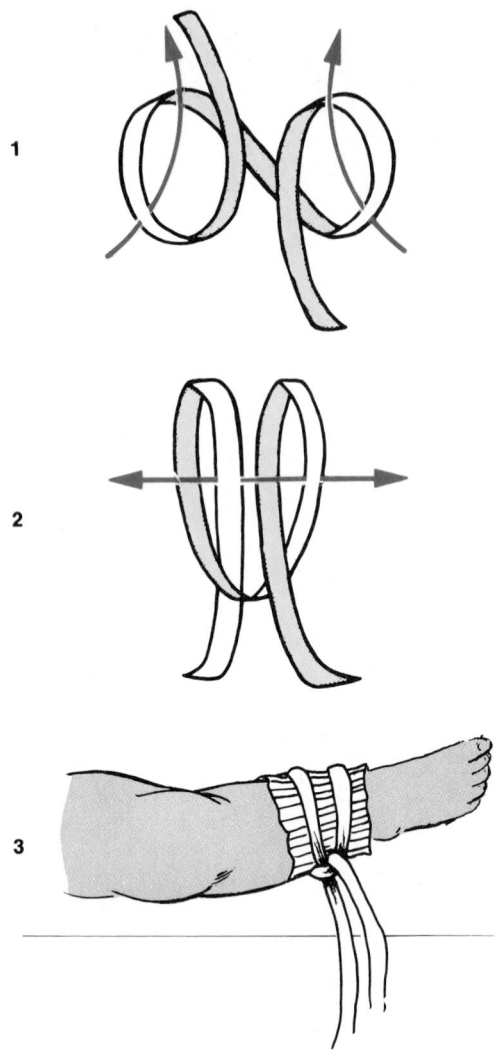

FIG. 22-10. Clove hitch restraint.

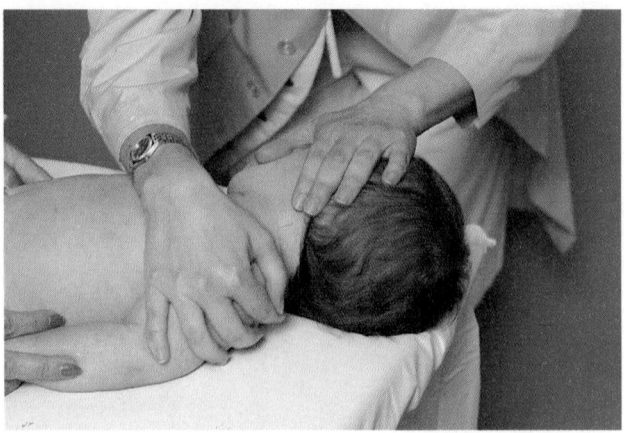

FIG. 22-11. Restraining child for jugular vein puncture.

frequently for signs of irritation and/or impairment of circulation. The ends of the restraints are never tied to the crib rails, since lowering the rail will disturb the extremity, frequently with a jerk that may hurt or injure the child.

The *clove hitch restraint* is fashioned from a length of gauze or muslin tape. When properly applied, the restraint should provide a snug fit with minimum danger of pulling too tightly. Fig. 22-10 illustrates the method of tying and applying a clove hitch restraint.

Elbow Restraint

Sometimes it is important to prevent the child from reaching the head or face (e.g., after lip surgery, when a scalp vein infusion is in place, or to prevent scratching in skin disorders). For this purpose, elbow restraints fashioned from a variety of materials function very well. The most common form of elbow restraint consists of a piece of muslin long enough to reach comfortably from just below the axilla to the wrist with a number of vertical pockets into which tongue depressors are inserted. The restraint is wrapped around the arm and secured with tapes or pins. It may be necessary to pin the top

of the restraint to the undershirt sleeve to prevent the restraint from slipping. Similar restraints can be made from commonly available products.

NURSING TIPS
Pad the ends of large-diameter towel rollers or appropriately sized plastic containers from which the tops and bottoms have been removed. Apply adhesive tabs to the top end and pin the tabs to the child's sleeves to prevent the restraint from slipping from the extremity.
Fashion adjustable restraints from tongue depressors placed vertically against strips of adhesive and then covered with adhesive; secure with adhesive tabs as described above.

POSITIONING FOR PROCEDURES

Jugular Venipuncture

The large, superficial external jugular vein may be used to obtain blood specimens from infants and young children. For easy access to the vein, the child is first placed in a mummy restraint in which the top edge of the restraint is low enough to permit access to the vein. The child is placed so that the head and shoulders extend over the edge of a table or a small pillow, with the neck extended and the head turned sharply to the side (Fig. 22-11). One alternate method for restraining arms and legs is with the nurse holding the child's arms and legs at the same time that the child's head is restrained and positioned. It is important for the nurse holding the infant to maintain control of the infant's head without interfering with the practitioner's approach to the vein. The infant's crying during the procedure increases intravenous pressure, which facilitates visualization of the vein. After venipuncture, digital pressure is applied to the site with a dry gauze square for 3 to 5 minutes or until bleeding stops. Care must be taken not to apply excessive pressure that might compromise circulation or breathing during or after the procedure.

Femoral Venipuncture

Other frequently used sites for venipuncture are the large femoral veins. The nurse restrains the infant by placing the child supine with the legs in a frog position to provide ex-

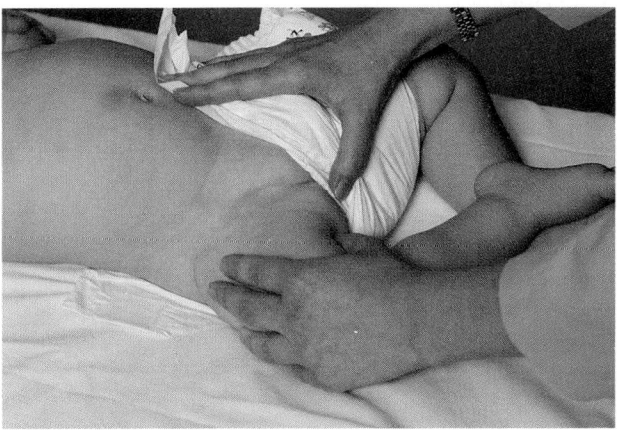

FIG. 22-12. Restraining infant for femoral vein puncture.

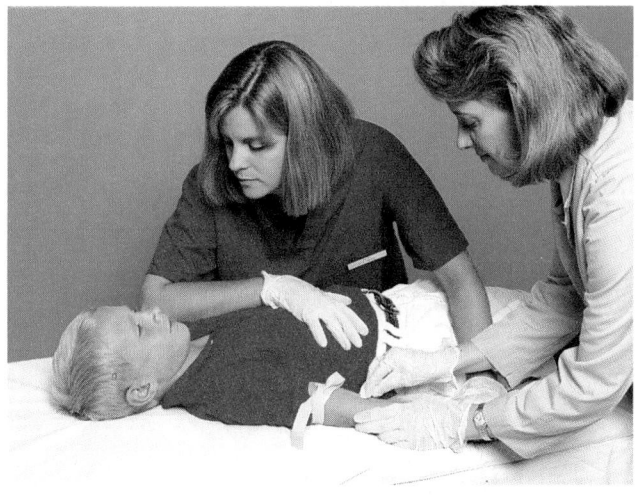

FIG. 22-13. Restraining child for extremity vein puncture.

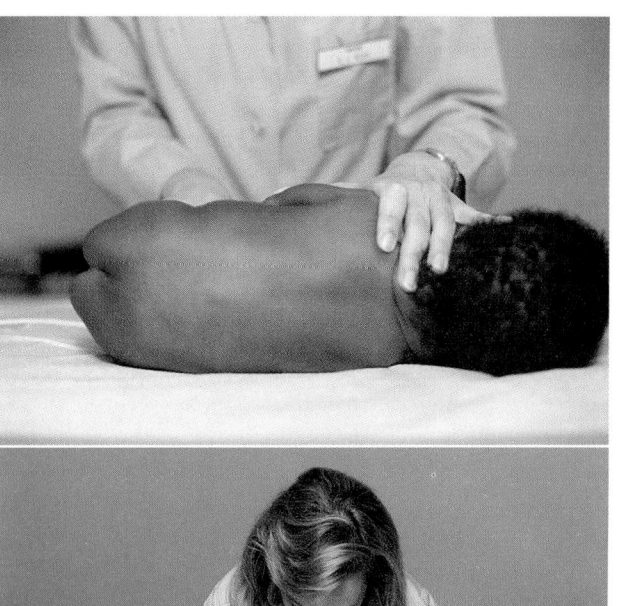

A

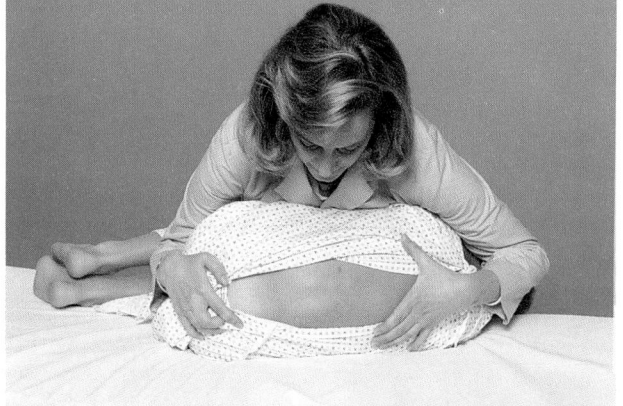

B

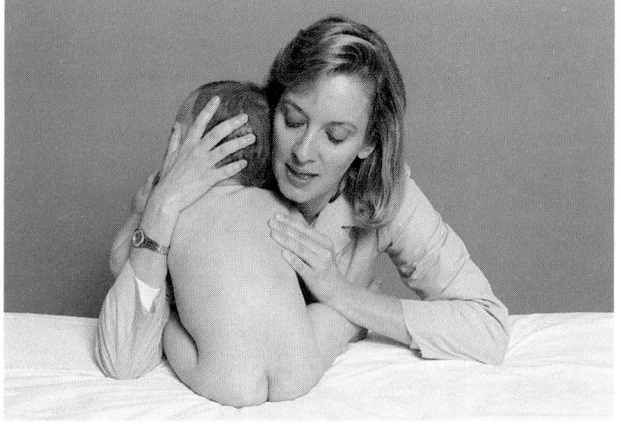

C

FIG. 22-14. A, Modified side-lying position for lumbar puncture. **B,** Older child in side-lying position. **C,** Infant sitting position allows for flexion of lumbar spine.

tensive exposure of the groin area. Both the arms and the legs of the infant can be effectively controlled by the nurse's forearms and hands (Fig. 22-12). Only the side used for the venipuncture is uncovered, so the practitioner is protected should the child urinate during the procedure. Pressure is applied to the site after the withdrawal of blood to prevent oozing from the site.

Extremity Venipuncture
The most common sites of venipuncture are the veins of the extremities, especially the arm and hand. A convenient position for restraint is having one person on either side of the bed. The child's outstretched arm is partially stabilized by the technician drawing the blood. The other person leans across the child's upper body, preventing its movement, and uses an arm to immobilize the venipuncture site. This type of restraint also comforts the child because of the close body contact and allows each person to maintain eye contact (Fig. 22-13).

Lumbar Puncture
The technique for lumbar puncture (LP) in infants and children is similar to that in the adult, although modifications

are suggested in neonates, who have less distress in a side-lying position with modified neck extension than in flexion or a sitting position (Fig. 22-14, A). Neonates tend to have more cardiorespiratory changes during an LP than older infants regardless of positioning; therefore oximetry and heart rate monitoring are advisable (Lehmann and others, 1990). Pediatric LP sets contain smaller spinal needles, but sometimes the practitioner will specify a particular size or type of needle that the nurse should make certain is placed on the tray.

Children are usually controlled best in the side-lying position, with the head flexed and the knees drawn up toward the chest. Even cooperative children need to be restrained to prevent possible trauma from unexpected, involuntary movement. They can be reassured that although they are trusted, the restraint will serve as a reminder to maintain the desired position. It also provides a measure of support and reassurance to them.

The child is placed on the side with the back close to the edge of the examining table on the side from which the practitioner is working. The nurse maintains the child's spine in a flexed position by holding the child with one arm behind the neck and the other behind the thighs (Fig. 22-14, *B*). The flexed position enlarges the spaces between the lumbar vertebral spines, which facilitates access to the spinal fluid space. It is helpful to wrap the legs before positioning to decrease leg movement.

An alternate position used with small infants and some older children is the sitting position. The child is placed with the buttocks at the edge of the table and with the neck flexed so that the chin rests on the chest. The infant's arms and legs are immobilized by the nurse's hands (Fig. 22-14, *C*).

> **Nursing ALERT** The sitting position may interfere with chest expansion and diaphragm excursion, and in infants the soft, pliable trachea may collapse. Therefore observe the child for difficulty with breathing.

Another position that employs close and comforting contact for the child involves holding the child upright against the nurse's (or parent's) chest with the child's legs wrapped around the adult's waist. The adult's arms are used to hug and restrain the child. For ease of the examiner, the adult should be standing. A small pillow is placed between the child's abdomen and the adult to help arch the child's back. If the pillow proves unsuccessful, a third person can place an arm in this space to achieve the desired position. Care should be taken that excessive pressure does not compromise circulation or breathing and that the nose and mouth are not covered by the restrainer's body.

Specimens and spinal fluid pressure are obtained, measured, and sent for analysis in the same manner as for the adult patient. Vital signs are taken as ordered, and the child is observed for any changes in level of consciousness, motor activity, or other neurologic signs. Post-LP headache may occur and is related to postural changes; this is less severe when the child lies flat. Headache is seen much less frequently in young children than in adolescents.

Bone Marrow Aspiration or Biopsy

Positioning for a bone marrow aspiration or biopsy depends on the location of the chosen site. In children the posterior or anterior iliac crest is most frequently used, although in infants the tibia may be selected because of easy access to the site and restraint of the child.

If the posterior iliac crest is used, the child is positioned prone. Sometimes a small pillow or folded blanket is placed under the hips to facilitate obtaining the bone marrow specimen. In children who have not received adequate analgesia or anesthesia, restraint is needed and is best applied with two people—one person to immobilize the upper body and a second person to immobilize the lower extremities. If the other sites are used, the child is placed supine and restraint is applied in a similar manner with modifications made for access to the tibia or anterior iliac crest.

Other Procedures

For subdural puncture through a fontanel or burr hole, the infant is wrapped in a mummy restraint and placed in the supine position with the head accessible to the examiner. To control the head, the nurse uses a firm hold on each side of it. Procedures for immobilizing the head for examining the ears, nose, or throat are discussed in Chapter 7.

COLLECTION OF SPECIMENS

URINE SPECIMENS

When children are admitted to the hospital or are seen in a clinic or office, a urine specimen may be needed. Older children and adolescents can use a bedpan or urinal or can be trusted to follow directions for collection in the bathroom. However, attention to their special needs and concerns is warranted. School-age children are cooperative but curious and are likely to ask questions regarding the disposition of their specimen and what one expects to discover from it. Self-conscious adolescents may be reluctant to carry a specimen bottle through a hallway or waiting room and appreciate a paper bag or other means for disguising the container. The presence of menses is sometimes an embarrassment or a concern to teenage girls; therefore it is a good idea to ask if they are menstruating and to make adjustments as necessary. The specimen can be delayed or a notation made on the laboratory slip to explain the presence of red blood cells.

Preschoolers and toddlers are usually unable to void on request. It is often best to offer them water or other liquids that they enjoy and wait about 30 minutes until they are ready to void voluntarily or to set a timer to alert them that they need to void shortly. The child will better understand what is expected if the nurse uses familiar terms, such as "pee-pee" or "tinkle." Some children will have difficulty voiding in an unfamiliar receptacle. Potty chairs or a potty hat placed on the toilet will usually prove satisfactory. Toddlers who have recently acquired bladder control may be especially reluctant, since they undoubtedly have been admonished for "going" in places other than those approved by parents. A useful approach is to enlist the help of parents; they are likely to be successful, and this helps them feel a part of the child's care.

For infants and toddlers who are not toilet trained, special urine collection devices may be used. These devices are clear, plastic, single-use bags with self-adhering material around the opening at the point of attachment. To prepare the infant, the genitalia, perineum, and surrounding skin are washed and dried thoroughly, since the adhesive will not stick to a moist, powdered, or oily skin surface. The collection bag is easiest to apply if attached first to the perineum, progressing to the symphysis (Fig. 22-15). With little girls the perineum is stretched taut during application to that area to ensure a leak-proof fit. With small boys the penis and scrotum are placed inside the bag. The adhesive portion of the bag must be firmly applied to the skin all around the genital area

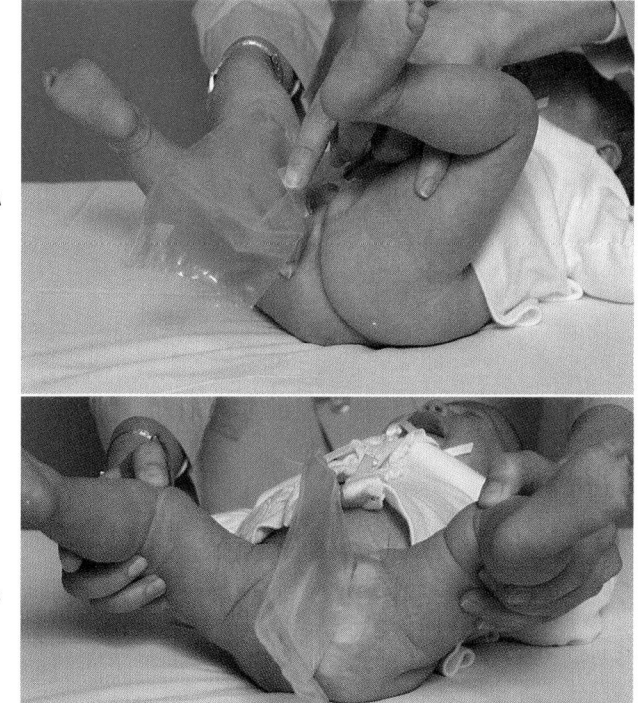

FIG. 22-15. Application of urine collection bag. **A,** On female infants, adhesive portion is applied to exposed and dried perineum first. **B,** Bag adheres firmly around perineal area to prevent urine leakage.

to avoid possible leakage. For low-birth-weight infants, small bags with adhesive that is gentle to the skin are available.* Anatomically correct urine collection bags are also available.†

The diaper is carefully replaced. The bag is checked frequently and removed as soon as the specimen is available, since the moist bag may become loosened on an active child. When urine is collected for culture, the bag is removed immediately. If the urine is not tested within 30 minutes, the specimen is refrigerated or placed in a sterile container with a preservative.

 Urine obtained from disposable diapers can be tested accurately for glucose, ketones, protein, blood, bilirubin, urobilinogen, nitrates, potassium, creatinine, and urea. Erythrocyte and leukocyte counts may be low. Superabsorbent disposable diapers may produce a false crystalluria. Specific gravity measurements are accurate for up to 4 hours provided that the disposable diapers are kept folded. The accuracy of these tests performed on urine obtained from cloth diapers is unknown (Wong and others, 1992). Traditionally, specific gravity refractometers have been used on nursing units to measure specific gravity. However, current regulations have limited the refractometer's use to the laboratory. Urine dipsticks can be used on the nursing unit with reasonable accuracy.

*Available from Hollister, Inc., 2000 Hollister Dr., Libertyville, IL 60048; (800) 323-4060.
†Available from ConvaTec, CN 5254, Princeton, NJ 08543-5254; (800) 422-8811.

NURSING TIPS
When using a urine collection bag, cut a small slit in the diaper and pull the bag through to allow room for urine to collect and to facilitate checking on the contents.
To obtain small amounts of urine, use a syringe without a needle to aspirate urine directly from the diaper; if diapers with absorbent gelling material that trap urine are used, place a small gauze dressing, some cotton balls, or a urine collection device* inside the diaper to collect urine and aspirate the urine with a syringe.
Wipe abdomen with alcohol pad and fan it dry; cooling effect often causes voiding within 2 minutes (Ellis, 1989). Apply pressure over suprapubic area or stroke paraspinal muscles (along spine) to elicit Perez reflex; in infants 4 to 6 months of age, reflex causes crying, extension of back, flexion of extremities, and urination.

At times parents may be requested to bring a urine sample to a health care facility for examination, especially when infants are unable to void during an outpatient visit. In this instance parents need instruction on applying the collection device and storage of the specimen.† Ideally the specimen should be brought to the designated place as soon as possible; if there is a delay, the sample is refrigerated and the lapsed time reported to the examiner.

Clean-Catch Specimens
The term *clean-catch specimen* traditionally refers to a urine sample obtained for culture after the urethral meatus is cleaned and the first few milliliters of urine are voided before the urine is collected *(midstream specimen).* The procedure consists of cleaning the perineum or tip of the penis with a soap- or antiseptic-soaked sterile pad, and in females wiping from front to back only once with each pad. This is repeated at least two times. The area may be wiped with sterile water to prevent accidental contamination of the urine with a solution that may destroy the pathogens, although minute amounts of antiseptic such as iodine do not alter bacterial counts.

 Although this traditional cleansing procedure is often practiced, studies have found that it does not significantly reduce contamination rates in infants, circumcised or uncircumcised males, or toilet-trained prepubertal children. Also, midstream collection does not significantly reduce contamination rates over nonmidstream specimens (Lohr, Donowitz, and Dudley, 1989; Saez-Llorens and others, 1989).

Twenty-Four–Hour Collection
Collection of urine voided over a 24-hour period creates a special challenge in infants and children. Collection bags and sometimes restraining methods are required to collect specimens from infants and small children. Older children require special instruction about notifying someone when they need to void or have a bowel movement so that urine can be collected separately and not discarded. Some older school-age children and adolescents can be trusted to take responsibility

*The Bard Sure Catch is available from Bard Urological Division, C.R. Bard, Inc., Covington, GA 30209; (770) 784-7754.
†Home care instructions on obtaining a urine sample are available in Wong DL: *Wong and Whaley's Clinical manual of pediatric nursing,* ed 4, St Louis, 1996, Mosby.

for collection of their own 24-hour specimens. They can keep output records and transfer each voiding to the 24-hour collection container if this is permitted.

As in any 24-hour urine collection, the collection period always starts and ends with an empty bladder. At the time the collection begins, the child is instructed to void and the specimen is discarded. All urine voided in the subsequent 24 hours is saved in a container with a preservative or is placed on ice. Twenty-four hours from the time the precollection specimen was discarded, the child is again instructed to void, the specimen is added to the container, and the entire collection is taken to the laboratory for examination.

Infants and small children who need a 24-hour urine collection require a special collection bag; frequent removal and replacement of adhesive collection devices can produce skin irritation. A thin coating of sealant, such as Skin-Prep, applied to the skin helps to protect it and aids adhesion, unless its use is contraindicated, such as in a premature infant or a child with irritated skin. Plastic collection bags with collection tubes attached are ideal when the container must be left in place for a time. These can be connected to a collecting device or emptied periodically by aspiration with a syringe. When such devices are not available, a regular bag with a feeding tube inserted through a puncture hole at the top of the bag serves as a satisfactory substitute. However, care must be taken to empty the bag as soon as the infant urinates to prevent leakage and loss of contents. An indwelling catheter may also be placed for the collection period.

Special Techniques

Catheterization or suprapubic aspiration is employed when a specimen is urgently needed or when the child is unable to void or otherwise provide an adequate specimen. *Catheterization* is most often used when urethral obstruction or anuria caused by renal failure is believed to be the cause of the child's failure to void. *Suprapubic aspiration* is useful in clarifying the diagnosis of suspected urinary tract infection in acutely ill infants.

Catheterizing a child requires aseptic technique, good light, and gentle, thorough cleansing of the vulva or glans penis. Most children, including female infants, accommodate a size 8 or 10 French catheter, but in male infants or when the larger catheters cannot be passed, a smaller, soft plastic feeding tube may be needed. Most children are frightened of this procedure, and few small children can be cooperative; therefore, even when the procedure is adequately explained, an assistant is needed to help restrain and reassure the child (see also Family Focus). Special care must be exercised when catheterizing young males to avoid trauma to the ductal and glandular openings into the urethra, which might result in sterility.

Suprapubic aspiration, which is performed by a practitioner skilled in the procedure, involves aspirating bladder contents by inserting a 20- or 21-gauge needle in the midline approximately 1 cm above the symphysis and directed vertically downward. The skin is prepared as for any needle insertion, but the bladder should contain an adequate volume of urine. This can be assumed if the infant has not voided for at least 1 hour or the bladder can be palpated above the symphysis. This technique is especially useful for obtaining clean specimens from young infants. The bladder is an abdominal organ at this time and is easily accessible.

Suprapubic aspiration is painful and has a higher failure rate than urethral catheterization; also, success depends more on the volume of urine in the bladder (Pollack, Pollack, and Andrew, 1994). (See Atraumatic Care and Family Focus boxes.)

STOOL SPECIMENS

Stool specimens are frequently collected in children to identify parasites and other organisms that cause diarrhea, to assess gastrointestinal function, and to check for occult (hidden) blood. Ideally, stool should be collected without contamination with urine, but in children wearing diapers, this is difficult unless a urine bag is applied. Children who are toilet trained should urinate first, flush the toilet, then defecate in the toilet, a bedpan (preferably one that is placed on the toilet to avoid embarrassment), or a commercial potty hat.

NURSING TIP To obtain a stool specimen, place plastic wrap over the toilet bowl to collect the stool. Use a tongue depressor or disposable spoon or knife to collect the stool and place the specimen in a covered cup or plastic bag.

Stool specimens should be large enough to obtain an ample sampling, not merely a fecal fragment. Specimens are placed in an appropriate container, which is covered and labeled. If several specimens are needed, the containers are marked with the date and time and kept in a specimen refrigerator. Special care is exercised in handling the specimen because of the risk of contamination.

BLOOD SPECIMENS

Although most blood specimens are obtained by the laboratory staff, nurses are increasingly responsible for specimen collection, especially if the child has an arterial or venous device. Whether the specimen is collected by the nurse or others, the nurse is responsible for making certain that specimens, such as serial examinations and fasting specimens, are

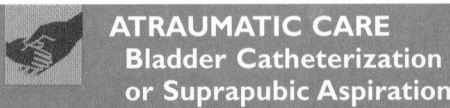

ATRAUMATIC CARE
Bladder Catheterization
or Suprapubic Aspiration

Use distraction to help the child relax (blowing bubbles, deep breathing, singing a song, etc.).

Use a water-soluble jelly to lubricate the catheter. Lidocaine jelly can be used to anesthetize the area before insertion.

FAMILY FOCUS
Bladder Catheterization

Parents may also be upset when their child is catheterized. Aside from the trauma the child experiences, some parents, especially those from different cultures, may fear that the procedure affects the daughter's virginity. To clarify this misconception, the family needs a detailed explanation of the genitourinary anatomy, preferably with a model that shows the separate vaginal and urethral openings.

collected on time and that the proper equipment is available, such as correct collection tubes and ice for blood gas samples.

Venous blood samples can be obtained by venipuncture or by aspiration from a peripheral or central access device. Withdrawing blood specimens through peripheral lock devices in small peripheral veins has met with varying degrees of success. Although it avoids an additional venipuncture for the child, attempting to aspirate blood from the peripheral lock may shorten the life of the device (see also p. 709). When using an intravenous infusion site for specimen collection, it is important to consider the type of fluid being infused. For example, a specimen collected for glucose determination would be inaccurate if removed from a catheter through which glucose-containing solution were being administered.

NURSING TIPS
To obtain a blood specimen from a central venous line or peripheral lock when the infusion solution may interfere with tests results, first aspirate a quantity of blood equal to the volume of fluid in the catheter and discard; then aspirate the blood sample.
For a blood culture, use the first sample of blood, since organisms are most likely to collect within the catheter itself (Schreiner, 1987).

Nursing ALERT On small or anemic children, keep track of the amount drawn and discarded over time. Frequent taking of blood specimens can rapidly decrease a child's blood count. Coordinate blood samples as much as possible to reduce the frequency.

Arterial blood samples are sometimes needed for blood gas measurement, although noninvasive techniques, such as transcutaneous oxygen/carbon dioxide monitoring and pulse oximetry, are used frequently. Arterial samples may be obtained by arteriopuncture using the radial, brachial, or femoral arteries; by deep heel puncture; or from indwelling

arterial catheters. Adequate circulation should be assessed before arterial puncture by observing capillary refill or performing the *Allen test,* a procedure that assesses the circulation of the radial, ulnar, or brachial arteries. Since unclotted blood is required, only heparinized collection tubes are used. In addition, no air bubbles should enter the tube, since they can alter blood gas concentration. Crying, fear, and agitation also affect blood gas values; therefore every effort is made to comfort the child. The blood samples are packed in ice to reduce blood cell metabolism and are taken to the laboratory for immediate analysis.

Capillary blood samples are taken from children by finger or earlobe stick methods, just as in the adult patient. The best method for taking peripheral blood samples from infants is by a heel stick. Before the blood sample is taken, the heel is warmed with warm, moist compresses for 5 to 10 minutes to dilate the vessels in the area. The area is cleansed with alcohol, and with the infant's foot firmly restrained with the free hand, the heel is punctured with a blade or an automatic lancet device. An automatic device, such as Tenderfoot,* delivers a more precise puncture depth (and possibly a less painful puncture) than that achieved with a blade or lance. Although obtaining capillary blood gases is a common practice, these measures may not accurately reflect arterial values (Courtney and others, 1990).

The most serious complication of infant heel puncture is necrotizing osteochondritis from lancet penetration of the underlying calcaneus bone. To avoid this, the puncture should be no deeper than 2.4 mm and should be made at the outer aspect of the heel. The boundaries of the calcaneus can be marked by an imaginary line extending posteriorly from a point between the fourth and fifth toes and running parallel to the lateral aspect of the heel and another line extending posteriorly from the middle of the great toe and running parallel to the medial aspect of the heel (Fig. 22-16).

The needed specimens are collected quickly, and then pressure is applied to the puncture site with a dry gauze square until bleeding stops. The arm is kept extended, not flexed, while pressure is applied for a few minutes after venipuncture in the antecubital fossa to reduce bruising. The site is then covered with an adhesive bandage. In young children, adhesive bandages pose an aspiration hazard; their use should be avoided or the adhesive bandage should be removed as soon as the bleeding stops. Applying warm compresses to ecchymotic areas increases circulation, helps remove extravasated blood, and decreases pain.

No matter how or by whom the specimen is collected, children, even some older ones, fear the loss of their blood. This is particularly true for children whose condition requires frequent blood specimens. They mistakenly believe that blood removed from their bodies is a threat to their lives. Explaining to them that their blood is continually being produced by their bodies provides them with a measure of reassurance regarding this aspect of the stress-provoking procedure. When the blood is drawn, a simple comment, such as "Just look how red it is. You're really making a lot of nice red blood," confirms this information and affords them an opportunity to express their concern. Covering the puncture

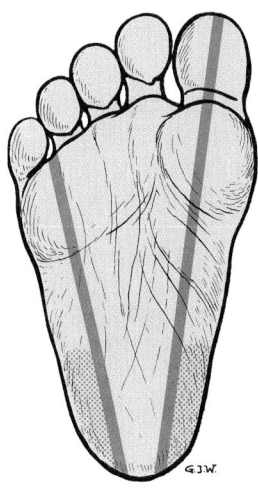

FIG. 22-16. Puncture site *(colored stippled area)* on sole of infant's foot.

*Available from International Technidyne Corp., 23 Nevsky St., Edison, NJ 08820; (908) 548-5700 or (800) 631-5945.

ATRAUMATIC CARE
Skin/Vessel Punctures and Multiple Blood Samples

To reduce the pain and distress associated with heel, finger, venous, or arterial punctures:

1. Apply EMLA topically over the site if time permits (at least 60 minutes) or use buffered lidocaine (injected intradermally near vein with 30-gauge needle) to numb the skin.
2. Use nonpharmacologic methods of pain and anxiety control (e.g., ask child to take a deep breath when the needle is inserted and again when the needle is withdrawn; ask child to count slowly and then faster and louder if pain is felt).
3. Emphasize that blood entering syringe or tube does not hurt.
4. Reassure young children that you did not "take their blood" away and that they have a lot more inside.
5. Keep arm extended, not flexed, while applying pressure for a few minutes after venipuncture in the antecubital fossa to reduce bruising (Dyson and Bogod, 1987).
6. Place *small* bandage over puncture site to make removal easy and less painful and to reassure young children that their blood will not leak out.

For multiple blood samples:

1. Use an intermittent infusion device to collect additional samples from existing intravenous line; consider peripherally inserted central catheters (PICCs) early, not as a last resort.
2. Coordinate care to allow several tests to be performed on one blood sample using micromethods of testing.
3. Anticipate tests (i.e., type and cross-match for blood transfusion) and ask laboratory to save blood for additional testing.

Contrary to popular belief, a study of children ages 3 to 6 years found that asking them not to look at the "finger stick" to avoid the sight of blood or applying a decorated bandage did not lessen their rating of pain intensity (Johnston, Stevens, and Arbess, 1993).

site with an adhesive bandage strip gives them added assurance that the vital fluids will not leak out.

Children also dislike the discomfort associated with venous, arterial, or capillary punctures. In fact, children have identified these procedures as the ones most frequently causing pain during hospitalization and arterial punctures as being one of the most painful of all procedures experienced (Wong and Baker, 1988). Consequently, nurses need to institute pain reduction techniques to lessen the discomfort of these procedures (see Atraumatic Care box). Younger children are more distressed by venipuncture than older children.

RESPIRATORY SECRETION AND THROAT SPECIMENS

Collection of sputum or nasal discharge is sometimes required for diagnosis of respiratory infections, especially tuberculosis and respiratory syncytial viruses (RSVs). Older children and adolescents are able to cough as directed and supply sputum specimens when given proper directions. It must be made clear to them that a coughed specimen is

needed, not mucus that is cleared from the throat. It is helpful to demonstrate a deep cough so that communication is clear. Infants and small children are unable to follow directions to cough and will swallow any sputum produced; therefore gastric washings (lavage) may be used to collect a sputum specimen. Sometimes it is possible to obtain a satisfactory specimen by using a suction device such as a mucus trap if the catheter is inserted into the trachea and the cough reflex is elicited. A catheter that is inserted into the back of the throat is not sufficient. For children with a tracheostomy, a specimen is easily aspirated from the trachea or major bronchi by attaching a collecting device to the suction apparatus.

Nasal washings are usually obtained to diagnose an infection of RSV. The child is placed supine, and 1 to 3 ml of sterile normal saline is instilled with a sterile syringe (without needle) into one nostril. The contents are aspirated using a small, sterile bulb syringe and are placed in a sterile container. To prevent any additional discomfort to the child, all the equipment should be ready before the procedure is begun.

Other respiratory secretion collection methods include nasopharyngeal swabs to diagnose *Bordetella pertussis* and throat cultures. The nurse swabs both the tonsils and the posterior pharynx when obtaining a throat culture. The swab stick is inserted into the culture tube. Some culture kits require squeezing an ampule to release the culture medium.

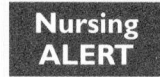

Nursing ALERT   Do not attempt to obtain a throat culture if acute epiglottitis is suspected. The trauma from the swab may increase edema, possibly occluding the airway.

ADMINISTRATION OF MEDICATION

PREPARATION FOR SAFE ADMINISTRATION

The safe administration of medication to children presents a number of problems that are not encountered when giving medication to adult patients. Children vary widely in age, weight, body surface area, and the ability to absorb, metabolize, and excrete medications. Nurses must be particularly alert when computing and administering drugs to infants and children.

Determination of Drug Dosage

It is the physician's responsibility to prescribe drugs in the correct dosage to achieve the desired effect without endangering the health of the child. However, nurses must have an understanding of the safe dosage of medications they administer to children, as well as the expected action, possible side effects, and signs of toxicity. Unlike with adult medications, there are few standardized pediatric dosage ranges, and with a few exceptions, drugs are prepared and packaged in average adult-dosage strengths.

Factors related to growth and maturation significantly alter an individual's capacity to metabolize and excrete drugs, and deficiencies associated with immaturity become more important with decreasing age. Immaturity or defects in any or all of the important processes of absorption, distribution, biotransformation, or excretion can significantly alter the effects of a drug. Newborn and premature infants with immature enzyme systems in the liver (where most drugs are broken down and detoxified), lower plasma concentrations of protein for binding with drugs, and immaturely functioning kidneys (where most drugs are excreted) are particularly vulnerable to the harmful effects of drugs. Beyond the newborn period, many drugs are metabolized more rapidly by the liver, necessitating larger doses or more frequent administration. This is particularly important in pain control, when the dosage may need to be increased or the interval between administering analgesics may need to be decreased.

Various formulas involving age, weight, and body surface area as the basis for calculations have been devised to determine children's drug dosage from a standard adult dose.

Since the administration of medication is a nursing responsibility, nurses need not only a knowledge of drug action and patient responses, but also some resources for estimating safe dosages for children. The method most often used to determine children's dosage is based on a specific dose per kilogram of body weight, such as 0.1 mg/kg.

Another method for determining children's dosage is to calculate the proportional amount of *body surface area (BSA)* to body weight. The ratio of BSA to weight varies inversely with length; therefore the infant who is shorter and weighs less than an older child or adult has relatively more surface area than would be expected from the weight. The usual determination of BSA requires the use of the West nomogram (Fig. 22-17). The BSA is estimated from the height and weight of the child.

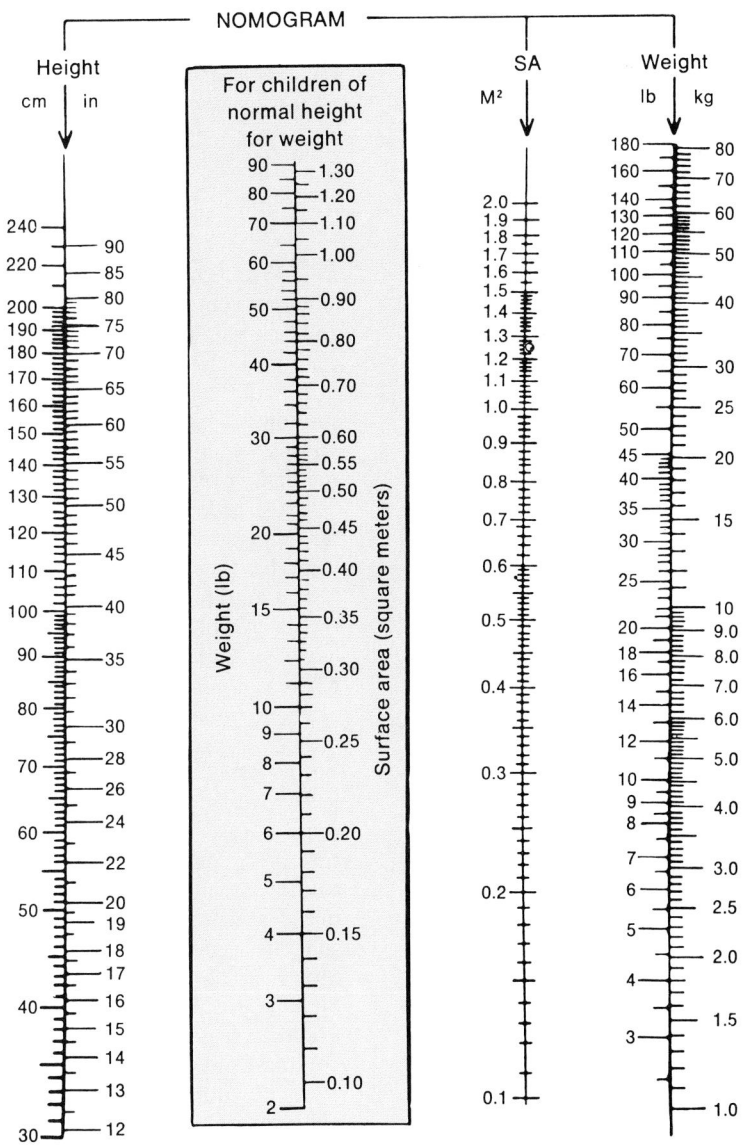

FIG. 22-17. West nomogram for estimation of surface areas. Surface area is indicated where a straight line connecting height and weight intersects surface area *(SA)* column or, if patient is approximately of normal proportion, from weight alone *(yellow area)*. (Nomogram modified from data of E. Boyd by C.D. West; from Behrman RE, Vaughan VC, editors: *Nelson textbook of pediatrics*, ed 14, Philadelphia, 1992, Saunders.)

Checking Dosage. Administering the correct dosage of a drug is a shared responsibility between the practitioner who orders the drug and the nurse who carries out that order. Children react with unexpected severity to some drugs, and ill children are especially sensitive to drugs. Therefore checking the dose if any doubt exists about its accuracy is a professional duty. When a dose is ordered that is outside the usual range or if there is some question regarding the preparation or the route of administration, the nurse should always check with the prescribing practitioner before proceeding with the administration, since the nurse is legally liable for any drug administered.

Administering some medications requires added safeguards. Even when it has been determined that the dosage is correct for a particular child, many drugs are potentially hazardous or lethal. Most hospital units or other facilities where medications are given to children have regulations requiring that specified drugs be double-checked by another nurse before they are given to the child. Among drugs that require such safeguards are digoxin, heparin, chemotherapeutic agents, and insulin. Others frequently included are epinephrine, opioids, and sedatives. Even if this precaution is not mandatory, nurses would be wise to take such precautions for their own sense of security. Errors in decimal point placement may easily occur and may result in a tenfold or more dosage error.

Identification

Before the administration of any medication, the child must be correctly identified, since children are not totally reliable in giving correct names on request. Infants are unable to give their name, a toddler or preschooler may admit to any name, and school-age children may deny their identity in an attempt to avoid the medication. Children sometimes exchange beds during play. Parents may be present to identify their child, but the only safe method for identifying children is to check their hospital identification band with the labeled medication or medication card.

Family Aspects

Parents can be useful sources of information regarding the child and his or her capabilities. Nearly all parents have given some kind of medication to their child and can describe approaches that they have found to be successful. In some cases it is less traumatic for the child if a parent gives the medication, provided that the nurse prepares the medication and supervises its administration and the practice is consistent with hospital or unit policy. Children being given daily medications at home are accustomed to the parent's functioning in this capacity and are less apt to object than they would if the medication were administered by a stranger.

Every child requires psychologic preparation for parenteral administration of medication and supportive care during the procedure (see p. 675). Even if children have received several injections, they rarely become accustomed to the discomfort and have as much right as any other child to understanding and patience from those involved in giving the injection. Safe administration of any drug requires meticulous attention to the safeguards discussed here.

ATRAUMATIC CARE
Encouraging a Child's Acceptance of Oral Medication

Give the child an ice pop or small ice cube to suck to numb the tongue before giving the drug.

Mix the drug with a small amount (about 1 tsp) of sweet-tasting substance, such as honey (except in infants because of the risk of botulism), flavored syrups, jam, fruit purees, sherbet, or ice cream; avoid essential food items, because the child may later refuse to eat them.

Give a "chaser" of water, juice, soft drink, or ice pop or frozen juice bar after the drug.

If nausea is a problem, give a carbonated beverage poured over finely crushed ice before or immediately after the medication.

When medication has an unpleasant taste, have the child pinch the nose and drink the medicine through a straw. Much of what we taste is associated with smell.

Another alternative is to have the pharmacist prepare the drug in a flavored, chewable troche or lozenge.*

*For information about compounding drugs in troches or suppositories, contact Technical Staff, Professional Compounding Centers of America (PCCA), P.O. Box 368, Sugarland, TX 77487; (800) 331-2498.

ORAL ADMINISTRATION

The oral route is preferred for administering medications to children whenever possible. Because of the ease of administration of oral medications, most are dissolved or suspended in liquid preparations. Although some children are able to swallow or chew solid medications at an early age, solid preparations are not recommended for young children because of the danger of aspiration.

Most pediatric medications come in palatable and colorful preparations for added ease of administration. However, some have a slightly unpleasant aftertaste. The nurse should taste a minute amount of an oral preparation to ascertain if it is palatable or bitter. In this way legitimate complaints of dislike from the child can be accepted and the taste camouflaged whenever possible. Most pediatric units have preparations available for this purpose (see Atraumatic Care box).

Preparation

Selecting a method to measure and administer a medication requires careful consideration. The devices available to measure medicines are not always sufficiently accurate for measuring the small amounts needed in pediatric nursing practice (Fig. 22-18). Disposable plastic calibrated cups offer reasonable accuracy in measuring moderate doses of liquids. However, the personal interpretation of a given measure is highly variable, and considerable amounts of thick medication may remain in the cup. Measures of less than a teaspoon are impossible to determine accurately with a cup.

Many liquid preparations are prescribed in measurements of teaspoons. However, the teaspoon is an inaccurate measuring device and is subject to error from a number of variables. For example, household teaspoons vary greatly in capacity, and different persons using the same spoon will pour different amounts. Therefore a drug ordered in teaspoons

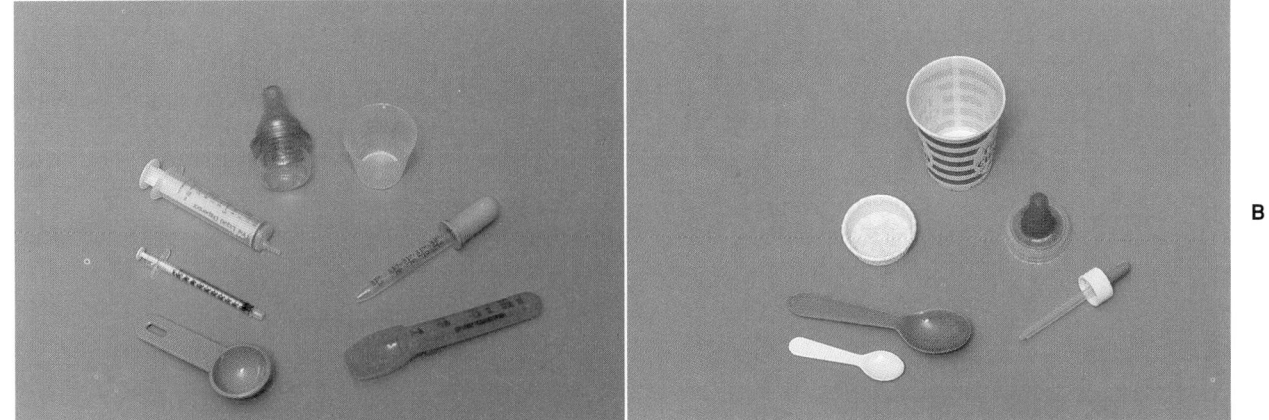

FIG. 22-18. **A,** Acceptable devices for measuring and administering oral medication to children *(clockwise):* measuring spoon, plastic syringes, calibrated nipple, plastic medicine cup, calibrated dropper, hollow-handled medicine spoon. **B,** Acceptable devices only for administering premeasured oral medication *(clockwise):* household teaspoons, paper cups, nipple, uncalibrated dropper.

should be measured in milliliters; the established standard is 5 ml per teaspoon. A convenient hollow-handled medicine spoon is available to accurately measure and administer the drug (Fig. 22-18). Household *measuring* spoons can also be used when other devices are not available.

Another unreliable device for measuring liquids is the dropper, which varies to a greater extent than the teaspoon or measuring cup. Droppers are available in numerous sizes, but even with the standard USP dropper, the volume of a drop will vary according to the viscosity of the liquid measured; viscid fluids produce much larger drops than thin liquids. Many medications are supplied with caps or droppers designed for measuring each specific preparation. These are accurate when used to measure that specific medication but are not reliable for measuring other liquids. Emptying dropper contents into a medicine cup invites additional error; since some of the liquid clings to the sides of the cup, a significant amount of the drug can be lost.

> **Nursing ALERT** Many pediatric medications are given by drops or dropper. A misunderstanding of these terms by parents can result in a potential overdose. In addition, many droppers that come with medications are marked in tenths of cubic centimeters. If a parent were to use a syringe instead of the dropper, 0.4 cc may be thought to be the same as 4 cc. Provide education to parents on correct methods for giving medication. Demonstrate the technique (Rudy, 1992).

The most accurate means for measuring small amounts of medication is the plastic disposable (never glass) syringe, especially the tuberculin syringe for volumes less than 1 ml. Not only does the syringe provide a reliable measure, but it also serves as a convenient means for transporting and administering the medication. The medication can be placed directly into the child's mouth from the syringe. For added safety, a short length of flexible tubing can be placed on the tip of the syringe to prevent injury to the mouth, although the tubing must be completely emptied of medication.

Young children and some older children as well have dif-

ficulty swallowing tablets or pills. Since a number of drugs are not available in pediatric preparations, the tablet needs to be crushed before it can be given to these children. Commercial devices* are available, or simple methods can be employed for crushing tablets.

NURSING TIP To minimize loss of the drug, crush the tablet between two spoons or place the tablet in either a medicine cup or between two small paper soufflé cups and use a pestle for crushing; collect the bits of pulverized medication that tend to cling to the sides of the cup or spoon and mix the crushed tablet with a palatable substance.

Not all drugs can be crushed (e.g., medication with an enteric or protective coating or medication formulated for slow release). For some children it may be possible to encourage swallowing the tablet or capsule by using a special glass designed with a shelf that holds the drug. The child drinks normally, and the tablet is carried to the back of the throat. For children who must take solid oral medication for an extended period, training sessions using progressively larger candy to teach the child to swallow can be beneficial (Funk, Mullins, and Olson, 1984).

Since pediatric doses often require dividing adult preparations of medication, the nurse may be faced with the dilemma of accurate dosage. With tablets, only those that are scored can be halved or quartered accurately. If the medication is soluble, the tablet or contents of a capsule can be mixed in a small, premeasured amount of liquid and the appropriate portion given. If half a dose is required, the tablet is dissolved in 5 ml of water or flavored liquid and 2.5 ml is given.

Administration

Although administering liquids to infants is relatively easy, the nurse must be careful to prevent aspiration. With the infant

---

*Trademark Medical manufactures a pill crusher and has compiled a list of more than 190 medications that should not be crushed or chewed. Both are available from Trademark Medical, 1053 Headquarters Park, Fenton, MO 63026-2033; (800) 325-9044.

held in a semireclining position, the medication is placed in the mouth from a spoon, plastic cup, plastic dropper, or plastic syringe (without needle). The dropper or syringe is best placed along the side of the infant's tongue, with the contents administered slowly in small amounts, allowing the child to swallow between deposits.

NURSING TIP In infants up to 11 months of age and children with neurologic impairments, blowing a small puff of air in the face frequently elicits a swallow reflex (Orenstein and others, 1988).

Medicine cups can be used effectively for older infants who are able to drink from a cup. Because of the natural outward tongue thrust in infancy, medications may need to be retrieved from the lips or chin and refed. Allowing the infant to suck medication that has been placed in an empty nipple or inserting the syringe or dropper into the side of the mouth, parallel to the nipple, while the infant nurses are other convenient methods for giving liquid medications to infants. Medication is not added to the infant's formula feeding. Dispose of any plastic covers that may be on the ends of syringes. These covers are small enough to be aspirated by young children.

The small child who refuses to cooperate or resists consistently despite explanation and encouragement may require mild physical coercion. If so, it is carried out quickly and carefully. Every effort is made to determine why the child resists,

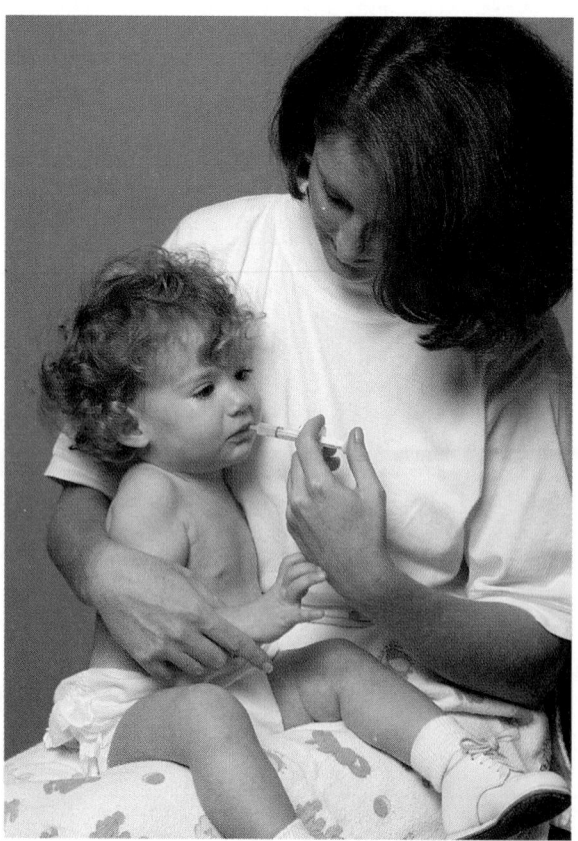

FIG. 22-19. Nurse partially restrains child for easy and comfortable administration of oral medication.

and the reasons for the coercion are explained to the child in such a way that the child will know that it is being carried out for his or her well-being and is not a form of punishment. There is always a risk in using even mild forceful techniques. A crying child can aspirate a medication, particularly when lying on the back. If the nurse holds the child in the lap with the child's right arm behind the nurse, the left hand firmly grasped by the nurse's left hand, and the head securely restrained between the nurse's arm and body, the medication can be slowly poured into the mouth (Fig. 22-19).

INTRAMUSCULAR (IM) ADMINISTRATION

Selecting the Syringe and Needle

The volume of medication prescribed for small children and the small amount of tissue for injection require that a syringe be selected that can measure very small amounts of solution. For volumes of less than 1 ml the tuberculin syringe, calibrated in one-hundredth increments, is appropriate. Very minute doses may require the use of a 0.5 ml, low-dose syringe. These syringes with specially constructed needles minimize the possibility of inadvertently administering incorrect amounts of a drug because of dead space, which allows fluid to remain in the syringe and needle after the plunger is pushed completely forward. A minimum of 0.2 ml of solution remains in a standard needle hub; therefore, when very small amounts of two drugs are combined in the syringe, such as mixtures of insulin, the ratio of the two drugs can be altered significantly. Measures that minimize the effect of dead space follow: (1) when two drugs are combined in the syringe, always draw them up in the same order to maintain a consistent ratio between the drugs; (2) use the same brand of syringe (dead space may vary); and (3) use one-piece syringe units (needle permanently attached to the syringe).

Dead space is also an important factor to consider when injecting medication, since flushing the syringe with an air bubble or parenteral fluid adds an additional amount of medication to the prescribed dose. This can be hazardous when very small amounts of a drug are given. For example, a tuberculin syringe filled to the 0.05 ml mark can deliver *more than twice* the calculated dose of medication when it is flushed with parenteral fluid from an intravenous line. Consequently, flushing is not advisable, especially when less than 1 ml of medication is given. Syringes are calibrated to deliver a prescribed drug dose, and the amount of medication left in the hub and needle is not part of the syringe barrel calibrations. However, the air-bubble technique (drawing up about 0.2 ml of air into the syringe after withdrawing the medication) may be beneficial with certain drugs, such as iron dextran and diphtheria and tetanus toxoid, to avoid tracking the drug through the tissue. Other techniques to minimize tracking include changing the needle after withdrawing the fluid from the vial (not always effective) and using the Z-track method.

The *needle length* must be sufficient to penetrate the subcutaneous tissue and deposit the medication in the body of the muscle. Although research is limited on adequate needle length for children, one study found that a 1-inch needle is necessary to adequately penetrate the vastus lateralis muscle in 4-month-old infants and probably is needed for 2-month-old infants (Hicks and others, 1989).

NURSING TIP To estimate the needle length for IM injection, first grasp the lateralis or deltoid muscle and choose a needle length that is approximately half the distance between the thumb and the index finger. With the ventrogluteal or dorsogluteal site, only subcutaneous tissue is grasped, so choose a needle length that is slightly more than half the distance. Choose a final needle length that allows for a small portion of the needle to be exposed at the skin surface as a precaution if the needle should break off from the hub.

Smaller-diameter (25 to 30 gauge) needles cause the least discomfort, but larger diameters are needed for viscous medication and prevention of accidental bending of longer needles.

Determining the Site

Factors that are considered when selecting a site for an IM injection on an infant or child include the following:

1. The amount and character of the medication to be injected
2. The amount and general condition of the muscle mass
3. The frequency or number of injections to be given during the course of treatment
4. The type of medication being given
5. Factors that may impede access to or cause contamination of the site
6. The child's ability to assume the required position safely

Older children and adolescents usually pose few problems in selecting a suitable site for IM injections, but infants, with their small and underdeveloped muscles, have fewer available sites. It is sometimes difficult to assess the amount of fluid that can be safely injected into a single site. Usually 1 ml is the maximum volume that should be administered in a single site to small children and older infants. The muscles of small infants may not tolerate more than 0.5 ml. As the child approaches adult size, volumes approaching those given to adults may be used. However, the larger the amount of solution, the larger the muscle must be into which it is injected.

Injections must be placed in muscles large enough to accommodate the medication; however, major nerves and blood vessels must be avoided. There is no universal agreement regarding the best IM injection site for children. The preferred site for infants is the vastus lateralis. A general recommendation for using the gluteal sites is to wait until after the child has been walking (length of suggested time varies), since the muscle develops with locomotion. Unfortunately, this recommendation is often applied to the ventrogluteal muscle site as well as the dorsogluteal site. However, significant differences exist between these two sites. The ventrogluteal site is relatively free of major nerves and blood vessels, is a relatively large muscle with less subcutaneous tissue than the dorsal site, has well-defined landmarks for safe site location, is less painful than the vastus lateralis, and is easily accessible in several positions (Beecroft and Redick, 1990). These advantages make it a preferred site over the dorsogluteal muscle and challenge the recommendation that the ventrogluteal site not be used until children have been walking. Although there are published recommendations regarding age, in clinical practice the ventrogluteal site has been used in children as young as newborns. Table 22-2 summarizes the four major injection sites and illustrates the location of the preferred IM injection sites for children.

Administration

Although injections that are executed with care are relatively safe, there have been reports of serious disability related to IM injections in children. Repeated use of a single site has been associated with fibrosis of the muscle with subsequent muscle contracture, and injections close to large nerves, such as the sciatic nerve, have been responsible for permanent disability, especially when potentially neurotoxic drugs are administered. There are several reports of tissue damage from penicillin; one of the difficulties in administering the opaque preparations, such as Bicillin, is that aspirated blood cannot be detected at the bottom of the syringe, thus increasing the risk of injecting into a blood vessel. When such drugs are injected, great care must be used in locating the correct site. When aspirating, the nurse should look for blood at the *top* of the syringe near the plunger, since blood may be drawn up through the column of penicillin (Stoller and Losey, 1985).

A reported potential hazard with medication in glass ampules is the presence of glass particles in the ampule after the container is broken. When the medication is withdrawn into the syringe, the glass particles may also be withdrawn and subsequently injected into the patient. As a precaution, medication from glass ampules should be drawn up only through a needle with a filter or injected intravenously through a site in the tubing that is distal to an intravenous filter. Other precautions related to needle use and disposal are on p. 699.

Children may be unpredictable and cannot be expected to cooperate totally when receiving an injection. Even children who appear to be relaxed and constrained can lose control under the stress of the procedure. It is advisable to have someone available to help restrain the child if needed. Since children often jerk or pull away unexpectedly, the nurse should carry an extra needle to exchange for a contaminated one so that the delay is minimal. The child, even a small one, is told that he or she is getting an injection (preferably using a phrase such as "putting medicine under the skin"), and then the procedure is carried out as quickly and skillfully as possible to avoid prolonging the stressful experience. Delay caused by lengthy explanations, attempts to hide the syringe from sight, or efforts to soothe the child only increase the anxiety. It must be kept in mind that intrusive procedures such as injections are especially anxiety provoking in preschool children and that small children usually associate any assault to the "behind" area with punishment. Since injections are painful, the nurse should employ excellent injection technique and effective pain reduction measures to reduce discomfort (see Guidelines box on p. 718).

Small infants offer little resistance to injections. Although they squirm and may be difficult to hold in position, they can usually be restrained without assistance. The body of a larger infant can be securely restrained between the nurse's elbow and body (Fig. 22-20, p. 719). To inject into the body of the muscle, the muscle mass is firmly grasped between the thumb and fingers to isolate and stabilize the site. In obese children, however, it is preferable first to spread the skin with the thumb and index finger to displace subcutaneous tissue and then grasp the muscle deeply on each side.

TABLE 22-2. Intramuscular (IM) injection sites in children

SITE	DISCUSSION

Vastus Lateralis
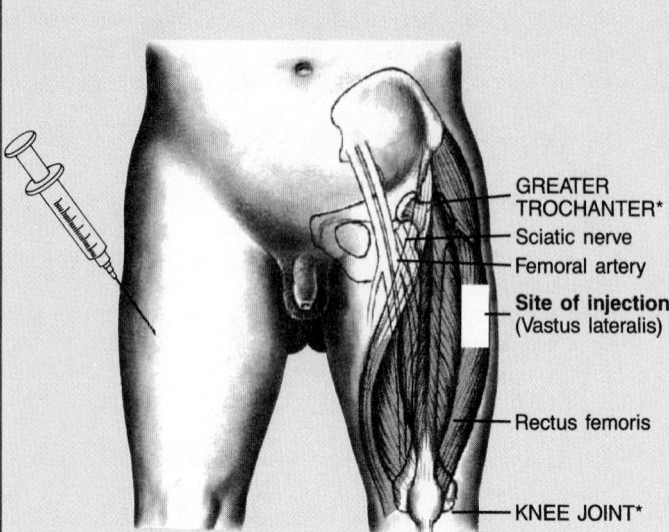
G.J.Wassilchenko
	Location*
	Palpate to find greater trochanter and knee joints; divide vertical distance between these two landmarks into thirds; inject into middle third
	Needle insertion and size
	Insert needle at 45-degree angle toward knee in infants and in young children or needle perpendicular to thigh or slightly angled toward anterior thigh
	22 to 25 gauge, ⅝ to 1 inch†
	  Advantages
	  Large, well-developed muscle that can tolerate larger quantities of fluid (0.5 ml [infant] to 2.0 ml [child])
	  No important nerves or blood vessels in this location
	  Easily accessible if child is supine, side lying, or sitting
	  A tourniquet can be applied above injection site to delay drug hypersensitivity reaction if necessary
	  Disadvantages
	  Thrombosis of femoral artery from injection in midthigh area
	  Sciatic nerve damage from long needle injected posteriorly and medially into small extremity

Labels on Vastus Lateralis illustration: GREATER TROCHANTER*, Sciatic nerve, Femoral artery, Site of injection (Vastus lateralis), Rectus femoris, KNEE JOINT*

Ventrogluteal

Labels on Ventrogluteal illustration: *ANTERIOR SUPERIOR ILIAC SPINE, POSTERIOR* ILIAC CREST, Site of injection (gluteus medius), PALM OVER GREATER TROCHANTER*, Iliac crest, Gluteus medius, Gluteus minimus, Greater trochanter, Ventrogluteal site of injection, G.J.Wassilchenko

Location*
Palpate to locate greater trochanter, anterior superior iliac tubercle (found by flexing thigh at hip and measuring up to 1 to 2 cm above crease formed in groin), and posterior iliac crest; place palm of hand over greater trochanter, index finger over anterior superior iliac tubercle, and middle finger along crest of ilium posteriorly as far as possible; inject into center of V formed by fingers

Needle insertion and size
Insert needle perpendicular to site but angled slightly toward iliac crest
22 to 25 gauge, ½ to 1 inch
  Advantages
  Free of important nerves and vascular structures
  Easily identified by prominent bony landmarks
  Thinner layer of subcutaneous tissue than in dorsogluteal site, thus less chance of depositing drug subcutaneously rather than intramuscularly
  Can accommodate larger quantities of fluid (0.5 ml [infant] to 2.0 ml [child])
  Easily accessible if child is supine, prone, or side lying
  Less painful than vastus lateralis
  Disadvantages
  Health professionals' unfamiliarity with site
  Not suitable for use of a tourniquet

*Locations are indicated by asterisks on illustrations.
†Research has shown that a 1-inch needle is needed for adequate muscle penetration in infants 4 months old and possibly in infants as young as 2 months (Hicks and others, 1989). Other recommendations for needle size and volume of fluid are based on traditional practice and have not been verified by research.

TABLE 22-2. Intramuscular (IM) injection sites in children—cont'd

SITE	DISCUSSION
Dorsogluteal 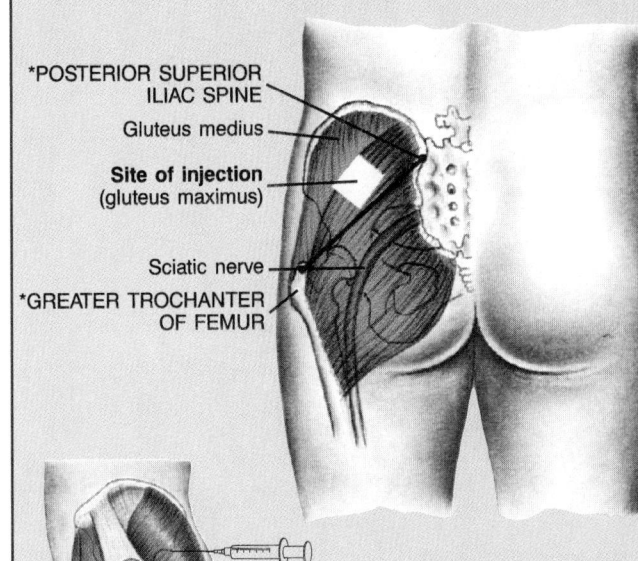	**Location*** Locate greater trochanter and posterior superior iliac spine; draw imaginary line between these two points and inject lateral and superior to line into gluteus maximus or medius muscle **Needle insertion and size** Insert needle perpendicular to surface on which child is lying when prone 20 to 25 gauge, ½ to 1½ inches **Advantages** In older child, large muscle mass; well-developed muscle can tolerate greater volume of fluid (up to 2.0 ml) Child does not see needle and syringe Easily accessible if child is prone or side lying **Disadvantages** Contraindicated in children who have not been walking for at least 1 year Danger of injury to sciatic nerve Thick, subcutaneous fat, predisposing to deposition of drug subcutaneously rather than intramuscularly Not suitable for use of a tourniquet Inaccessible if child is supine Exposure of site may cause embarrassment in older child

Labels on illustration: *POSTERIOR SUPERIOR ILIAC SPINE; Gluteus medius; Site of injection (gluteus maximus); Sciatic nerve; *GREATER TROCHANTER OF FEMUR

SITE	DISCUSSION
Deltoid 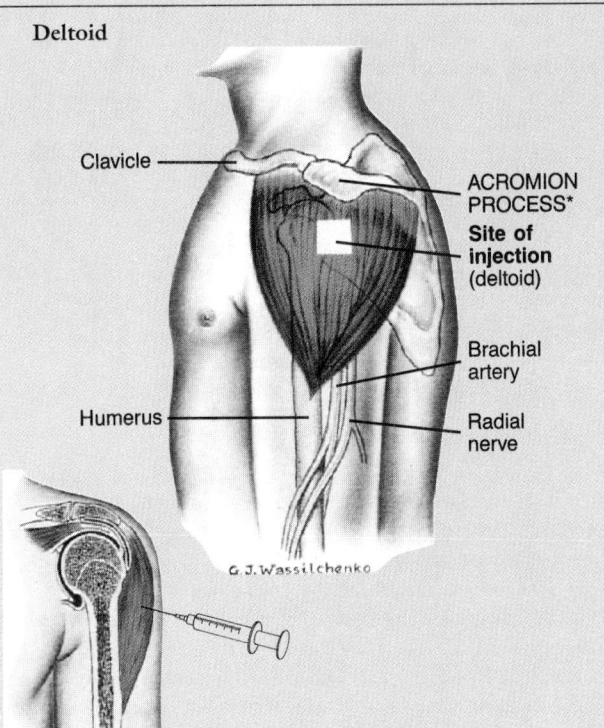	**Location*** Locate acromion process; inject only into upper third of muscle that begins about 2 fingerbreadths below acromion **Needle insertion and size** Insert needle perpendicular to site but angled slightly toward shoulder 22 to 25 gauge, ½ to 1 inch **Advantages** Faster absorption rates than gluteal sites Tourniquet can be applied above injection site Easily accessible with minimum removal of clothing Less pain and fewer local side effects from vaccines as compared with vastus lateralis **Disadvantages** Small muscle mass; only limited amounts of drug can be injected (0.5 to 1.0 ml) Small margins of safety with possible damage to radial nerve and axillary nerve (not shown, lies under deltoid at head of humerus)

Labels on illustration: Clavicle; ACROMION PROCESS*; Site of injection (deltoid); Brachial artery; Humerus; Radial nerve; G.J.Wassilchenko

*Locations are indicated by asterisks on illustrations.

GUIDELINES
Intramuscular (IM) Administration of Medication

Use safety precautions in administering medication (e.g., check child's identification).

Prepare medication.

Select needle and syringe appropriate to the following:

Amount of fluid to be administered (syringe size)

Viscosity of fluid to be administered (needle gauge)

Amount of tissue to be penetrated (needle length)

Maximum volume to be administered in a single site is 1 ml for older infants and small children.

Determine the site of injection (see Table 22-3); make certain muscle is large enough to accommodate volume and type of medication.

Older children: select site as with adult patient; allow child some choice of site, if feasible.

Following are acceptable sites for infants and small or debilitated children:

Vastus lateralis muscle

Ventrogluteal muscle

Dorsogluteal muscle is insufficiently developed to be a safe site for infants and small children.

Administer medication.

Provide for sufficient help in restraining child; children are often uncooperative, and their behavior is usually unpredictable.

Explain briefly what is to be done and, if appropriate, what child can do to help.

Expose injection area for unobstructed view of landmarks.

Select a site where skin is free of irritation and danger of infection; palpate for and avoid sensitive or hardened areas. With multiple injections, rotate sites.

Place child in a lying or sitting position; child is not allowed to stand because:

Landmarks are more difficult to assess.

Restraint is more difficult.

Child may faint and fall.

Use a new, sharp needle with smallest diameter that permits free flow of the medication.

Grasp muscle firmly between thumb and fingers to isolate and stabilize muscle for deposition of drug in its deepest part; in obese children, spread skin with thumb and index finger to displace subcutaneous tissue and grasp muscle deeply on each side.

Allow skin preparation to dry completely before skin is penetrated.

Have medication at room temperature.

Decrease perception of pain.

Distract child with conversation.

Give child something on which to concentrate (e.g., squeezing a hand or bed rail, pinching own nose, humming, counting, yelling "Ouch!").

Place a cold compress or wrapped ice cube on site about a minute before injection, or apply cold to contralateral site.

Say to child, "If you feel this, tell me to take it out, please."

Have child hold a small adhesive bandage and place it on puncture site after IM injection is given.

Apply EMLA topically over the site if time permits (at least 60 minutes, preferably 2 to 2½ hours for IM injection) (see Pain Management, Chapter 21).

Insert needle quickly, using a dartlike motion.

Use new needle, not one that has pierced rubber stopper on vial.

Avoid tracking any medication through superficial tissues:

Replace needle after withdrawing medication, or wipe medication from needle with sterile gauze.

If withdrawing medication from an ampule, use a needle equipped with a filter that removes glass particles; then use a new, nonfilter needle for injection.

Use the Z-track and/or air-bubble technique as indicated.

Avoid any depression of the plunger during insertion of the needle.

Aspirate for blood.

If blood is found, remove syringe from site, change needle, and reinsert into new location.

If no blood is found, inject into a relaxed muscle:

Dorsogluteal—place child on abdomen with legs and toes rotated inward.

Ventrogluteal—place child on side with upper leg flexed and placed in front of lower leg.

Inject medication slowly.

Remove needle quickly; hold gauze sponge firmly against skin near needle when removing it to avoid pulling on tissue.

Apply firm pressure to site after injection; massage site to hasten absorption unless contraindicated, as with irritating drugs and heparin.

Place a small adhesive bandage on puncture site; with young children decorate it by drawing a smiling face or other symbol of acceptance.

Hold and cuddle young child and encourage parents to comfort child; praise older child.

Allow expression of feelings.

Discard syringe and uncapped, uncut needle in puncture-resistant container located near site of use.

Record time of injection, drug, dose, and injection site.

The nurse should not try to administer an injection to a sleeping child, even though it may seem to be easier than waking the youngster. This practice can cause the child to fear going to sleep. When awakened first, the child knows that nothing will be done unless he or she is forewarned.

SUBCUTANEOUS AND INTRADERMAL ADMINISTRATION

Subcutaneous and intradermal injections are frequently administered to children, but the technique differs little from the method used with adults. Examples of *subcutaneous injections* include insulin, hormone replacement, allergy desen-

sitization, and some vaccines. Tuberculin (TB) testing, local anesthesia, and allergy testing are examples of frequently administered *intradermal injections.*

Techniques to minimize the pain associated with these injections include changing the needle if it pierced a rubber stopper on a vial, using 26- to 30-gauge needles, and injecting small volumes (up to 0.5 ml). The angle of the needle for the subcutaneous injection is typically 90 degrees. In children with little subcutaneous tissue, some practitioners insert the needle at a 45-degree angle. However, the benefit of using the 45-degree angle rather than the 90-degree angle remains controversial.

Although subcutaneous injections can be given anywhere

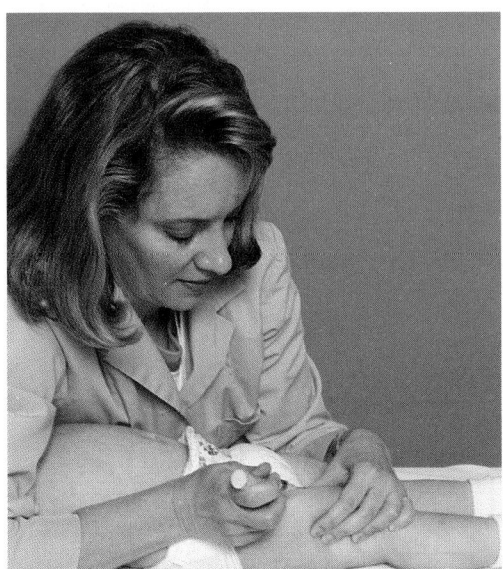

FIG. 22-20. Restraining small child for intramuscular (IM) injection. Note how nurse isolates and stabilizes muscle.

there is subcutaneous tissue, common sites include the center third of the lateral aspect of the upper arm, the abdomen, and the center third of the anterior thigh. Some practitioners believe it is not necessary to aspirate before injecting subcutaneously. For example, not aspirating is an accepted practice in the administration of insulin. Automatic injector devices do not aspirate before injecting.

When giving an intradermal injection into the volar surface of the forearm, the nurse should avoid the medial side of the arm, where the skin is more sensitive.

NURSING TIP Families often need to learn subcutaneous injection technique to administer medications, such as insulin, at home.* Begin teaching as early as possible to allow the family the maximum amount of practice time possible.

INTRAVENOUS (IV) ADMINISTRATION

The IV route for administering medications has gained widespread use in pediatric therapy. For some important drugs it is the only effective route of administration. This method is used for giving drugs to children who have poor absorption as a result of diarrhea, dehydration, or peripheral vascular collapse; children who need a high serum concentration of a drug; children with resistant infections that require parenteral medication over an extended time; children who need continuous pain relief; and children who require emergency treatment.

Insertion sites and observation of the IV infusion are discussed on p. 725. However, several factors need to be considered in relation to IV medication. When a drug is administered intravenously, the effect is almost instantaneous and further control is limited. Most drugs for IV administration

*Home care instructions on giving subcutaneous injections are available in Wong DL: *Wong and Whaley's Clinical manual of pediatric nursing,* ed 4, St Louis, 1996, Mosby.

require a specified minimum dilution and/or rate of flow, and many are highly irritating or toxic to tissues outside the vascular system. In addition to the precautions and nursing observations related to IV therapy, factors to consider when preparing and administering drugs to infants and children by the IV route include the following:

1. Amount of drug to be administered
2. Minimum dilution of drug and if child is fluid restricted
3. Type of solution in which drug can be diluted
4. Length of time over which drug can be safely administered
5. Rate of infusion that child and vessels can tolerate safely
6. Time that this or another drug is to be administered
7. Compatibility of all drugs that child is receiving intravenously

Before any IV infusion, the site of insertion is checked for patency. Medications are never administered with blood products. Only one antibiotic should be administered at a time.

IV infusion is suitable for children who can tolerate the necessary infusion rate and the extra fluid needed to administer the medication. For the very small infant or fluid-restricted child who is not able to tolerate the increased rate or fluids, other IV methods available are the direct technique and the retrograde technique. Although the medication must still be minimally diluted as recommended, the dose is administered closer to the child's vein, avoiding the need also to infuse the tubing volume.

In the ***direct technique,*** appropriately diluted medication is injected into the tubing at the site of the Y connection or through a stopcock in the direction of the child. A syringe pump may be used for a controlled rate. As syringe pumps become increasingly available, this method is being used more often for pediatric patients because of convenience, greater control over administration time, and the need to flush with less fluid when administering medications.

In the ***retrograde technique,*** appropriately diluted medication is injected into the IV tubing at the site of the Y connection or a stopcock in the direction away from (retrograde) the child. The tubing is clamped, or the stopcock to the child is turned off. After the medication is injected, the tubing is unclamped or the stopcock opened, and the infusion resumes, with subsequent administration of the medication. The rate may still need to be adjusted to deliver the medication in the specified time. This method does result in displacement of the fluid in the IV tubing, since the diluted medication is injected retrogradely. This fluid (but not more than 3 ml) can be accommodated by an empty drip chamber or by an empty syringe connected to an upper Y site or stopcock, which will accept the displaced fluid for discard. If the empty syringe method is used, the tubing volume between the two Y sites or stopcocks must be greater than the amount of diluted medication volume injected to avoid the medication reaching the discard syringe.

Nursing ALERT An often unrecognized source of contamination for vascular access lines (peripheral and central) is stopcock ports. Unaccessed ports should be covered at all times with a sterile cap or syringe, which is changed if contaminated during access for medication administration or blood collection (Brosnan and others, 1988).

Peripheral Venous Access Devices (VADs)

The *peripheral lock,* also known as an *intermittent infusion device, PRN adapter,* and *saline* or *heparin lock,* is used as an alternative for a keep-open infusion when extended access to a vein is required without the need for continuous fluid. It is most frequently employed for intermittent infusion of medication into a peripheral venous route. A short, flexible catheter (or occasionally a steel butterfly needle) is used as the lock device, and a site is selected where there will be minimum movement, such as the forearm. The needle/catheter device is inserted and secured in the same manner as any IV infusion device, but the hub is occluded with a stopper.

The type of device used may vary among medical establishments, and the care and use of the peripheral lock are carried out according to the specific protocol of the institution or unit. However, the general concept is the same. The needle or catheter remains in place and is flushed with saline or heparin (1:10 units/ml) after infusion of the medication. Either solution prevents blood from clotting in the device between infusions.

Heparin is incompatible with many drugs, so the peripheral lock must be flushed with saline before and after administering medication. Many studies show saline to be as effective in maintaining patency as heparin and to cause less pain during infusion (McMullen and others, 1993; Robertson, 1994). Children may be discharged with a peripheral lock in place in order to continue receiving medications without hospitalization; if so, this is usually reserved for children who require medications on a short-term basis and are referred to a home-based infusion company. Those with chronic illnesses who require repeated blood sampling or medications, long-term chemotherapy, or frequent hyperalimenation or antibiotic therapy are best managed with a central venous catheter.

NURSING TIP Using a positive-pressure technique, in which the flush syringe is slowly withdrawn from the peripheral lock as the last 0.5 ml of flush is being injected, may prevent backflow of blood into the infusion device, thus preventing clot formation in the catheter.

Central Venous Access Devices

Central VADs have several different characteristics. The practitioner has to consider the best type of catheter for the individual patient's needs. Factors that can influence the decision include the reason for placement of the catheter (diagnosis), length of therapy, risk to the patient in placement of the catheter, and availability of resources to assist the family in maintaining the catheter (Camp-Sorrell, 1990).

Short-term or *nontunneled catheters* are used in acute, emergency, and intensive care units. These catheters are made of polyurethane and are placed in large veins such as the subclavian, femoral, or jugular. A chest x-ray film should be taken to verify placement of the catheter tip before administration of fluids or medications.

Peripherally inserted central catheters (PICCs) can be used for short-term to moderate-length therapy. These catheters consist of silicone or polymer material and are placed by specially trained nurses (Brown, 1989). The most common insertion site is the antecubital area using the median, cephalic, or basilic vein. The catheter is threaded either with or without a guidewire into the superior vena cava. PICCs can be trimmed before insertion, and the decision can be made to insert the catheter "midline," which is considered between the insertion site and the head of the clavicle (Meares, 1992). If the catheter is threaded midline, total parenteral nutrition (TPN) should not be administered, since the high concentration of glucose makes it irritating to the vessel, and TPN should be infused through a central catheter.

The decision to insert a PICC needs to be made before several attempts at IV lines or blood sampling by phlebotomy. Once the antecubital veins have been punctured repeatedly, they are not considered to be a candidate for this type of catheter. Since this catheter is the least costly and has less chance of complications than other central VADs, it is an excellent choice for many pediatric patients. This catheter is also usually inserted either at the child's bedside or, more appropriately when available, in the unit's treatment room.

> **Nursing ALERT** Most PICC lines are not sutured into place, so care needs to be maintained when changing the dressing.

Long-term central VADs include tunneled and implanted infusion ports (Table 22-3). They may have single, double, or triple lumens. Several lumens (multilumen catheters) allow more than one therapy to be administered at the same time. Reasons to use multilumen catheters include repeated blood sampling, TPN, administration of blood products or infusion of large quantities and/or concentrations of fluids, ability to administer incompatible drugs or fluids at the same time (through different lumens), and central venous pressure (CVP) monitoring.

With any of the central venous catheters, instilling medication through the injection cap is easily accomplished. With the implanted device the port must be palpated for placement and stabilized, the overlying skin cleansed, and only special noncoring Huber needles used to pierce the port's diaphragm on the top or side, depending on the style. To avoid repeated skin punctures, a special infusion set with a Huber needle and extension tubing with Luer connection can be used (Fig. 22-21). With this attached, the injection procedure is the same as for the heparin device or venous catheters. To prevent infection, meticulous aseptic technique must be used anytime the devices are entered, including instillation of heparin or saline to prevent clotting.

The children and parents are taught the procedure for care of the VAD before discharge from the hospital, including preparation and injection of the prescribed medication, the flush, and dressing changes. A protective device may be recommended for some active children to prevent their accidentally dislodging the needle. Many children take responsibility for preparing and administering medications. Both verbal and written step-by-step instructions* are provided for the learners.

---

*Home care instructions for caring for peripheral or central infusion device are available in Wong DL: *Wong and Whaley's Clinical manual of pediatric nursing,* ed 4, St Louis, 1996, Mosby.

TABLE 22-3. Comparison of long-term central venous access devices (VADs)

DESCRIPTION	BENEFITS	CARE CONSIDERATIONS
Tunneled Catheter (e.g., Hickman/Broviac Catheter) Silicone, radiopaque, flexible catheter with open ends One or two Dacron cuffs or Vitacuffs (biosynthetic material impregnated with silver ions) on catheter(s) enhances tissue ingrowth May have more than one lumen	Reduced risk of bacterial migration after tissue adheres to Dacron cuff or Vitacuff Easy to use for self-administered infusions Removal requires pulling catheter from site (nonsurgical procedure)	Requires daily heparin flushes Must be clamped or have clamp nearby at all times Must keep exit site dry Heavy activity restricted until tissue adheres to cuff Risk of infection still present Protrudes outside body; susceptible to damage from sharp instruments and may be pulled out; may affect body image More difficult to repair Patient/family must learn catheter care
Groshong Catheter Clear, flexible, silicone, radiopaque catheter with closed tip and two-way valve at proximal end Dacron cuff or Vitacuff on catheter enhances tissue ingrowth May have more than one lumen	Reduced time and cost for maintenance care; no heparin flushes needed Reduced catheter damage: no clamping needed because of two-way valve Increased patient safety because of minimum potential for blood backflow or air embolism Reduced risk of bacterial migration after tissue adheres to Dacron cuff or Vitacuff Easily repaired Easy to use for self-administered IV infusions	Requires weekly irrigation with normal saline Must keep exit site dry Heavy activity restricted until tissue adheres to cuff Risk of infection still present Protrudes outside body; susceptible to damage from sharp instruments and may be pulled out; can affect body image Patient/family must learn catheter care
Implanted Ports (Port-A-Cath, Infus-A-Port, Mediport, Norport, Groshong Port) Totally implantable metal or plastic device that consists of self-sealing injection port with top or side access with preconnected or attachable silicone catheter that is placed in large blood vessel	Reduced risk of infection Placed completely under the skin; therefore cannot be pulled out or damaged No maintenance care and reduced cost for family Heparinized monthly and after each infusion to maintain patency (Groshong port only requires saline) No limitations on regular physical activity, including swimming Dressing only needed when port accessed with Huber needle that is not removed No or only slight change in body appearance (slight bulge on chest)	Must pierce skin for access; pain with insertion of needle; can use local anesthetic (EMLA) or intradermal buffered lidocaine before accessing port Special noncoring needle (Huber) with straight or angled design must be used to inject into port Skin preparation needed before injection Difficult to manipulate for self-administered infusions Catheter may dislodge from port, especially if child "plays" with port site (twiddler syndrome) Vigorous contact sports generally not allowed Removal requires surgical procedure

NURSING TIPS The use of a spandex-nylon bodysuit on active toddlers has successfully maintained central lines. One study showed that the suit could not be removed by the toddler and fit snugly over the catheter, its exit site, and its connections. The cost of two bodysuits per child, one for wearing while the other is being cleaned, is less than the costs and the risks of repeated central line insertions (Janik, Wayne, and Janik, 1995).

A pocket sewn on the inside of a T-shirt provides a place in which to coil the catheter line while the child is at play if a dressing is not used.

Infection and an occluded catheter are two of the most common complications of central venous catheters. Although neither is an emergency, both require treatment with antibiotics for infection and a fibrinolytic agent, such as urokinase, for clots. Uncapping can be prevented by taping the cap securely to the catheter and the clamped line to the dressing. Leaks can be prevented by using a smooth-edged clamp only. Parents are cautioned to keep scissors away from the child to prevent accidental cutting of the catheter. If the catheter leaks, they are instructed to tape it above the leak and then clamp the catheter at the taped site. The child should be taken

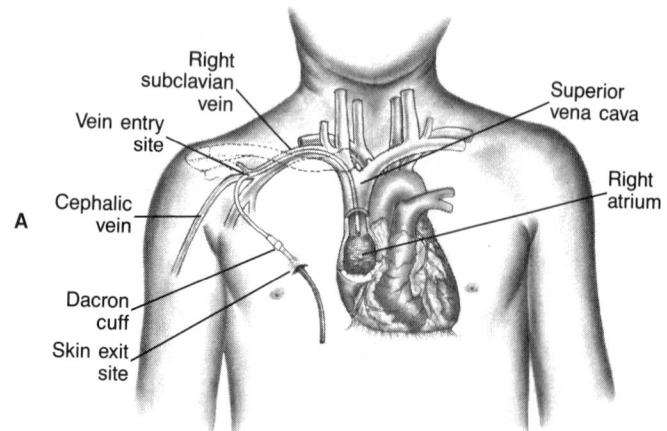
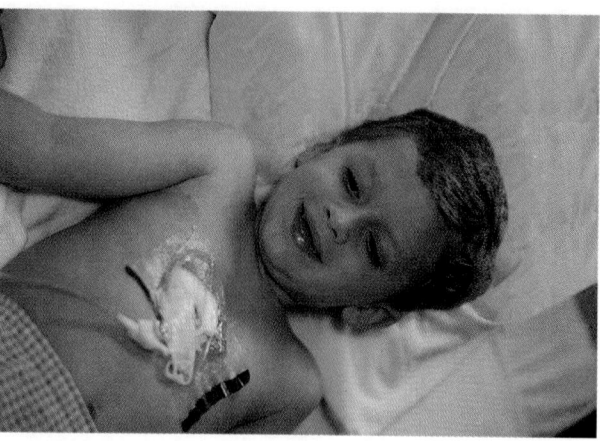

FIG. 22-21. Venous access devices (VADs). **A,** Central venous catheter insertion and exit site. **B,** Child receiving medication by way of an implantable port. Note needle and extension tubing inserted into port and secured with gauze dressings and a transparent dressing.

GUIDELINES
Nasogastric, Orogastric, or Gastrostomy Medication Administration in Children

Use elixir or suspension (rather than tablets) preparations of medication whenever possible.

Dilute viscous medication or syrup if possible with a small amount of water.

If administering tablets, crush tablet to a very fine powder and dissolve drug in a small amount of warm water.

  Never crush enteric-coated or sustained-release tablets or capsules.

Avoid oily medications because they tend to cling to side of tube.

Do not mix medication with enteral formula unless fluid is restricted. If adding a drug:

  Check with pharmacist for compatibility.

  Shake formula well and observe for any physical reaction (e.g., separation, precipitation).

  Label formula container with name of medication, dosage, date, and time infusion started.

Have medication at room temperature.

Measure medication in calibrated cup or syringe.

Check for correct placement of nasogastric or orogastric tube.

Attach syringe (with adaptable tip but without plunger) to tube.

Pour medication into syringe.

Unclamp tube and allow medication to flow by gravity.

Adjust height of container to achieve desired flow rate (e.g., increase height for faster flow).

As soon as syringe is empty, pour in water to flush tubing.

  Amount of water depends on length and gauge of tubing.

  Determine amount before administering any medication by using a syringe to fill completely an unused nasogastric or orogastric tube with water. The amount of flush solution is usually 1½ times this volume.

  With certain drug preparations (e.g., suspensions) more fluid may be needed.

If administering more than one drug at the same time, flush tube between each medication with clear water.

Clamp tube after flushing, unless tube is left open.

to the practitioner as soon as possible to prevent infection or clotting after a catheter leak.

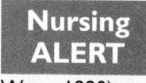

Nursing ALERT If a central venous catheter is accidentally removed, apply pressure to the *entry* site to the vein, not the exit site on the skin (Marcoux, Fisher, and Wong, 1990).

NASOGASTRIC, OROGASTRIC, OR GASTROSTOMY ADMINISTRATION

When a child has an indwelling feeding tube or a gastrostomy, oral medications are usually given via that route. An advantage of this method is the ability to administer oral medications around the clock without disturbing the child. A disadvantage is the risk of occluding or "clogging" the tube, especially when giving viscous solutions through small-bore feeding tubes. The most important preventive measure is adequate flushing after the medication is instilled. Guidelines for administration are presented in the box.

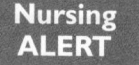

Nursing ALERT Sprinkle-type medication should be avoided. However, if there is no other option and the tube is large gauge (18 French or greater), but usually not a Foley catheter, it may be given by mixing the sprinkles with a small amount of pureed fruit and thinning with water. The fruit keeps the sprinkles suspended so they do not float to the top. Flush well. This procedure is not recommended for skin-level gastrostomy devices.

RECTAL ADMINISTRATION

The rectal route for administration is less reliable but is sometimes used when the oral route is difficult or contraindicated. Some of the drugs available in suppository form are aspirin, sedatives, analgesics (morphine), and antiemetics. The difficulty in using the rectal route is that unless the rectal ampulla is empty at the time of insertion, the absorption of the drug may be delayed, diminished, or prevented by the presence of feces. Sometimes the drug is later evacuated, securely surrounded by stool. However, the rectal route is used most frequently in children who are unable to take anything by mouth and are unlikely to have large amounts of stool. It is also used when oral preparations are unsuitable to control vomiting.

To insert a suppository, the wrapper is removed and the suppository lubricated with water-soluble jelly or warm water. A gloved finger is used to quickly but gently place the suppository into the rectum, beyond both the rectal sphincters. The buttocks are then held or taped together firmly to relieve pressure on the anal sphincter until the urge to expel the suppository has passed—5 to 10 minutes. Sometimes the amount of drug ordered is less than the dosage available. The irregular shape of most suppositories makes the process of dividing them into a desired dose difficult if not dangerous. If the suppository must be halved, it should be cut lengthwise. However, there is no guarantee that the drug is evenly dispersed throughout the petrolatum base.

 Rectal suppositories are usually inserted with the apex (pointed end) foremost. One study demonstrated easier insertion and a lower expulsion rate when the suppository was inserted with the base (blunt end) first. Reverse contractions or the pressure gradient of the anal canal may help the suppository to slip higher into the canal (Abd-El-Maeboud and others, 1991). This study, however, did not consider the issue of comfort on insertion.

If medication is administered via a retention enema, the same procedure is used. Drugs given by enema are diluted in the smallest amount of solution possible to minimize the likelihood of being evacuated.

OPTIC, OTIC, AND NASAL ADMINISTRATION

There are few differences in administering eye, ear, and nose medication to children or to adults. The major difficulty is in gaining children's cooperation or employing restraining techniques. The infant or young child's head is immobilized in the same manner as described in Fig. 7-22, *B*. Older children need only explanation and direction. Although the administration of optic, otic, and nasal medication is not painful, these drugs can cause unpleasant sensations that can be eliminated with various techniques.

NURSING TIPS To reduce unpleasant sensations, perform the following:
- **Eye**—Apply finger pressure to the lacrimal punctum at the inner aspect of the lid for 1 minute to prevent drainage of medication to the nasopharynx and the unpleasant "tasting" of the drug.
- **Ear**—Allow medications stored in the refrigerator to warm to room temperature before instillation.
- **Nose**—Position the child with the head hyperextended to prevent strangling sensations caused by medication trickling into the throat rather than up into the nasal passages.

To instill eye medication, the child is placed supine or sitting with the head extended, and the child is asked to look

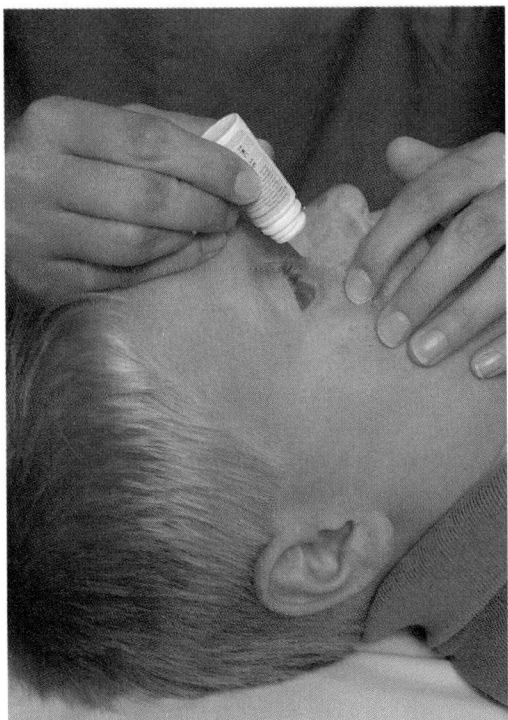

FIG. 22-22. Administering eye drops.

up. One hand is used to pull the lower lid downward; the hand that holds the dropper rests on the head so that it may move synchronously with the child's head, thus reducing the possibility of trauma to a struggling child or of dropping medication on the face (Fig. 22-22). As the lower lid is pulled down, a small conjunctival sac is formed; the solution or ointment is applied to this area, never directly on the eyeball. Another effective technique is to pull the lower lid down and out to form a cup, into which the medication is dropped. The lids are gently closed to prevent expression of the medication, and the child is asked to look in all directions to enhance even distribution of the preparation. Excess medication is wiped from the inner canthus outward to prevent contamination to the contralateral eye.

Instilling eye drops in infants can be most difficult, since they often clench the lids tightly closed. One approach is to place the drops in the nasal corner where the lids meet. The medication pools in this area, and when the child opens the lids, the medication flows onto the conjunctiva. For young children, playing a game can be helpful, such as instructing the child to keep the eyes closed until the count of 3, then to open them, at which time the drops are quickly instilled. Ointment can be applied when the child is sleeping by gently pulling down the lower lid and placing the ointment in the lower conjunctival sac.

Nursing ALERT If both eye ointment and drops are ordered, give drops first, wait 3 minutes, then apply the ointment to allow each drug to work. When possible, administer eye ointments before bedtime or naptime, since the child's vision will be blurred temporarily.

Ear drops are instilled with the child restrained in the supine position and the head turned to the appropriate side. For children younger than 3 years of age, the external auditory canal is straightened by gently pulling the pinna downward and straight back. The pinna is pulled upward and back in children older than 3 years of age (see Fig. 7-19). To place the drops deep in the ear canal without contaminating the tip of the dropper, place a disposable ear speculum in the canal and administer the drops through the speculum. After instillation, the child should remain lying on the unaffected side for a few minutes. Gentle massage of the area immediately anterior to the ear facilitates the entry of drops into the ear canal. The use of cotton pledgets prevents medication from flowing out of the external canal. However, the pledgets should be loose enough to allow any discharge to exit from the ear. Premoistening the cotton with a few drops of medication prevents the wicking action from absorbing the medication instilled in the ear.

Nose drops are instilled in the same manner as in the adult patient. Unpleasant sensations associated with medicated nose drops are minimized when care is taken to position the child with the head extended well over the edge of the bed or a pillow (Fig. 22-23). Depending on size, the infant can be positioned in the football hold (see Fig. 22-7, *B*), in the nurse's arm with the head extended and stabilized between the nurse's body and elbow and the arms and hands immobilized with the nurse's hands, or as in Fig. 22-23. After instillation of the drops, the child should remain in position for 1 minute to allow the drops to come in contact with the nasal surfaces.

Nasal spray dispensers are inserted into the nare vertically then angled nasally to avoid trauma to the septum and to direct medication toward the inferior turbinate.

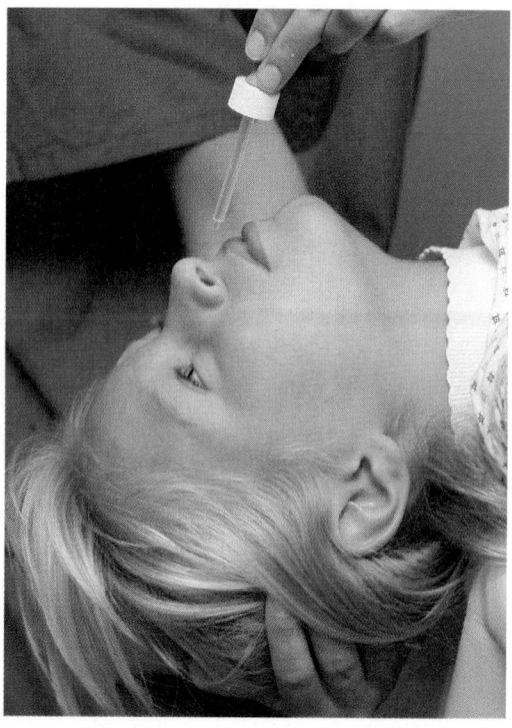

FIG. 22-23. Proper position for instilling nose drops.

FAMILY TEACHING AND HOME CARE

The nurse usually assumes the responsibility for preparing families to administer medications at home. The family should have an understanding of why the child is receiving the medication and the effects that might be expected, as well as the amount, frequency, and length of time the drug is to be administered. Instruction should be carried out in an unhurried, relaxed manner, preferably in an area away from busy ward or office routine, following the same guidelines for teaching as outlined on p. 688.

The caregiver is carefully instructed regarding the correct dosage, and the nurse is responsible for preparing parents for the specifics of the task. Some persons have difficulty understanding or interpreting terminology from the pharmacy, and just because they nod or otherwise indicate an understanding, it cannot be assumed that the message is clear. It is important to ascertain their interpretation of a teaspoon, for example, and to be certain they have acceptable devices for measuring the drug. If the drug is packaged with a dropper, syringe, or plastic cup, the nurse should show the point on the device that indicates the prescribed dose and demonstrate how the dose is drawn up into a dropper or syringe and measured and how the bubbles are eliminated. Also, the nurse must be certain that families understand that a prescription ordered in drops means single drops, not dropperfuls, a potential source of administration error (see Nursing Alert, p. 713). If the nurse has any doubts about the parent's ability to administer the correct dose, the parent should be asked to give a return demonstration. This verification is especially important when the drug has potentially serious consequences from incorrect dosage, such as insulin or digoxin, or when more complex administration is required, such as parenteral injections. When a parent is taught to give an injection, adequate time for instruction and practice must be allotted.

Home modifications are often necessary because the availability of equipment or assistance can differ from that of the hospital setting. For example, restraint is often necessary when giving medications to children, and the parent may need guidance in devising methods that allow for one person to restrain the child and safely give the drug. One successful method is described below.

NURSING TIP To administer oral, nasal, or optic medication when only one person is available to restrain the child, use the following procedure:
- Place child supine on flat surface (bed, couch, floor).
- Sit facing child so that his or her head is between operator's thighs and his or her arms are under operator's legs.
- Place lower legs over child's legs to restrain lower body, if necessary.
- To administer oral medication, place small pillow under child's head to reduce risk of aspiration.
- To administer nasal medication, place small pillow under child's shoulders to aid flow of liquid through nasal passages.

The time that the drug is to be administered is clarified with the parent. For instance, when a drug is prescribed in association with meals, the number of meals that the family is accustomed to eating influences the amount of drug the child receives; do they have meals twice a day or five times a day? When a drug is to be given several times during the day, together the nurse and parents can work out a schedule that accommodates the family's routine. This is particularly significant if the drug must be given at equal intervals throughout a 24-hour period. For example, telling parents that the child needs 1 teaspoon of medicine four times a day is subject to misinterpretation, since parents may routinely schedule the doses at incorrect times. Instead, a preplanned schedule based on 6-hour intervals should be set up with the number of days required for therapeutic dosage listed. Written instruction should accompany all drug prescriptions.*

NURSING TIP If parents have difficulty reading or understanding English, use colors to convey instructions. For example, mark each drug with a color and place the appropriate color on a calendar chart or on a drawing of a clock to identify when the drug needs to be given. If a liquid medication and syringe are used, also mark the syringe at the place the plunger needs to be with color-coded tape.

PROCEDURES RELATED TO MAINTAINING FLUID BALANCE

MEASUREMENT OF INTAKE AND OUTPUT (I & O)

One of the most important roles of the nurse in maintaining fluid balance is accurate measurement of fluid balance. Although the physician usually indicates when I & O are to be recorded, it is a nursing responsibility to keep an accurate I & O record on patients in the following situations:

- After major surgery
- Intravenous, diuretic, or corticosteroid therapy
- Severe thermal burns or injuries
- Renal disease or damage
- Congestive heart failure
- Dehydration (vomiting and diarrhea)
- Diabetes mellitus
- Oliguria
- Two years of age or younger

Infants or small children who are unable to use a bedpan or those who have bowel movements with every voiding require the application of a collecting device (p. 706). If collecting bags are not used, wet diapers or pads are carefully weighed to ascertain the amount of fluid lost. This includes liquid stool, vomitus, and other losses. The volume of fluid in milliliters is equivalent to the weight of the fluid measured in grams. The specific gravity as a measure of osmolality is determined with a urinometer or a refractometer and assists in assessing the degree of hydration (see FYI on p. 707).

The weighed-diaper method of fluid measurement has disadvantages, including (1) inability to differentiate one type of loss from another because of admixture, (2) loss of urine or liquid stool from leakage or evaporation (especially if the infant is under a radiant warmer), and (3) additional fluid in

diaper (superabsorbent disposable type) from absorption of atmospheric moisture (from high-humidity incubators). However, when several types of diapers, including cloth, conventional disposable, and superabsorbent disposable, were compared for accuracy in terms of evaporative effects, closed superabsorbent disposable diapers followed by open superabsorbent disposable diapers were affected the least (Fox, 1992). To avoid the problem of evaporative losses and leakage of excreta, diapers should be weighed as soon as possible after becoming soiled.

It is important to measure and record all intake—oral and parenteral—and output from all sources, including urine, stool, emesis, drainage tubes, fistulas, and wounds from which appreciable amounts of fluid are lost.

Special Needs When the Child Is NPO

Infants or children who are unable or not permitted to take fluids by mouth (NPO) have special needs. To ensure that they do not receive fluids, a sign can be placed in some obvious place, such as over their beds or on their shirts, to alert others to their status. To prevent temptation to drink, fluids should not be left at the bedside.

Oral hygiene, a part of routine hygienic care, is especially important when fluids are restricted or withheld (see p. 693). For the young child who cannot brush the teeth or rinse the mouth without swallowing fluid, the nurse can institute oral hygiene by wiping the teeth, gums, and tongue with a cloth moistened with saline.

NURSING TIP To keep the mouth feeling moist when the child is NPO, give ice chips (if this is permitted by the practitioner) or spray the mouth with a fine mist of cool water (a clean perfume atomizer works well).

The lips are kept moist with petrolatum (Vaseline) or another commercial lip aid. Lemon-glycerin swabs are avoided because they dry the skin, irritate open lesions, and can decay the teeth. To meet the need to suck, the infant is provided with a pacifier.

The child who is fluid restricted presents an equal challenge. Limiting fluids is often more difficult for the child than NPO, especially when IV fluids are also eliminated. To make certain the child does not drink the entire amount allowed early in the day, the daily allotment is calculated to provide fluids at periodic intervals throughout the child's waking hours. Serving the fluids in small containers gives the illusion of larger servings. No extra liquid is left at the bedside if compliance is a problem.

PARENTERAL FLUID THERAPY

Site and Equipment

The site selected for IV infusion depends on accessibility and convenience. In older children any accessible vein may be used. In small infants a scalp vein or a superficial vein of the wrist, hand, foot, or arm is usually most convenient and most easily stabilized (Fig. 22-24). Since superficial veins of the scalp have no valves, insertion is easier, and they can be used in infants up to about 9 months of age. For veins in the extremities, it is best to start with the most distal sites and to use the nondominant hand.

---

*Home care instructions on giving medications to children are available in Wong DL: *Wong and Whaley's Clinical manual of pediatric nursing,* ed 4, St Louis, 1996, Mosby.

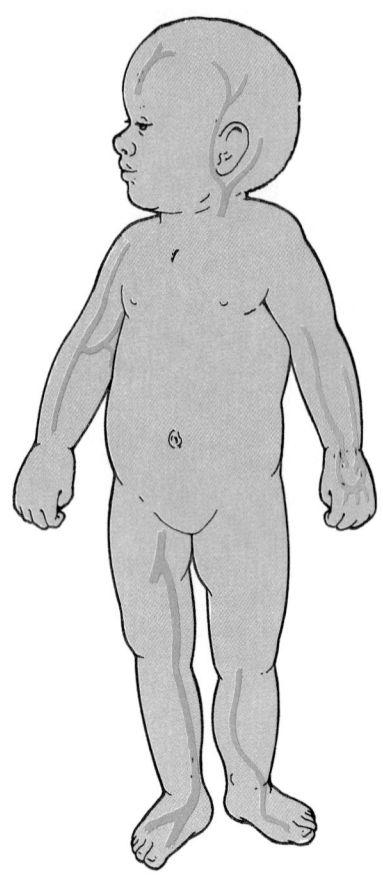

FIG. 22-24. Preferred sites for venous access in infants. (From Smith DP and others, editors: *Comprehensive child and family nursing skills*, St Louis, 1991, Mosby.)

For most IV infusions in children, an over-the-needle 20- to 24-gauge catheter or a scalp-vein size 21 or 23 needle with flexible winged tabs is used. In situations in which fluids are urgently needed and there is difficulty in entering a vein, a catheter inserted by the surgical cutdown procedure may be necessary. The vein of choice for this alternative is the internal saphenous vein located just anterior to the medial malleolus of the tibia. For long-term IV therapy a number of other devices may be used (see p. 720).

Other equipment needed includes an antiseptic swab to clean the site, a tourniquet, an appropriately sized padded armboard (when an extremity is used), rolled towels or small blankets for maintaining position of the head or extremity, tape (or dressing and bacteriostatic ointment if the hospital dictates), and a device to protect the IV site after insertion. The prescribed solution, tubing, filter, and infusion pump are prepared in advance, ready to connect to the needle after insertion.

Selection of a scalp vein as the venipuncture site requires shaving the area around the site to visualize the vein better and provide a smooth surface on which to tape the tubing. A rubber band slipped onto the head from brow to occiput will usually suffice as a tourniquet. Shaving off a portion of the infant's hair is very upsetting to parents; therefore they should be told what to expect and reassured that the hair will grow in again rapidly.

Situations may occur in which rapid establishment of a systemic access is vital and venous access may be hampered by peripheral circulatory collapse, cardiopulmonary arrest, burns, or other conditions. *Intraosseous infusion* provides an alternate route for administration of fluids and medications until intravascular access can be attained. A large-bore needle, such as a bone marrow needle, is inserted into the medullary cavity of a long bone, most often the distal femur, proximal tibia, and distal tibia. This procedure is usually reserved for children under 3 years of age who are unconscious or are receiving analgesics because the procedure is painful.

There are several modifications in equipment used for IV infusion for children. A gravity drainage apparatus used for children is much the same as that for adults except that it is designed to deliver a reduced drop size (60 drops/ml) and contains a calibrated volume control chamber (e.g., Buretrol or Solu-set) that regulates the amount of fluid that can be infused. A microdropper greatly facilitates calculation of flow rate because a prescribed number of milliliters per hour equals the number of drops per minute. For example, if the solution is to infuse at a rate of 30 ml per hour, the infusion is regulated to deliver 30 drops per minute.

A variety of infusion pumps are available that infuse a programmed amount of fluid from a bag hanging above the machine or from a syringe placed in the machine. Infusion devices are widely used in pediatrics because they can accurately infuse fluids, especially the syringe pumps, which infuse very small amounts of fluid. It is an important nursing responsibility to calculate the amount to be infused in a given length of time, set the infusion rate, and monitor the apparatus frequently (at least every 1 to 2 hours) to make certain that the desired rate is maintained, the integrity of the system remains intact, the site remains intact (free of infiltration or irritation), and the infusion does not stop.

Continuous infusion pumps, although convenient and efficient, are not without risks. Overreliance on the accuracy of the machine can cause either too much or too little fluid to be infused; therefore careful periodic assessment is essential. Excess pressure can build up if the machine is set at a rate faster than the vein is able to accommodate (or continues to pump when the needle is out of the lumen). This is especially true in very small infants and when circumstances necessitate the use of a capillary. No matter what device is used, a thorough understanding of the apparatus is essential for safe fluid administration.

Special Care Considerations

To maintain the integrity of the IV site, adequate protection of the site is required for the child. An attempt is made to position the extremity in a natural anatomic position with the use of gauze pads or rolls as needed. To prevent trauma to the skin from removal of tape, gauze or a barrier such as transparent film can be placed between the skin and the adhesive. Sometimes a covered board is taped to the extremities to prevent flexion of a foot, hand, or arm.

After insertion, the catheter or needle is firmly secured at the puncture site with nonallergenic tape and protected from becoming dislodged by immobilization of the extremity. The insertion site and about 1 inch of skin beyond the site are left uncovered for early detection of infiltration. Clear plastic dressings are ideal because they allow ready visualization of the insertion site. Some finger or toe areas are left unoccluded by dressings or tape to allow for assessment of circulation. The thumb is never immobilized because of the danger of contractures with limited movement later on. A commercial device, such as I.V. House,* or an improvised device, such as plastic or wax paper cup that is cut in half (with the rigid edges covered with tape), can be applied directly over the needle site for further protection. Some needle containers make excellent protective covers. A colorful and interesting sticker can be applied to the armboard or protecting device to add a positive note to the procedure.

Older children who are alert and cooperative can usually be trusted to protect the IV site. An IV infusion is not always a deterrent to mobility. When the child is feeling well and the insertion site is well secured, the child can be held or be walked, but precautions must be observed to preserve the integrity of the IV system.

Infants, small children, and uncooperative children require varying degrees of immobilization, and on rare occasions, complete restriction of movement may be needed to prevent removal of the IV infusion. The affected extremity is secured to the bed, and the remaining extremities that might be used to dislodge the needle are restrained. This includes feet, as well as hands, since most infants will attempt to brush away the offending attachment by rubbing it against another extremity or body part. Whenever possible, the infant or child should be held and cuddled to help meet emotional needs during this trying time (Fig. 22-25).

When an IV infusion must be discontinued, many children are distressed by the thought of needle removal. Therefore they need a careful explanation of the process and suggestions for helping. One way is to allow children to remove or help remove the tape from the site. This provides them with a measure of control and often encourages their cooperation. The procedure consists of turning off any pump apparatus, occluding the IV tubing, removing the tape, and pulling the needle or catheter out of the vessel while exerting firm pressure at the site. A dry dressing (adhesive bandage strip) is placed over the puncture site. If a catheter was used for the IV infusion, the tip is inspected to make certain the catheter is intact and no portion remains in the vein.

Complications. The same precautions regarding maintenance of asepsis, prevention of infection, and observation for infiltration are carried out with patients of any age. However, infiltration is more difficult to detect in infants and small children than in adults. The increased amount of subcutaneous fat and the amount of tape used to secure the needle often obscure the signs of early infiltration. When the fluid appears to be infusing too slowly or ceases, the usual assessment for obstruction within the apparatus—kinks, screw clamps, shutoff valve, and positioning interference (e.g., a bent elbow)—often locates the difficulty. When these actions fail to detect the problem, it may be necessary to remove carefully some of the tape and other material that obscure a clear view of the venipuncture site. Dependent areas, such as the

*Available from I.V. House, 7400 Foxmont Dr., Hazelwood, MO 63042; (800) 530-0400; Fax (314) 831-3863.

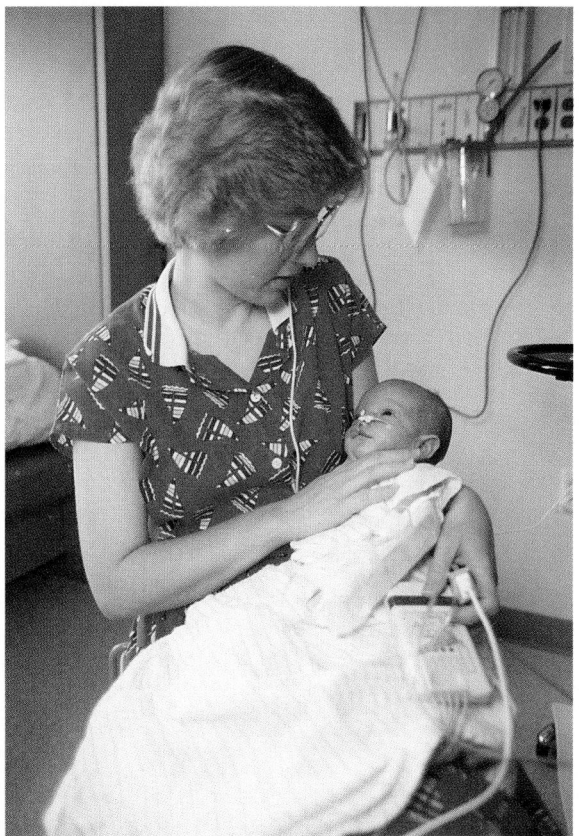

FIG. 22-25. Intravenous infusion, as well as other equipment, does not prevent infant from being picked up and cuddled.

palm and undersides of the extremity or the occiput and behind the ears, are examined.

Whenever possible, the IV infusion should be placed in an extremity to which the identification band (or bracelet) is not attached. Serious circulatory impairment can result from infiltrated solution distal to the band, which acts as a tourniquet preventing adequate venous return. To check for return blood flow through the needle, the bottle is lowered below the level of the infusion site. If the tubing is connected to an infusion pump, it must be removed from the pump before lowering.

Drugs are available to diffuse extravasated fluid or neutralize the extravasated medication. Hyaluronidase is used in severe cases to diffuse extravasated fluids rapidly through the tissue and increase the absorption rate. When used, the IV infusion is discontinued, and with the needle still in place, the drug is injected into the site. If the catheter is removed, the drug is then injected (as prescribed) into the area surrounding the insertion site. Assessment and documentation of the site continue until the infiltration has completely resolved. Staging of IV infiltrates may be performed to evaluate treatment options (Flemmer and Chan, 1993).

Prevention of infection is a major nursing function during IV therapy. The infusion site is protected from trauma and entry of bacteria. When an IV infusion continues for several days or longer, the tubing and bottle are changed at regular intervals according to hospital policy. Frequency ranges from every 24 to every 72 hours, most often every 48 hours. To ensure that the equipment is changed regularly, it is labeled with the date and time that the new bottle and tubing are attached. Any signs of inflammation, such as redness or pain, should be reported immediately. This usually requires removal of the infusion and restarting it at another site.

FAMILY TEACHING AND HOME CARE

Since maintaining fluid balance is so critical, especially in young children, families may need to continue some procedures, such as measuring intake, output, and daily weight, at home. These are simple skills, but families require time to learn and practice them before discharge. With the widespread use of superabsorbent disposable diapers, parents are advised that the diaper may be wet but still feel dry. Placing some cotton balls or tissues in the diaper facilitates checking for wetness. Also, the wet diaper may feel "doughy" and heavy.

IV therapy for fluid replacement is rarely carried out in the home, although parenteral administration of drugs or hyperalimentation is much more common. Home care of the child with home hyperalimentation is discussed on p. 741.

PROCEDURES FOR MAINTAINING RESPIRATORY FUNCTION

INHALATION THERAPY

The term *inhalation therapy* is an all-inclusive term that encompasses a variety of therapies that involve changing the composition, volume, or pressure of inspired gases. These therapies include primarily increasing the oxygen concentration of inspired gas (oxygen therapy), increasing the water vapor content of inspired gas (humidification), adding airborne particles with beneficial properties (aerosol therapy), and employing various means for controlling or assisting respiration (artificial ventilation, continuous positive airway pressure).

Oxygen Therapy

Oxygen (O_2) therapy is primarily carried out in the hospital, although increasing numbers of children are receiving oxygen in the home. O_2 delivered to the infant via the incubator is satisfactory when lower levels are adequate to prevent cyanosis, but the highest concentration (almost 100%) is supplied by way of a *plastic hood* (Fig. 22-26). The gas is not allowed to blow directly into the infant's face, and the hood should not rub against the infant's neck, chin, or shoulder. Older cooperative children can use a *nasal cannula* or *prongs,* which can supply a concentration of about 50%. A *mask* is not well tolerated by children.

For children beyond early infancy, the *oxygen tent* is a satisfactory means for administration of O_2 (Fig. 22-27). A tent does not require any device to come into direct contact with the face, but the concentration of O_2 within the tent is difficult to control and to maintain above 30% to 50%. A major difficulty with the use of the tent is keeping the tent closed so that O_2 concentration is maintained.

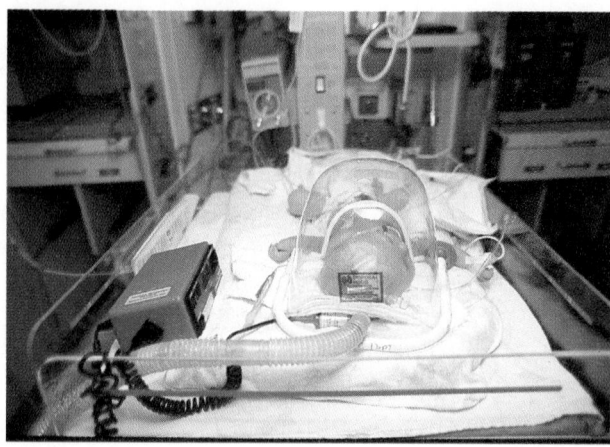

FIG. 22-26. Oxygen administered to infant by means of a plastic hood. Note oxygen analyzer (blue machine).

To reduce O_2 loss, nursing care is planned carefully so that the tent is opened as little as possible. Since O_2 is heavier than air, loss will be greater at the bottom of the tent; therefore the tent is tucked in snugly without open edges. The bottom of the tent should be examined more often when the child is restless and fussy and liable to pull the covers loose. Some tents are even open at the top. Because of the rapid diffusing qualities of carbon dioxide (CO_2), the levels of the gas do not build up within these enclosures.

After the tent has been opened for an extended period, it is flushed with O_2 by increasing the flow meter for a few minutes to raise quickly the O_2 and mist concentration. The flow meter is then reset to the prescribed number of liters.

The enclosed tent becomes very warm; therefore some type of cooling mechanism is provided. The temperature inside the tent must be checked periodically to be certain that it is maintained at the desired level. It is important to make certain that the child is kept warm and dry. Since O_2 is drying to the tissues, the gas is humidified, which causes moisture to condense on the tent walls.

> **Nursing ALERT** Keep the child warm and dry by checking the temperature inside the tent and the child's bedding and clothing frequently. Adjust the temperature and change clothing as often as needed.

The reactions of children to the O_2 tent are variable. Some, especially older children, feel comfortable in the tent and like the cozy, close privacy it affords. Others, more often younger children, may be frightened by the forced enclosure. The plastic walls distort their view of the world and constitute a barrier between them and their source of comfort, their parent. Their distress can be minimized if they are able to see someone nearby and are reassured that they will not be left alone. A favorite toy or object can accompany the child inside the tent. However, all toys should be inspected for safety and suitability. Other familiar items can be placed at the foot of the bed or otherwise in view.

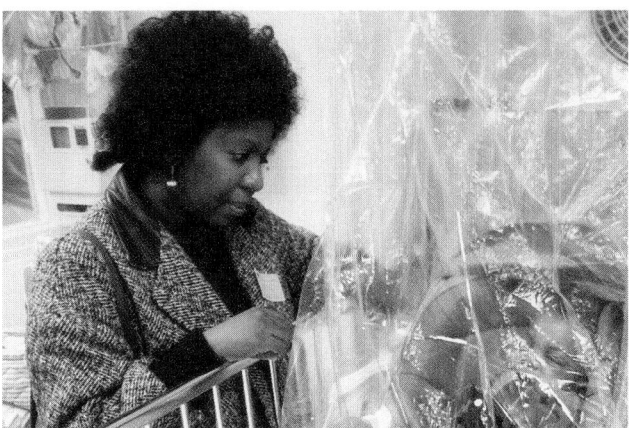

FIG. 22-27. The tent provides a comfortable method for oxygen administration. (From Wilson SF, Thompson JM: *Respiratory disorders*, St Louis, 1990, Mosby.)

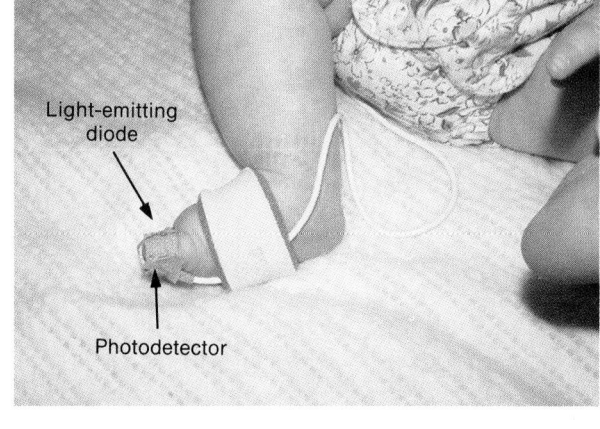

Light-emitting diode

Photodetector

FIG. 22-28. Oximeter sensor on great toe. Note that sensor is positioned with light-emitting diode opposite photodetector. Cord is secured to foot to minimize movement of sensor.

Nursing ALERT Inspect all toys for safety and suitability (e.g., vinyl or plastic, not stuffed items that absorb moisture and are difficult to keep dry). The high-level O_2 environment makes any source of sparks (e.g., mechanical or electrical toys) a potential fire hazard.

In most instances the child can be removed from the O_2 tent for activities such as feeding and bathing, whereas in other cases the child is placed in the tent only during periods of rest. Still other children may require O_2 continuously and can be removed from the tent or incubator only if an O_2 source is held close to the child's face. Any change in color, increased respiratory effort, or restlessness is an indication to return the child to the O_2 tent.

Oxygen Toxicity. O_2 is essential to life and a valuable therapeutic aid. However, prolonged exposure to high O_2 tensions can be damaging to some body tissues and functions. The organs most vulnerable to the adverse effects of excessive oxygenation are the retina of the premature infant and the lungs of persons at any age.

Oxygen-induced carbon dioxide narcosis is a physiologic hazard of O_2 therapy that may occur in persons with chronic pulmonary disease, such as cystic fibrosis. These children have chronic alveolar hypoventilation with a concomitant chronic CO_2 retention and hypoxemia. In these patients the respiratory center has adapted to the continuously higher arterial carbon dioxide tension ($Paco_2$) levels, and therefore hypoxia becomes the more powerful stimulus for respiration. When the arterial oxygen tension (Pao_2) level is elevated during O_2 administration, the hypoxic drive is removed, causing progressive hypoventilation and increased $Paco_2$ levels, and the child rapidly becomes unconscious.

Monitoring Oxygen Therapy

Pulse oximetry is a simple, continuous, noninvasive method of determining oxygen saturation (Sao_2) to guide O_2 therapy. A sensor comprising a light-emitting diode (LED) and a photodetector is placed in opposition around a foot, hand, finger, toe, or earlobe, with the LED placed on top of the nail when digits are used (Fig. 22-28). The LED emits red and infrared lights that pass through the skin to the photodetector. The photodetector measures the amount of each type of light absorbed by functional hemoglobins. Hemoglobin saturated with O_2 (oxyhemoglobin) absorbs more infrared light than does hemoglobin not saturated with O_2 (deoxyhemoglobin). Therefore pulsatile blood flow is the primary physiologic factor that influences accuracy of the pulse oximeter.

Another noninvasive method is *transcutaneous monitoring (TCM)*, which provides continual monitoring of transcutaneous partial pressure of oxygen in arterial blood ($tcPao_2$) and, with some devices, of carbon dioxide in arterial blood ($tcPaco_2$). An electrode is attached to the warmed skin to facilitate arterialization of cutaneous capillaries. The site of the electrode must be changed every 3 to 4 hours to prevent burning the skin, and the machine must be calibrated with every site change. TCM is used frequently in neonatal intensive care units, but it may not reflect Pao_2 in infants with impaired local circulation or in older infants whose skin is thicker.

The Pao_2 can be correlated with the Sao_2 by means of the *oxyhemoglobin dissociation curve* (Fig. 22-29). Most important, changes in Pao_2 do not cause identical changes in Sao_2. Rather, in the steep portion of the curve, small changes in Pao_2 result in large changes in Sao_2. In the flat portion of the curve, large changes in Pao_2 result in only small changes in Sao_2.

NURSING TIP A quick formula for calculating correlation of Pao_2 with Sao_2 is the 30-60, 60-90 rule. Assuming a normal pH, $Paco_2$, and body temperature, this rule can apply: when $Pao_2 = 30$ mm Hg, $Sao_2 = 60\%$; when $Pao_2 = 60$, $Sao_2 = 90\%$.

Also, oximetry is insensitive to hyperoxia because hemoglobin approaches 100% saturation for all Pao_2 readings greater than approximately 100 mm Hg, which is a dangerous situation for the premature infant at risk for developing retinopathy of prematurity (see Chapter 9). Therefore the premature infant being monitored with oximetry should have

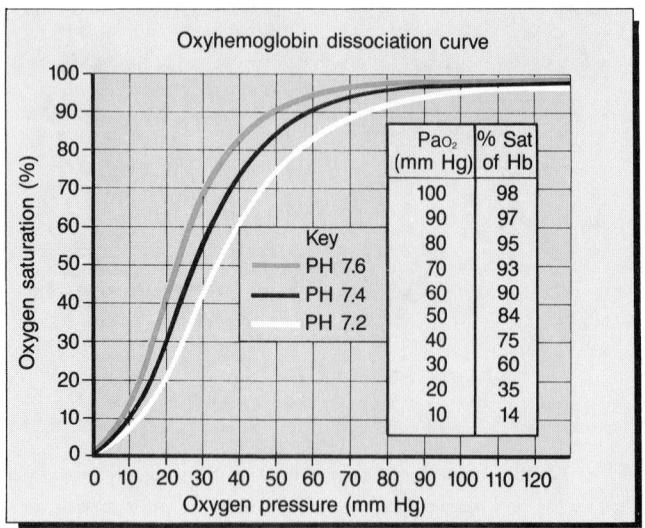

FIG. 22-29. Oxyhemoglobin dissociation curve. Changes in affinity of hemoglobin for oxygen shift position of curve. Shift to left *(colored line)* indicates increased affinity of hemoglobin for oxygen. Shift to right *(white line)* indicates decreased affinity of hemoglobin for oxygen.

upper limits identified, such as 90% to 95%, and a protocol established for decreasing O_2 when saturations are high.

The degree to which O_2 combines with hemoglobin is affected by several factors. A shift of the curve to the left causes an increased affinity of hemoglobin for O_2, but the O_2 is not easily released to the tissues. This represents an increase in the Sao_2 if it is measured against the same Pao_2 of the normal oxyhemoglobin dissociation curve. This left shift can be caused by an increase in blood pH or a decrease in $Paco_2$, body temperature, or 2,3-diphosphoglycerate (2,3-DPG), a substance in the red blood cells.

A shift of the curve to the right causes a decreased affinity of hemoglobin for O_2, but improved O_2 release to the tissues. This represents a lower Sao_2 if measured against the same Pao_2 of the normal oxyhemoglobin dissociation curve. This right shift can be caused by a decrease in blood pH or an increase in $Paco_2$, body temperature, or 2,3-DPG.

Oximetry offers several advantages over TCM. Oximetry (1) does not require heating the skin, thus reducing the risk of burns; (2) eliminates a delay period for transducer equilibration; and (3) maintains an accurate measurement regardless of the patient's age or skin characteristics or the presence of lung disease.

> **Nursing ALERT**
>
> It is important to make certain that sensory connectors and oximeters are compatible. Wiring that is incompatible can generate considerable heat at the tip of the sensor, causing second- and third-degree burns under the sensors. Pressure necrosis can also occur from sensors attached too tightly. Therefore inspect the skin under the sensor frequently.

Applying the sensor correctly is essential for accurate Sao_2 measurements. Since the sensor must identify every pulse beat to calculate the Sao_2, movement can interfere with sensing. Some devices synchronize the Sao_2 reading with the heart-

THINKING CRITICALLY ABOUT . . .
Mist Therapy

Continuous administration of mist, or aerosolized water, for the treatment of inflammatory conditions of the airways is a common practice that has no proven benefit (Alderson and Warren, 1984), although clinical improvement has been noted in some cases (e.g., the use of a mist tent or a very humid environment, such as a steamy bathroom, for the treatment of croup). For other pathologic conditions, however, mist therapy can be detrimental. For example, bronchoconstriction in children with asthma can be exacerbated by mist therapy.

The notion that inhaled mist can influence the viscosity of mucus in dehydrated children is erroneous; inhaled mist does not affect the water content of expectorated mucus. If dehydration is evident, oral or parenteral rehydration will normalize the water content of respiratory mucus.

beat, thereby reducing the interference caused by motion. Sensors are not placed on extremities used for blood pressure monitoring or with indwelling arterial catheters, since pulsatile blood flow can be affected.

NURSING TIPS

Infant: Tape the sensor securely to the great toe and tape the wire to the sole of the foot (or use a commercial holder that fastens with a self-adhering closure). Place a snugly fitting sock over the foot.

Child: Tape the sensor securely to the index finger and tape the wire to the back of the hand. Use self-adhering Ace-type wrap (e.g., Coban) around the finger and/or hand to further secure the sensor and wire.

Ambient light from ceiling lights and phototherapy, as well as high-intensity heat and light from radiant warmers, can interfere with readings. Therefore the sensor should be covered to block these light sources. Intravenous dyes; green, purple, or black nail polish; nonopaque synthetic nails; and possibly ink used for footprinting can also cause inaccurate Sao_2 measurements. The dyes should be removed or, in the case of porcelain nails, a different area used for the sensor. Skin color, thickness, and edema do not affect the readings.

Aerosol Therapy

Aerosol therapy can be effective in depositing medication directly into the airway. The value of aerosolized water or "mist therapy" is controversial (see Thinking Critically About . . . box). This route of administration can be useful in avoiding the systemic side effects of certain drugs and in reducing the amount of drug necessary to achieve the desired effect. Bronchodilators, steroids, and antibiotics can be suspended in particulate form and then inhaled so that the medication reaches the small airways. The use of aerosol therapy is particularly challenging in children who are too young to cooperate with controlling the rate and depth of breathing. Administration of this therapy requires skill, patience, and creativity.

Medications can be aerosolized or nebulized with air or with O_2-enriched gas. ***Hand-held nebulizers*** are the most frequently used equipment. The medicated "mist" is discharged into a small plastic mask, which the child holds over the nose and mouth. To avoid particle deposition in the nose and pharynx, the child is instructed to take slow, deep breaths through an open mouth during the treatment. For home use an air compressor is necessary to force air through the liquid medication to form the aerosol. Fairly compact, portable units can be rented from health equipment companies. The *metered-dose inhaler (MDI)* is a self-contained, hand-held device that allows for intermittent delivery of a specified amount of medication. Many bronchodilators are available in this form and are successfully used by children with asthma. For children under the age of 5 or 6 years, a *spacer device* attached to the MDI can help with coordination of breathing and aerosol delivery. It allows the aerosolized particles to remain in suspension longer. (See also Asthma, Chapter 23.)

A major nursing responsibility during aerosol therapy is to assess the effectiveness of the treatment and the patient's tolerance of the procedure. Assessments of breath sounds and work of breathing should be done before and after treatments. Small children who become upset with having a mask held close to the face may become fatigued with fighting the procedure and may actually appear worse during and immediately after the therapy. This takes careful assessment by the nurse and practitioner to determine if the treatment is worthwhile. It may be necessary to spend a few minutes calming the child after the procedure, and allowing the vital signs to return to baseline to accurately assess changes in breath sounds and work of breathing.

BRONCHIAL (POSTURAL) DRAINAGE

Bronchial drainage is indicated whenever excessive fluid or mucus in the bronchi is not being removed by normal ciliary activity and cough. Positioning the child to take maximum advantage of gravity facilitates removal of secretions. The effect is sometimes dramatic in children with chronic lung disease characterized by thick mucous secretions, such as asthma and cystic fibrosis.

Postural drainage is carried out three to four times daily and is more effective when it follows other respiratory therapy, such as bronchodilator and/or nebulization medication. Bronchial drainage is generally performed before meals (or 1 to 1½ hours after meals) to minimize the chance of vomiting and is repeated at bedtime. The length and duration of treatment depend on the child's condition and tolerance level, usually 20 to 30 minutes. There are positions to facilitate drainage from all major lung segments (Fig. 22-30), but all positions are not employed at each session. Children will usually cooperate for four to six positions, but more than six tend to exceed their limits of tolerance. Older children can be expected to tolerate longer periods.

In the hospital an older child can be positioned over an elevated knee rest. Small children and infants can be positioned with pillows or on the therapist's lap and legs (Fig. 22-31). Infants should not be placed in the Trendelenburg position because they do not have an autonomic regulation of blood flow to the head. Special modifications of the techniques are required in children whose conditions contraindicate the standard positioning, such as head injuries, some types of surgical incisions or burns, and casts or traction. At home small children can be positioned on a padded ironing board.* Children who require postural drainage over months or years may benefit from specially constructed tables padded and adjusted to their individual needs. The position used and the frequency and duration of treatment are individualized.

CHEST PHYSIOTHERAPY (CPT)

CPT usually refers to the use of postural drainage in combination with adjunctive techniques that are thought to enhance the clearance of mucus from the airway. These techniques include manual percussion, vibration, and squeezing of the chest; cough; forceful expiration; and breathing exercises. The efficacies of these techniques, both individually and combined, are controversial, however. Postural drainage in combination with forced expiration has been shown to be beneficial, but the benefit of the other techniques has yet to be demonstrated.

The most common technique used in association with postural drainage is manual percussion of the chest wall. Nurses are often responsible for this maneuver if a respiratory therapist is not available, so they should be skilled in the technique. The patient is dressed in a lightweight shirt and placed in a postural drainage position; then the nurse gently but firmly strikes the chest wall with a cupped hand (Fig. 22-32, *A*). For infants, special devices are available for percussing small areas (Fig. 22-32, *B*). A "popping," hollow sound should be the result, not a slapping sound. The procedure should be done over the rib cage only and should be painless. Percussion can be performed with a soft circular mask (adapted to maintain air trapping) or a percussion cup marketed especially for the purpose of aiding the loosening of secretions.

CPT is contraindicated when patients have pulmonary hemorrhage, pulmonary embolism, end-stage renal disease, increased intracranial pressure, osteogenesis imperfecta, or minimal cardiac reserves.

CPT should be used for patients who have increased sputum production. It is probably of no value to the uncomplicated postoperative patient or the patient with pneumonia. Forced expiration combined with postural drainage is more effective than cough alone, but percussion and vibration have no proven value. Appropriate use of bronchodilators before CPT therapy will enhance mucus clearance.

ARTIFICIAL VENTILATION

Artificial Airways

An artificial airway is usually used in association with artificial ventilation and in children with upper airway obstruction. Endotracheal intubation can be accomplished by the nasal (nasotracheal), oral (orotracheal), or direct tracheal (tracheostomy) routes. Although it is more difficult to place, nasotracheal intubation is preferred to orotracheal intubation because it facilitates oral hygiene and provides more stable fixation, which reduces the complication of tracheal erosion and the danger of accidental extubation. Uncuffed endotracheal tubes are almost always used with infants and children. Cuffed tubes may be used with adolescents to help provide

---

*Home care instructions on performing postural drainage are available in Wong DL: *Wong and Whaley's Clinical manual of pediatric nursing*, ed 4, St Louis, 1996, Mosby.

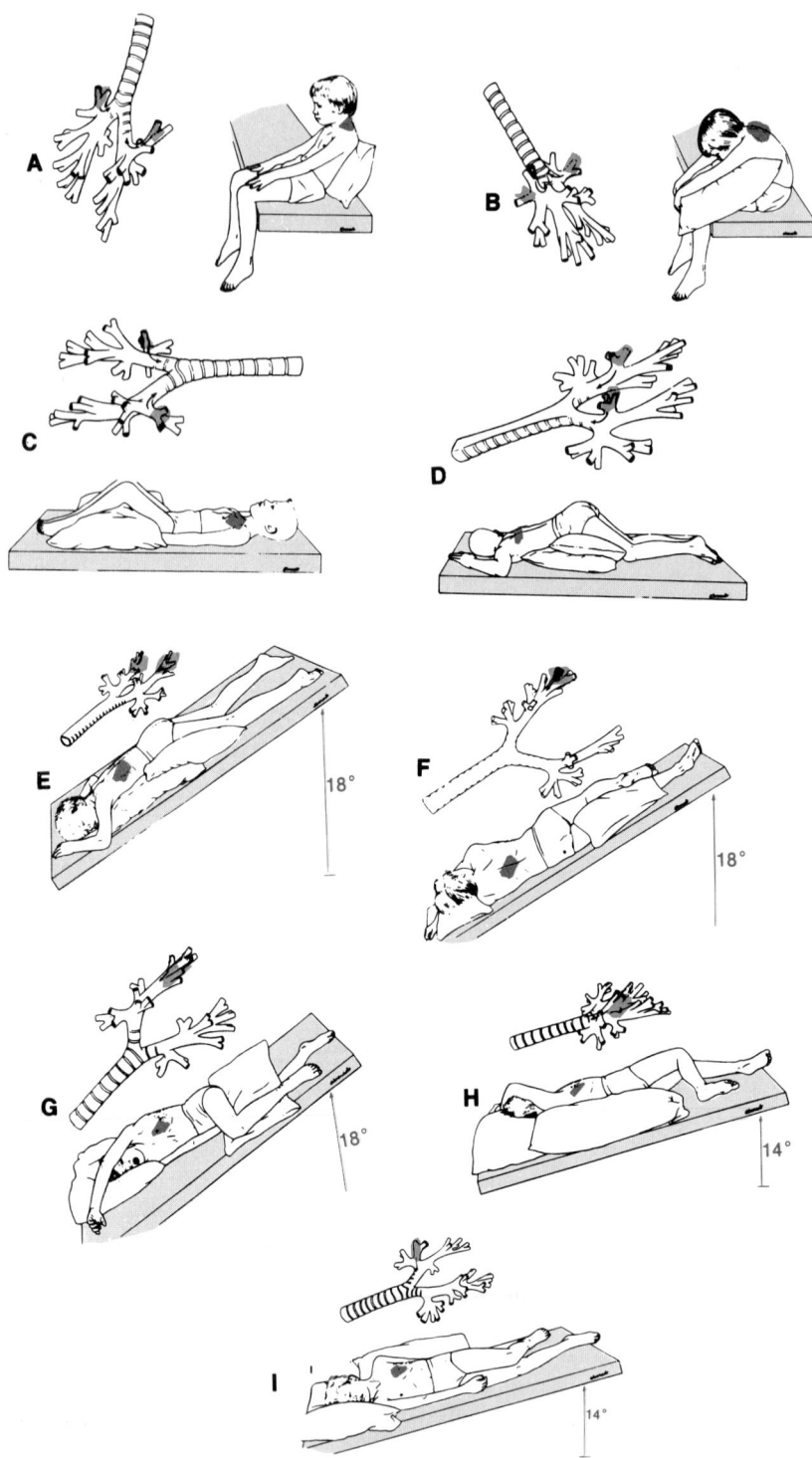

FIG. 22-30. Bronchial drainage positions for all major segments of child. For each position, model of tracheobronchial tree is projected beside child to show segmental bronchus *(striped)* being drained and pathway *(arrow)* of secretions out of bronchus. Drainage platform is horizontal unless otherwise noted. Striped area on child's chest indicates area to be cupped or vibrated by therapist. **A,** Apical segment of right upper lobe and apical subsegment of apical-posterior segment of left upper lobe. **B,** Posterior segment of right upper lobe and posterior subsegment of apical-posterior segment of left upper lobe. **C,** Anterior segments of both upper lobes; child should be rotated slightly away from side being drained. **D,** Superior segments of both lower lobes. **E,** Posterior basal segments of both lower lobes. **F,** Lateral basal segments of right lower lobe; left lateral basal segment would be drained by mirror image of this position (right side down). **G,** Anterior basal segment of left lower lobe; right anterior basal segment would be drained by mirror image of this position (left side down). **H,** Medial and lateral segments of right middle lobe. **I,** Lingular segments (superior and inferior) of left upper lobe (homologue of right middle lobe). (From Chernick V, editor: *Kendig's disorders of the respiratory tract of children*, ed 5, Philadelphia, 1990, Saunders.)

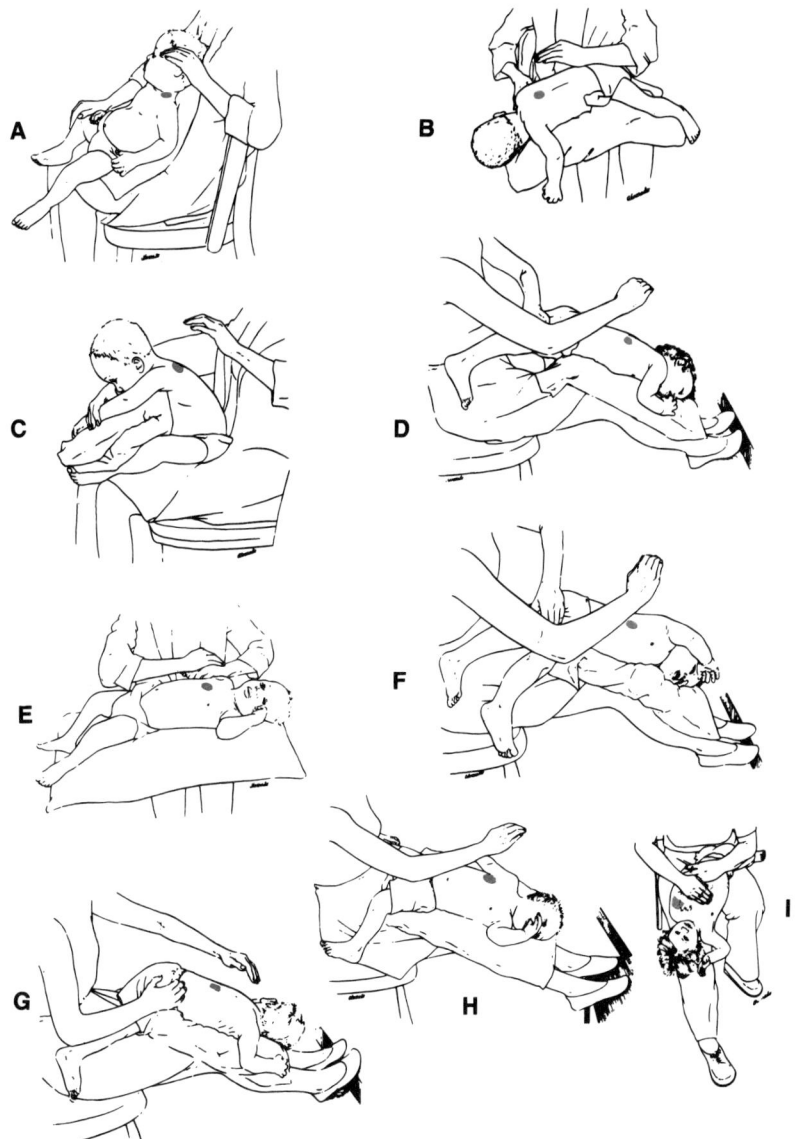

FIG. 22-31. Bronchial drainage positions for major segments of all lobes in infant. Procedure is most easily carried out in therapist's lap. Therapist's hand on chest indicates area to be cupped or vibrated. **A,** Apical segment of left upper lobe. **B,** Posterior segment of left upper lobe. **C,** Anterior segment of left upper lobe. **D,** Superior segment of right lower lobe. **E,** Posterior basal segment of right lower lobe. **F,** Lateral basal segment of right lower lobe. **G,** Anterior basal segment of right lower lobe. **H,** Medial and lateral segments of right middle lobe. **I,** Lingular segments (superior and inferior) of left upper lobe. (Modified from Cystic Fibrosis Foundation: *Infant segmental bronchial drainage,* Rockville, MD, The Foundation.)

an airtight seal. Air or gas delivered directly to the trachea must be humidified as in tracheostomy.

Tracheostomy

A tracheostomy is a surgical opening in the trachea; the procedure may be done on an emergency basis or may be an elective one, and it may be combined with mechanical ventilation.

Pediatric tracheostomy tubes are usually made of plastic or Silastic (Fig. 22-33). These tubes are constructed with a more acute angle than adult tubes, and they soften at body temperature, conforming to the contours of the trachea.

Since these materials resist the formation of crusted respiratory secretions, they are made without an inner cannula. Some children require a metal tracheostomy tube (usually made of sterling silver or stainless steel), which contains an inner cannula.

Children who have undergone a tracheostomy require a 7- to 10-day hospital stay. During this time the child is closely monitored for the development of complications such as hemorrhage, edema, aspiration, and the entrance of free air into the pleural cavity. The focus of postoperative nursing care is maintaining a patent airway, facilitating the removal of pulmonary secretions, providing humidified air or O_2, cleansing

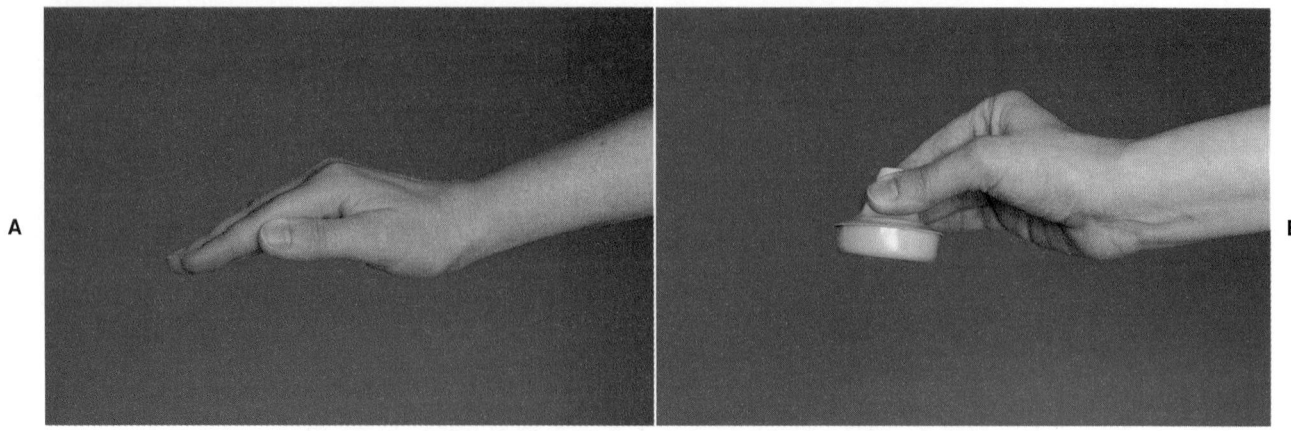

FIG. 22-32. A, Cupped hand position for percussion. **B,** Device for infant percussion.

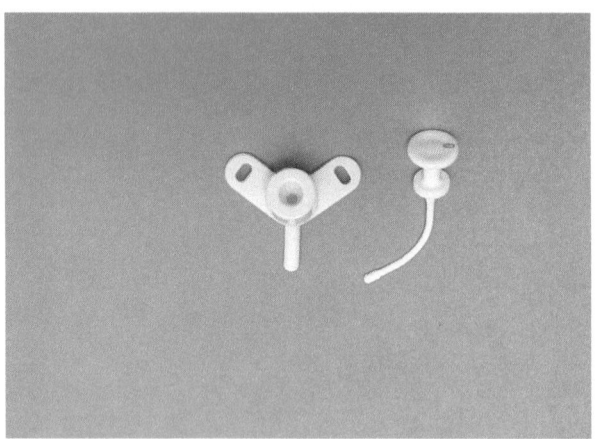

FIG. 22-33. Silastic pediatric tracheostomy tube and obdurator.

the stoma, monitoring the child's ability to swallow, and teaching while simultaneously preventing complications, the most dangerous being related to accidental decannulation and tube obstruction. Since the child may be unable to signal for help, direct observation and use of respiratory and cardiac monitors is essential. Respiratory assessments include breath sounds and work of breathing, vital signs, tightness of the tracheostomy ties, and the type and amount of secretions. Large amounts of bloody secretions are uncommon and should be considered a sign of hemorrhage. The practitioner should be notified immediately if this occurs.

The child is positioned with the head of the bed raised or in the position most comfortable to the child, with the call light easily available. Suction catheters, suction source, gloves, sterile saline, sterile gauze for wiping away secretions, scissors, an extra tracheostomy tube of the same size with ties already attached, another tracheostomy tube one size smaller, and the obturator are kept at the bedside. A source of humidification is provided, since the normal humidification and filtering functions of the airway have been bypassed. Intravenous fluids ensure adequate hydration until the child is able to swallow sufficient amounts of fluids.

Suctioning. The airway must remain patent and requires frequent suctioning during the first few hours after a tracheostomy to remove mucous plugs and excessive secretions. Proper vacuum pressure and suction catheter size are important to prevent atelectasis and decrease hypoxia from the suctioning procedure. Vacuum pressure should range from 60 to 100 mm Hg for infants and children and from 40 to 60 mm Hg for premature infants. Unless secretions are thick and tenacious, the lower range of negative pressure is recommended. Tracheal suction catheters are available in a variety of sizes. The catheter selected should have a diameter one-half the diameter of the tracheostomy tube. If the catheter is too large, it can block the airway. The catheter is constructed with a side port so that the catheter is introduced without suction and removed while simultaneous intermittent suction is applied by covering the port with the thumb (Fig. 22-34). The catheter is inserted to 0.5 cm beyond or just to the end of the tracheostomy tube. A small amount of sterile isotonic saline (a few drops to 0.5 to 2 ml, depending on the child's size) injected into the tube may help loosen secretions and crusts for easier aspiration, although the value of this practice is unproved. Only sterile saline without preservatives can be used (see Thinking Critically About . . . box).

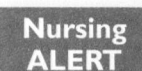 **Nursing ALERT** Suctioning should require no more than 5 seconds (Chandra and Hazinski, 1994).

Counting 1—one thousand, 2—one thousand, 3—one thousand, and so on while suctioning is a simple means for monitoring the time. Without a safeguard the airway may be obstructed for too long a period. Hyperventilating the child with 100% O_2 before and after suctioning (using a bag-valve-mask or increasing the FiO_2 [fraction of inspired oxygen concentration] ventilator setting) is also performed to prevent hypoxia. Closed tracheal suctioning systems that allow for uninterrupted O_2 delivery may also be used.

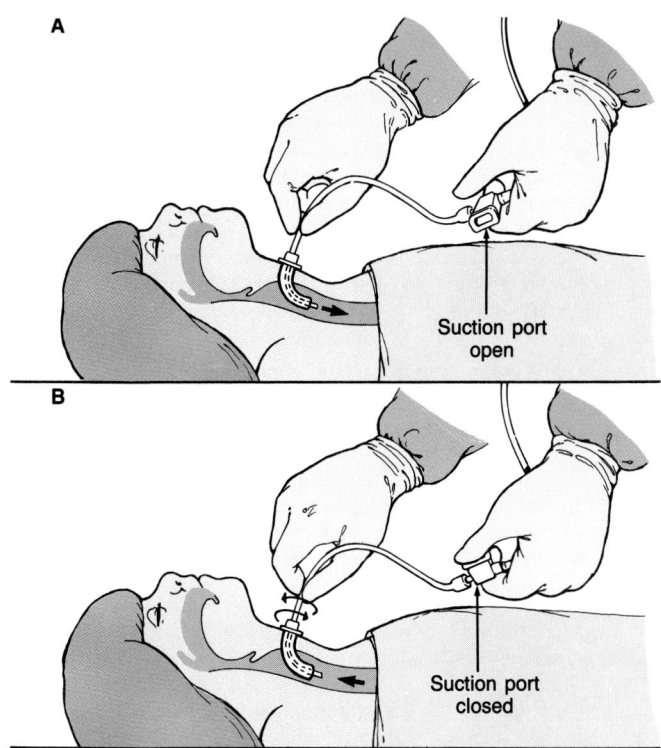

FIG. 22-34. Tracheostomy suctioning. **A,** Insertion, port open. **B,** Withdrawal, port occluded. Note that catheter is inserted just slightly beyond end of tracheostomy tube.

THINKING CRITICALLY ABOUT...
Suctioning, Catheter Length,
and Saline

Traditional technique for suctioning endotracheal (ET) or tracheostomy tubes recommends advancing a suction catheter into the tube until it meets resistance, then withdrawing it slightly and applying suction. However, studies indicate that this approach causes trauma to the tracheobronchial wall. This trauma can be avoided by inserting the catheter and advancing it to the premeasured depth of just to the tip (especially in infants) or no more than 0.5 cm beyond the tube (Kleiber, Krutzfield, and Rose, 1988).

Calibrated catheters are easier to use for premeasured suctioning technique, but unmarked catheters can also be used. To measure the length for catheter insertion, place the catheter near a sample ET or tracheostomy tube (same size as child's tube) with the end of the catheter at the correct position. Grasp the catheter with a sterile-gloved hand to mark the length, and insert the catheter until the hand reaches the stoma.

It has been common practice to instill a bolus of normal saline into the tube before suctioning. However, this technique may contribute to lower airway colonization and nosocomial pneumonia through repeated washing of organisms from the tube's surface into the lower airway (Hagler and Traver, 1994). Also, the use of saline has been shown to *decrease* the SaO_2 more than when it is not used in adults (Ackerman, 1993). In infants, one study showed that saline did not cause a significant change in SaO_2 (Shorten, Byrne, and Jones, 1991). More research is needed to demonstrate the value of instilling saline in the tube.

Nursing ALERT Suctioning is carried out *only as often as needed* to keep the tube patent. Signs of mucus partially occluding the airway include an increased heart rate, a rise in respiratory effort, a drop in SaO_2, cyanosis, or an increase in the positive inspiratory pressure (PIP) on the ventilator (Musser, 1992).

The child is allowed to rest for 30 to 60 seconds after each aspiration to allow O_2 tension to return to normal; then the process is repeated until the trachea is clear. Suctioning should be limited to about three aspirations in one period. Oximetry is used to monitor suctioning and prevent hypoxia.

In the acute care setting, aseptic technique is used during care of the tracheostomy. Secondary infection is a major concern, since the air entering the lower airway bypasses the natural defenses of the upper airway. Gloves are worn during the aspiration procedure, although a sterile glove is needed only on the hand touching the catheter. A new tube, gloves, and sterile saline solution are used each time (see Critical Thinking Exercise on p. 736).

Routine Care. The tracheostomy stoma requires daily care. Assessments of the stoma area include observations for signs of infection and breakdown of the skin. The skin is kept clean and dry, and secretions around the stoma may be gently removed with half-strength hydrogen peroxide. Hydrogen peroxide should not be used with sterling silver tracheostomy tubes because it tends to pit and stain the silver surface. The nurse should be aware of wet tracheostomy dressings, which can predispose the peristomal area to skin breakdown. Several products are available to prevent or treat excoriation. The Allevyn tracheostomy dressing is a hydrophilic sponge with a polyurethane back that is highly absorptive. Other possible barriers to help maintain skin integrity include the use of hydrocolloid wafers (e.g., Duoderm CGF, Hollister Restore) under the tracheostomy flanges, as well as use of extra-thin hydrocolloid wafers under the chin.

The tracheostomy tube is held in place with tracheostomy ties made of a durable, nonfraying material. The ties are changed daily and when soiled. New ties are looped through the flanges and tied snugly in a triple knot at the side of the neck *before* the soiled ties are cut and removed. Some nurses have found that threading the ties through a piece of ¼-inch surgical tubing cushions the ties; others have found the tubing to be irritating to the skin. The ties should be tight enough to allow just a fingertip to be inserted between the ties and the neck (Fig. 22-35). It is easier to ensure a snug fit if the child's head is flexed rather than extended while ties are being secured. Ties fastened with self-adhering closures are also available. These devices, such as the Dale tracheostomy tube holder, are made of a soft, cushioning, and slightly stretchy material that is very comfortable. They are becoming increasingly popular because of their ease of use and ability to maintain better skin integrity. One should still be aware, however, of the safety factor and use them on children who are unlikely to pull and undo the fastener.

Routine tracheostomy tube changes are usually carried out weekly after a tract has been formed to minimize formation of granulation tissue. The first change is usually performed by the surgeon; subsequent changes are performed by the

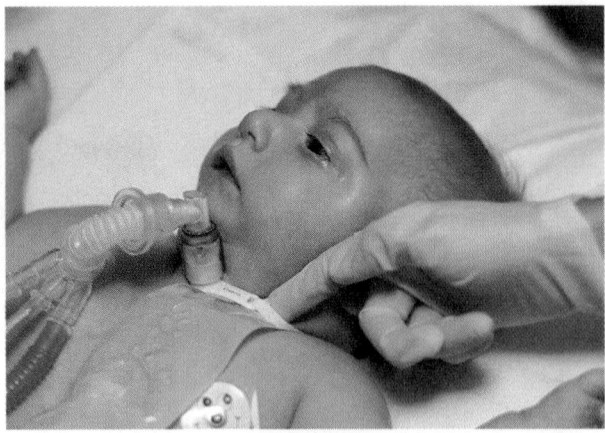

FIG. 22-35. Tracheostomy ties are snug but allow one finger to be inserted.

nurse and, if the child is discharged home with the tracheostomy, by either a parent or a visiting nurse. Ideally, two caregivers participate in the procedure to assist with positioning the child.

Changing the tracheostomy tube is accomplished using sterile technique. The new, sterile tube is prepared by inserting the obturator and attaching new ties. The child is suctioned before the procedure to minimize secretions, then restrained and positioned with the neck slightly extended. One caregiver cuts the old ties and removes the tube from the stoma. The new tube is inserted gently into the stoma (using a downward and forward motion that follows the curve of the trachea), the obturator is removed, and the ties are secured. The adequacy of ventilation must be assessed after a tube change because the tube can be inserted into the soft tissue surrounding the trachea; therefore breath sounds and respiratory effort are carefully monitored.

Supplemental O_2 is always delivered with a humidification system to prevent drying of the respiratory mucosa. Humidification of room air for an established tracheostomy can be intermittent if secretions remain thin enough to be coughed or suctioned from the tracheostomy. Direct humidification via tracheostomy mask can be provided during naps and at night so that the child is able to be up and around unencumbered during much of the day. Room humidifiers are also used successfully.

The inner cannula, if used, should be removed with each suctioning, cleaned with sterile saline and pipe cleaners to remove crusted material, dried thoroughly, and reinserted.

Emergency Care: Tube Occlusion and Accidental Decannulation. Occlusion of the tracheostomy tube is life-threatening, and infants and children are at greater risk than adults because of the smaller diameter of the tube. Maintaining patency of the tube is accomplished with suctioning and routine tube changes to prevent formation of crusts that can occlude the tube.

> **Nursing ALERT** Life-threatening occlusion is apparent when the child displays signs of respiratory distress and a suction catheter cannot be passed to the end of the tube despite several attempts and instillation of saline. This situation requires an immediate tube change.

Accidental decannulation also requires immediate tube replacement. Some children have a fairly rigid trachea, so the airway remains partially open when the tube is removed. However, others have malformed or flexible tracheal cartilage, which causes the airway to collapse when the tube is removed or dislodged. Since many infants and children with upper airway problems have little airway reserve, if replacement of the dislodged tube is impossible, a smaller-sized tube should be inserted. If the stoma cannot be cannulated with another tracheostomy tube, oral intubation should be performed.

FAMILY TEACHING AND HOME CARE

Some of the treatments families need to continue at home are often related to respiratory procedures. Some of these treatments, such as postural drainage, require less preparation than others, such as tracheostomy care. Regardless of the home therapy, the family needs ample time to learn the skills and demonstrate them before discharge; therefore instruction should begin as soon as it is identified that the child will go home with a tracheostomy. The more comfortable they are with all the aspects of care, the more confident and less anxious the family will be when faced with total care of the child at home. For example, the family may require many practice sessions before they feel comfortable with suctioning, cleaning, and changing a tracheostomy tube and performing cardiopulmonary resuscitation (CPR) in case of an emergency. Teaching sessions should be short, and written material must accompany instructions to reinforce what is being taught.* To facilitate the family's adjustment, supplies identical to the ones to which they are accustomed should be available in the home. In the event of substitution, parents need to be reassured that the unfamiliar equipment is safe to use on their child. The home should be properly equipped with all supplies and equipment needed before the child arrives.

A nurse from the public health department or other home care service should be available to the family and should periodically assess the family's ability to carry out the activities needed in care of the child. The parents may find it helpful to talk to other parents of children with similar needs. They also need to know whom to call and where they can get help and support in times of uncertainty or in an emergency.

To prepare for any emergency, the family must be taught infant or child CPR. The local utilities company and local emergency medical services (EMS) should be notified of the child's condition and the equipment used in the home. Prior notification allows for a quicker response if help is needed.

When a child has a tracheostomy, parents are encouraged to provide as normal a life as possible for their child and other family members. The child who is physically able (e.g., a child with a tracheostomy without respiratory disability such as recurrent laryngeal polyps) can usually be allowed to engage in most activities that are appropriate for the child's age. The child may play outdoors with a scarf or other protection to loosely cover the tracheostomy stoma. Both child and parents must be cautioned regarding play near any body of water, such as a swimming pool or stream, and informed about safety precautions in the bathtub. The child should not be exposed to noxious fumes (e.g., paint, varnish, hair spray) or talc (baby powder). Young children who may spill food near the stoma should wear a fabric bib (without plastic lining) or other device to prevent dribbled food or crumbs from being aspirated. The family should have a bag with routine and emergency supplies to take with the child at all times.

PROCEDURES RELATED TO ALTERNATIVE FEEDING TECHNIQUES

Some children are unable to take nourishment by mouth because of conditions such as anomalies of the throat, esophagus, or bowel; impaired swallowing capacity; severe debilita-

tion; respiratory distress; or unconsciousness. These children are frequently fed by way of a tube inserted orally or nasally into the stomach (**orogastric** or **nasogastric gavage**) or duodenum/jejunum (**enteral gavage**) or by a tube inserted directly into the stomach (**gastrostomy**) or jejunum (**jejunostomy**). Such feedings may be intermittent or by continuous drip. At times the entire alimentary tract must be bypassed, using intravenous (IV) feeding (total parenteral nutrition [TPN]). Because enteral feedings are used less often than gastric or IV feedings, the following discussion is limited to gastric gavage, gastrostomy, and TPN.

Feeding resistance, a problem that may result from any long-term feeding method that bypasses the mouth, is discussed in Chapter 9. During nonoral feedings, infants are given a pacifier; nonnutritive sucking has several advantages, such as increased weight gain and decreased crying. However, to prevent the possibility of aspiration, only pacifiers with a safe design may be used. Using improvised pacifiers made from bottle nipples is not a safe practice.

> **Nursing ALERT**
>
> When a child is concurrently receiving continuous-drip gastric or enteral feedings and parenteral (IV) therapy, the potential exists for inadvertent administration of the enteral formula through the circulatory system, especially when the parenteral solution is a fat emulsion, which looks milky. Safeguards to prevent this potentially serious error include the following (Garvin and Franck, 1989):
> Use a separate, specifically designed enteral feeding pump mounted on a separate pole for continuous-feeding solutions.
> Label all tubing for continuous enteral feeding with brightly colored tape or labels.
> Use specifically designed continuous-feeding bags to contain the solutions instead of parenteral equipment, such as a burette.

GAVAGE FEEDING

Infants and children can be fed simply and safely by a tube passed into the stomach through either the nares or the mouth. The tube can be left in place or inserted and removed with each feeding. In older children it is usually less traumatic to tape the tube securely in place between feedings. When this alternative is used, the tube should be removed and replaced with a new tube according to hospital policy, specific orders, and the type of tube used. Meticulous handwashing is practiced during the procedure to prevent bacterial contamination of the feeding, especially during continuous-drip feedings.

Preparation

The equipment needed for gavage feeding includes the following:

1. A suitable tube selected according to the size of the child and the viscosity of the solution being fed. Feeding tubes are available in silicone rubber, polyurethane, polyethylene, or polyvinylchloride. Polyurethane and silicone rubber tubes are smaller in diameter and more flexible than the others and are often referred to as small-bore tubes.
2. A receptacle for the fluid; for small amounts a 10 to 30 ml syringe barrel or Asepto syringe is satisfactory; for larger amounts a 50 ml syringe with a catheter tip is more convenient.
3. A syringe to aspirate stomach contents and/or to inject air after the tube has been placed.

---

*Home care instructions for tracheostomy care, postural drainage, and CPR are available in Wong DL: *Wong and Whaley's Clinical manual of pediatric nursing,* ed 4, St Louis, 1996, Mosby.

4. Water or water-soluble lubricant to lubricate the tube; sterile water is used for infants.
5. Paper or nonallergenic tape to mark the tube and to attach the tube to the infant's or child's cheek (and nose, if placed through the nares).
6. A stethoscope to determine the correct placement in the stomach.
7. The solution for feeding.

Not all feeding tubes are the same. Polyethylene and polyvinylchloride types lose their flexibility and need to be replaced frequently, usually every 3 to 4 days. The polyurethane and silicone rubber tubes are indwelling and remain flexible so that they can remain in place longer and afford more patient comfort. Use of these small-bore tubes for continuous feeding has greatly reduced the incidence of complications, such as pharyngitis, otitis media, and incompetence of the lower esophageal sphincter. Although the increased softness and flexibility of the tubes are advantages, they also cause disadvantages, such as difficult insertion (may require a stylet or metal guide wire), collapse of the tube during aspiration of gastric contents when testing for correct placement, dislodgment during forceful coughing, and unsuitability for thick feedings. Traditional methods for verifying placement are less reliable with the small-bore tubes.

Procedure

Infants will be easier to control if they are first wrapped in a mummy restraint (see Fig. 22-9). Even tiny infants with random movements can grasp and dislodge the tube. Premature infants do not ordinarily require restraint, but if they do, a small towel folded across the chest and secured beneath the shoulders is usually sufficient. Care must be taken so that breathing is not compromised.

Whenever possible, the infant should be held during the procedure to associate the comfort of physical contact with the feeding. When this is not possible, gavage feeding is carried out with the infant or child on the back or toward the right side and the head and chest elevated. Feeding the child

---

GUIDELINES
Nasogastric Tube Feedings in Children

Place the child supine with head slightly hyperflexed or in a sniffing position (nose pointed toward ceiling).

Measure the tube for approximate length of insertion, and mark the point with a small piece of tape.

Insert the tube that has been lubricated with sterile water or water-soluble lubricant through either the mouth or one of the nares to the predetermined mark. Since most young infants are obligatory nose breathers, insertion through the mouth causes less distress and helps to stimulate sucking. In older infants and children the tube is passed through the nose and alternated between nostrils. An indwelling tube is almost always placed through the nose.

When using the nose, slip the tube along the base of the nose and direct it straight back toward the occiput.

When entering through the mouth, direct the tube toward the back of the throat (Fig. 22-36, *B*).

If the child is able to swallow on command, synchronize passing the tube with swallowing.

Check the position of the tube by using *both* the following:

Attach the syringe to the feeding tube and apply negative pressure. Aspiration of stomach contents indicates proper placement, but aspiration of respiratory secretions may be mistaken for stomach contents. However, absence of fluid is not necessarily evidence of improper placement. The stomach may be empty, the tube may not be in contact with stomach contents, or a small-bore flexible tube may collapse. Note the amount and character of any fluid aspirated and return the fluid to the stomach.

With the syringe, inject a small amount of air (0.5 to 1 ml in premature or very small infants to 5 ml in larger children) into the tube while simultaneously listening with a stethoscope over the stomach area. Sounds of gurgling or growling will be heard if the tube is properly situated in the stomach, although it is possible to hear the air entering the stomach even when the tube is positioned above the gastroesophageal sphincter.

Stabilize the tube by holding or taping it to the cheek, not to the forehead, because of possible damage to the nostril. To maintain correct placement, measure and record the amount of tubing extending from the nose or mouth to the distal port when the tube is first positioned. Recheck this measurement before each feeding.

Warm the formula to room temperature. Pour formula into the barrel of the syringe attached to the feeding tube. To start the flow, give a gentle push with the plunger, but then remove the plunger and allow the fluid to flow into the stomach by gravity. The rate of flow should not exceed 5 ml every 5 to 10 minutes in premature and very small infants and 10 ml/minute in older infants and children to prevent nausea and regurgitation. The rate is determined by the diameter of the tubing and the height of the reservoir containing the feeding and is regulated by adjusting the height of the syringe. A usual feeding may take from 15 to 30 minutes to complete.

Flush the tube with sterile water (1 or 2 ml for small tubes to 5 to 15 ml or more for large ones), or see discussion of flushing for administering medication through nasogastric tubes in the Guidelines box on p. 722 to clear it of formula.

Cap or clamp indwelling tubes to prevent loss of feeding.

If the tube is to be removed, first pinch it firmly to prevent escape of fluid as the tube is withdrawn. Withdraw the tube quickly.

Position the child on the right side or abdomen for at least 1 hour in the same manner as following any infant feeding to minimize the possibility of regurgitation and aspiration. If the child's condition permits, bubble the youngster after the feeding.

Record the feeding, including the type and amount of residual, the type and amount of formula, and how it was tolerated. For most infant feedings, any amount of residual fluid aspirated from the stomach is refed to prevent electrolyte imbalance, and the amount is subtracted from the prescribed amount of feeding. For example, if the infant is to receive 30 ml and 10 ml is aspirated from the stomach before the feeding, the 10 ml of aspirated stomach contents is refed plus 20 ml of feeding. Another method can be used in children. If residual is more than one fourth of the last feeding, return the aspirate and recheck in 30 to 60 minutes. When residual is less than one fourth of the last feeding, give scheduled feeding. If high aspirates persist and the child is due for another feeding, notify the practitioner.

in a sitting position helps maintain the placement of the tube in the lowest position, thus increasing the likelihood of correct placement in the stomach.

The feeding tube can be passed through either the nose (nasogastric) or the mouth (orogastric). Since most young infants are obligatory nose breathers, insertion through the mouth causes less distress and helps to stimulate sucking. A tube passed through one of the nares in older infants and children is satisfactory once the tube is in place. An indwelling tube is almost always placed through the nose; the tube is alternated between nares with each insertion to minimize irritation, chance of infection, and possible breakdown of mucous membranes from pressure that occurs over time. The procedure for gavage feeding is described in the Guidelines box.

Two standard methods of measuring tube length for insertion are (1) measuring from the nose to the bottom of the earlobe and then to the end of the xiphoid process or (2) measuring from the nose to the earlobe and then to a point midway between the xiphoid process and the umbilicus (Fig. 22-36, *A*). However, research on using these methods in infants and children has cast serious doubt on their accuracy (Weibley and others, 1987). Studies have shown that height as a predictor of gastric tube insertion distance may provide a more valid measurement method (Ellett and others, 1992). For very-low-birth-weight infants, daily weight can be used to predict insertion length (Table 22-4).

Unfortunately, "bedside" methods used to verify the placement of the tube have serious shortcomings (see box). The only accurate method for testing tube placement is radi-

ography, but this practice is not feasible before each feeding. One method that appears promising is pH testing of aspirated fluid, since respiratory, gastric, and intestinal fluid have a different pH (Metheny and others, 1989). Until pH is studied further, especially in children, nurses need to use the traditional methods with an awareness of their limitations. If doubt exists regarding correct placement, the practitioner should be consulted.

GASTROSTOMY FEEDING

Feeding by way of a gastrostomy tube is a variation of tube feeding that is often used for children in whom passage of a tube through the mouth, pharynx, esophagus, and cardiac sphincter of the stomach is contraindicated or impossible. It is also used to avoid the constant irritation of a gastric tube in children who require tube feeding over an extended period. Placement of a gastrostomy tube may be performed with the patient under general anesthesia or percutaneously using an endoscope with the patient sedated and under local anesthesia. The tube is inserted through the abdominal wall into the stomach about midway along the greater curvature and when surgically placed is secured by a purse-string suture. The stomach is anchored to the peritoneum at the operative site. The tube used can be a Foley, wing-tip, or mushroom catheter.

Immediately after surgery the catheter is left open and attached to gravity drainage for 24 hours or more. Postoperative care of the wound site is directed toward prevention of infection and irritation. The area is cleansed at least daily or as often as needed to keep the area free of drainage. After

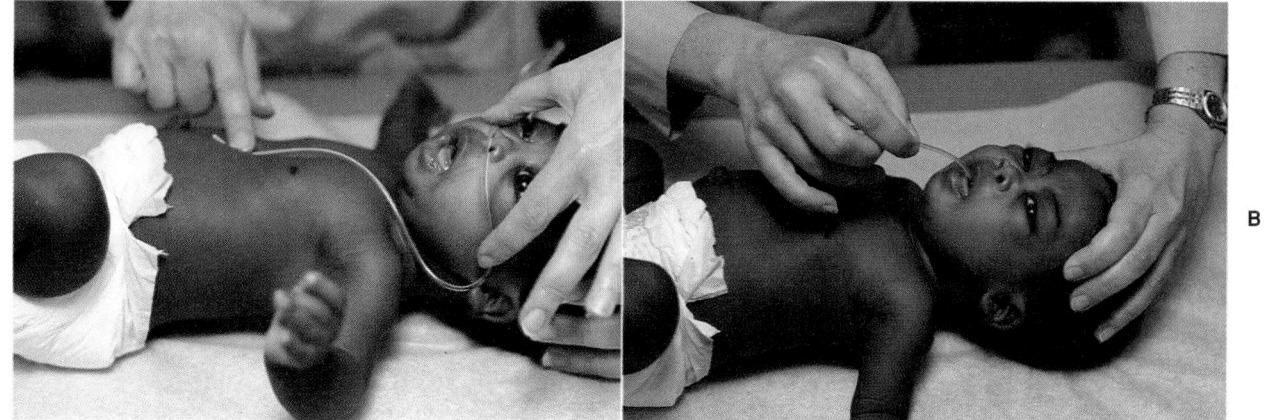

FIG. 22-36. Gavage feeding. **A,** Measuring tube for orogastric feeding from tip of nose to earlobe and to midpoint between end of xiphoid process and umbilicus. **B,** Inserting tube.

TABLE 22-4. Recommended minimum insertion lengths for orogastric tubes in very-low-birth-weight infants

	DAILY WEIGHT (g)			
	<750	750-999	1000-1249	1250-1499
Insertion length (cm)	13	15	16	17

From Gallaher KJ and others: Orogastric tube insertion length in very-low-birth-weight infants (<1500 grams), *J Perinatol* 13(2):128-131, 1993.

healing takes place, meticulous care is needed to keep the area surrounding the tube clean and dry to prevent excoriation and infection. Daily applications of antibiotic ointment or other preparations may be prescribed to aid in healing and prevention of irritation. Care is exercised to prevent excessive pull on the catheter that might cause widening of the opening and subsequent leakage of highly irritating gastric juices.

For children receiving long-term gastrostomy feeding, a skin-level device (e.g., MIC-KEY, Bard Button, Gastroport) offers several advantages. The small, flexible silicone device protrudes slightly from the abdomen, is cosmetically pleasing in appearance, affords increased comfort and mobility to the child, is easy to care for, and is fully immersible in water. The one-way valve at the proximal end minimizes reflux and eliminates the need for clamping. However, the button requires a well-established gastrostomy site and is more expensive than the conventional tube. In addition, the valve may become clogged. When functioning, the valve prevents air from escaping; therefore the child may require frequent bubbling. With some devices, during feedings the child must remain fairly still, since the tubing easily disconnects from the opening if the child moves. With other devices, extension tubing can be securely attached to the opening (Fig. 22-37). The feeding is instilled at the other end of the tubing in a manner similar to that for a regular gastrostomy. The extension tubing may also have a separate medication port. Both the feeding and the medication ports have plugs attached. Some skin-level devices require a special tube to allow one to decompress the stomach (to check residual or decompress air).

Positioning and feeding of water, formula, or pureed foods are carried out in the same manner and rate as in gavage feeding. After feedings the infant or child is positioned on the right side or in Fowler position, and the tube may be clamped, left open, and suspended between feedings, depending on the child's condition. A clamped tube allows more mobility but is appropriate only if the child can tolerate intermittent feedings without vomiting or prolonged backup of feeding into the tube. Sometimes a Y tube is used to allow for simultaneous decompression during feeding. If a Foley catheter is used as the gastrostomy tube, very slight tension is applied and the tube is securely taped to maintain the balloon at the gastrostomy opening and to prevent leakage of gastric contents and the tube's progression toward the pyloric sphincter, where it may occlude the stomach outlet. As a precaution, the length of the tube should be measured postoperatively and then remeasured each shift to be sure it has not slipped. A mark can be made above the skin level to further ensure its placement. When the gastrostomy tube is no longer needed, it is removed; the skin opening usually closes spontaneously by contracture.

TOTAL PARENTERAL NUTRITION (TPN)

TPN, also known as *intravenous alimentation* or *hyperalimentation,* provides for the total nutritional needs of infants or children whose lives are threatened because feeding by way of the gastrointestinal tract is impossible, inadequate, or hazardous.

Hyperalimentation therapy involves IV infusion of highly concentrated solutions of protein, glucose, and other nutrients. The hyperalimentation solution is infused through conventional tubing with a special filter attached to remove particulate matter or microorganisms that may have contaminated the solution. The highly concentrated solutions require infusion into a vessel with sufficient volume and turbulence to allow for rapid dilution. The wide-diameter vessels selected are the superior vena cava and innominate or intrathoracic subclavian veins approached by way of the external or internal jugular veins. The highly irritating nature of concentrated glucose precludes the use of the small peripheral veins in most instances. However, dilute glucose-protein hydrolysates that are appropriate for infusing into peripheral veins are being used with increasing frequency. When peripheral veins are used, intralipid becomes the major calorie source. For long-term alimentation, venous access devices (VADs) are usually used (see p. 720).

The major nursing responsibilities are the same as for any IV therapy: control of sepsis, monitoring of the infusion rate, and continuous observations. The TPN solution must be prepared under rigid aseptic conditions best accomplished by specially trained technicians. The solution and tubing are changed and the infusion site redressed by specially trained nurses using meticulous aseptic precautions. In some institutions this may be a nursing responsibility. If so, the procedure is carried out according to hospital protocol.

The infusion is maintained at a slow, uniform rate by means of a constant infusion pump to ensure the proper concentrations of glucose and amino acids. Accurate calculation of the rate is required to deliver a measured amount in a given length of time. Since alterations in flow rate are relatively common, the drip should be checked frequently to ensure

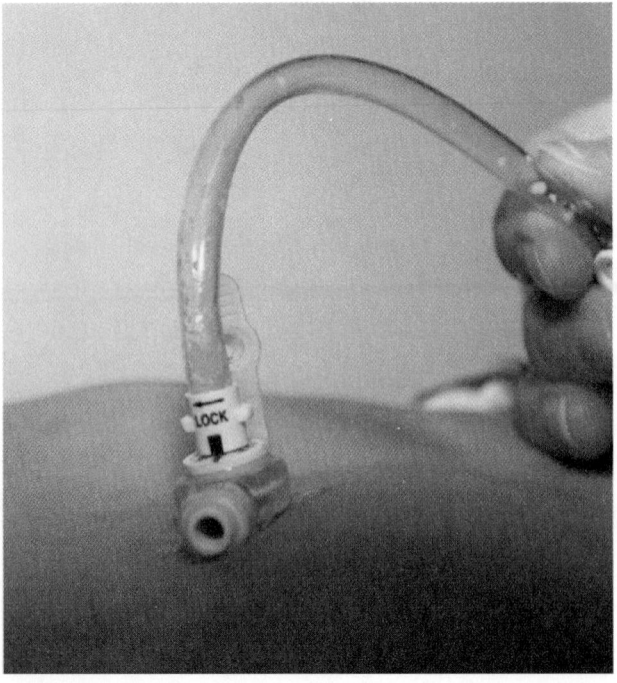

FIG. 22-37. Child with skin-level gastrostomy device (MIC-KEY), which provides for secure attachment of extension tubing to gastrostomy opening.

an even, continuous infusion. The hyperalimentation infusion rate should not be increased or decreased without the practitioner being informed, since alterations can cause hyperglycemia or hypoglycemia.

General assessments, such as vital signs, intake and output measurements, and checking results of laboratory tests facilitate early detection of infection or fluid and electrolyte imbalance. Additional amounts of potassium and sodium chloride are often required in hyperalimentation; therefore observation for signs of potassium or sodium deficit or excess is part of nursing care. This is rarely a problem except in children with reduced renal function or metabolic defects. Hyperglycemia may occur during the first day or two as the child adapts to the high-glucose load of the hyperalimentation solution. Although occurring infrequently, insulin may be required to assist the body's adjustment to the hyperglycemia. When this occurs, nursing responsibilities include blood glucose testing. To prevent hypoglycemia at the time the hyperalimentation is disconnected, the rate of the infusion and the amount of insulin are decreased gradually.

In addition to children's physical needs, their developmental needs must also be considered during the often long-term use of TPN. Regular assessment of development should be performed to assess the child's progress, and appropriate interventions should be instituted to encourage expected milestones. Delays in the areas of gross motor and language skills are found most often; therefore special attention should be directed to these areas.

FAMILY TEACHING AND HOME CARE

When alternative feedings are needed for an extended period, the family may need to learn how to feed the child with a nasogastric, gastrostomy, or TPN feeding regimen. The same principles discussed earlier in this chapter for compliance, especially in terms of education (see p. 687), and in Chapter 21 for discharge planning and home care are applied.* Because of the numerous skills the family must learn for home TPN, ample time must be planned for the family to learn and perform the procedures under supervision before assuming full responsibility for the child's care.

The family may be referred to community agencies that provide support and practical assistance. The **Oley Foundation**† is a nonprofit research and education organization that assists persons receiving enteral nutrition and home TPN.

PROCEDURES RELATED TO ELIMINATION

ENEMA

The procedure for giving an enema to an infant or child does not differ essentially from that for an adult, except for the type and amount of fluid administered and the distance for

---

*Home care instructions for gavage and gastrostomy feeding are available in Wong DL: *Wong and Whaley's Clinical manual of pediatric nursing,* ed 4, St Louis, 1996, Mosby.
†214 Hun Memorial, A23, Albany Medical Center, Albany, NY 12208; (800) 776-OLEY.

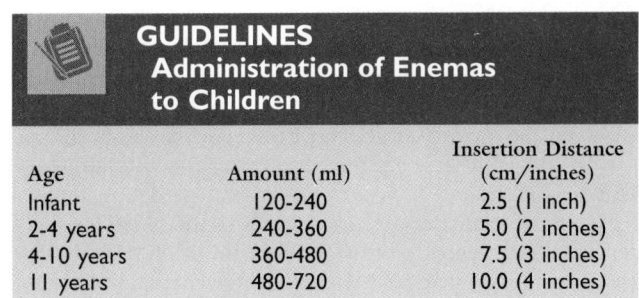

GUIDELINES
Administration of Enemas to Children

Age	Amount (ml)	Insertion Distance (cm/inches)
Infant	120-240	2.5 (1 inch)
2-4 years	240-360	5.0 (2 inches)
4-10 years	360-480	7.5 (3 inches)
11 years	480-720	10.0 (4 inches)

inserting the tube into the rectum. Depending on the volume, the nurse uses a syringe with rubber tubing, an enema bottle, or an enema bag (see Guidelines box).

Nursing ALERT Proper insertion of the catheter tip, especially in infants, is essential to prevent rectal damage and perforation (see Fig. 7-7, *B*). If insertion of the enema tip causes discomfort, remove the tip and notify the practitioner.

An isotonic solution is used in children. Plain water is not used because, being hypotonic, it can cause rapid fluid shift and fluid overload. The Fleet enema (pediatric or adult sized) is not advised for children because of the harsh action of its ingredients (sodium biphosphate and sodium phosphate). Commercial enemas can be dangerous to patients with megacolon and to dehydrated or azotemic children. The osmotic effect of the Fleet enema may produce diarrhea, which can lead to metabolic acidosis. Other potential complications are extreme hyperphosphatemia, hypernatremia, and hypocalcemia, which may lead to neuromuscular irritability and coma (McCabe, Sibert, and Routledge, 1991).

NURSING TIP If prepared saline is not available, it can be made by adding 1 tsp table salt to 500 ml (1 pint) tap water.

Since infants and young children are unable to retain the solution after it is administered, the buttocks must be held together for a short time to retain the fluid. The enema is administered and expelled while the child is lying with the buttocks over the bedpan and with the head and back supported by pillows. Older children are usually able to hold the solution if they understand what to do and if they are not expected to hold it for too long. The nurse should have the bedpan handy or, for the ambulatory child, ensure that the bathroom is readily available before beginning the procedure. An enema is an intrusive procedure and thus threatening to the preschool child; therefore a careful explanation is especially important to ease possible fear.

A preoperative bowel preparation solution given orally or through a nasogastric tube is increasingly being used instead of an enema. The polyethylene glycol–electrolyte lavage solution (Golytely) mechanically flushes the bowel without significant absorption, thereby avoiding potential fluid and electrolyte imbalances (Konings, 1989).*

---

*Home care instructions for giving an enema are available in Wong DL: *Wong and Whaley's Clinical manual of pediatric nursing,* ed 4, St Louis, 1996, Mosby.

OSTOMIES

Children may require stomas for various health problems. The most frequent causes are necrotizing enterocolitis and imperforate anus in the infant (less often, Hirschsprung disease). In the older child the most frequent causes are inflammatory bowel disease and ureterostomies for distal ureter or bladder defects.

Care and management of ostomies in the older child differ little from the care of ostomies in the adult patient. The major emphases in pediatric care are the preparation of the child for the procedure and teaching care of the ostomy to the child and family. The basic principles of preparation are the same as for any procedure (see p. 675). Simple, straightforward language is most effective, together with the use of illustrations and a replica model (e.g., drawing a picture of a child with a stoma on the abdomen and explaining it as "another opening where bowel movements [or any other term the child uses] will come out"). At another time the nurse can draw a pouch over the opening to demonstrate how the contents are collected. Using a doll to demonstrate the process is an excellent teaching strategy, and special books are available.*

All children with ileostomies are fitted immediately after surgery with an appliance to protect the skin from the proteolytic enzymes in the liquid stool. Parents are usually given a choice of caring for the colostomy with or without an appliance. Pediatric appliances are available in a variety of sizes to ensure an adequate fit.†

Ostomy equipment consists of a one- or two-piece system with a hypoallergenic skin barrier to maintain peristomal skin integrity. The pouch should be large enough to contain a moderate amount of stool and flatus but not so large as to overwhelm the infant or child. A backing helps minimize the risk of skin breakdown from moisture trapped between the skin and pouch. Small clips or rubber bands should be avoided to prevent choking in the young child. Granulation tissue may grow around an ostomy site (Fig. 22-38). This moist, beefy red tissue is not a sign of infection. However, if it continues to grow, the excess moisture can cause irritation of the surrounding skin.

Protection of the peristomal skin is a major aspect of stoma care. Well-fitting appliances are important to prevent leakage of contents. Before the appliance is applied, the skin is prepared with a skin sealant that is allowed to dry. Then stoma paste is applied around the base of the stoma. The sealant and paste work together to prevent peristomal breakdown.

In infants with a colostomy left unpouched, skin care is similar to that of any diapered child. However, the peristomal skin is protected with a wafer barrier, such as a hydrocolloid dressing (e.g., Duoderm) or a barrier substance (e.g., zinc oxide ointment [Desitin], karaya products, or a mixture of the zinc oxide ointment and karaya powder). If the skin becomes inflamed, denuded, or infected, the care is similar to the interventions used for diaper dermatitis (see Chapter 30). A product that helps protect healthy skin, heal excoriated skin, and minimize pain associated with skin breakdown is

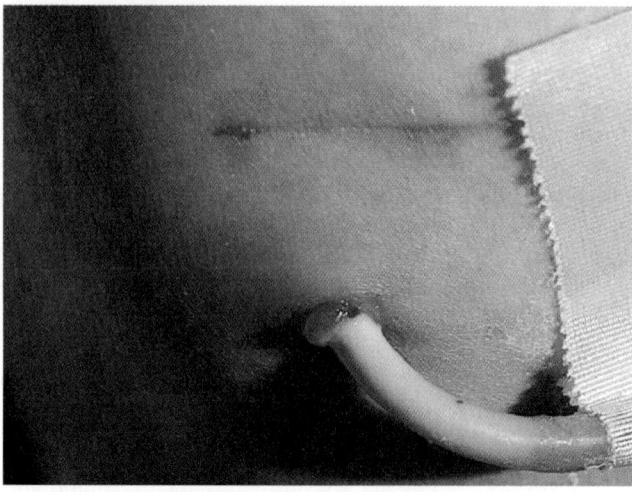

FIG. 22-38. Appearance of healthy granulation tissue around stoma.

Ilex Dermalytc Protective Barrier Ointment.* The ointment adheres to denuded weeping skin. It can be applied over topical antifungal and antibacterial agents if infection is present. If the infant is diapered, a coating of petrolatum is applied over the Ilex to prevent the gluteal creases and diaper from adhering to the ointment. When the area is cleaned, only the petrolatum is wiped off and reapplied. The Ilex is left intact to minimize trauma to the irritated skin. If Ilex is used under an appliance, an adhesive spray is applied over the ointment to help the appliance adhere.

With young children, protection of the pouch from being pulled off is also an important consideration. One-piece outfits keep exploring hands from reaching the pouch, and the loose waist prevents any pressure on the appliance. Keeping the child occupied with toys during the pouch change is also helpful. As children mature, their participation in ostomy care is encouraged. Even preschoolers can assist by holding supplies, pulling paper backings from the appliance, and helping clean the stoma area. Toilet training for bladder control needs to begin at the appropriate time as for any other child.

Older children and adolescents should eventually have total responsibility for ostomy care just as they would for usual bowel function. During adolescence, concerns for body image and the ostomy's impact on intimacy and sexuality emerge. The nurse should stress to teenagers that the presence of a stoma need not interfere with their activities. These youngsters can choose which ostomy equipment is best suited to their needs. Attractively designed and decorated pouch covers are well liked by teenagers.

FAMILY TEACHING AND HOME CARE

Since these children are almost always discharged with a functioning colostomy, preparation of the family should begin as early as possible in the hospital. The family is instructed in the application of the device (if used), care of the skin, and

---

Chris Has an Ostomy is available from **United Ostomy Association, Inc.,** 36 Executive Park, Suite 120, Irvine, CA 92714-6744; (800) 826-0826.
†Little Ones Ostomy Products, ConvaTec, CN 5254, Princeton, NJ 08543-5254; (800) 422-8811.

---

*Available from MEDCON Products, Inc., 50 Brigham Hill Rd., Grafton, MA 01519; (800) 443-6332.

instructions regarding appropriate action in case skin problems develop. Early evidence of skin breakdown or stomal complications, such as ribbonlike stools, excessive diarrhea, bleeding, prolapse, or failure to pass flatus or stool, is brought to the attention of the physician, the nurse, or the stoma specialist. The same principles are applied as discussed earlier in this chapter for compliance, especially in terms of education (see p. 687), and in Chapter 21 for discharge planning and home care.*

---

*Home care instructions on caring for a colostomy are available in Wong DL: *Wong and Whaley's Clinical manual of pediatric nursing,* ed 4, St Louis, 1996, Mosby.

KEY POINTS

- Informed consent is valid when the person is capable of giving consent (is over the age of majority and is competent), is supplied with information needed to make an intelligent decision, and acts voluntarily when exercising freedom of choice.
- Informed consent is needed for major surgery, minor surgery, and diagnostic tests and medical treatments with an element of risk.
- The major principles in psychologic preparation of the child for procedures are to establish trust, provide support, and give an explanation in easy-to-understand terms.
- In the performance of a procedure the nurse should expect success, involve the child when possible in the procedure, provide distraction, and allow for expression of feelings.
- In giving postprocedural support, the nurse should encourage the child to express feelings and praise the youngster for completion of the procedure.
- Assessment of compliance entails measuring factors that affect compliance through self-reporting, direct observation, monitoring appointments and therapeutic response, taking pill counts, and performing chemical assay.
- Compliance strategies may be classified as organizational, educational, treatment, and behavioral.
- Knowledge of the sick child's eating habits and favorite foods can help in maintaining adequate nutrition.
- Control of fever may be accomplished by pharmacologic means (administration of antipyretics); hyperthermia is controlled by environmental means (minimum clothing, increased air circulation, cool compresses).

- Infection control may be based on one of three basic systems: category-specific isolation precautions, disease-specific isolation precautions, or universal precautions. Only the system of universal precautions, especially body substance isolation, provides protection when the infected person is undiagnosed.
- Ensuring safety in the hospital setting is a major concern and can be achieved through environmental measures, limit-setting, and safe transportation.
- Common types of physical restraints for children are jacket, mummy, arm and leg, and elbow restraints.
- Factors that affect drug dosage determination are growth and maturation, difficulty in evaluating drug response, and body surface area.
- The preferred sites for intramuscular injection in children are the vastus lateralis and ventrogluteal areas.
- Intermittent venous access is accomplished by intermittent infusion device, central venous catheters, peripherally inserted catheters, or implanted ports.
- Nursing assessment of fluid and electrolyte disturbances entails observation of general appearance, vital signs, and intake and output measurement.
- Oxygen can be administered by hood, mask, nasal cannula, incubator, or oxygen tent.
- Tracheostomy suctioning involves premeasured insertion of the catheter, application of suction for 5 seconds when withdrawing the catheter, and supplemental oxygen before and after suctioning.
- Alternative forms of feeding include gavage feeding, gastrostomy feeding, and total parenteral nutrition.
- In the care of children with ostomies, nurses play an important role in family support and instruction in care of the stoma site.

REFERENCES

Abd-El-Maeboud K and others: Rectal suppository: common-sense and mode of insertion, *Lancet* 338(8770):798-800, 1991.

Ackerman MH: The effect of saline lavage prior to suctioning, *Am J Crit Care* 2(4):326-330, 1993.

Acute Pain Management Guideline Panel: *Acute pain management: operative or medical procedures and trauma: clinical practice guideline,* AHCPR Pub No 92-0032, Rockville, MD, 1992, Agency for Health Care Policy and Research, Public Health Service, US Department of Health and Human Services.

Alderson SH, Warren RH: Pediatric aerosol therapy guidelines, *Clin Pediatr* 23(10):553-557, 1984.

American Academy of Pediatrics, Committee on Drugs: Guidelines for monitoring and management of pediatric patients during and after sedation for diagnostic and therapeutic procedures, *Pediatrics* 86(6):1110-1115, 1992.

Arditi M, Killner M: Coma following use of rubbing alcohol for fever control, *Am J Dis Child* 141(3):237-238, 1987.

Bates T, Broome M: Preparation of children for hospitalization and surgery: a review of the literature, *J Pediatr Nurs* 1(4):230-239, 1986.

Beecroft P, Redick S: Intramuscular injection practices of pediatric nurses: site selection, *Nurse Educ* 15(4):23-28, 1990.

Brent NJ: The pediatric patient and consent for treatment, *Home Healthc Nurse* 9(5):10-12, 1991.

Broome ME: Preparation of children for painful procedures, *Pediatr Nurs* 16(6):537-541, 1990.

Brosnan KM and others: Contamination stopcock, *Am J Nurs* 88(3):320-323, 1988.

Brown JM: Peripherally inserted central catheters—use in home care, *J Intravenous Nurs* 12(3):144-150, 1989.

Bruce JL, Grove SK: Fever: pathology and treatment, *Crit Care Nurs* 12(1):40-55, 1992.

Bryant RA, editor: *Acute and chronic wounds: nursing management,* St Louis, 1992, Mosby.

Camp-Sorrell D: Advanced central venous access: selection, catheters, devices, and nursing management, *J Intravenous Nurs* 13(6):361-370, 1990.

Chandra NC, Hazinski MF, editors: *Textbook of basic life support for healthcare providers,* Dallas, 1994, American Heart Association.

Courtney SE and others: Capillary blood gases in the neonate: a reassessment and review of the literature, *Am J Dis Child* 144:168-172, 1990.

Cushing M: Demystifying informed consent, *Am J Nurs* 91(11):17-19, 1991.

Dyson A, Bogod D: Minimizing bruising in the antecubital fossa after venipuncture, *Br Med J* 294(6588):1659, 1987.

Ellett M and others: Predicting the distance for gavage tube placement in children using regression on height, *Pediatr Nurs* 18(2):119-121, 127, 1992.

Ellis R: Once more into the void, *Contemp Pediatr* 6(8):164, 1989.

Faber MM: A review of efforts to protect children from injury in crashes, *Fam Community Health* 4(3):25-41, 1986.

Fina DK: A chance to say goodbye, *Am J Nurs* 94(5):42-45, 1994.

Fox MD: Measurement of urine output volume: accuracy of diaper weights in neonatal environments, *Neonatal Network* 11(3):11-18, 1992.

Flemmer L, Chan JSL: A pediatric protocol for management of extravasation injuries, *Pediatr Nurs* 19(4):355-368, 1993.

Funk MJ, Mullins LL, Olson RA: Teaching children to swallow pills: a case study, *Child Health Care* 13(1):20-23, 1984.

Gablehouse BL, Gitterman BA: Maternal understanding of commonly used medical terms in a pediatric setting, *Am J Dis Child* 144:419, 1990.

Garvin G, Franck L: Preventing delivery of enteral formula via parenteral route, *Pediatr Nurs* 15(1):17-18, 1989.

Gribetz B, Cronley S: Underdosing of acetaminophen by parents, *Pediatrics* 80(5):630-633, 1987.

Hagelgans NA: Pediatric skin care issues for the home care nurse, *Pediatr Nurs* 19(5):499-507, 1993.

Hagler DA, Traver GA: Endotracheal saline and suction catheters: sources of lower airway contamination, *Am J Crit Care* 3(6):444-447, 1994.

Hall PA and others: Parents in the recovery room: survey of parental and staff attitudes, *Br Med J* 310(6973):163-164, 1995.

Hanna WJ, Sherlock H: Recall and fears of anaesthesia and surgery in 50 Jamaican paediatric patients, *West Indian Med J* 32:75-82, 1983.

Heiney SP: Helping children through painful procedures, *Am J Nurs* 91(11):20-24, 1991.

Hicks JF and others: Optimum needle length for diphtheria-inoculation of infants, *Pediatrics* 84(1):136-137, 1989.

Hogue EE: Informed consent: implications for critical care nurses, *Pediatr Nurs* 14(4):315-316, 1988.

Holtzclaw BJ: Control of febrile shivering during amphotericin B therapy, *Oncol Nurs Forum* 17(4):521-524, 1990.

Janik JP, Wayne ER, Janik JS: Securing central lines in rambunctious toddlers, *Pediatrics* 96(3):523-524, 1995.

Johannsen L: Adolescent abortion and mandated parental involvement, *Pediatr Nurs* 21(1):82-84, 1995.

Johnston CC, Stevens B, Arbess G: The effect of the sight of blood and use of decorative adhesive bandages on pain intensity ratings by preschool children, *J Pediatr Nurs* 8(3):147-151, 1993.

Joyner M: Hair care in the black patient, *J Pediatr Health Care* 2(6):281-287, 1988.

Kinmouth AL, Fulton Y, Campbell MJ: Management of feverish children at home, *Br Med J* 305(6862):1134-1136, 1992.

Kleiber C, Krutzfield N, Rose EF: Acute histologic changes in tracheobronchial tree associated with different suction catheter insertion techniques, *Heart Lung* 17:10-14, 1988.

Konings K: Preop use of Golytely in pediatrics, *Pediatr Nurs* 15(5):473-474, 1989.

Krouskop TA and others: Effectiveness of mattress overlays in reducing interface pressures during recumbency, *J Rehabil Res Dev* 22(3):7-10, 1985.

Krueger H, Osborn L: Effects of hygiene among the uncircumcised, *J Fam Pract* 22(4):353-355, 1986.

LaRosa-Nash PA and others: Implementing a parent-present induction program, *AORN J* 61(3):526-531, 1995.

Lehmann M and others: Upright or lying down: is one better for doing a lumbar puncture (LP)? *Am J Dis Child* 144:427, 1990.

Lohr J, Donowitz L, Dudley S: Bacterial contamination rates in voided urine collections in girls, *J Pediatr* 114(1):91-93, 1989.

Lynch P and others: Rethinking the role of isolation practices in the prevention of nosocomial infections, *Ann Intern Med* 107:243-246, 1987.

Marcoux C, Fisher S, Wong D: Central venous access devices in children, *Pediatr Nurs* 16(2):123-133, 1990.

McCabe M, Sibert JR, Routledge PA: Phosphate enemas in childhood: cause for concern, *Br Med J* 302(6784):1074, 1991.

McMullen A and others: Heparinized saline or normal saline: as a flush solution in intermittent intravenous lines in infants and children, *MCN Am J Matern Child Nurs* 18:78-85, 1993.

Meares C: PICC and MLC lines: options worth exploring, *Nursing '92* 22(10):52-55, 1992.

Metheny N and others: Effectiveness of pH measurements in predicting feeding tube placement, *Nurs Res* 38(5):280-285, 1989.

Musser V: How do you use shallow-suction technique in children? *Am J Nurs* 92(5):79-83, 1992.

Newman J: Evaluation of sponging to reduce body temperature in febrile children, *Can Med Assoc J* 132:641-642, 1985.

Nix KS: Obtaining informed consent. In Smith DP and others, editors: *Comprehensive child and family nursing skills,* St Louis, 1991, Mosby.

Olsen RJ and others: Examination gloves as barriers to hand contamination in clinical practice, *JAMA* 270(3):350-353, 1993.

Orenstein S and others: The Santmyer swallow: a new and useful infant reflex, *Lancet* 1(8581):345-346, 1988.

Pidgeon V: Compliance with chronic illness regimens: school-aged children and adolescents, *J Pediatr Nurs* 4(1):36-47, 1989.

Pollack CV, Pollack ES, Andrew ME: Suprapubic bladder aspiration versus urethral catheterization in ill infants: success, efficiency, and complication rates, *Ann Emerg Med* 23(2):225-230, 1994.

Robertson J: Intermittent intravenous therapy: a comparison of two flushing solutions, *Contemp Nurse* 3(4):174-179, 1994.

Rosenstock IM: Enhancing patient compliance with health recommendations, *J Pediatr Health Care* 2(2):67-72, 1988.

Rudy C: A drop or a dropper: the risk of overdose, *J Pediatr Health Care,* 6(1):40, 1992.

Saez-Llorens X and others: Bacterial contamination rates for non-clean catch and clean catch midstream urine collections in uncircumcised boys, *J Pediatr* 114(1):93-95, 1989.

Schreiner MS: Preoperative and postoperative fasting in children, *Pediatr Clin North Am* 41(1):111-120, 1994.

Schreiner V: Don't discard this specimen, *Nursing '87* 17(10):5, 1987.

Shorten DR, Byrne PJ, Jones RL: Infant responses to saline instillations and endotracheal suctioning, *J Obstet Gynecol Neonatal Nurs* 20(6):464-469, 1991.

Simon RE: Ibuprofen suspension: pediatric antipyretic, *Pediatr Nurs* 22(2):118-120, 1996.

Stoller KP, Losey R: Inadvertent intra-arterial injection of penicillin: an unseen danger, *Pediatrics* 75(4)785-786, 1985.

US Department of Labor, Occupational Safety and Health Administration: *Occupational exposure to bloodborne pathogen,* final rule, 29 DFR part 1910.1030, Washington DC, 1991, US Government Printing Office.

Van R and others: The effect of diaper type and overclothing on fecal contamination in day-care centers, *JAMA* 265(14):1840-1844, 1991.

Vessey J, Caserza L, Bogetz M: In my opinion . . . another Pandora's box? Parental participation in anesthetic induction, *Child Health Care* 19(2):116-118, 1990.

Villarreal P: Personal communication, University of Texas, San Antonio, 1992.

Weibley TT and others: Gavage tube insertion in the premature infant, *MCN Am J Matern Child Nurs* 12:24-27, 1987.

Wlody GS: Malignant hyperthermia, *Crit Care Nurs Clin North Am* 3(1):129-134, 1991.

Wong DL, Baker CM: Pain in children: comparison of assessment scales, *Pediatr Nurs* 14(1):9-17, 1988.

Wong DL and others: Diapering choices: a critical review of the issues, *Pediatr Nurs* 18(1):41-54, 1992.

Woolverton E: Practice pointers, *School Health Watch* 2(4):2, 1991.

BIBLIOGRAPHY

Informed Consent

Allen A: Informed consent: how far must it go? *J Post Anesth Nurs* 5(6):425-426, 1990.

Broome ME, Stieglitz KA: The consent process and children, *Res Nurs Health* 15(2):147-152, 1992.

Erlen JA: The child's choice: an essential component in treatment decisions, *Child Health Care* 15(3):156-160, 1987.

Hogue EE: Consent for minors, *Pediatr Nurs* 15(4):404, 1989.

Horton R: The context of consent, *Lancet* 344(8917):211-212, 1994.

Leikin S: A proposal concerning decisions to forgo life-sustaining treatment for young people, *J Pediatr* 115(1):17-22, 1989.

Rhodes AM: Consent for medical treatment, *MCN* 12(2):133, 1987.

Rhodes AM: A minor's refusal of treatment, *MCN Am J Matern Child Nurs* 15(4):261, 1990.

Rhodes AM: Obtaining consent to treat minors, *MCN* 12(3):209, 1987.

Rhodes AM: The rights of minors, *MCN* 13(4):281, 1988.

Rhodes AM: When parents refuse to consent, *MCN* 12(4):289, 1987.

Ruccione K and others: Informed consent for treatment of childhood cancer: factors affecting parents' decision making, *J Pediatr Oncol Nurs* 8(3):112-121, 1991.

Preparation for Procedures/Use of Play

Azarnoff P: Teaching materials for pediatric health professionals, *J Pediatr Health Care* 4(6):282-289, 1990.

Bauchner H, Vinci R, Waring C: Pediatric procedures: do parents want to watch? *Pediatrics* 84(5):907-909, 1989.

Cook BA and others: Sedation of children for technical procedures: current standard of practice, *Clin Pediatr* 31(3):137-142, 1992.

Cote CJ: Sedation for the pediatric patient: a review, *Pediatr Clin North Am* 41(1):31-58, 1994.

Emergency Nurses Association position statement: *Family presence at the bedside during invasive procedures and/or resuscitation,* Park Ridge, IL, 1994, The Association.

Goldberger J, Wolfer J: Helping children cope with health-care procedures, *Contemp Pediatr* 7(3):141-162, 1990.

LeVieux-Anglin L and others: Incorporating play interventions into nursing care, *Pediatr Nurs* 19(5):459-463, 1993.

Rollins J, Brantly D: Preparing the child for procedures. In Smith DP and others, editors: *Comprehensive child and family nursing skills,* St Louis, 1991, Mosby.

Zeltzer LK, Jay SM, Fisher DM: The management of pain associated with pediatric procedures, *Pediatr Clin North Am* 36(4):941-964, 1989.

Surgical Procedures

Ashby D: Malignant hyperthermia: a potential crisis in the postanesthesia care unit, *J Post Anesth Nurs* 5(4):279-281, 1990.

Avigne G, Phillips TL: Pediatric preoperative tours, *AORN J* 53(6):1458-1465, 1991.

Bender LH, Weaver K, Edwards K: Postoperative patient-controlled analgesia in children, *Pediatr Nurs* 16(6):549-554, 1990.

Cehaich K: Preparing the pediatric patient for surgery, *Plast Surg Nurs* 14(2):105-107, 1994.

Cote CJ: NPO after midnight for children—a reappraisal, *Anesthesiology* 72(4):589-592, 1990.

Davis JL and others: Perioperative care of the pediatric trauma patient, *AORN J* 60(4):561, 563-565, 1994.

Ellerton ML: Preparing kids and parents for surgery, *Can Nurs* 10(10):25-27, 1994.

Hannallah RS: Who benefits when parents are present during anaesthesia induction in their children? *Can J Anaesth* 41(4):271-275, 1994.

Heffline MS: A comparative study of pharmacological versus nursing interventions in the treatment of postanesthesia shivering, *J Post Anesth Nurs* 6(5):311-320, 1991.

Jones JG: Memory of intraoperative events, *Br Med J* 309(6960):967-968, 1994.

Kennedy CM, Riddle II: The influence of the timing of preparation on the anxiety of preschool children experiencing surgery, *Matern Child Nurs J* 18(2):117-132, 1989.

LaRosa-Nash PA, Murphy JM: A clinical case study: parent-present induction of anesthesia in children, *Pediatr Nurs* 22(2):109-111, 1996.

McIlvaine WB: Perioperative pain management in children: a review, *J Pain Symptom Manage* 4(4):215-229, 1989.

Meyer-Pahoulis E: Pediatric postanesthesia care, *Plast Surg Nurs* 14(2):92-98, 1994.

Moyer S, Howe C: Pediatric pain intervention in the PACU, *Crit Care Nurs Clin North Am* 3(1):49-57, 1991.

Noonan AT and others: Family-centered nursing in the postanesthesia care unit: the evaluation of practice, *J Post Anesth Nurs* 6(1):13-16, 1991.

Ogilvie L: Hospitalization of children for surgery: the parents' view, *Child Health Care* 19(1):49-56, 1990.

Pierce LA: Safety and care of children during surgery, *Plast Surg Nurs* 14(2):99-100, 1994.

Rivera WB: Practical points in the assessment and management of postoperative pediatric pain, *J Post Anesth Nurs* 6(1):40-42, 1991.

Tobias JD and others: Postoperative analgesia: use of intrathecal morphine in children, *Clin Pediatr* 29:44-48, 1990.

Vessey JA and others: Parental upset associated with participation in induction of anaesthesia in children, *Can J Anaesth* 41(4):276-280, 1994.

Compliance

Burckhardt CS: Ethical issues in compliance, *Top Clin Nurs* 7(4):9-16, 1986.

Clark SR: Compliance and health behaviors, *Top Clin Nurs* 7(4):39-46, 1986.

Connaway N: My patient won't follow the medical plan treatment. What should I do to protect myself—legally? . . . home health care, *Home Healthc Nurse* 3(4):6-8, 1985.

DiFlorio IA, Duncan PA: Design for successful patient teaching, *MCN Am J Matern Child Nurs* 11:246-249, 1986.

Friedman IM, Litt IF: Promoting adolescents' compliance with therapeutic regimens, *Pediatr Clin North Am* 33(4):955-973, 1986.

Gibson L: Patient education: effects of two teaching methods upon parental retention of infant feeding practices, *Pediatr Nurs* 21(1):78-80, 1995.

Kelloway JS and others: Comparison of patients' compliance with prescribed oral and inhaled asthma medications, *Arch Intern Med* 154:1349-1352, 1994.

Littlefield LC: Therapeutic drug monitoring in ambulatory pediatrics, *J Pediatr Health Care* 1(2):113-116, 1987.

McCord MA: Compliance: self-care or compromise? *Top Clin Nurs* 7(4):1-8, 1986.

McHatton M: A theory for timely teaching, *Am J Nurs* 85(7):798-800, 1985.

Miller A: When is the time ripe for teaching? *Am J Nurs* 85(7):801-804, 1985.

Padrick KP: Compliance: myths and motivators, *Top Clin Nurs* 7(4):17-22, 1986.

Sallis JF: Improving adherence to pediatric therapeutic regimens, *Pediatr Nurs* 11(2):118-120, 1985.

Spicher CM, Yund C: Effects of preadmission preparation on compliance with home care instructions, *J Pediatr Nurs* 4(4):255-262, 1989.

Stang H: Compliance: get parents in on the diagnosis, *Contemp Pediatr* 7(3):170, 1990.

Wright EC: A lesson in non-compliance, *Lancet* 343(8908):27, 1994.

General Hygiene and Care/Fever

American College of Emergency Physicians: Clinical policy for the initial approach to children under the age of 2 years presenting with fever, *Ann Emerg Med* 22:628-637, 1993.

Baraff LJ and others: Practice guideline for the management of infants and children 0 to 36 months of age with fever without source, *Ann Emerg Med* 22(7):108-120, 1993.

Barnett RI, Ablarde JA: Skin vascular reaction to standard patient positioning on a hospital mattress, *Adv Wound Care* 7(1):58-65, 1994.

Bedi A: A tool to fill the gap: developing a wound risk assessment chart for children, *Profess Nurs* 9(2), 1993.

Gildea JH: When fever becomes an enemy, *Pediatr Nurs* 18(2):165-167, 1992.

Gould KE and others: Therapeutic beds: the Trojan horses of the 1990s? *Lancet* 433(8914):65-66, 1994.

Herzog LW, Coyne LJ: What is fever? Normal temperature in infants less than 3 months old, *Clin Pediatr* 32(4):142-146, 1993.

Kleiman MB: Feverish children, frightened parents, *Contemp Pediatr* 6(3):161-167, 1989.

Marchand AC, Lidowski H: Reassessment of the use of genuine sheepskin for pressure ulcer prevention and treatment, *Decubitus* 6(1):44-47, 1993.

Reeves-Swift R: Rational management of a child's acute fever, *MCN Am J Matern Child Nurs* 15(2):82-85, 1990.

Singer L: When a sick child won't—or can't—eat, *Contemp Pediatr* 7(12):60-76, 1990.

Thurgood G: Nurse maintenance of oral hygiene, *Br J Nurs* 3(7):332-353, 1994.

Safety/Collection of Specimens/Infection Control

Amir J and others: The reliability of midstream urine culture from circumcised male infants, *Am J Dis Child* 147:969-970, 1993.

Blain-Lewis N: Comparative studies of bruising and healing after heelstick, *Neonatal Intensive Care* 5(5):18-21, 1992.

Brantly DK: Applying and maintaining restraints and restraining for procedures. In Smith DP and others, editors: *Comprehensive child and family nursing skills,* St Louis, 1991, Mosby.

Dennehy P: Heel blood sampling on older infants, *Neonatal Intensive Care* 5(5):21-23, 1992.

Fleischman AR: Clinical considerations for infant heel blood sampling, *Neonatal Intensive Care* 5(3):62-68, 1992.

Gleeson RM: Use of non-latex gloves for children with latex allergies, *J Pediatr Nurs* 10(1):64-65, 1995.

Jackson MM: Infection prevention and control for HIV and other infectious agents in obstetric, gynecologic and neonatal settings, *Clin Issues Perinat Women's Health Nurs* 1(1):115-121, 1990.

Jackson MM: Infection prevention and control. In Swearingen PL, Keen JH, editors: *Manual of critical care: applying nursing diagnoses to adult critical illness,* ed 3, St Louis, 1995, Mosby.

Korniewicz D, Kirwin M, Larson E: Do your gloves fit the task? *Am J Nurs* 91(6):38-40, 1991.

Larson E: Handwashing: it's essential—even when you use gloves, *Am J Nurs* 89(7):934-939, 1989.

Preusser BA and others: Quantifying the minimum discard sample required for accurate arterial blood gases, *Nurs Res* 38:276-279, 1989.

Schmitt BD: Protecting your child from infections, *Contemp Pediatr* 12(9):83-84, 1995.

Selekman J, Snyder B: Nursing perceptions of using physical restraints on hospitalized children, *Pediatr Nurs* 21(5):460-464, 1995.

Suri S: Simplifying urine collection from infants and children without losing accuracy, *MCN* 13(12):438-441, 1988.

Vernon S and others: Urine collection on sanitary towels, *Lancet* 344:612, 1994.

Weatherly KS, Young S, Andresky J: Needle stick injury in pediatric hospitals, *Pediatr Nurs* 17(1):95-99, 1991.

Whitehall J, Shvartzman P, Miller MA: A novel method for isolating and quantifying urine pathogens collected from gel-based diapers, *J Fam Pract* 40(5):476-479, 1995.

Administration of Medication

Beecroft PC, Redick S: Possible complications of intramuscular injections on the pediatric unit, *Pediatr Nurs* 15(4):333-376, 1989.

Beyea SC, Nicoll LH: Back to basics: administering IM injections the right way, *Am J Nurs* 96(1):34-35, 1996.

Bosserman G and others: Multidisciplinary management of vascular access devices, *Oncol Nurs Forum* 17(6):879-886, 1990.

Botash SA: Syringe caps: an aspiration hazard, *Pediatrics* 90(1):92-93, 1992.

Buckley T, Dudley SM, Donowitz LG: Defining unnecessary disinfection procedures for single-dose and multiple-dose vials, *Am J Crit Care* 3(6):448-451, 1994.

Dennis-Smithart R: Taking medication: the last straw, *Contemp Pediatr* 10(3):5, 1993.

Gahart BL: *Intravenous medications: a handbook for nurses and other allied health personnel,* ed 10, St Louis, 1994, Mosby.

Glassman SK, Measel CP: A makeshift mini-bottle: accurate small volume fluid or oral medication administration to infants, *Neonatal Network* 7(4):29-31, 1989.

Halperin D and others: Topical skin anesthesia for venous, subcutaneous drug reservoir and lumbar puncture in children, *Pediatrics* 84:281-284, 1989.

Intramuscular injections: a guide to sites and techniques, Philadelphia, 1985, Wyeth Laboratories.

Losek JD, Gyuro J: Pediatric intramuscular injections: do you know the procedure and complications? *Pediatr Emerg Care* 8(2):79-81, 1992.

Penatzer M and others: Common pediatric IV meds at a glance, *Pediatr Nurs* 14(1):56-58, 1988.

Raju TN and others: Medication errors in neonatal and paediatric intensive-care units, *Lancet* 2(8659):374-376, 1989.

Smith SE: Eyedrop instillation for reluctant children, *Br J Opthalmol* 75:480-481, 1991.

Thigpen J: Minimizing medication errors, *Neonatal Network* 14(2):85-86, 1995.

Wink DM: Giving infants and children drugs: precision + caution = safety, *MCN Am J Matern Child Nurs* 16(6):317-321, 1991.

Parenteral Therapy/Fluid Balance

Banta C: Hyaluronidase, *Neonatal Network* 11(6):103-105, 1992.

Baranowski L: Central venous access devices: current technologies, uses, and management strategies, *J Intravenous Nurs* 16(3):167-194, 1993.

Danek GD, Noris EM: Pediatric IV catheters: efficacy of saline flush, *Pediatr Nurs* 18(2):111-113, 1992.

Dick M and others: How to boost the odds of a painless IV start, *Am J Nurs* 92(6):49-50, 1992.

Gyr P and others: Double blind comparison of heparin and saline flush solutions in maintenance of peripheral infusion devices, *Pediatr Nurs* 21(4):383-389, 1995.

Hanrahan KS, Kleiber C, Fagan C: Evaluation of saline for IV locks in children, *Pediatr Nurs* 20(6):549-552, 1994.

Hastings-Tolsma MT and others: Effect of warm and cold applications on the resolution of IV infiltrations, *Res Nurs Health* 16(3):171-178, 1993.

Hodler C, Alexander J: A new and improved guide to IV therapy: protocols for intravenous therapy, *Am J Nurs* 90(2):43-47, 1990.

Kelly C and others: A change in flushing protocols of central venous catheters, *Oncol Nurs Forum* 19(4):599-605, 1992.

Kleiber C and others: Heparin vs. saline for peripheral IV locks in children, *Pediatr Nurs* 19:405-409, 1993.

Marcoux C, Fisher S, Wong D: Central venous access devices in children, *Pediatr Nurs* 16(2):123-133, 1991.

Moss JR, Craft MJ: Accurate assessment of infant emesis volume, *Pediatr Nurs* 16(5):455-457, 1990.

O'Brien R: Starting intravenous lines in children, *J Emerg Nurs* 17(4):225-231, 1991.

Orlowski JP: Emergency alternatives to intravenous access, *Pediatr Clin North Am* 41(6):1183-1199, 1994.

Pettit J, Hughes K: Intravenous extravasation: mechanisms, management, and prevention, *J Perinat Neonat Nurs* 6(4):69-79, 1993.

Ryder MA: Peripherally inserted central venous catheters, *Nurs Clin North Am* 28(4):937-971, 1993.

Tidwell B Jr, Parks BR Jr: Intraosseous infusions, *Pediatr Nurs* 17(1):56-57, 1991.

Tietjen SD: Starting an infant's IV, *Am J Nurs* 90:44-47, 1990.

Wilson D: Neonatal IVs: practical tips, *Neonatal Nurs* 11(2):49-53, 1992.

Zimerman E: The Landry vein light: increasing venipuncture success rates, *J Pediatr Nurs* 6(1):64-66, 1991.

Respiratory Therapy

AARC Clinical Practice Guideline: Endotracheal suctioning of mechanically ventilated adults and children with artificial airways, *Respir Care* 38(5):500-504, 1993.

Brown KA, Sauve RS: Evaluation of a caregiver education program: home oxygen therapy for infants, *J Obstet Gynecol Neonatal Nurs* 23(5):429-435, 1994.

Comer DM: Pulse oximetry: implications for practice, *J Obstet Gynecol Neonatal Nurs* 21(1):35-41, 1992.

Fitton CM: Nursing management of the child with a tracheotomy, *Pediatr Clin North Am* 41(3):513-523, 1994.

Giganti AW: Lifesaving tubes, lifetime scars? *MCN* 20:192-197, 1995.

Hodge D: Endotracheal suctioning and the infant: a nursing care protocol to decrease complications, *Neonatal Network* 9(5):7-15, 1991.

Noll ML, Hix C, Scott G: Closed tracheal suction systems: effectiveness and nursing complications, *AACN Clin Issues Crit Care Nurs* 1(2):327-328, 1990.

Ronczy NM, Beddome M: Preparing the family for home tracheotomy care, *AACN Clin Issues Crit Care Nurs* 1(2):367-377, 1990.

Runton N: Suctioning artificial airways in children: appropriate technique, *Pediatr Nurs* 18(2):115-118, 1992.

Russell R, Helms P: Comparative accuracy of pulse oximetry and transcutaneous oxygen in assessing arterial saturation in pediatric intensive care, *Neonatal Intensive Care* 5(1):38-40, 1992.

Salyer J, Lewis D: Pulse oximetry: application in the pediatric and neonatal critical care unit, *AACN Clin Issues Crit Care Nurs* 1(2):339-347, 1990.

Sobel DB: Burning of a neonate due to a pulse oximeter: arterial saturation monitoring, *Pediatrics* 89(1):154-155, 1992.

Stoneham MD, Saville GM, Wilson IH: Knowledge about pulse oximetry among medical and nursing staff, *Lancet* 334(8933):1339-1342, 1994.

Tolles CL, Stone KS: National survey of neonatal endotracheal suctioning practices, *Neonatal Network* 9(2):7-14, 1990.

Turner BS: Maintaining the artificial airway: current concepts, *Pediatr Nurs* 16(5):487-493, 1990.

Witham-Wilson MJ: Accidental breathing circuit disconnections in the neonatal or pediatric critical care setting, *Pediatr Nurs* 17(3):283-286, 293, 1991.

Alternative Feeding Techniques/Elimination

Boarini JH: Principles of stoma care for infants, *J Enterostom Ther* 16(1):21-25, 1989.

Bockus S: Troubleshooting your tube feedings, *Am J Nurs* 91(5):24-28, 1991.

Cady C, Yoshioka R: Using a learning contract to successfully discharge an infant on home total parenteral nutrition, *Pediatr Nurs* 17(1):67-71, 74, 1991.

Embon CM: Ostomy care for the infant with necrotizing enterocolitis: nursing considerations, *J Perinat Neonat Nurs* 4(3):56-63, 1990.

Ferraro AR, Huddleston KC: Safe administration of small-volume enteral feedings: an alternative to intravenous pumps, *J Pediatr Nurs* 6(5):352-354, 1991.

Garvin G: Caring for children with ostomies, *Nurs Clin North Am* 29(4):645-655, 1994.

Metheny N: Measures to test placement of nasogastric and nasointestinal feeding tubes: a review, *Nurs Res* 37(6):324-329, 1988.

Metheny N and others: Visual characteristics of aspirates from feeding tubes as a method for predicting tube location, *Nurs Res* 43(5):282-287, 1994.

Steele NF: The button: replacement gastrostomy device, *J Pediatr Nurs* 6(6):421-424, 1991.

Van Niel J: What's wrong with this peristomal skin? *Am J Nurs* 91(12):44-45, 1991.

Young RJ, Murray ND: Adapting intravenous pumps for enteral feeding, *MCN* 16:212-216, 1991.

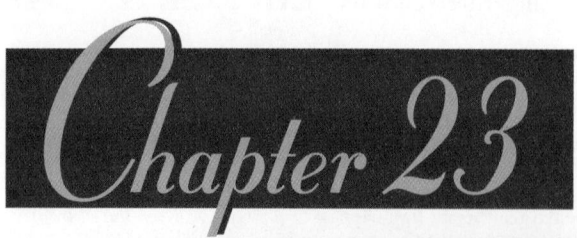

Chapter 23

THE CHILD WITH RESPIRATORY DYSFUNCTION

" Nintendo helps when you're in a chair or bed. You sit up better."

Charles "Aaron," age 7 years, asthma and pneumonia

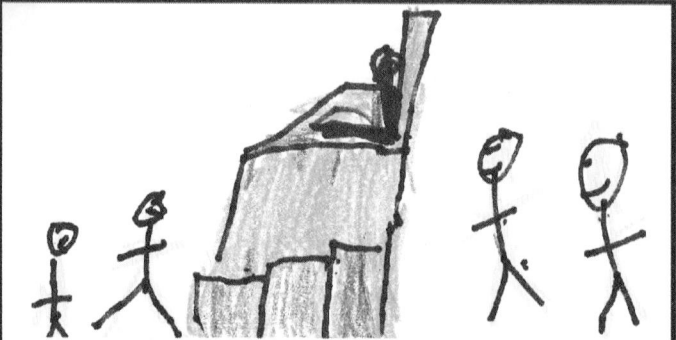

RELATED TOPICS

RESPIRATORY INFECTION

GENERAL ASPECTS OF RESPIRATORY INFECTIONS

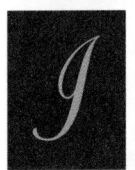nfections of the respiratory tract are described in a number of different ways according to the general areas of involvement in the more common infections. The *upper respiratory tract,* or *upper airway,* consists primarily of the nose and pharynx. The *lower respiratory tract* consists of the bronchi and bronchioles (which constitute the reactive portion of the airway because of their smooth muscle content and ability to constrict) and the alveoli. Authorities disagree about the designation for the structurally stable portion of the airway (including the epiglottis, larynx, and trachea). For this discussion, the trachea is considered with lower tract disorders, and infections of the epiglottis and larynx are categorized as croup syndromes. Respiratory infections seldom fall neatly into discrete anatomic areas. Infections tend to spread from one structure to another because of the contiguous nature of the mucous membrane lining the entire tract. Consequently, infections of the respiratory tract involve several areas rather than a single structure, although the effect on one may predominate in any given illness.

Etiology and Characteristics

Respiratory infections account for a large majority of acute illnesses in children. The etiology and course of these infections are influenced by a number of factors, including the age of the child, season, living conditions, and preexisting medical problems.

Infectious Agents.   The respiratory tract is subject to a wide variety of infective organisms, but the largest percentage of infections are caused by viruses, particularly in the upper respiratory passages. These infections account for many acute illnesses in children. Other agents that may be involved in primary or secondary invasion include group A β-hemolytic streptococci, staphylococci, *Haemophilus influ-*

enzae, Chlamydia trachomatis, Mycoplasma, and pneumococci.

Age.   The pattern of respiratory infection varies considerably with the child's age. Infants under age 3 months have a lower infection rate, presumably because of the protective function of maternal antibodies. The infection rate soars from age 3 to 6 months, the time between the disappearance of maternal antibodies and the infant's own antibody production. The viral infection rate continues to be high during the toddler and preschool years but drops steadily. By the time the child reaches 5 years of age, viral respiratory infections are much less frequent, but the incidence of *Mycoplasma pneumoniae* and group A β-streptococcal infections increases.

Some of the viral agents produce a mild illness in older children but cause severe lower respiratory tract illness or croup in infants. The amount of lymphoid tissue increases throughout middle childhood, and repeated exposure to organisms confers increasing immunity as the child grows older; thus older children have a greater resistance to most organisms. Whooping cough is a relatively harmless tracheobronchitis in childhood but a serious disease in infancy.

Size.   Anatomic differences influence the degree to which children respond to respiratory tract infections. The diameter of the airways is smaller in young children than in older children and is therefore subject to considerable narrowing from edematous mucous membranes and increased production of secretions. In addition, the distance between structures within the tract is shorter anatomically in the young child; therefore organisms move more rapidly down the respiratory tract for more extensive involvement. The relatively short and open eustachian tube in infants and young children allows pathogens easy access to the middle ear.

Resistance.   The ability to resist invading organisms depends on several factors. Deficiencies of the immune system place the child at risk for any infectious process. The general conditions that appear to decrease resistance to infection are malnutrition, anemia, fatigue, and chilling of the body. Conditions affecting the respiratory tract that weaken its defenses and predispose to infection include allergies (e.g., allergic rhinitis), asthma, cardiac anomalies that have a tendency to cause pulmonary congestion, and cystic fibrosis. Daycare atten-

David Wilson, MS, RNC, revised this chapter.

dance, especially if the caregivers smoke, also increases the likelihood of infection (Holberg, Wright, and Martinez, 1993).

Seasonal Variations. The most common respiratory tract pathogens appear in epidemics during the winter and spring months, but mycoplasma infections occur more often in autumn and early winter. Asthma occurs more frequently during cold weather.

Clinical Manifestations

Infants and young children, especially those between 6 months and 3 years of age, react more severely to acute respiratory tract infection than older children, and they are often more ill than their local manifestations would indicate. Young children display a number of generalized signs and symptoms, as well as local manifestations, that differ from those seen in older children and adults. An infant or child may display any or all of the signs and symptoms listed in the box below.

Nursing Considerations

❖ Assessment

The general assessment of the respiratory system follows the guidelines described in Chapter 7 (for nose, mouth and throat, chest, and lungs), and normal vital signs can be found on the inside back cover. In addition, special attention is given to the specific observations outlined in the box below using the components in the box on p. 751.

❖ Nursing Diagnoses

After a thorough assessment, a number of nursing diagnoses may be identified. The most likely diagnoses are outlined and discussed in the Nursing Care Plan on pp. 753-755. Others may be apparent in individual cases.

❖ Planning

The goals for the child with an acute respiratory infection and the family are as follows:

1. Child will exhibit normal respiratory efforts.
2. Child will receive adequate rest.

SIGNS AND SYMPTOMS ASSOCIATED WITH RESPIRATORY INFECTIONS IN INFANTS AND SMALL CHILDREN

Fever

May be absent in newborn infants, who may be hypothermic
Greatest at ages 6 months to 3 years
　Temperature may reach 39.5° to 40.5° C (103° to 105° F) even with mild infections
Often appears as first sign of infection
May be listless and irritable or somewhat euphoric and more active than normal, temporarily; some children talk with unaccustomed rapidity
Tendency to develop high temperatures with infection in certain families
　May precipitate febrile seizures (see Chapter 28)
　Febrile seizures uncommon after 3 or 4 years of age

Meningismus

Meningeal signs without infection of the meninges
Occurs with abrupt onset of fever
Accompanied by:
　Headache
　Pain and stiffness in the back and neck
　Presence of Kernig and Brudzinski signs
Subsides as the temperature decreases

Anorexia

Common with most childhood illnesses
Frequently the initial evidence of illness
Almost invariably accompanies acute infections in small children
Persists to a greater or lesser degree throughout febrile stage of illness; often extends into convalescence

Vomiting

Small children vomit readily with illness
A clue to the onset of infection
May precede other signs by several hours
Usually short-lived but may persist during the illness

Diarrhea

Usually mild, transient diarrhea but may become severe
Often accompanies respiratory infections, especially viral infections
Frequent cause of dehydration

Abdominal Pain

Common complaint
Sometimes indistinguishable from pain of appendicitis
Mesenteric lymphadenitis may be cause
Muscle spasms from vomiting may be a factor, especially in nervous, tense child

Nasal Blockage

Small nasal passages of infants easily blocked by mucosal swelling and exudation
Can interfere with respiration and feeding in infants
May contribute to the development of otitis media and sinusitis

Nasal Discharge

Frequently accompanies respiratory infections
May be thin and watery (rhinorrhea) or thick and purulent
　Depends on the type and/or stage of infection
Associated with itching
May irritate upper lip and skin surrounding the nose

Cough

Common feature of respiratory disease
May be evident only during the acute phase
May persist several months after a disease

Respiratory Sounds

Sounds associated with respiratory disease:
　Cough
　Hoarseness
　Grunting
　Stridor
　Wheezing
Auscultation:
　Wheezing
　Crackles
　Absence of air movement

Sore Throat

Frequent complaint of older children
Young children (unable to describe symptoms) may not complain even when highly inflamed
　Child will often refuse to take oral fluids or solids

COMPONENTS FOR ASSESSING RESPIRATORY FUNCTION

Respirations

The pattern of respirations is observed for rate, depth, ease, and rhythm of breathing:

Rate—Rapid *(tachypnea)*, normal, or slow for the particular child

Depth—Normal depth, too shallow *(hypopnea)*, too deep *(hyperpnea)*; usually estimated from the amplitude of thoracic and abdominal excursion

Ease—Effortless; labored *(dyspnea); orthopnea* (difficult breathing except in upright position); associated with intercostal and/or substernal retractions (inspiratory "sinking in" of soft tissues in relation to the cartilaginous and bony thorax); *pulsus paradoxus* (blood pressure falls with inspiration and rises with expiration); flaring nares; head bobbing (head of sleeping child with suboccipital area supported on caregiver's forearm bobs forward in synchrony with each inspiration); grunting; wheezing

Labored breathing—Continuous, intermittent, becoming steadily worse, sudden onset, at rest or on exertion, associated with wheezing or grunting, associated with pain

Rhythm—Variation in rate and depth of respirations

Other Observations

In addition to respirations, particular attention is addressed to the following:

Evidence of infection—Check for elevated temperature, enlarged cervical lymph nodes, inflamed mucous membranes, and purulent discharges from the nose, ears, or lungs (sputum)

Cough—Observe the characteristics of the cough (if present); for example, under what circumstances the cough is heard (e.g., night only, on arising), nature of the cough (paroxysmal with or without wheeze, "croupy" or "brassy"), frequency of cough, associated with swallowing or other activity, character of the cough (moist and dry), productivity

Wheeze—Expiratory or inspiratory, high-pitched or musical, prolonged, slowly progressive or sudden, associated with labored breathing

Cyanosis—Note distribution (peripheral, perioral, facial, trunk as well as face), degree, duration, associated with activity

Chest pain—May be a complaint of older children. Note location and circumstances: localized or generalized, referred to base of neck or abdomen, dull or sharp, deep or superficial, associated with rapid, shallow respirations or grunting

Sputum—Older children may provide sputum sample by coughing, whereas young children may need use of bulb suction to provide a sample; note volume, color, viscosity, and odor

Bad breath—May be associated with some lung infections

3. Child will remain comfortable.
4. Child will not spread primary infection to others.
5. Child's temperature will remain within normal limits.
6. Child will maintain normal hydration and adequate nutrition.
7. Child will experience no complications as a result of treatments and care.
8. Child and family will receive information, especially for home care, and support.

❖ Implementation

Ease Respiratory Efforts.   Most acute respiratory infections are mild and cause few distressing symptoms. Although children may feel uncomfortable and have a "stuffy" nose and some mucosal swelling, respiratory distress occurs infrequently. The interventions described in the remainder of the discussion are usually sufficient to relieve most minor discomfort and ease respiratory efforts. However, children with croup or epiglottitis may develop sufficient swelling to obstruct the airway. These children are hospitalized for observation and therapy (see discussions of specific disorders). Positioning for optimum respiration and observation for signs of respiratory distress are primary nursing interventions.

Warm or cool mist has been a common therapeutic measure for symptomatic relief of respiratory discomfort. The moisture soothes inflamed membranes and seems to be especially beneficial when there is hoarseness or any laryngeal involvement. However, use of steam vaporizers in the home should be discouraged because of the hazards related to their use and the little evidence to support their efficacy. Shallow pans with wide surface areas for evaporation increase humidity but should be placed where they do not pose a safety hazard.

A time-honored method of producing warm mist is the shower. Running a shower of hot water into the empty bathtub or open shower stall with the bathroom door closed produces a quick source of steam. Keeping a child in this environment for 10 to 15 minutes offers the same advantages as the mist tent without the fear and restraint often associated with the confines of a tent. A small child can be held on the lap of a parent or other adult. Older children can sit in the bathroom under the supervision of an adult.

NURSING TIP A large, wet beach towel hung with one end in shallow water in the bathtub will increase humidity if the bathroom door remains open.

Promote Rest.   Children who have an acute febrile illness should be placed on bed rest. This is usually not difficult while the temperature is elevated but may be difficult when children, particularly young children, feel fairly well. When parents take the advice seriously and consistently keep them in bed, most children learn to cooperate during illness. Often children are more apt to comply if they are allowed to lie quietly on a couch where they can watch television or participate in an alternate quiet activity. If children are difficult and expend an inordinate amount of energy in protest, allowing them to play quietly on the floor serves the purpose of rest better than allowing them to cry excessively in bed. A number of entertainment devices, based on individual interests and developmental stage, can be used to keep children quiet.

Promote Comfort.   Older children are usually able to manage nasal secretions with little difficulty. Parents are instructed about the correct administration of nose drops and throat irrigations, if ordered. For very young infants, who normally breathe through their noses, an infant nasal aspirator or a rubber ear syringe is helpful in removing nasal secretions before feeding. This practice, in conjunction with the instillation of saline nose drops, may be all that is necessary to clear nasal passages and promote feeding. Saline nose drops can be prepared at home by dissolving 1 teaspoon of salt in 1 pint of warm water.*

For older infants and children who can better tolerate decongestants, vasoconstrictive nose drops may be administered 15 to 20 minutes before feeding and at bedtime. Two drops are instilled, and since this shrinks only the anterior mucous membranes, 2 more drops are instilled 5 to 10 minutes later. Phenylephrine (Neo-Synephrine) 0.25% is the usual choice of decongestant nose drops, although others, such as ephedrine 1%, may be prescribed. Older cooperative children often prefer nasal sprays. They are taught to compress the plastic container at the moment of inspiration to gain relief. Spray bottles and bottles of nose drops should be used for one child only and only for one illness, since they become easily contaminated with bacteria. Nose drops or sprays should not be administered for more than 3 days to avoid rebound congestion.

Hot or cold applications sometimes provide relief for other children with painful cervical adenitis. An ice bag or heating pad applied to the neck may decrease the discomfort, but safety precautions must be observed to prevent burns. The ice bag or heating device must be covered, and the heating pad should not be set at high ranges.

Prevent Spread of Infection. Careful handwashing should be carried out when caring for children with respiratory infections. Children and families are taught the correct disposal of respiratory secretions and proper behavior related to airborne droplets (coughing and sneezing). They are taught to use a tissue or their hand to cover their nose and mouth when they cough or sneeze and to dispose of the tissues properly, as well as wash their hands.

| **Nursing ALERT** | To avoid contamination with respiratory viruses, wash hands and do not touch your eyes or nose. |

Every endeavor should be made to remove affected children from contact with other children. Parents are encouraged to keep affected children out of school and daycare settings to prevent the spread of infection. Ideally, ill children should be isolated in a separate bedroom at the first sign of illness. This is seldom a problem with an only child but is often difficult when living arrangements are crowded and there are several children in the family. If no separate bedroom is available, the other children perhaps could sleep on a couch or cot or with relatives or friends. An effort should be made to teach well children to stay away from ill children if the living conditions allow for separation, although this may be difficult or impossible to enforce.

Reduce Temperature. If the child has a significantly elevated temperature, controlling the fever becomes a major nursing task. The parent should know how to take a child's temperature and read the thermometer accurately. Most parents are able to do this, but nurses cannot make this assumption. An assessment of the parents' learning needs precedes teaching for measures such as taking the child's temperature.*

If the practitioner has prescribed acetaminophen, parents may need help administering the drug. Most parents can read the label and calculate the desired dose, but some have difficulty and will require careful instruction or precise direction.* It is important to emphasize accuracy in both the amount of drug given and the time intervals at which the drug is administered to avoid accumulation effects. Cool liquids are encouraged to help reduce the temperature and to minimize the chances of dehydration. (See Controlling Elevated Temperatures, Chapter 22).

Promote Hydration. Dehydration is always a hazard when children are febrile or anorexic, especially when vomiting or diarrhea is also present. Adequate fluid intake should be encouraged by offering small amounts of favorite fluids at frequent intervals. High-calorie liquids, such as colas, fruit juices, water flavored and sweetened with corn syrup, or similar drinks, help prevent catabolism and dehydration but should be avoided if diarrhea is present. Oral rehydration solutions, such as Infalyte or Pedialyte, should then be considered for infants, and sports drinks, such as Gatorade or Exceed, should be considered for older children. Fluids should not be forced, and children should not be awakened to take fluids. Forcing fluids may create the same difficulties as urging unwanted food. Gentle persuasion with preferred beverages usually is successful.

Parents should know how to assess their child's level of hydration (see Chapter 29). They are advised to observe the frequency of voiding and notify the nurse or practitioner if there appears to be insufficient voiding.

NURSING TIP Counting the number of wet diapers in a 24-hour period is a satisfactory method of assessing output in infants and toddlers.

Provide Nutrition. Loss of appetite is characteristic of children with acute infections, and in most cases, children can be permitted to determine their own need for food. Many children show no decrease in appetite, and others respond well to certain foods, such as gelatin, soup, and puddings (see also Feeding the Sick Child, Chapter 22). Since the illness is relatively short, the nutritional state is seldom compromised. In fact, urging foods on anorexic children may precipitate nausea and vomiting and in some cases even cause an aversion to the feeding situation that can extend into the convalescent period and beyond.

Support Family and Prepare for Home Care. Small children with respiratory infections are irritable and often difficult to comfort. Therefore the family needs support, encouragement, and practical suggestions for care. Since most care involves comfort measures and administration of medication, a primary goal of education is related to these activities.

In addition to antipyretics and nose drops, the child may require antibiotic therapy. It is usually the nurse who instructs the parents about continuing medication begun in the hospital or initiating medications at home, especially antibiotics.

---

*Home care instructions for administration of nose drops and nasal aspiration are available in Wong DL: *Wong and Whaley's Clinical manual of pediatric nursing,* ed 4, St Louis, 1996, Mosby.

*Home care instructions for measuring temperature and administration of medication are available in Wong DL: *Wong and Whaley's Clinical manual of pediatric nursing,* ed 4, St Louis, 1996, Mosby.

NURSING CARE PLAN
The Child with Acute Respiratory Infection

NURSING DIAGNOSIS: Ineffective breathing pattern related to inflammatory process

PATIENT GOAL 1: Will exhibit normal respiratory function

- **NURSING INTERVENTIONS/RATIONALES**

Position for maximum ventilation (i.e., open airway and permit maximum lung expansion)

Allow position of comfort (e.g., tripod position of child with epiglottitis or maintain head elevation of at least 30 degrees)

Check child's position frequently to ensure child does not slide down *to avoid compressing the diaphragm*

Avoid constricting clothing or bedding

Use pillows and padding to maintain open airway (e.g., in infant or child with hypotonia)

*Provide increased humidity and supplemental oxygen by placing child in small tent or hood (infant) or administer via nasal cannula or mask (preferred methods for children older than infants because of safety issues)

Promote rest and sleep by scheduling appropriate activity and rest periods

Encourage relaxation techniques

Teach child and family measures to ease respiratory efforts (i.e., appropriate positioning)

For most respiratory illnesses, use cool-mist humidifier in child's room

    For spasmodic croup, create warm mist by running hot water in a closed bathroom (warm mist, often used for children with spasmodic croup, may be helpful because of its relaxing effect, but mostly because child is being held upright in the shower)

- **EXPECTED OUTCOMES**

Respirations remain within normal limits (see inside back cover for normal variations)

Respirations are unlabored

Child rests and sleeps quietly

PATIENT GOAL 2: Will receive optimum oxygen supply

- **NURSING INTERVENTIONS**

Position for maximum ventilatory efficiency (see Goal 1, above)

Use pulse oximetry to monitor oxygen saturations

Place in a cool, humidified environment, using appropriate oxygen delivery system

*Provide oxygen as prescribed and/or needed

- **EXPECTED OUTCOMES**

Child breathes easily

Respirations remain within normal limits (see inside back cover for normal variations)

Oxygen saturation is 95% or higher

---

*Dependent nursing action.

NURSING DIAGNOSIS: Fear/anxiety related to difficulty breathing, unfamiliar procedures, and possibly environment (hospital)

PATIENT GOAL 1: Will experience reduction of fear/anxiety

- **NURSING INTERVENTIONS**

Explain unfamiliar procedures and equipment to child in developmentally appropriate terms

Establish rapport with child and parents

Remain with child during procedures

Use calm, reassuring manner

Provide frequent attendance during acute phase of illness

Provide comfort measures child prefers (e.g., rocking, stroking, music)

Provide attachment objects (e.g., familiar toy, blanket)

Encourage family-centered care with increased parental attendance and, when possible, involvement

Do nothing to make child more anxious or fearful

Instill confidence in both parents and child

Try to avoid any intrusive or painful procedures

Be aware of child's rest/sleep cycle or pattern in planning nursing activities

Assess and implement appropriate pain management therapy (i.e., sedatives and/or analgesics) (see Pain Assessment; Pain Management, Chapter 21).

Provide diversional activities appropriate to child's cognitive ability and condition

*Administer medications that promote improved ventilation (e.g., bronchodilators, expectorants) as prescribed

- **EXPECTED OUTCOMES**

Child exhibits no signs of respiratory distress or physical discomfort

Parents remain with child and provide comfort

Child engages in quiet activities appropriate for age, interest, condition, and cognitive level

---

NURSING DIAGNOSIS: Ineffective airway clearance related to mechanical obstruction, inflammation, increased secretions, pain

PATIENT GOAL 1: Will maintain patent airway

- **NURSING INTERVENTIONS/RATIONALES**

Position child in proper body alignment *to allow better lung expansion and improved gas exchange, as well as to prevent aspiration of secretions* (prone, semiprone, side lying)

Suction secretions from airway as needed

    Limit each suction attempt to 5 seconds with sufficient time between attempts to allow reoxygenation

Position supine with head in "sniffing" position with neck slightly extended and nose pointed to ceiling

    Avoid neck hyperextension

Continued.

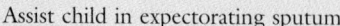

Nursing Care Plan

The Child with Acute Respiratory Infection—cont'd

Assist child in expectorating sputum
*Administer expectorants if prescribed
Perform chest physiotherapy
Give nothing by mouth *to prevent aspiration of fluids* (e.g., child with severe tachypnea)
*Administer appropriate pain management
Have emergency equipment available *to avoid delay in treatment if needed*
Avoid throat examination and culture with suspected epiglottitis *because it could cause airway obstruction*
Assist child in splinting any incisional/injured area *to maximize effects of coughing and chest physiotherapy*

• **EXPECTED OUTCOMES**

Airways remain clear
Child breathes easily; respirations are within normal limits (see inside back cover)

PATIENT GOAL 2: Will expectorate secretions adequately

• **NURSING INTERVENTIONS/**RATIONALES

Ensure adequate fluid intake *to liquefy secretions*
Provide humidified atmosphere *to prevent crusting of nasal secretions and drying of mucous membranes*
Explain importance of expectoration to child and family
Assist child in coughing effectively; provide tissues
Remove accumulated mucus; suction if needed
*Administer pain medications as indicated before attempt to clear airway
Provide nebulization with appropriate solution and equipment as prescribed
Assist with splinting *so child will experience minimal discomfort*
*Perform percussion, vibration, and postural drainage *to facilitate drainage of secretions*

• **EXPECTED OUTCOME**

Older child expectorates secretions without undue stress and fatigue; younger child is able to have a productive cough

NURSING DIAGNOSIS: High risk for infection related to presence of infective organisms

PATIENT GOAL 1: Will exhibit no signs of secondary infection

• **NURSING INTERVENTIONS/**RATIONALES

Maintain aseptic environment, using sterile suction catheters and good handwashing
Isolate child as indicated *to prevent nosocomial spread of infection*
Administer antibiotics as prescribed *to prevent or treat infection*

*Dependent nursing action.

Provide nutritious diet according to child's preferences and ability to consume nourishment *to support body's natural defenses*
Encourage good chest physiotherapy
Teach child and/or family manifestations of illness

• **EXPECTED OUTCOME**

Child exhibits evidence of diminishing symptoms of infection

PATIENT GOAL 2: Will not spread infection to others

• **NURSING INTERVENTIONS**

Use universal precautions (see Infection Control, Chapter 22)
Instruct others (parents, members of staff) in appropriate precautions
Teach affected children protective methods to prevent spread of infection (e.g., handwashing, disposal of soiled tissues)
Limit the number of visitors/family members/siblings and screen for any recent illness
Try to keep infants and small children from placing hands and objects in contaminated areas
Assess home situation and implement protective measures as feasible in individual circumstances
*Administer antimicrobial medications if prescribed

• **EXPECTED OUTCOME**

Others remain free from infection

NURSING DIAGNOSIS: Activity intolerance related to inflammatory process, imbalance between oxygen supply and demand

PATIENT GOAL 1: Will maintain adequate energy levels

• **NURSING INTERVENTIONS**

Assess child's level of physical tolerance
Assist child in those activities of daily living that may be beyond tolerance
Provide diversional activities appropriate to child's age, condition, capabilities, and interest
Provide diversional play activities that promote rest and quiet but prevent boredom and withdrawal
Provide rest and sleep periods appropriate to age and condition
Instruct child to rest when feeling tired
Balance rest and activity when ambulatory

• **EXPECTED OUTCOMES**

Child plays and rests quietly and engages in activities appropriate to age and capabilities (specify)
Child exhibits no evidence of increased respiratory distress
Child tolerates increasingly more activity

Nursing Care Plan
The Child with Acute Respiratory Infection—cont'd

PATIENT GOAL 2: Will receive optimum rest

• **NURSING INTERVENTIONS/RATIONALES**

Provide quiet environment
Organize activities for maximum sleep time
Do not perform nonessential treatments or procedures *to maximize rest*
Schedule visiting to allow for sufficient rest
Encourage parents to remain with child
Schedule treatments or other activities around child's needs *so that fatigue will be minimized.*
*Administer sedatives and analgesics as indicated if ordered for restlessness and pain
Encourage frequent rest periods and regular sleep times
Follow child's usual routine for bedtime and nap time
Implement measures to ensure sleep, such as quiet, darkened room

• **EXPECTED OUTCOMES**

Child remains calm, quiet, and relaxed
Child rests a sufficient amount (specify)

NURSING DIAGNOSIS: Pain related to inflammatory process, surgical incision

---

PATIENT GOAL 1: Will experience no pain or reduction of pain/discomfort to level acceptable to child

• **NURSING INTERVENTIONS**

Use local measures (gargles, troches, warmth or cold) to reduce throat pain
Apply heat or cold as appropriate to affected area

---
*Dependent nursing action.

---

*Administer analgesic as prescribed (see Pain Management, Chapter 21)
Assess response to pain control measures (see Pain Assessment, Chapter 21)
Encourage diversional activities appropriate to age, condition, capabilities

• **EXPECTED OUTCOME**

Child has no pain or acceptable level of pain

NURSING DIAGNOSIS: Altered family process related to illness and/or hospitalization of a child

---

PATIENT (FAMILY) GOAL 1: Will experience reduction of anxiety and increased ability to cope

• **NURSING INTERVENTIONS**

Recognize parental concern and need for information and support
Explore family's feelings and "problems" surrounding hospitalization and child's illness
Explain therapy and child's behavior
Provide support as needed
Encourage family-centered care and encourage family to become involved in child's care

• **EXPECTED OUTCOME**

Parents ask appropriate questions, discuss child's condition and care calmly, and become involved positively in child's care

See also:
Nursing Care Plan: The Family of the Ill or Hospitalized Child, Chapter 21
Nursing Care Plan: The Child in the Hospital, Chapter 21

Parents of children who are sent home with oral antibiotics need to understand the importance of regular administration and continuing the drug for the prescribed length of time, regardless of whether the child appears to be ill.

Parents are also cautioned against giving the child any medications that are not approved by the health practitioner. Adverse effects have been noted in children who have received some preparations intended for adults (e.g., some long-acting nose drops [Neo-Synephrine II] and dextromethorphan cough squares [mistaken for candy]). They are also cautioned about giving the child unprescribed antibiotics left over from a previous illness. Self-medication with unprescribed antibiotics is a significant problem. It should be emphasized that some drugs interact with others to produce serious side effects, and such a likelihood is increased when medications are administered to children without consulta-

tion with the practitioner. The nurse is in an excellent position to provide drug information to families. (See Chapter 22 for administration of medications and teaching parents.)

❖ Evaluation

The effectiveness of nursing interventions is determined by continual reassessment and evaluation of care based on the following observational guidelines and expected outcomes:

1. Observe child's respiratory effort and movement.
2. Observe signs and symptoms for progress toward health status before illness.
3. Observe child's behavior and activity.
4. Observe other family members and contacts for evidence of infection.
5. Take temperature.
6. Observe for signs of adequate hydration.

7. Observe eating behavior.
8. Assess child for evidence of complications, such as dehydration, weight loss, or spread of infection to other areas of the body.
9. Observe family's behavior and interview members regarding their feelings and concerns.

Expected outcomes:
See Nursing Care Plan, pp. 753-755.

ACUTE UPPER RESPIRATORY TRACT INFECTIONS (URIs)

NASOPHARYNGITIS

Acute nasopharyngitis (the equivalent of the "common cold") is caused by any of a number of different viruses, usually rhinoviruses, respiratory syncytial virus (RSV), adenovirus, influenza virus, or parainfluenza virus.

Symptoms of nasopharyngitis are more severe in infants and children than in adults. Fever is common, especially in young children. Older children have low-grade fevers, which appear early in the process. Other clinical manifestations are listed in the box.

Therapeutic Management

Children with nasopharyngitis are managed at home. There is no specific treatment, and effective vaccines are not available. Antipyretics are usually prescribed for mild fever and discomfort (see Chapter 28 for management of fever). Decongestants may be prescribed for children and infants older than 6 months in an effort to shrink swollen nasal passages. The decongestants that exert their effect by vasoconstriction are usually less effective when taken orally than when applied topically as nose drops. Since these drugs affect *all* vascular beds, they should be given with caution to children with diabetes.

Cough suppressants containing dextromethorphan may be prescribed for a dry, hacking cough. Some preparations contain up to 22% alcohol; they should not be administered to young children continuously and must be stored securely away from children.

Antihistamines are largely ineffective in treatment of nasopharyngitis. The drugs have a weak atropine-like effect that tends to dry secretions, but they can cause drowsiness and, paradoxically, have a stimulatory effect on children. There is no support for the usefulness of expectorants, and antibiotics are usually contraindicated because they can sensitize a child who may need the drugs in a severe illness.

Prevention. Nasopharyngitis is so widespread in the general population that it is difficult to prevent. In addition, children are more susceptible to colds because they have not yet developed resistance to many types of viruses. Very young infants are subject to relatively serious complications; therefore some attempt should be made to protect them from exposure. Rest is recommended until the child is afebrile for at least 1 day.

Nursing Considerations

A cold is often the parents' first introduction to an illness in their infants. Parents are assisted in managing the infant or child as described for general care. Most of the distress of nasopharyngitis is related to the nasal obstruction, especially in small infants. Placing the child in a prone position (unless respirations are compromised) and elevating the head of bed (assists with drainage of secretions), suctioning, and vaporization may help provide relief. Saline nose drops and gentle suction with a bulb syringe, particularly before feeding, are sometimes useful.

Maintaining adequate fluid intake is essential during any infectious process. Although a child's appetite for solid foods is usually diminished for several days, it is important to offer favorite fluids to prevent dehydration. Fluids can be cool or warm, depending on individual preference.

Because nasopharyngitis is spread from secretions, the best means for prevention is avoiding contact with affected persons. This goal is difficult in places where large numbers of people are confined in a small area for a long time, such as classrooms and daycare centers. Family members with a cold should try to "keep it to themselves" by carefully disposing of tissues; not sharing towels, glasses, or eating utensils; covering the mouth and nose with tissues when coughing or sneezing; and washing the hands thoroughly after nose blowing or sneezing. The most frequent carriers of infection are the human hands, which deposit viruses on doorknobs, faucets, and other everyday objects. Therefore children should be taught to wash their hands thoroughly before putting them near their eyes, nose, or mouth.

Family Support. Support and reassurance are important elements of care for families of young children with recurrent URIs. Because URIs are so frequent in children less than 3 years of age, families may feel they are on an endless roller coaster of illness. They can be reassured that frequent colds are a normal part of childhood and that by 5 years of age, their children will have developed immunity to many vi-

---

CLINICAL MANIFESTATIONS OF NASOPHARYNGITIS AND PHARYNGITIS

Nasopharyngitis	Pharyngitis
YOUNGER CHILD	**YOUNGER CHILD**
Fever	Fever
Irritability, restlessness	General malaise
Sneezing	Anorexia
Vomiting and/or diarrhea, sometimes	Moderate sore throat
	Headache
OLDER CHILD	**OLDER CHILD**
Dryness and irritation of nose and throat	Fever (may reach 40° C [104° F])
Sneezing, chilly sensation	Headache
	Anorexia
Muscular aches	Dysphagia
Cough, sometimes	Abdominal pain
	Vomiting
Physical Signs	*Physical Signs*
Edema and vasodilation of mucosa	**YOUNGER CHILD**
	Mild to moderate hyperemia
	OLDER CHILD
	Mild to fiery red, edematous pharynx
	Hyperemia of tonsils and pharynx; may extend to soft palate and uvula
	Often abundant follicular exudate that spreads and coalesces to form pseudomembrane on tonsils
	Cervical glands enlarged and tender

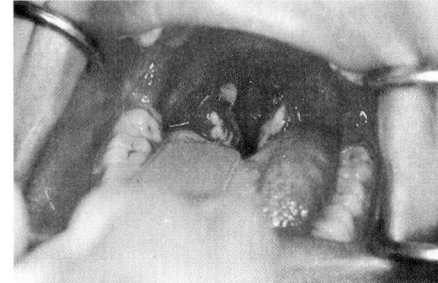

FIG. 23-1. Tonsillitis and pharyngitis. (From Thompson JM and others: *Clinical nursing,* St Louis, 1986, Mosby.)

ruses. Parents who work outside the home should expect to have to take time off to care for ill children during the fall and winter months. If the children are cared for routinely in daycare centers, the infection rate will be higher than if they were being cared for in the home. Parents should know the signs of respiratory complications and be counseled to notify a health professional if any signs of complications appear or if the child does not improve within 2 or 3 days (see box).

PHARYNGITIS

Group A β-hemolytic streptococci (GABHS) infection of the upper airway *(strep throat)* is not in itself a serious disease, but affected children are at risk for serious sequelae: *acute rheumatic fever (RF),* an inflammatory disease of heart, joints, and central nervous system (see Chapter 25), and *acute glomerulonephritis,* an acute kidney infection (see Chapter 27). Permanent damage can result from these sequelae, especially acute RF.

Clinical Manifestations

GABHS is generally a relatively brief illness that varies greatly in severity from subclinical (no symptoms) to comparatively severe toxicity. The onset is generally abrupt and characterized by pharyngitis, headache, fever, and (especially in small children) abdominal pain. The tonsils and pharynx may be inflamed and covered with exudate (Fig. 23-1), which usually appears by the second day of illness. Anterior cervical lymphadenopathy (30% to 50% of cases) usually occurs early, and the nodes are often tender. Pain can be relatively mild to severe enough to make swallowing difficult. Clinical manifestations usually subside in 3 to 5 days unless complicated by sinusitis or parapharyngeal, peritonsillar, or retropharyngeal abscess. Nonsuppurative complications may appear after the onset of GABHS—acute nephritis in about 10 days and RF in an average of 18 days.

Diagnostic Evaluation

Clinical diagnosis of GABHS infection can present difficulties. Although 80% to 90% of all cases of acute pharyngitis are viral, a throat culture should be performed to rule out GABHS and (in some cases) *Corynebacterium diphtheriae.*

Because some children normally harbor streptococci in their throats, a positive culture is not always conclusive evidence of active disease. Since most streptococcal infections are short-term illnesses, antibody (antistreptolysin O) responses do not appear until relatively late and are useful only for retrospective diagnosis.

Rapid identification of GABHS is possible with diagnostic test kits that can be used in the office or clinic setting. However, because of their questionable sensitivity, they are not yet considered to be a substitute for culture, especially if the organism is endemic in the community.

Therapeutic Management

If streptococcal sore throat infection is present, oral penicillin is prescribed in a dose sufficient to control the acute local manifestations and to maintain an adequate level for at least 10 days to eliminate any organisms that might remain to initiate RF symptoms. Penicillin does not appear to prevent the development of acute glomerulonephritis in susceptible children; however, it may prevent the spread of a nephrogenic strain of GABHS to others in the family. Penicillin usually produces a prompt response within 24 hours. Occasionally, patients require retreatment if the organism is not eradicated.

A combination of penicillin and rifampin is more effective in eradicating GABHS than penicillin alone and is recommended for carriers and persons resistant to penicillin. Erythromycin or a cephalosporin may be used for children who are sensitive to penicillin. Clinical manifestations are treated symptomatically.

Nursing Considerations

The nurse is often the person who performs a throat smear for culture and instructs the parents about administering penicillin and analgesics as prescribed. Most children prefer to remain in bed during the acute phase of the illness. Cold or warm compresses to the neck may provide relief. In children old enough to cooperate, warm saline gargles offer some relief of throat discomfort. Pain may interfere with oral intake, and the child should not be forced to eat. Cool liquids or ice chips are usually more acceptable than solids and are encouraged.

Special emphasis is placed on correct administration of oral medication and completing the course of antibiotic therapy (see Administration of Medication; Compliance, Chapter 22). If injections are required, they must be administered deep into a large muscle mass (e.g., vastus lateralis or gluteus muscle). Parents need to be aware of the residual tenderness, which may cause the child to limp for a day or two. Local applications of heat are helpful in relieving some of the discomfort.

TONSILLITIS

The tonsils are masses of lymphoid tissue located in the pharyngeal cavity. Their function is to filter and protect the respiratory and alimentary tracts from invasion by pathogenic organisms. They also may have a role in antibody formation. Although the size of tonsils varies, children generally have much larger tonsils than adolescents or adults. This difference is thought to be a protective mechanism at a time when young children are especially susceptible to URI.

Pathophysiology

Several pairs of tonsils are part of a mass of lymphoid tissue encircling the nasal and oral pharynx, known as *Waldeyer tonsillar ring* (Fig. 23-2). The *palatine,* or *faucial, tonsils* are located on either side of the oropharynx, behind and below the pillars of the fauces (opening from the mouth). A free surface of the palatine tonsils is usually visible during oral examination. The palatine tonsils are those removed during tonsillectomy. The *pharyngeal tonsils,* also known as the *adenoids,* are located above the palatine tonsils on the posterior wall of the nasopharynx. Their proximity to the nares and eustachian tubes causes difficulties in instances of inflammation. The *lingual tonsils* are located at the base of the tongue and only rarely are removed. The *tubal tonsils,* found near the posterior nasopharyngeal opening of the eustachian tubes, are not part of the Waldeyer tonsillar ring.

Etiology

Tonsillitis usually occurs in association with pharyngitis. Because of the abundant lymphoid tissue and the frequency of URIs, tonsillitis is a very common cause of morbidity in young children. The causative agent may be viral or bacterial.

Clinical Manifestations

The manifestations of tonsillitis are chiefly caused by inflammation. As the palatine tonsils enlarge from edema, they may meet in the midline (kissing tonsils), obstructing the passage of air or food. The child has difficulty swallowing and breathing. When enlargement of the adenoids occurs, the space behind the posterior nares may become blocked, making it difficult or impossible for air to pass from the nose to the throat. As a result, the child breathes through the mouth.

Therapeutic Management

Since tonsillitis is self-limiting, treatment of viral pharyngitis is symptomatic. Throat cultures positive for GABHS infection warrant antibiotic treatment. It is important to differentiate between viral and streptococcal infection in febrile exudative tonsillitis. Since most infections are of viral origin, early rapid tests can eliminate unnecessary antibiotic administration.

Tonsillectomy (removal of the palatine tonsils) is indicated for massive hypertrophy that results in difficulty breathing or eating (Derkay, Darrow, and LeFebvre, 1995). Absolute indications are malignancy and obstruction of the airway. *Adenoidectomy* (removal of the adenoids) is recommended for those children in whom hypertrophied adenoids obstruct nasal breathing. Their removal may be warranted in the child under 3 years of age and should be performed without a tonsillectomy. Contraindications to either tonsillectomy or adenoidectomy are (1) cleft palate, since both tonsils help minimize escape of air during speech; (2) acute infections at the time of surgery, since the locally inflamed tissues increase the risk of bleeding; and (3) uncontrolled systemic diseases or blood dyscrasias.

Nursing Considerations

Nursing care of the child with tonsillitis mainly involves providing comfort and minimizing activities or interventions that might precipitate bleeding. A soft to liquid diet is generally preferred. A cool-mist vaporizer helps keep the mucous membranes moist during periods of mouth breathing. Warm saltwater gargles, throat lozenges, and analgesic/antipyretic drugs such as acetaminophen (Tylenol) and codeine are useful to promote comfort.

If surgery is needed, the child requires the same psychologic preparation and physical care as for any other procedure (see Chapters 21 and 22). The following discussion focuses on postoperative nursing care for tonsillectomy and adenoidectomy (T & A), although both procedures may not be performed.

Until they are fully awake, children are placed on the abdomen or side to facilitate drainage of secretions, and any needed suctioning is performed carefully to avoid trauma to the oropharynx. When alert, children may prefer sitting up, although they should remain in bed for the remainder of the day. They are discouraged from coughing frequently, clearing their throat, and blowing their nose, activities that may aggravate the operative site.

Some secretions are common, particularly dried blood from surgery. All secretions and vomitus are inspected for evi-

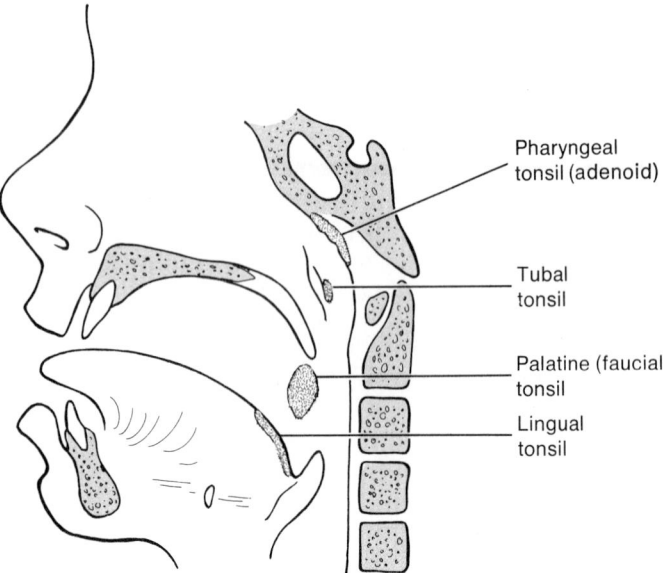

FIG. 23-2. Location of the various tonsillar masses.

Pharyngeal tonsil (adenoid)

Tubal tonsil

Palatine (faucial) tonsil

Lingual tonsil

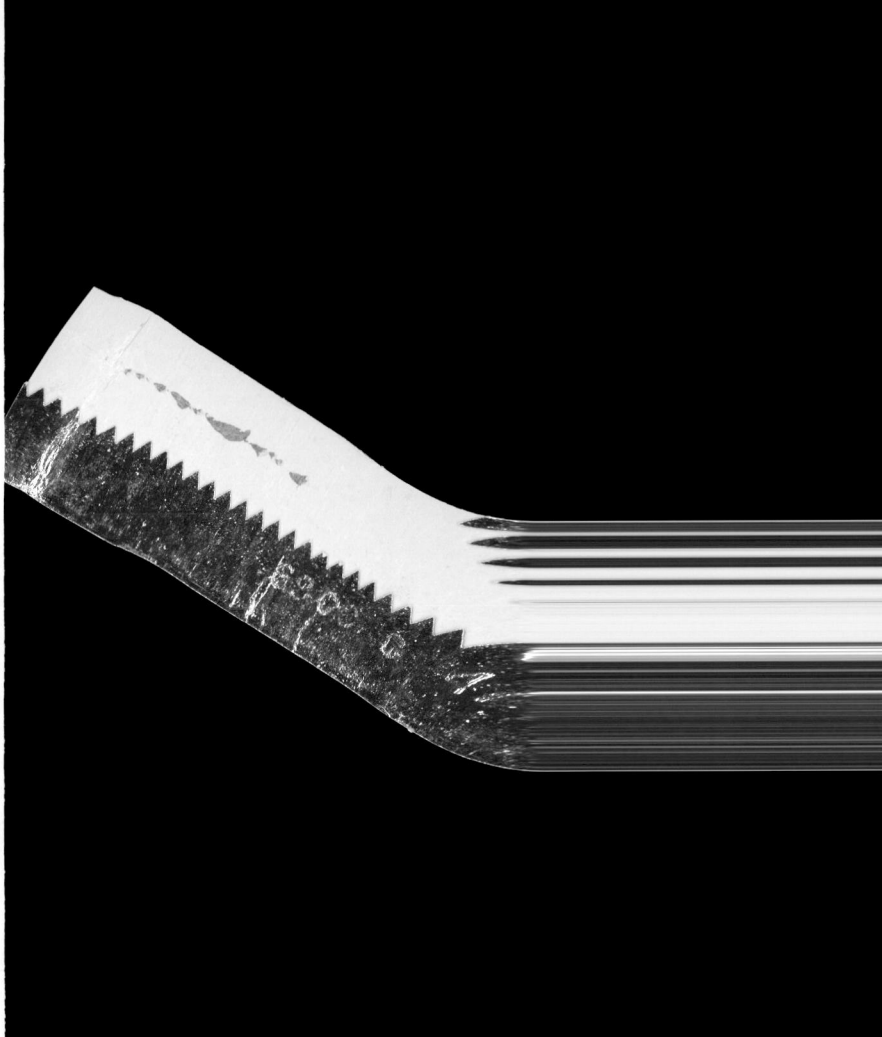

dence of fresh bleeding (some blood-tinged mucus is expected). Dark-brown (old) blood is usually present in the emesis, as well as in the nose and between the teeth. If parents do not expect this, they may be frightened at a time when they need to be calm and reassuring for their children.

The throat is very sore after surgery. An ice collar may provide relief, but many children find it bothersome and prefer not to have it. Most children experience considerable pain after a T &/or A and should receive pain medication for at least the first 24 hours. Analgesics are ordered but may need to be given rectally or intravenously to avoid the oral route. Since pain is continuous, pain control should be continuous or administered at regular intervals (see Pain Management, Chapter 21). Irritable children may require mild sedation to lessen crying, which irritates the operative site, increasing the chance of bleeding.

Food and fluid are restricted until children are fully alert and there are no signs of hemorrhage. Cool water, crushed ice, flavored ice pops, or dilute fruit juice is given first, although fluids with a red or brown color are avoided to distinguish fresh or old blood in emesis from the ingested liquid. Citrus juice may cause discomfort and is usually poorly tolerated. Soft foods, particularly gelatin, cooked fruits, sherbet, soup, and mashed potatoes, are started on the first or second postoperative day or as the child tolerates feeding. The pain from surgery often inhibits intake, reinforcing the need for adequate pain control.

> **F Y I**
> Traditionally, milk, ice cream, and pudding have not been offered, because milk products coat the mouth and throat, causing the child to clear the throat more often, which may initiate bleeding. However, when children were offered milk or apple juice, more youngsters chose the juice but over a third also drank the milk. The researchers concluded that children should be given an unrestricted diet postoperatively to increase their food and liquid consumption (Thomas, Moore, and Reilly, 1995).

Postoperative hemorrhage is unusual but can occur. Therefore the nurse observes the throat directly for evidence of bleeding, using a good source of light and, if necessary, carefully inserting a tongue depressor. Other signs of hemorrhage are increased pulse (greater than 120 beats/minute), pallor, frequent clearing of the throat or swallowing by a younger child, and vomiting of bright-red blood. Restlessness, an indication of hemorrhage, may be difficult to differentiate from general discomfort after surgery. Decreasing blood pressure is a much later sign of shock.

> **Nursing ALERT**
> The most obvious early sign of bleeding is the child's continuous swallowing of the trickling blood. While the child is sleeping, note the frequency of swallowing. If continuous bleeding is suspected, notify the surgeon immediately.

Family Support and Home Care. Discharge instructions include (1) avoiding foods that are irritating or highly seasoned, (2) avoiding the use of gargles or vigorous toothbrushing, (3) discouraging the child from coughing or clearing the throat or putting objects in the mouth, (4) using mild analgesics or an ice collar for pain, and (5) limiting activity to decrease the potential for bleeding. Hemorrhage may occur up to 10 days after surgery as a result of tissue sloughing from the healing process. Any sign of bleeding warrants immediate medical attention.

INFLUENZA

Influenza, or "flu," is caused by different viruses that may undergo significant changes from time to time. The disease is spread from one individual to another by direct contact (large-droplet infection) or by articles recently contaminated by nasopharyngeal secretions. There is no predilection for a specific age-group, but attack rates are highest in young children who have not had previous contact with a strain. [It is] frequently most severe in infants. During epidemics, inf[ection] among school-age children is believed to be a major [source] of transmission in a community. Influenza is more c[ommon] during the winter months. The disease has a 1- to 3-d[ay in]cubation period, and affected persons are most infectiou[s for] 24 hours before and after onset of symptoms.

Clinical Manifestations

The manifestations of influenza may be subclinical, mild, moderate, or severe. Most patients with overt illness have a dry throat and nasal mucosa, a dry cough, and a tendency toward hoarseness. A sudden onset of fever and chills is accompanied by flushed face, photophobia, myalgia, hyperesthesia, and sometimes prostration. Subglottal croup is common, especially in infants. The symptoms last for 4 to 5 days. Complications include severe viral pneumonia (often hemorrhagic), encephalitis, and secondary bacterial infections, such as otitis media, sinusitis, or pneumonia.

Therapeutic Management

Uncomplicated influenza in children usually requires only symptomatic treatment: acetaminophen for fever, dextromethorphan for cough (if needed), and sufficient fluids to maintain hydration. Amantadine hydrochloride (Symmetrel) has been effective in reducing symptoms associated with type A disease if administered within 24 to 48 hours after onset. It is ineffective against type B or C influenza or other viral diseases. It should not be given to children under 1 year of age but is recommended for unvaccinated high-risk children. Children with influenza (or other similar viruses) should not receive aspirin because of its possible link with Reye syndrome.

Prevention.   Inactivated influenza viral vaccines are safe and effective for prevention of influenza provided the antigens in the vaccine correlate with circulating influenza viruses. For information on immunization, see Chapter 10.

Nursing Considerations

Nursing care is the same as for any child with a URI, including helping the family to implement measures to relieve symptoms. The greatest danger to affected children is development of a secondary infection.

Nursing ALERT	Prolonged fever or appearance of fever during early convalescence is a sign of secondary bacterial infection and should be reported to the practitioner for antibiotic therapy.

OTITIS MEDIA (OM)

OM is one of the most prevalent diseases of early childhood. The incidence is highest in children ages 6 months to 2 years; it then gradually decreases with age, except for a small increase at age 5 or 6 years, the time of school entry. OM occurs infrequently in children over 7 years of age. Boys are affected more frequently than girls in children less than school age; later the sexes are affected equally. The incidence of acute otitis media (AOM) is highest in the winter months. Children living in households with many members (especially smokers) are more likely to have OM than those living with fewer persons, and children with siblings or parents who had a history of chronic OM have a higher incidence than those who do not.

OM has been defined in a variety of ways. The standard terminology that has been established to describe OM is outlined in the box below.

Etiology

AOM is most frequently caused by *Streptococcus pneumoniae* and *Haemophilus influenzae*. The etiology of the noninfectious type is unknown, although it is frequently the result of blocked eustachian tubes from the edema of URIs, allergic rhinitis, or hypertrophic adenoids. OME is frequently an extension of an acute episode. Passive smoking has been established as a significant factor in the development of OM. Tobacco smoke inhalation may increase the risk of a blocked eustachian tube by impairing mucociliary function, causing congestion of soft nasopharyngeal tissues, or by predisposing patients to URI. Daycare attendance is also a risk factor for OM (Alho and others, 1993).

Infants fed breast milk have a lower incidence of OM compared with formula-fed infants. Breast-feeding may protect infants against respiratory viruses and allergy by the presence of increased secretory immunoglobulin A (IgA) and limits the exposure of the eustachian tube and middle ear mucosa to microbial pathogens and foreign proteins. Also, reflux of milk up the eustachian tubes is less likely in breast-fed infants because of the semivertical positioning during breast-feeding compared with bottle-feeding. There is a definite link between the supine position during feeding and the reflux of

fluid into the middle ear (Tully, Bar-Haim, and Bradley, 1995).

Pathophysiology

OM is primarily the result of dysfunctioning eustachian tubes. The eustachian tube, which connects the middle ear to the nasopharynx, is normally closed and flat, preventing organisms from the pharyngeal cavity from entering the middle ear. It opens to allow drainage of secretions produced by the middle ear mucosa and to equalize air pressure between the middle ear and outside environment. Impaired drainage causes retention of secretions in the middle ear. Air, unable to escape through the obstructed tubes, is absorbed into the circulation, causing negative pressure within the middle ear. If the tube opens, this difference in pressure causes bacteria to be swept into the middle ear chamber, where the organisms quickly proliferate and invade the mucosa.

Diagnostic Evaluation

In AOM, otoscopy reveals an intact membrane that appears bright red and bulging, with no visible bony landmarks or light reflex. In OME, otoscopic findings may include a slightly inflamed, dull gray membrane, obscured landmarks, and a visible fluid level or meniscus behind the eardrum if air is present above the fluid. Diagnosis is usually based on clinical manifestations (see box below) and confirmed with **tympanometry,** which measures the change in air pressure in the external auditory canal from movement of the eardrum. The presence of fluid in the middle ear decreases membrane movement or compliance. *Pneumatic otoscopy* also provides an assessment of typanic membrane mobility. If purulent discharge is present, it should be cultured and a specific antibiotic selected for that organism. Hearing evaluation is recommended for a child who has had bilateral OME for a total of 3 months.

STANDARD TERMINOLOGY FOR OTITIS MEDIA

Otitis media (OM)—An inflammation of the middle ear without reference to etiology or pathogenesis

Acute otitis media (AOM)—A rapid and short onset of signs and symptoms lasting approximately 3 weeks

Otitis media with effusion (OME)—An inflammation of the middle ear in which a collection of fluid is present in the middle ear space

Chronic otitis media with effusion—Middle ear effusion that persists beyond 3 months

---

CLINICAL MANIFESTATIONS OF OTITIS MEDIA

Acute Otitis Media
Follows an upper respiratory infection
Otalgia (earache)
Purulent otorrhea may be present
Fever
Purulent discharge may or may not be present

Infant or Very Young Child
Crying
Fussy, restless, irritable
Tendency to rub, hold, or pull affected ear
Rolls head side to side
Difficulty comforting child
Loss of appetite

Older Child
Crying and/or verbalizes feelings of discomfort
Irritability
Lethargy
Loss of appetite

Chronic Otitis Media
Hearing loss
Difficulty communicating
Feeling of fullness, tinnitus, or vertigo may be present

Therapeutic Management

Treatment of AOM is administration of antibiotics, such as ampicillin, amoxicillin, sulfonamides, trimethoprim-sulfamethoxazole (Bactrim, Septra), erythromycin-sulfisoxazole (Pediazole), and the cephalosporins. With appropriate therapy most children improve within 48 to 72 hours. *Myringotomy* (surgical incision of the eardrum) may be required to relieve the symptoms in some children, especially those with acute suppuration who are in severe pain. Children with AOM should be seen after antibiotic therapy is complete to evaluate the effectiveness of the treatment and to identify potential complications, such as effusion or hearing impairment. Analgesic/antipyretic drugs are used to alleviate discomfort and reduce an elevated temperature.

The major goals in the management of OME are to establish and maintain an aerated middle ear free of fluid and with a normal mucosa and to achieve normal hearing. A trial of antibiotic therapy or simply observing the child may be tried first. The use of steroids, decongestants, and antihistamines to shrink the mucous membranes and increase eustachian tube function is not recommended. Surgical treatment involves tympanoplasty or insertion of ventilating tubes. Tympanostomy tubes (pressure-equalizer [PE] tubes or grommets) facilitate continued drainage of fluid and allow ventilation of the middle ear. Myringotomy with or without insertion of PE tubes should *not* be performed for initial management of OME in an otherwise healthy child. Adenoidectomy is not recommended for treatment of OME in a child ages 1 to 3 years without specific adenoid pathology. Tonsillectomy should not be performed, either alone or with adenoidectomy, for the treatment of OME in a child of any age (Stool and others, 1994).

Although the insertion of tympanostomy (PE) tubes is the number-one procedure performed in pediatrics, its use is highly controversial and considered unnecessary by many authorities.

In a study done to assess the appropriateness of using PE tubes, only about 40% of the proposed PE tube placements were defined as appropriate (Kleinman and others, 1994).

Although nurses do not make the decision regarding surgical intervention for OM, they do play an important role in counseling families about proposed treatments and assessing if parents are fully informed. The Agency for Health Care Planning and Research (AHCPR) has released federal guidelines for the treatment of OME. Nurses should be familiar with this publication, which may become an accepted standard of care.*

Nursing Considerations

❖ Assessment

Examination of the external auditory canal is an integral part of the physical assessment (see Chapter 7). Nurses should be alert to any child recovering from a URI who displays evidence of hearing difficulty (see Chapter 19).

---

*The *Managing Otitis Media with Effusion in Young Children* guidelines include an overview (AHCPR Pub. No. 94-0620), a quick reference guide (94-0623), and a parent guide (94-0624) that are available in English and Spanish from the AHCPR Publications Clearinghouse, OME/AAP, P.O. Box 8547, Silver Spring, MD 20907; (800) 358-9295.

NURSING DIAGNOSES: THE CHILD WITH ACUTE OTITIS MEDIA
Pain related to pressure caused by inflammatory process
High risk for impaired skin integrity related to drainage
Altered family processes related to ill child

❖ Nursing Diagnoses

Based on a careful assessment, several nursing diagnoses become evident (see box). Others may apply in specific situations and in the case of chronic OM or OME.

❖ Planning

Goals for the care of the child with AOM and the family include the following:

1. Child will experience no pain or a reduction of pain/discomfort to level acceptable to child.
2. Child will not experience recurrence of infection.
3. Child will not experience complications from illness or treatment modalities.
4. Family will receive adequate support and education.

❖ Implementation

Analgesics/antipyretics, such as acetaminophen, are helpful in reducing the severe earache and fever. The application of heat with a heating pad on low setting and wrapped in a towel may reduce the discomfort. Local heat should be placed over the ear with the child lying on the affected side. This position also facilitates drainage of the exudate if the eardrum has ruptured or if myringotomy was performed. An ice bag placed over the affected ear may also be beneficial, since it reduces edema and pressure. If the child is cooperative, either procedure can be tried to determine which offers maximum relief.

If the ear is draining, the external canal may be cleaned with sterile cotton swabs or pledgets soaked in hydrogen peroxide. If ear wicks or lightly rolled sterile gauze packs are placed in the ear after surgical treatment, they should be loose enough to allow accumulated drainage to flow out of the ear; otherwise the infection may be transferred to the mastoid process. The wicks need to stay dry during shampoos or baths. Occasionally, drainage is so profuse that the auricle and the skin surrounding the ear become excoriated from the exudate. This is prevented by frequent cleansing and application of various moisture barriers (e.g., Aloe Vesta, Proshield Plus) or petrolatum jelly (e.g., Vaseline).

Parents require anticipatory guidance regarding temporary hearing loss that accompanies OM. The nurse should caution parents not to assume that the child is ignoring them, but to realize that the child may be unaware of being spoken to. Parents are instructed to speak louder, at closer proximity, and facing the child. Persistent difficulty in hearing beyond the acute stage is evaluated.

A concern presented with the use of myringotomy tubes is the possibility of water entering the middle ear and introducing bacteria. Recommendations for the use of earplugs are inconsistent, but research indicates that swimming without earplugs poses no increased risk of infection. The question of whether or not bathwater is harmful remains unanswered.

Bathwater and shampoo water should be kept out of the ear, if possible, since soap reduces the surface tension of water, facilitating entry through the tube.

Parents should be aware of the appearance of a grommet (usually a tiny, white, plastic spool-shaped tube) so that they can observe if it falls out. They are reassured that this is normal and requires no immediate intervention, although they should notify the practitioner.

Prevention of recurrence requires adequate parent education regarding antibiotic therapy. Since the symptoms of pain and fever usually subside within 24 to 48 hours, nurses must emphasize that although the child appears well, the infection is not completely eradicated until all the prescribed medication is taken. Parents should be aware of the potential complications of OM that can occur with inadequate treatment, such as (1) conductive hearing loss; (2) a perforated and scarred eardrum; (3) *mastoiditis,* an inflammation of the mastoid air cell system; (4) *cholesteatoma,* a cystlike lesion that can invade and destroy surrounding auditory structures; and (5) intracranial infections, such as meningitis.

Nurses need to take an active role in teaching parents about the possibility of OM resulting from the supine feeding position when not followed by the infant sitting or walking. During bottle-feeding and breast-feeding the child should be semiupright. Propping bottles is discouraged both to avoid the supine position and to ensure human contact during feeding. Since infants have difficulty expressing themselves verbally, parents should be taught that some initial signs of OM may be irritability and ear pulling. Eliminating tobacco smoke and known allergens is also recommended.

❖ Evaluation

The efficacy of nursing intervention is determined by the following observational guidelines and expected outcomes:

1. Observe behaviors that indicate pain relief; seek verbal confirmation.
2. Observe skin in and around the external auditory canal.
3. Interview family regarding practices that prevent recurrence of infection.
4. Observe and interview family regarding their understanding of OM and therapies.
5. Interview family regarding their feelings and concerns.

Expected outcomes:

1. Child sleeps and rests quietly and exhibits no signs of discomfort.
2. Child exhibits no evidence of excoriated skin.
3. Child remains free of complications.
4. Family demonstrates the ability to care for child's condition.
5. Family and child express their feelings and concerns.

See also Nursing Care Plan: The Child with Acute Otitis Media.*

CROUP SYNDROMES

Croup is a general term applied to a symptom complex characterized by hoarseness, a resonant cough described as "bark-

---

*In Wong DL: *Wong and Whaley's Clinical manual of pediatric nursing,* ed 4, St Louis, 1996, Mosby.

---

ing" or "brassy" (croupy), varying degrees of inspiratory stridor, and varying degrees of respiratory distress resulting from swelling or obstruction in the region of the larynx. Acute infections of the larynx are of greater importance in infants and small children than they are in older children, in part because of the increased incidence in children in this age-group and the smaller diameter of the airway, which renders it subject to significantly greater narrowing with the same degree of inflammation.

Acute respiratory infections of the nonreactive airway involve all areas to some extent and are seldom restricted to one area. Croup syndromes affect to varying degrees the larynx, trachea, and bronchi. However, laryngeal involvement often dominates the clinical picture because of the severe effects on the voice and breathing. Croup syndromes are usually described according to the primary anatomic area affected (i.e., epiglottitis [or supraglottitis], laryngitis, laryngotracheobronchitis [LTB], and tracheitis). In general, LTB tends to occur in very young children, whereas epiglottitis is more characteristic of older children (see Table 23-1 for a comparison of croup syndromes).

ACUTE EPIGLOTTITIS

Acute epiglottitis, or *acute supraglottitis,* is a serious obstructive inflammatory process that occurs principally in children between 2 and 5 years of age but can occur from infancy to adulthood. The disorder requires immediate attention. The obstruction is supraglottic as opposed to the subglottic obstruction of laryngitis. The responsible organism is usually *Haemophilus influenzae;* LTB and epiglottitis do not occur together.

Clinical Manifestations

The onset of epiglottitis is abrupt, often preceded by a sore throat, and rapidly progressive to severe respiratory distress. The child usually goes to bed asymptomatic to awaken later, complaining of sore throat and pain on swallowing. The child has a fever, appears toxic out of proportion to the clinical findings, and presents a classic picture; the child generally insists on sitting upright and leaning forward, with chin thrust out, mouth open, and tongue protruding *(tripod position).* Drooling of saliva is common because of the difficulty or pain on swallowing and excessive secretions.

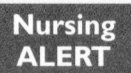 **Nursing ALERT**   Three clinical observations that indicate epiglottitis are absence of spontaneous cough, presence of drooling, and agitation.

The child is irritable and extremely restless and has an anxious, apprehensive, and frightened expression. The voice is thick and muffled, with a froglike croaking sound on inspiration. The child is not hoarse. Suprasternal and substernal retractions may be visible. The child seldom struggles to breathe, and slow, quiet breathing provides better air exchange. The sallow color of mild hypoxia may progress to frank cyanosis. The throat is red and inflamed, and a distinctive large, cherry-red, edematous epiglottis is visible on careful throat inspection. *Throat inspection should be attempted only when immediate intubation can be performed if needed.*

TABLE 23-1. Comparison of croup syndromes

	ACUTE EPIGLOTTITIS (SUPRAGLOTTITIS)	ACUTE LARYNGOTRACHEO-BRONCHITIS (LTB)	ACUTE SPASMODIC LARYNGITIS (SPASMODIC CROUP)	ACUTE TRACHEITIS
Age-group affected	1 to 8 years	3 months to 8 years	3 months to 3 years	1 month to 6 years
Etiologic agent	Bacterial, usually *Haemophilus influenzae*	Viral	Viral with allergic component	Bacterial, usually *Staphylococcus aureus*
Onset	Rapidly progressive	Slowly progressive	Sudden; at night	Moderately progressive
Major symptoms	Dysphagia	URI	URI	URI
	Stridor aggravated when supine	Stridor	Croupy cough	Croupy cough
	Drooling	Brassy cough	Stridor	Stridor
	High fever	Hoarseness	Hoarseness	Purulent secretions
	Toxic appearance	Dyspnea	Dyspnea	High fever
	Rapid pulse and respirations	Restlessness	Restlessness	No response to LTB therapy
		Irritability	Symptoms waken child	
		Low-grade fever	Symptoms disappear during day	
		Nontoxic appearance	Tends to recur	
Treatment	Antibiotics	Humidity	Humidity	Antibiotics
	Airway protection	Racemic epinephrine		

URI, Upper respiratory infection.

Therapeutic Management

The course of epiglottitis may be fulminant, with respiratory obstruction appearing suddenly. Progressive obstruction leads to hypoxia, hypercapnia, and acidosis followed by decreased muscular tone, reduced level of consciousness, and, when obstruction becomes more or less complete, a rather sudden death. A presumptive diagnosis of epiglottitis constitutes an emergency.

The child suspected of having epiglottitis should be examined where facilities are available for coping with this type of emergency. Examination of the throat with a tongue depressor is contraindicated until properly experienced personnel and equipment are at hand to proceed with immediate intubation or tracheostomy in the event that the examination precipitates further or complete obstruction.

If a lateral neck film is indicated, the same experienced personnel should accompany the child to the radiology department. Most practitioners prefer that the child not be transported but remain on the parent's lap in the examination area during portable radiology.

Endotracheal intubation or tracheostomy is usually considered for *H. influenzae* epiglottitis with severe respiratory distress. Whether or not there is an artificial airway, the child requires intensive observation by experienced personnel. The epiglottal swelling usually decreases after 24 hours of antibiotic therapy, and the epiglottis is near normal by the third day. Intubated children are generally extubated at this time.

Children with suspected bacterial epiglottitis are given antibiotics intravenously, followed by oral administration to complete a 7- to 10-day course. The use of corticosteroids for reducing edema may be beneficial during the early hours of treatment. Most intubated children will have had a course of corticosteroids for 24 hours before extubation.

Prevention. The American Academy of Pediatrics, Committee on Infectious Diseases (1996b) recommends that

all children beginning at 2 months of age receive the *H. influenzae* type B conjugate vaccine. Since administration of the vaccine has become a routine part of the regular immunization schedule, a decline in the incidence of epiglottitis has occurred. Patients now tend to be older and have disease caused by other organisms (See also Immunizations, Chapter 10.)

Nursing Considerations

Epiglottitis is a serious and frightening disease for the child and family. It is important to act quickly but calmly and provide support without unduly increasing anxiety. The child is allowed to remain in the position that provides the most comfort and security, and parents are reassured that everything possible is being done to obtain relief for their child.

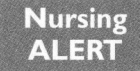 **Nursing ALERT** A nurse who suspects epiglottitis should not attempt to visualize the epiglottis directly with a tongue depressor or take a throat culture but should refer the child for medical evaluation immediately (see Critical Thinking Exercise on p. 764).

Acute care of the child is the same as that described for the child with LTB (see p. 765). Continuous monitoring of respiratory status, including pulse oximetry and blood gases, is part of nursing observations, and the intravenous (IV) infusion is maintained as described in Chapter 22.

ACUTE LARYNGITIS

Acute infectious laryngitis is a common illness in older children and adolescents. Infants and smaller children experience more generalized involvement (see following section on LTB). Viruses are the usual causative agents, and the principal complaint is hoarseness, which may be accompanied by

CRITICAL THINKING EXERCISE
Croup Syndrome

Kim Lee, 4 years old, is admitted to the emergency department with a sore throat, pain on swallowing, drooling, and a fever of 39° C (102.2° F). She looks ill, is agitated, and prefers to sit up and lean over. Which of the following medical orders should you question?

1. Obtain a complete blood count (CBC) and throat culture immediately.
2. Place child on oxygen saturation monitor.
3. Start an intravenous line of 5% dextrose in normal saline to run at 30 ml/hr.
4. Have pediatric-size tracheostomy tray available.

The correct answer is one. This child's symptoms suggest epiglottitis. The nurse should question the order for a throat culture because the procedure can precipitate obstruction of the airway. The CBC and other interventions are appropriate.

PROGRESSION OF SYMPTOMS IN LARYNGOTRACHEOBRONCHITIS (LTB)

Stage I
Fear
Hoarseness
Croupy cough
Inspiratory stridor when disturbed

Stage II
Continuous respiratory stridor
Lower rib retraction
Retraction of soft tissue of neck
Use of accessory muscles of respiration
Labored respiration

Stage III
Signs of anoxia and carbon dioxide retention
Restlessness
Anxiety
Pallor
Sweating
Rapid respiration

Stage IV
Intermittent cyanosis
Permanent cyanosis
Cessation of breathing

As described by Forbes. From Krugman S and others: *Infectious diseases of children,* ed 9, St Louis, 1992, Mosby.

---

other upper respiratory symptoms (e.g., coryza, sore throat, nasal congestion) and systemic manifestations (e.g., fever, headache, myalgia, malaise). Associated complaints vary with the infecting virus. Adenoviruses and influenza viruses are responsible for more systemic involvement; parainfluenza viruses, rhinoviruses, and RSV cause more mild illness.

Therapeutic Management and Nursing Considerations

The disease is almost always self-limited without long-term sequelae. Treatment is symptomatic with fluids and humidified air (see Nursing Care Plan on pp. 753-755).

ACUTE LARYNGOTRACHEOBRONCHITIS (LTB)

LTB is the most common of the croup syndromes and primarily affects children less than 5 years of age. Organisms usually responsible for LTB are the parainfluenza virus RSV, *H. influenzae* type B, and *Mycoplasma pneumoniae.* The disease is usually preceded by a URI, which gradually descends to adjacent structures. It is characterized by gradual onset of low-grade fever.

Inflammation of the mucosa lining the larynx and trachea causes a narrowing of the airway. When the airway is significantly narrowed, the child struggles to inhale air past the obstruction and into the lungs, producing the characteristic inspiratory stridor and suprasternal retractions. The typical child with LTB is a toddler who develops the classic barking or seallike cough and stridor after several days of coryza. When the child is unable to inhale a sufficient volume of air, symptoms of hypoxia become evident. Obstruction that is severe enough to prevent adequate exhalation of carbon dioxide causes respiratory acidosis, and eventually the child experiences respiratory failure (see progression of symptoms outlined in box).

Therapeutic Management

The major objective in medical management of infectious LTB is maintaining an airway and providing for adequate respiratory exchange. Children with mild croup (no stridor at rest) are managed at home. Parents are taught the signs of respiratory distress so that professional help can be summoned early if needed. Children who progress to serious respiratory symptoms should receive medical attention, usually with hospitalization.

High humidity with cool mist provides relief for most children. A cool-air vaporizer or a steamy bathroom can be used at home. In the hospital setting, hoods for infants or tents for toddlers are sometimes used to provide increased humidity and supplemental oxygen.

Nebulized epinephrine (racemic epinephrine) is often used in children with more severe disease, stridor at rest, retractions, or difficulty breathing. The α-adrenergic effects cause mucosal vasoconstriction and subsequent decreased subglottic edema. The onset of action is rapid, with detectable clinical improvement within 10 to 15 minutes, although symptoms frequently reappear—typically called "relapse"—within 2 hours. In a significant number of children, however, improvement persists and additional treatments are not necessary.

The use of corticosteroids is beneficial because the antiinflammatory effects decrease subglottic edema. The onset of action is clinically detectable as early as 6 hours after administration, with continued improvement over 12 to 24 hours.

It is essential to allow children with mild croup to continue to drink beverages they like and to encourage parents to try whatever comforting measures work best with their child (e.g., being held, rocked, walked, sung to). If the child is unable to take oral fluids, IV fluid therapy might be indicated.

> **Nursing ALERT**
>
> Children with severe respiratory distress (traditionally, for infants with a respiratory rate greater than 60 breaths/minute) should not be given anything by mouth to prevent aspiration and decrease the work of breathing.

Nursing Considerations

The most important nursing function in the care of children with LTB is continuous, vigilant observation and accurate assessment of respiratory status. Cardiac, respiratory, and non-invasive blood gas monitoring equipment supplement visual observations. Changes in therapy are frequently based on nurses' observations and assessment of a child's status, response to therapy, and tolerance of procedures. The trend away from early intubation of children with LTB emphasizes the importance of nursing observation and the ability to recognize impending respiratory failure so that intubation can be implemented without delay. Intubation equipment should be readily accessible and taken with the child during transport to other areas (e.g., radiology, operating room).

> **Nursing ALERT**
>
> Early signs of impending airway obstruction include increased pulse and respiratory rate; substernal, suprasternal, and intercostal retractions; flaring nares; and increased restlessness.

To conserve energy, children are given every opportunity to rest. Infants or small children find that being enclosed within a tent, coughing, having laryngeal spasms, and needing IV therapy are additional sources of distress. Infants and small children prefer sitting upright, and most want to be held. Children need the security of the parent's presence. Since crying increases respiratory distress and hypoxia, a child's individual tolerance for these therapies must be assessed. An extremely fussy child may do better when held in the parent's lap with cool mist directed toward the child's face.

The rapid progression of croup, the alarming sound of the cough and stridor, and the child's apprehensive behavior and ill appearance combine to create a very frightening experience for the parents. They need reassurance regarding the child's progress and an explanation of treatments. They may feel guilty for not having suspected the seriousness of the condition sooner. The family should be allowed to remain with their child as much as possible, especially when this decreases the child's distress.

The nurse can provide the parents with an opportunity to express their feelings, thus minimizing any blame or guilt. They need frequent reassurance provided in a calm, quiet manner and education regarding what they can do to make their child more comfortable. Fortunately, as the crisis subsides and the child responds to therapy, breathing becomes easier and recovery is generally prompt. Home care after discharge includes continued humidity, adequate hydration, and nourishment. Parents are encouraged to ask questions about home care and preparation for discharge. Referral to a public health agency for follow-up care may be advisable.

ACUTE SPASMODIC LARYNGITIS

Acute spasmodic laryngitis (*spasmodic croup,* "midnight croup," or "twilight croup") is distinct from laryngitis and LTB and is characterized by paroxysmal attacks of laryngeal obstruction that occur chiefly at night. Signs of inflammation are absent or mild, and there is frequently a history of previous attacks lasting 2 to 5 days, followed by uneventful recovery. It usually affects children ages 1 to 3 years. Some children appear to be predisposed to the condition; allergy and psychogenic factors are implicated in some cases.

The child goes to bed well or with some very mild respiratory symptoms but awakes suddenly with characteristic barking, metallic cough, hoarseness, noisy inspirations, and restlessness. The child appears anxious, frightened, and prostrated. Dyspnea is aggravated by excitement; but there is no fever, the attack subsides in a few hours, and the child appears well the next day.

Therapeutic Management and Nursing Considerations

Children with spasmodic croup are managed at home. Cool mist is recommended for the child's room. Warm mist provided by steam from hot running water in a closed bathroom may be helpful. Sometimes the spasm is relieved by sudden exposure to cold air (as when the child is taken out into the night air to see the practitioner). Parents are usually advised to have the child sleep in humidified air until the cough has subsided so that subsequent episodes may be prevented. Children with moderately severe symptoms may be hospitalized for observation and therapy with cool mist and racemic epinephrine, as for LTB. Patients may respond to corticosteroid therapy. The disease is usually self-limited.

BACTERIAL TRACHEITIS

Bacterial tracheitis, an infection of the mucosa of the upper trachea, is a distinct entity with features of both croup and epiglottitis. The disease is seen in children ages 1 month to 6 years and may be a serious cause of airway obstruction—severe enough to cause respiratory arrest. It is believed to be a complication of LTB, and although *S. aureus* is the most frequent organism responsible, group A β-hemolytic streptococci and *H. influenzae* have also been implicated.

Many of the manifestations of bacterial tracheitis are similar to those of LTB but are unresponsive to LTB therapy. There is a history of previous URI with croupy cough, stridor unaffected by position, toxicity, and high fever. A prominent manifestation is the production of thick, purulent tracheal secretions. Respiratory difficulties are secondary to these copious secretions.

Therapeutic Management and Nursing Considerations

Bacterial tracheitis requires vigorous management. Humidified oxygen, antipyretics, and antibiotics are prescribed. Most children require endotracheal intubation and frequent tracheal suctioning to prevent airway obstruction. The emphasis in this disorder is early recognition to prevent catastrophic airway obstruction.

INFECTIONS OF THE LOWER AIRWAYS

The *reactive portion* of the lower respiratory tract includes the bronchi and bronchioles in children. Cartilaginous support of the large airway is not fully developed until adolescence. Consequently, the smooth muscle in these structures represents a major factor in the constriction of the airway, particularly in the bronchioles, that portion that extends from the bronchi to the alveoli. Table 23-2 compares some of the major features of bronchial and bronchiolar infections.

BRONCHITIS

Bronchitis (sometimes referred to as *tracheobronchitis*) is inflammation of large airways (trachea and bronchi), which is almost invariably associated with a URI. Viral agents are the primary cause of the disease, although *Mycoplasma pneumoniae* is a common cause in children older than 6 years of age. The condition is characterized by a dry, hacking, and nonproductive cough that is worse at night and becomes productive in 2 to 3 days.

Bronchitis is a mild self-limiting disease that requires only symptomatic treatment, including analgesics, antipyretics, and humidity. Cough suppressants may be useful to allow rest but can interfere with clearance of secretions. Most patients recover uneventfully in 5 to 10 days.

RESPIRATORY SYNCYTIAL VIRUS (RSV)/BRONCHIOLITIS

Bronchiolitis is an acute viral infection with maximum effect at the bronchiolar level. The infection occurs primarily in winter and spring and is rare in children over 2 years of age. *Respiratory syncytial virus (RSV)* is responsible for more than half of all episodes of bronchiolitis. Adenoviruses and parainfluenza viruses may also cause acute bronchiolitis. The virus becomes epidemic in communities during the late fall and winter months and is easily spread by hand-to-nose or hand-to-eye transmission.

Pathophysiology

Bronchiole mucosa is swollen, and lumina are filled with mucus and exudate; the walls of the bronchi and bronchioles are infiltrated with inflammatory cells; and peribronchiolar interstitial pneumonitis is usually present. The variable degrees of obstruction produced in small air passages by these changes lead to hyperinflation, obstructive emphysema resulting from partial obstruction, and patchy areas of atelectasis. Dilation of bronchial passages on inspiration allows sufficient space for intake of air, but narrowing of the passages on expiration prevents air from leaving the lungs. Thus air is trapped distal to the obstruction and causes progressive overinflation *(emphysema)*.

TABLE 23-2. Comparison of conditions affecting the bronchi

	VIRAL-INDUCED ASTHMA*	BRONCHITIS	RESPIRATORY SYNCYTIAL VIRUS (RSV)/BRONCHIOLITIS
Description	Exaggerated response of bronchi to infection	Usually occurs in association with URI	A more common infectious disease of lower airways
	Bronchospasm, exudation, and edema of bronchi	Seldom an isolated entity	Maximum obstructive impact at bronchiolar level
Age-group affected	Late infancy and early childhood	Affects children in first 4 years of life	Usually children 2 to 12 months of age; rare after age 2
			Peak incidence at approximately age 6 months
Etiologic agents	Most often viruses but may be any of a variety of URI pathogens	Usually viral	Viruses, predominantly respiratory syncytial viruses; also adenoviruses, parainfluenza viruses, and *Mycoplasma pneumoniae*
		Other agents (e.g., bacteria, fungi, allergic disorders, airborne irritants) can trigger symptoms	
Predominant characteristics	Wheezing, productive cough	Persistent dry, hacking cough (worse at night) becoming productive in 2 to 3 days	Dyspnea, paroxysmal nonproductive cough, tachypnea with retractions and flaring nares, emphysema, may be wheezing
Treatment	Bronchodilators	Cough suppressants if needed	Oxygen mist
			Ribavirin if severe or for high-risk population

URI, Upper respiratory infection.
*See Asthma, p. 775.

Diagnostic Evaluation

Diagnosis of bronchiolitis is made on the basis of clinical findings, the child's age, season, and epidemiology of the community. Bronchiolitis begins as a simple URI with serous nasal discharge that may be accompanied by mild fever. The child gradually develops increasing respiratory distress with tachypnea, paroxysmal cough, and irritability. There may be wheezing. Chest radiographs show hyperaeration and areas of consolidation that are difficult to differentiate from bacterial pneumonia. Children may have considerable dyspnea but do not have the toxic appearance of children with bacterial infections (see box for signs and symptoms of RSV).

Apnea may be the first recognized indicator of RSV infection in very young infants. Severe disease may be followed by a rise in arterial carbon dioxide tension ($Paco_2$) (hypercapnia), leading to respiratory acidosis and hypoxemia. Positive identification of RSV is accomplished by enzyme-linked immunosorbent assay (ELISA) or rapid immunofluorescent antibody (IFA) from direct aspiration of nasal secretions or nasopharyngeal washings (see Respiratory Secretions Specimens, Chapter 22).

Therapeutic Management

Bronchiolitis is treated symptomatically with high humidity, adequate fluid intake, and rest. Most children with bronchiolitis can be managed at home. Hospitalization is usually recommended for children with complicating conditions, such as underlying lung or heart disease, associated debilitated states, or questionable adequacy of caregiver. The child should also be admitted who is tachypneic, has marked retractions, seems listless, or has a history of poor fluid intake. Mist therapy is generally combined with oxygen by hood or tent in concentrations sufficient to alleviate dyspnea and hypoxia, after which mist alone is continued for mild dyspnea. Fluids by mouth may be contraindicated because of tachypnea, weakness, and fatigue; therefore intravenous fluids are preferred until the acute crisis of the disease has passed.

Clinical assessments, noninvasive oxygen monitoring, and blood gas values guide therapy. Medical therapy for bronchiolitis is controversial. Bronchodilators, corticosteroids, cough suppressants, and antibiotics have not proved to be effective in uncomplicated disease and are not recommended for routine use. Corticosteroids, theophylline, and furosemide have all been used for intubated and ventilated infants and children.

Ribavirin, an antiviral agent, may be used to treat RSV infection. The drug is aerosolized and delivered via a small-particle aerosol generator (SPAG). It may be administered by hood, tent, or mask. Since the use of the drug is controversial, infection with RSV is usually self-limiting, the drug is very expensive, and recent studies failed to show a significant decrease in mortality when ribavirin was used, the Committee on Infectious Diseases of the American Academy of Pediatrics (1996a) now recommends that ribavirin aerosol therapy be considered for the following:

1. Infants at high risk for severe or complicated RSV infection (i.e., infants with complicated congenital heart disease, bronchopulmonary dysplasia, cystic fibrosis, and other chronic lung disease); some preterm infants (less than 37 weeks); and those less than 6 weeks of age
2. Infants hospitalized with RSV lower respiratory tract disease who are severely ill
3. Infants hospitalized with lower respiratory tract disease that is not initially severe, but who may be at some increased risk of progressing to a more complicated course (e.g., less than 6 weeks of age or those in whom prolonged illness might be particularly detrimental, such as multiple congenital anomalies, or neurologic or metabolic disease)
4. Infants with underlying immunosuppressive diseases or therapy, such as acquired immunodeficiency syndrome (AIDS), severe combined immunodeficiency disease (SCID), or organ transplantation, who have a high mortality and/or prolonged RSV illness

The first prophylactic drug for RSV has recently been approved. *RespiGam,* a hyperimmune gamma globulin, does not prevent RSV infections but reduces the severity of the disease (FDA OKs, 1996).

Prognosis. The disease lasts about 3 to 10 days, and the prognosis is generally good. Although most infants with RSV bronchiolitis appear to recover completely, severe disease is associated with recurrent pulmonary infection and bronchospasm. Infants with preexisting cardiopulmonary disease may have an increased incidence of death related to RSV infection. The recent development and use of an RSV immune globulin in combination with ribavirin has the potential for significantly decreasing morbidity and mortality from RSV.

Nursing Considerations

Children admitted to the hospital with suspect RSV infection may be assigned separate rooms or grouped with other RSV-infected children. A variety of infection control procedures have been employed over the years, the most important of which is consistent handwashing and not touching the nasal mucosa or conjunctiva. The routine use of gowns and masks has not been shown to be of additional benefit, although gowns may help diminish the potential for fomite spread during close contact when infectious secretions may contaminate

---

SIGNS AND SYMPTOMS OF RESPIRATORY SYNCYTIAL VIRUS (RSV)

Initial
Rhinorrhea
Pharyngitis
Coughing/sneezing
Wheezing
Possible ear infection or eye drainage
Fever

With Progression of Illness
Increased coughing and wheezing
Air hunger
Tachypnea and retractions
Cyanosis

Severe Illness
Tachypnea, greater than 70 breaths/minute
Listlessness
Apneic spells
Poor air exchange; poor breath sounds

clothing. Other isolation procedures of potential benefit are those aimed at diminishing the number of hospital personnel, visitors, and uninfected patients in contact with the child. Another measure includes making patient assignments so that nurses assigned to children with RSV are not taking care of other patients who may be considered high risk.

Patient care sometimes warrants opening the tent while the small-particle aerosol generator (SPAG) is still running; in these cases it is recommended that one first shut the machine off and wait a few moments before opening the tent. Gloves and gowns are not essential, since dermal absorption appears to be negligible. Scavenger devices are commercially available to help decrease the escape of aerosolized ribavirin.

> **Nursing ALERT**
> Pregnant health care providers should avoid caring for a child receiving ribavirin.

PNEUMONIAS

Pneumonia, inflammation of the pulmonary parenchyma, is common throughout childhood but occurs more frequently in infancy and early childhood. Clinically, pneumonia may occur either as a primary disease or as a complication of some other illness. Morphologically, pneumonias are recognized as follows:

Lobar pneumonia—all or a large segment of one or more pulmonary lobes is involved. When both lungs are affected, it is known as *bilateral* or *double pneumonia.*

Bronchopneumonia—begins in the terminal bronchioles, which become clogged with mucopurulent exudate to form consolidated patches in nearby lobules; also called *lobular pneumonia.*

Interstitial pneumonia—the inflammatory process is more or less confined within the alveolar walls (interstitium) and the peribronchial and interlobular tissues.

Pneumonitis is a localized acute inflammation of the lung without the toxemia associated with lobar pneumonia.

The pneumonias are more often classified according to morphology, clinical form and etiologic agent: viral, atypical (mycoplasma), bacterial, or aspiration of foreign substances (see p. 773). Less often pneumonia may be caused by histomycosis, coccidioidomycosis, and other fungi. The causative agent is identified largely from the clinical history, the child's age, the general health history, the physical examination, radiography, and the laboratory examination.

Viral Pneumonia

Viral pneumonias occur more frequently than bacterial pneumonias and are seen in children of all age-groups. They are often associated with viral URIs, and RSV accounts for the largest percentage in infants. There are few clinical symptoms to distinguish between the responsible organisms, and differentiations between viruses can be made only by laboratory examination (see box for clinical manifestations).

The prognosis is generally good, although viral infections of the respiratory tract render the affected child more susceptible to secondary bacterial invasion, especially when there is denuded bronchial mucosa. Treatment is usually symptomatic and includes measures to promote oxygenation and comfort, such as oxygen administration with cool mist, chest

---

CLINICAL MANIFESTATIONS OF VIRAL AND ATYPICAL PNEUMONIAS	
Viral Pneumonia	**Atypical Pneumonia**
May be acute or insidious	May be sudden or insidious
Symptoms variable	General systemic symptoms:
Mild: low-grade fever, slight cough, malaise	Fever
Severe: high fever, severe cough, prostration	Chills (older children)
	Headache
Cough usually unproductive early in disease	Malaise
A few wheezes or crackles heard on auscultation	Anorexia
	Myalgia
	Followed by:
	Rhinitis
	Sore throat
	Dry, hacking cough
	Nonproductive early, then seromucoid sputum, to mucopurulent or blood streaked
	Fine crepitant rales over various lung areas

---

physiotherapy and postural drainage, antipyretics for fever management, fluid intake, and family support. Although some authorities recommend antimicrobial therapy in hope of reducing or preventing secondary bacterial infection, it is usually reserved for children in whom the presence of such infection is demonstrated by appropriate cultures.

Primary Atypical Pneumonia

Approximately 10% to 20% of hospital admissions of children with pneumonia are caused by *M. pneumoniae.* It occurs principally in the fall and winter months and is more prevalent where there are crowded living conditions (see box).

Most affected persons recover from acute illness in 7 to 10 days with symptomatic treatment followed by a week of convalescence. Hospitalization is rarely necessary.

Bacterial Pneumonia

In children beyond the neonatal period, bacterial pneumonias display distinct clinical patterns that facilitate their differentiation from other forms of pneumonia, and individual microorganisms produce a distinct clinical picture. Onset is abrupt and is generally preceded by a viral infection that disturbs the natural defense mechanisms of the upper respiratory tract and allows the pathogenic bacteria normally harbored in the upper passages to increase in number.

Children with bacterial pneumonia appear ill and exhibit both general and localized physical findings. Symptoms and signs include fever, malaise, rapid and shallow respirations, cough, and chest pain that is often exaggerated by deep breathing. The pain may be referred to the abdomen and confused with appendicitis. Chills frequently occur, and meningeal symptoms *(meningism)* are also common.

Most older children with pneumococcal pneumonia can be treated at home, especially if the condition is recognized and treatment initiated early. Antibiotic therapy, bed rest, liberal oral intake of fluid, and administration of an antipyretic for fever and an antitussive for dry, hacking cough constitute the principal therapeutic measures. Hospitalization is indicated when pleural effusion or empyema accompanies the disease and is mandatory for children with staphylococcal pneumonia. Pneumonia in the infant or young child is best treated in the hospital, since the course of illness is more variable and complications are more common in very young patients. Fluids are usually given intravenously, and oxygen therapy may be required if the child is in respiratory distress.

At present the classic features and clinical course of pneumonia are rarely seen because of early and vigorous antibiotic and supportive therapy. However, a large number of children, especially infants, with staphylococcal pneumonia develop empyema, pyopneumothorax, or tension pneumothorax. Pleural effusion is not uncommon in children with lobar (pneumococcal) pneumonia. A thoracentesis may be performed to remove fluid in the pleural cavity, to obtain a culture of the fluid, and to instill antibiotics directly into the pleural space. Nonpurulent effusions, such as occur in pneumococcal pneumonia, do not require surgical drainage. Continuous closed-chest drainage is instituted when purulent fluid is aspirated, a frequent finding in staphylococcal infections.

Prognosis. The prognosis for pneumococcal infections is generally good, with rapid recovery when they are recognized and treated early. Streptococcal infections vary in duration but usually resolve spontaneously. The course of staphylococcal pneumonia is generally prolonged. The prognosis varies with the length of illness before treatment is begun, although early recognition and treatment are usually effective. Complications of bacterial pneumonia include pleural effusion, empyema, and tension pneumothorax.

Prevention. Use of pneumococcal polysaccharide vaccine is recommended for use in selected individuals, such as children over age 2 years who are at risk of acquiring pneumococcal infection or are at risk of serious disease (see Immunizations, Chapter 10). The infant or child with recurrent pneumonias should be further evaluated for cystic fibrosis.

Nursing Considerations

Nursing care of the child with pneumonia is primarily supportive and symptomatic but necessitates thorough respiratory assessment and administration of oxygen and antibiotics. The child's respiratory rate and status, as well as general disposition and level of activity, are frequently assessed. Isolation procedures are instituted according to hospital policy; rest and conservation of energy are encouraged by relief of physical and psychologic stress. The child is disturbed as little as possible by clustering care to encourage the child's regular sleep cycle. If the cough is disturbing, judicious use of antitussives, especially before rest times and meals, is often helpful. To prevent dehydration, fluids are frequently administered intravenously during the acute phase. Oral fluids, if allowed, are given cautiously to avoid aspiration and to decrease the possibility of aggravating a fatiguing cough.

Children may be placed in a mist tent with oxygen. Cool mist moistens the airways and provides a cool atmosphere that aids in temperature reduction. Children often require frequent clothing and linen changes to prevent chilling in the damp atmosphere. They are usually more comfortable in a semierect position but should be allowed to determine the position of comfort. Lying on the affected side (if pneumonia is unilateral) splints the chest on that side and reduces the pleural rubbing that often causes discomfort. Fever is usually controlled by administration of antipyretic drugs as prescribed, and temperature is monitored regularly.

Vital signs and breath sounds are monitored to assess the progress of the disease and to detect early signs of complications. Children with ineffectual cough or those with difficulty handling secretions, especially infants, will require suctioning to maintain a patent airway. A simple bulb syringe is usually sufficient for clearing the nares and nasopharynx of infants, but mechanical suction should be readily available if needed. Older children can usually handle secretions without assistance. Postural drainage and chest physiotherapy are generally prescribed every 4 hours or more often, depending on the child's condition.

The hospitalized child is apprehensive, and many of the treatments and tests are frightening and stress producing. Reducing anxiety and apprehension reduces psychologic distress in the child, and when the child is more relaxed, the respiratory efforts are lessened. Easing respiratory efforts makes the child less apprehensive, and encouraging the presence of the caregiver provides the child with a customary source of comfort and support.

The family also needs support. The child's dry, hacking cough can be tiring for the parents because it often disturbs the child's and family's sleep. Parents are kept informed of the child's progress and taught appropriate home care, such as use of a nasal aspirator and administration of antibiotics.*

OTHER INFECTIONS OF THE RESPIRATORY TRACT

PERTUSSIS (WHOOPING COUGH)

Pertussis (whooping cough) is an acute respiratory infection caused by *Bordetella pertussis* that occurs chiefly in children younger than 4 years of age who have not been immunized. It is highly contagious and is particularly threatening in young infants, in whom there are higher morbidity and mortality rates. (See Table 14-1 for signs, symptoms, and management of pertussis and Chapter 10 for immunization.) The incidence is highest in the spring and summer months, and a single attack confers lifetime immunity. Pertussis vaccine is effective, but the immunity diminishes with time after the initial infection or immunization. A small number of immunized adolescents may develop an asymptomatic case of pertussis.

TUBERCULOSIS (TB)

TB is an ancient disease that, although controlled in most developed countries, still remains a health hazard and a leading cause of death throughout many parts of the world. After decades of steady decline in the United States, the incidence of TB is increasing. The age-group affected most is 25 to 44 years old, but the disease has also increased significantly in children (Jackson, 1993). The increases are attributed in part to the interaction of foreign-born persons emigrating to the United States, the increase in homelessness, and the human

---

*Home care instructions for administration of medication and nasal aspiration are available in Wong DL: *Wong and Whaley's Clinical manual of pediatric nursing,* ed 4, St Louis, 1996, Mosby.

immunodeficiency virus (HIV) epidemic (Hoffman, Kelly, and Futterman, 1996).

TB is caused by *Mycobacterium tuberculosis.* Children are susceptible to both the human *(M. tuberculosis)* and the bovine *(M. bovis)* organisms, and in parts of the world where tuberculosis in cattle is not controlled or pasteurization of milk is not practiced, the bovine type is a common source of infection in children. Although the causative agent is the tubercle bacillus, other factors influence the degree to which the organism is able to produce an altered state in the host, including heredity (resistance to the infection may be genetically transmitted), sex (higher in adolescent girls), age (lower resistance in infants, higher incidence during adolescence), stress (emotional or physical), nutritional state, and intercurrent infection (especially measles and pertussis). Currently, infection with HIV is the most important risk factor for TB infection progressing to active disease.

The source of infection in children is usually an infected adult or a teenager, typically a member of the household. It can also be a baby-sitter, domestic worker, or a frequent visitor to the household. The lung is the usual portal of entry in human beings; the organism enters less often by ingestion. In the lungs a proliferation of epithelial cells surround and encapsulate the multiplying bacilli in an attempt to wall off the invading organisms, thus forming the typical tubercle. Extension of the primary lesion at the original site causes progressive tissue destruction as it spreads within the lung, discharges material from foci to other areas of the lungs (e.g., bronchi or pleura), or produces pneumonia. Erosion of blood vessels by the primary lesion can cause widespread dissemination of the tubercle bacillus to near and distant sites *(miliary tuberculosis).* Areas that are frequently affected include lymph nodes, meninges, and bone.

Diagnostic Evaluation

Several tests and procedures are used to establish a diagnosis. Diagnosis is based on information derived from physical examination, history, reaction to tuberculin tests, radiographic examinations, and organism cultures. In addition, it must be determined whether or not the lesion is in the active, quiescent, or healed stage (see box for clinical manifestations).

The *tuberculin test* is the most important test of whether a child has been infected with the tubercle bacillus. The recommended procedure is the **Mantoux test,** which uses purified protein derivative (PPD). The standard dose is 5 tuberculin units in 0.1 ml of solution, injected intradermally. Recommendations for TB skin testing of children are listed in the box on p. 771. Routine testing of children with no risk factors residing in communities with a low prevalence of TB is not indicated (American Academy of Pediatrics, 1996c).

A *positive reaction* indicates that the individual has been infected and has developed a sensitivity to the protein of the tubercle bacillus; however, it does not confirm the presence of active disease. Once individuals have reacted positively, they will always react positively. A previously negative reaction that becomes positive indicates that the person has been infected since the last test. Guidelines for interpreting the Mantoux skin test are listed in the box below.

Nursing ALERT   The American Academy of Pediatrics (1996c) recommends that Mantoux skin test results be read by health care professionals.

DEFINITION OF POSITIVE MANTOUX SKIN TEST (5 TU-PPD) IN CHILDREN*

Reaction ≥5 mm

Children in close contact with persons who have known or suspected infectious cases of tuberculosis (TB):
  Households with active or previously active cases if (1) treatment cannot be verified as adequate before exposure, (2) treatment was initiated after period of child's contact, or (3) reactivation is suspected
Children suspected to have TB disease:
  Chest x-ray film consistent with active or previously active tuberculosis
  Clinical evidence of TB
Children with immunosuppressive conditions† or human immunodeficiency virus (HIV) infection

Reaction ≥10 mm

Children at increased risk of dissemination:
  Young age: less than 4 years of age
  Other medical risk factors, including Hodgkin disease, lymphoma, diabetes mellitus, chronic renal failure, and malnutrition
Children with increased environmental exposure:
  Born, or whose parents were born, in regions of the world where TB is highly prevalent
  Frequently exposed to adults who are HIV infected, homeless, users of intravenous and other street drugs, poor and medically indigent city dwellers, residents of nursing homes, incarcerated or institutionalized persons, and migrant farm workers

Reaction ≥15 mm

Children 4 years of age or older without any risk factors

From American Academy of Pediatrics, Committee on Infectious Diseases: Update on tuberculin skin testing of children, *Pediatrics* 97(2):282-284, 1996.
*These recommendations should apply regardless of whether bacille Calmette-Guérin (BCG) has been previously administered.
†Including immunosuppressive doses of corticosteroids.

CLINICAL MANIFESTATIONS OF TUBERCULOSIS (TB)

Extremely variable
May be asymptomatic or produce a broad range of symptoms:
  Fever
  Malaise
  Anorexia
  Weight loss
  Cough may or may not be present (progresses slowly over weeks to months)
  Aching pain and tightness in the chest
  Hemoptysis (rare)
With progression:
  Respiratory rate increases
  Poor expansion of lung on the affected side
  Diminished breath sounds and rales
  Dullness to percussion
  Fever persists
  Generalized symptoms are manifested
  Develops pallor, anemia, weakness, and weight loss

REVISED TUBERCULIN SKIN TEST RECOMMENDATIONS*

Children for whom immediate skin testing is indicated:
  Contacts of persons with confirmed or suspected infectious tuberculosis (TB) (contact investigation); this includes children identified as contacts of family members or associates in jail or prison in the last 5 years
  Children with radiographic or clinical findings suggesting TB
  Children immigrating from endemic countries (e.g., Asia, Middle East, Africa, Latin America)
  Children with travel histories to endemic countries and/or significant contact with indigenous persons from such countries
Children who should be tested annually for TB†:
  Children infected with human immunodeficiency virus (HIV)
  Incarcerated adolescents
Children who should be tested every 2 to 3 years†:
  Children exposed to the following individuals: HIV infected, homeless, residents of nursing homes, institutionalized adolescents or adults, users of illicit drugs, incarcerated adolescents or adults and migrant farm workers; this would include foster children with exposure to adults in the above high-risk groups
Children who should be considered for tuberculin skin testing at ages 4 to 6 and 11 to 16 years:
  Children whose parents immigrated (with unknown tuberculin skin test status) from regions of the world with high prevalence of TB; continued potential exposure by travel to the endemic areas and/or household contact with persons from the endemic areas (with unknown tuberculin skin test status) should be an indication for repeat tuberculin skin testing
  Children without specific risk factors who reside in high-prevalence areas; in general, a high-risk neighborhood or community does not mean an entire city is at high risk; it is recognized that rates in any area of the city may vary by neighborhood, or even from block to block; physicians should be aware of these patterns in determining the likelihood of exposure; public health officials or local TB experts should help clinicians identify areas that have appreciable TB rates
Risk for progression to disease:
  Children with other medical risk factors, including diabetes mellitus, chronic renal failure, malnutrition, and congenital or acquired immunodeficiencies deserve special consideration; without recent exposure, these persons are not at increased risk of acquiring TB infection; underlying immune deficiencies associated with these conditions theoretically would enhance the possibility for progression to severe disease; initial histories of potential exposure to TB should be included for all these patients; if these histories or local epidemiologic factors suggest a possibility of exposure, immediate and periodic tuberculin skin testing should be considered in these patients; an initial Mantoux tuberculin skin test should be performed before initiation of immunosuppressive therapy in any child with an underlying condition that necessitates immunosuppressive therapy

Modified from American Academy of Pediatrics, Committee on Infectious Diseases: Update on tuberculosis skin testing of children, *Pediatrics* 97(2):282-284, 1996.
*Bacille Calmette-Guérin (BCG) immunization is not a contraindication to tuberculin skin testing.
†Initial tuberculin skin testing initiated at the time of diagnosis or circumstance.

Therapeutic Management

Medical management of TB lesions in children consists of adequate nutrition, chemotherapy, general supportive measures, prevention of unnecessary exposure to other infections that further compromise the body's defenses, prevention of reinfection, and sometimes surgical procedures. The need for hospitalization, except in acute illness, is usually required only for diagnostic tests, to obtain culture material, ascertain tolerance and compliance with medication, investigate household contacts for exposure, identify and initiate treatment for the index case, and remove active sources from the environment before returning the child to the home.

Chemotherapy. Chemotherapy is the most important therapeutic modality available for management of TB. A variety of chemical agents can be employed, and a regimen involving two or more drugs simultaneously has been found to be effective and is usually the mode of choice. The most frequently used combinations of drugs are isoniazid (INH) and rifampin, with the optional addition of pyrazinamide (PZA). Either a 6-month or a 9-month treatment regimen may be used. In either regimen, INH and rifampin are continued for at least 6 months after conversion of cultures. The HIV-infected child may require drug therapy for up to 12 months.

Surgical Procedures. Surgery may be required to remove the source of infection in tissues that are inaccessible to chemotherapy or that are destroyed by the disease. Orthopedic procedures for correction of bone deformities,

bronchoscopy for removal of a tuberculous granulomatous polyp, or resection of a portion of a diseased lung may also be performed.

Prognosis. Most children recover from primary TB infection and are often unaware of its presence. However, very young children have a higher incidence of disseminated disease. It is a serious disease during the first 2 years of life, during adolescence, and in children who are HIV positive. Except in cases of tuberculous meningitis, death seldom occurs in treated children. Antibiotic therapy has decreased the death rate and the hematogenous spread from primary lesions.

Prevention. The only certain means to prevent TB is to avoid contact with the tubercle bacillus. Maintaining an optimum state of health with adequate nutrition and avoidance of fatigue and debilitating infections promotes natural resistance but does not prevent infection.

Limited immunity can be produced by administration of the only successful vaccine to date, *bacille Calmette-Guérin (BCG),* a vaccine containing bovine bacilli with reduced virulence. The freshly prepared vaccine, injected intradermally, produces a definite although incomplete (about 50%) protection against TB. The distribution of the vaccine is controlled by local or state health departments, but the vaccine is not used extensively, even in areas with a high prevalence of disease. Greater protection is afforded by daily prophylactic administration of INH. The drug is given to children with a positive tuberculin test but no evidence of active disease.

Nursing Considerations

Most children with pulmonary TB almost always have non-infectious disease; therefore they seldom need to be isolated. There are few bacilli in the sputum, the amount of sputum produced is quite small, and sputum is swallowed rather than expectorated. Hospitalization is seldom necessary except for needed diagnostic tests; most children are managed satisfactorily at home. Therefore the major nursing care of children with TB involves nurses in ambulatory settings—outpatient departments, schools, and especially public health agencies.

Asymptomatic children are able to lead an essentially unrestricted life. They can and should attend school (or preschool), but older children are restricted from vigorous activities such as competitive games and contact sports during the active stage of primary TB. They should be protected from stresses, including parental anxieties, the tendency toward overprotection, and pressures regarding nutritional intake. The regular immunization schedule should be continued. Care should be exerted to maintain an optimum health status with proper diet, adequate rest, and avoidance of infection.

Nurses assume several important roles in management of the disease, including assisting with radiographic examinations, performing skin tests, and obtaining specimens for laboratory examination. Sputum specimens are difficult or impossible to obtain in an infant or young child, since they swallow any mucus coughed from the lower respiratory tract. Therefore the best means for obtaining material for smears or culture is by *gastric washing* (i.e., aspiration of lavaged contents from the fasting stomach). The procedure is carried out and the specimen obtained early in the morning before the customary breakfast time. Because the success of therapy depends on compliance with the drug regimen, parents are instructed regarding the importance of giving the medication as often and for as long as it is ordered (see Compliance, Chapter 22).

PULMONARY DYSFUNCTION CAUSED BY NONINFECTIOUS IRRITANTS

FOREIGN BODY (FB) ASPIRATION

Small children characteristically explore matter with their mouths and are therefore particularly prone to aspirate an FB into the air passages. Aspiration of an FB can occur at any age but is most seen in children under 3 years of age. The signs and changes produced depend on the degree of obstruction and the nature of the foreign body. For example, dry vegetable matter, such as a seed, nut, or piece of carrot or popcorn, that does not dissolve and that may swell when wet creates a particularly difficult problem. The high fat content of potato chips and peanuts may cause the added risk of lipoid pneumonia. "Fun foods" of any kind are among the worst offenders. Offending foods in the order of frequency of aspiration are as follows: hot dog, round candy, peanut or other nut, grape, cookie or biscuit, other meat, carrot, apple, and peanut butter.

Round foods are the most frequent offenders. The first four items together contribute more than 40% of all speci-fied food items. A sharp or irritating object produces irritation and edema. A round, pliable object that does not readily break apart is more likely to occlude an airway than an object with a different shape. Balloons are especially hazardous. A small object may cause little if any pathologic changes, whereas an object of sufficient size to obstruct a passage can produce various changes, including atelectasis, emphysema, inflammation, and abscess.

Diagnostic Evaluation

The diagnosis of FB aspiration is usually suspected on the basis of the history and physical signs. Initially a foreign body in the air passages produces choking, gagging, wheezing, or coughing. After the initial period there is often an interval of hours, days, or even weeks without symptoms. Secondary symptoms are related to the anatomic area in which the object is lodged and are usually caused by a persistent respiratory infection focused distal to the obstruction. An FB is always a possibility in acute or chronic pulmonary lesions. Often, by the time secondary symptoms appear, the parents have forgotten the initial episode of coughing and gagging.

The most common symptoms observed in children brought to medical attention are stridor, wheezing, sternal retraction, and cough. When the object is lodged in the larynx, there is inability to speak or breathe. An object in the bronchi produces cough, decreased airway entry, wheezing, and dyspnea. A nonobstructive, nonirritating object may cause few symptoms; an obstructive object quickly produces pathologic changes; a slight obstruction may be evidenced only by a wheeze.

Radiographic examination reveals opaque FBs but may be of limited use in localizing vegetable matter. Bronchoscopy is usually required for definitive diagnosis of an object in the larynx and trachea. Fluoroscopic examination is a valuable aid in detecting and localizing an object in the bronchi.

Therapeutic Management

FB aspiration may result in life-threatening airway obstruction, especially in infants because of the small diameters of their airways. Current recommendations for the emergency treatment of the choking child include the use of abdominal thrusts for children over 1 year of age and back blows and chest thrusts for children less than 1 year of age (see Cardiopulmonary Resuscitation [CPR]).

An FB is rarely coughed up spontaneously; therefore it must be removed instrumentally by direct laryngoscopy or bronchoscopy. This should be carried out as soon as possible, since the progressive local inflammatory process triggered by the foreign material hampers removal, a chemical pneumonia soon develops, and vegetable matter begins to macerate within a few days, causing it to be even more difficult to remove. After removal of the FB, the child is placed in a high-humidity atmosphere, and any secondary infection is treated with appropriate antibiotics.

Nursing Considerations

A major role of nurses caring for a child who has aspirated an FB is to recognize the signs of FB aspiration and implement immediate measures to relieve the obstruction.

All persons working with children should be prepared to deal effectively with aspiration of an FB. Choking on food or other material should not be fatal. Two very simple procedures, back blows and the Heimlich maneuver, which can be used by both health professionals and lay persons, can save lives. It is the obligation of nurses to learn the techniques and teach them to parents and other groups. (see Fig. 23-8).

To aid a child who is choking, nurses need to recognize the signs of distress. Not every child who gags or coughs while eating is truly choking.

> **Nursing ALERT**
>
> The child in distress (1) *cannot speak,* (2) *becomes cyanotic,* and (3) *collapses.* These three signs indicate that the child is truly choking and requires immediate action. The child can die within 4 minutes. Follow-up care after the FB is removed includes chest physiotherapy as indicated, monitoring for respiratory distress, and education of the parents.

Prevention. Small children should not be allowed access to enticing small objects that they might place in their mouth. Rubber balloons are high-risk items for children; Mylar balloons are the only safe variety for children. Unlikely items (e.g., foil tabs from soft drink containers, Band-Aids applied to fingers of infants or very small children, plastic tabs from protective coverings on containers and from price tags on clothing) can be hazardous. Peanut butter, a staple in the diet of children, should never be given to a child unless it is spread thinly on bread or a cracker. A spoonful of peanut butter can obstruct the airway and stick to mucous membranes, becoming difficult or impossible for the child to dislodge.

Nurses, as child advocates, are in a position to teach prevention in a variety of settings. They can educate parents singly or in groups about hazards of FB aspiration in relation to the developmental level of their children and encourage them to teach their children safety. Parents teach by example; therefore they should be cautioned about behaviors that their children might imitate, for example, holding foreign objects, such as pins, nails, and toothpicks, in their lips or mouth. Prevention based on the child's age is discussed in Chapters 10 and 12.

ASPIRATION PNEUMONIA

Aspiration of fluid or food substances is a particular hazard in the child who has difficulty with swallowing or is unable to swallow because of paralysis, weakness, debility, congenital anomalies, or absent cough reflex or who is force fed, especially while crying or breathing rapidly. In addition to fluids, food, vomitus, and nasopharyngeal secretions, other substances that cause pneumonia are hydrocarbons, lipids, talcum powder, and barium.

Nursing Considerations

Care of the child with aspiration pneumonia is the same as that described for the child with pneumonia from other causes. However, the major thrust of nursing care is aimed at prevention of aspiration. Proper feeding techniques should be carried out for weak, debilitated, and uncooperative children, and preventive measures are used to prevent aspiration of any material that might enter the nasopharynx.

Oily nose drops and oil-based vitamin preparations are not appropriate for infants and small children. Solvents, lighter fluid, and other hydrocarbon substances should be kept away from older infants and small children, who are apt to put anything in their mouths and who may be attracted by the slightly sweet smell. Talcum powder should not be used; if used, careful application (placing it on the caregiver's hand and then the child's skin) and proper storage are essential.

Infants and debilitated children should be positioned on the right side after feedings to minimize the possibility of aspirating vomitus or regurgitated feeding. Nurses play a major role in education for injury prevention (see Injury Prevention, Chapters 10 and 12).

ADULT RESPIRATORY DISTRESS SYNDROME (ARDS)

ARDS is now recognized in children, as well as in adults, and poses a major threat to a child recovering from a primary insult. It is characterized by respiratory distress and hypoxemia that occur within 72 hours of a serious injury or surgery in a person with previously normal lungs. It is a syndrome and not a disease; shock is the most common event associated with the onset of the syndrome.

The hallmark of ARDS is increased permeability of the alveolar-capillary membrane that results in pulmonary edema. The lungs become stiff, gas diffusion is impaired, and eventually there is bronchiolar mucosal swelling and congestive atelectasis. Surfactant secretion is reduced, and the atelectasis and fluid-filled alveoli provide an excellent medium for bacterial growth. The criteria for diagnosis of ARDS in children are an acute antecedent illness or injury, acute respiratory distress or failure, no evidence of prior cardiopulmonary disease, and diffuse bilateral infiltrates evidenced on chest radiography.

Treatment involves general supportive measures, such as prevention of infection, maintenance of vascular pressure and cardiac output, adequate nutrition, comfort measures, positioning to improve functional residual capacity, and psychologic support. Definitive therapy is primarily directed toward improvement of oxygenation. Recent developments in the treatment of ARDS include (1) medications to interrupt the formation or activation of mediators contributing to progression of intrapulmonary shunting and lung injury, such as nonsteroidal antiinflammatory drugs (NSAIDs); (2) immunotherapy with monoclonal antibodies that work against the specific toxins causing the lung injury; and (3) human and artificial surfactant to reduce the severity of and sequelae from RDS, which may be useful in treating lung disease associated with ARDS and near-drowning.

The prognosis for ARDS varies. Some children recover completely, whereas others are left with varying degrees of pulmonary dysfunction.

Nursing care involves careful monitoring of cardiac output, heart rate, perfusion, capillary filling, and urine output, as well as assessment of respiratory status. Blood gas analysis and pulse oximetry are important evaluation tools. Respiratory distress is a frightening situation for both the child and the parents, and attention to their psychologic needs is a major element in the care of these children.

INHALATION INJURY: SMOKE AND CARBON MONOXIDE

A number of noxious substances that may be inhaled are toxic to humans. They are primarily products of incomplete combustion and are believed to cause more deaths from fires than do flame injuries. The severity of the injury depends on the nature of the substances generated by the material being burned and whether the victim is confined in a closed space. Inhaled substances produce injuries (1) locally by irritation, inflammation, and damage to pulmonary tissues or (2) systemically.

Local Injury

A wide variety of gases may be generated during the combustion of materials such as clothing, furniture, and floor coverings. The synthetic materials are especially toxic. Irritant gases such as nitrous oxide or carbon dioxide combine with water in the lungs to form corrosive acids; aldehydes cause denaturation of proteins, cellular damage, and edema of pulmonary tissues.

Possible inhalation injury is suspected when there is a history of flames in a closed space whether burns are present or not. Sooty material around the nose or in the sputum, singed nasal hairs, or mucosal burns of the nose, lips, mouth, or throat are all signs that the affected person demands observation for possible pulmonary injury from inhalants. A hoarse voice and cough, inspiratory and expiratory stridor, and signs of respiratory distress are further evidence of airway involvement.

Systemic Injury

Gases that are nontoxic to the airways (e.g., carbon monoxide [CO] and hydrogen cyanide) can cause injury and death by interfering with or inhibiting cellular respiration. CO is an extremely dangerous gas and is responsible for more than half of all fatal inhalation poisonings in the United States. It is a colorless, odorless gas with an affinity for hemoglobin (Hb) 230 times greater than that of oxygen. When it enters the bloodstream, CO combines readily with hemoglobin to form carboxyhemoglobin (COHb) but is released less readily. Therefore tissue hypoxia reaches dangerous levels before oxygen is available to meet tissue needs.

> **Nursing ALERT**
>
> The oxygen saturation (Sao_2) obtained by pulse oximetry will be normal because the device measures only oxygenated and deoxygenated hemoglobin; it does not measure dysfunctional hemoglobin, such as COHb.

Accidental CO poisoning is most often the result of exposure to fumes of heaters or smoke from structural fires, although poorly ventilated recreational vehicles with improperly operated or maintained gas lamps or stoves and cooking in underventilated areas with charcoal grills or hibachis are also frequent causes. CO is produced by incomplete combustion of carbon or carbonaceous material such as wood or charcoal.

The signs and symptoms of CO poisoning are secondary to tissue hypoxia and vary with the level of COHb. Mild manifestations may produce headache, visual disturbances, irritability, and nausea, whereas more severe intoxication causes confusion, hallucinations, ataxia, and coma. The bright, cherry-red lips and skin often described are less often observed; pallor and cyanosis are seen more frequently.

Therapeutic Management

When smoke inhalation injury is suspected, the patient is given humidified 100% oxygen by mask, and blood is drawn to determine baseline arterial blood gases and COHb levels. Surprisingly, arterial oxygen partial pressure (Pao_2) may be within normal limits unless there is marked respiratory depression. If CO poisoning is confirmed, 100% oxygen is continued until COHb levels fall to the nontoxic range of about 10%, and artificial ventilation may be implemented in selected cases. Where a hyperbaric oxygen chamber is available, the breakdown of the COHb bond is greatly accelerated.

Respiratory distress may occur early in the course of smoke inhalation as a result of hypoxia, or patients who are breathing well on admission may later develop sudden respiratory distress. Therefore intubation and/or tracheostomy equipment should be available at the bedside. More often distress is related to transient edema of the airways, which can occur at any level in the tracheobronchial tree. Assessment and localization of the obstruction should be accomplished before severe swelling of the head, neck, or oropharynx occurs. Intubation is often necessary when (1) severe burns in the area of the nose, mouth, and face increase the likelihood of developing oropharyngeal edema and obstruction; (2) vocal cord edema causes obstruction; (3) the patient has difficulty handling secretions; and (4) progressive respiratory distress requires artificial ventilation. Much controversy surrounds tracheostomy, but many prefer this procedure when the obstruction is proximal to the larynx and reserve nasotracheal intubation for lower tract involvement.

Use of corticosteroids, although controversial, may be of value in reducing edema, and bronchodilators (usually isoproterenol) are often given intravenously or by nebulizer. A broad-spectrum antibiotic is sometimes administered prophylactically, but this, too, is controversial.

Nursing Considerations

Nursing care of the child with inhalation injury is the same as that for any child with respiratory distress. Vital signs and other respiratory assessments are performed frequently, and the pulmonary status is carefully observed and maintained. Pulmonary physiotherapy is usually part of the therapeutic program, as well as mechanical ventilation if needed.

In addition to the observation and management of the physical aspects of inhalation injury, the nurse also deals with the psychologic needs of a frightened child and distraught parents. As with any accidental injury, the parents feel overwhelming guilt, even when the injury occurred through no fault of their own. More often, however, the injury could have been prevented, which compounds their guilt feelings. They need much support, reassurance, and information regarding the child's condition, treatment, and progress.

PASSIVE SMOKING

Numerous researchers have investigated the effects of environmental pollution on children's health and have determined that the worst pollutant is parental smoking, especially maternal smoking. Children exposed to environmental tobacco smoke have an increased number of respiratory illnesses and may have reduced performance on pulmonary function tests. When compared with children of nonsmoking parents,

FAMILY HOME CARE
House Rules for Smoking Households

Do not smoke in same room with children.
Restrict smoking to an isolated, preferably outdoor, area.
Do not smoke in motor vehicles with children.
Do not smoke in rooms children use.

the number of illnesses is positively correlated with the number of cigarettes smoked.

Maternal cigarette smoking is associated with increased rates of respiratory illnesses (e.g., bronchitis, asthma, otitis media) decreased fetal growth, increased stillbirths and preterm deliveries, and greater incidence of sudden infant death syndrome (SIDS). Parental smoking may have a deleterious effect on children's growth, a finding that has important implications in disorders such as cystic fibrosis.

The American Academy of Pediatrics has renewed its statement on hazards of passive smoking (American Academy of Pediatrics, 1994a). The report states: "The dangers to children of both active and passive tobacco exposure, including smokeless forms, are so well established that pediatricians should make the elimination of this threat a major issue as they pursue the goal of a tobacco-free generation by the year 2000."

Nursing Considerations

Passive smoking during childhood may well be the most important precursor of chronic lung disease in the adult. Nurses and other health professionals need to be aware of the problem and include this information in all health assessments of children, especially those with respiratory and allergic illnesses. In families where smokers refuse to quit, house rules should be established for reducing smoke in the child's environment (see Family Home Care box). Nurses should also inform caregivers of the health hazards of children's exposure to environments of tobacco smoke, set an example for children and families, and become advocates for "no smoking" ordinances in public places, prohibition of advertising tobacco products in the media, and inclusion of health warnings of sidestream smoke on tobacco products.

LONG-TERM RESPIRATORY DYSFUNCTION

ASTHMA

Asthma is defined as "airway obstruction or a narrowing that is characterized by bronchial irritability after exposure to various stimuli" and that is reversible either spontaneously or with treatment. When the symptoms (shortness of breath, wheezing, and/or chest tightness) become worse, either abruptly or progressively, the child is experiencing an *exacerbation* (American Academy of Pediatrics, 1994b). Asthma can be *intermittent,* in which the child is symptom free for extended periods without medication, or *chronic,* in which the child requires frequent or continuous medical therapy.

TRIGGERS TENDING TO PRECIPITATE AND/OR AGGRAVATE ASTHMATIC EXACERBATIONS

Allergens
  Outdoor: trees, shrubs, weeds, grasses, molds, pollens, air pollution, spores
  Indoor: dust and/or dust mites, mold, cockroach antigen
Irritants: tobacco smoke, wood smoke, odors, sprays
Exposure to occupational chemicals
Exercise
Cold air
Changes in weather or temperature
Environmental change: moving to new home, starting new school, etc.
Colds and infections
Animals: cats, dogs, rodents, horses
Medications: aspirin, nonsteroidal antiinflammatory drugs (NSAIDs), antibiotics, beta blockers
Strong emotions: fear, anger, laughing, crying
Conditions: gastroesophageal reflux, tracheoesophageal fistula
Food additives: sulfite preservatives
Foods: nuts, milk/dairy products
Endocrine factors: menses, pregnancy, thyroid disease

The incidence, severity, and mortality associated with asthma have risen steadily throughout the world. The increasing numbers may result from increasing air pollution, poor access to medical care, and/or underdiagnosis and undertreatment. Asthma is the most common chronic disease of childhood, is the primary cause of school absences, and is responsible for a major proportion of pediatric admissions to emergency rooms and hospitals.

Etiology

Although the exact etiology of asthma remains equivocal, evidence suggests that the disease occurs from hypersensitivity to environmental substances that trigger an allergic reaction. A strong relationship exists between viral infections and asthma induction in infants, with allergens playing a less important role in this age-group because it takes time for allergic sensitivity to develop. Studies in children with asthma suggest, however, that allergy influences the persistence and severity of the disease. Important triggers that tend to induce exacerbations are listed in the box. There tends to be a family predisposition toward hyperactivity of the airways, but this relationship remains just one variable as a potential cause of asthma.

Although allergy does provide an explanation for triggering asthma, there are instances where no allergic process can be detected. Theories that attempt to explain the airway reaction include (1) a basic defect in the β-adrenergic receptors on leukocytes and (2) increased cholinergic activity in the airways (Duffs and Platts-Mills, 1992). Asthma is an extremely complex disorder involving biochemical, immunologic, infectious, endocrine, and psychologic factors.

Pathophysiology

There is general agreement that heightened airway reactivity is characteristic of children with asthma. The reasons for this are less clear, and most theories do not explain all types and causes of asthma. However, the mechanisms responsible for

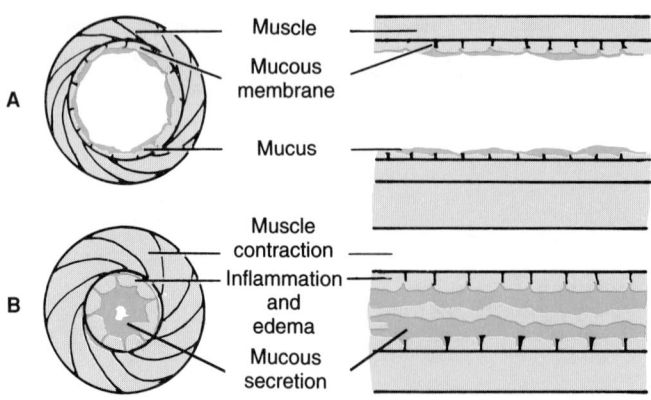

FIG. 23-3. Mechanisms of obstruction in asthma.

the obstructive symptoms of asthma (Fig. 23-3) are as follows:

1. Inflammation and edema of the mucous membranes
2. Accumulation of tenacious secretions from mucous glands
3. Spasm of the smooth muscle of the bronchi and bronchioles, which decreases the caliber of the bronchioles.

The role that each of these mechanisms plays varies from patient to patient and during the course of the disease in a given patient. In some patients, smooth muscle contraction is the major factor early in the episode, followed by mucosal inflammation and increased mucous secretion. In others the sequence of the responses is reversed.

Bronchial constriction is a normal reaction to foreign stimuli, but in the child with asthma it is abnormally severe, producing impaired respiratory function. The smooth muscle, arranged in spiral bundles around the airway, causes narrowing and shortening of the airway, which significantly increase airway resistance to airflow. Since the bronchi normally dilate and elongate during inspiration and contract and shorten on expiration, the respiratory difficulty is more pronounced during the expiratory phase of respiration. After the initial bronchial constrictions, an inflammatory process begins that causes the airways to obstruct and become more hyperresponsive to allergens. Recognition of the importance of this inflammatory response has made the use of antiinflammatory agents, especially inhaled steroids, a key component of treatment.

Increased resistance in the airway causes forced expiration through the narrowed lumen. The volume of air trapped in the lungs increases as airways are functionally closed at a point between the alveoli and the lobar bronchi by the combined mechanisms just described. This trapping of gas forces the individual to breathe at higher and higher lung volumes. Consequently, the person with asthma fights to inspire sufficient air. This expenditure of effort for breathing causes fatigue, decreased respiratory effectiveness, and increased oxygen consumption. Also, the inspiration occurring at higher lung volumes hyperinflates the alveoli and reduces the effectiveness of the cough. As the severity of obstruction increases, there is a reduced alveolar ventilation with carbon dioxide retention, hypoxemia, respiratory acidosis, and, eventually, respiratory failure.

CLINICAL MANIFESTATIONS OF ASTHMA

Cough
Hacking, paroxysmal, irritative, and nonproductive
Becomes rattling and productive of frothy, clear, gelatinous sputum in later stages

Respiratory-Related Signs
Shortness of breath
Prolonged expiratory phase
Audible wheeze
May have a malar flush and red ears
Lips deep, dark-red color
May progress to cyanosis of nail beds and/or circumoral cyanosis
Restlessness
Apprehension
Sweating may be prominent as the attack progresses
Older children may sit upright with shoulders in a hunched-over position, hands on the bed or chair, and arms braced
Speaks with short, panting, broken phrases

Chest
Hyperresonance on percussion
Coarse, loud breath sounds
Wheezes throughout the lung fields
Prolonged expiration
Crackles
Generalized inspiratory and expiratory wheezing; increasingly high pitched

With Repeated Episodes
Barrel chest
Elevated shoulders
Use of accessory muscles of respiration
Facial appearance: flattened malar bones, circles beneath the eyes, narrow nose, prominent upper teeth

---

Diagnostic Evaluation

Children with asthma may show signs and experience symptoms that range from acute episodes of shortness of breath, wheezing, and cough followed by a quiet period to a relatively continuous pattern of chronic symptoms that fluctuate in severity (see box). An attack may develop gradually or appear abruptly and may be preceded by a URI. The age of the child is often a significant factor, since the first attack in most cases occurs between ages 3 and 8 years. In infancy an attack usually follows a respiratory infection. Some children may experience a prodromal itching at the front of the neck or over the upper part of the back just before an attack.

The diagnosis is determined primarily on the basis of clinical manifestations, history, physical examination, and, to a lesser extent, laboratory tests. Radiographic examinations are used primarily to rule out other diseases and to evaluate coexisting disease. Generally, chronic cough in the absence of infection or diffuse wheezing during the expiratory phase of respiration is sufficient to establish a diagnosis.

Pulmonary function tests (PFTs) provide an objective and reproducible method of evaluating the presence and degree of lung disease, as well as the response to therapy. Spirometry can generally be performed reliably on children by the age of 5 or 6 years and includes either the traditional and simple mechanical spirometer often used in clinics, offices, and the home or the new computerized versions. One of the

GUIDELINES
Interpreting Peak Expiratory Flow Rates (PEFRs)*

- **Green (80% to 100% of personal best)** signals all clear. Asthma is under reasonably good control. No symptoms are present, and the routine treatment plan for maintaining control can be followed.
- **Yellow (50% to 80% of personal best)** signals caution. Asthma is not well controlled. An acute exacerbation may be present. Maintenance therapy may need to be increased. Call the practitioner if the child stays in this zone.
- **Red (below 50% of personal best)** signals a medical alert. Severe airway narrowing may be occurring. An immediate bronchodilator should be taken. Notify the practitioner if the PEFR measure does not return immediately and stay in yellow or green zones.

*These zones are guidelines only. Specific zones and management may be individualized for each child by the practitioner.

ATRAUMATIC CARE
Skin Testing

To help allay children's fears of skin tests, they need a careful and thorough explanation of what is to be done and how many "pricks" are involved (usually series of eight on each site, for a total of 30 tests). Very young, anxious patients may benefit from one prick on the arm to demonstrate how it feels. The skin is pierced with a stylet rather than a regular needle and syringe; then a drop of allergen is placed on the site. A helpful strategy is to have the child count off the number of pricks with the nurse as a distraction. For intradermal skin injection, EMLA, a topical anesthetic, reduces or eliminates pain without altering test results (Wolf and others, 1994).

key measurements is the *peak expiratory flow rate (PEFR)*, or the greatest flow velocity that can be obtained during a forced expiration using a *peak expiratory flow meter (PEFM)* (see p. 782). Three zones of measurement are typically used to interpret PEFR. The zone system is adapted to a traffic light so that the categories are easier to use and remember (see Guidelines box). Each child needs to establish his or her *personal best value.* A personal best value can be established during a 2- to 3-week period during which the child records PEFR at least twice a day. The present PEFR is then compared with the personal best (National Heart, Lung, and Blood Institute, 1991).

Skin testing is useful in identifying specific allergens, and those obtained by the puncture technique correlate better than intracutaneous tests with symptoms and measurements of specific immunoglobulin E (IgE) antibody (see Atraumatic Care box). *Provocative testing,* direct exposure of the mucous membranes to a suspected antigen in increasing concentrations, helps to identify inhaled allergens. The *radioallergosorbent test (RAST)* helps identify antigens against various foods and is often useful in determining appropriate therapy.

Therapeutic Management

The overall goal of asthma management is to prevent disability and to minimize physical and psychologic morbidity—to help the child live as normal and happy a life as possible. This includes facilitating the child's social adjustments in the family, school, and community and normal participation in recreational activities and sports. To accomplish these goals, efforts are directed toward recognizing acute episodes early and implementing appropriate therapy, identifying and eliminating irritant and allergic factors from the child's environment, educating parents to the long-term nature of the disease and how to manage exacerbations, and helping the child to deal constructively with the disease. Compliance to the prescribed regimen is essential to successful management.

Allergen Control. The goal of nonpharmacologic therapy is prevention and reduction of the child's exposure to airborne allergens and irritants. *House dust mites* and other components of house dust are the agents identified most of-

ten in children allergic to inhalants. The most important method to eliminate dust mites is to keep the humidity in the house under 50%, the level below which dust mites do not survive. Other recommendations for controlling allergens are in the Family Home Care box, p. 780.

Specific allergens are identified by skin testing, and steps are taken to eliminate or avoid the offending allergens. Often, simply removing the offending environmental factors will decrease the frequency of asthma episodes, for example, removal of a dog or cat from the home of a child sensitive to animal dander. Nonspecific factors that may trigger an episode, such as extremes of temperature, are sometimes controlled by dehumidifiers or air conditioners.

Drug Therapy. Most children do not require continuous medication. The goal is to control the acute exacerbation; therefore early recognition and treatment at the onset are most important. Promoting rapid relief of the bronchospasm reduces the need for drastic measures and increases the likelihood that relief will be complete. Several drugs are prescribed, often in combination, to reverse or prevent bronchospasm. Many of the medications are given by inhalation with a nebulizer or *metered-dose inhaler (MDI).* The MDI may have a spacing unit or reservoir attached, which makes it easier for young children to use. Children who have difficulty using the MDI can obtain effective relief with *nebulization.* The medication is mixed with saline and then nebulized with compressed air. Children are instructed to breathe normally with the mouth open to provide a direct route to the trachea.

Corticosteroids are the most effective antiinflammatory drugs for the treatment of reversible airflow obstruction and are highly effective in controlling symptoms and reducing bronchial hyperreactivity in chronic asthma. Corticosteroids may be administered parenterally, orally, or by aerosol. Oral medications are metabolized slowly, with an onset of action up to 3 hours after administration and peak effectiveness occurring within 6 to 12 hours. Acute short-term therapy is typically begun with high dosages, which can be maintained for 5 to 10 days. Long-term use is limited by the risk of significant adverse effects, such as osteoporosis, hypertension, Cushing syndrome, impaired immune mechanisms, and hypothalamic-pituitary-adrenal suppression (National Heart, Lung, and Blood Institute, 1991).

Inhaled corticosteroids should be attempted to determine whether oral corticosteroid treatment can be reduced or eliminated. Their use appears to result in a few side effects, such as oral or nasal irritation. However, the long-term effects of chronic inhalation of steroids remain unknown.

Cromolyn sodium is an NSAID for asthma. Although the exact mechanism of how it works is not known, it appears to act superficially to inhibit mast cell degranulation in both early-phase and late-phase allergen-induced airway narrowing and acute airway narrowing after exposure to exercise, cold dry air, and sulfur dioxide. There is no way to predict reliably whether a child will respond to the drug. Cromolyn sodium produces only minimal side effects, such as occasional coughing on inhalation of the powder formulation, and may be given via nebulizer or MDI. Another drug, *nedocromil sodium,* has both antiallergic and antiinflammatory properties. It is also being used with children.

β-*Adrenergic agonists,* primarily **albuterol, metaproterenol,** and **terbutaline,** are the medications of choice for treatment of acute exacerbations of asthma and for the prevention of exercise-induced asthma. They can be given via inhalation or as oral or parenteral preparations. The inhaled drug has a more rapid onset of action than the oral form but is more costly. Inhalation also reduces troublesome systemic side effects: irritability, tremor, nervousness, and insomnia.

Inhaled β-adrenergic agents can be taken two to four times daily for acute symptoms. *Salmeterol (Serevent)* is a long-acting bronchodilator that is used two times a day. Children with exercise-induced bronchospasm are advised to use the drug prophylactically 10 to 15 minutes before exercise.

Methylxanthines, principally *theophylline,* have been used for decades to relieve symptoms and prevent asthma attacks. Theophylline, however, is now considered as a third-line agent and perhaps even unnecessary for treating asthma exacerbations. When theophylline is used, it may be taken intravenously, intramuscularly, orally, or rectally (seldom used). The drug is also available in sustained-release form for oral ingestion. In addition to its bronchodilator effect, theophylline is also a central respiratory stimulant and increases respiratory muscle contractility.

Monitoring serum concentrations is an important component of both acute care and long-term management. Monitoring is required for children who fail to exhibit the expected bronchodilator effect, as well as for those who develop an adverse effect on the usual dose. Although theophylline has been accepted to have a therapeutic level of 10 to 20 μg/ml, a more conservative approach would be to aim for levels of 5 to 15 μg/ml (National Heart, Lung, and Blood Institute 1991). The signs and symptoms of theophylline intoxication involve many different organ systems, with gastrointestinal symptoms—nausea and vomiting—being the most common early events. Cardiopulmonary effects include tachycardia, dysrhythmias, and stimulation of the respiratory center (tachypnea), with diuresis, irritability, and even seizures possible. There have been reports that theophylline may cause behavior problems and poor school performance, but most research does not support these findings (Milgrom and Bender, 1995).

Exercise.   Airway obstruction often develops in children with asthma. *Exercise-induced bronchospasm,* or *exercise-induced asthma (EIA),* does not represent a unique syndrome but rather an example of the airway hyperactivity common to all persons with asthma. EIA is an acute, reversible, usually self-terminating airway obstruction that develops 5 to 15 minutes after strenuous exercise and lasts 15 to 60 minutes after the onset. Usually the episode subsides spontaneously in ½ to 1 hour. The severity of an attack increases as the exercise becomes increasingly strenuous. Patients with a history of EIA often have normal PFTs and are only symptomatic with exercise.

The problem is rare in activities that require only short bursts of energy (e.g., baseball, sprints, gymnastics, skiing) rather than those that involve endurance exercise (e.g., soccer, basketball, distance running). Swimming, even long-distance swimming, is well tolerated by children with EIA, partly because they are breathing air fully saturated with moisture, but the type of breathing required may also play a role. Exhaling under water is of benefit because it prolongs each expiration and increases the end-expiratory pressure within the respiratory tree (essentially pursed-lip breathing).

Children with asthma are often excluded from exercise by parents, teachers, and practitioners, as well as by the children themselves because they are reluctant to provoke an attack. This can seriously hamper peer interaction. Moderate or even strenuous exercise is advantageous for children with asthma. These children can participate in activities at school and in sports with minimum difficulty, provided that the asthma is under control. Participation should be evaluated on an individual basis in terms of tolerance for duration and intensity of effort. Appropriate prophylactic treatment with β-adrenergic agents or cromolyn sodium before exercise will usually permit full participation in strenuous exertion. Restrictions are invoked only when the child's condition makes it necessary.

Chest Physiotherapy (CPT).   CPT, a standard adjunct to treatment of chronic asthma, includes breathing exercises, physical training, and inhalation therapy. These therapies help produce physical and mental relaxation, improve posture, strengthen respiratory musculature, and develop more efficient patterns of breathing. For the motivated child, breathing exercises and controlled breathing are of value in preventing overinflation and improving the strength of respiratory muscles and the efficiency of the cough. Stretch exercises sometimes help increase the flexibility of the ribs. Sit-ups and leg exercises strengthen abdominal muscles and aid expiration.

Hyposensitization.   The role of hyposensitization in childhood asthma has not been clarified. In many cases the child demonstrates multiple sensitivities, which makes such therapy impractical. Moreover, the injections can be expensive and uncomfortable. When the allergen can be defined and cannot be avoided or controlled satisfactorily by drugs, specific hyposensitization is seriously considered.

Injection therapy is usually limited to clinically significant allergens, such as house dust, pollens, and molds. The initial dose of the offending allergen(s), based on the size of the skin reaction, is injected subcutaneously. The amount is increased at weekly intervals until a maximum tolerance is reached, after which a maintenance dose is given at 4-week intervals. This may be extended to 5- or 6-week intervals during the off-season for seasonal allergens. Successful treatment is continued for a minimum of 3 years and then stopped. If no symptoms appear, acquired immunity is said to be retained; if symptoms recur, treatment is reinstituted.

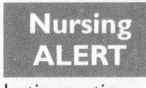

Nursing ALERT

Hyposensitization injections should be administered only with emergency equipment and medications readily available in the event of an anaphylactic reaction.

Prognosis. The outlook for children with asthma varies widely. Many children lose their symptoms at puberty, but no factor can predict which children will "outgrow" their asthma. Some develop other forms of allergy in adulthood, most frequently involving the nose.

The prognosis for control of or disappearance of symptoms will differ in children who have rare and infrequent attacks and in those who are constantly wheezing or who are subject to status asthmaticus. In general, the more severe and numerous the symptoms, the longer they have been present, and when there is a family history of allergy, the poorer is the prognosis for improvement. Many who outgrow their symptoms are subject to EIA as adults, and the associated disorders, such as growth impairment, chest deformity, and airway obstruction, are maintained throughout life.

Although death from asthma is rare, the death rate has increased 46% in the period 1980 to 1989 despite advances in therapy (American Academy of Pediatrics, 1994b). The adolescent age-group appears to be the most vulnerable, with the greatest increase occurring in ages 10 to 14 years. No reliable data exist to explain this increase. Factors that have been postulated include exposure of atopic persons to more allergens, change in severity of the disease, abuse of drug therapy (toxicity), failure of families and practitioners to recognize severity of asthma, and psychologic factors, such as denial or refusal to accept the disease. Risk factors for asthma deaths appear to be onset at an early age, frequent attacks, difficult-to-manage disease, adolescence, history of respiratory failure, psychologic problems (refusal to take medications), dependency on or misuse of drugs (high use), presence of physical stigmata (barrel chest, intercostal retractions), and abnormal PFTs (see Family Focus box).

Status Asthmaticus. Children who continue to display respiratory distress despite vigorous therapeutic measures, especially sympathomimetics, are considered to be in status asthmaticus. The condition may develop gradually or rapidly, often coincident with complicating conditions (e.g., pneumonia) that can influence the duration and treatment of the attack. These children are acutely ill and require hospi-

talization, preferably where pediatric intensive care is available. They need continuous nursing attendance with cardiorespiratory monitoring and vigilant observation.

Nursing ALERT

Status asthmaticus is a medical emergency that can result in respiratory failure and death if untreated. The child who sweats profusely, remains sitting upright, and refuses to lie down is in severe respiratory distress. Also, the child who suddenly becomes agitated, or the agitated child who suddenly becomes quiet and listless, may be seriously hypoxic and requires immediate intervention.

Therapy for status asthmaticus is directed toward improvement of ventilation, correction of dehydration and acidosis, and treatment of any concurrent infection. Bronchospasm is relieved by giving nebulized albuterol (either intermittent or continuous) along with corticosteroids (either oral or IV). For the child not responding to either of these therapies, subcutaneous epinephrine (1:1000) at a dose of 0.01 ml/kg, with a maximum dose of 0.3 ml, or subcutaneous terbutaline is administered.

The child is given IV fluids and nothing by mouth except liquids if the condition permits. The IV infusion provides a means for hydration and administering medications. The correction of dehydration, acidosis, hypoxia, and electrolyte derangements is guided by frequent determination of oxygenation (pulse oximetry), blood gases, and serum electrolytes.

Humidified oxygen is administered by tent, face mask, or cannula to maintain satisfactory oxygenation. Since oxygen is a stimulus for respiration, high levels may significantly depress respirations.

Administration of antibiotics is frequently advisable in therapy, since infection may be masked or may not always be evident and is always a threatening complication. As the attack subsides, fluids and medication are given orally and discharge plans are initiated, especially for follow-up care.

Nursing Considerations

❖ Assessment

Physical assessment of asthma involves the same observations and techniques described in the general discussion of assessment of respiratory infection (see p. 751) and physical assessment of the chest (see Chapter 7). In addition, some physical characteristics of chronic respiratory involvement are noted and evaluated. These include chest configuration, posturing, and type of breathing. The chest of a child with chronic obstructive respiratory disease often assumes a barrel shape from chronic hyperinflation.

Psychologic assessment consists of assessing the degree to which the disorder interferes with everyday activities, the child and the family cope with the condition, the disorder alters the child's self-concept, and the child and family comply with the therapeutic management.

❖ Nursing Diagnoses

Based on a thorough assessment, several nursing diagnoses are identified. The more common diagnoses for the child with asthma are included in the Nursing Care Plan on pp. 783-785. Others may apply in specific situations.

FAMILY FOCUS
Asthma: Factors Affecting Prognosis

Psychologic factors play an important role in children who die during an asthmatic episode. Those who die tend to have significant psychologic problems, such as extreme reactions to separation or loss, a history of family turmoil, and expressed hopelessness or despair that leads to depression. Their families are less likely to recognize the severity of the asthma and the need to comply with therapy. In this situation appropriate family education concerning the risks of the child's disease if treatment is inconsistent can be lifesaving (Klinnert, Miller, and Mrazek, 1990).

FAMILY HOME CARE
"Allergy-Proofing" the Home

Keep humidity between 40% and 50%; use dehumidifier if available.

Have carpets cleaned professionally frequently or remove them, including carpeting on concrete.

Avoid vacuuming carpets, which sends allergens into the air, although it does remove waste particles of dust mites.

If available, use central vacuum cleaner with collecting bag outside of home or use cleaner filters (e.g., high-efficiency particulate air [HEPA] filters).

Use chemical agents to kill mites or alter antigens in house.

Treating carpet with 3% tannic acid solution or benzylbenzoate (available in foam for mattresses and furniture and in powder for carpets) kills dust mites; keep child away from treated areas during and several hours after chemical application.*

If possible, use an air-cleaning device, such as electrostatic precipitator or with a HEPA filter; approximate-size units can be used in child's room.

Have air and heat ducts professionally cleaned annually; change or clean filters monthly.

Place airtight plastic, vinyl, or hypoallergenic covers on mattress, box spring, and pillows.*

Use foam rubber mattress and pillows or Dacron pillows and synthetic blankets.

Launder blankets and sheets in hot water (over 48.8° C [120° F]).

Store nothing under bed; keep closets and storage areas uncluttered.

Use washable shades rather than blinds or curtains.

Use child's bedroom for sleeping, not playing.

Remove from room unnecessary furniture, rugs, stuffed or real animals, toys, books, upholstered furniture, plants, aquariums, wall hangings, etc.

Cover or replace upholstered furniture; avoid rattan or wicker furniture.

Cover walls with washable paint or wallpaper.

Limit child's exposure to animals.

Change child's clothes after playing outdoors; wash hair nightly if outside and pollen count is high.

Keep child indoors while lawn is being mowed, bushes/trees are being trimmed, or pollen count is high.

Keep windows and doors closed during pollen season; use air conditioner if available.

Cover heating vents with filter material (e.g., cheesecloth) to prevent circulation of dust, especially when heat is turned on after summer.

Use smooth cotton or synthetic fabric for bedcovers, curtains, and scatter rugs and launder weekly.

Wet mop bare floors weekly.

Wet dust (or use Endust) and clean room weekly; child should not be present during housecleaning activities.

Encase wool or feather items in nonallergenic coverings.*

Limit or avoid child's exposure to tobacco and wood smoke.

Avoid odors or sprays (e.g., perfumes, talcum powder, room deodorizers, fresh paint).

Avoid cellar (basement) as play area and use dehumidifier in damp cellar.

Clean showers and tile areas; spray with antimold agent (e.g., Lysol).

Keep vaporizers and air conditioners (including automobile air conditioner) clean and free of mold.

*A source of information is **Allergy Control Products,** Inc., 96 Danbury Rd, Ridgefield, CT 06877; (800) 422-DUST.

❖ Planning

The goals for a child with asthma and the family include the following:

1. Child will not experience an asthmatic episode.
2. Child will exhibit improved ventilatory capacity.
3. Child will maintain optimum health.
4. Child will not develop complications.
5. Child will engage in normal activities for age.
6. Child and family will receive appropriate support and education regarding the disease and its management.

❖ Implementation

Avoid Allergens. The primary goal of asthma management is avoidance of an exacerbation. Parents need to know the nature of the disease and, when the allergens are determined, how they can avoid and/or relieve asthmatic episodes by modifying the environment to reduce contact with the offending allergen(s) (see Family Home Care box). The parents are cautioned to avoid exposing a sensitive child to excessive cold, wind, or other extremes of weather, smoke, sprays, or other irritants. Passive smoking has been associated with exacerbation of symptoms in children with hyperresponsive airways, especially in boys and older children.

Since approximately 2% to 6% of children with asthma are sensitive to aspirin, acetaminophen is recommended. Those children with aspirin-induced asthma may also be sensitive to NSAIDs and tartrazine (yellow dye number 5, a common food coloring).

Relieve Bronchospasm. Parents and older children need to learn how to use the medications prescribed to relieve bronchospasm. They are taught to recognize early signs and symptoms of an impending attack so that it can be controlled before symptoms become distressing. Most children can recognize prodromal symptoms well before an attack (about 6 hours) so that preventive therapy can be implemented. Some objective signs that parents may observe include rhinorrhea, cough, low-grade fever, irritability, itching (especially in front of neck and chest), apathy, anxiety, sleep disturbance, abdominal discomfort, and loss of appetite. A variety of easy-to-use, inexpensive PEFMs are available for use in the home to help assess the extent of the child's symptoms (see Family Home Care box on p. 781 [left]).

Older children who use a nebulizer or aerosol device to deliver adrenergic drugs need to learn how to use the device correctly. The MDI (Fig. 23-4) combines portability with a rapid and reliable dose for patients managed at home. The

FAMILY HOME CARE
Use of a Peak Expiratory Flow Meter (PEFM)

1. Before each use, make sure the sliding marker or arrow on the PEFM is at the bottom of the numbered scale.
2. Stand up straight.
3. Remove gum or any food from the mouth.
4. Close your lips tightly around the mouthpiece. Be sure to keep your tongue away from the mouthpiece.
5. Blow out as hard and as quickly as you can, a "fast hard puff."
6. Note the number by the marker on the numbered scale.
7. Repeat entire routine three times.
8. Record the *highest* of the three readings, not the average.
9. Measure your peak expiratory flow rate (PEFR) close to the same time and same way each day (i.e., morning and evening; before and/or 15 minutes after taking medication).
10. Keep a chart of your PEFRs.

FAMILY HOME CARE
Use of a Metered-Dose Inhaler*

Steps for Checking How Much Medicine Is in the Canister
1. If the canister is new, it is full.
2. If the canister has been used repeatedly, it might be empty. (Check product label to see how many inhalations should be in each canister.)
3. To check how much medicine is left in the canister, put the canister (not the mouthpiece) in a cup of water.
   a. If the canister sinks to the bottom, it is full.
   b. If the canister floats sideways on the surface, it is empty.

Steps for Using the Inhaler
1. Remove the cap and hold inhaler upright.
2. Shake the inhaler.
3. Tilt the head back slightly and breathe out.
4. With the inhaler in an upright position, insert the mouthpiece:
   a. About 3 to 4 cm from the mouth *or*
   b. Into an aerochamber *or*
   c. Into the mouth, forming an airtight seal between the lips and the mouthpiece
5. At the end of a normal expiration, depress the top of the inhaler canister firmly to release the medication (into either the aerochamber or the mouth), and breathe in slowly (about 3 to 5 seconds). Relax the pressure on the top of the canister.
6. Hold the breath for at least 5 to 10 seconds to allow the aerosol medication to reach deeply into the lungs.
7. Remove the inhaler and breathe out slowly through the nose.
8. Wait 1 minute between puffs (if additional one is needed).
9. To determine if child is using an inhaler properly, have child use the device in front of a mirror. If vapor does not appear on the mirror, the inhaler is being used correctly.

Adapted from National Heart, Lung, and Blood Institute, National Institutes of Health: *Guidelines for the diagnosis and management of asthma*, Pub No 91-3042, Bethesda, MD, 1991, The Institute.
*NOTE: Inhaled dry-powder capsules require a different inhalation technique. To use a dry-powder inhaler, it is important to close the mouth tightly around the mouthpiece of the inhaler and inhale rapidly.

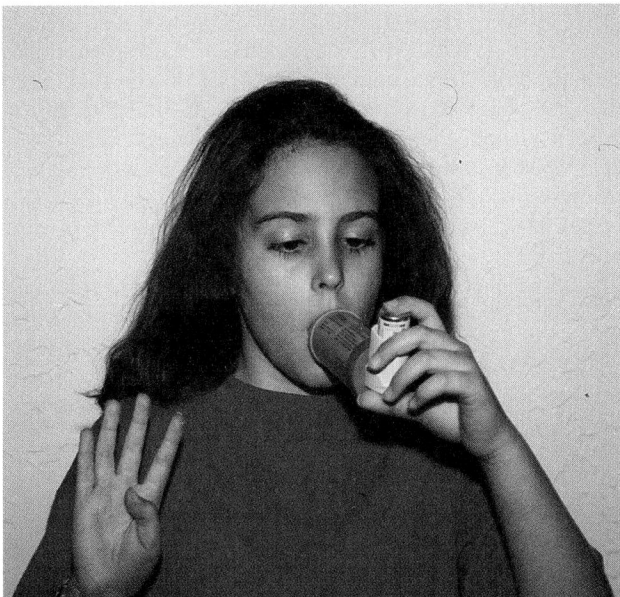

FIG. 23-4. Child using metered-dose inhaler (MDI) with spacer. Fingers are used for counting to 10 seconds.

objective of the device is to distribute the prescribed medication directly to the narrowed airways. It is important that the child learns to breathe slowly and deeply for better distribution to narrowed airways (see Family Home Care box).

Young children and those who are otherwise unable to manipulate the device or coordinate breathing with activation of the MDI are able to use special chambers called *spacers*. These permit an operator to deliver the medication from the MDI into the spacer from which the child inhales (see Critical Thinking Exercise).

The child and parents also need to be cautioned about the adverse effects of prescribed drugs and the dangers of overuse. They should know that it is important to use them when

CRITICAL THINKING EXERCISE
Asthma

Traditional thinking about the pathophysiology of asthma has changed in recent years. Which one of the following treatments reflects this better understanding of the mechanisms involved in an asthmatic episode?

1. Peak expiratory flow meter (PEFM)
2. Metered-dose inhaler (MDI)
3. Allergy hyposensitization
4. Chest physiotherapy

The correct answer is two. Inflammation of the bronchial airways is now recognized as a critical component in the pathophysiology of asthma. MDIs are used to deliver corticosteroids to decrease the inflammation. The PEFM is an assessment device; the other two choices have been used traditionally.

needed but not indiscriminately or as a substitute for avoiding the symptom-provoking allergen.

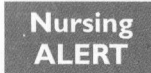 Side effects from theophylline include nausea, headache, irritability, and insomnia. Early signs of toxicity are nausea, tachycardia, and irritability; seizures and dysrhythmias occur at blood theophylline levels greater than 30 µg/ml.

The family can acquire a PEFM that measures the maximum PEFR to predict an acute exacerbation. This provides information for adjusting medication dosage.

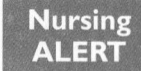 Long-acting β-adrenergic inhalers (salmeterol [Serevent]) should be used only as directed (usually every 12 hours) and not more frequently. They are not intended to relieve acute asthmatic symptoms.

The parents are cautioned to avoid exposing the child to excessive cold, wind, or other extremes of weather and to smoke, sprays, or other irritants. Although foods are an unusual cause of asthma, foods known to provoke symptoms should be eliminated from the diet. The foods most frequently allergenic are eggs, milk, grains, peanuts, and chocolate. Parents are advised to read labels on prepared foods and snacks to determine the presence of allergens. For example, a number of foods contain sodium caseinate or dried-milk products. Since approximately 2% to 6% of these children are sensitive to aspirin, nurses caution the parents to use other analgesic/antipyretic drugs for discomfort or fever.

The child should be protected from a respiratory infection that can trigger an attack or aggravate the asthmatic state, especially in young children. Their airways are mechanically smaller and more reactive; therefore edema from infection causes wheezing and other signs of respiratory obstruction. Also, the equipment used for the child, such as nebulizers, must be kept absolutely clean to decrease the chances of contamination with bacteria and fungi.

Breathing exercises and controlled breathing are taught and encouraged for motivated youngsters, and the nurse can help them select activities suitable to their capacity. Anything that promotes proper diaphragmatic breathing, side expansion, and generally improved mobility of the chest wall is encouraged. If the child requires postural drainage and percussion, someone in the family must assume responsibility for carrying out the procedure. It is the responsibility of the physical therapist or the nurse to teach the parent the proper technique.

NURSING TIP Play techniques that can be employed for younger children to extend their expiratory time and increase expiratory pressure include blowing cotton balls or a Ping-Pong ball on a table, blowing a pinwheel, or bubbles, or preventing a tissue from falling by blowing it against the wall.

Self-care is a hallmark of effective asthma management, and self-management programs are important in helping the child and family cope with the disease. The principles conveyed include the following:

1. Asthma is a very common disease, and to have asthma is annoying but not disgraceful.
2. Persons with asthma are able to live full and active lives.
3. It is much easier to prevent than to treat an asthmatic attack.
4. Individuals do not become addicted to asthma medication, but they do prefer to breathe more freely whenever possible.

Asthma camps have become popular in recent years as a means of encouraging physical activity in a more homogeneous, controlled, and less competitive environment. Although not all persons subscribe to this practice, some support the benefits, which are primarily that the denominator of asthma is removed as a factor. Everyone at the camp has asthma; therefore no child is different from the others.

Several organizations provide education and services for health professionals and families of children with asthma.* Asthma education and awareness are important aspects of asthma management. Although the principles of self-management are very general and the programs are designed for general use, each child and family have their own special needs that require individualized care and attention.

Provide Acute Asthma Care. Children who are admitted to the hospital with acute asthma are ill, anxious, and uncomfortable. In most instances the child is admitted on an emergency basis and is in acute distress. An IV infusion may be started to provide immediate access, and medications, usually nebulized albuterol and a corticosteroid, are administered to relieve bronchospasm. The child is monitored closely and continuously during therapy for relief of respiratory distress and signs of side effects.

It is especially important that the child receive sufficient fluid either orally or intravenously to replace losses through diaphoresis and hyperventilation. Cold liquids may trigger reflex bronchospasm and should be avoided. Nourishment is provided in small, frequent feedings to avoid abdominal distention that might interfere with diaphragmatic excursion.

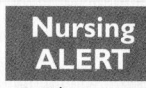 Dehydration should be corrected slowly; overhydration can increase the accumulation of interstitial pulmonary fluid to exacerbate small airway obstruction.

Older children usually prefer the high-Fowler position, although they may be more comfortable sitting upright or leaning slightly forward. When possible, the nurse communicates in such a way that a child need only reply in a few words to avoid fatigue. Shortness of breath makes talking difficult. Oxygen is indicated for relief of dyspnea and cyanosis; however, it is not administered indiscriminately but regulated according to the blood gas analysis, pulse oximetry, and objective observation of color, respiratory effort, and sensorium. Associated treatments such as intermittent positive-pressure breathing or postural drainage and tests (e.g., blood gases,

*Asthma and Allergy Foundation of America (AAFA), 1125 15th St. N.W., Washington, DC 20005, (202) 466-7643; American Lung Association, 1740 Broadway, New York, NY 10019, (212) 315-8700; Canadian Lung Association, 75 Albert St., Suite 908, Ottawa, Ontario K1P 5E7, (613) 237-1208; The Lung Association, 573 King St. East, Suite 201, Toronto, Ontario M5A 4L3, (416) 922-9440.

NURSING CARE PLAN
The Child with Asthma

NURSING DIAGNOSIS: High risk for suffocation related to interaction between individual and allergen(s)

PATIENT GOAL 1: Will experience no asthmatic episode

- **NURSING INTERVENTIONS/*RATIONALES***

Teach child and family how to avoid conditions or circumstances that precipitate asthmatic episode

Assist parents in eliminating allergens or other stimuli that trigger exacerbation (see box on p. 780), such as:
  Meal planning to eliminate allergenic foods
  Removal of pets
  Modification of environment: "allergy-proof" home, especially no smoking in home

Avoid extremes of environmental temperature
  When child is exposed to cold air, recommend breathing through nose (not mouth) and wearing a mask or scarf, or cupping hand over nose and mouth *to create a reservoir of warm air to breathe*

Assist parents in obtaining and/or installing device to control environment (dehumidifier, air conditioner, electronic air filter)

Teach child and family to recognize early signs and symptoms *so that an impending episode can be controlled before it becomes distressful*

Teach child and family correct use of bronchodilators and antiinflammatory drugs (e.g., corticosteroids, cromolyn sodium), adverse effects, and dangers of overuse or underuse of drugs

Teach child to understand how equipment works

Teach child correct use of inhalers, nebulizers, and peak expiratory flow meters (PEFMs)

Teach child and family prophylactic treatment when appropriate (e.g., prevent exercise-induced bronchospasm by using medication before exercise)

Explain to child and family possible benefits of hyposensitization therapy when allergen(s) can be defined and cannot be avoided (e.g., pollen, mold) or controlled satisfactorily by drugs

*Administer hyposensitization therapy if prescribed

- **EXPECTED OUTCOMES**

Family makes every effort to remove or avoid possible allergens or precipitating events

Child and family are able to detect signs of an impending episode early and implement appropriate actions

Child and family are able to administer medications and use inhalers and other equipment

---

*Dependent nursing action.

PATIENT GOAL 2: Will experience optimum health

- **NURSING INTERVENTIONS/*RATIONALES***

Encourage sound health practices *to support body's natural defenses:*
  Balanced, nutritious diet
  Adequate rest
  Good hygiene
  Appropriate exercise
  Follow-up care

Prevent respiratory infection *since it can trigger an attack or aggravate the asthmatic state*
  Avoid exposure to infection
  Take meticulous care of equipment *to avoid bacterial and/or fungal growth*
  Use good handwashing

- **EXPECTED OUTCOMES**

Child and parents practice sound health practices
Child exhibits no evidence of infection

NURSING DIAGNOSIS: Ineffective airway clearance related to allergenic response and inflammation in the bronchial tree

PATIENT GOAL 1: Will exhibit evidence of improved ventilatory capacity

- **NURSING INTERVENTIONS/*RATIONALES***

Instruct and/or supervise breathing exercises and controlled breathing *to promote proper diaphragmatic breathing, side expansion, and improved chest wall mobility*

Use play techniques for breathing exercises with young children (e.g., blow a pinwheel or blow cotton balls on table) *to extend expiratory time and increase expiratory pressure*

Teach correct use of prescribed medications

Teach correct use of PEFM, nebulizer, and metered-dose inhaler (MDI) if indicated

Teach family to perform percussion and postural drainage and to encourage coughing if indicated

Encourage physical exercise
  Recommend activities requiring short bursts of energy (e.g., baseball, sprints, skiing), *since they may be better tolerated than those requiring endurance exercise* (e.g., soccer, distance running)
  Recommend swimming *because child breathes air saturated with moisture, and exhaling underwater prolongs expiration and increases end-expiratory pressure*
  Restrict physical activity only when child's condition makes it necessary

Encourage good posture *for maximum lung expansion*

Assist child and family in selecting activities appropriate to child's capabilities and preferences

- **EXPECTED OUTCOMES**

Child breathes easily and without dyspnea
Child exhibits improved ventilatory capacity (specify)
Child engages in activities according to abilities and interest (specify)

Continued.

NURSING DIAGNOSIS: Activity intolerance related to imbalance between oxygen supply and demand

PATIENT GOAL 1: Will receive optimum rest

• **NURSING INTERVENTIONS**

Encourage activities appropriate to child's condition and capabilities (specify)
Provide ample opportunities for sleep, rest, and quiet activities, to conserve oxygen supply

• **EXPECTED OUTCOMES**

Child engages in appropriate activities (specify)
Child appears rested

NURSING DIAGNOSIS: Altered family processes related to having a child with a chronic illness

PATIENT/FAMILY GOAL 1: Will exhibit positive adaptation to the condition

• **NURSING INTERVENTIONS/RATIONALES**

Foster positive family relationships
Reinforce positive coping mechanisms of child and family
Use every opportunity to increase parents' and child's understanding of the disease and its therapies, *since adequate knowledge is related to family's timely use of preventive and emergency intervention*
Reinforce the need for responding to early signs of impending asthma episode using prescribed medications as needed *to decrease potential for a severe exacerbation*
Intervene appropriately if there is evidence of maladaptation
Be alert to signs of parental rejection or overprotection
Be alert to signs that child is depressed and make appropriate referral for psychologic support, *since depressed children, especially adolescents, may not comply with therapies as a means of passive suicide*
Teach child and family how to give respiratory treatments *to eliminate any confusion* regarding medication or inhalers/nebulizers
Encourage family to contact school personnel (e.g., nurse, teachers, coaches, principal) to develop a consistent plan of care for school setting
Refer family to appropriate support groups and community agencies

• **EXPECTED OUTCOMES**

Family copes with symptoms and effects of the disease and provides a normal environment for the child
See Nursing Care Plan: The Child with Chronic Illness or Disability, Chapter 18

Status Asthmaticus (Special Needs)

NURSING DIAGNOSIS: High risk for suffocation related to bronchospasm, mucus secretions, edema

PATIENT GOAL 1: Will experience cessation of bronchospasm

• **NURSING INTERVENTIONS/RATIONALES**

Establish intravenous (IV) infusion *for administration of medication and hydration*
*Administer aerolized bronchodilators, and either oral or IV corticosteroids with or without epinephrine as prescribed *to relieve bronchospasm*
Closely monitor vital signs before, during, and after administration *for maximum efficacy and minimum side effects*
Interview parents to determine medications given before admission to avoid possible overdose
Have emergency equipment and medications readily available *to prevent delay in treatment*

• **EXPECTED OUTCOMES**

Child breathes more easily
Child does not suffocate

PATIENT GOAL 2: Will exhibit normal respiratory function

• **NURSING INTERVENTIONS/RATIONALES**

Administer humidified oxygen by tent, face mask, or cannula *to maintain satisfactory oxygenation*
Closely monitor oxygen saturations and blood gases via pulse oximetry *to detect early or impending hypoxia*
Closely monitor percentage of oxygen delivered, *since high levels may depress respirations*
Position *for optimum lung expansion*
  High-Fowler position
  Provide overbed table with pillows on which to lean if more comfortable for child
Implement measures to reduce fear/anxiety *to decrease respiratory efforts and oxygen consumption*
Encourage relaxation techniques *to decrease anxiety and promote lung expansion*
Administer sedatives and tranquilizing agents, if prescribed, with extreme caution and when agitation is not caused by anoxia, *since these drugs can depress respirations and mask signs of anoxia*
Organize activities to allow for rest, sleep, and minimum expenditure of energy

• **EXPECTED OUTCOMES**

Child's respirations are unlabored and within normal limits (see inside back cover)
Child rests and sleeps comfortably
Child does not experience decreased oxygen saturations

PATIENT GOAL 3: Will successfully expel bronchial secretions

• **NURSING INTERVENTIONS/RATIONALES**

Provide adequate hydration, oral or IV, *to liquefy secretions for easier removal*
Maintain NPO (nothing by mouth), if necessary, *to prevent aspiration of fluids and food*
Provide humidified atmosphere *to prevent drying of mucous membranes*

---

*Dependent nursing action.

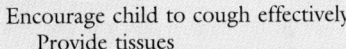

Encourage child to cough effectively
   Provide tissues
   Explain need to remove secretions
Suction, using correct technique, only when necessary
Do not use chest physiotherapy (CPT) during an acute episode since will only agitate an already anxious, dyspneic child and aggravate the episode; CPT may be started as soon as signs of airway obstruction significantly subside
Position, if necessary, *to prevent aspiration of secretions*
   Semiprone
   Side lying

• EXPECTED OUTCOMES

Secretions are adequately and easily expelled
Child coughs effectively
Child does not aspirate secretions, food, or fluids

> **NURSING DIAGNOSIS:** High risk for fluid volume deficit related to difficulty taking fluids, insensible fluid losses from hyperventilation, diaphoresis

PATIENT GOAL 1: Will exhibit adequate hydration

• NURSING INTERVENTIONS/*RATIONALES*

Maintain IV infusion at appropriate rate, *since fluid therapy will enhance liquefaction of secretions* (IV line usually run two-thirds to three-quarters maintenance [unless dehydration present] *to minimize the risk of pulmonary edema because of high inspiratory pressures*)
Encourage oral fluids
   Offer fluids when acute respiratory distress subsides *to decrease risk of aspiration*
   Avoid cold liquids, *since they can trigger reflex bronchospasm*
   Give fluids (and food) in small, frequent feedings *to avoid abdominal distention that might interfere with diaphragmatic excursion*
   Use play techniques appropriate to child's age *to encourage fluid intake*
Measure intake and output
Correct dehydration slowly, *since overhydration can increase the accumulation of interstitial pulmonary fluid, leading to increased airway obstruction*

• EXPECTED OUTCOME

Child exhibits adequate hydration

> **NURSING DIAGNOSIS:** High risk for injury (respiratory acidosis, electrolyte imbalance) related to hypoventilation, dehydration

PATIENT GOAL 1: Will not experience acidosis

• NURSING INTERVENTIONS/*RATIONALES*

Closely monitor blood pH, *since pH less than 7.25 impairs systemic, pulmonary, and coronary blood flow, and normal pH enhances effect of bronchodilators*

*Administer sodium bicarbonate as ordered *to prevent or correct acidosis*
Maintain IV infusion *for administration of emergency medications and to prevent dehydration*
Prevent vomiting and subsequent dehydration; initially, child will experience alkalosis, but if vomiting becomes severe or uncontrolled, can lead to acidosis
Implement measures to improve ventilation, *since hypoventilation may cause an accumulation of carbon dioxide, which will decrease pH*

• EXPECTED OUTCOME

Child exhibits no evidence of respiratory acidosis

PATIENT GOAL 2: Will exhibit normal serum electrolytes

• NURSING INTERVENTIONS/*RATIONALES*

Closely monitor serum electrolytes, *since dehydration, as well as medications, can alter normal serum electrolytes*
Maintain IV infusion at appropriate rate
Prevent dehydration and vomiting, *since they cause electrolyte imbalances*

• EXPECTED OUTCOME

Child exhibits normal serum electrolytes

> **NURSING DIAGNOSIS:** Altered family processes related to emergency hospitalization of child

PATIENT/FAMILY GOAL 1: Will experience reduction of anxiety

• NURSING INTERVENTIONS/*RATIONALES*

Keep parents informed of child's condition
Encourage expression of feelings, especially severity of condition and prognosis
Allow parents to be with child as much as possible by encouraging family-centered care concepts
Point out any evidence of improvement *to encourage positive coping behaviors*
If/when possible, schedule treatments and care to child's routines
Reduce sensory stimuli by maintaining quiet, relaxed environment

• EXPECTED OUTCOMES

Family verbalizes concerns and spends time with child
Family exhibits no signs of distress

See also:
   Nursing Care Plan: The Family of the Ill or Hospitalized Child, Chapter 21
   Nursing Care Plan: The Child in the Hospital, Chapter 21

---

*Dependent nursing action.

PFTs) may be performed by specialized personnel or may be the nurse's responsibility.

Children with acute asthma are apprehensive and anxious. The calm, efficient presence of a nurse helps to reassure them that they are safe and will be cared for during this stressful period. It is important to assure children that they will not be left alone and that their parents are allowed to be near and available when they need them.

Parents need reassurance, too. They want to be informed of their child's condition and the therapies being employed. Often they feel that they may have in some way contributed to the child's condition or could have prevented the attack. Reassurance regarding their efforts expended on the child's behalf and their parenting capabilities can help alleviate their stress. All efforts to reduce parental apprehension will, in turn, help reduce the child's distress. Anxiety is easily communicated to the child from parents and members of the staff.

Support Child and Family. The nurse working with children with asthma can provide them with support in a number of ways. Many children voice frustration about the ways their exacerbations interfere with their goal achievements and social lives. They need education about their disease, including what to do to prevent an episode and what to do during one. These children need reassurance from the health team and reinforcement of their coping mechanisms.

> **Nursing ALERT**
> Be aware of children, especially adolescents, who are depressed and may not comply with therapy as a means of passive suicide. Refer these youngsters for psychologic support.

Both short-term and long-term adaptation of affected children to the disease depends greatly on the family's acceptance of the disorder and compliance with therapy. The task of living day-to-day with affected children involves the family continually. There are periodic crises and the ever-present threat of a crisis, requiring parental vigilance, sleepless nights, frequent emergency trips to the hospital, and often overwhelming medical expenses. Throughout these stresses, parents are expected and encouraged to promote as normal a life as possible for their children without neglecting the needs of siblings.

❖ Evaluation

The effectiveness of nursing interventions is determined by continual reassessment and evaluation of care based on the following observational guidelines and expected outcomes:

1. Interview family about removal or avoidance of known allergens.
2. Observe child for evidence of respiratory symptoms.
3. Assess child's general health.
4. Observe child and interview family about any infections or other complications.
5. Interview child about daily activities.
6. Determine the degree to which the family and child understand the child's condition and the extent to which the therapies are carried out.

Expected outcomes:
See Nursing Care Plan, p. 783-785.

CYSTIC FIBROSIS (CF)

CF is inherited as an autosomal recessive trait; the affected child inherits the defective gene from both parents, with an overall incidence of 1:4 (see Appendix B). The mutated gene responsible for CF is located on the long arm of chromosome 7, along with its protein product, *cystic fibrosis transmembrane regulator (CFTR).* Almost 300 alterations that diverge from the original sequence of the gene have been reported; the ΔF508 is the most common alteration, found in about 70% of all known CF chromosomes (Tizzano and Buchwald, 1993).

Pathophysiology

With the discovery of the CFTR gene, research is continuing to determine its multisystemic effects on the body. CF is characterized by several apparently unrelated clinical features: increased viscosity of mucous gland secretions, a striking elevation of sweat electrolytes, an increase in several organic and enzymatic constituents of saliva, and abnormalities in autonomic nervous system function. Although both sodium and chloride are affected, the defect appears to be primarily a result of abnormal chloride movement; the CFTR appears to function as a chloride channel. Further evidence indicates that ΔF508 is closely related to pancreatic insufficiency. The role of CFTR, however, is not definitive.

The primary factor, and the one that is responsible for the multiple clinical manifestations of the disease, is mechanical obstruction caused by the increased viscosity of mucous gland secretions (Fig. 23-5). Instead of forming a thin, freely flowing secretion, the mucous glands produce a thick, inspissated mucoprotein that accumulates and dilates them. Small passages in organs such as the pancreas and bronchioles become obstructed as secretions precipitate or coagulate to form concretions in glands and ducts. The earliest manifestation of CF is *meconium ileus* in the newborn, in which the small intestine is blocked with thick, puttylike, tenacious, mucilaginous meconium.

In the pancreas the thick secretions block the ducts, eventually causing *pancreatic fibrosis.* This blockage prevents essential pancreatic enzymes from reaching the duodenum, which causes marked impairment in the digestion and absorption of nutrients. The disturbed function is reflected in bulky stools that are frothy from undigested fat and foul smelling from putrified protein. The islands of Langerhans may decrease in number as pancreatic fibrosis progresses, and in the liver, localized biliary obstruction and fibrosis are common and become more extensive with time.

The most common gastrointestinal complication associated with CF is *prolapse of the rectum,* which occurs most often in infancy and childhood. Affected children of all ages are subject to intestinal obstruction from inspissated or impacted feces.

Pulmonary complications are present in almost all children with CF and constitute the most serious threat to life. However, the time of appearance is variable. Most children show evidence before 1 year of age; others may not develop symptoms for weeks, months, or years. Bronchial and bronchiolar obstruction by the abnormally thick, tenacious mucus causes patchy atelectasis with hyperinflation. The child is unable to expectorate the mucus because of its increased viscosity. This retained mucus serves as an excellent medium for

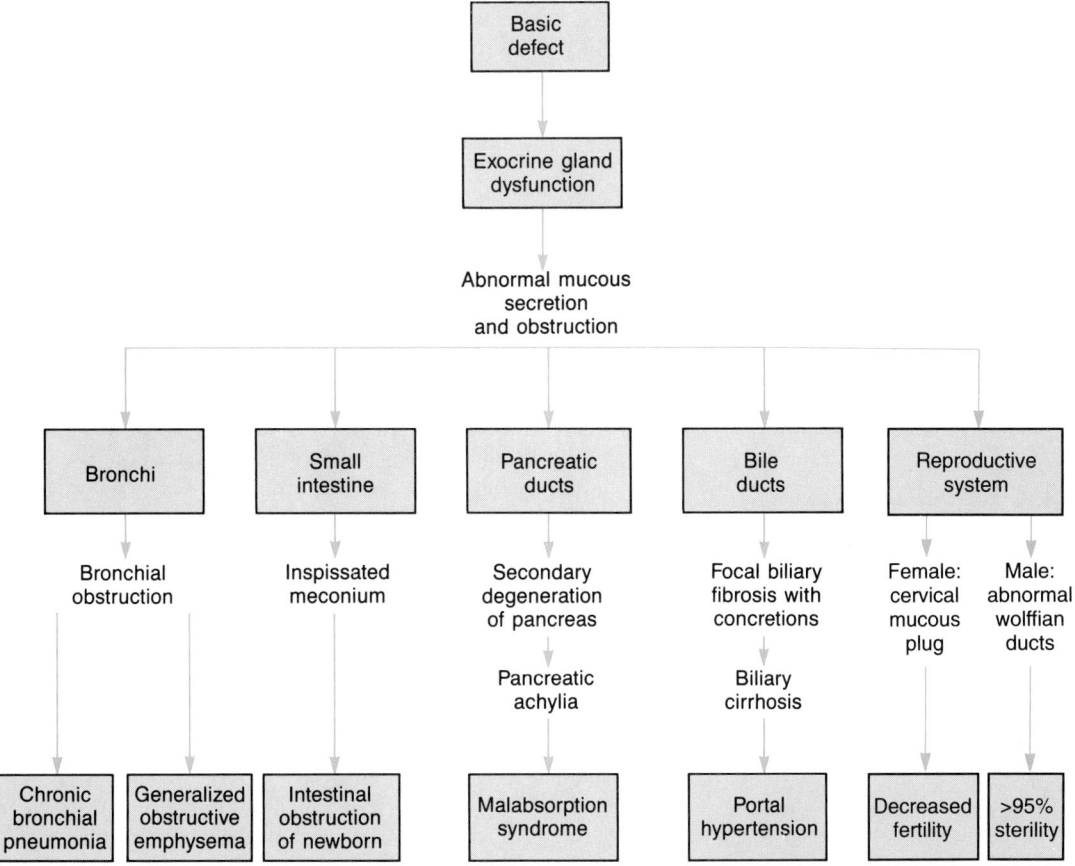

FIG. 23-5. Various effects of exocrine gland dysfunction in cystic fibrosis (CF).

any bacterial growth. Reduced oxygen–carbon dioxide exchange causes variable degrees of hypoxia, hypercapnia, and acidosis.

Diagnostic Evaluation

An initial evaluation is conducted with general appraisal in the areas of general activity, physical findings, nutritional status, and findings on chest radiograms (see box on p. 788 for clinical manifestations). The diagnosis of CF is established on the basis of (1) a history of the disease in the family, (2) absence of pancreatic enzymes, (3) increase in electrolyte concentration of sweat, and (4) chronic pulmonary involvement.

The consistent finding of abnormally high sodium and chloride concentrations in the sweat is a unique characteristic of CF. Parents frequently observe that their infants taste "salty" when they kiss them. For diagnostic purposes the quantitative *sweat chloride test* is performed on sweat obtained by iontophoresis of pilocarpine. Normally the sweat chloride content is less than 40 mEq/L; a chloride concentration greater than 60 mEq/L is diagnostic of CF.

Chest radiography reveals characteristic patchy atelectasis and obstructive emphysema. PFTs are sensitive indexes of lung function, providing evidence of abnormal small airway function in CF. Other diagnostic tools that may aid in diagnosis include stool fat and/or enzyme analysis. Stool analysis requires a 72-hour sample with accurate recording of food

intake during that time. Radiographs, including barium enema, are used for diagnosis of meconium ileus.

Therapeutic Management

The improved survival rate of patients with CF during the past two decades is attributable largely to antibiotic therapy and improved nutritional management. Goals of therapy therefore include the following: (1) to prevent or minimize pulmonary complications, (2) to ensure adequate nutrition for growth, and (3) to assist the child and family in adapting to a chronic disorder. In attempting to attain these, there is a multisystem approach to treatment modalities.

Management of Pulmonary Problems. Management of pulmonary problems is directed toward prevention and treatment of pulmonary infection by improving aeration, removing mucopurulent secretions, and administering antimicrobial agents. Most children will develop respiratory symptoms by 3 years of age. Young children normally have small airways and are predisposed to frequent viral infections. The large amounts and viscosity of respiratory secretions in children with CF contribute to the likelihood of infection. Once infection becomes established in relatively defenseless lungs, it is difficult to eradicate.

Prevention of infection involves a daily routine of CPT to maintain pulmonary hygiene (see Chapter 22). CPT is usually performed twice daily (on rising and in the evening) and

CLINICAL MANIFESTATIONS OF CYSTIC FIBROSIS

Meconium Ileus*

Abdominal distention
Vomiting
Failure to pass stools
Rapid development of dehydration

Gastrointestinal Manifestations

Large, bulky, loose, frothy, extremely foul-smelling stools
Voracious appetite (early in disease)
Loss of appetite (later in disease)
Weight loss
Marked tissue wasting
Failure to grow
Distended abdomen
Thin extremities
Sallow skin
Evidence of deficiency of fat-soluble vitamins A, D, E, K
Anemia

Pulmonary Manifestations

Initial signs:
  Wheezy respirations
  Dry, nonproductive cough
Eventually:
  Increased dyspnea
  Paroxysmal cough
  Evidence of obstructive emphysema and patchy areas of atelectasis
Progressive involvement:
  Overinflated, barrel-shaped chest
  Cyanosis
  Clubbing of fingers and toes
  Repeated episodes of bronchitis and bronchopneumonia

*In about 10% of cases.

more frequently if needed, especially during pulmonary infection. A new device, the *Flutter Mucus Clearance Device,** is a small, hand-held plastic pipe with a stainless-steel ball on the inside that facilitates removal of mucus. It has the advantage of increasing sputum expectoration and being used without an assistant (Davis, 1994).

Bronchodilator medication delivered in an aerosol helps open bronchi for easier expectoration and is administered before CPT when the patient exhibits evidence of reactive airway disease and/or wheezing. Another form of aerosolized medication is *recombinant human deoxyribonuclease* (rhDNase, known generically as dornase alfa [Pulmozyme]), which decreases the viscosity of mucus. It is well tolerated and has no major adverse effects; minor reactions are voice alterations and laryngitis. The drug causes slight improvement in PFTs and perceptions of well-being and dyspnea (Fuchs and others, 1994). However, its high cost may limit its use.

Physical exercise is an important adjunct to daily CPT. Exercise not only stimulates mucus secretion, it also provides a sense of well-being and increased self-esteem. In some instances, exercise can be substituted for CPT. Any aerobic exercise that is enjoyed by the patient should be encouraged.

*Manufactured by Scandipharm, Inc., 22 Inverness Center Parkway, Birmingham, AL 35242; (205) 991-8085.

The ultimate aim of exercise is to establish a good habitual breathing pattern.

Pulmonary infections are treated as soon as they are recognized. Some practitioners prefer to prescribe oral antibiotics prophylactically at the time of diagnosis; others begin therapy when pulmonary symptoms arise. Sputum culture and sensitivity guide the choice of antibiotic.

IV antibiotics are often administered at home as an alternative to hospitalization. Most children have central venous access devices for home administration of IV medications. When pulmonary function does not improve with outpatient management, hospitalization may be recommended for continued antibiotic therapy and vigorous CPT.

Oxygen administration is usually recommended for children with acute episodes, but since many of these children have chronic carbon dioxide retention, the unsupervised use of oxygen can be harmful (see Oxygen Toxicity, Chapter 21).

Pneumothorax is most often caused by rupture of subpleural blebs through the visceral pleura and usually occurs in patients with more advanced disease.

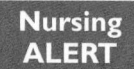 **Nursing ALERT** Signs of a pneumothorax are usually nonspecific and include tachypnea, tachycardia, dyspnea, pallor, and cyanosis.

Management of Gastrointestinal (GI) Problems. The principal treatment for pancreatic insufficiency is replacement pancreatic enzymes, which are administered with meals and snacks to ensure that digestive enzymes are mixed with food in the duodenum. Enteric-coated products prevent the neutralization of enzymes by gastric acids, thus allowing activation to occur in the alkaline environment of the small bowel. The amount of enzymes depends on the severity of the insufficiency, the response of the child to enzyme replacement, and the philosophy of the practitioner. Usually one to five capsules are administered with a meal, and a smaller amount is taken with snacks. Capsules can be swallowed whole or taken apart and the contents sprinkled on a small amount of food to be taken at the beginning of the meal. The amount of enzyme is adjusted to achieve normal growth and a decrease in the number of stools to one or two per day.

Children with CF require a well-balanced, high-protein, high-calorie diet (high calorie because of the impaired intestinal absorption). In fact, they often require up to 150% of the recommended daily allowances to meet their needs for growth. Breast-feeding with enzyme supplementation should be continued whenever possible for parents who prefer this method and, when necessary, supplemented with a higher-calorie-per-ounce formula. For formula-fed infants, commercial cow's milk formulas are usually adequate, although frequently a hydrolysate formula with medium-chain triglycerides (e.g., Pregestimil, Alimentum) may be recommended. Enzymes are mixed into cereal or fruit, such as applesauce. Since the uptake of fat-soluble vitamins is decreased, water-miscible forms of these vitamins (A, D, E, K) are given, along with multivitamins and the enzymes. When high-fat foods are eaten, the child is encouraged to add extra enzymes. Occasionally, patients will be placed on supplemental tube feedings or parenteral alimentation in an effort to build up nutritional reserves if there has been a history of inability to maintain weight.

Prognosis.   Despite more than 40 years of progress and a recent surge in new treatment modalities, CF remains a progressive and incurable disease. The pulmonary involvement ultimately determines the patient's outcome, since pancreatic enzyme deficiency is less of a problem if adequate nutrition is ensured. With advances in technology, parents and adolescents are now being challenged to set future goals that may include college, careers, social relationships, and marriage. Concurrently, they are faced with increasing morbidity and higher rates of CF complications as they grow older.

Screening.   The impact of genetic discoveries on understanding the etiology and treatment of CF is steadily unfolding at the same time that approaches to detection are changing to reflect new technologies. Although the standard method of diagnosis relies on detection of abnormal chloride secretions in sweat, genetic testing is now able to confirm the diagnosis. Carrier screening is available and reliable for siblings and family members of a child with CF.

Nursing Considerations

❖ Assessment

Assessment of the child with CF involves both pulmonary and GI observations. Pulmonary assessment is the same as that described for respiratory infection (see p. 751), with special attention to lung sounds, observation of cough, and evidence or degree of finger clubbing. GI assessment primarily involves observing the frequency and nature of the stools and abdominal distention. The observer is also alert to evidence of failure to thrive (e.g., weight loss, wasting, pallor, fatigue). Family members are interviewed to determine the child's eating and eliminating habits, to observe salty perspiration, and to confirm a history of frequent respiratory infections or bowel obstruction in infancy.

On initial contact, frequently in the hospital setting, nurses are involved in performing or assisting with diagnostic tests, primarily sweat for laboratory analysis of chloride content and, less often, stool specimens for trypsin and fat.

NURSING DIAGNOSES: THE CHILD WITH CYSTIC FIBROSIS (CF)

Ineffective airway clearance related to secretion of thick, tenacious mucus

Impaired gas exchange related to airway obstruction

Ineffective breathing pattern related to tracheobronchial obstruction

Altered nutrition: less than body requirements related to inability to digest nutrients, loss of appetite (advanced disease)

Altered growth and development related to inadequate digestion of nutrients

High risk for infection related to impaired body defenses, presence of mucus as medium for growth of organisms

Activity intolerance related to imbalance between oxygen supply and demand

Altered family processes related to situational crises

Impaired social interaction related to frequent hospitalizations, confinement to home, fatigue

Anticipatory grieving related to perceived potential loss of child

---

❖ Nursing Diagnoses

After a careful assessment numerous nursing diagnoses will become evident. The degree of both pulmonary and GI involvement varies among affected children; therefore nursing diagnoses will also vary according to the individual case (see box for the most common nursing diagnoses).

❖ Planning

The plan of care for the child with CF involves both the child and the family. Major goals include, but are not limited to, the following:

1. Child will demonstrate signs of adequate gas exchange.
2. Child will expectorate mucus.
3. Child will exhibit signs of adequate digestion.
4. Child will experience few or no complications.
5. Child will demonstrate adequate growth and development.
6. Child and family will receive adequate education of the disease and its management.
7. Child and family will receive adequate support.

❖ Implementation

Provide Hospital Care.   When the child is hospitalized for confirmation of the diagnosis or for pulmonary complications, aerosol therapy is instituted or continued. Respiratory therapy is usually initiated and supervised by a trained respiratory therapist or physiotherapist. In institutions with large support staffs, they may provide all treatments. Otherwise, it becomes the responsibility of the nurse to perform the prescribed aerosol therapy and CPT and to teach supervised breathing exercises. CPT should not be performed before or immediately after meals. Planning the activity so that it does not coincide with meals is difficult in the hospital situation. However, it is very important and is often overlooked by nursing personnel.

Oxygen is cautiously administered to children in respiratory distress, and the child requires frequent assessment. The hazard of *oxygen narcosis* is a constant threat in children with longstanding disease who receive oxygen (see Chapter 22). The child requires close observation to assist with cough and expectoration.

The diet is implemented for the newly diagnosed child or continued for the child who is hospitalized for pulmonary disease. Children in the early stages of the disease maintain a good appetite, and some will eat excessively. With infection and increased lung involvement, however, the appetite diminishes. Eventually it becomes a challenge to tempt failing appetites (see Feeding the Sick Child, Chapter 22). Some younger children may object to the extra fluids that are encouraged to prevent dehydration. Food is considered therapy for these patients. The caloric intake should be increased significantly. Pancreatic enzymes are supplied for each meal or snack, and adequate salt is provided, especially for febrile children.

Frequent skin care is carried out to prevent irritation and skin breakdown over bony prominences. Particular attention is necessary after use of the bedpan or when the diaper is changed. Careful cleansing helps to reduce irritation and odor from offensive stools, and the use of moisture barriers protects the skin.

The child will need support for the many treatments and tests that are a necessary part of the hospital therapy. IV fluids and blood tests are almost always a part of the treatment, and the child soon associates hospitalization with these stress-provoking procedures. Because these children are usually quite thin with little muscle mass, careful selection of injection sites is required.

Support to both child and family is a vital part of nursing care. The progressive nature of the disease makes each illness requiring hospitalization a potentially life-threatening event. Skilled nursing care and sympathetic attention to the emotional needs of the child and family help them cope with the stresses associated with repeated respiratory infections and hospitalization.

Prepare for Home Care. After the diagnosis is confirmed and a treatment program determined, preparation for home care is implemented. The plan of care should be flexible enough so that family activities are disrupted as infrequently as possible. Parents will need help in finding inhalation equipment available for home use that best meets their needs. They will need opportunities to learn about the practice the use of the equipment, as well as some of the problems they may encounter.

They need to learn about the preferred diet of nutritious meals with tolerated fat and ample protein and carbohydrate and the administration of pancreatic enzymes. Children usually adjust well to taking pancreatic enzymes. For infants and young children, the enzymes can be mixed with pureed fruit, such as applesauce, and fed with a spoon. Capsules are suitable for older children. It is important to stress to parents that the enzymes, in the amount regulated to the child's needs, should be administered about 30 minutes before all meals and snacks. They are cautioned about not restricting salt, especially during hot weather, and ensuring an adequate fluid intake, since dehydration aggravates the thick mucus secretions. Oral hygiene is important because of interference with salivation and the increased susceptibility to oral infections.

One of the most important aspects of educating parents for home care is teaching CPT and breathing exercises. The success of a therapy program depends on conscientious performance of these treatments regularly as prescribed. The number of times these therapies are performed each day is determined on an individual basis, and often parents readily learn to adjust the number and intensity of the treatments to the child's needs. When additional respiratory exercises are introduced to established routines, the family will need to be reeducated in new techniques, such as "huffing."

Postural drainage can be achieved with simple activities that are fun, such as hanging by the knees from a bar or low-hanging trapeze that can be easily built in the backyard (or indoors), turning somersaults, or playing "wheelbarrow" with the child suspended head down and propelling with the hands while the adult holds on to the feet. Most children respond to a challenge, such as "How long can you stand on your head?" Small children can "stand on their heads" with their heads on the cushion of a large chair with or without an adult holding on to their feet. Parents soon learn to respond to cues from their children and incorporate spontaneous activities into the treatment regimen.

The nurse can assist the family in contacting resources that provide help to families with affected children. The various special child health services, many local clinics, private agencies, service clubs, and other community groups often offer equipment and medications either free or at reduced rates. The **Cystic Fibrosis Foundation*** has chapters throughout the United States to provide education and services to families and professionals.

Support Family. One of the most important and difficult aspects of providing care for the family of a child with CF is coping with the emotional needs of the child and family. The diagnosis, treatment, and prognosis are fraught with many problems, frustrations, and feelings. The diagnosis with all its implications evokes feelings of guilt and self-recrimination in parents. These feelings may be particularly marked if the newly diagnosed child is the second affected child in the family, and the parents had been counseled about the 1:4 risk of such an event occurring.

The long-range problems are those encountered in the care of a child with a chronic illness (see Chapter 18). Both the child and the family must make many adjustments, the success of which depends on their ability to cope and also on the quality and quantity of support they receive from outside sources. Combined efforts of a variety of health professionals offer the most comprehensive services to families. It is often the responsibility of the nurse to organize and coordinate these services, to assess the home situation, and to collect the data needed to evaluate the effectiveness of the services in meeting the family's needs.

The persistent need for treatment several times daily also places a strain on the family. Someone must perform the procedures, such as percussion and vibration, even on older children who are able to assume responsibility for their own exercises and respiratory therapy. Children often balk at the treatments, and the parents are placed in the position of insisting on compliance. Sometimes the stress and anxiety related to this continual routine generate feelings of resentment, which are frequently focused on one aspect of the regimen, such as the diet or equipment. When possible, occasional trusted respite care should be made available to the parent or parents to allow them the opportunity to leave the situation for short periods without undue anxiety about the child's welfare.

The affected child also may become resentful about the disease, its relentless routine of therapy, and the necessary curtailment it places on activities and relationships. The child's activities are interrupted or built around treatment, medications, and diet that impose hardships (e.g., carrying medication to school and other places where the child may eat away from home), and the growth retardation associated with most chronic illnesses may be trying. Any of these aspects of the disease may be the cause of ridicule from other children. However, the child should be encouraged to attend school and join age-appropriate groups, such as scouting, to foster a life that is as normal and productive as possible.

---

*6931 Arlington Rd., Bethesda, MD 20814-3205; (800) FIGHT CF or (301) 951-4422. In Canada: **Canadian Cystic Fibrosis Foundation,** 586 Eglinton Ave., E., Suite 204, Toronto, Ontario M4P 1P2. Two excellent publications available from the Cystic Fibrosis Foundation are *What Everyone Should Know About Cystic Fibrosis* and *Cystic Fibrosis: A Summary of Symptoms, Diagnosis, and Treatment.* For information about specialized medications, especially Pulmozyne, and equipment for CF and other pulmonary diseases, contact **Cystic Fibrosis Pharmacy, Inc.,** H.H.C.S. Pharmacy Services, 633 E. Colonial Drive, Orlando, FL 32803; (800) 741-4427.

Families affected by CF have psychologic hurdles similar to those of all families coping with a child with a chronic illness, and a constant source of anxiety for both parents and child is the ever-present fear of death.

As the disease progresses, however, family stress should be expected, and the patient may become angry and noncompliant. It is important for the nurse to recognize the changing needs of the family. Families should be made aware of sources for counseling as stressful setbacks occur. Patients need to be guided into activities that enable them to express anger, sorrow, and fear without guilt.

As life expectancy continues to rise for children with CF, issues related to marriage, childbearing, and career choice become more pressing. Men must be informed at some point that they will be unable to produce offspring. It is important that the distinction be made between sterility and impotence. Normal sexual relationships can be expected. Female patients may be able to bear children but must be made aware of the possible deleterious effects on the respiratory system created by the burden of pregnancy. They need to know that their children will be carriers of the CF gene.

Life as an independent adult, the goal that most families have for their children, should be encouraged for children with CF. From the time that children can take partial responsibility for their own care (e.g., CPT and taking enzymes), independence and accountability should be fostered. Although the prognosis for these children has improved, many do not survive through the second decade of life. Anticipatory grieving and other aspects related to care of a child with a terminal illness are part of nursing care (see Chapter 18 and Family Focus box).

❖ Evaluation

Evaluation of the efficacy of nursing management can be determined by application of observational guidelines, which might include the following:

1. Monitor vital signs, especially respiratory parameters.
2. Monitor CPT and other procedures to assess the expected outcomes (e.g., expectoration of secretions, increased lung expansion).

FAMILY FOCUS
Children with Cystic Fibrosis (CF)

When I walk by Jeff's room, I still look in to see him, even though I know he will not be there. I took care of Jeff for 3 years, and during that time we became very close. He died of CF at 19 years of age. During his short life he did not have a normal childhood and he had no future, but he was very sensitive to people and their feelings. In addition to having CF, Jeff also had growth hormone deficiency; he had the body of a child and the mind of a young man. I miss Jeff, but I know that he can now breathe easier and is free of his disease.

Children with CF come from all walks of life. As nurses, we must recognize this fact and treat them as normally as the situation allows, never imposing our values on them. Let them know they are loved; their bodies may be affected, but their minds are not.

Imagene Smith, RN
The Children's Hospital at Saint Francis
Tulsa, OK

---

3. Monitor meals to ensure that enzymes are taken.
4. Monitor child for evidence of respiratory infection, GI dysfunction, and other complications.
5. Observe nutritional intake. For the child at home, interview the family regarding child's intake or have child maintain a log of nutritional intake. Obtain regular measurements of growth, and interview child and family regarding school attendance, interaction with peers, and participation in sports and other activities.
6. Explore family's understanding of the disease and its therapies and their ability to carry out the treatment plan.
7. Maintain contact with family (if feasible) at follow-up evaluations and during home care. Observe for readmissions. Interview child and family regarding involvement with agencies and services for children with CF.

Expected outcomes:

1. Child breathes easily and without dyspnea.
2. Child manages secretions with minimum distress.
3. Child takes pancreatic enzymes as prescribed.
4. Child displays no evidence of an infective process.
5. Child is well nourished, exhibits a satisfactory weight gain, and engages in appropriate activities.
6. Child and family demonstrate an understanding of the disease and comply with the therapeutic regimen (specify knowledge and method of demonstration).
7. Family maintains contact with health care providers.

See also Nursing Care Plan: The Child with Cystic Fibrosis.*

RESPIRATORY EMERGENCY

Nurses must be prepared to deal effectively with respiratory emergencies. Although the interventions are similar to those used for adults, there are some variations for infants and children.

RESPIRATORY FAILURE

In general, the term *respiratory insufficiency* is applied to two conditions: (1) children with increased work of breathing but with gas exchange function near normal (ventilatory insufficiency) and (2) children who are unable to maintain normal blood gases and develop hypoxemia and acidosis as a result of carbon dioxide retention.

Respiratory failure is defined as the inability of the respiratory apparatus to maintain adequate oxygenation of the blood, with or without carbon dioxide retention. *Respiratory arrest* is the cessation of respiration. *Apnea* is the absence of airflow (breathing).

Effective pulmonary gas exchange requires clear airways, normal lungs and chest wall, and adequate pulmonary circulation. Anything that affects these functions or their relationships can compromise respiration.

Diagnostic Evaluation

Respiratory failure that occurs as a result of acute obstruction of a major airway or cardiac arrest is sudden and readily apparent. Gradual or progressive deterioration of respiratory function is less easily recognized. Therefore nursing observa-

---

*In Wong DL: *Wong and Whaley's Clinical manual of pediatric nursing,* ed 4, St Louis, 1996, Mosby.

CLINICAL MANIFESTATIONS OF RESPIRATORY FAILURE

Cardinal Signs

Restlessness
Tachypnea
Tachycardia
Diaphoresis

Early but Less Obvious Signs

Mood changes, such as euphoria or depression
Headache
Altered depth and pattern of respirations
Hypertension
Exertional dyspnea
Anorexia
Increased cardiac output and renal output
Central nervous system symptoms (decreased efficiency, impaired judgment, anxiety, confusion, restlessness, irritability)
Flaring nares
Chest wall retractions
Expiratory grunt
Wheezing and/or prolonged expiration

Signs of More Severe Hypoxia

Hypotension or hypertension
Dimness of vision
Somnolence
Stupor
Coma
Dyspnea
Depressed respirations
Bradycardia
Cyanosis, peripheral or central

THINKING CRITICALLY ABOUT ... Parental Presence During CPR

Few acute care facilities allow parents to stay during CPR or a "code." Health professionals' reasons for this decision include believing the experience is too upsetting for the family, fearing the family will need care that will interfere with the staff's resuscitation efforts, experiencing discomfort being "watched" by the family, and fearing increased legal liability if the family knows what has been done or not done.

In reality, when parents do observe their child's CPR, these reasons are not supported. One study found that parents who were given the choice of staying during the code unanimously stated that they would choose this option again. Parents did not interfere with the resuscitation, they were assured that everything was done for their child, and they considered being present one of the most important memories of this difficult experience (Villarreal, 1992).

Of family members who stayed during CPR of an adult patient, 76% said their adjustment to death was easier and 64% thought their presence was beneficial to the dying person; 71% of staff members endorsed the policy (Hanson and Strawser, 1992). Also, the Emergency Nurses Association (1994) supports the option of family presence during invasive procedures and/or resuscitation efforts.

Based on these findings, we need to question the wisdom of excluding parents during CPR. All may not choose to be present, but shouldn't they be given the opportunity? Whose benefit is served by family exclusion? If the main reason is the staff's own fears and anxieties about being observed and possibly judged on their performance, is depriving the family of their wishes justified? Consider out-of-hospital arrests; emergency medical services personnel routinely perform CPR with family and strangers watching. Why is this public rescue attempt considered acceptable but an inhospital code considered a private event?

tion and judgment are vital to the recognition and early management of respiratory failure. Nurses must be able to assess a situation and initiate appropriate action within moments. Signs of respiratory failure are listed in the box.

Therapeutic Management

The interventions used in the management of respiratory failure are frequently dramatic, requiring special skills, and are often emergency procedures. Some of the techniques employed to assist ventilation include artificial ventilation, artificial airway, and cardiopulmonary resuscitation (CPR).

Artificial Ventilation.   There are a variety of methods for controlling or assisting ventilation. Temporary assistance can be provided by a manual self-inflating ventilation bag with a mask and nonreturnable valve to prevent rebreathing. With the mask placed over the child's nose and mouth (an open airway is established by correct positioning with the chin forward and the neck extended to the "sniffing" position), the bag is rhythmically compressed, forcing the gas from the bag into the child's lungs.

For more prolonged assistance, mechanical ventilation is employed to replace the bellows function of the diaphragm and thoracic wall muscles. The lungs are inflated by the application of either positive or negative pressure. The positive-pressure machine inflates the lung by increasing airway pressure above atmospheric pressure, and a negative-pressure ventilator creates a subatmospheric pressure around the chest wall, whereas airway pressure remains atmospheric. Application of positive pressure by mechanical means usually im-

proves the distribution of gas within the lung and often reinflates partially collapsed lung segments. The overall effect is the improvement of gas exchange.

Nursing Considerations

For those families whose child has a respiratory arrest, support focuses on keeping the family informed of the child's status and helping them cope with a near-death experience or an actual death (see Chapter 18). Knowing that their child requires CPR is a frightening and often overwhelming experience for parents. Uncertainty regarding outcome—both mortality and morbidity—is a primary concern. Traditionally, family members are not allowed to be present during resuscitation efforts (see Thinking Critically About . . . box). Nurses can serve as the family's advocate by either being present with them or making sure a support person, such as the clergy, is present. After the child's recovery or death, the family needs continued support and thorough medical information regarding lifesaving measures, the prognosis if the child survives, and the cause of death if the child dies.

CARDIOPULMONARY RESUSCITATION (CPR)

Cardiac arrest in the pediatric population is less often of cardiac origin than from prolonged hypoxemia secondary to inadequate oxygenation, ventilation, and circulation (shock). Some causes include injuries, suffocation (e.g., foreign body aspiration), smoke inhalation, SIDS, or infection. Respiratory arrest has been associated with a better survival than cardiac arrest. Once cardiac arrest occurs, the outcome of resuscitative efforts is poor.

Complete apnea signals the need for rapid and vigorous action to prevent cardiac arrest. In such situations, nurses must be prepared to initiate action immediately. Neurologically intact survival has occurred only in those children who receive immediate resuscitation and respond promptly. In the hospital, emergency equipment should be readily available in patient care centers, and the status of this resuscitation equipment should be checked at least once daily. Regardless of the cause of the arrest, some very basic procedures are carried out, modified somewhat according to the child's size.

Nursing ALERT	Rescuers who have infections that may be transmitted by blood or saliva should not perform mouth-to-mouth resuscitation if the circumstances allow other immediate or effective methods of ventilation.

Outside the hospital situation the first action in an emergency is to assess quickly the extent of any injury and determine whether the child is unconscious. A child who is struggling to breathe but conscious should be transported immediately to an *advanced life support (ALS)* facility, with the child maintaining whatever position affords the most comfort. However, attempting to transport a child by automobile wastes valuable time in obtaining help; transport by an *emergency medical service (EMS)* is recommended or preferable. Services in larger communities can institute ALS immediately or en route to a medical facility.

An unconscious child is managed with care to prevent additional trauma if a head or spinal cord injury has been sustained. The circumstances in which the child is found offer some clues to a possible injury. For example, a child who has been thrown from a bicycle or fallen from a tree is more likely to sustain trauma than a child who is discovered in bed. The child should be turned as a unit with firm support provided to the head and neck to prevent rolling, twisting, or tilting backward or forward.

Resuscitation Procedure

For effective CPR the victim is placed on the back on a firm flat surface, employing appropriate precautions (Fig. 23-6). With loss of consciousness the tongue, which is attached to the lower jaw, relaxes and falls back, obstructing the airway. To open the airway, the head is positioned with either the head tilt/chin lift or jaw thrust maneuver. Health professionals should be able to use both maneuvers. *Head tilt* is accomplished by placing one hand on the victim's forehead and applying firm, backward pressure with the palm to tilt the head back. The fingers of the free hand are placed under the bony portion of the lower jaw near the chin to lift and bring the chin forward *(chin lift)*. This supports the jaw and helps tilt the head back (Fig. 23-7, A).

The *jaw thrust* is accomplished by grasping the angles of the victim's lower jaw and lifting with both hands, one on each side, displacing the mandible upward and outward (Fig.

23-7, B). In suspected neck injuries the jaw thrust method should be used while the cervical spine is completely immobilized. After restoration of a patent airway by removal of foreign material and secretions (if indicated), and if the child is not breathing, continuation of the airway is maintained and rescue breathing is initiated. To ventilate the lungs in the infant (birth to 1 year of age), the operator's mouth is placed in such a way that both the mouth and the nostrils are covered (Fig. 23-7, C). Children (over 1 year of age) are ventilated through the mouth while the nostrils are firmly pinched for air-tight contact (Fig. 23-7, D).

The volume of air in an infant's lungs is small and the air passages are considerably smaller, with resistance to flow potentially higher than in adults. Therefore small puffs of air are delivered. Also, when a child requires CPR, consider the size, not just the age, of the child, since the guidelines for infants and for children ages 1 to 8 years may not always apply. For example, young children who can be placed on the rescuer's thigh should receive infant CPR. Since many older children with severe chronic illness or disability remain small in size, pediatric, not adult, CPR may be appropriate.

If air enters freely and the chest rises, the airway is assumed to be clear. Volume must be provided without causing abdominal distention. Gastric distention, which interferes with diaphragmatic excursion, frequently occurs when more volume than necessary is delivered and the breaths are delivered too rapidly.

After the initial two breaths, the pulse is palpated to ascertain the presence of a heartbeat. The carotid is the most central and accessible artery in children over 1 year of age (Fig. 23-7, E). However, the very short and often fat neck of the infant renders the carotid pulse difficult to palpate. Therefore it is preferable to use the brachial pulse in the infant, located on the inner side of the upper arm midway between the elbow and shoulder (Fig. 23-7, F). Absence of a carotid or brachial pulse is considered sufficient indication to begin external cardiac massage.

Chest Compression.   External chest compression consists of serial, rhythmic compressions of the chest to maintain circulation to vital organs until the child achieves spontaneous vital signs or ALS can be provided. *Chest compressions are always interspersed with ventilation of the lungs.* For optimum compressions, it is essential that the child's spine be supported on a firm surface during compressions of the sternum, and sternal pressure must be forceful but not traumatic. For an infant the hard surface can be the rescuer's hand or forearm, with the palm supporting the infant's back. The child's head is positioned for optimum airway opening using the head tilt/chin lift maneuver. It is essential to prevent overextension of the head of small infants, since this tends to close the flexible trachea.

The placement of the fingers for compression in infants is at a point on the lower sternum, one fingerbreadth below the intersection of the sternum and an imaginary line drawn between the nipples (Fig. 23-7, G). Compressions on the child 1 to 8 years of age are applied to the lower sternum two fingerbreadths above the sternal notch (Fig. 23-7, H). Sternal compression to infants is applied with two fingers on the sternum exerting a firm downward thrust; for children, pressure is applied with the heel of one hand. The depth of compression is also adapted to the child's size. The location, rate, and depth for children over 8 years of age are the same as for adults.

CPR is continued at the appropriate ratio of breaths/compressions for age until signs of recovery appear. These are evidenced by palpable peripheral pulses, return of pupils to normal size, the disappearance of mottling and cyanosis, and possibly return of spontaneous respiration.

Medications. Medications are an important adjunct to CRR, especially cardiac arrest, and are used during and after

resuscitation in children. Appropriate fluid therapy is initiated immediately to children in the hospital or by EMS personnel during transport (see Parenteral Fluid Therapy, Chapter 22, and Shock, Chapter 25). A complete supply of emergency medications is kept and maintained in all EMS vehicles and on all hospital units. The supply is checked on a regular basis (usually once on each 8-hour shift). Resuscitation medications are listed in Table 23-3.

	Objectives	ACTIONS		
		Adult (over 8 yr)	Child (1 to 8 yr)	Infant (under 1 yr)
A. AIRWAY	1. Assessment: Determine unresponsiveness.	Tap or gently shake shoulder.		
		Say, "Are you okay?"		Speak loudly.
	2. Get help.	Activate EMS.	Shout for help. If second rescuer available, have person activate EMS.	
	3. Position the victim.	Turn on back as a unit, supporting head and neck if necessary (4-10 seconds).		
	4. Open the airway.	Head-tilt/chin-lift.		
B. BREATHING	5. Assessment: Determine breathlessness.	Maintain open airway. Place ear over mouth, observing chest. Look, listen, feel for breathing (3-5 seconds).*		
	6. Give 2 rescue breaths.	Maintain open airway.		
		Seal mouth to mouth.		Mouth to nose/mouth.
		Give 2 slow breaths. Observe chest rise. Allow lung deflation between breaths.		
		1½ to 2 seconds each	1 to 1½ seconds each	
	7. Option for obstructed airway.	a. Reposition victim's head. Try again to give rescue breaths.		
			b. Activate EMS.	
		c. Give 5 subdiaphragmatic abdominal thrusts (the Heimlich maneuver).		c. Give 5 back blows.
				c. Give 5 chest thrusts.
		d. Tongue-jaw lift and finger sweep.	d. Tongue-jaw lift, but finger sweep only if you see a foreign object.	
		If unsuccessful, repeat a, c, and d until successful.		
C. CIRCULATION	8. Assessment: Determine pulselessness.	Feel for carotid pulse with one hand; maintain head-tilt with the other (5-10 seconds).		Feel for brachial pulse: keep head-tilt.
CPR	Pulse absent: Begin chest compressions: 9. Landmark check.	Run middle finger along bottom edge of rib cage to notch at center (top of sternum).		Imagine a line drawn between the nipples.
	10. Hand position.	Place index finger next to finger on notch:		Place 2-3 fingers on sternum. 1 finger's width below line. Depress ½ -1 in.
		Two hands next to index finger. Depress 1½ -2 in.	Heel of one hand next to index finger. Depress 1-1½ in.	
	11. Compression rate.	80-100 per minute	100 per minute	At least 100 per minute
	12. Compressions to breaths.	2 breaths to every 15 compressions	1 breath to every 5 compressions	
	13. Number of cycles.	4	20 (approximately 1 minute)	
	14. Reassessment.	Feel for carotid pulse.		Feel for brachial pulse.
		If no pulse, resume CPR, starting with compressions.	If alone, activate EMS. If no pulse, resume CPR, starting with compressions.	
	Pulse present; not breathing: Begin rescue breathing.	1 breath every 5 seconds (12 per minute)	1 breath every 3 seconds (20 per minute)	

FIG. 23-6. One-rescuer cardiopulmonary resuscitation (CPR). (Modified from Chandra NC, Hazinski MF, editors: *Textbook of basic life support for healthcare providers,* Dallas, 1994, American Heart Association.)

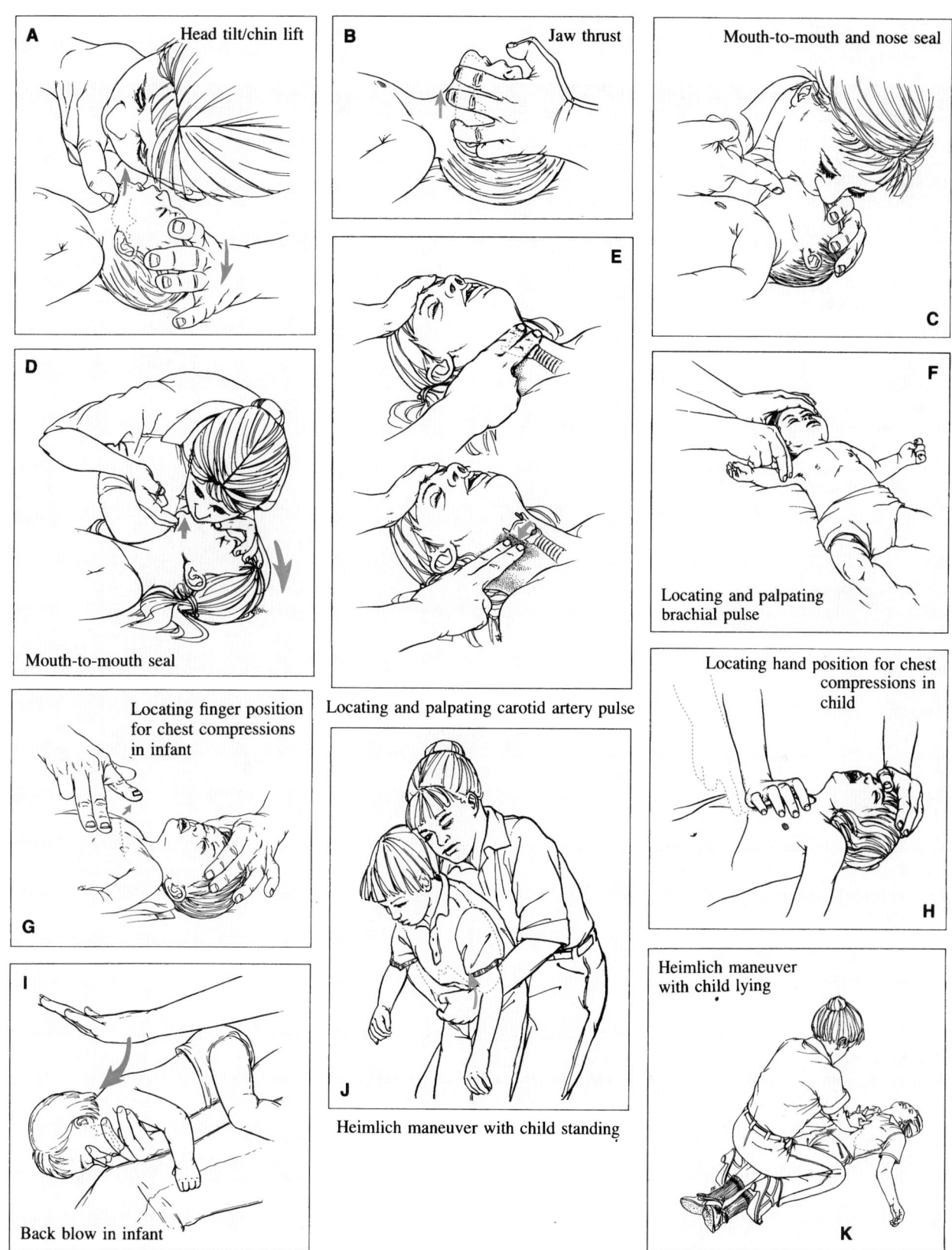

FIG. 23-7. Procedures for CPR, **A** to **H,** and airway obstruction, **I** to **K.** (From Chandra NC, Hazinski MF, editors: *Textbook of basic life support for healthcare providers,* Dallas, 1994, American Heart Association.)

TABLE 23-3. Drugs for pediatric cardiopulmonary resuscitation

DRUG/DOSE	ACTION	IMPLICATIONS
Epinephrine HCl IV/IO: 0.01 mg/kg (1:10,000)* ET: 0.1 mg/kg (1:1000)*	Adrenergic Acts on both alpha- and beta-receptor sites, especially heart and vascular and other smooth muscle	Most useful drug in cardiac arrest Disappears rapidly from bloodstream after injection May produce renal vessel constriction and decreased urine formation
Sodium bicarbonate 1 mEq/kg	Alkalinizer Buffers pH	Infuse slowly and only when ventilation is adequate
Atropine sulfate 0.02 mg/kg/dose Minimum dose: 0.1 mg Maximum single dose: infants and children, 0.5 mg; adolescents, 1.0 mg	Anticholinergic-parasympatholytic Increases cardiac output, heart rate by blocking vagal stimulation in heart	Used to treat bradycardia after ventilatory assessment
Calcium chloride 10% 20 mg/kg	Electrolyte replacement Needed for maintenance of normal cardiac contractility	Used only for hypocalcemia, calcium blocker overdose, hyperkalemia, or hypermagnesemia Administer slowly
Lidocaine HCl 1 mg/kg	Antidysrhythmic Inhibits nerve impulses from sensory nerves	Used for ventricular dysrhythmias only
Bretylium 5 mg/kg; may be increased to 10 mg/kg	Antidysrhythmic Inhibits release of norepinephrine in postganglionic nerve endings that control ventricular tachycardia	Used if lidocaine is not effective Administer rapidly
Adenosine 0.1 to 0.2 mg/kg Maximum single dose: 12 mg	Antidysrhythmic Causes a temporary block through the atrioventricular node and interrupts the reentry circuits	Administer rapidly Very effective Minimal side effects
Infusions *Epinephrine HCl infusion* 0.1-1.0 μg/kg/min	Adrenergic See above	Titrated to desired hemodynamic effect
Dopamine HCl infusion 2-20 μg/kg/min	Agonist Acts on alpha receptors, causing vasoconstriction Increases cardiac output	Titrated to desired hemodynamic response
Dobutamine HCl infusion 2-20 μg/kg/min	Adrenergic direct-acting beta₁ agonist Increases contractility and heart rate	Titrated to desired hemodynamic response Little vasoconstriction, even at high rates
Lidocaine HCl infusion 20-50 μg/kg/min	Antidysrhythmic Increases electrical stimulation threshold of ventricle	See above Lower infusion dose used in shock Used for ventricular tachycardia

*IV, Intravenous route; *IO,* intraosseous route; *ET,* endotracheal route.

Signs of life-threatening obstruction

The truly choking child *cannot speak*, *becomes cyanotic*, and *collapses*				
		Actions		
	Objectives	**Adult (over 8 yr)**	**Child (1 to 8 yr)**	**Infant (under 1 yr)**
CONSCIOUS VICTIM	1. Assessment: Determine airway obstruction.	Ask, "Are you choking?" Determine if victim can cough or speak.		Observe breathing difficulty, ineffective cough, no strong cry.
	2. Act to relieve obstruction.	Perform up to 5 subdiaphragmatic abdominal thrusts (Heimlich maneuver).		Give 5 back blows.
				Give 5 chest thrusts.
	Be persistent.	Repeat Step 2 until obstruction is relieved or victim becomes unconscious.		
VICTIM WHO BECOMES UNCONSCIOUS	3. Position the victim: call for help.	Turn on back as a unit, supporting head and neck, face up, arms by sides. Call out, "Help!" Activate EMS. If second rescuer available, have person activate EMS.		
	4. Check for foreign body.	Perform tongue-jaw lift and finger sweep.	Perform tongue-jaw lift. Remove foreign object only if you actually see it.	
	5. Give rescue breaths.	Open the airway with head-tilt/chin-lift. Try to give rescue breaths. If airway is obstructed, reposition head and try to ventilate again.		
	6. Act to relieve obstruction.	Perform up to 5 subdiaphragmatic abdominal thrusts (Heimlich maneuver).		Give 5 back blows.
				Give 5 chest thrusts.
	7. Be persistent.	Repeat steps 4-6 until obstruction is relieved.		
UNCONSCIOUS VICTIM	1. Assessment: Determine unresponsiveness.	Tap or gently shake shoulder. Shout, "Are you okay?"	Tap or gently shake shoulder.	
		If unresponsive, activate EMS.		
	2. Call for help: position the victim.	Turn on back as a unit, supporting head and neck, face up, arms by sides.		
			Call out for help.	
	3. Open the airway.	Head-tilt/chin-lift.		Head-tilt/chin-lift, but do not tilt too far.
	4. Assessment: Determine breathlessness.	Maintain an open airway. Ear over mouth; observe chest. Look, listen, feel for breathing. (3-5 seconds)		
	5. Give rescue breaths.	Make mouth-to-mouth seal.		Make mouth-to-nose-and-mouth seal.
		Try to give rescue breaths.		
	6. If chest is not rising, try again to give rescue breaths.	Reposition head. Try rescue breaths again.		
	7. Activate the EMS system.		If airway obstruction not relieved after about 1 minute, activate EMS as rapidly as possible.	
	8. Act to relieve obstruction.	Perform up to 5 subdiaphragmatic abdominal thrusts (Heimlich maneuver).		Give 5 back blows.
				Give 5 chest thrusts.
	9. Check for foreign body.	Perform tongue-jaw lift and finger sweep.	Perform tongue-jaw lift. Remove foreign object only if you actually see it.	
	10. Rescue breaths.	Open the airway with head-tilt/chin-lift. Try again to give rescue breaths. If airway is obstructed, reposition head and try to ventilate again.		
	11. Be persistent.	Repeat steps 8-10 until obstruction is relieved.		

FIG. 23-8. Foreign body (FB) airway obstruction management. (Modified from Chandra NC, Hazinski MF, editors: *Textbook of basic life support for healthcare providers*, Dallas, 1994, American Heart Association.)

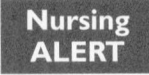 When administering drugs during CPR (or a "code"), use a saline flush between medications to prevent drug interactions. Document all drugs, dosages, and time and route of administration.

AIRWAY OBSTRUCTION

Attempts at clearing the airway should be considered for (1) children in whom FB aspiration is witnessed or strongly suspected and (2) unconscious, nonbreathing children whose airways remain obstructed despite the usual maneuvers to open them. When FB aspiration is strongly suspected, the child is encouraged to continue coughing as long as the cough remains forceful. If the cough becomes ineffective, mechanical maneuvers should be used in an attempt to dislodge the object.

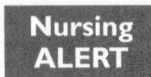 In a conscious choking child, attempt to relieve the obstruction only if:
> The child is unable to make any sounds.
> The cough becomes ineffective.
> There is increasing respiratory difficulty with stridor.

Blind finger sweeps are avoided in both infants and children. A combination of back blows (over the spine between the shoulder blades) and chest thrusts (on sternum, same location as chest compressions) are recommended to relieve FB obstruction in infants (Fig. 23-8).

Infants

A choking infant is placed face down over the rescuer's arm with the head lower than the trunk and the head supported (Fig. 23-7, *I*). For additional support the rescuer should support the arm firmly against the thigh. Up to five quick, sharp, back blows are delivered between the infant's shoulder blades with the heel of the rescuer's hand. Less force is required than would be applied to an adult. After delivery of the back blows, the rescuer's free hand is placed flat on the infant's back so that the infant is "sandwiched" between the two hands, making certain the neck and chin are well supported. While the rescuer maintains support with the infant's head lower than the trunk, the infant is turned and placed supine on the rescuer's thigh, where up to five quick downward chest thrusts are applied in rapid succession in the same location as external chest compressions described for CPR. Back blows and chest thrusts are continued until the object is removed or the infant becomes unconscious.

Children

The *Heimlich maneuver,* a series of *subdiaphragmatic abdominal thrusts,* is recommended for children over 1 year of age. The maneuver creates an artificial cough that forces air, and with it the foreign body, out of the airway. The procedure is carried out with the child in a standing, sitting, or lying position (Fig. 23-7, *J* and *K*). In the conscious choking child, upward thrusts are delivered to the upper abdomen with the fisted hand at a point just below the rib cage (Fig. 23-7, *J*). To prevent damage to the internal organs, the rescuer's hands should not touch the xiphoid process of the sternum or the lower margins of the ribs. Five thrusts are repeated in rapid succession until the foreign body is expelled.

It is neither necessary nor desirable to squeeze or compress the arms during the procedure. It is not a punch or a bear hug. The child may vomit after relief of the obstruction and should be positioned to prevent aspiration. After breathing is restored, the child should receive medical attention and be assessed for complications.

The success of the technique is primarily a result of the obstruction occurring at the end of a maximum respiration. The victim is most likely to choke on food during inspiration; therefore the tidal volume plus expiratory reserve volume is present in the lungs. When pressure is exerted on the diaphragm by the maneuver, the food bolus is ejected with considerable force by this trapped air.

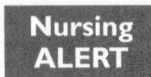 If victim is breathing or resumes effective breathing after emergency interventions, place in recovery position: (1) move head, shoulders, and torso simultaneously; (2) turn onto side; and (3) leg not in contact with ground may be bent and knee moved forward to stabilize victim (Fig. 23-9). Victim should not be moved in any way if trauma is suspected and should not be placed in recovery position if rescue breathing or CPR is required.

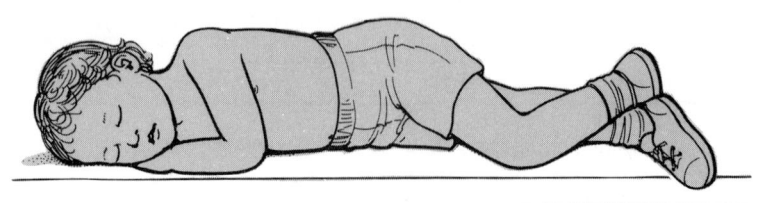

FIG. 23-9. Recovery position for child after respiratory emergency.

KEY POINTS

- Acute infection of the respiratory tract is the most common cause of illness in infancy and childhood.
- The incidence and severity of respiratory tract infections are influenced by the infectious agents involved, the child's age, and the child's natural defenses.
- Common respiratory tract infections of childhood include nasopharyngitis, pharyngitis (including tonsillitis), influenza, and otitis media.
- Croup syndromes involve acute inflammation and variable degrees of obstruction of the epiglottis, larynx, and/or trachea.
- The primary goals in the care of children with croup are observation for signs of respiratory distress and relief of laryngeal obstruction.
- Common infections of the lower airways are bacterial tracheitis, bronchitis, and respiratory syncytial virus (RSV)/bronchiolitis.
- Pneumonias are classified according to site (lobar, bronchial, or interstitial) or by etiologic agent (viruses, bacteria, mycoplasms, or associated with aspiration of foreign material).
- In tuberculosis, susceptibility to the bacillus can be influenced by heredity, age, stress, poor nutrition, and intercurrent infection.
- Passive inhalation of cigarette smoke is one of the primary environmental pollutants contributing to respiratory disease in children.

- Asthma is the leading cause of chronic illness in children.
- General therapeutic management of asthma includes allergen control, drug therapy, controlled exercise, physical therapy, and hyposensitization.
- Support for the family of the child with asthma includes education about the disease and its therapy and facilitation of self-management.
- Cystic fibrosis is the most common inherited disease in children.
- The diagnosis of cystic fibrosis is based on the family history, increased sweat electrolyte content, absent pancreatic enzymes, and chronic pulmonary involvement.
- Choking and respiratory failure are respiratory emergencies that necessitate immediate intervention.
- The Heimlich maneuver is reserved for children in whom foreign body aspiration is witnessed or strongly suspected. A combination of back blows and chest thrusts is used for infants with foreign body aspiration.
- In a conscious choking child, attempts to relieve the obstruction are used *only* if the child is unable to make any sounds; the cough becomes ineffective; or the child has increasing respiratory difficulty with stridor.

REFERENCES

Alho OP and others: Control of the temporal aspect when considering risk factors for acute otitis media, *Arch Otolaryngol Head Neck Surg* 119:444-449, 1993.

American Academy of Pediatrics, Committee on Infectious Diseases: Reassessment of the Indications for ribavirin therapy in respiratory syncytial virus infections, *Pediatrics* 97(1):137-140, 1996a.

American Academy of Pediatrics, Committee on Infectious Diseases: The recommended childhood immunization schedule for 1996, *Pediatrics* 97(1):143, 1996b.

American Academy of Pediatrics, Committee on Infectious Diseases: Update on tuberculin skin testing of children, *Pediatrics* 97(2):282-284, 1996c.

American Academy of Pediatrics, Committee on Substance Abuse: Tobacco-free environment: an imperative for the health of children and adolescents, *Pediatrics* 93(5):866-868, 1994a.

American Academy of Pediatrics, Provisional Committee on Quality Improvement: Practice parameter: the office management of acute exacerbations of asthma in children, *Pediatrics* 93(1):119-126, 1994b.

Colditz GA and others: Efficacy of BCG vaccine in the prevention of tuberculosis, *JAMA* 271(9):698-702, 1994.

Collins F: Cystic fibrosis: molecular biology and therapeutic implications, *Science* 256:774-779, 1992.

Davis PB: Evolution of therapy for cystic fibrosis, *NEJM* 331 (10):672-675, 1994.

Derkay CS, Darrow D, LeFebvre S: Pediatric tonsillectomy and adenoidectomy procedures, *AORN J* 62(6):887-904, 1995.

Duffs A, Platts-Mills T: Allergens and asthma, *Pediatr Clin North Am* 39(6):1277-1291, 1992.

Emergency Nurses Association Position Statement: family presence at the bedside during invasive procedures and/or resuscitation, Park Ridge, IL, 1994, The Association.

FDA OKs new RSV treatment, *Pediatr Alert* 12(2):1, 20, 1996.

Fuchs HJ and others: Effect of aerosolized recombinant human D Nase on exacerbations of respiratory symptoms and on pulmonary function in patients with cystic fibrosis, *NEJM* 331(10):637-642, 1994.

Hanson C, Strawser D: Family presence during cardiopulmonary resuscitation: Foote Hospital emergency department's nine-year perspective, *J Emerg Nurs* 18(2):104-106, 1992.

Hoffman N, Kelly C, Futterman D: Tuberculosis infection in human immunodeficiency virus–positive adolescents and young adults: a New York City cohort, *Pediatrics* 97(2):198-203, 1996.

Holberg CJ, Wright AL, Martinez FD: Child day care, smoking by caregivers, and lower respiratory tract illness in the first 3 years of life, *Pediatrics* 91:885-892, 1993.

Jackson M: Tuberculosis in infants, children and adolescents: new dilemmas with an old disease, *Pediatr Nurs* 19(5):437-442, 1993.

Kleinman LC and others: The medical appropriateness of tympanostomy tubes proposed for children younger than 16 years in the United States, *JAMA* 271(16):1250-1255, 1994.

Klinnert M, Miller B, Mrazek D: Asthma fatalities: who's at risk? *Contemp Pediatr* 7(11):81-98, 1990.

Milgram H, Bender B: Behavioral side effects of medications used to treat asthma and allergic rhinitis, *Pediatr Rev* 16(9):333-335, 1995.

National Heart, Lung, and Blood Institute, National Institutes of Health: *Guidelines for the diagnosis and Management of Asthma*, Pub No 91-3042, Bethesda, MD, 1991, The Institute.

Ott MJ, Horn M, McLaughlin D: Pediatric TB in the 1990s, *MCN Am J Matern Child Nurs* 20(1):16-20, 1995.

Stool SE and others: *Otitis media with effusion in young children: quick Managing Reference guide for clinicians*, AHCPR Pub No 94-0623, Rockville, MD, 1994, Agency for Health Care Policy and Research, Public Health Service, US Department of Health and Human Services.

Thomas PC, Moore P, Reilly JS: Child preferences for post-tonsillectomy diet, *Internat J Pediatr Otorhinolaryngol* 31:29-33, 1995.

Tizzano E, Buchwald M: Recent advances in cystic fibrosis research, *J Pediatr* 122(6):985-988, 1993.

Tully SB, Bar-Haim Y, Bradley RL: Abnormal tympanography after supine bottle feeding, *J Pediatr* 126:S105-S111, 1995.

Villarreal P: Personal communication, University of Texas, San Antonio, 1992.

Wolf SI and others: EMLA cream for painless skin testing: a preliminary report, *Ann Allergy* 73(1):40-42, 1994.

BIBLIOGRAPHY

Respiratory Infection

American Academy of Pediatrics, Committee on Rheumatic Fever, Endocarditis, and Kwashiorkor Disease of the Council on Cardiovascular Disease in the Young, and The American Heart Association: *Pediatrics* 96(4):758-764, 1995.

Buttaro TM, Ezell B, and Gray V: A care plan for children with tuberculosis, *Public Health Nurs* 12(3):181-188, 1995.

Clark G: Childhood tuberculosis cases escalate: disease makes comeback; new strains develop, *AAP News* 10(5):1, 8-9, 11, 1994.

Dajani A and others: Treatment of acute streptococcal pharyngitis and prevention of rheumatic fever: a statement for health professionals, *Pediatrics* 96(4):758-763, 1995.

Feldstein TJ and others: Ribavirin therapy: implementation of hospital guidelines and effect on usage and cost of therapy, *Pediatrics* 96(1):14-17, 1995.

Gaffney K, Dennis J, Carneiro C: Think TB: new focus for family assessment, *Pediatr Nurs* 20(1):37-38, 1994.

Gorelick MH, Baker MD: Epiglottitis in children, 1979 through 1992: effects of *Haemophilus influenzae* type b immunization, *Arch Pediatr Adolesc Med* 148(1):47-50, 1994.

Groothius JR and others: Prophylactic administration of respiratory syncytial virus immune globulin to high-risk infants and young children, *N Engl J Med* 329:1524-1530, 1993.

Hurwitz ES and others: Risk of respiratory illness associated with day-care attendance: a nationwide study, *Pediatrics* 87:62-69, 1991.

Kaiser and others: Effects of antibiotic treatment in the subset of common-cold patients who have bacteria in nasopharyngeal secretions, *Lancet* 347(9014):1507-1510, 1996.

Kitchens GG: Relationship of environmental tobacco smoke to otitis media in young children, *Laryngoscope* 105(5, pt 2, suppl 69):1-13, 1995.

LaVia W and others: Clinical profile of pediatric patients hospitalized with respiratory syncytial virus infection, *Clin Pediatr* 32(8):450-454, 1993.

Petrec CA: Sputum testing for TB: getting good specimens, *AJN* 96(2):14, 1996.

Pichichero ME, Pichichero CL: Persistent acute otitis media. I. Causative pathogens, *Pediatr Infect Dis J* 14(3):178-183, 1995.

Pichichero ME, Pichichero CL: Persistent acute otitis media. II. Antimicrobial treatment, *Pediatr Infect Dis J* 14(3):183-188, 1995.

Prows CA and others: Nature and prevalence of ribavirin aerosol administration in U.S. pediatric hospitals, *J Pediatr Nurs* 8(6):370-375, 1993.

Stamos JK, Rowley AH: Pediatric tuberculosis: an update, *Curr Probl Pediatr* 25(4):131-136, 1995.

Swanson DS, Starke JR: Drug-resistant tuberculosis in pediatrics, *Pediatr Clin North Am* 42(3):553-569, 1995.

Turcios NL: Gauging the severity of bronchiolitis, *J Respir Dis* 15(10):875-888, 1994.

Wolf SI and others: EMLA cream for painless skin testing: a preliminary report, *Ann Allergy* 73(1):40-42, 1994.

Otitis Media

Barnett ED, Klein JO: The problem of resistant bacteria for the management of acute otitis media, *Pediatr Clin North Am* 42(3):509-517, 1995.

Casselbrant M and others: Efficacy of antimicrobial prophylaxis and of tympanostomy tube insertion for prevention of recurrent acute otitis media, *Pediatr Infect Dis J* 11:278-286, 1992.

Duncan B and others: Exclusive breast-feeding for at least 4 months protects against otitis media, *Pediatrics* 91(5):867-872, 1993.

Etzel R and others: Passive smoking and middle ear effusion among children in day care, *Pediatrics* 90(2):228-232, 1992.

Heikkinen T, Ruuskanen O: Signs and symptoms predicting acute otitis media, *Arch Pediatr Adolesc Med* 149(1):26-29, 1995.

Isaacson G, Rosenfeld RM: Care of the child with tympanostomy tubes: a visual guide for the pediatrician, *Pediatrics* 93(6):924-929, 1994.

Mandel E and others: Antibiotic therapy for otitis media with effusion, *JAMA* 269(4):516-517, 1993.

Shurin P and others: Bacterial polysaccharide immune globulin for prophylaxis of acute otitis media in high-risk children, *J Pediatr* 123:801-810, 1993.

Williams R and others: Use of antibiotics in preventing recurrent acute otitis media and in treating otitis media with effusion, *JAMA* 270(11):1344-1351, 1993.

Zeisei SA and others: Prospective surveillance for otitis media with effusion among black infants in group child care, *J Pediatr* 127:875-880, 1995.

Noninfectious Irritants

Bakoula CG and others: Objective passive-smoking indicators and respiratory morbidity in young children, *Lancet* 346(8970):280-281, 1995.

Eliopoulos C and others: Hair concentrations of nicotine and cotinine in women and their newborn infants, *JAMA* 271:621-623, 1994.

Espeland K: Identifying the manifestations of inhalant abuse, *Nurse Pract* 20(5):49-50, 53, 1995.

Fitzpatrick JC, Cioffi WG Jr: Inhalation injury, *Trauma Q* 11(2):114-126, 1994.

Huston CJ: Carbon monoxide poisoning, *Am J Nurs* 96(1):48, 1996.

Mitchell A and others: Acute organophosphate pesticide poisoning in children, *MCN Am J Matern Child Nurs* 20(5):261-268, 1995.

Ruddy RM: Smoke inhalation injury, *Pediatr Clin North Am* 41(2):317-336, 1994.

Asthma

Bechler-Karsch A: Assessment and management of status asthmaticus, *Pediatr Nurs* 20(3):217-223, 238-239, 1994.

Buist AS, Vollmer WM: Preventing deaths from asthma, *New Engl J Med* 331(23):1584-1585, 1994 (editorial).

Capen CL and others: The team approach to pediatric asthma education, *Pediatr Nurs* 20(3):231-237, 1994.

Chou KJ, Cunningham SJ, Crain EF: Metered-dose inhalers with spaceres vs nebulizers for pediatric asthma, *Arch Pediatr Adolesc Med* 149(2):201-205, 1995.

Clark NK, Gotsch A, Rosenstock I: Patient, professional and public education on behavioral aspects of asthma: a review of strategies for change and needed research, *J Asthma* 39(4):241-255, 1993.

DiGiullo G and others: Hospital treatment of asthma: lack of benefit from theophylline given in addition to nebulized albuterol and intravenously administered corticosteroid, *J Pediatr* 122(3):464-466, 1993.

Ferrante S, Painter E: Continuous nebulization: a treatment modality for pediatric asthma patients, *Pediatr Nurs* 21(4):327-331, 1995.

Fitzpatrick MF and others: Effect of therapeutic theophylline levels on the sleep quality and daytime cognitive performance of normal subjects, *Am Rev Respir Dis* 145:1355-1358, 1992.

Handling the severe asthma attack: inhalers versus nebulizers, *Emerg Med* 25(13):49-51, 1993.

Karsch AB: Assessment and management of status asthmaticus, *Pediatr Nurs* 20(3):217-223, 1994.

Larter N, Kieckhefer G: Asthma. In Jackson P, Vessey J: *Primary care of the child with a chronic condition*, ed 2, St Louis, 1996, Mosby.

Morray B, Redding G: Factors associated with prolonged hospitalization of children with asthma, *Arch Pediatr Adolesc Med* 149(3):276-279, 1995.

Murphy S, Kelly W: Asthma, inflammation, and airway hyperresponsiveness in children, *Curr Opin Pediatr* 5:255-265, 1993.

Peter JFM and others: Long-term effect of inhaled corticosteroids on growth rate in adolescents with asthma, *Pediatrics* 91(3):1121-1126, 1993.

Rachelefsy G and others: An update on the diagnosis and management of pediatric asthma: based on the National Heart, Lung, and Blood Institute Expert Panel report, *Nurse Practitioner* 18(2):51-52+, 1993.

Ryan-Wenger N, Walsh M: Children's perspectives on coping with asthma, *Pediatr Nurs* 20(3):224-228, 1994.

Strauss RE and others: Aminophylline therapy does not improve outcome and increases adverse effects in children hospitalized with acute asthmatic exacerbations, *Pediatrics* 93(2):205-206, 1994.

Wenger NMR, Walsh M: Children's perspectives on coping with asthma, *Pediatr Nurs* 20(3):224, 1994.

Whatling J: Childhood asthma and passive smoking, *Nurs Standard* 8(46):25-27, 1994.

Cystic Fibrosis

Fulginiti V, Lewy J: Pediatrics: update on cystic fibrosis, *JAMA* 270(2):246-248, 1993.

Geller G: Cystic fibrosis and the pediatric caregiver: benefits and burdens of technology, *Pediatr Nurs* 21(1):57-61, 1995.

Gutteridge C, Kuhn RJ: Pulmozyme—dornase alfa, *Pediatr Nurs* 20(3):278-279, 1994.

Jedlicka-Köhler I, Gotz M, Eichler I: Parents' recollection of the initial communication of the diagnosis of cystic fibrosis, *Pediatrics* 97(2):204-209, 1996.

Loutzenhiser JL, Clark R: Physical activity and exercise in children with cystic fibrosis, *J Pediatr Nurs* 8(2):112-119, 1993.

Maynard LC: Pediatric heart-lung transplant for cystic fibrosis, *Heart Lung* 23(4):279-284, 1994.

McMullen AH: Cystic fibrosis. In Jackson PL, Vessey JA, eds: *Primary care of the child with a chronic condition*, ed 2, St Louis, 1996, Mosby.

Rosenstein BJ: Molecular basis, diagnosis, and treatment of cystic fibrosis, *Pediatr Rounds* 4(2):5-8, 1995.

Sawyer SM and others: The self-image of adolescents with cystic fibrosis, *J Adolesc Health* 16(3):204-208, 1995.

White K, Munro CL, Pickler R: Therapeutic implications of recent advances in cystic fibrosis, *MCN Am J Matern Child Nurs* 20(6):304-308, 1995.

Williams JK: Genetics and cystic fibrosis: a focus on carrier testing, *Pediatr Nurs* 21(5):444-448, 1995.

Respiratory Emergencies

Bledsoe BE: Pediatric respiratory emergencies, *J Emerg Med Serv* 19(2):38-41, 43-49, 1994.

Eichhorn DJ, Meyers TA, Guzzetta CE: Family presence during resuscitation: it is time to open the door, *Crit Care Nurs* 3(1):8-13, 1995.

Kabbani M, Goodwin SR: Traumatic epiglottitis following blind finger sweep to remove a pharyngeal foreign body, *Clin Pediatr* 34(9):495-497, 1995.

Leuthner SR, Jansen RD, Hageman JR: Cardiopulmonary resuscitation of the newborn, *Pediatr Clin North Am* 41(5):893-907, 1994.

Malinowski C: Neonatal resuscitation program and pediatric advanced life support, *Respir Care* 40(5):575-587, 1995.

Paediatric Life Support Working Party of the European Resuscitation Council: Guidelines for paediatric life support, *Br Med J* 308:1349-1355, 1994.

Poole Sr, Chetham M, Anderson M: Grunting respirations in infants and children, *Pediatr Emerg Care* 11(3):158-161, 1995.

Sarnaik AP, Lieh-Lai M: Adult respiratory distress syndrome in children, *Pediatr Clin North Am* 41(2):337-363, 1994.

Schroeder LL, Knapp JF: Recognition and emergency management of infectious causes of upper airway obstruction in children, *Semin Respir Infect* 10(1):21-30, 1995.

Walsh E, Ioli J: Childhood near-drowning: nursing care and primary prevention, *Pediatr Nurs* 20(3):265-269, 1994.

THE CHILD WITH GASTROINTESTINAL DYSFUNCTION

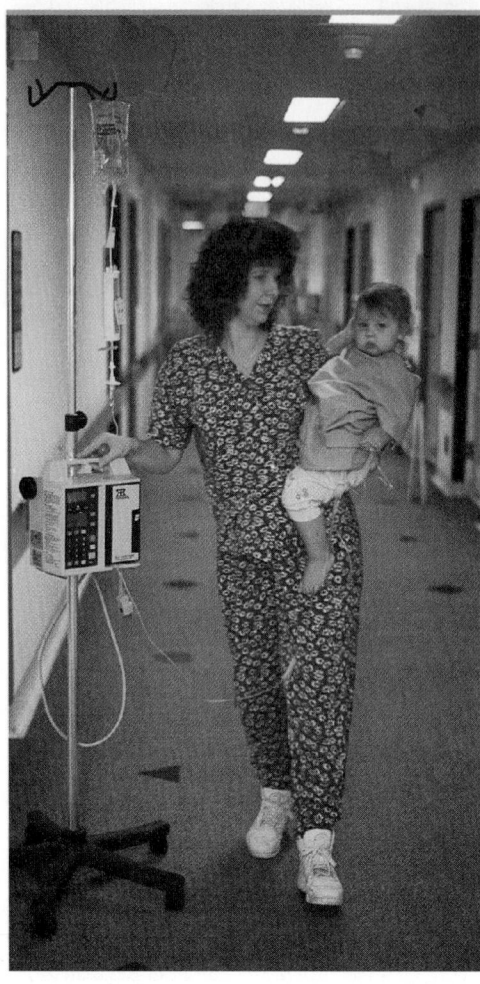

Chelsea, age 23 months, ascending cholangitis

RELATED TOPICS

GASTROINTESTINAL (GI) DYSFUNCTION

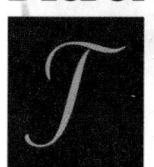

The extensive surface area of the GI tract and its digestive function represent the major means of exchange between the human organism and the environment. Inflammatory and malabsorptive disorders impair the functional integrity of the GI tract. In addition, since the immune system and mucosal barrier continue to mature after birth, the intestine of infants is extremely vulnerable to infection. Acute infectious diarrhea can cause significant alterations in fluid and electrolyte balance in infants and children.

Numerous general observations provide possible clues to specific GI problems (see box on p. 804). In any disorder that involves GI losses, particularly large amounts of fluid, dehydration poses a serious threat to life and demands immediate attention.

DEHYDRATION

Dehydration is a common body fluid disturbance in infants and children and occurs whenever the total output of fluid exceeds the total intake, regardless of the underlying cause. Dehydration may result from a number of diseases that cause insensible losses through the skin and respiratory tract, through increased renal excretion, and through the GI tract. Although dehydration can result from lack of oral intake (especially in elevated environmental temperatures), more often it is a result of abnormal losses, such as those that occur in vomiting or diarrhea, when oral intake only partially compensates for the abnormal losses. Other significant causes of dehydration are diabetic ketoacidosis and extensive burns.

Water Balance in Infants *more fat storage*

Because of several characteristics, infants and young children have a greater need for water and are more vulnerable to alterations in fluid and electrolyte balance. Compared with older children and adults, they have a greater fluid intake and output relative to size. Water and electrolyte disturbances occur more frequently and more rapidly, and children adjust less promptly to these alterations.

The fluid compartments in the infant vary significantly from those in the adult, primarily because of an expanded extracellular compartment. The *extracellular fluid (ECF)* compartment constitutes more than half the total body water at birth and has a greater relative content of extracellular sodium and chloride. The infant loses a large amount of fluid at birth and still maintains a larger amount of ECF than the adult until about 2 years of age. This contributes to greater and more rapid water loss during this age period.

Fluid losses create compartment deficits that reflect the duration of dehydration. In general, approximately 60% of fluid is lost from the ECF, and the remaining 40% comes from the *intracellular fluid (ICF)*. The amount of fluid lost from the ECF increases with acute illness and decreases with chronic loss.

Fluid losses may be divided into insensible, urinary, and fecal losses and vary with the patient's age. Approximately two thirds of insensible losses occur through the skin, and the remaining one third is lost through the respiratory tract. Insensible fluid loss is influenced by heat and humidity, body temperature, and respiratory rate. Infants and children have a much greater tendency to become highly febrile than do adults. Fever increases insensible water loss by approximately 7 ml/kg/24 hours for each degree rise in temperature above 99° F. Fever and increased surface area relative to volume are factors that contribute to greater insensible fluid losses in young patients.

Surface Area. The infant's relatively greater body surface area (BSA) allows larger quantities of fluid to be lost in insensible perspiration through the skin. It is estimated that the BSA of the premature neonate is five times as great, and that of the newborn is two to three times as great, as that of the older child or adult. The proportionately longer GI tract in infancy is also a source of relatively greater fluid loss, especially from diarrhea.

Metabolic Rate. The rate of metabolism in infancy is significantly higher than in adulthood because of the larger BSA in relation to the mass of active tissue. Consequently, there is a greater production of metabolic wastes that must be excreted by the kidneys. Any condition that increases metabolism causes greater heat production, with its concomitant insensible fluid loss and an increased need for water for excretion. The basal metabolic rate (BMR) in infants and children is higher to support growth.

Kidney Function. The kidneys of the infant are functionally immature at birth and are therefore inefficient in ex-

Lynn Mattis, MSN, RN, and Pamela DiVito-Thomas, MS, RN, revised this chapter.

CLINICAL MANIFESTATIONS OF GASTROINTESTINAL (GI) DYSFUNCTION IN CHILDREN

Failure to thrive—deceleration from established growth pattern or consistently below the 5th percentile for height and weight on standard growth charts; sometimes accompanied by developmental delays

Spitting up or regurgitation—passive transfer of gastric contents into the esophagus or mouth

Vomiting—forceful ejection of gastric contents; involves a complex process under central nervous system control that causes salivation, pallor, sweating, and tachycardia; usually accompanied by nausea

Projectile vomiting—vomiting accompanied by vigorous peristaltic waves and typically associated with pyloric stenosis or pylorospasm

Nausea—unpleasant sensation vaguely referred to the throat or abdomen with an inclination to vomit

Constipation—passage of firm or hard stools or infrequent passage of stool with associated symptoms such as difficulty expelling the stools, blood-streaked stools, and abdominal discomfort

Encopresis—overflow of incontinent stool causing soiling; often caused by fecal retention or impaction

Diarrhea—increase in the number of stools with an increased water content as a result of alterations of water and electrolyte transport by the GI tract; may be acute or chronic

Hypoactive, hyperactive, or absent bowel sounds—evidence of intestinal motility problems that may be caused by inflammation or obstruction

Abdominal distention—protuberant contour of the abdomen that may be caused by delayed gastric emptying, accumulation of gas or stool, inflammation, or obstruction

Abdominal pain—pain associated with the abdomen that may be localized or diffuse, acute or chronic; often caused by inflammation, obstruction, or hemorrhage

Gastrointestinal bleeding—may be from an upper or lower GI source and may be acute or chronic

Hematemesis—vomiting of bright-red blood or denatured blood that results from bleeding in the upper GI tract or from swallowed blood from the nose or oropharynx

Hematochezia—passage of bright-red blood per rectum, usually indicating lower GI tract bleeding

Melena—passage of dark-colored, "tarry" stools due to denatured blood, suggesting upper GI tract bleeding or bleeding from the right colon

Jaundice—yellow coloration of the skin and sclerae associated with liver dysfunction

Dysphagia—difficulty swallowing caused by abnormalities in the neuromuscular function of the pharynx or upper esophageal sphincter or by disorders of the esophagus

Dysfunctional swallowing—impaired swallowing caused by central nervous system defects or structural defects of the oral cavity, pharynx, or esophagus; can cause feeding problems or aspiration

Fever—common manifestation of illness in children with GI disorders; usually associated with dehydration, infection, or inflammation

DAILY MAINTENANCE FLUID REQUIREMENTS

1. Calculate weight of child in kilograms:

$$\frac{\text{Weight of child (in pounds)}}{2.2 \text{ lb/kg}} = \text{Weight in kilograms}$$

2. Allow 100 ml per kilogram for first 10 kg.
3. Allow 50 ml per kilogram for second 10 kg.
4. Allow 20 ml per kilogram for remainder of weight in kilograms.
5. Divide total amount by 24 hours to obtain rate in milliliters per hour.

Fluid Requirements. As a result of these characteristics, infants ingest and excrete a greater amount of fluid per kilogram of body weight than do older children. Since electrolytes are excreted with water and the infant has limited ability for conservation, maintenance requirements include both water and electrolytes. The daily exchange of ECF in the infant is greatly increased over that of older children, which leaves the infant little fluid volume reserve in dehydrated states. Fluid requirements depend on hydration status, size, environmental factors, and underlying disease. Daily maintenance fluid requirements are outlined in the box.

Types of Dehydration

The pathophysiology of dehydration can best be understood by recognizing that the distribution of water between the ECF and ICF spaces depends on active transport of potassium into and sodium out of cells by energy-requiring processes. Sodium is the chief solute in ECF and thus is the primary determinant of ECF volume. Potassium is primarily intracellular. When ECF volume is reduced in acute dehydration, the total body sodium content is almost always reduced as well, regardless of serum sodium measurements. Replacement of fluid volume should therefore be accompanied by sodium repletion. Sodium depletion in diarrhea occurs in two ways: out of the body in stool and into the ICF compartment to replace potassium in order to maintain electrical equilibrium.

Dehydration is classified into three categories on the basis of osmolality and depends primarily on the serum sodium concentration: (1) isotonic, (2) hypotonic, and (3) hypertonic. *most common*

Isotonic (isosmotic or *isonatremic) dehydration,* the most common form, occurs in conditions in which the electrolyte and water deficits are present in approximately balanced proportion; that is, salt and water are lost in equal amounts. Shock is the greatest threat to life in isotonic dehydration, and the child displays the symptoms characteristic of hypovolemic shock. Serum sodium remains within normal limits, between 130 and 150 mEq/L.

Hypotonic (hyposmotic or *hyponatremic) dehydration* occurs when the electrolyte deficit exceeds the water deficit, leaving the serum hypotonic. Since ICF is more concentrated than ECF in hypotonic dehydration, water moves from the ECF to the ICF to establish osmotic equilibrium. Therefore this further increases the ECF volume loss, and shock is a frequent finding. Since there is a greater proportional loss of

creting waste products of metabolism. Of particular importance for fluid balance is the inability of the infant's kidneys to concentrate or dilute urine, to conserve or excrete sodium, and to acidify urine. Therefore the infant is less able to handle large quantities of solute-free water than is the older child and is more apt to become dehydrated when given concentrated formulas or overhydrated when given excessive water or dilute formula.

ECF in hypotonic dehydration, the physical signs tend to be more severe with smaller fluid losses than with isotonic or hypertonic dehydration. Serum sodium concentration is less than 130 mEq/L.

Hypertonic (hyperosmotic or *hypernatremic) dehydration* results from water loss in excess of electrolyte loss and is usually caused by a proportionately larger loss of water and/or a larger intake of electrolytes. This sometimes occurs in infants with diarrhea who are given fluids by mouth that contain large amounts of solute, such as those receiving high-protein nasogastric tube feedings. In hypertonic dehydration, fluid shifts from the lesser concentration of the ICF to the ECF. Serum sodium concentration is greater than 150 mEq/L. Since the ECF volume is proportionately larger, hypertonic dehydration has a larger degree of water loss for the same intensity of physical signs. Shock is less apparent in hypertonic dehydration. However, neurologic disturbances, such as seizures, are more likely to occur. Cerebral changes are serious and may result in permanent damage.

Diagnostic Evaluation

Diagnosis of the type and degree of dehydration is made on the basis of clinical manifestations (Table 24-1). In infants, isotonic dehydration is usually described as 5% (mild), 10%

(moderate), or 15% (severe). A more accurate means of describing dehydration is to reflect acute loss (over 48 hours or less) in milliliters per kilogram of body weight (Finberg, 1990). Older children and adolescents, with proportionately less total body water, display smaller proportional losses; therefore the estimates of 3%, 6%, and 9% more nearly describe mild, moderate, and severe dehydration, respectively, in these age-groups (Table 24-2).

Shock is a common feature of severe depletion of ECF volume with tachycardia and very low blood pressure (see Shock, Chapter 25). Delayed capillary refill, cold extremities, acidosis, and coma are additional signs of severe dehydration, and in infants the anterior fontanel is depressed.

Therapeutic Management

See discussion on therapeutic management of diarrhea, p. 807.

Nursing Considerations

Nursing observation and intervention are essential to the detection and therapeutic management of dehydration. There are a wide variety of circumstances in which fluid loss may be precipitated, especially in infants, and changes can take place in a very short time. Therefore an important nursing respon-

TABLE 24-1. Clinical manifestations of dehydration

	ISOTONIC (LOSS OF WATER AND SALT)	HYPOTONIC (LOSS OF SALT IN EXCESS OF WATER)	HYPERTONIC (LOSS OF WATER IN EXCESS OF SALT)
Skin			
Color	Gray	Gray	Gray
Temperature	Cold	Cold	Cold or hot
Turgor	Poor	Very poor	Fair
Feel	Dry	Clammy	Thickened, doughy
Mucous membranes	Dry	Slightly moist	Parched
Tearing and salivation	Absent	Absent	Absent
Eyeball	Sunken	Sunken	Sunken
Fontanel	Sunken	Sunken	Sunken
Body temperature	Subnormal or elevated	Subnormal or elevated	Subnormal or elevated
Pulse	Rapid	Very rapid	Moderately rapid
Respirations	Rapid	Rapid	Rapid
Behavior	Irritable to lethargic	Lethargic to comatose; convulsions	Marked lethargy with extreme hyperirritability on stimulation

TABLE 24-2. Intensity of clinical signs associated with varying degrees of isotonic dehydration in infants

	DEGREE OF DEHYDRATION		
	MILD	MODERATE	SEVERE
Fluid volume loss	<50 ml/kg	50-90 ml/kg	≥100 ml/kg
Skin color	Pale	Gray	Mottled *gray marble looking*
Skin elasticity	Decreased	Poor	Very poor
Mucous membranes	Dry	Very dry	Parched
Urine output	Decreased	Oliguria	Marked oliguria and azotemia
Blood pressure	Normal	Normal or lowered	Lowered
Pulse	Normal or increased	Increased	Rapid and thready
Capillary filling time	<2 seconds	2-3 seconds	>3 seconds

more than 3 or 4 sec. - shock

sibility is perceptive observation for any signs of dehydration. Conditions in which changes can develop with surprising rapidity in young children include diarrhea; vomiting; sweating; fever; disorders such as diabetes, renal disease, and cardiac anomalies; administration of certain drugs, such as diuretics and steroids; and trauma, such as major surgery, burns, and other extensive injury.

The nursing assessment of suspected or potential fluid loss begins with the observation of general appearance and then proceeds with specific observations.

Intake and Output. Accurate measurements of fluid intake and output are vital to the assessment of dehydration. This includes oral and parenteral intake and losses from urine, stools, vomiting, fistulas, nasogastric suction, sweat, and wound drainage.

Urine—assess frequency, volume, color, and consistency of urine
Stools—assess frequency, volume, and consistency of stools
Vomitus—assess for volume, frequency, and type of vomitus
Sweating—can be only estimated from frequency of clothing and linen changes

NURSING TIP 1 g wet diaper weight = 1 ml urine

Other Observations. In addition to fluid intake and output, the following observations assist in assessment of dehydration:

Vital signs—temperature (normal, elevated, or lowered depending on degree of dehydration), pulse (tachycardia), respirations (tachypnea), and blood pressure (hypotension)
Skin—assess for color, temperature, turgor, presence or absence of edema, and capillary refill
Mucous membranes—assess for moisture, color, and presence of and consistency of secretions
Body weight—decreased in relation to degree of dehydration
Fontanel (infants)—sunken, soft, normal
Sensory alterations—presence of thirst

For nursing interventions, see discussion under specific disorders.

DISORDERS OF MOTILITY

ACUTE DIARRHEA

Diarrhea is a symptom that can result from disorders involving digestive, absorptive, and secretory functions. There are wide variations in colonic function among different individuals; therefore a precise definition and identification of what constitutes diarrhea pose a problem in terms of number or consistency of stools. For example, one infant may have one firm stool every second or third day, whereas another normally passes from five to eight small, soft stools daily. Important considerations are (1) a noticeable or sudden increase in the number of stools, (2) a change in their consistency with an increase in fluid content, and (3) a tendency for the stools to be greenish in color and contain mucus or blood.

Diarrhea may be acute or chronic, and inflammatory or noninflammatory; the physiologic consequences vary considerably in relation to its severity, duration, associated symptoms, the child's age, and the child's nutritional status be-

fore the onset of diarrhea. Diarrhea related to an inflammatory process is usually described as gastroenteritis, and the terms are often used interchangeably.

Etiology

Diarrhea can be attributed to a large number of specific causes, mechanisms, and predisposing factors. Factors that predispose a child to diarrhea and its physiologic consequences include the following: (1) the younger the child, the greater the susceptibility to diarrhea and the more severe the diarrhea is likely to be; (2) children who are malnourished or debilitated from disease are more susceptible to diarrhea, as are children who have an immune deficiency; and (3) lack of clean water and insufficient understanding of hygiene contribute to contamination, as does crowding and poor sanitation with inadequate facilities for food preparation and refrigeration.

Specific Causes. A variety of factors can produce diarrhea in the infant or child either as the presenting symptom or as an associated symptom. Often a specific etiologic diagnosis is lacking. **Acute diarrhea** is a leading cause of illness in children younger than 5 years of age; the dehydration that it causes is fatal for approximately 400 of these children a year in the United States (Kleinman, 1992). The sudden change in the frequency and consistency of the stools is more often caused by an inflammatory process of infectious origin but may also be the result of a toxic reaction to ingestion of poisons, dietary indiscretions, or infection outside the GI tract (e.g., communicable diseases, infections of the respiratory or urinary tracts, emotional tension). Most are self-limited and will ultimately subside without specific treatment if dehydration does not create a serious complication. Antibiotic therapy is also a common cause of diarrhea in children.

Chronic diarrhea, the passage of loose stools with increased frequency that lasts for more than 2 weeks, is more apt to be associated with disorders of malabsorption, anatomic defects, abnormal bowel motility, hypersensitivity (allergic) reaction, or a long-term inflammatory response.

Diarrheal disturbances can involve the stomach and intestine (**gastroenteritis**), the small intestine (**enteritis**), the colon (**colitis**), or the colon and intestine (**enterocolitis**). **Dysentery**, intestinal inflammation, especially of the colon, is accompanied by cramping abdominal pain and watery stools containing blood and mucus. Infectious organisms are frequent causes of diarrhea in infancy and childhood and are further discussed in relation to gastroenteritis (p. 812).

Common causes of diarrhea are dietary indiscretions (e.g., green apples or other fruits and fruit juices in large amounts), food sensitivities, and concentrated formulas. In some children, apple juice has been repeatedly demonstrated to cause or perpetuate nonspecific diarrhea. Studies indicate that "cloudy" apple juice, which is freshly pressed and unprocessed, is less likely to cause diarrhea than "clear" juice, which is processed (Hoekstra and others, 1995). Also, sorbitol, the sweetener used in some "sugar-free" gum and other products, is poorly absorbed in the GI tract and may produce osmotic diarrhea if ingested in large amounts.

Pathophysiology

Invasion of the GI tract by pathogens produces diarrhea by (1) production of enterotoxins that stimulate secretion of water and electrolytes, (2) direct invasion and destruction of intestinal epithelial cells, and (3) local inflammation and systemic invasion by the organisms. However, the most serious and immediate physiologic disturbances associated with severe diarrheal disease are (1) dehydration, (2) acid-base imbalance with acidosis, and (3) shock that occurs when dehydration progresses to the point that circulatory status is seriously impaired.

Diagnostic Evaluation

The history provides valuable information regarding exposure to infectious agents, personal contact, travel, or probable contact with contaminated foods. Allergic and dietary history may indicate food intolerances or allergies. Crowding and close person-to-person contact make epidemics with any enteric pathogen more likely.

The child's age provides clues to the cause of diarrheal disturbances. For example, milk allergy or intolerance of other formula constituents is suspected in early infancy. In later infancy, new foods added to the diet are frequent offenders. Most acute, inflammatory diarrheas are infectious, and the type of stools and the symptoms associated with the diarrhea provide clues to the organism (see p. 812).

The clinical manifestations of diarrhea are outlined in the box. Manifestations of severe diarrhea are primarily those of dehydration (see Dehydration, p. 803). Although vomiting may occur in all infectious diarrheas, it is not a major feature.

Although the child may not gain weight or may even show a slight loss in mild diarrhea, signs of dehydration are usually absent. If the diarrhea persists, if the child loses weight, if there is blood in the stools, or if the child develops associated signs such as deep breathing, listlessness, or reduced urine output that may signal complications, the child should be medically evaluated.

Laboratory Examination. Extensive laboratory evaluation is not indicated in a child with uncomplicated diarrhea and no evidence of dehydration. Laboratory tests are indicated when a child is moderately to severely dehydrated.

CLINICAL MANIFESTATIONS OF DIARRHEA

Mild diarrhea—a few loose stools each day without other evidence of illness
Moderate diarrhea—several loose or watery stools daily
  Normal or elevated temperature
  Vomiting
  Fretfulness and irritability
  Signs of dehydration usually absent, although may not gain weight or may even show weight loss
Severe diarrhea—numerous to continuous stools
  Signs of moderate to severe dehydration evident (see Table 24-1)
  Drawn, flaccid expressions
  Cry lacks vigor, is often whining and higher pitched than usual
  Irritable
  Seeks comfort and attention of parent
  Displays purposeless movements and inappropriate responses to people and familiar things
  May become lethargic, moribund, or comatose

Many cases of diarrhea are self-limiting, regardless of the cause.

Stool specimens should be examined in all children with diarrhea that persists for more than a few days. Examination of the stool for polymorphonuclear leukocytes ("polys") is the most widely used test to differentiate bacterial infections from viral ones. Cultures of the stool should be performed when blood or mucus is present in the stool, when abdominal cramps are severe, when there is a history of travel to a developing country, and when polys are found in the stool (indicating bacterial infection).

The stool should also be examined for ova and parasites when bacterial and viral cultures are negative and the diarrhea persists for more than a few days. Stool specimens to be tested for ova and parasites need to be preserved in a special solution to minimize false results. If there is a history of recent antibiotic use, the stool should be tested for the presence of *Clostridium difficile* toxin, and a sigmoidoscopy evaluation for pseudomembranous colitis may be indicated. A stool pH of less than 6 and the presence of reducing substances (determined with a Clinitest tablet and a small specimen of stool) suggests carbohydrate malabsorption or secondary lactase deficiency.

The urine specific gravity should be determined if dehydration is suspected. A complete blood count (CBC), serum electrolytes, creatinine, and blood urea nitrogen (BUN) should be obtained in the child who requires hospitalization. The hemoglobin, hematocrit, creatinine, and BUN levels are usually elevated in acute diarrhea and should also normalize with rehydration.

Therapeutic Management

Therapeutic management is directed at correcting the fluid imbalance and treating the underlying cause. Initial and regular ongoing evaluations are carried out to assess the patient's progress toward equilibrium and the effectiveness of therapy.

Mild or Moderate Diarrhea. Mild or moderate diarrhea is usually managed by simple measures and seldom requires hospitalization. When the moderate diarrhea becomes worse or does not respond to simple measures, hospitalization is indicated.

The major goals in the management of acute diarrhea include (1) assessment of the fluid and electrolyte imbalance, (2) rehydration, (3) maintenance fluid therapy, and (4) reintroduction of an adequate diet. Infants and children with acute diarrhea and dehydration should be treated first with *oral rehydration therapy (ORT)* or, in the few cases where this is not possible, with parenteral fluid therapy. ORT is effective, safer, less painful, and less costly than intravenous (IV) rehydration.

 ORT is one of the major worldwide health care advances of the past decade in underdeveloped, or Third World, countries. In developed countries, however, ORT has not been widely used because of the relative ease of access to IV fluids and entrenched patterns of care.

Oral rehydration solutions (ORS) are successful in treating infants with isotonic, hypotonic, and hypertonic dehydration. In a child with mild to moderate dehydration, 60 to 80 ml/kg should be administered over a 2-hour period (Johnson, 1993). After rehydration, ORS may be used during maintenance fluid therapy by alternating the solution with a low-sodium fluid such as water, breast milk, lactose-free formula, or half-strength lactose-containing formula. For older children, ORS can be given and a regular diet continued. Ongoing stool losses should be replaced on a 1:1 basis with ORS. If the stool output is not known, approximately 10 ml/kg or ½ to 1 cup of ORS should be given for each diarrheal stool.

Infants without clinical signs of dehydration do not need ORT. They should, however, receive the same fluids recommended for infants with signs of dehydration in the maintenance phase and for ongoing stool losses.

An ORS is useful in most cases of dehydration, and vomiting is not a contraindication. A child who is vomiting should be given ORS frequently in small amounts. The fluid may be given with a spoon or small syringe in 5 to 10 ml increments every 1 to 5 minutes by the child's caregiver. ORS may also be given through a nasogastric tube. In the United States, commercially prepared solutions, such as Pedialyte, Lytren, Ricelyte, and Resol, are used almost exclusively for oral rehydration. *Js . ā 10-15 min   if tolerated*

double
nothing carbonated - makes burp.

> **Nursing ALERT**
> Diarrhea is not managed by encouraging intake of clear fluids by mouth, such as fruit juices, carbonated soft drinks, and gelatin. These fluids usually have a high carbohydrate content, a very low electrolyte content, and a high osmolality (Avery and Snyder, 1990). Caffeinated soda is avoided, because caffeine is a mild diuretic and may lead to increased loss of water and sodium. Chicken or beef broth is not given, because it contains excessive sodium and inadequate carbohydrate.

Glucose-mediated enhanced sodium absorption forms the physiologic basis for the composition of ORS. Recent studies have evaluated the effectiveness of rice-based ORS. Results demonstrate that these nutrient-based solutions greatly reduced vomiting, decreased diarrhea volume loss, and shortened the duration of the disease (Santosham and Greenough, 1991).

Early reintroduction of normal nutrients is desirable and is gaining more widespread acceptance. Controversy still exists, however, regarding the best method of reintroducing feeding during recovery from diarrhea. Recent studies indicate that early reintroduction of a normal diet is beneficial because of its nutritional advantage and may reduce the number of stools, reduce weight loss, and shorten the duration of illness (Brown, 1991; Margolis and others, 1990). Continued feeding may protect against starvation-induced intestinal mucosal atrophy and enhance more rapid mucosal recovery following infectious diarrhea.

Breast-feeding, if being done, should be continued as a supplement to the ORS. Available evidence indicates that continued human milk feeding during diarrheal illness results in reduced severity and duration of the illness (Brown, 1991). Tolerance to human milk may result from its lower osmolality and its antimicrobial, enzymatic, and hormonal factors.

The use of nonhuman milk for infants and children with diarrhea remains controversial. This milk is of concern because maldigestion of lactose can occur in children with infectious diarrhea. However, evidence indicates that well-hydrated infants may resume full nonhuman milk feeding immediately without adverse reactions (Brown, Peerson, and Fontaine, 1994; Chew and others, 1993).

Many infants and children can be safely managed with a milk diet. Some practitioners advocate the use of a lactose-free formula only if milk or regular formula is not tolerated.

For older children a regular diet can generally be offered once rehydration has occurred. Bland foods may be better tolerated by some children. It is important to consider that recommendations to restrict infants' diets may be associated with significant noncompliance.

Parenteral fluid therapy is initiated whenever the child is unable to ingest sufficient amounts of fluid and electrolytes to (1) meet ongoing daily physiologic losses, (2) replace previous deficits, and (3) replace ongoing abnormal losses. Patients who usually require IV fluids are those with severe dehydration, those with uncontrollable vomiting, those who are unable to drink for any reason (e.g., extreme fatigue, coma), and those with severe gastric distention.

Severe Diarrhea. Severe diarrhea is largely a problem of infants and very young children, and regardless of the cause, successful management relies primarily on appropriate treatment of physiologic disturbances and is only secondarily concerned with specific treatment of the causative agent. Severe diarrhea warrants hospitalization, comprehensive evaluation, and parenteral fluid therapy. Fluid therapy is directed toward replacement of (1) the fluid deficit, as determined by weight loss and clinical signs; (2) ongoing normal losses from urine, lungs, and sweat; and (3) continued abnormal GI losses.

IV administration of fluid is begun immediately, and the solution is selected on the basis of what is known regarding the probable type and cause of the dehydration—usually a saline solution containing 5% dextrose in water. Sodium bicarbonate may be added, since acidosis is usually associated with severe dehydration. Although the initial phase of fluid replacement is rapid in both isotonic and hypotonic dehydration, it is contraindicated in hypertonic dehydration because of the risk of water intoxication, especially in the brain cells.

Once the severe effects of dehydration are under control, specific diagnostic and therapeutic measures are begun to detect and treat the cause of the diarrhea. This includes antimicrobial therapy where indicated and treatment of secondary effects of the illness or its therapy. For example, secondary bacterial growth may be countered with a short course of nonabsorbable antibiotics. *stay away from high fat*

Nursing Considerations

❖ Assessment

The nursing assessment of diarrhea begins with observation of the infant's or child's general appearance and behavior. The physical assessment includes all the parameters described for assessment of dehydration (p. 808). A history provides valuable information regarding probable etiologic agents, such as introduction of a new food, exposure to infectious agents, travel to an area of high susceptibility, contact with foods that might be contaminated, and contact with pets that are known to be sources of enteric infections. An allergic, drug, and dietary history may indicate food allergies.

❖ Nursing Diagnoses

Several nursing diagnoses become apparent on the basis of a thorough physical assessment. The major diagnoses appropriate for the infant or child are described in the Nursing Care Plan on pp. 810-811. Other diagnoses will be evident depending on the age, condition, and etiology of the diarrhea.

❖ Planning

The goals for the dehydrated infant or child and for the family are as follows:

1. Infant or child will maintain adequate hydration.
2. Infant or child will maintain appropriate nutrition for age.
3. Infant or child will not spread infection (if etiologic agent) to others.
4. Family will receive appropriate support and education, especially regarding home care.

❖ Implementation

Mild or moderate diarrhea is usually managed at home under the supervision of the nurse. The parents are allowed to give fluids to the child. Fluids are usually tolerated best at room temperature, and the parent is cautioned against giving other than those prescribed by the practitioner. The ORS is usually well accepted by infants, but older children find these solutions unpalatable. However, flavored solutions may be better accepted (see Critical Thinking Exercise).

Severe Diarrhea. The infant or child admitted to the hospital with diarrhea is usually isolated from children who do not have diarrhea, and appropriate precautions are implemented to prevent possible spread to other patients and personnel. Most infections that cause diarrhea are spread by the fecal-oral route or through contaminated food. Strict attention to disposal of soiled diapers, hygienic food preparation, not sharing toys, and proper handwashing will minimize transmission. The containment of feces is a key factor in infection control. Research indicates that superabsorbent paper diapers with elastic legs permit less fecal leakage than cloth diapers with plastic coverings (Kubiak and others, 1993). Each hospital has a policy regarding necessary precautions. (See Infection Control, Chapter 22.)

The child is weighed on admission and frequently during the initial rehydration period. Accurate intake and output measurement is imperative, and (if needed) a urine collection bag is placed to determine the volume of output, to measure specific gravity, and to determine if the renal blood flow is sufficient to permit administration of potassium. Unless urine is separated from stool, this essential information cannot be obtained.

Children who are sufficiently ill to require hospitalization may be placed on parenteral fluid therapy with nothing by mouth (NPO) for 12 to 48 hours. Monitoring the IV infusion is a primary nursing function, with careful attention given to ascertain that the correct fluid and electrolyte concentration is infused, the flow rate is adjusted to deliver the desired volume in a given time, and the IV site is maintained.

The nurse is responsible for examination of stools and collection of specimens for laboratory examination. Care should be exerted in obtaining and transporting stools to prevent possible spread of infection. Stool specimens should be transported to the laboratory in appropriate containers and media according to hospital policy. A clean tongue depressor can be

CRITICAL THINKING EXERCISE

Acute Diarrhea

An 8-month-old infant is evaluated in the primary care clinic because of fever, vomiting, and diarrhea of 12 hours' duration. The caregivers report that the infant had three times as many stools as usual, and the stools are watery in consistency. After the initial examination of the infant, it is apparent that the child is mildly dehydrated because of stool losses secondary to acute infectious diarrhea. Which of the following interventions would be indicated in this situation?

1. Recommend that the caregivers offer fruit juice only and delay reintroduction of food for 48 hours.
2. Administer antidiarrheal medications.
3. Educate the infant's caregivers regarding administration of oral rehydration solution (ORS).
4. Administer intravenous (IV) fluids and provide nothing by mouth for several hours.

The correct answer is three. The goals of management of acute diarrhea include assessment of hydration, provision of fluids for rehydration and maintenance, and reintroduction of an adequate diet. In this case, since the infant is mildly dehydrated, oral rehydration therapy (ORT) should be attempted. ORT is effective, safer, less painful, and less costly than IV rehydration. If ORS is administered at frequent intervals, vomiting can be minimized and IV hydration probably avoided.

Early reintroduction of normal nutrients is desirable, and delayed introduction of food may be harmful in terms of nutritional status and duration of illness. Breast-feeding generally should be continued, and most infants who receive cow's milk formulas may resume their usual feedings as soon as they are rehydrated. Occasionally a soy formula is recommended after an episode of acute infectious diarrhea if the infant demonstrates evidence of lactose malabsorption. Use of antidiarrheal medications should not be recommended for acute infectious diarrhea. These drugs may be harmful, because adverse effects such as slowed motility and ileus may occur.

used to obtain specimens for laboratory examination when a larger volume is needed or as an applicator for transfer to a culture medium. Tests for pH, blood, and reducing substance can be done on the nursing unit. (See Collection of Specimens, Chapter 22.)

Since diarrheal stools are highly irritating to the skin, extra care is needed to protect the skin of the diaper region from becoming excoriated. (See Diaper Dermatitis, Chapter 30.) Rectal temperatures are avoided because they can stimulate the bowel, increasing passage of stool.

Support for the child and family involves the same care and consideration as for all hospitalized children (see Chapter 21). Parents are kept informed of the child's progress and instructed in special care behaviors, such as handwashing and proper disposal of soiled diapers, clothes, and bed linen. Everyone caring for the child must be aware of "clean" areas and "dirty" areas, especially in the hospital, where the sink in the child's room is used for many purposes. For example, food, eating and drinking utensils, toothbrushes, pacifiers, toys, and other personal items are stored away from the sink, diaper-changing surface, and scale used to weigh diapers.

NURSING CARE PLAN

The Child with Acute Diarrhea (Gastroenteritis)

NURSING DIAGNOSIS: Fluid volume deficit related to excessive gastrointestinal (GI) losses in stool or emesis

PATIENT GOAL 1: Will exhibit signs of rehydration and maintain adequate hydration

• **NURSING INTERVENTIONS/*RATIONALES***

*Administer oral rehydration solutions (ORS) *for both rehydration and replacement of stool losses*
   Give ORS frequently in small amounts, especially if child is vomiting, *because vomiting, unless severe, is not a contraindication to using ORS*
*Administer and monitor intravenous fluids as prescribed *for severe dehydration and vomiting*
*Administer antimicrobial agents as prescribed *to treat specific pathogens causing excessive GI losses*
   After rehydration, offer child regular diet as tolerated *because studies show that early reintroduction of normal diet is beneficial in reducing number of stools and weight loss and shortening duration of illness*
   Alternate ORS with a low-sodium fluid such as water, breast milk, lactose-free formula, or half-strength lactose-containing formula *for maintenance fluid therapy*
   Maintain strict record of intake and output (urine, stool, and emesis) *to evaluate effectiveness of interventions*
   Monitor urine specific gravity every 8 hours or as indicated *to assess hydration*
   Weigh child daily *to assess for dehydration*
   Assess vital signs, skin turgor, mucous membranes, and mental status every 4 hours or as indicated *to assess hydration*
   Discourage intake of clear fluids such as fruit juices, carbonated soft drinks, and gelatin *because these fluids usually are high in carbohydrates, low in electrolytes, and have a high osmolality*
   Instruct family in providing appropriate therapy, monitoring intake and output, and assessing for signs of dehydration *to ensure optimum results and improve compliance with the therapeutic regimen*

• **EXPECTED OUTCOME**

Child exhibits signs of adequate hydration (specify)

NURSING DIAGNOSIS: Altered nutrition: less than body requirements related to diarrheal losses, inadequate intake

PATIENT GOAL 1: Will consume nourishment adequate to maintain appropriate weight for age

• **NURSING INTERVENTIONS/*RATIONALES***

After rehydration, instruct breast-feeding mother to continue feeding breast milk *because this tends to reduce severity and duration of illness*

*Dependent nursing action.

Avoid giving BRAT diet (bananas, rice, apples, and toast or tea) *because this diet is low in energy and protein, too high in carbohydrates, and low in electrolytes*
Observe and record response to feedings *to assess feeding tolerance*
Instruct family in providing appropriate diet *to gain compliance with therapeutic regimen*
Explore concerns and priorities of family members *to improve compliance with therapeutic regimen*

• **EXPECTED OUTCOME**

Child takes prescribed nourishment and exhibits a satisfactory weight gain

NURSING DIAGNOSIS: High risk for transmitting infection related to microorganisms invading GI tract

PATIENT (OTHERS) GOAL 1: Will not exhibit signs of GI infection

• **NURSING INTERVENTIONS/*RATIONALES***

Implement standard precautions or other hospital infection-control practices, including appropriate disposal of stool and laundry and appropriate handling of specimens, *to reduce risk of spreading infection*
Maintain careful handwashing *to reduce risk of spreading infection*
Apply diaper snugly *to reduce likelihood of fecal spread*
Use superabsorbent disposable diapers *to contain feces and decrease chance of diaper dermatitis*
Attempt to keep infants and small children from placing hands and objects in contaminated areas
Teach children, when possible, protective measures *to prevent spread of infection*, such as handwashing after using toilet
Instruct family members and visitors in isolation practices, especially handwashing, *to reduce risk of spreading infection*

• **EXPECTED OUTCOME**

Infection does not spread to others

NURSING DIAGNOSIS: Impaired skin integrity related to irritation caused by frequent, loose stools

PATIENT GOAL 1: Skin will remain intact

• **NURSING INTERVENTIONS/*RATIONALES***

Change diaper frequently *to keep skin clean and dry*
Cleanse buttocks gently with bland, nonalkaline soap and water or immerse child in a bath for gentle cleansing *because diarrheal stools are highly irritating to skin*
Apply ointment such as zinc oxide *to protect skin from irritation* (type of ointment may vary for each child and may require a trial period)

NURSING CARE PLAN

The Child with Acute Diarrhea (Gastroenteritis)—cont'd

Expose slightly reddened intact skin to air whenever possible *to promote healing;* apply protective ointment to very irritated or excoriated skin *to facilitate healing*

Avoid using commercial baby wipes containing alcohol on excoriated skin *because they will cause stinging*

Observe buttocks and perineum for infection, such as *Candida, so that appropriate therapy can be initiated*

*Apply appropriate antifungal medication *to treat fungal infection of skin*

• EXPECTED OUTCOME

Child has no evidence of skin breakdown

> **NURSING DIAGNOSIS:** Anxiety/fear related to separation from parents, unfamiliar environment, distressing procedures

PATIENT GOAL 1: Will exhibit signs of comfort

• NURSING INTERVENTIONS/*RATIONALES*

Provide mouth care and pacifier for infants *to provide comfort*

Encourage family visitation and participation in care as much as the family is able, *to prevent stress associated with separation*

Touch, hold, and talk to child as much as possible *to provide comfort and relieve stress*

Provide sensory stimulation and diversion appropriate for child's developmental level and condition *to promote optimum growth and development*

---

*Dependent nursing action.

• EXPECTED OUTCOMES

Child exhibits minimal signs of physical or emotional distress

Family participates in child's care as much as possible

> **NURSING DIAGNOSIS:** Altered family processes related to situational crisis, knowledge deficit

PATIENT (FAMILY) GOAL 1: Family will understand about child's illness and its treatment and will be able to provide care

• NURSING INTERVENTIONS/*RATIONALES*

Provide information to family about child's illness and therapeutic measures *to encourage compliance with therapeutic regimen, especially at home*

Assist family in providing comfort and support to child

Permit family members to participate in child's care as much as they desire, *to meet needs of both child and family*

Instruct family regarding precautions *to prevent spread of infection*

Arrange for posthospitalization health care *for continued assessment and treatment*

Refer family to a community health care agency *for supervision of home care as needed*

• EXPECTED OUTCOME

Family demonstrates ability to care for child, especially at home

---

Soiled diapers and linen should be discarded in receptacles close to the bedside.

NURSING TIP To remind caregivers to keep diapers and other soiled articles away from clean areas, place signs identifying "clean" (e.g., bed table) and "dirty" (e.g., sink, bathroom) areas in the room. List on each sign what articles should be stored in each area.

❖ Evaluation

The effectiveness of nursing interventions is determined by continued reassessment according to the following observational guidelines and expected outcomes:

1. Monitor fluid losses with careful intake and output measurements and daily weights.
2. Monitor food intake, especially calories.
3. Observe for evidence of complications from underlying disease (specify) and/or therapy.
4. Observe and interview family to determine extent and effectiveness of care.

Expected outcomes:
See Nursing Care Plan, pp. 810-811.

ACUTE INFECTIOUS DIARRHEA

Acute infectious diarrhea *(infectious gastroenteritis)* is caused by a wide variety of viral, bacterial, and parasitic pathogens. In the United States the incidence of acute infectious diarrhea is approximately 2½ episodes per person per year (Cohen, 1991). Infants and young children are at a high risk for the development of dehydration and malnutrition, the two major consequences of diarrhea.

Etiology/Epidemiology

Most organisms that cause diarrhea are spread by the fecal-oral route. Some are transmitted by direct person-to-person contact, especially where groups are in direct contact, such as in daycare centers. Viral disease occurs more frequently in winter months; bacterial disorders are more prevalent during summer and fall. Although acute gastroenteritis affects all age-groups, there is a greater frequency of diarrheal disease in younger children.

TABLE 24-3. Infectious causes of acute diarrhea

ORGANISM	PATHOLOGY	CHARACTERISTICS	COMMENTS
Viral Agents			
Rotavirus Incubation period: 1-3 days	Invade epithelium of small bowel mucosa Severely distorted mucosal architecture with atrophic mucosa and severe inflammatory changes Absorption of salt and water decreased	Abrupt onset Fever (38° C [100.4° F] or higher) lasting approximately 48 hours Nausea/vomiting Abdominal pain Associated upper respiratory tract infection Diarrhea may persist for more than a week	Incidence higher in cool weather (80% in winter) Affects all age-groups; 6- to 24-month-old infants more vulnerable Usually mild and self-limited Important cause of nosocomial infections in hospitals and gastroenteritis in children attending daycare centers
Norwalk-like organisms Incubation period: 1-3 days	Mechanism of effect unknown Blunting of villi and inflammatory changes in lamina propria Reduced enzymes	Fever Loss of appetite Nausea/vomiting Abdominal pain Diarrhea Malaise	Source of infection: drinking water, recreation water, food (including shellfish) Affects all ages Self-limited (2-3 days)
Bacterial Agents			
Pathogenic *Escherichia coli* Incubation period: highly variable, depends on strain	Usually caused by enterotoxin production (small bowel) Reduces absorption and increases secretion of fluids and electrolytes	Onset gradual or abrupt Variable clinical manifestations Most—green, watery diarrhea with blood and mucus; becomes explosive Vomiting may be present from onset Abdominal distention Diarrhea Fever, appears toxic	Incidence higher in summer Usually interpersonal transmission but may transmit via inanimate objects and undercooked meat, especially chopped beef Cause of nursery epidemics With symptomatic treatment only, may continue for weeks Full breast-feeding has a protective effect Symptoms generally subside in 3-7 days Relapse rate approximately 20%
Salmonella groups (nontyphoidal)—gram negative, nonencapsulated, nonsporulating Incubation period: 6-72 hours for gastroenteritis (usually less than 24); 3-60 days for enteric fever (usually 7-14)	Penetration of lamina propria (small bowel and colon) Local inflammation—no extensive destruction Stimulation of intestinal fluid excretion Systemic invasion of other sites	Rapid onset Variable symptoms—mild to severe Nausea/vomiting and colicky abdominal pain followed by diarrhea, occasionally with blood and mucus Fever Hyperactive peristalsis and mild abdominal tenderness Symptoms usually subside within 5 days May have headache and cerebral manifestations (e.g., drowsiness, confusion, meningismus, seizures) Infants may be afebrile and nontoxic May result in life-threatening septicemia and meningitis	Two thirds of patients are younger than 20 years of age; highest incidence in children younger than age 5 years, especially infants Highest incidence occurs from July through October, lowest from January through April Transmission primarily via contaminated food and drink—most from animal sources, including fowl, mammals, reptiles, and insects Most common sources are poultry and eggs In children—pets (e.g., dogs, cats, hamsters, and especially pet turtles) Communicable as long as organisms are excreted.
S. typhi	Rapid invasion of bloodstream from minor sites of inflammation Marked inflammation and necrosis of intestinal mucosa and lymphatics	Variable in infants Older children—irregular fever, headache, malaise, lethargy Diarrhea occurs in 50% at early stage Cough is common In a few days fever rises and is consistent; fatigue, cough, abdominal pain, anorexia, and weight loss develop; diarrhea begins	Decreased incidence in last decade Acute symptoms may persist for a week or more Transmitted by contaminated food or water (primary), infected animals (e.g., pet turtles)
Shigella groups—gram negative, nonmotile anaerobic bacilli	Enterotoxin Stimulates loss of fluids and electrolytes	Onset variable but usually abrupt Fever and cramping abdominal pain initially Fever—may reach 40.5° C (105° F)	Approximately 60% of cases in children younger than age 9 years with more than one third between ages 1 and 4 years

[handwritten annotation: "may have 2 or 3 wks. looser stools"]

[handwritten annotation in left margin: "meat"]

[handwritten annotation in left margin: "egg"]

TABLE 24-3. Infectious causes of acute diarrhea—cont'd

ORGANISM	PATHOLOGY	CHARACTERISTICS	COMMENTS
Shigella groups—cont'd Incubation period: 1-7 days, usually 2-4	Invasion of epithelium with superficial mucosal ulcerations *S. dysenteriae* forms exotoxin	Convulsions in about 10%—usually associated with fever Patient appears sick Headache, nuchal rigidity, delirium Watery diarrhea with mucus and pus starts about 12-48 hours after onset Stools preceded by abdominal cramps; tenesmus and straining follow Symptoms usually subside in 5-10 days	Peak incidence in late summer Transmitted directly or indirectly from infected persons Communicable for 1-4 weeks Self-limited disease Treat with antibiotics Severe dehydration and collapse can affect all patients Acute symptoms may persist for a week or more
Yersinia enterocolitica Incubation period: dose dependent, 1-3 weeks		Diarrhea—may be bloody Fever (>38.7° C [102° F]) Abdominal pain in right lower quadrant Vomiting, diarrhea	Seen more frequently in winter Majority in first 3 years of life Transmitted by food and pets Can resemble appendicitis May be relapsing and last for weeks
Campylobacter jejuni Incubation period: 1-7 days or longer	Precise mechanism unclear Jejunum, ileum, and colon involvement Extensive ulceration with hemorrhagic ileitis Broadening and flattening of mucosa	Fever Abdominal pain—often severe, cramping, periumbilical Watery, profuse, foul-smelling diarrhea with blood Vomiting	Person-to-person transmission May be transmitted by pets (e.g., cat, dog, hamster) Food (especially chicken) and water-borne transmission Relapse possible Most patients recover spontaneously Antibiotics may speed recovery Peak incidence in summer
Vibrio cholerae (cholera) groups Incubation period: usually 2-3 days; range from few hours to 5 days	Enterotoxin causes increased secretion of chloride and possibly bicarbonate Intestinal mucosa congested with enlarged lymph follicles Intact mucosal surface	Sudden onset of profuse watery diarrhea without cramping, tenesmus, or anal irritation, although children may complain of cramping Stools are intermittent at first, then almost continuous Stools are bloody with mucus	Rare in infants younger than 1 year old Mortality high in both treated and untreated infants and small children Transmitted via contaminated food and water Attack confers immunity
Clostridium difficile	Toxin stimulates colonic secretion by damaging epithelium	Diarrhea with blood in stools	May cause pseudomembranous colitis Follows antibiotic therapy
Food Poisoning *Staphylococcus* Incubation period: 4-6 hours	Produce heat-stable enterotoxin	Nausea, vomiting Severe abdominal cramps Profuse diarrhea Shock may occur in severe cases May be a mild fever	Transferred via contaminated food—inadequately cooked or refrigerated (e.g., custards, mayonnaise, cream-filled or cream-topped desserts) Self-limited; improvement apparent within 24 hours Excellent prognosis
Clostridium perfringens Incubation period: 8-24 hours, usually 8-12	Produces heat-resistant and heat-sensitive toxins	Moderate to severe crampy, midepigastric pain	Self-limited illness Transmission by commercial food products, most often meat and poultry
Clostridium botulinum Incubation period: 12-26 hours (range, 6 hours to 8 days)	Highly potent neurotoxin	Nausea, vomiting Diarrhea Central nervous system symptoms with curare-like effect Dry mouth, dysphagia	Transmitted by contaminated food products Variable severity—mild symptoms to rapidly fatal within a few hours Antitoxin administration

In young children in the United States and in other industrialized countries, most episodes of diarrhea are caused by viral pathogens. *Rotavirus* is the most important cause of dehydrating diarrhea in young children throughout the world. Its symptoms may range from no manifestations to death from dehydration. Rotavirus infection accounts for most hospitalizations for severe diarrhea in young children and is a significant nosocomial (hospital-acquired) pathogen. As of this writing, an oral vaccine is being tested that has been highly effective against very severe rotavirus gastroenteritis (Rennels and others, 1996). *Salmonella, Shigella,* and *Campylobacter* are the most frequently isolated bacterial pathogens, and *Giardia* and *Cryptosporidium* are the parasites that most often produce acute, infectious diarrhea (Table 24-3; see also Intestinal Parasitic Diseases, Chapter 14).

Diagnostic Evaluation

Infectious diarrheas have some features in common, such as vomiting, and frequently there is abdominal discomfort. Bacterial infections and some viral infections are accompanied by fever. The manifestations and severity are variable among the various forms (see Table 24-1). Laboratory confirmation of the specific organism confirms the diagnosis and serves as a guideline for appropriate therapeutic management.

Therapeutic Management

The primary concern in infectious gastroenteritis, as in all conditions in which fluid is lost in large amounts, is dehydration and the attendant physical deterioration. Fluid replacement, nutritional therapy, and monitoring of electrolyte status with replacement are the same as for any diarrheal disorder.

Treatment for acute infectious diarrhea should begin with effective preventive measures. Because spread of most of these organisms is fecal-oral, personal hygiene, water supplies, sewage control, and food preparation are important considerations (see Infection Control, Chapter 22).

Enteric infections are generally self-limited conditions. Antimicrobial therapy is not indicated in most children with acute diarrhea. Specific antimicrobial therapy is indicated only for culture-proven bacterial or parasitic infections in which this therapy can reduce the duration of the illness, severity of symptoms, shedding of organisms, and secondary spread of organisms (see also Intestinal Parasitic Diseases, Chapter 14). Effective antimicrobial therapy is not available for enteric viruses. Indiscriminate use of antibiotics may lead to pseudomembranous colitis and worsen the existing diarrhea.

Antidiarrheal drug therapy is usually not indicated in acute infectious diarrhea. Adverse side effects may occur, such as worsening of the diarrhea because of slowing of motility or prevention of absorption of medicines or nutrients in the intestine.

Nursing Considerations

Basic nursing care for the infant or child with infectious gastroenteritis is the same as for any diarrheal disease. However, appropriate isolation precautions are carried out to prevent the spread of the infection to others.

It may be necessary to obtain stool specimens from the child and other family members who are affected or suspected of being carriers of infectious organisms. The parents are provided with specimen containers and instructed in collection and disposition of stool samples.

Some medications appear to be safe for adults in preventing traveler's diarrhea; however, parents should be cautioned against giving any drugs to children. Until vaccines or other prophylactic measures are proved safe for children, the best prevention during travel to areas where the water supply may be contaminated is to allow children to drink only bottled water and carbonated beverages (from the container through a straw supply brought from home). Tap water, ice, unpasteurized dairy products, raw vegetables, and unpeeled fruits are avoided. Meats and seafoods may be risky as well and are best avoided or eaten fully cooked.

> **Nursing ALERT**
>
> To reduce the risk of bacteria transmitted via food, encourage parents to do the following:
> Quickly freeze or refrigerate all ground meat and other perishable foods.
> Never thaw food on the counter or let it sit out of the refrigerator for more than 2 hours.
> Wash hands, utensils, and work areas with hot soapy water after contact with raw meat to keep bacteria from spreading.
> Check meat with a fork to make sure no pink is showing before taking a bite.
> Cook all dishes made with ground meat until brown or gray inside or to an internal temperature of 71° C (160° F).

CONSTIPATION

Constipation is the infrequent passage of firm or hard stools or of small, hard masses with associated symptoms such as difficulty in expulsion of the stools, blood-streaked bowel movements, and abdominal discomfort. The frequency of bowel movements is not considered a diagnostic criterion, because it varies widely among children.

Constipation may arise secondary to a variety of organic disorders of the GI tract or in association with a wide range of systemic disorders. Structural disorders of the intestine may be found in association with constipation, such as strictures, ectopic anus, and Hirschsprung disease. A wide range of systemic disorders may be associated with constipation. Hypothyroidism disorders associated with hypercalcemia, such as hyperparathyroidism and vitamin D excess, are typically associated with chronic constipation in childhood. Chronic high-level lead poisoning may cause anorexia, vomiting, abdominal pain, and constipation. Constipation may also be associated with a wide range of drugs, such as antacids, diuretics, phenytoin (Dilantin), antihistamines, and opioids (narcotics), and iron supplementation. Spinal cord lesions may produce loss of rectal tone and sensation. These patients are therefore prone to chronic fecal retention and overflow incontinence. Having extremely long intervals between defecation is termed *obstipation.* Constipation with fecal soiling is called *encopresis.*

In the majority of children with chronic constipation, no underlying cause can be clearly identified. These children have idiopathic or functional constipation. Chronic constipation may be initiated by environmental or psychosocial factors. Transient illness, overzealous toilet-training attempts, personality, and emotional factors may play a role in the etiology of constipation.

Newborn Period

Normally the newborn infant passes a first meconium stool within 24 to 36 hours of birth. Any infant who does not do so should be assessed for evidence of intestinal atresia or stenosis, Hirschsprung disease (congenital aganglionic megacolon), hypothyroidism, meconium plugs, or meconium ileus. *Meconium plugs* are caused by meconium that has reduced water content and are usually evacuated following digital examination but may require irrigations of normal saline or the iodinated contrast medium.

Meconium ileus, the initial manifestation of cystic fibrosis, is the luminal obstruction of the distal small intestine by abnormal meconium. Treatment is the same as for a meconium plug. Rarely, surgical intervention may be needed.

Infancy

The onset of constipation frequently occurs during infancy and is often related to dietary practices. It is almost unknown in breast-fed infants. Constipation may accompany a change from human milk or modified cow's milk to whole cow's milk. Simple measures ordinarily correct the problem, such

---

CRITICAL THINKING EXERCISE

Constipation

A 6-month-old infant is referred to a pediatric gastroenterologist because of concerns about constipation. The infant usually has one hard stool every 4 to 5 days, which causes discomfort when the stool is passed. Abdominal distention and vomiting are not common occurrences, and growth has been normal. The infant's diet consists of cow's milk formula only. The infant's caregivers report that the infrequent passage of hard stools began approximately 1 month ago. It is determined that this infant likely has functional constipation because no underlying cause can be clearly identified. All the following early interventions would be indicated in this situation *except:*

1. Educate the infant's caregivers concerning normal bowel habits.
2. Administer two or three mineral oil enemas to cleanse the bowel.
3. Recommend that caregivers introduce food and fruit juice into the infant's diet.
4. Use several medications daily to maintain a loose consistency of stools.

The correct answer is four. The management of an infant with functional constipation should initially include education of the caregivers, simple measures to keep the bowel relatively empty of stool, and diet management to prevent further constipation. The caregivers should be educated that short periods of constipation are not uncommon and usually resolve as solid food is introduced into the diet. One or two offerings of fruit juice each day may be beneficial in preventing further constipation. If hard stools or anal fissures persist after initial bowel cleansing and diet management, medications such as malt extract or lactulose may be required.

---

as adding or increasing the amount of cereal, vegetables, and fruit in the diet of the older infant. Stool-withholding behavior may begin at this age in response to pain on defecation (see Critical Thinking Exercise).

Childhood

Children between 1 and 3 years of age are most likely to have constipation, usually as a result of environmental changes. It may be a result of some medications (e.g., iron or calcium supplements, diuretics, antacids, opioids, anticonvulsant agents). If there are associated manifestations, such as vomiting, abdominal distention or pain, and evidence of growth failure, the condition merits further investigation.

The management of simple constipation consists of a plan to keep the bowel relatively empty of stool and dietary management to prevent further constipation. There is not total agreement on the most effective means to clean the bowel, although most agree that the use of laxatives is not usually recommended because of their tendency to create dependency. Enemas are sometimes used to empty the bowel and repeated if voluntary evacuation does not occur within 48 hours. Treatment may also include the use of bisacodyl (Dulcolax) suppositories. Occasionally a polyethylene glycol–electrolyte solution (Golytely) by oral or nasogastric administration is necessary for severe fecal impaction.

Increasing the intake of fluids and implementing a high-fiber diet are advised. Any foods known to be constipating are eliminated. Sometimes a stool softener such as dioctyl sodium sulfosuccinate or mineral oil is of benefit.

Effective counseling is an essential element of the treatment plan for children with chronic constipation. Bowel function, the purpose of interventions, and the need for persistence should be explained to the child and family. Erroneous concepts concerning this condition need to be corrected. A child who has experienced discomfort during bowel movements may deliberately try to withhold stool. The rectum accommodates the stool accumulation, and the urge to defecate passes. When bowel contents are ultimately evacuated, the accumulated feces are passed with even greater pain, reinforcing the desire to withhold stool.

Retraining therapy involves habit training, reinforcement for toilet sitting and defecation, and emotional support. A regular toilet time is established once or twice a day, preferably after a meal. A reasonable amount of time (5 to 10 minutes) should be spent attempting to defecate completely. Biofeedback may be indicated as a form of behavioral modification. Children with chronic constipation and encopresis frequently experience inappropriate external anal sphincter contraction during defecation. Rectal biofeedback can teach children to relax the anal sphincter during defecation.

Constipation in school-age children may represent an ongoing chronic problem or may develop for the first time. The onset of constipation at this age often results from environmental changes, stresses, and changes in toileting patterns. A common cause of new-onset constipation at school entry is fear of using school bathrooms, which are noted for their lack of privacy. Also, early and hurried departure for school immediately after breakfast may impede bathroom use. Most schools will liberalize bathroom rules for individual children who have been identified and have a parent or health professional intervene on their behalf. Encopresis often causes ad-

HIGH-FIBER FOODS

Bread, Grains
Whole-grain bread or rolls
Whole-grain cereals
Bran
Pancakes, waffles, and muffins with fruit or bran
Unrefined (brown) rice

Vegetables
Raw vegetables, especially broccoli, cabbage, carrots, cauliflower, celery, lettuce, and spinach
Cooked vegetables, such as those listed above, and asparagus,
beans, brussels sprouts, corn, potatoes, rhubarb, squash,
string beans, and turnips

Fruits
Raw fruits, especially those with skins or seeds, other than ripe
banana or avocado
Raisins, prunes, or other dried fruits

Miscellaneous
Nuts, seeds, legumes, popcorn
High-fiber snack bars

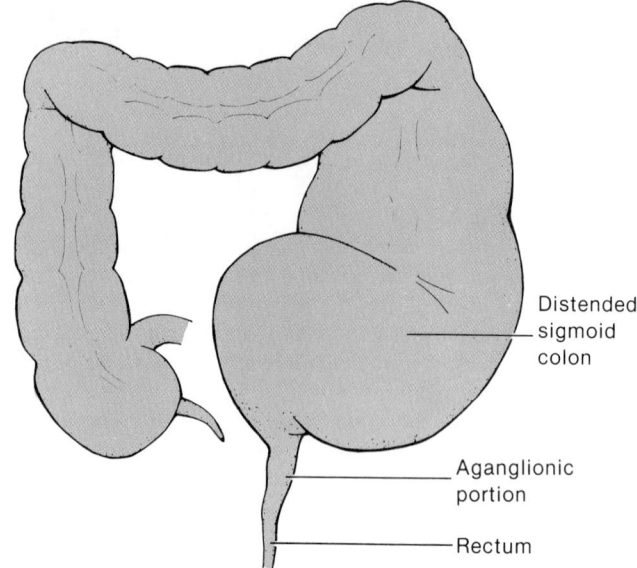

Distended
sigmoid
colon

Aganglionic
portion

Rectum

FIG. 24-1. Hirschsprung disease.

ditional emotional stress for the school-age child (see Chapter 17).

[handwritten: mineral oil – mix c̄ frozen OJ + Ice H₂O mix]

Nursing Considerations

Constipation, unfortunately, tends to be self-perpetuating. A child who has difficulty or discomfort when attempting to evacuate the bowels has a tendency to retain the bowel contents, and thus begins a vicious cycle. Nursing assessment begins with an accurate history of bowel habits, diet, events that may be associated with the onset of constipation, drugs or other substances that the child may be taking, and the consistency, color, frequency, and other characteristics of the stool. If there is no evidence of a pathologic condition that requires further investigation, the major task of the nurse is to educate the parents regarding normal stool patterns and to participate in the education and treatment of the child.

Dietary modifications are usually essential in preventing constipation. During infancy, simply increasing the carbohydrate (sugar or corn syrup) in the infant's formula will often relieve the problem. During childhood, the diet should contain increased amounts of fiber and fluid. Parents benefit from guidance in dietary planning, especially regarding foods that facilitate bowel movements (see box). They need reassurance concerning the benign nature of the condition. It is important to discuss with them their attitudes and expectations regarding toilet habits.

[handwritten left margin: APA recommend don't do]

HIRSCHSPRUNG DISEASE

Hirschsprung disease *(congenital aganglionic megacolon)* is a mechanical obstruction caused by inadequate motility of part of the intestine. It accounts for about one fourth of all cases of neonatal obstruction, although it may not be diagnosed until later in infancy or childhood. It is four times more common in males than in females, follows a familial pattern in a small number of cases, and is considerably more common in children with Down syndrome. The incidence is 1 in 5000 live births. Depending on its presentation, it may be an acute, life-threatening condition or a chronic disorder.

Pathophysiology

Hirschsprung disease results from failure of ganglion cells to migrate craniocaudally along the GI tract during gestation. The aganglionic segment almost always includes the rectum and a proximal portion of the large intestine. Rarely, "skip segments" or total intestinal aganglionosis may occur. Absence of propulsive movements (peristalsis) in the aganglionic bowel causes accumulation of intestinal contents and distention of the bowel proximal to the defect, thus the term *megacolon,* or large colon. In addition, the internal rectal sphincter fails to relax, which prevents evacuation of solids, liquids, and gas and thus contributes to the manifestations of obstruction (Fig. 24-1). Intestinal distention and ischemia may occur as a result of distention of the bowel wall, which contributes to the development of *enterocolitis* (inflammation of the small bowel and colon), the leading cause of death in children with Hirschsprung disease (Kirschner, 1991).

Diagnostic Evaluation

Clinical manifestations vary according to the age when symptoms are first recognized and the presence of complications, such as enterocolitis (see box). In the neonate, diagnosis is usually made on the basis of clinical signs of intestinal obstruction and failure to pass meconium. Radiographs, barium enema, and anorectal manometric examinations assist in the differential diagnosis, which is then confirmed by histologic examination of a full-thickness rectal biopsy demonstrating absence of ganglion cells in the myenteric and submucosal plexus.

Therapeutic Management

Treatment is primarily surgical to remove the aganglionic portion of the bowel in order to permit normal bowel motility and establish continence by improved functioning of the in-

CLINICAL MANIFESTATIONS OF HIRSCHSPRUNG DISEASE

Newborn Period

Failure to pass meconium within 24 to 48 hours after birth
Reluctance to ingest fluids
Bile-stained vomitus
Abdominal distention

Infancy

Failure to thrive
Constipation
Abdominal distention
Episodes of diarrhea and vomiting
Ominous signs (often signify the presence of enterocolitis)
　Explosive, watery diarrhea
　Fever
　Severe prostration

Childhood*

Constipation
Ribbonlike, foul-smelling stools
Abdominal distention
Visible peristalsis
Fecal masses easily palpable
Child usually poorly nourished and anemic

*Symptoms are more chronic.

ternal anal sphincter. In most cases this is accomplished in two stages. First, a temporary ostomy proximal to the aganglionic segment is performed to allow the normal bowel a period to rest and resume its normal caliber and tonicity. Second, complete correction is accomplished with a pull-through procedure of the bowel, which consists of "pulling" the end of functioning ganglionated bowel down through the muscular sleeve of the rectum. This procedure is referred to as the *Soave endorectal pull-through procedure.* The ostomy is usually closed at the time of the pull-through procedure. This surgery is typically delayed until the child weighs approximately 20 pounds (9 kg). Other definitive procedures that can be performed include the Swenson, Duhamel, and Boley procedures.

Prognosis.   Most children with Hirschsprung disease require surgery rather than medical therapy. Once the patient is stabilized with fluid and electrolyte replacement, if needed, the temporary colostomy is performed and has a high rate of success. After the later pull-through procedure, anal stricture and incontinence are potential complications that may occur, requiring further therapy, including dilatation or bowel-retraining therapy.

Nursing Considerations

Many of the nursing concerns depend on the child's age and the type of treatment. If the disorder is diagnosed during the neonatal period, the main objectives are (1) to help the parents adjust to a congenital defect in their child, (2) to foster infant-parent bonding, (3) to prepare them for the medical/surgical intervention, and (4) to assist them in colostomy care after discharge.

Preoperative Care.   Much of the child's preoperative care depends on the age and clinical condition. A child who is malnourished may not be able to withstand surgery until the physical status improves. Often this involves symptomatic treatment with enemas; a low-fiber, high-calorie, and high-protein diet; and in severe situations the use of total parenteral nutrition (TPN).

Physical preoperative preparation entails the same measures that are common to any surgery (see Surgical Procedures, Chapter 22). In the newborn, whose bowel is sterile, no additional preparation is necessary. However, in other children, in preparation for the pull-through procedure, emptying the bowel with repeated saline enemas and decreasing bacterial flora with systemic antibiotics and colonic irrigations using antibiotic solution are usually ordered. Oral antibiotics may also be prescribed.

Since progressive distention of the abdomen is a serious sign, the nurse measures abdominal circumference with a paper tape measure, usually at the level of the umbilicus or at the widest part of the abdomen. The point of measurement is marked with a pen to ensure reliability of subsequent measurements. Abdominal measurement can be performed at the same time that vital signs are taken and is recorded in serial order so that a change is readily apparent.

NURSING TIP To reduce any stress to the acutely ill child when frequent measurements of abdominal circumference are needed, the tape measure can be left in place beneath the child rather than removed each time.

The child's age dictates the type and extent of psychologic preparation necessary for child and parents. Since a colostomy is usually performed, the child who is of at least preschool age is told about the procedure in concrete terms, with the use of visual aids (see Chapter 22 for preparing a child for a colostomy). It is important to time explanations appropriately to prevent the anxiety and confusion that could result from too much information.

It is important to stress to parents and older children that the colostomy for Hirschsprung disease is temporary, unless so much bowel is involved that a permanent ileostomy must be performed. In most instances the extent of bowel resection is known before surgery, although the nurse should be aware of those instances when doubt exists concerning repair. The nurse should also keep in mind that although a temporary colostomy is favorable in terms of future health and adjustment, it also requires additional surgery, which may be very stressful to parents and children.

Postoperative Care.   Postoperative care is the same as for any child or infant with abdominal surgery (see Surgical Procedures, Chapter 22). When a colostomy is part of the corrective procedure, stomal care becomes a major nursing task (see Ostomies, Chapter 22). To prevent contamination of the abdominal wound with urine in the infant, the diaper should be pinned below the dressing. Sometimes a Foley catheter is used in the immediate postoperative period to divert the flow of urine away from the abdomen.

Discharge Care.   Postoperatively, parents need instruction concerning colostomy care. Even a preschooler can be included in the care by handing articles to the parent, rolling up the colostomy pouch after it is emptied, or applying barrier preparations to the surrounding skin. Although diagnosis of Hirschsprung disease is less frequent in school-age children or adolescents, if it is discovered in older children, they should be involved in colostomy care to the point of total responsibility.

Referral to a home health care agency establishes continuity of care, especially in relation to colostomy care and dietary management. The community nurse can also assist parents and children in anticipating subsequent surgery. Sometimes families require financial assistance and additional psychologic support. Therefore a referral to a social worker or other service agency may be necessary.*

See also Nursing Care Plan: The Child with Hirschsprung Disease (Megacolon).†

VOMITING

Vomiting, the forceful ejection of gastric contents through the mouth, is a well-defined, complex, coordinated process under central nervous system control. Often it is of a minor and temporary nature, but when vomiting is persistent and prolonged, the complications for the infant or child can be serious. Vomiting in childhood can be caused by numerous intrinsic and extrinsic factors but is usually the result of infections or psychologic causes.

viral agents - 12-36 hrs most

Therapeutic Management

Management is directed toward detection and treatment of the cause of the vomiting and prevention of complications from the loss of fluid. Fluids are administered in the same manner and in a similar electrolyte composition to those administered in diarrhea (see p. 807). Although most children respond well to these measures, antiemetic drugs may be needed. The specific antiemetic may block the receptors in the chemoreceptor trigger zone (ondansetron [Zofran], trimethobenzamide [Tigan]); enhance gastroduodenal peristalsis (metoclopramide [Reglan]); or compete for H_1-receptor sites (promethazine [Phenergan]). For children who are prone to motion sickness, it is often helpful to administer an appropriate dose of dimenhydrinate (Dramamine) before a trip.

Nursing Considerations

The major emphasis of nursing care of the vomiting infant or child is on observation and reporting of vomiting behavior and associated symptoms and the implementation of measures to reduce the vomiting. Accurate assessment of the type of vomiting, the appearance of the vomitus, and the child's behavior in association with the vomiting greatly aids in establishing a diagnosis of disorders that have vomiting as a clinical feature.

Nursing interventions are determined by the cause of the vomiting. When the vomiting is identified as a manifestation of improper feeding methods, establishing proper techniques through teaching and example will usually correct the situation. If the vomiting is assessed as a probable sign of a GI obstruction, food is usually withheld or special feeding techniques are implemented. In situations in which vomiting is related to concurrent infection, dietary indiscretion, or emo-

tional factors, efforts are directed toward maintaining hydration or preventing dehydration.

The thirst mechanism is the most sensitive guide to fluid needs, and ad libitum administration of a glucose-electrolyte solution to an alert child will restore water and electrolytes satisfactorily. It is important to include carbohydrate to spare body protein and to avoid ketosis resulting from exhaustion of glycogen stores. Once vomiting has abated, more liberal amounts of fluids can be offered, followed by simple foods such as gelatin, crackers, clear broth, and buttered toast in small portions, when the child desires, followed by gradual resumption of the regular diet.

The vomiting infant or child is positioned to prevent aspiration and observed for evidence of dehydration. It is important to emphasize the need for the child to brush the teeth or rinse the mouth after vomiting to dilute hydrochloric acid that comes in contact with the teeth. A flavored mouthwash or brushing also helps freshen the mouth. Careful monitoring of fluid and electrolyte status must be exercised to avoid the possibility of an electrolyte disturbance.

GASTROESOPHAGEAL REFLUX (GER)

GER can best be defined as the transfer of gastric contents into the esophagus. GER occurs in everyone; it is the frequency and persistence that make it abnormal. Approximately 1 in 300 to 1 in 1000 children have a significant problem. Earlier a great emphasis was placed on the resting or baseline *lower esophageal sphincter (LES) pressure.* Studies have been unable to show a relationship between baseline LES pressure and abnormal reflux. GER most likely occurs during transient and inappropriate relaxations of the LES. The exact cause is not known, but potential causes of this inappropriate relaxation of the LES may be related to the central nervous system (CNS) or to a developmentally exaggerated enteric reflex (Hillemeier, 1991). Several factors that cause the LES pressure to vary include gastric distention, increased abdominal pressure caused by coughing, CNS disease, delayed gastric emptying, hiatal hernia, and gastrostomy placement.

Some children are especially prone to developing GER. This condition may occur in children who have undergone tracheoesophageal or esophageal atresia repair, neurologic disorders, scoliosis, asthma, or cystic fibrosis.

Reflux of stomach contents to the esophagus predisposes to aspiration and the development of respiratory symptoms,

---

CLINICAL MANIFESTATIONS OF GASTROESOPHAGEAL REFLUX (GER)

Spitting up
Vomiting—can be quite forceful
Weight loss
Gagging, choking, at end of feeding
Respiratory problems
Hematemesis
Melena
Anemia
Heartburn/irritability
Apnea/acute life-threatening episode

---

*Home care instructions on caring for the child with a colostomy are available in Wong DL: *Wong and Whaley's Clinical manual of pediatric nursing,* ed 4, St Louis, 1996, Mosby.

†In Wong DL: *Wong and Whaley's Clinical manual of pediatric nursing,* ed 4, St Louis, 1996, Mosby.

Burned
Esophagel

particularly pneumonia. A particular concern is the association of life-threatening apnea with GER. Repeated irritation of the esophageal lining with gastric acid can lead to esophagitis and subsequent bleeding. Blood loss produces anemia and is seen as hematemesis or melena (blood in stools). Heartburn is also a frequent symptom in older children who are able to describe it, but it may go unrecognized in infants. (For a summary of clinical manifestations, see box.)

Diagnostic Evaluation

In addition to the history, several tests are available to establish the presence of reflux: observation of reflux following a barium swallow, 24-hour pH probe study, upper endoscopy, and scintigraphy (detects radioactive substances in the esophagus after a feeding of the compound and assesses gastric emptying).

Therapeutic Management

Therapeutic management of GER depends on its severity. No therapy is needed for the infant who is thriving and without respiratory complications. Some children require modification of feeding with small, frequent feedings of thickened formula and positioning therapy, which may help minimize the symptoms until the child grows and a normal physiologic barrier to reflux develops.

Controversies surround thickened feedings as a treatment for GER. Small, frequent feedings and frequent burping are generally accepted as reasonable strategies to minimize reflux. Constant nasogastric feedings may be necessary for the infant with severe reflux and failure to thrive. Feedings thickened with 1 teaspoon to 1 tablespoon of rice cereal per ounce of formula may be recommended as an initial measure to manage GER. The added calories may benefit the infant with GER.

Several studies have examined the effectiveness of positioning therapy for infants with GER. Traditionally, the upright position in an infant seat was recommended for infants with GER. Later, a head-elevated prone position maintained by use of an upper body harness was found to be superior (Fig. 24-2). However, another study found no significant dif-

ferences between the flat prone and head-elevated prone positions and concluded that the head-elevated prone position is probably not worth the extra effort required to maintain this position (Orenstein, 1990). At this time the available information suggests that either the flat prone or the head-elevated prone position after feeding and at night is a reasonable measure for treating infants with GER. The supine position is not used because GER worsens when the infant lies on the back. This is an exception to the recommended supine sleep position for healthy infants to decrease the risk of sudden infant death syndrome (SIDS) (Orenstein, 1994). (See Chapter 11.)

Pharmacologic therapy is sometimes used as an adjunct therapy to treat infants and children with GER. H_2 antagonists, such as cimetidine (Tagamet), ranitidine (Zantac), or famotidine (Pepcid), have proved effective in reducing the amount of acid present in gastric contents and may prevent esophagitis. Omeprazole (Prilosec) more completely suppresses gastric acid secretions than do H_2 blockers; however, the long-term effects are not known. Metoclopramide (Reglan) has been found to increase resting LES pressure mildly and to increase rates of gastric emptying. However, side effects, including restlessness, drowsiness, and extrapyramidal reaction, may occur, and in some patients, metoclopramide may actually increase the number of reflux episodes.

Cisapride (Propulsid) increases LES pressure, promotes gastric emptying, and has fewer CNS side effects than metoclopramide. It is often the preferred medication for GER (Orenstein, 1992). Bethanechol has also been shown to increase LES pressure greatly, but it has not been proved to decrease reflux by pH probe studies. Bethanechol also has side effects, including respiratory symptoms such as wheezing.

Surgical management as a treatment for GER is selected for children with severe complications, such as recurrent aspiration pneumonia, apnea, and severe esophagitis, and in whom medical therapy has failed. The *Nissen fundoplication,* which involves a 360-degree wrap of the fundus of the stomach around the distal esophagus, is the most common surgical procedure. Fundoplication combined with pyloroplasty may be performed in children with GER who also have delayed gastric emptying. Unfortunately, complications can occur following fundoplication; therefore the decision to perform this procedure should be carefully considered. Postoperative problems include small bowel obstruction, retching, gas-bloat syndrome, and dumping syndrome. For children with neurologic impairment who are continuously tube fed, an alternative to fundoplication with gastrostomy tube placement is a nonsurgical percutaneous gastrojejunostomy and placement of a jejunostomy tube (Albanese and others, 1993).

Prognosis. The majority of infants with GER have a mild problem that generally improves by about 1 year of age and requires only medical therapy. If GER is severe and remains unsuccessfully treated, multiple complications can occur. Esophageal strictures caused by persistent esophagitis with scarring is one of the most significant complications. Recurrent respiratory distress with aspiration pneumonia is another serious complication that is an indication for surgery. Failure to thrive caused by GER can often be managed with medical therapy and nutritional support.

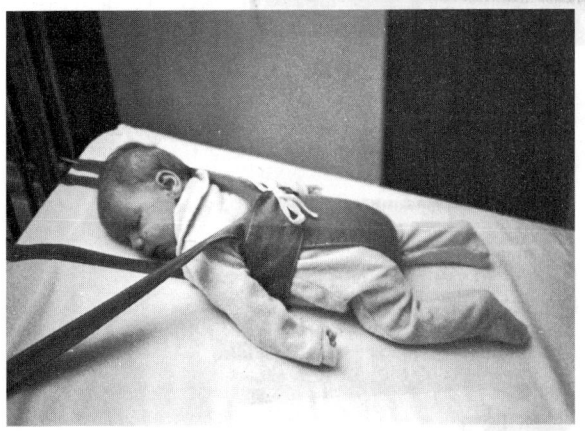

FIG. 24-2. Five-week-old infant positioned in harness. (From Orenstein SR, Whitington PF: Positioning for prevention of infant gastroesophageal reflux, *J Pediatr* 103:534-537, 1983.)

Nursing Considerations

Nursing care is directed at (1) identifying children with symptoms that suggest GER; (2) educating parents regarding home care, including feeding, positioning, and medications when indicated; and (3) if appropriate, providing care for the child undergoing surgical repair (see Surgical Procedures, Chapter 22).

To help parents cope with the inconvenience of dealing with a child who vomits frequently, simple measures such as using bibs and protective cloths during and after feeding are beneficial. The greatest challenge lies in maintaining the desired position for the child and adhering to a frequent feeding schedule. The 30-degree angle can be provided by elevating the head of the infant's crib with extra bedding, a wood or metal frame, or a wedge constructed from a cardboard box. An alternative is a specially constructed frame that can be moved about to allow the child a change of environment with minimum disturbance. The child is suspended from the head of the crib or frame in a prepared or improvised harness.

NURSING TIP An improvised harness can be made for the infant with GER using a baby blanket. The infant is placed prone on the blanket; the ends of the blanket are then brought up through the infant's legs, and all corners of the blanket are secured to the mattress with safety pins on either side of the infant's trunk.

When the infant is older and more mobile, maintaining correct positioning becomes increasingly difficult. An alternative frame has been described that consists of a cradle bed, bassinet, or board with a firm wooden base and a wooden spindle or large dowel that protrudes through the center of the mattress. To prevent undue pressure on areas such as the infant's knees and elbows, the mattress is covered with a sheepskin or soft blanket, and pressure areas are inspected for signs of redness.

Early in the treatment program, both parents and other available family members should be encouraged to participate in the feeding regimen, especially with alternate night shifts. Nurses need to be sensitive to the demands placed on the family and recognize those situations when hospitalization may be required to ensure continued treatment.

INFLAMMATORY DISORDERS

ACUTE APPENDICITIS

Appendicitis, inflammation of the *vermiform appendix* (blind sac at the end of the cecum), is the most common condition requiring abdominal surgery during childhood. Although uncommon in children younger than 2 years of age, it is associated with increased complications and mortality in this age-group. Primarily an acute condition, appendicitis rapidly progresses to perforation and peritonitis if it remains undiagnosed. It is a significant pediatric problem, because early diagnosis is frequently delayed as a result of the child's inability to verbalize symptoms; also, the clinical signs may be mistaken for other illnesses.

Etiology

The exact cause of appendicitis is poorly understood, but it is almost always a result of obstruction of the lumen, usually by a *fecalith* (hard fecal material). Sometimes a fold of peritoneum causes the appendix to adhere to the cecum, resulting in an obstructive kink. Other causes include lymphoid hyperplasia, fibrous stenosis from an earlier inflammation, and tumors. Parasites and microorganisms are potential etiologic agents. Pinworms have not been shown to be a cause of appendicitis. Dietary habits may play a role. Children with high-fiber diets have a lower incidence of appendicitis than those whose fiber intake is low (Shandling, 1991). Fiber increases the bulk and softness of the stool—a factor that minimizes the chance of obstruction and promotes evacuation.

Pathophysiology

With acute obstruction the outflow of mucus secretions is blocked and pressure builds within the lumen, resulting in compression of blood vessels. The resulting ischemia is followed by ulceration of the epithelial lining and bacterial invasion. Subsequent necrosis causes perforation or rupture with fecal and bacterial contamination of the peritoneal cavity. The resulting inflammation spreads rapidly throughout the abdomen (*peritonitis*), especially in young children who are unable to localize infection. Progressive peritoneal inflammation results in functional intestinal obstruction of the small bowel (*ileus*) because intense GI reflexes severely inhibit bowel motility. Since the peritoneum represents a major portion of total body surface, the loss of ECF to the peritoneal cavity leads to electrolyte imbalance and hypovolemic shock.

Diagnostic Evaluation

Diagnosis is based primarily on the history and physical examination (see box). The total white blood cell count (WBC) and the percentage of neutrophils are usually elevated. The WBC is seldom higher than 15,000 to 20,000/mm^3, and radiographic studies of the abdomen may reveal possible contributing causes of appendicitis, such as fecaliths or a foreign body.

Pain, the cardinal feature, is initially generalized (usually periumbilical); however, it usually descends to the lower right quadrant. The most intense site of pain may be at *McBurney point*, located at a point midway between the anterior superior iliac crest and the umbilicus. Rebound tenderness is not

---

CLINICAL MANIFESTATIONS OF APPENDICITIS

Right lower quadrant abdominal pain
Fever
Rigid abdomen
Decreased or absent bowel sounds
Vomiting (typically follows onset of pain)
Constipation or diarrhea may be present
Anorexia
Tachycardia, rapid shallow breathing
Pallor
Lethargy
Irritability
Stooped posture

a reliable sign and is extremely painful to the child. Referred pain, elicited by light percussion around the perimeter of the abdomen, indicates the presence of peritoneal irritation. Movement, such as riding over bumps in an automobile or gurney, aggravates the pain. In addition to pain, probably the most significant clinical manifestations are a change in behavior, anorexia, and vomiting.

Abdominal radiographs may aid in the diagnosis of appendicitis, such as the finding of a fecalith. Ultrasonography should be used to differentiate pediatric abdominal pain from other causes. Findings such as visualization of the appendix and presence of fluid around the appendix are important sonographic signs (Borowski, 1994).

Numerous infectious processes have features in common. For example, fever, vomiting, abdominal pain, and an elevated blood count are associated with inflammatory bowel disease, pelvic inflammatory disease, gastroenteritis, urinary tract infection, right lower lobe pneumonia, constipation, mesenteric adenitis, Meckel diverticulum, and intussusception. Fever is usually present, varying from 37.5° to 38.5° C (99.5° to 101.5° F). If the temperature is greater than 39° C (102.2° F), a viral illness or perforation is likely. Prolonged symptoms and delayed diagnosis may occur in preschool children, most likely because of their inability to verbalize their complaints clearly. Consequently, the risk of perforation is greater. *If pain stops abruptly think ruptured.*

> **Nursing ALERT**
> Signs of peritonitis in addition to fever include sudden relief from pain after perforation, subsequent increase in pain (usually diffuse and accompanied by rigid guarding of the abdomen), progressive abdominal distention, tachycardia, rapid shallow breathing, pallor, chills, and irritability.

Therapeutic Management

The definitive treatment of appendicitis before perforation is surgical removal of the appendix *(appendectomy)*. However, fluid and electrolyte imbalances need to be corrected before surgery, since the child is likely to be dehydrated as a result of the marked anorexia characteristic of appendicitis. Recovery is rapid, and if no complications occur, the child is discharged within 2 or 3 days.

Ruptured Appendix. Management of the child diagnosed with peritonitis caused by a ruptured appendix often begins preoperatively with IV administration of fluid and electrolytes, systemic antibiotics, and nasogastric (NG) suction. Postoperative management includes IV fluids, continued administration of antibiotics, and NG suction for abdominal decompression until intestinal activity returns. The child with peritonitis is given antibiotics, including ampicillin, gentamicin, and clindamycin, for 7 to 10 days.

In some instances the wound is closed following irrigation of the peritoneal cavity. Many surgeons, however, leave the wound open (delayed closure) to prevent wound infection. A Penrose drain may be used to permit transperitoneal drainage. When delayed closure is used, wound irrigations and wet-to-dry dressings are a routine part of postoperative care.

Prognosis. Complications occur infrequently after a simple appendectomy, and recovery is usually rapid and complete. The mortality rate from perforating appendicitis has improved from nearly certain death a century ago to 1% or less at present. Complications, however, do occur. Wound infection and intraabdominal abscess may complicate a perforated appendix. The key to reducing complications from appendicitis is the early recognition of the illness.

Nursing Considerations

❖ Assessment

Since abdominal pain is the most common childhood complaint with appendicitis, the nurse needs to make some preliminary evaluation of the severity of pain (see Chapter 21 for assessment of pain). One of the most reliable estimates is the degree of change in behavior. For example, a child who stays home from school and voluntarily lies down or refuses to play is much more likely to have considerable discomfort than the child who is absent from school but plays contentedly at home. The younger, nonverbal child will assume a rigid, motionless, side-lying posture with the knees flexed on the abdomen, and there is decreased range of motion of the right hip. Older children may exhibit all of these behaviors while complaining of abdominal pain. They can always indicate a point at which the pain is worse than at any other location.

❖ Nursing Diagnoses

Based on a thorough assessment, a number of nursing diagnoses become evident. The more likely diagnoses are listed in the box. Others will be apparent in specific circumstances.

❖ Planning

The goals of care for the child with a simple appendectomy include the following:

1. Child and family will be prepared for surgical intervention.
2. Child will receive postoperative care as described for the child undergoing surgery in Chapter 22.
3. Child with peritonitis will not experience postoperative complications, such as spread of infection.
4. Child and family will receive support and education.

❖ Implementation

Physical preparation of the child with appendicitis is the same as that for any child undergoing surgery.

> **Nursing ALERT**
> In any instance when severe abdominal pain is expected, be aware of the danger of administering laxatives or enemas or applying heat to the area. Such measures stimulate bowel motility and increase the risk of perforation.

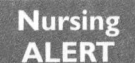

NURSING DIAGNOSES: THE CHILD WITH APPENDICITIS
Pain related to inflamed appendix
High risk for fluid volume deficit related to decreased intake and losses secondary to loss of appetite, vomiting
High risk for infection related to possibility of rupture
Altered family processes related to illness and hospitalization of a child

NURSING CARE PLAN
The Child with Appendicitis

Preoperative Care

NURSING DIAGNOSIS: Pain related to inflamed appendix

PATIENT GOAL 1: Will experience no pain or reduction of pain to level acceptable to child

- **NURSING INTERVENTIONS/*RATIONALES***

See Pain Assessment; Pain Management, Chapter 21
Allow position of comfort (usually with legs flexed) *because it may vary among children*
Provide small pillow *for splinting of abdomen*
*Administer analgesia *to provide pain relief*

- **EXPECTED OUTCOME**

Child rests quietly, reports and/or exhibits no evidence of discomfort

NURSING DIAGNOSIS: High risk for fluid volume deficit related to decreased intake and losses secondary to loss of appetite, vomiting

PATIENT GOAL 1: Will receive fluids for adequate hydration

- **NURSING INTERVENTIONS/*RATIONALES***

Maintain NPO *to minimize losses through vomiting and minimize abdominal distention*
Maintain integrity of infusion site *for intravenous (IV) fluids and electrolytes*
*Administer IV fluids and electrolytes as prescribed
Monitor intake and output *to assess hydration*

- **EXPECTED OUTCOMES**

Child receives sufficient fluids to replace losses
Child exhibits signs of adequate hydration (specify)

NURSING DIAGNOSIS: High risk for infection related to possibility of rupture

PATIENT GOAL 1: Will experience minimized risk of infection

- **NURSING INTERVENTIONS/*RATIONALES***

Closely monitor vital signs, especially for increased heart rate and temperature and rapid, shallow breathing, *to detect ruptured appendix*
Observe for other signs of peritonitis (e.g., sudden relief of pain [sometimes] at time of perforation, followed by increased, diffuse pain and rigid guarding of the abdomen, abdominal distention, bloating, belching [from accumulation of air], pallor, chills, and irritability) *for appropriate treatment to be initiated*
Avoid administering laxatives or enemas, *since these measures stimulate bowel motility and increase risk of perforation*
Monitor WBC *as indicator of infection*

- **EXPECTED OUTCOMES**

Child remains free of symptoms of peritonitis
Signs of peritonitis are recognized early (specify)

---
*Dependent nursing action.

Postoperative Care

See Postoperative Care in Nursing Care Plan: The Child Undergoing Surgery, Chapter 22

Ruptured Appendix

NURSING DIAGNOSIS: High risk for spread of infection related to presence of infective organisms in abdomen

PATIENT GOAL 1: Will experience minimized risk of spread of infection

- **NURSING INTERVENTIONS/*RATIONALES***

Provide wound care and dressing changes as prescribed *to prevent infection*
Monitor vital signs and WBC *to assess presence of infection*
*Administer antibiotics as prescribed

- **EXPECTED OUTCOME**

Child demonstrates resolution of peritonitis, as evidenced by lack of fever, clean wound, normal WBC

NURSING DIAGNOSIS: High risk for injury related to absence of bowel motility

PATIENT GOAL 1: Will not experience abdominal distention, vomiting

- **NURSING INTERVENTIONS/*RATIONALES***

Maintain NPO in early postoperative period *to prevent abdominal distention and vomiting*
Maintain nasogastric tube decompression *until bowel motility returns*
Assess abdomen for distention, tenderness, presence of bowel sounds *to assess presence of peristalsis*
Monitor passage of flatus and stool *as indicator of bowel motility*

- **EXPECTED OUTCOME**

Child does not exhibit signs of discomfort; abdomen remains soft and nondistended; child does not vomit

NURSING DIAGNOSIS: Altered family processes related to illness and hospitalization of child

PATIENT (FAMILY) GOAL 1: Will receive adequate support

- **NURSING INTERVENTIONS/*RATIONALES***

Encourage expression of feelings and concerns *to enhance coping*
Encourage child to discuss hospital admission and treatments *in order to clarify misconceptions*
See Nursing Care Plan: The Child in the Hospital, Chapter 21
See Nursing Care Plan: The Family of the Ill or Hospitalized Child, Chapter 21

- **EXPECTED OUTCOMES**

Child and family express feelings and concerns
Child and family demonstrate understanding of hospitalization and treatments

Postoperative Care.   Postoperative care for the non-perforated appendix is the same as for most abdominal procedures. Care of the child with a ruptured appendix and peritonitis involves more complex care. The course of recovery is considerably longer, usually 7 to 10 days of hospitalization.

The child is maintained on IV fluids, allowed nothing by mouth, and kept on low continuous gastric decompression until there is evidence of intestinal activity. Listening for bowel sounds and observing for other signs of bowel activity (e.g., passage of stool) are part of the routine assessment. Management of IV therapy is the same as for any child receiving fluids and parenteral antibiotics.

Frequent dressing changes are usually needed, as well as meticulous skin care to prevent excoriation of the area surrounding the surgical site. Often wound care includes irrigation with antibacterial solution.

Psychologic care of the child and parents is similar to that used in other emergency situations (see Emergency Admission, Chapter 21). Parents and older children need an opportunity to express their feelings and concerns regarding the events surrounding the illness and hospitalization. The nurse can provide important education and psychosocial support to promote adequate coping, with alleviation of anxiety for both the child and the family.

❖ Evaluation

The effectiveness of nursing interventions is determined by continual reassessment and evaluation of care based on the following observational guidelines:

1. Observe child preoperatively for reaction to the situation and compliance with care.
2. Observe for documentation regarding child's emotional and physical needs, especially assessment of pain and administration of analgesics.
3. Monitor child for evidence of infection.
4. Interview and observe child and family for evidence of their understanding of the condition, especially its sudden onset and the need for surgery.

Expected outcomes:
See Nursing Care Plan, p. 822.

MECKEL DIVERTICULUM

Meckel diverticulum is a remnant of the fetal omphalomesenteric duct that connects the yolk sac with the primitive midgut during fetal life. Normally this structure is obliterated by the seventh to eighth week of gestation, when the placenta replaces the yolk sac as the source of nutrition for the fetus. Failure of obliteration may result in an *omphalomesenteric fistula* (a fibrous band connecting the small intestine to the umbilicus, known as Meckel diverticulum).

Meckel diverticulum is a true diverticulum because it arises from the antimesenteric border of the small intestine, and all layers of the intestinal wall are present. The diverticulum is usually found within 100 cm (40 inches) of the ileocecal valve and averages 1 to 10 cm (⅖ to 4 inches) in length (Turgeon and Barnett, 1990).

Meckel diverticulum is the most common congenital malformation of the GI tract and is present in 1% to 3% of the population. It is twice as common in males as in females, and complications are several times more frequent in males. Most symptomatic cases are seen in childhood.

Pathophysiology

The symptomatic complications of Meckel diverticulum are caused by bleeding, obstruction, or inflammation. Gastric mucosa is the most common ectopic tissue found in Meckel diverticulum. Bleeding, which is the most common problem in children, is caused by peptic ulceration or perforation because of the unbuffered acidic secretion. Several mechanisms may cause obstruction. Intussusception may be led by the diverticulum. Obstruction may also be caused by entanglement of the small intestine around a fibrous cord, trapping of a loop of intestine under the band, incarceration within a hernia sac, or volvulus of the intestinal segment containing the diverticulum. Diverticulitis occurs when peptic ulceration or obstruction leads to inflammation.

Diagnostic Evaluation

Diagnosis is usually based on the history, physical examination, and radiographic studies. The signs and symptoms reflect the pathologic process as, for example, intestinal obstruction. Acute diverticulitis presents the same clinical picture as acute appendicitis, although the pain may be vague and recurrent (see box). In the pediatric population, bleeding most frequently appears as dark-red or "currant jelly" stools and is frequently severe enough to require transfusion. Abdominal radiographs, barium enema, and arteriography have generally been unsuccessful as aids to diagnosis. A specific nuclear scintigraphic study, which detects the presence of gastric mucosa, is the most sensitive and specific noninvasive test for Meckel diverticulum, with an overall diagnostic accuracy of 90% (Turgeon and Barnett, 1990). Blood studies are usually part of the general laboratory workup to rule out any bleeding disorders and to evaluate the severity of the anemia.

Therapeutic Management

The standard treatment is surgical removal of the diverticulum. When severe hemorrhage increases the surgical risk, medical intervention to correct hypovolemic shock, such as blood replacement, IV fluids, and oxygen, may be necessary. In diverticulitis, antibiotics may be used preoperatively to control infection. If intestinal obstruction has occurred, appropriate preoperative measures are used to reverse electrolyte imbalances and prevent abdominal distention.

CLINICAL MANIFESTATIONS OF MECKEL DIVERTICULUM

Abdominal Pain
Similar to appendicitis
May be vague and recurrent

Bloody Stools*
Painless
Bright or dark red with mucus ("currant jelly" stool)
In infants, bleeding may be accompanied by pain

Sometimes
Severe anemia
Shock

*Often a presenting sign.

Prognosis. If Meckel diverticulum is diagnosed and treated early, full recovery is likely. The mortality rate of untreated Meckel diverticulum has been reported to range from 2.5% to 15%. The serious complications of untreated Meckel diverticulum include GI hemorrhage and bowel obstruction.

Nursing Considerations

Nursing objectives are the same as for any child undergoing surgery (see Chapter 22). Since the onset is usually rapid, psychologic support parallels that for other conditions, such as appendicitis. It is important to remember that the massive intestinal bleeding is most often traumatic to both the child and the parent and may significantly affect their emotional reaction to hospitalization and surgery.

Specific preoperative considerations when intestinal bleeding is present include (1) frequent monitoring of vital signs and blood pressure for shock, (2) keeping the child on bed rest, and (3) recording the approximate amount of blood lost in stools. In the absence of frank hemorrhage, the nurse tests the stools for occult blood.

INFLAMMATORY BOWEL DISEASE (IBD)

The general term *inflammatory bowel disease* is used to designate two chronic intestinal disorders: *ulcerative colitis (UC)* and *Crohn disease (CD)*. Although these two diseases are classified as IBD because of their similar epidemiologic, immunologic, and clinical features, they are two distinct conditions with significant differences (Table 24-4). The most important reason for differentiating between the two is the prognosis. CD is considered the more serious and disabling disorder, and medical/surgical treatment is less effective than in UC. Growth failure is a unique and important feature of IBD in the pediatric population.

CD is now more common than UC. Between 25% and 40% of patients with CD and 15% and 40% of patients with UC are diagnosed in childhood and adolescence.

Etiology

The etiology of IBD is unknown, although there is evidence for a multifactorial etiology. The current hypothesis is that IBD is the result of a genetically determined susceptibility that may be promoted by one or more environmental influences. The inflammatory response is probably immunologically mediated. A primary role for psychologic factors in the pathogenesis of IBD has not been supported by evidence, although psychologic problems may occur secondary to IBD and may intensify symptoms and influence the course of the disease.

Several genetic and environmental factors influence the incidence of IBD: (1) there is a familial tendency in about 20% to 25% of patients; (2) more whites than nonwhites are affected; (3) the incidence is several times greater in Jews living in Europe and North America than in the general population; and (4) there is a higher occurrence of the disease in children living in urban settings than in those living in rural areas.

Pathophysiology: Ulcerative Colitis

The inflammation in UC is limited to the colon and rectum. The distal colon and rectum are often the most severely affected, producing bloody diarrhea or occult fecal blood, abdominal pain, and varying degrees of systemic manifestations and growth abnormalities (Jackson and Grand, 1991). Inflammation usually is limited to the mucosa and involves continuous segments along the length of the bowel, with varying degrees of ulceration, bleeding, and edema. In long-standing disease the bowel becomes narrowed, smooth, and inflexible with thin or absent mucosa heavily infiltrated by scar tissue.

Pathophysiology: Crohn Disease

CD is a chronic inflammatory process that may involve any part of the GI tract from mouth to anus but most often affects the terminal ileum. The disease characteristically involves all layers of the bowel wall (transmural). Acute edema and inflammation eventually progress to deep, transverse, or longitudinal ulcerations often associated with fissure formation. The inflammation may result in ulcerations, fibrosis, adhesions, stiffening of the bowel wall, stricture formation, and fistulas to other loops of bowel, bladder, vagina, or skin.

Diagnostic Evaluation

Diagnosis is suspected on the basis of the history and physical examination and is usually confirmed by endoscopic examination. A barium enema and small bowel series are often helpful, and mucosal biopsy is useful in demonstrating char-

---

TABLE 24-4. Clinical manifestations of inflammatory bowel diseases (IBDs)

CHARACTERISTICS	ULCERATIVE COLITIS	CROHN DISEASE
Rectal bleeding	Common	Uncommon
Diarrhea	Often severe	Moderate to absent
Pain	Less frequent	Common
Anorexia	Mild or moderate	Can be severe
Weight loss	Moderate	Severe
Growth retardation	Usually mild	Often marked
Anal and perianal lesions	Rare	Common
Fistulas and strictures	Rare	Common
Rashes	Mild	Mild
Joint pain	Mild to moderate	Mild to moderate

acteristic bowel changes. Stool examination is performed to rule out infections. Blood tests are completed and include a CBC with differential, serum iron, total protein, albumin, and erythrocyte sedimentation rate (ESR).

Therapeutic Management

The goals of therapy are as follows: (1) control the inflammatory process to reduce or eliminate the symptoms, (2) obtain long-term remission, (3) promote normal growth and development, and (4) allow as normal a life-style as possible. Treatment must be individualized and managed according to the severity of the disease, its location, and the response to therapy.

Medical Treatment. The drug sulfasalazine has proved useful in decreasing the frequency of recurrences in patients with mild cases of IBD. Because it interferes with the absorption and utilization of folic acid, daily supplements of folic acid are prescribed. Side effects of sulfasalazine include headache, nausea, vomiting, neutropenia, and oligospermia. Sulfasalazine is a combination of 5-aminosalicylate and sulfapyridine. Since many of the side effects are caused primarily by the sulfapyridine, alternative nonabsorbable salicylate drugs are being studied.

Corticosteroids are the most important and effective drugs for treating moderate and severe IBD. Among the newer corticosteroids, budesonide (Rhinocort) has emerged as the most promising (Sachar, 1994). High doses are administered for acute episodes and then are tapered according to the clinical response. Although high doses of corticosteroids can also interfere with growth, significant growth can be achieved with judicious management and maintenance of optimum nutrition. Sometimes steroid enemas are helpful in reducing the need for systemic administration for children with rectosigmoid involvement. Hospitalization and administration of IV corticosteroids are prescribed for severe disease. Some of the complications of high-dose steroid therapy include hypertension, osteoporosis, glaucoma, cataracts, hirsutism, diabetes, and altered body composition.

Other drugs include metronidazole for treatment of perianal CD; antispasmodic agents, which sometimes help relieve the discomfort of diarrhea and cramping; and immunosuppressive agents, which are effective in patients receiving high-dose corticosteroids. 6-Mercaptopurine, azathioprine, and cyclosporine A have been used with success in selected patients with IBD. The major risks of these drugs include immunosuppression and bone marrow suppression, which can cause leukopenia and opportunistic infections.

Nutritional Support. Increasing evidence supports the importance of nutritional therapy as an adjunctive, if not primary, therapy in children with IBD. Malnutrition is a common feature of IBD. The major complications of malnutrition in children and adolescents is the alteration in body composition and the disturbance in growth and sexual maturation. Nutritional deficiency is characterized by protein-energy malnutrition and multiple vitamin (vitamins B and D) and mineral (calcium, magnesium, iron, and zinc) deficiencies. Growth failure is characterized by weight deficits, alteration in body composition, linear growth retardation, and delayed sexual maturation. Growth failure affects approximately one third of pediatric patients with IBD and is significantly more common in children with CD than in those with UC.

The etiology of malnutrition is multifactorial and includes inadequate dietary intake, excessive GI losses, malabsorption, and increased nutritional requirements. Inadequate dietary intake results from the anorexia associated with chronic illness and episodes of increased inflammatory activity. Excessive losses of nutrients occur secondary to intestinal mucosal inflammation and diarrhea. Stool losses include protein, blood, electrolytes, and minerals. Malabsorption is common with IBD, particularly in CD, because of mucosal injury and bacterial overgrowth. Carbohydrate, lactose, fat, vitamin, and mineral malabsorption can occur. Vitamin B_{12} and folic acid deficiencies are common in patients with disease or resection of the terminal ileum. Nutritional requirements are increased with increased inflammatory activity, fever, and fistulas and during periods of rapid growth, such as adolescence.

The goals of nutritional support include (1) correction of specific nutrient deficits and replacement of ongoing losses, (2) provision of adequate energy and protein for healing, and (3) provision of adequate nutrients to promote normal growth. Nutritional support may include both enteral and parenteral nutrition. A well-balanced, high-protein, high-calorie diet is recommended for children whose symptoms do not prohibit an adequate oral intake. There is little evidence that avoiding specific foods influences the severity of the disease. Supplementation with multivitamins, iron, and folic acid is generally recommended.

Special enteral formulas, given either by mouth or by continuous NG infusion (often at night), may be required. Elemental formulas have been used successfully to improve nutritional status, as well as to induce remission in children and adolescents with CD. Elemental formulas are completely absorbed in the small intestine with almost no residue. Several studies have demonstrated that a diet consisting only of elemental formula not only improved nutritional status but also induced disease remission, either without steroids or with a diminished dosage of steroids required. An elemental diet is a safe and potentially effective primary therapy for patients with CD.

Total parenteral nutrition (TPN) has been shown to improve nutritional status in patients with IBD. Short-term remissions have been achieved following TPN, although complete bowel rest has not been proved to reduce inflammation or to add to the benefits of improved nutrition by TPN (Jackson and Grand, 1991). Nutritional support in patients with UC is less likely to induce a remission than in patients with CD. Improvement of nutritional status is important, however, in preventing deterioration of the patient's health status and in preparing the patient for surgery.

Surgical Treatment. UC can be cured by performance of a total colectomy. Surgery is indicated when medical and nutritional therapies fail to prevent significant complications. Surgical options include a *subtotal colectomy* and *ileostomy,* which leaves a rectal stump as a blind pouch; the *J-pouch or Kock pouch,* consisting of terminal ileum, which aids in continence; and an *ileoanal pull-through,* which preserves the normal pathway for defecation.

Surgery is required by children with CD when complications cannot be controlled by medical and nutritional therapy. Local resection is not curative, however, since the disease tends to recur, and further surgery may be needed.

Prognosis. IBD is a chronic disease. Relatively long periods of quiescent disease may follow exacerbations. The outcome of the disease process is influenced by the regions and severity of GI involvement, as well as by appropriate therapeutic management. Malnutrition, growth failure, and GI bleeding are serious complications of the disease. The overall prognosis for UC is good.

The development of carcinoma of the colon is a long-term complication of IBD. In UC, removal of the diseased bowel prevents development of carcinoma. In CD, however, surgical removal of the affected bowel does not prevent bowel cancer; therefore routine screening of stool specimens is needed for early detection.

Nursing Considerations

Many of the nursing considerations relate directly to the therapeutic management in treating IBD colitis. However, the scope of nursing responsibilities extends beyond the immediate period of hospitalization and involves (1) continued guidance of families in terms of dietary management, (2) coping with those factors that increase stress and emotional lability, (3) adjusting to a disease of remissions and exacerbations or one of chronic ill health, and (4) when indicated, preparing the child and parents for the possibility of diversionary bowel surgery.

Since diet therapy is very important, the nurse and nutritionist should collaborate to provide dietary counseling for the child and family members. Encouraging the anorexic child to consume sufficient quantities of this diet is of primary importance and is frequently a nursing challenge. An approach that is more likely to meet with success involves including the child in meal planning; encouraging small, frequent meals or snacks rather than three large meals a day; serving meals around medication schedules when diarrhea, mouth pain, and intestinal spasm are controlled; and preparing high-protein, high-calorie foods, such as eggnog, milkshakes, cream soups, puddings, or custard (if lactose is tolerated) (see also Feeding the Sick Child, Chapter 22). Foods that are known to aggravate the condition are avoided. The routine practice of using bran or a high-fiber diet for IBD is under question. Currently, bran, even in small amounts, has been shown to worsen the patient's condition (Francis and Whorwell, 1994). Occasionally the occurrence of aphthous stomatitis further complicates adherence to dietary management. Good mouth care before eating and the selection of bland foods help relieve the discomfort of mouth sores.

Nurses have an important role in preparing children and families to administer NG feedings or TPN when indicated. The purpose and the expected outcomes of these therapies should be carefully explained. The child's and family members' anxieties should be acknowledged, and they should be given adequate time to demonstrate the skills necessary to continue the therapy at home if needed.* (See Critical Thinking Exercise.)

The importance of continued drug therapy despite remission of symptoms must be stressed to the parents and child. Failure to adhere to the pharmacologic regimen can result in

---

*Home care instructions on gastrostomy feedings and caring for a central venous catheter (for TPN) are available in Wong DL: *Wong and Whaley's Clinical manual of pediatric nursing,* ed 4, St Louis, 1996, Mosby.

CRITICAL THINKING EXERCISE
Inflammatory Bowel Disease (IBD)

A 13-year-old girl is admitted to the hospital because of bloody diarrhea, abdominal pain, and weight loss. After a thorough evaluation, including laboratory tests, radiographic studies, and GI endoscopy procedures, the diagnosis of Crohn disease (CD) is made. Medical treatment, including corticosteroid drugs and nutritional support, is initiated in the hospital. Enteral formula administered by continuous nighttime nasogastric (NG) tube infusion and vitamin and mineral supplements will need to be continued at home after the hospitalization. All the following interventions are important preparations for successful home care *except:*

1. Educate the adolescent and family regarding the disease process.
2. Educate the adolescent and family regarding medication therapy and administration of NG tube feedings.
3. Provide psychosocial support to aid in the adjustment to a chronic disease of remissions and exacerbations.
4. Restrict school attendance and extracurricular activities for the duration of home therapy.

The correct answer is four. School absences or inability to compete with peers in some activities may occur during exacerbations of the disease, but self-esteem, positive school performance, and social interactions can be enhanced through support and guidance by the family and health care providers. Once the acute disease exacerbation is under control, the adolescent should be encouraged to resume school attendance and participate with peers in activities of interest. Important nursing responsibilities include educating the adolescent and her family regarding the disease process and therapeutic management and promoting adjustment to the chronic nature of the disease. The importance of continued drug therapy as prescribed despite remission of symptoms should be emphasized. The purpose and expected outcomes of nutrition support therapy should be explained thoroughly. The adolescent and her family members should be given adequate time to demonstrate skills necessary to continue therapy at home. Referral to a home health agency to ensure continuity of care is often beneficial.

---

exacerbation of the disease process (see Chapter 22 for a discussion of compliance).

Family Support. Attending to the emotional components of a chronic disease requires a thorough assessment of disease-related stress factors. Frequently the nurse can be instrumental in helping these children adjust to the problems of growth retardation, delayed sexual maturation, dietary restrictions, feelings of being "different" or "sickly," inability to compete with peers, and necessary absence from school during exacerbations of the illness (see Chapter 18).

If a permanent colectomy/ileostomy is required, the nurse can assist the child and family in accepting and adjusting to the change by teaching them how to care for the ileostomy; by emphasizing the positive aspects of surgery, particularly accelerated growth and sexual development, permanent recovery, and eliminated risk of colonic cancer in UC; and by stressing the normality of life despite bowel diversion. Introducing the child and parents to other ostomy patients, especially those of the child's age, can be the greatest therapeutic measure in fostering eventual acceptance. Whenever possible, the newer continent ostomies should be offered as options to the child, although they are not performed in all centers throughout the United States.

Because of the chronic and often lifelong nature of the disease, families benefit from many of the services provided by organizations such as the **Crohn's and Colitis Foundation of America, Inc. (CCFA),*** which has branches in many major communities and provides education regarding the management of IBD. If diversionary bowel surgery is indicated, the **United Ostomy Association†** and the **Wound Ostomy and Continence Nurses Society‡** are available to assist with ileostomy care and provides important psychologic support through its self-help groups. Adolescents often benefit by participating in peer-support groups, which are sponsored in some areas by the CCFA.

See also Nursing Care Plan: The Child with Inflammatory Bowel Disease.§

PEPTIC ULCER

A peptic ulcer, or *peptic ulcer disease (PUD),* is an erosion of the mucosal wall of the stomach, pylorus, or duodenum. *Gastric ulcers* affect the lining of the stomach, whereas *duodenal ulcers* involve the pylorus or duodenum. Although peptic ulcers are more common in adults, they are also a significant pediatric problem, occurring at any age.

Ulcers are described as either primary or secondary. *Primary ulcers* occur in the absence of a predisposing factor. *Secondary ulcers,* or *stress ulcers,* result from the stress of a severe underlying disease or injury (e.g., severe burns, sepsis, multisystem organ failure) or from ingestion of an ulcerogenic drug (e.g., salicylates, nonsteroidal antiinflammatory agents [NSAIDs], ferrous sulfate). Stress ulcers occur more frequently in infancy and early childhood. In older children and adolescents the majority of ulcers are primary. The incidence of ulcers in boys is two to three times greater than in girls, although this difference is less in very young children.

Etiology

The exact cause of peptic ulcer is not always known, although infectious, genetic, and environmental factors are important in the etiology of peptic ulcers. A strong relationship exists between *Helicobacter pylori* (formerly *Campylobacter pylori*) and upper GI disease. Nearly all patients with duodenal ulcers have *H. pylori* gastritis. Therefore infection with the organism may be a prerequisite for the occurrence of almost all duodenal ulcers in the absence of other precipitating factors (NIH Consensus Development Panel, 1994). *H. pylori* may cause ulcers by weakening the gastric mucosal barrier and allowing acid to damage the mucosa. Genetic factors play a role in the etiology of PUD, and a positive relationship to blood group O exists. Several drugs are known to contribute to ul-

cer formation, including aspirin, NSAIDs, steroids, and alcohol. Smoking has also been associated with PUD. Psychologic factors may also play a role in the development of PUD. Stressful life events, dependency, passiveness, and hostility have all been implicated as contributing factors in PUD.

Pathophysiology

Most likely, the pathogenesis of PUD is caused by an imbalance between destructive factors that promote the formation of peptic ulcers and protective factors that guard against ulcer formation (Ziller and Netchvolodoff, 1993). The gastroduodenal epithelium secretes a water-insoluble mucous gel that serves as a protective barrier. It is a barrier to hydrogen ions, which are neutralized by the bicarbonate within the mucous gel. Prostaglandins appear to play a role in mucosal defense because they stimulate both mucus and alkali secretion. Abnormalities of the mucus-bicarbonate barrier are likely to contribute to ulcer formation. As a result of either of these two conditions, the gastric mucosa is highly vulnerable to the digestive effects of gastric juice. Prolonged contact with the highly acidic contents of the stomach and duodenum causes an erosion of the mucosal wall, especially in those areas least protected, such as the cardiac and lesser curve of the stomach and the area immediately beyond the pylorus.

Diagnostic Evaluation

Diagnosis is based on the history (pattern of pain) (see box), physical examination, and diagnostic testing such as radiographs and barium studies. Upper endoscopy is the most reliable tool to diagnose PUD. Other tests include blood studies (anemia), stool samples (occult blood), and occasionally, gastric acid measurements (to identify hypersecretion).

CLINICAL MANIFESTATIONS OF PEPTIC ULCER

Neonates (Usually Gastric)
Usually perforation
Often massive hemorrhage
Almost the same as seen in stress ulcers

Infants to 2-Year-Old Children (Gastric or Duodenal, Primary or Secondary)
Poor eating, vomiting, crying spells after feeding, abdominal distention, tarry stools, melena
Vague discomfort
Irritability
Usually bleed rather than perforate

2- to 6-Year-Old Children (Gastric or Duodenal)
May have vomiting related to eating, generalized or periumbilical pain, melena, hematemesis
Wake at night or early morning, crying with pain
Perforation more likely in secondary ulcers

6- to 9-Year-Old Children (Usually Duodenal and Primary)
Pain—burning or gnawing sensation in epigastrium related to fasting state, melena, hematemesis, vomiting
Often with obstruction

Over 9 Years (Usually Duodenal)
Same as above
More typical of adult type

---

*444 Park Ave., South, New York, NY 10016; (212) 679-1570.
†36 Executive Park, Suite 120, Irvine, CA 92714-6744; (714) 660-8624.
‡2755 Bristol St., Suite 110, Costa Mesa, CA 92626; (714)476-0268. In Canada: **Canadian Foundation for Crohn's and Colitis,** 21 St. Clair Ave., East, Suite 301, Toronto, Ontario M4TL 1L9, (416) 920-5035; **United Ostomy Association, Canada,** 5 Hamilton Ave., Hamilton, Ontario L8V 2L3.
§In Wong DL: *Wong and Whaley's Clinical manual of pediatric nursing,* ed 4, St Louis, 1996, Mosby.

Therapeutic Management

The objectives of therapy for children with peptic ulcers are to relieve discomfort, promote healing, prevent complications, and prevent recurrence. The management of ulcers is primarily medical and consists of administration of medications that reduce or neutralize gastric acid secretion and, when possible, implementation of measures to eliminate or reduce stresses.

Antacids may be used in the initial treatment of peptic ulcers. The antacid of choice, usually a liquid aluminum or magnesium preparation, is administered every 1 and 3 hours after each meal and at bedtime. The dosage is determined by the size of the child. As healing progresses, the frequency of administration is gradually reduced but not usually discontinued for several weeks. Diarrhea may be a side effect of large amounts of magnesium-containing antacids.

One of the histamine (H_2) receptor antagonists—cimetidine (Tagamet), ranitidine (Zantac), or famotidine (Pepcid)—is usually prescribed for the treatment of PUD. Omeprazole (Prilosec), an extremely potent gastric acid antisecretory agent, is also used. The general course of therapy is 4 to 6 weeks. A nightly maintenance dose may be given for 6 months. Each of these drugs suppresses pepsin and gastric acid secretion and provides for greater compliance because of the reduced frequency of administration compared with antacids.

Sucralfate, an aluminum salt of sucrose octasulfate, forms a protective barrier for ulcerated mucosa against acid and pepsin. Sucralfate does not come in liquid form, although the pill can be mixed with water and given with a syringe or spoon. This drug may be given four times per day for 6 weeks. *Bismuth compounds* are sometimes prescribed for the relief of ulcers. The mechanism of their activity is poorly understood, but they do have an effect on inhibiting the growth of microorganisms. Bismuth demonstrates activity against *H. pylori,* and the eradication of *H. pylori* from GI tissue has been associated with improved healing of ulcers. Bismuth does not eradicate the organism in all cases, and antiinfective agents may be used.

The child is provided with a nutritious diet but advised to avoid caffeine and alcohol. Since aspirin is known to have a damaging effect on gastric mucosa, acetaminophen is recommended as a substitute. Psychologic assistance may be required for children with overlying anxiety problems.

A child with an acute ulcer who has developed complications, such as massive hemorrhage, requires emergency care. Administration of IV fluids, blood, or plasma depends on the amount of blood loss. Blood replacement with whole blood or packed cells may be necessary for significant loss.

Surgical intervention may be required in the management of complications of PUD, such as hemorrhage, perforation, or gastric outlet obstruction. Ligation of the source of bleeding or closure of a perforation may be performed. A vagotomy and pyloroplasty may be indicated in children with recurring ulcers despite aggressive medical treatment.

Prognosis. The long-term prognosis for PUD is variable. Many ulcers can be successfully treated with medical therapy; however, primary duodenal peptic ulcers frequently recur. A high incidence of complications, such as GI bleeding, can occur and extend into adult life. The effect of maintenance drug therapy on long-term morbidity remains to be established with further studies.

Nursing Considerations

The main nursing objective is to promote healing of the ulcer through compliance with the medication regimen. The diet is usually quite liberal, with avoidance of any food that causes the child discomfort. Substances that may irritate the gastric wall are alcohol, tobacco, tea, coffee, and aspirin. Use of alcohol and tobacco may be an issue in adolescents with ulcers.

Drug compliance is essential and can be a problem with frequent administration of antacids. Therefore strategies to improve compliance are instituted early in the course of therapy (see Chapter 22). For traveling and during school, the use of antacid tablets rather than liquid is more convenient.

Although the exact role stress plays in the pathogenesis of ulcers in children is unclear, especially since many ulcers occur secondary to other conditions, the nurse should be aware of those family and environmental conditions that may have precipitated or may aggravate the condition. Children may benefit from psychologic counseling and from learning how to cope more constructively with stresses in their lives.

See also Nursing Care Plan: The Child with Peptic Ulcer Disease.*

HEPATIC DISORDERS

ACUTE HEPATITIS

Hepatitis, or inflammation of the liver, is rapidly emerging as one of the major causes of morbidity and a significant cause of mortality in children. The discussion that follows is focused primarily on acute hepatitis, although the chronic disease may involve many of the same mechanisms.

Etiology

Hepatitis in children may be caused by a virus, a chemical or drug reaction, or some other disease process. The majority (90%) of cases of viral hepatitis are caused by five viruses, including the following:

- Hepatitis A virus (HAV, previously designated infectious hepatitis)
- Hepatitis B virus (HBV, previously designated serum hepatitis)
- Hepatitis C virus (HCV, previously designated parenterally transmitted non-A, non-B hepatitis virus [PT-NANB])
- Hepatitis D virus (HDV, delta agent)
- Hepatitis E virus (enterically transmitted non-A, non-B hepatitis virus [ET-NANB])

In addition, cytomegalovirus (CMV), Epstein-Barr virus (EBV), and herpes simplex virus (HSV) may occasionally cause hepatitis. The clinical symptoms of these viruses are similar. Epidemiologic features and serologic testing are used to differentiate the causes. Table 24-5 compares the features of HAV, HBV, and HCV.

Hepatitis A. HAV is highly contagious and is transmitted from one person to another primarily by the fecal-oral route, usually from ingestion of contaminated food or water.

---

*In Wong DL: *Wong and Whaley's Clinical manual of pediatric nursing,* ed 4, St Louis, 1996, Mosby.

TABLE 24-5. Clinical manifestations of types A, B, and C hepatitis

CHARACTERISTICS	TYPE A	TYPE B	TYPE C
Onset	Usually rapid, acute	More insidious	Usually insidious
Fever	Common and early	Less frequent	Less frequent
Anorexia	Common	Mild to moderate	Mild to moderate
Nausea and vomiting	Common	Less common	Mild to moderate
Rash	Rare	Common	Sometimes present
Arthralgia	Rare	Common	Rare
Pruritus	Rare	Sometimes present	Sometimes present
Jaundice	Sometimes present	Present	Present

This includes eating shellfish caught in contaminated water and swimming in this water. Hepatitis A is usually an acute and mild illness. There is no known carrier state. HAV can affect individuals at any age but often is found in children under 15 years of age. Additional sources for children are day-care centers (especially those that have children in diapers) and custodial care facilities. School contacts are considered a relatively low risk. The incubation period is approximately 4 weeks.

Hepatitis B. HBV can cause a wide spectrum of acute and chronic infection, ranging from asymptomatic limited infection to fatal fulminant hepatitis. Transmission is usually via the parenteral route through the exchange of blood or any bodily secretion or fluid. Intimate physical contact and spread from mother to infant are potential sources of infection. Contaminated fluids splashed into the mouth or eyes can cause infection. HBV infection from blood transfusion has been reduced as a result of blood product–screening procedures. Transplanted organs can also serve as a source of HBV. Adults whose occupations are associated with considerable exposure to blood or blood products, such as health care workers, are at an increased risk of exposure and may choose to receive HBV vaccination. HBV infection occurs in children and adolescents in specific high-risk situations: (1) infants of mothers who are chronic carriers, (2) children with hemophilia and others who have received multiple transfusions, (3) children involved in IV drug abuse, (4) institutionalized children, and (5) preschool children in endemic areas. The incubation period ranges from 50 to 180 days.

Most HBV in children is acquired perinatally. Newborns are at risk for hepatitis if the mother is infected with HBV or was a carrier of HBV during pregnancy. Possible routes of maternal-fetal (-infant) transmission include (1) leakage of virus across the placenta late in pregnancy or during labor, (2) ingestion of amniotic fluid or maternal blood, and (3) breast-feeding, especially if the mother has cracked nipples.

Hepatitis C. HCV has been called "non-A, non-B hepatitis" because of the absence of HAV and HBV serologic markers of infection. HCV transmission appears to be largely parenteral, although other routes may occasionally be responsible (Carey and Patel, 1992). HCV is the primary cause of posttransfusion hepatitis, and before heat treatment of clotting factor concentrates, patients with hemophilia who needed replacement therapy were at risk for acquiring HCV (Kanesaki and others, 1993). The clinical course is variable. The incubation period ranges from 14 days to 6 months. Some children may be asymptomatic, but HCV often

becomes a chronic condition and can cause cirrhosis and hepatocellular carcinoma. About 50% of individuals infected with HCV develop chronic disease (Carey and Patel, 1992). Although aplastic anemia is a rare complication of all forms of viral hepatitis, it is more common with HCV.

Hepatitis D. HDV infection occurs in patients already infected with HBV. HDV, which can result in chronic hepatitis, is a defective ribonucleic acid (RNA) virus that requires the function of HBV. HDV infection occurs primarily in hemophiliac patients and IV drug abusers. Usually more severe than hepatitis B, HDV infection can lead to cirrhosis and death. The incubation period is most likely several weeks.

Hepatitis E. Hepatitis E is epidemic or enterally transmitted non-A, non-B hepatitis. Transmission may occur via contaminated water. This illness is not chronic, and there is no carrier state. However, it can be a devastating disease among pregnant women, with a mortality rate of 10% to 20% (Krugman, 1992).

Pathophysiology

The pathologic changes occur primarily in the parenchymal cells of the liver and result in variable degrees of swelling, infiltration of liver cells by mononuclear cells, subsequent degeneration, necrosis, and autolysis. Structural changes within the hepatocyte are thought to account for altered liver functions.

Hepatitis can be self-limited, and complete regeneration of liver cells without scarring may occur within 2 to 3 months. However, some forms of hepatitis do not result in complete return of liver function. These include *fulminant hepatitis,* which is characterized by a severe, acute course with hepatic necrosis and death frequently occurring within 1 to 2 weeks, and *subacute* or *chronic active hepatitis,* which is characterized by progressive liver destruction and uncertain regeneration with the possibility of scarring.

The initial *anicteric* (absence of jaundice) *phase* symptoms include nausea and vomiting, extreme anorexia, malaise, easy fatigability, and slight to moderate fever. The child may have abdominal pain, especially epigastric or upper right quadrant; usually acts ill, preferring to rest in bed; and is fretful or irritable. This phase usually lasts 5 to 7 days and may be mistaken for influenza.

The *icteric* (jaundice) *phase* begins with darkening of the urine and the presence of light-colored stools, followed by yellowing of the sclera and skin. As jaundice worsens, the child usually begins to feel better, with improved appetite and behavior and the absence of nausea, vomiting, and fever, although pruritus can be a bothersome symptom. The icteric phase typically lasts less than 4 weeks. Complete recovery with return of normal liver function and a feeling of well-being with absence of fatigue or malaise may take 1 to 3 months.

Diagnostic Evaluation

The clinical manifestations for most types of viral hepatitis are similar except for a more rapid, acute onset in type A and a slower, more insidious onset in type B (Table 24-5). Types A and B may present with flulike symptoms. Some may never be recognized as actual cases of hepatitis.

Diagnosis of hepatitis is based on the history (especially regarding possible exposure to a hepatitis virus), physical examination, serologic markers, and liver function tests. The diagnosis is confirmed by detection of antibodies or antigens formed in response to the specific virus, such as HBsAg (the hepatitis B surface antigen). During the initial infective period, anti-HAV of the immunoglobulin M (IgM) class is present, but after about 3 to 6 months, this antibody declines and anti-HAV of the IgG class increases. Therefore detection of anti-HAV IgM indicates active infection, and anti-HAV IgG indicates past infection and immunity (Krugman, 1992). Antibodies to different HCV antigens can also be detected (Kanesaki and others, 1993).

No liver function test is specific for hepatitis. Serum aspartate and alanine aminotransferase (AST, ALT) levels are greatly elevated. Serum bilirubin levels peak 5 to 10 days after clinical jaundice appears.

Therapeutic Management

There is no specific treatment for viral hepatitis. Management primarily includes treatment of symptoms. The value of bed rest in promoting overall recovery is controversial. Since children feel ill and tired in the anicteric phase, they usually choose to stay in bed. However, once improvement of physical complaints begins, children usually prefer to resume normal activity gradually. The best approach is probably to allow children to regulate their own pace. Precautionary measures are implemented to prevent spread of the infection.

Children are allowed to choose foods they prefer, especially during the initial stage when anorexia is severe. A special diet is generally not of value. Hospitalization is required if coagulopathy or fulminant hepatitis develops.

Steroid therapy should not be used. Human alpha-interferon has been used with some success in the treatment of chronic HBV and chronic HCV infections (Bacon, 1991). Antiviral drugs are currently being studied.

Prevention. Proper handwashing and standard isolation precautions can prevent spread of hepatitis. Prophylactic use of standard immune globulin (IG) is effective in preventing HAV infection in situations of preexposure (e.g., anticipated travel to areas where HAV is prevalent) or in situations of postexposure during the early part of the incubation period. Hepatitis B immune globulin (HBIG) is effective in preventing HBV infection after exposure. IGs must be administered less than 2 weeks after exposure.

Active immunizations are not available against the non-A, non-B viruses. However, vaccines have been developed to prevent HBV and HAV infection. HBV vaccination is recommended for all newborns and for high-risk groups (see Immunizations, Chapter 10). It is possible to prevent HDV by preventing HBV (Lisanti and Talotta, 1992).

Prognosis. The prognosis for children with hepatitis is variable and depends on the type of virus causing the disease. HAV usually causes a mild and brief illness with no carrier state. HBV can cause a wide spectrum of acute and chronic illness. Chronic HBV infection leads to cirrhosis in 25% to 30% of cases (Ergun and Miskovitz, 1990). Hepatocellular carcinoma is a potentially fatal complication of HBV infection. HCV infection frequently becomes chronic, and cirrhosis may develop in as many as 20% of these patients. Fulminant hepatic failure occurs in approximately 1% to 2% of cases of viral hepatitis, regardless of the etiology, and is associated with a mortality rate of 60% to 90%, with higher mortality in older children (Krugman, 1992).

Nursing Considerations

Nursing objectives depend largely on the severity of the hepatitis, the medical management, and factors influencing the control and transmission of the disease. Since children with benign viral hepatitis are frequently cared for at home, the responsibility of explaining any medical therapies and control measures is frequently left to the clinic or office nurse. When further assistance is needed for parents to comply with such instructions, a public health nursing referral may be necessary.

The emphasis is on encouraging a well-balanced diet and a realistic schedule of rest and activity adjusted to the child's condition. Since HAV is not infectious within a week or so after the onset of jaundice, the child may feel well enough to resume school shortly thereafter. The parents are also cautioned about administering any medication to the child, since normal doses of many drugs may become dangerous because of the liver's inability to detoxify and excrete them.

Handwashing is the single most critical measure in reducing risk of hepatitis transmission in any setting. The nurse should explain to parents and children the usual ways in which HAV (oral-fecal route) and HBV (parenteral route) are spread.

Children who are hospitalized are not usually isolated in a separate room unless they are fecally incontinent or their toys and other items might become contaminated with feces. They are discouraged from sharing their toys. (For further discussion, see Infection Control, Chapter 22.)

In children with HBV infection who have a known or suspected history of illicit drug use, the nurse has the additional responsibility of helping them realize the associated dangers of drug abuse, stressing the parenteral mode of transmission of hepatitis and encouraging them to seek counseling through a drug program.

See also Nursing Care Plan: The Child with Acute Hepatitis.*

CIRRHOSIS

Cirrhosis occurs as the end stage of many chronic liver diseases. Liver damage can be caused by infectious, autoimmune, toxic, or structural factors. Cirrhosis occurs as a result of cell injury, tissue repair, and regeneration. A cirrhotic liver is irreversibly damaged.

---

*In Wong DL: *Wong and Whaley's Clinical manual of pediatric nursing,* ed 4, St Louis, 1996, Mosby.

Clinical manifestations of cirrhosis develop from the features typically seen with all chronic liver disorders. Children with cirrhosis often exhibit jaundice, poor growth, anorexia, muscle weakness, and lethargy. Ascites, edema, GI bleeding, anemia, and abdominal pain may be present in children with impaired intrahepatic blood flow. Pulmonary function may be impaired in children with cirrhosis because of pressure against the diaphragm from hepatosplenomegaly and ascites. Dyspnea and cyanosis may occur, especially on exertion. Intrapulmonary arteriovenous shunts may develop, which can also cause hypoxemia. Spider angiomas and prominent blood vessels on the upper torso are often present.

Therapeutic Management

Therapy is directed primarily toward (1) frequent assessment of liver status with physical examination and liver function tests and (2) management of specific complications. The only successful treatment for end-stage liver disease and liver failure may be *liver transplantation,* which has improved the prognosis substantially for many children with cirrhosis. Average 4-year survival rates are about 64% following orthotopic liver transplantation (Lloyd-Still, 1991). Unfortunately, many children die while waiting for a suitable donor.

Prognosis. The success of liver transplantation has revolutionized the approach to liver cirrhosis. Liver failure and cirrhosis are currently indications for transplantation. Liver transplantation reflects the failure of other medical and surgical measures to prevent or treat cirrhosis. Careful monitoring of the child's condition and quality of life are necessary to evaluate the need for and timing of transplantation (see Family Focus box).

Nursing Considerations

Nursing objectives in caring for the child with cirrhosis depend on several factors, including the precipitating cause of the cirrhosis, the severity of complications, and the prognosis. Overall, the last factor has the greatest impact, because the prognosis for life is poor unless successful liver transplantation can be performed. Therefore nursing care of this child is similar to that for any child with a life-threatening illness (Chapter 18). Hospitalization is usually required when complications occur.

BILIARY ATRESIA

Biliary atresia, now referred to as *extrahepatic biliary atresia (EHBA),* is the atresia or absence of the bile ducts outside of the liver. This disease is a progressive inflammatory process that causes both intrahepatic and extrahepatic bile

duct fibrosis, resulting in eventual ductal obstruction. The incidence of EHBA is between 1 in 10,000 and 1 in 25,000 live births. There does not seem to be a racial or genetic predilection, although there is a female predominance of 1.4:1 (Karrer and others, 1990). Associated malformations include polysplenia, intestinal atresia, and malrotation of the intestine. EHBA, if untreated, usually leads to cirrhosis, liver failure, and death in the first 2 years of life. EHBA is categorized as either correctable or noncorrectable, depending on the anatomy of the extrahepatic biliary system. Correctable lesions involve distal atresia with a patent proximal portion of the extrahepatic duct or patency of the gallbladder, cystic duct, and common bile duct. Noncorrectable EHBA involves obstruction at the porta hepatis. The majority of cases of EHBA are noncorrectable.

Etiology/Pathophysiology

EHBA is a progressive obliterative process. The pathologic process may occur in fetal life or early in the postnatal period. Reports have indicated that EHBA is not seen in the fetus or stillborn or newborn infant (Fanaroff and Martin, 1992). The exact cause is unknown, although immune mechanisms or viral injury may be responsible. Inflammation is progressive, causing both intrahepatic and extrahepatic bile duct fibrosis and obstruction. Surgery to obtain effective bile drainage must be achieved within 2 to 3 months after birth to diminish progressive liver damage.

Little is known regarding the development and maintenance of intrahepatic bile ducts; therefore the exact cause of intrahepatic biliary disease is unknown. Intralobular ducts are lost over months or years. Varying degrees of cholestasis occur. Cirrhosis may or may not occur. Irritants and toxins, such as bile acids, are retained, which often causes severe pruritus. There may be marked hypercholesterolemia.

Diagnostic Evaluation

Diagnosis of biliary disease is based on the history, physical examination, and a variety of tests. Growth parameters and nutritional status should be assessed, since many of these infants and children have nutritional deficiencies and poor growth. The disease is suspected on the basis of clinical signs (see box). Blood tests, including CBC, electrolytes, bilirubin,

FAMILY FOCUS
End-Stage Liver Disease

In many cases the child and family must cope with an uncertain progression of the disease. The only hope for long-term survival may be liver transplantation. Transplantation can be very successful, but the waiting period may be long, and there are many more children in need of organs than there are donors. The nurse should recognize the unique stresses of coping with end-stage liver disease and waiting for transplantation and assist the family in coping with these stressors. The assistance of social workers and support from other parents can be very beneficial.

CLINICAL MANIFESTATIONS OF EXTRAHEPATIC BILIARY ATRESIA

Jaundice
    Earliest manifestation and most striking feature of disorder
    First observed in sclera
    May be present at birth
    Usually not apparent until age 2 to 3 weeks
Urine dark and stains diaper
Stools lighter than expected or white or tan
Hepatomegaly and abdominal distention common
Splenomegaly occurs later
Poor fat metabolism results in:
    Poor weight gain
    General failure to thrive
Pruritus
Irritability
Difficult to comfort infant

and liver enzymes, are obtained. Additional laboratory analyses, including alpha$_1$-antitrypsin level, TORCHS titers (see Defects caused by infectious agents, Chapter 9, p. 272), hepatitis serology, urine cytomegalovirus, and a sweat test, may be indicated to rule out other conditions that cause persistent cholestasis and jaundice. Abdominal ultrasonography allows evaluation of the liver and biliary system. Biliary patency can be determined with hepatobiliary scintigraphy. Liver biopsy evaluates hepatic pathology. Definitive diagnosis of EHBA is obtained during an exploratory laparotomy and an intraoperative cholangiogram.

Therapeutic Management

The major hope in care of these children is that the condition will benefit from surgery. Although successful surgical correction is possible in only a few cases of EHBA, surgery is most successful when performed early; therefore diagnosis is urgent. The surgical procedure for EHBA is *hepatoportoenterostomy (Kasai procedure)*, in which a segment of intestine is anastomosed to the resected porta hepatis to attempt bile drainage. There are several variations of this procedure. In approximately 80% to 90% of infants with EHBA who undergo surgery when younger than 10 weeks of age, bile drainage is achieved (Ryckman and others, 1993). However, progressive cirrhosis still occurs in many children, and up to 80% may eventually require liver transplantation (Laurent and others, 1990).

Medical management is primarily supportive. It is the method of choice for intrahepatic disease and supplemental to surgical therapy in EHBA. Medical management consists of a high-calorie formula containing fats that can be digested without bile (Pregestimil), as well as water-soluble vitamins. Phenobarbital may be given to promote bile flow. A low-salt diet and diuretics may reduce ascites formation. Ursodeoxycholic acid has been used successfully to treat pruritus and hypercholesterolemia in children with liver disease. Prophylactic antibiotics are given after the Kasai procedure to prevent ascending cholangitis.

Prognosis. Untreated EHBA results in progressive cirrhosis and death in all children at a mean age of 19 months. The Kasai procedure does improve the prognosis, but it is not a cure. Biliary drainage can be achieved if the surgery is done before the intrahepatic bile ducts are destroyed, usually by 8 weeks of age. Long-term survival has been reported in children who received the Kasai procedure (Toyosaka and others, 1993). Despite successful bile drainage, many children ultimately develop liver failure.

Pediatric liver disorders can be cured with successful liver transplantation. The advances in surgical techniques and the development of cyclosporine A and other antirejection drugs have significantly improved the success of transplantation. The 1- to 4-year survival rate of pediatric liver transplantation is now 70% to 88% in most centers (Ryckman and others, 1993). The major obstacle remains the shortage of donor livers. Success with segmental size reduction of adult donor livers and increased public awareness may improve the availability of donor organs for children in the future.

Nursing Considerations

Nursing care of the infant with EHBA is primarily supportive. Initially the infant is not uncomfortable and requires care suited to any infant of the same age. As the disease progresses, the accumulation of toxic products causes the child to become irritable, restless, and difficult to comfort. Efforts are extended to allow as much sleep and rest as possible. The child is cared for when he or she awakes and is provided with comfort measures.

During the diagnostic phase of the illness the nurse assists with tests and procedures as ordered. The child who has undergone exploratory or corrective surgery is given the same care as any infant following abdominal surgery. Parental teaching includes administration of antibiotics and observation for signs of cholangitis. Families of children with liver disease can get help from the **Children's Liver Foundation,*** which provides educational materials, programs, and support systems for these families, who require special psychosocial support. The uncertain prognosis, discomfort, and waiting for transplantation all can produce considerable stress. In addition, as with any chronic illness, extended hospitalizations plus pharmacologic and nutritional therapy can impose significant financial burdens on the family. Parent support groups can be very helpful.

Early recognition and monitoring of the clinical signs of biliary disease is an important nursing responsibility. Nutritional support is an important task for the nurse and family. In cases of severe malnutrition and malabsorption, continuous nasogastric feedings or parenteral nutrition may be needed. The family should be educated about the purpose of these therapies and prepared to continue nutritional support at home if indicated.

STRUCTURAL DEFECTS

CLEFT LIP (CL) AND/OR CLEFT PALATE (CP)

Clefts of the lip and palate are facial malformations that occur during embryonic development, are common to all human populations, and can constitute a severe disability to the affected individual. They may appear separately or, more often, together. CL results from failure of the maxillary and median nasal processes to fuse; CP is a midline fissure of the palate that results from failure of the two sides to fuse. This discussion is concerned primarily with cleft lip and palate (CL/P).

CL may vary from a small notch to a complete cleft extending into the base of the nose (Fig. 24-3). Clefts can be unilateral or bilateral. Deformed dental structures are associated with CL. CP alone occurs in the midline and may involve the soft and hard palates. When associated with CL, the defect may involve the midline and extend into the soft palate on one or both sides.

The incidence of CL with or without CP is approximately 1 in 800 live births. The incidence of CP alone is 1 in 2000 live births. CL with or without CP is more common in males, and CP alone is more common in females. The defect appears more often in Orientals and certain tribes of Native Americans than in whites and less frequently in blacks.

*76 South Orange Ave., Suite 202, South Orange, NJ 07079.

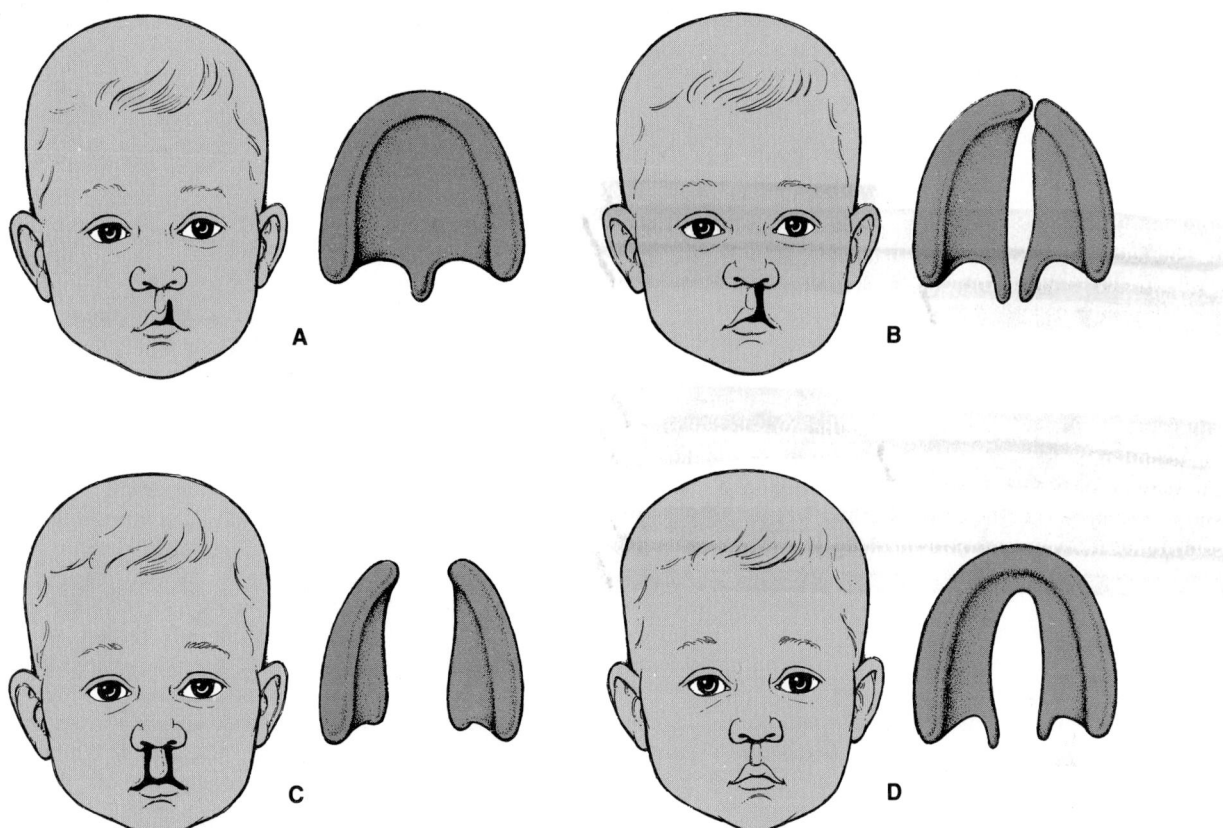

FIG. 24-3. Variations in clefts of lip and palate at birth. **A,** Notch in vermilion border. **B,** Unilateral cleft lip and palate. **C,** Bilateral cleft lip and palate. **D,** Cleft palate.

[handwritten: mild to moderate Breast feeding Best]

Etiology

The majority of cases appear to be consistent with the concept of multifactorial inheritance, as evidenced by an increased incidence in relatives and a higher concordance in monozygotic twins than in dizygotic twins. Many recognized syndromes include these defects as a feature and are the result of chromosomal abnormalities and environmental factors or teratogens that may be responsible for clefts at a critical point in embryonic development.

Pathophysiology

CL/P results from failure of the maxillary and premaxillary processes to come in contact during early embryonic life. Although often appearing together, CL and CP are distinct malformations embryologically, occurring at different times during the developmental process. Merging of the upper lip at the midline is completed between the seventh and eighth weeks of gestation. Fusion of the secondary palate (hard and soft palate) takes place later in development, between the seventh and twelfth weeks of gestation. In the process of migrating to a horizontal position, they are separated by the tongue for a short time. If there is delay in this movement, or if the tongue fails to descend soon enough, the remainder of development proceeds but the palate never fuses.

Diagnostic Evaluation

CL with or without CP is readily apparent at birth and is a defect that elicits severe emotional reactions in parents. Vary-ing degrees of nasal distortion usually accompany CL with or without CP. CP may occur as an isolated defect or in association with CL. Less obvious than CL, the defect may not be detected without a thorough assessment of the mouth. The deformity can be identified by placing the examiner's fingers directly on the palate. Clefts of the hard palate form a continuous opening between the mouth and the nasal cavity. The severity of the CP has an impact on feeding problems; the infant is unable to generate negative pressure and create suction in the oral cavity. This impairs feeding, even though in most cases the infant's ability to swallow is normal.

[handwritten: suck—air going through nose]

Therapeutic Management

Treatment of the child with CL/P involves the collaborative efforts of a number of specialists: pediatrician, nurses, plastic surgeon, orthodontist, prosthodontist, otolaryngologist, speech therapist, and sometimes a psychiatrist. Medical management is directed toward closure of the cleft(s), prevention of complications, and facilitation of normal growth and development of the child.

Surgical Correction: CL.   Closure of the lip defect precedes that of the palate, usually at 6 to 12 weeks of age. Surgical correction is performed when the infant is free of any oral, respiratory, or systemic infection. The method of repair of the CL involves one of several staggered suture lines (Z-plasty) to minimize notching of the lip from retraction of scar tissue.

Immediately after surgery the suture line is protected from

tension and trauma by a thin, arched metal device (the Logan bow) taped to the cheeks or by a butterfly-type adhesive restraint, and the arms are restrained at the elbows to prevent the infant from rubbing the incision with the hands. In the absence of infection or trauma, healing takes place with little scar formation.

Surgical Correction: CP.   CP repair is generally postponed until 12 to 18 months of age to take advantage of palatal changes that take place with normal growth. Most surgeons prefer to close the cleft at this time, before the child develops faulty speech habits.

Prognosis.   Even with good anatomic closure, the majority of children with CL/P have some degree of speech impairment that requires speech therapy. Physical problems result from inefficient functioning of the muscles of the soft palate and nasopharynx, improper tooth alignment, and varying degrees of hearing loss. Improper drainage of the middle ear, as a result of inefficient function of the eustachian tube, contributes to recurrent otitis media with scarring of the tympanic membrane, which leads to hearing impairment in many children with CP. Upper respiratory infections require immediate and meticulous attention, and extensive orthodontics and prosthodontics may be needed to correct problems of malposition of teeth and maxillary arches.

Some of the more difficult long-term problems are related to social adjustment of the child. The better the physical care, the better is the chance for emotional and social adjustment, although the presence of the defect and the degree of residual disability are not always directly related to a satisfactory adjustment. Physical defects are a threat to the self-image, and abnormal speech quality is an impediment to social expression.

Nursing Considerations

❖ Assessment
Since the lip defect is readily visible at birth, assessment consists of describing the location and extent of the defect, and the CP is estimated by visualization during crying. CP without CL is detected by palpating the palate with the finger during the newborn assessment.

The emotional impact of the birth of a child with a cosmetic, as well as a functional, disability is especially traumatic to the family. Consequently, the nursing assessment is also concerned with the emotional reaction of the family to the child and the defect.

❖ Nursing Diagnoses
Based on a thorough physical assessment, a number of nursing diagnoses are evident. These are described in the Nursing Care Plan on pp. 836-837.

❖ Planning
The goals of care for the infant with CL and CP are related to preoperative care, short-term postoperative care, and long-term management. The major goals of care for the infant and family include the following:

Preoperative care:
1. Family will cope with the impact of an infant with a defect.
2. Infant will receive optimum nutrition.
3. Infant will be prepared for surgery.

Postoperative care:
1. Infant will experience no trauma and minimal or no pain.
2. Infant will receive optimum nutrition.
3. Infant will experience no complications.
4. Infant and family will receive adequate support.
5. Family will be prepared for care at home and long-term needs of a child with CP.

❖ Implementation
The immediate nursing problems in the care of an infant with CL/P deformities are related to feeding the infant and dealing with the severe parental reaction to the defect. A CL is a disfiguring visible defect and one that may generate strong negative responses in both nurses and parents. It is especially important for nurses to emphasize the positive aspects of the infant's physical appearance and to be positive regarding surgical correction after acknowledging the parents' concerns. Sometimes showing parents a photograph of the possible cosmetic improvement as a result of surgery does much to relieve their anxiety. The manner of the nurse in handling the infant should convey to the parents that the infant is indeed a precious human being. (See Chapter 18 for interventions in assisting parents in accepting a birth defect.)

Throughout the course of therapy, parents need an explanation of the immediate and long-range problems frequently associated with CP. Often they are unaware that more is involved than merely repairing the defect. Whenever possible, they should be referred to a comprehensive CP team.

Feeding.   Feeding the infant offers a special challenge to nurses. Clefts of the lip or palate reduce the infant's ability to suck, which interferes with compression of the areola and renders breast-feeding and bottle-feeding difficult. Liquid taken into the mouth tends to escape via the cleft through the nose. Feeding is best accomplished with the infant's head in an upright position, either held in the caregiver's hand or cradled in the arm. Normal nipples are unsuitable for these infants, who are unable to generate the suction required; therefore special nipples or other feeding devices are needed. A variety of special "cleft palate" nipples have been devised and used with some success. However, large, soft nipples with large holes, Nursettes, or the long, soft lamb's nipples appear to offer the best means for nipple feeding (Fig. 24-4). The newer "gravity flow" nipple* attached to a squeezable plastic bottle allows formula to be deposited directly into the mouth in much the same manner as with a bulb syringe. Success has also been achieved by the modification of a standard nipple. A single small slit or cross-cut is made in the end of the nipple with a sharp surgical blade or a pair of scissors with sharp, thin blades. This allows the infant to swallow the formula easily, thereby bypassing the suction problem (Richard, 1991). The size of the slit is adjusted to the infant's needs.

Using these various types of nipples for feeding also has the advantage of helping to meet the infant's sucking needs. Muscle development is especially important for later development of speech. The nipple is positioned in such a way that it is compressed by the infant's tongue and existing palate. If a single-slit nipple is used, the slit is placed vertically so that the infant will be able to produce and stop a flow of milk by alternately opening and closing the opening. No matter which type of nipple is used, gentle, steady pressure on the

---

*Ross Laboratories, Columbus, OH 43216.

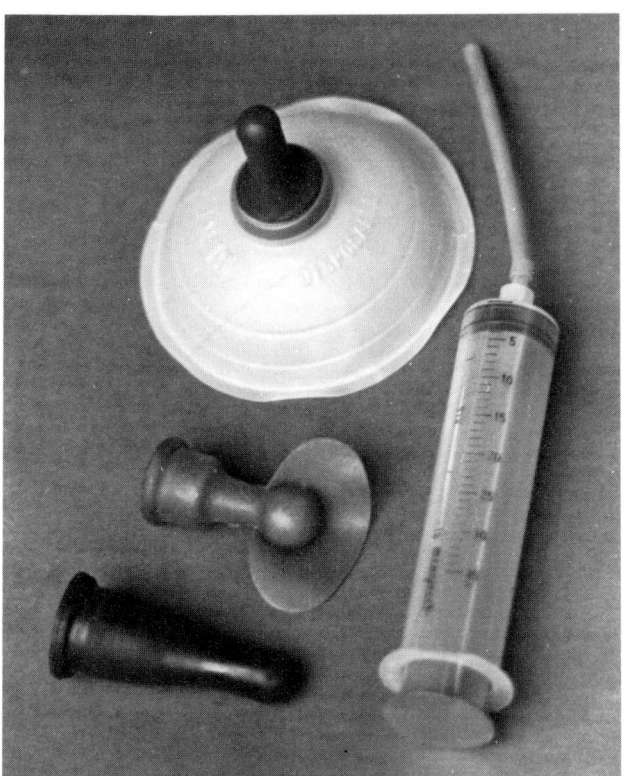

FIG. 24-4. Some devices used to feed an infant with a cleft lip and palate. *Clockwise*, Lamb's nipple, flanged nipple, special nurser, and syringe with rubber tubing (Breck feeder).

base of the bottle reduces the chance of choking or coughing, and the person feeding should resist the temptation to remove the nipple because of the noise the infant makes or for fear that the infant will choke. Since these infants have a tendency to swallow excessive amounts of air, they require frequent burping.

When the infant has trouble with nipple feeding, a rubber-tipped medicine dropper, Asepto syringe, or Breck feeder (a large syringe with soft rubber tubing) often provides an efficient, safe feeding device. The rubber extension should be sufficiently long to extend well back into the mouth to reduce the likelihood of regurgitation through the nose. The formula is deposited on the back of the tongue and the flow controlled by bulb or syringe compression that is adjusted to the infant's needs. With some infants, spoon feeding works best, especially if the formula is slightly thickened with cereal. After feeding, the infant is given water to rinse the mouth.

Breast-feeding is also an option. The nipple is positioned and stabilized well back in the oral cavity so that tongue action facilitates milk expression. However, the suction required to stimulate milk may be absent initially; therefore a breast pump may be useful before nursing to stimulate the let-down reflex.

Regardless of the feeding method used, the mother should begin to feed the infant as soon as possible, preferably after the initial nursery feeding. In this way she is able to help de-termine the method best suited to her and the infant and to become adept in the technique before they are discharged from the hospital.

Preoperative Care. In preparation for surgical repair, the parent is frequently instructed to accustom the infant to some of the needs of the early postoperative period, particularly if surgery is delayed for several months. Since it is mandatory for the infant to be positioned on the back or side postoperatively, it is helpful to train the infant to lie in these positions much of the time to reduce the irritability and resistance associated with any change in routine. It is also helpful to place the infant or child in arm restraints periodically before admission and, after admission, to feed him or her with a rubber-tipped Asepto syringe or other device in the manner to be used postoperatively.

Postoperative Care: CL. The major efforts in the postoperative period are directed toward protecting the operative site. Following CL repair *(cheiloplasty)*, a metal appliance or adhesive strips are securely taped to the cheeks to relax the surgical site and prevent tension on the suture line caused by crying or other facial movement. Elbow restraints are needed to prevent the infant from rubbing or otherwise disturbing the suture line and are usually applied immediately after surgery. It is advisable to pin the cuff of the restraints to the infant's clothing to keep the restraints in place. The older infant who is able to roll over will require a jacket restraint in addition to restricting arm movement to prevent rolling on the abdomen and rubbing the face on the sheet, especially if the repair involves the lip. It is important to remove the restraints periodically to exercise the arms, to provide relief from restrictions, and to observe the skin for signs of irritation. It is advisable to release the restraints one at a time, especially in a very vigorous, active infant. Removing restraints also offers an opportunity for cuddling and body contact. Sitting the infant in an infant seat provides a change of position and a different perspective of the environment. Sedation and appropriate analgesic medication are sometimes needed for a very restless, anxious infant. Rooming-in is always encouraged because preserving parent contact greatly increases the child's comfort.

Clear liquids are offered when the infant has fully recovered from the anesthesia, and formula feeding is usually resumed when tolerated. The Breck feeder is preferred in most cases. Care is taken to slip the rubber tip in from the side of the mouth to avoid the operative area and to prevent the infant from sucking on the tubing. This method is continued until the lip is well healed, after which bottle-feeding can be resumed if this has been the infant's mode of feeding. The mouth is rinsed with water after each feeding. The suture site is carefully cleansed of formula or serosanguineous drainage as needed with a cotton-tipped swab dipped in saline. A thin layer of antibiotic ointment is then applied to the suture line. Meticulous care of the suture line is a nursing responsibility, since inflammation or sloughing will interfere with optimum healing and the ultimate cosmetic effect of the surgical repair.

Gentle aspiration of mouth and nasopharyngeal secretions may be necessary to prevent aspiration and respiratory complications. An upright or infant seat position is helpful for the infant in the immediate postoperative period and for one who has difficulty in handling secretions.

Nursing Care Plan
The Child with Cleft Lip and/or Cleft Palate

Preoperative Care

> **NURSING DIAGNOSIS:** Altered nutrition: less than body requirements related to physical defect

PATIENT GOAL 1: Will consume adequate nourishment

• NURSING INTERVENTIONS/*RATIONALES*

Administer diet appropriate for age (specify)
Assist mother with breast-feeding if this is mother's preference, since the newborn with either defect can breast-feed
  Position and stabilize nipple well back in oral cavity *so that tongue action facilitates milk expression*
  Stimulate let-down reflex manually or with breast pump before nursing, *since suction required to stimulate milk may be absent initially*
Modify feeding techniques to adjust to defect, *since infant's ability to suck is reduced*
  Hold child in upright (sitting) position *to minimize risk of aspiration*
Use special feeding appliances *that compensate for infant's feeding difficulty*
  Try to nipple feed infant *to meet infant's need for sucking and to promote muscle development for speech*
  Position nipple between infant's tongue and existing palate *to facilitate compression of nipple*
  When using devices without nipples (e.g., Breck feeder, Asepto syringe), deposit formula on back of tongue *to facilitate swallowing* and adjust flow according to infant's swallowing *to prevent aspiration*
Bubble (burp) frequently *because of tendency to swallow excessive amounts of air*
Encourage parents to begin feeding infant as soon as possible *so that they become adept in feeding technique before discharge*
Monitor weight *to assess adequacy of nutritional intake*

• EXPECTED OUTCOMES

Infant consumes an adequate amount of nutrients (specify amount)
Infant exhibits appropriate weight gain

> **NURSING DIAGNOSIS:** High risk for altered parenting related to infant with a highly visible physical defect

PATIENT (FAMILY) GOAL 1: Will demonstrate acceptance of infant

• NURSING INTERVENTIONS/*RATIONALES*

Allow expression of feelings *to encourage family's coping*
Convey attitude of acceptance of infant and family *because parents are sensitive to affective attitudes of others*
Indicate by behavior that child is a valuable human being *to encourage acceptance of infant*
Describe results of surgical correction of defect
  Use photographs of satisfactory results *to encourage feeling of hope*

Arrange meeting with other parents who have experienced a similar situation and coped successfully

• EXPECTED OUTCOMES

Family discusses feelings and concerns regarding child's defect, its repair, and future prospects
Family exhibits an attitude of acceptance of infant
See also Nursing Care Plan: The Child Undergoing Surgery, Preoperative Care, Chapter 22

Postoperative Care

> **NURSING DIAGNOSIS:** High risk for trauma of the surgical site related to surgical procedure, dysfunctional swallowing

PATIENT GOAL 1: Will experience no trauma to operative site

• NURSING INTERVENTIONS/*RATIONALES*

Position on back or side or in infant seat (cleft lip, CL) *to prevent trauma to operative site*
Maintain lip protective device (CL) *to protect the suture line*
Use nontraumatic feeding techniques *to minimize risk of trauma*
Restrain elbows *to prevent access to operative site*
  Use jacket restraints on older infant *to prevent rolling onto abdomen and rubbing face on sheet*
  Avoid placing objects in the mouth after cleft palate (CP) repair (suction catheter, tongue depressor, straw, pacifier, small spoon) *to prevent trauma to operative site*
  Prevent vigorous and sustained crying, *which can cause tension on sutures*
  Cleanse suture line gently after feeding and as necessary in manner ordered by surgeon (CL), *since inflammation or infection will interfere with healing and the cosmetic effect of surgical repair*
Teach cleansing and restraining procedures, especially when infant will be discharged before suture removal, *to minimize complications after discharge*

• EXPECTED OUTCOME

Operative site remains undamaged

PATIENT GOAL 2: Will exhibit no evidence of aspiration

• NURSING INTERVENTION/*RATIONALES*

Position *to allow for drainage of mucus* (partial side-lying position, semi-Fowler position) and to *prevent aspiration of formula*

• EXPECTED OUTCOME

Child manages secretions and formula without aspiration

NURSING CARE PLAN

The Child with Cleft Lip and/or Cleft Palate—cont'd

NURSING DIAGNOSIS: Altered nutrition: less than body requirements related to difficulty eating following surgical procedure

PATIENT GOAL 1: Will consume adequate nourishment

- **NURSING INTERVENTIONS/*RATIONALES***

Monitor intravenous fluids (if prescribed)
Administer diet appropriate for age and as prescribed for postoperative period (specify)
Involve family in determining best feeding methods, *since family assumes feeding responsibility at home*
Modify feeding techniques *to adjust to defect and surgical repair*
  Feed in sitting position *to minimize risk of aspiration*
  Use special appliances *that compensate for feeding difficulties without causing trauma to operative site*
  Bubble frequently *because of tendency to swallow large amounts of air*
  Assist with breast-feeding if method of choice
Teach feeding and suctioning techniques to family *to ensure optimum home care*

- **EXPECTED OUTCOMES**

Infant consumes an adequate amount of nutrients (specify amounts)
Family demonstrates ability to carry out postoperative care
Infant exhibits appropriate weight gain

NURSING DIAGNOSIS: Pain related to surgical procedure

PATIENT GOAL 1: Will experience optimum comfort level

- **NURSING INTERVENTIONS/*RATIONALES***

Assess behavior and vital signs for evidence of pain
*Administer analgesics and/or sedatives as ordered
Remove restraints periodically while supervised *to exercise arms, provide relief from restrictions, and observe skin for signs of irritation*
Provide cuddling and tactile stimulation and other nonpharmacologic interventions *as needed for optimum comfort*
Involve parents in infant's care *to provide comfort and sense of security*

- **EXPECTED OUTCOME**

Infant appears comfortable and rests quietly

NURSING DIAGNOSIS: Altered family processes related to child with a physical defect, hospitalization

PATIENT (FAMILY) GOAL 1: Will receive adequate support

- **NURSING INTERVENTIONS/*RATIONALES***

See Nursing Care Plan: The Family of the Ill or Hospitalized Child, Chapter 21
Refer family to appropriate agencies and support groups

See also Nursing Care Plan: The Child with Chronic Illness or Disability, Chapter 18

*Dependent nursing action.

Postoperative Care: CP. The child with CP repair *(palatoplasty)* is allowed to lie on the abdomen, especially immediately postoperatively. Fluids are best taken from a cup. Young children are not given a pacifier, and children old enough to understand are cautioned against rubbing their tongue against the roof of the mouth. A blenderized diet is given postoperatively.

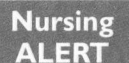 **Nursing ALERT** Avoid the use of suction or other objects in the mouth, such as tongue depressors, thermometers, spoons, or straws.

Usually, oral packing is secured to the palate after palatoplasty, which is left in place for 2 to 3 days. As with CL repair, the elbows are immobilized to keep the hands away from the mouth, and the parents are instructed to continue this

precaution at home until the palate is healed. They are instructed to remove the restraints (usually one at a time) at frequent intervals to allow the child to exercise the arms. It is important to stress that the child should be closely supervised during this time.

The child is generally discharged on a blenderized or soft diet, which parents are instructed to continue until the surgeon directs them otherwise. They are cautioned against allowing the child to eat hard items such as toast, hard cookies, and potato chips, which could damage the newly repaired palate. The nurse might suggest that the parents not offer the child any food harder than mashed potatoes.

Occasionally the child will have difficulty in breathing after surgery, especially the child with CP repair who must alter an established pattern of breathing and adjust to breathing through the nose. This is frustrating but seldom requires more than positioning and support. Sometimes the infant or child is placed in a mist tent for a short period after surgery.

The infant or child should be assessed for pain postoperatively. Opioids may be prescribed for the first 24 hours or more postoperatively and acetaminophen with or without codeine thereafter.

Long-Term Care. Children with CL/P often require a variety of services during the process of recovery. Secondary palate surgery may be required, including a pharyngeal flap procedure or palate bone grafting. Families of these children need support and encouragement by health professionals and guidance in activities that facilitate the most normal outcome for their children. With the combined efforts of the family and the health team, the majority of these children achieve a satisfactory outcome. Many children with CL/P have surgical correction that creates a near-normal-appearing lip and permits good function. Parents need to understand the function of therapy and the purpose and care of any appliance, as well as the importance of establishing good mouth care and proper brushing habits.

Throughout the child's development, an important goal is the development of a healthy personality and self-esteem. Many local areas have CP parents' groups who offer help and support to families. Several agencies provide services and information for children with CL/P and their families. These include the **American Cleft Palate Association** and **The Cleft Palate Foundation,** the **March of Dimes—Birth Defects Foundation,**† and state **Program for Children with Special Health Needs** (formerly Crippled Children's Services).

❖ Evaluation

The effectiveness of nursing interventions is determined by continual reassessment and evaluation of care based on the following observational guidelines and expected outcomes:

Preoperative care:
1. Observe and interview family members relative to their understanding, feelings, and concerns regarding the defect and anticipated surgery and their interactions with the infant.
2. Observe infant during feeding.
3. Complete preoperative checklist.

Postoperative care:
1. Inspect operative site, including the protective device.
2. Observe for behavioral and physiologic indicators of pain and response to analgesics.
3. Observe infant during feeding, measure intake and output, and weigh infant daily.
4. Observe operative site for evidence of infection, bleeding, sloughing, or irritation.
5. Observe and interview family regarding their understanding and concerns about the infant, including long-term needs.

Expected outcomes:
See Nursing Care Plan, pp. 836-837.

---

*1218 Grandview Ave., Pittsburgh, PA 15211; (800) 24-CLEFT or (412) 418-1376.
†1275 Mamaroneck Ave., White Plains, NY 10605; (914) 428-7100. In Canada: **Canadian Cleft Lip and Palate Family Association,** 170 Elizabeth St., Toronto, Ontario, Canada M5G 1E8; and **Aboutface,** 123 Edward St., Suite 1405, Toronto, Ontario, Canada M5G 1E2, (416) 928-0888.

ESOPHAGEAL ATRESIA WITH TRACHEOESOPHAGEAL FISTULA (TEF)

Congenital atresia of the esophagus and TEF are rare malformations that represent a failure of the esophagus to develop as a continuous passage. These defects may occur as separate entities or in combination (Fig. 24-5) and, without early diagnosis and treatment, are rapidly fatal.

Etiology

The cause of esophageal atresia and TEF is not known. The incidence has been estimated to be from 1 in 3000 to 1 in 3500 live births. There appears to be an equal sex incidence, but the birth weight of most affected infants is significantly lower than average and there is an unusually high incidence of prematurity in infants with esophageal atresia. Other congenital anomalies occur frequently. *VATER syndrome* describes the combination of vertebral, anorectal, and renal anomalies in addition to TEF.

Pathophysiology

In the most frequently encountered form of esophageal atresia and TEF (80% to 95% of cases), the proximal esophageal segment terminates in a blind pouch, and the distal segment is connected to the trachea or primary bronchus by a short fistula at or near the bifurcation (Fig. 24-5, *C*). The second most common variety (5% to 8%) consists of a blind pouch at each end, widely separated and with no communication to the trachea (Fig. 24-5, *A*). Less frequently an otherwise normal trachea and esophagus are connected by a common fistula (Fig. 24-5, *E*). Extremely rare anomalies involve a fistula from the trachea to the upper esophageal segment (Fig. 24-5, *B*) or to both the upper and the lower segments (Fig. 24-5, *D*).

Diagnostic Evaluation

The disorder is suspected on the basis of clinical manifestations (see box). Although the diagnosis is established on the basis of clinical signs and symptoms, the exact type of anomaly is determined by radiographic studies. A radiopaque catheter is inserted into the hypopharynx and advanced until it encounters an obstruction. Chest films are taken to ascertain esophageal patency or the presence and level of a blind pouch. Sometimes fistulas are not patent, which makes their presence more difficult to diagnose. Complete absence of air in the GI tract indicates esophageal atresia without TEF.

CLINICAL MANIFESTATIONS OF TRACHEOESOPHAGEAL FISTULA (TEF)
Excessive salivation and drooling
Three Cs of TEF:
Coughing
Choking
Cyanosis
Apnea
Increased respiratory distress after feeding
Abdominal distention

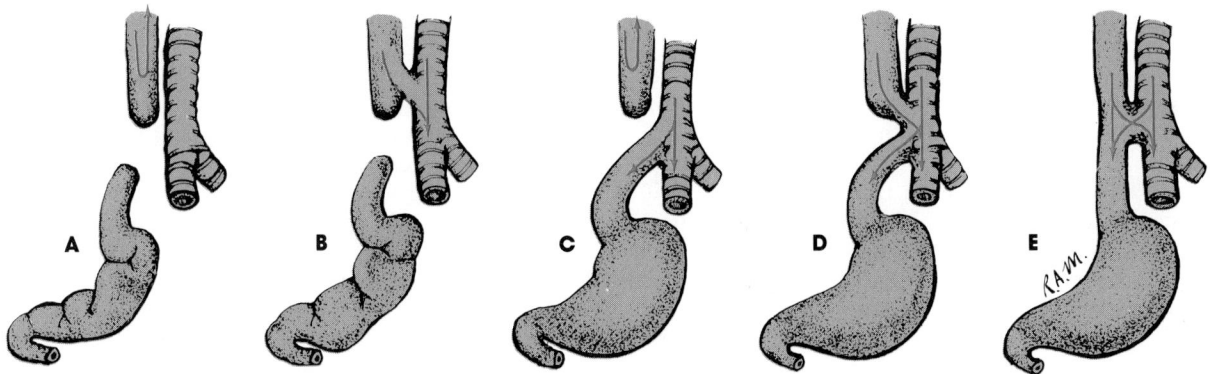

FIG. 24-5. Five most common types of esophageal atresia and tracheoesophageal fistula (TEF). (See text.)

Therapeutic Management

The treatment of esophageal atresia and TEF consists of prevention of pneumonia and surgical repair of the anomaly. When a TEF is suspected, the infant is immediately taken off oral intake, started on IV fluids, and placed in the position least likely to cause aspiration of either mouth or stomach secretions. Removal of secretions from the mouth and upper pouch requires frequent or continuous suction. Since aspiration pneumonia is almost inevitable and appears early, broad-spectrum antibiotic therapy is instituted.

Primary surgical correction consists of a thoracotomy with division and ligation of the TEF and an end-to-end anastomosis of the esophagus. For infants who are premature, have multiple anomalies, or are in very poor condition, a staged procedure is preferred that involves palliative measures, including gastrostomy, ligation of the TEF, and provision of constant drainage of the esophageal pouch. A delayed esophageal anastomosis is usually attempted after several weeks when the upper pouch elongates and the lower pouch undergoes hypertrophy. The technique of *bougienage* (the process whereby a blunt metal instrument is used to dilate a fistula or lengthen membranous tissue) of the upper pouch may be performed to elongate this segment. If an esophageal anastomosis still cannot be accomplished, a *cervical esophagostomy* (to allow drainage of saliva) and gastrostomy are performed.

There are rare instances in which a primary anastomosis cannot be accomplished because of insufficient length of the two segments of esophagus. In these cases the defect must be bridged with a colon interposition, gastric tube, or gastric interposition procedure. This esophageal replacement is usually deferred until the child is 16 to 24 months old. Endotracheal intubation may be required, since many of these infants may also have *tracheomalacia,* a weakness in the tracheal wall that occurs when a dilated proximal pouch compresses the trachea from early in fetal life or when the trachea does not develop normally because of a loss of intratracheal pressure.

Complications of a primary repair include an anastomotic leak, strictures due to tension or ischemia, esophageal motility disorders causing dysphagia, and gastroesophageal reflux. Motility disorders are common following esophageal atresia or TEF repair.

Prognosis. The prognosis for infants with esophageal atresia or TEF is related to the birth weight, associated congenital anomalies, and time of diagnosis. The survival rate is nearly 100% in full-term infants without severe respiratory distress or other anomalies. In premature low-birth-weight infants with associated anomalies, the incidence of complications is high. The overall mortality is 10% to 15% (Wright, 1991).

Nursing Considerations

Nursing responsibility for detection of this serious malformation begins *immediately* after birth. Ideally the condition is diagnosed before the initial feeding, but often it is not. If fed, the infant swallows normally but suddenly coughs and struggles, and the fluid is aspirated or returns through the nose and mouth. For this reason it is customary for the nurse to give the infant the first feeding of plain water or to be present when a parent feeds the child in order to observe the infant's response.

> **Nursing ALERT** Any infant who has an excessive amount of frothy saliva in the mouth or difficulty with secretions and unexplained episodes of cyanosis should be suspected of having a TEF.

Cyanosis is usually the result of laryngospasm caused by overflow of saliva into the larynx from the proximal esophageal pouch, and it normally clears after removal of the secretions from the oropharynx by suctioning. Any such suspicion is reported immediately. The infant is placed in an incubator or under a radiant warmer, and oxygen is administered to help relieve respiratory distress. Positive pressure is contraindicated, since it may add to air pressure in the stomach.

The most desirable position for a newborn who is suspected of having a TEF is supine with the head elevated on an inclined plane of at least 30 degrees. This positioning serves to minimize the reflux of gastric secretions up the distal esophagus into the trachea and bronchi.

It is imperative that the source of aspiration be removed at once. Oral fluids are withheld, and the infant's fluid needs are met parenterally or via gastrostomy. Until surgery the blind pouch is kept empty by intermittent or continuous suction through an indwelling nasal catheter that extends to the end of the pouch. The catheter needs attention, since it has a tendency to become clogged with mucus. It is usually replaced daily by the physician. In the event that a staged repair is performed, the gastrostomy tube is inserted and left open so that air entering the stomach through the fistula can escape, thus minimizing the danger that gastric contents will be regurgitated into the trachea. The tube empties by gravity drainage. It is imperative that any secretions that can be a source of aspiration be removed at once.

Postoperative Care. Postoperative care for these infants is essentially the same as the care of any high-risk newborn (see Nursing Care of the High-Risk Newborn and Family, Chapter 9). The infant is returned to the warm, high-humidity atmosphere of the incubator, and the gastrostomy tube is returned to gravity drainage until the infant can tolerate feedings, usually by the fifth to seventh postoperative day. At this time the tube is elevated and secured at a point above the level of the stomach. This allows gastric secretions to pass to the duodenum, whereas swallowed air can escape through the open tube. If tolerated, gastrostomy feedings are continued until the esophageal anastomosis is healed, on about the tenth to fourteenth day, after which oral feedings are initiated.

The initial attempt at oral feeding must be carefully observed to make certain that the infant is able to swallow without choking. Until the infant is able to take a sufficient amount by mouth, oral intake may need to be supplemented by gastrostomy feedings or parenteral nutrition. Ordinarily, infants are not discharged until they are taking oral fluids well and the gastrostomy tube has been removed. However, the infant who has undergone palliative surgery will be discharged with the gastrostomy tube in place. The nurse is responsible for making certain that the caregiver is educated and practiced in the care of the gastrostomy (see Chapter 22).*

Special Problems. Upper respiratory complications are a threat to life in both the preoperative and the postoperative period. In addition to pneumonia, there is a constant danger of respiratory distress resulting from atelectasis, pneumothorax, and laryngeal edema. Any persistent respiratory difficulty after removal of secretions is reported to the surgeon immediately. The infant is monitored for anastomotic leaks, as evidenced by purulent chest tube drainage, increased WBC, and temperature instability.

In the infant awaiting esophageal replacement surgery, the catheter is removed and the upper esophageal segment is drained through a cervical esophagostomy. This is a source of annoyance, since the skin may become irritated by moisture from the continual discharge of saliva. Frequent removal of drainage and application of a layer of protective ointment are usually sufficient treatment. A dressing or ostomy appliance may need to be applied to collect the drainage. An enterostomal therapist may provide helpful guidance in the prevention and/or treatment of skin breakdown.

Meeting the oral needs of infants who are unable to suck on a bottle should not be overlooked. A pacifier offered periodically is an acceptable substitute until oral feedings are instituted. The child who has corrective surgery delayed until 16 to 24 months of age may have a different problem. Children who have not been able to go through the process of eating in the normal manner often have difficulty with this new task and require patient guidance in learning the techniques of taking food into the mouth and swallowing. It is important to provide oral desensitization therapy to minimize this problem while the child is deprived of oral feeding.

As with any congenital anomaly, parents need support in adjusting to the child's condition (see Chapter 18). One of the difficulties in TEF is the immediate transfer of the sick newborn to the intensive care unit and sometimes lengthy hospitalization. The attachment process is facilitated by encouraging parents to visit the infant, participate in his or her care when appropriate, and express their feelings regarding the infant's condition. The nurse in the intensive care unit should assume responsibility for ensuring that the parents are kept fully informed of the infant's progress.

See also Nursing Care Plan: The Child with Esophageal Atresia and Tracheoesophageal Fistula.*

HERNIAS

A *hernia* is a protrusion of a portion of an organ or organs through an abnormal opening. The danger from herniation arises when the organ protruding through the opening is constricted to the extent that circulation is impaired or when the protruding organs encroach on and impair the function of other structures. A hernia that cannot be reduced easily is called an *incarcerated hernia.* A *strangulated hernia* is one in which the blood supply to the herniated organ is impaired. The herniations of concern are those that protrude through the diaphragm, the abdominal wall, or the inguinal canal (see also Genitourinary Tract Disorders/Defects, Chapter 27). The other hernias of significance to the pediatric age-groups are outlined in Table 24-6.

OBSTRUCTIVE DISORDERS

Obstruction of the bowel occurs when the passage of intestinal contents is mechanically impeded by a constricted or an occluded lumen or when there is interference with normal muscular contraction. The latter, commonly called *paralytic ileus,* occurs when there is motor dysfunction of the intestine. Intestinal obstruction from any cause is characterized by similar signs and symptoms (see box on p. 842), although the progression may vary greatly. For example, in acute conditions, such as intussusception, the clinical manifestations are apparent within a few hours of the onset of the disorder. In other conditions, such as pyloric stenosis, the signs and symptoms usually develop more gradually and can be missed in the early stages.

Mechanical obstructions may be congenital or acquired. Congenital obstructions, such as duodenal, jejunal, or ileal atresia, usually appear in the neonatal period. Malrotation,

---

*Home care instructions on giving gastrostomy tube feedings are available in Wong DL: *Wong and Whaley's Clinical manual of pediatric nursing,* ed 4, St Louis, 1996, Mosby.

*In Wong DL: *Wong and Whaley's Clinical manual of pediatric nursing,* ed 4, St Louis, 1996, Mosby.

TABLE 24-6. Summary outline of diaphragmatic and abdominal hernias

TYPE	MANIFESTATIONS/ DIAGNOSTIC EVALUATION	MANAGEMENT
Diaphragmatic Through foramen of Bochdalek: protrusion of part of the abdominal organs through an opening in the diaphragm	Symptoms—mild to severe respiratory distress within a few hours after birth; tachypnea, cyanosis, dyspnea, and severe acidosis Breath sounds absent in affected area; bowel sounds may be present Vomiting, abdominal pain Rarely asymptomatic Diagnosis made by radiographic study	Therapeutic: Supportive treatment of respiratory distress and correction of acidosis; possible use of extracorporeal membrane oxygenation Prophylactic antibiotic administration Surgical reduction of hernia and repair of defect Nursing: Preoperative Prevent crying Maintain suction, oxygen, and intravenous fluids Place in semi-Fowler position Assist with diagnostic and preoperative procedures Administer medications Postoperative Carry out routine postoperative care and observation Use comfort measures Support parents because child is seriously ill
Hiatal *Sliding:* protrusion of an abdominal structure (usually the stomach) through the esophageal hiatus	Symptoms—dysphagia, failure to thrive, vomiting, neck contortions, frequent unexplained respiratory problems, bleeding Diagnosis made by fluoroscopy	Therapeutic: surgical repair of defect Nursing: Be alert to significant signs Carry out routine postoperative care
Abdominal *Umbilical:* soft, skin-covered protrusion of intestine and omentum through a weakness in the abdominal wall around the umbilicus	Inspection and palpation of abdomen High incidence in black infants Spontaneous closure by age 1 to 2 years	Therapeutic: No treatment of small defects Operative repair if persists to age 2 to 5 years Strangulation requires immediate attention Nursing: Discourage use of home remedies (e.g., belly bands, coins) Reassure parents
Omphalocele: protrusion of intraabdominal viscera into the base of the umbilical cord; the sac is covered with peritoneum without skin *Gastroschisis:* protrusion of intraabdominal contents through a defect in the abdominal wall lateral to the umbilical ring; there is never a peritoneal sac	Obvious on inspection Observation for other malformations	Therapeutic: Surgical repair of defect Preoperative Large lesions—gradual reduction of abdominal contents Prophylactic antibiotic administration Nursing (preoperative): Keep sac or viscera moist with saline-soaked pads Use overhead warming unit Carry out routine care of intravenous line, nasogastric suction Give nothing by mouth Use comfort measures

duodenal web, and Hirschsprung disease often appear after the first few weeks of life.

HYPERTROPHIC PYLORIC STENOSIS (HPS)

HPS (obstruction at the pyloric sphincter by hypertrophy of the circular muscle of the pylorus) is one of the most common surgical disorders of early infancy. This functional anomaly is seen soon after birth with vomiting that becomes progressively more severe and projectile. It is five times more common in male infants than in female infants, affecting approximately 5 of every 1000 males and only 1 of every 1000 females. It is seen less frequently in black and Asian infants than in white infants. It is more likely to affect a full-term infant than a premature infant.

The cause of the increased size of the pyloric musculature is unknown. There is a genetic predisposition, and siblings

CLINICAL MANIFESTATIONS OF MECHANICAL/ PARALYTIC INTESTINAL OBSTRUCTION

Colicky abdominal pain—from peristalsis attempting to overcome the obstruction

Abdominal distention—as a result of accumulation of gas and fluid above the level of the obstruction.

Vomiting—often the earliest sign of a high obstruction; a later sign of lower obstruction (may be bilious or feculent)

Constipation and obstipation—early signs of low obstructions; later signs of higher obstructions

Dehydration—from losses of large quantities of fluid and electrolytes into the intestine

Rigid and boardlike abdomen—from increased distention

Bowel sounds—gradually diminish and cease

Respiratory distress—occurs as the diaphragm is pushed up into the pleural cavity

Shock—plasma volume diminishes as fluids and electrolytes are lost from the bloodstream into the intestinal lumen

Sepsis—caused by bacterial proliferation with invasion into the circulation

CLINICAL MANIFESTATIONS OF HYPERTROPHIC PYLORIC STENOSIS (HPS)

Projectile vomiting
  May be ejected 3 to 4 feet from the child when in a side-lying position, 1 foot or more when in a back-lying position
  Occurs shortly after a feeding (may not occur for several hours)
  May follow each feeding or appear intermittently
  Nonbilious vomitus; may be blood tinged
Infant hungry, avid nurser; eagerly accepts a second feeding after vomiting episode
No evidence of pain or discomfort except that of chronic hunger
Weight loss
Signs of dehydration
Distended upper abdomen
Readily palpable olive-shaped tumor in the epigastrium just to the right of the umbilicus
Visible gastric peristaltic waves that move from left to right across the epigastrium

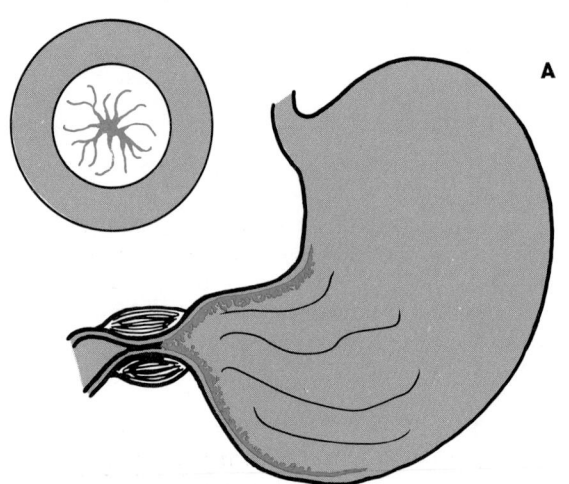
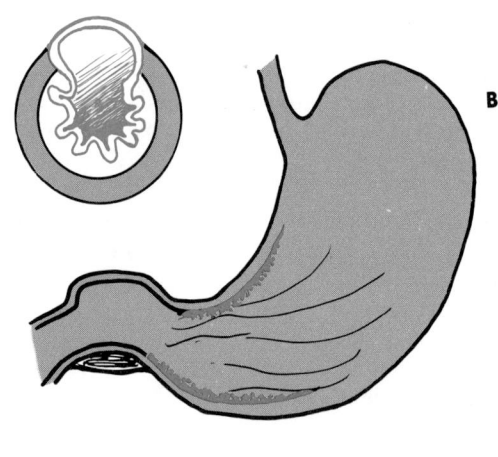

FIG. 24-6. Hypertrophic pyloric stenosis (HPS). **A,** Enlarged muscular area nearly obliterates pyloric channel. **B,** Longitudinal surgical division of muscle down to submucosa establishes adequate passageway.

and offspring of affected persons are at increased risk of developing HPS.

Pathophysiology

The circular muscle of the pylorus is grossly enlarged as a result of both hypertrophy (increased size) and hyperplasia (increased mass). This produces severe narrowing of the pyloric canal between the stomach and the duodenum. Consequently, the lumen at this point is partially obstructed. Over time, inflammation and edema further reduce the size of the opening until the partial obstruction may progress to complete obstruction. The muscle is thickened to as much as twice its usual size—2 to 3 cm long—and is almost cartilaginous in consistency. The distal portion ends abruptly and is externally distinct and easily palpated, but the proximal end

merges into the gastric antrum. The stomach is usually dilated (Fig. 24-6, *A*).

Evidence suggests that local innervation is involved in the pathogenesis. In most cases this is an isolated lesion; however, it may be associated with intestinal malrotation, esophageal and duodenal atresia, and anorectal anomalies.

Diagnostic Evaluation

The age of onset and pattern of vomiting are variable. Typically, infants with HPS are well during the first weeks of life. Initially there is only regurgitation or occasional nonprojectile vomiting that begins about the second to the fourth week after birth, although in a few infants symptoms begin at birth. Others do well for the first few weeks and then suddenly develop projectile vomiting that rapidly leads to dehydration.

feel over stomach
olive shaped mass

The projectile vomiting usually develops within a week and may lead to complete obstruction by 4 to 6 weeks. The emesis usually contains stale milk and is not bile stained. Often these infants become dehydrated and lethargic and appear significantly malnourished.

If the diagnosis is inconclusive from the history and physical signs (see box on p. 842), upper GI radiographic studies will reveal delayed gastric emptying and an elongated, threadlike pyloric channel. Ultrasound is accurate and less traumatic for diagnosis of HPS. Laboratory findings reflect the metabolic alterations created by severe depletion of both fluid and electrolytes from extensive and prolonged vomiting. There are decreased serum levels of both sodium and potassium, although these may be masked by the hemoconcentration from ECF depletion. Of greater diagnostic value are a decrease in serum chloride levels and increases in pH and bicarbonate (carbon dioxide content) characteristic of metabolic alkalosis.

Therapeutic Management

Surgical relief of the pyloric obstruction by *pyloromyotomy* (sometimes called *Fredet-Ramstedt procedure*) is the standard treatment for this disorder. The surgical procedure is performed through a right upper quadrant incision (laparotomy) and consists of a longitudinal incision through the circular muscle fibers of the pylorus down to, but not including, the submucosa (Fig. 24-6, *B*). The procedure has a very high success rate when infants receive careful preoperative preparation to correct fluid and electrolyte imbalances.

Feedings are usually begun 4 to 6 hours postoperatively, beginning with small, frequent feedings of glucose water or electrolyte solutions. If clear fluids are retained, about 24 hours after surgery formula is started in the same stepwise increments, with the amount and interval between feedings gradually increased until a full feeding schedule is reinstated, which usually takes about 48 hours. The infant is ready to be discharged from the hospital by about the second or third postoperative day.

Recently, another procedure, *laparoscopy,* has been found to be safe and successful for infants with HPS (Najmaldin and Tan, 1995). The use of a small incision for the laparoscope may result in a shorter surgical time, more rapid postoperative feeding, and quicker discharge.

Prognosis.   Most infants recover completely and rapidly following pyloromyotomy. Postoperative complications include persistent pyloric obstruction and wound dehiscence. Approximately 15% of infants with HPS also have gastroesophageal reflux (Milla, 1991).

Nursing Considerations

❖ Assessment

HPS should be considered as a possibility in the very young infant who appears alert but fails to gain weight and has a history of vomiting after meals. Assessment is based on observation of eating behaviors and evidence of other characteristic clinical manifestations.

❖ Nursing Diagnoses

Based on a thorough assessment, a number of nursing diagnoses are evident. The most typical are those listed in the box.

NURSING DIAGNOSES: THE INFANT WITH HYPERTROPHIC PYLORIC STENOSIS (HPS)

High risk for fluid volume deficit related to persistent vomiting
Altered nutrition: less than body requirements related to persistent vomiting
Altered family processes related to hospitalization of infant

---

❖ Planning

The goals of care for the child with HPS are primarily related to presurgical and postsurgical care of the infant, including the following:

1. Infant will consume sufficient amount of formula.
2. Infant will retain feedings.
3. Infant will experience no complications.
4. Family will receive adequate support and education.

❖ Implementation

Preoperative Care.   Preoperatively the emphasis is placed on restoring hydration and electrolyte balance. Infants with HPS are usually given no oral feedings and receive IV fluids with glucose and electrolyte replacement based on laboratory serum electrolyte values. Careful monitoring of the IV infusion and diligent attention to intake, output, and urine specific gravity measurements are important to the success of fluid replacement. Any vomiting, as well as the number and character of stools, is observed and recorded accurately.

Observations include assessment of vital signs, particularly those that might indicate fluid or electrolyte imbalances. These infants are especially prone to metabolic alkalosis from loss of hydrogen ions and to potassium, sodium, and chloride depletion. The skin and mucous membranes are assessed for alterations in hydration status, and daily weight provides added clues to water gain or loss.

When stomach decompression and gastric lavage are part of preoperative management, the nurse is responsible for ensuring that the tube is patent and functioning properly and for measuring and recording the type and amount of drainage. The infant is usually positioned flat or with the head slightly elevated. The infant who is receiving IV fluids and/or has an NG tube for continuous drainage must be adequately observed to prevent the needle and/or tube from becoming dislodged.

General hygienic care, with particular attention to the skin and mouth in dehydrated infants, is an important part of care. Protection from infection is also important, since infants with impaired nutritional status are even more susceptible than normal newborns. Parental involvement is encouraged and promoted.

Postoperative Care.   Postoperative vomiting may occur, and most infants, even with successful surgery, exhibit some vomiting during the first 24 to 48 hours. IV fluids are administered until the infant is taking and retaining adequate amounts by mouth. Therefore much of the same care that was instituted before surgery is continued postoperatively (i.e., observation of physical signs, monitoring of IV fluids, careful observation and recording of intake and output). In addition, the infant is observed for responses to the stress of surgery and for evidence of pain. Appropriate analgesics are given. The NG tube may be maintained after surgery for a variable time.

Feedings are usually instituted relatively soon, beginning with clear liquids containing glucose and electrolytes. They are offered slowly, in small amounts, and at frequent intervals as ordered by the practitioner. If the infant has been breast-fed, breast milk, expressed by the mother, is given by bottle when the infant is able to tolerate feedings, and breast-feeding is resumed as soon as feasible. Observation and recording of feedings and the infant's responses to feedings and feeding techniques are a vital part of postoperative care. Positioning with the head elevated is usually continued postoperatively. Care of the operative site consists of observation for any drainage or signs of inflammation and care of the incision as directed by the surgeon.

As with any child in the hospital, parents are encouraged to remain with their child and become involved in the child's care. Vomiting of a projectile nature is frightening to parents, and they often believe that they may have done something wrong or that surgery was not successful. Most parents need support and reassurance that the condition is caused by a structural problem and is in no way a reflection on their parenting skills and capacities.

❖ Evaluation

The effectiveness of nursing interventions is determined by reassessment based on the following observational guidelines and expected outcomes:

1. Observe feeding behavior, especially vomiting episodes.
2. Weigh infant daily.
3. Observe for evidence of complications.
4. Observe and interview family regarding feelings, understanding, and concerns.

Expected outcomes:

1. Infant consumes a sufficient amount of formula.
2. Infant takes and retains feedings.
3. Infant recovers with no evidence of complications.
4. Family members express their feelings and concerns, demonstrate an understanding of infant's condition, and are actively involved in infant's care.

See also Nursing Care Plan: The Child with Hypertrophic Pyloric Stenosis.*

INTUSSUSCEPTION

Intussusception is one of the most frequent causes of intestinal obstruction in children, generally between the ages of 3 months and 5 years. Half the cases occur in children younger than age 1 year; more often it occurs in children between 3 and 12 months of age, and most of the other cases occur in children during the second year. Intussusception is twice as common in males as in females and in children with cystic fibrosis. Although specific intestinal lesions can be found in a small percentage of these children, generally the cause is not known. More than 90% of intussusceptions do not have a pathologic lead point, such as a polyp, lymphoma, or Meckel diverticulum. The idiopathic cases are most likely a result of

*In Wong DL: *Wong and Whaley's Clinical manual of pediatric nursing,* ed 4, St Louis, 1996, Mosby.

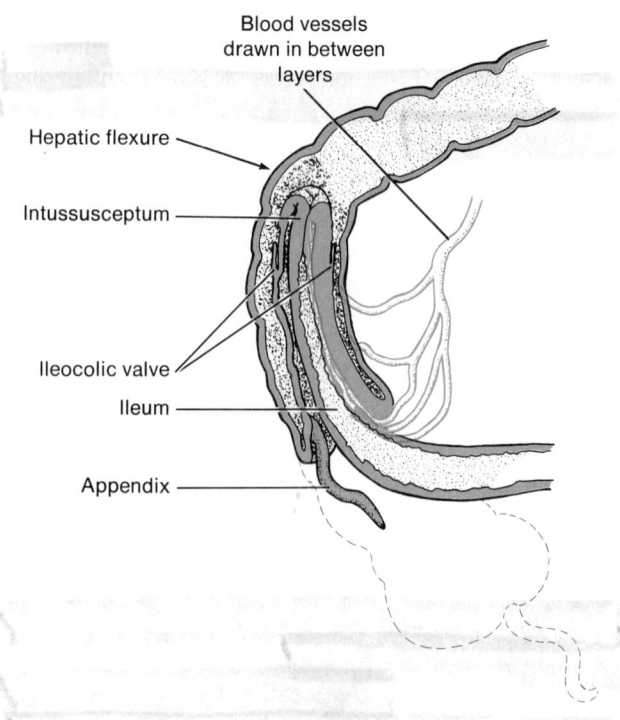

FIG. 24-7. Ileocolic intussusception.

hypertrophy of intestinal lymphoid tissue secondary to viral infection.

Pathophysiology

Intussusception is an invagination or telescoping of one portion of the intestine into another. The most common site is the *ileocecal valve,* where the ileum invaginates into the cecum and colon (Fig. 24-7), producing an obstruction to the passage of intestinal contents beyond the defect. In addition, the two walls of the intestine press against each other, causing inflammation, edema, and eventually decreased blood flow. Because fecal material is unable to move beyond the obstruction, the stools contain primarily blood and mucus, resulting in the "currant jelly" stools characteristic of the disorder. Ischemia, perforation, peritonitis, and shock are serious complications of intussusception. If left untreated, this condition is incompatible with life.

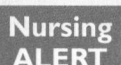 **Nursing ALERT** — A report of severe colicky abdominal pain in a child with vomiting and currant jelly–like stools is a significant clue to intussusception.

Diagnostic Evaluation

Frequently the diagnosis can be made on subjective findings alone (see box). The classic presentation of intussusception is a healthy, thriving child, usually between 3 and 12 months of age, who suddenly develops an episode of acute abdominal pain, vomiting, bloody stool, and a palpable abdominal mass. Definitive diagnosis is based on a barium enema, which clearly demonstrates the obstruction to the flow of barium. Initially, however, an abdominal radiograph is obtained to detect intraperitoneal air from a bowel perforation, which would contraindicate a barium enema. A rectal examination

---

**CLINICAL MANIFESTATIONS
OF INTUSSUSCEPTION**

Sudden acute abdominal pain
  Child screams and draws the knees onto the chest
  Child appears normal and comfortable during intervals be-
    tween episodes of pain
Vomiting
Lethargy
Passage of red, currant jelly–like stools (stool mixed with blood
  and mucus)
Tender, distended abdomen
Palpable sausage-shaped mass in upper right quadrant
Empty lower right quadrant (Dance sign)
Eventual fever, prostration, and other signs of peritonitis

---

reveals mucus, blood, and, occasionally, a low intussusception itself. With atypical cases, lethargy may be the primary presenting symptom (Hickey, Sodhi, and Johnson, 1990).

Therapeutic Management

In most cases the initial treatment of choice is nonsurgical hydrostatic reduction by barium enema at the time of diagnostic testing. The force exerted by the flowing barium is usually sufficient to push the invaginated portion of the bowel into its original position, similar to pushing an inverted "finger" out of a glove. This procedure is not recommended if there are clinical signs of shock or perforation. The use of barium as the contrast agent is becoming less routine. Presently a high percentage of radiologists use water-soluble contrast and air pressure to reduce intussusceptions (Meyer, 1992). Since this procedure may not always reduce the intussusception, the child is prepared for surgery. Fluid resuscitation, nasogastric decompression, and antibiotic therapy are often given before hydrostatic reduction attempts are made. Surgical intervention consists of reducing the invagination manually and, when indicated, resecting any nonviable intestine.

Prognosis. Many patients with intussusception can be successfully treated by hydrostatic reduction. Surgery is required for patients in whom the reduction was unsuccessful. If untreated, approximately 10% of children will have spontaneous reduction or chronic intussusception. The other 90% of untreated patients will worsen or die of complications such as perforation, peritonitis, and sepsis. With early diagnosis and treatment, serious complications and death occur infrequently.

Nursing Considerations

The nurse can help establish a diagnosis by carefully listening to the parent's description of the child's physical and behavioral symptoms. Parents are astute in detecting that something is wrong with their child, and it is not unusual for parents to express that they felt something was seriously wrong before others shared their concerns. The description of the child's severe colicky abdominal pain combined with vomiting is a significant sign of intussusception.

As soon as a possible diagnosis of intussusception is made, the nurse begins to prepare the parents for the immediate need for hospitalization, the usual nonsurgical technique of hydrostatic reduction, and the possibility of surgery. It is important at this time to explain the basic defect of intussusception.

NURSING TIP Intussusception is easily demonstrated by pushing the end of a finger on a rubber glove back into itself or using the example of a telescoping rod. The principle of reduction by hydrostatic pressure can be simulated by filling the glove with water, which pushes the "finger" into a fully extended position.

Since this hospitalization may be the child's first separation from the parents, it is especially important to preserve the parent-child relationship by encouraging rooming-in or extended visiting. It may also be the parents' first experience with hospital care for their child, necessitating their preparation for procedures such as IV therapy, frequent vital sign and blood pressure monitoring, dressings, and special orders, such as NPO. Because of the rapidity of the onset, diagnosis, and treatment, parents may be left with the feeling of stunned numbness. They may ask few questions, or they may constantly make inquiries, sometimes the same ones several times. If the nurse realizes the circumstances surrounding this condition, the parents' reactions are more likely to be understood and accepted.

Physical care of the child with intussusception differs little from that for any child undergoing abdominal surgery. Even though nonsurgical intervention may be successful, the usual preoperative procedures, such as withholding of fluids by mouth, routine laboratory testing (CBC and urinalysis), signed parental consent, and preanesthetic sedation, are carried out. For the child with signs of electrolyte imbalance, hemorrhage, or peritonitis, additional medical preparation such as replacement fluids, whole blood or plasma, and nasogastric suctioning may be performed. Before surgery the nurse monitors all stools.

> **Nursing
> ALERT**
> Passage of a normal brown stool usually indicates that the intussusception has reduced itself. This is immediately reported to the practitioner, who may choose to alter the diagnostic/therapeutic plan of care.

Postprocedural care includes the usual postoperative observations, such as vital signs, blood pressure, intact sutures and dressing, and the return of bowel sounds. After hydrostatic reduction or autoreduction, the nurse observes for passage of barium or water-soluble contrast material and the stool patterns, since there may be recurrences of the intussusception. Children may be admitted to the hospital or monitored closely on an outpatient basis. A recurrence of intussusception is usually treated with hydrostatic reduction. A laparotomy is considered for multiple recurrences.

See also Nursing Care Plan: The Child with Intussusception.*

ANORECTAL MALFORMATIONS

Malformations in the anorectal region of the GI tract are among the more common congenital malformations caused

---

*In Wong DL: *Wong and Whaley's Clinical manual of pediatric nursing,* ed 4, St Louis, 1996, Mosby.

by abnormal development. The incidence is approximately 1 in 5000 live births. All are classified as *imperforate anus.* However, distinction between these categories is important for planning therapy and determining a prognosis.

Clinically, anorectal malformations can be divided into the following three categories according to the relationship of the rectum to the puborectalis muscle:

Low anomalies. The rectum has descended normally through the puborectalis muscle, the internal and external sphincters are present and well developed with normal function, and there is no connection to the genitourinary tract (Fig. 24-8, *A* and *B*.)

Intermediate anomalies. The rectum is at or below the level of the puborectalis muscle; the anal dimple and external sphincter are positioned normally.

High anomalies. The rectum ends above the puborectalis muscle, and there is absence of the internal sphincter. This is usually associated with a genitourinary fistula: rectourethral (male) or rectovaginal (female) (Fig. 24-8, *F*).

Cloacal exstrophy is a rare form of imperforate anus. The bowel and the bladder open into the lower abdominal wall, and the common mucosa is composed of bladder epithelium and intestinal epithelium. The genitalia is ambiguous, and most of these children are raised as females.

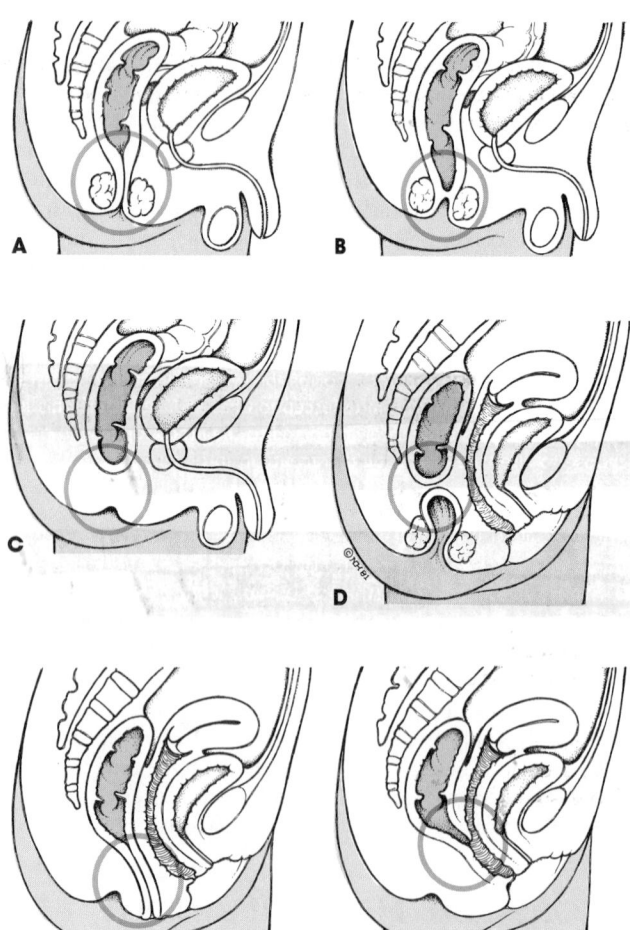

FIG. 24-8. Anorectal stenosis and imperforate anus. **A,** Congenital anal stenosis. **B,** Anal membrane atresia. **C,** Anal agenesis. **D,** Rectal atresia. **E,** Rectoperitoneal fistula. **F,** Rectovaginal fistula.

Diagnostic Evaluation

Inspection of the perineal area and checking for patency of the anus and rectum, as well as observation or inquiries regarding the passage of meconium, are a routine part of the newborn assessment. Failure to pass meconium is cause for investigation. Digital and endoscopic examinations identify constriction or the blind pouch of rectal atresia. Stenosis may not become apparent until 1 year of age or older, when the child has a history of difficult defecation, abdominal distention, and ribbonlike stools.

Fistulas associated with types B and C anomalies are not usually apparent at birth, but as peristalsis gradually forces the meconium through the fistula, they can be identified by careful examination. With a rectourinary fistula, meconium appears in the urine.

Definitive diagnosis of the extent and location of the rectal pouch is made by radiographic examination. With the infant inverted and an opaque marker at the anal dimple, air ascending into the rectum and lower bowel outlines the location of the pouch in relation to the anal depression.

Therapeutic Management

Successful treatment for anal stenosis is generally accomplished by manual dilations. The procedure, begun by the physician, is repeated on a regular basis by the nurses in the hospital and is continued at home by the parents after they are carefully instructed in the technique. An imperforate anal membrane is excised and followed by daily anal dilatations.

Reconstruction of an anus in the proper position is the goal of surgical treatment of other anorectal malformations. Malformations of the lower rectum often can be corrected in the neonatal period by way of simple dilatation or a minor perineal procedure. Infants with higher anomalies require a temporary colostomy in the newborn period. Final correction of higher defects is usually postponed for a year, when a pull-through procedure with *anorectoplasty* is performed.

Nursing Considerations

The first nursing responsibility is identification of undetected anorectal malformations. A newborn who does not pass a stool within 24 to 36 hours of birth requires further assessment, and meconium that appears at an inappropriate orifice is reported.

Postoperative nursing care usually presents few problems and is primarily directed toward healing of the anoplasty without infection or other complications. In situations where the infant has undergone a pull-through procedure with anoplasty, special nursing care involves maintaining the anal area as clean as possible with scrupulous perineal care. There may or may not be a temporary dressing and drain, but when the infant is passing stool, dressings are of little value. The preferred position is a side-lying prone position with the hips elevated or a supine position with the legs suspended at a 90-degree angle to the trunk to prevent pressure on perineal sutures.

The infant is administered regular infant formula as soon as peristalsis returns. In the meantime, there may be an NG tube for abdominal decompression and IV feedings. Care of the infant with a colostomy involves frequent dressing changes, meticulous skin care, and correct application of a collection device (see Chapter 22).

See also Nursing Care Plan: The Infant with an Anorectal Malformation.*

MALABSORPTION SYNDROMES

Malabsorption syndromes include a long list of disorders associated with some degree of impaired digestion and/or absorption. An important complication of malabsorption syndromes in children is failure to thrive. Most are classified according to the location of the supposed anatomic and/or biochemical defect. The term *celiac disease* is often used to describe a symptom complex that has four characteristics in common: (1) steatorrhea (fatty, foul, frothy, bulky stools), (2) general malnutrition, (3) abdominal distention, and (4) secondary vitamin deficiencies.

Digestive defects primarily are conditions in which the enzymes necessary for digestion are diminished or absent, such as (1) cystic fibrosis, in which pancreatic enzymes are absent; (2) biliary or liver disease, in which bile flow is affected; or (3) lactase deficiency, in which there is congenital or secondary lactose intolerance.

Absorptive defects are conditions in which the intestinal mucosal transport system is impaired. It may be because of a primary defect (e.g., celiac disease) or secondary to inflammatory disease of the bowel that results in impaired absorption because bowel motility is accelerated (e.g., ulcerative colitis). Obstructive disorders (e.g., Hirschsprung disease) can also cause secondary malabsorption from enterocolitis.

Anatomic defects, such as extensive resection of the bowel or "short bowel syndrome," affect digestion by decreasing the transit time of substances and affect absorption by severely compromising the absorptive surface.

CELIAC DISEASE (CD)

CD, also known as *gluten-induced enteropathy, gluten-sensitive enteropathy (GSE),* and *celiac sprue,* is second only to cystic fibrosis as a cause of malabsorption in children. The incidence is highly variable, being reported as 1 in 300 to 1 in 4000, and appears to be declining, possibly in relation to environmental factors. It is seen more frequently in Europe than in America and is rarely reported in Asians or blacks. The exact cause of CD is not known, but there appears to be an inherited predisposition with an influence by environmental factors.

Pathophysiology

The disease is characterized by an intolerance for *gluten,* one of the proteins found in wheat, barley, rye, and oats. Gluten consists of two factions: glutenin and gliadin. Although the pathologic process is still obscure, susceptible individuals are unable to digest the gliadin faction, resulting in an accumulation of a toxic substance that is damaging to the mucosal cells. Eventually villi atrophy, reducing the absorptive surface of the small intestine. There are two main theories regarding the damaging effect of gluten in CD: (1) the biochemical theory that a specific enzyme deficiency exists and (2) the

theory that the primary cause of the disease is an immunologic abnormality (Walker-Smith, 1991).

Diagnostic Evaluation

Symptoms of CD are first noted about 3 to 6 months after the introduction of gluten-containing grains into the diet, typically at 9 to 18 months of age, although it may not be evident until early childhood (see box). The clinical manifestations are usually insidious and chronic. The first evidence of the disease may be failure to thrive and diarrhea.

A definitive diagnosis is based on a jejunal biopsy, which demonstrates the atrophic changes in the mucosa of the small intestine. This procedure is performed by passing an endoscope through the mouth along the alimentary tract to the jejunum.

Another essential criterion of diagnosis is dramatic clinical improvement after adherence to a gluten-free diet. Within a day or two after instituting the diet, most children with CD demonstrate a favorable personality change. Weight gain, improved appetite, and disappearance of diarrhea and steatorrhea usually do not occur for several days or weeks. Diagnostic criteria for CD also usually include a histologic and/or clinical relapse following gluten reintroduction.

Therapeutic Management

Treatment of chronic CD is primarily dietary management. Although the diet is called "gluten free," it is actually *low* in gluten, since it is impossible to remove every source of this protein. Also, studies demonstrate that most patients are able to tolerate restricted amounts of gluten. Because gluten is found primarily in the grains of wheat and rye, but also in smaller quantities in barley and oats, these four foods are eliminated. Corn and rice become substitute grain foods.

In children with severe malnutrition, specific deficiencies

CLINICAL MANIFESTATIONS OF CELIAC DISEASE (CD)
Impaired Fat Absorption
Steatorrhea (excessively large, pale, oily, frothy stools)
Exceedingly foul-smelling stools
Impaired Absorption of Nutrients
Malnutrition
Muscle wasting (especially prominent in legs and buttocks)
Anemia
Anorexia
Abdominal distention
Behavioral Changes
Irritability
Fretfulness
Uncooperativeness
Apathy
Celiac Crisis*
Acute, severe episodes of profuse watery diarrhea and vomiting
May be precipitated by:
Infections (especially gastrointestinal)
Prolonged fluid and electrolyte depletion
Emotional disturbance
*In very young children.

*In Wong DL: *Wong and Whaley's Clinical manual of pediatric nursing,* ed 4, St Louis, 1996, Mosby.

may be treated with supplemental vitamins, iron, and calories.

Prognosis. CD is generally regarded as a chronic disease. The extent of the disease varies greatly among children. The most severe symptoms usually occur in early childhood and again in adult life. Strict dietary avoidance of gluten can prevent symptoms and may minimize the risk of developing lymphoma, one of the most serious complications of the disease.

Nursing Considerations

The main nursing consideration is helping the parents and child adhere to the prescribed diet. A considerable amount of time is involved in explaining the disease process, the specific role of gluten in aggravating the pathologic condition, and those foods that must be restricted. Although the chief source of grain is cereal and baked goods, grains are frequently added to processed foods as thickeners or fillers. To add to the difficulty, gluten is added to many foods but is obscurely listed on the label as "hydrolyzed vegetable protein." The nurse must advise parents to read carefully all ingredients on labels to avoid hidden sources of gluten. Many of the gluten-containing products can be eliminated from the infant's or young child's diet fairly easily, but monitoring the diet of a school-age child or adolescent is much more difficult. Many "favorite" foods, such as hot dogs, pizza, and spaghetti, are chief offenders. Luncheon preparation away from home is particularly difficult, since bread, luncheon meats, and instant soups are not allowed.

In addition to restricting gluten, other dietary alterations may be necessary in the beginning. For example, in some children who have more severe mucosal damage, the digestion of disaccharides is impaired, especially in relation to lactose. Therefore these children often need a temporary lactose-free diet, which necessitates eliminating all milk products.

Generally, management includes a diet high in calories and proteins, with simple carbohydrates, such as fruits and vegetables, but low in fats. Since the bowel is usually inflamed as a result of the pathologic processes in absorption, high-fiber foods, such as nuts, raisins, raw vegetables, and raw fruits with skin, are avoided until inflammation has subsided.

It is frequently recommended that the child continue the diet indefinitely. This is especially difficult for parents and children to understand when there have been no symptoms of the disease for an extended period and occasional dietary indiscretions, probably the result of increased tolerance to glutens, have not caused untoward effects. However, evidence demonstrates that the majority of individuals who relax their diet will experience a relapse of their disease and possibly exhibit growth retardation, anemia, or osteomalacia. There is also the risk of developing malignant lymphoma of the small intestine or other GI malignancies.

Several resources are available to assist parents in all aspects of coping with CD. The **American Celiac Society*** and the **Celiac Sprue Association/United States of America**† are organizations that provide support and guidance to families and supply educational materials concerning a gluten-free diet, food sources, recipes, and travel information.*

See also Nursing Care Plan: The Child with Celiac Disease.†

SHORT BOWEL SYNDROME (SBS)

SBS is a condition in which there is a loss of intestine resulting in a diminished ability to digest and absorb a regular diet normally. The most common causes of SBS in children include congenital anomalies (jejunal and ileal atresia, gastroschisis), ischemia (necrotizing enterocolitis), and trauma or vascular injury (volvulus [twisting of bowel on itself]). SBS occurs when a large part of gangrenous or atretic small intestine is resected.

Both the amount and the location of bowel lost are important in determining the severity of the condition. Preservation of the distal ileum and the ileocecal valve appears to be important to the infant's survival. Up to 50% of the intestine can be lost without affecting the child's health, unless the loss includes the distal ileum. A loss of greater than 70% of the small bowel results in severe malabsorption. However, the remaining intestine and stomach may adapt to the loss through compensatory growth, provided the child is kept alive with special nutritional support.

The small intestine has significant capacity for adaptation after resection. During the *adaptation process* the villus height increases (villus hyperplasia), which is the primary compensatory mechanism of the bowel. The cell number and absorptive surface area are also increased. A small amount of dilatation and lengthening of the small bowel occurs as well. As villus length and the number of enterocytes available for absorption per centimeter of bowel increase, nutrient absorption increases. Atrophy of the absorptive surface of the bowel occurs with nonuse (no enteral intake), even if nutrients are provided intravenously. Intraluminal enteral feedings stimulate the adaptation process and maintain the structural and functional integrity of the small intestine.

Therapeutic Management

The goals of treatment are (1) to preserve as much length of bowel as possible during surgery, (2) to maintain the child's nutritional status until adaptation to the altered bowel takes place, and (3) to stimulate the adaptation process of the bowel. For the severely affected child, total parenteral nutrition (TPN) is initially used with gradually increasing amounts of enteral feedings.

Enteral nutrition stimulates bowel adaptation. Elemental formulas are better tolerated than traditional infant formulas. Glucose or glucose polymers, medium-chain triglycerides, and hydrolyzed proteins require less digestion. Usually these formulas are better tolerated if provided by continuous slow infusion by either NG tube or gastrostomy. The transition to completely enteral feedings may take months or years. Home enteral and parenteral nutrition should be considered if it is anticipated that nutritional support will be required on a long-term basis.

---

*Dept. N83, 45 Gifford Ave., Jersey City, NJ 07304.
†3213 Rocklyn Dr., Des Moines, IA 50322. In Canada: **Canadian Celiac Association, Inc.,** L5N IA6; (905)567-7195. Mississauga, Ontario.

*A booklet, *Pointers for Parents: Coping with Celiac Sprue,* which provides information on shopping, cooking, and living with an affected child, is available from Clinical Dietetics Dept., Children's Memorial Hospital, 2300 Children's Plaza, Chicago, IL 60614; (312) 880-4000.
†In Wong DL: *Wong and Whaley's Clinical manual of pediatric nursing,* ed 4, St Louis, 1996, Mosby.

Numerous complications are associated with SBS and long-term TPN (see Chapter 22). Infectious, metabolic, and technical complications can occur secondary to TPN. Catheter sepsis can occur after improper care of the catheter. The GI tract can also be a source of microbial seeding of the catheter in children with SBS. Bowel atrophy may foster increased intestinal permeability of bacteria. A lack of adequate sites for central lines may become a significant problem for the child in need of long-term TPN. Hepatic dysfunction is also one of the common complications of TPN. Hepatomegaly with abnormal liver function tests and cholestasis may occur.

Chronic *bacterial overgrowth* is a common problem associated with SBS, which exacerbates malabsorption. Bacterial overgrowth often occurs when the ileocecal valve is absent, when a partial obstruction is present, or when a dilated segment of bowel with poor motility exists. These patients may respond to intermittent broad-spectrum antimicrobial therapy.

Many surgical interventions, including intestinal valves, antiperistaltic segments, recirculating loops, and intestinal lengthening procedures, have been attempted to delay intestinal transit time or increase absorptive surface area. None of these surgical procedures is sufficiently safe and successful to be used routinely (Thompson, 1993).

Transplantation of the small intestine may become a treatment option for selected children with SBS in the future. This procedure has recently been completed with success in children; however, the experience is limited, and the long-term results are unknown. Advancements in antirejection drugs have improved the outlook for this procedure. However, only children with severe disease and complications would be considered candidates for transplantation.

Prognosis. The prognosis for infants with SBS has improved with advances in TPN and with the understanding of the importance of intraluminal nutrition. Establishment of the prognosis depends in part on the length of the residual small intestine. An intact ileocecal valve improves the prognosis. Infants and children with SBS usually die of TPN-related problems, such as fulminant sepsis or severe TPN cholestasis. These TPN-related complications can be significant and life-threatening for many of these children.

Nursing Considerations

Nursing care is directed toward maintaining adequate nutrition. Once the child has reached the enteral feeding goal, transition is made to bolus or oral feedings if possible. Aversion to oral feedings can be a problem for children fed for an extended period with TPN or tube feedings. It has been suggested that lack of oral stimulation at the critical period of 6 to 12 months of age results in difficulty in eating solid food (Tuchman, 1991). In addition, the child may have an extreme sensitivity to anything placed in the mouth. An extensive training program with behavioral modification, using the expertise of speech-language and occupational therapists, may be necessary. To minimize later food aversion, early oral stimulation and nonnutritive sucking should be provided. In addition to a pacifier, occasionally it is acceptable to offer a few drops or tastes of liquids by mouth.

Every effort is made to prevent complications such as infection, especially in central venous access devices. When long-term parenteral nutrition is required, preparing the family for home care of the child is a major nursing responsibility that should be initiated early, whenever possible, to prevent a lengthy hospitalization with subsequent problems such as family dysfunction and developmental delays.* Many infants and children can be successfully cared for at home with enteral and parenteral nutrition if the family is thoroughly prepared and provided with adequate support services. Careful follow-up care by a multidisciplinary nutritional support service is essential. The nurse can have an active and important role in the success of a home nutrition program. Home infusion companies now provide portable equipment, which enables the child and family to maintain a more normal lifestyle.

When hospitalization is prolonged, the child's developmental and emotional needs must be met as well. This often requires special planning to promote normal family adjustment and adaptation of the hospital routines.

---

*Home care instructions on caring for a central venous catheter are available in Wong DL: *Wong and Whaley's Clinical manual of pediatric nursing,* ed 4, St Louis, 1996, Mosby.

KEY POINTS

- Infants are subject to fluid depletion because of their greater surface area relative to body mass, high rate of metabolism, and immature kidney function.
- Dehydration can be classified as isotonic, hypotonic, and hypertonic.
- Vomiting and diarrhea account for significant fluid depletion, especially in infants and small children.
- The amount, frequency, and characteristics of stool and vomitus are important nursing observations.
- Acute diarrhea can be caused by an inflammatory process of infectious origin, a toxic reaction to ingestion of poisonous substances, or dietary indiscretions or can be associated with infections outside the alimentary tract. The primary treatment of diarrhea is the use of oral rehydrating solution.
- Postoperative care of the child with abdominal surgery involves assessing the abdomen, providing hydration and nutrition, intravenous fluids, proper positioning, wound care, and psychologic support.
- Surgical correction in Hirschsprung disease is a two-stage approach: a temporary colostomy and reanastomosis at 8 months to 1 year of age with closure of the colostomy.
- Nursing care of gastrointestinal (GI) reflux is aimed

at identifying children with suggestive symptoms, helping parents with home care feeding and positioning, and caring for the child undergoing surgical intervention.

- Although the cause of appendicitis is poorly understood, it is typically a result of obstruction of the lumen, usually by a fecalith. Common signs and symptoms are right lower quadrant abdominal pain, tenderness, and fever.
- Meckel diverticulum, the most common congenital malformation of the GI tract, is characterized by bloody stools.
- Inflammatory bowel disease refers to ulcerative colitis and Crohn disease, of which persistent and recurring diarrhea is the most common feature. It is treated by dietary management and medication, although surgery is needed in a number of cases.
- Peptic ulcers are poorly understood, but one of two mechanisms probably reflects the basic defect: an increase in the rate of production of gastric juice or interference with the normal protective mechanisms of the mucosal lining.
- Viral hepatitis is caused by at least five types of virus: hepatitis A virus, hepatitis B virus, hepatitis D virus, and hepatitis C and E viruses (non-A, non-B viruses).
- Hepatitis A virus is spread by the fecal-oral route, whereas hepatitis B virus is transmitted primarily by the parenteral route. The most effective measure in prevention and control of hepatitis in any setting is handwashing and standard precautions.
- Structural disorders of the GI tract include cleft lip, cleft palate, esophageal atresia with tracheoesophageal fistula, anorectal malformations, and biliary atresia.
- Biliary atresia is a serious disorder, often causing progressive liver failure, which is an indication for liver transplantation.
- Cleft lip and palate, the most common facial malformation, may involve nutritional, dental, and speech problems.
- Hernias related to the GI tract can be minor (umbilical hernia) or life-threatening (hiatal, gastroschisis, omphalocele).
- General signs of obstruction include colicky abdominal pain, nausea and vomiting, abdominal distention, and decreased stool output.
- Hypertrophic pyloric stenosis is recognized by characteristic projectile vomiting, malnutrition, dehydration, and a palpable mass in the epigastrium and is relieved by pyloromyotomy.
- Intussusception is one of the most common causes of intestinal obstruction during infancy and is characterized by abdominal pain and blood in stools. Treatment is either nonsurgical hydrostatic reduction or surgical reduction.
- Malabsorption syndromes are disorders associated with some degree of impaired digestion and/or absorption. They include digestive defects, absorptive defects, and anatomic defects.
- Celiac disease, the second leading cause of malabsorption in children, is characterized by an intolerance for gluten. It is thought to be either an inborn error of metabolism or an immunologic response.
- Short bowel syndrome is characterized by a loss of intestine resulting in a diminished ability to digest and absorb a regular diet normally. Specialized enteral and parenteral nutrition is a major element of care for these children.

REFERENCES

Albanese CT and others: Percutaneous gastroenjunostomy versus Nissen fundoplication for enteral feeding of the neurologically impaired child with gastroesopageal reflux, *J Pediatr* 123:371-375, 1993.

Avery M, Snyder J: Oral therapy for acute diarrhea: the underused simple solution, *N Engl J Med* 323(13):891-894, 1990.

Bacon B: Managing chronic hepatitis, *Postgrad Med* 90(5):103-112, 1991.

Bishop W, Ulshen M: Bacterial gastroenteritis, *Pediatr Clin North Am* 35(1):69-87, 1988.

Borowski S: Common pediatric surgical problems, *Nurs Clin North Am* 29(4):551-562, 1994.

Brown K: Dietary management of acute childhood diarrhea: optimal timing of feeding and appropriate use of milks and mixed diets, *J Pediatr* 118(4):S92-S98, 1991.

Brown KH, Peerson JM, Fontaine O: Use of nonhuman milks in the dietary management of young children with acute diarrhea: a meta-analysis of clinical trials, *Pediatrics* 93(1):17-27, 1994.

Carey W, Patel G: Viral hepatitis in the 1990's. III. Hepatitis C, hepatitis E, and other viruses, *Cleve Clin J Med* 59(6):595-601, 1992.

Chew F and others: Is dilution of cows' milk formula necessary for dietary management of acute diarrhoea in infants aged less than 6 months? *Lancet* 341:194-197, 1993.

Cohen M: Etiology and mechanisms of acute infectious diarrhea in infants in the United States, *J Pediatr* 118(4):S34-S39, 1991.

Ergun G, Miskovitz P: Viral hepatitis, *Postgrad Med* 88(5):69-76, 1990.

Fanaroff AA, Martin RJ: Jaundice and liver disease. In Fanaroff AA, Martin RJ, editors: *Neonatal-perinatal medicine: diseases of the fetus and infant*, St Louis, 1992, Mosby.

Finberg L: Assessing the clinical clues to dehydration, *Contemp Pediatr* 7(4):45-57, 1990.

Francis CY, Whorwell PJ: Bran and irritable bowel syndrome: time for reappraisal, *Lancet* 344(8914):39-40, 1994.

Hickey R, Sodhi S, Johnson W: Two children with lethargy and intussusception, *Ann Emerg Med* 19(4):390-392, 1990.

Hillemeier A: Reflux and esophagitis. In Walker W and others, editors: *Pediatric gastrointestinal disease*, Philadelphia, 1991, Decker.

Hoekstra JH and others: Fluid intake and industrial processing in apple juice induced chronic non-specific diarrhoea, *Arch Dis Child* 73(2):126-130, 1995.

Jackson W, Grand R: Crohn's disease. In Walker W and others, editors: *Pediatric gastrointestinal disease*, Philadelphia, 1991, Decker.

Johnson K, editor (Johns Hopkins Hospital): *The Harriet Lane handbook*, ed 13, St Louis, 1993, Mosby.

Kanesaki T and others: Hepatitis C virus infection in children with hemophilia: characterization of antibody response to four different antigens and relationship of antibody response, viremia, and hepatic dysfunction, *J Pediatr* 123:381-387, 1993.

Karrer F and others: Congenital biliary tract disease, *Surg Clin North Am* 70(6):1403-1418, 1990.

Kirschner B: Hirschsprung's disease. In Walker W and others, editors: *Pediatric gastrointestinal disease,* Philadelphia, 1991, Decker.

Kleinman RE: We have the solution: now what's the problem? *Pediatrics* 90(1):113-155, 1992.

Krugman S: Viral hepatitis: A, B, C, D and E—infection, *Pediatr Rev* 13(6):203-212, 1992.

Kubiak M and others: Comparison of stool containment in cloth and single-use diapers using a simulated infant feces, *Pediatrics* 91(3):632-636, 1993.

Laurent J and others: Long-term outcome after surgery for biliary atresia, *Gastroenterology* 99(6):1793-1797, 1990.

Lisanti P, Talotta D: Hepatitis update: the delta virus, *AORN J* 55(3):790-800, 1992.

Lloyd-Still JD: Impact of orthotopic liver transplantation on mortality from pediatric liver disease, *J Pediatr Gastroenterol Nutr* 12:305-309, 1991.

Margolis P and others: Effects of unrestricted diet on mild infantile diarrhea, *Am J Dis Child* 144:162-164, 1990.

Meyer J: The current radiologic management of intussusception: a survey and review, *Pediatr Radiol* 22:323-325, 1992.

Milla P: Motor disorders including pyloric stenosis. In Walker W and others, editors: *Pediatric gastrointestinal disease,* Philadelphia, 1991, Decker.

Najmaldin A, Tan HL: Early experience with laparoscopic pyloromyotomy for infantile hypertrophic pyloric stenosis, *J Pediatr Surg* 30(1):37-38, 1995.

NIH Consensus Development Panel on *Helicobacter pylori* in peptic ulcer disease: *Helicobacter pylori* in peptic ulcer disease, *JAMA* 272(1):65-69, 1994.

Orenstein SR: Gastroesophageal reflux, *Pediatr Rev* 13(5):174-182, 1992.

Orenstein SR: The prone alternative, *Pediatrics* 94(1):104-105, 1994.

Orenstein S: Prone positioning in infant gastroesophageal reflux: is elevation of the head worth the trouble? *J Pediatr* 117(2):184-187, 1990.

Rennels MB and others: Safety and efficacy of high-dose rhesus-human reassortant rotavirus vaccines—Report of the National Multicenter Trial, *Pediatrics* 97(1):7-13, 1996.

Richard M: Feeding the newborn with cleft lip and/or palate: the enlargement, stimulate, swallow rest (ESSR) method, *J Pediatr Nurs* 6(5):317-321, 1991.

Ryckman F and others: Improved survival in biliary atresia patients in the present era of liver transplantation, *J Pediatr Surg* 28(3):382-386, 1993.

Sachar DB: Budesonide for inflammatory bowel disease: is it a magic bullet? *N Engl J Med* 331(13):873-874, 1994.

Santosham M, Greenough W: Oral rehydration therapy: a global perspective, *J Pediatr* 118(4):S44-S51, 1991.

Shandling B: Appendicitis. In Walker W and others, editors: *Pediatric gastrointestinal disease,* Philadelphia, 1991, Decker.

Thompson J: Surgical considerations in the short bowel syndrome, *Surg Gynecol Obstet* 176:89-101, 1993.

Toyosaka A and others: Outcome of 21 patients with biliary atresia living more than 10 years, *J Pediatr Surg* 28:1498-1501, 1993.

Tuchman D: Disorders of deglutition. In Walker W and others, editors: *Pediatric gastrointestinal disease,* Philadelphia, 1991, Decker.

Turgeon D, Barnett J: Meckel's diverticulum, *Am J Gastroenterol* 85(7):777-781, 1990.

Walker-Smith J: Celiac disease. In Walker W and others, editors: *Pediatric gastrointestinal disease,* Philadelphia, 1991, Decker.

Wright V: The esophagus: congenital anomalies. In Walker W and others, editors: *Pediatric gastrointestinal disease,* Philadelphia, 1991, Decker.

Ziller S, Netchvolodoff C: Uncomplicated peptic ulcer disease, *Postgrad Med* 93(4):126-138, 1993.

BIBLIOGRAPHY

Disorders of Motility

Booth IW: Dietary management of acute diarrhoea in childhood, *Lancet* 341(8851):996, 1993.

Clayden G: Management of chronic constipation, *Arch Dis Child* 67:340-344, 1992.

Dipalma J: Metoclopramide: a dopamine receptor antagonist, *Am Fam Physician* 41(3):919-921, 1990.

Ellett ML: Constipation/encopresis: a nursing perspective, *J Pediatr Health Care* 4(3):141-146, 1990.

Evans K: Pediatric management problems . . . chronic constipation, *Pediatr Nurs* 16(6):590-591, 1990.

Foster P, Cowan G, Wrenn E: Twenty-five years' experience with Hirschsprung's disease, *J Pediatr Surg* 25(5):531-534, 1990.

Hlusko D, McMurray J: Gastroesophageal reflux: treatment and nursing care, *Neonatal Network* 9(5):33-36, 1991.

Konings K: Preop use of Golytely in pediatrics, *Pediatr Nurs* 15:473-474, 1989.

Lifshitz F, Ament M: Role of juice carbohydrate malabsorption in chronic nonspecific diarrhea in children, *J Pediatr* 120(5):825-829, 1992.

Loening-Baucke V: Constipation in children, *Curr Opin Pediatr* 6:556-561, 1994.

Margolis P and others: Effects of unrestricted diet on mild infantile diarrhea, *Am J Dis Child* 144:162-164, 1990.

Orenstein SR and others: Reliability and validity of an infant gastroesophageal reflux questionnaire, *Clin Pediatr* 32(8):472-484, 1993.

Orenstein ST: Gastroesophageal reflux disease, *Semin Gastrointest Dis* 5(1):2-14, 1994.

Say B, Smith DP: Midline field defects and Hirschsprung disease, *Am J Med Genet* 61:293-294, 1996 (letter to editor).

Sterling C, Schaffer S, Jolley S: Home management related to medical treatment for childhood gastroesophageal reflux, *Pediatr Nurs* 19(2):167-173, 1993.

Sterling C and others: Nursing responsibility in the diagnosis, care, and treatment of the child with gastroesophageal reflux, *J Pediatr Nurs* 6(6):435-440, 1991.

Thorye SM: Mothers' internal working models with infants with gastroesophageal reflux, *Matern Child Nurs J* 22(2):39-48, 1994.

Treem W: Chronic nonspecific diarrhea of childhood, *Clin Pediatr,* 30(7):413-420, 1992.

Inflammatory Disorders

Anderson ML: *Helicobacter pylori* infection, *Postgrad Med* 96(6):40-50, 1994.

Andersson R and others: Indications for operation in suspected appendicitis and incidence of perforation, *Br Med J* 308(6921):107-110, 1994.

Christie PM, Hill GI: Effect of intravenous nutrition on nutrition and function in acute attacks of inflammatory bowel disease, *Gastroenterology* 99:730-736, 1990.

Cooke D: Inflammatory bowel disease: primary health care management of ulcerative colitis and Crohn's disease, *Nurse Pract* 16(8):27-39, 1991.

De Giacomo C and others: Omeprazole treatment of severe peptic disease associated with antral G cell hyperfunction and hyperpepsinogenemia I in an infant, *J Pediatr* 117(6):989-993, 1990.

Feagan BG and others: Low-dose cyclosporine for the treatment of Crohn's disease, *N Engl J Med* 330(26):1846-1851, 1994.

Ferguson A: Ulcerative colitis and Crohn's disease, *Br Med J* 309(6951):355-356, 1994.

Gamal R, Moore TC: Appendicitis in children aged 13 years and younger, *Am J Surg* 159:589-592, 1990.

Garretson DC, Frederich DO, Frederich ME: Meckel's diverticulum, *Am Fam Physician* 42(1):115-119, 1990.

Greenberger NJ, Miner PB: Is maintenance therapy effective in Crohn's disease? *Lancet* 344(8927):900-901, 1994.

Kisumoto and others: Complications and diagnosis of Meckel's diverticulum in 776 patients, *Am J Surg* 164:382-383, 1992.

Lichtiger S and others: Cyclosporine in severe ulcerative colitis refractory to steroid therapy, *N Engl J Med* 330(26):1841-1845, 1994.

McKenna CJ: Gastrointestinal bleeding in children: implications for nursing, *Nurs Clin North Am* 29(4):599, 1994.

Perrone-Pollack VE: Inflammatory bowel disease. In Jackson PL, Vessey JA: *Primary care of the child with a chronic condition*, ed 2, St Louis, 1996, Mosby.

Rothrock and others: Clinical features of misdiagnosed appendicitis in children, *Ann Emerg Med* 20(1):45-50, 1991.

Sherman PM: Peptic ulcer disease in children, *Gastroenterol Clin North Am* 23(4):707-725, 1994.

Hepatic Disorders

A-Kader HH: Hepatitis C virus: implications to pediatric practice, *Pediatr Infect Dis J* 12(10):853-866, 1993.

Beath S and others: Liver transplantation in babies and children with extrahepatic biliary atresia, *J Pediatr Surg* 28(8):1044-1047, 1993.

Beath SV and others: Successful liver transplantation in babies under 1 year, *Br Med J* 307:825-828, 1993.

Bodenhorn K: Hepatitis B: the challenge for nurses, *J Pediatr Health Care* 6(1):41-42, 1992.

Carey W, Patel G: Viral hepatitis in the 1990's. I. Current principles of management, *Cleve Clin J Med* 59(4):317-325, 1992.

Carey W, Patel G: Viral hepatitis in the 1990's. II. Hepatitis B and delta virus, *Cleve Clin J Med* 59(4):393-401, 1992.

Karrer FM and others: Congenital biliary tract disease, *Surg Clin North Am* 70(6):1403-1418, 1990.

Nowicki M, Balistreri W: Hepatitis A to E: building up the alphabet, *Contemp Pediatr* 9(11):118-128, 1992.

Pasquale M, Cerra F: Sengstaken-Blakemore tube placement, *Crit Care Clin* 8(4):743-753, 1992.

Poss JE: Hepatitis B virus infection in Southeast Asian children, *J Pediatr Health Care* 3:311-315, 1989.

Smith J: Hepatitis C: a major public health problem, *J Adv Nurs* 18:503-506, 1993.

Structural Defects

Borkowski S: Common pediatric surgical problems, *Nurs Clin North Am* 29(4):551-562, 1994.

Curtin G: The infant with cleft lip or palate: more than a surgical problem, *J Perinat Neonat Nurs* 3(3):80-89, 1990.

Dado DV: Experience with the functional cleft lip repair, *Plast Reconstr Surg* 86(5):872-881, 1990.

Eliason MJ: Cleft lip and palate: developmental effects, *J Pediatr Nurs* 6(2):107, 1991.

Filston HC: Fluid and electrolyte management in the pediatric surgical patient, *Surg Clin North Am* 72(6):1189-1200, 1992.

Kaufman FL: Managing the cleft lip and palate patient, *Pediatr Clin North Am* 38(5):1127-1147, 1991.

Kent PA, Curley MA: Challenges in nursing: infants with congenital diaphragmatic hernia, *Heart Lung* 21(4):381-389, 1992.

Laurent J and others: Long-term outcome after surgery for biliary atresia, *Gastroenterology* 99:1793-1797, 1990.

Levine AH: Fetal surgery: in utero repair of congenital diaphragmatic hernia, *AORN J* 54(1):16, 1991.

MacDonald CA: Biliary atresia, *J Pediatr Nurs* 6(6):374-383, 1991.

Moreno CN, Iovanne BA: Congenital diaphragmatic hernia. Part I, *Neonatal Network* 12(1):19, 1993.

Nyhus LM and others: Inguinal hernia repairs, *AORN J* 52(2):292-304, 1990.

Pate CMH: Care of the family following the birth of a child with a cleft lip and/or palate, *Neonatal Network* 5(6):30-37, 1987.

Puntis JW and others: Growth and feeding problems after repair of esophageal atresia, *Arch Dis Child* 65:84-88, 1990.

Ricketts R and others: Modern treatment of cloacal exstrophy, *J Pediatr Surg* 26(4):444-450, 1991.

Skinner M, Grosfeld J: Inguinal and umbilical hernia repair in infants and children, *Surg Clin North Am* 73(3):439-449, 1993.

Theorell CJ: Congenital diaphragmatic hernia: a physiologic approach to management, *J Perinat Neonat Nurs* 3(3):66-79, 1990.

Torfs C, Curry C, Roeper P: Gastroschisis, *J Pediatr* 116:1-6, 1990.

Van Meurs KP and others: Effect of extracorporeal membrane oxygenation on survival of infants with congenital diaphragmatic hernia, *J Pediatr* 117(6):954-960, 1990.

Obstructive Disorders/Malabsorption Syndromes

Anson O, Weizman Z, Zeevi N: Celiac disease: parental knowledge and attitudes of dietary compliance, *Pediatrics* 85:98-103, 1990.

Champoux AN, Beccaro MA, Nazar-Stewart V: Recurrent intussusception: risks and features, *Arch Pediatr Adolesc Med* 148(5):474-478, 1994.

Deluca S: Hypertrophic pyloric stenosis, *Am Fam Physician* 47(8):1771-1773, 1993.

Edes TE: Clinical management of short-bowel syndrome, *Postgrad Med* 88(4):91-95, 1990.

Guandalini S and others: Diagnosis of coeliac disease: time for a change? *Arch Dis Child* 64:1320-1325, 1989.

Horman SH: Pica as a presenting symptom in childhood celiac disease, *Am J Clin Nutr* 51:139-141, 1990.

Rollins MD and others: Pyloric stenosis: congenital or acquired? *Arch Dis Child* 64:138-147, 1989.

Saunderlin G: Celiac disease: a review, *Gastroenterol Nurs* 17(3):100-105, 1994.

Skipper R, Boeckman C, Klein R: Childhood intussusception, *Surg Gynecol Obstet* 171:151-153, 1990.

Trier J: Diagnosis and treatment of celiac sprue, *Hosp Pract* 30:41-54, 1993.

Wise B: Neonatal short bowel syndrome, *Neonatal Network* 11(7):9-15, 1992.

Zahr LK and others: The short bowel syndrome: an update and a case study, *J Pediatr Nurs* 7(3):189-195, 1992.

Chapter 25

THE CHILD WITH CARDIOVASCULAR DYSFUNCTION

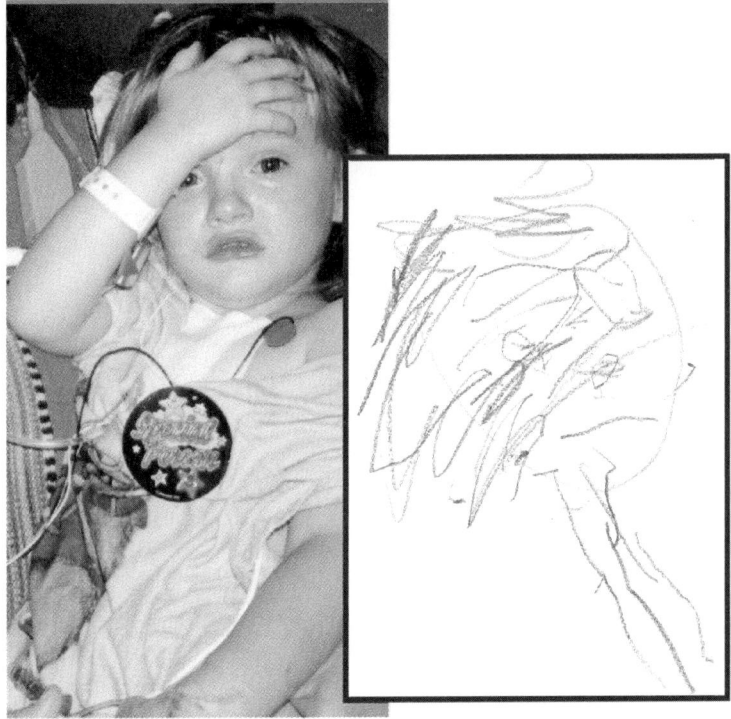

" *My heart is fixed now.* "

Lauren, age 3 years,
atrial septal defect repair

RELATED TOPICS

CARDIOVASCULAR DYSFUNCTION

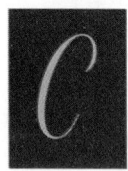ardiovascular disorders in children are divided into two major groups, congenital heart disease and acquired heart disorders. *Congenital heart disease* includes primarily anatomic abnormalities present at birth that result in abnormal cardiac function. The clinical consequences of congenital heart defects fall into two broad categories, congestive heart failure and hypoxemia. *Acquired cardiac disorders* refer to disease processes or abnormalities that occur after birth and can be seen in the normal heart or in the presence of congenital heart defects. They result from various factors, including infection, autoimmune responses, environmental factors, and familial tendencies.

ASSESSMENT OF CARDIAC FUNCTION

History and Physical Examination

Nursing assessment of children for evidence of cardiac dysfunction begins with a careful history to elicit information regarding possible causes of heart disease: (1) history of heart disease in other family members, such as a parent or sibling; (2) contact with known teratogens, such as rubella, during pregnancy; (3) presence of chromosomal abnormalities such as Down syndrome; (4) poor weight gain and/or feeding behavior; (5) frequent respiratory infections; (6) prior murmurs; (7) respiratory difficulties, such as tachypnea, dyspnea, and shortness of breath; or (8) recent streptococcal infection in the child. Exercise intolerance and fatigue (e.g., during feeding in the infant) are characteristic features of heart disease.

The physical assessment of suspected cardiac disease begins with observation of general appearance, then proceeds with more specific observations. The following are supplementary to the general assessment techniques described for physical assessment of the chest and heart in Chapter 7.

Patricia O'Brien, MSN, RN,C, PNP, revised this chapter.

Inspection

Nutritional state—failure to thrive or poor weight gain are associated with heart disease

Color—cyanosis is a common feature of congenital heart disease, and pallor is associated with poor perfusion

Chest deformities—an enlarged heart sometimes distorts the chest configuration

Unusual pulsations—visible pulsations of the neck veins are seen in some patients

Respiratory excursion—this refers to the ease or difficulty of respiration (e.g., tachypnea, dyspnea, presence of expiratory grunt)

Clubbing of fingers—this is associated with cyanosis

Palpation and Percussion

Chest—these maneuvers help discern heart size and other characteristics (e.g., thrills) associated with heart disease

Abdomen—hepatomegaly and/or splenomegaly may be evident

Peripheral pulses—rate, regularity, and amplitude (strength) may reveal discrepancies

Auscultation

Heart rate and rhythm—listen for fast heart rates (tachycardia), slow heart rates (bradycardia), or irregular rhythms

Character of heart sounds—listen for distinct or muffled sounds, murmurs, and additional heart sounds

Diagnostic Evaluation

A variety of invasive and noninvasive tests may be used in the diagnosis of heart disease (Table 25-1). Cardiac catheterization, which generates more anxiety than any other cardiac test, is discussed in detail.

CARDIAC CATHETERIZATION

Cardiac catheterization is a diagnostic procedure in which a radiopaque catheter is inserted through a peripheral blood vessel into the heart. The catheter is usually introduced through a cutdown procedure, in which a small incision is made to expose the vessel, or through a percutaneous technique, in which the catheter is threaded through a large-bore needle that is inserted into the vein. The catheter is guided through the heart with the aid of fluoroscopy. Once the tip of the catheter is within a heart chamber, contrast material is injected, and films are taken of the dilution and circulation

TABLE 25-1. Procedures for cardiac diagnosis

PROCEDURE	DESCRIPTION
Chest Radiograph (X-Ray)	Provides information on heart size and pulmonary blood flow patterns
Electrocardiography (ECG or EKG)	Graphic measure of the electrical activity of the heart
Holter Monitor	24-hour continuous ECG recording used to assess dysrhythmias
Echocardiography	Use of high-frequency sound waves obtained by a transducer to produce an image of cardiac structures
Transthoracic	Done with transducer on chest
M-mode	One-dimensional graphic view used to estimate ventricular size and function
Two-dimensional (2-D)	Real-time, cross-sectional views of heart used to identify cardiac structures and cardiac anatomy
Doppler	Identifies blood flow patterns and pressure gradients across structures
Fetal	Imaging fetal heart in utero
Transesophageal (TEE)	Transducer placed in esophagus behind the heart to obtain images of posterior heart structures or in patients with poor images from chest approach
Cardiac Catheterization	Imaging study using radiopaque catheters placed in a peripheral blood vessel and advanced into heart to measure pressures and oxygen levels in heart chambers and visualize heart structures and blood flow patterns
Hemodynamics	Measures pressures and oxygen saturations in heart chambers
Angiography	Use of contrast material to illuminate heart structures and blood flow patterns
Biopsy	Use of special catheter to remove tiny samples of heart muscle for microscopic evaluation; used in assessing infection, inflammation, or muscle dysfunction disorders; also to evaluate for rejection after heart transplant
Electrophysiology (EPS)	Special catheters with electrodes employed to record electrical activity from within heart; used to diagnose rhythm disturbances
Exercise Stress Test	Monitoring of heart rate, blood pressure, ECG, and oxygen consumption at rest and during progressive exercise on a treadmill or bicycle

of the material *(angiography)*. Types of cardiac catheterizations include the following:

1. **Diagnostic catheterizations**—used to diagnose congenital cardiac defects, particularly in symptomatic infants and before surgical repair. These are divided into right-sided catheterizations, in which the catheter is introduced through a vein (usually the femoral vein) and threaded to the right atrium (most common), and left-sided catheterizations, in which the catheter is threaded through an artery into the aorta and into the heart.
2. **Interventional catheterizations (therapeutic catheterizations)**—a balloon catheter or other device is used to alter the cardiac anatomy. Examples include dilating stenotic valves or vessels or closing abnormal connections.
3. **Electrophysiology studies**—catheters with tiny electrodes that record the impulses of the heart directly from the conduction system are used to evaluate dysrhythmias and sometimes destroy accessory pathways that cause some tachydysrhythmias.

Nursing Considerations

Cardiac catheterization has become a routine diagnostic procedure and may be done on an outpatient basis. However, it is not without risks, especially in neonates and seriously ill infants and children. Typical reactions include acute hemorrhage from the entry site (more likely with interventional procedures because larger catheters are used), low-grade fever, nausea, vomiting, loss of pulse in the catheterized extremity (usually transient, resulting from a clot, hematoma, or intimal tear), and transient dysrhythmias (generally catheter induced).

Preprocedural Care. A complete nursing assessment is necessary to ensure a safe procedure with minimum complications. This assessment should include accurate height (essential to correct catheter selection) and weight. Obtaining a history of allergic reactions is important, since some of the contrast agents are iodine based. Specific attention to signs and symptoms of infection is crucial. Severe diaper rash may be a reason to cancel the procedure if femoral access is required. Since assessment of pedal pulses is important after catheterization, the nurse should assess and mark pulses (dorsalis pedis, posterior tibial) before the child goes to the catheterization room. The presence and quality of pulses in both feet are clearly documented. Baseline oxygen saturation using pulse oximetry in children with cyanosis is also recorded.

Preparing the child and family for the procedure is the joint responsibility of the physician and nurse. The cardiologist usually explains the procedure to the parents, but nurses can reinforce and clarify the information. Many parents and older children who undergo both cardiac catheterization and cardiac surgery say, in retrospect, that they were more anxious about cardiac catheterization than about the surgery. Preparation for cardiac catheterization requires the same attention to the principles of preparation for procedures described in Chapter 22.

It is important to describe the catheterization ("cath") room because the x-ray machinery can appear frightening. Other aspects of the procedure that should be explained (using words the child understands) include, specifically, that (1) the groin (or sometimes the antecubital fossa) is cleansed with a special brown solution; (2) the child will receive some medicine (lidocaine) in that area so that the skin will go to sleep; (3) a tube will be placed in a blood vessel, and the child may feel a little pushing at times; (4) when a special "medicine" (referring to the contrast material) is put into the tubing, the child may feel warm for a few seconds; and (5) as soon as the medicine is put in, the lights will go off and a machine will begin to take pictures. The last point is important to stress because younger children may associate the lights going off with "causing" the warm feeling from the contrast agent. As a result, they may become fearful of the dark and the noise from the machines.

Methods of sedation vary among institutions and may include oral or intravenous (IV) medications (see Atraumatic Care box). The child's age, heart defect, clinical status, and type of catheterization procedure planned are considered when sedation is determined. Children are allowed nothing by mouth (NPO) for 2 or more hours before the procedure, and infants and patients with polycythemia may need IV fluids to prevent dehydration and hypoglycemia.

Postprocedural Care.   Essentially the care following cardiac catheterization is the same as general postoperative care. However, since children are not anesthetized during the procedure, they usually return directly to their room. Patients are usually placed on a cardiac monitor and a pulse oximeter for the first few hours of recovery. The most important nursing responsibility is observation of the following for signs of complications:

- Pulses, especially below the catheterization site, for equality and symmetry (pulse distal to the site may be weaker for the first few hours after catheterization but should gradually increase in strength)
- Temperature and color of the affected extremity, since coolness or blanching may indicate arterial obstruction

- Vital signs, which are taken as frequently as every 15 minutes, with special emphasis on heart rate, which is counted for 1 full minute for evidence of dysrhythmias or bradycardia
- Blood pressure, especially for hypotension, which may indicate hemorrhage from cardiac perforation or bleeding at the site of initial catheterization
- Dressing, for evidence of bleeding or hematoma formation in the femoral or antecubital area
- Fluid intake, both IV and oral, to ensure adequate hydration (blood loss in the catheterization laboratory, the child's NPO status, and diuretic actions of dyes used during the procedure put children at risk for hypovolemia and dehydration)
- Hypoglycemia, especially in infants who should receive dextrose-containing IV fluids; blood glucose levels should be checked

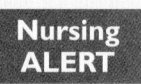 **Nursing ALERT** (Agamalian, 1986).   If bleeding occurs, direct continuous pressure is applied 2.5 cm (1 inch) above the percutaneous skin site to localize pressure over the vessel puncture

Depending on hospital policy, the child may be kept in bed with the affected extremity maintained straight for 4 to 6 hours after venous catheterization and 6 to 8 hours after arterial catheterization to facilitate healing of the cannulated vessel. If younger children have difficulty complying, they can be held in the parent's lap with the leg maintained in the correct position. The child's usual diet can be resumed as soon as tolerated, beginning with sips of clear liquids and advancing as the condition allows. The child is encouraged to void to clear the contrast material from the blood. Generally there is only slight discomfort at the percutaneous site. To prevent infection, the catheterization area is protected from possible contamination. If the child wears diapers, the dressing can be kept dry by covering it with a piece of plastic film and sealing the edges of the film to the skin with tape. However, the nurse must be careful to continue to observe the site for any evidence of bleeding (see Family Home Care box).

See also Nursing Care Plan: The Child Who Undergoes Cardiac Catheterization.*

---

*In Wong DL: *Wong and Whaley's Clinical manual of pediatric nursing,* ed 4, St Louis, 1996, Mosby.

ATRAUMATIC CARE
Cardiac Catheterization

To reduce the pain of the catheter insertion, apply EMLA topically to site for 60 minutes or use buffered lidocaine and 30-gauge needle for intradermal injection (see Pain Management, Chapter 21).

 FAMILY HOME CARE
Following Cardiac Catheterization

Remove pressure dressing the day after catheterization. Cover site with an adhesive bandage strip for several days.
Keep site clean and dry. Avoid tub baths for several days; may shower.
Observe site for redness, swelling, drainage, and bleeding. Monitor for fever. Notify practitioner if these occur.
Avoid strenuous exercise for several days. May attend school.
Resume regular diet without restrictions.
Use acetaminophen or ibuprofen for pain.
Keep follow-up appointments per practitioner's instruction.

Modified from Children's Hospital (Boston) Cardiovascular Program, 1994.

CONGENITAL HEART DISEASE (CHD)

GENERAL CONCEPTS

The incidence of CHD in children is generally believed to be 4 to 10 per 1000 live births and is the major cause of death in the first year (other than prematurity). The sexes are affected differently, depending on the defect. Children with CHD are also more likely to have extracardiac defects, such as tracheoesophageal fistula, renal agenesis, and diaphragmatic hernias.

The etiology of most congenital heart defects is not known. However, several factors are associated with a higher-than-normal incidence of the disease. These include prenatal factors such as (1) maternal rubella during pregnancy, (2) maternal alcoholism, (3) maternal age over 40 years, and (4) maternal insulin-dependent diabetes. Several genetic factors are also implicated, although the influence is multifactorial. For example, there is an increased risk of CHD in the child who (1) has a sibling with a heart defect, (2) has a parent with CHD, (3) has a chromosomal aberration, such as Down syndrome, or (4) is born with other, noncardiac congenital anomalies.

Circulatory Changes at Birth

During fetal life, blood carrying oxygen and nutritive materials from the placenta enters the fetal system through the umbilicus via the large umbilical vein. Oxygenated blood enters the heart by way of the inferior vena cava. Because of the higher pressure of blood entering the right atrium, it is directed posteriorly in a straight pathway across the right atrium and through the *foramen ovale* to the left atrium. In this way the better-oxygenated blood enters the left atrium and ventricle, to be pumped through the aorta to the head and upper extremities. Blood from the head and upper extremities entering the right atrium from the superior vena cava is directed downward through the tricuspid valve into the right ventricle. From here it is pumped through the pulmonary artery, where the major portion is shunted to the descending aorta via the *ductus arteriosus.* Only a small amount flows to and from the nonfunctioning fetal lungs (Fig. 25-1, *A*).

Before birth the high pulmonary vascular resistance created by the collapsed fetal lung causes greater pressures in the right side of the heart and the pulmonary arteries. At the same time the free-flowing placental circulation and the ductus arteriosus produce a low vascular resistance in the remainder of the fetal vascular system. With the cessation of placental blood flow from clamping of the umbilical cord and the expansion of the lungs at birth, the hemodynamics of the fetal vascular system undergo pronounced and abrupt changes (Fig. 25-1, *B*).

With the first breath, the lungs are expanded, and increased oxygen causes pulmonary vasodilation. Pulmonary pressures start to fall as systemic pressures, given the removal of the placenta, start to rise. Normally the foramen ovale closes as the pressure in the left atrium exceeds the pressure

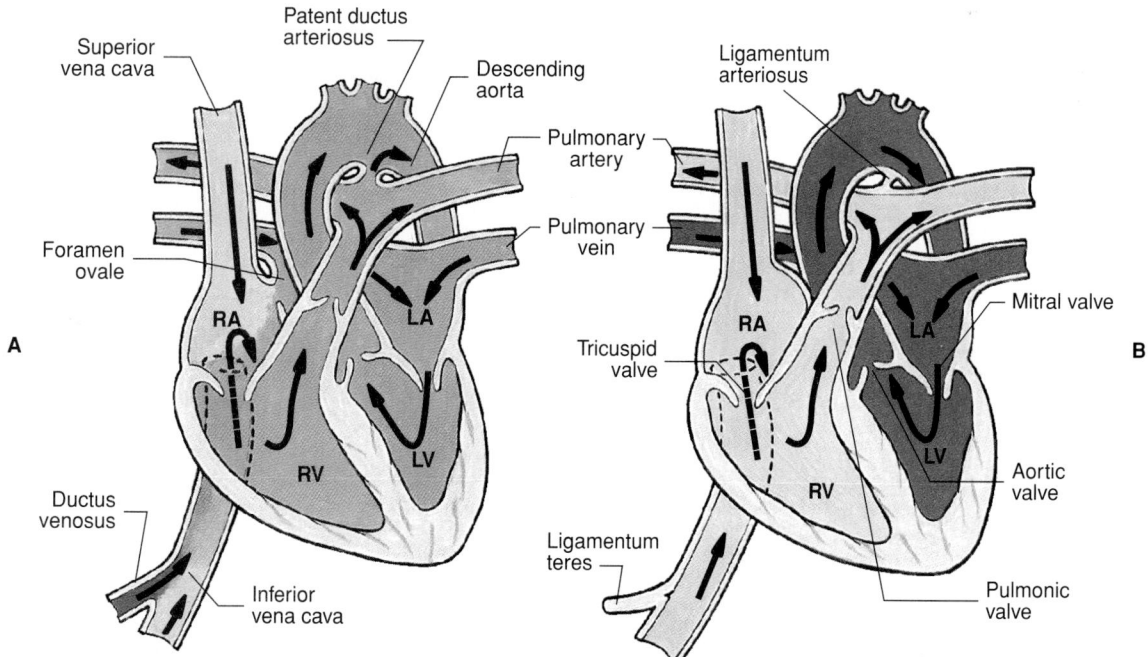

FIG. 25-1. Changes in circulation at birth. **A,** Prenatal circulation. **B,** Postnatal circulation. Arrows indicate direction of blood flow. Although four pulmonary veins enter the LA, for simplicity this diagram shows only two. *RA,* Right atrium; *LA,* left atrium; *RV,* right ventricle; *LV,* left ventricle.

in the right atrium. The ductus arteriosus starts to close in the presence of increased oxygen concentration in the blood and other factors.

Altered Hemodynamics

To appreciate the physiology of heart defects, it is necessary to understand the role of pressure gradients, flow, and resistance within the circulation. As with any fluid, blood flows from an area of high pressure to one of lower pressure and toward the path of least resistance in response to the pumping action of the heart. In general the higher the pressure gradient, the greater is the rate of flow; the higher the resistance, the less the rate of flow.

Normally the pressure on the right side of the heart is lower than that on the left side, and the resistance in the pulmonary circulation is less than that in the systemic circulation. Vessels entering or exiting these chambers have corresponding pressures. Therefore, if an abnormal connection exists between the heart chambers (such as a septal defect), blood will necessarily flow from an area of higher pressure (left side) to one of lower pressure (right side). Such a flow of blood is termed a *left-to-right shunt*. Anomalies resulting in cyanosis may result from a change in pressure so that the blood is shunted from the right to the left side of the heart *(right-to-left shunt)* because of either increased pulmonary vascular resistance or obstruction to blood flow through the pulmonic valve and artery. Cyanosis may also result from a defect that allows mixing of oxygenated and deoxygenated blood within the heart chambers or great arteries, such as occurs in truncus arteriosus.

CLASSIFICATION OF DEFECTS

Congenital heart defects have been divided into two categories. Traditionally, a physical characteristic, cyanosis, has been used as the distinguishing feature, dividing the anomalies into *acyanotic defects* and *cyanotic defects.* In clinical practice this system is problematic because children with acyanotic defects may develop cyanosis. Also, more often, those with cyanotic defects may be pink and have more clinical signs of congestive heart failure (CHF).

Another classification system, based on *hemodynamic characteristics,* also is used. The defining characteristic is blood flow patterns: (1) *increased pulmonary blood flow,* (2) *decreased pulmonary blood flow,* (3) *obstruction to blood flow* out of the heart, and (4) *mixed blood flow,* in which saturated and desaturated blood mix within the heart or great arteries. As a comparison, both classification systems are outlined in Fig. 25-2.

With the hemodynamic classification system, the clinical manifestations of each group are more uniform and predictable. Defects that allow blood flow from the high-pressure left side of the heart to the lower-pressure right side (left-to-right shunt) result in increased pulmonary blood flow and cause CHF. Obstructive defects impede blood flow out of the ventricles; obstruction on the left side of the heart results in CHF, whereas severe obstruction on the right side causes cyanosis. Defects that cause decreased pulmonary blood flow result in cyanosis. Mixed lesions present a variable clinical picture based on degree of mixing and amount of pulmonary blood flow; hypoxemia (with or without cyanosis) and CHF usually occur together. This system is used in the following discussion.

DEFECTS WITH INCREASED PULMONARY BLOOD FLOW

In this group of cardiac defects, intracardiac communications along the septum or an abnormal connection between the great arteries allows blood to flow from the high-pressure left side of the heart to the lower-pressure right side of the heart (Fig. 25-3). Increased blood volume on the right side of the heart increases pulmonary blood flow at the expense of sys-

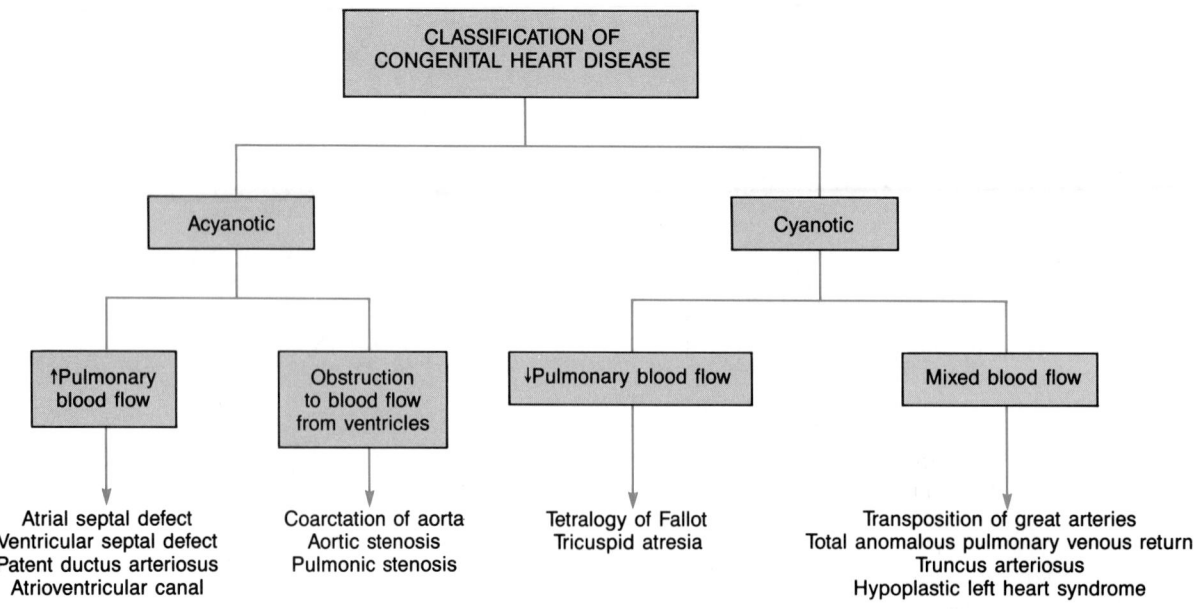

FIG. 25-2. Comparison of acyanotic-cyanotic and hemodynamic classification systems of congenital heart disease (CHD).

temic blood flow. Clinically patients demonstrate signs and symptoms of CHF. Atrial and ventricular septal defects and patent ductus arteriosus are typical anomalies in this group (see box on pp. 860-862).

OBSTRUCTIVE DEFECTS

Obstructive defects are those in which blood exiting the heart meets an area of anatomic narrowing *(stenosis)*, causing obstruction to blood flow. The pressure in the ventricle and in the great artery before the obstruction is increased, and the pressure in the area beyond the obstruction is decreased. The location of the narrowing is usually near the valve (Fig. 25-4), as follows:

Valvular—At the site of the valve itself
Subvalvular—Narrowing in the ventricle below the valve (also referred to as the *ventricular outflow tract*)
Supravalvular—Narrowing in the great artery above the valve

Coarctation of the aorta (narrowing of the aortic arch), aortic stenosis, and pulmonic stenosis are typical defects in this group (see box on pp. 862-864). Hemodynamically, there is a pressure load on the ventricle and decreased cardiac output. Clinically, infants and children exhibit signs of CHF. Children with mild obstruction may be asymptomatic. Rarely, as in severe pulmonic stenosis, hypoxemia may be seen.

DEFECTS WITH DECREASED PULMONARY BLOOD FLOW

In this group of defects, there is obstruction of pulmonary blood flow and an anatomic defect (atrial septal defect [ASD] or ventricular septal defect [VSD]) between the right and left sides of the heart (Fig. 25-5). Because blood has difficulty exiting the right side of the heart via the pulmonary artery, pressure on the right side increases, exceeding left-sided pressure. This allows desaturated blood to shunt right to left, causing desaturation in the left side of the heart and in the systemic circulation. Clinically these patients are hypoxemic and usually appear cyanotic. Tetralogy of Fallot and tricuspid atresia are the more common defects in this group (see box on pp. 864-865).

MIXED DEFECTS

Many complex cardiac anomalies are classified together in the *mixed* category (see box on pp. 866-868) because survival in the postnatal period depends on mixing of blood from the pulmonary and systemic circulations within the heart chambers. Hemodynamically, fully saturated systemic blood flow mixes with the desaturated pulmonary blood flow, causing a relative desaturation of the systemic blood flow. Pulmonary congestion occurs because the differences in pulmonary artery pressure and aortic pressure favor pulmonary blood flow. Cardiac output decreases because of a volume load on the ventricle. Clinically, these patients have a variable picture that combines some degree of desaturation (although cyanosis is not always visible) and signs of CHF. Some defects, such as transposition of the great arteries, cause severe cyanosis in the first days of life and later cause CHF. Others, such as truncus arteriosus, cause severe CHF in the first weeks of life and mild desaturation.

Text continued on p. 868.

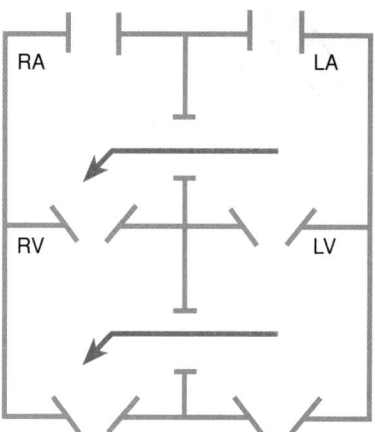

FIG. 25-3. Hemodynamics in defects with increased pulmonary blood flow.

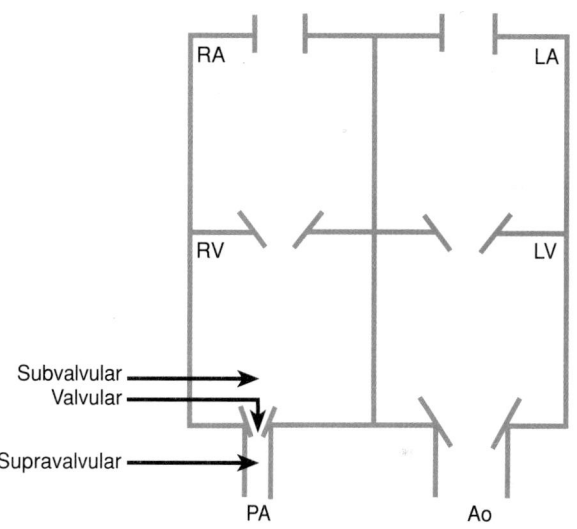

FIG. 25-4. Obstruction to ventricular ejection can occur at the valvular level (shown), below the valve (subvalvular), or above the valve (supravalvular). Pulmonic stenosis is shown here.

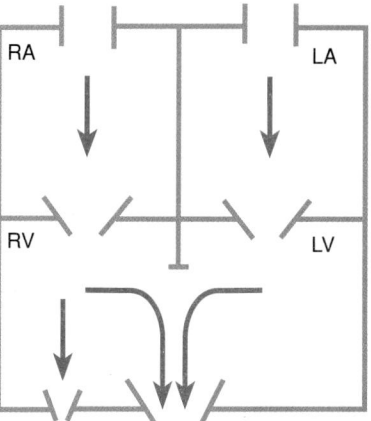

FIG. 25-5. Hemodynamic defects with decreased pulmonary blood flow. For abbreviations, see Fig. 25-1.

DEFECTS WITH INCREASED PULMONARY BLOOD FLOW

Atrial Septal Defect (ASD)

Description: Abnormal opening between the atria, allowing blood from the higher-pressure left atrium to flow into the lower-pressure right atrium. There are three types:

Ostium primum (ASD 1)—Opening at lower end of septum; may be associated with mitral valve abnormalities.

Ostium secundum (ASD 2)—Opening near center of septum.

Sinus venosus defect—Opening near junction of superior vena cava and right atrium; may be associated with partial anomalous pulmonary venous connection.

Pathophysiology: Because left atrial pressure slightly exceeds right atrial pressure, blood flows from the left to the right atrium, causing an increased flow of oxygenated blood into the right side of the heart. Despite the low pressure difference, a high rate of flow can still occur because of low pulmonary vascular resistance and the greater distensibility of the right atrium, which further reduces flow resistance. This volume is well tolerated by the right ventricle because it is delivered under much lower pressure than in a ventricular septal defect. Although there is right atrial and ventricular enlargement, cardiac failure is unusual in an uncomplicated atrial septal defect. Pulmonary vascular changes usually occur only after several decades if the defect is unrepaired.

Clinical manifestations: Patients may be asymptomatic. They may develop congestive heart failure (CHF). There is a characteristic murmur. Patients are at risk for atrial dysrhythmias (probably caused by atrial enlargement and stretching of conduction fibers) and pulmonary vascular obstructive disease and emboli formation later in life from chronic increased pulmonary blood flow.

Surgical treatment: Surgical Dacron patch closure of moderate to large defects similar to closure of ventricular septal defects. Open repair with cardiopulmonary bypass is usually performed before school age. In addition, the sinus venosus defect requires patch placement, so the anomalous right pulmonary venous return is directed to the left atrium with a baffle. The ASD 1 may require repair or, rarely, replacement of the mitral valve.

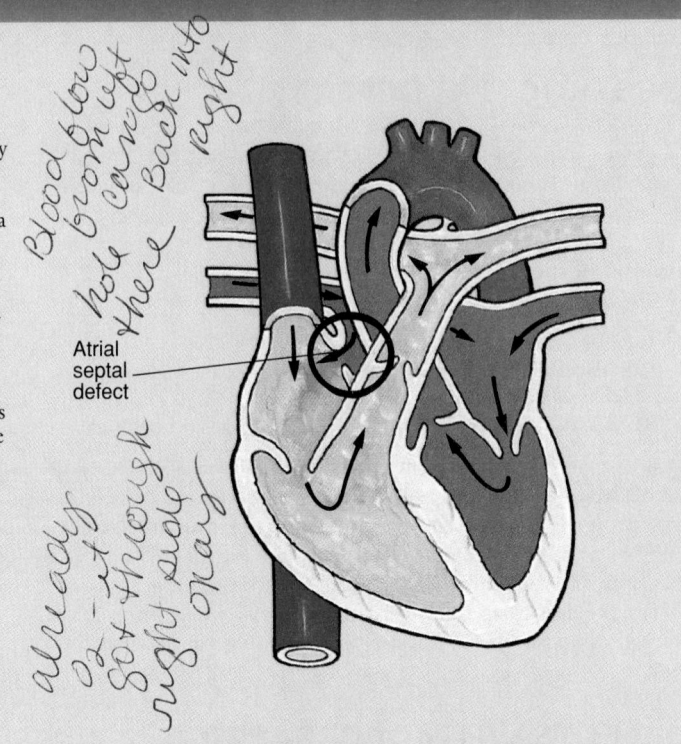

Atrial septal defect

Nonsurgical treatment: ASD 2 may also be closed using devices during cardiac catheterization. This technique is in clinical trials in some centers.

Prognosis: Very low operative mortality, less than 1%.

Ventricular Septal Defect (VSD)

Description: Abnormal opening between the right and left ventricles. May be classified according to location: membranous (accounting for 80%) or muscular. May vary in size from a small pinhole to absence of the septum, resulting in a common ventricle. Frequently associated with other defects, such as pulmonary stenosis, transposition of the great vessels, patent ductus arteriosus, atrial defects, and coarctation of the aorta. Many VSDs, especially those in infants with small defects, close spontaneously. Spontaneous closure is most likely to occur during the first year of life in children having small or moderate defects. A left-to-right shunt is caused by the flow of blood from the higher-pressure left ventricle to the lower-pressure right ventricle.

Pathophysiology: Because of the higher pressure within the left ventricle and because the systemic arterial circulation offers more resistance than the pulmonary circulation, blood flows through the defect into the pulmonary artery. The increased blood volume is pumped into the lungs, which may eventually result in increased pulmonary vascular resistance. Increased pressure in the right ventricle as a result of left-to-right shunting and pulmonary resistance causes the muscle to hypertrophy. If the right ventricle is unable to accommodate the increased workload, the right atrium may also enlarge as it attempts to overcome the resistance offered by incomplete right ventricular emptying. In severe defects, Eisenmenger syndrome may develop.

Clinical manifestations: CHF is common. There is a characteristic murmur. Patients are at risk for bacterial endocarditis and pulmonary vascular obstructive disease. In severe defects, Eisenmenger syndrome may develop.

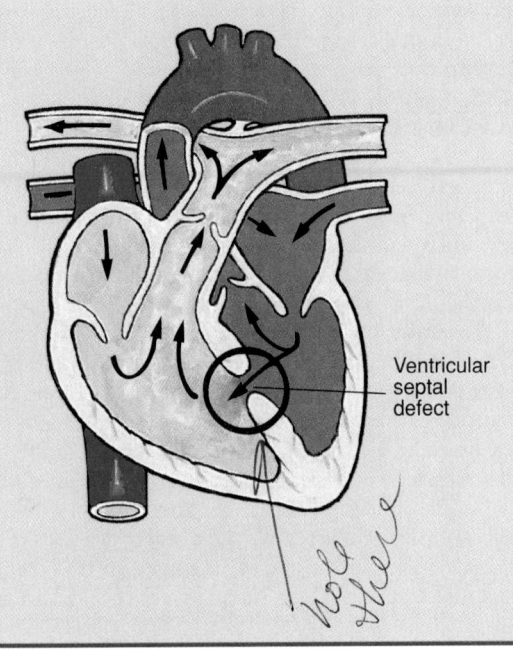

Ventricular septal defect

DEFECTS WITH INCREASED PULMONARY BLOOD FLOW—cont'd

Ventricular Septal Defect (VSD)—cont'd

Surgical treatment

Palliative: Pulmonary banding in symptomatic infants. Although palliation using a pulmonary artery band is used in some institutions, data suggest that complete primary repair can be performed without an increased risk during the first year of life. Age alone has little influence on the outcome of the repair, although younger infants are frequently sicker in the postoperative period.

Complete repair: Small defects are repaired with a purse-string approach. Large defects usually require a knitted Dacron patch sewn over the opening. Both procedures are performed via cardiopulmonary bypass. The repair is generally approached through the right atrium and the tricuspid valve. Postoperative complications include residual VSD and conduction disturbances.

Nonsurgical treatment: Device closure during cardiac catheterization is under clinical trials in some centers for closure of muscular defects that carry a high operative risk.

Prognosis: Risks depend on the location of the defect, number of defects, and other associated cardiac defects. Single membranous defects have a low mortality (less than 5%); multiple muscular defects can have a risk of more than 20%.

Atrioventricular Canal (AVC) Defect

Description: Incomplete fusion of endocardial cushions. Consists of a low atrial septal defect that is continuous with a high ventricular septal defect and clefts of the mitral and tricuspid valves, creating a large central atrioventricular (A-V) valve that allows blood to flow between all four chambers of the heart. The directions and pathways of flow are determined by pulmonary and systemic resistance, left and right ventricular pressures, and the compliance of each chamber, although flow is generally from left to right. It is the most common cardiac defect in children with Down syndrome.

Pathophysiology: The alterations in the hemodynamics depend on the defect's severity and the child's pulmonary vascular resistance. Immediately after birth, while the newborn's pulmonary vascular resistance is high, there is minimum shunting of blood through the defect. Once this resistance falls, left-to-right shunting occurs and pulmonary blood flow increases. The resultant pulmonary vascular engorgement predisposes to development of CHF.

Clinical manifestations: Patients usually have moderate to severe CHF. There is a characteristic murmur. There may be mild cyanosis that increases with crying. Patients are at high risk for developing pulmonary vascular obstructive disease.

Surgical treatment

Palliative: Pulmonary artery banding for infants with severe symptoms that are caused by increased pulmonary blood flow in some centers. Other centers believe complete repair can be performed in infants.

Complete repair: Surgical repair consists of patch closure of the septal defects and reconstruction of the A-V valve tissue (either repair of the mitral valve cleft or fashioning two A-V valves). If the mitral valve defect is severe, a valve replacement may be needed. Postoperative complications include heart block, CHF, mitral regurgitation, dysrhythmias, and pulmonary hypertension.

Prognosis: Operative mortality is about 10%. Potential later problem is mitral regurgitation, which may require valve replacement.

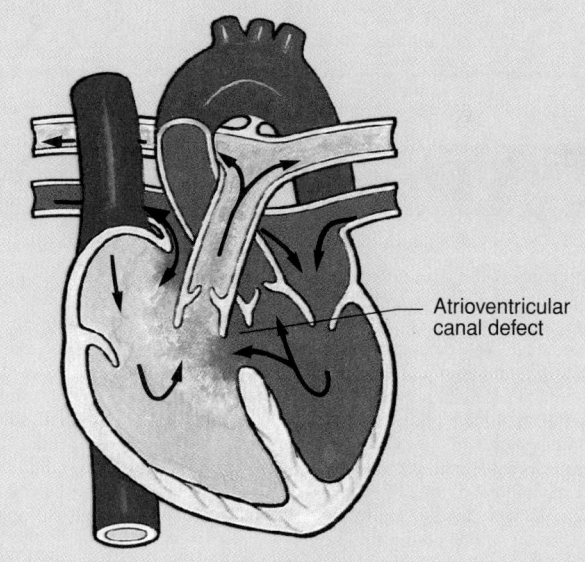

Atrioventricular canal defect

Patent Ductus Arteriosus (PDA)

Description: Failure of the fetal ductus arteriosus (artery connecting the aorta and pulmonary artery) to close within the first weeks of life. The continued patency of this vessel allows blood to flow from the higher-pressure aorta to the lower-pressure pulmonary artery, causing a left-to-right shunt.

Pathophysiology: The hemodynamic consequences of PDA depend on the size of the ductus and the pulmonary vascular resistance. At birth the resistance in the pulmonary and systemic circulations is almost identical, thus equalizing the resistance in the aorta and pulmonary artery. As the systemic pressure exceeds the pulmonary pressure, blood begins to shunt from the aorta, across the duct, to the pulmonary artery (left-to-right shunt).

The additional blood is recirculated through the lungs and returned to the left atrium and left ventricle. The effect of this altered circulation is increased workload on the left side of the heart, increased pulmonary vascular congestion and possibly resistance, and potentially increased right ventricular pressure and hypertrophy.

Clinical manifestations: Patients may be asymptomatic or show signs of CHF. There is a characteristic machinery-like murmur. A widened pulse pressure and bounding pulses result from runoff of blood from the aorta to the pulmonary artery. Patients are at risk for bacterial endocarditis and pulmonary vascular obstructive disease in later life from chronic excessive pulmonary blood flow.

Continued.

DEFECTS WITH INCREASED PULMONARY BLOOD FLOW—cont'd

Patent Ductus Arteriosus (PDA)—cont'd

Medical management: Administration of indomethacin (prostaglandin inhibitor) has proved successful in closing a patent ductus in premature infants and some newborns.

Surgical treatment: Surgical division or ligation of the patent vessel via a left thoracotomy. A newer technique, visually assisted thoracoscopic surgery (VATS), uses a thoracoscope and instruments placed through three small incisions on the left side of the chest to place a clip on the ductus. It is used in some centers and eliminates the need for a thoracotomy, thereby speeding postoperative recovery.

Nonsurgical treatment: Closure with placement of an occluder device during cardiac catheterization is done in some institutions.

Prognosis: Both procedures can be done at low risk with less than 1% mortality.

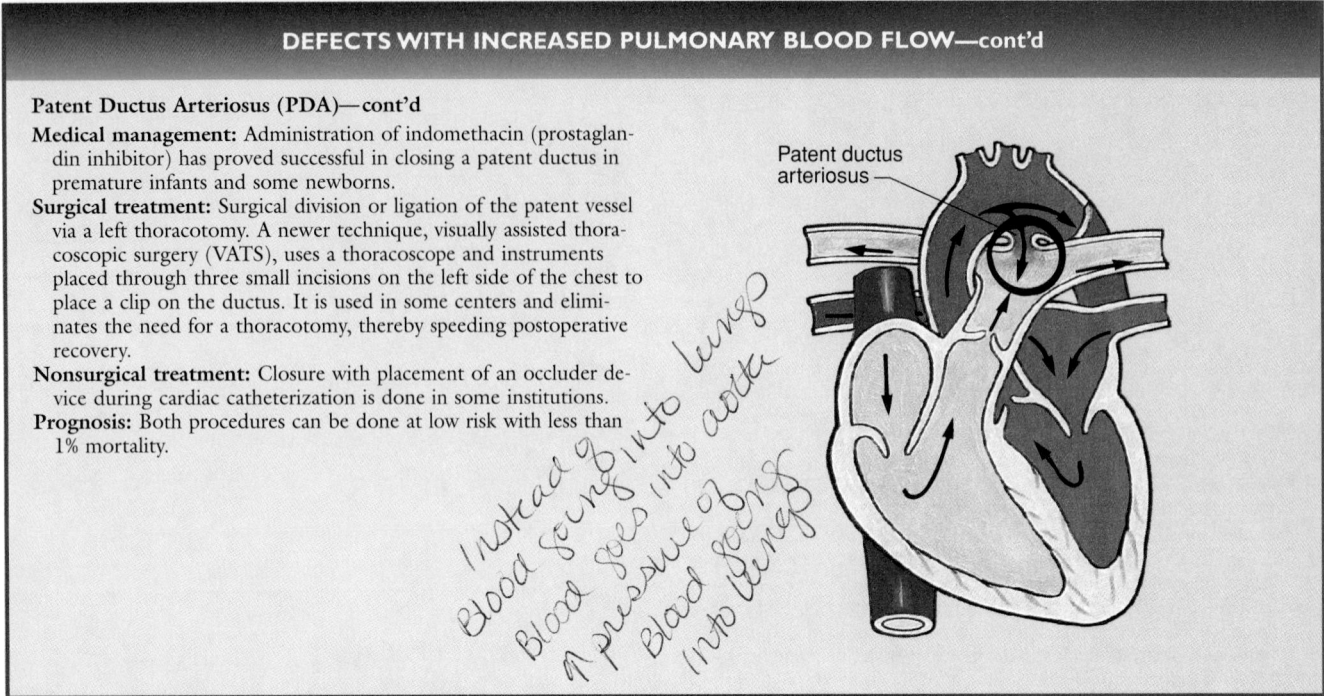

Patent ductus arteriosus

[Handwritten note: Instead of blood going into lungs, Blood goes into aorta. ↑ pressure of Blood going into lungs]

OBSTRUCTIVE DEFECTS

Coarctation of the Aorta (COA)

Description: Localized narrowing near the insertion of the ductus arteriosus, resulting in increased pressure proximal to the defect (head and upper extremities) and decreased pressure distal to the obstruction (body and lower extremities).

Pathophysiology: The effect of a narrowing within the aorta is increased pressure proximal to the defect and decreased pressure distal to it. In the preductal type of COA, the lower half of the body is supplied with blood by the right ventricle through the ductus arteriosus. In the postductal type, right ventricular outflow cannot maintain blood flow to the descending aorta. Therefore collateral circulation develops during fetal life to maintain flow from the ascending to the descending aorta.

Clinical manifestations: There may be high blood pressure and bounding pulses in arms, weak or absent femoral pulses, and cool lower extremities with lower blood pressure. There are signs of congestive heart failure (CHF) in infants. Often these patients' hemodynamic condition deteriorates rapidly, and they are admitted to the intensive care unit near death, usually severely acidotic and hypotensive. Mechanical ventilation and inotropic support are often necessary before surgery. Older children may experience dizziness, headaches, fainting, and epistaxis resulting from hypertension. Patients are at risk for hypertension, ruptured aorta, aortic aneurysm, or cerebrovascular accident (stroke).

Surgical treatment: Either resection of the coarcted portion with an end-to-end anastomosis of the aorta or enlargement of the constricted section using a graft of prosthetic material or a portion of the left subclavian artery. Because this defect is outside the heart and pericardium, cardiopulmonary bypass is not required and a thoracotomy incision is used. Postoperative hypertension (greater than 160 mm Hg) is treated with intravenous sodium nitroprusside or amrinone, followed by oral medications, such as captopril, hydralazine, and/or propranolol. Residual permanent hypertension after repair of COA seems to be related to age and time of repair. To prevent both hypertension at rest and exercise-provoked systemic hypertension after repair, elective surgery for COA is advised within the first 2 years of life. There is a small risk of recurrent

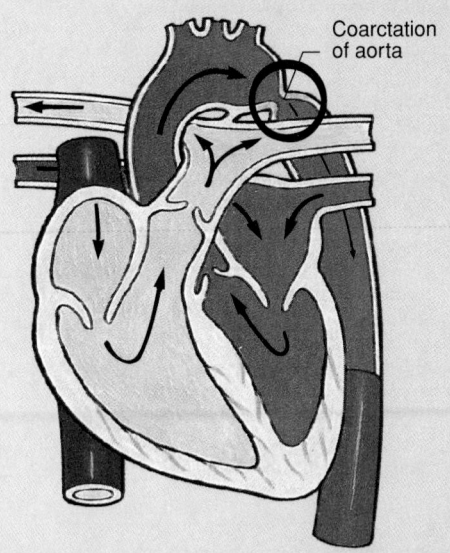

Coarctation of aorta

narrowing in patients who underwent surgical repair as infants. Percutaneous balloon angioplasty techniques have proved very effective in relieving residual postoperative coarctation gradients.

Nonsurgical treatment: Balloon angioplasty as a primary intervention for COA is being performed in some centers, but concerns about inadequate relief of gradients, risk of aneurysm formation, and restenosis have limited its widespread use. More clinical experience and longer follow-up are needed (Friedman, 1992).

Prognosis: Less than 5% mortality in patients with isolated coarctation; increased risk in infants with other complex cardiac defects.

OBSTRUCTIVE DEFECTS—cont'd

Aortic Stenosis (AS)

Description: Narrowing or stricture of the aortic valve, causing resistance to blood flow in the left ventricle, decreased cardiac output, left ventricular hypertrophy, and pulmonary vascular congestion. The prominent anatomic consequence of AS is the hypertrophy of the left ventricular wall, which eventually will lead to increased end-diastolic pressure, resulting in pulmonary venous and pulmonary arterial hypertension. Left ventricular hypertrophy also interferes with coronary artery perfusion and may result in myocardial infarction or scarring of the papillary muscles of the left ventricle, causing mitral insufficiency. *Valvular stenosis,* the most common type, is usually caused by malformed cusps resulting in a bicuspid rather than tricuspid valve or fusion of the cusps. *Subvalvular stenosis* is a stricture caused by a fibrous ring below a normal valve. *Supravalvular stenosis* occurs infrequently. Valvular AS is a serious defect for the following reasons: (1) the obstruction tends to be progressive; (2) sudden episodes of myocardial ischemia, or low cardiac output, can result in sudden death; and (3) surgical repair rarely results in a normal valve. This is one of the rare instances in which strenuous physical activity may be curtailed because of the cardiac condition.

Pathophysiology: A stricture in the aortic outflow tract causes resistance to ejection of blood from the left ventricle. The extra workload on the left ventricle causes hypertrophy. If left ventricular failure develops, left atrial pressure will increase; this causes increased pressure in the pulmonary veins, resulting in pulmonary vascular congestion (pulmonary edema).

Clinical manifestations: Infants with severe defects demonstrate signs of decreased cardiac output with faint pulses, hypotension, tachycardia, and poor feeding. Children show signs of exercise intolerance, chest pain, and dizziness when standing for long periods. There is a characteristic murmur. Patients are at risk for bacterial endocarditis, coronary insufficiency, and ventricular dysfunction.

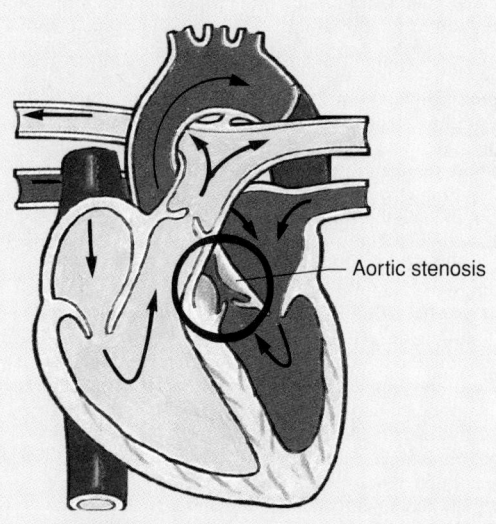

Aortic stenosis

Valvular Aortic Stenosis

Surgical treatment: Aortic valvotomy under inflow occlusion.

Prognosis: Aortic valvotomy in critically ill neonates and infants still carries a mortality of 10% to 20% in major medical centers. Results of aortic valvotomy in older children are very good, with mortality close to 0%. However, aortic valvotomy remains a palliative procedure, and approximately 25% of patients require additional surgery within 10 years for recurrent stenosis. A valve replacement may be required at the second procedure.

Nonsurgical treatment: Dilating narrowed valve with balloon angioplasty in the catheterization laboratory.

Prognosis: The incidence of side effects and complications, including aortic insufficiency or valvular regurgitation, tearing of the valve leaflets, loss of pulse in the catheterized limb, or serious dysrhythmias, is about 40%. In critically ill neonates the mortality rate is similar to that of surgery.

Subvalvular Aortic Stenosis

Surgical treatment: May involve incising a membrane if one exists or cutting the fibromuscular ring. If the obstruction results from narrowing of the left ventricular outflow tract and a small aortic valve annulus, a patch may be required to enlarge the entire left ventricular outflow tract and annulus and replace the aortic valve, an approach known as the *Konno procedure.* An aortic homograft with a valve may also be used *(extended aortic root replacement),* or the pulmonic valve may be moved to the aortic position and replaced with a homograft valve *(Ross procedure).*

Prognosis: Mortality from surgical repairs of subvalvular AS is less than 2% in major centers; however, about 10% of these patients develop recurrent subaortic stenosis and require additional surgery. All procedures to replace the aortic root and enlarge the left ventricular outflow tract require further evaluation.

Continued.

OBSTRUCTIVE DEFECTS—cont'd

Pulmonic Stenosis (PS)

Description: Narrowing at the entrance to the pulmonary artery. Resistance to blood flow causes right ventricular hypertrophy and decreased pulmonary blood flow. *Pulmonary atresia* is the extreme form of PS in that there is total fusion of the commissures and no blood flows to the lungs. The right ventricle may be hypoplastic.

Pathophysiology: When PS is present, resistance to blood flow causes right ventricular hypertrophy. If right ventricular failure develops, right atrial pressure will increase and may result in reopening of the foramen ovale, shunting of unoxygenated blood into the left atrium, and systemic cyanosis. If PS is severe, CHF occurs, and systemic venous engorgement will be noted. An associated defect such as a PDA partially compensates for the obstruction by shunting blood from the aorta to the pulmonary artery and into the lungs.

Clinical manifestations: Patients may be asymptomatic; some have mild cyanosis or CHF. Newborns with severe narrowing will be cyanotic. There is a characteristic murmur. Cardiomegaly is evident on chest x-ray film. Patients are at risk for bacterial endocarditis, with progressive narrowing causing increased symptoms.

Surgical treatment: In infants, transventricular (closed) valvotomy *(Brock procedure)*. In children, pulmonary valvotomy with cardiopulmonary bypass.

Nonsurgical treatment: Balloon angioplasty in the cardiac catheterization laboratory to dilate valve. A catheter is inserted across the stenotic pulmonic valve into the pulmonary artery, and a balloon at the end of the catheter is inflated and rapidly passed through the narrowed opening (see figure below, right). The procedure is associated with few complications and has proved highly effective, with a significant reduction in pressure gradient across the pulmonic valve and a low rate of complications. It is the treatment of choice for discrete PS in most centers and can be done safely in neonates.

Prognosis: Low risk for both procedures; less than 2% mortality. Both balloon dilation and surgical valvotomy leave the pulmonic valve incompetent because they involve opening the fused valve leaflets; however, these patients are clinically asymptomatic. Long-term problems with restenosis or valve incompetence may occur.

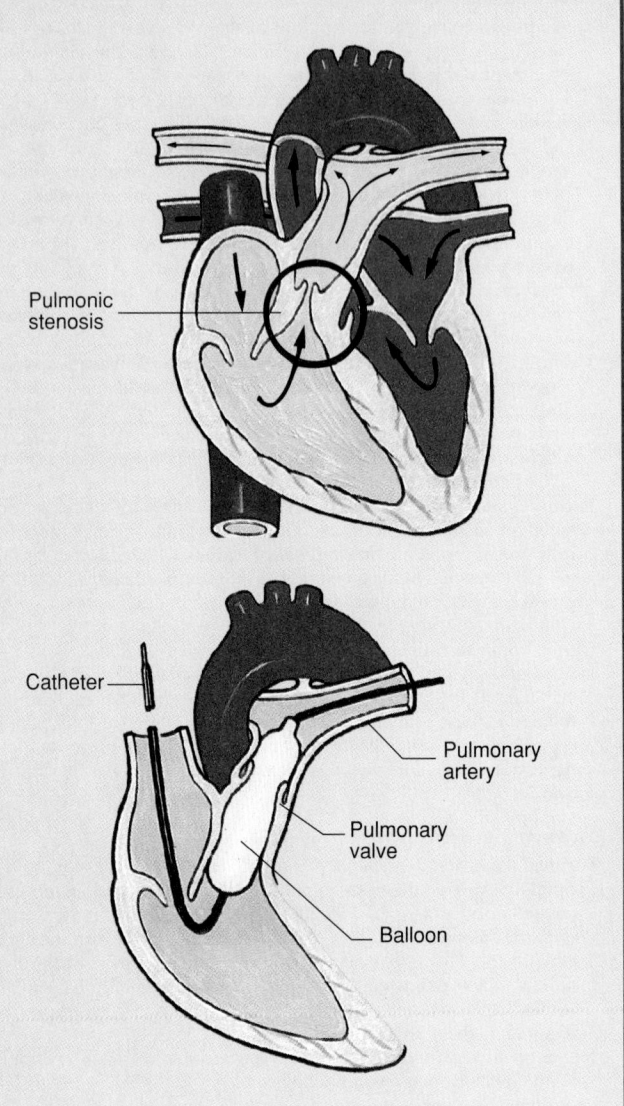

Pulmonic stenosis

Catheter

Pulmonary artery

Pulmonary valve

Balloon

DEFECTS WITH DECREASED PULMONARY BLOOD FLOW

Tetralogy of Fallot (TOF)

Description: The classic form includes four defects: (1) ventricular septal defect (VSD), (2) pulmonic stenosis (PS), (3) overriding aorta, and (4) right ventricular hypertrophy.

Pathophysiology: The altered hemodynamics vary widely, depending primarily on the degree of PS, but also on the size of the VSD and the pulmonary and systemic resistance to flow. Because the VSD is usually large, pressures may be equal in the right and left ventricles. Therefore the shunt direction depends on the difference between pulmonary and systemic vascular resistance. If pulmonary vascular resistance is higher than systemic resistance, the shunt is from right to left. If systemic resistance is higher than pulmonary resistance, the shunt is from left to right. PS decreases blood flow to the lungs and consequently the amount of oxygenated blood that returns to the left heart. Depending on the position of the aorta, blood from both ventricles may be distributed systemically.

Clinical manifestations

Infants: Some infants may be acutely cyanotic at birth; others have mild cyanosis that progresses over the first year of life as the PS worsens. There is a characteristic murmur. There are acute episodes of cyanosis and hypoxia, called blue spells or tet spells. Anoxic spells occur when the infant's oxygen requirements exceed the blood supply, usually during crying or after feeding.

DEFECTS WITH DECREASED PULMONARY BLOOD FLOW—cont'd

Tetralogy of Fallot (TOF)—cont'd

Children: With increasing cyanosis, there may be clubbing of the fingers, squatting, and poor growth.

Patients are at risk for emboli, cerebrovascular disease, brain abscess, seizures, and loss of consciousness or sudden death following an anoxic spell.

Surgical treatment

Palliative shunt: In infants who cannot undergo primary repair, a palliative procedure to increase pulmonary blood flow and increase oxygen saturation may be performed. The preferred procedure is the ***modified Blalock-Taussig shunt,*** which provides blood flow to the pulmonary arteries from the left or right subclavian artery (see Table 25-3). In general, however, shunts are avoided because they may result in pulmonary artery distortion.

Complete repair: Elective repair is usually performed in the first year of life. Indications for repair include increasing cyanosis and the development of hypercyanotic spells. Complete repair involves closure of the VSD and resection of the infundibular stenosis, with a pericardial patch to enlarge the right ventricular outflow tract. The procedure requires a median sternotomy and the use of cardiopulmonary bypass.

Prognosis: The operative mortality for total correction of TOF is less than 5%. With improved surgical techniques there is a lower incidence of dysrhythmias and sudden death; surgical heart block is rare. Congestive heart failure (CHF) may occur postoperatively.

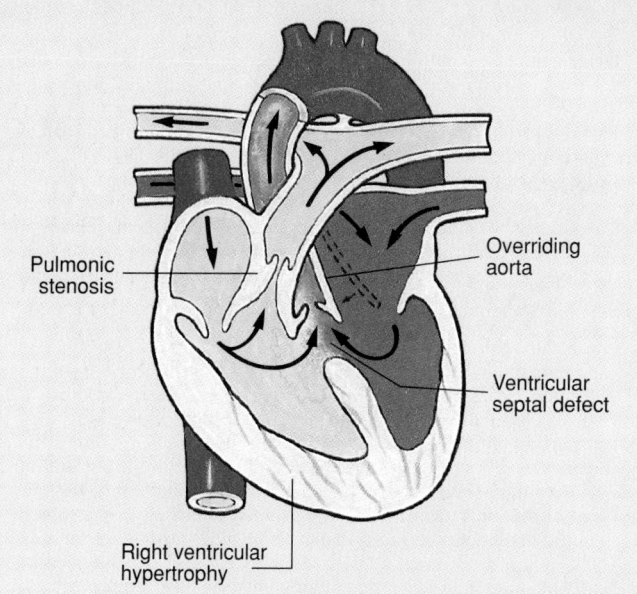

Pulmonic stenosis

Overriding aorta

Ventricular septal defect

Right ventricular hypertrophy

Tricuspid Atresia

Description: Failure of the tricuspid valve to develop, consequently no communication from right atrium to right ventricle. Blood flows through an atrial septal defect (ASD) or a patent foramen ovale to the left side of the heart and through a VSD to the right ventricle and out to the lungs. It is often associated with PS and transposition of the great arteries. There is complete mixing of unoxygenated and oxygenated blood in the left side of the heart, resulting in systemic desaturation and varying amounts of pulmonary obstruction, causing decreased pulmonary blood flow.

Pathophysiology: At birth the presence of a patent foramen ovale (or other atrial septal opening) is required to permit blood flow across the septum into the left atrium; the patent ductus arteriosus allows blood flow to the pulmonary artery into the lungs for oxygenation. A VSD allows a modest amount of blood to enter the right ventricle and pulmonary artery for oxygenation. Pulmonary blood flow usually is diminished.

Clinical manifestations: Cyanosis is usually seen in the newborn period. There may be tachycardia and dyspnea. Older children have signs of chronic hypoxemia with clubbing. Patients are at risk for bacterial endocarditis, brain abscess, and stroke.

Therapeutic management: For the neonate whose pulmonary blood flow depends on the patency of the ductus arteriosus, a continuous infusion of prostaglandin E$_1$ is started until surgical intervention can be arranged.

Surgical treatment: *Palliative* treatment is the placement of a shunt *(systemic to pulmonary artery)* to increase blood flow to the lungs. If the ASD is small, an atrial septostomy is done during cardiac catheterization. Some children have increased pulmonary blood flow and require ***pulmonary artery banding*** to lessen the volume of blood to the lungs. A ***bidirectional Glenn shunt*** (cavopulmonary anastomosis) may be performed at 6 to 9 months as a second stage (see Table 25-3).

Modified Fontan procedure—Systemic venous return is directed to the lungs without a ventricular pump through surgical connections between the right atrium and the pulmonary artery. A fenestration (opening) in the right atrial baffle is sometimes done to relieve pressure. Patient must have normal ventricular function and a low pulmonary vascular resistance for the procedure to be successful. The modified Fontan procedure separates oxy-

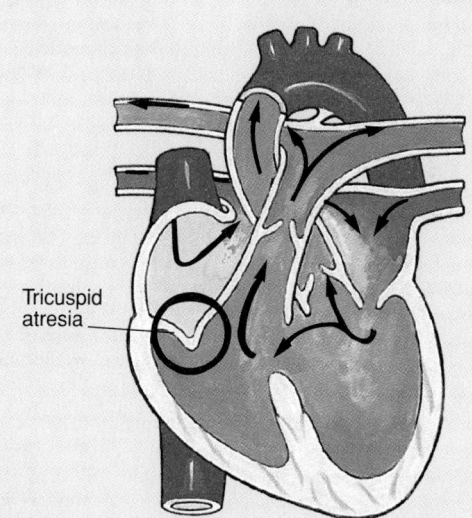

Tricuspid atresia

genated and unoxygenated blood inside the heart and eliminates the excess volume load on the ventricle but does not restore normal anatomy or hemodynamics.

Prognosis: Surgical mortality is greater than 10%. Postoperative complications include dysrhythmias, systemic venous hypertension, pleural and pericardial effusions, elevated pulmonary vascular resistance, and ventricular dysfunction. Although initial results have been encouraging, long-term survival and morbidity must await future studies.

MIXED DEFECTS

Transposition of the Great Arteries (TGA) or Transposition of the Great Vessels (TGV)

Description: The pulmonary artery leaves the left ventricle, and the aorta exits from the right ventricle, with no communication between the systemic and pulmonary circulations.

Pathophysiology: Associated defects such as septal defects or patent ductus arteriosus (PDA) must be present to permit blood to enter the systemic circulation and/or the pulmonary circulation for mixing of saturated and desaturated blood. The most common defect associated with TGA is a patent foramen ovale. At birth there is also a PDA, although in most instances this closes after the neonatal period. Another associated anomaly may be ventricular septal defect (VSD). Presence of these defects increases the risk of congestive heart failure (CHF), since they often produce high pulmonary blood flow under high pressure. For example, a large VSD permits blood to flow from the right to the left ventricle, into the pulmonary artery, and finally to the lungs. However, it also produces high pulmonary blood flow under high pressure, which can result in pulmonary vascular resistance. The same series of events occurs with a large PDA, since blood directly from the aorta flows under high pressure into the pulmonary artery and lungs.

Clinical manifestations: Depend on the type and size of the associated defects. Children with minimum communication are severely cyanotic and depressed at birth. Those with large septal defects or a PDA may be less severely cyanotic but may have symptoms of CHF. Heart sounds vary according to the type of defect present. Cardiomegaly is usually evident a few weeks after birth.

Therapeutic Management

To provide intracardiac mixing: The administration of intravenous prostaglandin E_1 may be initiated to temporarily increase blood mixing if systemic and pulmonary mixing is inadequate to provide an oxygen saturation of 75% or to maintain cardiac output. During cardiac catheterization a balloon atrial septostomy *(Rashkind procedure)* may also be performed to increase mixing and maintain cardiac output over a longer period.

Surgical treatment

Arterial switch procedure: Procedure of choice performed in first weeks of life. Involves transecting the great arteries and anastomosing the main pulmonary artery to the proximal aorta (just above the aortic valve) and anastomosing the ascending aorta to the proximal pulmonary artery. The coronary arteries are switched from the proximal aorta to the proximal pulmonary artery, creating a new aorta. Reimplantation of the coronary arteries is critical to the infant's survival, and they must be reattached without torsion or kinking to provide the heart with its supply of oxygen. The advantage of the arterial switch procedure is the reestablishment of normal circulation, with the left ventricle acting as the systemic pump. Potential complications of

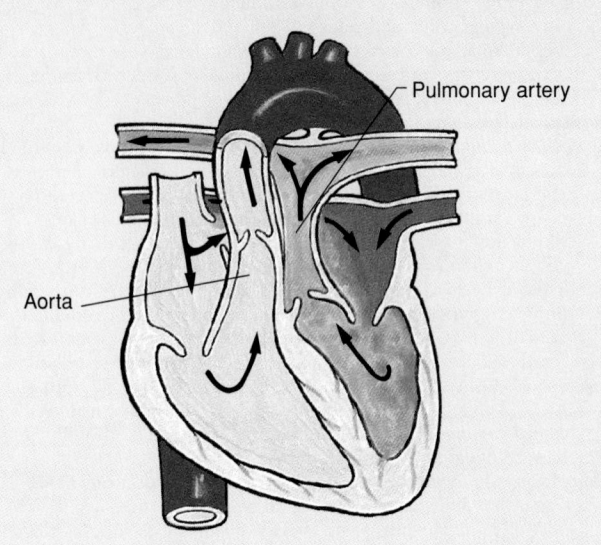

Pulmonary artery

Aorta

the arterial switch include narrowing at the great artery anastomoses or coronary artery insufficiency.

Creation of an intraatrial baffle to divert venous blood to the mitral valve and pulmonary venous blood to the tricuspid valve using the patient's atrial septum *(Senning procedure)* or a prosthetic material *(Mustard procedure)*. Performed in first year of life. A disadvantage is the continuing role of the right ventricle as the systemic pump and the late development of right ventricular failure and rhythm disturbances. Other potential postoperative complications include loss of normal sinus rhythm, baffle leaks, and ventricular dysfunction.

Rastelli procedure: Operative choice in infants with TGA, VSD, and severe PS. It involves closure of the VSD with a baffle, directing left ventricular blood through the VSD into the aorta. The pulmonic valve is then closed, and a conduit is placed from the right ventricle to the pulmonary artery, creating a physiologically normal circulation. Unfortunately, this procedure requires multiple conduit replacements as the child grows.

Prognosis: Operative mortality is about 5% to 10% with all procedures; with atrial level repairs there is a later risk of dysrhythmias and ventricular dysfunction.

Total Anomalous Pulmonary Venous Connection (TAPVC)

Description: Rare defect characterized by failure of the pulmonary veins to join the left atrium. Instead, the pulmonary veins are abnormally connected to the systemic venous circuit via the right atrium or various veins draining toward the right atrium, such as the superior vena cava. The abnormal attachment results in mixed blood being returned to the right atrium and shunted from the right to the left through an atrial septal defect (ASD). The type of TAPVC is classified according to the pulmonary venous point of attachment as:

Supracardiac—Attachment above the diaphragm, such as to the superior vena cava (most common form).

Cardiac—Direct attachment to the heart, such as to the right atrium or coronary sinus.

Infracardiac—Attachment below the diaphragm, such as to the inferior vena cava (most severe form).

TAPVC is also called *total anomalous pulmonary venous return* (TAPVR) or *total anomalous pulmonary venous drainage* (TAPVD).

Pathophysiology: The right atrium receives all the blood that normally would flow into the left atrium. As a result, the right side of the heart hypertrophies, whereas the left side, especially the left atrium, may remain small. An associated ASD or patent foramen ovale allows systemic venous blood to shunt from the higher-pressure right atrium to the left atrium and into the left side of the heart. As a result, the oxygen saturation of the blood in both sides of the heart (and ultimately, in the systemic arterial circulation) is the same. If the pulmonary blood flow is large, pulmonary venous return is also large and the amount of saturated blood is relatively high. However, if there is obstruction to pulmonary venous drainage, pulmonary venous return is impeded, pulmonary venous pressure rises, and pulmonary interstitial edema develops and eventually contributes to CHF. Infracardiac TAPVC is often associated with obstruction to pulmonary venous drainage and is a surgical emergency.

MIXED DEFECTS—cont'd

Total Anomalous Pulmonary Venous Connection (TAPVC)—cont'd

Clinical manifestations: Most infants develop cyanosis early in life. The degree of cyanosis is inversely related to the amount of pulmonary blood flow: the more pulmonary blood, the less cyanosis. Children with unobstructed TAPVC may be asymptomatic until pulmonary vascular resistance decreases during infancy, increasing pulmonary blood flow, with resulting signs of CHF. Cyanosis becomes worse with pulmonary vein obstruction; once obstruction occurs, the infant's condition usually deteriorates rapidly. Without intervention, cardiac failure will progress to death.

Surgical treatment: Corrective repair in early infancy. The surgical approach varies with the anatomic defect. In general, however, the common pulmonary vein is anastomosed to the left atrium, the ASD is closed, and the anomalous pulmonary venous connection is ligated. The cardiac type is most easily repaired; the infracardiac type has the highest morbidity and mortality because of the higher incidence of pulmonary vein obstruction. Potential postoperative complications include reobstruction; bleeding; dysrhythmias, particularly heart block; pulmonary artery hypertension; and persistent heart failure.

Prognosis: The cardiac type has a surgical mortality of less than 5%; the incidence of morbidity is greater with the other types and increases with the presence of pulmonary vein obstruction.

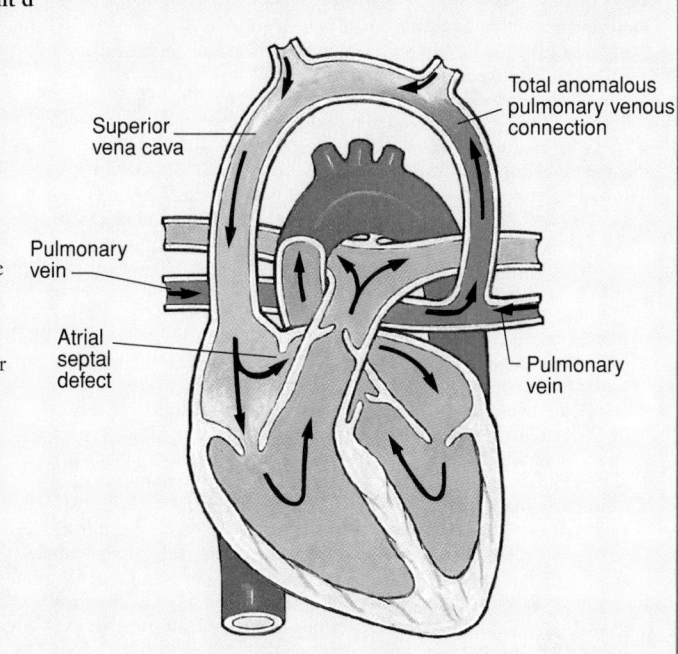

Truncus Arteriosus (TA)

Description: Failure of normal septation and division of the embryonic bulbar trunk into the pulmonary artery and the aorta, resulting in a single vessel that overrides both ventricles. Blood from both ventricles mixes in the common great artery, causing desaturation and hypoxemia. Blood ejected from the heart flows preferentially to the lower-pressure pulmonary arteries, causing increased pulmonary blood flow and reduced systemic blood flow. There are three types:

Type I—A single pulmonary trunk arises near the base of the truncus and divides into the left and right pulmonary arteries.

Type II—The left and right pulmonary arteries arise separately from the posterior aspect of the truncus.

Type III—The pulmonary arteries arise independently from the lateral aspect of the truncus.

Pathophysiology: Blood ejected from the left and right ventricles enters the common trunk, mixing pulmonary and systemic circulations. Blood flow is distributed to the pulmonary and systemic circulations according to the relative resistances of each system. The amount of pulmonary blood flow depends on the size of the pulmonary arteries and the pulmonary vascular resistance. Generally, resistance to pulmonary blood flow is less than systemic vascular resistance, resulting in preferential blood flow to the lungs. Pulmonary vascular disease develops at an early age in patients with truncus arteriosus.

Clinical manifestations: Most infants are symptomatic with moderate to severe CHF and variable cyanosis, poor growth, and activity intolerance. There is a characteristic murmur. Patients are at risk for brain abscess and bacterial endocarditis.

Surgical treatment: Early repair in the first few months of life. Corrective repair involves closing the VSD so that the truncus arteriosus receives the outflow from the left ventricle, excising the pulmonary arteries from the aorta, and attaching them to the right ventricle by means of a homograft. Currently, homografts (segments of cadaver aorta and pulmonary artery that are treated with antibiotics and cryopreserved) are preferred over synthetic con-

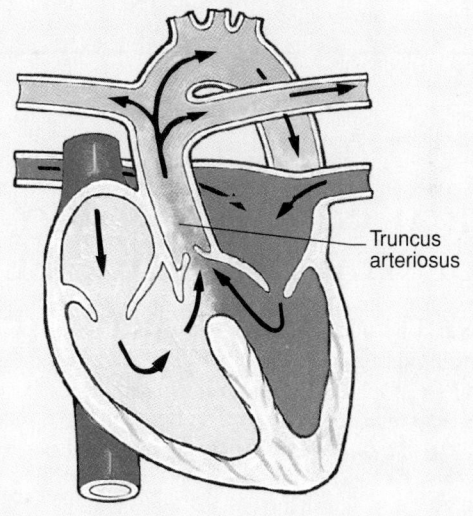

duits to establish continuity between the right ventricle and pulmonary artery. Homografts are more flexible and easier to use during the procedure and appear less prone to obstruction. Postoperative complications include persistent heart failure, bleeding, pulmonary artery hypertension, dysrhythmias, and residual VSD.

Prognosis: Mortality is greater than 10%; future procedures are required to replace the conduits.

Continued.

MIXED DEFECTS—cont'd

Hypoplastic Left Heart Syndrome (HLHS)

Description: Underdevelopment of the left side of the heart, resulting in a hypoplastic left ventricle and aortic atresia. Most blood from the left atrium flows across the patent foramen ovale to the right atrium, to the right ventricle, and out the pulmonary artery. The descending aorta receives blood from the PDA supplying systemic blood flow.

Pathophysiology: An ASD or patent foramen ovale allows saturated blood from the left atrium to mix with desaturated blood from the right atrium and to flow through the right ventricle and out into the pulmonary artery. From the pulmonary artery the blood flows to the lungs, then through the ductus arteriosus into the aorta and out to the body. The amount of blood flow to the pulmonary and systemic circulations depends on the relationship between the pulmonary and systemic vascular resistances. The coronary and cerebral vessels receive blood by retrograde flow through the hypoplastic ascending aorta.

Clinical manifestations: There is mild cyanosis and signs of CHF until the PDA closes, then progressive deterioration with cyanosis and decreased cardiac output, leading to cardiovascular collapse. It is usually fatal in the first months of life without intervention.

Therapeutic management: Neonates require stabilization with mechanical ventilation and inotropic support preoperatively. A prostaglandin E_1 infusion is needed to maintain ductal patency, ensuring adequate systemic blood flow.

Surgical treatment: Several-staged approach. First stage is *Norwood procedure*—anastomosis of the main pulmonary artery to the aorta to create a new aorta, shunting to provide pulmonary blood flow, and creation of a large ASD. Postoperative complications include imbalance of systemic and pulmonary blood flow, bleeding, low cardiac output, and persistent heart failure. Second stage is often a *bidirectional Glenn shunt* (see Table 25-3) done at 6 to 9 months of age to relieve cyanosis and reduce the volume load on the right ventricle. The final repair is a *modified Fontan procedure* (see Tricuspid Atresia in box on p. 865).

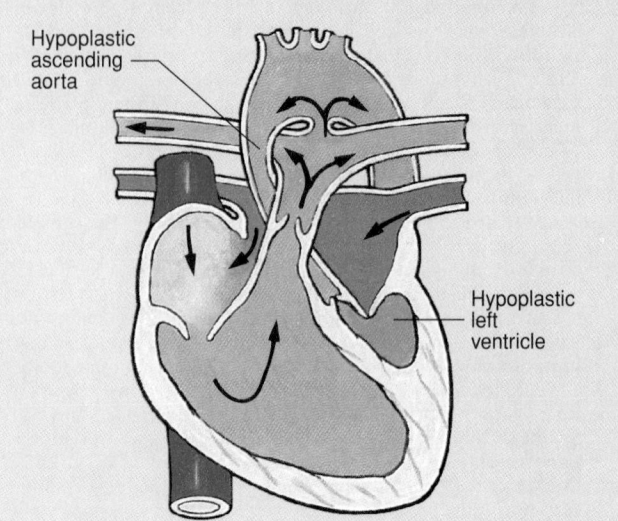

Hypoplastic ascending aorta

Hypoplastic left ventricle

Transplantation: Some programs believe that heart transplantation in the newborn period is the best option for these infants. Problems include the shortage of newborn organ donors, risk of rejection, long-term problems with chronic immunosuppression, and infection (see Heart Transplantation, p. 899).

Prognosis: Mortality risks of more than 25% with both surgery and transplantation. Because of the high-risk nature of both surgical palliation and neonatal heart transplantation, some cardiologists continue to recommend no treatment for this defect.

CLINICAL CONSEQUENCES OF CONGENITAL HEART DISEASE

CONGESTIVE HEART FAILURE (CHF)

CHF is the inability of the heart to pump an adequate amount of blood to the systemic circulation to meet the metabolic demands of the body. In children, CHF most frequently occurs secondary to structural abnormalities that result in increased blood volume and pressure. CHF is a symptom caused by an underlying cardiac defect, not a disease in itself, since it is usually the result of an excessive workload imposed on a normal myocardium. CHF is most common in infants.

Pathophysiology

Heart failure is often separated into two categories, right-sided and left-sided failure. In *right-sided failure* the right ventricle is unable to pump blood effectively into the pulmonary artery, resulting in increased pressure in the right atrium and systemic venous circulation. Systemic venous hypertension causes hepatosplenomegaly and occasionally edema. In *left-sided failure* the left ventricle is unable to pump blood

into the systemic circulation, resulting in increased pressure in the left atrium and pulmonary veins. The lungs become congested with blood, causing elevated pulmonary pressures and pulmonary edema.

Although each type of heart failure produces different signs and symptoms, clinically it is unusual to observe solely right- or left-sided failure in children. Since each side of the heart depends on adequate function of the other side, failure of one chamber causes a reciprocal change in the opposite chamber.

If the abnormalities precipitating CHF are not corrected, the heart muscle becomes damaged. Despite compensatory mechanisms, the heart is unable to maintain an adequate cardiac output. Decreased blood flow to the kidneys continues to stimulate sodium and water reabsorption, leading to hypervolemia, increased workload on the heart, and congestion in the pulmonary and systemic circulations (Fig. 25-6).

The signs and symptoms of CHF can be divided into three groups: (1) impaired myocardial function, (2) pulmonary congestion, and (3) systemic venous congestion (see box). Because these hemodynamic changes occur from different causes and at differing times, the clinical presentation may vary among children.

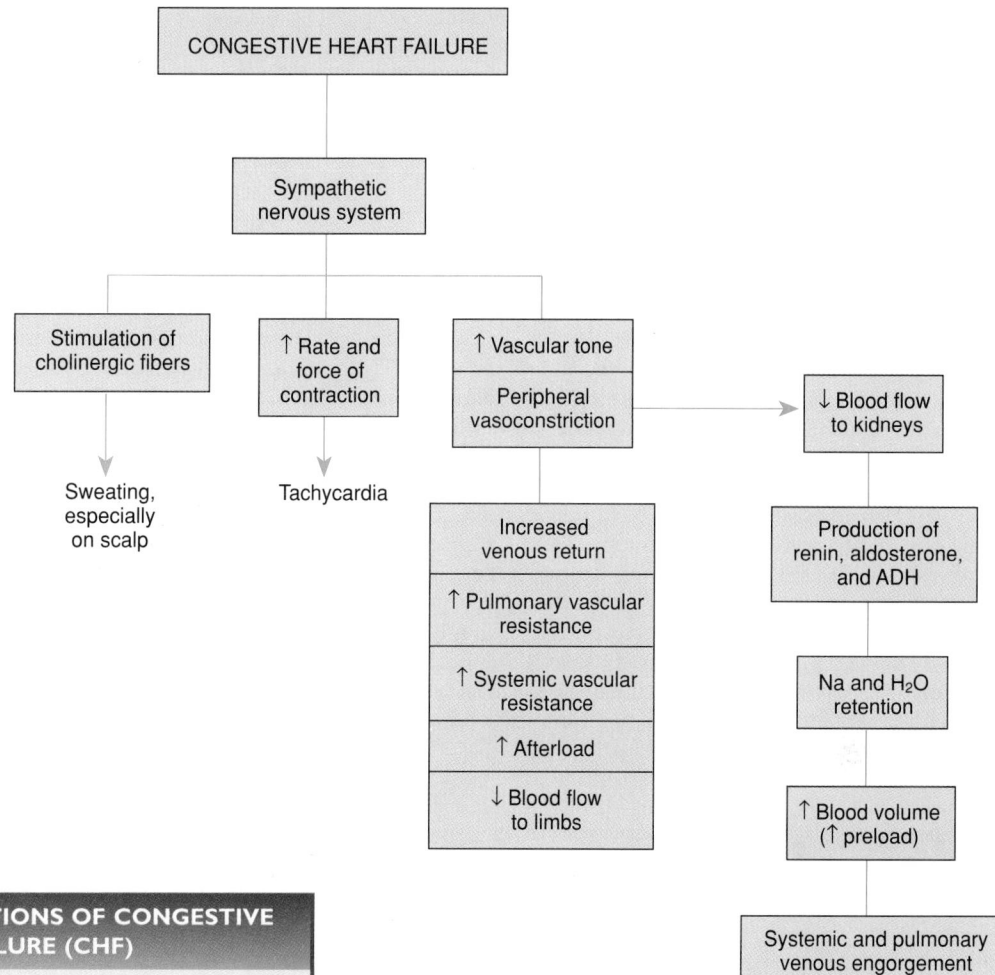

FIG. 25-6. Pathophysiology of congestive heart failure (CHF).

Diagnostic Evaluation

Diagnosis of CHF is made on the basis of clinical manifestations (see box). A chest x-ray film demonstrates cardiomegaly and increased pulmonary vascular markings caused by increased pulmonary blood flow. Ventricular hypertrophy appears on the electrocardiogram (ECG).

Therapeutic Management

The goals of treatment are to (1) improve cardiac function, (2) remove accumulated fluid and sodium, (3) decrease cardiac demands, and (4) improve tissue oxygenation and decrease oxygen consumption.

Improve Cardiac Function. Myocardial efficiency is improved through administration of digitalis glycosides. The beneficial effects are increased cardiac output, decreased heart size, decreased venous pressure, and relief of edema. In pediatrics, *digoxin (Lanoxin)* is used almost exclusively because of its more rapid onset. It is available as an elixir (0.05 mg/ml) for oral administration. For infants the dose is calculated in micrograms (1000 µg = 1 mg).

Treatment consists of a digitalizing dose, given orally or

intravenously in divided doses over 24 hours to produce optimum cardiac effects, and a maintenance dose, given orally twice a day to maintain blood levels. During digitalization the child is monitored by means of an ECG to observe for the desired effects (prolonged P-R interval and reduced ventricular rate) and detect side effects, especially dysrhythmias.

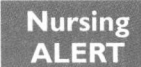 Therapeutic serum digoxin levels range from 0.8 to 2.0 µg/L.

A newer group of drugs used in the treatment of CHF are the **angiotensin-coverting enzyme (ACE) inhibitors.** As their name implies, these drugs inhibit the normal function of the renin-angiotensin system in the kidney. The ACE inhibitors block the conversion of angiotensin I to angiotensin II so that instead of vasoconstriction, vasodilation occurs. Vasodilation results in decreased pulmonary and systemic vascular resistance, decreased blood pressure, and a reduction in afterload. Two ACE inhibitors are currently used in pediatrics: **captopril (Capoten),** given three times a day, and **enalapril (Vasotec),** given twice a day. Captopril is used in infants and young children because it can be given in smaller doses; its principal side effects are hypotension, renal dysfunction, and cough.

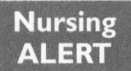 Because ACE inhibitors also block the action of aldosterone, the addition of potassium supplements or spironolactone (Aldactone) to the drug regimen of patients taking diuretics is usually not needed and may cause hyperkalemia.

Remove Accumulated Fluid and Sodium. Treatment consists of diuretics, possible fluid restriction, and possible sodium restriction. Diuretics are the mainstay of therapy to eliminate excess water and salt to prevent reaccumulation. The most frequently used agents are **furosemide (Lasix),** the **thiazides (chlorothiazide suspension** or **hydrochlorothiazide tablets),** and **spironolactone (Aldactone)** (Table 25-2). Since furosemide and the thiazides are potassium-losing diuretics, potassium supplements may be prescribed, and rich sources of the electrolyte are encouraged in the diet.

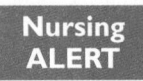 A fall in the serum potassium level enhances the effects of digitalis, increasing the risk of digoxin toxicity. Therefore serum potassium levels must be carefully monitored.

Fluid restriction may be required in the acute states of CHF and must be carefully calculated to avoid dehydrating

TABLE 25-2. Diuretics used in congestive heart failure (CHF)		
ACTION	COMMENTS	NURSING CONSIDERATIONS
Furosemide (Lasix) Blocks reabsorption of sodium and water in proximal renal tubule and interferes with reabsorption of sodium	Drug of choice in severe CHF Causes excretion of chloride and potassium (hypokalemia may precipitate digitalis toxicity)	Begin to record output as soon as drug is given Observe for dehydration caused by profound diuresis Observe for side effects (nausea and vomiting, diarrhea, ototoxicity, hypokalemia, dermatitis, postural hypotension) Encourage foods high in potassium and/or give potassium supplements Monitor chloride and acid-base balance with long-term therapy Observe for signs of digoxin toxicity
Chlorothiazide (Diuril) Acts directly on distal tubules to decrease sodium, water, potassium, chloride, and bicarbonate absorption	Less frequently used drug Causes hypokalemia, acidosis from large doses May be given on alternate days or for 4 or 5 days and stopped for 2 days to allow for reabsorption of potassium	Observe for side effects (nausea, weakness, dizziness, paresthesia, muscle cramps, skin eruptions, hypokalemia, acidosis) Encourage foods high in potassium and/or give potassium supplements
Spironolactone (Aldactone) Blocks action of aldosterone, which promotes retention of sodium and excretion of potassium	Weak diuretic Has potassium-sparing effect; frequently used with thiazides, furosemide Poorly absorbed from gastrointestinal tract Takes several days to achieve maximum actions	Observe for side effects (skin rash, drowsiness, ataxia, hyperkalemia) Do not administer potassium supplements

the child, especially if cyanotic CHD and significant polycythemia are present. Infants rarely need fluid restrictions because CHF makes feeding so difficult that they struggle to take maintenance fluids.

Sodium-restricted diets are used less often in children than in adults to control CHF because of their potential negative effects on appetite. If salt intake is restricted, the diet usually consists of avoiding additional table salt and highly salted foods.

Decrease Cardiac Demands. The workload on the heart is reduced when metabolic needs are kept to a minimum. This is accomplished by limiting physical activity (bed rest), preserving body temperature, treating any infections, reducing the effort of breathing (semi-Fowler position), and using medication to sedate an irritable child.

Improve Tissue Oxygenation and Decrease Oxygen Consumption. All the preceding measures serve to increase tissue oxygenation, either by improving myocardial function or by lessening tissue oxygen demands. Supplemental cool humidified oxygen is usually provided to increase the amount of available oxygen during inspiration. Oxygen is a vasodilator that decreases pulmonary vascular resistance. The amount of cool humidity is carefully regulated to prevent chilling.

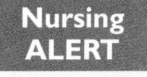 **Nursing ALERT** Oxygen is a drug and is only administered with an appropriate order. In some uncommon circumstances in patients with complex hemodynamics, oxygen can be detrimental.

Nursing Considerations

The infant or child with CHF is usually admitted to the hospital where intensive nursing care is available. The child is positioned for optimum ventilation and administered oxygen by the most effective means, IV access is established, and cardiac and respiratory function is monitored continuously using a cardiac monitor and pulse oximeter to monitor oxygen saturation. Urinary output and serum electrolytes are evaluated frequently.

❖ Assessment

Nurses need to be alert to signs of CHF in infants and children with suspected or known congenital defects. Signs of CHF indicate a worsening clinical condition; the earlier they are detected, the sooner treatment can be begun.

Nursing ALERT The early signs of CHF are the following:
Tachycardia, especially during rest and slight exertion
Tachypnea
Profuse scalp sweating, especially in infants
Fatigue and irritability
Sudden weight gain
Respiratory distress

❖ Nursing Diagnoses

A number of nursing diagnoses are identified after a thorough assessment. Some of these are included in the Nursing Care

Plan on pp. 874-875. Others may become apparent in special circumstances and with children in different age-groups.

❖ Planning

The goals for the infant or child with CHF and the family are as follows:

1. Child will exhibit improved cardiac output.
2. Child will experience decreased cardiac demands.
3. Child will exhibit improved respiratory function.
4. Child will maintain adequate nutritional status.
5. Child will exhibit no evidence of fluid excess.
6. Child and family will receive adequate support and education.

❖ Implementation

Although the objectives of nursing care are the same, the interventions differ depending on the child's age. Interventions for infants are quite different from those for older children.

Assist in Measures to Improve Cardiac Function. The nurse's responsibility in administering digoxin includes observing for signs of toxicity, calculating and administering the correct dosage, and instituting parental teaching regarding drug administration at home. The child's apical pulse is always checked before administering digoxin. As a general rule the drug is not given if the pulse is below 90 to 110 beats/minute in infants and young children or below 70 beats/minute in older children (the cutoff point for adults is 60). However, since the pulse rate varies in children in different age-groups, the written drug order should specify at what heart rate the drug is withheld. The nurse should also use judgment in evaluating the pulse rate. If it is significantly lower than the previous recording, the dose should be withheld until the practitioner is notified.

The apical rate is taken because a pulse deficit (radial pulse rate lower than apical) may be present with decreased cardiac output. It is auscultated for 1 full minute to evaluate alterations in rhythm. If the child is monitored by means of an ECG, a rhythm strip is obtained and attached to the chart for rate and rhythm analysis, such as abnormal lengthening of the P-R interval (more than a 50% increase over predigitalization interval) and dysrhythmias.

Digoxin is a potentially dangerous drug because the margin of safety of therapeutic, toxic, and lethal doses is very narrow. Many toxic responses are extensions of its therapeutic effects. Therefore the nurse must maintain a high index of suspicion for signs of toxicity when administering digoxin (see box).

Since digoxin toxicity can occur from accidental overdose, great care must be taken in properly calculating and measuring the dosage. When converting milligrams to micrograms to milliliters, the nurse carefully checks the placement of the decimal point, since an error causes a significant change in

COMMON SIGNS OF DIGOXIN TOXICITY IN CHILDREN	
Gastrointestinal	**Cardiac**
Nausea	Bradycardia
Vomiting	Dysrhythmias
Anorexia	

FAMILY HOME CARE
Administering Digoxin

Give digoxin at regular intervals, usually every 12 hours, such as 8 AM and 8 PM.

Plan the times so that the drug is given *1 hour before* or *2 hours after* feedings.

Use a calendar to mark off each dose that is given, or post a reminder, such as a sign on the refrigerator.

Have the prescription refilled *before* the medication is completely used.

Administer the drug carefully by slowly directing it on the side and back of the mouth.

Do not mix it with other foods or fluids, since refusal to consume these results in inaccurate intake of the drug.

If the child has teeth, give water after administering the drug; whenever possible, brush the teeth to prevent tooth decay from the sweetened liquid.

If a dose is missed and more than 4 hours has elapsed, withhold the dose and give the next dose at the regular time; if less than 4 hours has elapsed, give the missed dose.

If the child vomits, do not give a second dose.

If more than two consecutive doses have been missed, notify the practitioner.

Do not increase or double the dose for missed doses.

If the child becomes ill, notify the practitioner immediately.

Keep digoxin in a safe place, preferably a locked cabinet.

In case of accidental overdose of digoxin, call the nearest Poison Control Center immediately; the number is usually listed in the front of the telephone directory.

CRITICAL THINKING EXERCISE
Digoxin Toxicity

You are visiting a 3-month-old infant at home who began receiving digoxin and Lasix 5 days ago for management of CHF. The infant seems well. The mother mentions the infant vomited several times yesterday and again this morning. Your assessment reveals an irregular heartbeat at 104 beats/minute.

You should:

1. Give the digoxin and instruct the mother to call the cardiologist in a few days if the vomiting persists.
2. Explain that vomiting and a slow heart rate are common side effects of digoxin.
3. Calm the infant and check the heart rate again.
4. Notify the health care provider of your findings before giving digoxin.

The correct answer is four. A slow and irregular heartbeat and intermittent vomiting are common signs of digoxin toxicity in infants. This medication was started only 5 days ago. The practitioner should be notified for further assessment and management. The margin of safety for digoxin blood levels is narrow. Continuing to give the digoxin can cause a fatal toxic reaction.

dosage. For example, 0.1 mg is 10 times the dosage of 0.01 mg.

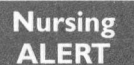

Nursing ALERT   Infants rarely receive more than 1 ml (50 μg or 0.05 mg) in one dose; a higher dose is an immediate warning of a dosage error. To ensure safety, compare the calculation with another staff member before giving the drug.

These same principles are taught to parents in preparation for discharge, although the correct dose in milliliters is usually specified on the container, thus reducing potential errors in calculation. The nurse observes the parent measure the elixir in the dropper and stresses the level mark as the meniscus of the fluid that is observed at eye level. Other instructions for administering digoxin are listed in the Family Home Care box and the Critical Thinking Exercise.

Parents are also advised of the signs of toxicity. According to the practitioner's preference, they may be taught to take the pulse before giving the drug. A return demonstration of the procedure from both parents or other principal caregiver is included as part of the teaching plan. Their level of anxiety in counting the pulse is assessed, since overconcern about the heart rate may result in excessive withholding of the drug.

Afterload Reduction.   For patients receiving ACE inhibitors for afterload reduction, the nurse should carefully monitor blood pressure before and after dose administration, observe for symptoms of hypotension, and notify the practitioner if blood pressure is low. Numerous medications affecting the kidney can potentiate renal dysfunction, so children taking multiple diuretics along with an ACE inhibitor require careful assessment of serum electrolytes and renal function.

Decrease Cardiac Demands.   The infant requires rest and conservation of energy for feeding. Every effort is made to organize nursing activities to allow for uninterrupted periods of sleep. Whenever possible, parents are encouraged to stay with their infant to provide the holding, rocking, and cuddling that help children sleep more soundly. To minimize disturbing the infant, changing bed linen and complete bathing are done only when necessary. Feeding is planned to accommodate the infant's sleep and wake patterns. The child is fed when hungry, such as when sucking on fists rather than when crying for a bottle, since the stress of crying exhausts the limited energy supply. Since infants with CHF tire easily and may sleep through feedings, smaller feedings every 3 hours may be helpful. Gavage feedings may be instituted to provide adequate nutrition and allow the infant to rest.

Every effort is made to minimize unnecessary stress. Older children need an explanation of what is happening to them to decrease anxiety about their illness and necessary treatments such as cardiac monitoring, oxygen administration, and medications. Outlining a plan for the day, preparation for tests and procedures, providing quiet activities, and providing adequate rest periods are all helpful interventions with older children. Some infants and children require sedation during the acute phase of illness to allow them to rest.

Temperature is carefully monitored because hyperthermia or hypothermia increases the need for oxygen. Febrile states are reported to the physician, since infection must be promptly treated. Maintaining body temperature is of special importance in children who are receiving cool, humidified oxygen and in infants who tend to be diaphoretic and lose heat by way of evaporation.

Skin breakdown from edema is prevented with a change of position every 2 hours (from side to side while in semi-Fowler position) and use of a pressure-relieving mattress or bed. The skin, especially over the sacrum, is checked for evidence of redness from pressure.

Reduce Respiratory Distress. Careful assessment, positioning, and oxygen administration can reduce respiratory distress. Respirations are counted for 1 full minute during a resting state. Any evidence of increased respiratory distress is reported, since this may indicate worsening CHF.

Infants are positioned to encourage maximum chest expansion, with the head of the bed elevated; they should sit up in an infant seat or be held at a 45-degree angle. Children prefer to sleep on several pillows and remain in a semi-Fowler or high Fowler position during waking hours. Shirts and diapers are pinned loosely to allow maximum chest expansion. Safety restraints, such as those used with infant seats, are applied low on the abdomen and loosely enough to provide both safety and maximum expansion.

The infant or child is often given humidified supplemental oxygen via oxygen hood or tent, nasal cannula, or mask. The child's response to oxygen therapy is carefully evaluated by noting respiratory rate, ease of respiration, color, and especially oxygen saturations, as measured by oximetry.

Respiratory infections can exacerbate CHF and should be appropriately treated and prevented if possible. The child should be protected from persons with respiratory infections and have a noninfectious roommate. With an older child, it is advantageous to choose a roommate who is also confined to bed and relatively quiet in order to promote a restful environment. Good handwashing is practiced before and after caring for any hospitalized child. Antibiotics may be given to combat respiratory infection. The nurse ensures that the drug is given at equally divided times over a 24-hour schedule to maintain high blood levels of the antibiotic.

Maintain Nutritional Status. Meeting the nutritional needs of infants with CHF or serious cardiac defects is a nursing challenge. The metabolic rate of these infants is greater because of poor cardiac function and increased heart and respiratory rates. Their caloric needs are greater than those of the average infant because of their increased metabolic rate, yet their ability to take in adequate calories is hampered by their fatigue. Feeding for a fragile infant with serious CHD is similar to exercise in an adult, and they often do not have the energy or cardiac reserve to do extra work. The nurse seeks measures to enable the infant to feed easily without excess fatigue and to increase the caloric density of the formula.

The infant should be well rested before feeding and fed soon after awakening so as not to expend energy on crying. A 3-hour feeding schedule works well for many infants. (Feeding every 2 hours does not provide enough rest between feedings, and a 4-hour schedule requires an increased volume of feeding, which many infants are unable to take.) The feeding schedule should be individualized to the infant's needs. A soft preemie nipple or a slit in a regular nipple to enlarge the opening decreases the energy expenditure of the infant while sucking. Infants should be well supported and fed in a semiupright position. The infant may need to rest frequently and may need to have the jaw and cheeks stroked to encourage sucking. Generally, giving an in-

fant about a half hour to complete a feeding is reasonable. Prolonging the feeding time can exhaust the infant and decrease the rest period between feedings.

Infants with feeding difficulties are often gavage fed using a nasogastric tube to supplement their oral intake and ensure adequate calories. If they are very stressed and fatigued, in respiratory distress, or tachypneic to 80 to 100 breaths/minute, oral feedings may be withheld and all nutrition given by gavage feedings. Gavage feedings are usually a temporary measure until the infant's medical status improves and nutritional needs can be met through oral feedings. Some infants with severe CHF, neurologic deficits, or significant gastroesophageal reflux may need placement of a gastrostomy tube to allow adequate nutrition.

Increasing the caloric density of formulas by concentration and then adding corn, medium-chain triglycerides (MCT Oil), or polycose is frequently done. Infant formulas provide 20 calories per ounce, and the use of additives can increase the calories to 30 calories or more per ounce. This allows the infant to obtain more calories despite a smaller volume intake of formula. The caloric density of the formula needs to be increased slowly (by 2 calories per ounce per day) to prevent diarrhea or formula intolerance. Breast-feeding mothers are encouraged to provide the infant with alternating feedings of breast milk and high-calorie formulas. Some lactating mothers will prefer to feed the child expressed breastmilk that has been fortified with Similac or Enfamil powder, polycose, or corn oil to increase caloric intake. A supplemental nurser may also be helpful. A diet plan specific to the individual infant's needs is calculated and prescribed by the nutritionist in collaboration with the other health personnel. The nurse needs to reinforce this information with the parents as necessary.

Assist in Measures to Promote Fluid Loss. When diuretics are given, the nurse records fluid intake and output and monitors body weight at the same time each day to evaluate benefit from the drug. Since profound diuresis may cause dehydration and electrolyte imbalance (loss of sodium, potassium, chloride, bicarbonate), the nurse observes for signs indicating either complication, as well as signs and symptoms suggesting reactions to the drugs. Diuretics should be given early in the day to children who are toilet trained to avoid the need to urinate at night. If potassium-losing diuretics are given, the nurse encourages foods high in potassium, such as bananas, oranges, whole grains, legumes, and leafy vegetables, and administers prescribed supplements. Serum potassium levels are checked frequently.

NURSING TIP Mix the elixir with fruit juice (red punch or grape juice works well) to disguise the bitter taste and to prevent intestinal irritation from a concentrated solution.

Fluid restriction is rarely necessary in infants because of their difficulty in feeding. However, if fluids are restricted, the nurse plans fluid intake schedules for a 24-hour period, allowing for most fluids during waking hours. Toddlers and preschoolers should be given small amounts of liquid in small cups so the containers appear full. Suitable utensils are decorated medicine cups, paper cups, doll-sized teacups, or measuring cups. It is also important to avoid leaving extra fluids at the bedside, since older children may help themselves to

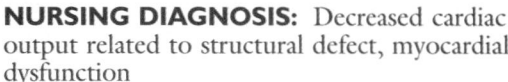

NURSING CARE PLAN
The Child with Congestive Heart Failure

NURSING DIAGNOSIS: Decreased cardiac output related to structural defect, myocardial dysfunction

PATIENT GOAL 1: Will exhibit improved cardiac output

- **NURSING INTERVENTIONS/*RATIONALES***

*Administer digoxin (Lanoxin) as ordered, using established precautions *to prevent toxicity*
  Make certain dosage is within safe limits
  Infants rarely receive more than 1 ml (50 µg or 0.05 mg) in one dose; *a higher dose is an immediate warning of a dosage error*
  Ascertain correct preparation for route
  Check dosage with another nurse *to ensure safety*
  Count apical pulse for 1 full minute before giving drug
    Withhold medication and notify practitioner if pulse rate is less than 90 to 110 beats/minute (infants) or 70 to 85 beats/minute (older children), depending on previous pulse readings
  Recognize signs of digoxin toxicity (nausea, vomiting, anorexia, bradycardia, dysrhythmias)
  Often an ECG rhythm strip is taken *to assess cardiac status before administration*
  Ensure adequate intake of potassium
  Observe for signs of hypokalemia (muscle weakness, hypotension, dysrhythmias, tachycardia or bradycardia, irritability, drowsiness) or hyperkalemia (muscle weakness, twitching, bradycardia, ventricular fibrillation, oliguria, apnea)
  Monitor serum potassium levels *because decrease enhances digoxin toxicity*
*Administer medications to decrease afterload, as ordered
  Check blood pressure
    Observe for signs of hypotension
  Monitor electrolyte levels
Attach cardiac monitor if ordered

- **EXPECTED OUTCOMES**

Heartbeat is strong, regular, and within normal limits for age (see inside front cover)
Peripheral perfusion is adequate

NURSING DIAGNOSIS: Ineffective breathing pattern related to pulmonary congestion

PATIENT GOAL 1: Will exhibit improved respiratory function

- **NURSING INTERVENTIONS/*RATIONALES***

Place in inclined posture of 30 to 45 degrees *to encourage maximum chest expansion;* tilt mattress support of incubator: place older infant in infant seat
Avoid any constricting clothing or restraints around abdomen and chest

*Administer humidified oxygen as prescribed
Assess respiratory rate, ease of respiration, color, and oxygen saturations as measured by oximetry

- **EXPECTED OUTCOME**

Respirations remain within normal limits, color is good, and child rests quietly (see inside front cover for normal variations in respirations)

PATIENT GOAL 2: Will experience reduction of anxiety

- **NURSING INTERVENTIONS/*RATIONALES***

Employ flexible feeding schedule *that reduces fretfulness associated with hunger*
Handle child gently
Hold and comfort infant
Employ comfort measures found effective for individual child
Encourage family to provide comfort and solace
Explain equipment and procedures to child *to decrease anxiety*

- **EXPECTED OUTCOME**

Child rests quietly and breathes easily

NURSING DIAGNOSIS: Fluid volume excess related to fluid accumulation (edema)

PATIENT GOAL 1: Will exhibit no evidence of fluid excess

- **NURSING INTERVENTIONS/*RATIONALES***

*Administer diuretics as prescribed
Maintain accurate intake and output
Weigh daily at same time and on same scale *to assess fluid gain or loss*
Assess for evidence of increased or decreased edema
Maintain fluid restriction, if ordered
Provide skin care for children with edema
Change position frequently *to prevent skin breakdown associated with edema*
  Use alternating-pressure mattress

- **EXPECTED OUTCOME**

Infant exhibits evidence of fluid loss (frequent urination, weight loss)

NURSING DIAGNOSIS: Activity intolerance related to imbalance between oxygen supply and demand

PATIENT GOAL 1: Will exhibit no additional respiratory or cardiac stress

- **NURSING INTERVENTIONS/*RATIONALES***

Maintain neutral thermal environment *because hypothermia or hyperthermia increases need for oxygen*
  Place newborn in incubator or under warmer
  Keep infant warm
  Treat fever promptly

---

*Dependent nursing action.

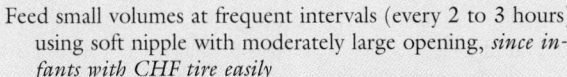

NURSING CARE PLAN
The Child with Congestive Heart Failure—cont'd

Feed small volumes at frequent intervals (every 2 to 3 hours) using soft nipple with moderately large opening, *since infants with CHF tire easily*

Implement gavage feeding if infant becomes fatigued before taking an adequate amount

Time nursing activities to disturb child as little as possible

Implement measures to reduce anxiety

Respond promptly to crying or other expressions of distress

• **EXPECTED OUTCOME**

Child rests quietly

NURSING DIAGNOSIS: High risk for infection related to reduced body defenses, pulmonary congestion

---

See Infection Control, Chapter 22

See Nursing Care Plan: The Child with Congenital Heart Disease, pp. 884-885

NURSING DIAGNOSIS: Altered family processes related to a child with a life-threatening illness

---

PATIENT (FAMILY) GOAL 1: Will receive adequate support

• **NURSING INTERVENTIONS/*RATIONALES* AND EXPECTED OUTCOMES**

See Nursing Care Plan: The Family of the Ill or Hospitalized Child, Chapter 21

PATIENT (FAMILY) GOAL 2: Will be prepared for home care

• **NURSING INTERVENTIONS/*RATIONALES***

Teach family:
  Medication administration and side/toxic effects
  Signs and symptoms of CHF and to report them to designated practitioner
  Feeding techniques and nutritional requirements
  Positioning
  Need for rest
  Growth and developmental considerations
    Growth is slowed
    Gross motor skills may be delayed more than fine motor skills
Refer to outpatient services and community resources as needed *for ongoing support*

• **EXPECTED OUTCOMES**

Family demonstrates an understanding of the condition and required care at home
Family uses appropriate community resources

---

additional servings. Older children's cooperation is gained by placing them in charge of recording fluid intake.

If salt is limited, the nurse discusses food sources of sodium with the family and discourages their bringing salt-containing treats to the child. At mealtime the child's tray is checked to make sure the appropriate diet is given.

Support Child and Family. CHF is a serious complication of heart disease. Parents and older children are usually acutely aware of the critical nature of the condition. Since stress places additional demands on cardiac function, the nurse should focus on reducing anxiety through anticipatory preparation, frequent communication with the parent regarding the child's progress, and constant reassurance that everything possible is being done.

Home care involves many of the same interventions discussed under Plan for Discharge and Home Care (see p. 883). The nurse teaches the family about the medications that need to be administered and alerts them to the signs of worsening CHF that require medical attention, such as increased sweating, decreased urine output (noted in fewer wet diapers or infrequent use of the toilet), or poor feeding. Compliance is a major issue, and every effort is extended to improve the

family's adherence to the medication schedule (see Chapter 22). Written instructions regarding correct administration of digoxin are essential (see Family Home Care, p. 872), including an explanation regarding signs of toxicity.

If CHF is the end stage of a severe heart defect, the nurse cares for this child as for any child who is terminally ill, using the principles discussed in Chapter 18.

❖ Evaluation

The effectiveness of nursing interventions for the family and the child with CHF is determined by continual reassessment and evaluation of care based on the following observational guidelines and expected outcomes:

1. Monitor heart rate and quality, respiratory rate and efforts, and color, and observe behaviors that provide clues to expended effort.
2. Observe nutritional intake, feeding behaviors, and weight.
3. Monitor intake, output, and weight.
4. Interview and observe behaviors of family.

Expected outcomes:
See Nursing Care Plan, pp. 874-875.

HYPOXEMIA

Hypoxemia refers to an arterial oxygen tension (or pressure, Pao_2) that is less than normal and can be identified by a decreased arterial saturation or a decreased Pao_2. *Hypoxia* is a reduction in tissue oxygenation that results from low oxygen saturations and Pao_2 and results in impaired cellular processes. *Cyanosis* is a blue discoloration in the mucous membranes, skin, and nail beds of the child with reduced oxygen saturation. It results from the presence of deoxygenated hemoglobin (hemoglobin not bound to oxygen) in a concentration of 5 g/dl of blood or more. Cyanosis is usually apparent when arterial oxygen saturations are 80% to 85%. Determination of cyanosis is subjective. It can vary depending on skin pigment, quality of light, color of the room, or clothing worn by the child. The presence of cyanosis may not accurately reflect arterial hypoxemia because both oxygen saturation and amount of circulating hemoglobin are involved. Children with severe anemia may not be cyanotic despite severe hypoxemia because the hemoglobin level may be too low to produce the characteristic blue color. Conversely, patients with polycythemia may appear cyanotic despite a near normal Pao_2. Heart defects that cause hypoxemia and cyanosis result from desaturated venous blood (blue blood) entering the systemic circulation without passing through the lungs.

Adolescents and young adults may become cyanotic because of unrepaired septal defects in which the increased pulmonary blood flow over many years results in pulmonary vascular changes. *Eisenmenger complex (syndrome)* refers to the clinical situation in which a left-to-right shunt becomes a right-to-left shunt because of a progressive increase in pulmonary vascular resistance. With increasing pulmonary vascular thickening, the resistance in the pulmonary circulation can exceed or equal that in the systemic circulation, causing a reversal of blood flow from the right to the left ventricle.

Clinical Manifestations

Over time, two physiologic changes occur in the body in response to chronic hypoxemia: polycythemia and clubbing. *Polycythemia,* an increased number of red blood cells, increases the oxygen-carrying capacity of the blood. However, anemia may result if iron is not readily available for the formation of hemoglobin. Polycythemia increases the viscosity of the blood and crowds out clotting factors. *Clubbing,* a thickening and flattening of the tips of the fingers and toes, is thought to occur because of chronic tissue hypoxemia and polycythemia (Fig. 25-7). Infants with mild hypoxemia may be asymptomatic except for cyanosis and exhibit near-normal growth and development. Those with more severe hypoxemia may exhibit fatigue with feeding, poor weight gain, tachypnea, and dyspnea. Severe hypoxemia resulting in tissue hypoxia is manifested by clinical deterioration and signs of poor perfusion.

Squatting, most characteristic of children with tetralogy of Fallot, is seen in toddlers and older children as an unconscious attempt to relieve chronic hypoxia, especially during exercise. Because of early surgical intervention during infancy, squatting is rarely seen.

Hypercyanotic spells, also referred to as *blue spells* or *tet spells* because they are often seen in infants with tetralogy of Fallot, may occur in any child whose heart defect includes obstruction to pulmonary blood flow and communication between the ventricles. The infant becomes acutely cyanotic and hyperpneic because sudden infundibular spasm decreases pulmonary blood flow and increases right-to-left shunting (the proposed mechanism in tetralogy of Fallot). Spells, rarely seen before 2 months of age, occur most frequently in the first year of life. They occur more often in the morning and may be preceded by feeding, crying, defecation, or stressful procedures (see Critical Thinking Exercise). Because profound hypoxemia causes cerebral hypoxia, hypercyanotic spells require prompt assessment and treatment to prevent brain damage or possibly death.

Persistent cyanosis as a result of cyanotic cardiac defects places the child at risk for significant *neurologic complications.* Cerebrovascular accident (CVA, stroke), brain abscess,

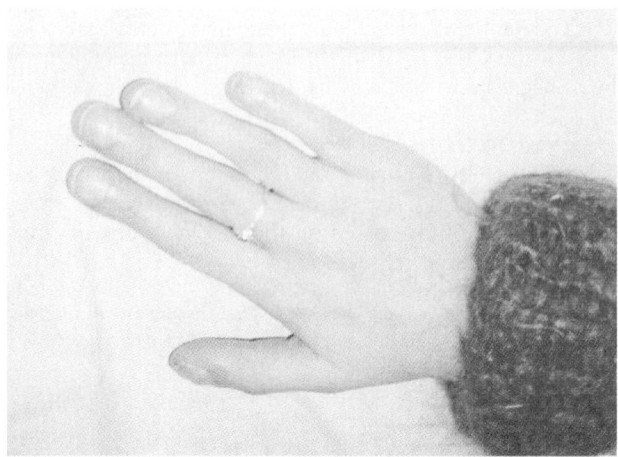

FIG. 25-7. Clubbing of fingers.

CRITICAL THINKING EXERCISE
Hypercyanotic Spell

A 4-month-old infant known to have tetralogy of Fallot is seen in the emergency department because of a 2-day history of diarrhea, low-grade fever, and poor oral intake. When blood tests are done, he becomes acutely cyanotic with rapid shallow respirations. You would:

1. Begin cardiopulmonary resuscitation (CPR).
2. Calm the infant, place in the knee-chest position and administer blow-by oxygen, and call for assistance.
3. Continue the procedure; this is expected for an infant with tetralogy of Fallot.
4. Stop the procedure and wait for color to improve before completing the blood test.

The correct answer is two. The infant is having a hypercyanotic or "tet" spell, and the first actions should be to calm the infant, place in the knee-chest position, and give supplemental oxygen. A hypercyanotic spell will likely worsen without intervention, so prompt action is needed. CPR is inappropriate at this time because the infant has an adequate heart rate and effective respirations. A severe hypercyanotic spell may require IV medications, hydration, and resuscitative measures to stabilize the infant.

and developmental delays, especially in motor and cognitive development, may result from chronic hypoxia.

Therapeutic Management

Hypercyanotic spells occur suddenly, and prompt recognition and treatment are essential. In the hospital setting, spells are often seen during blood drawing or IV insertion, when the child is highly agitated, or after cardiac catheterization. Treatment of a hypercyanotic spell is outlined in the Guidelines box. Morphine, administered subcutaneously or through an existing IV line, helps to reduce infundibular spasm. Generally, a spell indicates the need for prompt surgical treatment if possible (Driscoll, 1990). In infants with defects not amenable to surgical repair, a shunt may be created surgically to increase blood flow to the lungs. Currently used types of shunts are described in Table 25-3.

The cyanotic infant and child are well hydrated to keep the hematocrit and blood viscosity within acceptable limits to reduce the risk of CVAs. Fevers are carefully evaluated because bacteremia can result in bacterial endocarditis. The infant is monitored closely for anemia because of the risk of CVAs and the reduced arterial oxygen-carrying capacity that occurs. Iron supplementation and possibly blood transfusion are used as needed.

Respiratory infections or reduced pulmonary function from any cause can worsen hypoxemia in the cyanotic child. Aggressive pulmonary hygiene, chest physiotherapy, administration of antibiotics, and use of oxygen to improve arterial saturations are important interventions.

Nursing Considerations

The general appearance of infants and children with significant cyanosis poses unique concerns. Blue lips and fingernails are obvious signs of their hidden cardiac defect. Clubbing and

GUIDELINES
Treating Hypercyanotic Spells

Place infant in knee-chest position (Fig. 25-8).
Employ calm, comforting approach.
Administer 100% oxygen by face mask.
Give morphine subcutaneously or through existing IV line.
Begin IV fluid replacement and volume expansion if needed.
Repeat morphine administration.

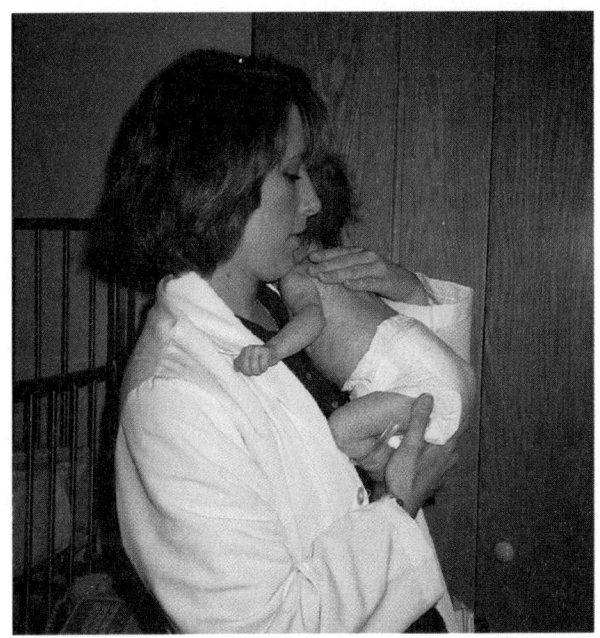

FIG. 25-8. Infant held in knee-chest position.

TYPE OF SHUNT/LOCATION	COMMENTS
Modified Blalock-Taussig (BT) Subclavian artery to pulmonary artery using Gore-Tex or Impra tube graft	Shunt flow sometimes excessive, requiring use of diuretics Possibility of thrombosis; antiplatelet therapy may be used postoperatively Easy to ligate at time of definitive correction Shunt size fixed and may become too small as child grows
Central Ascending aorta to main pulmonary aorta using Gore-Tex graft	Length of shunt acts to restrict blood flow, limiting symptoms of CHF; may require diuretics Uncommon; used when modified BT shunt cannot be done Easy to perform and remove at time of repair
Glenn Superior vena cava to side of right pulmonary artery, which is ligated from main pulmonary artery Blood flow to right lung only	Used as a second shunt procedure if complete repair not possible High mortality in infants under age 6 months Superior vena cava syndrome may occur Pulmonary arteriovenous fistulas may occur many years later Difficult to take down at time of definitive repair
Bidirectional Glenn (Cavopulmonary Anastomosis) Superior vena cava to side of right pulmonary artery Blood flow to both lungs	Done as a second shunt; often as a staging step to a Fontan procedure Can be incorporated into eventual modified Fontan procedure Relieves cyanosis and decreases volume overload on ventricle

TABLE 25-3. Selected shunt procedures for children with cardiac defects

small, thin stature in older children further indicate severe heart disease. Adolescents are especially concerned about their body image; children with cyanosis are often teased about their appearance and singled out as different. Many children, when asked what surgery will do, reply, "Make me pink." Their joy and excitement following surgery are evident when they see their pink fingers. Accentuating the normal and positive and being careful not to call attention to their cyanosis are helpful interventions. Meeting other children who are cyanotic in the clinic or hospital reassures them that they are not the only ones who are blue.

Parents are often fearful of their child's bluish color, since cyanosis is usually associated with lack of oxygen and severe illness. They also must deal with comments from relatives, friends, and strangers about their child's abnormal color. They need a simple explanation of hypoxemia and cyanosis and reassurance that cyanosis does not imply a lack of oxygen to the brain. Their questions and fears need to be addressed in a calm, supportive manner, and positive aspects of their child's growth and development are emphasized. They are taught the treatment for hypercyanotic spells (see box on p. 877).

Dehydration must be prevented in hypoxemic children because it potentiates the risk of CVAs. Fluid status is carefully monitored, with accurate intake and output and daily weight measurements. Maintenance fluid therapy is the minimum requirement, supplemental fluids should be readily available, and gavage feeding or IV hydration is given to children unable to take adequate oral fluids. Fever, vomiting, and diarrhea can cause dehydration and require prompt treatment. Parents are instructed in the importance of adequate fluid intake and measures to prevent dehydration. An oral electrolyte solution should be available at home in the event the infant is unable to tolerate the usual formula. The practitioner should be notified of fever, vomiting, diarrhea, or other problems.

Preventive measures and accurate assessment of respiratory infection are important nursing considerations. Any compromise in pulmonary function will increase the infant's hypoxemia. Good handwashing and protection from individuals with an obvious respiratory infection are important. Aggressive pulmonary hygiene, treatment with antibiotics or antiviral agents as indicated, and supplemental oxygen to decrease hypoxemia are necessary measures. Infants may need to be gavage fed or given parenteral hydration if respiratory distress prevents oral feeding.

Nursing ALERT	Intracardiac shunting of blood from the right side (desaturated) to the left side of the heart allows air in the venous system to go directly to the brain, resulting in an air embolism. Therefore all IV lines should have filters in place to prevent air from entering the system, the entire tubing should be checked for air, all connections should be taped securely, and any air should be removed.

NURSING CARE OF THE FAMILY AND CHILD WITH CONGENITAL HEART DISEASE

❖ Assessment

Nursing care of the child with CHD begins as soon as the diagnosis is suspected. However, in many instances symptoms that suggest a cardiac anomaly are not present at birth or, if manifest, are so subtle that they are easily overlooked (see box).

Many heart defects are not evident until the child's growth and/or energy expenditure exceeds the ability of the heart to supply oxygenated blood. Since the onset is gradual, the child may curtail activity so that the signs of exercise intolerance are less obvious.

A vital component of nursing assessment is related to the impact of the disorder on the family, especially the parents. Therefore the reactions, coping, and concerns of the family are also included in the assessment process (see Chapter 18).

❖ Nursing Diagnoses

Many nursing diagnoses are apparent after a thorough assessment of the child and family. Some of these are developed in the Nursing Care Plan on pp. 884-885. Others will be evident based on assessment of individual cases.

❖ Planning

The goals for the infant with CHD and the family include the following:

1. Family and child (if appropriate) will adjust to the diagnosis.
2. Family will be knowledgeable regarding symptoms of the disease and their management.

CLINICAL MANIFESTATIONS OF CONGENITAL HEART DISEASE

Infants

Cyanosis—generalized, especially mucous membranes, lips and tongue, conjunctiva; highly vascularized areas
Cyanosis during exertion such as crying, feeding, straining, or when immersed in water; peripheral or central
Dyspnea, especially after physical effort such as feeding, crying, straining
Fatigue
Poor growth and development (failure to thrive)
Frequent respiratory tract infections
Feeding difficulties
Hypotonia
Excessive sweating
Syncopal attacks such as paroxysmal hyperpnea, anoxic spells

Older Children

Impaired growth
Delicate, frail body build
Fatigue
Effort dyspnea
Orthopnea
Digital clubbing
Squatting for relief of dyspnea
Headache
Epistaxis
Leg fatigue

3. Family will cope with effects of the disorder.
4. Child (if appropriate) and family will be prepared for surgical repair of a defect.
5. Child undergoing cardiac surgery will receive appropriate care.
6. Family will receive adequate emotional support.
7. Family will be prepared for home care.

❖ Implementation

Help Family Adjust to the Disorder

Once parents learn of the heart defect, whether it is soon after the child's birth or at a later period in life, they are initially in a period of shock, followed by high anxiety, especially fear of the child's death. The family needs time to grieve before they can assimilate the meaning of the defect. Unfortunately the demands for medical treatment may not allow this, necessitating that the parents immediately give informed consent for diagnostic/therapeutic procedures. The nurse can be instrumental in supporting parents in their loss, assessing their level of understanding, supplying information as needed, and helping other members of the health team to understand the parents' reactions (see Family Focus box).

Severely distressed newborns usually remain in the hospital. This can seriously affect parent-infant attachment unless parents are encouraged to hold, touch, and look at their child. Every effort must be made by health personnel to foster attachment. (See Chapter 8 for suggestions on promoting attachment between parents and their hospitalized newborn.)

The effect of a child with a serious heart defect on the family is complex. No member, regardless of the degree of positive adjustment, is unaffected. Mothers frequently feel inadequate in their mothering ability because they gave birth to a child with a defect and are unable to keep the child well. They often feel constantly exhausted from the pressures of caring for these children and the other family members. Fathers and siblings may feel neglected and resentful, a reaction similar to the feelings of family members toward other chronic conditions (see Chapter 18). Often, parents do not feel confident leaving the child in another's care. This often sets up a trap for parents, especially mothers, who become locked into the child's care with no relief. Although the fears are justified, they can be minimized by gradually teaching someone (a reliable relative or neighbor) how to care for the child.

The need to maintain discipline and set consistent limits cannot be overemphasized. Using behavior modification techniques, either in the form of concrete awards (e.g., a favorite activity) or social reinforcement (e.g., approval), can be effective. However, it is most beneficial if employed *before* the child learns to control the family. Therefore it is necessary to guide parents toward the need for discipline while the child is in infancy to prevent later problems. Use of behavior modification techniques also teaches these children how to tolerate frustration and delayed gratification (this ability often is lacking because all their needs are satisfied immediately).

Another issue that may develop within family relationships is the child's overdependency. This is often the result of parental fear that the child may die. The best approach to dealing with this dilemma is prevention. Parents need guidance to recognize the eventual hazards of continuing dependency and protectiveness as the child grows older, and the nurse can assist parents in learning ways to foster optimum development. Unless parents are shown what activities the child can do, they may focus on physical limitations and encourage dependency.

The child also needs opportunities for social development. These children do not need to be prevented from playing with other children because of concern regarding overexertion. Such practices foster increased dependency in the home environment. Parents need to be encouraged to seek appropriate social activity, especially before kindergarten.

A child with CHD may constitute a long-term family crisis. Frequently the continuing unremitting stresses of care—physical exhaustion, financial costs, emotional upset, fear of death, and concern for the child's future—are not fully appreciated by those caring for the family. Even when the child's condition is stabilized or corrected, the family may need to make new adjustments in their life-style. Introducing them to other families with similarly affected children can help them adjust to the daily stresses.*

Educate Family About the Disorder

Once parents are ready to hear about the heart condition, it is essential that they be given a clear explanation based on their level of understanding. Lack of familiarity with the cardiovascular system may be a major reason for lack of parental understanding, and it is usually helpful to review the basic structure and function of the heart before describing the defect. A simple diagram, pictures, or a model of the heart can be most helpful in visualizing the heart and the congenital defect. Parents appreciate receiving written information about the specific condition.† Parents also require informa-

---

FAMILY FOCUS
The Diagnosis of Heart Disease

Remember, we don't have your experience. We don't see children everyday who have heart disease. We would have been upset finding out our child had to have his tonsils out. How could we ever be prepared for this? Please remember, we only know people who have trivial heart murmurs. How could we ever expect this to happen? And to us, this is the worst problem we've ever heard of.

We still fear most what we don't know and understand. Be honest with us. If you don't know either, tell us. But at least don't leave us wondering about what you know and we don't. Not knowing anything really can be worse than knowing something bad. Be honest, but don't strip us of hope. . . .

Please, remember we are trying to learn complex information in a moment of time. And trying to learn it in a context of great pain and emotional investment. This is our lives you're talking about. Please be thorough, but keep it simple. Tell us again, maybe even again and again, when we can hear better.

From Schrey C, Schrey M: A parent's perspective: our needs and our message, *Crit Care Nurs Clin North Am* 6(1):113-119, 1994.

---

*Some local chapters of the **American Heart Association** have organized parent groups.

†A booklet that can be given to parents is *If Your Child Has a Congenital Heart Defect: A Guide for Parents*, available from the American Heart Association, 7272 Greenville Ave., Dallas, TX 75231; (214) 373-6300.

tion on the treatment options for the cardiac condition and the prognosis.

Another fact to remember is that different health personnel may convey the same information using different diagrams and medical terms. To prevent this from becoming a problem, which often happens when several health team members work with a family, the same type of diagram should be used, and the parents should write down any unclear terms or ask for clarification. Sometimes it is helpful to provide the family with a glossary of frequently used words for reference.

Infants and children with CHD require good nutrition. Providing infants with adequate nutrition is especially difficult because of their high caloric requirements and inability to suck effectively because of fatigue and tachypnea. Instructing parents in feeding methods that decrease the work of the infant and giving high-calorie formula are important interventions. (See p. 873 for a discussion on feeding the infant with CHF.)

Children with severe cardiac defects are often anorexic. Encouraging them to eat can be a tremendous challenge. Because of the parents' concern over eating, children learn early to manipulate parents through eating, such as making unrealistic demands for foods that are not available. The nurse advises parents of this potential problem, since prevention yields greater success than intervention. For example, the child should be given a choice of available high-quality foods. Suggestions for feeding sick children are discussed in Chapter 22.

The family also needs to be knowledgeable regarding the therapeutic management of the disorder, especially in terms of the medications that the child is receiving. Parents are taught the correct procedure for giving drugs* and cautioned to keep them in a safe area to prevent accidental ingestion (see Family Home Care box, p. 880).

Children of various ages have different ideas about their heart. Children between ages 4 and 6 years have heard about the heart, know its approximate anatomic location in the chest or back, illustrate it as valentine shaped, and characterize it by sounds such as *tick-tock* and *thump*. Children ages 7 to 10 have a clearer concept of the heart, realizing that it is not shaped like a valentine and that it has vital functions, such as "It makes you live." However, their knowledge of its integrated functions to pump blood through a system of vessels to all parts of the body is still hazy. By the age of 10 or 11 children have a much more involved concept of the heart, with knowledge of veins, valves, pumping action, and circulation. They are beginning to appreciate why death occurs when the heart stops.

Information given to the child must be tailored to the child's developmental age. As the child matures, the level of information is revised to meet the child's new cognitive level. Preschoolers need basic information about what they will experience more than what is actually occurring physiologically. School-age children benefit from a concrete explanation of the defect. Preadolescents and adolescents often appreciate a more detailed description of how the defect affects their heart. Children of all ages need to express their feelings concerning the diagnosis.

---

*Home care instructions on giving medications to children are available in Wong DL: *Wong and Whaley's Clinical manual of pediatric nursing,* ed 4, St Louis, 1996, Mosby.

Help Family Cope with Effects of the Disorder

Parents also need an explanation regarding the symptoms of the disease. Many children have few symptoms but may develop CHF. Therefore parents should be aware of early signs of worsening physical status, such as sweating, sudden weight gain, decreased exercise tolerance, poor feeding, and increased breathing effort. These symptoms need medical evaluation, but the family is assured that the symptoms usually respond quickly to therapeutic intervention.

Another area of parental concern is the child's level of physical activity. Children do not need to restrict activity, and the best approach is to treat the child normally and allow self-limited activity. Deliberately attempting to prevent crying should be avoided because it can establish a maladaptive parental pattern of relating to the infant. Exceptions to self-determined activity primarily involve strenuous recreational and competitive sports.

> **Nursing ALERT** Although decisions regarding activity restrictions are made on an individual basis on the cardiologist's advice, children with aortic stenosis or insufficiency are usually not permitted to engage in strenuous activity (Fyler, 1992).

Prepare Child and Family for Surgery

Few surgical procedures demand as much planning for preoperative preparation and postoperative care as heart surgery. The reader is urged to review the general principles for preparing children for procedures, such as surgery, discussed in Chapter 22. This discussion focuses on those measures specific to cardiovascular procedures. The child is usually admitted to the hospital 1 day before surgery or the day of surgery. Preoperative preparation is often done in the outpatient setting.

Introduce Child and Family to the Environment. Ideally, when the child is admitted, a plan should be made to provide consistent caregivers. In some institutions the nurse who will care for the child postoperatively in the intensive care unit (ICU) is also assigned to the child at admission to facilitate forming a relationship with the family and to share preoperative teaching, such as introduction to the recovery room and ICU. To increase familiarity, all nurses should call the child and parents by name and refer to themselves by name. Wearing a name tag reinforces this point. Postoperatively the family will feel more at ease recognizing familiar names, faces, and voices.

If a visit to the recovery room and/or ICU is planned, it should take place when there is least activity in the area, the parents can accompany the child, and the child is well rested. Usually a day before surgery is ample time to allow the child to ask questions and to prevent undue fantasizing about the experience. If a visit is included in the teaching plan, the nurse can use a book, preferably with pictures or photographs of the actual rooms, to explain the environment to the child.

During the visit to the ICU, the child and parents should experience everything that directly affects the child's care, such as the sounds of ECG monitors, oxygen tents, and placement of the bed. All positive, nonfrightening aspects of the environment are emphasized, such as the play area, visitors' section, pictures or mobiles in the room, or television. If it is a pediatric ICU, the nurse can introduce the family to other children who may be recovering from surgery. The child should be protected from the frightening sights in the unit, and equipment not in view postoperatively, such as equipment located behind or below the bed, needs less attention. The child and parents are encouraged to ask questions or to explore further any equipment in the room, but they should not be pushed to assimilate more information than they appear to be tolerating.

Familiarize Child and Family with Equipment. Some of the equipment, such as the stethoscope, blood pressure apparatus, and thermometer, will already be familiar to the child and parents. However, the nurse emphasizes that procedures involving such equipment will be done more frequently. If monitoring devices, such as blood pressure or oximetry, are used, the child is told about the placement of the sensor on the skin.

Types of equipment new to many families are the oxygen mask, suction, chest tubes, endotracheal tubes, incentive spirometers, nasogastric tube, and IV tubing. Each of these is shown and demonstrated either on the child or on a doll, if he or she appears ready. With a younger child, miniaturized equipment suitable for use with a doll or puppet is often less anxiety producing than the actual samples. If other children in the unit have an IV infusion or are in oxygen tents, the older child may benefit from seeing them, but this must be planned carefully to avoid frightening the child.

Several IV lines are inserted perioperatively: (1) an ordinary line for infusion of fluids, inserted in a peripheral vein; (2) a venous pressure line, inserted into the right subclavian or jugular vein; and (3) an arterial line for direct measurement of arterial pressure. Younger children need only know the location of each tubing. Older children may appreciate knowing the reason for each infusion. Since the lines are inserted during surgery, they are not painful; they only cause discomfort because movement is restricted.

The type and size of incision the child will have after surgery are discussed and can be shown on a doll. Usually one of two types of incisions is made: a *median sternotomy,* which splits the sternum, or a *lateral thoracotomy,* which extends from the midaxillary line to the scapula. Frequently no sutures are visible because subcuticular, absorbable sutures may be used. If this is done, it should be pointed out to the child and parents, who may fear the incision will open.

The child may be told about chest tubes and their purpose in draining fluid from around the heart and lungs. An endotracheal (ET) tube is inserted during surgery and may be left in place for ventilatory assistance and tracheobronchial suctioning. However, it may be best to prepare older children for the ET tube only if *prolonged* ventilatory support is planned. The ET tube can be presented as a "breathing tube" that is placed in the nose or mouth. The nurse explains that while the tube is in, the child will feel it in the throat and will not be able to talk, but nothing is wrong. The child can express desires by pointing or using a picture communication board. At this point, communicating the amount of discomfort from the surgery can also be discussed, especially using measurement tools such as numbers or faces (see Pain Assessment, Chapter 21). The nurse stresses that the tube will

be removed as soon as possible, often during the first postoperative day.

Preoperative physical care differs little, if any, from that for any other surgery and is discussed in Chapter 22. The child should be assured that the parents will be there when he or she wakes up; parents should be allowed to accompany their child as far as possible to the operating suite. After all the equipment and procedures have been explained, it is important to talk about "getting well" and going home. If a doll was used during the preparatory session, the tubes can be removed, and the doll can be dressed in regular clothes in anticipation of discharge.

Provide Postoperative Care

Immediate postoperative care is usually provided by specially trained nurses in ICUs. Many of the procedures, such as arterial pressure and central venous pressure (CVP) monitoring and the observations related to vital functions, require advanced educational training (the reader should refer to critical care texts for further information). However, nurses caring for the child before surgery and during the convalescent period need to be familiar with the major principles of care. Selected complications that may occur postoperatively are described in the box.

SELECTED COMPLICATIONS AFTER CARDIAC SURGERY AND TREATMENT APPROACHES

Cardiac
Congestive heart failure: digoxin, diuretics, etc. (see p. 868)
Low cardiac output: intravenous inotropes (see shock, p. 895)
Dysrhythmias: identification, drug treatment, possible pacing, cardioversion (see p. 890)
Tamponade (blood or fluid in the pericardial space constricting the heart): Prompt removal of fluid by pericardiocentesis

Respiratory
Atelectasis: chest physiotherapy, coughing, deep breathing, ambulation
Pulmonary edema: diuretics
Pleural effusions: diuretics, possible chest tube drainage
Pneumothorax: possible chest tube drainage

Neurologic
Seizures: assessment, antiepileptic drugs
Cerebrovascular accident (stroke), cerebral edema, neurologic deficits: assessment and treatment

Infectious Disease
Infections, especially wound, pneumonia, otitis media, and sepsis: antibiotics

Hematologic
Anemia: iron supplementation, possible transfusion
Postoperative bleeding: initially, clotting factors, blood products; may need repeat surgery to locate and ligate source of bleeding

Other
Postpericardiotomy syndrome (syndrome of fever, leukocytosis, friction rub, pericardial and pleural effusions, lethargy seen about 7 to 21 days after cardiac surgery; possible viral or autoimmune etiologies): antipyretics, diuretics, antiinflammatory medications

Observe Vital Signs.   Vital signs and blood pressure are recorded frequently until stable. Heart rate and respirations are counted for 1 full minute, compared with the ECG monitor, and recorded with activity. The heart rate is normally increased after surgery. The nurse observes cardiac rhythm and notifies the practitioner of any changes in regularity. Dysrhythmias may occur postoperatively secondary to anesthetics, acid-base and electrolyte imbalance, hypoxia, surgical intervention, or trauma to conduction pathways (see also p. 889).

At least hourly the lungs are auscultated for breath sounds. Diminished or absent sounds most likely indicate an area of atelectasis, which necessitates further medical assessment.

Temperature changes are typical during the early postoperative period. Hypothermia is expected immediately after surgery from hypothermia procedures, effects of anesthesia, and loss of body heat to the cool environment. During this period the child is kept warm to prevent additional heat loss. Infants may be placed under radiant heat warmers. During the next 24 to 48 hours the body temperature may rise to 37.7° C (100° F) or slightly higher as part of the inflammatory response to tissue trauma. After this period an elevated temperature is most likely a sign of infection and warrants immediate investigation for probable cause.

Maintain Respiratory Status.   The child is generally maintained on mechanical ventilation in the immediate postoperative period. When weaning and extubation are completed, humidified oxygen is delivered by mask or hood. The child is kept warm and dry, since excessive chilling from wet linens causes an increased metabolic need and consequent increased cardiac demand. The child is encouraged to turn and deep breathe at least hourly. Every measure is used to enhance ventilation and decrease pain, such as splinting of the operative site and judicious use of analgesics.

Suctioning is performed *only* as needed and maintained for no more than 5 seconds at a time to prevent depleting the oxygen supply. Supplemental oxygen is administered with a manual resuscitation bag before and after the procedure to prevent hypoxia. Heart rate is monitored after suctioning to detect changes in rhythm or rate, especially bradycardia. The child should be positioned facing the nurse to permit assessment of the child's color and tolerance to the procedure.

> **Nursing ALERT**   During suctioning, observe for signs and symptoms of respiratory distress, such as tachypnea, use of accessory muscles for breathing, restlessness, and changes in oxygen saturation on the pulse oximeter.

Drainage from chest tubes is checked hourly for color and quantity. Immediately after surgery the drainage may be bright red, but afterward it should be serous. The largest volume of drainage occurs in the first 12 to 24 hours and is greater in extensive heart surgery.

> **Nursing ALERT**   Chest tube drainage greater than 3 ml/kg/hour for more than 3 consecutive hours is excessive and may indicate postoperative hemorrhage (Hazinski, 1992). The surgeon is notified immediately, since cardiac tamponade can develop rapidly and is life-threatening.

Chest tubes are usually removed on the first to third postoperative day. Removal of chest tubes is a painful, frightening experience. Analgesics such as morphine sulfate, often combined with midazolam (Versed), should be given before the procedure. Older children are forewarned that they will feel a sharp, momentary pain. After the suture is cut, the tubes are quickly pulled out at the end of full inspiration to prevent intake of air into the pleural cavity. A purse-string suture (placed when the tubes were inserted) is pulled tight to close the opening. A petrolatum-covered gauze dressing is immediately applied over the wound and securely taped on all four sides to the skin so that an airtight seal is formed. The dressing is checked for signs of drainage and any evidence of infection.

Monitor Fluids.   Intake and output of all fluids must be accurately calculated. Intake is primarily IV fluids; however, a record of fluid used to flush the arterial and CVP lines or to dilute medications is also kept. Output includes hourly recordings of urine (usually a Foley catheter is inserted and attached to a closed collecting device), drainage from chest and nasogastric tubes, and blood drawn for analysis. Urine is analyzed for specific gravity to assess the concentrating ability of the kidneys and to assess approximately the body's degree of hydration. Renal failure is a potential risk from a transient period of low cardiac output.

> **Nursing ALERT**   The signs of renal failure are decreased urine output (less than 1 ml/kg/hour) and elevated levels of blood urea nitrogen and serum creatinine.

Fluids are restricted during the immediate postoperative period to prevent hypervolemia, which places additional demands on the myocardium, predisposing to cardiac failure. To monitor fluid retention, the child is weighed daily, and the same scale is used at approximately the same time each day to avoid errors in measurement. The child is usually given nothing by mouth for the first 24 hours. If an ET tube is inserted, oral fluids are usually withheld until the child is extubated. Fluid restriction may be imposed even when oral fluids are given. The nurse calculates the distribution over a 24-hour period based on the child's preoperative weight and drinking habits. The distribution should allow for most fluid to be given during the child's most wakeful and active periods.

Provide Rest and Progressive Activity.   After heart surgery, rest should be provided to decrease the workload of the heart and promote healing. The simplest way to ensure individualized, efficient, high-quality care is to plan at the beginning of the shift the nursing procedures to be done, with periods of rest identified. The schedule should be shared with parents to allow them to visit at the most advantageous times, such as after a rest period when no special treatments are anticipated.

A progressive schedule of ambulation and activity is planned, based on the child's preoperative activity patterns and postoperative cardiovascular and pulmonary function. Ambulation is initiated early, usually by the second postoperative day, when chest tubes, arterial lines, and assisted ventilatory equipment may be removed. Activity progresses from sitting on the edge of the bed and dangling the legs to standing up and to sitting in a chair. Heart rate and respirations are carefully monitored to assess the degree of cardiac demand imposed by each activity. Tachycardia, dyspnea, cyanosis, desaturation, progressive fatigue, or dysrhythmias indicate the need to limit further energy expenditure.

Provide Comfort and Emotional Support. Heart surgery is both painful and frightening for children, and comfort is a primary nursing concern. Continuous IV opioid infusions, particularly morphine and fentanyl, are safe and effective analgesics (Maguire and Maloney, 1988). Patient-controlled analgesia may be used with children old enough to understand the concept. Nonsteroidal antiinflammatory drugs (NSAIDs) such as ketorolac (Toradol) may be used intravenously. Epidural morphine may be another option, since it affords very good pain control when a thoracotomy is performed. Paralyzing agents such as pancuronium (Pavulon) or metocurine (Metubine) may also be used with the analgesics for children who are very agitated or hemodynamically unstable.

Most patients need IV analgesics for pain control during the immediate postoperative period. After extubation and removal of lines and tubes, pain can be satisfactorily controlled with oral medications such as ibuprofen, codeine with acetaminophen (Tylenol), or oxycodone and acetaminophen (Tylox). Acetaminophen alone provides adequate pain relief for most children at discharge. Sternotomy incisions are usually well tolerated, with some discomfort when walking and coughing. Thoracotomy incisions are usually more painful because the incision is through muscle; a more aggressive pain management plan with round-the-clock medications for several days is often necessary to allow for adequate rest, ambulation, and pulmonary hygiene.

In addition to pharmacologic pain control, every effort is made to minimize the discomfort of procedures, such as using a firm pillow or favorite stuffed animal placed against the chest incision during movement and performing treatments *after* pain medication is given, preferably at a time that coincides with the drug's peak effect. Nonpharmacologic measures are used to lessen the perception of pain, and parents are encouraged to comfort their child as much as possible. (See also Pain Assessment; Pain Management, Chapter 21.)

Children may also be angry and uncooperative after surgery as a response to the physical pain and to the loss of control imposed by the surgery and treatments. They need an opportunity to express feelings, either verbally or through activity. Children also may express feelings of anger or rejection toward parents. The nurse must reassure parents that this is normal and that with continued support the anger will subside.

The nurse can support the parents by being available for information and explaining all the procedures to them. The first few postoperative days are particularly difficult because parents see their child in pain and realize the potential risks from surgery. They often are overwhelmed by the physical environment of the ICU and feel useless because they can do so little for their child. The importance of their presence in making the child feel more secure is stressed, even if they do not provide physical care.

Plan for Discharge and Home Care

Ideally, discharge planning begins on admission for cardiac surgery and includes an assessment of the parents' adjustment

FAMILY HOME CARE
Topics to Include in Discharge Teaching After Cardiac Surgery

Medication teaching (for digoxin, see p. 872)
Activity restrictions
Diet and nutrition
Wound care (include dressings if any, suture removal, bathing)
Bacterial endocarditis prophylaxis (see p. 886)
Follow-up appointments (cardiologist, primary care provider)
   Community agencies as needed (visiting nurse service, early developmental intervention)
When to call practitioner; signs and symptoms of postoperative problems
Review of cardiac defect and surgical repair

to the child's altered state of health. As mentioned earlier, one of the most common parental reactions is overprotection, and the nurse needs to be aware of times when the family may need help in recognizing the child's improved health status. With surgical correction of heart anomalies occurring during infancy, there is less likelihood of this pattern of over-dependency developing.

The family will need both verbal and written instructions on medication, nutrition, activity restrictions, subacute bacterial endocarditis, return to school, wound care, and signs and symptoms of infection or complications (see Family Home Care box). Referrals to community agencies may be warranted to assist parents in the transition from hospital to home and to reinforce the teaching.

The parents will also need clear instructions on when to seek medical care, such as for a change in the child's behavior or an unexplained fever. Follow-up with the cardiologist is also arranged before discharge. Appropriate identification, such as a Medic-Alert device, is indicated for children with a pacemaker or a heart transplant and for those receiving anticoagulation therapy or antidysrhythmic medication.

The nurse also discusses common behavior disturbances that may occur after discharge, such as nightmares, sleep disturbances, separation anxiety, and overdependence. A supportive, consistent response is essential to allow the child to overcome the surgical experience. The child should be encouraged to work out feelings and fears through therapeutic play.

Although surgical correction of heart defects has improved dramatically, it is still not possible to reverse totally many of the complex anomalies. For many children, repeat procedures are required to replace conduits or grafts or to manage complications, such as restenosis. Consequently the long-term prognosis is uncertain, and full recovery is not always possible. For these families, medical follow-up and continued emotional support are essential. The nurse can often serve as an important primary health professional and as a resource for referrals when needed.

❖ Evaluation

The effectiveness of nursing interventions for the family and the child with CHD is determined by continual reassessment and evaluation of care based on the following observational guidelines and expected outcomes:

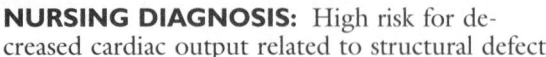

Nursing Care Plan
The Child with Congenital Heart Disease

NURSING DIAGNOSIS: High risk for decreased cardiac output related to structural defect

PATIENT GOAL 1: Will exhibit improved cardiac output

• **NURSING INTERVENTIONS/*RATIONALES***

*Administer digoxin as ordered, using established precautions *to prevent toxicity* (see p. 871 and Family Home Care box, p. 872)
*Administer afterload reduction medications as ordered (see p. 873)
*Administer diuretics as ordered (see p. 870)

• **EXPECTED OUTCOMES**

Heart rate, blood pressure, and peripheral perfusion are normal for age (see inside front cover)
Urine output is adequate (between 0.5 to 2 ml/kg, depending on age)

NURSING DIAGNOSIS: Activity intolerance related to imbalance between oxygen supply and demand

PATIENT GOAL 1: Will maintain adequate energy levels without additional stresses

• **NURSING INTERVENTIONS/*RATIONALES***

Allow for frequent rest periods and uninterrupted periods of sleep
Encourage quiet games and activities
Help child select activities appropriate to age, condition, and capabilities
Avoid extremes of environmental temperature *because hyperthermia or hypothermia increases the need for oxygen*
Implement measures to reduce anxiety
Respond promptly to crying or other expressions of distress

• **EXPECTED OUTCOMES**

Child determines and engages in activities commensurate with capabilities
Child receives appropriate amount of rest/sleep (specify)

NURSING DIAGNOSES: Altered growth and development related to inadequate oxygen and nutrients to tissues; social isolation

PATIENT GOAL 1: Will follow growth curve for weight and height

• **NURSING INTERVENTIONS/*RATIONALES***

Provide well-balanced, highly nutritious diet *to achieve adequate growth*
Monitor height and weight; plot on growth charts *to determine growth trend*

*Dependent nursing action.

May administer iron supplements *to correct anemia,* if ordered

• **EXPECTED OUTCOME**

Child achieves adequate growth (specify)

PATIENT GOAL 2: Will have opportunity to participate in age-appropriate activities

• **NURSING INTERVENTIONS/*RATIONALES***

Encourage age-appropriate activities
Emphasize that child has same need for socialization as other children
Allow child to set own pace and activity limits *because child will rest when tired*

• **EXPECTED OUTCOMES**

Child engages in age-appropriate activities
Child does not experience social isolation

NURSING DIAGNOSIS: High risk for infection related to debilitated physical status

PATIENT GOAL 1: Will exhibit no evidence of infection

• **NURSING INTERVENTIONS/*RATIONALES***

Avoid contact with infected persons
Provide for adequate rest
Provide optimum nutrition *to support body's natural defenses*

• **EXPECTED OUTCOME**

Child remains free of infection

NURSING DIAGNOSIS: Altered family processes related to having a child with a heart condition

See Nursing Care Plan: The Child with Chronic Illness or Disability, Chapter 18

PATIENT/FAMILY GOAL 1: Will experience reduction of fear and anxiety

• **NURSING INTERVENTIONS/*RATIONALES***

Discuss with parents and child (if appropriate) their fears and concerns regarding child's cardiac defects and physical symptoms, *since these frequently cause anxiety and fear*

• **EXPECTED OUTCOME**

Family discusses their fears and anxieties

PATIENT GOAL 2: Will exhibit positive coping behaviors

• **INTERVENTIONS/*RATIONALES***

Encourage family to participate in care of child while hospitalized *to facilitate better coping at home*
Encourage family to include others in child's care *to prevent their own exhaustion*

NURSING CARE PLAN
The Child with Congenital Heart Disease—cont'd

Assist family in determining appropriate physical activity and disciplining methods for child

- **EXPECTED OUTCOME**

Family copes with child's symptoms in a positive way

PATIENT (FAMILY) GOAL 3: Will demonstrate knowledge of home care

- **NURSING INTERVENTIONS/***RATIONALES*

Teach skills needed for home care:
  Administration of medications
  Feeding techniques
  Interventions for conserving energy and those directed toward relief of frightening symptoms
  Signs that indicate complications
  Where and whom to contact for help and guidance
Anticipate need for further information and support
Refer family to local chapter of the American Red Cross *for instruction in cardiopulmonary resuscitation (CPR)*

- **EXPECTED OUTCOMES**

Family demonstrates ability and motivation for home care
Family members learn CPR technique

NURSING DIAGNOSIS: High risk for injury (complications) related to cardiac condition and therapies

---

PATIENT (FAMILY) GOAL 1: Will recognize signs of complications early

- **NURSING INTERVENTIONS/***RATIONALES*

Teach family to recognize signs of complications
  Congestive heart failure (CHF) (for complete list, see box on p. 871)
  Early signs:
    Tachycardia, especially during rest and slight exertion
    Tachypnea
    Profuse scalp sweating, especially in infants
    Fatigue and irritation

    Sudden weight gain
    Respiratory distress
  Digoxin toxicity
    Vomiting (earliest sign)
    Nausea
    Anorexia
    Bradycardia
    Dysrhythmias
  Increased respiratory effort—retraction, grunting, cough, cyanosis
  Hypoxemia—cyanosis, restlessness
  Cardiovascular collapse—pallor, cyanosis, hypotonia
Teach family to intervene during hypercyanotic spells because cerebral hypoxin can cause brain damage or death
  Place child in knee-chest position (see Fig. 25-8)
  Remain calm
  Administer 100% oxygen by face mask if available
  Call practitioner

- **EXPECTED OUTCOME**

Family recognizes signs of complications and institutes appropriate action

PATIENT/FAMILY GOAL 2: Will demonstrate understanding of diagnostic tests and surgery

- **NURSING INTERVENTIONS**

Explain or clarify information presented to family by the practitioner and surgeon
Prepare child and parents for the procedure
Assist with family's decision regarding surgery
Explore feelings regarding surgical options

- **EXPECTED OUTCOME**

Family demonstrates an understanding of procedures (e.g., tests, surgery) (specify learning and manner of demonstration)

See also:
  Nursing Care Plan: The Child in the Hospital, Chapter 21
  Nursing Care Plan: The Family of the Ill or Hospitalized Child, Chapter 21
  Nursing Care Plan: The Child Undergoing Surgery, Chapter 22

---

1. Interview family and observe their behavior with infant or child.
2. Encourage family to discuss their feelings and concerns; observe their response to education.
3. Interview child and observe his or her behavior and concerns; encourage verbal child to express feelings.
4. Interview family and observe family interactions and relationships.
5. Interview family regarding their understanding of the condition and the proposed surgery.
6. Monitor and observe infant or child and family preoperatively and postoperatively.
7. Observe and interview child and family regarding their understanding of home care needs, ability to carry out care, and compliance with the plan of care.

Expected outcomes:
See Nursing Care Plan, pp. 884-885.

ACQUIRED CARDIOVASCULAR DISORDERS

BACTERIAL (INFECTIVE) ENDOCARDITIS (BE)

BE, or infective endocarditis (IE), also referred to as *subacute bacterial endocarditis* (SBE), is an infection of the valves and inner lining of the heart. Although it can occur without underlying heart disease, BE most often is a sequela of bacteremia in the child with acquired or congenital anomalies of the heart or great vessels. It especially affects children with valvular abnormalities, prosthetic valves, recent cardiac surgery with invasive lines, and rheumatic heart disease with valve involvement. In addition, a growing problem is endocarditis associated with drug abuse (Dajani and Taubert, 1995). The most common causative agent is *Streptococcus viridans;* other causative agents are *Staphylococcus aureus,* gram-negative bacteria, and fungi such as *Candida albicans.*

Pathophysiology

Organisms may enter the bloodstream from any site of localized infection. The most common portals of entry are oral from dental work *(S. viridans);* urinary tract, such as from urinary tract infection after catheterization (gram-negative bacilli); heart, from cardiac surgery, especially if synthetic material is used (valves, patches, conduits); and the bloodstream from long-term indwelling catheters. The microorganisms grow on the endocardium, forming vegetations (verrucae), deposits of fibrin, and platelet thrombi. The lesion may invade adjacent tissues, such as aortic and mitral valves, and may break off and embolize elsewhere, especially in the spleen, kidney, and central nervous system.

Diagnostic Evaluation

The diagnosis of IE is suspected on the basis of clinical manifestations (see box). Several laboratory findings may suggest IE, for example, ECG changes (prolonged P-R interval), radiographic evidence of cardiomegaly, anemia, elevated erythrocyte sedimentation rate, leukocytosis, and microscopic hematuria. Vegetations on the valve and abnormal valve function can often be visualized by echocardiography. Definitive diagnosis rests on growth and identification of the causative agent in the blood.

Therapeutic Management

Treatment should be instituted immediately and consists of administration of high doses of appropriate antibiotics intravenously and/or intramuscularly for at least 4 weeks. Blood cultures are taken periodically to evaluate response to antibiotic therapy.

BE in susceptible children is prevented by administering prophylactic antibiotic therapy both before and for a short period after procedures known to increase the risk of entry of organisms, including dental work and any manipulation of the respiratory, genitourinary, or gastrointestinal tract. In female adolescents this includes childbirth (see box).

Nursing Considerations

Ideally the objective of nursing care is prevention through counseling parents of high-risk children about the need for prophylactic antibiotic therapy before procedures such as dental work. Unless parents are aware of the risk inherent in exposing their child to these procedures, they may not be inclined to seek medical treatment beforehand. The family's regular dentist should be advised of existing cardiac problems in the child as an added precaution and to ensure that preventive treatment is carried out.

Treatment of BE requires hospitalization for the institution of parenteral drug therapy. In many patients, IV antibiotics may be administered at home with nursing supervision to complete the course of treatment. Nursing goals during this period are (1) preparation of the child for continuous IV infusion, possibly for several venipunctures for blood cultures; (2) observation for side effects of antibiotics; and (3) observation for complications, especially from embolism, and the possibility of heart failure. For specific interventions see Nursing Care Plan: The Child with Congestive Heart Failure, pp. 874-875.

RHEUMATIC FEVER (RF)

RF, or acute RF, is an inflammatory disease affecting the heart, joints, central nervous system, and subcutaneous tissue. It derives its name from involvement of joints and the presence of fever in the acute stage. The most significant sequela of RF is *rheumatic heart disease,* especially damage to and scarring of the mitral valve. Although the disease has declined during the past 30 years, recent outbreaks have been reported in several areas, causing concern among health professionals.

Etiology

Strong evidence supports a relationship between upper respiratory infection with group A streptococci and subsequent development of RF (usually within 2 to 6 weeks). In almost all cases of RF a previous infection with group A streptococci can be documented by laboratory evidence of rising antibody titers. Prevention or treatment of group A streptococcal infection prevents RF.

CLINICAL MANIFESTATIONS OF INFECTIVE ENDOCARDITIS (IE)

Onset usually insidious
Unexplained fever (low grade and intermittent)
Anorexia
Malaise
Weight loss
Characteristic findings caused by extracardiac emboli formation:
    Splinter hemorrhages (thin black lines) under the nails
    Osler nodes (red, painful intradermal nodes found on pads of phalanges)
    Janeway lesions (painless hemorrhagic areas on palms and soles)
    Petechiae on oral mucous membranes
May be present:
    Congestive heart failure
    Cardiac dysrhythmias
    New murmur or change in previously existing one

PROCEDURES REQUIRING PROPHYLAXIS FOR BACTERIAL ENDOCARDITIS (BE)

All dental procedures likely to induce gingival or mucosal bleeding, including professional teeth cleaning (not simple adjustment of orthodontic appliances or shedding of deciduous teeth)
Tonsillectomy and/or adenoidectomy
Surgical procedures or biopsy involving respiratory or intestinal mucosa
Bronchoscopy with a rigid bronchoscope
Incision and drainage of infected tissue
Genitourinary and gastrointestinal procedures, including most diagnostic and therapeutic procedures that are invasive (sclerotherapy for esophageal varices, esophageal dilation, cystoscopy, urethral dilation, urethral catheterization or surgery if urinary tract infection is present, prostatic surgery, vaginal hysterectomy, and vaginal delivery in presence of infection)

Data from Dajani AS and others: Prevention of bacterial endocarditis: recommendations by the American Heart Association, *JAMA* 264(22):2919-2922, 1990.

Diagnostic Evaluation

Diagnosis is based on a set of guidelines recommended by the American Heart Association. These guidelines, known as *modifications of the Jones criteria,* suggest that the presence of two major manifestations or one major and two minor manifestations, such as fever and arthralgia, with supportive evidence of recent streptococcal infection, indicates a high probability of RF (see box).

Children suspected of having RF are tested for streptococcal antibodies. The most reliable and best standardized test is an elevated or rising *antistreptolysin-O (ASO* or *ASLO) titer,* which occurs in 80% of children with RF. Others include anti-DNAse B and anti-DPNase tests, erythrocyte sedimentation rate, and C-reactive protein. ECGs and radiographs are obtained to detect any evidence of heart involvement.

Therapeutic Management

The goals of medical management are (1) eradication of hemolytic streptococci, (2) prevention of permanent cardiac damage, (3) palliation of the other symptoms, and (4) prevention of recurrences of RF. Penicillin is the drug of choice, with erythromycin as a substitute in penicillin-sensitive children. Salicylates are used to control the inflammatory process, especially in the joints, and reduce the fever and discomfort. Bed rest is recommended during the acute febrile phase but need not be strict.

Prophylactic treatment against recurrence of RF is started after the acute therapy and involves monthly intramuscular injections of benzathine penicillin G (1.2 million U), two daily oral doses of penicillin (200,000 U), or one daily dose of sulfadiazine (1 g). The duration of long-term prophylaxis is uncertain. Because of the risk of BE in rheumatic heart disease, the same prophylaxis discussed earlier is implemented. The antibiotic regimens used to prevent recurrences of RF are inadequate for the prevention of BE.

Children who have had acute RF are susceptible to recurrent RF for the rest of their lives and should be followed medically for at least 5 years. Children and families must be aware of the need for continuing antibiotic prophylaxis for dental work, infection, and invasive procedures.

Nursing Considerations

The objectives of nursing care for the child with RF are to (1) encourage compliance with drug regimens, (2) facilitate recovery from the illness, (3) provide emotional support, and (4) prevent the disease. Since compliance is a major concern in long-term drug therapy, every effort is made to encourage adherence to the therapeutic plan (see Compliance, Chapter 22). When compliance is poor, monthly injections may be substituted for daily oral administration of antibiotics, and children need preparation for this often dreaded procedure.

Interventions during home care are primarily concerned with providing rest and adequate nutrition. Usually, once the febrile stage is over, children can resume moderate activity, and their appetite improves. If carditis is present, the family must be aware of any activity restrictions and may need help in choosing less strenuous activities for the child.

One of the most disturbing and frustrating manifestations of the disease is *chorea.* The onset is gradual and may occur weeks to months after the illness; it sometimes even occurs

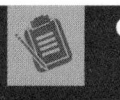

GUIDELINES
Diagnosis of Initial Attack of Rheumatic Fever (RF) (Jones Criteria, 1992 Update)*

Major Manifestations
Carditis
Tachycardia out of proportion to degree of fever
Cardiomegaly
New murmurs or change in preexisting murmurs
Muffled heart sounds
Precardial friction rub
Precordial pain
Changes in ECG (especially prolonged P-R interval)

Polyarthritis
Swollen, hot, red, painful joint(s)
After 1 to 2 days affects different joint(s)
Favors large joints—knees, elbows, hips, shoulders, wrists

Erythema Marginatum
Erythematous macules with clear center and wavy, well-demarcated border
Transitory
Nonpruritic
Primarily affects trunk and extremities (inner surfaces)

Chorea (St. Vitus Dance, Sydenham Chorea)
Sudden aimless, irregular movements of extremities
Involuntary facial grimaces
Speech disturbances
Emotional lability
Muscle weakness (can be profound)
Muscle movements exaggerated by anxiety and attempts at fine motor activity; relieved by rest

Subcutaneous Nodes
Nontender swelling
Located over bony prominences
May persist for some time, then gradually resolve

Minor Manifestations
Clinical findings
    Arthralgia
    Fever
Laboratory findings
    Elevated acute-phase reactants
        Erythrocyte sedimentation rate
        C-reactive protein

Supporting Evidence of Antecedent Group A Streptococcal Infection
Positive throat culture or rapid streptococcal antigen test
Elevated or rising streptococcal antibody titer

From Special Writing Group of the Committee on Rheumatic Fever, Endocarditis, and Kawasaki Disease of the Council on the Cardiovascular Disease in the Young of the American Heart Association: Guidelines for the diagnosis of rheumatic fever: Jones criteria, 1992 (update), *JAMA* 268:2069-2073, 1992.
*If supported by evidence of preceding group A streptococcal infection, the presence of two major manifestations or of one major and two minor manifestations indicates a high probability of acute RF.

in children who have not been diagnosed with RF. It may be mistaken for nervousness, clumsiness, behavioral changes, inattentiveness, and learning disability. It is usually a source of great frustration to the child because the movements, incoordination, and weakness severely limit physical ability. The child needs an opportunity to verbalize feelings. Of utmost importance is stressing to parents and schoolteachers the involuntary, sudden nature of the movements, that the chorea is transitory, and that all manifestations eventually disappear.

Nurses also have a role in prevention, primarily in screening school-age children for sore throats caused by group A streptococci. This may involve actively participating in throat culture screening programs or in referring children with a possible streptococcal infection for testing.

See also Nursing Care Plan: The Child with Rheumatic Fever.*

HYPERLIPIDEMIA (HYPERCHOLESTEROLEMIA)

Hyperlipidemia is a general term for excessive lipids (fat and fatlike substances); *hypercholesterolemia* refers to excessive cholesterol in the blood. High lipid or cholesterol levels are believed to play an important role in producing atherosclerosis (fatty plaques on the arteries), which eventually can lead to coronary artery disease, a primary cause or morbidity and mortality in the adult population. Current research indicates that a presymptomatic phase of atherosclerosis begins in childhood.

Cholesterol is part of the lipoprotein complex in plasma that is essential for cellular metabolism. Triglycerides, natural fats synthesized from carbohydrates, are used for energy. Both are major lipids transported on *lipoproteins*, a combination of lipids and proteins, which include the following:

Low-density lipoproteins (LDLs)—contain low concentrations of triglycerides, high levels of cholesterol, and moderate levels of protein. LDL is the major carrier of cholesterol to the cells. Cells use cholesterol for synthesis of membranes and steroid production. Elevated circulating LDL is a strong risk factor in cardiovascular disease.

High-density lipoproteins (HDLs)—contain very low concentrations of triglycerides, relatively little cholesterol, and high levels of protein. They transport free cholesterol to the liver for excretion in the bile. High levels of HDL are thought to protect against cardiovascular disease.

Diagnostic Evaluation

Hyperlipidemia is diagnosed on the basis of analysis of blood for a full lipid profile. Two samples drawn in the fasting state (12 hours) should be analyzed, and the average of the values used for diagnosis. Blood samples should be collected after having the child sit for 5 minutes, and the tourniquet should be applied immediately before the needle puncture, since posture and vascular stasis may affect results. Diagnostic values for acceptable, borderline, and high total cholesterol and LDL cholesterol levels are listed in Table 25-4.

Screening children for hypercholesterolemia is a controversial issue, with some authorities advocating universal screening and others proposing selective screening (see Thinking Critically About . . . box). Current guidelines recommended by the National Cholesterol Education Program (NCEP) (1992) recommend a strategy that combines two complementary approaches: (1) a population approach that

*In Wong DL: *Wong and Whaley's Clinical manual of pediatric nursing,* ed 4, St Louis, 1996, Mosby.

TABLE 25-4. Classification of total and low-density lipoprotein (LDL) cholesterol levels in children and adolescents from families with hypercholesterolemia or premature cardiovascular disease

CATEGORY	TOTAL CHOLESTEROL (mg/dl)	LDL CHOLESTEROL (mg/dl)
Acceptable	<170	<110
Borderline	170-199	110-129
High	≥200	≥130

From National Cholesterol Education Program: Report of the Expert Panel on Blood Cholesterol Levels in children and adolescents, *Pediatrics* 89(3, pt 2):527, 1992.

aims to lower the average levels of blood cholesterol among all American children through population-wide changes in nutrient intake and eating patterns and (2) an individualized approach that targets children and adolescents for screening who have a family history of premature cardiovascular disease or at least one parent with high blood cholesterol (240 mg/dl or higher).

Therapeutic Management

Treatment of high cholesterol is primarily dietary. Children with borderline LDL cholesterol are advised to follow the same nutrient intake recommended for the general population (i.e., less than 10% of total calories from saturated fatty acids, no more than 30% of calories from total fat, less than 300 mg/day of cholesterol, and adequate calories to support growth and development and to reach or maintain desirable body weight). Children with high LDL cholesterol levels initially are placed on this diet. If these dietary modifications fail to achieve satisfactory levels of LDL after 3 months of therapy, dietary restrictions include a further reduction of saturated fatty acid intake to 7% of calories and of cholesterol intake to less than 200 mg/day.

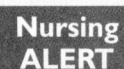 **Nursing ALERT** The Report of the Expert Panel on Blood Cholesterol Levels in Children and Adolescents regarding recommendations for fat intake are not intended for infants from birth to 2 years of age, whose fast growth requires a higher percentage of calories from fat. Toddlers 2 to 3 years of age may safely make the transition to the recommended eating pattern as they begin to eat with the family. No treatment recommendations are made for any child younger than 2 years of age.

For children with severe hypercholesterolemia who fail to respond to dietary modifications, drug therapy may be necessary. Two drugs recommended for treatment are the bile acid sequestrants *cholestyramine* and *colestipol.* These two drugs act by binding bile acids in the intestinal lumen. Because they are not absorbed by the intestine, they do not produce systemic toxicity and are safe for children. Cholestyramine and colestipol are both powders that are mixed with water or juice just before ingestion. The most common side effects of the bile acid sequestrants are gastrointestinal symp-

THINKING CRITICALLY ABOUT . . .
Cholesterol Screening

The American Heart Association, the American Academy of Pediatrics, and the National Institutes of Health recommend selected screening for children with a family history of hyperlipidemia, xanthomas, sudden death, early angina, or myocardial infarction (less than 50 years of age for males, less than 60 years for females) in siblings, parents, uncles, aunts, or grandparents. In addition, children with nonfamilial risk factors, such as obesity, diabetes, and Kawasaki disease, should be screened.

Those favoring universal screening believe that selective screening is too limited and overlooks many children with hyperlipidemia. Although universal screening would identify most children with hyperlipidemia, whether long-term survival would increase with early treatment to lower blood lipid levels is unknown. For the present, nurses play an important role in identifying children who meet the criteria for selective screening.

toms, such as constipation, nausea, bloating, epigastric fullness, and flatulence. The bile acid sequestrants may also prevent absorption of fats, fat-soluble vitamins, and folic acid. Therefore, in addition to monitoring children's height and weight during therapy, attention should be paid to a sufficient intake of fat-soluble vitamins and folic acid to prevent deficiencies.

Niacin (nicotinic acid), a B vitamin, may be given in therapeutic doses to older children. Although available without a prescription, niacin is treated as a prescription medicine in children. Its use is monitored closely by a health care professional with clinical and laboratory monitoring, especially liver function tests (Colletti and others, 1993).

Nursing Considerations

Nurses play an important role in the screening, education, and support of children with hyperlipidemia and their families. When a child is referred to a lipid clinic, it is essential that the family be adequately prepared for the first visit. Generally the parents will be asked to keep a dietary history of the child before this visit. Sometimes they will need to complete a questionnaire regarding the child's normal dietary habits over the preceding year. Families should be instructed to keep their child fasting for at least 12 hours before screening. Therefore it is important to schedule the blood test early in the morning and to arrange for nourishment immediately thereafter. At the visit a full family history should be taken, including the health of both parents and all first-degree relatives. Specific questions should be asked regarding early heart disease, hypertension, strokes (CVAs), sudden death, hyperlipidemia, diabetes, and endocrine abnormalities. Nurses may also uncover risk factors when obtaining a health history for other purposes. It is therefore important that nurses be familiar with current screening practices and the availability of resources for children with positive family histories.

Parents and extended families should be informed about cholesterol and hyperlipidemia. This education should include a brief introduction to the different lipoprotein categories, including cholesterol, HDL, LDL, and triglycerides. Also, behavioral risk factors for heart disease, such as smoking and exercise, should be reviewed. For management to be effective, parents need to understand the rationale for dietary

and/or pharmacologic intervention. The key is prevention of future cardiovascular disease.

Stringent dietary guidelines may become an issue of control and a source of great stress for many families. Children should not be viewed as having a disease. Rather, the positive aspects of healthy eating, regular exercise, and avoiding smoking should be emphasized. Basic dietary changes should be encouraged for the whole family so that the affected sibling is not singled out. Cultural differences must be considered and recommendations individualized. Substitution rather than elimination needs to be emphasized. Visual aids are often helpful, especially for the children (e.g., test tubes depicting the amount of fat in a hot dog). Diets should be flexible and individually tailored by a nutritionist experienced in combining recommendations that meet both the nutritional demands of the growing child and the lipid modifications. Parents are encouraged to participate in dietary and educational sessions, ask questions, and share ideas and experiences.

Parents often feel guilty about the hereditary component of hyperlipidemia. Many also believe they have failed if the diet alone is not making a significant difference in their child's lipid profile. They need to be reassured that a dietary approach alone is often not sufficient, especially for children with LDL values greater than 130 mg/dl.

Parents of children who require pharmacologic therapy need to understand the purpose, dosage, and possible side effects of the various drugs. Medication schedules should remain flexible and should not interfere with the child's daily activities. For example, children of elementary school age may have better compliance if they take a resin-binding agent (e.g., cholestyramine, colestipol) twice a day (i.e., before school and at night) rather than the standard three times a day. Follow-up phone calls by the nurse between visits allow parents to discuss their concerns and ask any questions that have arisen.

CARDIAC DYSRHYTHMIAS

Cardiac *dysrhythmias,* or abnormal heart rhythms, occur less frequently in children than in adults. However, they are not rare, and the incidence is rising. The survival rate of children undergoing complex cardiac surgical procedures is higher, and conduction system damage may be a complication. Practitioners are also more aware that certain cardiac dysrhythmias in otherwise normal children are important.

The basic diagnostic procedure is the ECG, including 24-hour Holter monitoring. *Electrophysiologic cardiac catheterization* allows for identification of the conduction disturbance and immediate investigation of drugs that may control the dysrhythmia. Another procedure that may be employed is *transesophageal recording.* An electrode catheter is passed to the lower esophagus and, when in position at a point proximal to the heart, is used to stimulate and record dysrhythmias.

Classification

Dysrhythmias can be classified according to various criteria, such as effect on heart rate and rhythm, as follows:

Bradydysrhythmias—abnormally slow rate
Tachydysrhythmias—abnormally rapid rate
Conduction disturbances—irregular heart rate

Before classifying an infant or child with an abnormal rate, nurses must be familiar with the standards of normal heart rate for the particular age-group (see inside front cover). Heart rate variations considered normal for a particular child can vary tremendously.

Bradydysrhythmias. The most common bradydysrhythmia in children is *complete atrioventricular block (A-V block),* also referred to as *complete heart block.* This can be either congenital or acquired, as seen in postoperative patients after surgery in the area of the A-V valves and ventricular septum.

Sinus bradycardia in children can be caused by the influence of the autonomic nervous system, as with hypervagal tone, or in response to hypoxia and hypotension. *Junctional* or *nodal rhythms* are common in the postoperative patient. The impulse for these rhythms originates further down the conduction system, in the A-V node. Identification is marked by absence of P waves on the ECG, and often little change occurs in the heart rate or cardiac output. If there is no significant compromise to the patient's cardiac status, no treatment is necessary.

Tachydysrhythmias. *Sinus tachycardia* caused by fever, anxiety, pain, anemia, dehydration, or any other etiologic factor requiring increased cardiac output should be ruled out first before diagnosing an increased heart rate as pathologic. *Supraventricular tachycardia (SVT)* is one of the most common dysrhythmias found in children and refers to a rapid regular heart rate of 200 to 300 beats/minute. The onset of SVT is often sudden, and the duration is variable. Infants and young children with SVT may be unable to communicate the rapid heart rate, and the clinical course can progress to CHF. Important signs in the infant and young child are poor feeding, extreme irritability, and pallor.

Conduction Disturbances. Most rhythm disturbances are seen postoperatively in the child undergoing cardiac surgery and are of little significance. A-V blocks are most often related to edema around the conduction system and resolve without treatment. Temporary epicardial wires are placed in most patients at surgery; if a rhythm disturbance occurs, temporary pacing can be employed. Just before discharge, the health practitioner removes the wires by pulling slowly and deliberately down on them from the site of insertion.

Premature contractions can occur from an atrial, ventricular, or junctional focus. Their significance depends on the degree of compromise and the presence or absence of underlying CHD.

Therapeutic Management

Treatment of dysrhythmias depends on the cause and severity. Whenever possible, the underlying cause is treated. However, in some cases it is necessary to use antidysrhythmic drugs, with the goal being control, not cure. A permanent *pacemaker* may be needed in some children, such as those with postsurgical A-V block or, less frequently, congenital A-V block. The pacemaker takes over or assists in the conduction function of the heart. The surgical implantation of a pacemaker is usually a low-risk procedure. Once the wire has been introduced, a small incision is made, and a pocket formed under the muscle to house and protect the generator. Continuous ECG monitoring is necessary during the recovery phase to assess pacemaker function. The nurse should be aware of the programmed rate and expected individual generator variations. A baseline ECG strip should be documented for future comparison.

The treatment of SVT depends on the degree of compromise imposed by the dysrhythmia. In some instances, *vagal maneuvers,* such as applying ice to the face, massaging the carotid artery (on *one* side of the neck only), or having an older child perform a Valsalva maneuver (e.g., exhaling against a closed glottis, blowing on the thumb as if it were a trumpet for 30 to 60 seconds), have reversed the SVT. When vagal maneuvers fail, adenosine may be used to end the episode of SVT by impairing A-V node conduction. If the infant or child is minimally symptomatic, digitalization should be undertaken, with careful monitoring of vital signs and patient response to the intervention. If cardiac output is significantly compromised or signs of CHF exist, esophageal overdrive pacing or synchronized cardioversion can be employed in the intensive care setting.

Nursing Considerations

An initial nursing responsibility is recognition of an abnormal heartbeat, either in rate or rhythm. When a dysrhythmia is suspected, the apical rate is counted for 1 full minute and compared with the radial rate. Consistently high or low heart rates should be regarded as suspicious. Accurate nursing assessment, especially in regard to cardiac output, is essential.

The onset and diagnosis of a cardiac dysrhythmia are frightening experiences for parents and the older child. Sometimes the dysrhythmia rapidly leads to heart failure and an emergency medical crisis. In this situation parents need much support to express their feelings, understand the diagnosis, and comply with home therapy, such as daily drug administration. Often an unspoken fear of potential death exists even if the dysrhythmia is benign, and repeated explanations are needed to allay the anxiety.

A primary focus of nursing care is education of the family regarding the specific treatment of the dysrhythmia. After the first episode of SVT, parents should be taught to take a pulse for 1 full minute. If medication is prescribed, instructions regarding accurate dosage and the importance of administering the correct dose at specified intervals are stressed.

When a pacemaker is implanted, the education of the parents and child includes an explanation of the device, a description of the component parts and the surgical procedure, and discharge teaching. For example, discharge teaching includes information about the signs and symptoms of infection, general wound care, and any specific limitations to activity. Instructions for telephone transmission of ECG readings are also given. Children with pacemakers should wear a Medic-Alert device, and their parents should have a pacer identification card with specific pacer data in case of an emergency.

VASCULAR DYSFUNCTION

SYSTEMIC HYPERTENSION

Hypertension is defined as the consistent elevation of blood pressure (BP) beyond values considered to be the upper limits of normal. The National Heart, Lung, and Blood Institute's report (1987) on blood pressure control in children defines BP as the following:

Normal BP—systolic and diastolic pressure below the 90th percentile for age and sex

Normal high BP—average systolic and/or average diastolic BP between 90th and 95th percentiles for age and sex

High BP—average systolic and/or average diastolic BP at or greater than the 95th percentile for age and sex with measurements obtained on at least three occasions

The two major categories are *essential hypertension* (no identifiable cause) and *secondary hypertension* (subsequent to an identifiable cause). Hypertension is a primary risk for CVAs and a major risk factor for myocardial infarction in adults. In recent years there has been increasing interest in this disorder in adolescents and children, particularly in terms of prevention of later morbidity and mortality.

Routine BP measurements have detected hypertension with surprising frequency in asymptomatic children, especially teenagers. Although the prevalence of the condition in adolescents is difficult to evaluate, evidence is accumulating to indicate that the essential hypertension of adulthood may have its origin in childhood; thus its early detection has significance for prevention and treatment.

Etiology

Most instances of hypertension observed in young children occur secondary to a structural abnormality or an underlying pathologic process, although this is being challenged by screening programs of relatively healthy children. The most common cause of secondary hypertension is renal disease, followed by cardiovascular, endocrine, and some neurologic disorders.

The causes of essential hypertension are undetermined, but evidence indicates that both genetic and environmental factors play a role. The incidence of hypertension has been shown to be higher in children whose parents are hypertensive. American blacks have a higher incidence of hypertension than whites, and in these persons it develops earlier, is frequently more severe, and results in mortality at an earlier age. Environmental factors that contribute to the risk of developing hypertension include obesity, salt ingestion, smoking, and stress.

Diagnostic Evaluation

From the increasing numbers of hypertensive or potentially hypertensive children and adolescents being identified, a BP determination should be a routine part of annual assessment in children. Although clinical manifestations associated with

---

CLINICAL MANIFESTATIONS OF HYPERTENSION

Adolescents and Older Children
Frequent headaches
Dizziness
Changes in vision

Infants or Young Children
Irritability
Head-banging or head-rubbing
May wake up screaming in the night

---

hypertension depend largely on the underlying cause, some observations can provide clues to the examiner that an elevated BP may be a factor (see box). In infants and very young children who cannot communicate symptoms, observation of behavior provides clues, although gross behavioral changes may not be apparent until complications are present.

No definitive cutoff values are used in the diagnosis of hypertension in the pediatric patient. The suggested classification is in Table 25-5. *Significant hypertension* is a BP persistently between the 95th and 99th percentiles for age and sex. *Severe hypertension* is a BP persistently at or above the 99th percentile for age and sex. It is important to note that a child who is large for age may normally have a higher BP than a child who is of average size. Before a diagnosis is made, BP should be measured on at least three separate occasions.

In children with suspected primary hypertension, initial laboratory data are also obtained. This generally includes a urinalysis, renal function studies such as creatinine and blood urea nitrogen, a lipid profile, complete blood count, and electrolytes. More intensive tests may be indicated for those with probable secondary hypertension.

Therapeutic Management

Therapy for secondary hypertension involves diagnosis and treatment of the underlying cause. In cases amenable to surgical repair, the nature of the condition, the type of surgery, and the age of the child are all important considerations. Children or adolescents with consistently elevated BP readings from no known cause or those with secondary hypertension not amenable to surgical correction may be treated with a combination of nonpharmacologic and pharmacologic interventions. Dietary practices and life-style changes are important in the control of hypertension both for children and for adults. Nonpharmacologic measures, such as limitation of dietary salt, weight control, increased exercise, and avoidance of stress and smoking, carry no risk and should be instituted first, except in severe cases. Since the long-term effects of antihypertensive agents on children are not known, drug treatment of asymptomatic children with mild or borderline hypertension is not recommended.

Drug therapy is instituted with caution in children with significant elevations of BP resistant to nonpharmacologic intervention. The treatment should begin with one drug and should add other drugs only if control is not obtained. Compliance with antihypertensive drug regimens is extremely difficult. The oral antihypertensive drugs used most often in children include the beta blockers (propranolol), ACE inhibitors, diuretics, and occasionally a vasodilator (hydralazine). The goal is to achieve a normotensive state throughout the day without accompanying drug side effects.

Nursing Considerations

The nurse is active in detection, diagnosis, and therapy in many settings. Nurses are frequently the persons who operate well-child care and follow-up units and are usually the primary contact between health services and the child and family.

BP measurement should always be a part of the routine assessment of infants and children. To obtain an accurate reading, care is taken to quiet the child or relax the adolescent while the measurement is recorded to avoid false readings caused by excitement. The chief cause of falsely elevated

TABLE 25-5. Classification of hypertension by age-group

AGE-GROUP	SIGNIFICANT HYPERTENSION (mm Hg)	SEVERE HYPERTENSION (mm Hg)
Newborn (7 d)	Systolic BP ≥96	Systolic BP ≥106
(8-30 d)	Systolic BP ≥104	Systolic BP ≥110
Infant (<2 yr)	Systolic BP ≥112	Systolic BP ≥118
	Diastolic BP ≥74	Diastolic BP ≥82
Children (3-5 yr)	Systolic BP ≥116	Systolic BP ≥124
	Diastolic BP ≥76	Diastolic BP ≥84
Children (6-9 yr)	Systolic BP ≥122	Systolic BP ≥130
	Diastolic BP ≥78	Diastolic BP ≥86
Children (10-12 yr)	Systolic BP ≥126	Systolic BP ≥134
	Diastolic BP ≥82	Diastolic BP ≥90
Adolescents (13-15 yr)	Systolic BP ≥136	Systolic BP ≥144
	Diastolic BP ≥86	Diastolic BP ≥92
Adolescents (16-18 yr)	Systolic BP ≥142	Systolic BP ≥150
	Diastolic BP ≥92	Diastolic BP ≥98

From National Heart, Lung, and Blood Institute: Report of the Second Task Force on Blood Pressure Control in Children, 1987, *Pediatrics* 79(1):1-25, 1987.

BP readings is the use of improperly fitting, narrow cuffs. Therefore attention to correct measurement technique is essential (see Blood Pressure, Chapter 7).

Nursing counseling and guidance of affected children are challenges. Education aimed at understanding hypertension and its implication over the life span is essential in promoting patient and family compliance with both nonpharmacologic and pharmacologic therapies (see Compliance, Chapter 22).

Home BP measurements can facilitate surveillance in youngsters with chronic hypertension and can document effectiveness of therapy. A family member can be instructed in how to take and record accurate BP measurements, thus decreasing the number of trips to a health care facility. This individual needs to understand when to contact the practitioner regarding elevated values. The school nurse can often be a valuable resource in monitoring BPs.

The nurse plays an important role in assessing individual families and providing targeted information regarding nonpharmacologic modes of intervention, such as diet, weight loss, smoking, and exercise programs. If extensive dietary counseling is required, the child should be referred to a nutritionist with expertise in working with children and adolescents. Exercise regimens should be individualized. School children and young adolescents generally prefer team sports rather than individual training, which they may view as a burden rather than an enjoyable activity. If peers and family members can be encouraged to participate in any of the management strategies, the child's compliance is likely to be greater.

Young hypertensive women should avoid oral contraceptives because of their pressor effects. Other options need to be presented before this form of birth control is discontinued (see Contraception, Chapter 17).

If drug therapy is prescribed, the nurse needs to provide information to the family regarding the reasons for it, how the drug works, and possible side effects. General instructions for all the antihypertensive drugs include the following:

- Rise slowly from a horizontal position and avoid sudden position changes.
- Take drug as prescribed.
- Notify practitioner if unpleasant side effects occur, but do not discontinue drug.
- Avoid alcohol and stay on prescribed diet.

The need for follow-up is stressed, especially since antihypertensive therapy can sometimes be safely discontinued if BP remains under control over time.

KAWASAKI DISEASE (KD) (MUCOCUTANEOUS LYMPH NODE SYNDROME)

KD is an acute systemic vasculitis. It is seen in every racial group, and about 80% of the cases occur in children under the age of 5 years, with peak incidence in the toddler age-group. The acute disease is self-limited. Without treatment, however, approximately 1 in 5 children develop cardiac sequelae. Infants less than 1 year of age are most seriously affected by KD and are at the greatest risk for heart involvement.

The etiology of KD remains a mystery. Although it is not spread by person-to-person contact, several factors support infectious etiologic factors. It is often seen in geographic and seasonal outbreaks, with the most cases reported in the late winter and early spring.

Pathophysiology

The principal area of involvement is the cardiovascular system. During the initial stage of the illness, extensive inflammation of the arterioles, venules, and capillaries occurs, which later progresses to the formation of coronary artery aneu-

DIAGNOSTIC CRITERIA FOR KAWASAKI DISEASE

The child must exhibit five of the following six criteria, including fever:
1. Fever for 5 or more days (often diagnosed with shorter duration of fever if other symptoms are present)
2. Bilateral conjunctival injection (inflammation) without exudation
3. Changes in the oral mucous membranes, such as erythema, dryness, and fissuring of the lips; oropharyngeal reddening; or "strawberry tongue" (large papillae are exposed)
4. Changes in the extremities, such as peripheral edema, erythema of the palms and soles, and periungual desquamation (peeling) of the hands and feet
5. Polymorphous rash
6. Cervical lymphadenopathy (one lymph node >1.5 cm)

rysms in some children. When death occurs, it is usually the result of coronary thrombosis or severe scar formation and stenosis of the main coronary artery.

Clinical Manifestations

Since no specific diagnostic test exists for KD, the diagnosis is established on the basis of clinical findings and associated laboratory results (see box). KD manifests in three phases: acute, subacute, and convalescent. The *acute phase* begins with the abrupt onset of high fever that is unresponsive to antibiotics and antipyretics. The child then develops the remaining diagnostic symptoms. During this stage the child is typically *very* irritable. The *subacute phase* begins with resolution of the fever and lasts until all clinical signs of KD have disappeared. During this phase the child is at greatest risk for the development of coronary artery aneurysms. Echocardiograms are used to monitor myocardial and coronary artery status. A baseline echocardiogram should be obtained at the time of diagnosis for comparison with future studies. Irritability persists during this phase. In the *convalescent phase,* all the clinical signs of KD have resolved, but the laboratory values have not returned to normal. This phase is complete when all blood values are normal (6 to 8 weeks after onset). At the end of this stage the child has regained his or her usual temperament, energy, and appetite.

Therapeutic Management

The current treatment of KD includes high-dose IV gamma globulin along with salicylate therapy. Gamma globulin has been demonstrated to be effective at reducing the incidence of coronary artery abnormalities when given within the first 10 days of the illness. A single large infusion of 2 g/kg over 8 to 12 hours is safe and effective in reducing fever and aneurysm formation (Newburger and others, 1991).

Aspirin is given initially in an antiinflammatory dose (80 to 100 mg/kg/day in divided doses every 6 hours) to control fever and symptoms of inflammation. Once fever has subsided, aspirin is continued at an antiplatelet dose (3 to 5 mg/kg/day). Low-dose aspirin is continued in patients without echocardiographic evidence of coronary abnormalities until the platelet count has returned to normal (6 to 8 weeks). If the child develops coronary abnormalities, salicylate therapy

is continued indefinitely. Additional anticoagulation with coumadin may be indicated in children with giant aneurysms.

Prognosis. Most children with KD recover fully after treatment. However, when cardiovascular complications occur, serious morbidity may result. Death occurs rarely and almost always results from coronary thrombosis.

Nursing Considerations

In the initial phase the nurse must monitor the child's cardiac status carefully. Intake and output and daily weight measurements are recorded. Although the child may be reluctant to eat and therefore may be partially dehydrated, fluids need to be administered with care because of the usual finding of myocarditis. The child should be assessed frequently for signs of CHF, including decreased urine output, gallop rhythm (an additional heart sound), tachycardia, and respiratory distress.

Administration of gamma globulin should follow the same guidelines as for any blood product, with frequent monitoring of vital signs. Patients must be watched for allergic reactions (see Table 26-4). Cardiac status must be monitored because of the large volume being administered to patients with myocarditis and diminished left ventricular function.

Most nursing care focuses on symptomatic relief. To minimize skin discomfort, cool cloths, nonscented lotions, and soft, loose clothing are helpful. During the acute phase, mouth care, including lubricating ointment to the lips, is important for the mucosal inflammation. Clear liquids and soft foods can be offered.

Patient irritability is perhaps the most challenging problem. These children need a quiet environment that promotes adequate rest. Their parents need to be supported in their efforts to comfort an often inconsolable child. They may need time away from their child, and nurses can often provide respite care for the family. Parents need to understand that irritability is a hallmark of KD and that they need not feel guilty or embarrassed about their child's behavior.

Discharge Teaching. Parents need accurate information about the progression of KD, including the importance of follow-up monitoring and when they should contact their practitioner. Irritability is likely to persist for up to 2 months after the onset of symptoms. Peeling of the hands and feet is painless and occurs primarily in the second and third weeks. Arthritis, especially of the larger weight-bearing joints, may persist for several weeks. Children are typically most stiff in the mornings, during cold weather, and after naps. Passive range of motion in the bathtub is often helpful in increasing flexibility. Any live immunizations (e.g., measles-mumps-rubella) should be deferred for 3 months after the administration of gamma globulin, since the body might not produce the appropriate amount of antibodies. The decision to give the varicella (chickenpox) vaccine while the child is receiving aspirin therapy is made individually by the practitioner. Temperature should be recorded after discharge until the child has been afebrile for several days.*

All parents should understand the unlikely but real possibility of myocardial infarction as well as the signs and symptoms of cardiac ischemia in a child. At discharge the ultimate

---

*Home care instructions for measuring a child's temperature and for infant and child cardiopulmonary resuscitation are available in Wong DL: *Wong and Whaley's Clinical manual of pediatric nursing,* ed 4, St Louis, 1996, Mosby.

cardiac sequela is generally not known, since changes occur up to a month after the onset of KD. In addition, the parents of children with known severe coronary artery sequelae may be taught cardiopulmonary resuscitation.*

SHOCK

Shock, or *circulatory failure,* is a complex clinical syndrome characterized by inadequate tissue perfusion to meet the metabolic demands of the body, resulting in cellular dysfunction and eventual organ failure. Although the causes are different, the physiologic consequences are the same: hypotension, tissue hypoxia, and metabolic acidosis.

Circulatory failure in children is the result of hypovolemia, altered peripheral vascular resistance, or pump failure. Types of shock are outlined in the accompanying box.

---

*See footnote on p. 893.

TYPES OF SHOCK

Hypovolemic Shock
Characteristics

Reduction in size of vascular compartment
Falling blood pressure
Poor capillary filling
Low central venous pressure (CVP)

Most Frequent Causes

Blood loss (hemorrhagic shock)—trauma, gastrointestinal bleeding, intracranial hemorrhage
Plasma loss—increased capillary permeability associated with sepsis and acidosis, hypoproteinemia, burns, peritonitis
Extracellular fluid loss—vomiting, diarrhea, glycosuric diuresis, sunstroke

Distributive Shock
Characteristics

Reduction in peripheral vascular resistance
Profound inadequacies in tissue perfusion
Increased venous capacity and pooling
Acute reduction in return blood flow to the heart
Diminished cardiac output

Most Frequent Causes

Anaphylaxis (anaphylactic shock)—extreme allergy or hypersensitivity to a foreign substance
Sepsis (septic shock, bacteremic shock, endotoxic shock)—overwhelming sepsis and circulating bacterial toxins
Loss of neuronal control (neurogenic shock)—interruption of neuronal transmission (spinal cord injury)
Myocardial depression and peripheral dilation—exposure to anesthesia or ingestion of barbiturates, tranquilizers, narcotics, antihypertensive agents, or ganglionic blocking agents

Cardiogenic Shock
Characteristic

Decreased cardiac output

Most Frequent Causes

After surgery for congenital heart disease
Primary pump failure—myocarditis, myocardial trauma, biochemical derangements, congestive heart failure
Dysrhythmias—paroxysmal atrial tachycardia, atrioventricular block, and ventricular dysrhythmias; secondary to myocarditis or biochemical abnormalities (occasionally)

Pathophysiology

A healthy child's circulatory system is able to transport oxygen and metabolic substrates to body tissues, which require a constant source for these essential needs. The cardiac output and distribution to the various body tissues can change very rapidly in response to intrinsic (myocardial and intravascular) or extrinsic (neuronal) control mechanisms. In shock states these mechanisms are altered or challenged.

Reduced blood flow, as in hypovolemic shock, causes diminished venous return to the heart, low central venous pressure (CVP), low cardiac output, and hypotension. Vasomotor centers in the medulla are signaled, causing a compensatory increase in the force and rate of cardiac contraction and constriction of arterioles and veins, thereby increasing peripheral vascular resistance. Simultaneously the lowered blood volume leads to the release of large amounts of catecholamines, antidiuretic hormone, adrenocorticosteroids, and aldosterone in an effort to conserve body fluids. This causes reduced blood flow to the skin, kidneys, muscles, and viscera in order to shunt the available blood to the brain and heart. Consequently, the skin feels cold and clammy, there is poor capillary filling, and glomerular filtration and urine output are significantly reduced.

As a result of impaired perfusion, oxygen is depleted in the tissue cells, causing them to revert to anaerobic metabolism, producing lactic acidosis. The acidosis places an extra burden on the lungs as they attempt to compensate for the metabolic acidosis by increased respiratory rate to remove excess carbon dioxide. Prolonged vasoconstriction results in fatigue and atony of the peripheral arterioles, which leads to vessel dilation. Venules, less sensitive to vasodilator substances, remain constricted for a time, causing massive pooling in the capillary and venular beds, which further depletes blood volume.

Complications of shock create further hazards. Central nervous system hypoperfusion may eventually lead to cerebral edema, cortical infarction, or intraventricular hemorrhage. Renal hypoperfusion causes renal ischemia with possible tubular or glomerular necrosis and renal vein thrombosis. Reduced blood flow to the lungs can interfere with surfactant secretion and result in adult respiratory distress syndrome (ARDS), characterized by sudden pulmonary congestion and atelectasis with formation of a hyaline membrane. Gastrointestinal tract bleeding and perforation are always a possibility following splanchnic ischemia and necrosis of intestinal mucosa. Metabolic complications of shock may include hypoglycemia, hypocalcemia, and other electrolyte disturbances.

Diagnostic Evaluation

The etiology of shock can be discerned from the history and the physical examination. The severity of the shock is determined by measurements of vital signs, including CVP and capillary filling (see box on p. 895). Shock can be regarded as a form of compensation for circulatory failure. Because of the progressive nature of shock, it can be divided into the following three stages or phases:

Compensated shock. Vital organ function is maintained by intrinsic compensatory mechanisms; blood flow is usually normal or increased but generally uneven or maldistributed in the microcirculation.

CLINICAL MANIFESTATIONS OF SHOCK	
Compensated	**Uncompensated**
Apprehensiveness	Confusion and somnolence
Irritability	Tachypnea
Unexplained tachycardia	Moderate metabolic acido-
Normal blood pressure	sis
Narrowing pulse pressure	Oliguria
Thirst	Cool, pale extremities
Pallor	Decreased skin turgor
Diminished urine output	Poor capillary filling
Reduced perfusion of ex-	
tremities	**Irreversible**
	Thready, weak pulse
	Hypotension
	Periodic breathing or apnea
	Anuria
	Stupor or coma

EMERGENCY TREATMENT
Shock

Ventilation
Establish airway—be prepared for intubation.
Administer oxygen, usually 100% by mask.

Fluid Administration
Restore blood or fluid volume as ordered.

Cardiovascular Support
Administer vasopressors, especially epinephrine in dose of 0.01 mg/kg until maximum dose of 0.5 ml of 1:1000 dilution subcutaneously; may repeat in 30 minutes.

General Support
Keep child flat with legs raised above level of heart.
Keep child warm and calm.

In Addition:
Septic shock: Administer broad-spectrum antibiotics intravenously.
Anaphylaxis: Remove allergen if possible; may place tourniquet above site of injection.

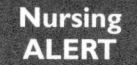

Nursing ALERT
Unexplained mild tachycardia and a decrease in perfusion of the hands and feet are differentiating features of compensated shock.

Uncompensated shock. Efficiency of the cardiovascular system gradually diminishes, until perfusion in the microcirculation becomes marginal despite compensatory adjustments. The outcomes of circulatory failure that progress beyond the limits of compensation are tissue hypoxia, metabolic acidosis, and eventual dysfunction of all organ systems.

Nursing ALERT
Tachycardia is pronounced; BP is maintained, but pulse pressure (difference between systolic and diastolic BP) becomes narrowed; there is poor capillary filling; and the child in uncompensated shock exhibits decreased responsiveness, confusion, and sleepiness.

Irreversible, or terminal, shock. Damage to vital organs, such as the heart or brain, of such magnitude that the entire organism will be disrupted regardless of therapeutic intervention. Death occurs even if cardiovascular measurements return to normal levels with therapy.

At all stages the principal differentiating signs are observed in the (1) degree of tachycardia and perfusion to extremities, (2) level of consciousness, and (3) blood pressure (BP). Additional signs or modifications of these more universal signs may be present depending on the type and cause of the shock. Initially the child's ability to compensate is effective; therefore, early signs are subtle. As the shock state advances, signs are more obvious and indicate early decompensation.

Additional signs may be present, depending on the type and etiology of the shock. In early septic shock there are chills, fever, and vasodilation, with increased cardiac output that results in warm, flushed skin (hyperdynamic or "hot" shock). A later and ominous development is disseminated intravascular coagulation (see Chapter 26), the major hematologic complication of septic shock. Anaphylactic shock is frequently accompanied by urticaria and angioneurotic edema, which is life-threatening when it involves the respiratory passages (see p. 896).

Laboratory tests that assist in assessment are blood gas measurements, pH, and sometimes liver function tests. Coagulation tests are evaluated when there is evidence of bleeding, such as oozing from a venipuncture site, bleeding from any orifice, or petechiae. Cultures of blood and other sites are indicated when there is a high suspicion of sepsis. Renal function tests are performed when impaired renal function is evident.

Therapeutic Management

Treatment of shock consists of three major thrusts: (1) ventilation, (2) fluid administration, and (3) improvement of the pumping action of the heart (vasopressor support). The first priority is to establish an airway and administer oxygen. Once the airway is assured, circulatory stabilization is the major concern.

Ventilatory Support. The lung is the organ most sensitive to shock. Decreased or redistribution of blood flow to respiratory muscles plus the increased work of breathing can rapidly lead to respiratory failure. Critically ill patients are unable to maintain an adequate airway. To place the lung at rest and improve ventilation, tracheal intubation is initiated early with positive-pressure ventilation. Supplemental oxygen is always given as soon as possible. Blood gases and pH are monitored frequently.

Increased extravascular lung water caused by edema contributes to the development of respiratory complications. Therapy is directed toward maintaining normal arterial blood gas measurements, normal acid-base balance, and circulation. Efforts are made to remove fluid and prevent its accumulation with the use of diuretics.

Cardiovascular Support. In most cases, rapid restoration of blood volume is all that is needed for resuscitation of the child in shock. An isotonic crystalloid solution (normal saline or Ringer's lactate) is the fluid of choice; colloids such as albumin are also used. Successful resuscitation is reflected by an increase in BP and a reduction in heart rate;

increased cardiac output will result in improved capillary circulation and skin color. CVP measurements of right atrial pressure help guide fluid therapy, and urine output measurement is an important indicator of adequacy of circulation. Correction of acidosis, hypoxemia, and any metabolic derangements is mandatory.

Temporary pharmacologic support may be required to enhance myocardial contractility, to reverse metabolic or respiratory acidosis, and/or to maintain arterial pressure. The principal agents used to improve cardiac output and circulation are the sympathetic amines administered by constant infusion pump. Those given most often are catecholamines, such as dopamine (Intropin), epinephrine (Adrenalin), and isoproterenol (Isuprel). Vasodilators that are sometimes used include nitroprusside (Nipride) and hydralazine (Apresoline).

Acidosis is corrected with adequate ventilatory support, including oxygen, and the administration of sodium bicarbonate. Calcium chloride may be administered to improve cardiac function. Appropriate antibiotics are administered to patients with septic shock. In cases of septic shock caused by gram-negative organisms, corticosteroids are of value. Other complicating disorders are treated appropriately.

Nursing Considerations
When shock is a likely complication, the child is observed carefully for any early signs, which are reported immediately for further medical evaluation.

| **Nursing ALERT** | Early clinical signs include apprehension, irritability, normal BP, narrowing pulse pressure (difference between diastolic and systolic BP), thirst, pallor, diminished urine output, unexplained mild tachycardia, and a decrease in perfusion of the hands and feet. |

The child who is in shock requires intensive observation and care. *The initial action is to ensure adequate tissue oxygenation.* The nurse should be prepared to administer oxygen by the appropriate route and to assist with any intubation and ventilatory procedures indicated. Other procedures and activities that require immediate attention are establishing an IV line, weighing the child, obtaining baseline vital signs, placing an indwelling catheter, obtaining blood gas and other measurements, and administering medications as indicated. The child is best positioned flat with the legs elevated.

The nurse's responsibilities are to monitor the IV infusion, intake and output, vital signs (including CVP), and general systems assessments on a routine basis. IV medications are titrated according to patient responses, and vital signs are taken every 15 minutes during the critical periods and thereafter as needed. Urine output is measured hourly; blood gases, hematocrit, pH, and electrolytes are monitored frequently to assess the status of the child and the efficacy of therapy. An apnea and cardiac monitor is attached and monitored continuously. In the initial stages of acute shock the care of the child often requires the attendance of more than one nurse in order to manage all the necessary activities that must be carried out simultaneously (see Emergency Treatment box on p. 895).

Throughout the intense activity the family must not be overlooked. Someone should contact family members at frequent intervals to inform them about what is being done and if there is any progress. Ideally, someone should remain with the parents to serve as liaison between them and the intensive care team. However, this is not always feasible in such a critical situation. As soon as possible they should be allowed to see the child. A member of the clergy may be called to help provide comfort and support.

See also Nursing Care Plan: The Child in Circulatory Failure (Shock).*

ANAPHYLAXIS
Anaphylaxis is the acute clinical syndrome resulting from the interaction of an allergen and a patient who is hypersensitive. When the antigen enters the circulatory system, a generalized reaction rapidly takes place. Vasoactive amines (principally histamine or a histamine-like substance) are released and cause vasodilation, bronchoconstriction, and increased capillary permeability.

Severe reactions are immediate in onset, are often life-threatening, and frequently involve multiple systems, primarily the cardiovascular, respiratory, gastrointestinal, and integumentary. Exposure to the antigen can be by ingestion, inhalation, skin contact, or injection. Examples of common allergens associated with anaphylaxis include drugs (e.g., antibiotics, chemotherapeutic agents, radiologic contrast media), latex, foods, venoms from bees or snakes, and biologic agents (antisera, enzymes, hormones, blood products).

| **Nursing ALERT** | Penicillin allergy is associated with immediate onset (within an hour of administration) or accelerated onset (1 to 72 hours after administration) of skin eruption, especially a urticarial rash, or more serious symptoms such as laryngeal edema or anaphylactic shock. |

Clinical Manifestations
The onset of clinical symptoms usually occurs within seconds or minutes of exposure to the antigen, and the rapidity of the reaction is directly related to its intensity: the sooner the onset, the more severe the reaction. The reaction may be preceded by symptoms of uneasiness, restlessness, irritability, severe anxiety, headache, dizziness, paresthesia, and disorientation. The patient may lose consciousness. Cutaneous signs of flushing and urticaria are common early signs, followed by angioedema, most notable in the eyelids, lips, tongue, hands, feet, and genitalia.

Bronchiolar constriction may follow, causing narrowing of the airway; pulmonary edema and hemorrhage also may occur. Laryngeal edema with severe acute upper airway obstruction may be life-threatening and requires rapid intervention. Shock occurs as a result of mediator-induced vasodilation, which causes capillary permeability and loss of intravascular fluid into the interstitial space. Sudden hypotension and impaired cardiac output with poor perfusion are seen.

Therapeutic Management
Successful outcome of anaphylactic reactions depends on rapid recognition and institution of treatment. The goals of

---
*In Wong DL: *Wong and Whaley's Clinical manual of pediatric nursing,* ed 4, St Louis, 1996, Mosby.

treatment are to provide ventilation, restore adequate circulation, and prevent further exposure by identifying and removing the cause when possible.

A mild reaction with no evidence of respiratory distress or cardiovascular compromise can be managed with subcutaneous administration of antihistamines, such as diphenhydramine (Benadryl) and epinephrine.

Moderate or severe distress presents a potentially life-threatening emergency. Establishing an airway is the first concern, as with all shock states. Epinephrine is given subcutaneously or intravenously as an antihistamine and to support the cardiovascular system and increase blood pressure. Other routes for giving epinephrine are intramuscular and via the airway, either nebulized or injected through an ET tube. In severe anaphylaxis, epinephrine by any route is better than none (Fisher, 1992). Fluids are given to restore blood volume. Additional vasopressors may be given to improve cardiac output. Children with serious anaphylaxis should be hospitalized and monitored for at least 24 hours, since relapses may occur (Bochner and Lichtenstein, 1991).

Prevention of a reaction is preferable. Preventing exposure is more easily accomplished in children known to be at risk, including those with (1) a history of previous allergic reaction to specific antigen, (2) a history of atopy, (3) a history of severe reactions in immediate family members, and (4) a reaction to a skin test, although skin tests are not available for all allergens. Desensitization may be recommended in certain cases.

Nursing Considerations

The major nursing responsibility in anaphylaxis is anticipating which children are likely to develop a reaction, recognizing the early signs, and intervening appropriately. When an anaphylactic reaction is suspected, both immediate intervention and preparation for medical therapy are nursing responsibilities. Ventilation is ensured by placing the child in a head-elevated position, unless contraindicated by hypotension, to facilitate breathing and administer oxygen. If the child is not breathing, cardiopulmonary resuscitation (CPR) is initiated, and emergency medical services are summoned.

If the cause can be determined, measures are implemented to slow the spread of the offending substance. For example, a tourniquet is applied above the point of entry (e.g., sting, injection), or IV medication or dye infusion is discontinued. An IV infusion is established immediately. Emergency medications are given intravenously whenever possible; however, epinephrine may be given subcutaneously (see Emergency Treatment box). Vital signs and urine output are monitored frequently. Medications are administered as prescribed, with regular assessment to monitor effectiveness and to detect signs of side effects of medication and fluid overload.

To prevent an anaphylactic reaction, parents are always asked about possible allergic responses to foods, latex, medications, and environmental conditions. (See Guidelines box, Taking an Allergy History, p. 120). These are displayed prominently on the patient's chart. The specific allergen is noted, as well as the type and severity of the reaction. Parents are excellent historians, especially when the child has displayed a pronounced reaction to a substance. Drugs, including related drugs (e.g., penicillin, nafcillin), and other items, such as latex, that have produced a reaction previously are

never used. If the child is allergic to insect venom, the family is instructed to purchase an emergency kit to be kept with the child at all times. Both the family and the child, if the child is old enough, are taught how to use the equipment. Medical identification should be carried by the patient at all times.

TOXIC SHOCK SYNDROME (TSS)

TSS is a relatively rare disease that occurs predominantly (but not exclusively) in previously healthy young women during their menstrual periods. The organism implicated is the phage group-1 *Staphylococcus aureus,* which is believed to produce an epidermal toxin. The disease has been observed primarily in women who use tampons during a menstrual period. The tampons may carry the organism from the fingers or the vulva into the vagina during insertion, the tampon might traumatize the vaginal wall and provide a focus of infection, or the tampon itself may provide a favorable environment for growth of the organism or elaboration of its toxin.

Diagnostic Evaluation

Diagnosis is established on the basis of the criteria established by the Centers for Disease Control and Prevention's toxic case definition (see box). A history of tampon use contributes to the diagnosis. Additional laboratory tests include cultures from blood, vagina, cervix, and any discharge. Other laboratory tests are those that facilitate the management of shock.

CASE DEFINITION OF TOXIC SHOCK SYNDROME

1. Fever (temperature at or above 38.9° C, or 102° F)
2. Rash (diffuse macular erythroderma)
3. Desquamation 1 to 2 weeks after onset of illness, particularly of the palms and soles
4. Hypotension (systolic blood pressure at or below 90 mm Hg for adults or below the fifth percentile for age for children younger than 16 years of age, or orthostatic syncope)
5. Involvement of three or more of the following organ systems:
   a. Gastrointestinal (vomiting or diarrhea at onset of illness)
   b. Muscular (severe myalgia or creatine phosphokinase level above two times the upper limits of normal)
   c. Mucous membrane (vagina, oropharyngeal, or conjunctival hyperemia)
   d. Renal (blood urea nitrogen or creatinine levels above two times the upper limits of normal or above 5 white blood cells per high-power field—in the absence of a urinary tract infection)
   e. Hepatic (total bilirubin, serum glutamic oxaloacetic transaminase [SGOT], or serum glutamic pyruvic transaminase [SGPT] above two times the upper limits of normal)
   f. Hematologic (platelets below $100,000/mm^3$)
   g. Central nervous system (disorientation or alterations in consciousness without focal neurologic signs when fever and hypotension are absent)
6. Negative results on the following tests, if obtained:
   a. Blood, throat, or cerebrospinal fluid cultures
   b. Serologic tests for Rocky Mountain spotted fever, leptospirosis, or measles

From Centers for Disease Control: *MMWR* 29:442, 1980.

Therapeutic Management

The management of TSS is the same as management of shock of any etiology and may involve supportive care in mild cases to hospitalization and intensive care in severe cases. Appropriate parenteral antibiotics are usually administered after cultures are obtained.

Nursing Considerations

Nursing care and observation of the acutely ill patient are the same as those described for shock of any etiology. Since the disease is relatively rare, the major efforts of nursing are directed toward prevention. The association between the disease and the use of tampons provides some direction for education. Avoiding the use of tampons offers the most certain preventive measure, although this approach is probably unacceptable to most adolescent girls, who prefer the freedom, comfort, and inconspicuousness that tampons afford.

Adolescent girls who use tampons can be taught general hygiene measures, such as handwashing before insertion of the tampon and not to use a tampon that has been dropped or otherwise soiled. Tampons should be inserted carefully to avoid vaginal abrasion. Also, it is wise to modify their use. For example, tampons may be used intermittently during the menstrual cycle, alternating with sanitary napkins—perhaps using the napkins during the night, when at home during the day, and when flow is slight. Young girls are advised not to use superabsorbent tampons and not to leave any tampon in the body for more than 4 to 6 hours.

Patients who use tampons need to understand that they should remove the tampon and consult their health professional if they develop a sudden high fever, vomiting, diarrhea, muscle pain, dizziness, fainting or near fainting when standing up, or rash that resembles a sunburn.

HENOCH-SCHÖNLEIN PURPURA (HSP)

HSP *(Schönlein-Henoch vasculitis, allergic purpura, anaphylactoid purpura)* is a relatively common acquired disorder in children characterized by a nonthrombocytopenic purpura and variable joint and visceral abnormalities. The etiology is unknown, but the disease often follows an upper respiratory infection, and allergy or drug sensitivity plays a role in some instances. The disease occurs in children ages 6 months to 16 years but more frequently in children between ages 2 to 8 years. It is observed more often in white children and in boys three times more often than in girls.

Pathophysiology

The disease is characterized by inflammation of small blood vessels, and the manifestations observed are influenced by the size and distribution of the affected vessels. A generalized vasculitis of dermal capillaries (and to a lesser extent small arterioles and veins) causing extravasation of red blood cells produces the petechial skin lesions. Inflammation and hemorrhage may also occur in the gastrointestinal (GI) tract, synovium, glomeruli, and central nervous system.

Diagnostic Evaluation

Diagnosis is usually established on the basis of clinical manifestations (see box). The onset of the disease may be abrupt, with simultaneous appearance of several manifestations, or

---

CLINICAL MANIFESTATIONS OF HENOCH-SCHÖNLEIN PURPURA

Primary feature: symmetric purpura
 Involves buttocks and lower extremities
 May extend to include extensor surfaces of upper extremities; less often, upper trunk and face
 May be associated with maculopapular lesions and variable elements of urticaria and erythema
 Often marked edema of scalp, eyelids, lips, ears, and dorsal surfaces of hands and feet, especially in infants and younger children
Arthritic effects (two thirds of affected children)
 Asymptomatic swelling around a single joint
 Painful tender swelling of several joints, most often the knees and ankles
Gastrointestinal involvement (two thirds of affected children)
 Recurrent colicky midabdominal pain
 Often associated with nausea and vomiting
 Stools contain gross or occult blood and mucus
Renal involvement (up to one half of affected children)
 Hematuria
 Casts
 Proteinuria

---

gradual, with sequential appearance of different manifestations. Laboratory tests are used to assess GI and renal involvement and to determine adequacy of hematostatic function.

Therapeutic Management

Management is primarily supportive, with close observation for signs of renal or GI manifestations. Edema, rash, malaise, and arthralgia are usually managed with appropriate analgesics, such as acetaminophen, and mild sedation if necessary. Corticosteroids may be prescribed for relief of more severe edema, arthralgia, and colicky abdominal pain but are not warranted in all cases.

Prognosis. Most children recover without the need for hospitalization, and in most instances a single acute episode clears spontaneously within a month. Others may have periodic recurrences for as long as 2 to 3 years before permanent remission from symptoms. Rarely, death occurs from severe GI complications, acute renal failure, or central nervous system involvement.

Nursing Considerations

Nursing care of the child hospitalized with HSP is primarily supportive, with vigilant observation for signs of complications. Vital signs are taken and recorded at regular intervals, specimens obtained for laboratory examination, and medication administered as prescribed. Urine and stools are carefully observed for fresh and occult blood.

If the child has joint pain with positioning, careful movement and administration of analgesics help reduce discomfort. Analgesics also relieve the discomfort of fever and malaise. More severe involvement, such as GI symptoms and nephritis, is managed as for any such disorder.

Concern about the unsightly appearance of the rash is common. The child and parents are reassured that it is only a temporary phenomenon, and the child can be encouraged to wear clothing that helps to hide the rash, such as long sleeves, pants, and robe. Emphasizing good grooming and attractive apparel helps promote a more positive self-image.

HEART TRANSPLANTATION

Heart transplantation has become a treatment option for infants and children with worsening heart failure and a limited life expectancy despite maximum medical and surgical management. Indications for cardiac transplantation in children are cardiomyopathy and end-stage CHD. An important and controversial group of patients with CHD are infants with hypoplastic left heart syndrome who undergo heart transplantation as their initial treatment.

In a study of infants from 3 hours to 12 months of age, the overall survival was 83%, with the best results in very young infants (Bailey and others, 1993). In the short term, after successful transplantation, children are able to return to full participation in age-appropriate activities and appear to adapt well to their new life-style. The long-term prognosis is unknown.

The heart transplant procedure may be orthotopic or heterotopic. *Orthotopic heart transplantation* refers to removing the recipient's own heart and implanting a new heart from a donor who has had brain death but a healthy heart. The donor and recipient are matched by weight and blood type. *Heterotopic heart transplantation* refers to leaving the recipient's own heart in place and implanting a new heart to act as an additional pump or "piggyback" heart; this type of transplant is rarely done in children.

Before transplantation, potential recipients are carefully evaluated to identify problems in other organ systems that might preclude or increase the risk of transplantation. A psychosocial evaluation of the patient and family is done to identify possible problems in complying with the complex medical regimen following transplantation and in providing needed support systems. Patients are listed on a national computer network organized by the *United Network for Organ Sharing (UNOS)* to match donors and recipients. Because of the limited donor supply, some infants waiting for heart transplants will die before receiving a donor heart (see also Tissue Donation/Autopsy, Chapter 18).

Nursing Considerations

Nursing care following transplantation is demanding and complex, with careful attention to both the physical needs of the child and the emotional needs of the child and family. Care of a child after a heart transplant requires the expertise and dedication of many members of the health care team. Nurses play vital roles in assessment, coordination of care, psychosocial support, and patient and family education.

Transplantation raises a number of ethical issues, including the use of newborns with anencephaly as organ donors, use of animal hearts in human transplantation, scarcity of donors, and donor allocation issues. Other factors, often unique to pediatrics, involve the patient's status as a minor, specifically issues of informed consent and parental responsibility and authority.

KEY POINTS

- Congenital heart disease (CHD) is the most common form of cardiac disease in children.
- Major categories to investigate in the cardiac history are poor weight gain, poor feeding habits, and fatigue during feeding; frequent respiratory infections and difficulties; and evidence of exercise intolerance.
- The most common tests used in assessing cardiac function are radiography, electrocardiography, echocardiography, and cardiac catheterization.
- Cardiac catheterization procedures can be divided into three groups: (1) diagnostic procedures, including angiography, that measure pressures and saturations to establish cardiac diagnosis; (2) interventional procedures, in which catheters or balloon devices are used to correct cardiac defects; and (3) electrophysiology studies, in which catheters with electrodes are used to evaluate dysrhythmias.
- Diagnostic cardiac catheterization provides important information about oxygen saturation of blood within the chambers and great vessels, pressure changes, changes in cardiac output or stroke volume, and anatomic abnormalities.
- Several prenatal factors may predispose children to CHD: maternal rubella during pregnancy, maternal alcoholism, maternal age above 40 years, and maternal insulin-dependent diabetes.
- Congenital heart defects can be divided into four main groups, as determined by hemodynamic patterns: (1) defects that result in increased pulmonary blood flow, (2) obstructive defects, (3) defects that result in decreased pulmonary blood flow, and (4) mixed defects.
- Clinical consequences of congenital heart defects include congestive heart failure (CHF) and hypoxemia. A child can have both hypoxemia and CHF, although usually they occur independently.
- Clinical manifestations of CHF are impaired myocardial function (tachycardia, cardiomegaly), pulmonary congestion (dyspnea, tachypnea, orthopnea, cyanosis), and systemic congestion (hepatosplenomegaly, edema, distended veins).
- Nursing measures in the care of a child with CHF are to assist in improving cardiac function, decrease cardiac demands, reduce respiratory distress, maintain nutritional status, promote fluid loss, and provide family support.
- Clinical manifestations of hypoxemia are cyanosis, polycythemia, clubbing, and delayed growth and development. The child is at increased risk for hypercyanotic spells, cerebrovascular accidents, brain abscess, and bacterial endocarditis.

- Caring for the child with CHD and the family requires helping them to adjust to the disorder and to cope with the effects of the defect and fostering growth-promoting family relationships.
- Preoperative care of the child with a congenital heart defect involves introducing the child and family to the hospital and preparing them for preoperative and postoperative procedures.
- Providing postoperative care includes observing vital signs and arterial/venous pressures, maintaining respiratory status, allowing maximum rest, providing comfort, monitoring fluids, planning for progressive activities, giving emotional support, observing for complications of surgery, and planning for discharge and home care.
- Acquired cardiovascular disorders include bacterial endocarditis, rheumatic fever, hyperlipidemia (hypercholesterolemia), and cardiac dysrhythmias.
- Prevention of bacterial endocarditis in certain children with CHD involves administration of prophylactic antibiotics when specific procedures are performed.
- Acute rheumatic fever is a systemic inflammatory disease that can damage the cardiac valves and is associated with previous group A streptococcal infection. Its incidence has increased in some areas of the United States.
- Cholesterol screening in children is controversial; currently, children with known risk factors for hyperlipidemia are screened and treated as needed. The influence of childhood cholesterol levels on later development of coronary artery disease is under investigation.

- Common dysrhythmias in children include slow rhythms (bradycardias, heart block) and fast rhythms (sinus tachycardia, supraventricular tachycardia).
- Education of the child with hypertension and the family focuses on drug therapy, diet control, and appropriate exercise.
- Kawasaki disease is an extensive inflammation of small vessels and capillaries that may progress to involve the coronary arteries, causing aneurysm formation. The administration of gamma globulin is an important aspect of treatment.
- Emergency treatment for shock includes ensuring ventilation; administering vasopressors, fluids/blood, and antibiotics as needed; and providing supportive measures, such as correct positioning, warmth, and psychologic reassurance to the child and family.
- Persons at risk for anaphylaxis may be identified by a history of previous allergic reaction, history of atopy, history of severe reactions in family, and positive skin test to the allergen.
- Nursing management of the patient with toxic shock syndrome focuses on prevention primarily through education concerning safe tampon use.
- Henoch-Schönlein purpura is characterized by a nonthrombocytic purpura and variable joint and visceral abnormalities. Nursing care is primarily supportive, with observation for complications and provision of comfort being key nursing goals.
- Heart transplantation has been extended to infants and children with cardiomyopathy and complex congenital heart defects involving ventricular dysfunction, such as hypoplastic left heart syndrome.

REFERENCES

Agamalian B: Pediatric cardiac catheterization, *J Pediatr Nurs* 1(2):73-79, 1986.

Bailey LL and others: Bless the babies: one hundred fifteen late survivors of heart transplantation during the first year of life, *J Thorac Cardiovasc Surg* 105(5):805-815, 1993.

Bochner BS, Lichtenstein LM: Anaphylaxis, *N Engl J Med* 324(25):1785-1790, 1991.

Colletti RB and others: Niacin treatment of hypercholesterolemia in children, *Pediatrics* 92(1):78-82, 1993.

Dajani AS, Taubert RA: Infective endocarditis. In Emmanulides GC and others, editors: *Moss and Adams heart disease in infants, children, and adolescents,* ed 5, Baltimore, 1995, Williams & Wilkins.

Driscoll DJ: Evaluation of the cyanotic newborn, *Pediatr Clin North Am* 37(1):1-23, 1990.

Fisher M: Treating anaphylaxis with sympathomimetic drugs, *Br Med J* 305:1107-1108, 1992.

Fyler DC: *Nadas' pediatric cardiology,* Philadelphia, 1992, Hanley and Belfus.

Hazinski MF: Cardiovascular disorders. In Hazinski MF, editor: *Nursing care of the critically ill child,* ed 2, St Louis, 1992, Mosby.

Maguire DP, Maloney P: A comparison of fentanyl and morphine use in neonates, *Neonatal Network* 7(1):27-35, 1988.

National Cholesterol Education Program: Report of the expert panel on blood cholesterol levels in children and adolescents, *Pediatrics* 89(3, pt 2):525-584, 1992.

National Heart, Lung, and Blood Institute: Report of the Second Task Force on Blood Pressure Control in Children, 1987, *Pediatrics* 79:1-25, 1987.

Newburger J and others: A single intravenous infusion of gamma-globulin as compared with four infusions in the treatment of acute Kawasaki syndrome, *N Engl J Med* 324(23):1623-1639, 1991.

Radtke W, Lock JE: Balloon dilation, *Pediatr Clin North Am* 37(1):193-214, 1990.

BIBLIOGRAPHY

Cardiac Diagnosis

Apple S, Thurkauf GE: Preparing for and understanding transesophageal echocardiography, *Crit Care Nurse* 12:29-34, 1992.

Driscoll DJ: Evaluation of the cyanotic newborn, *Pediatr Clin North Am* 37(1):1-23, 1990.

Fabius DB: Understanding heart sounds: solving the mystery of heart murmurs, *Nursing '94* 24(7):39-44, 1994.

Fabius DB: Understanding heart sounds: uncovering the secrets of snaps, rubs, and clicks, *Nursing '94* 24(7):45-50, 1994.

Gardner RM, Hujes M: Fundamentals of physiologic monitoring, *AACN Clin Issues Crit Care Nurs* 4(1):11-24, 1993.

Monett Z, Moynihan P: Cardiovascular assessment of the neonatal heart, *J Perinat Neonat Nurs* 5(2):50-59, 1991.

Monett Z, Roberts P: Patient care for interventional cardiac catheterization, *Nurs Clin North Am* 29(2):333-346, 1995.

Pederson C: Children's and adolescents' experiences while undergoing cardiac catheterization, *Matern Child Nurs J* 23(1):15-25, 1995.

Roberts PJ: Caring for patients undergoing therapeutic cardiac catheterization, *Crit Care Nurs Clin North Am* 1(2):275-288, 1989.

Sondheimer HM: Cardiac catheterization—a new role in the 90s, *Contemp Pediatr* 7(3):91-106, 1990.

Vargo L: Evaluation of cardiac size on the neonatal chest x-ray, *Neonatal Network* 12(3):65-67, 1993.

Webster H, Chellis MJ: Physiologic monitoring of infants and children, *AACN Clin Issues Crit Care Nurs* 4(1):180-197, 1993.

Congenital Heart Disease

Abbott K: Therapeutic use of play in the psychological preparation of preschool children undergoing cardiac surgery, *Issues Compr Pediatr Nurs* 13(4):265-277, 1990.

Cardiovascular health and disease in children: current status, *Circulation* 89(2):923-930, 1994.

Combs VL, Marino BL: A comparison of growth patterns in breast and bottle fed infants with congenital heart disease, *Pediatr Nurs* 19(2):175-179, 1993.

Craig J: The postoperative cardiac infant: physiologic basis for neonatal nursing interventions, *J Perinat Neonat Nurs* 5(2):60-70, 1991.

Cullen S, Celermajer DS, Deanfield JE: Exercise in congenital heart disease, *Cardiol Young* 1(2):129-135, 1991.

Johnson AB, Davis JS: Treatment options for the neonate with hypoplastic left heart syndrome, *J Perinat Neonat Nurs* 5(2):84-92, 1991.

Kulik L and others: Pharmacologic interventions for the neonate with compromised cardiac function, *J Perinat Neonat Nurs* 5(2):71-84, 1991.

Lobo ML: Parent infant interactions during feeding with infants with congenital heart defects, *J Pediatr Nurs* 7(2):97-105, 1992.

Moynihan P, Naclerio L, Kiley K: Parent participation, *Nurs Clin North Am* 29(2):231-242, 1995.

Norris MKG, editor: Pediatric and neonatal cardiology, *Crit Care Nurs Clin North Am* 9(2):111-236, 1994.

Norris MKG, Hill CS: Nutritional issues in infants and children with congenital heart disease, *Crit Care Nurs Clin North Am* 9(2):153-164, 1994.

O'Brien P, Boisvert JT: Discharge planning for children with heart disease, *Crit Care Nurs Clin North Am* 1(2):297-305, 1989.

Smith JB, Vernon-Levett P: Care of infants with HLHS, *AACN Clin Issues Crit Care Nurs* 4(2):329-339, 1993.

Swanson LT: Treatment options for hypoplastic left heart syndrome: a mother's perspective, *Crit Care Nurse* 15(3):70-79, 1995.

Tong E, Sparacino P: Special management issues for adolescents and young adults with congenital heart disease, *Crit Care Nurs Clin North Am* 9(2):199-214, 1994.

Uzark K: Counseling adolescents with congenital heart disease, *J Cardiovasc Nurs* 6(3):65-73, 1992.

Congestive Heart Failure/Hypoxemia

Brown KK: Boosting the failing heart with inotropic drugs, *Nursing '93* 23(6):34-44, 1993.

Dahlmann AR: Captopril, *Neonatal Network* 7(5):41-43, 1989.

Delgizzi LJ, Ueda JN: Using inotropic and vasodilating agents in pediatric patients with cardiac disease, *AACN Clin Issues Crit Care Nurs* 1(1):131-147, 1990.

Hagedorn MI, Gardner SL: Physiologic sequelae of prematurity: the nurse practitioner's role. Part III, *J Pediatr Health* 4(5):229-236, 1990.

Kaplan S: New drug approaches to the treatment of heart failure in infants and children, *Drugs* 39(3):388-393, 1990.

Kohr L, O'Brien P: Current management of congestive heart failure in infants and children, *Nurs Clin North Am* 29(2):261-290, 1995.

Noerr B: Captopril, *Neonatal Network* 9(5):69-71, 1991.

O'Brien P, Smith P: Chronic hypoxemia in children with cyanotic heart disease, *Crit Care Nurs Clin North Am* 9(2):215-226, 1994.

Werner NP: Congestive heart failure: pathophysiology and management throughout infancy, *J Perinat Neonat Nurs* 7(3):59-76, 1993.

Cardiac Surgery

Callow LB: Postoperative nursing management of the infant with TAPVC, *DCCN* 10(3):140-149, 1991.

Callow LB: Current strategies in the nursing care of infants with HLHS undergoing 1st stage palliation with the Norwood procedure, *Heart Lung* 21(5):463-470, 1992.

Cohen DM: Surgical management of congenital heart disease in the 1990's, *Am J Dis Child* 146:1447-1452, 1992.

Craig J: The postoperative cardiac infant: physiologic basis for neonatal nursing interventions, *J Perinat Neonat Nurs* 5(2):60-70, 1991.

Jensen CA: Nursing care of a child following an arterial switch procedure for transposition of the great arteries, *Crit Care Nurs* 12(8):51-57, 1992.

Johnston J: Cardiac transplant in early infancy, *Crit Care Nurs Clin North Am* 4(3):521-535, 1992.

Ludwick F and others: Examining management of pain for infants following cardiac surgery, *DCCN* 14(3):136-143, 1995.

Medicus L and others: Preventing pulmonary hypertensive crisis in the pediatric patient after cardiac surgery, *Am J Crit Care* 4(1):49-55, 1995.

Muirhead J: Heart transplantation in children: indications, complications, and management, *J Cardiovasc Nurs* 6(3):44-55, 1992.

Noonan DM and others: Nursing considerations for neonates awaiting heart transplant for HLHS, *J Pediatr Nurs* 6(5):327-330, 1991.

O'Brien P, Elixson M: The child following the Fontan procedure: nursing strategies, *Clin Issues Crit Care Nurs* 1(1):46-58, 1990.

O'Brien P, Hanley FH: New directions in pediatric heart transplantation, *Crit Care Nurs Clin North Am* 4:193-203, 1992.

Rotondi P, editor: Neonatal and pediatric cardiovascular nursing, *Crit Care Nurs Clin North Am* 1(2):195-305, 1989.

Stinson J and others: Mother's information needs related to caring for infants at home following cardiac surgery, *J Pediatr Nurs* 10(1):48-57, 1995.

Tong E: An overview of artificial heart valve replacement in infants and children, *J Cardiovasc Nurs* 6(3):30-43, 1992.

Uzark K: Caring for families of pediatric transplant recipients: psychosocial implications, *Crit Care Nurs Clin North Am* 4:255-263, 1992.

Bacterial Endocarditis

Dajani AS and others: Prevention of bacterial endocarditis: recommendations by the American Heart Association, *JAMA* 264(22):2919-2911, 1990.

Kaplan EL: Bacterial endocarditis prophylaxis, *Pediatr Ann* 21(4):249-255, 1992.

Saiman L, Prince A, Gersony W: Pediatric infective endocarditis in the modern era, *J Pediatr* 122(6):847-853, 1993.

Scrima DA: Infective endocarditis: nursing considerations, *Crit Care Nurse* 7:47-56, 1987.

Snelson C, Cline BA, Luby C: Infective endocarditis: a challenging diagnosis, *Dimens Crit Care Nurs* 12(1):4-16, 1993.

Rheumatic Fever

Bisno AL: Group A streptococcal infections and acute rheumatic fever, *N Engl J Med* 325(11):783-793, 1991.

Forster J, editor: Rheumatic fever: keeping up with the Jones criteria, *Contemp Pediatr* 10:51-60, 1993.

Freund B and others: Acute rheumatic fever revisited, *J Pediatr Nurs* 8:167-176, 1993.

Griffiths SP: Rheumatic fever. In Hoekelman RA and others, editors: *Primary pediatric care,* ed 2, St Louis, 1992, Mosby.

Grimes DE, Woolbert LF: Facts and fallacies about streptococcal infection and rheumatic fever, *J Pediatr Health Care* 4(4):186-192, 1990.

Special Writing Group of the Committee on Rheumatic Fever, Endocarditis, and Kawasaki Disease of the Council on the Cardiovascular Disease in the Young of the American Heart Association: Guidelines for the diagnosis of rheumatic fever: Jones Criteria, 1992 (update), *JAMA* 268:2069-2073, 1992.

Veasy LG, Tani LY, Hill HR: Persistence of acute rheumatic fever in the intermountain area of the United States, *J Pediatr* 124:9-16, 1994.

Hyperlipidemia (Hypercholesterolemia)

Bakir A, Roberts C, Gothing C: Dyslipidemias in childhood: an overview, *Nurs Clin North Am* 29(2):243-260, 1995.

Davidson DM, Smith RM, Qaqundah PY: Cholesterol screening in children during office visits, *J Pediatr Health Care* 4(1):11-17, 1990.

Gillman MW: Screening for familial hypercholesterolemia in childhood, *Am J Dis Child* 147(4):393-396, 1993.

Mietus-Snyder M and others: Effects of nutritional counseling on lipoprotein levels in a pediatric lipid clinic, *Am J Dis Child* 147(4):378-381, 1993.

Mistretta EF, Stroudy S: Hypercholesterolemia in children: risk and management, *Pediatr Nurs* 16(2):152-154, 1990.

Neufeld EJ, Newburger JW: How should children with hypercholesterolemia be managed? *Choices Cardiol* 7:233-236, 1993.

Nolan R: Child hypercholesterolemia: implications for nurse practitioners, *Pediatr Nurs* 20(11):46-50, 1994.

Schifman V, Hannaman KN: Cholesterol: a practical teaching plan for children and adolescents, *Issues Compr Pediatr Nurs* 12(5):359-369, 1989.

Cardiac Dysrhythmias

Alpern D, Uzark K, Dick M: Psychosocial responses of children to cardiac pacemakers, *J Pediatr* 114(3):494-501, 1989.

Boisvert J, Reidy S, Lulu J: Overview of pediatric arrhythmias, *Nurs Clin North Am* 29(2):365-380, 1995.

Cox DM: Complete heart block in the pediatric patient, *J Emerg Nurs* 18(6):497-500, 1992.

Farrington E: Adenosine, *Pediatr Nurs* 17(6):590, 1991.

Hanisch DG and others: Complex dysrhythmias in infants and children, *AACN Clin Issues Crit Care Nurs* 3(1):255-269, 1992.

Moulton L and others: Radiofrequency catheter ablation for supraventricular tachycardia, *Heart Lung* 22:3-14, 1993.

Philich LM and others: A pediatric case study: use of adenosine in the treatment of SVT, *Am J Crit Care* 3(3):228-231, 1994.

Suddaby E, Riker S: Defibrillation and cardioversion in children, *Pediatr Nurs* 17(5):477-481, 1991.

Zeigler V: Adenosine in the pediatric population: nursing implications, *Pediatr Nurs* 17(6):600-602, 1991.

Zeigler V: Postoperative rhythm disturbances, *Crit Care Nurs Clin North Am* 9(2):227-236, 1994.

Systemic Hypertension

Carmon M and others: Cardiovascular screening programs: implications for school nurses, *Pediatr Nurs* 16(5):509-511, 1990.

Daniels SR: Primary hypertension in childhood and adolescence, *Pediatr Ann* 21(4):224-234, 1992.

Falkner B: Essential hypertension in children, *Curr Opin Pediatr* 1(1):131-134, 1989.

Gillman MW and others: Identifying children at high risk for the development of essential hypertension, *J Pediatr* 122:837-846, 1993.

Jung FF, Ingelfinger JR: Hypertension in childhood and adolescence, *Pediatr Rev* 14(5):169-179, 1993.

Rocchini A, editor: Childhood hypertension, *Pediatr Clin North Am* 40(1):entire issue, 1993.

Kawasaki Disease

American Academy of Pediatrics, Committee on Infectious Diseases: Intravenous γ-globulin use in children with Kawasaki disease, *Pediatrics* 82(1):122, 1988.

Baker A: Acquired heart disease in infants and children, *Crit Care Nurs Clin North Am* 9(2):175-186, 1994.

Fujita Y and others: Kawasaki disease in families, *Pediatrics* 84(4):666-669, 1989.

Gersony WM: Long-term issues in Kawasaki disease, *J Pediatr* 121(5):731-733, 1992.

McEnhill M, Vitale K: Kawasaki disease: new challenges in care, *MCN* 14:406-410, 1989.

Shreve B: Kawasaki disease: early treatment/positive results, *Pediatr Nurs* 19(6):607-610, 1993.

Shock

Barry W and others: Intravenous immunoglobulin therapy for toxic shock syndrome, *JAMA* 267(24):3315-3316, 1992.

Berro EA, Bechler-Karsch A: A closer look at septic shock, *Pediatr Nurs* 19:289-297, 1993.

Brown KK: Critical interventions in septic shock. Part 2, *Am J Nurs* 94(10):20-26, 1994.

Brown KK: Septic shock: how to stop the deadly cascade. Part 1, *Am J Nurs* 94(9):20-27, 1994.

Pamillo JE: Pathogenetic mechanisms of septic shock, *N Engl J Med* 328:1471-1477, 1993.

Rice V: Shock, a clinical syndrome: an update. Part 1, *Crit Care Nurse* 11:20-27, 1991.

Rice V: Shock, a clinical syndrome: an update. Part 2, *Crit Care Nurse* 11:74-82, 1991.

Rice V: Shock, a clinical syndrome, an update. Part 3, *Crit Care Nurse* 11:34-39, 1991.

Rice V: Shock, a clinical syndrome, an update. Part 4, *Crit Care Nurse* 11:28-32, 35-43, 1991.

Strodtbeck F, Joyce B: Shock in newborns and children, *Crit Care Nurs Q* 11:75-83, 1988.

Wynn SR: Anaphylaxis at school, *J School Nurs* 9:5-11, 1993.

Chapter 26

THE CHILD WITH HEMATOLOGIC OR IMMUNOLOGIC DYSFUNCTION

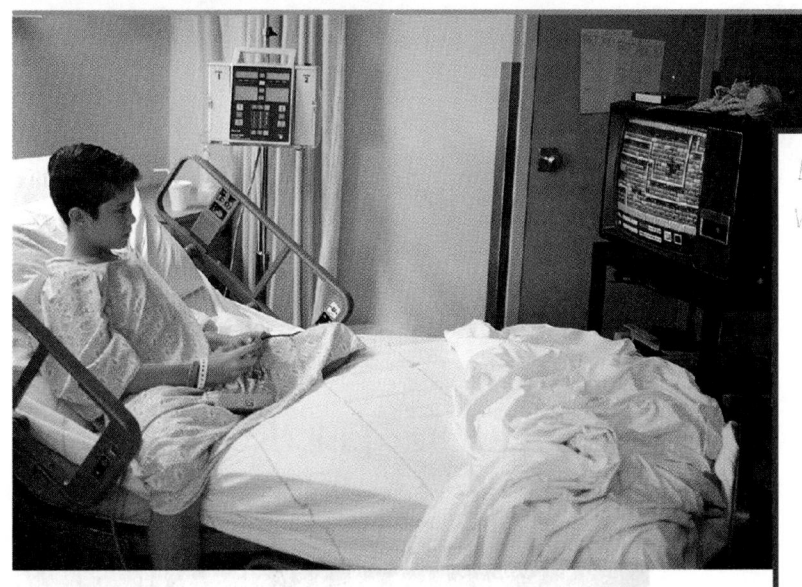

Dual Channel Volumetric Infusion Pump

Jason, age 13 years, anemia

" It's boring to be in the hospital. You just watch TV and play Nintendo and sleep. "

RELATED TOPICS

903

HEMATOLOGIC/IMMUNOLOGIC DYSFUNCTION

ASSESSMENT OF HEMATOLOGIC FUNCTION

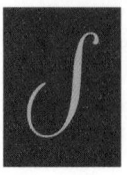everal tests can be performed to assess hematologic function, including additional procedures to identify the cause of the dysfunction. The following discussion is limited to a description of the most common and one of the most valuable tests, the *complete blood count (CBC)*. Other procedures, such as those related to iron, coagulation, and immune status, are discussed throughout the chapter as appropriate. The nurse should be familiar with the significance of the findings from the CBC (see Table 26-1) and aware of normal values for age, which are listed in Appendix E.

As with any disorder, the history and physical examination are essential to identification of hematologic dysfunction, and the nurse is often the first person to suspect a problem based on information from these sources. Comments by the parent regarding the child's lack of energy, food diary of poor sources of iron, frequent infections, and bleeding that is difficult to control offer clues to the more common disorders affecting the blood. A careful physical appraisal, especially of the skin, can reveal findings such as pallor, petechiae, or bruising that may indicate minor or serious hematologic conditions. Nurses need to be aware of the clinical manifestations of blood diseases to assist in recognizing symptoms and establishing a diagnosis.

 A common term used in describing an abnormal CBC is *shift to the left,* which refers to the presence of immature cells in the peripheral blood from hyperfunction of the bone marrow, as seen during an infection.

Christina Algiere Kasprisin, MS, RN, revised this chapter.

RED BLOOD CELL (RBC) DISORDERS

ANEMIA

The term *anemia* describes a condition in which the number of RBCs and/or the hemoglobin (Hgb or Hb) concentration is reduced below normal. As a result of this decrease, the oxygen-carrying capacity of the blood is diminished, causing a reduction in the oxygen available to the tissues. Anemia is the most common hematologic disorder of infancy and childhood and is not a disease itself but an indication or manifestation of an underlying pathologic process.

Classification

Anemias are classified in relation to (1) *etiology* or *physiology,* manifested by erythrocyte and/or Hgb depletion, and (2) *morphology,* the characteristic changes in RBC size, shape, and/or color. Although the morphologic classification is more useful in terms of laboratory evaluation of anemia, the etiologic approach provides direction for planning nursing care. For example, anemia with reduced Hb concentration may be caused by a dietary depletion of iron, and the principal intervention is replenishing iron stores. Etiologic factors responsible for anemia are described in the box on p. 905.

Consequences of Anemia

The basic physiologic defect caused by anemia is a decrease in the oxygen-carrying capacity of blood and consequently a reduction in the amount of oxygen available to the cells. When the anemia has developed slowly, the child usually adapts to the declining Hgb level.

The effects of anemia on the circulatory system can be profound. Because the viscosity of blood depends almost entirely on the concentration of RBCs, the resulting hemodilution of severe anemia decreases peripheral resistance, causing greater quantities of blood to return to the heart. The increased circulation and turbulence within the heart may produce a murmur. Since the cardiac workload is greatly increased, especially

<table>
<tr><td colspan="2">

CLASSIFICATION OF ANEMIA

Etiology/Pathophysiology

Excessive blood loss—from acute or chronic hemorrhage (internal or external); until stores are replaced, there is usually a normocytic (normal size), normochromic (normal color) anemia, provided that there are sufficient iron stores for hemoglobin (Hb) synthesis

Destruction (hemolysis) of erythrocytes—as a result of an intracorpuscular defect within the red blood cell (RBC) (e.g., sickle cell anemia) or an extracorpuscular factor (e.g., infectious agents, chemicals, immune mechanisms) that causes destruction to outpace production

Decreased or impaired production of erythrocytes or their components—as a result of bone marrow failure (caused by factors such as neoplastic diseases, irradiation, chemicals, or disease) or deficiency of essential nutrients (e.g., iron)

Morphology

Size—cell size; for example, *normocytes* (normal), *microcytes* (smaller than normal), or *macrocytes* (larger than normal)

Shape—irregularly shaped RBCs; for example, *poikilocytes* (irregularly shaped cells), *spherocytes* (globular cells), and *drepanocytes* (sickle cells)

Staining characteristics or color—reflects the hemoglobin concentration; for example, *normochromic* (sufficient or normal amount) or *hypochromic* (reduced amount)

</td>
<td colspan="2">

CLINICAL MANIFESTATIONS OF ANEMIA

General Manifestations

Muscle weakness
Easy fatigability
  Frequent resting
  Shortness of breath
  Poor sucking (infants)
Pale skin
  Waxy pallor seen in severe anemia
Pica—eating clay, ice, paste

Central Nervous System Manifestations

Headache
Dizziness
Lightheadedness
Irritability
Slowed thought processes
Decreased attention span
Apathy
Depression

Shock (Blood Loss Anemia)

Poor peripheral perfusion
Skin moist and cool
Low blood pressure and central venous pressure
Increased heart rate

</td></tr>
</table>

during exercise, infection, or emotional stress, cardiac failure may ensue.

Children seem to have a remarkable ability to function quite well despite low levels of Hgb. *Cyanosis* (the result of the quantity of deoxygenated Hgb in arterial blood) is typically not evident. Growth retardation, resulting from decreased cellular metabolism and coexisting anorexia, is a common finding in chronic severe anemia and is frequently accompanied by delayed sexual maturation in the older child.

Diagnostic Evaluation

In general, anemia may be suspected from findings on the history and physical examination, such as lack of energy, easy fatigability, and pallor, but unless the anemia is severe, the first clue to the disorder may be alterations in the CBC, such as decreased RBCs, and decreased Hgb and hematocrit (Hct) levels (see box). Although anemia is sometimes defined as an Hgb below 10 or 11 g/dl, this arbitrary cutoff is inappropriate for all children, because Hgb levels normally vary with age (see Table 26-1 and Appendix E).

Other tests specific to a particular type of anemia are employed to determine the underlying cause of anemia. These are discussed in relation to the particular disorder.

Therapeutic Management

The objective of medical management is to reverse the anemia by treating the underlying cause and to make up for any deficiency of blood, blood component, or substance the blood needs for normal functioning. For example, blood or blood cells are replaced after hemorrhage; in nutritional anemias the specific deficiency is replaced.

In patients with severe anemia, supportive medical care may include oxygen therapy, bed rest, and replacement of intravascular volume with intravenous (IV) fluids. See Table 26-2 for medical management of selected anemias. The prognosis for anemia depends on the correction of the cause.

Nursing Considerations

❖ Assessment

The assessment of anemia includes the basic techniques that are applicable to any condition. The age of the infant or child provides some clues regarding the possible etiology of the anemia. For example, iron deficiency anemia occurs more frequently in infants between 6 and 24 months of age and during the growth spurt of adolescence.

Racial or ethnic background is significant. For example, the anemias related to abnormal Hb levels are found in Southeast Asians and persons of African or Mediterranean ancestry. These same groups may be genetically deficient in the enzyme lactase after the period of infancy. Affected individuals are unable to tolerate lactose in the diet, with consequent intestinal irritation and chronic blood loss.

Special emphasis is placed on a careful history to elicit any information that might help identify the cause of the anemia. For example, a statement such as "The baby drinks lots of milk" is a frequent finding in infants with iron deficiency anemia. An episode of diarrhea may have precipitated a temporary lactose intolerance in infants.

Stool examination for occult (invisible) blood (Hemacult test) can identify chronic intestinal bleeding that results from a primary or secondary lactase deficiency. It is also important to understand the significance of various blood tests. Blood loss from overt hemorrhage may be manifested as shock.

TABLE 26-1. Tests performed as part of the complete blood count

TEST (AVERAGE VALUE)*	DESCRIPTION/COMMENTS
Red blood cell (RBC) count (4.5-5.5 million/mm³)	Number of RBCs/mm³ of blood Indirectly estimates Hgb content of blood Reflects function of bone marrow
Hemoglobin (Hgb) determination (11.5-15.5 g/dl)	Amount of Hgb/dl of whole blood Total blood Hgb primarily depends on number of circulating RBCs, but also on amount of Hgb in each cell
Hematocrit (Hct) (35%-45%)	Percentage or volume of packed RBCs to whole blood Indirectly measures Hgb content Is approximately three times Hgb content
RBC indices	MCV and MCH depend on accurate counts of RBCs, whereas MCHC does not; therefore MCHC is often more reliable All indices depend on *average* cell measurements and do not show anisocytosis (individual RBC variations)
Mean corpuscular volume (MCV) (77-95 μm³)	Average of mean volume (size) of a single RBC MCV values expressed as cubic microns (μm³) or femtoliters (fl)
Mean corpuscular hemoglobin (MCH) (25-33 pg/cell)	Average or mean quantity (weight) of Hgb of a single RBC MCH values expressed as picograms (pg) or micromicrograms (μμg)
Mean corpuscular hemoglobin concentration (MCHC) (31%-37% Hgb [g]/dl RBC)	Average concentration of Hgb in a single RBC MCHC values expressed as % Hgb (g)/cell or Hgb (g)/dl RBC
RBC volume distribution width (RDW) 13.4% ± 1.2%	Average size of RBCs
Reticulocyte count (0.5%-1.5% erythrocytes)	% Reticulocytes to RBCs Index of production of mature RBCs by red bone marrow Decreased count indicates depressed bone marrow function Increased count indicates erythrogenesis in response to some stimulus When reticulocyte count is extremely high, other forms of immature RBCs (normoblasts, even erythroblasts) may be present Indirectly estimates hypochromic anemia Usually elevated in patients with chronic hemolytic anemia
White blood cell (WBC) count (4.5-13.5 × 10³ cells/mm³)	Number of WBCs/mm³ of blood Total number of WBCs less important than differential count
Differential WBC count	Inspection and quantification of WBC types present in peripheral blood Values are expressed as percentages; to obtain absolute number of any type of WBCs, multiply its respective percentage by total number of WBCs
Neutrophils (polys) (54%-62%) (3.0-5.8 × 10³ cells/mm³)	Primary defense in bacterial infection; capable of phagocytizing and killing bacteria
Bands (3%-5%) (0.15-0.4 × 10³ cells/mm³)	Immature neutrophil Increased numbers in bacterial infection Also capable of phagocytosis and killing
Eosinophils (1%-3%) (0.05-0.25 × 10³ cells/mm³)	Named for their staining characteristics with eosin dye Increased in allergic disorders, parasitic diseases, certain neoplasms, and other diseases
Basophils (0.075%) (0.015-0.030 cells/mm³)	Named for their characteristic basophilic stippling Contain histamine, heparin, and serotonin; believed to cause increased blood flow to injured tissues while preventing excessive clotting
Lymphocytes (25%-33%) (1.5-3.0 × 10³ cells/mm³)	Involved in development of antibody and delayed hypersensitivity
Monocytes (3%-7%)	Large phagocytic cells that are involved in early stage of inflammatory reaction

*See Appendix E for normal values according to ages.

TABLE 26-1. Tests performed as part of the complete blood count—cont'd

TEST (AVERAGE VALUE)*	DESCRIPTION/COMMENTS
Absolute neutrophil count (ANC) (>1000)	% Neutrophils × WBC Indicates body's capability to handle bacterial infections
Platelet count (150-400 × 10³/mm³)	Cellular fragments that are necessary for clotting to occur
Stained peripheral blood smear	Visual estimation of amount of Hgb in RBCs and overall size, shape, and structure of RBCs Various staining properties of RBC structures may be evidence of immature forms of erythrocyte Shows variation in size and shape of RBCs: microcytic, macrocytic, poikilocytic (variable shapes)

TABLE 26-2. Description and management of selected anemias

TYPE OF ANEMIA	DESCRIPTION	MANAGEMENT
Blood loss anemia	Until 20% or more of blood volume is lost with normal vital signs	No therapy needed
	Altered vital signs with losses of 30% to 40% of blood volume and signs of shock	Blood replacement Plasma or plasma protein product until blood is available
Iron deficiency anemia	Decreased RBC production	See discussion in text
Anemia of renal disease	Usually not until symptomatic and Hb is less than 7 to 8 mg/dl	Transfusion of packed RBCs
Hemolytic anemias Spherocytosis Elliptocytosis	Shortened survival of RBCs	Splenectomy
Sickle cell anemia	Shortened survival of RBCs	See discussion in text
Thalassemia	Shortened survival of RBCs	See discussion in text

❖ Nursing Diagnoses

A variety of nursing diagnoses may be evident following assessment of anemia. Some of the general aspects of nursing management are included in the Nursing Care Plan on pp. 908-909. Others become apparent in specific situations.

❖ Planning

The goals of care for the infant or child with anemia depend on the severity of the condition and the cause. Most children tolerate mild anemia well, and a priority goal is preparing them for diagnostic tests and possible blood transfusion (see p. 943). Other goals of care are as follows:

1. Child and family will receive adequate support and education.
2. Child will exhibit minimal physical or emotional exertion.
3. Child will experience no complications from anemia or its treatment.

❖ Implementation

Prepare Child and Family for Laboratory Tests. Usually, several blood tests are ordered, but since they are generally done sequentially rather than at one time, the child is subjected to multiple finger or heel punctures and/or venipunctures. Laboratory technicians frequently are not aware of the trauma that repeated punctures represent to a child. However, these invasive procedures need not be painful (see Blood Specimens, Chapter 22). For example, the topical application of *EMLA (eutectic mixture of local anesthetics)* before needle punctures can eliminate any pain (see Pain Management, Chapter 21). Therefore the nurse is responsible for preparing the child and family for the tests by (1) explaining the significance of each test, particularly why the tests are not done at one time; (2) encouraging parents or another supportive person to be with the child during the procedure; and (3) allowing the child to play with the equipment on a doll and/or participate in the actual procedure (e.g., by cleansing the finger with an alcohol swab). Older children may appreciate the opportunity to observe the blood cells under a microscope or in photographs. This experience is an especially important consideration if a serious blood disorder, such as leukemia, is suspected, since it serves as a foundation for explaining the pathophysiology of the disorder.

Bone marrow aspiration is not a routine hematologic test

NURSING CARE PLAN
The Child with Anemia

NURSING DIAGNOSIS: Anxiety/fear related to diagnostic procedures/transfusion

PATIENT/FAMILY GOAL 1: Will become knowledgeable about the disorder, diagnostic tests, and treatment

- **NURSING INTERVENTIONS/RATIONALES**

Prepare child for tests *to relieve anxiety/fear*
Remain with child during tests and initiation of transfusion *to provide support and observe for possible complications*
Explain purpose of blood components *to increase understanding of disorder, diagnostic tests, and treatment*

- **EXPECTED OUTCOMES**

Child and family display minimal anxiety
Child and family demonstrate an understanding of the disorder, diagnostic tests, and treatment

NURSING DIAGNOSIS: Activity intolerance related to generalized weakness, diminished oxygen delivery to tissues

PATIENT GOAL 1: Will receive adequate rest

- **NURSING INTERVENTIONS/RATIONALES**

Observe for signs of physical exertion (tachycardia, palpitations, tachypnea, dyspnea, shortness of breath, hyperpnea, breathlessness, dizziness, lightheadedness, sweating, change in skin color) and fatigue (sagging, limp posture; slow, strained movements; inability to tolerate additional activity) *to plan appropriately for rest*
Anticipate and assist in those activities of daily living that may be beyond child's tolerance *to prevent exertion*
Provide diversional play activities *that promote rest and quiet but prevent boredom and withdrawal*
Choose appropriate roommate of similar age and interests who requires restricted activity *to encourage compliance with need for rest*
Plan nursing activities *to provide sufficient rest*
Assist with activities requiring exertion

- **EXPECTED OUTCOMES**

Child plays and rests quietly and engages in activities appropriate to capabilities
Child does not exhibit signs of physical exertion or fatigue

PATIENT GOAL 2: Will exhibit normal respirations

- **NURSING INTERVENTIONS/RATIONALES**

Maintain high-Fowler position *for optimum air exchange*
Administer supplemental oxygen if needed *to increase oxygen to tissues*
Take vital signs during periods of rest *to establish baseline for comparison during periods of activity*

- **EXPECTED OUTCOME**

Patient breathes easily; respiratory rate and depth are normal (see inside back cover)

PATIENT GOAL 3: Will experience minimal emotional stress

- **NURSING INTERVENTIONS/RATIONALES**

Anticipate child's irritability, short attention span, and fretfulness by offering to assist child in activities rather than waiting for request for help
Encourage parents to remain with child *to minimize stress of separation*
Provide comfort measures (e.g., pacifier, rocking, music) *to minimize stress*
Encourage child to express feelings *to minimize anxiety/fear*
See also Nursing Care Plan: The Child in the Hospital, Chapter 21

- **EXPECTED OUTCOME**

Child remains calm and quiet

PATIENT GOAL 4: Will receive appropriate blood elements

- **NURSING INTERVENTIONS/RATIONALES**

*Administer blood, packed cells, platelets as prescribed
*Administer hematopoetic growth factors as prescribed *to stimulate blood cell formation*

- **EXPECTED OUTCOME**

Child receives appropriate blood elements without incident

NURSING DIAGNOSIS: Altered nutrition: less than body requirements related to reported inadequate iron intake (less than RDA); knowledge deficit regarding iron-rich foods

PATIENT GOAL 1: Will receive adequate supply of iron

- **NURSING INTERVENTIONS/RATIONALES**

Provide diet counseling to caregiver, especially in regard to:
    Food sources of iron (e.g., meat, liver, fish, egg yolks, green leafy vegetables, legumes, nuts, whole grains, iron-fortified infant cereal and dry cereal) (see also Chapter 11) *to ensure that child receives adequate supply of iron*
Feed milk as supplemental food in infant's diet after solids are begun *because overingestion of milk decreases child's intake of iron-rich solid foods*
Teach older child about importance of adequate iron in the diet *to encourage compliance*

- **EXPECTED OUTCOME**

Child receives at least minimum daily requirement of iron

*Dependent nursing action.

NURSING CARE PLAN
The Child with Anemia—cont'd

PATIENT GOAL 2: Will consume iron supplements

- **NURSING INTERVENTIONS/*RATIONALES***

*Administer iron preparations as prescribed
Instruct family regarding correct administration of oral iron preparation
  Give in divided doses (specify) *for maximum absorption*
  Give between meals *to increase absorption in upper gastro-intestinal tract*
  Administer with fruit juice or multivitamin preparation *because vitamin C appears to facilitate absorption of iron*
  Do not give with milk or antacids, *since they decrease absorption*

*Administer liquid preparation with dropper, syringe, or straw *to avoid contact with teeth and possible staining*
Assess characteristics of stools *because adequate dosage of oral iron turns stool a tarry green color*

- **EXPECTED OUTCOMES**

Family relates a diet history that verifies child's compliance with these suggestions
Child is given iron supplement as evidenced by green, tarry stools
Child takes medication appropriately

See also Nursing Care Plan: The Family of the Ill or Hospitalized Child, Chapter 21

*Dependent nursing action.

---

but is essential for definitive diagnosis of the leukemias, lymphomas, and certain anemias. Suggested explanations in teaching children about blood components are as follows:

NURSING TIP
Red blood cells—carry the oxygen you breathe from your lungs to all parts of your body.
White blood cells—help keep germs from causing infection.
Platelets—small parts of cells that help to make bleeding stop; platelets help your body stop bleeding by forming a clot (scab) over the hurt area.
Plasma—the liquid portion of blood; has clotting factors that help make the bleeding stop.

Decrease Tissue Oxygen Needs. Since the basic pathology in anemia is a decrease in oxygen-carrying capacity, an important nursing responsibility is to assess the child's energy level and minimize excess demands. The child's level of tolerance for activities of daily living and play is assessed, and adjustments are made to allow as much self-care as possible without undue exertion. During periods of rest the nurse takes vital signs and observes behavior to establish a baseline of nonexertion energy expenditure. During periods of activity the nurse repeats these measurements and observations to compare them with resting values.

| Nursing ALERT | Signs of exertion include tachycardia, palpitations, tachypnea, dyspnea, shortness of breath, hyperpnea, breathlessness, dizziness, lightheadedness, diaphoresis, and change in skin color. The child looks fatigued (sagging, limp posture; slow, strained movements; inability to tolerate additional activity). |

Diversional activities are planned that promote rest but prevent boredom and withdrawal. Since short attention span, irritability, and restlessness are common in anemia and increase stress demands on the body, appropriate activities are planned, such as listening to music; using a tape recorder; watching television; reading or listening to stories or comics; continuing a favorite hobby, such as stamp collecting, coloring, or drawing; playing board and card games; or being wheeled in a carriage or chair. Choosing the appropriate roommate, such as a child of similar age with a diagnosis that also requires restricted activity, is a helpful intervention.

If infants or young children are hospitalized, the importance of preventing separation from parents must be considered. Crying and fretfulness place increased stress demands on the body, which increases oxygen needs. Parents need help in understanding the importance of their presence, even though the child may be less responsive than usual. The nurse also explains the reason for mood changes and the necessity of allowing the child's dependency.

Prevent Complications. Children who are so severely anemic that they are hospitalized may require oxygen to prevent or reduce tissue hypoxia. Since these children are susceptible to infection, every effort is expended to prevent exposure to infectious agents. All the usual precautions are taken to prevent infection, such as practicing thorough handwashing, selecting an appropriate room in a noninfectious area, restricting visitors or hospital personnel with active infection, and maintaining adequate nutrition. The nurse also observes for signs of infection, particularly temperature elevation and leukocytosis.

Support Family. See Nursing Care Plan on pp. 908-909 for other supportive and educative strategies.

❖ Evaluation
The effectiveness of nursing interventions is determined by continual reassessment and evaluation of care based on the following observational guidelines and expected outcomes:

1. Interview child and family regarding their understanding of diagnostic procedures and the blood disorder, as well as regarding their feelings and concerns.

2. Monitor therapeutic interventions and child's tolerance for activity.
3. Assess child for evidence of complications of therapies.

Expected outcomes:
See Nursing Care Plan, pp. 908-909.

IRON DEFICIENCY ANEMIA

Anemia caused by an inadequate supply of dietary iron is the most prevalent nutritional disorder in the United States and the most common mineral disturbance. Almost 16% of lower-income children 6 to 24 months of age are anemic (Wimberly and Parks, 1991). However, the prevalence has decreased, probably in part because of families' participation in the Women, Infants, and Children (WIC) program, which provides iron-fortified formula for the first year of life (Oski, 1993). Premature infants are especially at risk because of their reduced fetal iron supply. Adolescents are also at risk because of their rapid growth rate combined with poor eating habits.

Pathophysiology

Iron deficiency anemia can be caused by any number of factors that decrease the supply of iron, impair its absorption, increase the body's need for iron, or affect the synthesis of Hb. Although the clinical manifestations and diagnostic evaluation are quite similar regardless of the cause, the therapeutic and nursing considerations depend on the specific reason for the iron deficiency. The following discussion is limited to iron deficiency anemia resulting from inadequate iron in the diet.

During the last trimester of pregnancy, iron is transferred from mother to fetus. Most of the iron is stored in the circulating erythrocytes of the fetus, with the remainder stored in the fetal liver, spleen, and bone marrow. These iron stores are usually adequate for the first 5 to 6 months in a full-term infant but for only 2 to 3 months in premature infants or multiple births. If dietary iron is not supplied to meet the infant's growth demands once the fetal iron stores are depleted, iron deficiency anemia results.

Although most infants with iron deficiency anemia are underweight, many are overweight because of excessive milk ingestion (known as *milk babies*). These children become anemic for two reasons. Milk, a poor source of iron, is given almost to the exclusion of solid foods, and some infants fed cow's milk have an increased fecal loss of blood.

Therapeutic Management

Once the diagnosis of iron deficiency anemia is made, therapeutic management focuses on increasing the amount of supplemental iron the child receives. This is usually done through dietary counseling and the administration of oral iron supplements.

In formula-fed infants the most convenient and best sources of supplemental iron are iron-fortified commercial formula and iron-fortified infant cereal. Iron-fortified formula provides a relatively constant and predictable amount of iron and is not associated with an increased incidence of gastrointestinal (GI) symptoms, such as colic, diarrhea, or constipation. Infants under 12 months of age should *not* be given fresh cow's milk to decrease the possibility of iron deficiency from GI blood loss occurring from allergy to the milk protein. Dietary addition of iron-rich foods is usually inad-

equate as the sole treatment of iron deficiency anemia, because the iron is poorly absorbed and provides insufficient supplemental quantities of iron.

If dietary sources of iron cannot replace body stores, oral iron supplements are prescribed for approximately 3 months. Ferrous iron, more readily absorbed than ferric iron, results in higher Hgb levels. Ascorbic acid (vitamin C) appears to facilitate absorption of iron and may be prescribed in addition to the iron preparation.

If the Hgb level is very low or if levels fail to rise after 1 month of oral therapy, intramuscular (IM) or IV iron is administered. Transfusions are indicated for the most severe anemia and in cases of serious infection, cardiac dysfunction, or surgical emergency when anesthesia is required. Packed RBCs, not whole blood, are used to minimize the chance of circulatory overload. Supplemental oxygen is administered when tissue hypoxia is severe.

Prognosis. The prognosis for a child with this condition is very good. However, there is some evidence that if the iron deficiency anemia is longstanding, mild cognitive impairment may result (Idjradinata and Pollitt, 1993).

Nursing Considerations

An essential nursing responsibility is instructing parents in the administration of iron. Oral iron should be given as prescribed in three divided doses between meals, when the presence of free hydrochloric acid is greatest, because more iron is absorbed in the acidic environment of the upper GI tract. A citrus fruit or juice taken with the medication aids in absorption.

An adequate dosage of oral iron turns the stools a tarry green color. The nurse advises parents of this normally expected change and inquires about its occurrence on follow-up visits. Absence of the greenish black stool may be a clue to poor administration of iron, either in schedule or in dosage. Vomiting and/or diarrhea can occur with iron therapy. If the parents report these symptoms, the iron can be given with meals and the dosage reduced and then gradually increased until tolerated.

Liquid preparations of iron may temporarily stain the teeth. If possible, the medication should be taken through a straw or given through a syringe or medicine dropper placed toward the back of the mouth. Brushing the teeth after administration of the drug lessens the discoloration.

If parenteral iron preparations are prescribed, iron dextran must be injected deeply into a large muscle mass using the Z-tract method. The injection site is *not* massaged after injection to minimize skin staining and irritation. Since no more than 1 ml should be given in one site, the IV route should be considered to avoid multiple injections. Careful observation is required because of the risk of adverse reactions, such as anaphylaxis with IV administration. A test dose is recommended before routine use.

Diet. A primary nursing objective is to prevent nutritional anemia through family education. The nurse discusses with parents the importance of using iron-fortified formula and the introduction of solid foods at the appropriate age. The best solid food source of iron is commercial infant cereals. It may be difficult at first to teach the infant to accept foods other than milk. The same principles are applied as those for introducing new foods (see Nutrition, Chapter 10), especially feeding the solid food before the milk. Predominantly milk-fed infants rebel against solid foods, and parents are cautioned about this and the need to be firm in not relinquishing control to the child. It may require intense problem solving on the part of both the family and the nurse to overcome the child's resistance.

A difficulty encountered in discouraging the parents from feeding milk to the exclusion of other foods is dispelling the popular myth that milk is a "perfect food." Many parents believe that milk is best for the infant and equate the weight gain with a "healthy child" and "good mothering." They are not concerned about providing other foods as long as the child continues to take milk. The nurse can also stress that overweight is not synonymous with good health.

Diet education of teenagers is especially difficult, especially since teenage girls are particularly prone to following weight-reduction diets. Emphasizing the effect of anemia on appearance (pallor) and energy level (difficulty maintaining popular activities) may be useful. (See Chapter 11—Mineral Disturbances and Table 11-2—for sources of iron-rich foods.)

SICKLE CELL ANEMIA (SCA)

SCA is one of a group of diseases collectively termed *hemoglobinopathies,* in which normal adult hemoglobin (hemoglobin A [HbA]) is partly or completely replaced by abnormal sickle hemoglobin (HbS). *Sickle cell disease (SCD)* includes all those hereditary disorders whose clinical, hematologic, and pathologic features are related to the presence of HbS. Even though SCD is sometimes used to refer to SCA, this use is incorrect. Other correct terms for SCA are *SS* and *homozygous sickle cell disease.*

In the United States the most common forms of SCD are the following:

1. **Sickle cell trait,** the heterozygous form of the disease (HbA and HbS, HbAS, or SA)
2. **Sickle cell anemia,** the homozygous form of the disease (HbSS or SS)
3. **Sickle cell–C disease,** a heterozygous variant of SCD, including both HbS and HbC (SC)
4. **Sickle cell–hemoglobin E disease,** a variant of SCD in which glutamic acid has been substituted for lysine in the number-26 position of the β-chain (SE)
5. **Sickle thalassemia disease,** a combination of sickle cell trait and β-thalassemia trait (Sβthal)

Of the SCDs, SCA is the most common form in African Americans, followed by sickle cell–C disease and sickle β-thalassemia.

SCA infrequently affects Caucasians, especially those of Mediterranean descent. The incidence of the disease varies in different geographic locations. Among African Americans the incidence of sickle cell trait is about 8%. In West Africa the incidence is reported to be as high as 40% among native blacks. The high incidence of sickle cell trait in West Africans is believed by some to be the result of selective protection afforded trait carriers against one type of malaria.

The gene that determines the production of HbS is situated on an autosome and, when present, is always detectable and therefore dominant. Heterozygous persons who have hemoglobin containing both normal HbA and abnormal HbS are said to have *sickle cell trait.* Persons who are homozygous have predominantly HbS and have *sickle cell anemia.*

The inheritance pattern is essentially that of an autosomal recessive disorder (see Appendix B). Therefore, when both parents have sickle cell trait, there is a 25% chance of their producing an offspring with SCA.

Although the defect is inherited, the sickling phenomenon is usually not apparent until later in infancy because of the presence of fetal hemoglobin (HbF). As long as HbF persists, sickling does not occur because there is less HbS. The newborn has from 60% to 80% HbF, but this rapidly decreases during the first year, so the child is at risk for sickle cell–related complications (Sickle Cell Disease Guideline Panel, 1993).

Pathophysiology

The clinical features of SCA are primarily the result of (1) *obstruction* caused by the sickled RBCs and (2) increased RBC *destruction* (Fig. 26-1). The entanglement and enmeshing of rigid sickle-shaped cells with one another intermittently block the microcirculation, causing vaso-occlusion. The resultant absence of blood flow to adjacent tissues causes local hypoxia, leading to tissue ischemia and infarction (cellular death). Most of the complications seen in SCA can be traced to this process and its impact on various organs of the body.

CLINICAL MANIFESTATIONS OF SICKLE CELL ANEMIA (SCA)

General
Possible growth retardation
Chronic anemia (Hgb 6 to 9 g/dl)
Possible delayed sexual maturation
Marked susceptibility to sepsis

Vaso-occlusive Crisis
Pain in area(s) of involvement
Manifestations related to ischemia of involved areas:
  Extremities: painful swelling of hands and feet (sickle cell dactylitis, or "hand-foot syndrome"), painful joints
  Abdomen: severe pain resembling acute surgical condition
  Cerebrum: stroke, visual disturbances
  Chest: symptoms resembling pneumonia, protracted episodes of pulmonary disease
  Liver: obstructive jaundice, hepatic coma
  Kidney: hematuria
  Genital: priapism (painful constant penile erection)

Sequestration Crisis
Pooling of large amounts of blood:
  Hepatomegaly
  Splenomegaly
  Circulatory collapse

Effects of Chronic Vaso-occlusive Phenomena
Heart: cardiomegaly, systolic murmurs
Lungs: altered pulmonary function, susceptibility to infections, pulmonary insufficiency
Kidneys: inability to concentrate urine, progressive renal failure, enuresis
Liver: hepatomegaly, cirrhosis, intrahepatic cholestasis
Spleen: splenomegaly, susceptibility to infection, functional reduction in splenic activity progressing to autosplenectomy
Eyes: intraocular abnormalities with visual disturbances, sometimes progressive retinal detachment and blindness
Extremities: skeletal deformities, especially lordosis and kyphosis, chronic leg ulcers, susceptibility to osteomyelitis
Central nervous system: hemiparesis, seizures (acute, not chronic)

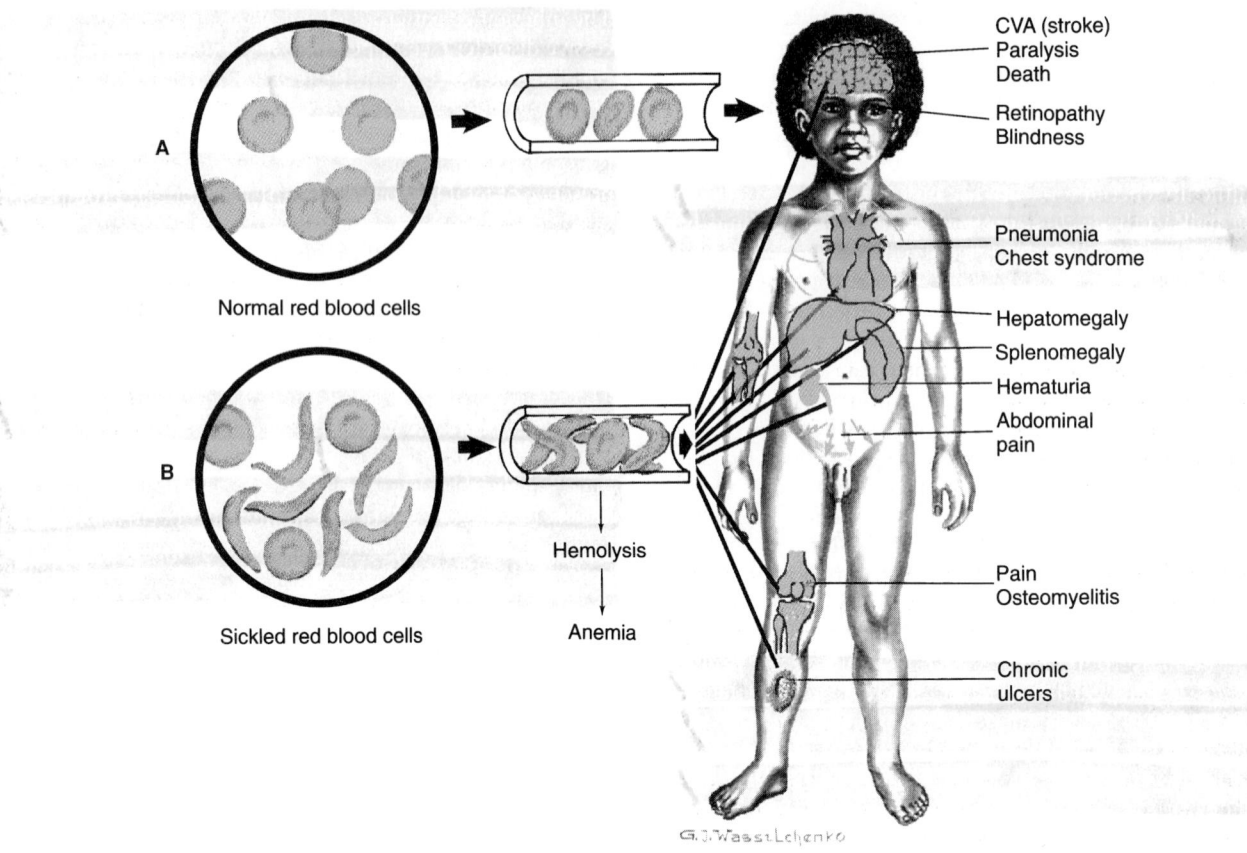

Normal red blood cells

Sickled red blood cells

Hemolysis

Anemia

CVA (stroke)
Paralysis
Death

Retinopathy
Blindness

Pneumonia
Chest syndrome

Hepatomegaly
Splenomegaly
Hematuria
Abdominal
pain

Pain
Osteomyelitis

Chronic
ulcers

G.J.Wassilchenko

FIG. 26-1. Differences between normal and sickled blood cells.

The effect of sickling and infarction on organ structures occurs in the following sequence (see also consequences in the box on p. 911):

1. Stasis with enlargement
2. Infarction with ischemia and destruction
3. Replacement with fibrous tissue (scarring)

Clinical Manifestations

The clinical manifestations of SCA vary greatly in severity and frequency. The most acute symptoms of the disease occur during periods of exacerbation called *crises.* There are several types of episodic crises: vaso-occlusive, acute splenic sequestration, aplastic, hyperhemolytic, cerebrovascular accident (stroke), chest syndrome, and infection. The crises may occur individually or concomitantly with one or more other crises. The episode may be a *vaso-occlusive crisis,* preferably called a "painful episode," characterized by distal ischemia and pain; *sequestration crisis,* a pooling of blood in liver and spleen with decreased blood volume and shock; *aplastic crisis,* diminished RBC production resulting in profound anemia; or *hyperhemolytic crisis,* an accelerated rate of RBC destruction characterized by anemia, jaundice, and reticulocytosis. This complication frequently suggests other coexisting conditions, such as viral illness, or glucose-6-phosphate dehydrogenase (G6PD) deficiency, which is also common in African Americans.

Another serious complication is *chest syndrome,* which is clinically similar to pneumonia. It is associated with chest pain, fever, pneumonia-like cough, and associated anemia. A *cerebrovascular accident (CVA, stroke)* is a sudden and severe complication, often with no related illnesses. Sickled cells block the major blood vessels in the brain, resulting in cerebral infarction, which causes variable degrees of neurologic impairment. Repeat CVAs causing progressively greater brain damage occur in 60% of children who have already experienced one stroke.

Diagnostic Evaluation

Newborn screening for SCA is mandatory in most of the United States so that infants can be identified before symptoms occur. At birth the infant has up to 80% of HbF, which does not carry the defect. During the first months of life the infant begins production of RBCs with HbA and with HbS if the gene is present. At this point the child may become symptomatic. Since levels of HbS are low at birth, hemoglobin electrophoresis or other tests that measure Hgb concentrations are indicated. Early diagnosis (before 3 months of age) enables initiation of appropriate interventions to minimize complications. The family is taught to administer prophylactic antibiotics and identify early signs of *infection* in order to seek medical therapy as soon as possible.

If SCA is not diagnosed in early infancy, it is likely to manifest symptoms during the toddler and preschool years. SCA is occasionally first diagnosed during a crisis that follows an acute respiratory or GI infection. Routine hematologic tests are done to evaluate the anemia. Several specific tests detect the presence of the abnormal Hb in the heterozygote and/or the homozygote. For screening purposes the *sickle-turbidity test (Sickledex)* is frequently used, since it can be performed on blood from a finger stick and yields accurate results in 3 minutes. However, if the test is positive, Hgb electrophoresis is necessary to distinguish between those children with the trait and those with the disease. *Hemoglobin electrophoresis* ("finger-printing" of the protein) is an accurate, rapid, and specific test for detecting the homozygous and heterozygous forms of the disease, as well as the percentages of the various hemoglobins.

Therapeutic Management

There is no cure for SCA. The aims of therapy are (1) to prevent conditions that enhance sickling phenomena, which are responsible for the pathologic sequelae, and (2) to treat the medical emergencies of sickle cell crisis. Prevention consists of maintaining hemodilution. The successful implementation of this goal depends more often on nursing interventions than on medical therapies.

Medical management of a crisis is usually directed at supportive and symptomatic treatment. The main objectives are to provide (1) bed rest to minimize energy expenditure and oxygen use, (2) hydration through oral and IV therapy, (3) electrolyte replacement, (4) analgesics for the severe abdominal and joint pain, (5) blood replacement to treat anemia, and (6) antibiotics to treat any existing infection.

Administration of pneumococcal and meningococcal vaccines beginning at 2 years of age is recommended for these children because of their susceptibility to infection as a result of functional asplenia. With the likelihood of transfusion therapy for individuals with SCA, hepatitis B vaccine is recommended for those children who have not received it as part of their routine immunization schedule. (See Immunizations, Chapter 10.) Oral penicillin prophylaxis is also recommended twice daily (Sickle Cell Disease Guideline Panel, 1993).

Short-term oxygen therapy may be helpful if a child has symptoms of respiratory difficulty. Severe hypoxia must be prevented because this causes massive systemic sickling that can be fatal. Although oxygen may prevent more sickling, it usually is not effective in reversing sickling, since the oxygen is unable to reach the enmeshed sickled erythrocytes in clogged vessels. In addition, prolonged administration can depress bone marrow, further aggravating the anemia.

Exchange transfusion, which reduces the number of circulating sickle cells and slows down the vicious cycle of hypoxia, thrombosis, tissue ischemia, and injury, has been successful. The procedure is sometimes advocated as a possible preventive technique. However, multiple transfusions carry the risk of hepatitis, hemosiderosis, and transfusion reactions. Once a CVA has occurred, blood transfusions are usually given every 4 to 5 weeks to help prevent a repeat stroke. To reduce iron overload, home subcutaneous chelation therapy may be started (see p. 916).

In children with recurrent splenic sequestration, splenectomy may be a lifesaving measure. However, since the spleen usually atrophies on its own through progressive fibrotic changes *(functional asplenia)*, routine splenectomy is not recommended. Any procedure that requires anesthesia has increased risk for these children. *Painful priapism (continual erection)* may be treated by aspiration of the corpora cavernosum. This complication is particularly frequent in vaso-occlusive crises.

The most frequent problem for patients with SCA is *vaso-occlusive pain*. The chronic nature of this pain can greatly affect the child's development. A multidisciplinary approach is best for its management. When mild to moderate pain is reported, ibuprofen or acetaminophen is used initially. If these drugs are not effective alone, codeine can be added. The dosages of both drugs are titrated (adjusted) to a therapeutic level. Opioids such as immediate- and sustained-release morphine, oxycodone, hydromorphone (Dilaudid), and methadone are administered intravenously or orally for severe pain and are given around the clock. Patient-controlled analgesia (PCA) has been used successfully for sickle cell–related pain. PCA reinforces the patient's role and responsibility in managing the pain and provides flexibility in dealing with pain, which may vary in severity over time. The use of high-dose IV methylprednisolone has decreased the duration of severe pain in children (Griffin, McIntire, and Buchanan, 1994). (See Pain Management, Chapter 21.)

Nursing ALERT	Meperidine (pethidine [Demerol]) is not recommended. Normeperidine, a metabolite of meperidine, is a central nervous system stimulant that produces anxiety, tremors, myoclonus, and generalized seizures when it accumulates with repetitive dosing. Patients with SCD are particularly at risk for normeperidine-induced seizures (American Pain Society, 1992).

Prognosis. The prognosis varies. Most of the time, children are without symptoms and participate in normal activities without restrictions. The greatest risk is usually in children between 1 and 3 years of age, and the majority of deaths in these children and individuals under age 20 are caused by overwhelming infection. Consequently, SCA is a chronic illness with a potentially terminal outcome.

Individuals with low levels of HbF are more likely to die earlier than those with higher levels (Platt and others, 1994). Research is investigating hydroxyurea and erythropoietin, which may increase the concentration of HbF and ultimately reduce complications (Charache, 1994). Bone marrow transplant may be a possible cure for SCD (Johnson and others, 1994; Vermylen and Cornu, 1994) (see p. 945).

Nursing Considerations

❖ Assessment

Many nurses are involved in screening programs for SCA to identify persons with the abnormal Hb in order to implement therapy for homozygotes and provide genetic counseling for heterozygotes. Young children from families of at-risk racial or geographic origins who exhibit any of the signs previously described are advised to seek medical attention immediately.

Assessment of the child in sickle cell crisis involves all areas and systems that can be affected by circulatory obstruction, including vital signs, neurologic signs, vision, and hearing assessment, as well as assessment of the respiratory, GI, renal, and musculoskeletal systems. It is also important to assess the location and intensity of pain (see Pain Assessment, Chapter 21).

NURSING DIAGNOSES: THE CHILD WITH SICKLE CELL ANEMIA

High risk for infection related to decreased or absent splenic function

Impaired physical mobility related to tissue ischemia, generalized weakness

Altered family processes related to child with a chronic condition

Sickle Cell Crisis

Pain related to tissue ischemia (sickle cell crisis)

Altered tissue perfusion related to impaired arterial blood flow

---

 FAMILY FOCUS
Fear of Addiction

Although pain is usually severe and opioids are warranted, many families fear that their child will become addicted to the narcotic. Unfortunately, misinformed health professionals may foster this unfounded fear, resulting in needless suffering. Few, if any, children who receive opioids for severe pain become behaviorally addicted to the drug (Morrison, 1991). Families and older children, especially adolescents, need to be reassured that opioids are medically indicated, high doses may be needed, and addiction is rare.

❖ Nursing Diagnoses

Nursing diagnoses are derived from observation and assessment of children with the disease or those in crisis (see box). Others will be apparent depending on the state of the child's health, the organs involved, and the individual needs of the child and family.

❖ Planning

The primary goals are as follows:

1. Family and child (when appropriate) will receive education regarding the sickling phenomenon and possible consequences and early recognition of crises and infection.
2. Child will receive supportive therapies during crises.
3. Child and parents will adjust to a lifelong, potentially fatal hereditary disease.
4. Family members will receive genetic counseling.

❖ Implementation

Educate Family and Child. Family education begins with an explanation of the disease and its consequences. Following this explanation, the most important issues to teach the family are to (1) seek early intervention for problems, such as fever of 38.5° C (101.5° F) or greater; (2) give penicillin as ordered; (3) recognize signs and symptoms of splenic sequestration, as well as respiratory problems that can lead to hypoxia; and (4) treat child normally. The nurse tells families that the child is normal but can get sick in ways that other children cannot.

NURSING TIP One simple yet graphic way to demonstrate the effect of sickling is to roll rounded objects, such as marbles or beads, through a tube to simulate normal circulation and then roll pointed objects, such as screws or jacks, through the tube. The effect of sickling and clumping of the pointed objects is especially noticeable at a bend or slight narrowing of the tube.

The nurse emphasizes the importance of adequate hydration to prevent sickling and to delay the stasis-thrombosis-ischemia cycle in a crisis. It is not sufficient to advise parents to "force fluids" or "encourage drinking." They need specific instructions on how many daily glasses or bottles of fluid are required. Many foods are also a source of fluid, particularly soups, popsicles, ice cream, sherbet, gelatin, and puddings.

heat will help
never ice

Nursing ALERT Advise parents to be particularly alert to situations where dehydration may be a possibility, such as hot weather, and to recognize early signs of reduced intake, such as decreased urine output (e.g., fewer wet diapers) and increased thirst.

Increased fluids combined with impaired kidney function result in the problem of *enuresis*. Parents who are unaware of this fact frequently employ the usual measures to discourage bed-wetting, such as limiting fluids at night, and may resort to punishment and shame to force bladder control. Enuresis is treated as a complication of the disease, such as joint pain or some other symptom, in order to alleviate parental pressure on the child.

Promote Supportive Therapies During Crises. The success of many of the medical therapies relies heavily on nursing implementation. Management of pain is an especially difficult problem and often involves experimenting with various analgesics, including opioids, and schedules before relief is achieved. Unfortunately, these children tend to be undermedicated, resulting in their "clock watching" and demands for additional doses sooner than might be expected. Often this incorrectly raises suspicions of drug addiction, when in fact the problem is one of improper dosage (see Family Focus box). In choosing and scheduling analgesics, the goal should be *prevention* of pain.

Any pain program should be combined with psychologic support to help the child deal with the depression, anxiety, and fear that may accompany the disease. This includes regular visits with the child to discuss any concerns during the hospitalization and positive reinforcement of coping skills, such as successful methods of dealing with the pain and compliance with treatment prescriptions.

Frequently, heat to the affected area is soothing. Cold compresses are not applied to the area because this enhances sickling and vasoconstriction. Bed rest is usually well tolerated during a crisis, although actual rest depends greatly on pain alleviation and organized schedules of nursing care. Some activity, particularly passive range-of-motion exercises, is beneficial to promote circulation. Usually the best course of action is to let children dictate their activity tolerance.

If blood transfusions or exchange transfusions are given, the nurse has the responsibility of observing for signs of transfusion reaction (see Table 26-4). Since hypervolemia from too rapid transfusion can increase the workload of the heart, the nurse also is alert to signs of cardiac failure.

In splenic sequestration the size of the spleen is gently measured by abdominal palpation (see Abdomen, Chapter 7). The nurse should be aware of spleen size because an increasing splenomegaly is an ominous sign. A decreasing spleen size denotes response to therapy. Vital signs and blood pressure are also closely monitored for impending shock. Anemia is typically not a presenting complication in vaso-occlusive crises but is a critical problem in other types of crises. The nurse monitors for evidence of increasing anemia and institutes appropriate nursing intervention (see p. 908). If oxygen is ordered, pulse oximetry values for blood oxygen saturation are monitored for evidence of the oxygen's benefit. No improvement in oxygen saturation is especially important to report. The drug oxygen can have side effects, such as decreasing RBC production.

Intake, especially of IV fluids, and output are recorded. The child's weight should be taken on admission, since it serves as a baseline for evaluating hydration. Since diuresis can result in electrolyte loss, the nurse also observes for signs of hypokalemia and should be familiar with normal serum electrolyte values to report changes.

Recognize Other Complications. Nurses also need to be aware of the signs of chest syndrome and CVA, both potentially fatal complications.

Support Family. Families need the opportunity to discuss their feelings regarding transmitting a potentially fatal, chronic illness to their child. Because of the widely publicized prognosis for children with SCA, many parents express their prevalent fear of the child's death. Since there is no way to predict which child will follow a favorable course, nursing care for the family should be the same as for any family with a child with a life-threatening illness. Particular emphasis is placed on the siblings' reactions, the stress on the marital relationship, and the childrearing attitudes displayed toward the child (see Chapter 18). Several resources are available to the family with a sickling disorder.*

The nurse advises parents to inform all treating personnel of the child's condition. The use of medical identification, such as a bracelet, is another way of ensuring awareness of the disease.

If family members have the SCD trait and/or SCA, genetic counseling is necessary. A primary goal is informing parents who carry the trait, in language they can understand, of the 1-in-4 risk of having a child with the disease.

❖ Evaluation

The effectiveness of nursing interventions is determined by continual reassessment and evaluation of care based on the following observational guidelines and expected outcomes:

1. Interview family regarding their understanding of the disease, the sickling phenomena, its consequences, and early recognition of complications.

---

*A Sickle Cell Home Study Kit For Families is available from the **National Association for Sickle Cell Disease, Inc.,** 3345 Wilshire Blvd., Suite 1106, Los Angeles, CA 90010-1880; (800) 421-8453. Additional resources are **Howard University, Center for Sickle Cell Disease,** 2121 Georgia Ave., N.W., Washington, DC 20059, (202) 806-7930; **National Sickle Cell Disease Program, National Heart, Lung, and Blood Institute,** Bldg 31, Room 4A-21, Rockville Pike, Bethesda, MD 20205, (301) 496-4236; and **Sickle Cell Association of Ontario,** 1076 Bathurst St., Suite 305, Toronto, Ontario M5R 3G9, (416) 789-2855.

| **Nursing ALERT** | Report signs of the following immediately: |

Chest syndrome:
    Severe chest pain, sometimes spreading to abdomen
    Fever of 38.8° C (102° F) or higher
    Very congested cough
    Dyspnea, tachypnea
    Retractions
    Declining oxygen saturation (oximetry)
Cerebrovascular accident (CVA, stroke):
    Jerking or twitching of the face, legs, or arms
    Seizures
    Strange, abnormal behavior
    Inability to move an arm and/or a leg
    Stagger or an unsteady walk
    Stutter or slurred speech
    Weakness in the hands, feet, or legs
    Changes in vision
    Severe, unrelieved headaches
    Severe vomiting

2. Observe child for any evidence of sickling; monitor preventive strategies and therapies, especially pain assessment and management.
3. Interview and observe child and family regarding the way the disease has affected their lives.
4. Interview the family to determine their understanding of the risk of having another child with SCA.
5. Ensure that medical attention is sought appropriately.

Expected outcomes:

1. Family demonstrates an understanding of the disease and its consequences and verbalizes symptoms to report (specify knowledge and method of demonstration).
2. Family gives antibiotic on a consistent basis.
3. Child exhibits few episodes of sickling; pain is effectively controlled.
4. Family takes advantage of genetic counseling services and medical care.
5. Child and family express their feelings and concerns regarding the disease.

See also Nursing Care Plan: The Child with Sickle Cell Disease.*

β-THALASSEMIA (COOLEY ANEMIA)

The term *thalassemia,* which is derived from the Greek word *thalassa,* meaning "sea," is applied to a variety of inherited blood disorders characterized by deficiencies in the rate of production of specific globin chains in hemoglobin. The name appropriately refers to descendants of or those people living near the Mediterranean sea who have the highest incidence of the disease, namely, Italians, Greeks, and Syrians. Evidence suggests that the high incidence of the disorders among these groups is a result of selective advantage of the trait to malaria, as is postulated in sickle cell disease.

β-Thalassemia is the most common of the thalassemias and occurs in three forms: a heterozygous form, *thalassemia minor* or *thalassemia trait,* which produces a mild microcytic

---

*In Wong DL: *Wong and Whaley's Clinical manual of pediatric nursing,* ed 4, St Louis, 1996, Mosby.

anemia; *thalassemia intermedia,* which is manifested as splenomegaly and moderate to severe anemia; and a homozygous form, *thalassemia major* (also known as *Cooley anemia*), which results in a severe anemia that would lead to cardiac failure and death in early childhood without transfusion support.

Pathophysiology

Normal postnatal hemoglobin is composed of 2 α- and 2 β-polypeptide chains. In β-thalassemia there is a partial or complete deficiency in the synthesis of the β-chain of the Hgb molecule. Consequently, there is a compensatory increase in the synthesis of α-chains, and γ-chain production remains activated, resulting in defective Hgb formation. This unbalanced polypeptide unit is very unstable; when it disintegrates, it damages RBCs, causing severe anemia.

To compensate for the hemolytic process, an overabundance of erythrocytes is formed unless the bone marrow is suppressed by transfusion therapy. Excess iron from hemolysis of supplemental RBCs in transfusions and from the rapid destruction of defective cells is stored in various organs *(hemosiderosis).*

Diagnostic Evaluation

The onset of thalassemia major may be insidious and not recognized until the latter half of infancy. The clinical effects of thalassemia major are primarily attributable to (1) defective synthesis of hemoglobin A, (2) structurally impaired RBCs, and (3) shortened life span of erythrocytes (see box).

Hematologic studies reveal the characteristic changes in RBCs and immature erythrocytes. Low Hgb and Hct levels are seen in severe anemia, although they are typically lower than the reduction in RBC count because of the prolifera-

---

CLINICAL MANIFESTATIONS OF β-THALASSEMIA

Anemia (Before Diagnosis)
Unexplained fever
Poor feeding
Greatly enlarged spleen

With Progressive Anemia
Signs of chronic hypoxia
    Headache
    Precordial and bone pain
    Decreased exercise tolerance
    Listlessness
    Anorexia

Other Features
Small stature
Delayed sexual maturation
Bronzed, freckled complexion (if not chelated)

Bone Changes (Older Children if Untreated)
Enlarged head
Prominent frontal and parietal bosses
Prominent malar eminences
Flat or depressed bridge of the nose
Enlarged maxilla
Protrusion of the lip and upper central incisors and eventual
   malocclusion
Oriental appearance of eyes

---

tion of immature erythrocytes. Hemoglobin electrophoresis confirms the diagnosis, and radiographs of involved bones reveal characteristic findings.

Therapeutic Management

The objective of supportive therapy is to maintain sufficient Hb levels to prevent bone marrow expansion and the resulting bony deformities, as well as to provide sufficient RBCs to support normal growth and normal physical activity. Transfusions are the foundation of medical management. Recent studies have evaluated the benefits of maintaining the child's Hb level above 10 g/dl, a goal that may require transfusions as often as every 3 weeks. The advantages of this therapy include (1) improved physical and psychologic well-being because of the ability to participate in normal activities, (2) decreased cardiomegaly and hepatosplenomegaly, (3) fewer bone changes, and (4) normal or near-normal growth and development until puberty.

One of the potential complications of frequent blood transfusions is iron overload. Since the body has no effective means of eliminating the excess iron, the mineral is deposited in body tissues. To minimize the development of hemosiderosis, deferoxamine (Desferal), an iron-chelating agent, is given with small oral supplements of vitamin C. Deferoxamine is given intravenously or subcutaneously, often at home using a portable infusion pump, over 8 to 24 hours on a daily basis. Creative strategies such as behavioral contracting have been used to assist the child in complying with the deferoxamine regimen (Koch and others, 1993).

In some children with severe splenomegaly who demonstrate increased transfusion requirements, a splenectomy may be necessary. Over time the spleen may accelerate the rate of RBC destruction and thus increase transfusion requirements. After a splenectomy, children generally require fewer transfusions, although the basic defect in Hb synthesis remains unaffected. A major postsplenectomy complication is severe and overwhelming infection. Therefore these children are kept on prophylactic antibiotics with close medical supervision for many years and should receive the pneumococcal and meningococcal vaccines (see Immunizations, Chapter 10).

> **Nursing ALERT** Ensure family/patient understands the need to notify health professional of all fevers of 38.5° C (101.5° F) or greater because of risk of sepsis in a child with asplenia.

Prognosis. Most children treated with blood transfusion and early chelation therapy survive well into adulthood. The most common cause of death is iron-induced heart disease, followed by infection, liver disease, and malignancy (Zurlo and others, 1989). A promising treatment for some children is bone marrow transplantation (see p. 945). In one study, children under 16 years of age who underwent allogeneic bone marrow transplantation had a 59% to 98% rate of complication-free survival (Lucarelli and others, 1990).

Nursing Considerations

The objectives of nursing care are to (1) promote compliance with transfusion and chelation therapy, (2) assist the child in coping with the anxiety-provoking treatments and the effects of the illness, and (3) foster the child's and family's adjustment to a chronic illness. Basic to each of these goals is explaining to parents and older children the defect responsible for the disorder, its effect on RBCs, and the potential effects of untreated iron overload, such as diabetes and heart disease. Since the prevalence of this condition is high among families of Mediterranean descent, the nurse also inquires about the family's previous knowledge about thalassemia. All families with a child with thalassemia should be tested for the trait and referred for genetic counseling.

As with any chronic illness, the needs of the family must be met for optimum adjustment to the stresses imposed by the disorder (see Chapter 18). One source of information for the family is the **Cooley's Anemia Foundation.*** Genetic counseling for the parents and fertile offspring is mandatory, and both prenatal diagnosis using amniocentesis at 10 weeks of gestation or fetal blood sampling at 20 weeks and screening for thalassemia trait are available.

APLASTIC ANEMIA

Aplastic anemia refers to a condition in which all formed elements of the blood are simultaneously depressed. The peripheral blood smear demonstrates pancytopenia or the triad of profound anemia, leukopenia, and thombocytopenia. *Hypoplastic anemia* is characterized by a profound depression of RBCs, but normal or slightly decreased white blood cells (WBCs) and platelets.

Etiology

Aplastic anemia can be *primary (congenital)* or *secondary (acquired).* The best-known congenital disorder of which aplastic anemia is an outstanding feature is *Fanconi syndrome,* a rare hereditary disorder characterized by pancytopenia, hypoplasia of the bone marrow, and patchy brown discoloration of the skin due to the deposition of melanin and associated with multiple congenital anomalies of the musculoskeletal and genitourinary systems. The syndrome appears to be inherited as an autosomal recessive trait with varying penetrance; therefore affected siblings may demonstrate several different combinations of defects.

Several factors contribute to the development of acquired

*129-09 26th Ave., Flushing, NY 11354; (718) 321-2873 or (800) 522-7222.

COMMON CAUSES OF ACQUIRED APLASTIC ANEMIA

Infection with the human parvovirus (HPV), hepatitis, or overwhelming infection

Irradiation

Drugs such as the chemotherapeutic agents and several antibiotics, one of the most notable being chloramphenicol

Industrial and household chemicals, including benzene and its derivatives, which are found in petroleum products, dyes, paint remover, shellac, and lacquers

Infiltration and replacement of myeloid elements, such as in leukemia or the lymphomas

Idiopathic, in which no identifiable precipitating cause can be found

---

hypoplastic anemia. The most common causes of acquired aplastic anemia are listed in the box. The following discussion focuses on acquired aplastic anemia, which carries a poorer prognosis and follows a more rapidly fatal course than do the primary types.

Diagnostic Evaluation

The onset of clinical manifestations, which include anemia, leukopenia, and decreased platelet count, is usually insidious, not unlike that seen in leukemia. Definitive diagnosis is determined from bone marrow aspiration, which demonstrates the conversion of red bone marrow to yellow, fatty bone marrow.

Therapeutic Management

The objectives of treatment are based on the recognition that the underlying disease process is failure of the bone marrow to carry out its hematopoietic functions. Therefore therapy is directed at restoring function to the marrow and involves two main approaches: (1) immunosuppressive therapy to remove the presumed immunologic functions that prolong aplasia and/or (2) replacement of the bone marrow through transplantation. Bone marrow transplantation is the treatment of choice for severe aplastic anemia when a suitable donor exists.

Currently, *antilymphocyte globulin (ALG)* or *antithymocyte globulin (ATG)* is the principal drug treatment for aplastic anemia. The rationale for using ATG is based on the theory that aplastic anemia may be the result of autoimmunity. ATG suppresses T-cell-dependent autoimmune responses but does not cause bone marrow suppression. The optimum schedule for ATG administration is still under investigation. It is usually given intravenously over 12 to 16 hours, after a test dose to check for hypersensitivity. Subsequent doses are given depending on the reduction in circulating lymphocytes.

Colony-stimulating factors (CSFs), given parenterally, may be used to enhance bone marrow production. Androgens may be used with ATG to stimulate erythropoiesis, although the exact mechanism of erythropoietic action is unclear. Cyclosporine may also be administered in children who fail to respond to ATG, and success has also been achieved using high-dose methylprednisolone. IV immunoglobulin has been used with success in aplastic anemia of infectious origin (Dwyer, 1992).

Because of the relatively poor prognosis in aplastic anemia treated with drug therapy, bone marrow transplantation should be considered *early* in the course of the disease if a compatible donor can be found. Transplantation is more successful when performed before multiple transfusions have sensitized the child to leukocyte and HLA antigens. Bone marrow transplantation is associated with a 63% 5-year survival rate (Pinkel, 1993; Sanders and others, 1994).

Nursing Considerations

The care of the child with aplastic anemia is similar to that of the child with leukemia (p. 922)—specifically, preparing the child and family for the diagnostic and therapeutic procedures, preventing complications from the severe pancytopenia, and emotionally supporting them in terms of a potentially fatal outcome. Since each of these nursing considerations is discussed in the section on leukemia, only the exceptions are presented here.

The drug ATG is usually administered by way of a central vein. If not, vigilant care must be directed to the IV infusion to prevent extravasation. Meticulous care of the venous access is essential because of the child's susceptibility to infection. CSFs are usually given by subcutaneous injection over several days. The typical anesthetic cream EMLA minimizes the puncture pain.

Testosterone produces several undesirable effects that, when combined with the effects of steroid therapy, such as moon face, result in dramatic body image alterations. The virilizing effects of testosterone include deepening of the voice, hirsutism, growth of pubic hair, enlargement of the penis in males, flushing of the skin, and acne. Potentially, testosterone can cause muscular and skeletal maturation, resulting in severely retarded height in a young child. Not only are these changes difficult to accept, but they also are especially difficult to explain to children not approaching puberty. Parents may feel embarrassed because they are unprepared for the sexual changes. Information and support are available from the **Aplastic Anemia Foundation of America.***

Since chemotherapeutic agents may be used, many of the reactions, such as nausea and vomiting, alopecia, and painful mucosal ulceration, can be encountered. In addition, extensive ecchymotic areas of the oral mucosa that result from thrombocytopenia require meticulous mouth care to prevent breakdown, bleeding, and infection. Local anesthetics are usually not necessary, but anorexia is still a consequence because of the edematous nature of the lesions. Liquid, bland, and soft diets are usually tolerated best (see Feeding the Sick Child, Chapter 22). Specialized care is required for children who have a bone marrow transplant (see p. 945).

DEFECTS IN HEMOSTASIS

Hemostasis is the process that stops bleeding when a blood vessel is injured. Vascular and plasma clotting factors, as well as platelets, are required. A complex system of clotting, anticlotting, and clot breakdown *(fibrinolysis)* exists in equilibrium to ensure clot formation only in the presence of blood vessel injury and to limit the clotting process to the site of vessel wall injury. Dysfunction in these systems will lead to bleeding or abnormal clotting. Although the coagulation process is complex, clotting depends on three factors: (1) vascular influence, (2) platelet role, and (3) clotting factors.

HEMOPHILIA

The term *hemophilia* refers to a group of bleeding disorders in which there is a deficiency of one of the factors necessary for coagulation of the blood. Although the symptomatology is similar regardless of which clotting factor is deficient, the identification of specific factor deficiencies allows definitive treatment with replacement agents.

In about 80% of all cases of hemophilia, the inheritance pattern is demonstrated as X-linked recessive (see Appendix B). The two most common forms of the disorder are *factor*

VIII deficiency (hemophilia A or *classic hemophilia)*, and *factor IX deficiency (hemophilia B* or *Christmas disease)*. The following discussion is primarily concerned with factor VIII deficiency, which accounts for about 75% of all cases.

Pathophysiology

The basic defect of hemophilia A is a deficiency of *factor VIII (antihemophilic factor [AHF])*. AHF is produced by the liver and is necessary for the formation of thromboplastin in phase I of blood coagulation. The less AHF found in the blood, the more severe is the disease. Individuals with hemophilia have two of the three factors required for coagulation, vascular influence, and platelets. Therefore they may bleed for longer periods, but not a faster rate.

Bleeding into tissue can occur anywhere, but hemorrhage into joint cavities and muscles is the most frequent type of internal bleeding. Bony changes and crippling deformities occur after repeated bleeding episodes over several years. Bleeding in the neck, mouth, or thorax is serious, since the airway can become obstructed. Intracranial hemorrhage can result in fatal consequences. Hemorrhage anywhere along the GI tract can lead to anemia, and hematomas in the spinal cord can cause paralysis.

Diagnostic Evaluation

Overt, prolonged hemorrhage is readily apparent; bleeding into tissues is less apparent (see box). The diagnosis is usually made from a history of bleeding episodes, evidence of X-linked inheritance (only one third of the cases are new mutations), and laboratory findings. The tests specific for hemophilia plasma depend on specific factors for a reaction to occur, such as the partial thromboplastin time (PTT). Specific determination of factor deficiencies requires assay procedures normally performed in specialized laboratories.

Therapeutic Management

The primary therapy for hemophilia is replacement of the missing clotting factor. The products currently available are (1) *factor VIII concentrate* from pooled plasma or a genetically engineered recombinant, to be reconstituted with sterile water immediately before use; (2) *cryoprecipitate,* a concentrated form of AHF plus fibrinogen; and (3) *DDAVP (1-deamino-8-D-arginine vasopressin),* a synthetic form of vasopressin that may be the treatment of choice in mild hemophilia if the child shows an appropriate response. Vigorous therapy is instituted to prevent chronic crippling effects from joint bleeding.

---

*P.O. Box 22689, Baltimore, MD 21203; (800) 747-2820.

CLINICAL MANIFESTATIONS OF HEMOPHILIA

Prolonged bleeding anywhere from or in the body
Hemorrhage from any trauma—loss of deciduous teeth, circumcision, cuts, epistaxis, injections
Excessive bruising—even from a slight injury, such as a fall
Subcutaneous and intramuscular hemorrhages
Hemarthrosis (bleeding into the joint cavities), especially the knees, ankles, and elbows
Hematomas—pain, swelling, and limited motion
Spontaneous hematuria

Other drugs may be included in the therapy plan, depending on the source of the hemorrhage. Corticosteroids are used judiciously to treat inflammation in the joints. Nonsteroidal antiinflammatory drugs (NSAIDs), such as aspirin, indomethacin (Indocin), and phenylbutazone (Butazolidin), should not be used because they inhibit platelet function. Ibuprofen (Motrin, Advil, Nuprin) has been demonstrated to be safe despite its antiplatelet aggregation effect. Oral administration and/or local application of epsilon-aminocaproic acid (Amicar) prevents clot destruction; however, its use is limited to mouth or trauma surgery.

A regular program of exercise and physical therapy is an important aspect of management. Physical activity within reasonable limits strengthens muscles around joints, which will help retard or confine bleeding in the area.

Treatment without delay results in more rapid recovery and a decreased likelihood of complications; therefore most children are treated at home. The family is taught the technique of venipuncture and to administer the AHF to children over 3 years of age. The child learns the procedure for self-administration at 9 to 12 years of age. Home treatment is highly successful, and the rewards, in addition to the immediacy, are less disruption of family life, fewer school or work days missed, and enhancement of the child's self-esteem.

Prognosis. Although there is no cure for hemophilia, its symptoms can be controlled and its potentially crippling deformities greatly reduced or even avoided. Today many children with hemophilia function with minimal or no joint damage. They are normal children with an average life expectancy in every respect but one: they have a tendency to bleed, which is a significant inconvenience but not necessarily a life-threatening event.

Unfortunately, those individuals with hemophilia who were treated before current purification techniques for factor VIII concentrate may have been exposed to human immunodeficiency virus (HIV). One estimate is that 70 to 90% of these patients have seroconverted to HIV positive and a significant number have acquired immunodeficiency syndrome (AIDS). As these individuals become sexually active, the issue of sexual transmission of HIV becomes increasingly important. The adolescent must be knowledgeable regarding high-risk sexual behavior. Individuals with hemophilia diagnosed and treated with factor concentrates since 1985 are at virtually no risk for developing HIV infection. Current manufacturing techniques have also greatly reduced the risk of hepatitis transmission.

Nursing Considerations

❖ Assessment

The earlier a bleeding episode is recognized, the more effectively it can be treated. Signs that indicate internal bleeding are especially important to recognize. Children are aware of internal bleeding and are very reliable in telling the examiner where an internal bleed is. In addition to the manifestations described (see box on p. 918), the nurse maintains a high level of suspicion when a child with hemophilia demonstrates unlikely signs, such as headache, slurred speech, loss of consciousness (from cerebral bleeding), and black tarry stools (from GI bleeding).

NURSING DIAGNOSES: THE CHILD WITH HEMOPHILIA
High risk for injury (trauma)
Pain related to bleeding into tissues
Impaired physical mobility related to hemorrhages into joints and other tissues
Altered family processes related to child with a chronic illness

❖ Nursing Diagnoses

Nursing diagnoses for the child with hemophilia include but are not limited to the diagnoses listed in the box.

❖ Planning

The objectives of care can be divided into immediate needs and long-term goals. The patient and family goals for nursing care include the following:

1. Family and child will receive education regarding hemophilia and early recognition of bleeding episodes.
2. Child and family will recognize and control bleeding episodes, and child will receive supportive therapy.
3. Child and parents will adjust to a chronic hereditary disease.
4. Family members will receive genetic counseling.

❖ Implementation

Prevent Bleeding. The goal of prevention of bleeding episodes is directed toward decreasing the risk of injury. Prophylactic administration of factor VIII concentrates is reserved for troublesome target joints in an effort to break the bleeding cycle. The cost of the factor concentrate is prohibitive for routine administration. Prevention of bleeding episodes is geared mostly toward appropriate exercises to strengthen muscles and joints and to allow age-appropriate activity. During infancy and toddlerhood the normal acquisition of motor skills creates innumerable opportunities for falls, bruises, and minor wounds. Restraining the child from mastering motor development can herald more serious long-term problems than allowing the behavior. However, the environment should be made as safe as possible, with close supervision maintained during playtime, to minimize incidental injuries.

For older children the family usually needs assistance in preparing for school. A nurse who knows the family can be instrumental in discussing the situation with the school nurse and in jointly planning an appropriate schedule of activity. Since almost all persons with hemophilia are boys, the physical limitations in regard to active sports may be a difficult adjustment, and activity restrictions must be tempered with sensitivity to the child's emotional, as well as physical, needs. Use of protective equipment, such as padding and helmets, is particularly important, and noncontact sports, especially swimming, are encouraged.

To prevent oral bleeding, some readjustment in terms of dental hygiene may be needed to minimize trauma to the gums, such as use of a water irrigating device, softening the toothbrush in warm water before brushing, or using a sponge-tipped disposable toothbrush. A regular toothbrush should be soft bristled and small in size.

Since any trauma can lead to a bleeding episode, all persons caring for these children must be aware of their disorder. These children should wear medical identification, and older children should be encouraged to recognize situations in which disclosing their condition is important, such as during dental extraction or injections. Health personnel need to take special precautions to prevent the use of procedures that may cause bleeding, such as IM injections or venipunctures. The IV and subcutaneous routes are substituted for IM injections whenever possible. Neither aspirin nor any aspirin-containing compound should be used. Acetaminophen (Tylenol) is a suitable aspirin substitute, especially for use during control of pain at home.

Recognize and Control Bleeding. As noted, the earlier a bleeding episode is recognized, the more effectively it can be treated. Factor replacement therapy should be instituted according to established medical protocol, and supportive measures may be implemented, such as (1) applying pressure to the area for at least 10 to 15 minutes to allow clot formation, (2) immobilizing and elevating the area above the level of the heart to decrease blood flow, and (3) applying cold to promote vasoconstriction. When parents and older children are taught such measures beforehand, they can be prepared to initiate immediate treatment. Plastic bags of ice or cold packs should be kept in the freezer for such emergencies. However, such measures do not take the place of factor replacement.

Prevent Crippling Effects of Bleeding. As a result of repeated episodes of hemarthrosis, incompletely absorbed blood in the joints, and limitation of motion, bone and muscle changes occur that result in flexion contractures and joint fixation. During bleeding episodes the joint is elevated and immobilized. Active range-of-motion exercises are usually instituted after the acute episode. This allows the child to control the degree of exercise and discomfort. If an exercise program is instituted in the home, a physical therapist or public health nurse may need to supervise compliance with the regimen. Diet is also an important consideration, since excessive body weight can increase the strain on affected joints, especially the knees, and predispose to hemarthrosis. Consequently, calories need to be supplied in accordance with energy requirements.

Support Family and Prepare for Home Care. Genetic counseling is essential as soon as possible after diagnosis. Unlike many other disorders in which both parents carry the trait, the feeling of responsibility for this condition usually rests with the mother. Without an opportunity to discuss her feelings, the marital relationship can suffer. Technology is now available to identify carriers in approximately 80% of cases and may reduce the anxiety regarding childbearing in females who may be at risk of carrying the defective gene, such as sisters or maternal aunts of an affected male. The discovery of factor concentrates has greatly changed the outlook for these children. Bleeding can be minimized, and the child can live a much more normal, unrestricted life. Children are taught to take responsibility for their disease at an early age. They learn their limitations and other preventive measures, as well as self-administration of the prophylactic AHF.

The needs of families who have children with hemophilia are best met through a comprehensive team approach of physicians (pediatrician, hematologist, orthopedist), nurse, social worker, and physical therapist. Parent-group discussions are

beneficial in meeting those needs often best met by similarly affected families. For example, with the improved prognosis for these children, parents and adolescents with hemophilia are faced with vocational and financial problems, in addition to concern over future childbearing. Once children reach 21 years of age, many insurance companies will no longer carry them. This can be disastrous in terms of the cost of treatment. The **National Hemophilia Foundation*** and the **Canadian Hemophilia Society†** provide numerous services and publications for both health providers and families. Financial support is particularly important. A person with severe hemophilia may require factor replacement therapy and other medical treatments that cost in excess of $70,000 to $90,000 a year.

Children who have become infected with HIV through transfusions and factor replacement products are faced with the consequences of this dreaded disease. Consequently, they need the support of health professionals, especially in the area of public education, regarding AIDS and ways to deal with public reactions to persons who have AIDS (see p. 941).

❖ Evaluation

The effectiveness of nursing interventions is determined by continual reassessment and evaluation of care based on the following observational guidelines and expected outcomes:

1. Interview child and family regarding preventive measures implemented and any bleeding episodes the child suffers.
2. Observe child for evidence of bleeding episodes; monitor preventive strategies and therapies, especially pain assessment and management.
3. Observe and interview family regarding treatments and schedule of prophylactic administration of AHF.
4. Interview family and/or consult the genetic counseling service regarding the carrier status of other members of the family.

Expected outcomes:

1. Child exhibits no evidence of bleeding.
2. Child exhibits no evidence of tissue damage.
3. Child and family discuss their feelings and concerns and demonstrate an understanding of the disease and its therapy (specify knowledge and method of demonstration).
4. Family seeks genetic counseling.

See also Nursing Care Plan: The Child with Hemophilia.‡

IDIOPATHIC THROMBOCYTOPENIC PURPURA (ITP)

ITP is an acquired hemorrhagic disorder characterized by (1) *thrombocytopenia,* excessive destruction of platelets, and (2) *purpura,* a discoloration caused by petechiae beneath the skin. Although the cause is unknown, it is believed to be an autoimmune response to disease-related antigens. It is the most frequently occurring thrombocytopenia of childhood.

The disease occurs in one of two forms: an acute, self-limiting course or a chronic condition interspersed with

*110 Green St., Room 303, New York, NY 10012; (212) 219-8180 or (800) 42HANDI.
†1450 City Councillors, Bureau 840, Montreal, Quebec H3A 2E6; (514) 848-0503.
‡In Wong DL: *Wong and Whaley's Clinical manual of pediatric nursing,* ed 4, St Louis, 1996, Mosby.

90,000 yr for factor

remissions. The acute form is most often seen after upper respiratory infections or after the childhood diseases measles, rubella, mumps, and chickenpox.

Diagnostic Evaluation

The diagnosis is suspected on the basis of clinical manifestations (see box). In ITP the platelet count is reduced to below 20,000 mm^3; therefore tests that depend on platelet function are abnormal, such as the tourniquet test, bleeding time, and clot retraction. Although there is no definitive test on which to establish a diagnosis of ITP, several are usually performed to rule out other disorders in which thrombocytopenia is a manifestation, such as systemic lupus erythematosus, lymphoma, or leukemia.

Therapeutic Management

Management is primarily supportive, since the course of ITP is self-limited in most patients. Activity is restricted at the onset while the platelet count is low and while active bleeding or progression of lesions is occurring. This restriction is most easily accomplished in the hospital. Corticosteroids are employed for children with the highest risk for serious bleeding, for chronic cases with increased bleeding tendencies, as an adjunct to life-threatening hemorrhage, or before splenectomy to decrease the risk of surgical bleeding. Administration of IV gamma globulin has proved successful in increasing the platelet count of children with chronic disease. Children with chronic ITP have also experienced and sustained a rise in platelet count when treated with ascorbate (a product of ascorbic acid [vitamin C]) (Cohen and others, 1993). Splenectomy is reserved for symptomatic children with chronic disease or as an emergency measure in the event of life-threatening hemorrhage. Packed RBCs may be given to replace blood lost in symptomatic children. Platelets are seldom administered.

Prognosis. The majority of children have a self-limited course without major complications. Some children will develop chronic ITP and require ongoing therapy. A splenectomy may modify the disease process, and the child will be asymptomatic.

Nursing Considerations

Nursing care is largely supportive. Children with ITP and parents need careful explanations of the rationale behind the

therapies employed and support in their efforts to comply. The nursing considerations of controlling bleeding and preventing bruising are similar to those discussed in the section on leukemia. The harmful effects of using aspirin and NSAIDs to control pain are critical for these children; therefore substitutes such as acetaminophen (paracetamol) are used.

DISSEMINATED INTRAVASCULAR COAGULATION (DIC)

DIC, also known as *consumption coagulopathy,* is a secondary disorder of coagulation that occurs as a complication of a number of pathologic processes, such as hypoxia, acidosis, shock, and endothelial damage. It can result from many severe systemic diseases, such as congenital heart disease, necrotizing enterocolitis, gram-negative bacterial sepsis, rickettsial infections, and some severe viral infections. The disorder is characterized by inappropriate systemic activation and acceleration of the normal clotting mechanism.

Pathophysiology

DIC occurs when the first stage of the coagulation process is abnormally stimulated. Although no well-defined sequence of events occurs, two distinct phases can be identified. First, when the clotting mechanism is triggered in the circulation, thrombin is generated in greater amounts than can be neutralized by the body. Consequently, there is rapid conversion of fibrinogen to fibrin with aggregation and destruction of platelets. If local and widespread fibrin deposition in blood vessels takes place, obstruction and eventual necrosis of tissues occur. Second, the fibrinolytic mechanism is activated, causing extensive destruction of clotting factors. With a deficiency of clotting factors the child is vulnerable to uncontrollable hemorrhage into vital organs. An additional complication is damage and hemolysis of RBCs (Fig. 26-2).

Diagnostic Evaluation

DIC is suspected when the patient has an increased tendency to bleed (see box on p. 922). Hematologic findings include

---

CLINICAL MANIFESTATIONS OF IDIOPATHIC THROMBOCYTOPENIC PURPURA (ITP)

Easy bruising
  Petechiae
  Ecchymoses
  Most often over bony prominences
Bleeding from mucous membranes
  Epistaxis
  Bleeding gums
  Internal hemorrhage evidenced by:
    Hematuria
    Hematemesis
    Melena
    Hemarthrosis
    Menorrhagia
Hematomas over lower extremities

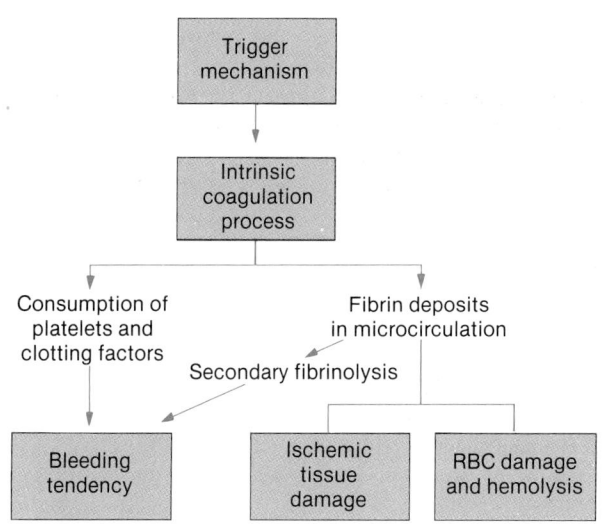

FIG. 26-2. Effects of disseminated intravascular coagulation (DIC).

CLINICAL MANIFESTATIONS OF DISSEMINATED INTRAVASCULAR COAGULATION

Petechiae
Purpura
Bleeding from openings in the skin
  Venipuncture site
  Surgical incision
Bleeding from umbilicus, trachea (newborn)
Evidence of gastrointestinal bleeding
Hypotension
Organ dysfunction from infarction and ischemia

---

prolonged prothrombin time (PT), partial thromboplastin time (PTT), and thrombin time (TT). There is a profoundly depressed platelet count, fragmented RBCs, and depleted fibrinogen.

Therapeutic Management
Treatment of DIC is directed toward control of the underlying or initiating cause, which in most instances stops the coagulation problem spontaneously. Platelets and fresh-frozen plasma may be needed to replace lost plasma components, especially in the child whose underlying disease remains uncontrolled. The extremely ill newborn infant may require exchange transfusion with fresh blood. The IV administration of heparin to inhibit thrombin formation is most often restricted to severe cases.

Nursing Considerations
The goals of nursing care are to be aware of the possibility of DIC in the severely ill child and to recognize signs that might indicate its presence. The skills needed to monitor IV infusion and blood transfusions and to administer heparin are the same as for any child receiving these therapies (see p. 943). See Chapter 18 for care of the child with a life-threatening illness.

EPISTAXIS (NOSEBLEEDING)
Isolated and transient episodes of epistaxis, or nosebleeding, are common in childhood. The nose, especially the septum, is a highly vascular structure, and bleeding usually results from direct trauma, including blows to the nose, foreign bodies, and nose picking, or from mucosal inflammation associated with allergic rhinitis and upper respiratory infections. The bleeding ordinarily stops spontaneously or with minimum pressure and requires no medical evaluation or therapy.

Recurrent epistaxis and severe bleeding may indicate an underlying disease, particularly vascular abnormalities, leukemia, thrombocytopenia, and clotting factor deficiency diseases, such as hemophilia and von Willebrand disease. Nosebleeds are sometimes associated with administration of aspirin, even in normal amounts. Persistent episodes of epistaxis require medical evaluation.

Nursing Considerations
In the event of a nosebleed, an essential intervention is to remain calm. Otherwise the child will become more agitated, the blood pressure will increase, and the child will not cooperate. Although in most instances a nosebleed is not serious,

it can be very upsetting to family members as well. They need reassurance that the loss of blood is not serious and that the bleeding usually stops within 10 to 15 minutes.

To control the bleeding, the child is instructed to sit up and lean forward (not to lie down) to avoid aspiration of blood. Most of the nosebleeding originates in the anterior part of the nasal septum and can be controlled by applying pressure to the soft lower portion of the nose with the thumb and forefinger (see Emergency Treatment box on p. 923). During this time the child breathes through the mouth.

In the event that hemorrhage continues, the child should be evaluated by a practitioner, who may pack the nose with epinephrine-soaked gauze. After a nosebleed, petroleum or water-soluble jelly can be inserted into each nostril to prevent crusting of old blood and to lessen the likelihood of the child's picking at the nose and restarting the hemorrhage. If a child has numerous nosebleeds, factors believed to increase the likelihood of bleeds are eliminated, such as discouraging nose picking or altering the household humidity by placing a cool-mist humidifier in the child's room. Repeated bleeding episodes may be an indication to refer the child for evaluation for the possibility of a bleeding disorder.

NEOPLASTIC DISORDERS*

Neoplastic disorders are the leading cause of death from disease in children past infancy, and almost half of all childhood cancers involve the blood or blood-forming organs. Leukemias and lymphomas are discussed here. Malignant solid tumors of childhood are discussed elsewhere in relation to the tissues or organs involved.

LEUKEMIAS
Leukemia, cancer of the blood-forming tissues, is the most common form of childhood cancer. The annual incidence is 4.2 per 100,000 population in white children under 15 years of age and 2.4 per 100,000 population in black children (Poplack, 1993). It occurs more frequently in males than in females after age 1 year, and the peak onset is between 2 and 6 years of age. It is one of the forms of cancer that has demonstrated dramatic improvements in survival rates. Current 4-year survival rates for children with acute lymphoblastic leukemia exceed 80% in major research centers, and a majority of these children may be cured (Pediatric Oncology Group, 1992). (See also Prognosis, p. 924.)

Classification
Leukemia is a broad term given to a group of malignant diseases of the bone marrow and lymphatic system. Current research has revealed that it is a complex disease of varying heterogeneity. Consequently, classification has become increasingly complex, sophisticated, and essential, since identification of the subtype of leukemia has therapeutic and prognostic implications (see p. 923). The following is a brief overview of the major classification systems currently being used.

---

*Marilyn Hockenberry-Eaton, PhD, RN, C, PNP, and Nancy E. Kline, MS, RN, CPNP, revised this section.

Morphology. Leukemia is classified according to its predominant cell type and level of maturity, as described by the following:

Lympho—for leukemias involving the lymphoid or lymphatic system
Myelo—for those of myeloid (bone marrow) origin
Blastic and acute—for those involving immature cells
Cytic and chronic—for those involving mature cells

In children, two forms are generally recognized: *acute lymphoid leukemia (ALL)* and *acute nonlymphoid (myelogenous) leukemia (ANLL or AML)*. Synonyms for ALL include lymphatic, lymphocytic, lymphoblastic, and lymphoblastoid leukemia. Usually the terms *stem cell* or *blast cell leukemia* also refer to the lymphoid type of leukemia. Synonyms for the AML type include granulocytic, myelocytic, monocytic, myelogenous, monoblastic, and monomyeloblastic. Also, much rarer forms of leukemia are named for the specific cell involved, such as basophilic or eosinophilic leukemia.

Cytochemical Markers. Leukemic cells demonstrate different reactions when they are exposed to certain chemicals. For example, terminal deoxynucleotidyl transferase is able to provide excellent differentiation between ALL and AML.

Chromosomal Studies. Chromosomal analysis has become an important tool in the diagnosis of acute lymphoblastic leukemia. For example, children with trisomy 21 have 15 times the risk of other children for developing ALL. Children who are hyperdiploid (more chromosomes) have a better prognosis. Translocation of chromosomes 4 and 10 also is associated with a better prognosis (Poplack, 1993).

Cell-Surface Immunologic Markers. Cell-surface antigens have permitted differentiation of ALL into three broad classes: non-T, non-B ALL (also called early pre–B cell); B-cell ALL; and T-cell ALL. Children with non-T, non-B ALL have the best prognosis, especially if they have

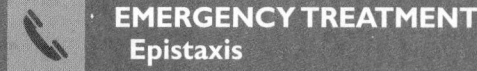

EMERGENCY TREATMENT
Epistaxis

Have child sit up and lean forward (not lying down).
Apply continuous pressure to nose with thumb and forefinger for at least 10 minutes.
Insert cotton or wadded tissue into each nostril, and apply ice or cold cloth to bridge of nose if bleeding persists.
Keep child calm and quiet.

the common acute lymphocytic leukemia antigen, known as CALLA positive, on their cell surfaces (Poplack, 1993).

Pathophysiology

Leukemia is an unrestricted proliferation of immature WBCs in the blood-forming tissues of the body. Although not a "tumor" as such, the leukemic cells demonstrate the same neoplastic properties as solid cancers. Therefore the resulting pathologic condition and clinical manifestations are caused by infiltration and replacement of any tissue of the body with nonfunctional leukemic cells. Highly vascular organs, such as the spleen and liver, are the most severely affected.

To understand the pathophysiology of the leukemic process, it is important to clarify two common misconceptions. First, although leukemia is an overproduction of WBCs, most often in the acute form the leukocyte count is low (thus the term *leukemia*). Second, these immature cells do not deliberately attack and destroy the normal blood cells or vascular tissues. Cellular destruction takes place by infiltration and subsequent competition for metabolic elements (Table 26-3).

In all types of leukemia the proliferating cells depress the production of formed elements of the blood in bone marrow by competing for and depriving the normal cells of the essential nutrients for metabolism. The most frequent pre-

TABLE 26-3. Pathology and related clinical manifestations of leukemia

ORGAN OR TISSUE	CONSEQUENCES	MANIFESTATIONS
Bone marrow dysfunction	Decreased RBCs—anemia	Pallor, fatigue
	Neutropenia—infection	Fever
	Decreased platelets—bleeding tendencies	Hemorrhage (petechiae)
	Invasion of bone marrow—bone weakness; invasion of periosteum	Tendency toward fractures
		Pain
Liver	Infiltration, enlargement, eventual fibrosis	Hepatomegaly
Spleen		Splenomegaly
Lymph glands		Lymphadenopathy
Central nervous system: meninges	Increased intracranial pressure, ventricular enlargement	Severe headache
		Vomiting
		Irritability, lethargy
		Papilledema
	Meningeal irritation	Eventual coma
		Pain
		Stiff neck and back
Hypermetabolism	Cell deprivation of nutrients by invading cells	Muscle wasting
		Weight loss
		Anorexia
		Fatigue

senting signs and symptoms of leukemia are a result of infiltration of the bone marrow. The three main consequences are (1) *anemia* from decreased RBCs, (2) *infection* from neutropenia, and (3) *bleeding tendencies* from decreased platelet production. The invasion of the bone marrow with leukemic cells gradually causes a weakening of the bone and a tendency toward fractures. As leukemic cells invade the periosteum, increasing pressure causes severe pain.

The spleen, liver, and lymph glands demonstrate marked infiltration, enlargement, and eventually fibrosis. Hepatosplenomegaly is typically more common than lymphadenopathy. The next most important site of involvement is the central nervous system (CNS). The usual effect of leukemic infiltration is increased intracranial pressure, which causes the signs and symptoms normally associated with this condition. Cranial nerves may be involved as well, and the signs and symptoms observed reflect the area affected (see Table 7-12).

Leukemic cells may also invade the testes, kidneys, prostate, ovaries, GI tract, and lungs. With long-term survivors becoming more common, such sites of leukemia invasion, especially the testes, are becoming more important clinically.

The immense metabolic needs of proliferating leukemic cells eventually deprive all body cells of nutrients necessary for survival. In addition to the risk of death from infection and hemorrhage, uncontrolled growth of leukemic cells can also terminate in metabolic starvation.

Diagnostic Evaluation

Leukemia is usually suspected by the history, physical manifestations (Table 26-3), and a peripheral blood smear that contains immature forms of leukocytes, frequently combined with low blood counts. Definitive diagnosis is based on bone marrow aspiration or biopsy. Typically the bone marrow is hypercellular, with primarily blast cells. Once the diagnosis is confirmed, a lumbar puncture is performed to determine if there is any CNS involvement, although a very small number of children have CNS involvement at the time of diagnosis, and most are asymptomatic.

Therapeutic Management

Treatment of leukemia involves the use of chemotherapeutic agents, with or without cranial irradiation, in three phases: (1) *induction therapy*, which achieves a complete remission or disappearance of leukemic cells; (2) *CNS prophylactic therapy*, which prevents leukemic cells from invading the CNS; and (3) *maintenance with intensification therapy* (consolidation), which serves to maintain the remission phase. Although the combination of drugs and radiation may vary according to institutions, the prognostic or risk characteristics of the patient, and the type of leukemia being treated, the following general principles for each phase are quite consistently employed.

Remission Induction.   Almost immediately after confirmation of the diagnosis, induction therapy is begun and lasts for 4 to 6 weeks. The principal drugs used for induction in ALL are corticosteroids (especially prednisone), vincristine, and L-asparaginase, with or without doxorubicin. Drug therapy for AML includes doxorubicin or daunorubicin (daunomycin) and cytosine arabinoside; various other drugs may be used.

Since many of the drugs also cause myelosuppression of normal blood elements, the period immediately following a remission can be critical. The body is defenseless against and highly susceptible to infection and spontaneous hemorrhage. Consequently, supportive therapy during this time is essential.

CNS Prophylactic Therapy.   Treatment of the CNS consists of prophylactic therapy using intrathecal chemotherapy with methotrexate, cytarabine, and hydrocortisone. Because of the concern regarding late effects of cranial irradiation, this treatment is reserved for high-risk patients and those with CNS disease.

Once complete remission is obtained, a period of intensified treatment is administered to reduce further the leukemia burden. Drugs typically used during consolidation include methotrexate, cytosine arabinoside, and L-asparaginase.

Maintenance Therapy.   Maintenance therapy is begun after completion of successful induction and consolidation therapy to preserve the remission and further lessen the number of leukemic cells. As with induction therapy, combined drug regimens have been more successful in maintaining remissions and preventing drug resistance. Also, during maintenance therapy, periodic CBCs are taken to evaluate the marrow's response to the drugs.

Reinduction Following Relapse.   When the presence of leukemic cells are observed in the bone marrow, CNS, or testes, the child has relapsed. Therapy for the child who has relapsed includes reinduction with prednisone and vincristine, along with a combination of other drugs not previously used. CNS preventive therapy and maintenance therapy follow as outlined before, once remission occurs.

Bone Marrow Transplantation (BMT).   Bone marrow transplants have been used successfully for treating children who have ALL and AML. BMT is *not* recommended for children with ALL during the first remission because of the excellent results possible with chemotherapy. Because of the poorer prognosis in children with AML, BMT may be considered during the first remission (Johnson, 1991).

A small number of hematopoietic stem cells circulate in the peripheral blood. These *peripheral blood stem cells (PBSCs)* are capable of differentiating into the specialized cells of the hematologic system, including RBCs, WBCs, and platelets. PBSC transplantation may be used either as an alternative to or in conjunction with BMT to restore bone marrow function after myeloablative therapy (Hooper and Santas, 1994). Patients receiving PBSC transplantation are hospitalized for a shorter time because engraftment occurs much sooner. This therapy is undergoing research to learn more about its usefulness.

Prognosis.   The most important prognostic factors for determining long-term survival for children with ALL (in addition to treatment) are (1) the initial WBC count, (2) the child's age at the time of diagnosis, (3) the type of cell involved, (4) the sex of the child, and (5) karyotype analysis. Children with a normal or low WBC count and who have non-T, non-B ALL and are CALLA positive have a much better prognosis than those with a high count or other cell types. Children diagnosed between 2 and 9 years of age have consistently demonstrated a better outlook than those diagnosed before 2 or after 10 years of age, and females appear to have a more favorable prognosis than males. Children with a deoxyribonucleic acid (DNA) index greater than 1.16 (hyper-diploid) and translocation of chromosomes 4 and 10 have a better prognosis (Poplack, 1993). In addition, it appears that the more rapid the induction of a remission in AML, the better the chance for an ultimate long-term continuous remission.

Late Effects of Treatment.   Although vigorous treatment of childhood cancers has resulted in dramatically improved survival rates, increasing concern surrounds late effects—adverse changes related to treatment modalities—and recurrence of the disease process. Almost no organ is exempt, and almost every antineoplastic agent, including and especially irradiation, is responsible for some adverse effect. There is a substantially increased risk of developing secondary cancers.

In children with leukemia, impairment caused by treatment with cranial irradiation and intrathecal chemotherapy is of particular concern, especially the risk of developing CNS tumors (Allen, 1993). In addition, intellectual and motor function may be impaired because of interference with neural development before maturation of the brain is complete. Children under the age of 5 years are at the highest risk for these complications.

Nursing Considerations

Nursing care of the child with leukemia is directly related to the regimen of therapy. General psychologic interventions during each phase of therapy are discussed in Chapter 18.

❖ Assessment

The history and physical examination often yield the first clues to the presence of neoplastic disease. Vague complaints, such as fatigue, pain in a limb, night sweating, lack of appetite, headache, and general malaise, may be the earliest clues and need to be taken seriously. Most children have great energy and, if sick with a cold or other childhood affliction, recover quickly and completely. Any evidence of a lingering disorder is often the first sign of leukemia.

❖ Nursing Diagnoses

A number of nursing diagnoses become apparent following an assessment of the child with leukemia and the family. Some are considered in the Nursing Care Plan on pp. 933-938. Others will be identified in specific situations.

❖ Planning

The goals of nursing care of the child with leukemia and the family include the following:

1. Child will receive appropriate primary health care.
2. Child and family will be prepared for diagnostic and therapeutic procedures.
3. Child will experience minimal complications of myelosuppression.
4. Problems of irradiation and drug toxicity will be managed.
5. Child and family will receive adequate support and education.

❖ Implementation

Nursing care of the child with leukemia is directly related to the regimen of therapy. Nurses working with families of children with cancer have a significant supportive role in helping them understand the various therapies, preventing or managing expected side effects or toxicities, observing for late effects of treatment, and helping the child and family live as normal a life as possible and cope with the emotional aspects of the disease. Education is a constant feature of the nursing role, especially in terms of new treatments, clinical trials, and home care.

Because of the anxiety generated by the diagnosis of leukemia, some families may resort to unproven methods of therapy that are frequently referred to as "cancer quackery." These unorthodox approaches are a threat to every cancer family. Nurses can be instrumental in working against cancer quackery by being aware of factors that increase a family's likelihood of seeking unproven remedies, by communicating effectively with families about the diagnosis and forms of therapy, and by providing all possible support and reassurance during treatment.

Prepare Child and Family for Diagnostic and Therapeutic Procedures.   From the time before diagnosis to cessation of therapy, children must undergo several tests, the most traumatic of which are bone marrow aspiration or biopsy and lumbar punctures. Multiple finger sticks and venipunctures for blood analysis and drug infusion are common occurrences for several years after the diagnosis. Therefore the child needs an explanation of why each procedure is done and what can be expected. In addition, effective pharmacologic measures, including conscious and unconscious sedation, and nonpharmacologic strategies are used to reduce discomfort associated with these painful procedures.

Relieve Pain.   The effective use of analgesia is especially important when the malignant process is uncontrolled and causes pain. Bone pain is particularly acute. Dosages of opioids (narcotics) are adjusted or *titrated to the child's needs* and administered *around the clock* for optimum pain control. Nonpharmacologic strategies should be implemented as needed but are not substitutes for pharmacologic management. The reader is encouraged to review the principles of pain assessment and management presented in Chapter 21 and Preparation for Procedures in Chapter 22 when caring for a child with leukemia.

Prevent Complications of Myelosuppression. The leukemic process and most of the chemotherapeutic agents cause myelosuppression. The reduced numbers of blood cells result in secondary problems of infection, bleeding tendencies, and anemia. Supportive care involves both medical and nursing management. Because these are so closely linked, they are discussed together rather than separately.

Infection.   A frequent complication of treatment for childhood cancer is overwhelming infection secondary to neutropenia. The child is most susceptible to overwhelming infection during three phases of the disease: (1) at the time of diagnosis and relapse when the leukemic process has replaced normal leukocytes, (2) during immunosuppressive therapy, and (3) after prolonged antibiotic therapy that predisposes to the growth of resistant organisms. However, the use of granulocyte colony–stimulating factor (GCSF) has reduced the incidence and duration of infection in children receiving treatment for cancer.

The first defense against infection is prevention. When the child is hospitalized, the nurse employs all measures to control transfer of infection. These typically include the use of a private room, restriction of all visitors and health personnel with active infection, and strict handwashing technique with an antiseptic solution. In some research centers, special germ-free environments are available during complete myelosuppression from intensive chemotherapy or for bone marrow transplant.

> **Nursing ALERT** Because the usual viral infections of childhood are particularly dangerous, the child is *not* immunized against these diseases (measles, rubella, mumps, and polio) until the immune system is capable of responding appropriately to the vaccine. If given when the immune system is depressed, the attenuated virus can result in an overwhelming infection. The child can receive the Salk (inactivated) vaccine for poliomyelitis. The varicella (chickenpox) vaccine is being given to certain children with ALL who have not received it as part of their routine immunizations (see Immunizations, Chapter 10).

The child is evaluated for potential sites of infection (e.g., mucosal ulceration, skin abrasion or tear, such as a hangnail) and observed for any elevation in temperature. To identify the source of infection, chest radiographs and blood, stool, urine, and nasopharyngeal cultures are taken. IV antibiotics are administered, and if this therapy is prolonged, a venous access device, such as a peripherally inserted central catheter (PICC), intermittent infusion device (saline lock or PRN adaptor), catheter, or implanted infusion port, is used to maintain IV access.

Prevention of infection continues to be a priority after discharge from the hospital. Ordinarily the child is allowed to return to school when the WBC count is at a satisfactory level, usually an absolute neutrophil count (ANC) greater than 500/mm³ (see Guidelines box). At all times family members are encouraged to practice good handwashing to prevent introducing pathogens into the home. The child may need to be isolated from school contacts in the event of an outbreak of a childhood disease, especially chickenpox.

Nutrition is another important component of infection prevention. An adequate protein-caloric intake provides the child with better host defenses against infection and increased tolerance to chemotherapy and irradiation. However, providing optimum nutrition during periods of anorexia and vomiting from chemotherapy is a tremendous challenge (see Feeding the Sick Child, Chapter 22).

Hemorrhage. Before the use of transfused platelets, hemorrhage was a leading cause of death in patients with leukemia. Now most bleeding episodes can be prevented or con-

trolled with the administration of platelet concentrates or platelet-rich plasma.

Since infection increases the tendency toward hemorrhage, and since bleeding sites become more easily infected, skin punctures are avoided whenever possible. When finger sticks, venipunctures, IM injections, and bone marrow aspirations are performed, aseptic technique must be employed, as well as continued observation for bleeding. Meticulous mouth care is essential, since gingival bleeding with resultant mucositis is a frequent problem. Since the rectal area is prone to ulceration from various drugs, feces and urine are removed immediately, and the perianal area is washed. Rectal temperatures are avoided to prevent trauma. Children are advised to avoid activities that might cause injury or bleeding, such as riding bicycles or skateboards, climbing trees or playground equipment, and playing contact sports.

Platelet transfusions are generally reserved for active bleeding episodes that do not respond to local treatment and that may occur during induction or relapse therapy. Epistaxis and gingival bleeding are the most common. The nurse teaches parents and older children measures to control nosebleeding (see p. 923). Pressure at the site without disturbing clot formation is the general rule.

During bleeding episodes the parents and child need much emotional support. The sight of oozing blood is very upsetting. Often parents will request a platelet transfusion, unaware of the need for trying local measures first. The nurse can be instrumental in allaying anxiety by acknowledging the feelings of the child and family and explaining the reason for delaying a platelet transfusion until absolutely necessary.

Anemia. Initially, anemia may be profound from complete replacement of the bone marrow by leukemic cells. During induction therapy blood transfusions with packed RBCs may be necessary to raise the hemoglobin to levels approaching 10 g/dl. The usual precautions in caring for the child with anemia are instituted (see p. 908).

Use Precautions in Administering and Handling Chemotherapeutic Agents. Many chemotherapeutic agents are vesicants (sclerosing agents) that can cause severe cellular damage if even minute amounts of the drug infiltrate surrounding tissue. Only nurses experienced with chemotherapeutic agents should administer vesicants. Guidelines are available* and must be followed exactly to prevent tissue damage to patients. Interventions for extravasation vary, but each nurse should be aware of the institution's policies and implement them at once.

> **Nursing ALERT** Chemotherapeutic drugs must be given through a free-flowing IV line. The infusion is stopped *immediately* if any sign of infiltration (pain, stinging, swelling, or redness at the cannulation site) occurs.

In addition to extravasation, a potentially fatal complication is anaphylaxis, especially from L-asparaginase, teniposide (VM-26), etoposide (VP-16), bleomycin, and cisplatin. Nursing responsibilities include prevention of, recognition of, and preparation for serious reactions. Prevention begins with a careful history for known allergy.

> **GUIDELINES**
> **Calculating the Absolute Neutrophil Count (ANC)**
>
> Determine the total percent of neutrophils ("polys" or "segs" and "bands").
> Multiply white blood cell (WBC) count by percent of neutrophils.
> ***Example:*** WBC = 1000, neutrophils = 7%, nonsegmented
> neutrophils (bands) = 7%
> Step 1: 7% + 7% = 14%
> Step 2: 0.14 × 1000 = 140 ANC

Cancer Chemotherapy Guidelines can be obtained from the **Oncology Nursing Society,** 501 Holiday Dr., Pittsburgh, PA 15220-2749; (412) 921-7373.

Nursing ALERT

When chemotherapeutic and immunologic agents are given, the child must be observed for 20 minutes after the infusion for signs of anaphylaxis (cyanosis, hypotension, wheezing, severe urticaria). Emergency equipment (especially blood pressure monitor and bag-valve-mask) and emergency drugs (especially oxygen, epinephrine, antihistamine, aminophylline, corticosteroids, and vasopressors) must be available. If a reaction is suspected, the drug is discontinued, the IV line is flushed with saline, and the child's vital signs and subsequent responses are monitored.

In addition to the many responsibilities nurses must have in regard to the child and family, they must also use safeguards to protect themselves. Handling chemotherapeutic agents may present risks to handlers and to their offspring, although the exact degree of risk is not known.

Some children have a venous access device, which facilitates administration of IV drugs. During treatment and remission, many drugs are taken orally at home. Compliance with the medication schedule is essential, and nurses play an important role in educating the family about the drugs and encouraging adherence to the plan.*

Manage Problems of Drug Toxicity. Chemotherapy presents several nursing challenges. The complexity of the treatment protocols is often overwhelming to families. In addition, each therapy is associated with a number of predictable side effects. Nurses must be aware of these side effects and use judgment in recognizing which are normal reactions and which indicate toxicity (see box on pp. 928-930).

Nausea and Vomiting. The nausea and vomiting that occur shortly after administration of several of the drugs and from cranial or abdominal radiation can be profound. The serotonin-receptor antagonists (e.g., ondansetron [Zofran]) are effective in the control of nausea and vomiting occurring after emetogenic chemotherapy and radiation therapy. When combined with dexamethasone, these agents are the treatment of choice in the prevention of cisplatin-induced emesis (Tonato, Roila, and Del Favero, 1994).

The most beneficial regimen for antiemetic control has been the administration of the antiemetic *before* the chemotherapy begins. The goal is to prevent the child from ever experiencing nausea or vomiting, thus preventing development of anticipatory symptoms (the conditioned response of developing nausea and vomiting before receiving the drug) (Hockenberry-Eaton and Benner, 1990).

Anorexia. Loss of appetite is a direct consequence of the chemotherapy and/or irradiation. It is a major problem for parents because it is the one area they feel responsible for, particularly when so many other facets of care are outside their control. There are no universally successful techniques for encouraging a sick child to eat. However, the guidelines in Chapter 22 can be helpful during the anorexic period and can prevent additional problems during the remission.

Some children still do not eat despite these approaches. When loss of appetite and weight persist, the nurse should investigate the family situation to determine if any factors (e.g., conditioned aversion to food, environmental stress related to eating, controlling behavior, anger) might be contributing to the problem. Nasogastric tube feedings or total parenteral nutrition may be implemented for children with significant nutritional problems.

Mucosal Ulceration. One of the most distressing side effects of several drugs is GI mucosal cell damage, which can produce ulcers anywhere along the alimentary tract. Oral ulcers greatly compound anorexia because eating is extremely uncomfortable, but the following interventions may be helpful: (1) provide a bland, moist, soft diet appropriate for the child's age and preferences; (2) use a soft sponge toothbrush (Toothettes)* or cotton-tipped applicator; (3) provide frequent mouthwashes with normal saline (using a solution of 1 teaspoon of table salt and 1 pint of water) or sodium bicarbonate mouthrinses (using a solution of 1 teaspoon of baking soda in 1 quart of water); and (4) use local anesthetics (e.g., Chloraseptic lozenges) or nonprescription preparations without alcohol (e.g., Orabase, Ulcerase). Although local anesthetics are effective in temporarily relieving the pain, many children dislike the taste and numb feeling they produce.

Nursing ALERT

Viscous lidocaine is not recommended for young children; if applied to the pharynx, it may depress the gag reflex, increasing the risk of aspiration. Seizures have been rarely associated with the use of oral viscous lidocaine (Hess and Walson, 1988).

Other preparations that may be used to prevent or treat mucositis include chlorhexidine gluconate (Peridex) because of its dual effectiveness against candidal and bacterial infections, antifungal troches (lozenges) or mouthwash, and lip balm (e.g., Aquaphor) to keep the lips moist. Agents that should not be used are lemon glycerine swabs (irritate eroded tissue and can decay teeth), hydrogen peroxide (delays healing by breaking down protein), and milk of magnesia (dries mucosa) (Galbraith and others, 1991).

Stomatitis may cause such difficulty with eating that the child may require hospitalization for hydration, parenteral nutrition, and pain control (often with IV morphine). The child will usually choose the foods that are best tolerated, and the nurse should encourage parents to relax any eating pressures. Since the stomatitis is a temporary condition, the child can resume good food habits once the ulcers heal. Dental hygiene can become a serious problem for children with orthodontic appliances. Sometimes it may be necessary to remove the braces to allow chemotherapy to continue.

Rectal ulcers are managed by meticulous toilet hygiene and use of an occlusive ointment or dressing applied to the ulcerated area to promote epithelialization. Exposing the denuded skin to air, heat, or supplemental oxygen delays healing. (See Maintaining Healthy Skin, Chapter 22, and Process of Wound Healing, Chapter 30.) Parents are advised to record bowel movements, since the child may voluntarily avoid defecation to prevent discomfort. Rectal temperatures and suppositories are contraindicated because the thermometer may further traumatize the area.

---

*Home care instructions on caring for a venous access device and administering medications to children are available in Wong DL: *Wong and Whaley's Clinical manual of pediatric nursing*, ed 4, St Louis, 1996, Mosby.

*Manufactured by Halbrand, Inc., Willoughby, OH.

SUMMARY OF SELECTED CHEMOTHERAPEUTIC AGENTS USED IN THE TREATMENT OF CHILDHOOD LEUKEMIAS AND LYMPHOMAS*

Bleomycin (Blenoxane)
Administration

IV, IM, SC†

Side Effects and Toxicity

Allergic reaction—fever, chills, hypotension, anaphylaxis
Fever (nonallergic)
N/V (mild)‡
Stomatitis
Cumulative dose effects include:
  Skin—rash, hyperpigmentation, thickening, ulceration, peeling, nail changes, alopecia
  Lungs—pneumonitis with infiltrate that can progress to fatal fibrosis

Comments and Specific Nursing Considerations

Should give test dose (SC) before therapeutic dose administered
Have emergency drugs at bedside
Hypersensitivity occurs with first one to two doses
May give acetaminophen before drug to reduce likelihood of fever
Concentration of drug in skin and lungs accounts for toxic effects

Corticosteroids (Prednisone)
Administration

PO; IM or IV rarely used

Side Effects and Toxicity, Short-Term

For short-term use, no acute toxicity
Usual side effects are mild: moon face, fluid retention, weight gain, mood changes, increased appetite, gastric irritation, insomnia, susceptibility to infection

Comments and Specific Nursing Considerations

Explain expected effects, especially in terms of body image, increased appetite, and personality changes
Monitor weight gain
Recommend moderate salt restriction
Administer with antacid and early in morning (sometimes given every other day to minimize side effects)
May need to disguise bitter taste (crush tablet and mix with syrup, jam, ice cream, or other highly flavored substance; use ice to numb tongue before administration; place tablet in gelatin capsule if child can swallow it)
Observe for potential infection sites; usual inflammatory response and fever are absent

Side Effects and Toxicity, Long-Term

Long-term effects of chronic steroid administration are mood changes, hirsutism, trunk obesity (buffalo hump), thin extremities, muscle wasting and weakness, osteoporosis, poor wound healing, bruising, potassium loss, gastric bleeding, hypertension, diabetes mellitus, growth retardation

Comments and Specific Nursing Considerations

Same as for short-term use; in addition, encourage foods high in potassium (bananas, raisins, prunes, coffee, chocolate)
Test stools for occult blood
Monitor blood pressure
Test blood for sugar and urine for acetone
Observe for signs of abrupt steroid withdrawal: flulike symptoms, hypotension, hypoglycemia, shock

Daunorubicin (Daunomycin, Rubidomycin) and Doxorubicin (Adriamycin, Doxyrubicin)
Administration

IV

Side Effects and Toxicity

N/V (moderate)
Stomatitis
BMD§ (7-14 days later)
Fever, chills
Local phlebitis
Alopecia
Cumulative-dose toxicity includes:
  Cardiac abnormalities
  Electrocardiographic changes
  Heart failure

Comments and Specific Nursing Considerations

Vesicant‖ (extravasation may *not* cause pain)
Use only sterile distilled water as a diluent
Observe for any changes in heart rate or rhythm and signs of failure
Cumulative dose must not exceed 400 mg/m^2
Warn parents that drug causes urine to turn red (for up to 12 days after administration); this is normal, not hematuria

L-Asparaginase (Elspar)
Administration

IM, IV

Side Effects and Toxicity

Allergic reactions (including anaphylactic shock)
Fever
N/V (mild)
Anorexia
Weight loss
Arthralgia
Toxicity:
  Liver dysfunction
  Hyperglycemia
  Renal failure
  Pancreatitis

Comments and Specific Nursing Considerations

Have emergency drugs at bedside
Record signs of allergic reaction, such as urticaria, facial edema, hypotension, or abdominal cramps
Check weight daily
Normally, blood urea nitrogen (BUN) and ammonia levels rise as a result of drug; not evidence of liver damage
Check urine for sugar and blood amylase

Mechlorethamine (Nitrogen Mustard, Mustargen)
Administration

IV, IT

Side Effects and Toxicity

N/V (½-8 hours later) (severe)
BMD (2-3 weeks later)
Alopecia
Local phlebitis

---

*Includes principal drugs used in the treatment of childhood leukemias and lymphomas. Several other conventional and investigational chemotherapeutic agents may be employed in the treatment regimen.
†*IV*, Intravenous; *IT*, intrathecal; *PO*, by mouth; *IM*, intramuscular; *SC*, subcutaneous.
‡*N/V*, Nausea and vomiting. Mild = <20% incidence; moderate = 20% to 70% incidence; severe = >75% incidence.
§*BMD*, Bone marrow depression.
‖Vesicants (sclerosing agents) can cause severe cellular damage if even minute amounts of the drug infiltrate surrounding tissue.

SUMMARY OF SELECTED CHEMOTHERAPEUTIC AGENTS USED IN THE TREATMENT OF CHILDHOOD LEUKEMIAS AND LYMPHOMAS—cont'd

Mechloretamine—cont'd
Comments and Specific Nursing Considerations
Vesicant

Mercaptopurine (6-MP, Purinethol)
Administration
PO

Side Effects and Toxicity
N/V (mild)
Diarrhea
Anorexia
Stomatitis
BMD (4-6 weeks later)
Immunosuppression
Dermatitis
Less often may be hepatic dysfunction

Comments and Specific Nursing Considerations
6-MP is an analog of xanthine; therefore allopurinol (Zyloprim) delays its metabolism and increases its potency, necessitating a lower dose (⅓ to ¼) of 6-MP

Methotrexate (MTX, Amethopterin)
Administration
PO, IV, IM, IT
May be given in conventional doses (mg/m²) or high doses (g/m²)

Side Effects and Toxicity
N/V (severe at high doses)
Diarrhea
Mucosal ulceration (2-5 days later)
BMD (10 days later)
Immunosuppression
Dermatitis
Photosensitivity
Alopecia (uncommon)
Toxic effects include:
   Hepatitis (fibrosis)
   Osteoporosis
   Nephropathy
   Pneumonitis (fibrosis)
Neurologic toxicity with IT use—pain at injection site, meningismus (signs of meningitis without actual inflammation), especially fever and headache; potential sequelae—transient or permanent hemiparesis, convulsions, dementia, death

Comments and Specific Nursing Considerations
Side effects and toxicity are dose related
Potency and toxicity are increased by reduced renal function, salicylates, sulfonamides, and aminobenzoic acid; avoid use of these substances, such as aspirin
Avoid exposure to sun
High-dose therapy:
   Citrovorum factor (folinic acid or leucovorin) decreases cytotoxic action of MTX; used as an antidote for overdose and to enhance normal cell recovery after high-dose therapy; avoid use of vitamins containing folic acid during MTX therapy unless prescribed by physician
IT therapy:
   Drug *must* be mixed with preservative-free diluent
   Report signs of neurotoxicity immediately

Procarbazine (Matulane)
Administration
PO

Side Effects and Toxicity
N/V (moderate)
BMD (3-4 weeks later)
Lethargy
Dermatitis
Myalgia
Arthralgia
Less often:
   Stomatitis
   Neuropathy
   Alopecia
   Diarrhea

Comments and Specific Nursing Considerations
Central nervous system (CNS) depressants (phenothiazines, barbiturates) enhance CNS symptoms
Monoamine oxidase (MAO) inhibition sometimes occurs; therefore all other drugs are avoided unless medically approved; red wine, fava beans, and broad bean pods are avoided

Vincristine (Oncovin) and Vinblastine (Velban)
Administration
IV

Side Effects and Toxicity
Neurotoxicity (less severe with vinblastine)—paresthesia (numbness); ataxia; weakness; footdrop; hyporeflexia; constipation (dynamic ileus); hoarseness (vocal cord paralysis); abdominal, chest, and jaw pain; mental depression
Fever
N/V (mild)
BMD (minimal; 7-14 days later)
Alopecia

Comments and Specific Nursing Considerations
Vesicant
Report signs of neurotoxicity because may necessitate cessation of drug
Individuals with underlying neurologic problems may be more prone to neurotoxicity
Monitor stool patterns closely; administer stool softener
Excreted primarily by liver into biliary system; administer cautiously to anyone with biliary disease

Cytosine Arabinoside (Ara-C, Cytosar, Cytarabine, Arabinosyl Cytosine)
Administration
IV, IM, SC, IT

Side Effects and Toxicity
N/V (mild)
BMD (7-14 days later)
Mucosal ulceration
Immunosuppression
Hepatitis (usually subclinical)

Comments and Specific Nursing Considerations
Crosses blood-brain barrier
Use with caution in patients with hepatic dysfunction

Cyclophosphamide (Cytoxan, CTX, Neosar)
Administration
PO, IV, IM

Side Effects and Toxicity
N/V (3-4 hours later) (severe at high doses)
BMD (10-14 days later)
Alopecia

Continued.

SUMMARY OF SELECTED CHEMOTHERAPEUTIC AGENTS USED IN THE TREATMENT OF CHILDHOOD LEUKEMIAS AND LYMPHOMAS—cont'd

Hemorrhagic cystitis Severe immunosuppression Stomatitis (rare) Hyperpigmentation Transverse ridging of nails Infertility ***Comments and Specific Nursing Considerations*** BMD has platelet-sparing effect Give dose early in day to allow adequate fluids afterward Force fluids before administering drug and for 2 days after to prevent chemical cystitis; encourage frequent voiding even during night Warn parents to report signs of burning on urination or hematuria to practitioner	**Dacarbazine (DTIC-Dome)** ***Administration*** IV ***Side Effects and Toxicity*** N/V (especially after first dose) (severe) BMD (7-14 days later) Alopecia Flulike syndrome Burning sensation in vein during infusion (not extravasation) ***Comments and Specific Nursing Considerations*** Vesicant (less sclerosive) Must be given cautiously in patients with renal dysfunction Decrease IV rate or use warm moist towels on IV site to decrease burning

Neuropathy. Vincristine and, to a lesser extent, vinblastine can cause various neurotoxic effects. Nursing interventions for management of these effects include (1) administering stool softeners or laxatives for severe constipation caused by decreased bowel innervation; (2) maintaining good body alignment and, if on bedrest, using a footboard or high-top shoes to minimize or prevent footdrop; (3) carrying out safety measures during ambulation because of weakness and numbing of the extremities, which may cause difficulty in walking or fine hand movement; and (4) providing a soft or liquid diet for severe jaw pain.

Hemorrhagic Cystitis. Sterile hemorrhagic cystitis, a side effect of chemical irritation to the bladder from cyclophosphamide, can be decreased and often prevented by (1) a liberal fluid intake (at least one and a half times the recommended daily fluid requirement); (2) frequent voiding immediately after feeling the urge, before bed, and after arising; (3) administering the drug early in the day to allow for sufficient oral intake and voiding; and (4) administering mesna as ordered, an agent that provides protection to the bladder. If oral home administration is prescribed, the family needs *specific* instructions regarding exactly how much fluid the child must have.

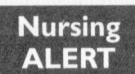 **Nursing ALERT**   If signs of cystitis occur, such as burning on urination, prompt medical evaluation is needed.

Alopecia. Hair loss is a common side effect of several chemotherapeutic drugs and cranial irradiation, although not all children lose their hair during drug therapy. It is better to warn children and parents of this side effect than to allow them to think that it is only a remote possibility. A soft cotton cap is the most comfortable head wear for children. Polyester increases perspiration and causes itching. Other options include scarves, hats, or a wig.

NURSING TIP If the child chooses to wear a wig, encouraging a child to select one similar to the child's own hairstyle and color before the hair falls out is helpful in fostering later adjustment to hair loss.

The nurse should also inform the family that hair regrows in 3 to 6 months and may be of a different color and texture. Frequently the hair is darker, thicker, and curlier than before. If the child chooses not to wear a wig, attention to some type of head covering, especially in cold climates and during exposure to sun, and scalp hygiene are important. The scalp should be washed like any other body part.

Moon Face. Short-term steroid therapy produces no acute toxicities and produces two beneficial reactions: increased appetite and a sense of well-being. However, it does produce alterations in body image, which, although not clinically significant, can be extremely distressing to older children. One of these is moon face, in which the child's face becomes rounded and puffy. It is not unusual for other children to make fun of the child with such remarks as "Miss Piggy," "Porky Pig," or "fat face." It is helpful to reassure children who experience such name-calling that after cessation of the drug the facial changes will return to normal. Unlike hair loss, little can be done to camouflage this obvious change. If the child resumes activity early in the course of treatment, the change may be less noticeable to peers than after a long absence.

Mood Changes. Shortly after beginning steroid therapy, children experience a number of mood changes that range from feelings of well-being and euphoria to depression and irritability. If parents are unaware of these drug-induced changes, they may become unduly concerned. Therefore the nurse should warn them of the reactions and encourage them to discuss the behavioral changes with each other and the child.

Provide Continued Physical Care and Emotional Support. Because of the improved survival of these children, continued monitoring of physical and intellectual growth and development is essential. Nurses should stress the importance of regular follow-up care.

An important aspect of continued emotional support involves the prognosis. Although leukemia is no longer invariably fatal, it must be remembered that survival statistics are only average estimates and apply to those children treated with the latest protocols since diagnosis. For the low-risk child the chances may be better, but for the high-risk child they may be significantly poorer. Of those who do survive after discontinuing therapy, some will relapse. Therefore, at present, only the passage of time is positive confirmation of the child's being ultimately "cured" of the disease. Remission, even in excess of 5 years, cannot be equated with a cure. With increasing concern regarding late effects of treatment, continued surveillance of the child's health status is needed. The nurse who is working with family members must individualize information regarding the "numbers" and the potential risks. An understanding of each member's emotional needs, as well as competent care of physical ones, is essential to the positive, growth-promoting support of the family. Comprehensive emotional support for the family of the child with a potentially fatal illness is discussed in Chapter 18.

❖ Evaluation

The effectiveness of nursing interventions is determined by continual reassessment and evaluation of care based on the following observational guidelines and expected outcomes:

1. Compare number of visits for primary health with recommended schedule of health supervision.
2. Monitor growth, development, and other aspects of regular health assessment; check mouth for adequacy of dental hygiene; review immunization record for age-appropriate vaccines and use of non–live virus preparations.
3. Interview child and family regarding their understanding of treatments and diagnostic tests.
4. Employ pain assessment techniques for procedural pain.
5. Make careful observations of physical status:
   a. Take vital signs regularly.
   b. Observe for evidence of bleeding, infection, neuropathy, cystitis, and mucosal ulceration.
   c. Observe and record intake and output.
6. Interview child and family and observe behaviors as a result of complications of therapies.
7. Interview child and family and observe behaviors that provide clues to their response to the disease, its therapy, and nursing interventions.

Expected outcomes:
See Nursing Care Plan, pp. 933-938.

LYMPHOMAS

The lymphomas are a group of neoplastic diseases that arise from the lymphoid and hemopoietic systems. They are usually divided into Hodgkin disease and non-Hodgkin lymphoma (NHL) and subdivided according to tissue type and extent of disease (staging). Before adolescence, NHL is more common than Hodgkin disease.

HODGKIN DISEASE

Hodgkin disease is a neoplastic disease that originates in the lymphoid system and primarily involves the lymph nodes. Although Hodgkin disease is extremely rare before 5 years of age, there is a striking increase in children 15 to 19 years of age, when it occurs with almost the same frequency as leukemia. The malignancy originates in the lymphoid system and primarily involves the lymph nodes. It predictably metastasizes to nonnodal or extralymphatic sites, especially the spleen, liver, bone marrow, and lungs, although no tissue is exempt from involvement (Fig. 26-3). *Most vascular*

The disease is usually classified according to four histologic types: (1) lymphocytic predominance, (2) nodular sclerosis, (3) mixed cellularity, and (4) lymphocytic depletion. Accu-

Blood flow

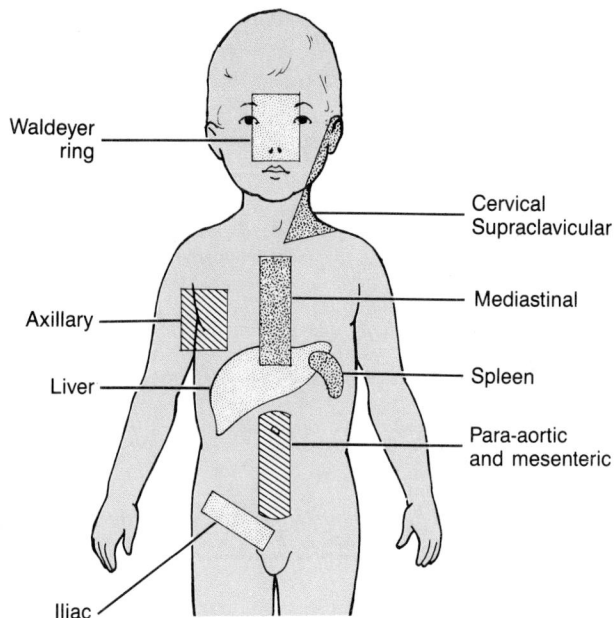

FIG. 26-3. Main areas of lymphadenopathy and organ involvement in Hodgkin disease.

rate staging of the extent of disease is the basis for treatment protocols and expected prognoses. The specific classification for each patient is derived from the history, physical examination, radiographic studies, laboratory tests, and biopsy findings. The staging system proceeds from stages I to IV, or from most to least favorable prognosis, respectively.

Diagnostic Evaluation

The diagnosis is often suspected on the basis of clinical manifestations and detection of enlarged lymph nodes during a physical examination (see box on p. 932). Because of the multiple organs that can become involved, diagnosis consists of several tests to confirm the presence of Hodgkin disease and to assess the extent of involvement for accurate staging. Tests include CBC, uric acid levels, liver function tests, urinalysis, and erythrocyte sedimentation rate. Computed tomography (CT) of the chest, liver, and spleen and bone scans are performed to detect metastasis.

Although used less frequently, *lymphangiography* may be performed. This is the visualization of lymphatic circulation of the lower extremities, groin, ileopelvic and abdominal-aortic regions, and the thoracic duct by way of a radiopaque medium injected in the feet or hands.

Lymph node biopsy is essential to diagnosis and staging. A bone marrow aspiration or biopsy also is performed. A laparotomy is recommended for definitive pathologic staging, and the spleen is removed, although this remains a controversial practice because of the risk of overwhelming infections from asplenia.

Therapeutic Management

The primary modalities of therapy are radiation and chemotherapy. Each may be used alone or in combination based on the clinical staging. Radiation may involve only the involved field (IF), an extended field (EF) (involved areas plus adja-

CLINICAL MANIFESTATIONS OF HODGKIN DISEASE

Painless enlargement of the lymph nodes:
  Enlarged, firm, nontender, movable nodes in the cervical area are most common
  "Sentinel" node located near the left clavicle may be first enlarged node
  Axillary and inguinal lymph nodes less frequently
Other signs and symptoms of lymphadenopathy:
  Enlarged mediastinal nodes cause persistent nonproductive cough
  Enlarged retroperitoneal nodes produce unexplained abdominal pain
Systemic symptoms (usually indicate advanced involvement):
  Low-grade and/or intermittent fever
  Anorexia
  Nausea
  Weight loss
  Night sweats
  Pruritus

cent nodes), or total nodal irradiation (TNI), depending on the extent of involvement. The most widely used chemotherapeutic regimen is *MOPP (mechlorethamine [Mustargen], vincristine [Oncovin], prednisone, and procarbazine)*, which is alternated with *adriamycin, bleomycin, vinblastine, and dacarbazine (ABVD)*.

Follow-up care of children no longer receiving therapy is essential to identify relapse and secondary cancers. In children with asplenia, prophylactic antibiotics are administered for an indefinite period, and immunizations against pneumococci and meningococci are recommended.

Prognosis. Long-term survival for all stages of Hodgkin disease is excellent. Early-stage disease can have survival rates greater than 90%, with advanced stages having rates between 65% and 75%. The most serious consequence of curative therapy is the development of secondary cancer, especially leukemia (AML) and solid tumors (Urba and Longo, 1992).

Nursing Considerations

Nursing care involves the same objectives as for patients with other types of cancer—specifically, (1) preparation for diagnostic and operative procedures, (2) explanation of treatment side effects (see box on pp. 928-930), and (3) child and family support (see Chapter 18). Since this is most often a disease of adolescents and young adults, the nurse must have an appreciation of their psychologic needs and reactions during the diagnostic and treatment phases. (See also Nursing Care Plan, pp. 933-938.)

Once the child is hospitalized for suspected Hodgkin disease, a battery of diagnostic tests is ordered. The family needs an explanation of why each test is performed, since many of them, such as bone marrow aspiration, are not routine. The one test that deserves special explanation is lymphangiography.

The child needs to be prepared for the lymphangiogram and especially told that the length of the procedure frequently averages 4 to 5 hours. Although the feet are anesthetized, the initial injections are painful. The use of EMLA cream and/or buffered lidocaine reduces or eliminates the pain (see

Pain Management, Chapter 21). Immobilization of the feet or hands during lymphatic vessel catheterization may be uncomfortable and tiresome, especially since the child must remain still for long periods. Whenever possible, the child is encouraged to sleep, or diversions should be provided, such as listening to music, reading, or talking. Ideally a family member should be allowed to accompany the child. Fluids and food are not necessarily restricted. If allowed, provisions are made for the child to have a favorite drink or snack.

The procedure is not without complications, the most serious of which is pulmonary embolism from the oil-based contrast media. The child and family need considerable reassurance. The contrast medium also turns the urine and skin of the feet and/or hands bluish green. Although the urine clears rapidly, the discoloration of the skin may last for months. Adolescents may be very self-conscious about the staining, especially in the hands.

Nursing ALERT Signs of pulmonary embolism include apprehension, cyanosis, distended neck veins, hypotension, liver tenderness, and edema in the lower extremities from increased venous resistance. Emergency medical treatment usually involves supplemental oxygen and antihypotensive drugs.

The most common side effect of irradiation is fatigue, which may last for a year after treatment. This is particularly difficult for active, outgoing school-age children and adolescents, because it prevents them from keeping up with their peers. Sometimes adolescents will push themselves to the point of physical exhaustion rather than admit and succumb to the decreased activity tolerance. The nurse cautions parents to observe for such behavior, such as extreme fatigue at the end of the day, falling asleep at the dinner table, inability to concentrate on homework, or an increased susceptibility to infection. A regular bedtime and scheduled rest periods are important for these children, especially during chemotherapy, when myelosuppression increases the risk of infection and debilitation. Prior to discharge the nurse should discuss a feasible school schedule with the parents and child.

An area of concern for adolescents is the high risk of sterility from irradiation and chemotherapy. Both irradiation to the gonads and drugs, particularly procarbazine and alkylating agents, can lead to infertility. Adolescents should be informed of these side effects early in the course of the diagnosis and treatment. Sperm banking is now offered at many cancer centers before the initiation of treatment in adolescent males. Sexual function is not altered, although the appearance of secondary sexual characteristics and menstruation may be delayed in the pubescent child. Delayed sexual maturation may be an extremely sensitive and stressful issue for children (see Chapter 17). It is important for the nurse to respect their concern and refrain from casually placating them with expressions such as "You'll catch up someday."

NON-HODGKIN LYMPHOMA (NHL)

NHL in children is strikingly different from Hodgkin disease and adult NHL in several aspects, including the following (Sandlund, Hutchison, and Crist, 1991):

Text continued on p. 938.

NURSING CARE PLAN
The Child with Cancer

NURSING DIAGNOSIS: High risk for injury related to malignant process, treatment

PATIENT GOAL 1: Will experience partial or complete remission from disease

- **NURSING INTERVENTIONS**

*Administer chemotherapeutic agents as prescribed
Assist with radiotherapy as ordered
Assist with procedures for administration of chemotherapeutic agents (e.g., lumbar puncture for intrathecal administration)
†Prepare child and family for surgical procedure if appropriate

- **EXPECTED OUTCOME**

Child achieves a partial or complete remission from disease

PATIENT GOAL 2: Will not experience complications of chemotherapy

- **NURSING INTERVENTIONS/RATIONALES**

Follow guidelines for administration of chemotherapeutic agents
Observe for signs of infiltration at intravenous (IV) site: pain, stinging, swelling, redness
Immediately stop infusion if any sign of infiltration occurs *to prevent severe tissue damage*
Implement policies of institution *to treat infiltration*
Obtain careful history for known allergies *to prevent anaphylaxis*
Observe child for 20 minutes after infusion *for signs of anaphylaxis* (cyanosis, hypotension, wheezing, severe urticaria)
Stop infusion of drug and flush IV line with normal saline if reaction is suspected
Have emergency equipment (especially blood pressure monitor and manual resuscitation bag and mask) and emergency drugs (especially oxygen, epinephrine, antihistamine, aminophylline, corticosteroids, and vasopressors) readily available *to prevent delay in treatment*

- **EXPECTED OUTCOMES**

Child will not experience complications of chemotherapy
Child will receive prompt, appropriate treatment of complications

---

NURSING DIAGNOSIS: High risk for infection related to depressed body defenses

PATIENT GOAL 1 : Will experience minimized risk of infection

- **NURSING INTERVENTIONS/RATIONALES**

Place child in private room *to minimize exposure to infective organisms*
Advise all visitors and staff to use good handwashing technique *to minimize exposure to infective organisms*

Screen all visitors and staff for signs of infection *to minimize exposure to infective organisms*
Use scrupulous aseptic technique for all invasive procedures
Monitor temperature *to detect possible infection*
Evaluate child for any potential sites of infection (e.g., needle punctures, mucosal ulceration, minor abrasions, dental problems)
Provide nutritionally complete diet for age *to support body's natural defenses*
Avoid giving live attenuated virus vaccines (e.g., measles, mumps, rubella, oral poliovirus) to child with depressed immune system *because these vaccines can result in overwhelming infection*
*Give inactivated virus vaccines (e.g., varicella [chickenpox], Salk polio, influenza) as prescribed and indicated *to prevent specific infections*
Administer antibiotics as prescribed
*Administer granulocyte colony–stimulating factor (GCSF) as prescribed

- **EXPECTED OUTCOMES**

Child does not come in contact with infected persons or contaminated articles
Child consumes diet appropriate for age (specify)
Child does not exhibit signs of infection

NURSING DIAGNOSIS: High risk for injury (hemorrhage, hemorrhagic cystitis) related to interference with cell proliferation

PATIENT GOAL 1: Will exhibit no evidence of bleeding

- **NURSING INTERVENTIONS/RATIONALES**

Use all measures to prevent infection, especially in ecchymotic areas, *because infection increases tendency toward bleeding*
Use local measures (e.g., apply pressure, ice) to stop bleeding
Restrict strenuous activity *that could result in accidental injury*
Involve child in responsibility for limiting activity when platelet count drops *to encourage compliance*
Avoid skin punctures when possible *to prevent bleeding*
Observe for bleeding after procedures such as venipuncture, bone marrow aspiration
Turn frequently and use pressure-reducing or pressure-relieving mattress *to prevent decubitus ulcers*
Teach parents and older child measures to control nosebleeding
Prevent oral and rectal ulceration *because ulcerated skin is prone to bleeding*
Avoid aspirin-containing medications *because aspirin interferes with platelet function*
*Administer platelets as prescribed *to raise platelet count*

- **EXPECTED OUTCOME**

Child exhibits no evidence of bleeding

---

*Dependent nursing action.
†Indicates content that is specific to a particular malignancy.

Continued.

PATIENT GOAL 2: Will exhibit no evidence of hemorrhagic cystitis

- **NURSING INTERVENTIONS/RATIONALES**

Observe for signs of cystitis (e.g., burning and pain on urination)

Report signs of cystitis to practitioner, *since prompt medical evaluation is needed*

Give liberal (3000 ml/m²/day) fluid intake (meters squared is calculated from West nomogram, see Administration of Medication, Chapter 22)

Encourage frequent voiding, including during nighttime, *to minimize metabolites' contact with bladder mucosa*

Administer drugs irritating to bladder early in the day *to allow for sufficient fluid intake and voiding*

- **EXPECTED OUTCOMES**

Child voids without discomfort
No hematuria is present

PATIENT GOAL 3: Will experience minimal effects of anemia

- **NURSING INTERVENTIONS/RATIONALES** AND EXPECTED OUTCOMES

See Nursing Care Plan: The Child with Anemia, p. 908

NURSING DIAGNOSIS: High risk for fluid volume deficit related to nausea and vomiting

---

PATIENT GOAL 1: Will experience no nausea or vomiting

- **NURSING INTERVENTIONS/RATIONALES**

*Administer initial dose of antiemetic before chemotherapy begins *to prevent child from ever experiencing nausea and vomiting, thus preventing an anticipatory response*

*Administer antiemetic around the clock for as long as nausea and vomiting typically last *to prevent any episodes from occurring*

Assess child's response to antiemetic, *since no antiemetic drug is uniformly successful*

Avoid foods with strong odors *that may induce nausea and vomiting*

Uncover hospital food tray outside of child's room *to reduce food odors that may induce nausea*

Encourage frequent intake of fluids in small amounts, *since small portions are usually better tolerated*

*Administer IV fluid, as prescribed, *to maintain hydration*

- **EXPECTED OUTCOMES**

Child retains food and fluid
Child does not experience nausea or vomiting

---

*Dependent nursing action.

NURSING DIAGNOSIS: Altered mucous membranes related to administration of chemotherapeutic agents

---

PATIENT GOAL 1: Will not develop oral mucositis

- **NURSING INTERVENTIONS/RATIONALES**

Inspect mouth daily for oral ulcers; report evidence of ulcers to practitioner *for early treatment*

Avoid oral temperatures *to prevent trauma*

Institute meticulous oral hygiene as soon as a drug is used that causes oral ulcers

  Use soft sponge toothbrush, cotton-tipped applicator, or gauze-wrapped finger *to avoid trauma*

  Administer frequent (at least every 4 hours and after meals) mouthwashes (normal saline with or without sodium bicarbonate solution) *to promote healing*

Apply local anesthetics to ulcerated areas before meals and as needed *to relieve pain*

  Avoid using viscous lidocaine for young children, *because if applied to pharynx, it may depress gag reflex, increasing risk of aspiration, and may cause seizures*

Apply lip balm *to keep lips moist and prevent cracking or fissuring*

Serve bland, moist, soft diet; offer food best tolerated by child

Encourage fluids; use a straw *to help bypass painful areas*

Encourage parents to relax any eating pressures, *since stomatitis is a temporary condition*

Avoid juices containing ascorbic acid and hot or cold or spicy foods if they cause further discomfort

Avoid using lemon glycerin swabs (*irritate eroded tissue and can decay teeth*), hydrogen peroxide (*delays healing by breaking down protein*), and Milk of Magnesia (*dries mucosa*)

Explain to parents that child may require hospitalization *for hydration, parenteral nutrition, and pain control (often with IV morphine)* if stomatitis interferes with food and fluid intake

*Administer antiinfective medication as ordered *to prevent or treat mucositis*

*Administer analgesics, including opioids, *to control pain*

- **EXPECTED OUTCOMES**

Mucous membranes remain intact
Ulcers show evidence of healing
Child reports and/or exhibits no evidence of discomfort

PATIENT GOAL 2: Will not develop rectal ulceration

- **NURSING INTERVENTIONS/RATIONALES**

Wash perianal area after each bowel movement *to lessen irritation*

Use warm sitz baths or tub baths *to promote healing*

Expose reddened but not ulcerated areas to air *to keep skin dry*

Apply protective skin barriers (transparent film dressings, occlusive ointment) to perineal area *to protect skin from direct contact with urine or feces and to promote healing*

Observe for constipation *resulting from child's voluntary refusal to defecate or from chemotherapy*

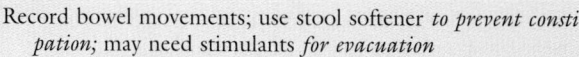

Record bowel movements; use stool softener *to prevent constipation;* may need stimulants *for evacuation*

Avoid rectal temperatures and suppositories *to prevent rectal trauma*

• EXPECTED OUTCOMES

Rectal mucosa remains clean and intact

Ulcerated areas heal without complications

Child has regular bowel movements

NURSING DIAGNOSIS: Altered nutrition: less than body requirements related to loss of appetite

---

PATIENT GOAL 1: Will receive adequate nutrition

• NURSING INTERVENTIONS/*RATIONALES*

Encourage parents to relax pressures placed on eating; explain that loss of appetite *is a direct consequence of nausea and vomiting and chemotherapy*

Allow child *any* food tolerated; plan to improve quality of food selections when appetite increases

Explain expected increase in appetite from steroids *to prepare child and parents for this change*

Take advantage of any hungry period: serve small "snacks," *since small portions are usually better tolerated*

Fortify foods with nutritious supplements, such as powdered milk or commercial supplements, *to maximize quality of intake*

Allow child to be involved in food preparation and selection *to encourage eating*

Make food appealing

Remember usual food practices of children in each age-group, such as food jags in toddlers or normal occurrence of physiologic anorexia, *to distinguish these expected changes from actual refusal to eat*

Assess family for additional problems (e.g., use of food by child as a control mechanism if appetite does not improve despite improved physical status) *to identify areas that require intervention*

• EXPECTED OUTCOME

Nutritional intake is adequate

NURSING DIAGNOSIS: Impaired skin integrity related to administration of chemotherapeutic agents, radiotherapy, immobility

---

PATIENT GOAL 1: Will maintain skin integrity

• NURSING INTERVENTIONS/*RATIONALES*

Provide meticulous skin care, especially in mouth and perianal regions, *because they are prone to ulceration*

Change position frequently *to stimulate circulation and relieve pressure*

Encourage adequate caloric-protein intake *to prevent negative nitrogen balance*

• EXPECTED OUTCOME

Skin remains clean and intact

PATIENT GOAL 2: Will experience minimal negative effects of therapy

• NURSING INTERVENTIONS/*RATIONALES*

Select loose-fitting clothing over irradiated area *to minimize additional irritation*

Protect area from sunlight and sudden changes in temperature (avoid ice packs, heating pads) during radiotherapy or administration of methotrexate

• EXPECTED OUTCOME

Child and family comply with suggestions (specify)

NURSING DIAGNOSIS: Impaired physical mobility related to neuromuscular impairment (neuropathy)

PATIENT GOAL 1: Will experience minimal negative effects of peripheral neuropathy

• NURSING INTERVENTIONS/*RATIONALES*

Encourage ambulation when child is able

Alter activity, including school attendance, *to prevent injuries if weakness occurs*

Use footboard or high-top shoes *to prevent footdrop*

Provide fluids and soft foods *to lessen chewing movements with jaw pain*

• EXPECTED OUTCOME

Child ambulates without incident or difficulty

NURSING DIAGNOSIS: Body image disturbance related to loss of hair, moon face, debilitation

---

PATIENT/FAMILY GOAL 1: Will exhibit positive coping behaviors

• NURSING INTERVENTIONS/*RATIONALES*

Introduce idea of wig before hair loss

    Encourage child to select a wig similar to child's own hairstyle and color before hair falls out *to foster later adjustment to hair loss*

Provide adequate covering during exposure to sunlight, wind, or cold, *since natural protection is lost*

Suggest keeping thin hair clean, short, and fluffy *to camouflage partial baldness*

Explain that hair begins to regrow in 3 to 6 months and may be a slightly different color or texture *to prepare child and family for changes in appearance of new hair*

Explain that alopecia during a second treatment with same drug may be less severe

Encourage good hygiene, grooming, and sex-appropriate items (e.g., wig, scarves, hats, makeup, attractive sex-appropriate clothing) *to enhance appearance*

• EXPECTED OUTCOMES

Child verbalizes concern regarding hair loss

Child helps determine methods to reduce effects of hair loss and applies these methods

Child appears clean, well groomed, and attractively dressed

Continued.

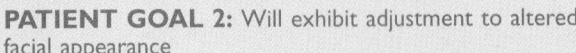

NURSING CARE PLAN
The Child with Cancer—cont'd

PATIENT GOAL 2: Will exhibit adjustment to altered facial appearance

- **NURSING INTERVENTIONS/RATIONALES**

Encourage rapid reintegration with peers *to lessen contrast of changed facial appearance*

Stress that this reaction is temporary *to provide reassurance that usual appearance will return*

Evaluate weight gain carefully *(with weight gain resulting from administration of steroids, extremities remain thin)*

Encourage visits from friends before discharge *to prepare child for reactions and questions*

- **EXPECTED OUTCOMES**

Family demonstrates understanding of consequences of therapies

Child resumes former activities and relationships within capabilities

PATIENT GOAL 3: Will express feelings

- **NURSING INTERVENTIONS**

Provide opportunities for child to discuss feelings and concerns

Provide materials for nonverbal expression (e.g., play, art)

- **EXPECTED OUTCOME**

Child expresses feelings regarding altered body in words, play, art (specify)

NURSING DIAGNOSIS: Pain related to diagnosis, treatment, physiologic effects of neoplasia

---

PATIENT GOAL 1: Will experience no pain or reduction of pain to level acceptable to child

- **NURSING INTERVENTIONS/RATIONALES**

Whenever possible, make use of procedures (e.g., noninvasive temperature monitoring, venous access device) *to minimize discomfort*

Assess need for pain management (see Chapter 21)

Evaluate effectiveness of pain relief with degree of alertness vs sedation *to determine need for change in dosage, time of administration, or drug*

Implement appropriate nonpharmacologic pain reduction techniques *as adjunct to analgesics*

*Administer analgesics as prescribed

    Avoid aspirin or any of its compounds (e.g., other nonsteroidal antiinflammatory agents) *because aspirin increases bleeding tendency*

*Administer drugs on preventive schedule (around the clock) *to prevent pain from recurring*

Monitor effectiveness of therapy on pain assessment record

- **EXPECTED OUTCOME**

Child rests quietly, reports and/or exhibits no evidence of discomfort, and verbalizes no complaints of discomfort

---

NURSING DIAGNOSIS: Fear related to diagnostic tests, procedures, treatments

---

PATIENT GOAL 1: Will exhibit reduced fear related to diagnostic procedures and tests

- **NURSING INTERVENTIONS/RATIONALES**

Explain procedure carefully at child's level of understanding *to reduce fear of the unknown*

Explain what will take place and what child will feel, see, and hear *to increase sense of control*

Use recall of each step *as method of distraction*

Explain special requests of child (e.g., need to remain motionless during test and/or radiotherapy) *to encourage cooperation*

Provide child with some means for involvement with procedure (e.g., holding a piece of equipment, such as bandage or tape, counting with the operator, answering questions) *to promote sense of control, encourage cooperation, and support child's coping skills*

Implement distracting techniques and pain reduction techniques as indicated

See also Preparation for Procedures, Chapter 22

- **EXPECTED OUTCOMES**

Child readily responds to verbal directives

Child repeats information accurately

NURSING DIAGNOSIS: Fear related to diagnosis, prognosis

See Nursing Care Plan: The Child Who Is Terminally Ill or Dying, Chapter 18

NURSING DIAGNOSIS: Diversional activity deficit related to restricted environment (private room)

PATIENT GOAL 1: Will have opportunity to participate in diversional activities

- **NURSING INTERVENTIONS/RATIONALES**

Provide age-appropriate toys that can be properly cleaned *to provide diversion without risk of infection*

Involve child-life specialist or other supportive services in planning diversional activities

- **EXPECTED OUTCOMES**

Child engages in activities appropriate for age and interests

Suitable toys are provided

NURSING DIAGNOSIS: Altered family processes related to having a child with a life-threatening disease

---

*Dependent nursing action.

NURSING CARE PLAN
The Child with Cancer—cont'd

PATIENT/FAMILY GOAL 1: Will demonstrate knowledge about diagnostic/therapeutic procedures

• **NURSING INTERVENTIONS/RATIONALES**

Explain reason for each test and procedure
Explain reason for radiotherapy, chemotherapy
Explain operative procedure honestly (if appropriate)
Avoid overemphasis on benefits, which may not be immediately evident (applies primarily to brain tumors) *to avoid unrealistic expectations*
See also Preparation for Procedures, Chapter 22

• **EXPECTED OUTCOME**

Child and family demonstrate understanding of procedures (specify learning and manner of demonstration)

PATIENT (FAMILY) GOAL 2: Will receive adequate support

• **NURSING INTERVENTIONS/RATIONALES**

Teach parents about disease process
Explain all procedures that will be done to child
Schedule time for family to be together, without interruptions from staff, *to encourage communication and expression of feelings*
Help family plan for future, especially for helping child live a normal life, *to promote child's optimum development*
Encourage family to discuss feelings regarding child's course before diagnosis and child's prognosis
Discuss with family how they will tell child about outcome of treatment and need for additional treatment (if appropriate) *to maintain open and honest communication*
Refer to local chapter of American Cancer Society or other organizations

• **EXPECTED OUTCOMES**

Family demonstrates knowledge of child's disease and treatments (specify methods of learning and evaluation)
Family expresses feelings and concerns and spends time with child
See also:
    Nursing Care Plan: The Child in the Hospital, Chapter 21
    Nursing Care Plan: The Family of the Ill or Hospitalized Child, Chapter 21

> **NURSING DIAGNOSIS:** Altered family processes related to a child undergoing therapy

PATIENT (FAMILY) GOAL 1: Will demonstrate understanding of side effects and/or complications of treatment

• **NURSING INTERVENTIONS/RATIONALES**

Advise family of expected side effects vs toxicities; clarify which demand medical evaluation (mucosal ulceration, hemorrhagic cystitis, peripheral neuropathy, evidence of infection or dehydration) *to prevent delay in treatment*
Reassure family that such reactions are not caused by return of cancer cells *to minimize undue concern*

Interpret prognostic statistics carefully, realizing family's temporary need to interpret them as they see necessary, *to present a realistic, but hopeful, future*
Prepare family for expected mood changes from steroids
Interpret mood changes based on drugs or reactions to disease/treatment *to prevent any unwarranted negative reaction to child (e.g., punishment)*

• **EXPECTED OUTCOMES**

Family demonstrates knowledge of instructions (specify methods of learning and evaluation)
Family demonstrates understanding of behavior changes

PATIENT GOAL 2: Will receive adequate support during treatment

• **NURSING INTERVENTIONS/RATIONALES**

Explain reason for antibiotics and/or transfusions, particularly why platelets are reserved for acute, uncontrolled bleeding episodes
Observe for signs of transfusion reaction (see Table 26-4)
Record appropriate time for hemostasis to occur after administration of platelets *to determine if transfusions are becoming less effective*

• **EXPECTED OUTCOME**

Child demonstrates understanding of procedures and tests (specify methods of learning and evaluation)

PATIENT (FAMILY) GOAL 3: Will be prepared for home care

• **NURSING INTERVENTIONS/RATIONALES**

Teach preventive measures at discharge (e.g., handwashing, isolation from crowds) *to prevent infection*
Stress importance of isolating child from any known cases of chickenpox or other childhood diseases; work with school nurse and physician to determine optimum time for school reattendance *to prevent unnecessary absences or risk of infection*
Teach home care instructions specific to child's needs

• **EXPECTED OUTCOME**

Family demonstrates ability to provide home care for child (specify)

> **NURSING DIAGNOSIS:** Anticipatory grief related to perceived potential loss of a child

PATIENT (FAMILY) GOAL 1: Will acknowledge and cope with possibility of child's death

• **NURSING INTERVENTIONS/RATIONALES**

Provide consistent contact with family *to establish a trusting relationship that encourages communication*
Clarify, refocus, and supply information as needed
Help family plan care of child, especially at terminal stage (e.g., extent of extraordinary lifesaving measures) *to ensure their wishes are implemented*

Continued.

NURSING CARE PLAN
The Child with Cancer—cont'd

Provide or arrange for hospice care if family desires it

Arrange for spiritual support in accordance with family's beliefs and/or affiliations

- **EXPECTED OUTCOMES**

Family remains open to counseling and nursing contact

Family and child discuss their fears, concerns, needs, and desires at terminal stage

Family investigates hospice care

Appropriate religious representative is contacted (specify)

PATIENT (FAMILY) GOAL 2: Will receive adequate support

- **NURSING INTERVENTIONS/*RATIONALES* AND EXPECTED OUTCOMES**

See Nursing Care Plan: The Child Who Is Terminally Ill or Dying, Chapter 18

---

1. The disease is usually diffuse rather than nodular.
2. The cell type is either undifferentiated or poorly differentiated.
3. Dissemination occurs early, more often, and rapidly.
4. Mediastinal involvement and invasion of meninges are common.

NHL exhibits a variety of morphologic, cytochemical, and immunologic features, not unlike the diversity seen in leukemia. Classification is based on the histologic pattern: (1) lymphoblastic, (2) Burkitt or non-Burkitt, or (3) large cell (Huizdala, 1991). Immunologically these cells are also classified as T-cells, B-cells, or null cells (lacking immunologic properties).

The clinical staging system used in Hodgkin disease is of little value in NHL, although it has been modified and other systems have been developed.

Diagnostic Evaluation

Because the clinical presentation of most children with NHL is widespread disseminated disease, thorough pathologic staging is unnecessary. Clinical manifestations depend on the anatomic site and extent of involvement. These manifestations include many of those seen in Hodgkin disease and leukemia, as well as organ symptoms related to pressure from enlargement of adjacent lymph nodes, such as intestinal or airway obstruction, cranial nerve palsies, and spinal paralysis.

Current recommendations for staging include a surgical biopsy of an enlarged node, histopathologic confirmation of disease with cytochemical and immunologic evaluation, bone marrow examination, radiographic studies (especially tomograms of the lungs and GI organs), and lumbar puncture.

Therapeutic Management

The present treatment protocols for NHL include aggressive use of irradiation and chemotherapy. Similar to leukemic therapy, the protocols include induction, consolidation, and maintenance phases, some with intrathecal chemotherapy. Several drug combinations are employed, most of which contain several antineoplastic agents.

Prognosis.   The prognosis is excellent for children with localized disease, and long-term remissions are possible in many patients, even in those with disseminated disease. Since relapse after 2 years is rare, survival after 24 months is considered a cure.

Nursing Considerations

Nursing care of the child with NHL is very similar to that required for children with leukemia. Many of the same drugs are employed, although the schedules differ. Because of the intense chemotherapy, nursing care is primarily directed toward managing the side effects of these agents and providing supportive care to the child and family. (See also Nursing Care Plan, pp. 933-938.)

IMMUNOLOGIC DEFICIENCY DISORDERS

A number of disorders can cause profound, often life-threatening alterations within the body's immune system. The most serious are those conditions that completely depress immunity, such as severe combined immunodeficiency disease. However, the one disorder that generates the most anxiety, within both the family and the community at large, is acquired immunodeficiency syndrome (AIDS).

Several classifications of immune dysfunction exist. *AIDS, severe combined immunodeficiency syndrome (SCIDS),* and *Wiskott-Aldrich syndrome* are syndromes wherein the body is unable to mount an immune response. The immune response can also be misdirected. In *autoimmune disorders,* antibodies, macrophages, and lymphocytes attack healthy cells.

MECHANISMS INVOLVED IN IMMUNITY

In simple terms, the function of the immune system is to recognize "self" from "nonself" and to initiate responses to eliminate the nonself or the foreign substance known as *antigen.* However, the specific processes involved in this function are complex and interrelated, and advances in the understanding of immunologic mechanisms are helping to explain further the complexities of this system.

Intact skin serves as the first line of protection for the body. Body secretions such as mucus, saliva, sweat, and tears contain chemicals that can kill many organisms. The stomach contains acids that can destroy swallowed pathogens as they adhere to the mucus of the nose and mouth. Organisms trapped in these areas are expelled by sneezing or coughing. If the foreign substance has penetrated these barriers, cellular elements are mobilized to provide further protection.

The immune system includes the primary lymphoid organs (thymus, bone marrow, and probably liver) and the secondary lymphoid organs (lymph nodes, spleen, and gut-associated lymphoid tissue [GALT]). The functions of the immune system are basically of two types: nonspecific and specific. *Nonspecific immune defenses* are activated on exposure to any foreign substance but react similarly regardless of the type of antigen; they are unable to identify the antigen, except to know that it is "nonself." The principal activity of this system is *phagocytosis,* the process of ingesting and digesting foreign substances. Phagocytic cells include neutrophils and monocytes.

Specific (adaptive) defenses have the ability to recognize the antigen and respond selectively. Adaptive immunity consists of (1) *humoral immunity,* which includes antibodies in the form of immunoglobulin and which is concerned primarily with response to foreign antigens, and (2) *cell-mediated immunity,* which provides protection against most invading organisms. Conditions that cause interference with any or all of these protective mechanisms leave the body vulnerable to disease.

ACQUIRED IMMUNODEFICIENCY SYNDROME (AIDS)

AIDS is a disorder that has generated intense medical investigation and even greater public concern and fear. *Human immunodeficiency virus (HIV)* causes AIDS. The virus has been found in blood and almost all body fluids (semen, saliva, vaginal secretions, urine, breast milk, tears), but the evidence to date is that the virus is transmitted primarily through direct contact with blood or blood products, including sharing of intravenous needles for drug use and intimate sexual contact. There is no evidence that *casual* contact between affected and unaffected individuals can spread the virus (Caldwell and Rogers, 1991).

People with AIDS (PWA) make up a diverse group. In the pediatric age-group, three populations are primarily affected: children who are exposed in utero to an infected mother (referred to as "vertical transmission"; maternal transmission can also occur at delivery or through breast-feeding); children who have received blood products, such as children with hemophilia; and adolescents who are infected because of sexual activity with an infected partner and other high-risk behaviors. Each group has unique needs relative to the origin of the infection. The majority of children with AIDS are less than 2 years of age and constitute a small percentage of the total AIDS population.

Diagnostic Evaluation

HIV infection has spread beyond the previously identified risk groups and geographic areas. With the prevalence of the virus, the American Academy of Pediatrics Provisional Committee on Pediatric AIDS (1995) recommends maternal and/or newborn HIV testing. Perinatal transmission of HIV has been significantly reduced in those pregnant women who take zidovudine during pregnancy. The current testing procedures enable 50% of affected infants to be identified at birth, and 95% can be diagnosed by 1 to 3 months of age. This allows prophylaxis for *Pneumocystis carinii* pneumonia (PCP), the most frequent opportunistic infection associated with HIV, to begin within the first few months of life (see boxes).

Therapeutic Management

There is currently no cure for pediatric HIV disease. Treatment is primarily supportive, although some drugs have increased the life span for these children. *AZT (zidovudine)* and *DDI (dideoxyinosine)* are the current drugs used to treat pediatric HIV disease. A combination of these drugs is effective in delaying symptoms of AIDS. These children also receive prophylaxis for PCP infection with *trimethoprim-sulfamethoxazole (TMP/SMZ).*

Bactrim [handwritten]

CLINICAL MANIFESTATIONS OF AIDS IN CHILDREN

All
Failure to thrive
Hepatosplenomegaly
Chronic interstitial pneumonitis

Infants
Oral candidiasis
Failure to thrive
Hepatosplenomegaly
Respiratory distress secondary to *Pneumocystis carinii* pneumonia (PCP)

Toddlers
Parotitis
Generalized lymphadenopathy
Recurrent bacterial infections
Neurologic disease
Developmental abnormalities

RISK FACTORS FOR AIDS IN CHILDREN

Maternal Factors
Intravenous drug use
Maternal promiscuity
Diagnosis of AIDS in mother
Haitian or sub-Saharan African origin

High-Risk Groups
Intravenous drug abusers
Sexual partners of risk-group
Sexually active homosexual males
Bisexual males
Disadvantaged, out-of-school youth, especially females

Disease prevention is of great importance for these children, and immunization against common childhood illnesses is recommended for all children with HIV infection. The only change in the schedule is the avoidance of varicella (chickenpox) vaccine and the use of inactivated poliovirus (IPV) rather than oral poliovirus (OPV) for these children and their close contacts (American Academy of Pediatrics, 1995). For children with AIDS the pneumococcal and influenza vaccines are recommended. These children must be evaluated for their response to the immunizations.

Prognosis. Early recognition and improved medical care have changed HIV disease from a rapidly fatal to a chronic, but terminal, disease of childhood. The ultimate prognosis for perinatal HIV infection depends on the age of the child at diagnosis and the types of secondary diseases. Children diagnosed with AIDS in early infancy are more likely to die at an earlier age. Secondary diseases that are associated with more rapid death include severe bacterial infections, progressive encephalopathy, anemia, fever, and diarrhea. Children with recurrent respiratory tract infections, hepatosplenomegaly, lymphadenopathy, parotitis, and skin diseases have a better prognosis (Tovo and others, 1992). However, most develop progressive encephalopathy, which is manifested by delayed development or loss of milestones in infants (Joshi, 1991) and by progressive cognitive impairment in older children (Spiegel and Mayers, 1991). A serious issue for AIDS patients is pain management. These individuals report significant pain that is often undertreated (see Pain Management, Chapter 21).

Nursing Considerations

Nursing considerations are primarily directed at caring for the child with AIDS, preventing the transmission of HIV, and educating the public regarding the *realistic* concerns in terms of communicability of the virus. Recommendations for preventing spread of the virus consist of the use of universal precautions (see Infection Control, Chapter 22, and Nursing Care Plan, pp. 941-942).*

The nurse's role is central to the child and family. The nurse serves as educator, direct care provider, case manager, and advocate. As with all chronic illnesses, these children will have much involvement with the health care system. The physiologic care of the AIDS patient is directed at minimum exposure to infections, nutritional support, comfort measures, and assessment and recognition of changes in status that may indicate impending sepsis or other complications. The psychologic interventions will vary with the unique circumstances of the child and family.

The family of the child with perinatal transmission usually is faced with multiple problems, since the mother is infected. The nurse must encourage the mother to receive regular health care. Assistance should be offered to help parents care for a child with a chronic illness. Grandparents or other relatives may have to assume responsibility for the care of the child. These surrogate parents should be given support for their role. If no extended family is available, the child may be placed in a foster home or group home.

Since these children are frequently ill, they may have multiple hospitalizations (Boland and Santacroce, 1994). Foster care is difficult to arrange because of the nature of the illness and the fear of disease transmission. These children have many symptoms, including diarrhea, lung infections, failure to thrive, and encephalopathy. They are often irritable, with a shrill cry, and difficult to console. If there is family involvement, nursing considerations are directed at supporting the family. Whenever possible, social services and home health and nutritional services such as Women, Infants, and Children (WIC) should be made available. Nurses in community-based systems of care have impacted greatly on the quality of life for these children. The nurses assist with placement and school attendance. Since the disease is congenitally acquired, the parents must deal with feelings of guilt. They will need support during the disease progression and terminal phase (see Family Focus box).

Another group of individuals increasingly infected with HIV is adolescents. As young people engage in the high-risk behaviors associated with AIDS, the possibility of infection increases. Adolescents must be taught about the risk factors, including injection drug use and high-risk sexual practices, such as anal intercourse and sex with multiple partners (see Human Immunodeficiency Virus Infection and Acquired Immunodeficiency Syndrome, Chapter 17). Numerous AIDS educational materials are available.*

One of the most pressing concerns in caring for PWA is protection for the caregiver. Although children with HIV infection can be held, cuddled, and fed safely, standard precautions (see Chapter 22) must be used in caring for all patients. Unfortunately, the public is also very fearful of contracting the disease from AIDS victims, and criticism and ostracism of the child and family are common. In an effort to protect the child and deal with the community's fear, the family may keep the child at home in an atmosphere of overprotection.

---

*Information is available from the AIDS hotline: (800) 342-2437 (AIDS); and from the **National Pediatric HIV Resource Center**, 15 S. 9th St., Newark, NJ 07107, (201) 268-8251 or (800) 362-0071.

 FAMILY FOCUS
Caregivers and the Infant with AIDS

Unlike other fatal pediatric diseases, AIDS is associated with special family alterations. The infant infected in utero faces multiple physical and parental problems. Because the mother is infected, she may be ill or dying and therefore unable to care for the child. If possible, grandparents or other relatives may assume care. Foster care is often difficult to arrange because of the nature of the disease, especially in relation to the social stigma and the child's multiple medical needs. When extended family members or foster care is not available, the child may become a ward of the state or a "boarder" in an acute care hospital. Because these children are frequently ill, they may spend most of their lives in the hospital. When children remain in the hospital, the importance of consistent caregivers, especially primary nurses, who attend to the youngsters' physical, developmental, and emotional needs cannot be overemphasized. However, primary nurses may face the risk of overinvolvement and must be aware of the boundaries of a therapeutic relationship.

---

*Home care instructions on preventing HIV and hepatitis infection are available in Wong DL: *Wong and Whaley's Clinical manual of pediatric nursing*, ed 4, St Louis, 1996, Mosby.

NURSING CARE PLAN

The Child with Human Immunodeficiency Virus (HIV)

NURSING DIAGNOSIS: High risk for infection related to impaired body defenses, presence of infective organisms

PATIENT GOAL 1: Will experience minimized risk of infection

- **NURSING INTERVENTIONS/*RATIONALES***

Use thorough handwashing technique *to minimize exposure to infective organisms*

Advise visitors to use good handwashing technique *to minimize exposure to infective organisms*

Place child in room with noninfectious children or in private room

Restrict contact with persons who have infections, including family, other children, friends, and members of staff; explain that child is highly susceptible to infection *to encourage cooperation and understanding*

Observe medical asepsis as appropriate *to decrease risk of infection*

Encourage good nutrition and adequate rest *to promote body's remaining natural defenses*

Explain to family and older child importance of contacting health professional if exposed to childhood illnesses (e.g., chickenpox, measles) *so that appropriate immunizations can be given*

*Administer appropriate immunizations as prescribed *to prevent specific infections*

*Administer antibiotics as prescribed

- **EXPECTED OUTCOMES**

Child does not come in contact with infected persons or contaminated articles

Child and family apply good health practices

Child exhibits no evidence of infection

PATIENT GOAL 2: Will not spread disease to others

- **NURSING INTERVENTIONS/*RATIONALES***

Implement and carry out standard precautions, *to prevent spread of virus* (see Infection Control, Chapter 22)

Instruct others (e.g., family, members of staff) in appropriate precautions; clarify any misconceptions about communicability of virus, *since this is a frequent problem and may interfere with use of appropriate precautions*

Teach affected children protective methods *to prevent spread of infection* (e.g., handwashing, handling genital area, care after using bedpan or toilet)

Endeavor to keep infants and small children from placing hands and objects in contaminated areas

Place restrictions on behaviors and contacts for affected children who bite or who do not have control of their bodily secretions

Assess home situation and implement protective measures as feasible in individual circumstances

- **EXPECTED OUTCOME**

Others do not acquire the disease

NURSING DIAGNOSIS: Altered nutrition: less than body requirements related to recurrent illness, diarrheal losses, loss of appetite, oral candidiasis

PATIENT GOAL 1: Will receive optimum nourishment

- **NURSING INTERVENTIONS/*RATIONALES***

Provide high-calorie, high-protein meals and snacks *to meet body requirements for metabolism and growth*

Provide foods child prefers *to encourage eating*

Fortify foods with nutritional supplements (e.g., powdered milk or commercial supplements) *to maximize quality of intake*

Provide meals when child is most likely to eat well

Use creativity to encourage child to eat (see Feeding the Sick Child, Chapter 22)

Monitor child's weight and growth *so that additional nutritional interventions can be implemented if growth begins to slow or weight drops*

*Administer antifungal medication as ordered *to treat oral candidiasis*

- **EXPECTED OUTCOME**

Child consumes a sufficient amount of nutrients (specify)

NURSING DIAGNOSIS: Impaired social interaction related to physical limitations, hospitalizations, social stigma toward HIV

PATIENT GOAL 1: Will participate in peer group and family activities

- **NURSING INTERVENTIONS/*RATIONALES***

Assist child in identifying personal strengths *to facilitate coping*

Educate school personnel and classmates about HIV *so that child is not unnecessarily isolated*

Encourage child to participate in activities with other children and family

Encourage child to maintain phone contact with friends during hospitalization *to lessen isolation*

- **EXPECTED OUTCOME**

Child participates in activities with peer group and family

NURSING DIAGNOSIS: Altered sexuality pattern related to risk of disease transmission

PATIENT GOAL 1: Will exhibit healthy sexual behavior

---

*Dependent nursing action.

Continued.

NURSING CARE PLAN

The Child with Human Immunodeficiency Virus (HIV)—cont'd

- **NURSING INTERVENTIONS/*RATIONALES***

Educate adolescent about the following *so that adolescent has adequate information to identify safe, healthy expressions of sexuality:*
Sexual transmission
Risk of perinatal infection
Dangers of promiscuity
Abstinence, use of condoms
Avoidance of high-risk behaviors
Encourage adolescent to talk about feelings and concerns related to sexuality *to facilitate coping*

- **EXPECTED OUTCOMES**

Adolescent exhibits a positive sexual identity
Adolescent does not infect other individuals

> **NURSING DIAGNOSIS:** Pain related to disease process (e.g., encephalopathy, treatments)

PATIENT GOAL 1: Will exhibit minimal or no evidence of pain or irritability

- **NURSING INTERVENTIONS/*RATIONALES***

Assess pain (see Pain Assessment, Chapter 21)
Use nonpharmacologic strategies *to help child manage pain*
    For infants, may try general comfort measures (e.g., rocking, holding, swaddling, reducing environmental stimuli [may or may not be effective because of encephalopathy])
*Use pharmacologic strategies (see Pain Management, Chapter 21)
    Plan preventive schedule if analgesics are effective in relieving continuous pain

---

*Dependent nursing action.

Encourage use of premedication for painful procedures *to minimize discomfort*
Child may benefit from use of adjunctive analgesics (e.g., antidepressants) that are effective against neuropathic pain
Use pain assessment record *to evaluate effectiveness of pharmacologic and nonpharmacologic interventions*

- **EXPECTED OUTCOME**

Child exhibits absence of or minimal evidence of pain or irritability

> **NURSING DIAGNOSIS:** Altered family processes related to having a child with a dreaded and life-threatening disease

PATIENT (FAMILY) GOAL 1: Will receive adequate support and will be able to meet needs of child

- **NURSING INTERVENTIONS/*RATIONALES* AND EXPECTED OUTCOMES**

See Nursing Care Plan: The Family of the Ill or Hospitalized Child, Chapter 21

> **NURSING DIAGNOSIS:** Anticipatory grief related to having a child with a potentially fatal illness

See Nursing Care Plan: The Child Who Is Terminally Ill or Dying, Chapter 18

Although certain precautions are justified in limiting exposure to sources of infection, they must be tempered with concern for the child's normal developmental needs. Both the family and the community need education about HIV to dispel many of the myths that have been perpetuated by uninformed persons.

Of major concern for both family and community has been school attendance for children with AIDS. Both the Centers for Disease Control and Prevention (1985) and the American Academy of Pediatrics (1986) have published guidelines regarding school attendance, which include the following:

1. Unrestricted school attendance for most school-age children and adolescents, including those with AIDS or who have antibody to the virus, with the approval of their personal physician, is recommended.
2. Students who do not have control of their bodily secretions, who

display behaviors such as biting, or who have open sores that cannot be covered may present a greater risk and should be given a more restricted school environment until more is known about the disease.

SEVERE COMBINED IMMUNODEFICIENCY DISEASE (SCID)

SCID is a defect characterized by absence of both humoral and cell-mediated immunity. The terms *Swiss-type lymphopenic agammaglobulinemia,* an autosomal recessive form of the disease, and *X-linked lymphopenic agammaglobulinemia* have been used to describe this disorder, which, as the names imply, can follow either mode of inheritance.

Susceptibility to infection occurs early in life, most often by 3 months of age, when prenatal acquired immunity is exhausted. The child suffers from chronic infection, fails to completely recover from an infection, is frequently reinfected, and is infected with unusual agents. Failure to thrive is a consequence of the persistent illnesses.

Diagnosis is usually based on a history of recurrent, severe infections from early infancy and specific laboratory findings, which include lymphopenia, lack of lymphocyte response to antigens, and absence of plasma cells in the bone marrow. Documentation of immunoglobulin (Ig) deficiency is difficult during infancy because of the normally delayed response of infants to producing their own immunoglobulins and material transfer of IgG.

Therapeutic Management
The only definitive treatment for SCID is a bone marrow transplant from a histocompatible donor, usually a sibling. If a compatible sibling is not available, a parent's marrow can be used after the T-lymphocytes have been depleted. Intravenous Ig can be used to augment the humoral immunity until the transplant is performed.

Nursing Considerations
Nursing care focuses on the prevention of infection and supporting the child and family. If bone marrow transplantation is attempted, the care is consistent with that needed for bone marrow transplantation for any condition (see p. 945). Since the prognosis for SCID is very poor if a compatible bone marrow donor is not available, nursing care is directed at supporting the family in caring for a child with a life-threatening illness (Chapter 18). Genetic counseling is essential because of the modes of transmission in either form of the disorder.

WISKOTT-ALDRICH SYNDROME
The Wiskott-Aldrich syndrome is an X-linked recessive disorder characterized by a triad of abnormalities: (1) thrombocytopenia, (2) eczema, and (3) immunodeficiency of selective functions of B- and T-lymphocytes. At birth the major effect of the disorder is bleeding as a result of the thrombocytopenia. As the child grows older, recurrent infection and eczema become more severe, and the bleeding becomes less frequent.

Eczema is typical of the allergic type and easily becomes superinfected. Chronic infection with herpes simplex is a frequent problem and may lead to chronic keratitis of the eye with loss of vision. Chronic pulmonary disease, sinusitis, and otitis media result from repeated infections. In those children who survive the bleeding episodes and overwhelming infections, malignancy presents an additional risk to survival.

Specific tests for immunologic function confirm the diagnosis. Medical treatment involves (1) counteracting the bleeding tendencies with platelet transfusions, (2) providing gamma globulin to provide passive immunity, and (3) administering prophylactic antibiotics to prevent and control infection. Bone marrow transplants have been attempted but, even if successful, do not reverse all the defects of this disorder.

Nursing Considerations
Because of the poor prognosis for these children, the main nursing consideration is supporting the family in the care of a fatally ill child (see Chapter 18). Physical care is directed at

controlling the problems imposed by the disorder. The measures used to control bleeding are similar to those for hemophilia. Another major goal is prevention or control of infection. Since eczema is a troublesome problem, nursing measures specific to this condition are especially important (see Chapter 30). The genetic implications of this X-linked recessive disorder differ little from those of any other X-linked disorder.

TECHNOLOGIC MANAGEMENT OF HEMATOLOGIC/ IMMUNOLOGIC DISORDERS

BLOOD TRANSFUSION THERAPY
Technologic advances in blood banking and transfusion medicine enable the administration of only the blood component needed by the child, such as packed RBCs in anemia or platelets for bleeding disorders. However, regardless of the blood component infused, all transfusions have some risks. Therefore nurses need to be aware of the possible complications and the appropriate interventions. Table 26-4 summarizes the major hazards of transfusions, the signs and symptoms typically associated with each, and nursing responsibilities. General guidelines that apply to all transfusions include the following:

- Take vital signs, including blood pressure, *before* administering blood to establish baseline data for intratransfusion and posttransfusion comparison, then every 15 minutes for 1 hour while blood is infusing.
- Check the identification of the recipient with the donor's blood group and type, regardless of the blood product used.
- Administer the first 50 ml of blood or ⅕ the volume (whichever is smaller) *slowly* and stay with the child.
- Administer with normal saline on a piggyback setup.
- Administer blood through an appropriate filter to eliminate particles in the blood and prevent the precipitation of formed elements; gently shake container frequently.
- Use blood within 30 minutes of its arrival from the blood bank; if it is not used, return to blood bank—do not store in regular unit refrigerator.
- Infuse a unit of blood (or the specified amount) within 4 hours. If the infusion will exceed this time, the blood should be divided into appropriate-size quantities by the blood bank and the unused portion refrigerated under controlled conditions.
- If a reaction of any type is suspected, take vital signs, stop the transfusion, maintain a patent IV line with normal saline and new tubing, notify the physician, and do not restart the transfusion until the child's condition has been medically evaluated.

Although hemolytic reactions are rare, ABO incompatibility remains the most common cause of death from blood transfusion, and human error is usually responsible (administration of the wrong type to the patient or mislabeling of the blood product). Hemolysis can also cause the release of large quantities of phospholipids, which are capable of stimulating disseminated intravascular coagulation (DIC). Acute kidney shutdown and eventual renal failure are a result of renal vasoconstriction from antigen-antibody complexes derived from the RBC surface.

Blood is usually administered to children by infusion pump; therefore the usual precautions and management re-

TABLE 26-4. Nursing care of the child receiving blood transfusions

COMPLICATION	SIGNS/SYMPTOMS	PRECAUTIONS/NURSING RESPONSIBILITIES
Immediate Reactions		
Hemolytic Reactions		
Most severe type, but rare	Chills	Identify donor and recipient blood types and groups before transfusion is begun; verify with another nurse or practitioner
Incompatible blood	Shaking	
Intradonor incompatibility in multiple transfusions	Fever	
	Pain at needle site and along venous tract	Transfuse blood slowly for first 15 to 20 minutes and/or initial ⅕ volume of blood; remain with patient
	Nausea/vomiting	Stop transfusion immediately in event of signs or symptoms, maintain patent intravenous line, and notify practitioner
	Sensation of tightness in chest	
	Red or black urine	Save donor blood to re-crossmatch with patient's blood
	Headache	Monitor for evidence of shock
	Flank pain	Insert urinary catheter and monitor hourly outputs
	Progressive signs of shock and/or renal failure	Send sample of patient's blood and urine to laboratory for presence of hemoglobin (indicates intravascular hemolysis)
		Observe for signs of hemorrhage resulting from disseminated intravascular coagulation (DIC)
		Support medical therapies to reverse shock
Febrile Reactions		
Leukocyte or platelet antibodies	Fever	May give acetaminophen for prophylaxis
Plasma protein antibodies	Chills	Leukocyte-poor red blood cells (RBCs) are less likely to cause reaction
		Stop transfusion immediately; report to practitioner for evaluation
Allergic Reactions		
Recipient reacts to allergens in donor's blood	Urticaria	Give antihistamines for prophylaxis to children with tendency toward allergic reactions
	Flushing	
	Asthmatic wheezing	Stop transfusions immediately
	Laryngeal edema	Administer epinephrine for wheezing or anaphylactic reaction
Circulatory Overload		
Too rapid transfusion (even a small quantity)	Precordial pain	Transfuse blood slowly
	Dyspnea	Prevent overload by using packed RBCs or administering divided amounts of blood
Excessive quantity of blood transfused (even slowly)	Rales	
	Cyanosis	Use infusion pump to regulate and maintain flow rate
	Dry cough	Stop transfusion immediately if signs of overload
	Distended neck veins	Place child upright with feet in dependent position to increase venous resistance
Air Emboli		
May occur when blood is transfused under pressure	Sudden difficulty in breathing	Normalize pressure before container is empty when infusing blood under pressure
	Sharp pain in chest	Clear tubing of air by aspirating air with syringe at nearest Y connector if air is observed in tubing; disconnect tubing and allow blood to flow until air has escaped only if a Y connector is not available
	Apprehension	
Hypothermia	Chills	Allow blood to warm at room temperature (less than 1 hour)
	Low temperature	Use approved mechanical blood warmer or electric warming coil to warm blood rapidly; never use microwave oven
	Irregular heart rate	
	Possible cardiac arrest	Take temperature if patient complains of chills; if subnormal, stop transfusion
Electrolyte Disturbances		
Hyperkalemia (in massive transfusions or in patients with renal problems)	Nausea, diarrhea	Use washed RBCs or fresh blood if patient is at risk
	Muscular weakness	
	Flaccid paralysis	
	Paresthesia of extremities	
	Bradycardia	
	Apprehension	
	Cardiac arrest	

TABLE 26-4. Nursing care of the child receiving blood transfusions—cont'd

COMPLICATION	SIGNS/SYMPTOMS	PRECAUTIONS/NURSING RESPONSIBILITIES
Delayed Reactions		
Transmission of Infection	Signs of infection (e.g., jaundice)	Blood is tested for antibodies to human immunodeficiency virus (HIV), hepatitis C virus (HCV), and hepatitis B core antigen (HBcAg); in addition, blood is tested for hepatitis B surface antigen (HBsAg) and alanine aminotransferase (ALT), and a serology test is performed for syphilis; positive units are destroyed; individuals at risk for carrying certain viruses are deferred from donation
Hepatitis		
AIDS	Toxic reaction: high fever, severe headache or substernal pain, hypotension, intense flushing, vomiting/diarrhea	
Malaria		
Syphilis		
Bacteria or viruses		Report any sign of infection and, if occurring during transfusion, stop transfusion immediately, send sample for culture and sensitivity tests, and notify physician
Other		
Alloimmunization	Increased risk of hemolytic, febrile, and allergic reactions	Use limited number of donors
(Antibody formation)		Observe carefully for signs of reactions
Occurs in patients receiving multiple transfusions		
Delayed Hemolytic Reaction	Destruction of RBCs and fever 5 to 10 days after transfusion	Observe for posttransfusion anemia and decreasing benefit from successive transfusion

lated to pumps apply. When the blood is started with a standard transfusion set, the filter chamber is filled to allow the total filter to be used. The drip chamber is partially filled with blood to permit counting of the drops. In adjusting the flow rate, it is important to remember that blood administration sets do not use microdrops (60 drops/ml) but regular drops (usually 10 or 15 drops/ml). Therefore this must be considered when calculating the flow rate.

BONE MARROW TRANSPLANTATION (BMT)

Advances in the selection of bone marrow donors and prevention of posttransplant complications have offered the hope of a cure to children with a variety of sometimes fatal disorders. BMT may be used to replace nonfunctioning marrow (aplastic anemia), dysfunctioning marrow (sickle cell disease or thalassemia), or malignant marrow (leukemia, lymphoma).

At present, the following three types of BMT may be done:

Allogeneic, which involves the matching of a histocompatible donor, usually a sibling, with the recipient; may also involve an unmatched donor

Autologous, which uses the patient's own marrow that was collected from disease-free tissue and frozen or uses stem cells that were collected from peripheral blood through apheresis (also referred to as *peripheral blood cell transplantation*) (see p. 924)

Syngeneic, which uses marrow from an identical twin

The most common type of BMT is allogeneic. Finding a suitable donor involves matching antigens from the *human leukocyte antigen (HLA)* system. Siblings have a 25% chance of being a match.

The importance of HLA matching is to minimize the serious complication known as *graft-versus-host disease (GVHD),* which is characterized by a hardening of organ tissues and drying of the mucous membranes. The donor's marrow may contain antigens not matched to the recipient's antigens, which begin attacking body cells. The more closely the HLA systems match, the less likely GVHD is to develop. However, it can occur even with a perfect HLA match, because there are as yet unidentified and thus unmatched antigens. GVHD is not a complication in autologous BMT.

The pretransplant procedure depends on the reason for the BMT. In most instances, lethal doses of chemotherapy, often combined with total-body radiotherapy, are given to kill malignant cells, prepare the host marrow cavity for donor engraftment, and reduce the risk of rejection. The actual transplant procedure involves harvesting several bone marrow specimens from the donor (which is done with the patient under general anesthesia) and administering diluted marrow intravenously to the recipient.

The posttransplant period involves a long stay in a protected environment. Before the marrow begins to function (engrafts), the child is extremely susceptible to infections, as well as to the risk of GVHD. During the posttransplant period the child's and family's emotional needs are equally important. Nurses can offer much support and encouragement to the family through the stages of the transplant (see Family Focus box on p. 946).

APHERESIS

Apheresis is the removal of blood from an individual, separation of the blood into its components, retention of one or more of these components, and reinfusion of the remainder of the blood into the individual. Apheresis is most often used to remove large quantities of platelets from healthy adult donors. These transfusion products have greatly prolonged the survival of patients with hematologic and oncologic diseases.

This technique is used to remove peripheral blood stem

cells (PBSCs) from children before they receive bone marrow transplants or high-dose chemotherapy and/or radiation therapy, which is severely toxic to the bone marrow. These PBSCs can then be used to restore the child's bone marrow. Apheresis is also used as a therapeutic modality. The blood component that is diseased or toxic is separated from the blood, and the remainder is returned to the individual. Therapeutic apheresis is considered part of standard therapy for many diseases. Plasma is selectively removed from individuals with hyperviscosity, life-threatening complications of myasthenia gravis, Guillain-Barré syndrome, thrombotic thrombocytopenic purpura, and certain drug overdoses. WBCs are removed from individuals with high-WBC-count leukemia.

Nursing Considerations

Difficult venous access and small blood volume can limit the ability to use this therapy in the infant and young child. Education of the family and child focuses on the purposes of the therapy as well as the technology.

Specially trained individuals perform the apheresis procedure. Attention focuses on rate of removal, blood component separation, and reinfusion of blood into the child. Vital signs are monitored, and the child is continuously observed for any adverse reactions secondary to the circulatory volume changes and the anticoagulant used.

When apheresis components are infused, nursing measures will differ if the product is autologous (blood component from the child) or allogeneic (blood component from another individual). Autologous components are the child's own blood; therefore a major precaution is proper identification to ensure the correct component. The rate of infusion should be adjusted to the child's tolerance. If the product is allogeneic, all precautions for blood transfusions apply.

KEY POINTS

- Anemia is defined as reduction of red blood cell volume or hemoglobin concentration to levels below normal; disorders are classified either by etiology/physiology or by morphology.
- The role of the nurse in treatment of anemia is to assist in establishing a diagnosis, prepare the child for laboratory tests, administer prescribed medications, decrease tissue oxygen needs, implement safety precautions, and observe for complications.
- The main nursing goal in prevention of nutritional anemia is parent education regarding optimum feeding practices to ensure adequate sources of iron.
- Sickle cell anemia is a hereditary hemoglobinopathy affecting primarily African Americans.
- Nursing care of the child with sickle cell anemia is aimed at teaching the family how to prevent and recognize sickling, managing pain during crises, and helping the child and parents adjust to a lifelong, potentially fatal disease.
- Nursing care of the child with thalassemia involves observing for complications of multiple blood transfusions, assisting the child in coping with the effects of illness, and fostering parent-child adjustment to long-term illness.

- Causes of acquired aplastic anemia include irradiation, drugs, industrial and household chemicals, infections, infiltration and replacement of myeloid elements, and idiopathic conditions.
- The human body controls bleeding through three processes: vascular spasm, platelet aggregation, and coagulation and clot formation.
- Nursing care of the child with hemophilia involves preventing bleeding by decreasing the risk of injury, recognizing and managing bleeding with factor replacement, preventing the crippling effects of joint degeneration, and preparing and supporting the child and family for home care.
- Goals in the care of the child with leukemia are to prepare the family for diagnostic and therapeutic procedures, prevent complications of myelosuppression, manage problems of irradiation and drug toxicity, and provide continued emotional support.
- The lymphomas include Hodgkin and non-Hodgkin lymphoma and are disorders involving the lymph glands.
- Immunodeficiency disorders are those that in some way render the affected individual unable to fight infectious organisms.

- Pediatric AIDS is acquired primarily from a parent with AIDS and in adolescents from engaging in high-risk behaviors. Blood transfusions are no longer a source of HIV infection but were responsible for AIDS in children treated with multiple blood transfusions, especially those with hemophilia.
- Blood transfusions supply needed blood components.

- Bone marrow transplantation replaces the diseased or malfunctioning bone marrow with viable blood stem cells.
- Apheresis is the selective removal of a blood component. It can be used to supply cellular elements needed for therapy (i.e., platelets or stem cells) or to remove diseased components.

REFERENCES

Allen JC: What we learn from infants with brain tumors, *N Engl J Med* 328(24):1780-1781, 1993.

American Academy of Pediatrics, Committee on Infectious Diseases: Recommendations for the use of live attenuated varicella vaccine, *Pediatrics* 95:791-796, 1995.

American Academy of Pediatrics, Committee on School Health, Committee on Infectious Disease: School attendance of children and adolescents with human T-lymphotropic virus III/lymphadenopathy-associated virus infection, *Pediatrics* 77:430-432, 1986.

American Academy of Pediatrics, Provisional Committee on Pediatric AIDS: Perinatal human immunodeficiency virus testing, *Pediatrics* 95:303-307, 1995.

American Pain Society: *Principles of analgesic use in the treatment of acute pain and chronic cancer pain,* ed 3, Skokie, IL, 1992, The Society.

Boland MG, Santacroce SJ: Case management: nursing care roles in the care of the child and family. In Pizzo PA, Wilfert CM: *Pediatric AIDS: the challenge of HIV infection in infants, children, and adolescents,* ed 2, Baltimore, 1994, Williams & Wilkins.

Caldwell MB, Rogers MF: Epidemiology of pediatric HIV infection, *Pediatr Clin North Am* 38(1):1-16, 1991.

Centers for Disease Control and Prevention: Education and foster care of children infected with human T-lymphotropic virus type III/lymphadenopathy-associated virus, *MMWR* 34:517-521, 1985.

Charache S: Experimental therapy of sickle cell disease, *Am J Pediatr Hematol Oncol* 16(1):62-66, 1994.

Cohen HA and others: Treatment of chronic idiopathic thrombocytopenic purpura with ascorbate, *Clin Pediatr* 32(5):300, 1993.

Dwyer JM: Manipulating the immune system with immune globulin, *N Engl J Med* 326(2):107-116, 1992.

Galbraith LK and others: Treatment for alteration in oral mucosa related to chemotherapy, *Pediatr Nurs* 17(3):233-236, 1991.

Griffin TC, McIntire D, Buchanan, GR: High-dose intravenous methylprednisolone therapy for pain in children and adolescents with sickle cell disease, *N Engl J Med* 330(11):733-737, 1994.

Hess G, Walson P: Seizures secondary to oral viscous lidocaine, *Ann Emerg Med* 17:725-727, 1988.

Hockenberry-Eaton M, Benner A: Patterns of nausea and vomiting in children: assessment and intervention, *Oncol Nurs Forum* 17(4):574-584, 1990.

Hooper PJ, Santas ED: Peripheral blood stem cell transplantation, *Oncol Nurs Forum* 20:1215-1220, 1994.

Huizdala EV: Nonlymphoblastic lymphoma in children, *J Clin Oncol* 9:1189-1195, 1991.

Idjradinata P, Pollitt E: Reversal of developmental delays in iron-deficient anaemic infants treated with iron, *Lancet* 341:1-4, 1993.

Johnson FL: Bone marrow transplantation. In Fernbach DJ, Vietti TJ, editors: *Clinical pediatric oncology,* ed 4, St Louis, 1991, Mosby.

Johnson FL and others: Bone marrow transplantation for sickle cell disease: the United States experience, *Am J Pediatr Hematol Oncol* 16(1):22-26, 1994.

Joshi VV: Pathology of childhood AIDS, *Pediatr Clin North Am* 38(1):97-120, 1991.

Koch DA and others: Behavioral contracting to improve adherence in patients with thalassemia, *J Pediatr Nurs* 8(2):106-111, 1993.

Lucarelli G and others: Bone marrow transplantation in patients with thalassemia, *N Engl J Med* 322(7):417-421, 1990.

Morrison R: Update on sickle cell disease: incidence of addiction and choice of opioid in pain management, *Pediatr Nurs* 17(5):503, 1991.

Pediatric Oncology Group: Progress against childhood cancer: the Pediatric Oncology Group experience, *Pediatrics* 89(4):597-600, 1992.

Pinkel D: Bone marrow transplantation in children, *J Pediatr* 122(3):331, 1993.

Platt OS and others: Mortality in sickle cell disease—life expectancy and risk factors for early death, *N Engl J Med* 330(23):1639-1644, 1994.

Poplack DG: Acute lymphoblastic leukemia. In Pizzo PA, Poplack DG: *Principles and practice of pediatric oncology,* ed 2, Philadelphia, 1993, Lippincott.

Sanders JE and others: Marrow transplant experience for children with severe aplastic anemia, *Am J Pediatr Hematol Oncol* 16(1):43-49, 1994.

Sandlund JT, Hutchison RE, Crist WM: Non-Hodgkin's lymphoma. In Fernback DJ, Vietti TJ, editors: *Clinical pediatric oncology,* ed 4, St Louis, 1991, Mosby.

Sickle Cell Disease Guideline Panel, Agency for Health Care Policy and Research: Sickle cell disease: screening, diagnosis, management, and counseling in newborns and infants, AHCPR Pub No 93-0562, Rockville, MD, 1993, The Agency.

Spiegel L, Mayers A: Psychosocial aspects of AIDS in children and adolescents, *Pediatr Clin North Am* 38(1):153-168, 1991.

Tonato M, Roila F, Del Favero A: Are there differences among the serotonin antagonists? *Support Care Cancer* 2(5):293-296, 1994.

Tovo PA and others: Prognostic factors and survival in children with perinatal HIV-1 infection, *Lancet* 339:1249-1253, 1992.

Urba WJ, Longo DL: Hodgkin's disease, *N Engl J Med* 326(10):678-687, 1992.

Vermylen C, Cornu G: Bone marrow transplantation for sickle cell disease: the European experience, *Am J Pediatr Hematol Oncol* 16(1):18-21, 1994.

Wimberley TH, Parks BR: Iron preparations it's elementary, my dear, *Pediatr Nurs* 17:274-275, 1991.

Zurlo MG and others: Survival and causes of death in thalassemia major, *Lancet* 1(8653):27-29, 1989.

BIBLIOGRAPHY

Anemia/Iron Deficiency Anemia

Francis EE, Williams D, Yarandi H: Anemia as an indicator of nutrition in children enrolled in a Head Start program, *J Pediatr Health Care* 7:156-160, 1993.

Fuchs G and others: Gastrointestinal blood loss in older infants: impact of cow milk versus formula, *J Pediatr Gastroenterol Nutr* 16(1):4-9, 1993.

Furman WL, Crist WM: Biology and clinical applications of hemopoietins in pediatric practice, *Pediatrics* 90(5):716, 1992.

Gavin MW, McCarthy DM, Garry PJ: Evidence that iron stores regulate iron absorption—a setpoint theory, *Am J Clin Nutr* 59:1376-1380, 1994.

Groopman JE, Molina JM, Scadden DT: Hematopoietic growth factors: biology and clinical applications, *N Engl J Med* 321(21):1449-1459, 1989.

Idjradinata P, Watkins WE, Pollitt E: Adverse effect of iron supplementation on weight gain of iron replete young children, *Lancet* 343:1252-1254, 1994.

Lozoff B, Jimenez E, Wolf AW: Long-term developmental outcome of infants with iron deficiency, *N Engl J Med* 325:687-694, 1991.

Raunikar RA, Sabio H: Anemia in the adolescent athlete, *Am J Dis Child* 146(10):1201-S, 1992.

Shannon KM: Recombinant erythropoietin in pediatrics: a clinical perspective, *Pediatr Ann* 19(3):197-206, 1990.

Walter T and others: Effectiveness of iron-fortified infant cereal in prevention of iron deficiency anemia, *Pediatrics* 91:976-982, 1993.

Sickle Cell Disease

Balkaran B and others: Stroke in a cohort of patients with homozygous sickle cell disease, *J Pediatr* 120(3):360-366, 1992.

Bray GL and others: Assessing clinical severity in children with sickle cell disease: preliminary results from a cooperative study, *Am J Pediatr Hematol Oncol* 16(1):50-54, 1994.

Carroll BA: Sickle cell disease. In Jackson PL, Vessey JA: *Primary care of the child with a chronic condition,* ed 2, St Louis, 1996, Mosby.

Cohen AR and others: Increased blood requirements during long-term transfusion therapy for sickle cell disease, *J Pediatr* 118(3):405-407, 1991.

Day S, Brunson G, Wang W: A successful education program for parents of infants with newly diagnosed sickle cell disease, *J Pediatr Nurs* 17(1):52-57, 1992.

Day S and others: Iron overload? In sickle cell disease? *MCN* 18:330, 1993.

Evans JPM, Rogers DW: Sickle cell disease and thalassemia, *Curr Opin Pediatr* 2(1):121-123, 1990.

Howard RJ, Lillis C, Tuck SM: Contraceptives, counseling, and pregnancy in women with sickle cell disease, *Br Med J* 306:1735-1737, 1993.

Mankad VN: Growth and development in sickle hemoglobinopathies, *Am J Pediatr Hematol Oncol* 14(4):283-284, 1992 (editorial).

Mentzer WB and others: Availability of related donors for bone marrow transplantation in sickle cell anemia, *Am J Pediatr Hematol Oncol* 16(1):27-29, 1994.

Milne RIG: Assessment of care of children with sickle cell disease: implications for neonatal screening programmes, *Br Med J* 300:371-374, 1990.

Resar LM, Oski FA: Cold water exposure and vaso-occlusive crises in sickle cell anemia, *J Pediatr* 118(3):407-409, 1991.

Vichinsky EP: A comparison of conservative and aggressive transfusion regimens in perioperative management of sickle cell disease, *N Engl J Med* 333(4):206-213, 1995.

Wang WC and others: High risk of recurrent stroke after discontinuance of five to twelve years of transfusion therapy in patients with sickle cell disease, *J Pediatr* 118(3):377-382, 1991.

Ware RE, Filston HC: Surgical management of children with hemoglobinopathies, *Surg Clin North Am* 72(6):1223-1231, 1992.

Zipursky A and others: Oxygen therapy in sickle cell disease, *Am J Pediatr Hematol Oncol* 14(3):222-228, 1992.

Thalassemia

Bhambhani K, Aronow R: Lead poisoning and thalassemia trait or iron deficiency, *Am J Dis Child* 144(11):1231-1233, 1990.

Brittenham GM and others: Efficacy of deferoxamine in preventing complications of iron overload in patients with thalassemia major, *N Engl J Med* 331(9):557-573, 1994.

Butler RB and others: β-Thalassemia major and sickle cell disease, *NAACOG Clin Issues Perinat Women's Health Nurs* 2(3):345-356, 1991.

Esposito NW: Thalassemias: simple screening for hereditary anemias, *Nurse Pract* 17(2):50, 53-56, 61, 1992.

Giardina PJ, Hilgartner MW: Update on thalassemia, *Pediatr Rev* 13(2):55-62, 1992.

Giardini C: Bone marrow transplantation for thalassemia: experience in Pesaro, Italy, *Am J Pediatr Hematol Oncol* 16(1):6-10, 1994.

Martin MB, Butler RB: Understanding the basics of β-thalassemia major, *Pediatr Nurs* 19(2):143-145, 1993.

Maurer HS and others: A prospective evaluation of iron chelation therapy in children with severe beta-thalassemia: a six-year study, *Am J Dis Child* 142(3):287-292, 1988.

Olivieri N and others: Survival in medically treated patients with homozygous beta thalassemia, *N Engl J Med* 331(9):574-578, 1994.

Uysal Z and others: Desferrioxamine and urinary zinc excretion in β-thalassemia major, *Pediatr Hematol Oncol* 10:257-260, 1993.

Walters MC, Thomas ED: Bone marrow transplantation for thalassemia: the USA experience, *Am J Pediatr Hematol Oncol* 16(1):11-17, 1994.

Aplastic Anemia

Glader BE: Red blood aplasias in children, *Pediatr Ann* 19(3):168-176, 1990.

Werner EJ and others: Immunosuppressive therapy versus bone marrow transplantation for children with aplastic anemia, *Pediatrics* 83(1):61-65, 1989.

Defects in Hemostasis

Aledort LM: New approaches to management of bleeding disorders, *Hosp Pract* 24(2):207-226, 1989.

Brubaker DB, Simpson MB, editors: *Dynamics of hemostasis and thrombosis,* Bethesda, MD, 1995, American Association of Blood Banks.

Bussel JB: Thrombocytopenia in newborns, infants, and children, *Pediatr Ann* 19(3):181-193, 1990.

Cohen HA and others: Treatment of chronic idiopathic thrombocytopenic purpura with ascorbate, *Clin Pediatr* 32(5):300, 1993.

Conway JH, Hilgartner MW: Initial presentations of pediatric hemophiliacs, *Arch Pediatr Adolesc Med* 148:589-594, 1994.

Dragone MA, Karp S: Bleeding disorders In Jackson PL, Vessey JA: *Primary care of the child with a chronic condition,* ed 2, St Louis, 1996, Mosby.

Dwyer JM: Manipulating the immune system with immune globulin, *N Engl J Med* 326(2):107-116, 1992.

George JN, El-Harake MA, Raskob GE: Chronic idiopathic thrombocytopenic purpura, *N Engl J Med* 331(18):1207-1211, 1994.

Lusher JM and others: Recombinant factor VIII for the treatment of previously untreated patients with hemophilia A: safety, efficacy, and development of inhibitors, *N Engl J Med* 328:453-459, 1993.

Manno CS: Difficult pediatric diagnoses: bruising and bleeding, *Pediatr Clin North Am* 38(3):637, 1991.

Spitzer A: Children's knowledge of illness and treatment experiences in hemophilia, *J Pediatr Nurs* 7(1):43-51, 1992.

Leukemias/Lymphomas

Boice J, Linet M: Chernobyl, childhood cancer, and chromosome 21, *Br Med J* 309(8917):139-140, 1994.

Bucholtz J: Issues concerning the sedation of children for radiation therapy, *Oncol Nurs Forum* 19(4):649-655, 1992.

Cooley ME and others: Cisplatin: a clinical review. Part I. Current uses of cisplatin and administration guidelines, *Cancer Nurs* 17(3):173-184, 1994.

Cooley ME and others: Cisplatin: a clinical review. Part II. Nursing assessment and management of side effects of cisplatin, *Cancer Nurs* 17(4):283-293, 1994.

Frankiewicz V, Farrington E: Ondansetron HCl (Zofran), *Pediatr Nurs* 18(4):385-386, 1992.

Galbraith L and others: Treatment for alteration in oral mucosa related to chemotherapy, *Pediatr Nurs* 17(3):233-236, 1991.

General recommendations on immunization: recommendations of the Advisory Committee on Immunization Practices (ACIP), *MMWR* 43(RR-1):22, 1994.

Jankovic M and others: Association of 1800 cGy cranial irradiation with intellectual function in children with acute lymphoblastic leukaemia, *Lancet* 344:224-227, 1994.

Kapelushnik J and others: Evaluating the efficacy of EMLA in alleviating pain associated with lumbar puncture: comparison of open and double-blinded protocols in children, *Pain* 41:31-34, 1990.

Kennedy BJ: Hodgkin's disease, *CA Cancer J Clin* 43(6):325-326, 1993.

Mack TM and others: Concordance for Hodgkin's disease in identical twins suggesting genetic susceptibility to the young adult form of the disease, *N Engl J Med* 332(7):413-418, 1995.

McCalla JL, Santacroce SJ, Woolery-Antill M: Nursing support of the child with cancer. In Pizzo PA, Poplack DG, editors: *Principles and practice of pediatric oncology,* ed 2, Philadelphia, 1993, Lippincott.

Moore BD III and others: Cognitive deficits in long-term survivors of childhood cancer, *Arch Neurol* 49:809-817, 1992.

Mulvihill J: Clinical genetics of pediatric oncology. In Pizzo PA, Poplack DG: *Principles and practice of pediatric oncology,* ed 2, Philadelphia, 1993, Lippincott.

National Cancer Institute: Bone marrow transplantation, NIH Pub No 92-1178, Bethesda, MD, 1991, National Institutes of Health.

Pui CH: Medical progress: childhood leukemia, *N Engl J Med* 332(24):1618-1630, 1995.

Ramsay NK: Bone marrow transplantation in pediatric oncology. In Pizzo PA, Poplack DG, editors: *Principles and practice of pediatric oncology,* ed 2, Philadelphia, 1993, Lippincott.

Rivera GK and others: Treatment of acute lymphoblastic leukemia, *N Engl J Med* 329(18):1289-1295, 1993.

Robertson CM, Hawkins MM, Kingston JE: Late deaths and survival after childhood cancer: implications for cure, *Br Med J* 309(6948):162-166, 1994.

Schecter N, Altman A, Weisman S: Report of the consensus conference on the management of pain in childhood cancer, *Pediatrics* 86(5):entire issue, 1990.

Smith MC, Holcombe JK, Stullenbarger E: A meta-analysis of intervention effectiveness for symptom management in oncology nursing research, *Oncol Nurs Forum* 21(7):1201-1210, 1994.

Immunologic Deficiency Disorders

American Academy of Pediatrics: Guidelines for human immunodeficiency virus (HIV)–infected children and their foster families, *Pediatrics* 89(4):681-683, 1992.

Armstrong FD, Seidel JF, Swales TP: Pediatric HIV infection: a neuropsychological and educational challenge, *J Learn Disabil* 26(2):92-103, 1993.

Bale JF: The neurologic complications of AIDS in infants and young children, *Inf Young Child* 3(2):15-23, 1990.

Boland MJ, Conviser R: Nursing care of the child. In Pizzo PA, Wilfert CM: *Pediatric AIDS: the challenge of HIV infection in infants, children, and adolescents,* Baltimore, 1991, Williams & Wilkins.

Butz AM and others: Care of HIV-risk infants: nursing outreach by PNPs, *J Pediatr Health Care* 6(3):138-145, 1992.

Chaisson RE, Keruly JC, Moore RD: Race, sex, drug use, and progression of human immunodeficiency virus disease, *N Engl J Med* 333(12):751-756, 1995.

Cohen DG: Similarities between the nursing care needs of children with cancer and children with human immunodeficiency virus infection, *J Pediatr Oncol Nurs* 7(4):149-153, 1990.

Connor EM and others: Reduction of maternal-infant transmission of human immunodeficiency virus type 1 with zidovudine treatment, *N Engl J Med* 331(18):1173-1180, 1994.

Czarniecki L, Oleske J: Pain in children with HIV infection, *J Pain Symptom Manage* 6(3):177, 1991.

Edelson PJ, editor: Childhood AIDS, *Pediatr Clin North Am* 38(1):entire issue, 1991.

Edlin BR and others: Intersecting epidemics: crack cocaine use and HIV infection among inner-city young adults, *N Engl J Med* 331(21):1422-1427, 1994.

Fahrner R, Benson M: Pediatric HIV infection and AIDS. In Jackson PL, Vessey JA: *Primary care of the child with a chronic condition,* ed 2, St Louis, 1996, Mosby.

Flaskerud JH: *AIDS/HIV infection: a reference guide for nursing professionals,* Philadelphia, 1989, Saunders.

Fry-Revere S: A bioethics consultant's thoughts on caring for pediatric patients with HIV, *Pediatr Nurs* 20(2):177-180, 1994.

Graham BS, Wright PF: Drug therapy: candidate AIDS vaccines, *N Engl J Med* 333(20):1331-1339, 1995.

Greene WC: AIDS and the immune system, *Sci Am* 269(3):99-105, 1993.

Guidelines for prevention of transmission of human immunodeficiency virus and hepatitis B virus to health-care and public-safety workers, *MMWR* 38(S-6), June 23, 1989.

Hutto C and others: A hospital-based prospective study of perinatal infection with human immunodeficiency virus type 1, *J Pediatr* 118(3):347-353, 1991.

Janeway Jr CA: How the immune system recognizes invaders, *Sci Am* 269(3):73-79, 1993.

Majer LS: HIV-infected students in school: who really "needs to know"? *J School Health* 62(6):243, 1992.

Marrack P, Kappler JW: How the immune system recognizes the body, *Sci Am* 269(3):81-89, 1993.

Mugrditchian L and others: The nutrition of the HIV infected child. II. Care management, *Top Clin Nutr* 7(2):11-20, 1992.

Murphy JM, Famolare NE: Caring for pediatric patients with HIV: personal concerns and ethical dilemmas, *Pediatr Nurs* 20(2):171-176, 180, 1994.

National Pediatric HIV Resource Center in cooperation with the Region II Head Start Resource Center: *Getting a head start on HIV: a resource manual for enhancing services to HIV-affected children in Head Start,* Newark, NJ, 1992, National Pediatric HIV Resource Center.

Nicholas SW: Management of the HIV-positive child with fever, *J Pediatr* 119(1):21-24, 1991.

1993 revised classification system for HIV infection and expanded surveillance case definition for AIDS among adolescents and adults, *MMWR* 41(RR-17):2, 1992.

Nossal GJV: Life, death and the immune system, *Sci Am* 269(3):53-62, 1993.

Pantaleo G, Graziosi C, Fauci AS: The immunopathogenesis of human immunodeficiency virus infection, *N Engl J Med* 328(5):327-335, 1993.

Pekham C, Gibb D: Mother to child transmission of the immunodeficiency virus, *N Engl J Med* 333(5):298-306, 1995.

Peterson K: Iatrogenic immune suppression, *Pediatr Nurs* 21(1):11-26, 98, 1995.

Projections of the number of persons diagnosed with AIDS and the number of immunosuppressed HIV-infected persons—United States, 1992-1994, *MMWR* 41(RR-18):1-29, 1992.

Recommendations for HIV testing services for inpatients and outpatients in acute-care hospital settings and technical guidance on HIV counseling, *MMWR* 42(RR-2):1-6, 1993.

Santelli JS, Birn AE, Linde J: School placement for human immunodeficiency virus–infected children: the Baltimore City experience, *Pediatrics* 89:843-848, 1992.

St Louis ME and others: Human immunodeficiency virus infection in disadvantaged adolescents, *JAMA* 266(17):2387-2391, 1991.

Schvaneveldt JD: Children's understanding of AIDS: a developmental viewpoint, *Fam Relations* 39(3):330-335, 1990.

Spector SA and others: A controlled trial of intravenous immune globulin for the prevention of serious bacterial infections in children receiving zidovudine for advanced human immunodeficiency virus infection, *N Engl J Med* 331(18):1181-1187, 1994.

Stiehm ER, Vink P: Transmission of human immunodeficiency virus infection by breast-feeding, *J Pediatr* 118(3):410-412, 1991.

Task Force on Pediatric AIDS: Adolescents and human immunodeficiency virus infection: the role of the pediatrician in prevention and intervention, *Pediatrics* 92(4):626-630, 1993.

Todd J: A most intimate foe: how the immune system can betray the body it defends, *Science* 30(2):20-27, 1990.

Turner BJ and others: Survival experience of 789 children with the acquired immunodeficiency syndrome, *Pediatr Infect Dis J* 12(4):310-320, 1993.

US Public Health Service task force on anti-*Pneumocystis* prophylaxis for patients with human immunodeficiency virus infection Recommendations for prophylaxis against *Pneumocystis carinii* pneumonia for adults and adolescents infected with human immunodeficiency virus, *MMWR* 41(4), 1992.

Weissman IL, Cooper MD: How the immune system develops, *Sci Am* 269(3):65-71, 1993.

Wiener L, Fair C, Pizzo PA: *Care for the child with HIV infection and AIDS,* Bethesda, MD, 1993, Pediatric Branch National Cancer Institute and Social Work Department, The Clinical Center, National Institutes of Health.

Wigzell H: The immune system as a therapeutic agent, *Sci Am* 269(3):127-134, 1993.

Working Group on Antiretroviral Therapy: National Pediatric HIV Resource Center: Antiretroviral therapy and medical management of the human immunodeficiency virus–infected child, *Pediatr Infect Dis J* 12:513-522, 1993.

Blood Transfusion/Bone Marrow Transplantation (General)

Armstrong TS: Stomatitis in the bone marrow transplant patient—an overview and proposed oral care protocol, *Cancer Nurs* 17(5):403-410, 1994.

Finfer S and others: Managing patients who refuse blood transfusions: an ethical dilemma, *Br Med J* 308:1423-1426, 1994.

Ford REN: Psychosocial and ethical issues in bone marrow transplantation. In Kasprisin CA, Snyder EL, editors: *Bone marrow transplantation: a nursing perspective,* Arlington, VA, 1990, American Association of Blood Banks.

Holyoake TL: Bone marrow transplants from peripheral blood, *Br Med J* 309:6946-6947, 1994.

Hooper PF, Santas EJ: Peripheral blood stem cell transplantation, *Oncol Nurs Forum* 20(8):1215-1223, 1993.

Jassak PF, Riley MB: Autologous stem cell transplant, *Cancer Pract* 2(2):141-145, 1995.

Lasky LC and others: Collection and use of peripheral blood stem cells in very small children, *Bone Marrow Transplant* 7(4):281-284, 1991.

Leibundgut K and others: Autotransplants with peripheral bleed stem cells and clinical results obtained in children: a review, *Eur J Pediatr* 152(7):546-554, 1993.

Linden JV, Paul B, Dressler KP: A report of 104 transfusion errors in New York State, *Transfusion* 32:601-606, 1992.

Quintero C: Blood administration in pediatric Jehovah's Witnesses, *Pediatr Nurs* 19(1):46-48, 1993.

Rockwood MT, Graham-Pole J: Development of an art program on a bone marrow transplant unit, *Cancer Nurs* 17(3):185-192, 1994.

Secundy MG: Psychosocial issues: unanswered questions in the use of bone marrow transplantation for treatment of hemoglobinopathies, *Am J Pediatr Hematol Oncol* 16(1):76-79, 1994.

Tong MJ and others: Clinical outcomes after transfusion associated hepatitis C, *N Engl J Med* 332:1463-1466, 1995.

Walker F and others: Guiding patients and their families through peripheral stem cell transplantation with the help of a teaching booklet, *Oncol Nurs Forum* 21(3):585-591, 1994.

Walker F and others: An overview of the rationale, process, and nursing implications of peripheral blood stem cell transplantation, *Cancer Nurs* 17(2):141-148, 1994.

Winters G and others: Provisional practice: the nature of psychosocial bone marrow transplant nursing, *Oncol Nurs Forum* 21(7):1147-1154, 1994.

Chapter 27

THE CHILD WITH GENITOURINARY DYSFUNCTION

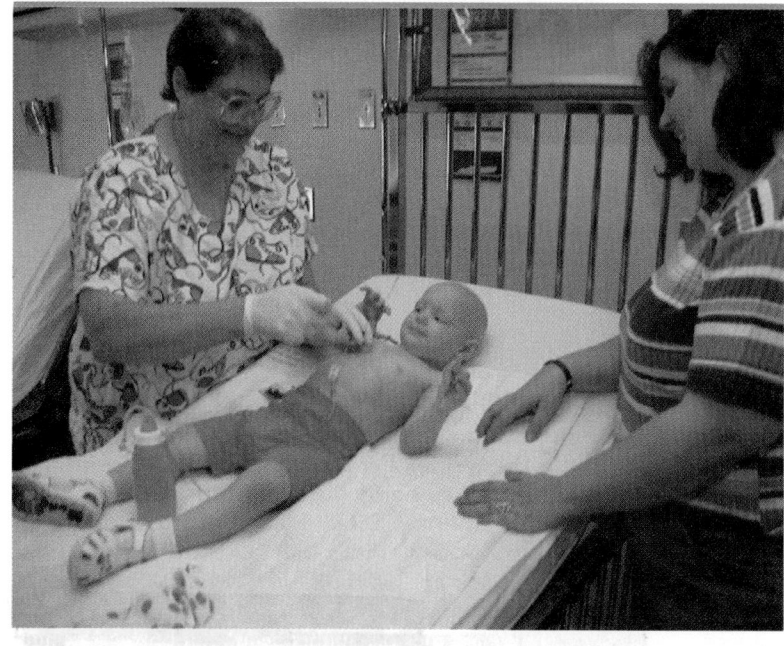

" I'm less worried about her, knowing the nurses all take such good care of her. They all know her; they check on her a lot."

Erika, mother of Skylar, age 2 years, Wilms tumor

RELATED TOPICS

LEARNING OBJECTIVES
On completion of this chapter the reader will be able to:

- Describe the various factors that contribute to urinary tract infections in infants and children
- Discuss the preoperative preparation of the child and parents when the child has a structural defect of the genitourinary tract
- Demonstrate an understanding of the causes and mechanisms of edema formation in nephrotic syndrome
- Outline a nursing care plan for a child with nephrotic syndrome
- Compare the child with minimal-change nephrotic syndrome and the child with

acute glomerulonephritis in terms of clinical manifestations and nursing care
- Contrast the causes, complications, and management of acute and chronic renal failure
- List the types of renal dialysis
- Recognize signs of kidney transplant rejection

951

GENITOURINARY DYSFUNCTION

ASSESSMENT OF RENAL FUNCTION

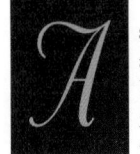ssessment of kidney and urinary tract integrity and diagnosis of renal or urinary tract disease are based on several evaluative tools. Physical examination, history taking, and observation of symptoms are the initial procedures. In suspected urinary tract diseases or disorders, further assessment by laboratory, radiologic, and other evaluative methods is carried out.

Clinical Manifestations

As in most disorders of childhood, the incidence and type of kidney or urinary tract dysfunction change with the age and maturation of the child. In addition, the presenting complaints and the significance of these complaints vary with maturation. For example, a complaint of enuresis has greater significance at age 8 years than at age 4. In the newborn, urinary tract disorders are associated with a number of obvious malformations of other body systems, including the curious and unexplained but frequent association between malformed or low-set ears and urinary tract anomalies.

Many of the clinical manifestations of renal disease are common to a variety of childhood disorders, but their presence is an indication to obtain further information from the past history, family history, and laboratory studies as part of a complete physical examination. Suspected renal disease can be further evaluated by means of radiographic studies and renal biopsy (Table 27-1).

Laboratory Tests

Both urine and blood studies contribute vital information for detection of renal problems. The single most important test is probably routine urinalysis. Specific urine and blood tests provide additional information. Since nurses are usually the persons who collect the specimens for examination and who often perform many of the screening tests, they should be familiar with the test, its function, and factors that can alter or distort the results of the test. The major urine and blood tests are outlined in Tables 27-2 and 27-3.

Nursing Considerations

Nursing responsibilities in assessment of genitourinary disorders and/or diseases begin with observation of the child for any manifestations that might indicate dysfunction. Many conditions have specific characteristics that distinguish them from other disorders. These are discussed as appropriate throughout the chapter.

The nurse is generally the one who is responsible for preparing infants, children, and parents for tests and for collection of urine and (sometimes) blood specimens (see Preparation for Procedures, Chapter 22, and Collection of Specimens, Chapter 22) for observation and laboratory analysis. An important nursing responsibility is to maintain careful *intake and output* measurements and *blood pressure* on most children with genitourinary dysfunction and those who might be at risk for developing renal complications (e.g., children

in shock, postoperative patients). For example, any significant degree of renal disease can diminish the glomerular filtration rate, a measure of the amount of plasma from which a given substance is totally cleared in 1 minute. A number of substances can be used, but the most useful clinical estimation of glomerular filtration is the clearance of *creatinine,* an end product of protein metabolism in muscle and a substance that is freely filtered by the glomerulus and secreted by renal tubular cells. The nurse's responsibility in this test is collection of urine, usually a 12- or 24-hour specimen.

GENITOURINARY TRACT DISORDERS/DEFECTS

URINARY TRACT INFECTION (UTI)

Infection of the genitourinary tract is one of the most common conditions of childhood. UTIs may involve the urethra, bladder (lower urinary tract), and/or the ureters, renal pelvis, calyces, and renal parenchyma (upper urinary tract). Because it is often impossible to localize the infection, the broad designation UTI is applied to the presence of significant numbers of microorganisms anywhere within the urinary tract, except the distal one third of the urethra, which is usually colonized with bacteria. The peak incidence of UTIs not caused by structural anomalies occurs between 2 and 6 years of age, and except for the neonatal period, females have 10 to 30 times the risk of males for developing UTI. An increased incidence of UTIs is observed in adolescents, especially those who are sexually active.

Classification

Infection of the urinary tract may be present with or without clinical symptoms. As a result, the site of infection is often difficult to pinpoint with any degree of accuracy. Various terms used to describe urinary tract disorders include the following:

Bacteriuria—Presence of bacteria in the urine
Asymptomatic bacteriuria—Significant bacteriuria with no evidence of clinical infection (usually defined as greater than 100,000 colony-forming units [CFUs])
Symptomatic bacteriuria—Bacteriuria accompanied by physical signs of urinary infection (dysuria, suprapubic discomfort, hematuria, fever)
Recurrent UTI—Repeated episode of bacteriuria or symptomatic UTI
Persistent UTI—Persistence of bacteriuria despite antibiotic treatment
Febrile UTI—Bacteriuria accompanied by fever and other physical signs of urinary infection; presence of a fever typically implies a pyelonephritis
Cystitis—Inflammation of the bladder
Urethritis—Inflammation of the urethra
Pyelonephritis—Inflammation of the upper urinary tract and kidneys
Urosepsis—Febrile urinary tract infection coexisting with systemic signs of bacterial illness; blood culture reveals presence of urinary pathogen

Etiology

A variety of organisms can be responsible for UTI. *Escherichia coli* (80% of cases) and other gram-negative enteric organisms

Natalie Cloutman Arnold, MSN, RN, PNP, and Teresa Hall, MS, RN, revised this chapter.

TABLE 27-1. Radiologic and other tests of urinary system function

TEST	PROCEDURE	PURPOSE	COMMENTS AND NURSING RESPONSIBILITIES
Renal Biopsy	Removal of kidney tissue by open or percutaneous technique for study by light, electron, or immunofluorescent microscopy	Yields histologic and microscopic information about glomeruli and tubules; helps to distinguish between types of nephrotic syndromes Distinguishes other renal disorders	Give nothing orally 4-6 hours before test* Premedicate as ordered Prepare setup for procedure Assist with procedure Take vital signs Apply pressure to area with pressure dressing and, if feasible, a sandbag Bed rest for 24 hours Observe for abdominal pain, tenderness Monitor input and output; surgical incision may be required in infants
Renal/Bladder Ultrasound	Transmission of ultrasonic waves through renal parenchyma, along ureteral course, and over bladder	Allows visualization of renal parenchyma, renal pelvis without exposure to external beam radiation or radioactive isotopes Visualization of dilated ureters and bladder wall also possible	Noninvasive procedure
Testicular (Scrotal) Ultrasound	Transmission of ultrasonic waves through scrotal contents and testis	Allows visualization of scrotal contents, including testis Testicular ultrasound is used to identify masses, and Doppler-enhanced ultrasound is used to differentiate hyperemia of epididymo-orchitis from ischemia of torsion	Noninvasive procedure
Computed Tomography (CT)	Narrow-beam x-rays and computer analysis provide precise reconstruction of area	Visualizes vertical or horizontal cross section of kidney Especially valuable to distinguish tumors and cysts	Noncontrast scan is noninvasive Contrast enhanced CT scan preparation is similar to intravenous pyelogram (IVP)
Urine Culture and Sensitivity	Collection of sterile specimen	Determines presence of pathogens and the drugs to which they are sensitive	Does not require specific parental permission Send specimen to laboratory immediately after collection Catherization, clean-catch, or suprapubic specimen
Urodynamics	Set of tests designed to measure bladder filling, storage, and evacuation functions *Uroflowmetry* is a test to determine efficiency of urination *Cystometrogram* is a graphic comparison of bladder pressure as a function of volume *Sphincter electromyogram* (EMG) is a test of pelvic muscle function during bladder filling and evacuation *Voiding pressure study* is a comparison of detrusor contraction pressure, sphincter EMG, and urinary flow	Determine characteristics of voiding dysfunction Used to identify type (cause) of incontinence or urinary retention Especially valuable for voiding dysfunction complicated by urinary infection, urinary retention, or neurogenic bladder dysfunction	Prepare child for catheterization Insertion of a rectal tube will produce feelings of rectal fullness or pressure Insertion of needles may be required for sphincter EMG
Whitaker Perfusion Test	Injection of contrast material through renal pelvis and ureters Pressures are measured in renal pelvis and urinary bladder	Determine presence of obstruction causing upper urinary tract dilation	Prepare child for insertion of a spinal needle or perfusion catheter in renal pelvis (anesthesia often required)

*Current research supports oral intake of clear fluids up to 2 hours before test.

TABLE 27-2. Urine tests of renal function

TEST	NORMAL RANGE	DEVIATIONS	SIGNIFICANCE OF DEVIATIONS
Physical Tests			
Volume	Age related	Polyuria	Osmotic factors (urinary glucose level in diabetes mellitus)
		Oliguria	Retention caused by obstructive disease
			Inadequate bladder emptying caused by neurogenic bladder or obstructive disorder
		Anuria	Obstruction of urinary tract; acute renal failure
Specific gravity	With normal fluid intake: 1.016-1.022	High	Dehydration
			Presence of protein or glucose
	Newborn: 1.001-1.020		Presence of radiopaque contrast medium after radiologic examinations
	Others: 1.001-1.030	Low	Excessive fluid intake
			Distal tubular dysfunction
			Insufficient antidiuretic hormone
			Diuresis
		Fixed at 1.010	Chronic glomerular disease
Osmolality	Newborn: 50-600 mOsm/L	High or low	Same as for specific gravity
	Thereafter: 50-1400 mOsm/L		More sensitive index than specific gravity
Appearance	Clear pale yellow to deep gold	Cloudy	Contains sediment
		Cloudy reddish pink to reddish brown	Blood from trauma or disease
			Myoglobin after severe muscle destruction
		Light	Dilute
		Dark	Concentrated
		Red	Trauma
Chemical Tests			
pH	Newborn: 5-7	Weak acid or neutral	If associated with metabolic acidosis, suggests tubular acidosis
	Thereafter: 4.8-7.8		If associated with metabolic alkalosis, suggests potassium deficiency
	Average: 6		Urinary infection
			Metabolic alkalosis
		Alkaline	Metabolic alkalosis
Protein level	Absent	Present	Abnormal glomerular permeability (e.g., glomerular disease, changes in blood pressure)
			Most kidney disease
			Orthostatic in some individuals
Glucose level	Absent	Present	Diabetes mellitus
			Infusion of concentrated glucose-containing fluids
			Glomerulonephritis
			Impaired tubular reabsorption
Ketone levels	Absent	Present	Conditions of acute metabolic demand (stress)
			Diabetic ketoacidosis
Leukocyte esterase	Absent	Present	Can identify both lysed and intact white blood cells via enzyme detection
Nitrites	Absent	Present	Most species of bacteria convert nitrates to nitrites in the urine
Microscopic Tests			
White blood cell count	Less than 1 or 2	More than 5 polymorphonuclear leukocytes/field	Urinary tract inflammatory process
		Lymphocytes	Allograft rejection
			Malignancy

TABLE 27-2. Urine tests of renal function—cont'd

TEST	NORMAL RANGE	DEVIATIONS	SIGNIFICANCE OF DEVIATIONS
Red blood cell count	Less than 1 or 2	4-6/field in centrifuged specimen	Trauma Stones Glomerular injury Infection Neoplasms
Presence of bacteria	Absent to a few	More than 100,000 organisms/ml in centrifuged specimen	Urinary tract infection
Presence of casts	Occasional	Granular casts Cellular casts White blood cell Red blood cell Hyaline casts	Tubular or glomerular disorders Degenerative process in advanced renal disease Pyelonephritis Glomerulonephritis Proteinuria; usually transient

TABLE 27-3. Blood tests of renal function

TEST	NORMAL RANGE (mg/dl)	DEVIATIONS	SIGNIFICANCE OF DEVIATIONS
Blood Urea Nitrogen (BUN)	Newborn: 4-18 Infant, child: 5-18	Elevated	Renal disease—acute or chronic (the higher the BUN, the more severe the disease) Increased protein catabolism Dehydration Hemorrhage High protein intake Corticosteroid therapy
Uric Acid	Child: 2.0-5.5	Increased	Severe renal disease
Creatinine	Infant: 0.2-0.4 Child: 0.3-0.7 Adolescent: 0.5-1.0	Increased	Severe renal impairment

are most frequently implicated; these organisms are usually found in the anal and perineal region. Other organisms associated with UTI include *Proteus, Pseudomonas, Klebsiella, Staphylococcus aureus, Haemophilus,* and coagulase-negative *Staphylococcus.* Several factors contribute to the development of UTI in childhood.

Anatomic and Physical Factors. The structure of the lower urinary tract is believed to account for the increased incidence of bacteriuria in females. The short urethra, which measures about 2 cm (¾ inch) in young girls and 4 cm (1½ inches) in mature women, provides a ready pathway for invasion of organisms. In addition, the closure of the urethra at the end of micturition may return contaminated bacteria to the bladder. The longer male urethra (as long as 20 cm [8 inches] in an adult) and the antibacterial properties of prostatic secretions inhibit the entry and growth of pathogens.

 Considerable evidence suggests that there is a higher incidence of UTI in uncircumcised male infants than in circumcised male infants (Wiswell and Hachey, 1993; Craig and others, 1996). However, other research suggests that the uncircumcised male infant is not at increased risk for UTI (Fleiss, 1995).

The single most important host factor influencing the occurrence of UTI is **urinary stasis**. Ordinarily, urine is sterile, but at 37° C (98.6° F) it provides an excellent culture medium. Under normal conditions the act of completely and repeatedly emptying the bladder flushes away any organisms before they have an opportunity to multiply and invade surrounding tissue. However, urine that remains in the bladder allows bacteria from the urethra to rapidly become established in the rich medium. Incomplete bladder emptying (stasis) may result from *reflux* (see below for a discussion of reflux), anatomic abnormalities (especially those involving the ureters), dysfunction of the voiding mechanism, or extrinsic ureteral or bladder compression that may be caused by constipation.

Altered Urine and Bladder Chemistry. Several mechanical and chemical characteristics of the urine and bladder mucosa help maintain urinary sterility. An increased fluid intake promotes flushing of the normal bladder and lowers the concentration of organisms in the infected bladder. Diuresis also seems to enhance the antibacterial properties of the renal medulla.

Most pathogens favor an alkaline medium. Normally, urine is slightly acidic, but it can be made more acidic by diet (apple juice, cranberry juice, and large amounts of ascorbic acid) or acid-forming drugs. A urine pH of about 5 hampers bacterial multiplication, although the acidification rarely eliminates the bacteriuria. However, it may enhance the therapeutic effectiveness of drugs and of the natural defense mechanisms, as well as help relieve some of the symptoms.

Diagnostic Evaluation

The clinical manifestations of UTIs depend on the age of the child (see box). Diagnosis of UTI is confirmed by detection of bacteriuria in urine culture, but urine collection is often difficult, especially in infants and very small children. Several factors may alter a urine specimen, and contamination of a specimen by organisms from sources other than the urine, such as perineal and perianal flora in bag specimens, is the most frequent cause of false-positive results. Unless the specimen is a first morning sample, a recent high fluid intake may indicate a falsely low organism count. Therefore children should not be encouraged to drink large volumes of water in an attempt to obtain a specimen quickly.

More accurate estimates of bacterial content are obtained from *suprapubic aspiration* (in children younger than 2 years of age) and properly performed bladder catheterization (as long as the first few milliliters are excluded from collection). The specimen should be taken directly to the laboratory for culture immediately.

Tests to detect bacteriuria are being used with increased frequency in screening for UTI. The dipstick tests that test for leukocyte esterase or nitrite are quick and inexpensive methods for detecting infection before obtaining final culture results.

Localization of the infection site may involve more specific tests, including ureteral catheterization and bladder washout procedures. Other tests, such as ultrasonography, voiding cystourethrogram (VCUG), intravenous pyelogram (IVP), and DSMA (dimercaptosuccinic acid) scan, may be performed after the infection subsides to identify anatomic abnormalities contributing to the development of infection and existing kidney changes from recurrent infection.

Therapeutic Management

The objectives of treatment of children with UTI are (1) to eliminate current infection, (2) to identify contributing factors to reduce the risk of recurrence, (3) to prevent systemic spread of the infection, and (4) to preserve renal function. Antibiotic therapy should be initiated on the basis of identification of the pathogen, the child's history of antibiotic use, and the location of the infection. A variety of antimicrobial

---

SIGNS AND SYMPTOMS OF URINARY TRACT DISORDERS OR DISEASE AT DIFFERENT AGES

Neonatal Period (Birth to 1 Month)

Poor feeding
Vomiting
Failure to gain weight
Rapid respiration (acidosis)
Respiratory distress
Spontaneous pneumothorax or pneumomediastinum
Frequent urination
Screaming on urination
Poor urine stream
Jaundice
Seizures
Dehydration
Other anomalies or stigmata
Enlarged kidneys or bladder

Infancy (1 to 24 Months)

Poor feeding
Vomiting
Failure to gain weight
Excessive thirst
Frequent urination
Straining or screaming on urination

Foul-smelling urine
Pallor
Fever
Persistent diaper rash
Seizures (with or without fever)
Dehydration
Enlarged kidneys or bladder

Childhood (2 to 14 Years)

Poor appetite
Vomiting
Growth failure
Excessive thirst
Enuresis, incontinence, frequent urination
Painful urination
Swelling of face
Seizures
Pallor
Fatigue
Blood in urine
Abdominal or back pain
Edema
Hypertension
Tetany

---

drugs are available for treating UTI, but all of them can occasionally be ineffective because of resistance of organisms. Common antiinfective agents used for UTI include the penicillins, sulfonamide (including trimethoprim and sulfisoxazole in combination), the cephalosporins, nitrofurantoin, and the tetracyclines. All antibiotics may cause side effects.

If anatomic defects such as primary reflux or bladder neck obstruction are present, surgical correction of these abnormalities may be necessary to prevent recurrent infection. Follow-up study is an important component of medical management, since the relapse rate is high and recurrent infection tends to occur 1 to 2 months after termination of treatment. The aim of therapy and careful follow-up is to reduce the chance of renal scarring. However, recurrent infection of the urinary bladder predisposes the individual to transient episodes of vesicoureteral reflux.

Vesicoureteral Reflux (VUR). VUR refers to the retrograde flow of bladder urine into the ureters. During voiding, urine is swept up the ureters and then flows back into the empty bladder, where it acts as a reservoir for bacterial growth until the next void. Therefore reflux increases the chances for and perpetuates infection. *Primary reflux* results from congenitally abnormal insertion of ureters into the bladder; *secondary reflux* occurs as a result of an acquired condition.

VUR is managed conservatively with low-dose antibacterial therapy and frequent urine cultures and requires a motivated, reliable, and cooperative family. Indications for surgical intervention include significant anatomic abnormality at the ureterovesical junction, recurrent UTIs, severe forms of VUR, noncompliance with medical therapy, intolerance to antibiotics, and VUR after puberty in females.

Prognosis. With prompt and adequate treatment at the time of diagnosis, the long-term prognosis for UTIs is usually excellent. However, the hazard of progressive renal injury is greatest when infection occurs in young children (especially under 2 years of age) and is associated with congenital renal malformations and reflux. Therefore early diagnosis of children at risk is particularly important during infancy and toddlerhood.

Nursing Considerations

❖ Assessment

Since children are not a captive population, mass screening is difficult. However, annual health examinations should include a routine urinalysis. In addition, nurses should instruct parents to observe regularly for clues suggesting UTI. Unfortunately, the signs of UTI are not as evident as those of upper respiratory tract infection. Therefore many cases go undetected because no one thought to investigate this very common problem.

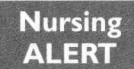 **Nursing ALERT** A child who exhibits the following should be evaluated for UTI:
Incontinence in a toilet-trained child
Strong-smelling urine
Frequency and/or urgency

Since infants and young children are unable to express their feelings and sensations verbally, it is difficult to detect discomfort they may be experiencing from dysuria. A careful history regarding voiding habits, stooling pattern, and episodes of unexplained irritability may assist in detecting less obvious cases of UTI. Consequently, parents should be cautioned to observe for specific clues of UTI in suspected cases.

NURSING TIP Check the diaper every ½ hour. This increases the opportunity for observing the stream for such findings as straining or fretting before voiding begins, signs of discomfort before and during urinating, starting and stopping the stream intermittently, and frequent dripping of small amounts of urine.

When infection is suspected, collecting an appropriate specimen is essential. It is the nurse's responsibility to take every precaution to obtain acceptable clean-voided specimens to avoid the use of other collecting procedures except when absolutely indicated.

❖ Nursing Diagnoses

Based on a thorough assessment, a number of nursing diagnoses become evident. They include but are not limited to those listed in the box.

NURSING DIAGNOSES: THE CHILD WITH URINARY TRACT INFECTION

High risk for injury related to possibility of kidney damage from chronic infection
Anxiety related to unfamiliar procedures
Altered family processes related to illness of a child

❖ Planning

The goals of care for the child with UTI and family are as follows:

1. Child and family will be prepared properly for needed tests and procedures.
2. Parents and child will receive appropriate education regarding prevention and treatment of infection.

❖ Implementation

Frequently, additional tests are performed to detect anatomic defects. Children are prepared for these tests as appropriate for their age. This includes an explanation of the procedure, its purpose, and what the children will experience (see Preparation for Procedures, Chapter 22). Sometimes a simple description of the urinary system is helpful. Especially for preschool children, the nurse must clarify that the urinary tract is separate from any sexual function and that the test is for a problem that they did not cause. Children may associate blame for perceived wrongdoing (e.g., masturbation) or unacceptable thoughts with the reason for the illness or the tests. For young children under 3 to 4 years of age, the procedure can be explained on a doll. For those who are older, a simple drawing of the bladder, urethra, ureters, and kidneys makes the explanation more understandable.

Children may be treated as outpatients to avoid overnight separation from home for some procedures. In such cases, nurses must be careful not to overlook the need for adequate preparation. If surgery is subsequently indicated, the child will be able to encounter the impending procedure with facts and understanding of the procedures that will help to decrease his or her fear and anxiety concerning more extensive medical-surgical intervention.

Since antibacterial drugs are indicated in UTI, the nurse advises parents of proper dosage and administration. When antiseptics such as nitrofurantoin are used for prolonged therapy to maintain urine sterility, parents need an explanation of the drug's continued necessity when no signs of infection are present.* For all children an adequate or increased fluid intake is encouraged.

Prevention. Prevention is the most important goal in both primary and recurrent infection, and most preventive measures are simple hygienic habits that should be a routine part of daily care (see Guidelines box on p. 958). For example, parents are taught to cleanse their infant's genital areas from front to back to avoid contaminating the urethral area with fecal organisms. Female children are taught to wipe from front to back after voiding or defecating. Children should void as soon as they feel the urge. (See Critical Thinking Exercise on p. 958.)

Sexually active adolescent females are advised to urinate as soon as possible after intercourse to flush out bacteria introduced during the activity. Children with disabilities involving the bladder are frequently on a prophylactic regimen, such as acidifying agents and prescribed fluid intake. The nurse should reinforce the importance of compliance to parents and responsible children.

---

*Home care instructions for giving medications to children and collecting a urine sample are available in Wong DL: *Wong and Whaley's Clinical manual of pediatric nursing*, ed 4, St Louis, 1996, Mosby.

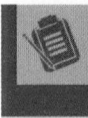

GUIDELINES
Prevention of Urinary Tract Infection

Factors Predisposing to Development	Measures of Prevention
Short female urethra close to vagina and anus	Perineal hygiene: wipe from front to back.
	Avoid tight clothing or diapers; wear cotton panties rather than nylon.
	Check for vaginitis or pinworms, especially if child scratches between legs.
Incomplete emptying (reflux) and overdistention of bladder	Avoid "holding" urine; encourage child to void frequently, especially before a long trip or other circumstances where toilet facilities are not available.
	Empty bladder completely with each void.
	Avoid straining during defecation and avoid constipation.
Concentrated and alkaline urine	Encourage generous fluid intake.
	Acidify urine with juices such as cranberry and a diet high in animal protein.

CRITICAL THINKING EXERCISE
Recurrent Urinary Tract Infections (UTIs)

Joyce, 10 years old, has been hospitalized for acute pyelonephritis. She has a history of urinary tract infection (UTI) and vesicoureteral reflux. As the nurse assigned to Joyce, you are obtaining a detailed history of Joyce's voiding pattern and fluid intake. Her mother reports that when she does laundry, Joyce's underwear frequently smells strongly of urine. The mother denies any problem with enuresis or accidental urination. When describing Joyce's fluid intake, both she and her mother agree on her consumption of 8 to 10 ounces of juice after school each day, 8 ounces of milk with the evening meal, and 8 ounces of water or juice in the evening. Joyce eats both breakfast and lunch at school. On Saturday and Sunday, she routinely consumes 46 ounces of fluid per day. Joyce's weight is 26 kg.

In continuing this interaction, you should do which of the following?

1. Ask about Joyce's bowel elimination pattern.
2. Develop an intervention strategy to increase Joyce's fluid intake to 54 ounces per day.
3. Develop an intervention strategy to decrease fluid intake in the evening.
4. Develop a line of inquiry about Joyce's fluid and elimination pattern at school.

The correct answer is four. All the actions are appropriate except three. The relationship of chronic constipation to recurrent UTIs is well documented. Joyce's calculated fluid requirement per day is 54 ounces; decreasing her fluid intake is not warranted. Of most concern now, however, is the information related to Joyce's behavior at school. It is not unusual for both boys and girls to avoid using the restrooms at school. Some children are known to omit drinking during the daytime to avoid needing to use the school restroom. They sometimes lose small amounts of urine into their underwear as they attempt to "hold" their urine until they get home. This may or may not be true for Joyce, but your inquiry should elicit school behavior before changing lines of inquiry or moving to interventions.

❖ Evaluation

The effectiveness of nursing interventions is determined by continual reassessment and evaluation of care based on the following.

Observational guidelines:

1. Question children and families regarding their understanding of the disease and the diagnostic measures required for identifying the presence of infection and/or physical abnormalities.
2. Observe and interview family and child regarding preventive practices and observe laboratory reports of urinalyses and cultures for evidence of treatment efficacy.

Expected outcomes:

1. Child and family demonstrate an understanding of the illness and diagnostic tests (specify knowledge and means of demonstration).
2. Child and family demonstrate an understanding of preventive practices (specify means of demonstration).

OBSTRUCTIVE UROPATHY

Structural or functional abnormalities of the urinary system that obstruct the normal flow of urine can produce renal disorders. When there is interference with urine flow, the back up of urine above the obstruction causes *hydronephrosis* (the collection of urine in the renal pelvis to the point of cyst formation from the distention) with eventual pressure destruction to renal parenchyma, although the dilating ureters form a reservoir that reduces the effect on the kidneys for a long time.

Obstruction may be congenital or acquired, unilateral or bilateral, complete or incomplete, and the manifestations may be acute or chronic. The obstruction can occur at any level of the upper or lower urinary tract (Fig. 27-1). Partial obstruction may not be symptomatic unless there is a water or solute diuresis. Boys are affected more frequently than girls, and malformations should be suspected when patients have some other congenital defects (e.g., prune belly syndrome, chromosome anomalies, hypospadias, anorectal malformations, or defects of the pinna of the ear).

Damage to distal nephrons in chronic uropathy alters the ability to concentrate urine, contributing to increased urine flow and metabolic acidosis occurring from decreased excretion of acid secondary to impaired ability of the distal nephron to secrete hydrogen ions. Partial obstruction results in progressive loss of renal function as a result of irreversible damage to the nephrons. Pooled urine serves as a medium for bacterial growth; therefore UTIs further increase the extent of renal damage.

Early diagnosis and surgical correction or procedures that divert the flow of urine to bypass the obstruction, such as

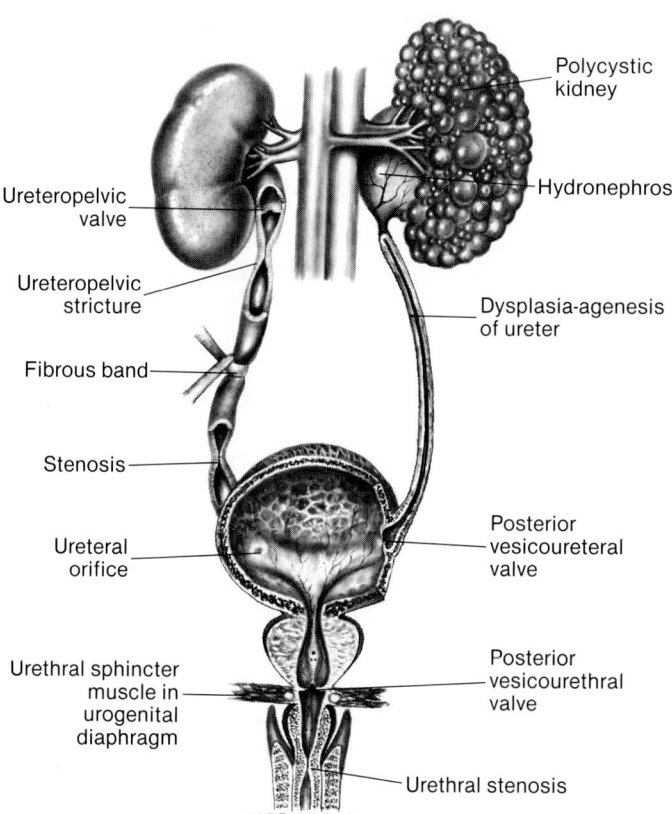

FIG. 27-1. Major sites of urinary tract obstruction.

Labels:
Polycystic kidney
Hydronephrosis
Ureteropelvic valve
Dysplasia-agenesis of ureter
Ureteropelvic stricture
Fibrous band
Stenosis
Posterior vesicoureteral valve
Ureteral orifice
Urethral sphincter muscle in urogenital diaphragm
Posterior vesicourethral valve
Urethral stenosis

ileal conduit or *cutaneous ureterostomy,* are essential to prevent progressive renal damage. Medical complications of acute or chronic renal failure and/or infection are managed as described for those disorders.

Nursing Considerations

Nursing goals in urinary tract obstruction include helping to identify cases, assisting with diagnostic procedures, and caring for children with complications (described elsewhere). Preparing parents and children for procedures is a major nursing responsibility. Preparation for urinary diversion procedures is of special importance. (see Preparation for Procedures, Chapter 22).

Parents and children need emotional support and counseling during the lengthy management of these disorders. Many children are discharged with ureteral drainage systems in place that must be protected from damage, and the danger of infection is a constant concern. Parents are taught to care for the equipment and recognize the signs of possible obstruction or infection within the system.

Children with external diversional systems will need psychologic support and guidance, especially as they reach adolescence and body image concerns assume more prominence. Those with progressive renal deterioration may face the prospect of dialysis and/or transplantation and the emotional aspects that accompany these procedures.

EXTERNAL DEFECTS

Defects of the external genitourinary tract are serious conditions primarily because of the psychologic impact on the child. Satisfactory surgical repair is successful for the more common disorders and is carried out or initiated as early as possible. The major anomalies of the lower genitourinary tract, their description, and their management are outlined in Table 27-4.

Psychologic Problems Related to Genital Surgery

Surgery involving sexual organs can be particularly disruptive to children, especially preschoolers fearing punishment, retaliation, body mutilation, or castration. Some of the problems of hospitalization, separation, and anxiety can be eased by hospital practices that are sensitive to the needs of the child (see Chapter 21).

The body image of a child is largely derived as a result of feedback from the primary caregivers, and parental anxiety regarding an acceptable physical appearance and adequate future sexual competency is readily communicated to an affected child. Therefore children with birth defects are at risk for developing a distorted body image that reflects the caregiver's subtly communicated evaluation of their bodies. The trend toward repair of visible genital defects is based in large part on these psychologic variables. The earlier a repair can be achieved, the more likely the possibility that the child will develop a normal body image.

During the years from 3 to 6, the phallic-oedipal period, children show a strong interest and concern about the genital area, sex differences, and genital normality or its lack. It is also a time when children are frightened of what they perceive to be threats to their body and bodily function. They also view any untoward happening as a punishment for real or imagined wrongdoing or unacceptable sexual feelings, such as masturbation, sex play, or erotic feelings. Surgical repair is recommended before these fears and anxieties develop (see Critical Thinking Exercise on p. 961).

Nursing Considerations

Preparing children and their families for diagnostic and surgical procedures (see Preparation for Procedures, Chapter 22) and for home care are major nursing functions. Most postoperative care involves care of the surgical site. Tub baths are discouraged for 1 week following simple surgeries, and the surgical site is kept clean and otherwise protected from infection and inspected for signs of infection. Dressings, if any, are inspected regularly. More complex surgeries require additional care and observation (e.g., catheter care for urethral reconstruction and care of urinary diversion stomas and collection devices).

Some older children's activities, such as pushing, lifting, playing with straddle toys, or in sandboxes, swimming, and rough activities, may be restricted for some types of surgical repairs. Precise restrictions depend on the specific type of surgery. Activities of infants and toddlers are not limited.

In most cases the results of surgery are quite satisfactory. However, in some of the more severe defects, such as exstrophy and those that require stomas, additional emotional interventions may be needed. A major concern of parents and children is related to surgery affecting the genitals directly. Concerns about penile size, appearance of the genitalia, potential ability to procreate, and rejection by peers (especially the opposite sex) are potential fears that require psychologic adjustment, particularly during adolescence.

TABLE 27-4. Defects of the genitourinary tract

DEFECT	THERAPEUTIC MANAGEMENT	DEFECT	THERAPEUTIC MANAGEMENT
Inguinal Hernia Protrusion of abdominal contents through inguinal canal into scrotum	Detected as painless inguinal swelling of variable size Surgical closure of inguinal defect	**Cryptorchidism** Failure of one or both testes to descend normally through inguinal canal	Detected by inability to palpate testes within scrotum Medical: administration of human chorionic gonadotropin (older child) Surgical: orchiopexy Objectives of therapy: Prevent damage to undescended testicle Decrease incidence of malignant tumor formation Avoid trauma and torsion Close inguinal canal Prevent cosmetic and psychologic disability from empty scrotum
Hydrocele Fluid in scrotum	Surgical repair indicated if spontaneous resolution not accomplished in 1 year		
Phimosis Narrowing or stenosis of preputial opening of foreskin	Mild cases: manual retraction of foreskin and proper cleansing of area Severe cases: circumcision or vertical division and transverse suturing of foreskin		
Hypospadias Urethral opening located behind glans penis or anywhere along ventral surface of penile shaft	Objectives of surgical correction: To enable child to void in standing position and direct stream voluntarily in usual manner Improve physical appearance of genitalia Produce a sexually adequate organ	**Exstrophy of Bladder** Eversion of posterior bladder through anterior bladder wall and lower abdominal wall; associated with open pubic arch (a severe defect)	Potential objectives of surgical correction: Preserve renal function Attain urinary control Adequate reconstructive repair Improve sexual function (especially in males)
		Ambiguous Genitalia Types: Masculinized female (female pseudohermaphrodite) Incompletely masculinized male (male pseudohermaphrodite)	Assignment of gender sex Surgical correction if needed; gender assignment—female Gender assignment—female
Chordee Ventral curvature of penis, often associated with hypospadias	Surgical release of fibrous band causing the deformity		
Epispadias Meatal opening located on dorsal surface of penis	Surgical correction, usually including penile and urethral lengthening and bladder neck reconstruction (if necessary)	True hermaphrodite (both ovaries and testes) Mixed gonadal dysgenesis	Gender assignment depends on predominant characteristics Gender assignment depends on predominant characteristics

GLOMERULAR DISEASE

NEPHROTIC SYNDROME

Nephrotic syndrome is a clinical state that includes massive proteinuria, hypoalbuminemia, hyperlipemia, and edema. The disorder can occur as (1) a primary disease known as *idiopathic nephrosis, childhood nephrosis,* or *minimal-change nephrotic syndrome (MCNS);* (2) a secondary disorder that occurs as a clinical manifestation after or in association with glomerular damage of known or presumed etiology; or (3) a congenital form inherited as an autosomal recessive disorder. The disorder is characterized by increased glomerular permeability to plasma protein, which results in massive urinary protein loss. The glomerulus is responsible for the initial step in formation of urine, and filtration rate depends on an intact

glomerular membrane. This discussion is devoted to MCNS because it constitutes 80% of nephrotic syndrome cases.

Pathophysiology

The onset of MCNS can occur at any age but predominantly occurs in children between the ages of 2 and 7 years. It is rare in children younger than 6 months of age, uncommon in infants younger than 1 year of age, and unusual after the age of 8.

The pathogenesis of MCNS is not understood. There may be a metabolic, biochemical, physiochemical, or immune-mediated disturbance that causes the basement membrane of the glomeruli to become increasingly permeable to protein, but the cause and mechanisms are only speculative.

The glomerular membrane, normally impermeable to albumin and other proteins, becomes permeable to proteins, especially albumin, which leak through the membrane and are lost in urine *(hyperalbuminuria)*. This reduces the serum albumin level *(hypoalbuminemia)*, decreasing the colloidal osmotic pressure in the capillaries. As a result, the vascular hydrostatic pressure exceeds the pull of the colloidal osmotic pressure, causing fluid to accumulate in the interstitial spaces *(edema)* and body cavities, particularly in the abdominal cavity *(ascites)*. The shift of fluid from the plasma to the interstitial spaces reduces the vascular fluid volume *(hypovolemia)*, which in turn stimulates the renin-angiotensin system and the secretion of antidiuretic hormone and aldosterone. Tubular reabsorption of sodium and water is increased in an attempt to increase intravascular volume. The elevation of serum lipids is unexplained. The sequence of events in nephrotic syndrome is diagrammed in Fig. 27-2.

Diagnostic Evaluation

The disease is suspected on the basis of clinical manifestations (see box on p. 962), especially when weight gain in a previously well child increases slowly over days or weeks. The generalized edema may develop rapidly or gradually but eventually prompts the family to seek medical attention (Fig. 27-3). Parents usually give a history of the child being well but steadily gaining weight and then becoming anorexic, irritable, and less active.

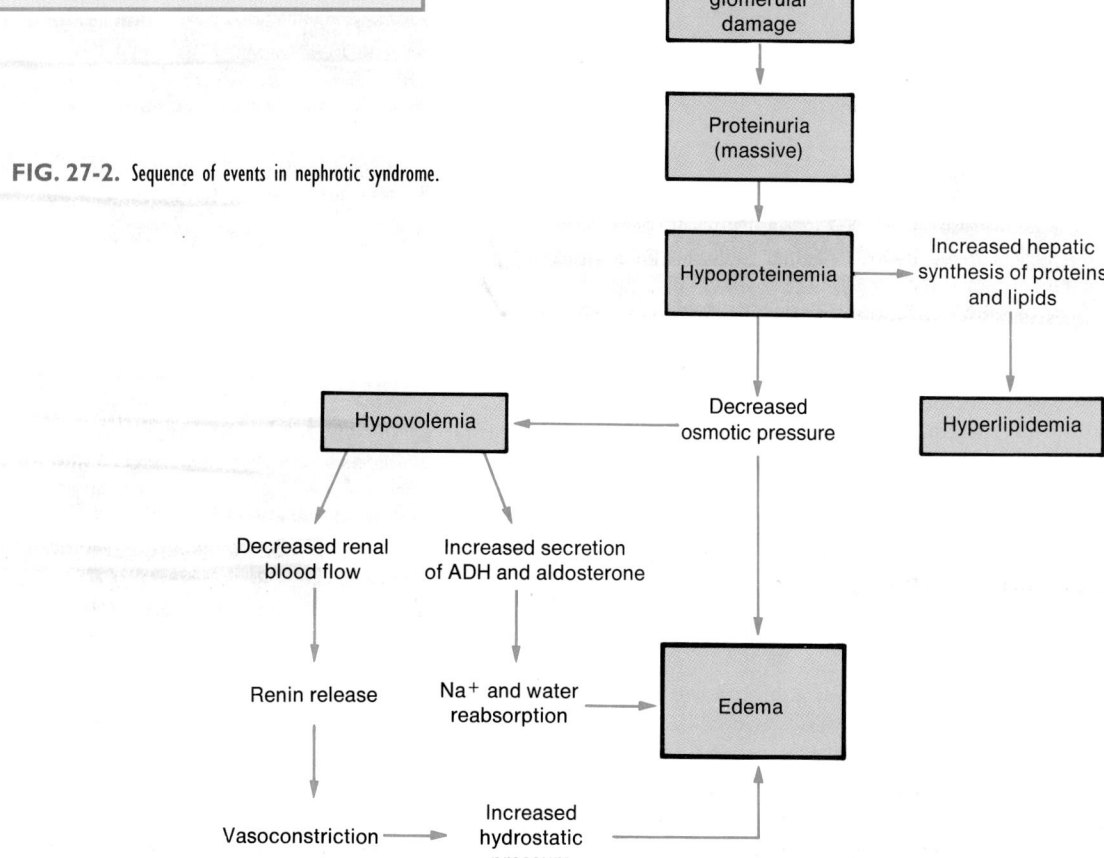

FIG. 27-2. Sequence of events in nephrotic syndrome.

CLINICAL MANIFESTATIONS OF NEPHROTIC SYNDROME

Weight gain
Edema
Puffiness of face:
    Especially around the eyes
    Apparent on arising in the morning
    Subsides during the day
Abdominal swelling (ascites)
Respiratory difficulty (pleural effusion)
Labial or scrotal swelling
Edema of intestinal mucosal causes:
    Diarrhea
    Anorexia
    Poor intestinal absorption
Extreme skin pallor (often)
Irritability
Easily fatigued
Lethargic
Blood pressure normal or slightly decreased
Susceptibility to infection
Urine alterations:
    Decreased volume
    Darkly opalescent
    Frothy

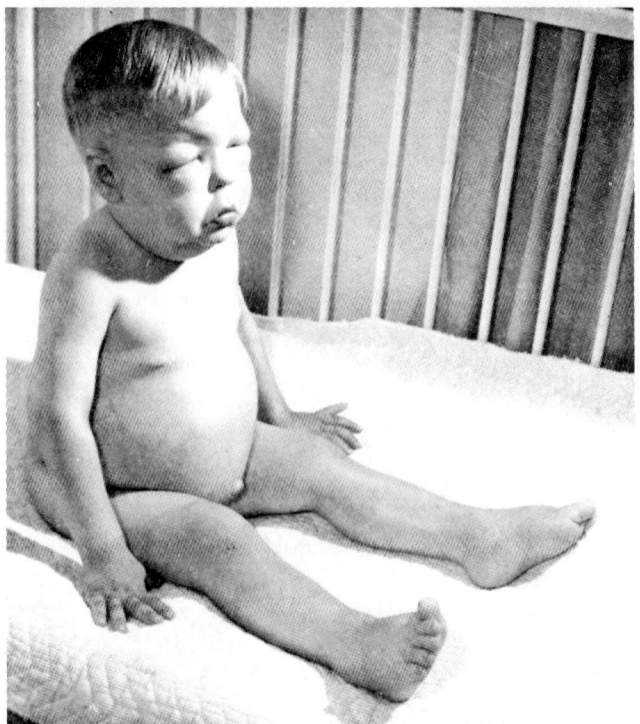

FIG. 27-3. Child with nephrotic syndrome. (From Bentz GS: *Pediatric nursing*, ed 5, St Louis, 1964, Mosby. Courtesy University of Minnesota Photographic Laboratory.)

Nursing ALERT A child who exhibits the following should be evaluated for the possibility of nephrotic syndrome:

Weight gain over that expected based on previous pattern
Parent observation that the child's clothes fit tightly
Decreased urine output
Pallor, fatigue

The diagnosis of MCNS is made on the basis of the history and clinical manifestations (edema, proteinuria, hypoalbuminemia, and hypercholesterolemia in the absence of hematuria and hypertension) in children between the ages of 2 and 8 years.

Massive proteinuria is reflected in urinary excretion of protein with high specific gravity proportionate to the concentration of protein. Hyaline casts, fat bodies, and a few red blood cells can be found in the urine of most affected children, although there is seldom gross hematuria. If hypovolemia is not significant and if the child is well hydrated, the glomerular filtration rate is usually normal.

Total serum protein concentrations are lowered, with the albumin fractions significantly reduced and plasma lipids elevated. Hemoglobin and hematocrit are usually normal or elevated and the platelet count is high as a result of hemoconcentration. Serum sodium concentration is usually low.

A renal biopsy may be performed to distinguish between types of nephrotic syndrome in order to predict the probable disease course and response to drugs. The biopsy of children with MCNS is remarkable for fusion of the foot processes of the basement membrane and otherwise normal kidney tissue.

Therapeutic Management

Objectives of therapeutic management include (1) reducing excretion of urinary protein, (2) reducing fluid retention in the tissues, (3) preventing infection, and (4) minimizing complications related to therapies. If edema is not incapacitating, ambulation is encouraged. Dietary restrictions include a *low-salt diet* during periods of generalized edema. If complications of edema develop (severe gastrointestinal upset, ascites, or respiratory distress), diuretic therapy including plasma expanders may be initiated to provide temporary relief from edema. Acute and intercurrent infections are treated with appropriate antibiotics, and efforts are made to eliminate possible infection.

Corticosteroids have been found to have a therapeutic value in treating MCNS, although the success of the treatment depends on the individual child's response to the medication (*prednisone*). In most children this response occurs within 7 to 21 days. The medication is then tapered over several weeks and eventually stopped if the child remains asymptomatic. A relapse wherein proteinuria returns requires immediate repeated courses of high-dose steroid therapy. Side effects of the medication include rounding of the face, increased appetite, abdominal distention, hirsutism, growth retardation, cataracts, hypertension, gastrointestinal bleeding, bone demineralization, infection, and hyperglycemia. Children who do not respond to steroid therapy, those who have frequent relapses, and those in whom the side effects threaten their growth and general health may be considered for a course of therapy using other immunosuppressant medications (cyclophosphamide, chorambucil, or cyclosporine).

Complications of nephrotic syndrome include relapse, infection, circulatory insufficiency secondary to hypovolemia, and thromboembolism. Relapses can be triggered by many factors, such as viruses, allergies, bacterial infections, and occasionally immunizations. Relapses in children with MCNS occur two to four times per year and continue over many years. Infections that may be seen in children with nephrotic syndrome include peritonitis, cellulitis, and pneumonia and require prompt recognition and vigorous treatment with appropriate antibiotic therapy. (See Critical Thinking Exercise.)

Prognosis. The prognosis for ultimate recovery in most cases is good. It is a self-limiting disease, and in children who respond to steroid therapy the tendency to relapse decreases with time. With early detection and prompt implementation of therapy to eradicate proteinuria, progressive basement membrane damage is minimized, so that when the tendency to exacerbations is past, renal function is usually normal or near normal. It is estimated that approximately

---

CRITICAL **T**HINKING **E**XERCISE

Nephrotic Syndrome

Jerome is an 8-year-old boy with relapsing nephrotic syndrome who has become steroid dependent. During your initial assessment in the outpatient clinic you identify the following: (1) weight has increased 2 kg in the last 2 weeks; (2) blood pressure is 100/70; (3) mother reports that Jerome is not urinating very much and she does not know how much he has been drinking; (4) while you are measuring Jerome's abdominal girth, he guards his abdomen and complains of stomachache; and (5) his temperature is 38° C (100.4° F) orally. Of the following correct actions, you should first do which of the following?

1. Examine Jerome's abdomen more thoroughly while eliciting a 24-hour recall of illness symptoms from his mother.
2. Elicit a 24-hour recall of food and fluid intake from Jerome and his mother together.
3. Obtain a clean-catch urine specimen. Divide the specimen so that you can perform a dipstick analysis immediately and retain the other specimen for possible urinalysis and culture after consultation with the primary health practitioner.
4. Explore the mother's understanding of Jerome's illness and its relationship to his current condition to begin outlining your teaching plan for this family.

The correct response is one. One of the complications of severe nephrotic syndrome is peritonitis, which can occur secondary to migration of intestinal bacteria across the bowel wall and into the protein-rich acidic fluid. Jerome's mother has already said that she does not know what he has been drinking. Therefore your only possibility of assessing his intake is to elicit the recall while they are together. Although his weight gain and reduced urine output are major concerns, they are secondary to peritonitis. (It should be recognized that children on strict fluid restrictions are prone to obtain fluids from unauthorized sources.) Obtaining a urine specimen for dipstick analysis is part of the initial assessment for Jerome. In this instance the fever and abdominal pain are the first priority. As with option three, the fourth choice must be addressed, along with evaluation of the current stress level in the home, after the fever and pain have been addressed.

80% of affected children have this favorable prognosis, although half the children have relapses even after 5 years.

Nursing Considerations

❖ Assessment

Continuous monitoring of fluid retention or excretion is an important nursing function. Strict intake and output records are essential but may be difficult to obtain from very young children. Application of collection bags is highly irritating to edematous skin that is readily subject to breakdown. Application of diapers or weighing wet pads may be necessary. Other methods of monitoring progress include urine examination for specific gravity and albumin, daily weight, and measurement of abdominal girth. Assessment of edema (e.g., increased or decreased swelling around the eyes and dependent areas), the degree of pitting (if noted), and the color and texture of skin are part of nursing care. Vital signs are monitored to detect any early signs of complications such as shock or an infective process.

❖ Nursing Diagnoses

Constant reassessment and evaluation reveal a number of nursing diagnoses that are relevant to the care of these children and their families (see Nursing Care Plan, pp. 964-965). Others will be apparent in specific situations.

❖ Planning

The goals of care of the child with nephrotic syndrome and family are as follows:

1. Child will exhibit no evidence of fluid accumulation.
2. Child will exhibit no evidence of skin breakdown or infection.
3. Child will receive optimum nutrition.
4. Child and family will express feelings and concerns.

❖ Implementation

Children hospitalized with MCNS may be placed on bed rest during the edema phase of the disease. They seldom offer resistance, since they are usually lethargic and easily fatigued, and their cumbersome edematous bulk is not conducive to movement.

Reducing the excretion of urinary protein primarily involves the administration of corticosteroids. Nurses must be aware of the problems associated with these drugs and be alert to complications from their use.

Infection is a constant source of danger to edematous children and those receiving corticosteroid therapy. These children are particularly vulnerable to upper respiratory infection; therefore they must be kept warm and dry, turned frequently, and protected from contact with infected roommates, visitors, and personnel. Vital signs are monitored to detect any early signs of an infective process.

Loss of appetite accompanying active nephrosis creates a perplexing problem for nurses. During this time the combined efforts of nurse, dietitian, parents, and the child are needed to formulate a nutritionally adequate and attractive diet. Salt is usually restricted (but not eliminated) during the edema phase, and fluid restriction (if prescribed) is limited to short-term use during massive edema. Every effort should be made to serve attractive meals with preferred foods and a minimum of fuss, but it usually requires a considerable

NURSING CARE PLAN
The Child with Nephrotic Syndrome

NURSING DIAGNOSIS: Fluid volume excess (total body) related to fluid accumulation in tissues and third spaces

PATIENT GOAL 1: Will exhibit no or minimal evidence of fluid accumulation

- **NURSING INTERVENTIONS/*RATIONALES***

Assess intake relative to output
    Measure and record intake and output accurately
    Weigh daily (or more often, if indicated) *to assess fluid retention*
Assess changes in edema
    Measure abdominal girth at umbilicus *to assess ascites*
    Monitor edema around eyes and dependent areas *because these are common sites of edema*
    Note degree of pitting, if present
    Note color and texture of skin
Test urine for specific gravity, albumin *because hyperalbuminuria is manifestation of nephrotic syndrome*
Collect specimens for laboratory examination
*Administer corticosteroids as prescribed *to reduce excretion of urinary protein*
*Administer diuretics if ordered *to provide temporary relief from edema*
Limit fluids as indicated *during massive edema*

- **EXPECTED OUTCOME**

Child exhibits no or minimal evidence of fluid accumulation (specify parameters)

PATIENT GOAL 2: Will receive appropriate volume of fluid

- **NURSING INTERVENTIONS/*RATIONALES***

Regulate fluid intake carefully *so that child does not receive more than prescribed amount*
Monitor intravenous infusion *to maintain prescribed intake*
Employ strategies to prevent undesired intake
    Use small containers for fluid intake *so that volume does not appear so restricted*
    Divide allowed intake into small volumes spread over entire day
    Spray mouth with atomizer (mist) *to prevent feeling of dryness*
    Offer chewing gum and sugarless hard candies
Keep lips lubricated *for comfort and to prevent cracking*

- **EXPECTED OUTCOME**

Child receives no more fluid than prescribed

NURSING DIAGNOSIS: High risk for (intravascular) fluid volume deficit related to protein and fluid loss, edema

PATIENT GOAL 1: Will exhibit no or minimal evidence of intravascular fluid loss or hypovolemic shock

- **NURSING INTERVENTIONS/*RATIONALES***

Monitor vital signs *to detect physical evidence of fluid depletion*
Assess pulse quality and rate *for signs of hypovolemic shock*
Measure blood pressure *to detect hypovolemic shock*
Report any deviations from normal *so that prompt treatment is instituted*
*Administer salt-poor albumin if prescribed *as a plasma expander*

- **EXPECTED OUTCOME**

Child exhibits no or minimal evidence of intravascular fluid loss or hypovolemic shock

NURSING DIAGNOSIS: High risk for infection related to lowered body defenses, fluid overload

PATIENT GOAL 1: Will exhibit no evidence of infection

- **NURSING INTERVENTIONS/*RATIONALES***

Protect child from contact with infected persons *to minimize exposure to infective organisms*
    Place in room with noninfectious children
    Restrict contact with persons who have infections, including family, other children, friends, and staff members
    Teach visitors appropriate preventive behaviors (e.g., handwashing)
Observe medical asepsis
Use good handwashing
Keep child warm and dry *because of vulnerability to upper respiratory infection*
Monitor temperature *for early evidence of infection*
Teach parents signs and symptoms of infections

- **EXPECTED OUTCOMES**

Child and family apply good health practices
Child exhibits no evidence of infection

---

*Dependent nursing action.

NURSING CARE PLAN
The Child with Nephrotic Syndrome

NURSING DIAGNOSIS: High risk for impaired skin integrity related to edema, lowered body defenses

PATIENT GOAL 1: Will maintain skin integrity

- **NURSING INTERVENTIONS/*RATIONALES***

Provide meticulous skin care
Avoid tight clothing *that may cause pressure areas*
Cleanse and powder opposing skin surfaces several times per day *to prevent skin breakdown*
Separate opposing skin surfaces with soft cotton *to prevent skin breakdown*
Support edematous organs, such as scrotum, *to relieve pressure areas*
Cleanse edematous eyelids with warm saline wipes
Change position frequently; maintain good body alignment *because child with massive edema is usually lethargic, easily fatigued, and content to lie still*
Use pressure-relieving or pressure-reducing mattresses or beds as needed *to prevent ulcers* (see Maintaining Healthy Skin, Chapter 22)

- **EXPECTED OUTCOME**

Child's skin displays no evidence of redness or irritation

NURSING DIAGNOSIS: Altered nutrition: less than body requirements related to loss of appetite

PATIENT GOAL 1: Will receive optimum nutrition

- **NURSING INTERVENTIONS/*RATIONALES***

Offer nutritious diet
Restrict sodium during edema and steroid therapy
*Administer supplementary vitamins and iron as ordered
Enlist aid of child, parents, and dietitian in formulation of diet *to encourage optimum nutrition despite loss of appetite*
Provide cheerful, clean, relaxed atmosphere during meals *so that child is more likely to eat*
Serve small quantities initially *to stimulate appetite;* encourage seconds
Provide special and preferred foods *to encourage child to eat*
Serve foods in an attractive manner *to stimulate appetite*
See also Feeding the Sick Child, Chapter 22

- **EXPECTED OUTCOME**

Child consumes an adequate amount of nutritious food

NURSING DIAGNOSIS: Body image disturbance related to change in appearance

PATIENT GOAL 1: Will express feelings and concerns

- **NURSING INTERVENTIONS/*RATIONALES***

Explore feelings and concerns regarding appearance *to facilitate coping*
    Point out positive aspects of appearance and evidence of diminished edema *so that child feels encouraged*
    Explain to child and family that symptoms associated with steroid therapy will subside when medication is discontinued
Encourage activity within limits of tolerance
Encourage socialization with persons without active infection *so that child is not lonely and isolated*
Provide positive feedback *so that child feels accepted*
Explore areas of interest and encourage their pursuit

- **EXPECTED OUTCOMES**

Child discusses feelings and concerns
Child engages in activities appropriate to interests and abilities

NURSING DIAGNOSIS: Activity intolerance related to fatigue

PATIENT GOAL 1: Will receive adequate rest

- **NURSING INTERVENTIONS**

Maintain bed rest initially if severely edematous
Balance rest and activity when ambulatory
Plan and provide quiet activities
Instruct child to rest when he or she begins to feel tired
Allow for periods of uninterrupted sleep

- **EXPECTED OUTCOMES**

Child engages in activities appropriate to capabilities
Child receives adequate rest and sleep

NURSING DIAGNOSIS: Altered family processes related to a child with a serious disease

PATIENT (FAMILY) GOAL 1: Will receive adequate support

- **NURSING INTERVENTIONS/*RATIONALES* AND EXPECTED OUTCOMES**

See Nursing Care Plan: The Family of the Ill or Hospitalized Child, Chapter 21

See also Nursing Care Plan: The Child in the Hospital, Chapter 21

*Dependent nursing action.

amount of ingenuity and enticement to get the child to eat (see Feeding the Sick Child, Chapter 22).

As the edema subsides, children are allowed increased activity. Although easily fatigued, children usually adjust activities according to their tolerance level. However, they may require guidance in selecting play activities. Suitable recreational and diversional activities are an important part of their care. Once edema fluid has been lost, children are allowed to resume their usual activities with discretion. Irritability and mood swings that accompany the inactivity, disease process, and steroid therapy are not unusual manifestations in these children, and they create an additional challenge to the nurse and the family.

Family Support and Home Care.   Continuous support of the child and family is one of the major nursing considerations. Many children are treated at home during exacerbations. Parents are taught to detect signs of relapse and to bring the child for treatment at the earliest indications. Unless the edema and proteinuria are severe or the parents, for some reason, are unable to care for the ill child, *home care is preferred.* Parents are instructed in testing urine for albumin, administration of medications, and general care. Parents are also instructed regarding avoiding contact with infected playmates, but the child should attend school.

The prolonged course of the relapsing form of nephrotic syndrome is taxing to both the child and the family. The up-and-down course of remissions and exacerbations with periodic disruption of family life by hospitalization places a severe strain on the child and the family, both psychologically and financially. Parents and children over 5 or 6 years of age need reassurance regarding this characteristic of the course of the disease, with emphasis on the importance of long-term care to gain their cooperation. A satisfactory response is more likely when relapses are detected and therapy is instituted early, and remissions are prolonged when instructions are carried out faithfully. Continuous support of the child and family is one of the major nursing considerations (see Chapter 18).

❖ Evaluation

The effectiveness of nursing interventions is determined by continual reassessment and evaluation of care based on the following observational guidelines and expected outcomes:

1. Measure intake and output and examine urine for albumin.
2. Monitor vital signs and assess the skin for evidence of breakdown or infection.
3. Assess appetite and eating behaviors.
4. Observe and interview child and family regarding their understanding of the disease, therapies, and compliance with the prescribed regimen.

Expected outcomes:
See Nursing Care Plan, pp. 964-965.

ACUTE GLOMERULONEPHRITIS (AGN)

AGN may be a primary event or a manifestation of a systemic disorder that can range from minimal to severe. Common features include oliguria, edema, hypertension and circulatory congestion, hematuria, and proteinuria. Most cases are postinfectious and have been associated with pneumococcal, streptococcal, and viral infections. *Acute poststreptococcal glomerulonephritis (APSGN)* is the most common of the postinfectious, associated renal diseases in childhood and the one for which a cause can be established in the majority of cases. APSGN can occur at any age but affects primarily early school-age children, with a peak age of onset of 6 to 7 years. It is uncommon in children younger than 2 years of age, and males outnumber females 2:1.

Etiology

APSGN is an immune-complex disease that occurs as a byproduct of an antecedent streptococcal infection with certain strains of the group A β-hemolytic streptococcus. Most streptococcal infections *do not* cause APSGN. A latent period of 10 to 14 days occurs between the streptococcal infection and the onset of clinical manifestations. The peak incidence of disease corresponds to the incidence of streptococcal infection. Disease secondary to streptococcal pharyngitis is more common in the winter or spring, but when it is associated with pyoderma (principally **impetigo**), it may be more prevalent in later summer or early fall, especially in warmer climates. Multiple cases tend to occur in families. Second episodes of AGN are rare.

Pathophysiology

The mechanism by which the reaction takes place is still speculative; one explanation is that the streptococcal infection is followed by the release of a membranelike material from the specific organism into the circulation. Because it is antigenic, antibody is formed, and after the appropriate period of time, an immune-complex reaction occurs. The glomeruli become edematous and infiltrated with polymorphonuclear leukocytes, which occlude the capillary lumen. The resulting decrease in plasma filtration results in an excessive accumulation of water and retention of sodium that expands plasma and interstitial fluid volumes, leading to circulatory congestion and edema. It is unclear whether the decreased glomerular filtration rate, increased capillary permeability, or vascular spasm is responsible for these various manifestations. The cause of the hypertension associated with acute glomerulonephritis is also unexplained.

Diagnostic Evaluation

Typically, affected children are in good health until they experience the streptococcal infection. In some instances there is no history of an infection, or it is only described as a mild cold. The onset of nephritis appears after an average latent period of about 10 days (see box). Since the child appears to be well during this time, the association is not recognized by the parents. The edema is relatively moderate and may not be appreciated by someone unfamiliar with the child's normal appearance.

Urinalysis during the acute phase characteristically shows hematuria, proteinuria, and increased specific gravity. The specific gravity is moderately elevated and seldom exceeds 1.02. Proteinuria generally parallels the hematuria, and the content usually shows 3+ or 4+ but is not the massive proteinuria seen in nephrotic syndrome. Gross discoloration of the urine reflects its red blood cell and hemoglobin content. Microscopic examination of the sediment shows many red blood cells, leukocytes, epithelial cells, and granular and red

CLINICAL MANIFESTATIONS OF ACUTE POSTSTREPTOCOCCAL GLOMERULONEPHRITIS

Edema:
  Especially periorbital
  Facial edema more prominent in the morning
  Spreads during the day to involve extremities and abdomen
Anorexia
Urine:
  Cloudy, smoky brown (resembles tea or cola)
  Severely reduced volume
Pallor
Irritability
Lethargy
Child appears ill
Child seldom expresses specific complaints
Older children may complain of:
  Headaches
  Abdominal discomfort
  Dysuria
Vomiting possible
Mild to moderately elevated blood pressure

blood cell casts. Bacteria are not seen, and urine cultures are negative.

Azotemia that results from impaired glomerular filtration is reflected in elevated blood urea nitrogen and creatinine levels in at least 50% of cases. When proteinuria is excessive, there may be changes associated with nephrotic syndrome (i.e., transient hypoproteinemia and hyperlipidemia).

Cultures of the pharynx are positive for streptococci in only a few cases, and the numbers are not significantly greater than the normal carrier incidence in many communities. Positive cultures help to establish a diagnosis. Cultures should be obtained from other household members, and persons positive for group A streptococci should receive a course of antistreptococcal therapy.

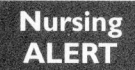 **Nursing ALERT**
A child who exhibits the following should be evaluated for possible AGN:
  Orbital edema, which parents report is worse in the morning
  Loss of appetite
  Decreased output
  Dark-colored urine
  Antecedent streptococcal infection

Some serologic tests may help in the diagnosis of AGN. The *antistreptolysin O (ASO) titer* is the most familiar and readily available test for streptococcal infection. It is used to detect the presence of antibodies, which documents a recent infection, especially a rising titer in two samples taken a week apart. Other serologic tests that may aid in diagnosis following streptococcal skin infections are elevated antihyaluronidase (AHase), antideoxyribonuclease B (ADNase-B), and antinicotyladenine dinucleotidase (ANADase) titers.

Since AGN is an immune-complex disease, there is reduced total serum complement activity in the early stages of the disease. Rising complement levels (C_3, C_4) are used as a guide to indicate improvement of the disease. Other studies that are employed include a chest x-ray examination, which shows characteristic generalized cardiac enlargement, pulmonary congestion, and pleural effusion during the edematous phase of acute disease. Renal biopsy for diagnostic purposes is seldom required but may be useful in the diagnosis of atypical cases.

Therapeutic Management

Management consists of general supportive measures and early recognition and treatment of complications. Children who have normal blood pressure and a satisfactory urine output can generally be treated at home. Those with substantial edema, hypertension, gross hematuria, and/or significant oliguria should be hospitalized because of the unpredictability of complications.

Bed rest may be recommended during the acute phase, but ambulation does not seem to have an adverse effect on the course of the disease once the symptoms have resolved. Dietary restrictions depend on the stage and severity of the disease, especially the extent of edema. Moderate sodium restriction is usually instituted for children with hypertension and edema. Foods with substantial amounts of potassium are generally restricted during the period of oliguria.

Regular measurement of vital signs, body weight, and intake and output is essential in order to monitor the progress of the disease and to detect complications that may appear at any time during the course of the disease. *A record of daily weight is the most useful means for assessing fluid balance.* Rarely, children with AGN will develop acute renal failure with oliguria that significantly alters the fluid and electrolyte balance (resulting in hyperkalemia, acidosis, hypocalcemia, and/or hyperphosphatemia). These children require careful management that may include peritoneal dialysis or hemodialysis.

Acute hypertension must be anticipated and identified early. Blood pressure measurements are taken every 4 to 6 hours. A variety of antihypertensive medications, as well as diuretics, are used to control mild to moderate hypertension. Seizure activity associated with hypertensive encephalopathy requires anticonvulsant therapy, as well as antihypertensive agents.

Antibiotic therapy is indicated only for those children with evidence of persistent streptococcal infections. It is used to prevent transmission of nephritogenic streptococci to other family members.

Prognosis. Almost all children correctly diagnosed as having APSGN recover completely, and specific immunity is conferred so that subsequent recurrences are uncommon. Deaths from complications still occur but are fortunately rare. A few of these children may develop chronic disease, but many of these cases are believed to be (probably) different glomerular diseases misdiagnosed as poststreptococcal disease.

Nursing Considerations

❖ Assessment

Vital signs provide clues to the severity of the disease and early signs of complications. They are carefully measured, and any deviations are reported and recorded. The volume and character of urine are noted, and the child is weighed daily. Children with restricted fluid intake, especially those who are not severely edematous or those who have lost weight, are observed for signs of dehydration.

Assessment of the child's appearance for signs of cerebral

complications is an important nursing function, since the severity of the acute phase is variable and unpredictable. The child with edema, hypertension, and gross hematuria may be subject to complications, and anticipatory preparations such as seizure precautions and intravenous equipment are included in the nursing care plan.

❖ Nursing Diagnoses

Based on assessment, several nursing diagnoses become obvious (see box). Others may be evident in specific situations.

❖ Planning

The goals of care for the child with AGN and family include the following:

1. Child will receive optimum rest.
2. Child will receive sufficient nutrition.
3. Child will exhibit no evidence of complications.
4. Child and family will receive appropriate support and education regarding child's condition.

❖ Implementation

During the acute phase, children are generally quite content to lie in bed. Activities should be those that require little expenditure of energy. Since they are generally listless and experience fatigue and malaise, most children voluntarily restrict their activities during the most active phase of the disease. As they begin to feel better and as their symptoms subside, activities are planned to allow for frequent rest periods and avoidance of fatigue.

For most children a regular diet is allowed, but it should contain no added salt. Foods high in sodium and salted treats are eliminated, and parents and friends are advised not to bring items such as potato chips or pretzels. However, the total amount of salt ingested is usually less than prescribed because of the child's poor appetite. Fluid restriction, if prescribed, is more difficult, and the amount permitted should be evenly divided throughout the waking hours and served in small cups to give the illusion of larger servings. Meal preparation and service require special attention, since the child is indifferent to meals during the acute phase. Again, collaboration with parents and the dietitian and special consideration for food preferences facilitate meal planning.

Children who have mild edema and no hypertension, as well as convalescent children who are being treated at home, need follow-up care. Parents are instructed regarding general measures, including activity, diet, and prevention of infection. Strenuous activity is usually restricted until there is no evidence of proteinuria or macroscopic hematuria, which may persist for months.

Health supervision is continued with weekly, followed by monthly, visits for evaluation and urinalysis. Parent education and support in preparation for discharge and home care include education in home management and the need for follow-up care and health supervision.

❖ Evaluation

The effectiveness of nursing interventions is determined by continual reassessment and evaluation of care based on the following observational guidelines and expected outcomes:

1. Observe child's behavior.
2. Monitor dietary and fluid intake; interview family regarding child's diet and appetite.
3. Monitor vital signs, intake and output, and observe for signs of complications, such as hypertension, increased intracranial pressure, and infection.
4. Observe behaviors and interview child and family regarding reaction to the disease and therapies.

Expected outcomes:

1. Child plays and rests quietly.
2. Child consumes a sufficient amount of appropriate foods.
3. Child exhibits no evidence of complications.
4. Child and family demonstrate an understanding of the disease and its therapy (specify learnings and methods of demonstration), and they express their feelings and concerns.

MISCELLANEOUS RENAL DISORDERS

HEMOLYTIC-UREMIC SYNDROME (HUS)

HUS is an uncommon, acute renal disease that occurs primarily in infants and small children between the ages of 6 months and 5 years. It occurs worldwide but is recognized predominantly in white children. HUS is the most frequent cause of acquired acute renal failure in children (Brandt and others, 1994). The clinical features of the disease include acquired hemolytic anemia, thrombocytopenia, renal injury, and central nervous system symptoms. The etiology of HUS is thought to be associated with bacterial toxins, chemicals, and viruses. The appearance of the disease has been associated with *Rickettsia*, viruses (especially coxsackie virus, echovirus, and adenovirus), *Escherichia coli*, pneumococci, *Shigella*, and *Salmonella* and may represent an unusual response to these infections. Multiple cases of HUS caused by enteric infection of the *E. coli* 0157:H7 serotype have been traced to undercooked meat. The clinical presentation is usually a history of a prodromal illness (most often gastroenteritis or an upper respiratory infection) followed by the sudden onset of hemolysis and renal failure.

Pathophysiology

The primary site of injury appears to be the endothelial lining of the small glomerular arterioles, which become swollen and occluded with deposits of platelets and fibrin clots (intravascular coagulation). Red blood cells are damaged as they attempt to move through the partially occluded blood vessels. These damaged cells are removed by the spleen, causing acute hemolytic anemia. The platelet aggregation within the

CLINICAL MANIFESTATIONS OF HEMOLYTIC-UREMIC SYNDROME

Vomiting
Irritability
Lethargy
Marked pallor
Hemorrhagic manifestations:
    Bruising
    Petechiae
    Jaundice
    Bloody diarrhea
Oliguria or anuria
Central nervous system involvement:
    Convulsions
    Stupor/coma
Signs of acute heart failure (sometimes)

CLINICAL MANIFESTATIONS OF WILMS TUMOR

Abdominal swelling or mass:
    Firm
    Nontender
    Confined to one side
Hematuria (less than one fourth of cases)
Fatigue/malaise
Hypertension (occasionally)
Weight loss
Fever
Manifestations resulting from compression of tumor mass
Secondary metabolic alterations from tumor or metastasis
If metastasis, symptoms of lung involvement:
    Dyspnea
    Cough
    Shortness of breath
    Chest pain (sometimes)

damaged blood vessels or the damage and removal of platelets produce the characteristic thrombocytopenia.

Diagnostic Evaluation

The triad of anemia, thrombocytopenia, and renal failure is sufficient for diagnosis (see box). Renal involvement is evidenced by proteinuria, hematuria, and the presence of urinary casts; blood urea nitrogen and serum creatinine levels are elevated. A low hemoglobin and hematocrit and a high reticulocyte count confirm the hemolytic nature of the anemia.

Therapeutic Management

The goals of therapy are early diagnosis and aggressive, supportive care of the acute renal failure and hemolytic anemia. The most consistently effective treatment of HUS is hemodialysis or peritoneal dialysis, which is instituted in any child who has been anuric for 24 hours or who demonstrates oliguria with uremia or hypertension and seizures. Other treatments include use of pharmacologic agents, fresh-frozen plasma, and plasma pheresis. Blood transfusions with fresh, washed packed cells are administered for severe anemia but are used with caution to prevent circulatory overload from added volume.

Prognosis. With prompt treatment the recovery rate is about 95%, but residual renal impairment ranges from 10% to 50% in various areas. Long-term complications include chronic renal failure, hypertension, and central nervous system disorders. Death is usually caused by residual renal impairment or central nervous system injury.

Nursing Considerations

Nursing care is the same as that provided in acute renal failure and, for children with continued impairment, includes management of chronic disease.

WILMS TUMOR*

Wilms tumor, or nephroblastoma, is the most common primary malignant tumor of the kidney in children. Its frequency

---

*Marilyn Hockenberry-Eaton, PhD, RNC, PNP, and Nancy E. Kline, MS, RN, CPNP, revised this section.

is estimated to be 1 per 125,000 white children less than 15 years of age. Wilms tumor occurs about three times more often in blacks than in East Asians in the United States. The peak age at diagnosis is approximately 3 years, and occurrence is slightly more frequent in boys than in girls. Wilms tumor is one of the childhood cancers that may be genetically inherited. Unfortunately, there is no method of identifying gene carriers at this time.

Etiology

Wilms tumor probably arises from a malignant, undifferentiated cluster of primordial cells capable of initiating the regeneration of an abnormal structure. Its occurrence slightly favors the left kidney, which is advantageous because surgically this kidney is easier to manipulate and remove. In about 10% of cases both kidneys are involved. Although the tumor may become quite large, it remains encapsulated for an extended time. Studies have shown that development of Wilms tumor involves both genetic and somatic mosaicism and not germ-line mutation (Green and others, 1996).

Diagnostic Evaluation

In a child suspected of having Wilms tumor, special emphasis is placed on the history and physical examination for the presence of congenital anomalies, a family history of cancer, and signs of malignancy, such as weight loss, size of liver and spleen, indications of anemia, and lymphadenopathy. Most children with Wilms tumor are brought to the practitioner because of abdominal swelling or an abdominal mass (see box). Specific tests include radiographic studies, including abdominal ultrasound, computed tomography, hematologic studies (polycythemia is sometimes present if the tumor secretes excess erythropoietin), biochemical studies, and urinalysis. Studies to demonstrate the relationship of the tumor to the ipsilateral kidney and the presence of a normal functioning kidney on the contralateral side are essential. If a large tumor is present, an inferior venacavagram is necessary to demonstrate possible tumor involvement adjacent to the vena cava. A bone marrow aspiration may be performed to rule out metastasis, which is rare in children with Wilms tumor.

Therapeutic Management

Combined treatment of surgery and chemotherapy with or without radiation is based on the clinical stage and histologic pattern.

Surgery is scheduled as soon as possible after confirmation of a renal mass, usually within 24 to 48 hours of admission. A large transabdominal incision is performed for optimum visualization of the abdominal cavity. The tumor, affected kidney, and adjacent adrenal gland are removed. Great care is taken to keep the encapsulated tumor intact, since rupture can seed cancer cells throughout the abdomen, lymph channel, and bloodstream. The contralateral kidney is carefully inspected for evidence of disease or dysfunction. Regional lymph nodes are inspected, and a biopsy is performed when indicated. Any involved structures, such as part of the colon, diaphragm, or vena cava, are removed. Metal clips are placed around the tumor site for exact marking during radiotherapy.

If both kidneys are involved, the child may be treated with radiotherapy and/or chemotherapy before surgery to decrease the size of the tumor, allowing more conservative surgery. If may be possible to perform a partial nephrectomy on the less affected kidney, with a total nephrectomy on the opposite side. When a transplant is feasible, such as from a twin, sibling, or parent, bilateral nephrectomy is considered.

Postoperative radiation therapy is indicated for children with large tumors, metastasis, residual postoperative disease, unfavorable histology, or recurrence. Chemotherapy is indicated for all stages. The most effective agents for treating Wilms tumor are actinomycin D (dactinomycin), vincristine, and adriamycin. The duration of therapy varies, ranging from 6 to 15 months.

Prognosis. Survival rates for Wilms tumor are the highest among all childhood cancers. Children with localized tumor (stages I and II) have a 90% chance of cure with multimodal therapy. Factors that favorably affect the success of further therapy include initial treatment with only vincristine and dactinomycin, relapse to the lungs only, relapse in the abdomen of a patient who received no prior abdominal irradiation, and relapse more than 12 months after diagnosis. Wilms tumor may recur, especially in the lungs. Both chemotherapy and radiation therapy can induce second tumors, usually in areas that have been irradiated (Green and others, 1996).

Nursing Considerations

Do not palpate Abdomen

Nursing care of the child with Wilms tumor is similar to that of children with other cancers treated with surgery, irradiation, and chemotherapy. However, there are some significant differences; these are discussed for each phase of nursing intervention.

Preoperative Care. The preoperative period is one of swift diagnosis. The nurse is faced with the challenge of preparing the child and parents for all laboratory and operative procedures. Because of the little time available, explanations are kept simple, focused on what the child will experience, and repeated often. In addition to the usual preoperative observations, blood pressure is monitored, since hypertension from excess renin production is a possibility.

There are several special preoperative concerns, the most important of which is that the _tumor is not palpated unless absolutely necessary,_ since manipulation of the mass may cause dissemination of cancer cells to adjacent and distant sites.

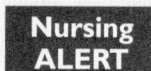

Nursing ALERT To reinforce the need for caution, it may be necessary to post a sign on the bed that reads "DO NOT PALPATE ABDOMEN." Careful bathing and handling are also important in preventing trauma to the tumor site.

Since radiotherapy and chemotherapy are usually begun immediately after surgery, parents need an explanation of what to expect, such as major benefits and side effects. The timing of the information should be considered to avoid overwhelming the family. Ideally the nurse should be present during physician-parent conferences to answer questions as they arise. It is usually better to reserve telling the child about these side effects until after surgery. Alopecia, usually of most concern to older children, does not occur until 2 weeks after the initial treatment regimen. Therefore the child can be prepared for the hair loss postoperatively.

Postoperative Care. Despite the extensive surgical intervention necessary in many children with Wilms tumor, the recovery is usually rapid. The major nursing responsibilities are the same as those after any abdominal surgery (see Surgical Procedures, Chapter 22). Since these children are at risk for intestinal obstruction from vincristine-induced adynamic ileus, radiation-induced edema, and postsurgical adhesion formation, gastrointestinal activity, such as bowel movements, bowel sounds, distention, vomiting, and pain, are carefully monitored.

The nurse also monitors blood pressure for a possible drop after removal of the tumor, urine output to assess functioning of the remaining kidney, and signs of infection, especially during chemotherapy. Because of the myelosuppression from the drugs, pulmonary hygiene measures are instituted in the immediate postoperative period to prevent lung involvement.

Nursing ALERT Because the child is left with one kidney, certain precautions, such as avoiding contact sports, are recommended to prevent injury to the remaining organ. Prompt detection and treatment of any genitourinary signs or symptoms are mandatory.

Family Support. The postoperative period is frequently difficult for parents. The shock of seeing their child immediately after surgery may be the first realization of the seriousness of the diagnosis. It also marks the confirmation of the stage of the tumor. Again, during this period, the nurse should be with the parents to assure them of the child's recovery after surgery and to assess the parent's understanding of the operative report. They need an opportunity to express their feelings and to realize that their feelings are normal and realistic. The same emotional care discussed in Chapter 18 for families who have a child with a life-threatening disorder is applied to these individuals.

Older children need an opportunity to deal with their feelings concerning the many procedures to which they have been subjected in rapid succession. Play therapy with dolls or puppets or through drawing can be extremely beneficial in helping them adjust to the surgery and hair loss. It is not unusual for children to feel angry because they were not adequately prepared for the extent of surgery, the need for additional therapy, or the seriousness of the disorder.

RENAL FAILURE

Renal failure is the inability of the kidneys to excrete waste material, concentrate urine, and conserve electrolytes. It can occur suddenly *(acute renal failure)* in response to inadequate perfusion, kidney disease, or urinary tract obstruction, or it can develop slowly *(chronic renal failure)* as a result of longstanding kidney disease or an anomaly.

Azotemia and uremia are terms often used in relation to renal failure. *Azotemia* is the accumulation of nitrogenous waste within the blood. *Uremia* is a more advanced condition in which retention of nitrogenous products produces toxic symptoms. Azotemia is not life threatening, whereas uremia is a serious condition that often involves other body systems.

ACUTE RENAL FAILURE (ARF)

ARF is said to exist when the kidneys suddenly are unable to regulate the volume and composition of urine appropriately in response to food and fluid intake and the needs of the organism. The principal feature of ARF is oliguria* associated with azotemia, metabolic acidosis, and diverse electrolyte disturbances. ARF is not common in childhood, but the outcome depends on the cause, associated findings, and prompt recognition and treatment.

The pathologic conditions that produce ARF caused by glomerulonephritis and hemolytic-uremic syndrome have been discussed in relation to those disorders. ARF can also develop as a result of a large number of related or unrelated clinical conditions: poor renal perfusion, urinary tract obstruction, acute renal injury, or the final expression of chronic, irreversible renal disease. The most common cause in children is transient renal failure resulting from severe dehydration or other causes of poor perfusion that may respond to restoration of fluid volume.

Pathophysiology

ARF is usually reversible, but the deviations of physiologic function can be extreme, and mortality in the pediatric age-group remains high. There is severe reduction in the glomerular filtration rate, an elevated blood urea nitrogen level, and a significant reduction in renal blood flow.

The clinical course is variable and depends on the cause. In reversible ARF there is a period of severe oliguria, or a low-output phase, followed by an abrupt onset of diuresis, or a high-output phase, and then a gradual return to, or toward, normal urine volumes.

Diagnostic Evaluation

In many instances of ARF the infant or child is already critically ill with the precipitating disorder, and the explanation for development of oliguria may or may not be readily apparent (see box). When a previously well child develops ARF without obvious cause, a careful history is taken to reveal symptoms that may be related to glomerulonephritis or obstructive uropathy, or exposure to nephrotoxic chemicals, such as ingestion of heavy metals, or inhalation of carbon tetrachloride or other organic solvents or drugs known to be toxic to the kidneys. Significant laboratory measurements

---

CLINICAL MANIFESTATIONS OF ACUTE RENAL FAILURE
Specific:
Oliguria
Anuria uncommon (except in obstructive disorders)
Nonspecific (may develop):
Nausea
Vomiting
Drowsiness
Edema
Hypertension
Manifestations of underlying disorder or pathologic condition

---

during renal shutdown that serve as a guide for therapy are blood urea nitrogen, serum creatinine, pH, sodium, potassium, and calcium.

Therapeutic Management

Treatment of ARF is directed toward (1) treatment of the underlying cause, (2) management of the complications of renal failure, and (3) provision of supportive therapy within the constraints imposed by the renal failure.

Treatment of poor perfusion resulting from dehydration consists of volume restoration, as described in Chapter 24 in treatment of dehydration. If oliguria persists after restoration of fluid volume or if the renal failure is caused by intrinsic renal damage, the physiologic and biochemical abnormalities that have resulted from kidney dysfunction must be corrected or controlled. Initially a Foley catheter is inserted to rule out urine retention, to collect available urine for analysis, and to monitor results of diuretic administration. The catheter may or may not be removed during the oliguric phase.

The amount of exogenous water provided should not exceed the amount needed to maintain zero water balance. It is calculated on the basis of estimated endogenous water formation and losses from sensible (primarily gastrointestinal) and insensible sources. No allotment is calculated for urine as long as oliguria persists.

When the output begins to increase, either spontaneously or in response to diuretic therapy, the intake of fluid, potassium, and sodium must be monitored and adequate replacement provided to prevent depletion and its consequences. Some patients pass enormous amounts of electrolyte-rich urine.

Complications. The child with ARF has a tendency to develop water intoxication and hyponatremia, which make it difficult to provide calories in sufficient amounts to meet the needs of the child and reduce the tissue catabolism, metabolic acidosis, hyperkalemia, and uremia. If the child is able to tolerate oral foods, food sources high in concentrated carbohydrate and fat but low in protein, potassium, and sodium may be provided. However, many children have functional disturbances of the gastrointestinal tract, such as nausea and vomiting; therefore the intravenous route is generally preferred and usually consists of essential amino acids or a combination of essential and nonessential amino acids administered by the central venous route.

Control of water balance in these patients requires careful monitoring of feedback information, such as accurate intake and output, body weight, and electrolyte measurements. In

---

*The definition of oliguria varies extensively in the literature, from 1.8 to 4 dl/m²/24 hours.

general, during the oliguric phase, no sodium, chloride, or potassium is given unless there are other large, ongoing losses. Regular measurement of plasma electrolyte, pH, blood urea nitrogen, and creatinine levels is required to assess the adequacy of fluid therapy and to anticipate complications that require specific treatment.

Hyperkalemia is the most immediate threat to the life of the child with ARF. Hyperkalemia can be minimized and sometimes avoided by eliminating potassium from all food and fluid, by reducing tissue catabolism, and by correcting acidosis. Measures employed for the reduction of serum potassium levels are oral or rectal administration of an ion-exchange resin such as sodium polystyrene sulfonate (Kayexalate) and peritoneal dialysis or hemodialysis (see p. 978). The resin produces its effect by exchange of its sodium for the potassium, thus binding potassium for removal from the body. This increased sodium concentration may contribute to fluid overload, hypertension, and cardiac failure. Dialysis removes potassium and other waste products from the serum by diffusion through a semipermeable membrane.

> **Nursing ALERT**
> Any of the following signs of hyperkalemia constitute an emergency and are reported immediately:
> Serum potassium concentrations in excess of 7 mEq/L
> Presence of electrocardiographic abnormalities, such as prolonged QRS complex, depressed ST segment, high peaked T waves, bradycardia, or heart block

Hypertension is a frequent and serious complication of ARF, and, to detect it early, blood pressure measurements are made every 4 to 6 hours. The most common cause of hypertension in ARF is overexpansion of extracellular fluid and plasma volume together with activation of the renin-angiotensin system. Hypertension is controlled with antihypertensive drugs. Other measures that may be used include limiting fluids and salt.

Anemia is frequently associated with ARF, but transfusion is not recommended unless the hemoglobin drops below 6 g/dl. Transfusions, if used, consist of fresh, packed red blood cells given slowly to reduce the likelihood of increasing blood volume, hypertension, and hyperkalemia.

Seizures occur rather often when renal failure progresses to uremia and are also related to hypertension, hyponatremia, and hypocalcemia. Treatment is directed to the specific cause when known. More obscure causes are managed with antiepileptic drugs.

Cardiac failure with pulmonary edema is almost always associated with hypervolemia. Treatment is directed toward reduction of fluid volume, with water and sodium restriction and administration of diuretics.

Prognosis. The prognosis of ARF depends largely on the nature and severity of the causative factor or precipitating event and the promptness and competence of management. The outcome is least favorable in children with rapidly progressive nephritis and cortical necrosis. Children in whom ARF is a result of hemolytic-uremic syndrome or acute glomerulitis may recover completely, but residual renal impairment or hypertension is more often the rule. Complete recovery is usually expected in children whose renal failure is a result of dehydration, nephrotoxins, or ischemia. ARF following cardiac surgery is less favorable. It is often impossible to assess the extent of recovery for several months.

Nursing Considerations

❖ Assessment

Meticulous attention to fluid intake and output is mandatory and includes all the physical measurements discussed previously in relation to problems of fluid balance. Monitoring fluid balance and vital signs is a continuous process, and observers are constantly on the alert for signs of complications so that appropriate interventions can be implemented. Because these children require intensive observation and, often, specialized treatment, such as dialysis, they are usually admitted to an intensive care unit in which needed equipment and trained personnel are available.

> 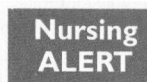 **Nursing ALERT**
> Diminished urine output and lethargy in a child who is dehydrated, in shock, or recently postoperative should be evaluated for possible acute kidney failure.

❖ Nursing Diagnoses

A number of nursing diagnoses are evident after a thorough assessment of the child with ARF (see box). Others will be noted depending on the age of the child, the cause of the renal failure, and any concomitant complications.

❖ Planning

The major goals for the child with ARF and the family are as follows:

1. Child will maintain appropriate fluid volume.
2. Child will maintain normal electrolyte levels.
3. Child will maintain blood pressure within acceptable limits.
4. Child will experience minimized risk of infection.
5. Child and family will receive adequate support.

❖ Implementation

The major nursing task in the care of the infant or child with ARF is monitoring and assessing fluid and electrolyte balance. Limiting fluid intake requires ingenuity on the part of caregivers to cope with the child who is thirsty. Rationing the daily intake in small amounts of fluid served in containers that give the impression of larger volumes is one strategy. Older children who understand the rationale of fluid limits can help determine how their daily ration should be distributed.

> **NURSING DIAGNOSES: THE CHILD WITH ACUTE RENAL FAILURE**
>
> Fluid volume excess related to failure of or compromised renal regulatory mechanisms
> High risk for injury related to accumulated electrolytes and waste products
> High risk for infection related to lowered body defenses, fluid overload
> Altered family processes related to a child with a serious disorder

Meeting nutritional needs is sometimes a problem; the
child may be nauseated, and encouraging concentrated foods
without fluids may be difficult. When nourishment is provided by the intravenous route, careful monitoring is essential to prevent fluid overload. In addition, nursing measures,
such as maintaining an optimum thermal environment, reducing any elevation of body temperature, and reducing restlessness and anxiety, are employed to decrease the rate of tissue catabolism.

The nurse must be continually alert for changes in behavior that indicate the onset of complications. Infection from
reduced resistance, anemia, and general morbidity is a constant threat. Fluid overload and electrolyte disturbances can
precipitate cardiovascular complications such as hypertension
and cardiac failure. Fluid and electrolyte imbalances, acidosis, and accumulation of nitrogenous waste products can produce neurologic involvement manifested by coma, seizures,
or alterations in sensorium (see Critical Thinking Exercise).

Although children with ARF are usually quite ill and voluntarily diminish their activity, infants may become restless
and irritable, and children are often anxious and frightened.
There are frequent, painful, and stress-producing treatments
and tests that must be performed. The presence of a supportive, empathetic nurse can provide comfort and stability in a
threatening and unnatural environment.

Family Support. Providing support and reassurance
to parents is among the major nursing responsibilities. The
seriousness and emergency nature of ARF are stressful to parents, and most feel some degree of guilt regarding the child's
condition, especially when the illness is the result of ingestion of a toxic substance, dehydration, or a genetic disease.
They need reassurance and a sympathetic listener. They also
need to be kept informed of the child's progress and provided explanations regarding the therapeutic regimen. The

equipment and the child's behavior are sometimes frightening and anxiety provoking. Nurses can do much to help parents comprehend and deal with the stresses of the situation.

❖ Evaluation

The effectiveness of nursing interventions is determined by
continual reassessment and evaluation of care based on the
following.

Observational guidelines:

1. Carry out frequent assessment of vital signs and behaviors.
2. Observe eating behaviors and energy expenditure; monitor intake
   of protein and calories; carefully monitor intake and output; weigh
   daily or more often as prescribed.
3. Monitor vital signs, sensorium, and other neurologic signs; evaluate laboratory results and observe for signs of electrolyte imbalance.
4. Observe and interview child and family regarding their understanding of the disease and therapies; encourage child and family
   to express their feelings and concerns.

Expected outcomes:

1. Alterations in vital signs and behavior are detected.
2. Child consumes a sufficient amount of appropriate nutrients without evidence of fluid gain or waste product accumulation.
3. Child exhibits no evidence of infection.
4. Evidence of complications is detected early, and appropriate interventions are implemented.
5. Child and family express their feelings and concerns and demonstrate their understanding of the condition and the therapies
   (specify knowledge and method of demonstration).

See also Nursing Care Plan: The Child with Acute Renal
Failure.*

CHRONIC RENAL FAILURE (CRF)

The kidneys are able to maintain the chemical composition
of fluids within normal limits until more than 50% of functional renal capacity is destroyed by disease or injury. Chronic
renal insufficiency or failure begins when the diseased kidneys can no longer maintain the normal chemical structure
of body fluids under normal conditions. Progressive deterioration over months or years produces a variety of clinical and
biochemical disturbances that eventually culminate in the
clinical syndrome known as *uremia.*

A variety of diseases and disorders can result in CRF. The
most frequent causes are congenital renal and urinary tract
malformations, vesicoureteral reflux associated with recurrent
urinary tract infection, chronic pyelonephritis, hereditary disorders, chronic glomerulonephritis, and glomerulonephropa-
thy associated with systemic diseases such as anaphylactoid
purpura and lupus erythematosus.

Pathophysiology

Early in the course of progressive nephrotic destruction, the
child remains asymptomatic with only minimal biochemical
abnormalities. Unless the presence of CRF is detected in the
process of routine assessment, signs and symptoms that indicate advanced renal damage frequently emerge only late in
the course of the disease. Midway in the disease process, as
increasing numbers of nephrons are totally destroyed and

---

*In Wong DL: *Wong and Whaley's Clinical manual of pediatric nursing,* ed
4, St Louis, 1996, Mosby.

most others are damaged to varying degrees, the few that remain intact are hypertrophied but functional. These few normal nephrons are able to make sufficient adjustments to stresses to maintain reasonable degrees of fluid and electrolyte balance. Definitive biochemical examination at this time will reveal restricted tolerance to excesses or restrictions. As the disease progresses to the end stage, because of a severe reduction in the number of functioning nephrons, the kidneys are no longer able to maintain fluid and electrolyte balance, and the features of uremic syndrome appear.

The accumulation of various biochemical substances in the blood, those that result from diminished renal function, produces complications such as the following:

> *Retention of waste products,* especially the blood urea nitrogen and creatinine
> *Water and sodium retention,* which contributes to edema and vascular congestion
> *Hyperkalemia* of dangerous levels
> *Metabolic acidosis* of a sustained nature because of continual hydrogen ion retention and bicarbonate loss
> *Calcium and phosphorus disturbances,* resulting in altered bone metabolism, which in turn causes growth arrest or retardation, bone pain, and deformities known as *renal osteodystrophy*
> *Anemia* caused by hematologic dysfunction, including shortened life span of red blood cells, impaired red blood cell production related to decreased production of erythropoietin, prolonged bleeding time, and nutritional anemia
> *Growth disturbance,* probably caused by such factors as renal osteodystrophy, poor nutrition associated with dietary restrictions and loss of appetite, and biochemical abnormalities

Children with CRF seem to be more susceptible to infection, especially pneumonia, urinary tract infection, and septicemia, although the reason for this is unclear. These children become extraordinarily sensitive to changes in vascular volume that may cause pulmonary overload, central nervous system symptoms, hypertension, and cardiac failure.

Diagnostic Evaluation

The diagnosis of CRF is usually suspected on the basis of any number of clinical manifestations, a history of prior renal disease, and/or biochemical findings. The onset is usually gradual, and the initial signs and symptoms are vague and nonspecific (see box).

Laboratory and other diagnostic tools and tests are of value in assessing the extent of renal damage, biochemical disturbances, and related physical dysfunction (see Tables 27-1, 27-2, and 27-3). Often they can help establish the nature of the underlying disease and differentiate between other disease processes and the pathologic consequences of renal dysfunction.

Therapeutic Management

In irreversible renal failure the goals of medical management are (1) to promote maximal renal function, (2) to maintain body fluid and electrolyte balance within safe biochemical limits, (3) to treat systemic complications, and (4) to promote as active and normal a life as possible for the child for as long as possible. The child is allowed unrestricted activity and is allowed to set his or her own limits regarding rest and extent of exertion. School attendance is encouraged as long as the child is able. When the effort is too great, home tutoring is arranged.

Diet regulation is the most effective means, short of dialysis, for reducing the quantity of materials that require renal excretion. The goal of the diet in renal failure is to provide sufficient calories and protein for growth while limiting the excretory demands made on the kidney, to minimize metabolic bone disease *(osteodystrophy),* and to minimize fluid and electrolyte disturbances. Dietary protein intake is limited only to the recommended daily allowance (RDA) for the child's age. Restriction of protein intake below the RDA is believed to impact growth and neurodevelopment negatively (Raymond and others 1990).

Sodium and water are not usually limited unless there is evidence of edema or hypertension, and potassium is not usually restricted. However, restrictions of any or all three may be imposed in later stages or at any time that abnormal serum concentrations are evident.

CLINICAL MANIFESTATIONS OF CHRONIC RENAL FAILURE

Early signs:
  Loss of normal energy
  Increased fatigue on exertion
  Pallor, subtle (may not be noticed)
  Elevated blood pressure (sometimes)
As the disease progresses:
  Decreased appetite (especially at breakfast)
  Less interest in normal activities
  Increased or decreased urine output with compensatory intake of fluid
  Pallor more evident
  Sallow, muddy appearance of skin
Child may complain of:
  Headache
  Muscle cramps
  Nausea
Other signs and symptoms:
  Weight loss
  Facial edema
  Malaise
  Bone or joint pain
  Growth retardation
  Dryness or itching of the skin
  Bruised skin
  Sensory or motor loss (sometimes)
  Amenorrhea (common in adolescent girls)
Uremic syndrome (untreated):
  Gastrointestinal symptoms
    Anorexia
    Nausea and vomiting
  Bleeding tendencies
    Bruises
    Bloody diarrheal stools
    Stomatitis
    Bleeding from lips and mouth
  Intractable itching
  Uremic frost (deposits of urea crystals on skin)
  Unpleasant "uremic" breath odor
  Deep respirations
  Hypertension
  Congestive heart failure
  Pulmonary edema
  Neurologic involvement
    Progressive confusion
    Dulled sensorium
    Coma (ultimately)
    Tremors
    Muscular twitching
    Seizures

Dietary phosphorus is controlled to prevent or correct the calcium/phosphorus imbalance by the reduction of protein and milk intake. Phosphorus levels can be further reduced by oral administration of calcium carbonate preparations that combine with the phosphorus to decrease gastrointestinal absorption and thus the serum levels of phosphate. At the same time serum calcium levels are increased from the calcium carbonate, vitamin D therapy is begun to increase calcium absorption.

Metabolic acidosis is alleviated through administration of alkalizing agents such as sodium bicarbonate or a combination of sodium and potassium citrate.

Growth failure is one major consequence of CRF, especially in the preadolescent. These children grow poorly both before and after the initiation of hemodialysis. The use of recombinant human growth hormone to accelerate growth in children with growth retardation secondary to CRF has been successful (Hokken-Koelega and others, 1994). *Osseous deformities* that result from renal osteodystrophy, especially those related to ambulation, are troublesome and require correction if they occur. *Dental defects* are common in children with CRF, and the earlier the onset of the disease, the more severe are the dental manifestations (including hypoplasia, hypomineralization, tooth discolorization, alteration in size and shape of teeth, malocclusion, and ulcerative stomatitis). Therefore regular dental care is especially important in these children.

Anemia in children with CRF is related to decreased production of erythropoietin. Recombinant human erythropoietin (rHuEPO) is being offered to these children as thrice-weekly or weekly subcutaneous injections and is replacing the need for frequent blood transfusions. The drug corrects the anemia and in turn increases appetite, activity, and general well-being in the children who receive it.

Hypertension of advanced renal disease may be managed initially by cautious use of a low-sodium diet, fluid restriction, and perhaps diuretics, such as hydrochlorothiazide or furosemide. Severe hypertension requires the use of antihypertensive agents, singly or in combinations.

Intercurrent infections are treated with appropriate antimicrobials at the first sign of infection; however, any drug eliminated through the kidneys is administered with caution. Other complications are treated symptomatically (e.g., central-acting antiemetics for *nausea,* antiepileptics for *seizures,* and diphenhydramine [Benadryl] for *pruritus*).

Once evidence of *end-stage renal disease (ESRD)* appears in a child, the disease runs its relentless course and results in death in a few weeks, unless waste products and toxins are removed from body fluids by dialysis and/or kidney transplantation. Since these techniques have been adapted for infants and small children, these alternatives have been implemented in most cases of renal failure once conservative management is no longer effective (see p. 978).

Prognosis.   Dialysis and transplantation are the only treatments currently available for children with ESRD. Although children may survive on dialysis, it is not an ideal long-term modality. Complications include infection of access sites, growth failure, and disruption of normal socialization. Many pediatric centers encourage families of children with ESRD to consider renal transplantation. The overall graft survival rate for kidneys from living related donors is 89% at 1 year and 80% at 3 years. For cadaver kidneys the graft survival rate is 74% at 1 year and 62% at 3 years (McEnery and others, 1992). Posttransplant complications include infection, hypertension, steroid toxicity, hyperlipidemia, aseptic necrosis, malignancy, and growth retardation (Suthanthiran and Strom, 1994). Long-term graft survival is not guaranteed, and many children require a second or third transplant. Successful renal transplantation does improve rehabilitation of children with CRF, both educationally and psychologically. Increasing use of primary or preemptive renal transplants without a prior course of dialysis is being recommended in many pediatric centers (Fine, Tejani, and Sullivan, 1994).

Nursing Considerations

❖ Assessment

Assessment of the child with CRF is primarily one of observation for signs of complications and evidence of improvement through therapy. Some of the first changes observed are growth failure, developmental delay, bone disease, and hypertension.

❖ Nursing Diagnoses

A number of nursing diagnoses become evident on assessment of the child. The most relevant in the majority of cases are outlined in the Nursing Care Plan on pp. 976-977. Others will be appropriate for individual children and their families.

❖ Planning

The goals of care for the child with CRF, especially one in ESRD, and family are as follows:

1. The child will receive encouragement in his or her normal growth and development, minimizing the impact of the disease process.
2. The child will remain free of complications.
3. The child and family will receive appropriate support, guidance, and education.

❖ Implementation

The multiple complications of ESRD are managed according to medical protocols prescribed for the care of those specific problems. However, progressive disease places a number of stresses on the child and family, including those of a potentially fatal illness (see Chapter 18). There is a continuing need for repeated examinations that often entail painful procedures, side effects, and frequent hospitalizations. Diet therapy becomes progressively more restricted and intense, and the child is required to take a variety of medications. Ever present in all aspects of the treatment regimen is the agonizing realization that without treatment, death is inevitable.

Some specific stresses related to ESRD and its treatment are predictable. When it first becomes apparent that ESRD is inevitable, both parents and child experience depression and anxiety. Acceptance is particularly difficult if renal failure progresses rapidly after diagnosis. Denial and disbelief are usually pronounced, especially among the parents. Once the kidney failure is established and symptoms become progressively more distressing, the initiation of hemodialysis is usually perceived as a positive experience, and after experiencing initial concerns regarding the treatment, the child begins to feel better and parental anxiety is relieved for a time.

Initiating a hemodialysis regimen is a traumatic and anxiety-provoking experience for most children, since it in-

NURSING CARE PLAN
The Child with Chronic Renal Failure (CRF)

NURSING DIAGNOSIS: High risk for injury related to accumulated electrolytes and waste products

PATIENT GOAL 1: Will maintain near-normal electrolyte levels

- **NURSING INTERVENTIONS/*RATIONALES***

*Assist with dialysis *to maintain excretory function*
*Administer Kayexalate as prescribed *to reduce serum potassium levels*
Provide diet low in protein, potassium, sodium, and phosphorus, if prescribed, *to reduce excretory demand on kidneys*
Observe for evidence of accumulated waste products (hyperkalemia, hyperphosphatemia, uremia) *to ensure prompt treatment*

- **EXPECTED OUTCOME**

Child exhibits no evidence of waste product accumulation

NURSING DIAGNOSIS: Fluid volume excess related to failure of renal regulatory mechanisms

PATIENT GOAL 1: Will maintain appropriate fluid volume

- **NURSING INTERVENTIONS/*RATIONALES***

*Assist with dialysis *to maintain excretory function*
Monitor progress *to assess adequacy of therapy and detect possible complications*

- **EXPECTED OUTCOME**

Child exhibits no evidence or complications of accumulated fluid between dialysis sessions

PATIENT GOAL 2: Will maintain appropriate fluid volume through regulation of fluid intake

- **NURSING INTERVENTIONS/*RATIONALES***

*Administer oral fluids as prescribed
Employ strategies to prevent undesirable intake
 Review daily fluid restrictions with parents and child *to encourage cooperation*
 Suggest ways to divide total volume of fluid into small quantities to be spread over entire day
 Keep mouth moist by other means, such as hard candy, ice chips, fine mist spray of cool water *to prevent feeling of dryness*

- **EXPECTED OUTCOME**

Child exhibits no evidence of fluid gain

NURSING DIAGNOSIS: Altered nutrition related to restricted diet

PATIENT GOAL 1: Will consume appropriate diet

- **NURSING INTERVENTIONS/*RATIONALES***

Provide dietary instructions for foods *that reduce excretory demands on kidney and provide sufficient calories and protein for growth*
 *Limit protein, phosphorus, salt, and potassium as prescribed
 Encourage intake of carbohydrates, *to provide calories for growth,* and foods high in calcium, *to prevent bone demineralization*
 Recommend foods that are rich in folic acid and iron *because anemia is a complication of CRF*
 Arrange for renal dietitian to meet with family to review allowable foods and assist in dietary planning *so that family understands dietary needs of child*
Help hemodialysis patients to fill out menu requests for meals (to be eaten while on dialysis)

- **EXPECTED OUTCOMES**

Child consumes an adequate amount of appropriate foods
Child shows no evidence of deficiencies or weight loss

NURSING DIAGNOSIS: Body image disturbance related to chronic illness, impaired growth, and perception of being "different"

PATIENT GOAL 1: Will develop positive self-esteem and understanding of disease

- **NURSING INTERVENTIONS/*RATIONALES***

Provide education about CRF, including management, treatment, and long-term outcome
Encourage child's independence with care and management of CRF, *since independence helps child develop positive self-esteem*
 Allow child to participate in dialysis procedures
 Allow child to participate in making decisions when appropriate
Promote self-esteem in child with CRF
 Organize patient support group or suggest counseling as needed
 Provide positive reinforcement during dialysis procedures and follow-up visits

- **EXPECTED OUTCOMES**

Child demonstrates an understanding of CRF and complies with therapies
Child exhibits signs of positive self-esteem

---

*Dependent nursing action.

NURSING CARE PLAN
The Child with Chronic Renal Failure (CRF)—cont'd

NURSING DIAGNOSIS: Altered family processes related to a child with a chronic disease

PATIENT (FAMILY) GOAL I: Will exhibit positive coping behaviors

- **NURSING INTERVENTIONS/RATIONALES**

Assist parents in diet planning and support their efforts to adjust diet to meet needs of all family members

Provide anticipatory guidance regarding probable and expected events, such as symptoms, diet, and effects of medications

Assist parents in decision making regarding dialysis and transplantation, *since these are the alternatives once palliative care is no longer effective*

Prepare child and family for hemodialysis and/or kidney transplantation *because preparation is essential for positive coping*

Prepare child and family for home hemodialysis or continuous home peritoneal dialysis

Maintain periodic contact with family *for ongoing support*

Refer family to special agencies and support groups *for long-term support*

- **EXPECTED OUTCOME**

Child and family demonstrate ability to cope with stresses of illness (specify)

See also:
Nursing Care Plan: The Child with a Chronic Illness or Disability, Chapter 18
Nursing Care Plan: The Child in the Hospital, Chapter 21
Nursing Care Plan: The Family of the Ill or Hospitalized Child, Chapter 21

---

volves surgery for implantation of a graft, fistula, or peritoneal catheter. The initial experience with the hemodialysis procedure is frightening to most children. They need reassurance about the nature of the preparations for hemodialysis and the conduct of the treatment.

Both the graft and the fistula require needle insertions at each dialysis. The goal is to perform pain-free venipuncture. Using buffered lidocaine or one of the more rapid-onset novacaines (e.g., procaine) with a small-gauge needle (30 gauge) to anesthetize the area before venipuncture of the graft/fistula is one method. Using an anesthetizing topical preparation such as EMLA (eutetic mixture of local anesthetics [lidocaine and prilocaine]) 1 hour before venipuncture is another approach (see Pain Management Chapter 21).

External dual-lumen venous access devices eliminate the need for needles but are more prone to infection and other central line complications.

Adolescents, with their increased need for independence and their urge for rebellion, usually adapt less well. They resent the control and enforced dependence imposed by the rigorous and unrelenting therapy program. They resent being dependent on hemodialysis technology, their parents, and the professional staff. Depression and/or hostility are common in adolescents undergoing hemodialysis.

The availability of home dialysis has offered a greater degree of freedom for persons undergoing long-term dialysis. The nurse is responsible for teaching the family about (1) the disease, its implications, and the therapeutic plan; (2) the possible psychologic effects of the disease and the treatment; and (3) the technical aspects of the procedure. The family learns to manage the various aspects of the dialysis procedure, how to maintain accurate records, and how to observe for signs of complications that need to be reported to the proper persons.

Body changes related to the disease process, such as skin color, growth retardation, and lack of sexual maturation, are stress provoking. Dietary restrictions are particularly burdensome for both children and parents. Children feel deprived when they are unable to eat foods previously enjoyed and that are unrestricted for other family members. Consequently, failure to cooperate may occur. Diet restrictions may be interpreted as punishment. Some children, unable to understand fully the purpose of restrictions, will sneak forbidden food items at every opportunity. Allowing children, especially adolescents, maximum participation in and responsibility for their own treatment program is helpful.

After months or years of dialysis, the parents and child feel anxiety associated with the prognosis and continued pressures of the treatment. The relentless need for treatment interferes with family plans. The time spent in transportation to and from the dialysis unit and the time spent undergoing dialysis treatments cut into time for outside activities, including school. Graft and fistula problems, as well as peritoneal catheter exit site infections, may develop and present a common source of aggravation (see Family Focus box on p. 978).

The possibility of renal transplantation often provides hope for relief from the rigors of hemodialysis and peritoneal dialysis. Most children and families respond well to a kidney transplant, and most children can be successfully rehabilitated.

The **National Kidney Foundation*** and other agencies provide a number of services and information for families of children with renal disease.

---

*30 E. 33rd St., New York, NY 10016; (212) 889-2210 or (800) 622-9010. In Canada: the **Kidney Foundation of Canada,** 5160 Boulevard Decarie, Bureau 780, Montreal, Quebec H3X 2H9; (514) 369-4806.

❖ Evaluation

The effectiveness of nursing interventions is determined by continual reassessment and evaluation of care based on the following observational guidelines and expected outcomes:

1. Observe and interview family regarding their compliance with the medical and dietary regimen.
2. Monitor vital signs, growth measurements, laboratory reports, behavior, and appearance.
3. Observe and interview child and family regarding their feelings, concerns, and fears; observe reactions to therapies and prognosis.

Expected outcomes:
See Nursing Care Plan, pp. 976-977.

TECHNOLOGIC MANAGEMENT OF RENAL FAILURE

DIALYSIS

Dialysis is the process of separating colloids and crystalline substances in solution by the difference in their rate of diffusion through a semipermeable membrane. Methods of dialysis currently available for clinical management of renal failure are *peritoneal dialysis,* wherein the abdominal cavity acts as a semipermeable membrane through which water and solutes of small molecular size move by osmosis and diffusion according to their respective concentrations on either side of the membrane, and *hemodialysis,* in which blood is circulated outside the body through artificial membranes that permit a similar passage of water and solutes. A third type of dialysis is *hemofiltration,* in which blood filtrate is circulated outside the body by hydrostatic pressure exerted across a semipermeable membrane with simultaneous infusion of a replacement solution. Types of hemofiltration include *continuous arteriovenous hemofiltration (CAVH), continuous arteriovenous hemodialysis (CAVHD)* and *continuous venovenous hemofiltration (CVVH).* CAVH, CAVHD, and CVVH are used primarily in acute conditions, such as to remove fluid overload, rather than in ESRD.

Peritoneal dialysis is the preferred form of dialysis for children/parents who wish to remain independent, families who live a long distance from the medical center, and children who prefer fewer dietary restrictions and a gentler form of dialysis. Chronic peritoneal dialysis is most often performed at home. The two types of peritoneal dialysis are *continuous ambulatory peritoneal dialysis (CAPD)* and *continuous cycling peritoneal dialysis (CCPD).* In both methods, commercially available sterile dialysate is instilled into the peritoneal cavity through a surgically implanted indwelling catheter tunneled subcutaneously and sutured into place. The warmed solution is allowed to enter the peritoneal cavity by gravity and remains a variable length of time according to the procedure used. The care and management of the procedure are the responsibility of the parents of young children. Use of home health nurses to give parents respite from care has been initiated in some centers (Cascio and others, 1994). Older children and adolescents can carry out the procedure themselves, which provides them with some control and less dependency. This is especially important for adolescents.

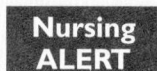

Nursing ALERT   Observe for changes in the color of the dialysate draining from the child. The solution should be straw color. If the color is pink, bright yellow, or brown, or if the solution is cloudy, notify the practitioner immediately.

Hemodialysis requires the creation of a vascular access and the use of special dialysis equipment—the hemodialyzer, or so-called artificial kidney. Vascular access may be one of three types: fistulas, grafts, or external vascular access devices. An *atriovenous fistula* is an access in which a vein and artery are connected surgically. The preferred site is the radial artery and a forearm vein. An alternative is the creation of a subcutaneous (internal) *arteriovenous graft* by anastomosing a segment of a saphenous vein autograft or a bovine arterial xenograft to the brachial artery and brachiocephalic vein, which produces dilation and thickening of the superficial vessels of the forearm to provide easy access for repeated venipuncture. Both the graft and the fistula require needle insertions at each dialysis.

For external vascular access devices, percutaneous catheters are inserted in the femoral, subclavian, or internal jugular veins, even in very small children. A more permanent form of external access is available via a central catheter inserted surgically into the subclavian vein or internal jugular vein. This catheter has a dual lumen, which allows differentiation between arterial and venous blood. Catheters eliminate the need for skin punctures but require some home care.*

Hemodialysis is best suited to children who do not have someone in the family who is capable of learning to perform home dialysis and to those who live close to a dialysis center. The procedure is usually performed three times a week for 4 to 6 hours, depending on the size of the child. Hemodialysis achieves rapid correction of fluid and electrolyte abnormalities but can cause problems in association with this rapid change, such as muscle cramping and hypotension. Disadvantages include school absence during dialysis and strict fluid and dietary restrictions between dialysis sessions. Boredom for the child and family is often a problem during dialysis,

---

*Home care instructions on central venous catheters are available in Wong DL: *Wong and Whaley's Clinical manual of pediatric nursing,* ed 4, St Louis, 1996, Mosby.

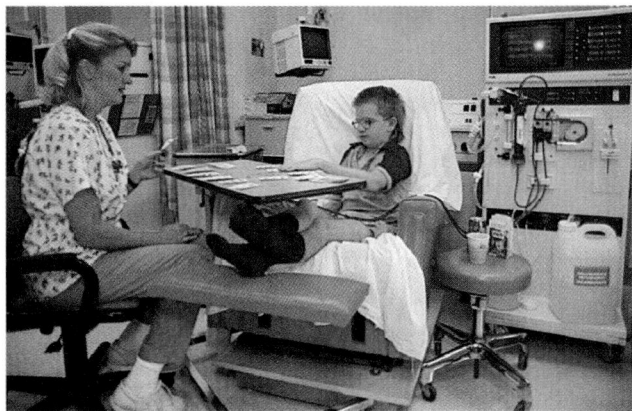

FIG. 27-4. Diversional activities help lessen the boredom children can experience during hemodialysis.

and planned quiet activities should be introduced (Fig. 27-4).

Most children show rapid clinical improvement with the implementation of dialysis, although it is directly related to the duration of uremia before dialysis and the extent to which dietary regulations are followed. Growth rate and skeletal maturation improve, but recovery of normal growth occurs infrequently. In many cases, sexual development, although delayed, progresses to completion.

TRANSPLANTATION

Renal transplantation is now an acceptable and effective means of therapy in the pediatric age-group. Although peritoneal dialysis and hemodialysis are life-preserving, both require major alterations in life-style. Transplantation offers the opportunity for a relatively normal life and is the preferred form of treatment for children with CRF. Primary or preemptive transplants maintain the greatest amount of normalcy in the family's life.

Kidneys for transplant are available from two sources: a *living related donor (LRD),* usually a parent or a sibling, or a *cadaver donor (CAD),* wherein the family of a dead or brain-dead patient consents to donation of a healthy kidney. The criteria for selection of kidney recipients are quite liberal, with no limit regarding age. Retransplantation occurs frequently.

The primary goal in transplantation is the long-term survival of grafted tissue by securing tissue that is antigenically similar to that of the recipient and by suppressing the recipient's immune mechanism. The immunosuppressant therapy of choice has been corticosteroids (Prednisone) in conjunction with cyclosporine and azathioprine. Other therapies include antilymphoblast globulin or monoclonal antibodies. New immunosuppressant medications are rapidly coming into clinical trials and into use in large transplant centers. It is important for the nurse to learn about the medications and their side effects used in the antirejection protocol(s). Since the immunosuppressant medications are taken indefinitely, transplant patients experience many side effects of the drugs, including hypertension, growth retardation, cataracts, risk of infection, obesity, characteristics of Cushing syndrome, and hirsutism.

Rejection of the transplanted kidney is the most common cause of transplant failure. Rejection is treated aggressively with immunosuppressant medications and can often be reversed. Some patients do not respond to treatment of acute rejection or develop chronic rejection and must eventually return to dialysis or undergo another kidney transplant.

Nursing ALERT The child with a recent kidney transplant (a few days) or one who was grafted approximately 6 months previously who exhibits any of the following should be evaluated immediately for possible rejection:

Fever
Swelling and tenderness over graft area
Diminished urine output
Elevated blood pressure

KEY POINTS

- Common inflammatory disorders of the genitourinary tract include urinary tract infection, nephrotic syndrome, and acute glomerulonephritis.
- Management of urinary tract infections is directed at eliminating infection, detecting and correcting functional or anatomic abnormalities, preventing recurrences, and preserving renal function.
- Vesicoureteral reflux is the retrograde flow of bladder urine into the ureters.
- Obstructive uropathy is a result of structural or functional abnormalities of the urinary system that obstruct the normal flow of urine.
- The more common defects of the genitourinary tract include phimosis, cryptorchidism, inguinal hernia, hydrocele, and hypospadias.

- Body image concerns and castration anxiety are particularly intense in children with defects in the genital area.
- Nephrotic syndrome is characterized by increased glomerular permeability to protein, with massive urinary loss of protein resulting in hypoproteinemia and edema.
- Management of nephrotic syndrome is aimed at reducing excretion of protein, reducing or preventing fluid retention by tissues, and preventing infection and other complications.
- Common features of acute glomerulonephritis are oliguria, edema, hypertension, circulatory congestion, hematuria, and proteinuria.

- Therapeutic management of acute glomerulonephritis is maintenance of fluid balance, treatment of hypertension, and antibiotic therapy.
- Management of hemolytic-uremic syndrome is aimed at control of complications and hematologic manifestations of renal failure.
- Wilms tumor is the most common malignant neoplasm of the kidney in infants and children.
- In acute renal failure, management is directed at determining treatment of the underlying cause, management of complications of renal failure, and supportive therapy.
- Abnormalities in chronic renal failure are waste product retention, water and sodium retention, hyperkalemia, acidosis, calcium and phosphorus disturbance, anemia, and growth disturbances.
- The types of dialysis used in end-stage renal disease (ESRD) are peritoneal dialysis and hemodialysis.
- When the child will need home dialysis, the nurse educates the family on the disease, its implications, the therapeutic plan, possible psychologic effects of the disease, and the treatment and technical aspects of the procedure.
- The major concerns in renal transplantation are tissue matching and prevention of rejection; psychologic concerns involve self-image as related to possible body changes as a result of the effects of corticosteroid therapy.

REFERENCES

Brandt JR and others: More on *E. coli*-induced hemolytic-uremic syndrome, *J Pediatr* 125(4):519-526, 1994.

Cascio C and others: Use of private duty nurses for daily CCPD and family relief in pediatric PD patients, *Adv Perit Dial* 10:304-306, 1994.

Craig JC and others: Effect of circumcision on incidence of urinary tract infection in preschool boys, *J Pediatr* 128(1):23-27, 1996.

Fine RN, Tejani A, Sullivan EK: Pre-emptive renal transplantation in children: report of the North American Pediatric Renal Transplant Cooperative Study, *Clin Transplant* 8(5):474-478, 1994.

Fleiss PM: Explanation for false-positive urine cultures obtained by bag technique, *Arch Pediatr Adolesc Med* 149(9):1041-1042, 1995.

Green DM and others: Wilms tumor, *CA Cancer J Clin* 46:46-63, 1996.

Hokken-Koelega ACS and others: Growth hormone treatment in growth-retarded adolescents after renal transplant, *Lancet* 343:1313-1317, 1994.

McEnery PT and others: Renal transplantation in children, *N Engl J Med* 326(26):1727-1732, 1992.

Raymond NG and others: An approach to protein restriction in children with renal insufficiency, *Pediatr Nephrol* 4:145-148, 1990.

Suthanthiran M, Strom TB: Renal transplantation, *N Engl J Med* 331(6):365-376, 1994.

Wiswell TE, Hachey W: Urinary tract infections and the uncircumcised state: an update, *Clin Pediatr* 32(4):130-134, 1993.

BIBLIOGRAPHY

General

Collecting a 24-hour urine sample, *Patient Care* 24(17):99, 1990.

Gibbs T: Genitourinary embryology and congenital malformations: the kidneys and ureters. Part I, *Urol Nurs* 10(3):16-24, 1990.

Gillenwater JY and others, editors: *Adult and pediatric urology*, vol 3, ed 3, St Louis, 1969, Mosby.

Gray ML: *Genitourinary disorders*, St Louis, 1992, Mosby.

Jacobson H, Striker GE, Klahr S, editors: *The principles and practice of nephrology*, ed 2, St Louis, 1995, Mosby.

Kaplan WE: Summary of the urologic section, *Pediatrics* 93(5):845-849, 1994.

Kelalis PP, King LR, Belman AB, editors: *Clinical pediatric urology*, Philadelphia, 1992, Saunders.

Kenner C, Brueggemeyer A: Assessment and management of genitourinary dysfunction. In Kenner C and others: *Comprehensive neonatal nursing: a physiologic perspective*, Philadelphia, 1993, Saunders.

McCance KL, Huether SE: *Pathophysiology: the biologic basis for diseases in adults and children*, St Louis, 1994, Mosby.

Perelstein EM: Renal tubular acidosis, *Int Pediatr* 8(3):326-333, 1993.

Raymond NG and others: An approach to protein restriction in children with renal insufficiency, *Pediatr Nephrol* 4:145-148, 1990.

Rowe PC and others: Epidemiology of hemolytic-uremic syndrome in Canadian children from 1986-1988, *J Pediatr* 119(2):218-224, 1994.

Tanagho EA: Anatomy of the genitourinary tract. In Tanagho EA, McAnnich JW, editors: *Smith's general urology*, Los Altos, CA, 1992, Lange.

Urinary Tract Infection/Reflux

Andrich MP, Majd M: Diagnostic imaging in the evaluation of the first urinary tract infection in infants and young children, *Pediatrics* 90(3):436-441, 1992.

Avorn J and others: Reduction of bacteriuria and pyuria after ingestion of cranberry juice, *JAMA* 271(10):751-754, 1994.

Brindle M: Urinary tract infection in children, *Br Med J* 309(6954):609, 1994.

Burns M: Pediatric urinary tract infection: diagnosis, classification and significance, *Pediatr Clin North Am* 34:1111-1120, 1988.

Cepero-Akselrad A, Ramirez-Seijas F, Castaneda A: Urinary tract infection in children, *Int Pediatr* 8(3):314-325, 1993.

Conway JJ, Cohn RA: Evolving role of nuclear medicine for the diagnosis and management of urinary tract infection, *J Pediatr* 124(1):87-90, 1994.

Dick PT, Feldman W: Routine diagnostic imaging for childhood urinary tract infections: a systemic overview, *J Pediatr* 128(1):15-22, 1996.

Edelmann CM Jr: Urinary tract infection and vesicoureteral reflux, *Pediatr Ann* 17:568-582, 1988.

Fussell EN and others: Adherence of bacteria to human foreskins, *J Urol* 140:997-1001, 1988.

Heldrich FJ: UTI diagnosis: getting it right the first time, *Contemp Pediatr* 12(2):110-133, 1995.

Kramer SA: Vesicoureteral reflux. In Kelalis PP, King LR, Belman AB, editors: *Clin pediatric urology*, Philadelphia, 1992, Saunders.

Rosenfeld DL and others: Current recommendations for children with urinary tract infections, *Clin Pediatr* 261-264, 1995.

Schlager TA and others: Explanation for false-positive urine cultures obtained by bag technique, *Arch Pediatr Adolsc Med* 149:170-173, 1995.

Todd JK: Management of urinary tract infections: children are different, *Pediatr Rev* 16(5):190-196, 1995.

When to rely on the urine dipstick in children, *Emerg Med* 24(2):224-225, 1992.

Winberg J: What hygiene measures are advisable to prevent recurrent urinary tract infection and what evidence is there to support this advice? *Pediatr Nephrol* 8(6):652, 1994.

Wiswell TE, Geschke DW: Risks from circumcision during the first month of life compared with those for uncircumcised boys, *Pediatrics* 83:1011-1015, 1989.

Structural Defects of the Urinary Tract

Castiglia PT: Ambiguous genitalia, *J Pediatr Health Care* 3(6):319-321, 1989.

Forest-Lalande L: Teaching nonsterile intermittent catheterization in a pediatric setting, *CAET J* 9(6):7-10, 1990.

Horton H and others: Hypospadias: when baby boys need surgery, *RN* 53(6):48-52, 1990.

Rajput A, Gauderer MWL, Hack M: Inguinal hernias in very low birth weight infants: incidence and timing of repair, *J Pediatr Surg* 27(10):1322-1324, 1992.

Skinner M, Grosfeld J: Inguinal and umbilical hernia repair in infants and children, *Surg Clin North Am* 73(3):439-449, 1993.

Smoyer WE: Urinary tract obstruction in children, *Clin Pediatr* 31(2):109-119, 1992.

Steele BT, De Maria J: A new perspective on the natural history of vesicoureteric reflux, *Pediatrics* 90(1):30-32, 1992.

Stylianos L, Jacir NN, Harris BH: Incarceration of inguinal hernia in infants prior to elective repair, *J Pediatr Surg* 28(4):582-583, 1993.

Van Gool JD and others: Historical clues to the complex of dysfunctional voiding, urinary tract infection and vesicorureteral reflux, *J Urol* 148:1699-1702, 1992.

Renal Diseases and Tumors

Andrews PE, Kelalis PP, Haase GM: Extrarenal Wilms' tumor: results of the National Wilms' Tumor Study, *J Pediatr Surg* 27(9):1181-1184, 1992.

Brodeur FA, Brodeur GM: Abdominal masses in children; neuroblastoma, Wilms Tumor and other considerations, *Pediatr Rev* 12(7):196-207, 1991.

Canpolat C, Pearson P, Jaffe N: Cisplatin-associated hemolytic uremic syndrome, *Cancer,* 74(11):3059-3062, 1994.

D'Angio G and others: Wilms' tumor: status report, *J Clin Oncol* 9:877-887, 1991.

Haws RM, Baum M: Efficacy of albumin and diuretic therapy in children with nephrotic syndrome, *Pediatrics* 91(6):1142-1146, 1993.

Kelsch RC, Sedman AB: Nephrotic syndrome, *Pediatr Rev* 14(1):30-38, 1993.

Klee KM, AcAfee N, Greefleaf K: Pediatric case study: hemolytic uremic syndrome, *ANNA J* 20(4):505-506, 1993.

Ruccione KS: Wilms' tumor: a paradigm, a parallel and a puzzle, *Semin Oncol Nurs* 8(4):241-251, 1992.

Sakarcan A, Timmons C, Seikaly MG: Reversible idiopathic acute renal failure in children with primary nephrotic syndrome, *J Pediatr* 125(5):723-727, 1994.

Renal Failure

Doolittle RF: Biotechnology—the enormous cost of success, *N Engl J Med* 324(19):1360-1362, 1991.

Frauman A and others: Care of the family of the child with end stage renal disease, *ANNA J* 17(5):383-396, 1990.

Kling PJ and others: Pharmacogenetics and pharmacodynamics of erythropoietin during therapy in an infant with renal failure, *J Pediatr* 121(5):822-825, 1992.

Obrecht JA, Gallo AM, Knafl KA: A case of illustration of family management style in childhood end stage renal disease, *ANNA J* 19(3):255-260, 1992.

Dialysis/Transplantation

Alexander SR, Honda M: Continuous peritoneal dialysis for children: a decade of worldwide growth and development, *Kidney Int Suppl* 40:S65-S74, 1993.

Avner ED and others: Renal transplantation and chronic dialysis in children and adolescents: the 1993 annual report of the North American Pediatric Renal Transplant Cooperative Study, *Pediatr Nephrol* 9(1):61-73, 1995.

Bunchman TE and others: Continuous venovenous hemodiafiltration in infants and children, *Am J Kidney Dis* 25(1):17-21, 1995.

Cohen B and others: Children's compliance to dialysis, *Pediatr Nurs* 17(4):359-365, 420, 1991.

Currier H: Ethical issues in the neonatal patient with end-stage renal disease, *J Perinat Neonat Nurs* 8(1):74-78, 1994.

Doyle CL, Flanigan MJ, Mabe C: Tidal peritoneal dialysis vs continuous cyclic peritoneal dialysis: children's preference, *ANNA J* 19(3):249-254, 1992.

Ellis D, and others: Comparison of FK-506 and cyclosporine regimens in pediatric renal transplantation, *Pediatr Nephrol* 8(2):193-200, 1994.

Gorynski L, Knight F: A peer group for adolescent dialysis patients, *ANNA J* 19(3):262-264, 1992.

Gutch CF, Stoner MH, Corea AL: *Review of hemodialysis for nurses and dialysis personnel,* ed 5, St Louis, 1992, Mosby.

Hendrix B: Dialysis therapies in critically ill children, *ACCN Clin Issues Crit Care Nurs* 3(3):605-613, 1992.

Iglesias JH, Richard GA: Pediatric renal transplantation, *Int Pediatr* 8(3):373-785, 1993.

Knight F and others: Hemodialysis of the infant or small child with chronic renal failure, *ANNA J* 20(3):315-323, 1993.

Kurtin PS, Landgraf JM, Abetz L: Patient-based health status measurements in pediatric dialysis: expanding the assessment of outcome, *Am J Kidney Dis* 24(2):376-382, 1994.

Miller D: Immunosuppression in pediatric transplant patients, *Pediatr Nurs* 21(1):21-26, 1995.

Peterson K: Iatrogenic immune suppression, *Pediatr Nurs* 21(1):11-15, 1995.

Suddaby EC, Bell SB, Murphy KJ: Continuous hemofiltration in infants and children, *Pediatr Nurs* 16:79-82, 1990.

Tejani A and others: Analysis of rejection outcomes and implications—a report of the North American Pediatric Renal Transplant Cooperative Study, *Transplantation* 59(4):500-504, 1995.

Tejani A and others: Factors predictive of sustained growth in children after renal transplantation, *J Pediatr* 122(3):397-402, 1993.

Tejani A, Fine RN: Cadaver renal transplantation in children, *Clin Pediatr* 32(4):194-202, 1993.

Uzark K: Caring for families of pediatric transplant recipients: psychosocial implications, *Crit Care Nurs Clin North Am* 4(2):255-261, 1992.

Weichler NK: Caretakers' informational needs after their children's renal or liver transplant, *ANNA J* 20(2):135-139, 1993.

Wise BV: Advances in pediatric solid organ transplantation, *Nurs Clin North Am* 29(4):615-629, 1994.

Chapter 28

THE CHILD WITH CEREBRAL DYSFUNCTION

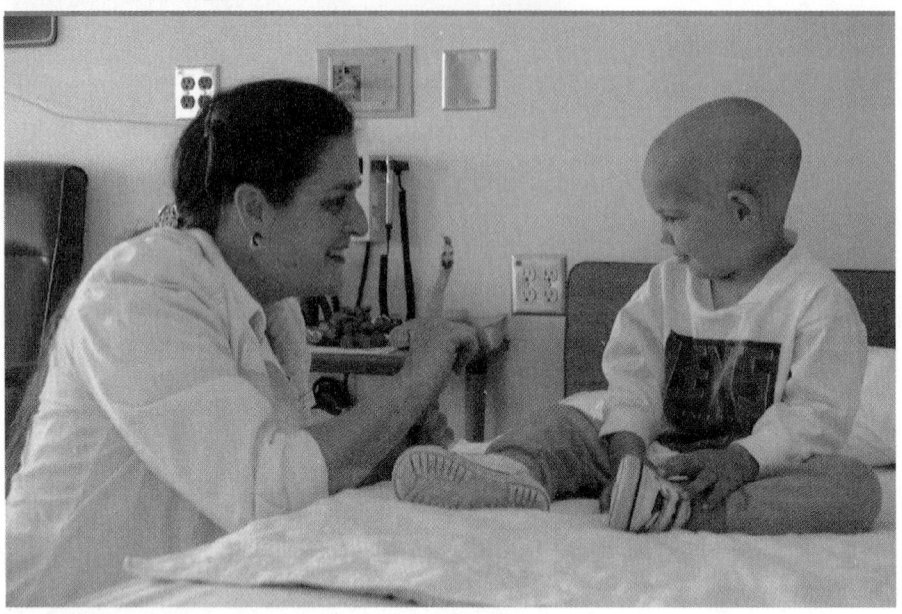

" *When we pull up to the hospital, he knows and says 'owie' and holds his port.* "

Jan, mother of Colton, age 2½ years, brain tumor

RELATED TOPICS

CEREBRAL DYSFUNCTION

ASSESSMENT OF CEREBRAL FUNCTION

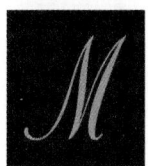

ost of the information about the status of the brain is obtained by indirect measurements. Some of these measurements are discussed in relation to numerous aspects of child care (e.g., as part of assessments of health [Chapter 7], newborn status [Chapter 8], mental retardation [Chapter 19], hypoxic injury [cerebral palsy, Chapter 32], and attainment of developmental milestones at each stage of development). Since increased intracranial pressure and altered states of consciousness have such prominent places in neurologic dysfunction, they are described here, followed by techniques for neurologic assessment and diagnostic tests.

General Aspects

Children younger than 2 years of age require special evaluation, since they are unable to respond to directions designed to elicit specific responses in infants neurologically. Early neurologic responses in infants are primarily reflexive; these responses are gradually replaced by meaningful movement in the characteristic cephalocaudal direction of development. This evidence of progressive maturation reflects more extensive myelinization and changes in neurochemical and electrophysiologic properties.

Most information about infants and small children is gained by observing their spontaneous and elicited reflex responses as they develop increasingly complex locomotor and fine motor skills and by eliciting progressively sophisticated communicative and adaptive behaviors. Delay or deviation from expected milestones helps identify high-risk children. Persistence or reappearance of reflexes that normally disappear indicates pathology. In evaluating the infant or young child, it is also important to obtain the pregnancy and delivery history to determine the possible effect of intrauterine environmental influences known to affect the orderly maturation of the central nervous system (CNS). These influences include maternal infections, chemicals, trauma, and metabolic insults.

Jeanne O'Connor Egan, MSN, RN, revised this chapter.

General aspects of assessment that provide clues to the etiology of dysfunction include:

Family history—sometimes offers clues regarding possible genetic disorders with neurologic manifestations
Health history—may provide valuable clues regarding the cause of dysfunction (e.g., an injury, short febrile illness, encounter with an animal or insect, ingestion of neurotoxic substances, inhalation of chemicals, a past illness, or known diabetes mellitus)
Physical evaluation of infants—includes observation of the following:

Size and shape of the head
Spontaneous activity and postural reflex activity
Sensory responses
Attitude—normal flexed posture, extreme extension, opisthotonos, hypotonia
Symmetry in movement of extremities
Excessive tremulousness or frequent twitching movements
Altered expiratory cycle:
Prolonged apnea
Ataxic breathing
Paradoxic chest movement
Hyperventilation
Skin and hair texture
Distinctive facial features
Presence of a high-pitched, piercing cry
Abnormal eye movements
Inability to suck or swallow
Lip smacking
Asymmetric contraction of facial muscles
Yawning (may indicate cranial nerve involvement)
Muscular activity and coordination
Level of development

Increased Intracranial Pressure (ICP)

The brain, tightly enclosed in the solid bony cranium, is well protected but highly vulnerable to pressure that may accumulate within the enclosure. Its total volume—brain, cerebrospinal fluid (CSF), and blood—must remain approximately the same at all times. A change in the proportional volume of one of these components (e.g., increase or decrease in intracranial blood) must be accompanied by a compensatory change in another. In this way the volume and pressure normally remain constant. Examples of compensatory changes are reduction in blood volume, decrease in CSF production, increase in CSF absorption, or shrinkage of brain mass by displacement of intracellular and extracellular fluid.

CLINICAL MANIFESTATIONS OF INCREASED INTRACRANIAL PRESSURE IN INFANTS AND CHILDREN

Infants
Tense, bulging fontanel; lack of normal pulsations
Separated cranial sutures
Macewen (cracked-pot) sign
Irritability
High-pitched cry
Increased occipital-frontal circumference
Distended scalp veins
Changes in feeding
Cries when held or rocked
"Setting sun" sign *eyes get very wide + looking up*

Children
Headache
Nausea
Vomiting—often without nausea
Diplopia, blurred vision
Seizures

Personality and Behavior Signs
Irritability (toddlers), restlessness
Indifference, drowsiness, or lack of interest
Decline in school performance
Diminished physical activity and motor performance
Increased complaints of fatigue, tiredness; increased time devoted to sleep
Significant weight loss possible from anorexia and vomiting
Memory loss if pressure is markedly increased
Inability to follow simple commands
Progression to lethargy and drowsiness

Late Signs
Lowered level of consciousness
Decreased motor response to command
Decreased sensory response to painful stimuli
Alterations in pupil size and reactivity
Sometimes decerebrate or decorticate posturing
Cheyne-Stokes respirations
Papilledema

LEVELS OF CONSCIOUSNESS

Full consciousness—Awake and alert, oriented to time, place, and person—behavior appropriate for age
Confusion—Impaired decision making
Disorientation—Disorientation to time and place, decreased level of consciousness
Lethargy—Limited spontaneous movement, sluggish speech
Obtundation—Arousable with stimulation
Stupor—Remains in a deep sleep, responsive only to vigorous and repeated stimulation
Coma—No motor or verbal response to noxious (painful) stimuli
Persistent vegetative state (PVS)—the permanently lost function of the cerebral cortex—eyes follow objects only by reflex or when attracted to the direction of loud sounds; all four limbs are spastic, but can withdraw from painful stimuli; hands show reflexive grasping and groping; the face can grimace, some food may be swallowed, and the child may groan or cry but utter no words

Modified from Hazinski MF, editor: *Care of the critically ill child*, ed 2, St Louis, 1992, Mosby.

Children with open fontanels compensate by skull expansion and widened sutures. However, at any age the capacity for spatial compensation is limited. An increase in ICP may be caused by tumors or other space-occupying lesions, accumulation of fluid within the ventricular system, bleeding, or edema of cerebral tissues. Once compensation is exhausted, any further increase in volume will result in a rapid rise in ICP.

Early signs and symptoms of increased ICP are often subtle and assume many patterns (see box above). As pressure increases, signs and symptoms become more pronounced, and the level of consciousness deteriorates.

 Up until 5 years of age, a child's suture line may open again with increased ICP.

Altered States of Consciousness

Consciousness implies awareness—the ability to respond to sensory stimuli and have subjective experiences. There are two components of consciousness: *alertness,* an arousal-waking state including the ability to respond to stimuli, and *cognitive power,* including the ability to process stimuli and produce verbal and motor responses.

An altered state of consciousness usually refers to varying states of unconsciousness that may be momentary or may extend for hours, days, or indefinitely. *Unconsciousness* is depressed cerebral function—the inability to respond to sensory stimuli and have subjective experiences. *Coma* is defined as a state of unconsciousness from which the patient cannot be aroused even with powerful stimuli.

Levels of Consciousness (LOC). Assessment of LOC remains the earliest indicator of improvement or deterioration in neurologic status. LOC is determined by observations of the child's responses to the environment. Other diagnostic tests, such as motor activity, reflexes, and vital signs, are more variable and do not necessarily directly parallel the depth of the comatose state. The most consistently used terms are described in the box.

Coma Assessment. Several scales have been devised in an attempt to standardize the description and interpretation of the degree of depressed consciousness. The most popular of these is the *Glasgow Coma Scale (GCS),* which consists of a three-part assessment: eye opening, verbal response, and motor response (Fig 28-1). When LOC is being assessed in young children, it is often useful to have a parent present to help elicit a desired response. An infant or child may not respond in an unfamiliar environment or to unfamiliar voices. Children over 3 years of age should be able to give their name, although they may not be cognizant of place or time.

Numeric values are assigned to the levels of response in each category, and the sum of these numeric values provides an objective measure of the patient's LOC. The lower the score, the deeper the coma. A person with an unaltered LOC would score the highest, 15; a score of 7 or below is generally accepted as a definition of coma; the lowest score, 3, indicates deep coma. In cases of irreversible coma, the Task

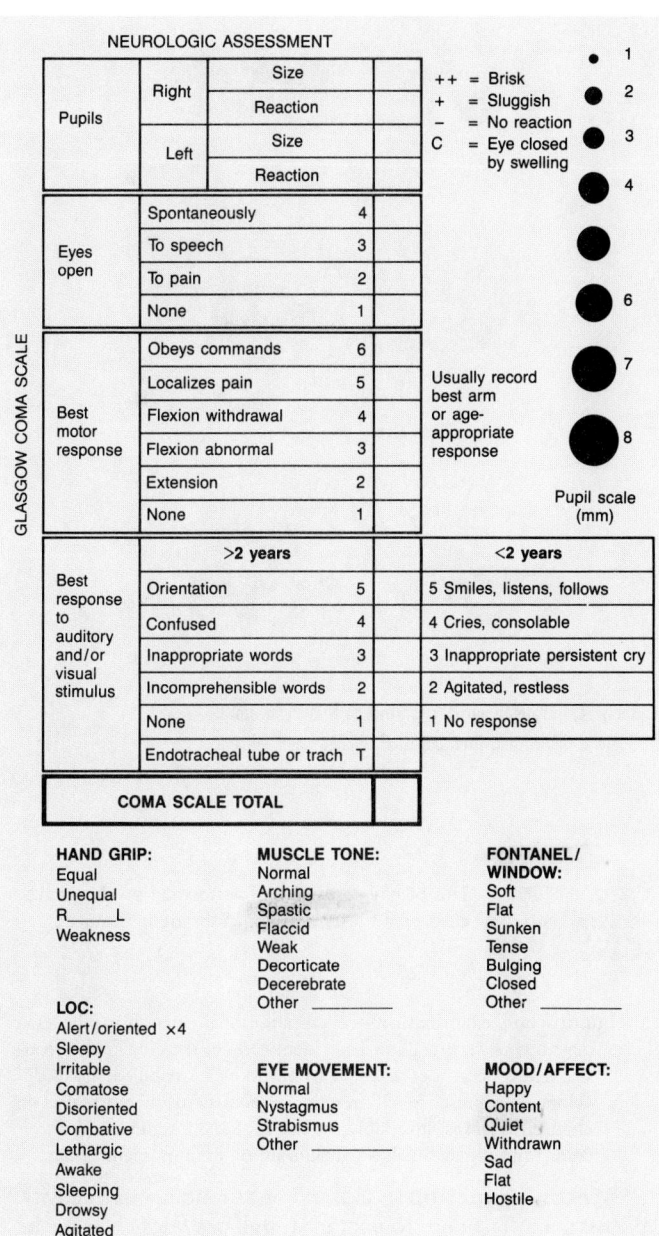

NEUROLOGIC ASSESSMENT

Pupils	Right	Size		++	= Brisk
		Reaction		+	= Sluggish
	Left	Size		−	= No reaction
		Reaction		C	= Eye closed by swelling

Eyes open	Spontaneously	4
	To speech	3
	To pain	2
	None	1

Best motor response	Obeys commands	6
	Localizes pain	5
	Flexion withdrawal	4
	Flexion abnormal	3
	Extension	2
	None	1

Usually record best arm or age-appropriate response

Pupil scale (mm)

Best response to auditory and/or visual stimulus	>2 years		<2 years
	Orientation	5	5 Smiles, listens, follows
	Confused	4	4 Cries, consolable
	Inappropriate words	3	3 Inappropriate persistent cry
	Incomprehensible words	2	2 Agitated, restless
	None	1	1 No response
	Endotracheal tube or trach	T	

COMA SCALE TOTAL	

HAND GRIP:
Equal
Unequal
R____L
Weakness

LOC:
Alert/oriented ×4
Sleepy
Irritable
Comatose
Disoriented
Combative
Lethargic
Awake
Sleeping
Drowsy
Agitated

MUSCLE TONE:
Normal
Arching
Spastic
Flaccid
Weak
Decorticate
Decerebrate
Other ____

EYE MOVEMENT:
Normal
Nystagmus
Strabismus
Other ____

FONTANEL/WINDOW:
Soft
Flat
Sunken
Tense
Bulging
Closed
Other ____

MOOD/AFFECT:
Happy
Content
Quiet
Withdrawn
Sad
Flat
Hostile

FIG. 28-1. Pediatric coma scale.

Force for the Determination of Brain Death in Children has established physical examination criteria.

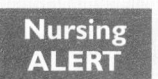 **Nursing ALERT** Lack of response to painful stimuli is abnormal and is reported immediately.

Neurologic Examination

The purpose of the neurologic examination is to establish an accurate, objective baseline of neurologic information. It is essential that the neurologic examination be documented in a fashion that is able to be reproduced by others. Descriptions of behaviors should be simple, objective, and easily interpreted: "Drowsy but awake and conversationally rational/

oriented"; "Sleepy but arousable with vigorous physical stimuli. Pressure to nail base of right hand results in upper extremity flexion/lower extremity extension."

Vital Signs. Pulse, respiration, and blood pressure provide information regarding the adequacy of circulation and the possible underlying cause of altered consciousness. Autonomic activity is most intensively disturbed in deep coma and in brainstem lesions.

Body temperature is often elevated, and sometimes the elevation may be extreme. Coma of a toxic origin may produce hypothermia. High temperature is most frequently a sign of an acute infectious process or heat stroke but may be caused by ingestion of some drugs (especially salicylates, alcohol, and barbiturates) or intracranial bleeding, especially subarachnoid hemorrhage. A fever sometimes follows a cerebral seizure.

The *pulse* is variable and may be rapid, slow and bounding, or feeble. *Blood pressure* may be normal, elevated, or at shock levels. The Cushing reflex or pressor response that causes a slowing of the pulse and an increase in blood pressure is uncommon in children; when it occurs, it is a very late sign. Vital signs are also affected by medications. For assessment purposes *changes* in pulse and blood pressure are more important than the direction.

Respirations are often slow, deep, and irregular. Slow, deep breathing is often seen in the heavy sleep caused by sedatives, after seizures, or in cerebral infections. Slow, shallow breathing may result from sedatives or opioids (narcotics). Hyperventilation (deep and rapid respirations) is usually the result of metabolic acidosis or abnormal stimulation of the respiratory center in the medulla caused by salicylate poisoning, hepatic coma, or Reye syndrome.

Breathing patterns have been described with a number of terms (e.g., apneustic, cluster, ataxic, Cheyne-Stokes). However, it is better to describe what is being observed rather than placing a label on it. The terms are often used and interpreted incorrectly. Periodic or irregular breathing is an ominous sign of brainstem (especially medullary) dysfunction that often precedes complete apnea. The *odor* of the breath may provide additional clues (e.g., the fruity, acetone odor of ketosis, the foul odor of uremia, the fetid odor of hepatic failure, or the odor of alcohol).

Skin. The skin may offer clues to the cause of unconsciousness. The body surface should be examined for the presence of injury, needle marks, petechiae, bites, and ticks. Evidence of toxic substances may be found on the hands, face, mouth, and clothing—especially in small children.

Eyes. Pupil size and reactivity are assessed (Figs. 28-1 and 28-2). Pinpoint pupils are commonly observed in poisoning, such as opiate or barbiturate poisoning, or in brainstem dysfunction. Widely dilated and reactive pupils are often seen after seizures and may involve only one side. Dilated pupils may also be caused by eye trauma. Widely dilated and fixed pupils suggest paralysis of cranial nerve III secondary to pressure from herniation of the brain through the tentorium. A unilateral fixed pupil usually suggests a lesion on the same side. Bilateral fixed pupils usually imply brainstem damage if present for more than 5 minutes. Dilated and unreactive pupils are also seen in hypothermia, anoxia, ischemia, poisoning with atropine-like substances, or prior instillation of mydriatic drugs.

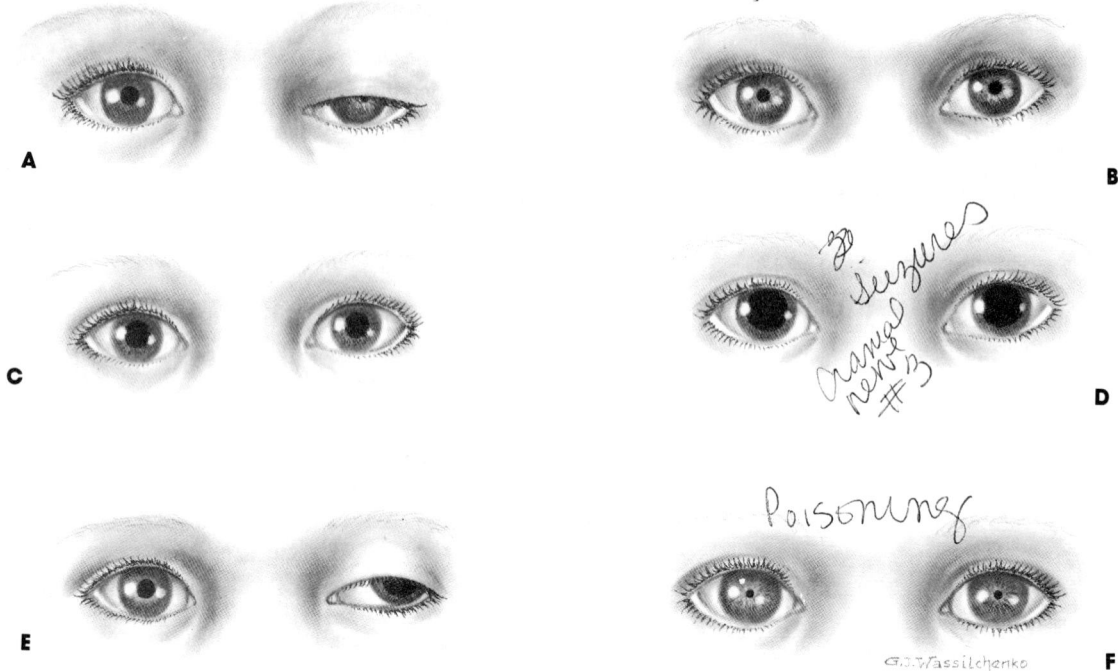

FIG. 28-2. Variations in pupil size with altered states of consciousness. **A,** Ipsilateral pupillary constriction with slight ptosis. **B,** Bilateral small pupils. **C,** Midposition; light fixed to all stimuli. **D,** Bilateral dilated and fixed pupils. **E,** Dilated pupil; left eye abducted with ptosis. **F,** Pinpoint pupils.

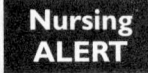 The sudden appearance of a fixed and dilated pupil(s) is a neurosurgical emergency.

The description of eye movements should indicate whether one or both eyes are involved and how the reaction was elicited. The parents should be asked about preexisting strabismus, which will cause the eyes to appear normal under compromise. A posttraumatic strabismus indicates cranial nerve VI damage.

Special tests, usually performed by qualified persons, include the following:

Doll's head maneuver—the child's head is rotated quickly to one side and then to the other. Conjugate (paired or working together) movement of the eyes in the direction opposite to the head rotation is normal. Absence of this response suggests dysfunction of the brainstem or oculomotor nerve (cranial nerve III).

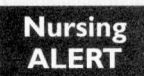 This assessment is not attempted until after cervical spine injury has been ruled out.

Caloric test, or oculovestibular response—elicited with the child's head up by irrigating the external auditory canal with ice water, which normally causes conjugate movement of the eyes toward the side of stimulation. This is lost when the pontine centers are impaired, thus providing important information in assessment of the comatose patient.

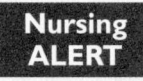 This painful test is never performed on the awake child or if the tympanic membrane is ruptured.

Funduscopic examination—reveals additional clues. If papilledema develops at all, it will not be evident early in the course of unconsciousness because it takes 24 to 48 hours for papilledema to develop. The presence of preretinal (subhyaloid) hemorrhages in children is almost invariably the result of acute trauma with intracranial bleeding, usually subarachnoid or subdural hemorrhage.

Motor Function. Observing spontaneous activity, posture, and response to painful stimuli provides clues to the location and extent of cerebral dysfunction. Even subtle movements (e.g., the outward rotation of a hip) should be noted, and the child observed for other signs. Asymmetric movements of the limbs or absence of movement suggests paralysis. In hemiplegia the affected limb lies in external rotation and will fall uncontrollably when lifted and allowed to drop. These observations should be described rather than labeled.

In the deeper comatose states there is little or no spontaneous movement, and the musculature tends to be flaccid. There is considerable variability in the motor behavior in lesser degrees of coma. For example, the child may be relatively immobile or restless and hyperkinetic; muscle tone may be increased or decreased. Tremors, twitching, and spasms of muscles are common observations. The patient may display purposeless plucking or tossing movements. Combative or negativistic behavior is not uncommon. Hyperactivity is more common in acute febrile and toxic states than in cases

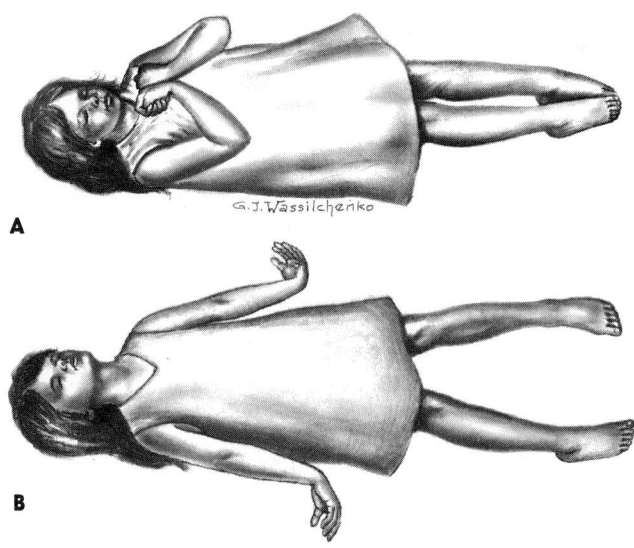

A

B

FIG. 28-3. A, Decorticate posturing. **B,** Decerebrate posturing.

of increased ICP. Convulsions are common in children and may be present in coma from any cause. Any repetitive or convulsive movements should be described.

Posturing. Since cortical control over motor function is lost in brain dysfunction, primitive postural reflexes emerge. These are evident in posturing and motor movements directly related to the area of the brain involved. *Decorticate posturing* (Fig. 28-3, *A*), is seen when there is severe dysfunction of the cerebral cortex. Typical decorticate posturing includes adduction of arms at the shoulders, flexion of the arms on the chest with the wrists flexed and the hands fisted, and extension and adduction of the lower extremities. *Decerebrate posturing* (Fig. 28-3, *B*), a sign of dysfunction at the level of the midbrain, is characterized by rigid extension and pronation of the arms and legs. The posturing may not be evident when the child is quiet but can usually be elicited by applying painful stimuli, such as a blunt object pressed on the base of the nail.

Reflexes. Testing of some reflexes may be of limited value. In general, the corneal, pupillary, muscle-stretch, superficial, and plantar reflexes tend to be absent in deep coma. The state of reflexes is variable in lighter grades of unconsciousness and depends on the underlying pathologic process and the location of the lesion. Absence of corneal reflexes and presence of a tonic neck reflex are associated with severe brain damage. The Babinski reflex (see Extremities, Chapter 7) may be of value if it is found to be present consistently in children older than 18 months. A positive Babinski reflex is significant in assessment of pyramidal tract lesions when it is unilateral and associated with other pyramidal signs.

Nursing ALERT	Three key reflexes that demonstrate neurologic health in young infants are the Moro, tonic neck, and withdrawal reflexes.

Special Diagnostic Procedures

Numerous diagnostic procedures are used for assessment of cerebral function. Laboratory tests that may help to determine the cause of unconsciousness include blood glucose, urea nitrogen, and electrolyte (pH, sodium, potassium, chloride, calcium, and bicarbonate) tests; clotting studies, hematocrit, and a complete blood count; liver function tests; blood cultures if there is fever; and sometimes studies to detect lead or other toxic substances, such as drugs.

Highly sophisticated tests are carried out with specialized equipment by skilled personnel. Most of these tests are outlined in the accompanying box. Because such tests can be threatening to children, a child will need preparation for, and support and reassurance during, the tests. (See also Preparation for Procedures, Chapter 22.)

Children who are old enough to understand require careful explanation of the procedure, why it is being done, what they will experience, and how they can help. School-age children usually appreciate a more detailed description of why contrast material is injected. The importance of lying still for tests, particularly tomography, needs to be stressed. Children unfamiliar with the machines can be shown a picture beforehand. Although radiographic examinations are not painful, the machinery is often so frightening in appearance that the child protests because of anxiety.

Tests such as computed tomography (CT) and magnetic resonance imaging (MRI) require that children be immobilized. Chin and cheek pads are sometimes used to prevent the slightest head movement, and straps are applied to the body to prevent a slight change in body position. The nurse can explain these events to a frightened child by comparing them to an astronaut's preparation for a space flight. It is very important to emphasize to the child that at no time is the procedure painful.

Developmentally, the nurse should not expect cooperation from a young child. Conscious sedation will be required. Drugs commonly used are intravenous pentobarbital or oral chloral hydrate. Chloral hydrate may be the drug of choice for children under 2 years of age. The suggested oral dosage is (Barkovich, 1990):

<10 kg: 75 to 100 mg/kg, or
>10 kg: 75 to 100 mg/kg plus 50 mg/kg for each kg of weight >10 kg (to a maximum dose of 2 g)
If child is still awake after 20 minutes, supplementary doses may be given up to a total dose of 2 g.
The drug should be given 35 to 45 minutes before the anticipated imaging time.

It is helpful for nurses to become acquainted with the equipment and the general environment in which the test will take place so that they can better explain the procedure to children at their level of understanding. Equipment is often strange and ominous to a child and may be perceived as a frightening monster. They need constant reassurance from a trusted companion. Since children are particularly frightened of needles, they need to be informed of any medication or contrast media to be administered intravenously.

Physical preparation may involve administering a sedative or providing an intravenous access for infusion of contrast material. If so, children should be helped through the preparation and administration and assured that someone will re-

PROCEDURES USED IN CEREBRAL ASSESSMENT

Lumbar Puncture (LP)

Diagnostic—measures spinal fluid pressure, obtains CSF for visualization and laboratory analysis

Subdural Tap

Helps rule out subdural effusions
Relieves ICP

Electroencephalography (EEG)

Measures electric activity of cerebral cortex
Detects electric abnormalities—diagnosis of seizures
Used to determine brain death

Video EEG

Split-screen simultaneous visualization of whole body, facial, and EEG recording

Computed Tomography (CT) Scan

Visualizes horizontal and vertical cross section of brain at any axis
Distinguishes density of various intracranial tissues and structures—congenital abnormalities, hemorrhage, tumors, and demyelinating and inflammatory processes

Nuclear Brain Scan

Test material accumulates in areas where blood-brain barrier is defective
Identifies focal brain lesions (e.g., tumors, abscesses)
Positive uptake of material with encephalitis and subdural hematoma
Visualizes CSF pathways

Transillumination

Varying degrees of localized glowing may be seen in abnormal fluid accumulation in various areas of head

Echoencephalography

Identifies shifts in midline structures from their normal positions as a result of intracranial lesions
May show ventricular dilation

Radiography

Shows fractures, dislocations, spreading suture lines, and craniostenosis
Shows degenerative changes, bone erosion, and calcifications

Magnetic Resonance Imaging (MRI)

Permits visualization of morphologic features of target structures
Permits tissue discrimination unavailable with many techniques

Positron Emission Transaxial Tomography (PETT) or Positron Emission Tomography (PET)

Detects and measures such functions as blood volume and flow in brain, metabolic activity, and biochemical changes within tissues

Real-Time Ultrasonography (RTUS)

Allows high-resolution anatomic visualization in variety of imaging planes

Digital Subtraction Angiography (DSA)

Visualizes vasculature of target tissue
Visualizes finite vascular abnormalities

CRITICAL THINKING EXERCISE
Conscious Sedation

Brian, 4 weeks old, is returned to his room after a CT scan to evaluate a seizure episode. Upon examination you find a sleepy infant arousable with vigorous stimulation, with pale, dusky colored skin and mucous membranes. The vital signs are temperature of 35.8° C, pulse of 110, respiratory rate of 20, and blood pressure of 82/40; the oxygen saturation is 89%-92%. His weight is 5 kg and he received 500 mg of chloral hydrate (<10 kg: 75-100 mg/kg dosage) as ordered before leaving for the CT. During the report the CT nurse reviews the conscious sedation record and you note it does not include the infant's temperature. An additional dosage of 250 mg of chloral hydrate was administered in CT to achieve sleep for Brian. The best intervention is to:

1. Monitor the vital signs and cover the infant
2. Place a radiant warmer over the infant and notify the physician
3. Fill out a medication error report
4. Allow the infant to sleep

The correct answer is two. Brian is experiencing thermoregulation problems compounded by administration of too much chloral hydrate for conscious sedation. The maximum dosage of sedation was exceeded for this infant. Conscious sedation flow sheets to record vital signs often do not include temperature measurement, an essential observation in infants because of their inability to maintain body temperature.

---

main with them (if this is possible). Children will need continual support and reinforcement during procedures in which they remain conscious. Vital signs and physiologic response to the procedure are monitored throughout. Conscious sedation records become part of the child's chart. Many diagnostic procedures performed on an outpatient basis require sedation, and children need recovery time and observation. Written instructions should be reviewed with parents if the child is discharged to home following a procedure (see Critical Thinking Exercise).

Children who have undergone a procedure while under general anesthesia require postanesthesia care, including positioning to prevent aspiration of secretions and frequent assessment of vital signs and LOC. In addition, other neurologic functions, such as pupillary responses, motor strength, and movement, are tested at regular intervals. Any surgical wound resulting from the test is checked for bleeding, CSF leakage, and other complications. Children who undergo repeated subdural taps should have their hematocrit measured daily to detect any blood loss from the procedure.

Children's emotional reactions to procedures are also considered. They should be allowed to express their feelings about their experiences through verbal expression and the use of therapeutic play. Parents also seek and are entitled to an explanation of results of tests and procedures performed on their children. Nurses are in a unique position to provide support and education to parents regarding procedures.

NURSING CARE OF THE UNCONSCIOUS CHILD

The unconscious child requires continuous nursing attendance with observation, recording, and evaluation of changes in objective signs. These observations provide valuable information regarding the patient's progress. Often they serve as a guide to diagnosis and treatment. Therefore, careful and detailed observations are essential for the patient's welfare. In addition, vital functions must be maintained, and complications prevented through conscientious and meticulous nursing care. The outcome of unconsciousness may be early with complete recovery, death within a few hours or days, persistent and permanent unconsciousness, or recovery with varying degrees of residual mental and/or physical disability. The outcome and recovery of the unconscious child may depend on the level of nursing care and observational skills.

Emergency measures are directed toward assuring a patent airway, treatment of shock, and reduction of ICP (if present). Delayed treatment often leads to increased damage. As soon as emergency measures have been implemented—in many cases concurrently—therapies for specific causes are begun. Because nursing care is closely related to the medical management, both are considered here.

❖ Assessment

Continual observation of LOC, pupillary reaction, and vital signs is essential to management of CNS disorders. Regular assessment of neurologic signs is a vital part of nursing comatose children. Vital signs are taken and recorded regularly. The frequency depends on the cause of coma, the status, and the progression of cerebral involvement. Intervals may be as frequent as every 15 minutes or as long as every 2 hours. Significant alterations are reported immediately. Temperature is taken every 2 to 4 hours, depending on the patient's condition.

An elevated temperature may occur in children with CNS dysfunction; therefore a light covering is sufficient. Vigorous efforts, such as tepid sponge baths or application of a hypothermia blanket, are needed to prevent brain damage if temperature exceeds 40° C (104° F) rectally.

The LOC is assessed periodically, including size, equality, and reaction of pupils to light and signs of meningeal irritation, such as nuchal rigidity. This also includes response to vocal commands, spontaneous behavior, resistance to care, and response to painful stimuli. Motions of any type, changes in muscle tone or strength, and body position are noted. Seizure activity is described according to the type and length of seizure and body areas involved (see box on p. 1021).

Pain management for the comatose child requires astute nursing observation and management. Signs of pain include changes in behavior (e.g., increased agitation and rigidity, and alterations in physiologic parameters); usually increased heart rate, respiratory rate, and blood pressure; and decreased oxygen saturation. Since these findings are not specific for pain, the nurse should observe for their appearance during times of induced or suspected pain and their disappearance following the inciting procedure or the administration of analgesia. A pain assessment record should be used to document indications of pain and the effectiveness of interventions (see Pain Assessment, Chapter 21).

The use of opioids, such as morphine, to relieve pain is controversial because they may mask signs of altered consciousness or depress respirations. However, unrelieved pain activates the stress response, which can elevate ICP. To block the stress response, some authorities advocate the use of analgesics, sedatives, and, in some cases such as head injury, paralyzing agents via continuous intravenous infusion. A frequently used combination is fentanyl, midazolam (Versed), and vecuronium. If there are concerns about assessing the LOC or respiratory depression, naloxone can be used to reverse the opioid effects. Acetaminophen and codeine may also be effective analgesics for mild to moderate pain. Regardless of the drugs used, adequate dosage and regular administration are essential to providing optimum pain relief.

Other measures to relieve discomfort include providing a quiet, dimly lit environment, limiting visitors to a minimum, preventing any sudden jarring movement, such as banging into the bed, and preventing an increase in ICP. The last is most effectively achieved by proper positioning and prevention of straining, such as during coughing, vomiting, or defecating. (See Pain Management, Chapter 21.)

> **Nursing ALERT**
> When opioids are used, bowel elimination must be closely monitored because of their constipating effect. A stool softener should be given regularly with laxatives as needed to prevent constipation.

Antiepileptic drugs, such as phenytoin (Dilantin) or phenobarbital, are ordered for control of seizure activity.

❖ Nursing Diagnoses

Based on a thorough assessment, several nursing diagnoses are identified. The more common diagnoses for the unconscious child are included in the Nursing Care Plan on pp. 994-996. Others may apply in specific situations.

❖ Planning

Goals for the unconscious child and family include the following:

1. Child will maintain respiratory integrity.
2. Child will not experience increasing ICP.
3. Child will have basic needs (hygiene, nutrition, hydration, elimination) met.
4. Child will not experience complications of immobility.
5. Family will receive adequate support and education.

❖ Implementation

Respiratory Management

Respiratory effectiveness is the primary concern in care of the unconscious child, and establishment of an adequate airway is *always* the first priority. Carbon dioxide has a potent vasodilating effect and will increase cerebral blood flow (CBF) and ICP. Cerebral hypoxia that lasts longer than 4 minutes nearly always causes irreversible brain damage.

> **Nursing ALERT**
> Respiratory obstruction leads to cardiac arrest. Always maintain an adequate airway.

Children in lighter states of coma may be able to cough and swallow, but those in deeper states are unable to handle secretions, which tend to pool in the throat and pharynx. Dysfunction of cranial nerves IX and X place the child at risk for aspiration and cardiac arrest; therefore, the child is positioned to prevent aspiration of secretions, and the stomach is emptied to reduce the likelihood of vomiting. In infants blockage of air passages from secretions can happen in seconds. In addition, upper airway obstruction from laryngospasm is a frequent complication in comatose children.

An oral airway can be used for the child who is suffering a temporary loss of consciousness, such as after a contusion, seizure, or anesthesia. For children who remain unconscious for a time, a nasotracheal or orotracheal tube is inserted to maintain the open airway and facilitate removal of secretions. A tracheostomy is performed in cases in which laryngoscopy for introduction of an endotracheal tube would be difficult or dangerous. Suctioning is used only as needed to clear the airway, exerting care to prevent increasing ICP. Respiratory status is observed and evaluated regularly. Signs of respiratory embarrassment may be an indication for ventilatory assistance.

When the respiratory center is involved, mechanical ventilation is usually indicated (see Chapter 22). Blood gas analysis is performed regularly, and oxygen is administered when indicated. Moderately severe hypoxia and respiratory acidosis are often present but not always evident from clinical manifestations. Hyperventilation frequently accompanies unconsciousness and may lead to respiratory alkalosis, or it may represent the body's attempt to compensate for metabolic acidosis. Therefore blood gas and pH determinations are essential guides for electrolyte therapy. Chest physiotherapy is carried out on a regular basis, and the child's position is changed at least every 2 hours to prevent pulmonary complications.

Increased ICP Monitoring

Management of the child with increased ICP is possibly the most formidable task and the most controversial subject in pediatric critical care. It appears that the outcome in pediatric neurologic injury may reflect more the initial cerebral damage than subsequent intracranial hypertension.

When increased ICP is the result of accumulation of CSF from obstruction of CSF flow, a ventricular tap will provide relief quickly and effectively. Evacuation of a hematoma reduces pressure from this source. Indications for inserting an ICP monitor are (1) Glasgow Coma Scale evaluation of less than 7, (2) Glasgow Coma Scale evaluation of less than 8 with respiratory assistance, (3) deterioration of condition, and (4) subjective judgment regarding clinical appearance and response.

Four major types of ICP monitors are (1) intraventricular catheter with fibroscopic sensors attached to a monitoring system, (2) subarachnoid bolt (Richmond screw), (3) epidural sensor, and (4) anterior fontanel pressure monitor. Transducers for both ventricular and subarachnoid monitoring should be set up without the use of a flush device. Direct ventricular pressure measurement remains the gold standard of ICP monitoring.

The catheter method involves introduction of a catheter into the lateral ventricle on the nondominant side, if known, or placement in the subdural space. The catheter has the advantage of providing a means of extraventricular (or continuous) drainage to reduce pressure. A drainage bag attached to the system is kept at the level of the ventricles and can be lowered to decrease ICP (see Critical Thinking Exercise).

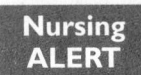

Nursing ALERT If the external ventricular drain (EVD) is unclamped for CSF drainage, carefully monitor the level of the collection container. If the container is too low, improper CSF decompression could lower ICP too rapidly, causing bleeding and pain.

In the bolt method the end of the bolt is placed into the subarachnoid space. The bolt cannot be adequately secured in a small child's pliant skull, although special modifications have been developed for children under 6 years of age.

Nursing ALERT The bolt is stabilized with dressings, but these are not changed or disturbed, even to check the site.

The placement of the bolt is not adjusted by anyone except the neurosurgeon who placed the device. The neurosurgeon is notified if a satisfactory wave form is not observed.

An epidural sensor can be placed between the dura and the skull through a burr hole and connected to a stopcock assembly and a transducer, which provides a readout of the pressure. Correlation of pressure readings is less invasive but may be inconsistent. In infants a fontanel transducer can be used to detect impulses from a pressure sensor and convert them to electrical energy. The electrical energy is then converted to visible waves or numeric readings on an oscillo-

---

CRITICAL THINKING EXERCISE

Hydrocephalus

Three-year-old Emma is 5 days postoperative for removal of a posterior fossa tumor. Although an external ventricular drain (EVD) was placed to treat her hydrocephalus, she continues to demonstrate signs of increased ICP, including holding the back of her head, anorexia, crying when moved or when strangers enter room, and lethargy. On examination, fluid drainage is noted on the mother's clothes, and Emma is experiencing repetitive, rapid eyelid blinking. The best intervention is to:

1. Lower the EVD drain.
2. Check the EVD dressing site, do a neurologic exam, and notify the practitioner.
3. Change the dressing to a transparent adhesive.
4. Request a CT Scan.

The correct answer is two. The EVD is not draining properly but is taking the path of least resistance through the insertion site. Lowering the EVD may cause rapid drainage of the CSF resulting in subdural complications. The dressing may need to be changed to a clear adhesive so that the site can be observed. A CT may be required, but the priority is to stabilize Emma, who is demonstrating signs of increased ICP and cranial neuropathy.

scope. ICP measurement from the anterior fontanel is non-invasive but may prove to be inaccurate if the equipment is poorly placed or inconsistently recalibrated. The intraparenchymal pressure monitoring device (e.g., Camino) is a result of fiberoptic technology and has a reliable performance.

ICP can be increased by instillation of solutions; therefore antibiotics are administered sytemically if a positive CSF culture is obtained. However, intravenous ICP monitoring rarely causes infection. Since CSF is a body fluid, standard precautions are implemented according to hospital policy (see Infection Control, Chapter 22).

Nurses caring for patients with intracranial monitoring devices must be acquainted with the system, assist with insertion, interpret the monitor readings, and be able to distinguish between danger signals and mechanical dysfunction.

For increased ICP resulting from cerebral edema, several medical measures are available. Osmotic diuretics may provide rapid relief in emergency situations. Although their effect is transient, lasting only about 6 hours, they can be life-saving in emergencies. These substances are rapidly excreted by the kidneys and carry with them large quantities of sodium and water. Mannitol (or sometimes urea) administered intravenously is the drug most frequently used for rapid reduction. The infusion is generally given slowly but may be pushed rapidly if there is herniation or impending herniation. Because of the profound diuretic effect of the drug, an indwelling catheter is inserted to ensure bladder emptying. Adrenocorticosteroids are not recommended for cerebral edema secondary to head trauma. $Paco_2$ should be maintained at 25 to 30 mm Hg to produce vasoconstriction, which reduces CBF, thereby decreasing ICP.

Nursing Activities. In cases of high levels of increased ICP, nursing procedures tend to trigger reactive pressure waves in many patients. For example, increased intrathoracic or abdominal pressure will be transmitted to the cranium. Particular care should be taken in positioning these patients to avoid neck vein compression, which may further increase ICP by interfering with venous return.

> **Nursing ALERT**
> The head of the bed is elevated 15 to 30 degrees, and the child is positioned so that the head is maintained in midline to facilitate venous drainage and avoid jugular compression. Turning side to side is contraindicated because of the risk of jugular compression.

The child can be propped to one side or the other, and the use of an alternating-pressure mattress reduces the chance of prolonged pressure to vulnerable areas. Frequent clinical assessment of the child cannot be replaced by an ICP monitoring device.

It is important to avoid activities that may increase ICP by causing pain, emotional stress, or crying or those that might trigger a convulsive seizure. Gentle range-of-motion exercises can be carried out but should not be performed vigorously. Nontherapeutic touch can cause an increase in ICP. Any disturbing procedures to be performed should be scheduled to take advantage of therapies that reduce ICP, such as osmotherapy and sedation. Efforts are taken to minimize or eliminate environmental noise. Assessment and intervention to relieve pain are important nursing functions to decrease ICP.

> **NURSING TIP** Placing earphones over a child's ears has been shown to lower the ICP, heart rate, and blood pressure significantly. A greater net decline was achieved when soothing music was played through the earphones (Wincek, as reported by Wong, 1988).

Suctioning. Suctioning and percussion are poorly tolerated and are therefore contraindicated unless there are concurrent respiratory problems. Hypoxia and the Valsalva maneuver associated with cough both acutely elevate ICP. Vibration, which does not increase ICP, accomplishes excellent results and should be tried first if treatment is needed. If suctioning is necessary, it should be brief and preceded by hyperventilation with 100% oxygen, which can be monitored during suctioning with a pulse oxygen sensor reading to determine oxygen saturation.

Nutrition and Hydration

Fluids and calories are supplied initially by the intravenous route (see Chapter 22). An intravenous infusion is started early, and the type of fluid administered is determined by the general condition of the patient. Fluid therapy requires careful monitoring and adjustment based on neurologic signs and electrolyte determinations. Often comatose children are unable to cope with the same amounts of fluid they could tolerate at other times, and overhydration must be avoided to prevent fatal cerebral edema.

Later, nutrition is provided in a balanced formula given by nasogastric or gastrostomy tube. The nasogastric tube is usually taped in place with care to prevent pressure on the nares. Most children have continuous feedings, but if bolus feedings are used, the tube is rinsed with water after each feeding. Tubes are replaced according to unit policy. Nostrils are alternated with each replacement to prevent nasal irritation and pressure. Overfeeding should be avoided to prevent vomiting with its attendant danger of aspiration. Stomach contents are aspirated and measured before feeding to ascertain the amount remaining in the stomach. If the residual volume is excessive (depending on the size of the child), the dietitian and physician should be consulted regarding alteration of the formula composition to provide the needed calories and nutrients in a smaller volume. The aspirated contents should always be refed.

Hydration is maintained in the same manner. When cerebral edema is a threat, fluids may be restricted to reduce the chance of fluid overload. Skin and mucous membranes are examined for signs of dehydration. Observation for signs of altered fluid balance related to abnormal pituitary secretions is a part of nursing care.

Altered Pituitary Secretion. An altered ability to handle fluid loads is attributed in part to the syndrome of inappropriate antidiuretic hormone (SIADH) and diabetes insipidus (DI) resulting from hypothalamic dysfunction (see Chapter 29). SIADH frequently accompanies CNS diseases such as head injury, meningitis, encephalitis, brain abscess, brain tumor, and subarachnoid hemorrhage. In the patient with SIADH, scant quantities of urine are excreted, electrolyte analysis reveals hyponatremia and hyposmolality, and manifestations of overhydration are evident. It is important to evaluate all parameters, since the reduced urine output might be erroneously interpreted as a sign of dehydration.

TABLE 28-1. Effects of altered pituitary secretion		
MEASUREMENT	DI	SIADH
Urine output	Increased	Decreased
Specific gravity	Decreased	Increased
Serum sodium	Increased (hypernatremia)	Decreased (hyponatremia)

The treatment of SIADH consists of restriction of fluids until serum electrolytes and osmolality return to normal levels. Since SIADH frequently occurs with meningitis in children, fluid restriction is often prescribed. Likewise, DI may occur following intracranial trauma. There is increased urine volume and the accompanying danger of dehydration (see Table 28-1 for comparison of fluid changes in SIADH and DI). Adequate replacement of fluids is essential, and observation of electrolyte balance is necessary to detect signs of hypernatremia and hyperosmolality. Exogenous vasopressin may be administered.

Medications

The cause of unconsciousness determines specific drug therapies. Children with infectious processes are given antibiotics appropriate to the disease and the infecting organism, and corticosteroids are prescribed for inflammatory conditions and edema. Cerebral edema is an indication for osmotherapy with osmotic diuretics. Sedatives or antiepileptics are prescribed for seizure activity. Sedation in the combative child provides amnesic and anxiolytic properties in conjunction with a paralytic agent. The combination decreases ICP and allows treatment of cerebral edema. Usual drugs include morphine, midazolam (Versed), and pancuronium. Midazolam is attractive because of its short half-life.

> **Nursing ALERT** When used for seizures, phenytoin should be administered slowly by direct IV push at a rate not to exceed 50 mg/min. Since phenytoin precipitates in the presence of glucose, only normal saline is used for flushing the needle or catheter.

Deep coma, induced by administration of barbiturates, is controversial in the management of ICP. Barbiturates are currently reserved for the reduction of increased ICP when all else has failed. Barbiturates decrease the cerebral metabolic rate for oxygen and protect the brain during times of reduced CPP. Barbiturate coma requires extensive monitoring, cardiovascular and respiratory support, and ICP monitoring to assess response to therapy. Paralyzing agents, such as pancuronium (Pavulon) also may be needed to aid in performing diagnostic tests, improving effectiveness of therapy, and reducing risks of secondary complications. Elevation of ICP and/or heart rate of patients who are being given paralyzing agents or are under sedation may indicate the need for another dose of either or both medications.

Thermoregulation

Hyperthermia often accompanies cerebral dysfunction; if it is present, measures are implemented to reduce the temperature to prevent brain damage and to reduce metabolic demands generated by the increased body temperature. Antipyretics are the method of choice for fever reduction; cooling devices are used for hyperthermia. Laboratory tests and other methods are used in an attempt to determine the cause, if any, of the hyperthermia. Shivering responses triggered by a cooling blanket can often be alleviated by keeping the child warm. Treatment with hypothermia and barbiturates increases the risk of iatrogenic complications.

Elimination

A retention catheter is usually inserted in the acute phase, although diapers may be used and weighed to record urinary output. The child who formerly had bowel and bladder control is generally incontinent. If the child remains comatose for a long period, the indwelling catheter may be removed and periodic bladder emptying accomplished by intermittent catheterization. Stool softeners are usually sufficient to maintain bowel function, but suppositories or enemas may be needed occasionally for adequate elimination and to prevent an impaction. The passage of liquid stool after a period of no bowel activity is usually a sign of an impaction. To avoid this preventable problem, daily recording of bowel activity is essential.

Hygienic Care

Routine measures for cleansing and maintaining skin integrity are an integral part of nursing care of the unconscious child. Skinfolds require special attention to prevent excoriation. The child who is unable to move is prone to develop tissue breakdown and pressure necrosis; therefore the child may be placed on a pressure-reducing or pressure-relieving device to prevent pressure on prominent areas of the body. The goal is prevention by regular change of position and inspection of vulnerable areas, such as the ankle, trochanter, and shoulder. Since unconscious children undergo numerous invasive procedures, these skin sites require special assessment and intervention to promote healing and to prevent infection. Bed linen and any clothing are kept dry and free of wrinkles. If the child requires surgery or radiography, the nurse checks all dressings, bony sites, catheters, and intravenous access lines (See also Maintaining Healthy Skin, Chapter 22).

Mouth care is performed at least twice daily, since the mouth tends to become dry or coated with mucus. The teeth are carefully brushed with a soft toothbrush or cleaned with gauze saturated with saline. Commercially prepared cleansing devices, such as Toothettes, are convenient for cleansing the mouth and teeth. Lips are coated with ointment or other preparations to protect them from drying, cracking, or blistering.

The deeply comatose child is also prone to eye irritation. The corneal reflexes are absent; therefore the eyes are easily irritated or damaged by linen, dust, or other substances that

> **Nursing ALERT** The eyes should be examined regularly and carefully for early signs of irritation or inflammation. Artificial tears (methylcellulose) are placed in the eyes every 1 to 2 hours. Sometimes eye dressings may be needed to protect the eyes from possible damage.

may come in contact with them. There is excessive dryness as a result of decreased secretions, especially if the child is undergoing osmotherapy to reduce or prevent brain edema, and incomplete closure of the eyes.

The hair is combed and styled neatly. Long hair is usually braided and secured with rubber bands. The scalp should be kept clean with dry or wet shampoos as needed. The child's head may be shaved for tests or surgical procedures. If so, the hair is saved if possible and given to the family.

Positioning and Exercise

The unconscious child is positioned to prevent aspiration of saliva, nasogastric secretions, and vomitus and to minimize ICP. The head of the bed is elevated, and the child is placed in a side-lying or semiprone position. A small, firm pillow is placed under the head, and the uppermost limbs are flexed and supported with pillows. The weight of the body should not rest on the dependent arm. In the semiprone position the child lies with the dependent arm at the side behind the body, the opposite side supported on pillows, and the uppermost arm and leg flexed and resting on the pillows. This position prevents undue pressure on the dependent extremities. The dependent position of the face encourages drainage of secretions and prevents the flaccid tongue from obstructing the airway.

Normal range of motion exercises help to maintain function and prevent contractures of joints. Exercises should be done gently and with full range of motion. A small rolled pad can be placed in the palms to help maintain proper position of fingers; footboards or boots can be used to help prevent footdrop; splinting may be needed to prevent severe contractures of wrist, knee, or ankle in decerebrate children.

Stimulation

Sensory stimulation is important in the care of the unconscious child, just as it is in the care of the alert child. For the temporarily unconscious or semiconscious child, sensory stimulation helps to arouse the child to the conscious state and orient the child in terms of time and place. Auditory and tactile stimulation are especially valuable. Tactile stimulation is not appropriate for the child in whom it may elicit an undesirable response. However, for other children tactile contact often has a relaxing and calming effect. When the child's condition permits, holding or rocking has a soothing effect and provides the body contact needed by young children.

The auditory sense is often present in a state of coma. Hearing is the last sense to be lost and the first one to be regained; therefore the child should be spoken to as any other child. Conversation around the child should not include thoughtless or derogatory remarks. A radio playing soft music, a music box, or a record player is frequently used to provide auditory stimulation. Singing the child's favorite songs or reading a favorite story is a tactic used to maintain the child's contact with a familiar world. Having parents tape songs or stories provides a continuous source of familiar stimulation. Above all, it is important to remember that this is a child who has all the needs of any ill child.

Regaining Consciousness. Awakening from a coma is a gradual process; however, sometimes children regain consciousness within a short time. Regaining orientation involves knowing person, place, and time, in that order.

Certain behaviors have been observed when children awaken from the unconscious state. The stress and anxiety they appear to feel in a strange and unfamiliar environment are consistently expressed in silent and withdrawn behavior. Children respond to basic questioning but usually do not display their prehospitalization personality and social behavior until they are transferred from the critical care area.

Family Support

Helping parents of an unconscious child cope with the situation is especially difficult. They may demonstrate all the guilt, fear, hostility, and anxiety of any parent of a seriously ill child (see Chapter 18). In addition, these parents are faced with the uncertain outcome of the cerebral dysfunction. The fear of death, mental retardation, or other permanent disability is present. Nursing intervention with parents depends on the nature of the pathologic condition, the personality of the parents, and the parent-child relationship before injury or illness.

If there is little or no residual effect, the child will be dismissed to home care fairly soon. The parents need the most intensive nursing intervention during the period of crisis and uncertainty. During the recovery phase they are given information, information is clarified, and they are encouraged to become involved in the child's care. Often the child's hospitalization is brief; however, some children require extended hospitalization for intensive therapy and rehabilitation.

The parents of children who die within hours or days require the support and guidance that the parents of any dying child would need in coping with the reality of the death and resolving their grief (see Chapter 18).

Probably the most difficult situations are those that involve children who are unconscious permanently or for an indefinite period. Unlike parents who lose a child through death, the finality is lacking for these parents, often leaving them in a state of suspended grief. The presence of the child renders the parents unable to resolve the loss. Like parents of dying children, parents of the comatose child search for any signs of hope. Well-meaning friends and relatives relate instances of miraculous recoveries. The parents seek confirmation and support for such possibilities and assign erroneous meanings to any sign in the child, such as reflexive muscle contractions, that might be interpreted as evidence of recovery.

At these times nurses need to respond with compassion and gentle honesty. They can acknowledge that miraculous recoveries do occur, but they are rare. The important message is to maintain open communication with the family.

Like parents who lose a child through death, the parents of the child lost to their world attempt to reconstitute a representation of the child. They bring items that belong to the child, such as favorite toys, music, and other objects cherished by the child. This is interpreted as an attempt to provide stimulation for the child in the hope of eliciting a response, to let the hospital staff know the child as the unique individual he or she was so that the parents' distress can be better appreciated, and to reconstitute an image of the child "lost" to them and for whom they mourn. An awareness of these behaviors and coping mechanisms provides nurses with the understanding that helps them support the parents in their grief process.

Superimposed on the process of grieving for the "lost" child, parents may be faced with difficult decisions. When the

NURSING DIAGNOSIS: High risk for suffocation (aspiration): ineffective airway clearance related to depressed sensorium, impaired motor function

PATIENT GOAL 1: Will maintain patent airway

• **NURSING INTERVENTIONS/*RATIONALES***

Position for optimum ventilation
　Insert oral airway if indicated
　Position with neck slightly extended and nose in "sniffing" position *to open trachea fully*
　Avoid neck hyperextension, *which can block airway*
　Place in semiprone or side-lying position *to prevent aspiration*
Remove accumulated secretions promptly *to prevent aspiration*
Administer care of endotracheal tube or tracheostomy if appropriate; have equipment available for emergency insertion if indicated for respiratory distress *to prevent delay in treatment*
Monitor artificial ventilation

• **EXPECTED OUTCOME**

Airway remains patent

NURSING DIAGNOSIS: High risk for injury related to physical immobility, depressed sensorium, intracranial pathology

PATIENT GOAL 1: Will maintain stable ICP

• **NURSING INTERVENTIONS/*RATIONALES***

Elevate head of bed 15 to 30 degrees with child's head in midline position *to facilitate venous drainage and avoid jugular compression*
Avoid positions or activities that increase ICP
　Pressure on neck veins
　　Turning side-to-side is contraindicated *because of risk of jugular compression*
　Flexion or hyperextension of neck
　Head rotation
　Valsalva maneuver
　Painful stimuli
　Respiratory procedures (especially suctioning, percussion)
Prevent constipation *because Valsalva maneuver increases ICP*
　*Administer stool softener as prescribed
　Closely monitor bowel elimination when child is receiving codeine *because of its constipating effect*
Minimize emotional stress and crying *because they cause increased ICP*
　Provide quiet, subdued environment
　Reduce environmental noise (e.g., placing earphones over child's ears *has been shown to lower ICP, heart rate, and blood pressure*)
　Provide pleasant auditory experiences
　Use therapeutic touch
　Avoid emotionally stressful conversation (e.g., about pain, condition, prognosis)

　*Administer sedation, if ordered, for extreme agitation or restlessness
Prevent or relieve pain, *since pain causes increased ICP*
　Closely observe child for signs of pain, especially changes in behavior (e.g., agitation); increased heart rate, respiratory rate, and blood pressure *(usually increase with pain);* decreased oxygen saturation
　Observe child's response during times of induced or suspected pain
　Observe child's response following a painful procedure or the administration of analgesia
　Use pain assessment record (see Chapter 21)
　*Administer paralyzing and analgesic agents if prescribed
Schedule disturbing procedures to take advantage of therapies that reduce ICP (e.g., bathe child after sedation or osmotherapy)
Monitor ICP monitoring device

• **EXPECTED OUTCOMES**

ICP remains within safe limits
Child shows no evidence of sustained increased ICP

PATIENT GOAL 2: Will exhibit no signs of cerebral hypoxia

• **NURSING INTERVENTIONS/*RATIONALES***

Maintain patent airway *because respiratory obstruction leads to cardiac arrest, and cerebral hypoxia lasting longer than 4 minutes nearly always causes irreversible brain damage*
Provide oxygen as indicated by objective signs or as ordered
*Hyperventilate at prescribed intervals if ordered
Monitor blood gases and pH
If child is on mechanical ventilation:
　Monitor for correct settings, proper functioning
　Prepare to provide artificial ventilation in case of ventilatory failure; have manual resuscitation bag at bedside
*Administer medications as ordered *to prevent cerebral edema and improve cerebral circulation*

• **EXPECTED OUTCOME**

Child breathes easily; respirations are within normal limits (see inside back cover)

PATIENT GOAL 3: Will exhibit no evidence of cerebral edema

• **NURSING INTERVENTIONS/*RATIONALES***

Elevate head of bed to 15 to 30 degrees *to facilitate venous drainage*
Maintain intravenous fluids as prescribed
　Avoid overhydration *to prevent cerebral edema*
Monitor intake and output
Monitor electrolyte balance and specific gravity *to detect signs of hypernatremia and hyperosmolality because diabetes insipidus and the syndrome of inappropriate antidiuretic hormone frequently occur with CNS diseases and trauma*
*Administer hyperosmolar fluids as prescribed
*Administer corticosteroids as ordered

• **EXPECTED OUTCOME**

Child exhibits no signs of sustained increased ICP

---

*Dependent nursing action.

PATIENT GOAL 4: Will experience no seizures

- **NURSING INTERVENTIONS/***RATIONALES*

Avoid stimulation that precipitates undesirable responses
Schedule nursing activities for minimum disturbance
*Administer antiepileptic drugs as prescribed
    Carefully administer phenytoin (Dilantin) if prescribed
    Administer drug slowly; *too-rapid administration may
    cause cardiac dysrhythmias*
    Infuse completely in 1 hour *because drug tends to precipi-
    tate*
    Never mix phenytoin with 5% dextrose; *drug will precipi-
    tate*
    Dilute phenytoin with normal saline *to decrease vein irrita-
    tion and pain*

- **EXPECTED OUTCOME**

Child exhibits no seizure activity or undue restlessness and
    agitation

PATIENT GOAL 5: Will exhibit stable body temperature

- **NURSING INTERVENTIONS/***RATIONALES*

Closely monitor child's temperature *because elevations often
    occur with CNS dysfunction*
Remove excess coverings
*Administer antipyretics if prescribed for fever
Give tepid sponge bath, if indicated, only for hyperthermia,
    not for fever, *because it may induce shivering*
Apply and monitor hypothermia blanket if indicated and or-
    dered; administer antishivering agents, if ordered, *because
    shivering increases ICP and metabolic rate*

- **EXPECTED OUTCOME**

Body temperature remains within safe limits (see inside back
    cover)

PATIENT GOAL 6: Will exhibit no evidence of respiratory tract infection

- **NURSING INTERVENTIONS/***RATIONALES*

Turn frequently—at least every 2 hours, as tolerated, unless
    contraindicated by increased ICP
Keep persons with upper respiratory tract infection away from
    child
Use good handwashing technique
Keep all equipment in contact with child clean or sterile
Provide good oral hygiene *to decrease presence of infective or-
    ganisms*
Perform chest physiotherapy if prescribed and as tolerated;
    avoid percussion, *since it can increased ICP*

- **EXPECTED OUTCOME**

Child exhibits no evidence of pulmonary dysfunction

PATIENT GOAL 7: Will experience no corneal irritation

- **NURSING INTERVENTIONS/***RATIONALES*

Patch eye, if indicated, *for protection*
Keep lids completely closed *to protect corneas when corneal
    reflexes are absent*

Instill "artificial tears" *to lubricate eyes*
Assess eyes carefully for early signs of irritation or inflammation

- **EXPECTED OUTCOME**

Corneas remain clear and moist

PATIENT GOAL 8: Will exhibit no breakdown in mucous membrane integrity

- **NURSING INTERVENTIONS/***RATIONALES*

Provide meticulous mouth care, *since mouth tends to become
    dry or coated with mucus*
Avoid drying products (e.g., lemon and glycerin swabs)

- **EXPECTED OUTCOME**

Mucous membranes remain clear, moist, and free of irritation

PATIENT GOAL 9: Will experience no physical injury

- **NURSING INTERVENTIONS/***RATIONALES*

Keep siderails up *to prevent falls*
Pad hard surfaces *that may injure extremities during spontane-
    ous or involuntary movements*

- **EXPECTED OUTCOME**

Child remains free of physical injury

PATIENT GOAL 10: Will maintain limb flexibility and
full range of motion

- **NURSING INTERVENTIONS/***RATIONALES*

Perform passive range-of-motion exercises *to prevent contrac-
    tures*
Position *to reduce contractures*
    Place small, rolled pad in palms to *maintain proper posi-
    tion of fingers*
    Use footboard or ankle-high shoes to *prevent footdrop*
    Splint joints, if needed, *to prevent severe contractures of
    wrists, knees, and ankles*

- **EXPECTED OUTCOME**

Joints remain flexible and retain full range of motion

> **NURSING DIAGNOSIS:** High risk for im-
> paired skin integrity related to immobility, body
> secretions, invasive procedures

PATIENT GOAL 1: Will maintain skin integrity

- **NURSING INTERVENTIONS/***RATIONALES*

Place child on pressure-reducing surface *to prevent tissue
    breakdown and pressure necrosis*
Change position frequently unless contraindicated by in-
    creased ICP
Protect pressure points (e.g., trochanter, sacrum, ankle, heels,
    shoulder, occiput)
Inspect skin surfaces regularly for signs of irritation, redness,
    evidence of pressure
Cleanse skin regularly, at least once daily
Protect skinfolds and surfaces that rub together *to prevent
    excoriation*
Keep clothing and linen clean, dry, and free of wrinkles
Carry out good perineal care

---

*Dependent nursing action.

Gently massage skin with lotion or other lubricating substance, unless on existing reddened pressure areas, *to stimulate circulation and prevent drying*

Protect lips with cream or ointment *to prevent drying and cracking*

- **EXPECTED OUTCOME**

Skin remains clean, intact, and free of irritation

> **NURSING DIAGNOSIS:** Feeding, bathing/ hygiene, toileting self-care deficits (level 4) related to physical immobility, perceptual and cognitive impairment

PATIENT GOAL 1: Will receive optimum nutrition

- **NURSING INTERVENTIONS/RATIONALES**

Provide nourishment in manner suitable to child's condition
Monitor intravenous feedings when ordered
Record intake and output
*Feed prescribed formula by means of nasogastric or gastrostomy tube
Weigh daily or as ordered *to monitor nutritional adequacy*

- **EXPECTED OUTCOME**

Child obtains sufficient nourishment

PATIENT GOAL 2: Will receive proper hygienic care

- **NURSING INTERVENTIONS/RATIONALES**

Bathe daily or more often if indicated
Dress appropriately
Keep hair clean, combed, and styled

- **EXPECTED OUTCOME**

Child appears clean and as well groomed as possible within limitations of condition

PATIENT GOAL 3: Will void and defecate adequately

- **NURSING INTERVENTIONS/RATIONALES**

Provide sufficient liquid intake, unless contraindicated by cerebral edema or if overhydration is a threat
Apply urine-collecting device or insert indwelling catheter (if ordered)
Provide proper care of catheter
Clean skin well after each elimination *to prevent skin irritation*
Diaper as needed *to contain stool and urine*
Check abdomen for evidence of distention
  Measure abdominal girth *to detect enlargement*
*Administer stool softener *to prevent constipation*
*Administer suppositories or enema as indicated *to promote evacuation*

- **EXPECTED OUTCOMES**

Child eliminates sufficient urine (specify)
Bowel is evacuated daily
Child's diaper area remains clean and free of irritation

*Dependent nursing action.

> **NURSING DIAGNOSIS:** Sensory/perceptual alterations (visual, auditory, kinesthetic, gustatory, tactile, olfactory) related to central nervous system impairment, bed rest

PATIENT GOAL 1: Will receive appropriate sensory stimulation

- **NURSING INTERVENTIONS/RATIONALES**

Provide tactile stimulation as tolerated
Provide auditory stimulation (e.g., by voice, radio, music box)
Provide visual stimuli appropriate for age
Provide proprioceptive stimulation (e.g., by rocking, cuddling)
Encourage family to participate in stimulation program
Demonstrate for family how and where to touch child

- **EXPECTED OUTCOMES**

Child receives sensory stimulation appropriate to age and condition
Child appears relaxed and rests quietly
Stimulation does not induce seizures or increase ICP

PATIENT GOAL 2: Will exhibit no evidence of pain

- **NURSING INTERVENTIONS/RATIONALES**

Assess for evidence of pain
Use pain assessment record *to document effectiveness of interventions*
Administer pain medication as needed

- **EXPECTED OUTCOME**

Child exhibits no evidence of pain

> **NURSING DIAGNOSIS:** Altered family processes related to a child hospitalized with a potentially fatal condition or permanent disability

PATIENT (FAMILY) GOAL 1: Will receive adequate support

- **NURSING INTERVENTIONS/RATIONALES AND EXPECTED OUTCOMES**

See Nursing Care Plan: The Family of the Ill or Hospitalized Child, Chapter 21

PATIENT (FAMILY) GOAL 2: Will express feelings and concerns

- **NURSING INTERVENTIONS/RATIONALES**

Provide needed information
Answer family's questions; encourage expression of feelings
Refer to persons or agencies for further information and clarification
Support parents' decisions

- **EXPECTED OUTCOME**

Family verbalizes feelings and concerns

child's brain is so severely damaged that vital functions must be maintained by artificial means, the parents must make the final decision to remove life-support systems. Since the decision is so difficult for parents, the practitioner is frequently placed in a position of making the decision indirectly. After providing the parents with all the information, the practitioner will suggest that the child be removed from the life support to "see if the child can make it without help." The approach relieves the parents of the decision and can be effective, but it is based on an evaluation of the parents' intellectual level and emotional state. Sometimes parents may even choose to refuse treatment if they believe it to be best for the child and the family (informed dissent). At other times parents request that "everything possible" be done for the child.

The nurses can be instrumental in providing guidance and clarifying information—a valued but demanding undertaking. It is not unusual for the family to ask the same questions and to compare responses elicited from different staff members. A child's death is an intensely personal issue that deserves direct involvement by the nurse and auxiliary support systems.

When the child has survived the illness or injury that produced the brain damage but is left unconscious permanently, the parents must decide whether to place the child in a chronic care facility or make arrangements to care for the child at home. The nurse can listen to the parents' discussions regarding alternatives, provide information where appropriate, and support the family in their decision. The nurse can help the family prepare for the transfer of the child and make referrals to persons or agencies that can provide additional assistance.

When the child has survived the cerebral insult and is not comatose, but physical and/or mental capacity is limited, either minimally or severely, families must cope with the long and tedious rehabilitation process and uncertain outcome. The drain on financial, emotional, and social resources can be enormous.

For parents who choose to care for their child at home, planning for home care begins early in the process of recovery. The family should become involved with the care of the child as soon as they indicate an interest and ability to do so. They need education and support in learning to care for the child, regular follow-up observation and assessment of the home management, and planning for some respite care of the child. Parents need to understand that it is important to plan for periodic relief from the continual care of the child (see Prepare for Discharge and Home Care, Chapter 21, and Home Care in Chapter 20).

❖ Evaluation

The effectiveness of nursing interventions for the unconscious child is determined by continual reassessment and evaluation of care based on the following observational guidelines and expected outcomes:

1. Monitor child's neurologic signs, vital signs, and behavior.
2. Observe child's response to nursing activities, therapies, and diagnostic procedures; monitor ICP.
3. Observe child's color, position, and motor activity; measure fluid and nutritional intake and output.
4. Monitor status of child's respiratory, renal, and gastrointestinal systems and skin.
5. Observe family behaviors and interview members regarding their understandings and their feelings and concerns.

Expected outcomes:
See Nursing Care Plan, pp. 994-996.

CEREBRAL TRAUMA

HEAD INJURY

Head injury is a pathologic process involving the scalp, skull, meninges, or brain as a result of mechanical force. According to national statistics and the **Safe Kids Campaign,*** injuries are the number one health risk for children and the leading cause of death in children older than 1 year of age. Yearly, one child in four in the United States will suffer an injury serious enough to require medical attention. Tragically, 8000 children are killed every year by injuries. It has been estimated that 300 per 100,000 children per year have a traumatic brain injury and that 10 per 100,000 children per year die as a result of the brain injury. Studies indicate that as many as three fourths of the childhood deaths caused by mechanical trauma are the direct result of a brain injury.

Etiology

The three major causes of brain damage in childhood in order of importance are falls, motor vehicle injuries, and bicycle injuries. Neurologic injury accounts for the highest mortality, with boys usually affected twice as often as girls. In motor vehicle accidents children less than 2 years of age are almost exclusively injured as passengers, whereas older children may also be injured as pedestrians or cyclists. The majority of deaths from brain trauma caused by bicycle injuries occur between the ages of 5 and 15 years. With the advent of bike helmet laws, this should be a decreasing trend.

The exposed nature of the head renders it particularly vulnerable to external violence, and many of the physical characteristics of children predispose them to craniocerebral trauma. For example, infants are frequently left unattended on beds, in high chairs, and in other places from which they can fall. Because the head of an infant or toddler is proportionately large and heavy in relation to other body parts, it is the most likely to be injured. Incomplete motor development contributes to falls at young ages, and the natural curiosity and exuberance of children increase their risk of an injury.

Pathophysiology

The pathology of brain injury is directly related to the force of impact. Intracranial contents (brain, blood, CSF) are damaged because the force is too great to be absorbed by the skull and musculoligamentous support of the head. The elastic, pliable skulls of infants and young children absorb much of the direct energy of physical impact to the head and afford some protection to intracranial structures. Although nervous tissue is delicate, it usually requires a severe blow to cause significant damage.

---

*SAFE KIDS, 111 Michigan Ave., N.W., Washington, DC 20010-2970; (202)884-4993.

A child's response to head injury is different from that of adults. The larger head size and insufficient musculoskeletal support render the very young child particularly vulnerable to acceleration-deceleration injuries. The surface area of the child's scalp is large with remarkable vascularity; therefore a child can bleed to death from a severe scalp laceration.

Primary head injuries are those that occur at a time of trauma and include skull fracture, contusions, intracranial hematoma, and diffuse injury. Subsequent complications include hypoxic brain damage, ICP, infection, and cerebral edema. The predominant feature of a child's brain injury is the diffuse amount of swelling that occurs. Hypoxia and hypercapnia threaten the energy requirements of the brain and increase cerebral bloodflow (CBF). The added volume across the blood-brain barrier plus the loss of autoregulation exacerbates cerebral edema. Pressure inside the skull greater than arterial pressure results in inadequate perfusion.

Cerebral hyperemia occurs more often in children, and this volume expansion may account for their tendency to develop intracranial hypertension (Ward, 1994). However, because the cranium of very young children has the ability to expand and the thin skull is more compliant, they may tolerate increases in ICP better than older children and adults. Children have a significantly higher percentage of good outcomes and a lower mortality rate, as well as a lower incidence of surgical mass lesions after severe head trauma. However, their thinner, softer brain may sustain greater long-term damage than previously suggested.

Physical forces act on the head through *acceleration, deceleration,* or *deformation.* Acceleration or deceleration is more descriptive of the circumstances responsible for most head injuries. When the stationary head receives a blow, the sudden acceleration causes deformation of the skull and mass movement of the brain. Continued movement of the intracranial contents allows the brain to strike parts of the skull (e.g., the sharp edges of the sphenoid or the irregular surface of the anterior fossa) or the edges of the tentorium.

Although the brain volume remains unchanged, significant distortion takes place as the brain changes shape in response to the force of impact to the skull. This movement can cause bruising at the point of impact *(coup)* and/or at a distance as the brain collides with the unyielding surfaces far removed from the point of impact *(contrecoup)* (Fig. 28-4). Thus a blow to the occipital region can cause severe injury to the frontal and temporal areas of the brain. Sudden deceleration, such as takes place during a fall, causes the greatest cerebral injury at the point of impact. Children with an acceleration/deceleration injury demonstrate diffuse generalized cerebral swelling produced by increased blood volume or a redistribution of cerebral blood volume (cerebral hyperemia) rather than by increased water content (edema), as seen in adults.

Another effect of brain movement is shearing stresses, which may tear small arteries and cause subdural hemorrhages. Another source of damage occurs when severe compression of the skull causes the brain to be forced through the tentorial opening. This can produce irreparable damage to the brainstem (Figs. 28-5 and 28-6).

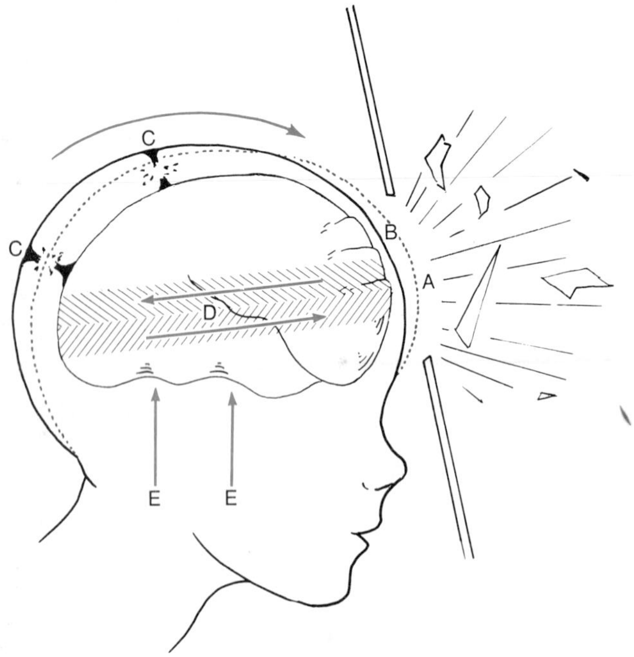

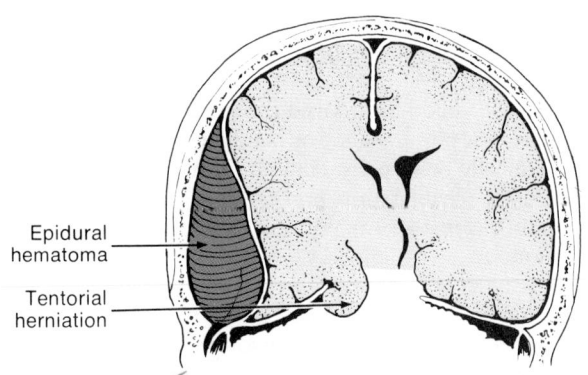

FIG. 28-5. Epidural (extradural) hematoma and compression of portion of temporal lobe through tentorial hiatus.

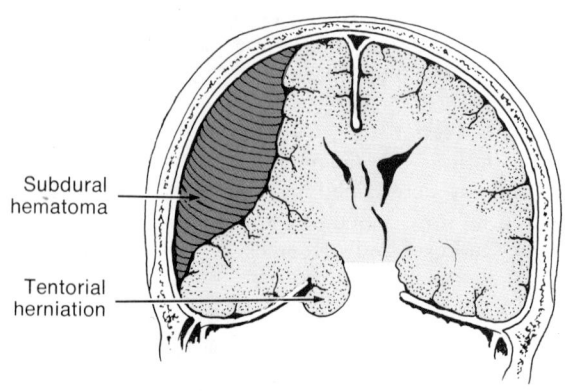

FIG. 28-6. Subdural hematoma.

FIG. 28-4. Mechanical distortions of cranium during closed head injury. **A,** Preinjury contour of skull; **B,** immediate postinjury contour of skull; **C,** torn subdural vessels; **D,** shearing forces; **E,** trauma from contact with floor of cranium. (Redrawn from Grubb RL, Coxe WS: Central nervous system trauma: cranial. In Eliasson SG, Prensky AL, Hardin WB Jr, editors: *Neurological pathophysiology,* New York, 1974, Oxford University Press.)

Concussion. The most common head injury is *concussion,* a transient and reversible neuronal dysfunction, with instantaneous loss of awareness and responsiveness, that results from trauma to the head and persists for a relatively short time, usually minutes or hours. It is generally followed by amnesia for the moment of the injury and a variable period before the injury. The common misconception that loss of consciousness is the hallmark of concussion is not true, especially for children. Concussion is correctly defined as "a traumatically induced alteration in mental status." Confusion and amnesia following head impact are the hallmarks of concussion.

The pathogenesis of concussion is still unclear but may be a result of shearing forces that cause stretching, compression, and tearing of nerve fibers, particularly in the area of the central brainstem, the seat of the reticular activating system. It has also been suggested that the anatomic alterations of nerve fibers cause the release of large quantities of acetylcholine into the CSF and a reduction in oxygen consumption with increased lactate production.

Contusion and Laceration. The terms *contusion* and *laceration* are used to describe visible bruising and tearing of cerebral tissue. Contusions represent petechial hemorrhages along the superficial aspects of the brain at the site of impact (coup injury) and/or a lesion remote from the site of direct trauma (contrecoup injury). In serious accidents there may be multiple sites of injury.

The major areas of the brain susceptible to contusion or laceration are the occipital, frontal, and temporal lobes. Also, the irregular surfaces of the anterior and middle fossae at the base of the skull are capable of producing bruises or lacerations on forceful impact. Contusions may cause focal disturbances in strength, sensation, or visual awareness. The degree of brain damage in the contused areas varies according to the extent of vascular injury. Signs will vary from mild, transient weakness of a limb to prolonged unconsciousness and paralysis. However, the signs and symptoms may be clinically indistinguishable from concussion.

The lower incidence of cerebral contusion in infancy has been attributed to the infant's pliable skull with less convolutional markings of the inner space between brain tissue and bone. Also, the infant's brain tissue has a softer consistency, which also reduces surface injury. However, infants who are roughly shaken (shaken baby syndrome) can sustain profound neurologic impairment, seizures, retinal hemorrhages, and intracranial subarachnoid or subdural hemorrhages. In addition to these classic injuries, high cervical spinal cord hemorrhages and contusions can occur.

Cerebral lacerations are generally associated with penetrating or depressed skull fractures. However, they may occur without fracture in small children. When brain tissue is actually torn, with bleeding into and around the tear, usually more severe and prolonged unconsciousness and paralysis occur, leaving permanent scarring and some degree of disability.

Fractures. Because of its flexibility, the immature skull is able to sustain a greater degree of deformation than the adult skull before it incurs a fracture. A great deal of force is required to produce a fracture in the skull of an infant. However, the undersurface of the skull contains grooves in which the meningeal arteries lie. A fracture that runs through one of these grooves may tear the artery and produce severe and damaging hemorrhage. Hypovolemic hypotension can occur in infants with skull fractures.

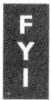 A fracture may occur with little or no brain damage, or severe and fatal brain injury can take place without fracture.

The types of fractures that occur are as follows:

Linear fractures are those in which the lines of the fracture are predetermined by the site and velocity of the impact, as well as by the strength of the bone. These are uncommon before 2 to 3 years of age but constitute the majority of childhood skull fractures.

Depressed fractures are those in which the bone is locally broken, usually into several irregular fragments that are pushed inward, causing pressure on the brain. The inner portion of the bone is more extensively fragmented than the outer portion, which almost invariably produces tears in the dura. These are uncommon before 2 to 3 years of age. In infants and very young children, the soft, malleable bone may become dented in a peculiar rounded or ping-pong ball depression, without laceration of either skin or dura.

Compound fractures consist of laceration of skin that extends to the site of the bony fracture, which can be linear, depressed, or comminuted.

Basilar fractures involve the basilar portion of the frontal, ethmoid, sphenoid, temporal, or occipital bones. Because of the proximity of the fracture line to structures surrounding the brainstem, this is a serious head injury.

Diastatic fractures are traumatic separations of cranial sutures. These most frequently affect the lambdoid suture and are rarely seen beyond the first 4 years of life. They require no specific treatment but should be observed for "growing fractures," development of a fluid-filled cyst.

Complications

The major complications of trauma to the head are hemorrhage, infection, edema, and herniation through the tentorium. Infection is always a hazard in open injuries, and edema is related to tissue trauma. Vascular rupture may occur even in minor head injuries, causing hemorrhage between the skull and cerebral surfaces. Compression of the underlying brain produces effects that can be rapidly fatal or insidiously progressive.

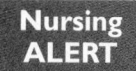 Posttraumatic meningitis should be suspected in children with increasing drowsiness and fever who also have basilar skull fractures.

Epidural Hemorrhage. The blood accumulates between the dura and the skull to form a hematoma, which, because of the difficulty with which dura is stripped from bone, forces the underlying brain contents downward and inward as the brain expands (see Fig. 28-5). Since bleeding is generally arterial, brain compression occurs rapidly. Most often the expanding hematoma is located in the parietotemporal region, forcing the medial portion of the temporal lobe under the edge of the tentorium, where it causes pressure on nerves and blood vessels. The lower incidence of epidural hematoma in childhood has been attributed to the fact that the middle meningeal artery is not embedded in the bone surface of the skull until approximately 2 years of age. Therefore a fracture of the temporal bone is less likely to lacerate the artery. Second, the dura closely adheres to the inner table of the skull, especially at the level of the sutures, making separation from bleeding less likely. However, a child's skull can be indented with sufficient force to tear the middle meningeal artery and the rebound intact without causing a fracture. Hemorrhage can also derive from dural veins or the dural sinuses, especially in infants and small children, in whom fracture is less likely to occur. In 20% to 40% of children a skull fracture is not detectable.

The classic clinical picture of epidural hemorrhage (momentary unconsciousness followed by a normal period, then lethargy or coma) is seldom evident in children (see box below for clinical manifestations). The period of impaired consciousness is frequently lacking, and the symptom-free period is atypical because of nonspecific complaints such as irritability, headache, and vomiting. The symptom-free period frequently lasts longer than 48 hours. Clinically significant epidural hematomas are uncommon in children younger than 4 years of age. These differences may be caused by the decreased tendency of the resilient skull to fracture; the ability of blood to escape through widened sutures, an open fontanel, or a fracture; bleeding from smaller vessels with less rapid and massive bleeding; lower systolic blood pressure in children; and possibly the decreased susceptibility of the child's brain to pressure changes.

Subdural Hemorrhage. A subdural hemorrhage is bleeding between the dura and the cerebrum, usually as a result of rupture of cortical veins that bridge the subdural space (see Fig. 28-6). Subdural hematomas are 10 times more fre-

quent than epidural hematomas, occurring most often in infancy, with a peak incidence at 6 months.

Unlike epidural hemorrhage, which develops inwardly against the less resistant brain tissue, subdural hemorrhage tends to develop more slowly and spreads thinly and widely until it is limited by the dural barriers—the falx and tentorium. Subdural hematoma is fairly common in infants, frequently as a result of birth trauma, falls, assaults, or violent shaking. The small subdural space and dura firmly attached to the skull in this area are highly vulnerable to increased ICP.

> **Nursing ALERT**
> Children with a subdural hematoma and retinal hemorrhages should be evaluated for the possibility of child abuse, especially shaken baby syndrome (SBS).

Repeated subdural taps often provide relief in the infant, as revealed by follow-up CT scans, improved neurologic status, and a flat anterior fontanel. Surgical evacuation of the hematoma is the treatment of choice in the older child and is frequently required in infants.

Cerebral Edema. Some degree of brain edema is expected, especially 24 to 72 hours after craniocerebral trauma. Cerebral edema caused by direct cellular injury or vascular injury induces vascular stasis, anoxia, and further vasodilation. If the progression continues unchecked, ICP exceeds arterial pressure and fatal anoxia ensues, and/or the pressure causes herniation of a portion of the brain over the edge of the tentorium, compressing the brainstem and occluding the posterior cerebral arteries. Diffuse cerebral swelling and changes in CBF are common patterns following head injury in children.

> **Nursing ALERT**
> If a child loses consciousness or vomits more than three times, medical attention should be sought.

Diagnostic Evaluation

A detailed history, especially a health history, both past and present, is essential in evaluating the child with a craniocerebral trauma. Certain disorders, such as drug allergies, hemophilia, diabetes mellitus, or epilepsy, may produce similar symptoms. Furthermore, even minor traumatic injury can aggravate a preexisting disease process. Events surrounding the injury often supply significant data. It must be determined whether the infant or child exhibited alterations in consciousness, and any other signs and behaviors exhibited by the child must be noted. Since head injuries are frequently accompanied by injuries in other areas, the examination is performed with care to avoid further damage.

> **Nursing ALERT**
> Stabilize a child's spine after head injury until a spinal cord injury is confirmed or ruled out.

Initial Assessment. Priorities in the initial phase in the care of a child with a head injury include assessment of the ABCs (airway, breathing, circulation); evaluation for shock;

CLINICAL MANIFESTATIONS OF ACUTE HEAD INJURY

Minor Injury
May or may not lose consciousness
Transient period of confusion
Somnolence
Listlessness
Irritability
Pallor
Vomiting (one or more episodes)

Signs of Progression
Altered mental status (e.g., difficulty rousing child)
Mounting agitation
Development of focal lateral neurologic signs (see p. 984)
Marked changes in vital signs

Severe Injury
Signs of increased ICP (see box on p. 984)
 Increased head size (infant)
 Bulging fontanel (infant)
Retinal hemorrhage
Extraocular palsies (especially cranial nerve VI)
Hemiparesis
Quadriplegia
Elevated temperature (sometimes)
Unsteady gait (older child)
Papilledema (older child)

Associated Signs
Skin injury (to area of head sustaining injury)
Other injuries (e.g., to extremities)

a neurologic examination, especially LOC; pupillary symmetry and response to light; and seizures. The assessment is carried out quickly in relation to vital signs (see Emergency Treatment). Excited and irritable children may have a rapid pulse, hyperventilate, appear pale, and feel clammy shortly after an injury.

> **Nursing ALERT**
> Deep, rapid, periodic, or intermittent and gasping respirations, wide fluctuations or noticeable slowing of the pulse, and widening pulse pressure or extreme fluctuations in blood pressure are signs of brainstem involvement. It is important to note that marked hypotension may represent internal injuries.

Ocular signs such as fixed and dilated pupils, fixed and constricted pupils, and pupils that are poorly reactive or unreactive to light and accommodation indicate increased ICP or brainstem involvement. It is important to remain with the child who demonstrates fixed and dilated pupils, since these are ominous signs, with the probability of respiratory arrest. Dilated, nonpulsating blood vessels indicate increased ICP before the appearance of papilledema. Retinal hemorrhages are seen in acute head injuries.

> **Nursing ALERT**
> Observation of asymmetric pupils or one dilated, unreactive pupil in a comatose child is a neurosurgical emergency that may require evacuation of an epidural hematoma.

Less urgent but important additional assessments include examination of the scalp for lacerations and palpation for other abnormalities. However, a significant amount of blood loss can occur from scalp lacerations.

> **Nursing ALERT**
> Bleeding from the nose or ears needs further evaluation, and a watery discharge from the nose (rhinorrhea) that is positive for glucose (as tested with Dextrostix) suggests leaking of CSF from a skull fracture.

An accurate assessment of clinical signs provides baseline information. Serial evaluations, preferably by a single observer, help to detect changes in the neurologic status. Alterations in mental status, evidenced by increased difficulty in rousing the child, mounting agitation, development of focal lateral neurologic signs, or marked changes in vital signs, usually indicate extension or progression of the basic pathologic process.

Special Tests. After a thorough clinical examination, a variety of diagnostic tests are helpful in providing a more definitive diagnosis of the type and extent of the trauma. The severity of a head injury may not be apparent on clinical examination of a child, but it will be detectable on a CT scan. Whenever the child has a history consistent with a serious head injury (unrestrained occupant in a severe motor vehicle accident or a fall from a significant height), it is important that a scan be performed even if the child initially appears alert and oriented. All children with head injuries who have any alteration of consciousness, headache, vomiting, skull

EMERGENCY TREATMENT
Head Injury

Assess child:
  A—airway
  B—bleeding
  C—circulation
Stabilize neck and spine
Clean any abrasions with soap and water.
  Apply clean dressing.
  If bleeding, apply ice for 1 hour to relieve pain and swelling.
Give only clear liquids until no vomiting for at least 6 hours.
Assess pain.
Check pupil reaction every 4 hours (including twice during night) for 48 hours.
Awaken twice during night to check level of consciousness.
Seek medical attention if there is any of the following:
  Injury sustained
    • at high speed (e.g., auto)
    • fall from a significant distance (e.g., roof, tree)
    • from great force (e.g., baseball bat)
    • under suspicious circumstances
  Child younger than 6 months of age
  Unconscious more than 5 seconds
  Discomfort (crying) more than 10 minutes after injury
  Headache that is severe, worsening, interferes with sleep
  Vomiting three or more times
  Swelling in front of or above earlobe or swelling that increases in size
  Confused or not behaving normally
  Difficult to rouse from sleep
  Difficulty with speaking
  Blurring of vision or seeing double
  Unsteady gait
  Difficulty using upper extremities
  Neck pain
  Pupils dilated or fixed
  Infant with bulging fontanel

fracture, seizure, or a predisposing medical condition should also undergo CT scanning.

MRI and neurobehavioral assessment following early head injury may be useful in documenting cognitive impairment in relation to structural alterations in the young brain. MRI provides details of soft tissues better than any other noninvasive device. Electroencephalography is not particularly helpful for early diagnosis but is useful for defining seizure activity or focal destructive lesions after the acute phase of illness. Lumbar puncture is rarely used in craniocerebral trauma and is contraindicated in the presence of increased ICP. In some centers monitoring ICP is part of the assessment.

Posttraumatic Syndromes. Posttraumatic syndromes can be clinically manifested because of structural complications resulting from a head injury and through the signs and symptoms demonstrated by the child. Structural complications can include hydrocephalus and focal deficits such as optic atrophy, cranial nerve palsies, motor deficits, diabetes insipidus, aphasia, and seizures. Behavioral disturbances include sleep disturbances, phobias, emotional lability, altered school performance, and changes related to aggressiveness or withdrawal. *Postconcussion syndrome* is a common sequela to brain injury and occurs within minutes to an hour after a minimum head injury. The manifestations vary with the age of the child. The syndrome occurs very frequently in children under 1 year of age. The syndrome in adolescents is similar to that in adults. The duration of manifestations can vary from several days to several months. Death from concussion is preventable unless overwhelming secondary brain injury has occurred (Bruce, 1993).

Posttraumatic seizures occur in a number of children who survive a head injury. The onset may be in the first 24 hours, usually within the first year, and in most cases within 2 years after the injury. *Structural complications* may occur, and the type of residual effect depends on the location and nature of the trauma. True mental retardation occurs only after severe injuries.

Therapeutic Management

The majority of children with mild to moderate concussion who have not lost consciousness can be cared for and observed at home after careful examination reveals no serious intracranial injury. Nurses should provide parents with clear explanations and instructions and should encourage them to ask questions both before and after leaving the medical facility if clarification is needed (see Family Focus box below). The parents are instructed to check the child every 2 hours to determine any changes in responsiveness. The sleeping child should be wakened to see if he or she can be roused normally. Parents are advised to maintain contact with the health professional, who usually wishes to examine the child again in 1 or 2 days. The manifestations of epidural hematoma in children do not generally appear until 24 hours or more after injury.

Children with severe injuries, those who have lost consciousness for more than a few minutes, and those with prolonged and continued seizures or other focal or diffuse neurologic signs must be hospitalized until their condition is stable and their neurologic signs have diminished.

The child is maintained on nothing by mouth or restricted to clear liquids, if able to take fluids by mouth, until it is determined that vomiting will not occur. Intravenous fluids are indicated in the child who is comatose or displays dulled sensorium and/or in the child with persistent vomiting. Fluid balance is closely monitored by daily weights, accurate intake and output measurements, and serum osmolality to detect early signs of water retention, excessive dehydration, and states of hypertonicity or hypotonicity.

The volume of intravenous fluid is carefully monitored to avoid aggravating any cerebral edema and to minimize the possibility of overhydration in case of SIADH. However, damage to the hypothalamus or pituitary gland may produce diabetes insipidus with its accompanying hypertonicity and dehydration.

Restlessness can be satisfactorily managed, if necessary, with mild sedation, and headache is usually controlled with acetaminophen (Tylenol). Antiepileptics are used for seizure control and frequently in cases of suspected contusion or laceration. Antibiotics may be administered if there are lacerations, CSF leakage, or excessive cerebral tissue damage. Prophylactic tetanus toxoid is given as appropriate. Cerebral edema is managed as described for the unconscious child. Hyperthermia is controlled with tepid sponges or a hypothermia blanket.

Surgical Therapy. Scalp lacerations are sutured after the underlying bone is carefully examined (see Atraumatic Care box). Depressed fractures require surgical reduction and removal of bone fragments. Torn dura is sutured. "Ping-pong ball" skull fractures in very young infants ordinarily correct themselves within a few weeks and do not require specific treatment, although they can be reduced by pressure against the bone.

Prognosis. The outcome of craniocerebral trauma depends on the extent of injury and complications. However, the outlook is generally more favorable for children than for adults. Over 90% of children with concussions or simple linear fractures recover without symptoms after the initial period. The incidence of fatalities and neurologic sequelae is lower in children, even in those with severe head injuries. The prognosis for recovery is primarily related to the duration of coma and the degree of injury. The combination of impaired consciousness and skull fracture carries the highest risk of complication.

The concern regarding outcome is increasingly focused on cognitive, emotional, and/or mental problems. Recent studies indicate that children experience a higher frequency of psychologic disturbances following head injury, whereas adults are more prone to complaints of a physical nature.

Children may be more vulnerable than adults to long-term cognitive and behavioral dysfunction after diffuse brain injury. Even with recovery, the effects of brain injury on a child's potential can never be known.

True coma (not obeying commands, eyes closed, and not speaking) usually does not last more than 2 weeks. A child's eventual outcome can range from brain death to a persistent vegetative state to complete recovery. However, even the best recovery may be associated with personality changes, including mood lability and loss of confidence, impaired short-term memory, headaches, and subtle cognitive impairments. Many

---

FAMILY FOCUS
Maintaining Contact

Maintaining contact with parents for continued observation and reevaluation of the child, when indicated, facilitates early diagnosis and treatment of possible complications from head injury, such as hematoma, hydrocephalus, cysts, and posttraumatic seizures. Children are generally hospitalized for 24 to 48 hours' observation if their family lives far from medical facilities or lacks transportation or a telephone that would provide access to immediate help. Other circumstances, such as language or other communication barriers, or even emotional trauma, may hinder learning and make it difficult for families to feel confident in caring for their child at home.

ATRAUMATIC CARE
Noninvasive Local Anesthesia

The use of topical lidocaine, adrenalin, and tetracaine (LAT) adrenaline and cocaine (TC), or TC with tetracaine (TAC) provides noninvasive anesthesia for suturing lacerations (Bonadio and Wagner, 1992; Ernst and others, 1995).

children are left with significant disabilities after head injury that appear months later as learning difficulties, behavioral changes, or emotional disturbances (Reynolds, 1992). Generally, within 6 months to 1 year after the injury, 90% of the long-term neurologic outcome has been achieved.

Nursing Considerations

The hospitalized child requires careful neurologic assessment and evaluation (including vital signs) repeated at frequent intervals to provide information needed to establish a correct diagnosis, to reveal signs and symptoms of increased ICP, to determine clinical management, to prevent many complications, and to provide support to the child and family during the recovery phases.

The child is placed on bed rest, usually with the head of the bed elevated slightly, and appropriate safety measures, such as siderails kept up for older children and seizure precautions for children of all ages, are implemented. For the extremely restless child, hard surfaces may have to be padded and restraint used to prevent the possibility of further injury. Care is individualized according to the specific needs of the child. The unconscious child is managed as described in the previous section, but most childhood head injuries are those causing momentary stunning or temporary unconsciousness. Children may be restless and irritable, but more often their reaction is to fall asleep when left undisturbed. A quiet environment helps reduce the restlessness and irritability. Shining bright lights directly into the child's face is irritating and often makes checking the ocular responses more difficult to perform and more aggravating to the child.

Frequent examinations of vital signs, neurologic signs, and LOC are extremely important nursing observations. When possible, they should be performed by a single observer to better detect subtle changes that may indicate worsening of neurologic status. Pupils are checked for size, equality, reaction to light, and accommodation. After the initial elevations usually seen after injury, the vital signs generally return to normal unless there is brainstem involvement. An axillary measurement of temperature is the safest method, since seizures are not uncommon and vomiting is a frequent response in children, especially when the child is disturbed.

The most important nursing observation is assessment of the child's LOC. Alterations in consciousness appear earlier in the progression of an injury than alterations of vital signs or focal neurologic signs. Some expected responses may be misinterpreted as deviations from the normal. Frequent examinations of alertness are fatiguing to the child; therefore the child often desires to fall asleep, which may be confused with depressed consciousness. When left alone, the child promptly dozes. It is not uncommon to observe ocular divergence through the partially closed eyelids.

A key nursing role is to provide sedation and analgesia for the child. The conflict between the need to promote comfort and relieve anxiety in the child versus the need to be able to assess for neurologic changes presents a dilemma. However, both goals can be achieved with close observation of the child's LOC and response to analgesics, use of a pain assessment record, and effective communication with the practitioner. To differentiate between sedation from an opioid or the injury, naloxone (Narcan) can be given *slowly* to reverse the opioid's sedative effect. Decreasing restlessness after administration of an analgesic most likely reflects pain control rather than a decreasing LOC.

Observations of position and movement provide additional information. Any abnormal posturing is noted, as well as whether or not it occurs continuously or intermittently. Are the child's handgrips strong and equal in strength? Are there any signs of decerebrate or decorticate posturing? What is the child's response to stimulation? Is movement purposeful, random, or absent? Are movement and/or sensation equal on both sides or restricted to one side only?

The child may complain of headache or other discomfort. The child who is too young to describe a headache will be fussy and resist being handled. The child who suffers from vertigo will often assume a position and vigorously resist efforts to be moved. Forcible movement causes the child to vomit and display spontaneous nystagmus. Seizures, relatively common in children with craniocerebral trauma, may be of any type but are more often generalized, regardless of the type of injury. Any seizure activity should be carefully observed and described in detail. Children in postictal (postseizure) states are more lethargic, with sluggish pupils.

Drainage from any orifice is noted. Bleeding from the ear suggests the possibility of a basal skull fracture. The amount and characteristics of the drainage are observed, and since the auditory canal may be a source of infection, dry, sterile cotton can be placed loosely at the orifice and changed when soiled.

> **Nursing ALERT**
> Suctioning through the nares or passing a nasogastric tube is contraindicated, since there is a high risk of secondary infection and the probability of the catheter entering the brain substance through the fracture.

Head trauma is frequently accompanied by other undetected injuries; therefore any bruises, lacerations, or evidence of internal injuries or fractures of the extremities is noted and reported. Associated injuries are evaluated and treated appropriately.

The child with normal LOC is usually allowed clear liquids unless fluid is restricted. If the child has an intravenous infusion, it is maintained as prescribed. The diet is advanced to that appropriate for the child's age as soon as the condition permits. Intake and output are measured and recorded, and any incontinence of bowel or bladder is noted in the child who has been toilet trained.

The child should be observed for any unusual behavior, but behavior should be interpreted in relation to the child's normal behavior. For example, urinary incontinence during sleep would be of no consequence in a child who routinely wets the bed but would be highly significant for one who is always dry. In addition, a child who is subject to nightmares might cry out and demonstrate agitated behavior at night. Parents are valuable resources. Information obtained from parents at or shortly after admission is helpful in evaluating the child's behavior; for example, the ease with which the child is roused normally, the usual sleeping position, how much the child sleeps during the day, motor activity the child is capable of (rolling over, sitting up, climbing), hearing and visual acuity, appetite, and manner of eating (spoon, bottle, cup). There would be less concern about a child who falls asleep several times during the day if this particular type of behavior is consistent with the child's usual behavior.

Family Support. The emotional and educational support of the family of children who have suffered head injury presents a formidable, challenging aspect to nursing care. Witnessing the parents' ordeal of grief and helplessness on seeing their child in an intensive care unit connected to monitoring equipment in an altered state evokes empathy. The nurse can encourage the family to be involved in the child's care, to bring in familiar belongings, or to make a tape recording of familiar voices and sounds. Parents may need a demonstration on how to touch or cuddle their child and may want to talk about their grief. The nurse can listen attentively, reinforce what is being done to assist the child, and direct parents toward signs and symptoms of recovery to instill hope without promises. A common phenomenon is for families to seek information from all health care providers, asking, "What will she be like? What do you know?" as they search for some clue that the child is recovering. Honesty and kindness, along with competent care, distinguish excellent nursing abilities.

When the child is discharged, the parents are advised of probable posttraumatic symptoms that may be expected, such as behavioral changes, sleep disturbances, phobias, and seizures. They should understand observations that should be made and how to contact the physician, nurse, or health facility in case the child develops any unusual signs or symptoms. The importance of follow-up evaluation should be emphasized. It is often advisable to refer the family to a public health agency for home follow-through to be certain that the child receives posthospital evaluation.

Rehabilitation. The rehabilitation and management of the child with permanent brain injury are essential aspects of care. Rehabilitation of brain-injured children is begun as soon as feasible and usually involves the family and a rehabilitation team. Careful assessment of the child's capabilities, limitations, and probable potential is made as early as possible and appropriate interventions are implemented to maximize the residual capacities. The *National Head Injury Foundation** "arose from the mutual frustration and sense of hopelessness experienced by families in their search for appropriate facilities and support to return head-injured loved ones to their maximum functioning potential." It provides information and listings of rehabilitation services and support groups throughout the country.

Pediatric trauma rehabilitation is a national concern. Coordinating care and services for early rehabilitation involves identifying the child and family's response to the traumatic injury and disability, securing available resources, and recognizing the parental role in the process.

The child with a disability resulting from head trauma requires assessment on a physical, cognitive, emotional, and social level. The child has experienced separation, pain, sensory deprivation and overload, changes in circadian cycle, and fear of the unknown. Recovery and transition require new coping strategies at the same time that regressive and acting-out behavior may start. Parents and children need honest communication for decision making. Rehabilitation is advocated when the child is making progress beyond what can be provided in a hospital setting. The Rancho Los Amigos Scale provides a systematic assessment of the progress a child with a severe head injury may achieve.

Prevention. Tremendous strides have been taken in the prevention of cerebral damage after head injury in children. New developments requiring research point to the prevention of cellular injury or the primary insult. However, the greatest benefit lies in prevention of head injuries. Nurses can exert a valuable influence on behalf of children through education. The reason injuries remain preventable is that unnecessary risks go unchecked. Inadequate supervision combined with a child's natural sense of indestructibility and exploration can lead to lethal results. Nurses are in the unique position of influencing caregivers in terms of growth and development. Banning the use of infant walkers is an example. This equipment does not help develop motor skills but places infants at risk for head and neck injuries from falls, especially down steps. Public education, coupled with legislative support, can prevent childhood injuries.

(For extensive discussions of childhood injuries, see the discussions on injury prevention in Chapters 10, 12, 13, 15, and 16. See also Childhood Mortality in Chapter 1 and Nursing Care Plan: The Child with a Head Injury*.)

NEAR-DROWNING

Drowning ranks second as a cause of accidental death in children. Most cases of drowning are accidental, usually involving children who are helpless in water, such as inadequately attended children in or near swimming pools or infants in bathtubs; small children who fall into ponds, streams, and flooded excavations, usually near home; occupants of pleasure boats who fail to wear life preservers; children who have diving accidents; and children who are able to swim but overestimate their endurance. Accidental drowning occurs five times more often in boys than in girls; 50% of children are under the age of four and 90% occur in private swimming pools (Kyriacou Arcinue, and Peek, 1994).

Drowning can take place in any body of water, including such unlikely places as a pail of water. Top-heavy toddlers fall head first into a pail of water, their arms become trapped, and they are unable to free themselves. Hot tubs and whirlpool spas have been implicated in childhood drowning injury. The suction created at the outlet is strong enough to trap even larger children underwater. Drowning as a form of fatal child abuse has also been recognized as a problem. Homicidal drownings are unwitnessed, usually occur in the home, and the victims are either infants or toddlers. However, with expeditious treatment many children can be and are being saved. For purposes of this discussion, two terms need clarification:

Drowning—death from asphyxia while submerged, regardless of whether fluid has entered the lungs
Near-drowning—survival at least 24 hours after submersion in a fluid medium

Pathophysiology

The major pulmonary changes that occur in drowning are directly related to the length of submersion (regardless of the

---

*1140 Connecticut Ave., N.W., Suite 812, Washington, DC 20036; (202) 296-6443 or (800) 444-6443 (Family Helpline).

*In Wong DL: *Wong and Whaley's Clinical manual of pediatric nursing*, ed 4, St Louis, 1996, Mosby.

type and amount of fluid aspirated), the physiologic response of the victim, and the development and degree of immersion hypothermia. In addition, cerebral recovery depends on the effectiveness of initial resuscitation and subsequent critical care measures to support cerebral salvage.

Physiologic factors that influence the extent of damage from immersion include resistance to asphyxia and anoxia, which shows some individual variation. There is greater resistance with diminishing age; young children can withstand longer periods of submersion. More important is the drowning, or diving, reflex. This neurologic response is triggered by immersion of the face in cold water. Blood is shunted away from the periphery, and the flow is concentrated to the brain and heart predominantly.

The problems created by near-drowning are (1) hypoxia and asphyxiation, (2) aspiration, and (3) hypothermia (except near-drowning in hot tubs). Cardiopulmonary arrest is secondary to asphyxia.

Hypoxia is the primary problem because it results in global cell damage, and different cells tolerate variable lengths of anoxia. Neurons, especially cerebral cells, sustain irreversible damage after 4 to 6 minutes of submersion. The heart and lungs can survive up to 30 minutes. Regardless of the amount of water aspirated, there is arterial hypoxemia (resulting from atelectasis with shunting of blood through the nonventilated alveoli) and a combined respiratory acidosis (resulting from retained carbon dioxide) and metabolic acidosis (caused by buildup of acid metabolites from anaerobic metabolism). The pathologic events are directly related to the duration of submersion. The major difficulty is acute ventilatory insufficiency. Approximately 10% of drowning victims die without aspirating fluid but succumb from acute asphyxia as a result of prolonged reflex laryngospasm.

Aspiration of fluid occurs in the majority of drownings. The aspirated fluid results in pulmonary edema, atelectasis, airway spasm, and pneumonitis, which aggravates the hypoxia. It was previously thought that submersion in salt water or fresh water altered the physiologic response to near-drowning. However, there is no clinically significant difference in the response of human survivors, and the submersion does not alter the therapy or outcome.

Hypothermia occurs rapidly in infants and children partly because of their large surface area relative to body mass and partly as a result of the cold water itself. Water is an excellent heat conductor, and the contact with the skin is increased by struggling. Hypothermia may make resumption or maintenance of cardiac function possible if body temperature is less than 30° C (86° F). Profound hypothermia is usually evidence of lengthy submersion.

Therapeutic Management

Resuscitative measures should begin at the scene of a drowning, and the victim should be transported to the hospital with maximum ventilatory and circulatory support. Many victims need care for some time after aspiration of fluid. In the hospital, intensive pulmonary care is implemented and continued according to the needs of the patient.

In general, the management of the near-drowning victim is based on the degree of cerebral insult (see box). The first priority is to restore oxygen delivery to the cells and prevent further hypoxic damage. A spontaneously breathing child will

---

CLINICAL MANIFESTATIONS OF NEAR-DROWNING

Directly related to the degree of consciousness following rescue and resuscitation:

Category A: Awake (minimum injury)
- Fully conscious
- May have mild hypothermia
- Mild chest radiographic changes
- Mild arterial blood gas abnormalities

Category B: Blunted sensorium (moderate injury)
- Obtunded
- Stuporous
- Purposeful response to painful stimuli
- Mild to moderate hypothermia
- Respiratory distress (frequently)
- Chest radiographs abnormal
- Arterial blood gas abnormalities

Category C: Comatose (severe anoxia)
- Patient unarousable
- Abnormal response to pain
- Abnormal respiratory pattern
- Seizures
- Shock
- Marked arterial blood gas abnormalities
- Abnormal chest radiographs
- Dysrhythmias
- Metabolic acidosis
- Hyperkalemia, hyperglycemia
- Disseminated intravascular coagulation

Also:
- **C1:** Decorticate, Cheyne-Stokes respirations
- **C2:** Decerebrate, central hyperventilation
- **C3:** Flaccid, apneustic, or cluster breathing
- **C4:** Flaccid, apneic, no detectable circulation

---

do well in an oxygen-enriched atmosphere; the more severely affected child will require endotracheal intubation and mechanical ventilation. Blood gases and pH are monitored frequently as a guide to oxygen, fluid, and electrolyte therapies.

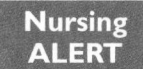 **Nursing ALERT** All children experiencing near-drowning should be admitted to the hospital for observation. Complications of respiratory distress and cerebral edema may occur 24 hours after the incident.

Aspiration pneumonia is a frequent complication that occurs about 48 to 72 hours after the episode. Bronchospasm, alveolar-capillary membrane damage, atelectasis, abscess formation, and hyaline membrane disease are other complications that occur after aspiration of fluid.

Prognosis. Studies report that the best predictors of a good outcome were length of submersion in non-icy water (>5° C [41° F]) for less than 5 minutes and the presence of sinus rhythm, reactive pupils, and neurologic responsiveness at the scene. The worst prognoses—for death or severe neurologic impairment—were in children submerged for more than 10 minutes and not responding to advanced life support within 25 minutes. All children without spontaneous, purposeful movement and normal brainstem function 24 hours after near drowning suffered severe neurologic deficits or death (Bratton, Jardine, and Morray, 1994).

Nursing Considerations

Nursing care depends on the condition of the child. A child who survives may need intensive respiratory nursing care with attention to vital signs, mechanical ventilation and/or tracheostomy, blood gas determination, chest therapy, and intravenous infusion. Frequently the child is comatose for an indefinite period and requires the same care as an unconscious child.

A difficult aspect in the care of the child victim of near-drowning is helping the parents cope with severe guilt reactions. The magnitude of the event is so great that efforts to provide comfort and support are of only limited success. Parents need to hear that everything possible is being done to treat the child, and this message needs to be repeated often.

The parents of the child who is saved from death are also faced with the anxiety of not knowing what the outcome will be, and sometimes they wish for the death of the child. Because their situation generates such intense feelings of loneliness, it is important for families to know that they are not alone. They need to be reminded frequently that there are caring people to assist them both during the crisis and later. Additional sources of support that can be recommended are psychiatric and social work consultants, community services, and religious support. Self-help groups are excellent if these are available in the community.

Nurses often have difficulty relating to the parents if obvious neglect has precipitated the accident and subsequent problems; therefore it is important for those who care for these children and their families to assess their own feelings about the situation, as well as the coping abilities and resources of the family. Caring for near-drowning victims and their families requires nurses to be sensitive to the needs of the child and the family and to recognize their own reactions and emotions.

Prevention. Most drownings, particularly of infants or small children, can be prevented with adequate supervision. Water safety and survival training should be required for all school-age children, and nurses can be active advocates in their communities. Nurses are also in a position to emphasize the importance of adequate adult supervision when children are in the water. Young children should never be left unattended when in or near the water. Parents with pools should know cardiopulmonary resuscitation (CPR) techniques.* See also Injury Prevention, Chapters 10, 12, 13, 15 and 16.

CENTRAL NERVOUS SYSTEM TUMORS[†]

Two major forms of childhood cancer—brain tumors and neuroblastomas—are derived from neural tissue. Both these tumors are difficult to treat and have not demonstrated the dramatic improvements in survival seen in may other forms of childhood cancer. Neuroblastomas, tumors that usually arise in the autonomic nervous system or adrenal medulla,

*Home care instructions for CPR are in Wong DL: *Wong and Whaley's Clinical manual of pediatric nursing,* ed 4, St Louis, 1996, Mosby.
[†]Marilyn Hockenberry-Eaton, PhD, RN,C, PNP, and Nancy E. Kline, MS, RN, CPNP, revised this section.

are not cerebral tumors but are included here for convenience.

BRAIN TUMORS

Brain tumors are the most common solid tumors that occur in children and are second only to leukemia as a form of cancer. They may be benign or malignant. The majority of tumors (about 60%) are *infratentorial* (below the tentorium cerebelli). They occur in the posterior third of the brain, primarily in the cerebellum or brainstem. This anatomic distribution accounts for the frequency of symptoms resulting from increased ICP. A smaller number are *supratentorial,* or

---

CLINICAL MANIFESTATIONS OF BRAIN TUMORS

Headache
Recurrent and progressive
In frontal or occipital areas
Worse on arising, less during day
Intensified by lowering head and straining, such as during bowel movement, coughing, sneezing

Vomiting
With or without nausea or feeding
Progressively more projectile
More severe in morning
Relieved by moving about and changing position

Neuromuscular Changes
Incoordination or clumsiness
Loss of balance (use of wide-based stance, falling, tripping, banging into objects)
Poor fine motor control
Weakness
Hyporeflexia or hyperreflexia
Positive Babinski sign
Spasticity (in child older than 1 year of age)
Paralysis

Behavioral Changes
Irritability
Decreased appetite
Failure to thrive
Fatigue (frequent naps)
Lethargy
Coma

Cranial Nerve Neuropathy
Cranial nerve involvement varies according to tumor location
Most common signs
    Head tilt
    Visual defects (nystagmus, diplopia, strabismus, episodic "greying out" of vision, and visual field defects)

Vital Sign Disturbances
Decreased pulse and respiration
Increased blood pressure
Widened pulse pressure
Hypothermia or hyperthermia

Other Signs
Seizures
Cranial enlargement*
Tense, bulging fontanel at rest*
Nuchal ridigity
Papilledema (edema of optic nerve)

*Present only in infants and young children.

within the anterior two thirds of the brain, mainly the cerebrum.

Neoplasms can arise from any cell within the cranium, and the type of cell in which the tumor has its origin provides a histologic classification for major tumors. The major infratentorial tumors of childhood are medulloblastoma, cerebellar astrocytoma, brainstem glioma, and ependymomas. Gliomas, arising from glial cells (the supporting structures of the brain), are the most common brain tumors in children. Astrocytomas, the most common glial tumor, arise from astrocytes, cells that form most of the supportive tissues for the neurons.

Diagnostic Evaluation

The signs and symptoms of brain tumors are those of increased ICP and are directly related to their anatomic location and size and to some extent the age of the child. In infants, whose cranial sutures are still open, virtually no early detectable symptoms develop. It is not until spinal fluid obstruction causes markedly increased head size that a lesion may be suspected. Even in older children, clinical manifestations are nonspecific. However, the most common symptoms are headache, especially on awakening, and vomiting that is not related to feeding. The common clinical manifestations of brain tumors are presented in the box on p. 1006.

Diagnosis of a brain tumor is based subjectively on presenting clinical signs (see box) and objectively on neurologic tests. Because the signs and symptoms are vague and easily overlooked, early diagnosis necessitates a high index of suspicion during history taking. A number of tests may be used in the neurologic evaluation, but the most common diagnostic procedure is magnetic resonance imaging (MRI), which determines the location and extent of the tumor. Other tests that may be used include computed tomography (CT), angiography, electroencephalography, or lumbar puncture, although lumbar puncture is dangerous in the presence of increased ICP because of the possibility of brainstem herniation following a sudden release of pressure.

Therapeutic Management

Treatment may involve the use of surgery, radiotherapy, and chemotherapy. All three may or may not be used, depending on the type of tumor. The treatment of choice is total removal of the tumor without residual neurologic damage. Patients with the most complete tumor removal have the greatest chance of survival. Radiotherapy is used to treat most tumors and to shrink the size of the tumor before attempting surgical removal. Chemotherapy is being used with increased

---

frequency and is helpful in delaying the timing of radiation (Duffner and others, 1993).

Prognosis. The prognosis for the child with a brain tumor depends on the type of brain tumor, the size of the tumor, the extent of the disease, and the age of the child. Problems associated with treatment and relatively poor prognosis, primarily in infants and young children, are compounded by serious late effects of therapy (Duffner and Cohen, 1991). A decline in incidence of children with medulloblastoma has been significantly linked with a protective effect of maternal folate, iron, and multivitamin supplementation. The introduction of periconceptional multivitamin supplementation in the 1980s may have caused this significant decline of medulloblastoma (Thorne, Pearson, and Nicoll, 1994).

Nursing Considerations

medulloblastoma most common

❖ Assessment

A child admitted to the hospital with neurologic dysfunction is often suspected of having a brain tumor, although the actual diagnosis is as yet unconfirmed. Establishing a baseline of data on which to compare preoperative and postoperative changes is an essential step toward planning physical care and preventing complications. It also allows the nurse to assess the degree of physical incapacity and the family's emotional reaction to the diagnosis.

Vital signs, including blood pressure and pulse pressure (the difference between systolic and diastolic pressures), are taken routinely and more often when any change is noted. Any sudden variations are reported immediately. It is especially important to note a change in vital signs during or following diagnostic procedures. A routine neurologic assessment is also performed at the same time as vital signs, and head circumference is measured on infants and very young children.

The child is observed for evidence of headache, vomiting, and any seizure activity. The location, severity, and duration of the headache are noted, as well as its relationship to activity and time of day. Behaviors such as lying flat and facing away from light or refusing to engage in play are clues to discomfort in the nonverbal child. The child's gait is observed at least once daily. Head tilt and other changes in posturing are always noted.

❖ Nursing Diagnoses

A number of nursing diagnoses will be evident following a thorough assessment of the child and family. Some of these are outlined in the accompanying box; others may be determined in individual cases.

❖ Planning

Goals of care for the child with a brain tumor are as follows:

1. Child and family will be prepared for diagnostic/operative procedures.
2. Child will experience no postoperative complications.
3. Child and family will receive adequate support.
4. Child will return to normal functioning.

❖ Implementation

The suspected diagnosis of a brain tumor is always a crisis event. Despite the fact that some tumors are removed with

---

> **NURSING DIAGNOSES: THE CHILD WITH A BRAIN TUMOR**
>
> Sensory/perceptual alterations (visual, auditory, kinesthetic, gustatory, tactile, olfactory related to altered sensory reception, transmission, and/or integration)
> Pain related to increased ICP
> Altered family processes related to situational crisis (child with a serious illness)
> Anxiety related to diagnosis, diagnostic and treatment procedures
> Anticipatory grieving related to potential loss of child

excellent results, the physician can rarely give definitive answers regarding prognosis until after surgery. Therefore parents and older children require much emotional support to face the diagnostic procedures and a craniotomy.

Prepare Child and Family for Diagnostic/Operative Procedures. How children are prepared for the diagnostic tests depends on their age and previous experience. Since most of the tests involve x-ray equipment, the child may be familiar with the procedure. By the time most children are late preschoolers, they know that the head and brain are important parts of their bodies. It may be helpful to have them draw their concept of the brain in order to clarify misconceptions and base the explanation on their level of understanding.

Although the temptation is to justify the need for surgery by stating that removing the tumor will take away various symptoms, the nurse should refrain from emphasizing this point too strenuously. Postsurgery headaches and cerebellar symptoms, such as ataxia, may be aggravated rather than improved. Surgery may not improve vision. With optic gliomas the child will be blind in one eye. Finally, surgical removal of the mass may be impossible, and after surgery there may be temporary deterioration of functioning. Being honest before surgery most often makes honesty after the operation easier because no false hopes were created.

However, honesty does not negate instilling hope. A truthful explanation regarding the operation is: "The surgeon will see exactly where the tumor is. If it is small and in one place, it will be removed. If it is large, as much of it as possible will be removed so that some of your symptoms will go away." It is best to deliver information in small amounts to let the child pursue additional answers. For example, some children will ask about what happens when part of the tumor is left in. An honest reply is that, after surgery, a special radiation machine and/or drugs may be used to make the tumor smaller. A further explanation of radiation or chemotherapy should be delayed until a decision regarding these treatments is made.

The hair is shaved in the operating room just before surgery, or in the child's room, usually the night before surgery. When shaving is done with the child awake, the procedure is approached in a sensitive, positive way. If the child's hair is long, it should be braided so that the long swatch can be saved. Showing children how they look at different stages of the process helps them prepare for the final appearance.

Once the hair is clipped very short or shaved, the child can be given a cap or scarf to wear to camouflage the baldness. Every precaution is taken to provide privacy during the procedure and to protect the child from teasing or ridicule by other children before surgery. It is also emphasized that the hair will regrow shortly after surgery. Depending on the child's immediate adjustment to the hair loss, the nurse may introduce the idea of wearing a wig until the hair is grown in, particularly if additional irradiation or chemotherapy is anticipated.

The child is also told about the size of the dressing. Usually the entire scalp is covered to maintain a tight wound closure, even if a small incision is made. Infratentorial head dressings may be attached to the upper back and extend forward on the neck to maintain slight extension and alignment as a precaution against wound rupture. Applying a similar

dressing or "special hat" to a doll is often a less traumatic way of demonstrating the physical appearance.

The child also needs a brief explanation of how he or she will feel after surgery and where he or she will be. Ordinarily children will return to a special intensive care unit, which they may visit beforehand, depending on hospital policy. The child should be aware that he or she may be sleepy for some time after surgery and that a headache is likely, although it should last only a few days.

Parents need similar explanations before surgery, especially in terms of special equipment used in the intensive care unit, dressings, and their child's behavior. For example, they should know that it is not unusual for the child to be comatose or lethargic for a few days after surgery. The nurse may wish to encourage less frequent visiting during this period so that parents can rest and be able to support their child when he or she awakens.

It is also advisable for the nurse to participate in preoperative conferences with the physician and parents. The nurse needs to know what information the parents have been given in order to be able to give further explanations or emotional support when necessary.

Prevent Postoperative Complications. Usually the surgeon will prescribe specific orders for vital signs, neurologic checks, positioning, fluid regulation, and medication. These vary somewhat, depending on the location of the craniotomy. The following are general principles of care for infratentorial or supratentorial surgery. Additional aspects of care that are discussed elsewhere may include care of the child with seizures and care of the unconscious child in terms of neurologic assessment.

Vital signs are taken as frequently as every 15 to 30 minutes until stable. Temperature measurement is particularly important because of hyperthermia resulting from surgical intervention in the hypothalamus or brainstem and from some types of general anesthesia. To prepare for this reaction, a cooling blanket should be placed on the bed *before* the child returns to the unit so that it is ready for use when needed. The temperature is monitored carefully when any cooling measures are taken because hypothermia can occur suddenly. Observations for signs of other complications include increased ICP, meningitis, and respiratory tract infection.

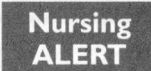 When temperature is elevated, an infectious process must always be suspected, particularly if the febrile state occurs 1 to 2 days after surgery.

Neurologic checks are an essential aspect of care, and include pupillary reaction to light, LOC, sleep patterns, and response to stimuli. Although children may be comatose for a few days, once they regain consciousness there should be a steady increase in alertness. Regression to a lethargic, irritable state indicates increasing pressure, possibly caused by meningitis or cerebral edema.

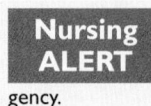 Sluggish, dilated, or unequal pupils are reported immediately because they may indicate increased ICP and potential brainstem herniation, a medical emergency.

Observations for function are not instituted until the child regains consciousness. However, as soon as possible the nurse should begin testing reflexes, handgrip, and functioning of the cranial nerves. Muscle strength is usually diminished as a result of general weakness after surgery but should improve daily. Ataxia may be significantly worse with cerebellar intervention, but it will slowly improve. Edema near the cranial nerves may depress important functions such as the gag, blink, or swallowing reflex.

Dressings are observed for evidence of drainage. If soiled, the dressing is not removed but reinforced with dry sterile gauze. The approximate amount of drainage is estimated and recorded. A drain may be placed in the operative site.

> **Nursing ALERT**
>
> To keep an accurate account of drainage, the soiled area is circled with a pen every hour or so. In this way continuous bleeding is easily recognized. The presence of colorless drainage is reported immediately, since it most likely is CSF from the incisional area. A foul odor from the dressing may indicate an infection. Such a finding is reported, and a culture is taken.

Once the younger child is alert, the arms may need to be restrained to preserve the dressing. Even a child who has been cooperative before surgery must be closely supervised during the initial stages of regaining consciousness, when disorientation and restlessness are common. Correct positioning after surgery is critical to prevent pressure against the operative site, reduce ICP, and avoid the danger of aspiration. If a large tumor was removed, the child is not placed on the operative site, since the brain may suddenly shift to that cavity, causing trauma to the blood vessels, linings, and the brain itself. The nurse confers with the surgeon to be certain of the correct position, including degree of neck flexion. The first 24 to 48 hours after brain surgery are critical. If position is restricted, notice of this is posted above the head of the bed. When the child is turned, every precaution is used to prevent jarring or malalignment in order to prevent undue strain on the sutures. Two nurses, one supporting the head and the other the body, are needed. The use of a turning sheet may facilitate turning a heavy child.

The child with an infratentorial procedure is usually positioned flat and on either side. Pillows should be placed against the child's back, not head, to maintain the desired position. Ordinarily the head and neck are kept in midline with the body and slightly extended. In a supratentorial craniotomy the head is usually elevated above the heart to facilitate CSF drainage and decrease excessive blood flow to the brain to prevent hemorrhage.

> **Nursing ALERT**
>
> The Trendelenburg position is contraindicated in both infratentorial and supratentorial surgeries because it increases ICP and the risk of hemorrhage. If shock is impending, the practitioner is notified immediately, before the head is lowered.

With an infratentorial craniotomy the child is allowed nothing by mouth for at least 24 hours, or longer if the gag and swallowing reflexes are depressed or the child is comatose. With a supratentorial operation, feeding may be resumed soon after the child is alert, sometimes within 24 hours. If the child vomits, oral liquids are stopped. Vomiting not only predisposes to aspiration, but increases ICP and the potential for incisional rupture.

The child should be fed to conserve energy and minimize movement. If there is any sign of facial paralysis, the child is fed slowly to prevent choking or aspiration. Sometimes gavage feeding is necessary when bodily functions are too depressed to permit safe oral feedings or when the child refuses to eat or drink. Intravenous fluids are continued until fluids are well tolerated. Because of the cerebral edema postoperatively and danger of increased ICP, fluids are carefully monitored.

Headache may be severe and is largely the result of cerebral edema. Measures to relieve some of the discomfort include providing a quiet, dimly lit environment, restricting visitors to a minimum, preventing any sudden jarring movement, such as banging into the bed, and preventing an increase in ICP. The last is most effectively achieved by proper positioning and prevention of straining, such as during coughing, vomiting, or defecating. The use of opioids, such as morphine, to relieve pain is controversial because it is thought that they may mask signs of altered consciousness or depress respirations. However, they can be given safely, since naloxone can be used to reverse opioid effects, such as sedation or respiratory depression. Acetaminophen and codeine are also effective analgesics for mild to moderate pain. Regardless of the drugs used, adequate dosage and regular administration are essential to providing optimum pain relief. (See also Pain Assessment; Pain Management, Chapter 21.)

Bowel movements are monitored to prevent constipation. Stool softeners may be given as soon as liquids are tolerated to facilitate easy passage of stool. Placing an ice bag on the forehead may also provide some headache relief, especially if facial edema is severe. Saline drops, or artificial tears, may be needed if the eyelids do not close completely, to prevent corneal ulceration.

Support Child and Family. The emotional needs of the family are great when the diagnosis is a brain tumor, and feelings are influenced by the extent of surgery, any neurologic deficits, expected prognosis, and additional therapy. Since few definitive answers can be given before surgery, the surgeon's report is a significant finding that can vary from a completely benign, resected neoplasm to a highly malignant, invasive, and only partially removed tumor. Although parents try to prepare themselves for a potentially fatal diagnosis, it is a shock for them.

Ideally a nurse should be with the family when the physician visits with them to discuss with parents the expected prognosis and plan of therapy. Although parents may hear only a fraction of what they are told, they can begin to put the future into perspective. While some children will be cured, those with residual tumor may die within a relatively short period of time or live for several years. Regardless of the future prospects, the parents' thinking must be directed toward helping the child recover and resume a normal life to his or her maximum potential.

It is also a time to encourage parents to verbalize their feelings about the diagnosis. Often they express tremendous guilt for attributing the insidious onset of symptoms, such as ataxia, visual difficulty, or headache, to "minor complaints" by the child. Any comments that insinuate that the parents should have sought medical advice sooner are avoided, since such remarks only add to the parents' guilt feelings.

During this period the nurse should also discuss with parents what they plan to tell the child. If the child was prepared honestly, the diagnosis can be expressed in a similar manner, such as "The physician removed most of the tumor; the rest will be treated with special medicine and x-ray treatments." As the child improves, additional explanation about the treatment (similar to that discussed for leukemia), as well as the reason for any residual neurologic effects, such as ataxia or blindness, may be needed.

Promote Return to Optimum Functioning. The ultimate goal is a cured child who has maximum functioning. As soon as possible the child should resume usual activities within tolerable limits, especially returning to school.* Until the skull is completely healed, the child may need to wear a helmet when engaging in any active sport. The school nurse and teacher should confer with the parents to discuss activity restrictions, such as physical education and the reactions of schoolmates to the child's appearance. Since children often equate brain surgery with "going crazy," it is important to prepare the child for possible remarks to this effect. As one child told a classmate, "It's *your* head they should have fixed, because you're crazy. Can't you see that I'm all better?"

After discharge, the family needs continuing medical and emotional support from health personnel. Children who are long-term survivors after treatment for a brain tumor may have residual disabilities, such as growth retardation, cranial nerve palsies, sensory defects, motor abnormalities, especially ataxia, intellectual deficits, memory loss, dysphagia, dysgraphia, and behavioral problems. The high frequency of late effects requires follow-up care despite successful treatment of the tumor (Heideman and others, 1993).

❖ Evaluation
The effectiveness of nursing interventions is determined by continual reassessment and evaluation of care based on the following observational guidelines and expected outcomes:

1. Interview child and family regarding their understanding of scheduled tests and procedures; observe child's behavior during procedures.
2. Monitor child's vital signs, neurologic signs, and dressing.
3. Interview child and family and observe their behaviors during hospitalization and recovery.
4. Interview child and family regarding activities and interests.

Expected outcomes:

1. Child is able to demonstrate an understanding of the tests and procedures and copes with a minimum of stress.
2. Child exhibits no evidence of complications.
3. Child and family demonstrate evidence of healthy coping.
4. Family devises and carries out a realistic activity schedule, and child attends school with reasonable regularity (specify).

See also Nursing Care Plan: The Child with Cancer, Chapter 26; and Nursing Care Plan: The Child with a Brain Tumor.†

---

*Excellent publications, including the pamphlet *When Your Child Is Ready to Return to School*, are available from the **Association for Brain Tumor Research,** 3725 N. Talman Ave., Chicago, IL 60618; (312) 684-1400.
†In Wong DL: *Wong and Whaley's Clinical manual of pediatric nursing,* ed 4, St Louis, 1996, Mosby.

NEUROBLASTOMA

Neuroblastomas are the most common malignant tumors of infancy and are second only to brain tumors as the type of solid malignancy seen during the first 10 years. They occur in about 1 per 10,000 live births, with a slightly higher incidence in males. About half the cases occur in children under 2 years of age, and another fourth occur in children under age 4 years. These tumors originate from embryonic neural crest cells that normally give rise to the adrenal medulla and the sympathetic ganglia. Consequently, the majority of tumors develop in the adrenal gland or the retroperitoneal sympathetic chain. Other sites may be in the head, neck, chest, or pelvis.

Neuroblastoma is a "silent" tumor. In more than 70% of cases, diagnosis is made after metastasis occurs, with the first signs caused by involvement in the nonprimary site, usually the lymph nodes, bone marrow, skeletal system, skin, or liver.

Diagnostic Evaluation
The objective of diagnosis is to locate the primary site and areas of metastasis. The signs and symptoms of neuroblastoma depend on the location and stage of the disease. Most presenting signs are caused by compression of adjacent structures (see box). Skeletal survey; skull, neck, chest, abdominal, and bone CT scans; and a bone marrow test are used to locate a tumor mass and/or metastasis. An intravenous pyelogram may provide evidence of renal involvement.

Urinary excretion of catecholamines is increased in children with adrenal or sympathetic tumors. A 24-hour urine collection analyzed for breakdown products of catecholamine metabolism permits detection of a suspected tumor both before and after therapeutic intervention.

CLINICAL MANIFESTATIONS OF NEUROBLASTOMA

Abdominal Tumors
Firm, nontender, irregular mass
Crosses the midline
Compression of kidney, ureter, or bladder may cause urinary frequency or retention

Distant Metastasis
Ocular:
  Supraorbital ecchymosis
  Periorbital edema
  Proptosis (exophthalmos) from invasion of retrobulbar soft tissue
Lymphadenopathy, especially cervical and supraclavicular
Skeletal: bone pain may or may not be present
Intracranial: neurologic impairment
Thoracic: respiratory obstruction
Spinal cord: varying degrees of paralysis
Adrenal:
  Increased catecholamine excretion
  Flushing
  Hypertension
  Tachycardia
  Diaphoresis

Widespread Metastasis—Vague Symptoms
Pallor
Weakness
Irritability
Anorexia
Weight loss

In recent years considerable controversy has developed regarding the use of mass screening for neuroblastoma in infants by measuring catecholamine metabolites (vanillymandelic acid [VMA] and homovanillic acid [HVA]). However, the effectiveness of mass screening in terms of reducing mortality from the tumor remains unproved (Murphy and others, 1991).

Therapeutic Management

Accurate clinical staging is important for establishing initial treatment. Therefore surgery is used both to remove as much of the tumor as possible and to obtain biopsies. In early stages, complete surgical removal of the tumor is the treatment of choice. If the tumors are large, partial resection is attempted, with a course of irradiation postoperatively to shrink the tumor in the hope of complete removal at a later date. Radiation therapy also offers palliation for metastatic lesions in bones, lung, liver, or brain. Chemotherapy, administered in a variety of combinations, is the mainstay of therapy for extensive local or disseminated disease.

Prognosis. Because of the frequency of invasiveness, the prognosis for neuroblastoma is poor. Generally, the younger the child at diagnosis (especially under 1 year of age), the better the survival rates. Also, neuroblastoma is one of the few tumors that demonstrates spontaneous regression, possibly as a result of maturity of the embryonic cell or the development of an active immune system.

Nursing Considerations

Nursing considerations are similar to those discussed for leukemia and brain tumors, including psychologic and physical preparation for diagnostic and operative procedures, prevention of postoperative complications for abdominal, thoracic, or cranial surgery, and explanation of chemotherapy and radiotherapy and their side effects.

Since this tumor carries a poor prognosis for many children, every consideration must be given the family in terms of coping with a life-threatening illness (see Chapter 18). Because of the high degree of metastasis at the time of diagnosis, many parents suffer much guilt for not having recognized signs earlier. Often the guilt is expressed as anger toward practitioners for not diagnosing it sooner. Parents need much support in dealing with these feelings and expressing them to the appropriate people.

INTRACRANIAL INFECTIONS

The nervous system and its coverings are subject to infection by the same organisms that affect other organs of the body. However, the nervous system is limited in the ways in which it responds to injury. Infectious processes share virtually the same clinical and pathologic features. They differ primarily in the growth and virulence of the specific organism. It is generally difficult to distinguish between the various etiologic agents by looking at clinical manifestations. Laboratory studies are needed to identify the causative agent. The inflammatory process can affect the meninges *(meningitis)*, the brain *(encephalitis)*, or the spinal cord *(myelitis)*.

The most common infection of the CNS is meningitis. It can be caused by a variety of organisms, but the three main types are the following:

1. **Bacterial,** or pyogenic, caused by pus-forming bacteria, especially the meningococcus, pneumococcus, and influenza bacillus
2. **Tuberculous,** caused by the tubercle bacillus
3. **Viral,** or aseptic, caused by a wide variety of viral agents

BACTERIAL MENINGITIS

Bacterial meningitis is a potentially fatal disease, and although the advent of antimicrobial therapy has had a marked effect on the course and prognosis, it remains a significant cause of illness in the pediatric age-groups. Its importance lies primarily in the frequency with which it occurs in infancy and childhood and the unnecessarily high death rates and residual damage caused by undiagnosed and untreated or inadequately treated cases. Ninety percent of all cases appear before 5 years of age with infants demonstrating the greatest risk (Booy and Kroll, 1994).

Bacterial meningitis can be caused by any of a variety of bacterial agents. *Haemophilus influenzae* (type B), *Streptococcus pneumoniae,* and *Neisseria meningitidis* (meningococcal) organisms are responsible for bacterial meningitis in 95% of children older than 2 months of age. The leading causes of neonatal meningitis are the group B streptococci and *Escherichia coli* organisms. *E. coli* infection is seldom seen beyond infancy. Meningococcic (epidemic cerebrospinal) meningitis occurs in epidemic form and is the only form readily transmitted to others. It is transmitted by droplet infection from nasopharyngeal secretions. Although it may develop at any age, the risk of meningococcal infection increases with the number of contacts; therefore it occurs predominantly in school-age children and adolescents.

Pathophysiology

Meningitis appears to occur as an extension of a variety of bacterial infections, probably as a result of the lack of acquired resistance to the various causative organisms. The most common route of infection is by vascular dissemination from a focus of infection elsewhere. Organisms also gain entry by direct implantation after penetrating wounds, skull fractures that provide an opening into the skin or sinuses, lumbar puncture or surgical procedures, and anatomic abnormalities such as spina bifida or foreign bodies such as a ventricular shunt. Once implanted, the organisms spread into the CSF, which serves as a conduit for spread of infection throughout the subarachnoid space.

The infective process is that seen in any bacterial infection—inflammation, exudation, white blood cell accumulation, and varying degrees of tissue damage. The brain becomes hyperemic and edematous, and the entire surface of the brain is covered with a layer of purulent exudate. As infection extends to the ventricles, thick pus, fibrin, or adhesions may occlude the narrow passages, obstructing the flow of CSF.

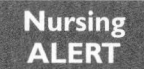 **Nursing ALERT** Any child who is acutely ill and develops a purpuric rash (petechiae and ecchymoses) must receive medical evaluation immediately for the possibility of fulminant (overwhelming) meningococcemia (see box).

Diagnostic Evaluation

A lumbar puncture (LP) is the definitive diagnostic test. The fluid pressure is measured, and samples are obtained for cul-

CLINICAL MANIFESTATIONS OF BACTERIAL MENINGITIS

Children and Adolescents

Usually abrupt onset
Fever
Chills
Headache
Vomiting
Alterations in sensorium
Seizures (often the initial sign)
Irritability
Agitation
May develop:
  Photophobia
  Delirium
  Hallucinations
  Aggressive or maniacal behavior
  Drowsiness
  Stupor
  Coma
Nuchal rigidity
  May progress to opisthotonos
Positive Kernig and Brudzinski signs
Hyperactive but variable reflex responses
Signs and symptoms peculiar to individual organisms:
  Petechial or purpuric rashes (meningococcal infection), especially when associated with a shocklike state
  Joint involvement (meningococcal and *H. influenzae* infection)
  Chronically draining ear (pneumococcal meningitis)

Infants and Young Children

Classic picture rarely seen in children between 3 months and 2 years of age (above)
Fever
Poor feeding
Vomiting
Marked irritability
Frequent seizures (often accompanied by a high-pitched cry)
Bulging fontanel
Nuchal rigidity may or may not be present [*handwritten: not usually under 18 mos.*]
Brudzinski and Kernig signs are not helpful in diagnosis
  Difficult to elicit and evaluate in this age-group
Subdural empyema (*H. influenzae* infection)

Neonates: Specific Signs

Extremely difficult to diagnose
Manifestations vague and nonspecific
Well at birth but within a few days begins to look and behave poorly
Refuses feedings
Poor sucking ability
Vomiting or diarrhea
Poor tone
Lack of movement
Poor cry
Full, tense, and bulging fontanel may appear late in course of illness
Neck usually supple

Neonates: Nonspecific Signs That May Be Present

Hypothermia or fever (depending on the maturity of the infant)
Jaundice
Irritability
Drowsiness
Seizures
Respiratory irregularities or apnea
Cyanosis
Weight loss

---

ture, Gram stain, blood cell count, and determination of glucose and protein content. The findings are usually diagnostic. Culture and stain are needed to identify the causative organism. Spinal fluid pressure is usually elevated, but interpretation is often difficult when the child is crying. Sedation with meperidine (Demerol) or fentanyl and midazolam (Versed) can alleviate the child's pain and fear associated with this procedure. EMLA, a topical anesthetic cream applied to the spinal area one hour before LP reduces pain for children undergoing this procedure. The site of application is usually at lumbar vertebrae 2 and 3.

There is generally an elevated white blood cell count, predominantly polymorphonuclear leukocytes, but it may be extremely variable. The glucose level is reduced, generally in proportion to the duration and severity of the infection. A blood culture is advisable for all children suspected of having meningitis and occasionally proves positive when results of CSF culture are negative. Nose and throat cultures may provide helpful information in some cases.

Therapeutic Management

Acute bacterial meningitis is a medical emergency that requires early recognition and immediate institution of therapy to prevent death and avoid residual disabilities. The initial therapeutic management includes the following:

- Isolation precautions
- Initiation of antimicrobial therapy
- Maintenance of optimum hydration
- Maintenance of ventilation
- Reduction of increased ICP
- Management of bacterial shock
- Control of seizures
- Control of extremes of temperature
- Correction of anemia
- Treatment of complications

The child is isolated from other children, usually in an intensive care unit for close observation. An intravenous infusion is started as soon as the lumbar puncture has been completed in order to facilitate the administration of antimicrobial agents, fluids, anticonvulsant drugs, and blood if needed. The child is placed on a cardiac monitor.

Until the causative organism is identified, antibiotics such as chloramphenicol, ampicillin, ceftriaxone, gentamycin, or tobramycin may be used afterward, the choice of antibiotic is based on the known sensitivity of the organism. Except under special circumstances, the drugs are administered intravenously throughout the course of treatment. They are given in large doses, and the period of therapy is determined by CSF findings (normal glucose level and negative culture) and the child's clinical condition. Appropriate antibiotics are administered following identification of the causative organism. The use of dexamethasone as an anti-inflammatory agent to reduce hearing loss and/or neurologic sequelae is controversial (Wald and others, 1995).

Maintaining hydration is a prime concern, and the decision to administer intravenous fluids and the type and amount of fluid are determined by the patient's condition. The optimum hydration involves correction of any fluid deficits followed by maintenance of low levels to prevent cerebral edema. Cerebral edema and electrolyte disturbances are complications associated with poor neurologic outcomes (Brown and Feigin, 1994). If indicated, measures are taken to reduce ICP as described previously (see p. 990).

Complications are treated appropriately, such as aspiration of subdural effusion in infants and heparin therapy for children who develop disseminated intravascular coagulation syndrome. If shock occurs, it is managed by restoration of blood volume and maintenance of electrolyte balance. Seizures, which occur in a large number of children, are controlled with anticonvulsants.

Lumbar puncture is carried out as needed to determine the effectiveness of therapy. The patient is evaluated neurologically during the convalescent period and at regular intervals during the succeeding year.

Prognosis. The age of the child, the type of organism, the severity of the infection, the duration of the illness before the onset of therapy, and the sensitivity of the organism to antimicrobial drugs are important factors in determining the prognosis. Sequelae are most commonly seen when the disease occurs in the first 2 months of life and least often in children with meningococcal meningitis. The residual deficits in infants are primarily a result of communicating hydrocephalus and the greater effects of cerebritis on the immature brain. In older children the residual effects are related to the inflammatory process itself or result from vasculitis associated with the disease. Evaluation of cranial nerve VIII is needed for at least a 6-month follow-up period to assess for possible hearing loss.

Prevention. Vaccines are available for types A, C, Y, and W-135 meningococci and *H. influenzae* type b. Routine meningococcal vaccination of children is not recommended. However, routine vaccinations for *H. influenzae* type b is recommended for all children beginning at 2 months of age (see Immunizations, Chapter 10). A declining incidence of *H. influenzae* type b disease has occurred since the introduction of the Hib vaccination (Murphy and others, 1993).

Nursing Considerations

Nurses should take necessary precautions to protect themselves and others from possible infection. Parents are taught the proper procedures and supervised in their application.

Nursing ALERT	The first priority of nursing care of a child suspected of having meningitis is to administer the antibiotic as soon as it is ordered. The child is also placed on respiratory isolation for at least 24 hours after implementation of antimicrobial therapy.

The room should be kept as quiet as possible, and environmental stimuli kept at a minimum, since most affected children are sensitive to noise, bright lights, and other external stimuli. Most children are more comfortable without a pillow and with the head of the bed slightly elevated. A side-lying position is more often assumed because of nuchal rigidity. The nurse should avoid actions, such as lifting the child's head, that cause pain or increase discomfort. Measures are taken to ensure safety, since the child is often restless and subject to seizures.

The nursing care of the child with meningitis is determined by the child's symptoms and treatment. Observation of vital signs, neurologic signs, LOC, urine output, and other

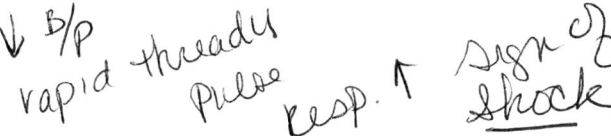

↓ B/P
rapid thready pulse
resp. ↑
sign of shock

pertinent data is carried out at frequent intervals. The child who is unconscious is managed as described previously (see p. 989), and all children are observed carefully for signs of complications just described, especially signs of increased ICP, shock, or respiratory distress. Head circumference is measured on the infant because subdural effusions and obstructive hydrocephalus can develop as a complication of meningitis.

Fluids and nourishment are determined by the child's status. The child with dulled sensorium is usually given nothing by mouth. Other children are allowed clear liquids initially and progressed to a diet suitable for their age. Careful monitoring and recording of intake and output are needed to determine deviations that might indicate impending shock or increasing fluid accumulation, such as cerebral edema or subdural effusion.

One of the problems in nursing care of children with meningitis is maintaining the intravenous infusion for the length of time needed to provide adequate antimicrobial therapy (usually 10 days). Since continuous intravenous fluids are usually not necessary, an intermittent infusion device is used. In some cases, children who are recovering uneventfully are sent home with the device, and parents are taught intravenous drug administration.*

See also Nursing Care Plan: The Child with Acute Bacterial Meningitis.†

Family Support. The sudden nature of the illness makes emotional support of the child and parents extremely important. Parents are very upset and concerned about their child's condition and frequently feel guilty for not having suspected the seriousness of the illness sooner. They need much reassurance that the natural onset of meningitis is sudden and that they acted responsibly in seeking medical assistance when they did. The nurse encourages them to openly discuss their feelings to minimize blame and guilt. They also are kept informed of the child's progress and of all procedures and treatments. In the event that the child's condition worsens, they need the same psychologic care as parents facing the possible death of their child (see Chapter 18; see also Family Focus).

---

*Home care instructions for caring for an intermittent infusion device are available in Wong DL: *Wong and Whaley's Clinical manual of pediatric nursing,* ed 4, St Louis, 1996, Mosby.
†In Wong DL: *Wong and Whaley's Clinical manual of pediatric nursing,* ed 4, St Louis, 1996, Mosby.

NONBACTERIAL (ASEPTIC) MENINGITIS

Aseptic meningitis is caused by a number of agents, principally viruses, and is frequently associated with other diseases, such as measles, mumps, herpes, and leukemia. Enteroviruses and mumps viruses account for a large number of cases.

The onset may be abrupt or gradual. The initial manifestations are headache, fever, malaise, gastrointestinal symptoms, and signs of meningeal irritation that develop a day or two after the onset of illness. Abdominal pain and nausea and vomiting are common; back and leg pain, sore throat, chest pain, photophobia, and generalized muscular aches or pains are found occasionally. There may be a maculopapular rash. These symptoms usually subside spontaneously and rapidly, and the child is well in 3 to 10 days with no residual effects.

Diagnosis is based on clinical features and CSF findings, which include increased lymphocytes, predominantly mononuclear cells. It is important to differentiate this self-limited disorder from the more serious form of meningitis and to diagnose and treat any disease of which it is a manifestation.

Treatment is primarily symptomatic, such as acetaminophen for headache and muscle pain and positioning for comfort. Antimicrobial agents may be administered and isolation enforced until a definitive diagnosis is made as a precaution against the possibility that the disease might be of bacterial origin.

Nursing care is similar to nursing care of the child with bacterial meningitis.

ENCEPHALITIS

Encephalitis is an inflammatory process of the CNS producing altered function of various portions of the brain and spinal cord. Encephalitis can be caused by a variety of organisms, including bacteria, spirochetes, fungi, protozoa, helminths, and viruses. Most infections are associated with viruses, and this discussion will be limited to these etiologic agents.

Etiology

Encephalitis can occur as a result of (1) direct invasion of the CNS by a virus or (2) postinfectious involvement of the CNS after a viral disease. Often the specific type of encephalitis in a particular child may not be identified for some time or at all. The majority of cases of known etiology are associated with the childhood viral diseases. Most other viral infections are those involved with arthropod vectors and those associated with hemorrhagic fevers. The vector reservoir for most agents pathogenic for humans and detected in the United States are mosquitos and ticks; therefore most cases of encephalitis appear during the hot summer months.

Herpes simplex encephalitis is an uncommon disease, but 30% of cases involve children. The initial clinical findings are nonspecific (fever, altered mental status), but most cases evolve to demonstrate focal neurologic signs and symptoms. Children may experience focal seizures. The CSF is abnormal in most cases. Because of a rise in the number of children with herpes simplex virus encephalitis, suspected cases require prompt attention, especially since the diagnosis can be difficult. The clinical diagnosis can be confirmed by the rapid appearance of IgM antibody to herpes simplex virus

type 1 in CSF and serum. The early use of intravenous acyclovir reduces mortality and morbidity.

Diagnostic Evaluation

The clinical features are similar, regardless of the agent involved. Manifestations can range from a mild, benign form that resembles aseptic meningitis, lasting a few days and followed by rapid and complete recovery, to a fulminating encephalitis with severe CNS involvement (see box).

The diagnosis is made on the basis of clinical findings, circumstances associated with the disease, and (where possible) identification of the specific virus. A diagnostic evaluation of encephalitis may include a brain biopsy, usually from the temporal lobe area. Togaviruses (some of which were formerly labeled arboviruses) are rarely detected in the blood or spinal fluid, but viruses of herpes, mumps, measles, and enteroviruses may be found in CSF. Serologic diagnosis may be reached by means of a variety of antibody tests. The first should be drawn as soon after onset as possible, and the second 2 or 3 weeks later. Laboratory detection of herpes simplex virus—DNA in CSF may be used to expedite diagnosis of herpes simplex encephalitis.

Therapeutic Management

Patients suspected of having encephalitis are hospitalized promptly for skilled nursing care and observation. Treatment is primarily supportive, including conscientious nursing care, control of cerebral manifestations, and adequate nutrition and hydration, with observations and management as for other disorders involving cerebral injury. Follow-up care with periodic reevaluation and rehabilitation are important requisites to survivors with residual effects of the disease.

Prognosis. The prognosis for the child afflicted with encephalitis depends on the child's age, the type of organism, and residual neurologic damage. Very young children, younger than 2 years of age, may exhibit increased neurologic disability, including learning difficulties and seizure disorders.

Nursing Considerations

Nursing care of the child with encephalitis is the same as for any unconscious child and the child with meningitis. Neurologic monitoring, administration of medications, and support to the child and parents are the major aspects of care.

CLINICAL MANIFESTATIONS OF ENCEPHALITIS

Onset: Sudden or Gradual	Severe Cases
Malaise	High fever
Fever	Stupor
Headache	Seizures
Dizziness	Disorientation
Apathy	Spasticity
Neck stiffness	Coma (may proceed to death)
Nausea and vomiting	Ocular palsies (may occur)
Ataxia	Paralysis (may occur)
Tremors	
Hyperactivity	
Speech difficulties	

REYE SYNDROME (RS)

RS is a disorder defined as toxic encephalopathy associated with other characteristic organ involvement. It is characterized by fever, profoundly impaired consciousness, and disordered hepatic function.

The etiology of the disorder is obscure, but most cases of RS follow a common viral illness, most frequently influenza or varicella. The link between aspirin and RS is possible but has not been firmly established as a cause-and-effect relationship. However, aspirin and non-steroidal antiinflammatory drugs (NSAIDs), such as ibuprofen, are not recommended for children with varicella or those suspected of having influenza.

Pathophysiology

RS has been defined by the Centers for Disease Control and Prevention as an acute noninflammatory encephalopathy and hepatopathy, with no reasonable explanation for the cerebral and hepatic abnormalities. The pathology of RS is a mitochondrial insult induced by different viruses, drugs, exogenous toxins, and genetic factors.

Diagnostic Evaluation

Elevated ammonia levels tend to correlate with the clinical manifestations and prognosis. Definitive diagnosis is established by liver biopsy (see box). Children who in the past would have been diagnosed with RS are now given other diagnoses such as metabolic disorders, as a result of improved diagnostic techniques.

Therapeutic Management

The most important aspect of successful management of the child with RS is early diagnosis and aggressive therapy. Rapid progression through coma stages and high peak ammonia concentrations are associated with a more serious prognosis. Cerebral edema with increased ICP represents the most immediate threat to life. Recovery from RS is rapid and usually without sequelae if there has been early diagnosis and implementation of therapy.

Prognosis. Although the incidence of Reye syndrome is declining, survivors may have subtle neuropsychologic deficits. Generally recovery is good given the gravity of the disease (Quam, 1994).

Nursing Considerations

The child who is acutely ill with RS requires continuous and intensive nursing care. In addition to an appraisal of vital functions and neurologic status, the nurse assists with a lumbar puncture, obtains blood for laboratory examination, and inserts various intravenous lines such as peripheral, arterial, and central venous pressure. A retention catheter and a nasogastric tube are inserted, and when respirations are compromised, an endotracheal tube is inserted and attached to a respirator for controlled respirations.

Care and observations are implemented as for any child with an altered state of consciousness (see p. 989) and increasing ICP. Accurate and frequent monitoring of intake and output is essential for adjusting fluid volumes to prevent both dehydration and cerebral edema. The child who is paralyzed and in a drug-induced coma is totally dependent on the caregivers, and meticulous vigilance and attention to all biologic needs are mandatory. Since hypovolemic shock is a constant danger in children with controlled fluid intake and osmotic diuresis, vital signs, including central venous pressure and/or cardiac output (Swan-Ganz catheter), are monitored frequently. Because of related liver dysfunction, the nurse must observe for signs of impaired coagulation such as prolonged bleeding time.

Family Support. Parents of children with RS need a great deal of emotional support. They are usually frightened by the child's appearance, the treatment, and the life-threatening severity and suddenness of the illness. Their distress is increased if they believe that their actions may have contributed to a delay in diagnosis. They need to be kept informed regarding the child's progress, to have diagnostic procedures and therapeutic management explained, and to be given concerned and sympathetic support.

The **National Reye's Syndrome Foundation*** has been established by the parents of a child who died of this disease in hope of encouraging research on the disease and of educating parents and health professionals.

HUMAN IMMUNODEFICIENCY VIRUS (HIV) ENCEPHALOPATHY

About 2000 infants are born each year with HIV. It is the seventh leading killer of young children. Documented routine HIV education and routine testing with consent for all pregnant women in the United States is recommended (American Academy of Pediatrics, 1995). The use of zidovudine (ZDV) by HIV-infected pregnant women significantly reduces the chance that a mother will infect the infant.

Children with HIV encephalopathy, a complication of acquired immunodeficiency syndrome (AIDS), present a nursing challenge. Progressive encephalopathy occurs in 30% to

---

STAGING CRITERIA FOR REYE SYNDROME	
Stage I	Vomiting, lethargy, and drowsiness; liver dysfunction; type I EEG, follows commands, pupillary reaction brisk
Stage II	Disorientation, combativeness, delirium, hyperventilation, hyperactive reflexes, appropriate responses to painful stimuli; evidence of liver dysfunction; type I EEG, pupillary reaction sluggish
Stage III	Obtunded, coma, hyperventilation, decorticate rigidity, preservation of pupillary light reaction and oculovestibular reflexes (although sluggish); type II EEG
Stage IV	Deepening coma, decerebrate rigidity, loss of oculocephalic reflexes, large and fixed pupils, loss of doll's eye reflex, loss of corneal reflexes; minimum liver dysfunction; type III or IV EEG, evidence of brainstem dysfunction
Stage V	Seizures, loss of deep tendon reflexes, respiratory arrest, flaccidity; type IV EEG; usually no evidence of liver dysfunction

---

*P.O. Box 829, Bryan, OH 43506; (419) 636-2679.

50% of infants and children infected with HIV; 82% are younger than 5 years of age.

Neurologic manifestations in children suggest that the progressive encephalopathy is the result of primary and persistent infection of the brain with the virus. Unexplained neurodevelopmental regression and focal seizures are the dominant clinical features of the disorder. Others include progressive motor dysfunction and atypical CNS infections. These manifestations indicate a poor prognosis and, almost invariably, a fatal outcome. However, earlier implementation of therapies for AIDS may allow for slower progression of these neurologic complications.

Appropriate precautions are practiced by nurses when caring for these children. Careful handling of the child is a hallmark of excellent nursing, since these children may experience pain, isolation, social stigma, susceptibility to infection, and abandonment resulting in less than minimum sensorimotor stimulation. Nursing assessment and intervention warrant planning time to meet developmental needs, especially if it means holding, rocking, and comforting the child. (See Chapter 26 for a more extensive discussion of AIDS.)

RABIES

Rabies is an acute infection of the nervous system caused by a virus that is almost invariably fatal if left untreated. It is transmitted to humans by the saliva of an infected mammal introduced through a bite or skin abrasion. After entry into a new host, the virus multiplies in muscle cells and is spread through neural pathways without stimulating a protective host immune response.

Approximately 88% of rabies cases come from wild animals, and 12% from domestic animals. Cats are now the most common domestic animals and should be the target of rabies vaccination programs. Carnivorous wild animals (especially raccoons, skunks, and foxes) and bats are the animals most often infected with rabies and the cause of most indigenous cases of human rabies in the United States (Raccoon Rabies, 1994). The likelihood of human exposure to a rabid domestic animal has decreased greatly. The circumstances of a biting incident are important. An unprovoked attack is

more likely to indicate a rabid animal than a provoked attack. Bites inflicted on a child attempting to feed or handle an apparently healthy animal can generally be regarded as provoked. Any child bitten by a wild animal is assumed to be exposed to rabies.

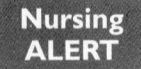 **Nursing ALERT**   Unusual behavior in an animal is cause for suspicion; children should be warned to beware of wild animals that appear friendly.

The disease is uncommon in humans, but the highest incidence occurs in children under 15 years of age. The incubation period usually ranges from 1 to 3 months but may be as short as 10 days or as long as 8 months. Only 10% to 15% of persons bitten develop the disease, but once symptoms are present, rabies progresses inexorably to a fatal outcome. Diagnosis is made on the basis of the history and clinical features (see box). Although treatment is of little avail once symptoms appear, the long incubation period allows time for induction of active and passive immunity before the onset of illness.

Therapeutic Management

Two types of immunizing products are available for use in humans: (1) the *inactivated rabies vaccines,* which induce an active immune response, and (2) the *globulins,* which contain preformed antibodies. The two types of products should be used concurrently for rabies postexposure treatment when prophylaxis is indicated.

The current therapy for a rabid animal bite consists of thorough cleansing of the wound and passive immunization with *human rabies immune globulin (HRIG)* as soon as possible after exposure to provide rapid, short-term passive immunity (Baevsky and Bartfield, 1993).

Postexposure active immunity is conferred by administration of the *human diploid cell rabies vaccine (HDCV).* The first dose of the vaccine is given at the same time as the immune globulin and followed by intramuscular injections at 3, 7, 14, and 28 days after the first dose. An additional dose in 90 days is recommended by the World Health Organization. Before antirabies prophylaxis is initiated, the local or state health department is consulted.

Nursing Considerations

Both parents and children are frightened by the urgency and seriousness of the situation. They need anticipatory guidance for the therapy and support and reassurance regarding the efficacy of the preventive measures for this dreaded disease. EMLA cream, a topical anesthetic, can be placed on the injection site 2 hours before the procedure to reduce the pain.

Mass immunization is unnecessary and unlikely to be implemented. Certain circumstances may warrant vaccination, such as when a child is being taken to an area of the world where rabies in stray dogs is still a problem.

SEIZURE DISORDERS

Seizures are brief malfunctions of the brain's electrical system resulting from cortical neuronal discharge. The manifes-

---

CLINICAL MANIFESTATIONS OF RABIES

Initial Signs
General malaise
Fever
Sore throat

Excitement Phase
Hypersensitivity
Increased reaction to external stimuli
Convulsions
Maniacal behavior
Choking

Severe Spasm of Respiratory Muscles*
Apnea
Cyanosis
Anoxia

*From attempts at swallowing (characteristics from which the term "hydrophobia" was derived).

tations of seizures are determined by the site of origin and may include unconsciousness or altered consciousness, involuntary movements, and changes in perception, behaviors, sensations, and posture. Seizures are the most frequently observed neurologic dysfunction in children and can occur with a wide variety of conditions involving the CNS.

EPILEPSY*

Seizures result from paroxysmal discharges in cortical neurons and are symptoms of abnormal brain function. They are considered to be a symptom of an underlying disease process. Once it is determined that the child has had a seizure, it is important to distinguish whether the episode was an epileptic or a nonepileptic seizure. Seizures are the indispensable characteristic of epilepsy; however, not every seizure is epileptic. Epilepsy is a chronic seizure disorder with recurrent and unprovoked seizures.

Etiology

Seizure disorders have numerous and varied causes (e.g., tumors, infections, neoplasms). Most are *idiopathic*. Although the cause of idiopathic epilepsy is unknown, genetic factors may in some way alter the seizure threshold to influence neuronal discharge. A seizure disorder also can be *acquired* as a result of brain injury during prenatal, perinatal, or postnatal periods. This injury may be caused by trauma, hypoxia, infections, exogenous or endogenous toxins, and a variety of other factors. Biochemical events (e.g., hypoglycemia, hypocalcemia, and certain nutritional deficiencies) produce seizure activity.

The incidence of causative factors associated with childhood seizures is frequently related to the age of the child. Seizures are more common during the first 2 years of life than during any other period of childhood. In very young infants the most frequent causes are birth injuries, such as intracranial trauma, hemorrhage, or anoxia, and congenital defects of the brain. Acute infections are a frequent cause of seizures in late infancy and early childhood but become an infrequent cause in middle childhood. In children older than 3 years of age the most common factor is idiopathic epilepsy.

Seizure activity is believed to be caused by spontaneous electric discharge initiated by a group of hyperexcitable cells referred to as the *epileptogenic focus*. These cells display increased electric excitability in response to any of a variety of physiologic stimuli, such as cellular dehydration, abnormal blood sugar levels, electrolyte imbalance, fatigue, emotional stress, and endocrine changes. When neuronal excitation from the epileptogenic focus spreads to the brainstem, a generalized seizure develops. Seizures are designated as *focal (localized)*, *focal with rapid generalization*, and *generalized*, on the basis of the characteristic neuronal discharges. In a large proportion of children focal seizures spread to other areas, ultimately becoming generalized with loss of consciousness.

Classification

There are many different types of epileptic seizures, and each has unique characteristics. The onset of a seizure is abrupt, paroxysmal, and transitory, and signs are highly variable. The current classification system divides seizures into two major categories: partial and generalized seizures (see box). Some of these are described in the following segment.

Partial seizures are caused by abnormal electric discharges from epileptogenic foci limited to a more or less circumscribed region of the cerebral cortex. Focal seizures may arise from any area of the cerebral cortex, but the frontal, temporal, and parietal lobes are the ones most often affected. The area of cerebral involvement is reflected by clinical manifestations. Partial seizures are subdivided into three types. *Simple partial seizures* have elementary or simple symptoms and no alteration of consciousness (also called an *aura*). *Complex partial seizures* involve complex symptoms and impairment of consciousness. These seizures may begin with an *aura*, a simple partial seizure that is usually a sensation or sensory phenomenon that reflects the complicated connections and integrative functions of that area of the brain. The aura is part of the seizure event and is associated with EEG changes (Van Donselaar, Geerts, and Schimscheimer, 1990). *Simple* or *complex seizures secondarily generalized* develop into generalized seizures, usually a tonic-clonic event

Generalized seizures without a focal onset appear to arise in the reticular formation, and the clinical observations indicate that the initial involvement is from both hemispheres. Frequently loss of consciousness occurs and is the initial clinical manifestation. Unlike partial seizures that become generalized, there is no aura. Episodes occur at any time, day or night, and the interval between episodes may be minutes, hours, weeks, or even years. Most affected persons first experience seizures in childhood, and children whose seizures begin before age 4 years have mental retardation and behavioral and learning problems more frequently than those whose seizures begin after age 4.

Diagnostic Evaluation

Up to 20% of children have been misdiagnosed as having epilepsy (Sagraves, 1990). The careful diagnosis of epilepsy should be made and substantiated with clinical evidence because of the important prognostic and therapeutic implications, which also involve the identification and treatment of the etiology.

Establishing a diagnosis is critical. The process of diagnosis in a child with a seizure disorder has two major foci: (1) to ascertain the type of seizure the child has experienced and (2) to attempt to understand the cause of the events. The assessment and diagnosis rely heavily on a thorough history, skilled observation, and use of several diagnostic tests.

During the assessment process it is unusual to observe the child having a seizure; therefore, a complete, accurate, and detailed history should be obtained from a reliable and knowledgeable informant. This history involves prenatal, perinatal, and neonatal periods, including any instances of infection, apnea, colic, or poor feeding, and information regarding any previous accidents or serious illnesses.

History of the seizure(s) should be equally detailed, including the type of seizure or description of the child's behavior during the event(s), the age at onset, and the time at which the seizure occurs (i.e., early morning, before meals, while awake, or during sleep). Any factors that may have precipitated the seizure are important, including fever, infection, falls that may have caused trauma to the head, anxiety, fa-

---

*Ellen F. Johnsen, BA, RN,C, revised this section.

CLASSIFICATION AND CLINICAL MANIFESTATIONS OF SEIZURES

Partial Seizures

Simple Partial Seizures with Motor Signs

Characterized by:
  Localized motor symptoms
  Somatosensory, psychic, autonomic symptoms
  Combination of these
  Abnormal discharges remain unilateral
Manifestations:
  Aversive seizure (most common motor seizure in children)
    Eye or eyes and head turn away from the side of the focus
    Awareness of movement or loss of consciousness
  Rolandic (Sylvan) seizure
    Tonic-clonic movements involving the face
    Salivation
    Arrested speech
    Most common during sleep
  Jacksonian march (rare in children)
    Orderly, sequential progression of clonic movements beginning in a foot, hand, or face and moving or "marching" to adjacent body parts

Simple Partial Seizures With Sensory Signs

Characterized by various sensations, including:
  Numbness, tingling, prickling, paresthesia, or pain originating in one area (e.g., face or extremities) and spreading to other parts of the body
  Visual sensations or formed images
  Motor phenomena such as posturing or hypertonia
  Uncommon in children under 8 years of age

Complex Partial Seizures (Psychomotor Seizures)

Observed more often in children from 3 years through adolescence
Characterized by:
  Period of altered behavior
  Amnesia for event (no recollection of behavior)
  Inability to respond to environment
  Impaired consciousness during event
  Drowsiness or sleep usually follows seizure
  Confusion and amnesia may be prolonged
  Complex sensory phenomena (aura)
    Most frequent sensation—strange feeling in the pit of the stomach that rises toward the throat
    Often accompanied by:
      Odd or unpleasant odors or tastes
      Complex auditory or visual hallucinations
      Ill-defined feelings of elation or strangeness (e.g., deja vu, a feeling of familiarity in a strange environment)
  May be strong feelings of fear and anxiety, distorted sense of time and self
  Small children may emit a cry or attempt to run for help
Patterns of motor behavior:
  Stereotypic
  Similar with each subsequent seizure
  May suddenly cease activity, appear dazed, stare into space, become confused and apathetic, and become limp or stiff or display some form of posturing
  May be confused
  May perform purposeless, complicated activities in a repetitive manner (automatisms), such as walking, running, kicking, laughing, or speaking incoherently, most often followed by postictal confusion or sleep; may be oropharyngeal activities, such as smacking, chewing, drooling, swallowing, and nausea or abdominal pain followed by stiffness, a fall, and postictal sleep; rarely manifests such as rage or temper tantrums; aggressive acts uncommon during seizure

Generalized Seizures

Tonic-Clonic Seizures (Formerly Known as Grand Mal)

Most common and most dramatic of all seizure manifestations
Occur without warning
Tonic phase: lasts approximately 10 to 20 seconds
Manifestations:
  Eyes roll upward
  Immediate loss of consciousness
  If standing, falls to floor or ground
  Stiffens in generalized, symmetric tonic contraction of entire body musculature
  Arms usually flexed
  Legs, head, and neck extended
  May utter a peculiar piercing cry
  Apneic, may become cyanotic
  Increased salivation and loss of swallowing reflex
Clonic phase: lasts about 30 seconds but can vary from only a few seconds to a half hour or longer
Manifestations:
  Violent jerking movements as the trunk and extremities undergo rhythmic contraction and relaxation
  May foam at the mouth
  May be incontinent of urine and feces
As event ends, movements become less intense, occur at longer intervals, then cease entirely
Status epilepticus: series of seizures at intervals too brief to allow the child to regain consciousness between the time one event ends and the next begins
  Requires emergency intervention
  Can lead to exhaustion, respiratory failure, and death
Postictal state:
  Appears to relax
  May remain semiconscious and difficult to rouse
  May awaken in a few minutes
  Remains confused for several hours
  Poor coordination
  Mild impairment of fine motor movements
  May have visual and speech difficulties
  May vomit or complain of severe headache
  When left alone, usually sleeps for several hours
  On awakening is fully conscious
  Usually feels tired and complains of sore muscles and headache
  No recollection of entire event

Absence Seizures (Formerly Called Petit Mal or Lapses)

Characterized by:
  Onset usually between 4 and 12 years of age
  More common in girls than in boys
  Usually cease at puberty
  Brief loss of consciousness
  Minimal or no alteration in muscle tone
  May go unrecognized because little change in child's behavior
  Abrupt onset; suddenly develops 20 or more attacks daily
  Event often mistaken for inattentiveness or daydreaming
  Events can be precipitated by hyperventilation, hypoglycemia, stresses (emotional and physiologic), fatigue, or sleeplessness
Manifestations:
  Brief loss of consciousness
  Appear without warning or aura
  Usually last about 5 to 10 seconds
  Slight loss of muscle tone may cause child to drop objects
  Able to maintain postural control; seldom falls
  Minor movements such as lip smacking, twitching of eyelids or face, or slight hand movements
  Not accompanied by incontinence
  Amnesia for episode
  May need to reorient self to previous activity

CLASSIFICATION AND CLINICAL MANIFESTATIONS OF SEIZURES—cont'd

Atonic and Akinetic Seizures (Also Known As Drop Attacks)

Characterized by:

Onset usually between 2 and 5 years of age

Sudden, momentary loss of muscle tone and postural control

Events recur frequently during the day, particularly in the morning hours and shortly after awakening

Manifestations:

Loss of tone causes child to fall to floor violently

Unable to break fall by putting out hand

May incur a serious injury to the face, head, or shoulder

Loss of consciousness only momentary

Myoclonic Seizures

A variety of convulsive episodes

May be isolated as benign essential myoclonus

May occur in association with other seizure forms

Characterized by:

Sudden, brief contractures of a muscle or group of muscles

Occur singly or repetitively

No postictal state

May or may not be symmetric

May or may not be loss of consciousness

Infantile Spasms

Also called: infantile myoclonus, massive spasms, hypsarrhythmia, salaam episodes or infantile myoclonic spasms

Most commonly occur during the first 6 to 8 months of life

Twice as common in males as in females

Child may have numerous seizures during the day without postictal drowsiness or sleep

Outlook for normal intelligence poor

Manifestations:

Possible series of sudden, brief, symmetric, muscular contractions

Head flexed, arms extended, and legs drawn up

Eyes may roll upward or inward

May be preceded or followed by a cry or giggling

May or may not be loss of consciousness

Sometimes flushing, pallor, or cyanosis

Infants who are able to sit but not stand:

Sudden dropping forward of the head and neck with trunk flexed forward and knees drawn up—the "salaam" or "jack-knife" seizure

Less often: alternate clinical forms observed

Extensor spasms rather than flexion of arms, legs, and trunk and head nodding

Lightning events involving a single, momentary, shocklike contraction of the entire body

---

tigue, activity (e.g., hyperventilation), and environmental events (exposure to strong stimuli such as bright, flashing lights or loud noises). If the child can describe any sensory phenomena, these are recorded. The duration and progression of the seizure (if any) and the postictal feelings and behavior, such as confusion, inability to speak, amnesia, headache, and sleep, are recorded. The ability to identify seizure types accurately has resulted from the technologic advances in video recording and long-term electroencephalogram (EEG) monitoring.

A complete physical and neurologic examination, including developmental assessment of language, learning, behavior, and motor abilities, often provides clues to neurologic disturbances. A family history can offer clues to paroxysmal disorders such as migraine, breath-holding spells, febrile seizures, or neurologic diseases that may be related to the seizure disorder.

Laboratory studies that may prove to be of value include a complete blood cell count (for evidence of lead poisoning) and white blood cell count (for signs of infection). Blood and CSF glucose may give evidence of hypoglycemic episodes; and serum electrolytes, blood urea nitrogen, calcium, and other blood studies might indicate metabolic disturbances. Lumbar puncture can confirm a suspected diagnosis of cerebrospinal infection or trauma.

Skull radiographs, CT scans, echoencephalograms, brain scans, and other studies help to identify skull abnormalities, separation of sutures, and intracranial calcifications. Focal seizures in children younger than 1 year of age are indications for a diagnostic CT scan to rule out supratentorial tumor. The EEG is obtained for all children with seizure manifestations and is the most useful tool for evaluating seizure disorders. The EEG is carried out under varying conditions—with the child asleep, awake, awake with provocative stimulation

(flashing lights, noise), and hyperventilating. Stimulation elicits abnormal electrical activity, which is recorded on the EEG.

Variations of the EEG are video recordings and simultaneous polygraphs of the patient during waking and/or sleeping. These techniques can be used concurrently and are especially valuable in differentiating epileptic activity from paroxysmal behavior or nonepileptic motor events. *Magnetic resonance imaging (MRI)* can identify skull abnormalities, separation of sutures, and intracranial calcifications.

Therapeutic Management

The objectives of treatment of seizure disorders are to (1) control the seizures or reduce their frequency, (2) discover and correct the cause when possible, and (3) help the child who has recurrent seizures to live as normal a life as possible. Seizures of a recurrent nature are treated as soon as the diagnosis is established. If the seizure activity is a manifestation of an infectious, traumatic, or metabolic process, the seizure therapy is instituted as a part of the general therapeutic regimen. Seizure control is considered to prevent secondary brain cell injury from the neuronal discharge and hypoxia.

It is known that persons predisposed to epilepsy have seizures when their basal level of neuronal excitability exceeds a critical point or threshold; no event occurs if the excitability is maintained below this threshold. The administration of antiepileptic drugs serves to raise this threshold and prevent seizures. Consequently, the primary therapy for seizure disorders is the administration of the appropriate antiepileptic drug or combination of drugs in a dosage that provides the desired effect without causing undesirable side effects or toxic reactions.

Numerous drugs are available for control of seizures. The primary drugs prescribed for partial seizures and/or generalized tonic-clonic seizures are carbamazepine (Tegretol), phenytoin (Dilantin), and valproic acid (Depakote or Depakene). The drug of choice for absence seizures is ethosuximide (Zarontin) and valproic acid. The dosage is determined by monitoring serum drug levels. Complete control can be achieved in only 50% to 75% of affected children, however, even with careful attention to details of therapy.

A present breakthrough in drug management is the realization that polypharmacy confers no benefit over monotherapy in about 90% of individuals with epilepsy (Brodie, 1990). There is increasing evidence that diminishing polypharmacy can bring about a better quality of life; therefore single-drug therapy is recommended. Several new drugs have also increased seizure control for many children. These include gabapentin, lamotrigine, and felbamate. The use of felbamate is controversial because of the side effects of aplastic anemia or hepatic failure.

Once seizures are controlled, the drug or drugs are continued for a prolonged time. However, periodic reevaluation of the drug is important to assess the continued effectiveness and to alter the dosage if indicated. The dosage will need to be increased as the child grows.

Withdrawal of antiepileptic therapy follows a predesigned protocol, usually begun when the child has been seizure free for at least 2 years with a normal EEG. Relapse in children may be related to factors such as neurologic deficit or a positive family history for epilepsy. Recurrence is most likely within the first year after discontinuance of the medication. When a medication is discontinued, the dosage should be reduced gradually over 1 to 2 weeks. Sudden withdrawal of a drug can cause an increase in the number and severity of seizures, often precipitating status epilepticus. If the time for reducing the medication coincides with puberty or, in younger children, occurs during periods when the child is subject to frequent infections, the drug is continued for a longer period. Repeat EEGs are generally obtained every ½ to 2 years.

When seizure activity is determined to be caused by a hematoma, tumor, or other progressive cerebral lesion, surgical removal is the treatment. Surgery also may be indicated for those who suffer from repetitive, incapacitating seizures that are caused by a focal brain abnormality, if removal of the lesion does not result in significant loss of vital functions, such as speech and movement. The risks of brain surgery cannot be underestimated. Also, the costs of surgical interventions must be taken into consideration, as well as the numerous tests necessary to assess the child before surgery.

Status Epilepticus. Status epilepticus is a continuous seizure that lasts more than 30 minutes or a series of seizures from which the child does not regain a premorbid level of consciousness. The initial treatment is directed toward support and maintenance of vital functions, including maintaining an adequate airway, administration of oxygen, and hydration, and followed by intravenous administration of either diazepam (Valium) or phenobarbital. Rectal diazepam is a

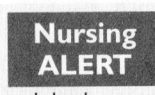

Nursing ALERT Diazepam is incompatible with many drugs. To give intravenously, inject slowly directly into the vein or through tubing as close as possible to the vein insertion site. To decrease the burning sensation, dilute with normal saline.

simple, effective, and safe treatment for prehospital management (Dieckmann, 1994). Lorazepam (Ativan) may be replacing intravenous diazepam as the drug of choice. It has a longer duration of action and causes less respiratory distress in children over 2 years of age.

The child must be closely monitored during administration to detect early alterations in vital signs that may indicate impending cardiac arrest or respiratory depression. When diazepam is ineffective, phenobarbital, often in extremely high levels that may require respiratory support, is given intravenously as the initial medication. Patients who do not respond to drug therapy may require the use of intravenous lidocaine, general anesthesia, or a potent skeletal muscle relaxant such as curare. This should be administered by an anesthesiologist.

Nursing ALERT Status epilepticus is a medical emergency requiring immediate intervention to prevent permanent injury to the brain, exhaustion, respiratory failure, and death.

Equally imperative to halting the tonic-clonic movement is correct diagnosis of the underlying problem. The outcome is related to the etiology and duration of the status epilepticus. *The younger the age the worse prog*

Prognosis. The course and prognosis for children with seizures depend on the etiology, type of seizure, age at onset, and family and medical histories. In one study of children with epilepsy (excluding those with generalized absence, myoclonus, akinetic, atonic, and infantile seizures), 55% of children "outgrew" the disorder and remained seizure-free without medication during an average 7-year follow-up period. At diagnosis the best predictors of remission were age under 12 years at onset, normal intelligence, no prior neonatal seizures, and fewer than 21 seizures before treatment (Camfield and Camfield, 1993).

Risk factors associated with recurrence of epilepsy include being 16 years of age or older, taking more than one antiepileptic drug, having seizures after starting drug treatment, having a history of primary or secondarily generalized tonic-clonic seizures or an EEG showing myoclonic seizures; and having an abnormal EEG. The risks of seizures recurring decreases with increasing time without seizures (Medical Research Council, 1993).

The prognosis following treatment for status epilepticus is more favorable than previously reported. The majority of children will probably have no intellectual impairment. Children who do have cognitive deficits or who die are likely to have preceding developmental delay, neurologic abnormality, or concurrent serious illness (Verity, Ross, and Golding, 1993).

Nursing Considerations

❖ Assessment

An important nursing function during a seizure is observing the seizure and describing its pertinent features. Any alterations in behavior and characteristics of the seizure such as sensory-hallucinatory phenomena (e.g., an aura), motor effects (e.g., eye movements, muscular contractions, laterality,

ASSESSMENT OF THE CHILD DURING A TONIC-CLONIC SEIZURE

Observe Seizure
Describe
Only what is actually observed
Order of events
Duration of seizure

Onset
Significant preseizure events—bright lights, noise, excitement, emotional outbursts
Behavior
    Change in facial expression, such as of fear
    Cry or other sound
    Stereotyped or automatous movements
    Random activity
Position of head, body, extremities
    Unilateral or bilateral posturing of one or more extremities
    Body deviation to side
Time of onset

Movement
Change of position, if any
Site of commencement—hand, thumb, mouth, generalized
Tonic phase, if present—length, parts of body involved
Clonic phase—twitching or jerking movements, parts of body involved, sequence of parts involved, generalized, change in character of movements
Lack of movement of any extremity

Face
Color change—pallor, cyanosis, flushing
Perspiration
Mouth—position, deviating to one side, teeth clenched, tongue bitten, frothing at mouth, flecks of blood or bleeding

Eyes
Position—straight ahead, deviation upward, deviation outward, conjugate or divergent
Pupils (if able to assess)—change in size, equality, reaction to light and accommodation

Respiratory Effort
Presence and length of apnea
Presence of stertor

Other
Involuntary urination
Involuntary defecation

Observe Postictally
Method of termination
State of consciousness—unresponsiveness, drowsiness, confusion
Orientation to time, place, persons, and so on
Sleeping but able to be aroused
Record length of postictal sleep
Motor ability
    Any change in motor power
    Ability to move all extremities
    Any paresis or weakness
    Ability to whistle (if appropriate to age)
Speech—changes, peculiarities, type and extent of any difficulties
Sensations
    Complaint of discomfort or pain
    Any sensory impairment of hearing, vision
    Recollection of preseizure sensations, warning of event
    Awareness that event was beginning

---

and complex activities), alterations in consciousness, and postictal state are noted and recorded (see box above).

Generalized seizures and others with dramatic manifestations are easily detected, but absences may be more difficult to detect. They are easily misinterpreted as inattention. Any unusual behavior, even seemingly inconsequential behavior such as a momentary interruption of activity, staring, or mental blankness, should be described. The more detailed these descriptions, the more valuable they are for assessment. The nurse notes the time that the seizure began and times the length of the seizure. This is especially important if the child becomes cyanotic.

History taking is a vital tool for helping to identify factors that are valuable in establishing a cause of the seizures. Interviewing the child and family helps to elicit problems related to the psychologic impact of the disorder on their lives.

NURSING DIAGNOSES: THE CHILD WITH EPILEPSY

High risk for injury related to sudden and unexpected loss of consciousness
Body image disturbance related to perception of seizure disorder
Altered family processes related to chronic disease of a child

❖ Nursing Diagnoses
Several nursing diagnoses that become apparent following an assessment of the child with a seizure disorder are listed in the box below. Others may be identified in specific cases.

❖ Planning
The goals for the child with a seizure disorder and the family include the following:

1. Child will be protected during a seizure.
2. Child will experience as few seizures as possible.
3. Child and family will cope with the challenges associated with the disorder.
4. Child will develop a positive self-image.
5. Child and family will identify triggering factors.

❖ Implementation
When they first witness a child in a generalized cerebral seizure, nurses are often frightened, puzzled, and immobilized. These reactions are normal but can reduce the effectiveness of care for the child and interfere with observations of the event. The child must be protected from injury during the seizure, and nursing observations made during the event provide valuable information for diagnosis and management of the disorder (see Emergency Treatment box on p. 1023).

It is impossible to halt a seizure once it has begun, and no attempt should be made to do so. The nurse must remain calm, stay with the child, and prevent the child from sustaining any harm during the seizure. If possible, the child should be isolated from the view of others by closing a door or pulling screens. A seizure can be very upsetting to the child, other visitors, and their families. If other persons are present, they should be assured that everything is being done for the child. After the seizure, they can be given a simple explanation about the event as needed.

> **Nursing ALERT** Do not move or forcefully restrain the child during a tonic-clonic seizure and do not place a solid object between the teeth.

If the nurse is able to reach the child in time, a child who is standing or is seated in a chair (including a wheelchair) is eased to the floor immediately. During and sometimes after the tonic-clonic seizure, the swallowing reflex is lost, salivation increases, and the tongue is hypotonic. Therefore the child is at risk for aspiration and airway occlusion. Placing the child on the side facilitates drainage and helps to maintain a patent airway. After the seizure the child is kept on the side in bed or a similar place to allow the youngster to sleep. If the child is at school or away from home, the child is allowed to rest. When feasible, the child is integrated into the environment as soon as possible. Sending a child with a chronic seizure disorder home is not necessary, unless the parents request this.

Children who are known to have seizures or who are under observation for seizures will require some precautions. The extent of these measures depends on the type and frequency of the seizure (see box).

Long-Term Care. Care of the child with a recurrent convulsive disorder involves physical care and instruction regarding the importance of the drug therapy and, probably more significant, the problems related to the emotional aspects of the disorder. There are few diseases that generate as much anxiety among relatives as epilepsy. Fears and misconceptions about the disease and its treatment abound in the lay person's mind. For many it represents the archetype of severe hereditary affliction. Therefore the foci of nursing care are directed toward helping the child and the family to deal with the psychologic and sociologic problems related to the

---

SEIZURE PRECAUTIONS

Extent of precautions depends on type, severity, and frequency of seizures

May include the following:
  Siderails raised when child is sleeping or resting
  Siderails and other hard objects padded
  Waterproof mattress/pad on bed/crib
  Appropriate precautions during potentially hazardous activities:
    Swimming with a companion
    Use of protective helmet and padding during bicycle riding, skate-boarding, in-line skating
    Supervision during use of hazardous machinery/equipment
Have child carry or wear medical identification
Alert other caregivers to need for any special precautions
Identify and avoid triggering factors whenever possible

---

disorder and educating the child, the family, peers, and the public toward a more realistic and liberal view of the disease.

Children subject to seizures are placed on some type of drug therapy. The nurse can help the parents plan the administration of the medication at convenient times to minimize disruption to the family routine. The most convenient times for administration seem to be with meals or at bedtime. Although antiepileptic drugs are available in liquid extracts or emulsions, the tablet form is preferred by neurologists. The unequal distribution of the drug in the solute and the increased likelihood of inaccurate measurements make liquid medication less desirable. For small children the tablet of the proper dosage can be crushed and administered in syrup, jelly, or other palatable substances.

> **Nursing ALERT** Children taking phenobarbital and/or phenytoin should receive adequate vitamin D and folic acid, since deficiencies of both have been associated with these antiepileptics. Phenytoin should not be taken with milk.

It is important to impress on the family the need to continue the medication regularly without interruption for as long as required. The parents and the child will need to know the common side effects of the drug prescribed and observe for signs that might indicate unfavorable reactions.

Parents need to be warned of possible behavioral changes as the seizures are controlled in children taking primidone, phenobarbital, or phenytoin. Changes in personality, indifference to school activities and family, hyperactivity, or even psychotic behavior may sometimes be observed. The potential effects of antiepileptics on learning and behavior should be considered. Progressive intellectual deterioration in a child with epilepsy requires investigation of present medication plus the role of the underlying cerebral pathology. Parents should notify the health professional if the child has an illness, including vomiting or fever. Vomiting can interfere with drug absorption; fever may increase metabolic requirements; both can precipitate seizure activity.

Rectal preparations of some medications are highly useful and effective when a child is unable to take oral medications because of repeated vomiting, gastrointestinal surgery, or status epilepticus. Administration of rectal drugs can be learned by parents for home treatment during a seizure.* Rectal ativan is useful adjunctive home treatment for children at risk for prolonged seizures. Hospitalization is minimized, and parental confidence enhanced (Camfield and others, 1989).

The degree to which activities are restricted is individualized for each child and depends on the type, frequency, and severity of the seizures, the child's response to therapy, and the length of time the seizures have been controlled. Normal healthy activities are encouraged for children, and participation in competitive sports is determined on an individual basis. With encouragement most older children can accept the restrictions placed on activities. Only essential restrictions should be placed on children regarding sports and peer activity to reduce the likelihood of needlessly accentuating differences.

---

*Home care instructions for administering oral and rectal medications are available in Wong DL: *Wong and Whaley's Clinical manual of pediatric nursing*, ed 4, St Louis, 1996, Mosby.

CRITICAL THINKING EXERCISE
Seizures

Since age 2 years, Jane Little has had epilepsy that is well controlled with medication. However, now that she has begun elementary school, her seizures have returned. On the way home Jane usually has a seizure on the bus; however, on weekends and holidays she is seizure-free. As the school nurse, you advise Jane's parents to:

1. Take her for medical reevaluation.
2. Increase her antiepileptic medication.
3. Drive her home from school.
4. Ride with her on the school bus.

The correct answer is four. Your first priority is to help the family identify triggering events. At your suggestion, Mrs. Little rode the school bus home with Jane. As the child began to seize, the mother noted that they had just passed a white picket fence, the triggering factor. Once the child was seated on the other side of the bus, the seizure episodes stopped.

With the consistent pattern and abrupt onset of the seizures, seeking medical reevaluation should be advised only if no triggering event is identified. It is not within the scope of nursing practice for you to change the dosage of the medication. Even if the child rides home in a car, the seizures may occur if Jane sits in the same position as on the school bus.

Because the child is encouraged to attend school, camp, and other normal activities, the school nurse and the teacher should be made aware of the child's condition and therapy. They can help to ensure regularity of medication and any special care the child might need. Teachers, child care providers, camp counselors, youth organization leaders, coaches, and other adults who assume responsibility for children should be instructed regarding care of the child during a seizure so that they can act in a calm manner for the welfare of the child and to influence the attitude of the child's peers.*

Triggering Factors. Careful and detailed documentation of seizures over a period of time may reveal a pattern. When this occurs, the nurse or responsible adult may intervene to identify the triggering factors and make changes in the environment that may prevent or decrease seizure frequency. Frequently the necessary changes are very simple and cost-free but can make an enormous difference in the child's and family's lives (see Critical Thinking Exercise box).

Factors that may trigger seizures in children include changes in dark-light patterns, such as those that occur with a flash on a camera, automobile headlights, walking by a picket fence, reflections of light on snow or water, or rotating blades on a fan; sudden loud noises; specific voices, songs, or nursery rhymes; startling or sudden movements; extreme or drastic changes in temperature; dehydration; fatigue; hyperventilation; hypoglycemia; caffeine; and insufficient protein in the diet (protein is needed to metabolize some antiepileptic drugs). Although there have been reports of seizures triggered by flashing video games, this relationship has not

*An excellent resource is *Students with seizures: a manual for school nurses* by N. Santilli, W.E. Dodson, and A.V. Walton (1991, Epilepsy Foundation of America).

Tonic-Clonic Seizure
During the Seizure
Time seizure episode.
Approach calmly.
If child is standing or seated, ease child down.
Place pillow or folded blanket under child's head. If no bedding is available, place own hands under child's head.
Do not:
   Attempt to restrain child or use force
   Put anything in child's mouth
   Give any food or liquids.
Loosen restrictive clothing.
Remove eyeglasses.
Clear area of any hazards or hard objects.
Allow seizure to end without interference.
If vomiting occurs, try to turn child to one side as a unit.

After the Seizure
Time postictal period.
Check for breathing. Check position of head and tongue. Reposition if head is hyperextended. If breathing is not present, give rescue breathing and call EMS.
Check around mouth for evidence of burns or suspicious substances that might indicate poisoning.
Keep child on side.
Remain with child until full recovery.
Do not give food or liquids until fully alert and swallowing reflex has returned.
Call EMS when necessary.
Look for medical identification and determine what factors occurred before onset of seizure and which may have been triggering factors.
Check head and body for possible injuries and fractures. Check inside of mouth to see if tongue or lips have been bitten.

Complex Partial Seizure
During the Seizure
Do not restrain unless in danger.
Remove harmful objects from path.
Redirect to safe area.
Do not agitate; instead, talk in calm, reassuring manner.
Do not expect child to follow instructions.
Watch to see if seizure generalizes to tonic-clonic type.

After the Seizure
Stay with child and reassure until fully conscious.

• • •

Call Emergency Medical Service (EMS) if:
Child stops breathing.
There is evidence of injury or youngster is diabetic or pregnant.
Seizure lasts for more than 5 minutes (unless duration of seizure is typically longer than 5 minutes as specified in medical orders).
Status epilepticus occurs.
Pupils are not equal in size after seizure.
Child vomits continuously 30 minutes after seizure has ended (sign of possible acute problem).
Child cannot be awakened and is unresponsive to pain after seizure has ended.
Seizure occurs in water (shock and aspiration may be delayed).
This is child's first seizure.

Modified from *Seizure recognition and first aid*, Landover, MD, 1989, Epilepsy Foundation of America.

been confirmed by controlled studies. Seizures may be caused by the length of playing time, which may cause sleep deprivation, fatigue, excitement, or photosensitivity (Ferrie and others, 1994). On the basis of current knowledge, the overwhelming majority of children with seizures can play video games without the risk of seizures.*

If a child is photosensitive, avoiding such things as wallpaper with stripes, a ceiling fan, blinking lights, viewing the TV screen from a distance of at least 2 yards and covering one eye may be necessary.

Family Support. Parental attitudes and management of a child with a seizure disorder are as varied as those of other parents of children with a chronic disorder, and they are subject to the same long-term problems (see Chapter 18). Whether the seizures result from illness, injury, or unknown etiology, the parents may feel guilt, anxiety, and often humiliation. They want to know if it will affect the child's mental capacities. To many persons epilepsy is erroneously associated with mental deficiency. Seizures do frequently accompany other manifestations of severe brain damage from disease or injury, but the majority of children with seizures, like any population of healthy children, display a wide range of intelligence.

Parents also wonder how the illness will affect the child's future and need reassurance that it will not shorten the life of the child and that the child can attend school, marry, and elect to have children. The child will need vocational guidance, and the parents should become familiar with the laws in their state regarding any limitations that might be imposed on the child because of the disorder. It should be emphasized that seizures can be controlled or greatly reduced in the majority of children and that new studies hold the promise of progress in future treatment. Parents also need reassurance that in this enlightened day and age there is less stigma attached to the disease than there has been in the past.

It is important to encourage a healthy attitude toward the child and the disease and to help the parents feel competent in their ability to meet their responsibilities. The child should be reared as any normal child, with natural concern tempered by the understanding of the need not to be overprotected. Many parents refrain from correcting or punishing the child, especially if they have had the experience of such an emotional stress precipitating a seizure. The child must not be made to feel different in any way. Parents should be encouraged to be honest and open about the disorder with the child and to others. Some parents are tempted to try to conceal the nature of the child's illness because of their belief that the disorder is shameful or a disgrace to the family.

Restrictions on the child's activities will be necessary for safety, but this area can be approached in a positive way in terms of what the child *can* do rather than what the child cannot do. Sometimes parents curtail the child's activities more than necessary. The child needs to experience the maturing influences of play and work. The **Epilepsy Foundation of America**[†] is a national organization that works to-

ward and for the welfare of persons with epilepsy and their families, helps with employment and legal problems, and provides education to patients, families, and communities.

The Child with Epilepsy. The child who is provided the security of a loving family, rewards and punishments no different from those of other children, and support in acquiring self-esteem is more apt to have a positive attitude toward the disease. Children derive their self-concept and self-esteem from observations of others' reactions to them and their own perception of their capabilities. The suddenness and unpredictability of seizures and the reactions of others further influence their feelings. When others consider children to be different, inferior, or objects of ridicule, they come to view themselves as different, inferior, and incapable.

Behavioral problems are common in children with epilepsy and can become more serious than the seizures. Much of the behavior difficulty, especially aggressive or delinquent behaviors, has been attributed to the child's reaction to parental rejection. Feelings of guilt, frustration, depression, and self-negation can contribute to antisocial behaviors. Behavioral problems and school difficulties, such as dependency and underachievement, are common in children with epilepsy and can become more serious than the seizures (Vining, 1990).

Children with epilepsy need to learn about their disease and the role that the medication plays in contributing to their prolonged well-being. As soon as they are old enough, children should assume responsibility for taking their own medication and be advised to carry medical identification with pertinent information about their condition. Planning activities with children and emphasizing those in which they can engage rather than those in which they cannot participate help them succeed and gain satisfaction in their achievements. They should be offered opportunities and encouraged to exercise judgment in their daily lives.

The adolescent period may prove to be a trying time for the child with epilepsy. Limits imposed on the young person's activities at a time when freedom and independence are desired may bring the disability into sharp focus. For example, some states do not allow persons with epilepsy to obtain a driver's license, even when the disease is controlled; in others there are restrictions on employment insurance.

Epilepsy should not be a severe impairment to most youngsters, and the nurse, by assuming the role of patient advocate, helping to educate the public regarding the disease, working toward making opportunities available to persons with the disorder, and lobbying for legislation that recognizes the needs of the individual with a seizure disorder, can help to erase the stigma that still remains regarding the disease.

❖ Evaluation

The effectiveness of nursing interventions for the child with epilepsy is determined by continual reassessment and evaluation of care based on the following observational guidelines and expected outcomes:

1. Observe child's behavior for evidence of seizure activity and assess the environment for situations that could cause injury to child in the event of a seizure; interview family regarding management of child during a seizure.
2. Interview child and family regarding compliance with the medication regimen and identification of triggering factors.
3. Observe and interview family regarding their feelings and concerns and their understanding of child's condition.

---

*For more information on video games and epilepsy, contact the Epilepsy Foundation of America.
[†]4351 Garden City Drive, Landover, MD 20785; (301) 459-3700. In Canada: **Epilepsy Canada,** 1470 Peel St., Suite 745, Montreal, Quebec H3A 1T1; (514) 845-7855.

4. Observe child's interactions with others and interview child about any feelings or concerns about own health.

Expected outcomes:

1. Child exhibits no evidence of physical injury.
2. Family complies with instructions; child remains free of seizure activity.
3. Child exhibits no or minimal complications from medication.
4. Child and family identify triggering factors and make adjustments that diminish the frequency of seizure episodes.
5. Child expresses feelings and concerns and has a positive self-image.
6. Child and family demonstrate a healthy view of the disorder and alterations in life-style that it imposes.

See also Nursing Care Plan: The Child with Epilepsy.*

FEBRILE SEIZURES

Febrile seizures are transient disorders of children that occur in association with a fever. They are one of the most common neurologic disorders of childhood, affecting about 4% of children. Most febrile seizures occur after 6 months of age and usually before age 3 years, with increased frequency in children younger than 18 months. They are unusual after 5 years of age. Boys are affected about twice as often as girls, and there is an increased susceptibility in families, indicating a possible genetic predisposition. Most febrile seizures are generalized and last less than 5 minutes (Farwell and others, 1994). About 30% to 40% of children will have one recurrence.

The cause of febrile seizures is still uncertain. In most children the height but not the rapidity of the temperature elevation seems to be a factor. The fever usually exceeds 38.8° C (101.8° F) and occurs during the temperature rise rather than after a prolonged elevation. Sometimes it constitutes the dramatic beginning of an illness. Febrile seizures usually accompany an upper respiratory or gastrointestinal infection. Although pertussis vaccine does not cause febrile seizures, this immunization is a precipitating factor in initial episodes of febrile seizures in children prone to having seizures (Cherry and others, 1993).

Most febrile seizures have stopped by the time the child is taken to a medical facility. However, if the seizure continues, treatment consists of controlling the seizure with diazepam (Valium) and reducing the temperature by administration of acetaminophen. Antiepileptic prophylaxis may be considered for children experiencing (1) a focal or prolonged seizure, (2) neurologic abnormalities, (3) afebrile seizures in a first-degree relative, (4) age younger than 1 year, and (5) multiple seizures occurring within 24 hours. The febrile seizure tendency may be a fundamental marker of an individual's seizure threshold (Camfield, Camfield, and Gordon, 1994). Little risk of neurologic deficit, epilepsy, mental retardation, or altered behavior has been observed as sequelae of febrile seizures.

Parents need reassurance of the *benign* nature of febrile seizures (almost 95% of children with febrile seizures will not develop epilepsy or any neurologic damage). They should be told that their child is in no danger of dying during a febrile seizure. They also need education regarding protecting the

child from harm and observing exactly what happens to the child during the event. Attempts to lower the temperature with acetaminophen or to use diazepam to prevent a seizure are of no benefit in most children (Uhari and others, 1995). Tepid sponge baths are ineffective in significantly lowering the temperature, the shivering effect further increases metabolic output, and cooling causes discomfort in the child.

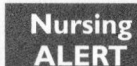 **Nursing ALERT** If a febrile seizure lasts more than 10 minutes, parents should seek medical attention right away. Encourage them to drive carefully; a few extra minutes will not make any significant difference (Camfield and Camfield, 1993).

CEREBRAL MALFORMATIONS

CRANIAL DEFORMITIES

In the normal newborn the cranial sutures are separated by membranous seams several millimeters wide. For the first few hours to 1 to 2 days after birth, the cranial bones are highly mobile, which allows them to mold and slide over one another, adjusting the circumference of the head to accommodate to the changing shape and character of the birth canal. The principal sutures in the infant's skull are the sagittal, coronal, and lambdoidal sutures, and the major soft areas at the juncture of these sutures are the anterior and posterior fontanels (see Fig. 8-6).

Following birth, growth of the skull bones occurs in a direction *perpendicular* to the line of the suture, and normal closure occurs in a regular and predictable order. Although there are wide variations in the age at which closure takes place in individual children, normally all sutures and fontanels are ossified by the following ages:

8 weeks: Posterior fontanel closed
6 months: Fibrous union of suture lines and interlocking of serrated edges
18 months: Anterior fontanel closed
12 years: Sutures unable to be separated by increased ICP

Solid union of all sutures is not completed until very late childhood.

Closure of a suture before the expected time inhibits the perpendicular growth. Since normal increase in brain volume requires expansion, the skull is forced to grow in a direction *parallel* to the fused suture. This alteration in skull growth always produces a distortion of the head shape when the underlying brain growth is normal. The small head with closed and normal shape is the result of deficient brain growth; the suture closure is secondary to this brain growth failure. Failure of brain growth is not secondary to suture closure.

Various types of cranial deformities are encountered in early infancy. These include the enlarged head with frontal protrusion (bossing) characteristic of hydrocephalus, the parietal bossing that is seen in chronic subdural hematoma, the small head, and a variety of skull deformities (see box on p. 1026). Some occur during prenatal development; in others, head circumference is usually within normal limits at birth, and the deviation from normal development becomes apparent with advancing age.

---

*In Wong DL: *Wong and Whaley's Clinical manual of pediatric nursing,* ed 4, St Louis, 1996, Mosby.

CRANIAL DEFORMITIES

Microcephaly—head circumference more than 2 standard deviations below average for age, sex, and gestation; caused by failure of brain development
Management—no treatment available
Craniosynostosis—premature closure of single or multiple sutures of the cranial vault, face, and base of skull
Scaphocephaly—premature closure of sagittal suture causes skull to become elongated in an anteroposterior direction with a high cranial vault and a subnormal transverse diameter
Brachycephaly—premature closure of the coronal sutures causes skull to become shortened in an anteroposterior direction with flattening of occiput and forehead
Oxycephaly—premature closure of both coronal and sagittal sutures causes an excessively high and narrow skull that tapers upward on all sides
Plagiocephaly—unilateral closure of one coronal or lambdoidal suture causes skull to become asymmetric
Craniofacial dysostosis (Crouzon disease)—premature closure of any or all cranial sutures, most frequently the coronal, and a typical facial deformity (widely spaced eyes, hypoplastic maxilla, and beaklike nose; tongue appears large and protruding; frequently with exophthalmos)
Management—surgical release of closed sutures; Crouzon disease—surgical correction of major facial deformities

FAMILY FOCUS
Blood Donation

Parents may wish to provide a compatible blood donor for their infant undergoing a planned surgical correction for craniosynostosis. Nurses need to inform and guide parents through this blood bank procedure.

Prognosis. The majority of infants presenting with craniosynostosis have normal brain development. The exceptions are those genetic disorders that involve brain pathology.

Nursing Considerations

Nursing care of families in which there is a child with a cranial defect involves identifying children with deformities and referring them for evaluation. Since there is no therapy available for children with microcephaly, nursing care is directed toward helping parents adjust to rearing a child with brain damage (see Chapter 19).

Caring for infants who benefit from surgery requires special emphasis on observation for signs of decreased hematocrit and hemoglobin because of the large blood loss during surgery (see Family Focus box). A cardiac monitor may demonstrate a resting heart rate of 200. Nursing care includes observation for signs of hemorrhage, infection, pain, and swelling and parental education for suture care and safety. Surgical sutures should remain dry and intact. Parents need to observe for any signs of redness, drainage, or swelling and report any temperature greater than 38.4° C (101° F).

Early surgical management of craniosynostosis allows proper expansion of the brain and the creation of an acceptable appearance. Parents require special support and education during this time, especially from other parents whose infants have undergone similar operations. (Richards, 1994). The nurse can serve as a liasion for this type of parental support.

HYDROCEPHALUS

Hydrocephalus is a condition caused by an imbalance in the production and absorption of CSF in the ventricular system. When production is greater than absorption, CSF accumulates within the ventricular system, usually under increased pressure, producing passive dilation of the ventricles.

Pathophysiology

The two mechanisms by which CSF is formed include secretion by the choroid plexuses and lymphatic-like drainage by the extracellular fluid of the brain. CSF circulates throughout the ventricular system, then is absorbed within the subarachnoid spaces by a mechanism that is not entirely clear. Prenatal diagnosis is undoubtedly having an impact on the current prevalence at birth of hydrocephalus. The advent of MRI and CT scanning has provided valuable information about the pathophysiology of various diseases. The causes are diverse; they are either congenital (maldevelopment or intrauterine infection) or acquired (neoplasm, hemorrhage, or infection).

Hydrocephalus is a symptom of an underlying brain pathology resulting in either (1) impaired absorption of CSF within the subarachnoid space (ventricles communicate; communicating hydrocephalus) or (2) obstruction to the flow of CSF within the ventricles (ventricles do not communicate; noncommunicating hydrocephalus). Any imbalance of secretion and absorption causes an increased accumulation of CSF in the ventricles, which become dilated and compress the brain substance against the surrounding rigid bony cranium. When this occurs before fusion of the cranial sutures, it produces enlargement of the skull, as well as dilation of the ventricles (Fig. 28-7). In children under 10 to 12 years of age, previously closed suture lines, especially the sagittal suture, may become diastatic or opened (Swaiman, 1994).

Most cases of noncommunicating hydrocephalus are a result of developmental malformations. Although the defect usually is apparent in early infancy, it may become evident at any time from the prenatal period to late childhood or early adulthood. Other causes include neoplasms, infections, and trauma. An obstruction to the normal flow can occur at any point in the CSF pathway to produce increased pressure and dilation of the pathways proximal to the site of obstruction.

Developmental defects—for example, Arnold-Chiari malformations (ACMs), aqueduct stenosis, aqueduct gliosis, and atresia of the foramina of Luschka and Magendie (Dandy-Walker syndrome)—account for most cases of hydrocephalus from birth to 2 years of age. Hydrocephalus is so often associated with myelomeningocele that all such infants should be observed for its development. In the remainder of cases there is a history of intrauterine infection, perinatal hemorrhage, and neonatal meningoencephalitis. In older children hydrocephalus is most often the result of space-occupying lesions, intracranial infections, hemorrhage, or preexisting developmental defects, such as aqueduct stenosis or the ***Arnold-Chiari malformation*** (a congenital anomaly in which the

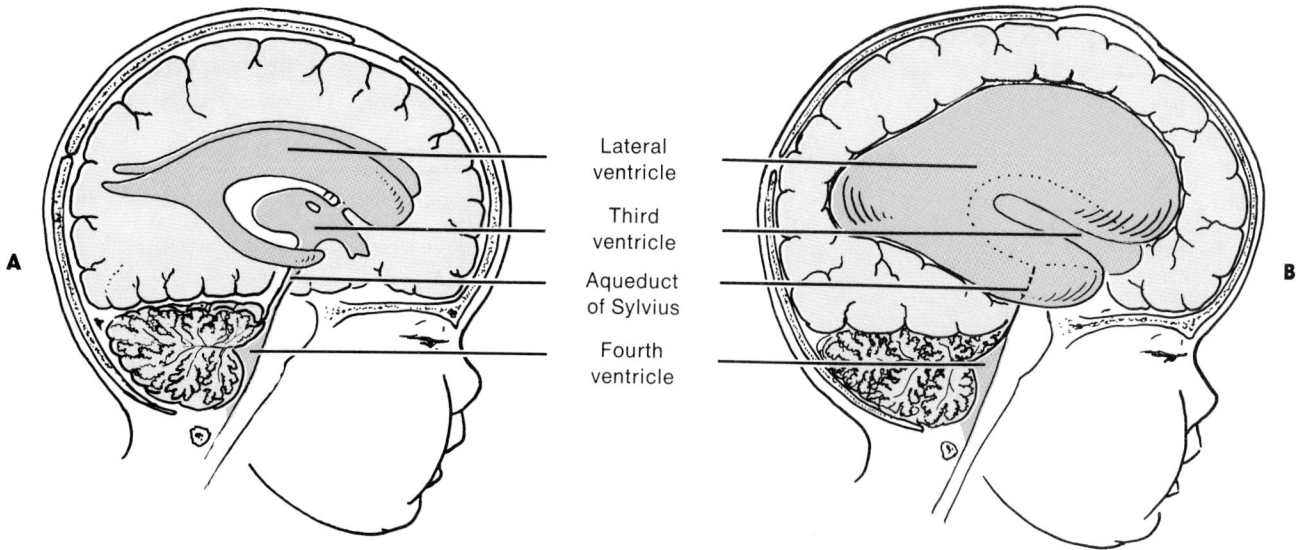

FIG. 28-7. Hydrocephalus: a block in the flow of CSF. **A,** Patent cerebrospinal fluid circulation. **B,** Enlarged lateral and third ventricle caused by obstruction of circulation—stenosis of the aqueduct of Sylvius.

Lateral ventricle

Third ventricle

Aqueduct of Sylvius

Fourth ventricle

cerebellum and medulla oblongata extend down through the foramen magnum).

Diagnostic Evaluation

The two factors that influence the clinical picture in hydrocephalus are the time of onset and the presence of preexisting structural lesions. In infancy, before closure of the cranial sutures, head enlargement is the predominant sign, whereas in older infants and children the lesions responsible for hydrocephalus produce other neurologic signs through pressure on adjacent structures before causing CSF obstruction (see box on p. 1028).

In infancy the diagnosis of hydrocephalus is based on head circumference that crosses one or more grid lines on the measurement chart within a period of 2 to 4 weeks and on associated neurologic signs that are present and progressive. However, other diagnostic studies are needed to localize the site of CSF obstruction. Routine daily head circumference measurements are carried out in infants with myelomeningocele and intracranial infections. In evaluation of a premature infant, specially adapted head circumference charts are consulted to distinguish abnormal head growth from rapid head growth that takes place normally.

The signs and symptoms in early to late childhood are caused by increased ICP, and specific manifestations are related to the focal lesion. Most commonly resulting from posterior fossa neoplasms and aqueduct stenosis, the clinical manifestations are primarily those associated with space-occupying lesions.

The primary diagnostic tools for detecting hydrocephalus are CT and MRI. Sedation is required, since the child must remain absolutely still for an accurate picture to be produced. Diagnostic evaluation of children who have symptoms of hydrocephalus after infancy is similar to that used in those with suspected intracranial tumor. In the neonate echoencephalography is useful in comparing the ratio of lateral ventricle to cortex.

Therapeutic Management

The treatment of hydrocephalus is directed toward (1) relief of the hydrocephalus, (2) treatment of complications, and (3) management of problems related to the effect of the disorder on psychomotor development. The treatment is, with few exceptions, surgical. This is accomplished by direct removal of an obstruction (such as a tumor) or a shunt procedure that provides primary drainage of the CSF from the ventricles to an extracranial compartment, usually the peritoneum (ventricular peritoneal [VP] shunt) (Fig. 28-8).

Most shunt systems consist of a ventricular catheter, a flush pump, a unidirectional flow valve, and a distal catheter. In all models the valves are designed to open at a predetermined

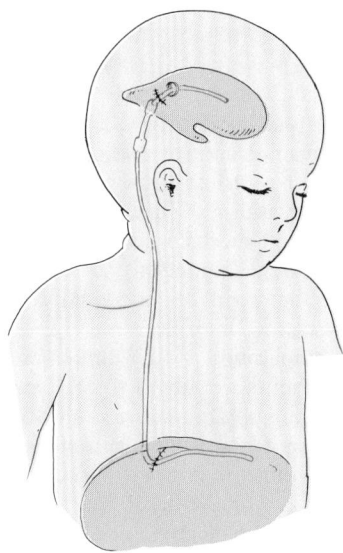

FIG. 28-8. Ventricular peritoneal shunt. Catheter is threaded subcutaneously from small incisions at the sites of ventricular and peritoneal insertions.

CLINICAL MANIFESTATIONS OF HYDROCEPHALUS

Infancy, Early

Abnormally rapid head growth
Bulging fontanels (especially anterior) sometimes without head enlargement:
    Tense
    Nonpulsatile
Dilated scalp veins
Separated sutures
Macewen sign ("cracked-pot" sound) on percussion
Thinning of skull bones

Infancy, Later

Frontal enlargement or "bossing"
Depressed eyes
"Setting sun" sign (sclera visible above the iris)
Pupils sluggish, with unequal response to light

Infancy, General

Irritability
Lethargy
Infant cries when picked up or rocked and quiets when allowed to lie still
Early infantile reflex acts may persist
Normally expected responses fail to appear
May display:
    Change in level of consciousness
    Opisthotonos (often extreme)
    Lower-extremity spasticity
Advanced cases:
    Difficulty in sucking and feeding
    Shrill, brief, high-pitched cry
    Cardiopulmonary embarrassment

Childhood

Headache on awakening; improvement following emesis or upright posture
Papilledema
Strabismus
Extrapyramidal tract signs (e.g., ataxia)
Irritability
Lethargy
Apathy
Confusion
Often incoherence

NURSING DIAGNOSES: THE CHILD WITH HYDROCEPHALUS

High risk for altered neurologic function related to increased ICP
High risk for infection related to presence of mechanical drainage system
High risk for impaired skin integrity related to pressure areas, paralysis, relaxed anal sphincter
Altered family processes related to situational crisis (child with a physical defect)

The most serious complication, shunt infection, can occur at any time, but the period of greatest risk is 1 to 2 months following placement. The infection is generally the result of intercurrent infections at the time of shunt placement. Infections include septicemia, bacterial endocarditis, wound infection, shunt nephritis, meningitis, and ventriculitis. Meningitis and ventriculitis are of greatest concern, since any complicating CNS infection is a significant predictor of intellectual outcome. Infection is treated with massive doses of antibiotics administered by the intravenous route. A persistent infection requires removal of the shunt until the infection is controlled. External ventricular drainage (EVD) is used until CSF is sterile.

Prognosis. The prognosis of children with treated hydrocephalus depends largely on the rate at which hydrocephalus develops, the duration of raised ICP, the frequency of complications, and the cause of the hydrocephalus. For example, malignant tumors may have a high mortality regardless of other complicating factors.

Surgically treated hydrocephalus with continued neurosurgical and medical management has a survival rate of about 80%, with the highest incidence of mortality occurring within the first year of treatment. Of the surviving children approximately one third are both intellectually and neurologically normal, and one half have neurologic disabilities.

Nursing Considerations

❖ Assessment

Preoperatively the infant with diagnosed or suspected hydrocephalus is observed carefully for signs of increasing ICP. In infants the head is measured daily at the point of largest measurement—the occipitofrontal circumference (OFC) (see Head Circumference, Chapter 7, for technique). Fontanels and suture lines are gently palpated for size, signs of bulging, tenseness, and separation. An infant with normal ICP will display bulging under certain circumstances such as straining or crying; therefore such accompanying behavior should be noted. Irritability, lethargy, or seizure activity, as well as altered vital signs and feeding behavior, may indicate an advancing pathologic condition.

In older children, who are usually admitted to the hospital for elective or emergency shunt revision, the most valuable indicator of increasing ICP is an alteration in the child's LOC and the way in which the child interacts with the environment. Changes are identified by observation and by comparison of present behavior with customary behavior, sleep patterns, developmental capabilities, and habits, all obtained

intraventricular pressure and close when the pressure falls below that level, thus preventing backflow of secretions.

The initial shunt is placed when necessary to relieve CSF obstruction, and revisions are needed when there are signs of malfunction. In all mechanisms the initial success rate is relatively high; however, shunts are associated with complications that interfere with continued shunt function or that threaten the life of the child.

The major complications of VP shunts are infection and malfunction. All shunts are subject to mechanical difficulties, such as kinking, plugging, or separation or migration of the tubing. Malfunction is most often caused by mechanical obstruction either within the ventricles from particulate matter (tissue or exudate) or at the distal end from thrombosis or displacement as a result of growth. The child with a shunt obstruction is often first seen in an emergency room with clinical manifestations of increased ICP, frequently accompanied by worsening neurologic status.

through a detailed history and a baseline assessment. This baseline information serves as a guide for postoperative assessment and evaluation of shunt function.

❖ Nursing Diagnoses

Following a thorough assessment, nursing diagnoses become apparent. These include, but are not limited to, those listed in the accompanying box.

❖ Planning

The goals of care of the child with hydrocephalus and family include the following:

1. Child will experience no complications of hydrocephalus and/or corrective surgery.
2. The family will receive adequate education and emotional support.

❖ Implementation

General nursing care of the infant with hydrocephalus may present special problems. Maintaining adequate nutrition often requires flexible feeding schedules to accommodate diagnostic procedures, since feeding before or after handling can precipitate an episode of vomiting. Small feedings at more frequent intervals are often better tolerated than are larger ones spaced farther apart. These infants are often difficult to feed and require extra time and innovation.

The nurse is responsible for preparing the child for diagnostic tests such as tomography and for assisting the physician with procedures such as a ventricular tap, which is often performed to relieve excessive pressure during the preoperative period and for CSF examination. Sedation is required, since the child must remain absolutely still during diagnostic testing. Intravenous pentobarbital or oral chloral hydrate is commonly used for these procedures. (See Chapter 22 for preparing children for procedures.)

> **Nursing ALERT**
> If surgery is anticipated, intravenous infusions should not be placed in a scalp vein on a child with hydrocephalus.

Fortunately, almost all affected children are recognized, and treatment is begun early. For those children with significant head enlargement, care must be exercised to see that the head is well supported when the infant is fed or moved to prevent extra strain on the infant's neck, and measures must be taken to prevent development of pressure areas. As the hydrocephalus progresses, untreated children become increasingly helpless and prone to the multiple problems of immobility (e.g., pressure sores and contracture deformities). Not infrequently, infants with irreversible brain damage or with severe developmental defects such as hydranencephaly, in which both cerebral hemispheres fail to develop and are replaced with a membranous sac filled with cerebrospinal fluid, are placed in long-term care facilities.

Postoperative Care. Routine postoperative care and observation are instituted. In addition, the infant or child is positioned carefully on the unoperated side to prevent pressure on the shunt valve and pressure areas. The child is kept flat to help avert complications resulting from too rapid reduction of intracranial fluid. When the ventricular size is reduced too rapidly, the cerebral cortex may pull away from the dura and tear the small interlacing veins, producing a subdural hematoma. This is not a problem in children with elective shunt revision, since their intraventricular size and pressure have been normal. The surgeon indicates the position to be maintained and the extent of activity allowed. If there is increased ICP, the surgeon will prescribe elevation of the head of the bed and/or that the child be allowed to sit up to enhance gravity flow through the shunt. Pain management can usually be achieved with acetaminophen with or without codeine for mild to moderate pain and opioids for severe pain (see Chapter 21 for pain management).

Observation for signs of increased ICP, which indicates obstruction of the shunt, is continued. Neurologic assessment includes evaluation of pupil dilation (pressure causes compression or stretching of the oculomotor nerve, producing dilation on the same side as the pressure) and blood pressure (hypoxia to the brainstem causes variability in these vital signs).

> **Nursing ALERT**
> Never pump the shunt to assess function, because this may pull choroid plexuses into the ventricular slits, resulting in blockage; cause headache by decreasing CSF; or obstruct the peritoneal end of the catheter.

The child is also observed for abdominal distention, because CSF may cause peritonitis or a postoperative ileus as a complication of distal catheter placement. In addition, intake and output are carefully monitored. Children may be placed on fluid restriction with nothing by mouth for 24 hours. The intravenous infusion is closely monitored to prevent fluid overload. Routine feeding is resumed after the prescribed NPO period, but the presence of bowel sounds is determined before feeding children with VP shunts.

Since infection is the greatest hazard of the postoperative period, nurses are continually on the alert for the usual manifestations of CSF infection, which may include elevated vital signs, poor feeding, vomiting, decreased responsiveness, and seizure activity. There may be signs of local inflammation at the operative sites and along the shunt tract. The child's diaper should be kept off the peritoneal dressing site or suture line. Antibiotics are administered by the intravenous route as ordered, and the nurse may also need to assist the practitioner with intraventricular instillation. The incision site is inspected for leakage, and any suspected drainage is tested for glucose, an indication of cerebrospinal fluid.

Meticulous skin care is continued postoperatively, with extra care taken to prevent tissue damage from pressure. A pressure-reducing mattress or overlay pad underneath the child helps prevent pressure on prominent areas. Skin is inspected regularly for any signs of pressure, irritation, or infection.

Family Support. Specific needs and concerns of parents during periods of hospitalization are related to the reason for the child's hospitalization (shunt revision, infection, diagnosis) and the diagnostic and/or surgical procedures to which the child must be subjected. Often parents have very little understanding of anatomy; therefore, they need further exploration and reinforcement of information that was given to them by the physician and neurosurgeon, as well as information about what they can expect. They are especially frightened of any procedure that involves the brain, and the fear of retardation or brain damage is very real and pervasive. Nurses can do much to allay their anxiety by explaining the rationale underlying the various nursing and medical activities such as positioning or testing, and by simply being available and willing to listen to their concerns.

To prepare for the child's discharge and home care, the parents are instructed on how to recognize signs that indicate shunt malfunction or infection and how to pump the shunt, if necessary. Active children may have accidents, such as a fall, that can damage the shunt, and the tubing may pull out of the distal insertion site or become disconnected during normal growth.

Safe transportation is an essential issue to discuss with parents. The tendency for the enlarged head to fall forward and to turn to the side, combined with poor head control, influences the type of child restraint system needed. Small infants can be restrained reclining in an approved car restraint bed.*

The management of hydrocephalus in a child is a demanding task for both family and health professionals, and helping a family cope with the child is an important nursing responsibility. It is important to emphasize that hydrocephalus is a lifelong problem and that the child will require evaluation on a regular basis. The overall aim is to establish realistic goals and an appropriate educational program that will assist the child to achieve his or her optimum potential.

Anticipatory guidance will prepare parents for possible problems and help them to avoid being overprotective of the child. There need be few restrictions (mainly contact sports) placed on the child's activities, and the child should be encouraged to live as would any other child of the same age and abilities. Parents need support and encouragement in coping with the child and with problems the child may encounter in relationships with peers and others. Reactions of other children when the child has a noticeably enlarged head or requires shaving at the times of revision are stress situations for both child and parents. (See Chapter 18 for a discussion on problems and coping with the child with a disability.)

Families can be referred to community agencies for support and guidance. The **National Hydrocephalus Foundation (NHF)*** provides information on the condition for families and assists interested groups in establishing local organizations. Helpful booklets are available from this and other sources.

❖ Evaluation

The effectiveness of nursing interventions is determined by continual reassessment and evaluation of care based on the following.

Observational guidelines:

1. Monitor child's neurologic status (physical signs and behavior), take temperature, examine skin at points of pressure.
2. Interview family regarding their feelings and concerns.

Expected outcomes:

1. Child remains free from complications of the disorder and surgical correction.
2. Family discusses their feelings and concerns regarding child's condition.

See also Nursing Care Plan: The Child with Hydrocephalus.†

---

*Information on restraints for children with special needs is available from Automotive Safety for Children Program, Riley Hospital for Children, 534 N. Clinical Dr., Rm. 118, Indianapolis, IN 46202-5109; (317) 274-2977 or (800) KID-N-CAR (in Indiana).

*Route 1, River Rd., Box 210 A, Joliet, IL 60436; (800) 431-8093.
†In Wong DL: *Wong and Whaley's Clinical manual of pediatric nursing*, ed 4, St Louis, 1996, Mosby.

KEY POINTS

- Level of consciousness (LOC) is the most important indicator of neurologic health; altered levels include full consciousness, confusion, disorientation, lethargy, obtundation, stupor, coma, and persistent vegetative state.
- Complete neurologic examination includes LOC; posture; motor, sensory, cranial nerve, and reflex testing; and vital signs.
- Nursing care of the unconscious child focuses on respiratory management, neurologic assessment, intracranial pressure (ICP) monitoring, supplying adequate nutrition and hydration, drug therapy, promoting elimination, hygienic care, positioning and exercise, stimulation, and family support.
- Fractures resulting from head injuries may be classified as depressed, compound, basilar, and diastatic.
- Primary head injury involves features that occur at the time of trauma, including fractured skull, contusions, intracranial hematoma, and diffuse injury. Secondary complications include hypoxic brain damage, increased ICP, infection, cerebral edema, and posttraumatic syndromes.
- The young child's response to head injury is different because of the following features: larger head size; expandable skull; larger amount of blood volume to the brain; small subdural spaces; and thinner, softer brain tissue.
- Problems resulting from near-drowning include hypoxia and asphyxiation, aspiration, and hypothermia.
- Nursing care of the child with a brain tumor includes observing for signs and symptoms related to the tumor, preparing the child and family for diagnostic tests and operative procedures, preventing postoperative complications, planning for discharge, and promoting a return to optimum health.
- Nursing care of the child with meningitis includes ad-

ministration of antibiotics, prevention of self-infection, removal of environmental stimuli, correct positioning, vital signs monitoring, intravenous therapy, and promoting fluid, nutritional status, and supportive care of the family.

- Routine immunization of infants against *H. influenzae* type B infection has reduced the incidence of bacterial meningitis.
- Encephalitis may result from direct invasion of the central nervous system by a virus or from involvement of the central nervous system after viral disease.
- A seizure is a symptom of underlying pathology and may be manifest by sensory-hallucinatory phenomena, motor effects, sensorimotor effects, and loss of consciousness.
- Partial seizures are categorized as simple (without associated impairment of consciousness) or complex (with impaired consciousness); both types may become generalized.
- Generalized seizures are categorized as tonic-clonic

convulsive absence, atonic and akinetic, myoclonic, and infantile spasms.

- Long-term care of the child with recurrent seizure disorders includes physical care and education regarding the importance of drug therapy and problems related to emotional aspects of the disorder.
- Febrile seizures are frightening to parents but are usually benign events that do not require antipyretic or antiepileptic therapy.
- Many cranial deformities are amenable to surgical correction.
- Hydrocephalus is a symptom of an underlying brain pathology, demonstrated by impaired absorption of cerebrospinal fluid (CSF) or obstruction to the flow of CSF within the ventricles.
- Therapy for hydrocephalus involves relief of the hydrocephalus, treatment of the underlying brain pathology if possible, prevention and/or treatment of complications, and management of problems related to psychomotor development.

REFERENCES

American Academy of Pediatrics: Perinatal human immunodeficiency virus testing, *Pediatrics* 95(2):303-307, 1995.

Baevsky RH, Bartfield JM: Human rabies: a review, *Am J Emerg Med* 11(3):279-86, 1993.

Barkovich AJ: Techniques and methods in pediatric imaging. In Barkovich AJ: *Pediatric neuroimaging*, New York, 1990, Raven Press.

Bonadio W, Wagner V: Adrenaline-cocaine gel topical anesthetic for dermal laceration repair in children, *Ann Emerg Med* 21(12):1435-1438, 1992.

Booy R, Kroll S: Bacterial meningitis in children, *Curr Opin Pediatr* 6(1):29-35, 1994.

Bratton SL, Jardine DS, Morray JP: Serial neurological examinations after near drowning and outcome, *Arch Pediatr* 148(2):167-170, 1994.

Brown LW, Feigin RD: Bacterial meningitis: fluid balance and therapy, *Pediatr Ann* 23(2):93-98, 1994.

Bruce D: Head trauma. In Eichelberger MR: *Pediatric trauma: prevention, acute care, and rehabilitation*, St Louis, 1993, Mosby.

Camfield CS and others: Home use of rectal diazepam to prevent status epilepticus in children with convulsive disorders, *J Child Neurol* 4:125-126, 1989.

Camfield CS, Camfield PR: Febrile seizures: an Rx for parent fears and anxiety, *Contemp Pediatr* 10(4):26-44, 1993.

Camfield PR, Camfield CS, Gordon K: What types of epilepsy are preceded by febrile seizures, *Dev Med Child Neurol* 36(10):887-892, 1994.

Cherry JD and others: Pertussis immunization and characteristics related to first seizures in infants and children, *J Pediatr* 122(6):900-903, 1993.

Dieckmann RA: Rectal diazepam for prehospital pediatric status epilepticus, *Ann Emerg Med* 23:216-224, 1994.

Duffner PK, Cohen ME: The long-term effects of CNS therapy on children with brain tumors, *Neurol Clin* 9:479-495, 1991.

Duffner PK and others: Postoperative chemotherapy and delayed radiation in children less than three years of age with malignant brain tumors, *N Engl J Med* 328:1725-1733, 1993.

Ernst AA and others: Lidocaine adrenaline tetracaine gel versus tet-

racaine adrenaline cocaine gel for topical anesthesia in linear scalp and facial lacerations in children aged 5 to 17 years, *Pediatrics* 95(2):255-258, 1995.

Farwell JR and others: First febrile seizures: characteristics of the child, the seizure, and the illness, *Clin Pediatr* 33(5):263-267, 1994.

Ferrie CD and others: Video-game epilepsy, *Lancet* 344(8938): 1710-1711, 1994.

Heideman RL and others: Tumors of the central nervous system. In Pizzo PA, Poplack DG: *Principles and practice of pediatric oncology*, ed 2, Philadelphia, 1993, JP Lippincott.

Kyriacou DN, Arcinue EL, Peek C: Effects of immediate resuscitation on children with submersion injury, *Pediatrics* 123:137-142, 1994.

Medical Research Council Antiepileptic Drug Withdrawal Study Group: Prognostic index for recurrence of seizures after remission of epilepsy, *Br Med J* 306:1374-1378, 1993.

Murphy SB and others: Consensus statement from the American Cancer Society Workshop on Neuroblastoma Screening: Do children benefit from mass screening for neuroblastoma? *CA* 41(4):227-230, 1991.

Murphy TV and others: Declining incidence of *Haemophilus influenzae* type b disease since introduction of vaccination, *JAMA* 269(2):246-248, 1993.

Quam DA: Recognizing a case of Reye's syndrome, *Am Fam Phy* 15(7):1491-1496, 1994.

Raccoon rabies epizootic—United States, 1993, *MMWR* 43(15):269-270, 1994.

Reynolds E: Controversies in caring for the child with a head injury, *MCN* 17:246-251, 1992.

Richards MD: Common pediatric craniofacial reconstructions, *Nurs Clin North Am* 29(4):791-799, 1994.

Sagraves R: Antiepileptic drug therapy for pediatric generalized tonic-clonic seizures, *J Pediatr Health Care* 4(6):314-319, 1990.

Swaiman KF: *Pediatric neurology: principles and practice*, ed 2, St Louis, 1994, Mosby.

Thorn RN, Pearson AD, Nicoll JA: Decline in incidence of medulloblastoma in children, *Cancer* 74(12):4350-4354, 1994.

Uhari M and others: Effect of acetaminophen and of low intermittent doses of diazepam on prevention of recurrences of febrile seizures, *J Pediatr* 126(6):991-995, 1995.

van Donselaar CA, Geerts AT, Schimscheimer RJ: Usefulness of an aura for classification of a first generalized seizure, *Epilepsia* 31(5):529-535, 1990.

Verity CM, Ross EM, Golding J: Outcome of childhood status epilepticus and lengthy febrile convulsions: findings of national cohort study, *Br Med J* 307:225-228, 1993.

Vining E: The psychosocial impact of epilepsy in children and their families, *Int Pediatr* 5(2):186-188, 1990.

Wald E and others: Dexamethasone therapy for children with bacterial meningitis, *Pediatrics* 95(1):21-28, 1995.

Ward JD: Pediatric head injury: a further experience, *Pediatr Neurosurg* 20(30):1883-1885, 1994.

Wong D: Changing what children hear in the ICU can lower intracranial pressure, *Am J Nurs* 88:279-280, 1988.

BIBLIOGRAPHY

General

Ashwal S, Eyman Rk, Call TL: Life expectancy of children in a persistent vegetative state, *Pediatr Neurol* 10(1):27-33, 1994.

Blevins SH, Benson S: A better way to get kids through scans, *RN* 55(10):40-44, 1992.

Fields AI, Coble DH, Pollack MM: Outcomes of children in a persistent vegetative state *Crit Care Med* 21(12):1890-1894, 1993.

Hollman GA, Elderbrook MK, VanDenLangenberg B: Results of a pediatric sedation program on head MRI scan success rates and procedure duration times, *Clin Pediatr* 34:300-305, 1995.

Multi-Society Task Force on PVS: Medical aspects of the persistent vegetative state, *New Engl J Med* 330(22):1572-1579, 1994.

Rushton CH, Hogue EE: When parents demand everything, *Pediatr Nurs* 19(2):180-183, 1993.

Sips HJ, Catsman-Berrevoets CE, van Dongen HR: Measuring right-hemisphere dysfunction in children, *Dev Med Child Neurol* 36(1):57-63, 1994.

Increased Intracranial Pressure

Cotton MR, Donald PR, Schoeman JF: Raised intracranial pressure, the syndrome of inappropriate ADH, *Childs Nerv Syst* 9(1):10-15, 1993.

Gambardella G, Zaccone C, Cardia E: Intracranial pressure monitoring in children: comparison of external ventricular device with fiberoptic system, *Childs Nerv Syst* 9(8):470-473, 1993.

Longatti PL, Carteri A: Active singling out of shunt independence, *Childs Nerv Syst* 10(5):334-336, 1994.

Shankaran S, Woldt E, Bedard MP: Feasibility of invasive monitoring of intracranial pressure, *Brain Dev* 16(2):121-125, 1994.

Taylor GA, Phillips JD, Ichord RN: Intracranial compliance in infants, *Radiology* 191(3):787-791, 1994.

Zaritsky A: Outcome of pediatric cardiopulmonary resuscitation, *Crit Care Med* 21(9):325-327, 1993.

Head Injury

Appleton R: Head injury rehabilitation of children, *Nurs Times* 90(22):39-31, 1994.

Brown JK, Minns RA: Non-accidental head injury, *Dev Med Child Neurol* 35(10):849-869, 1993.

Davis RL, Mullen N, Makela M: Cranial CT scans in children after minimal head injury with loss of consciousness, *Ann Emerg Med* 24(4):640-645, 1994.

Greenspan AI, MacKenzie EJ: Functional outcome after pediatric head injury, *Pediatrics* 94(4):425-432, 1994.

Hoekelman RA: A pediatrician's view: why deaths from head injuries are on the decline, *Pediatr Ann* 23(1):8-10, 1994.

Kaufman BA, Dacey RG: Acute care management of closed head injury in childhood, *Pediatr Ann* 23(1):18-20, 1994.

Kaufman PM, Fletcher JM, Levin HS: Attentional disturbance after pediatric closed head injury, *J Child Neurol* 8(4):348-353, 1993.

Mitchel KA, Fallat ME, Raque GH: Evaluation of minor head injury in children, *J Pediatr Surg* 29(7):851-854, 1944.

Nazarian LF: When parents become critical observers, *Pediatr Rev* 14(8):299-301, 1993.

Weiss BS: Bicycle-related head injuries, *Clin Sports Med* 13(1):99-112, 1994.

Near-Drowning

Fredrickson JM, Fauer W, Arellano D: Emergency nurses' perceived knowledge and comfort levels regarding pediatric patients, *J Emerg Nurs* 20(1):13-7, 1994.

Kallas HJ, O'Rourke PP: Drowning and immersion injuries in children, *Curr Opin Pediatr* 5(3):295-302, 1993.

Kemp AM, Mott AM, Sibert JR: Accidents and child abuse in bathtub submersions, *Arch Dis Child* 70(5):435-438, 1994.

Kriel RL, Krach LE, Luxenberg MG: Outcome of severe anoxic—ischemic brain injury in children, *Pediatr Neurol* 10(3):207-212, 1994.

Lavell JM, Shaw KN: Near drowning, *Crit Care Med* 21(3):368-373, 1993.

Norris MK: Pediatr near drowning, *Nursing* 23(5):33, 1993.

Walsh EA, Ioli JG: Childhood near-drowning: nursing care and primary prevention, *Pediatr Nurs* 20(3):265-269; 292, 1994.

Central Nervous System Tumors

Allen JC: What we learn from infants with brain tumors, *N Engl J Med* 328(24):1780-1781, 1993.

Bucholtz J: Issues concerning the sedation of children for radiation therapy, *Oncol Nurs Forum* 19(4):649-655, 1992.

Cullen PM: Pharmacologic supportive care of children with central nervous system tumors, *J Pediatr Oncol Nurs* 12(4):230-232, 1995.

Green DM, D'Angio GJ: Late effects of treatment for childhood cancer, *J Pediatr Oncol Nurs* 10(1):40-42, 1993.

Lew CM, LaVally B: The role of stereotactic radiation therapy in the management of children with brain tumors, *J Pediatr Oncol Nurs* 12(4):212-222, 1995.

Moore IM: Central nervous system toxicity of cancer therapy in children, *J Pediatr Oncol Nurs* 12(4):203-210, 1995.

Shiminski-Maher T, Shields M: Pediatric brain tumors: diagnosis and management, *J Pediatr Oncol Nurs* 12(4):188-198, 1995.

Intracranial Infections

American Academy of Pediatrics, Committee on Infectious Disease: Dexamethasone therapy for bacterial meningitis in infants and children, *Pediatrics* 86(1):130-133, 1990.

Ashwal S, Perkin RM, Thompson JR: Bacterial meningitis in children, *Adv Pediatr* 40:185-215, 1993.

Carno M: Meningococcemia: Recognizing and reducing complications in pediatric patients, *AACN Clin Iss Crit Care Nurs* 5(3):278-288, 1994.

Dodge PR: Neurological sequelae of acute bacterial meningitis, *Pediatr Ann* 23(2):101-106, 1994.

Green PA, Singh KV, Murray BE: Recurrent group B streptococcal infections in infants *J Pediatr* 125(6):931-938, 1994.

Jenkins T: Fulminant meningococcemia in pediatric patients: nursing considerations *Pediatr Nurs* 18:629-634, 1992.

Klein JO: Antimicrobial treatment and prevention of meningitis, *Pediatr Ann* 23(2):76-81, 1994.

Oliver LG, Harwood-Nuss AL: Bacterial meningitis in infants and children: a review, *J Emerg Med* 11(5):555-564, 1993.

Pavlakis SG, Frank Y, Nocyze M: Acquired immunodeficiency syndrome and the developing nervous system, *Adv Pediatr* 41:427-451, 1994.

Poss WB, Vernon DD, Dean JM: A reemergence of Reye's syndrome, *Arch Pediatr Adolesc Med* 148(8):879-882, 1994.

Epilepsy

Austin JK: Predicting parental anticonvulsant medication compliance, *J Pediatr Nurs* 4:88-95, 1989.

Austin JK, McDermott N: Parental attitude and coping behavior in families of children with epilepsy, *J Neurosci Nurs* 20:174-179, 1988.

Carter JR: The use of new antiepileptic medications in pediatric patients with epilepsy, *J Pediatr Health Care* 8(6):277-282, 1994.

Commission on Classification and Terminology of the International League Against Epilepsy, *Epilepsia* 30:389-399, 1989.

Maytal J and others: Low morbidity and mortality of status epilepticus in children, *Pediatrics* 83:323-331, 1989.

Meldrum BS: Anatomy, physiology, and pathology of epilepsy, *Lancet* 336:231-234, 1990.

National Institutes of Health Consensus Conference: Surgery for epilepsy, *JAMA* 264(6):729-733, 1990.

Pellock JM: Efficacy and adverse effects of antiepileptic drugs, *Pediatr Clin North Am* 36:435-448, 1989.

Pellock JM: Recent advances concerning status epilepticus, *Int Pediatr* 5(2):189-196, 1990.

Santilli N, Dodson WE, Walton AV: *Students with seizures: a manual for school nurses,* Landover, MD, 1991, Epilepsy Foundation of America.

Scheuer ML, Pedley TA: The evaluation and treatment of seizures, *N Engl J Med* 323(21):1468-1474, 1990.

Shorvon SD: Epidemiology, classification, natural history, and genetics of epilepsy, *Lancet* 336:93-96, 1990.

Status epilepticus—the first hour is critical, *Emerg Med* 24(8):181-184, 1992.

Vining EP: Educational, social, and life-long effects of epilepsy, *Pediatr Clin North Am* 36:449-461, 1989.

Ziemba SK: Seizures, *Am J Nurs* 95(2):32-33, 1995.

Febrile Seizures

Berg AT: Are febrile seizures provoked by a rapid rise in temperature? *Am J Dis Child* 147:1101-1103, 1993.

Camfield PR and others: Prevention of recurrent febrile seizures, *J Pediatr* 126(6):929-930, 1995.

Farwell JR, Blackner G, Sulzbacher S: First febrile seizures, *Clin Pediatr* 33(5):263-267, 1994.

Offringa M, Bossuyt PM, Lubsen J: Risk factors for seizure recurrence in children with febrile seizures, *J Pediatr* 124(4):574-584, 1994.

Smith MC: Febrile seizures: recognition and management, *Drugs* 47(6):933-944, 1994.

Stenklyft PH, Carmona M: Febrile seizures, *Emerg Med Clin North Am* 12(4):989-999, 1994.

Van-Esch A, Steyerberg EW, Berger MY: Family history and recurrence of febrile seizures, *Arch Dis Child* 70(5):395-399, 1994.

Cranial Deformities/Hydrocephalus

Bragg CL, Edwards-Beckett J, Eckle N: Shunt dysfunction and constipation, *J Neurosci Nurs* 26(2):91-94, 1994.

Hockley AD: Craniosynostosis, *Lancet* 342(8865):189-190, 1993.

Jackson PL: Primary care needs of children with hydrocephalus, *J Pediatr Health Care,* 4:59-71, 1990.

Kontny U, Hofling B, Gutjahr P: CSF shunt infections in children, *Infection* 21(2):89-92, 1993.

Lee M, Wisofff JH, Abbot R: Management of hydrocephalus in children with medulloblastoma, *Pediatr Neurosurg* 20(4):240-247, 1994.

McCallum JE, Turbeville D: Cost and outcome in a series of shunted premature infants with intraventricular hemorrhage, *Pediatr Neurosurg* 20(1):63-67, 1994.

Richard ME: Common pediatric craniofacial reconstructions, *Nurs Clin North Am* 29(4):791-799, 1994.

Ryan JA, Shiminski-Maher T: Hydrocephalus and shunts in children with brain tumors, *J Pediatr Oncol Nurs* 12(4):223-229, 1995.

Sainte-Rose C: Shunt obstruction: a preventable complication? *Pediatr Neurosurg* 19(3):156-164, 1993.

Scheinblum DT, Hammond M: The treatment of children with shunt infections: extraventricular drainage system care, *Pediatr Nurs* 16:139-143, 1990.

Sloan ES: Face value: trends and advances in craniofacial surgery, *Todays OR Nurse* 12:17-22, 1990.

Tilem D, Greenberg CS: Nursing care of the child with a ventriculostomy, *J Pediatr Nurs* 3:188-193, 1988.

THE CHILD WITH ENDOCRINE DYSFUNCTION

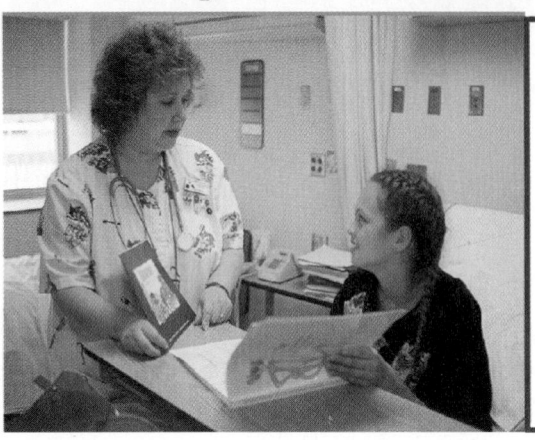

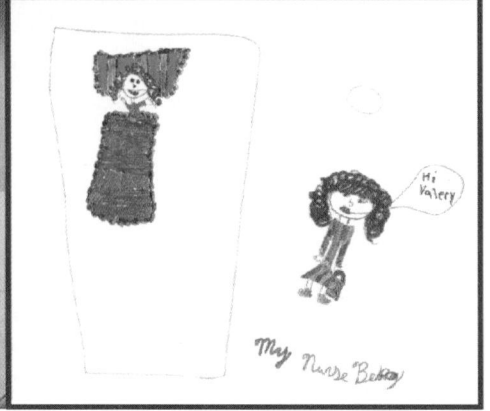

" *My nurse Becky is funny and I like her. She makes me laugh.* "

Valery, age 11 years, diabetes

RELATED TOPICS

LEARNING OBJECTIVES
On completion of this chapter the reader will be able to:

- Differentiate between the disorders caused by hypopituitary and hyperpituitary dysfunction
- Describe the manifestations of thyroid hypofunction and hyperfunction and the management of children with the disorders

- Distinguish between the manifestations of adrenal hypofunction and hyperfunction
- Differentiate among the various categories of diabetes mellitus
- Discuss the management and nursing care of the child with diabetes mellitus in the acute care setting

- Distinguish between a hypoglycemic and a hyperglycemic reaction
- Design a teaching plan for a child with diabetes mellitus
- Formulate a teaching plan for instructing parents of a child with diabetes mellitus

DISORDERS OF PITUITARY FUNCTION

T he *pituitary gland,* or *hypophysis,* is often referred to as the *master gland* because of its role in regulating other endocrine glands. Under the influence of secretions from the hypothalamus, the anterior lobe of the pituitary (adenohypophysis) releases or withholds seven hormones (Table 29-1). These hormones control the secretion of hormones from other endocrine glands and influence somatic and sexual development. Because of this relationship, a dysfunction observed in target tissues can be the result of malfunction of

the hypothalamus, the pituitary gland, or the target gland. If the tropic hormones are involved, the resulting disorder reflects the altered stimulus to the target gland. For example, if thyroid-stimulating hormone is deficient, thyroid hormone is also deficient, and the child displays the manifestations of hypothyroidism. Overproduction of pituitary hormone is thought to be caused by hyperplasia of the pituitary cells or by a primary hypothalamic defect that results in excess production of the hormone's releasing factor.

Deficiencies of the anterior pituitary hormones may be the result of organic defects or of idiopathic etiology and may occur as a single hormonal problem or in combination with other hormonal deficiencies. The clinical manifestations depend on the hormones involved and the age of onset. This discussion is limited to dysfunction related primarily to the secretion of growth hormone.

Susan B. Zekauskas, MSN, RN, PNP, revised this chapter.

TABLE 29-1. Endocrine glands and their function

GLAND/HORMONE	PRIMARY EFFECT	GLAND/HORMONE	PRIMARY EFFECT
Adenohypophysis (Anterior Pituitary)		**Adrenal Cortex**	
Growth hormone (GH)	Promotes growth of bone and soft tissues	Aldosterone	Regulates sodium retention and excretion
Thyroid-stimulating hormone (TSH)	Stimulates thyroid hormone secretion	Sex hormones	Influence development of bones, reproductive organs, and secondary sex characteristics
Adrenocorticotropic hormone (ACTH)	Stimulates adrenal cortex to secrete glucocorticoids and androgens	Glucocorticoids	Promote metabolism
Gonadotropins	Stimulate gonads to mature		Mobilize body defenses during stress
Follicle-stimulating hormone (FSH)	and produce sex hormones and germ cells		Suppress inflammatory reaction
Luteinizing hormone (LH)		**Adrenal Medulla**	
Prolactin	Stimulates milk secretion	Catecholamines	Produce a sympathetic response
Melanocyte-stimulating hormone (MSH)	Promotes pigmentation of skin		Increase blood pressure and blood glucose levels
Neurohypophysis (Posterior Pituitary)		**Islands of Langerhans of Pancreas**	
Antidiuretic hormone (ADH)	Acts on kidney tubules to reabsorb water	Insulin	Promotes utilization of glucose by cells; decreases blood glucose levels
Oxytocin	Stimulates uterine contractions	Glucagon	Increases blood glucose levels
	Causes milk-ejection reflex		Accelerates glyconeogenesis
		Somatostatin	Inhibits secretion of insulin and glucagon
Thyroid Gland			
Thyroid hormones	Regulate metabolic rate	**Ovaries**	
	Control rate of body cell growth	Estrogen	Stimulates ripening of ova
Thyrocalcitonin	Influences ossification and development of bone		Produces female secondary sex characteristics
			Promotes epiphyseal closure of bones
Parathyroid Glands		Progesterone	Prepares uterus for fertilization
Parathyroid hormone (PTH)	Regulates calcium metabolism		
		Testes	
		Testosterone	Stimulates spermatogenesis
			Produces male secondary sex characteristics
			Promotes epiphyseal closure of bones

height retarded more than [handwritten annotation]

Nursing ALERT	Children with panhypopituitarism should wear medical identification such as a bracelet.

HYPOPITUITARISM: GROWTH HORMONE (GH) DEFICIENCY

Hypopituitarism is primarily a disorder associated with deficient secretion of *GH (somatotropin)*. It may be caused by a variety of conditions: developmental defects; destructive lesions such as tumors, trauma, vascular abnormalities, or surgery; certain hereditary disorders; or functional disorders such as anorexia nervosa or psychosocial dwarfism. In more than half of children with hypopituitarism, no lesion is evident and the cause is unknown—*idiopathic hypopituitarism* or *idiopathic pituitary growth failure.*

GH deficiency inhibits somatic growth in all body cells (Fig. 29-1). The primary site of dysfunction in the syndrome appears to be in the hypothalamus. The extent of idiopathic GH deficiency may be complete or partial, but the cause is unknown. It is frequently associated with other pituitary hormone deficiencies and is treated more frequently in boys than in girls.

Diagnostic Evaluation

Only a small number of children with delayed growth or short stature have hypopituitary dwarfism. In the majority of instances the cause is constitutional delay (see Chapter 17). Although children with hypopituitarism are normal at birth, they show growth patterns that progressively deviate from the normal growth rate, often beginning in infancy. The chief complaint in most instances is short stature (see box).

A complete diagnostic evaluation should include a family history, a history of the child's growth patterns and previous health status, physical examination, radiographic surveys, and endocrine studies. Definitive diagnosis is based on radioimmunoassay of plasma GH levels stimulated pharmacologically with two or more agents. GH levels below 10 ng/ml after two provocative tests establish the diagnosis.

Radiographic examination of the hand and wrist for centers of ossification is an important procedure in evaluating growth. Endocrine studies to detect tropic hormone deficiencies are also performed if there is evidence of hypothyroidism, hypersecretion of cortisol, or gonadal aplasia.

Therapeutic Management

Treatment of GH deficiency caused by organic lesions is directed toward correction of the underlying disease process (e.g., surgical removal or irradiation of a tumor). The definitive treatment of GH deficiency is replacement of GH. *Biosynthetic GH* prepared by recombinant DNA technology is the therapy of choice. Children with other hormone deficiencies require replacement therapy to correct the specific disorders. This may involve administration of thyroid extract, cortisone, testosterone, or estrogens and progesterone. The sex hormones are usually begun during adolescence to promote normal sexual maturation.

Prognosis. GH replacement is successful in 80% of affected children. Children who respond to therapy typically increase their growth rate from 3.5 to 4 cm/year before treatment to 8 to 10 cm/year during the first year of therapy. Young children, obese children, and severely GH-deficient children respond best. Although treated children display initial rapid catch-up growth, treatment does not appear to make up a deficit in the *prognosis* of eventual height that is already present at diagnosis, indicating that the dosage of GH is not sufficient to override genetic predisposition (Moore and others, 1992). Therefore early diagnosis is important to successful therapy.

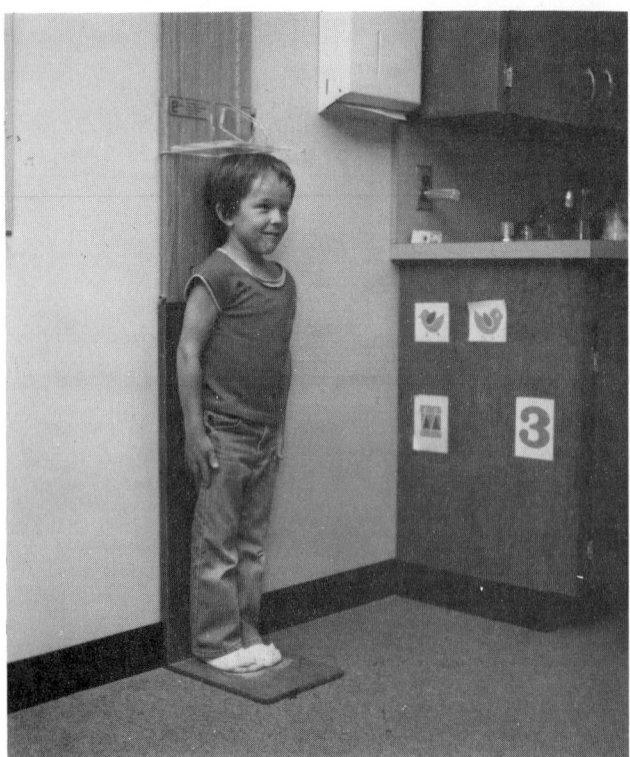

FIG. 29-1. Ten-year-old child with growth hormone deficiency—height is 42.5 inches.

CLINICAL MANIFESTATIONS OF HYPOPITUITARISM

Presenting complaint—short stature
  Usually normal growth first year
  Growth during second year drops below established percentile
  Growth measurements below 5th percentile
Premature aging common in later life
Height may be retarded more than weight
Appear well-nourished
Skeletal proportions normal
Tend to be relatively inactive
Less apt to participate in aggressive, sporting-type activities
Bone age nearly always retarded but closely related to height age
Usually primary teeth appear at expected age; eruption of permanent teeth delayed
Teeth are overcrowded and malpositioned (because of underdeveloped jaw)
Sexual development usually delayed but normal

Creutzfeldt-Jakob disease (CJD), a rare neurodegenerative condition, was reported in some patients after administration of cadaver-derived human growth hormone (HGH), but does not occur with the use of biosynthetic GH. Circumstances make it likely that HGH contaminated with CJD, a slow-growing, virus-like particle, may have been responsible for fatalities in patients treated with HGH. Blood banks do not accept donation from former HGH recipients because of the inability to test for infection with CJD (Zekauskas and others, 1990). Currently much controversy exists over the use of GH in children who are short but not GH deficient.

Nursing Considerations

Nursing care is primarily directed toward assisting in establishing the diagnosis and providing emotional support to the child and family (see also Chapter 17). Since these children appear younger than their chronologic age, others frequently relate to them in childish ways. Parents and teachers benefit from guidance directed toward realistic expectations of the child based on age and abilities (Stabler, 1993).

Children undergoing hormone replacement require additional support, such as preparation for daily subcutaneous injections and education for self-management during the school-age years* (see Critical Thinking Exercise).

*Home care instructions on giving subcutaneous injections are available in Wong DL: *Wong and Whaley's Clinical manual of pediatric nursing*, ed 4, St Louis, 1996, Mosby.

CRITICAL THINKING EXERCISE
Growth Hormone Deficiency

Kevin, an 11-year-old male, is being treated for GH deficiency. A work-up was initiated after Kevin's mother noticed that his pants size had not changed in 2 years and that his 8-year-old brother was rapidly becoming taller than Kevin. Kevin has become increasingly hostile to his brother and is refusing to attend school on a regular basis. Kevin's mother is administering the daily injections of GH. Which of the following interventions should be initiated first to allow Kevin to regain feelings of mastery and control over his environment?

1. Preparation for home schooling.
2. Family counseling related to sibling rivalry.
3. Education and support related to self administration of GH.
4. Encouragement and assurance that the therapy is temporary and will maximize his adult height.

The correct answer is three. Children with GH deficiency may develop behaviors related to feelings of inadequacy and loss of control. Often families, teachers, and peers relate to the child relative to his short height rather than his chronologic age. A child of 11 years is competent to draw up and administer daily injections of GH, which will allow the child increased control over his environment and a feeling that he is responsible for treatment of his growth deficit.

Option one is incorrect; these children must remain in regular school. At this point option two is probably not necessary, since increasing Kevin's control may reduce his hostility. Although option four is always appropriate, it does not address the principle issue—that Kevin should be independently responsible for his therapy.

Even when hormone replacement is successful, these children attain their eventual adult height at a slower rate than their peers; thus they need assistance in setting realistic expectations regarding improvement. Professionals and families may find education and support from the *Human Growth Foundation.** The treatment is expensive—up to $20,000 to $30,000 per year depending on dosage.

Nursing ALERT Injections are given at bedtime to most closely approximate physiologic release of GH.

PITUITARY HYPERFUNCTION

Excess GH prior to closure of the epiphyseal shafts results in proportional overgrowth of long bones until the individual reaches a height of 8 feet or more. Vertical growth is accompanied by rapid and increased development of muscles and viscera. Weight is increased but is usually in proportion to height. Proportional enlargement of head circumference also occurs and may result in delayed closure of the fontanels. Children with a pituitary-secreting tumor may also demonstrate signs of increasing intracranial pressure, especially headache.

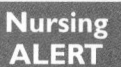 *long faces*

If hypersecretion of GH occurs after epiphyseal closure, growth is in the transverse direction, producing a condition known as *acromegaly*. Typical facial features include overgrowth of the head, lips, nose, tongue, jaw, and paranasal and mastoid sinuses; separation and malocclusion of the teeth in the enlarged jaw; disproportion of the face to the cerebral division of the skull; increased facial hair; and thickened, deeply creased skin.

Diagnostic Evaluation

Diagnosis is based on a history of excessive growth during childhood and evidence of increased levels of GH. Radiologic studies may reveal a tumor in an enlarged sella turcica; normal bone age; enlargement of bones, such as the paranasal sinuses; and evidence of joint changes. Endocrine studies to confirm excess of other hormones, such as cortisol and sex hormones, are also included in the differential diagnosis.

Therapeutic Management

If a lesion is present, surgical treatment, including cryosurgery or hypophysectomy, may be warranted to remove the tumor whenever feasible. Other therapies that destroy pituitary tissue include external irradiation and radioactive implants. Depending on the extent of surgical extirpation and the degree of pituitary insufficiency, hormone replacement with thyroid extract, cortisone, and sex hormones may be necessary.

Nursing Considerations

The primary nursing consideration is early identification of children with excessive growth rates. Although medical management does not diminish the height already attained, it can retard further growth. The earlier the treatment is begun, the better the chance to attain a normal adult height.

Children with excessive growth rates require as much

*7777 Leesburg Pike, Falls Church, VA 22043; (800) 451-6434.

emotional support as those with short stature. However, girls may suffer from the effects of excessive height much more than boys, who may find their height an asset when pursuing sports such as basketball. A compassionate nurse can be very supportive to these children, especially prior to adolescence, when they are larger than their peers. The nurse can emphasize to a tall girl that as boys grow older, they become taller and she will not always be looking down at them. Since early adolescence is a time of idol worship, the nurse can point out marriages of celebrities in which the woman is taller than the man to help the girl gain a perspective that not all heterosexual relationships must follow stereotypic models.

PRECOCIOUS PUBERTY

Manifestations of sexual development before age 9 years in boys or age 8 years in girls are considered precocious and should be investigated. Early sexual development can have a number of causes and may result from a disorder of the gonad, the adrenal gland, or the hypothalamic-pituitary gonadal axis. The disorder occurs far more frequently in girls than in boys. No causative factor can be found in 80% to 90% of girls and 50% of boys with the condition (DiGeorge, 1992).

True, or *complete, precocious puberty* is always isosexual and results from premature activation of the hypothalamic pituitary-gonadal axis, which produces early maturation and development of the gonads with secretion of sex hormones, development of secondary sex characteristics, and sometimes production of mature sperm or ova. Precocious puberty is explained only as an unusually early activation of the maturation process regarded as a normal course of events at a later age. There is early acceleration of linear growth with early epiphyseal fusion and ultimate height less than what would have been anticipated with later pubertal onset. *Precocious pseudopuberty,* or *incomplete puberty,* differs from true sexual precocity in that there is no early secretion of gonadotropin. Most cases result from early overproduction of sex hormone, usually caused by a tumor of the ovary or testis, a tumor or hyperplasia of the adrenal gland, or exogenous sources of androgens or estrogens.

Therapeutic Management

Treatment of precocious pseudopuberty is directed toward the specific cause when known. Precocious puberty of central origin is managed with monthly subcutaneous injections of a synthetic analog of *luteinizing hormone-releasing hormone (LHRH; Lupron),* which regulates pituitary secretions. This therapy slows the prepubertal growth to normal rates in affected children. Treatment is discontinued at a chronologically appropriate time, allowing pubertal changes to resume.

Nursing Considerations

Psychologic support and guidance of the child and family are the most important aspects of management. Parents need a detailed explanation and reassurance of the benign nature of the condition. Dress and activities for the physically precocious child should be appropriate to the chronologic age.

Despite the early sexual development, maturation of the gonads and the appearance of secondary sexual characteristics proceed in the usual order. After puberty, physical differences from peers are no longer present. Although the child's

heterosexual behavior is appropriate for the chronologic age, the nurse should emphasize to parents that the child is fertile. No form of contraception is necessary, however, unless the child is sexually active.

Children receiving LHRH therapy need preparation for the subcutaneous injections. Both parents and children should be taught the injection procedure.*

DIABETES INSIPIDUS (DI)

The principal disorder of posterior pituitary hypofunction is DI, also known as *neurogenic DI.* The disease is the result of hyposecretion of *antidiuretic hormone (ADH),* or *vasopressin,* which produces a state of uncontrolled diuresis. Primary causes are familial or idiopathic; secondary causes include trauma (accidental or surgical), tumors, granulomatous disease, infections (meningitis or encephalitis), or vascular anomalies (aneurysm). The disorder is not to be confused with nephrogenic DI, a rare hereditary disorder caused by unresponsiveness of the renal tubules to the hormone.

Clinical Manifestations

The cardinal signs of DI are polyuria and polydipsia. In the older child excessive urination accompanied by a compensatory insatiable thirst may be so intense that the child does little other than drink fluids and void. Not infrequently, the first sign is enuresis. In the infant the initial symptom is irritability that is relieved with feedings of water but not milk. The infant is also prone to dehydration, electrolyte imbalance, hyperthermia, azotemia, and potential circulatory collapse.

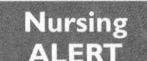 **Nursing ALERT** The child with DI complicated by congenital absence of the thirst center must be encouraged to drink sufficient quantities of liquid to prevent electrolyte imbalance.

Diagnostic Evaluation

The simplest test used to diagnose this condition is restriction of oral fluids and observation of consequent changes in urine volume and concentration. In DI fluid restriction has little or no effect on urine formation but causes weight loss from dehydration. If this test is positive, the child should be given a test dose of injected *aqueous vasopressin (Pitressin),* which should alleviate the polyuria and polydipsia. Unresponsiveness to exogenous vasopressin usually indicates nephrogenic DI.

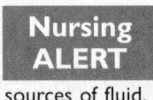 **Nursing ALERT** Small children require close supervision during fluid restriction to prevent them from drinking even from toilet bowls, plants, or other unlikely sources of fluid.

Therapeutic Management

The usual treatment is hormone replacement with either an intramuscular or a subcutaneous injection of *vasopressin tannate* in peanut oil or via *aqueous vasopressin* nasal spray. The

---

*Home care instructions on giving subcutaneous injections are available in Wong DL: *Wong and Whaley's Clinical manual of pediatric nursing,* ed 4, St Louis, 1996, Mosby.

injectable form has the advantage of lasting 48 to 72 hours, which affords the child a full night's sleep. However, it has the disadvantages of requiring frequent injections and proper preparation of the drug.

Desmopressin acetate (DDAVP) is available and administered intranasally by way of a flexible tube to achieve adequate control. It is usually administered twice daily. The response pattern of the child is variable, with duration ranging from 8 to 20 hours (Gildea, 1993). Children receiving DDAVP need to be observed for a possible overdose of the drug. The signs of overdosage are those of water intoxication and are similar to manifestations of inappropriate secretion of antidiuretic hormone.

Nursing Considerations

The initial objective of care is identification of the disorder. After confirmation of the diagnosis, parents need a thorough explanation of the condition, with special emphasis on distinguishing the difference between diabetes insipidus and diabetes mellitus. The parents must realize that treatment is lifelong. If the child is to receive the injectable vasopressin, ideally both parents, as well as children who are over 7 years of age, should be taught the correct procedure for preparation and administration of the drug.* Once children are old enough, they should be encouraged to assume full responsibility for care.

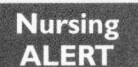 To be effective, vasopressin must be thoroughly resuspended in the oil by being held under warm running water for 10 to 15 minutes and shaken vigorously before being drawn into the syringe. If this is not done, the oil may be injected without the antidiuretic hormone. Small brown particles, which indicate drug dispersion, must be seen in the suspension.

For emergency purposes these children should wear medical alert identification. Older children are advised to carry the nasal vasopressin spray with them for temporary relief of symptoms. School personnel should be made aware of the problem so that the child is granted unrestricted use of the lavatory and drinking water. Failure to permit this may result in embarrassing accidents that often result in the child's unwillingness to attend school.

SYNDROME OF INAPPROPRIATE ANTIDIURETIC HORMONE SECRETION (SIADH)

Hypersecretion of the posterior pituitary *antidiuretic hormone (ADH, vasopressin)* produces the disorder known as the syndrome of inappropriate ADH secretion (SIADH). SIADH is observed with increased frequency in a variety of conditions, especially those involving infections, tumors, and trauma of the central nervous system.

The manifestations observed are directly related to fluid retention and hypotonicity. Increased secretion of ADH causes the kidneys to reabsorb water, which increases the fluid

volume and decreases serum osmolality. When serum sodium levels are lowered to 120 mEq/L, the child displays anorexia, nausea (sometimes vomiting), stomach cramps, irritability, and personality changes. With progressive reduction in sodium, other neurologic signs, stupor, and seizures may be evident. The symptoms disappear when the underlying disorder is corrected. Immediate management consists of restricting fluids.

Nursing Considerations

The first goal of nursing management is recognizing the presence of SIADH from symptoms described in patients at risk. Accurately measuring intake, output, and daily weight, and observing for signs of fluid overload are primary nursing functions, especially in the child receiving intravenous fluids.

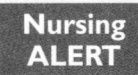 Children with SIADH develop an expanded circulatory volume but do not form edema, which is an excess of both water and sodium (Gildea, 1993).

Seizure precautions are implemented, and the child and family need education regarding the rationale for fluid restriction. The rare child with chronic SIADH will be placed on a long-term regimen of ADH-antagonizing medication and will require instructions for its administration.

DISORDERS OF THYROID FUNCTION

The thyroid gland secretes two types of hormones: *thyroid hormone,* which consists of the hormones *thyroxine (T_4)* and *triiodothyronine (T_3),* and *thyrocalcitonin.* The secretion of thyroid hormones is controlled by *thyroid-stimulating hormone (TSH)* from the anterior pituitary. Hypothyroidism or hyperthyroidism may result from a defect in the target gland or from a disturbance in secretion of TSH or its releasing factor in the hypothalamus.

Since the functions of T_3 and T_4 are qualitatively the same, the term *thyroid hormone (TH)* is used throughout this discussion.

The synthesis of TH depends on available sources of dietary iodine and tyrosine. The thyroid is the only endocrine gland capable of storing excess amounts of hormones for release as needed. The main physiologic action of TH is to regulate the basal metabolic rate and thereby control the processes of growth and tissue differentiation.

Thyrocalcitonin helps maintain blood calcium levels by decreasing the calcium concentration. Its effect is the opposite of parathormone; it inhibits skeletal demineralization and promotes calcium deposition in the bone.

JUVENILE HYPOTHYROIDISM

Hypothyroidism is one of the most common endocrine problems of childhood. It may be either congenital (see Chapter 9) or acquired and represents a deficiency in secretion of TH. Hypothyroidism from dietary insufficiency of iodine is rare in the United States because iodized salt is a readily available

CLINICAL MANIFESTATIONS OF JUVENILE HYPOTHYROIDISM	

Decelerated growth
  Less when acquired at later age
Myxedematous skin changes
  Dry skin
  Puffiness around eyes
  Sparse hair
	Constipation
	Sleepiness
	Mental decline

source of the nutrient. This discussion is limited to the juvenile form of hypothyroidism.

Beyond infancy, primary hypothyroidism may be caused by a number of defects. For example, a congenital hypoplastic thyroid gland may provide sufficient amounts of TH during the first year or two but be inadequate when rapid body growth increases demands on the gland. A partial or complete thyroidectomy for cancer or thyrotoxicosis can leave insufficient thyroid tissue to furnish hormones for body requirements. Irradiation for Hodgkin disease or other malignancies or infectious processes may be a cause of hypothyroidism. A high risk for thyroid disease, including thyroid cancer and Graves disease, persists for more than 25 years after patients have received radiation therapy (Hancock, Cox, and McDougall, 1991).

Clinical manifestations depend on the extent of dysfunction and the age of the child at the onset (see box). Since brain growth is nearly complete by 2 to 3 years of age, mental retardation or neurologic sequelae are not associated with juvenile hypothyroidism.

Therapy is oral TH replacement, the same as for hypothyroidism in the infant, although the prompt treatment needed for brain growth in the infant is not required in the child. In children with severe symptoms, the restoration of euthyroidism is achieved more gradually, with administration of increasing amounts of L-thyroxine over 4 to 8 weeks to avoid symptoms of hyperthyroidism that can occur with treatment of chronic hypothyroidism.

Nursing Considerations

The importance of early recognition in the infant is discussed in Chapter 9. Cessation or retardation of growth in a child whose growth has previously been normal should alert the observer to the possibility of hypothyroidism. Following diagnosis and implementation of thyroxine therapy, the importance of compliance and periodic monitoring of the response to therapy should be stressed to the parents. Children should learn to take responsibility for their health as soon as they are old enough, at about 9 to 10 years of age.

GOITER

A goiter is an enlargement or hypertrophy of the thyroid gland. It can be congenital or acquired. Congenital disease usually occurs as a result of antithyroid drugs and/or iodides administered to the mother during pregnancy. The acquired disease can result from increased secretion of pituitary thyrotropic hormone in response to decreased circulating levels of TH, neoplastic or inflammatory processes, or dietary iodine deficiency.

Enlargement of the thyroid gland may be mild and noticeable only when there is an increased demand for TH (e.g., during periods of rapid growth). Enlargement of the thyroid at birth can be sufficient to cause severe respiratory distress. TH replacement is necessary to treat the hypothyroidism and reverse the TSH effect on the gland.

Nursing Considerations

Large goiters are identified by their obvious appearance. Smaller nodules may be evident only on palpation. Nurses in ambulatory settings need to be aware of the possibility of neck enlargement from goiters and report such findings.

Nursing ALERT If an infant is born with a goiter, immediate precautions are instituted for emergency ventilation, such as supplemental oxygen and a tracheostomy set. Positioning the child with the neck hyperextended often facilitates breathing.

Immediate surgery to remove part of the gland may be lifesaving. When thyroid replacement is necessary, parents have the same needs regarding its administration as discussed for the parents of children who have hypothyroidism (Chapter 9).

LYMPHOCYTIC THYROIDITIS

Lymphocytic thyroiditis *(Hashimoto disease, juvenile autoimmune thyroiditis)* is the most common cause of thyroid disease in children and adolescents, and it accounts for the largest percentage of juvenile hypothyroidism. It also accounts for many of the enlarged thyroid glands formerly designated as thyroid hyperplasia of adolescence, or "adolescent goiter." The disease is more common in girls than in boys and in white persons than in black persons. It occurs more frequently after age 6, reaching a peak incidence at adolescence; there is evidence that the disease is self-limited.

Pathophysiology

There is a strong genetic predisposition to the development of autoimmune thyroiditis, although no mode of inheritance has been delineated and the basic stimulus or autoimmune defect is unknown. The disease is characterized by lymphocytic infiltration of the gland, inflammation, and, in many patients, replacement with fibrous tissue. In the early stages there may be only hyperplasia.

Diagnostic Evaluation

The enlarged thyroid gland may be detected by the practitioner during a routine examination, although it may be noted by parents when the youngster swallows. Most children are euthyroid, but some display symptoms of hypothyroidism. Others have signs that suggest hyperthyroidism (see box).

Thyroid function tests are usually normal, although TSH levels may be slightly or moderately elevated. With progressive disease the T_4 decreases, followed by a decrease in T_3 levels and an increase in TSH. A variety of abnormalities in radioactive iodine uptake may be noted. The majority of children have serum antibody titers to thyroid antigens, but fewer children have a positive red blood cell hemagglutination test.

CLINICAL MANIFESTATIONS OF LYMPHOCYTIC THYROIDITIS	
Enlarged Thyroid Gland Usually symmetrical Firm Freely movable Nontender **Tracheal Compression** Sense of fullness Hoarseness Dysphagia	**Hyperthyroidism (Possible)** Nervousness Irritability Increased sweating Hyperactivity

CLINICAL MANIFESTATIONS OF HYPERTHYROIDISM (GRAVES DISEASE)

Cardinal Signs
 Emotional lability
 Physical restlessness, characteristically at rest
 Decelerated school performance
 Voracious appetite with weight loss in 50% of cases.
 Fatigue
 	
 Physical Signs
 Tachycardia
 Widened pulse pressure
 Dyspnea on exertion
 Exophthalmos (protruding eyeballs)
 Wide-eyed, staring expression with lid lag
 Tremor
 Goiter (hypertrophy and hyperplasia)
 Warm, moist skin
 Accelerated linear growth
 Heat intolerance (may be severe)
 Hair fine and unable to hold a curl
 Systolic murmurs
 	
 Thyroid Storm
 Acute onset:
   Severe irritability and restlessness
   Vomiting
   Diarrhea
   Hyperthermia
   Hypertension
   Severe tachycardia
   Prostration
 May progress rapidly to:
   Delirium
   Coma
   Death

When both tests are used, almost all children with thyroid autoimmunity are detected.

Therapeutic Management

In many cases the goiter is transient and asymptomatic and regresses spontaneously within a year or two. Therapy of non-toxic diffuse goiter is usually simple, uncomplicated, and effective. Oral administration of TH depresses TSH, thus decreasing the size of the gland significantly. Surgery is contraindicated in this disorder.

Nursing Considerations

Nursing care consists of identifying the youngster with thyroid enlargement, reassuring the child that the condition is probably only temporary, and reinforcing instructions for thyroid therapy.

HYPERTHYROIDISM (GRAVES DISEASE)

The largest percentage of hyperthyroidism in childhood is caused by Graves disease, which is usually associated with an enlarged thyroid gland and exophthalmos. The peak incidence of the disease occurs between 12 and 14 years of age, but it may be present at birth in children of thyrotoxic mothers. The incidence is five times higher in girls than in boys. The disease is apparently caused by a serum thyroid-stimulating immunoglobulin, but no specific etiology has been identified. There is definitive evidence for familial association; a large number of persons with the disease possess the histocompatibility antigen HLA-B8.

Diagnostic Evaluation

The development of manifestations is highly variable (see box). Manifestations develop gradually with an interval between onset and diagnosis of approximately 6 to 12 months. Diagnosis is established on the basis of increased levels of T_4 and T_3. Thyrotropin (TSH) is suppressed to unmeasurable levels. Other tests are rarely indicated.

Therapeutic Management

Therapy for hyperthyroidism is controversial, but all methods are directed toward retarding the rate of hormone secretion. The three acceptable modes available are (1) the antithyroid drugs, which interfere with the biosynthesis of TH, including propylthiouracil (PTU) and methimazole (MTZ,

Tapazole); (2) subtotal thyroidectomy; and (3) ablation with radioiodine (^{131}I-iodide). When affected children exhibit signs and symptoms of hyperthyroidism their activity should be limited. Vigorous exercise is restricted until thyroid levels are decreased to normal or near normal values.

Thyrotoxicosis (thyroid "crisis" or thyroid "storm") may occur from sudden release of the hormone. Although it is unusual in children, a crisis can be life-threatening. A crisis may be precipitated by acute infection, surgical emergencies, or discontinuation of antithyroid therapy. Treatment, in addition to antithyroid drugs, is administration of β-adrenergic blocking agents (propranolol), which provide relief from the disturbing side effects of the reaction.

Nursing Considerations

The initial nursing objective is identification of children with hyperthyroidism. Since the clinical manifestations often appear gradually, the goiter and ophthalmic changes may not be noticed, and the excessive activity may be attributed to behavioral problems. Nurses in ambulatory settings, particularly those caring for children in school, need to be alert to signs that suggest this disorder, especially weight loss despite an excellent appetite, academic difficulties resulting from a short attention span and inability to sit still, unexplained fatigue and sleeplessness, and difficulty with fine motor skills, such as writing. Exophthalmos may develop long before the onset of signs and symptoms of hyperthyroidism and may be the only presenting sign (Tallstedt and others, 1992).

Much of the care during diagnosis and initial medical therapy is related to the physical symptoms. The child needs a quiet, unstimulating environment that is conducive to rest, and sometimes hospitalization is necessary during the immediate treatment phase. A regular routine is beneficial, with frequent rest periods, minimizing the stress of coping with unexpected demands, and meeting the child's needs promptly. Physical activity is restricted. For example, school physical education classes are discontinued. Despite the excessive activity of these children, they tire easily, experience muscle weakness, and are unable to relax to recoup their strength.

Emotional lability is often manifested by sudden episodes of crying or elation. Such behavior, together with irritability, disrupts interpersonal relationships, creating difficulties within and outside the home. Heat intolerance may produce considerable family conflict. Since a cooler environment is preferred, the child is likely to open windows, complain about the heat, wear minimum clothing, and kick off blankets while sleeping. Hygiene should be stressed because of excessive sweating.

Dietary requirements are regulated to meet the child's increased metabolic rate. Although the need for calories is increased, these should be provided in wholesome foods rather than "junk" foods. Vitamin supplements may be needed to meet daily requirements. Rather than three large meals, the child's appetite may be better satisfied by five or six moderate meals throughout the day.

Once therapy is instituted, the nurse explains the drug regimen, emphasizing the importance of observing for side effects of antithyroid drugs. Untoward effects of propylthiouracil and related compounds include skin rash, drug fever, enlargement of the salivary and cervical lymph glands, diminished sense of taste, hepatitis, and edema of the lower extremities. (See Critical Thinking Exercise.)

> **Nursing ALERT** Children being treated with propylthiouracil must be carefully monitored for side effects of the drug. Since sore throat and fever accompany the grave complication of leukopenia, these children should be seen by a practitioner if such symptoms occur. Parents and children should be taught to recognize and report symptoms immediately.

Parents should also be aware of the signs of hypothyroidism, which can occur from overdose of the drugs. The most common indications are lethargy and somnolence.

Surgical Care. If surgery is anticipated, iodine is usually administered for a few weeks before the procedure. Since oral iodine preparations are unpalatable, they should be mixed with a strong-tasting fruit juice, such as grape or punch flavors, and be given through a straw. Compliance with iodine therapy is essential to avoid the danger of thyroid crisis after sudden discontinuation.

Psychologic preparation of children for thyroidectomy is similar to that for any other surgical procedure (see Chapter 22). However, of special consideration is the site of the incision. The fear of having the throat cut is very real and in older children is associated with death. The nurse should explain that the throat is not cut, only the skin, to allow for removal of the gland. Showing children a picture of the anatomic location of the thyroid around the trachea is often helpful. Children should be prepared for the dressing around the neck and the possibility of an endotracheal or "breathing" tube after surgery.

Postoperative care involves positioning with the neck slightly flexed to avoid strain on the sutures and observation for bleeding and complications. The children are taught to support the neck in this position when they sit up. Damage to the recurrent laryngeal nerve is evidenced by severe stridor and/or hoarseness, although some hoarseness is expected. Observation for signs of hypoparathyroidism, which causes hypocalcemia, should be implemented in the immediate postoperative period.

> **Nursing ALERT** The earliest indication of hypoparathyroidism may be anxiety and mental depression, followed by paresthesia and evidence of heightened neuromuscular excitability, such as
>
> **Chvostek sign**—facial muscle spasm elicited by tapping the facial nerve in the region of the parotid gland
> **Trousseau sign**—carpal spasm elicited by pressure applied to nerves of the upper arm
> **Tetany**—carpopedal spasm (sharp flexion of wrist and ankle joints), muscle twitching, cramps, seizures, and sometimes stridor

---

CRITICAL THINKING EXERCISE
Graves Disease

Susie, 15 years old, has noticed a racing pulse, ravenous appetite with continued weight loss, heat intolerance, sensitivity, and eyes that appear to be bulging from their sockets. After a diagnosis of Graves disease Susie is started on a therapeutic dose of propylthiouracil. Because of tachycardia, Susie is cautioned to participate in sedentary activities only and to discontinue school physical education classes. Environmental temperature and appropriate dress related to heat sensitivity, as well as dietary adjustments to meet increased metabolic needs, are addressed by the nurse. Susie is shown that exopthalmus can be minimized with artful application of cosmetics. Episodic emotional lability is discussed with Susie and her family. The drug regimen is explained with special emphasis on its side effects. After 6 weeks of treatment Susie presents with a sore throat and fever. Which of the following interventions is most appropriate?

1. Immediate follow-up by the practitioner.
2. Further instruction related to heat sensitivity.
3. Instruction related to symptomatic relief of the common cold.
4. Psychosocial interventions related to somatization of emotional lability.

The correct answer is one. Therapeutic levels of propylthiouracil can be accompanied by the grave complication of leukocytopenia. Any indication of infection must be promptly evaluated and appropriate therapy instituted. None of the other options addresses the immediate problem.

DISORDERS OF PARATHYROID FUNCTION

The parathyroid glands secrete *parathormone (PTH),* whose main function, along with vitamin D, is to maintain homeostasis of blood calcium concentration. PTH exerts its effect by (1) increasing the release of calcium and phosphate from the bone (bone demineralization), (2) increasing the absorption of calcium and the excretion of phosphate by the kidneys, and (3) promoting calcium absorption in the gastrointestinal tract. The net result of these actions is to increase the plasma calcium concentration while lowering the plasma phosphate concentration.

HYPOPARATHYROIDISM

Two classic forms of hypoparathyroidism are observed during childhood. *Autoimmune hypoparathyroidism,* in which there is deficient production of PTH, may occur as a component of multiglandular failure, usually in relation to autoimmune phenomena. Familial hypoparathyroidism is inherited as an autosomal recessive trait, with early onset, usually in the first month of life. In *pseudohypoparathyroidism* production of PTH is increased but end-organ responsiveness to the hormone is deficient. Pseudohypoparathyroidism is also thought to be inherited as an X-linked dominant trait with variable expressivity. Transient hypoparathyroidism may also be observed in infants born to mothers with the disease or in infants fed a milk formula with a high phosphate/calcium ratio (Chapter 9).

Diagnostic Evaluation

The diagnosis of hypoparathyroidism is made on the basis of clinical manifestations associated with *decreased serum calcium* and *increased serum phosphorus levels* (see box). Levels of plasma PTH are low in idiopathic hypoparathyroidism but high in pseudohypoparathyroidism. End-organ responsiveness is tested by the administration of PTH with measurement of urinary cyclic AMP. Kidney function tests are included in the differential diagnosis to rule out renal insufficiency. Although bone radiographs are usually normal, they may demonstrate increased bone density and suppressed growth.

Therapeutic Management

The objective of treatment is to maintain normal serum calcium and phosphate levels with minimum complications. Acute or severe tetany is corrected immediately by intravenous and oral administration of calcium gluconate and follow-up daily doses to achieve normal levels. When the diagnosis is confirmed, *vitamin D therapy* is begun. Long-term management consists of administration of massive doses of vitamin D; oral calcium supplementation may be useful, although it is not essential.

Nursing Considerations

The initial objective is recognition of hypocalcemia. Unexplained seizures, irritability (especially to external stimuli), gastrointestinal symptoms (e.g., diarrhea, vomiting, abdominal cramps), and positive signs of tetany should lead the nurse to suspect this disorder. Much of the initial nursing care is

CLINICAL MANIFESTATIONS OF HYPOPARATHYROIDISM

Pseudohypoparathyroidism

Short stature
Round face
Short, thick neck
Short, stubby fingers and toes
Dimpling of skin over knuckles
Subcutaneous soft tissue calcifications
Mental retardation a prominent feature

Idiopathic Hypoparathyroidism

None of the above physical characteristics observed
Papilledema may be seen
May be mental retardation

Both Types

Dry, scaly, coarse skin with eruptions
Hair often brittle
Nails thin and brittle with characteristic transverse grooves
Dental and enamel hypoplasia
Muscle contractions:
  Tetany
  Carpopedal spasm
  Laryngospasm (laryngeal stridor)
  Muscle cramps and twitching
  Positive Chvostek and/or Trousseau signs (see p. 1042)
Paresthesias, tingling
Neurologic:
  Headache
  Seizures (generalized, absence, or focal)
  Swings of emotion
  Loss of memory
  Depression
  Confusion can occur
Gastrointestinal:
  Muscle cramps
  Diarrhea
  Vomiting
Retarded skeletal growth

related to the physical manifestations and includes institution of seizure and safety precautions, reduction of environmental stimuli (e.g., sudden noises or movements, bright lights), and observation for signs of laryngospasm.

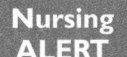 **Nursing ALERT** Signs of *laryngospasm* are stridor, hoarseness, and a feeling of tightness in the throat. A tracheostomy set and injectable calcium gluconate should be placed near the bedside for emergency use. The intravenous administration of calcium gluconate requires precautions against extravasation of the drug and tissue destruction.

After initiation of treatment, the nurse discusses with the parents the need for continuous daily administration of calcium salts and vitamin D. Because vitamin D toxicity can be a serious consequence of therapy, parents are advised to watch for signs, which include weakness, fatigue, lassitude, headache, nausea, vomiting, and diarrhea. Early renal impairment is manifested by polyuria, polydipsia, and nocturia.

HYPERPARATHYROIDISM

Hyperparathyroidism is rare in childhood but can be primary or secondary. The most common cause of primary hyperparathyroidism is adenoma of the gland. The most common causes of secondary hyperparathyroidism are chronic renal disease, renal osteodystrophy, and congenital anomalies of the urinary tract. The common factor is hypercalcemia.

Diagnostic Evaluation

Blood studies to confirm the presence of *elevated calcium* and *lowered phosphorus levels* are routinely performed. Measurement of PTH, as well as several tests to isolate the cause of the hypercalcemia, such as renal function studies, should be included. Other procedures employed to substantiate the physiologic consequences of the disorder include electrocardiography and radiographic bone surveys (see box).

Therapeutic Management

Treatment depends on the cause. The treatment of primary hyperparathyroidism is surgical removal of the tumor or hyperplastic tissue. Treatment of secondary hyperparathyroidism is directed at the underlying contributing cause, thus subsequently restoring the serum calcium balance. However, in some instances the underlying disorder is irreversible, such as in chronic renal failure (see Chapter 27). In this instance treatment is the same as the treatment for renal osteodystrophy.

CLINICAL MANIFESTATIONS OF HYPERPARATHYROIDISM

Gastrointestinal
Nausea
Vomiting
Abdominal discomfort
Constipation

Central Nervous System
Delusions
Confusion
Hallucinations
Impaired memory
Lack of interest and initiative
Depression
Varying levels of consciousness

Neuromuscular
Weakness
Easy fatigability
Muscle atrophy (especially proximal muscles of lower limbs)
Tongue twitching
Paresthesias in extremities

Skeletal
Vague bone pain
Subperiosteal resorption of phalanges
Spontaneous fractures
Absence of lamina dura around teeth

Renal
Polyuria
Polydipsia
Renal colic
Hypertension

Nursing Considerations

Since surgical exploration is the major treatment modality, nursing care is similar to that discussed for the child with hyperthyroidism (see p. 1041). Since hypocalcemia is a potential complication, observation for signs of tetany, institution of seizure precautions, and having calcium gluconate available for emergency use are part of the nursing care.

DISORDERS OF ADRENAL FUNCTION

The *adrenal cortex* secretes three main groups of hormones collectively called *steroids* and classified according to their biologic activity: (1) *glucocorticoids* (cortisol, corticosterone), (2) *mineralocorticoids* (aldosterone), and (3) *sex steroids* (androgens, estrogens, and progestins). Alterations in the levels of these hormones produce significant dysfunction in a variety of body tissues and organs. Since the adrenocortical cells are capable of producing any of the steroids, pathologic conditions may result in a deficiency or an excess of more than one type of hormone. However, most are rare in children.

The *adrenal medulla* secretes the *catecholamines epinephrine* and *norepinephrine*. Both hormones have essentially the same effects on various organs as those caused by direct sympathetic stimulation, except that the hormonal effects last several times longer. Catecholamine-secreting tumors are the primary cause of adrenal medullary hyperfunction.

ACUTE ADRENOCORTICAL INSUFFICIENCY

The acute form of adrenocortical insufficiency (*adrenal crisis*) may result from a number of causes during childhood. Although a rare disorder, some of the more common etiologic factors include hemorrhage into the gland from trauma, which may be caused by a prolonged, difficult labor; fulminating infections, such as meningococcemia, which result in hemorrhage and necrosis (Waterhouse-Friederichsen syndrome); abrupt withdrawal of exogenous sources of cortisone or failure to increase exogenous supplies during stress; or congenital adrenogenital hyperplasia of the salt-losing type.

Diagnostic Evaluation

There is no rapid, definitive test for confirmation of acute adrenocortical insufficiency. Routine procedures such as measurement of plasma cortisol levels are too time-consuming to be practical. Therefore diagnosis is usually based on clinical symptoms (see box). Improvement with cortisol therapy confirms the diagnosis.

Therapeutic Management

Treatment involves replacement of cortisol, replacement of body fluids to correct dehydration and hypovolemia, administration of glucose solutions to correct hypoglycemia, and specific antibiotic therapy in the presence of infection. If hemorrhage has been severe, whole blood may be replaced. In the event that these measures do not reverse the circulatory collapse, vasopressors are used for immediate vasoconstriction and elevation of blood pressure. Once the child's condition is stabilized, oral doses of cortisone, fluids, and salt are given, similar to the regimen used for chronic adrenal insufficiency.

Nursing Considerations

Because of the abrupt onset and potentially fatal outcome of this condition, prompt recognition is essential. Vital signs and blood pressure are measured often to monitor the hyperpyrexia and shocklike state. Seizure precautions are instituted, since seizures from the elevated temperature are not uncommon. As soon as therapy is instituted, the nurse monitors the child's response to fluid and cortisol replacement, being alert to too-rapid administration of fluids and drugs. Overtreatment with cortisol and sodium chloride can precipitate complications, such as an ascending flaccid paralysis. The nurse should observe for signs of hypokalemia and should evaluate serum electrolyte levels. The condition is rapidly corrected with intravenous and oral potassium replacement. Intake and urinary output are measured and recorded.

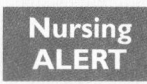 **Nursing ALERT** Monitor serum electrolyte levels and observe for signs of hypo- or hyperkalemia, (e.g., weakness, poor muscle control, paralysis, cardiac dysrhythmias, and apnea).

NURSING TIP When the oral preparation is given, potassium supplement should be mixed with a small amount of strongly flavored fruit juice to disguise its bitter taste.

The sudden, severe nature of this disorder requires considerable emotional support for the child and family. The child is usually in an intensive care unit, where the surroundings are strange and frightening. Since recovery within 24 hours is often dramatic, the nurse should keep the parents apprised of the child's condition, emphasizing signs of improvement, such as a lowered temperature and elevated blood pressure. If paralysis occurs, the nurse should assure them that this condition is temporary and quickly reversed.

CHRONIC ADRENOCORTICAL INSUFFICIENCY (ADDISON DISEASE)

Chronic adrenocortical insufficiency is rare in children. When it does occur, it is usually caused by a destructive lesion of the adrenal glands or a neoplasm, or it has an idiopathic cause.

Evidence of this disorder is usually gradual in onset, since 90% of adrenal tissue must be nonfunctional before signs of insufficiency are manifested (see box). However, during periods of stress, when demands for additional cortisol are increased, symptoms of acute insufficiency may appear in a previously well child (see box).

CLINICAL MANIFESTATIONS OF ACUTE ADRENOCORTICAL INSUFFICIENCY

Early Symptoms
Increased irritability
Headache
Diffuse abdominal pain
Weakness
Nausea and vomiting
Diarrhea

Generalized Hemorrhagic Manifestations (Waterhouse-Friderichsen Syndrome)
Fever—increases as condition worsens
Central nervous system signs
   Nuchal rigidity
   Seizures
   Stupor
   Coma

Shocklike State
Weak, rapid pulse
Decreased blood pressure
Shallow respirations
Cold, clammy skin
Cyanosis
Circulatory collapse (terminal event)

Newborn
Hyperpyrexia
Tachypnea
Cyanosis
Seizures
Gland may be evident as palpable retroperitoneal mass (hemorrhagic)

CLINICAL MANIFESTATIONS OF CHRONIC ADRENOCORTICAL INSUFFICIENCY

Neurologic Symptoms
Muscular weakness
Mental fatigue
Irritability, apathy, and negativism

Pigmentary Changes
Previous scars
Palmar creases
Mucous membranes
Hair
Hyperpigmentation over pressure points (elbows, knees, or waist)
Less frequently, vitiligo (loss of pigmentation)

Gastrointestinal Symptoms
Dehydration
Anorexia
Weight loss

Hypotension and Small Heart Size
Dizziness
Syncopal (fainting) attacks

Hypoglycemia
Headache
Hunger
Weakness
Trembling
Sweating

Other Signs (Seen in Some Children)
Recurrent, unexplained seizures
Intense craving for salt
Acute abdominal pain

Definitive diagnosis is based on measurements of functional cortisol reserve. The cortisol and urinary 17-hydroxycorticosteroid levels are low and fail to rise, whereas plasma adrenocorticotropic hormone (ACTH) levels are elevated with corticotropin stimulation, the definitive test for the disease.

Therapeutic Management

Treatment involves replacement of *glucocorticoids (cortisol)* and *mineralocorticoids (aldosterone).* Some children are able to be maintained solely on oral supplements of cortisol (cortisone or hydrocortisone preparations) with a liberal intake of salt. Other forms of therapy include monthly injections of desoxycorticosterone acetate or implantation of desoxycorticosterone acetate pellets subcutaneously every 9 to 12 months. During stressful situations, such as infection, emotional upset, or surgery, the dosage must be tripled to accommodate the body's increased need for glucocorticoids. Failure to meet this requirement will precipitate an acute crisis. Overdosage produces cushingoid signs (see Fig. 29-2).

Nursing Considerations

Once the disorder is diagnosed, parents need guidance concerning drug therapy. They must be aware of the continuous need for cortisol replacement. Sudden termination of the drug because of inadequate supplies or inability to ingest the oral form because of vomiting places the child in danger of an acute adrenal crisis. Ideally, the parents should have a prefilled syringe of hydrocortisone in the home, and should be taught the proper technique for intramuscular administration of the drug in case of a crisis.* Unnecessary administration of cortisone will not harm the child but, if needed, may be lifesaving. Any evidence of acute insufficiency is reported to the practitioner immediately.

Since the body cannot supply endogenous sources of cortical hormones during times of stress, the home environment should be stable and relatively unstressful. Parents need to be aware that during periods of emotional or physical crisis the child requires additional hormone replacement. The child should wear a medical alert identification tag to permit medical personnel to adjust the requirements during emergency care.

CUSHING SYNDROME

Cushing syndrome is a characteristic group of manifestations caused by excessive circulating free cortisol. It can result from a variety of etiologies, which generally fall into one of four categories:

Pituitary, with adrenal hyperplasia, usually attributed to an excess of ACTH

Adrenal, with hypersecretion of glucocorticoids, generally the result of adrenocortical neoplasms

Ectopic, with autonomous secretion of ACTH, most often caused by extrapituitary neoplasms

Iatrogenic, frequently the result of administration of large amounts of exogenous corticosteroids

Food dependent, inappropriate sensitivity of adrenal glands to nor-

---

*Home care instructions on giving intramuscular injections are available in Wong DL: *Wong and Whaley's Clinical manual of pediatric nursing,* ed 4, St Louis, 1996, Mosby.

CLINICAL MANIFESTATIONS OF CUSHING SYNDROME
Centripetal fat distribution
Truncal obesity
Supraclavicular fat pads
Fat pads on neck and back ("buffalo hump")
Rounded or "moon" face
Muscular wasting
Thin extremities
Pendulous abdomen
Muscle weakness
Thin skin and subcutaneous tissue
Poor wound healing
Increased susceptibility to infection
Decreased inflammatory response
Excessive bruising
Petechial hemorrhages
Facial plethora ("red cheeks")
Reddish purple abdominal striae
Hypertension
Hypokalemia
Alkalosis
Osteoporosis
Compression fractures of vertebrae
Kyphosis
Backache
Retarded linear growth
Hypercalciuria-renal calculi
Psychoses
Irritability
Insomnia
Euphoria
Depression
Frank psychoses
Peptic ulcer
Hyperglycemia
Glycosuria
Latent or overt diabetes
Virilization
Hirsutism (excessive body hair)
Acne
Deepening of voice
Clitoral enlargement
Tendency toward male physique in female
Amenorrhea
Impotence

mal postprandial increases in secretion of gastric inhibitory polypeptide (Bertagna, 1992)

Cushing syndrome is uncommon in children. When seen, it is often caused by excessive or prolonged steroid therapy, which produces a cushingoid appearance (see box above and Fig. 29-2). This condition is reversible once steroids are discontinued. Abrupt withdrawal may precipitate acute adrenal insufficiency; gradual withdrawal of exogenous supplies is necessary to allow the anterior pituitary an opportunity to secrete increasing amounts of ACTH to stimulate the adrenals to produce cortisol.

Diagnostic Evaluation

Several tests are helpful in confirming excess cortisol levels. These include fasting blood glucose levels for hyperglycemia, serum electrolyte levels for hypokalemia and alkalosis, 24-hour urinary levels of elevated 17-hydroxycorticoids and 17-ketosteroids, and radiographic studies of bone for evidence

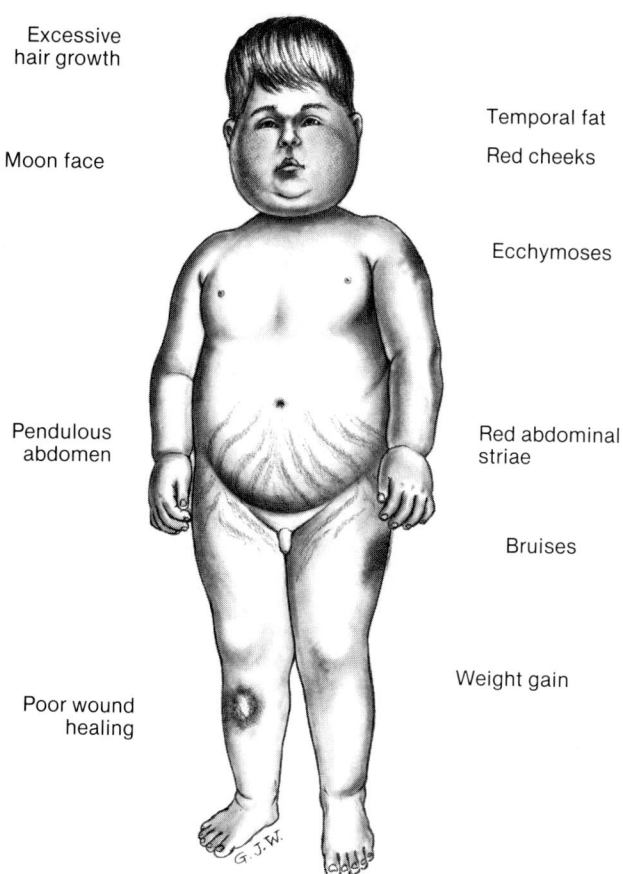

Excessive hair growth

Moon face

Pendulous abdomen

Poor wound healing

Temporal fat
Red cheeks

Ecchymoses

Red abdominal striae

Bruises

Weight gain

FIG. 29-2. Characteristics of Cushing syndrome.

of osteoporosis and of the skull for enlargement of the sella turcica. Administration of an exogenous supply of cortisone normally suppresses ACTH production. However, in individuals with Cushing syndrome, cortisol levels remain elevated. This test is helpful in differentiating between children who are obese and those who appear to have cushingoid features.

Therapeutic Management

Treatment depends on the cause. In most cases surgical intervention involves bilateral adrenalectomy and postoperative replacement of the cortical hormones (the therapy for this is the same as that outlined for chronic adrenal insufficiency). If a pituitary tumor is found, surgical extirpation or irradiation may be chosen. In either of these instances treatment of panhypopituitarism with replacement of growth hormone, thyroid extract, antidiuretic hormone, gonadotropins, and steroids may be necessary for an indefinite period.

Nursing Considerations

Nursing care also depends on the cause. When cushingoid features are caused by steroid therapy, the effects may be lessened with administration of the drug early in the morning and on an alternate-day basis. Giving the drug early in the day maintains the normal diurnal pattern of cortisol secretion. If given during the evening, the drug is more likely to produce symptoms, because endogenous cortisol levels are al-

ready low and the additional supply exerts more pronounced effects. An alternate-day schedule allows the anterior pituitary an opportunity to maintain more normal hypothalamic-pituitary-adrenal control mechanisms.

If an organic cause is found, nursing care is related to the treatment regimen. Although a bilateral adrenalectomy permanently solves one condition, it also produces another syndrome. Before surgery, parents need to be adequately informed of the operative benefits and disadvantages. Postoperative teaching regarding drug replacement is a nursing function.

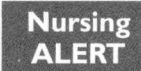 **Nursing ALERT** Postoperative complications of adrenalectomy are related to the sudden withdrawal of cortisol. Observe for signs of a shocklike state, especially hypotension and hyperpyrexia.

CONGENITAL ADRENOGENITAL HYPERPLASIA (CAH)

Disorders caused by excessive secretion of androgens by the adrenal cortex are known variously as *congenital adrenogenital hyperplasia (CAH)*, *adrenocortical hyperplasia (ACH)*, *adrenogenital syndrome (AGS)*, and *congenital adrenocortical hyperplasia (CAH)*. Although hyperfunction of the adrenal gland can occur from a number of causes, such as a virilizing adrenal tumor, in children the most common cause is congenital adrenogenital hyperplasia (CAH), an inborn deficiency of various enzymes necessary for the biosynthesis of cortisol. CAH is inherited as an autosomal-recessive disorder or may result from a tumor or maternal ingestion of steroids.

Pathophysiology

Interference in the biosynthesis of cortisol during fetal life results in an increased production of ACTH, which stimulates hyperplasia of the adrenal gland. Depending on the enzymatic defect, increased quantities of cortisol precursors and androgens are secreted. There are six major types of biochemical defects. In each there is excess production of androgens, which causes ambiguous genitalia in females and precocious genital development in males. In both sexes, linear growth is accelerated, and epiphyseal closure is premature, ultimately resulting in short stature. Other forms of CAH do not result in excess production of androgens but cause various degrees of hypoaldosteronism or hyperaldosteronism.

The most common biochemical defect is partial or complete *21-hydroxylase deficiency*. With partial deficiency, enough aldosterone is produced to preserve sodium, and adequate cortisol is produced to prevent signs of adrenocortical insufficiency. In the complete or salt-losing form, insufficient amounts of aldosterone and cortisol are produced, so that circulatory collapse occurs without immediate replacement of the mineralocorticoids and glucocorticoids.

Diagnostic Evaluation

Clinical diagnosis is initially based on congenital abnormalities that lead to difficulty in assigning sex to the newborn (see box on p. 1048) and on signs and symptoms of adrenal insufficiency or hypertension. Definitive diagnosis is confirmed

CLINICAL MANIFESTATIONS OF ADRENOGENITAL HYPERPLASIA

Female: Masculinization
    Enlarged clitoris (appears as small phallus)
    Fusion of labia (saclike structure resembling a scrotum)
    Vaginal orifice usually closed by fused labia
Male: Precocious genital development
    Genital enlargement (macrogenitosomia precox)
    Frequent erections
Untreated: Early sexual maturation
    Enlargement of external sexual organs
    Development of axillary, pubic, and facial hair
    Deepening of voice
    Acne
    Marked increase in musculature (changes toward an adult
        male physique)
    Accelerated linear growth
    Premature epiphyseal closure (short stature by end of pu-
        berty)
    Female:
        No breast development
        Females remain amenorrheic and infertile
    Male:
        Testes remain small

FAMILY FOCUS
Parents of a Child With Congenital Adrenal Hyperplasia (CAH)

The first question asked of parents of a newborn is, "Is it a boy or a girl?" For the parents of a child born with ambiguous genitalia, the answer, "We are not sure," can be extremely upsetting. It is important for the nurse to keep in mind the social stigmata the parents of a child with CAH face. Parents need to be told immediately of the diagnosis and be given an adequate explanation of the condition. Chromosome typing for positive sex determination is always done and can facilitate acceptance of the child's true sex. The nurse should refer to the child as "infant" or "baby" until identification of sex is known. Suggestions of ways to avoid questioning remarks from visitors, such as diapering the child in a separate room, are also helpful. If surgery is anticipated, showing parents pictures of reconstruction may reinforce a positive acceptance of the child.

Families can be creative in how they handle questions of gender. One family told only their close relatives that the newborn's sex was unclear until tests were done. To others, they stated that they had had twins—a boy and a girl. When the gender was confirmed, they said that the opposite sex twin had died. Nurses must be sensitive to parents' and other family members' difficulty in revealing the diagnosis and respect their ways of coping.

by evidence of increased 17-ketosteroid levels in most types of CAH. Blood electrolytes demonstrate loss of sodium and chloride and elevation of potassium. A karyotype for positive sex determination should always be done in any case of ambiguous genitalia.

Ultrasonography can also be used to visualize the presence of pelvic structures. It is especially useful in CAH to identify the absence or presence of female reproductive organs in a newborn or child with ambiguous genitalia. Because it yields immediate results, it has the advantage of determining the child's gender long before the more complex laboratory results for chromosomal analysis or steroid levels are available.

Therapeutic Management

The initial medical objective is to confirm the diagnosis and assign a sex to the child, usually according to the genotype. In both sexes cortisone is administered to suppress the abnormally high secretions of ACTH. Cortisone depresses the secretion of ACTH by the adenohypophysis, which in turn inhibits the secretion of adrenocorticosteroids, which stems the progressive virilization. If cortisol is given early enough, the signs and symptoms of masculinization in the female gradually disappear, and excessive early linear growth is slowed. Puberty occurs normally at the appropriate age.

Since these children are unable to produce cortisol in response to stress, the dosage is increased during episodes of infection, fever, or other stresses. Acute emergencies require immediate intravenous or intramuscular administration. Children with the salt-losing type of CAH require aldosterone replacement and supplementary dietary salt.

Depending on the degree of masculinization in the female, reconstructive surgery may be required to reduce the size of the clitoris, separate the labia, and create a vaginal orifice. This should be done after the infant is physically able to tolerate the procedure and before she is old enough to be aware of the abnormal genitalia. Plastic surgery is generally done in

stages and yields excellent cosmetic results. The capacity for orgasm and sexual gratification is not necessarily impaired.

Unfortunately, not all children with CAH are diagnosed at birth and raised in accordance with their genetic sex. Particularly in the case of affected females, masculinization of the external genitalia may have led to sex assignment as a male. In these situations it is advisable to continue rearing the child as a male in accordance with the assigned sex and phenotype. Hormone replacement may be required to permit linear growth and to initiate male pubertal changes. Surgery is usually indicated to remove the female organs and reconstruct the phallus for satisfactory sexual relations. These individuals are not fertile. In males diagnosis is usually delayed until early childhood, when signs of virilism appear.

Nursing Considerations

The nursing care of the child with CAH and family is concerned primarily with identifying the condition, and providing support and assistance. Of major importance is recognition of ambiguous genitalia in newborns. If there is any question regarding assignment of sex, the parents need to be told immediately to prevent the embarrassing situation of informing family members of the child's sex and then having to change the announcement (see Family Focus box). As with any congenital defect, the parents require an adequate explanation of the condition and a period of time to grieve for the loss of perfection. Parents need an explanation regarding this disorder that facilitates their explaining it to others. The external genitalia are referred to as sex organs, and the similarity between the penis/clitoris and scrotum/labia during fetal development is emphasized to help parents understand that too much male hormone secretion caused some organs to overdevelop. Using a correct vocabulary allows parents to explain the abnormalities to others in a straightforward manner, just as if the defect involved the heart or an extremity. As soon as the sex is determined, parents are informed of the findings and encouraged to choose an appropriate name, and the child is identified as a male or female, with no reference to ambiguous sex. If the appearance of the enlarged genitalia in a female child concerns the parents, they are encouraged to discuss their feelings.

Nursing considerations regarding cortisol and aldosterone replacement are the same as those for chronic adrenocortical insufficiency. A follow-up visit by a public health nurse may be desirable to ensure that parents understand and comply with the treatment regimen. Likewise, nurses in well-child facilities should assume responsibility for guidance and supervision regarding this aspect of care during each visit.

Since these infants are especially prone to dehydration and salt-losing crises, parents need to be aware of signs of dehydration and the urgency of immediate medical intervention to stabilize the child's condition. Parents, and later the child, need to understand that the medical regimen must be a lifelong commitment; therefore, they should be provided with the education and counseling that is most likely to ensure informed and willing compliance. They also need to know that growth retardation that may have occurred before therapy cannot be overcome and that normal stature is not a realistic expectation, even though growth velocity may improve with medication. The parents are also taught to give necessary injections (see Chapter 22).*

| Nursing ALERT | The parents should be advised that there is no physical harm in treating for suspected adrenal insufficiency that is not present whereas the consequence of not treating acute adrenal insufficiency can be fatal (Ruble, 1992). |

In the unfortunate situation in which the sex is erroneously assigned and the correct sex determined later, parents need a great deal of help in understanding the reason for the incorrect sex identification and the options for sex reassignment and/or medical/surgical intervention. Since children become aware of their sexual identity by 18 months to 2 years of age, it is believed that any reassignment after this period can cause tremendous psychologic conflicts in the child. Therefore sex rearing should be continued as previously established with medical/surgical intervention as required.

A dilemma often arises regarding what these children should know about their condition, especially concerning gender identification. Because the knowledge that one has been reared opposite to the genetic gender can initiate profound psychologic problems, it is recommended that children not be told this fact but rather be given an explanation regarding their physical disabilities, such as infertility, and the need for hormone replacement and plastic surgery. Parents, in turn, must believe that these children have been raised according to their "true sex," which is absolutely honest, since sex is not solely a biologic entity but an expression of multiple environmental influences.

Since the hereditary form of adrenogenital hyperplasia is an autosomal-recessive disorder, parents should be referred

for genetic counseling before conceiving another child. Affected offspring also require genetic counseling, since both sexes are generally able to reproduce. (See genetic counseling in Chapter 9 and Appendix B.)

HYPERALDOSTERONISM

Excessive secretion of aldosterone may be caused by an adrenal tumor; also, in some types of adrenogenital syndromes, symptoms are caused by increased sodium levels, water retention, and potassium loss. The clinical diagnosis is suspected when there are findings of hypertension, hypokalemia, and polyuria that fail to respond to antidiuretic hormone administration.

Therapeutic Management

Temporary treatment of the disorder involves replacement of potassium and administration of spironolactone (Aldactone), a diuretic that blocks the effects of aldosterone.

Nursing Considerations

An important nursing consideration is recognition of the syndrome, particularly in children who demonstrate high blood pressure. After the diagnosis, nursing care is related to the treatment regimen, such as education about the diuretic and potassium supplements. Parents need to be aware of the signs of hypokalemia and hyperkalemia. (See Nursing Tip and Nursing Alert, p. 1045.)

PHEOCHROMOCYTOMA

Pheochromocytoma is an adrenal tumor characterized by secretion of catecholamines. In children this type of tumor is most frequently bilateral or multiple and is generally benign. Often there is a familial transmission of the condition as an autosomal-dominant trait that tends to favor males. The clinical manifestations of pheochromocytoma are caused by an increased production of catecholamines, and they mimic those of other disorders, such as hyperthyroidism, diabetes mellitus, or functional hyperventilation (see box).

Therapeutic Management

Definitive treatment consists of surgical removal of the tumor. In children the tumors may be bilateral, requiring a bilateral adrenalectomy and lifelong glucocorticoid and mineralocorticoid therapy.

Nursing Considerations

An initial nursing objective is identification of children with this disorder. Outstanding clues are hypertension and hyper-

---

CLINICAL MANIFESTATIONS OF PHEOCHROMOCYTOMA

Hypertension	Polyuria
Tachycardia	Polydipsia
Headache	Hyperventilation
Decreased gastrointestinal activity	Nervousness
Resultant constipation	Diaphoresis
Anorexia	Signs of congestive heart failure in severe cases
Weight loss	
Hyperglycemia	

---

*Home care instructions for giving injections are available in Wong DL: *Wong and Whaley's Clinical manual of pediatric nursing,* ed 4, St Louis, 1996, Mosby.

tensive attacks. Preoperative nursing care involves frequent monitoring of vital signs and observing for evidence of hypertensive attacks and congestive heart failure. Urine should be tested at least daily for sugar and ketones. Any signs of hyperglycemia are noted and reported immediately.

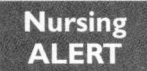 **Nursing ALERT** DO NOT PALPATE MASS. Preoperative palpation may facilitate release of catecholamines, which can stimulate severe hypertension and tachyarrythmias.

The environment should be conducive to rest and free of emotional stress. This requires adequate preparation during hospital admission and before surgery. Parents are encouraged to room-in with their child and to participate in the care. Play activities need to be tailored to the child's energy level but should not be overly strenuous or challenging, since these can increase the metabolic rate and promote frustration and anxiety.

After surgery the child is observed for signs of shock from removal of excess catecholamines. If a bilateral adrenalectomy was performed, the nursing interventions are those discussed for chronic adrenocortical insufficiency.

DISORDERS OF PANCREATIC HORMONE FUNCTION

The islands of Langerhans of the pancreas have three major functioning cells:

1. The *alpha cells* produce *glucagon,* which increases the blood glucose levels by stimulating the liver and other cells to release stored glucose (glycogenolysis).
2. The *beta cells* produce *insulin,* which lowers blood glucose levels by facilitating the entrance of glucose into the cells for metabolism.
3. The *delta cells* produce *somatostatin,* which is believed to regulate the release of insulin and glucagon.

The discussion of disorders of pancreatic hormone secretion is limited to diabetes mellitus.

DIABETES MELLITUS (DM)

DM is a disease of metabolism characterized by a total or partial deficiency of the hormone *insulin,* resulting in a metabolic adjustment or physiologic change in almost all areas of the body. It is the most frequent endocrine disorder of childhood, with the peak incidence reached during early adolescence.

DM can be classified into three major groups:

Insulin-dependent (IDDM), or type I—characterized by catabolism and the development of ketosis in the absence of insulin replacement therapy; onset is typically in childhood and adolescence but can be at any age

Non-insulin-dependent (NIDDM), or type II—appears to involve resistance to insulin action and defective glucose-mediated insulin secretion; onset is usually after age 40, and there appears to be considerable heterogeneity; affected persons may or may not require daily insulin injections

Maturity-onset diabetes of youth (MODY)—transmitted as an autosomal-dominant disorder in which there is formation of structurally abnormal insulin that has decreased biologic activity

Because DM of childhood is, with few exceptions, the IDDM form, the remainder of this discussion is devoted to this important cause of long-term health problems. However, NIDDM is included as is appropriate for comparison throughout. Also, Native American children invariably develop NIDDM.

Etiology

The clinical syndrome of DM results from a large variety of etiologic and pathogenic mechanisms. IDDM is now believed to be an autoimmune disease that arises when a person with a genetic predisposition is exposed to a precipitating event, such as a viral infection.

Genetic Factors. IDDM is not inherited, but heredity is unquestionably a prominent factor in the etiology. A variety of genetic mechanisms have been proposed, but most authorities favor a multifactorial inheritance or a recessive gene somehow linked to the human lymphocyte antigen (HLA). However, the genetic influence in NIDDM and IDDM appears to differ in several ways. Studies of NIDDM in identical twins demonstrate a 100% concordance throughout the lifespan, whereas studies of IDDM in identical twins demonstrate a 30% to 50% concordance rate. The lower rate suggests that environmental and genetic factors are important in the genesis of IDDM (Winters, Chihara, and Schatz, 1993).

Autoimmune Mechanisms. An autoimmune process is involved in persons who develop IDDM. The current theory is that the presence of the HLA genes causes a defect in the immune system that renders the possessor susceptible to a trigger event that can be a dietary source, a virus, bacterium, or chemical irritant. The predisposing event initiates an autoimmune process that gradually destroys beta cells. Without beta cells no insulin can be produced. There is also a strong association between IDDM and other autoimmune endocrine disorders, such as thyroiditis and Addison disease.

Pathophysiology

Insulin is needed to support the metabolism of carbohydrates, fats, and proteins, primarily by facilitating the entry of these substances into the cell, with the exception of nerve cells and vascular tissue. With a deficiency of insulin, glucose is unable to enter the cell, and its concentration in the bloodstream *(hyperglycemia)* increases. The increased concentration of glucose produces an osmotic gradient that causes the movement of body fluid from the intracellular space to the extracellular space; from there the body fluid is excreted by the kidneys. When the serum glucose level exceeds the renal threshold (± 180 mg/dl), glucose "spills" into the urine *(glycosuria),* along with an osmotic diversion of water *(polyuria),* a cardinal sign of diabetes. The urinary fluid losses cause the excessive thirst *(polydipsia)* observed in diabetes. As might be expected, this water washout results in a depletion of other essential chemicals.

Protein is also wasted during insulin deficiency. Since glucose is unable to enter the cells, protein is broken down and converted to glucose by the liver *(glucogenesis);* this glucose then contributes to the hyperglycemia. Without the use of carbohydrates for energy, fat and protein stores are depleted as the body attempts to meet its energy needs. The hunger mechanism is triggered, but the increased food intake

↑osmotic gradient
H₂O from intracellular to extracellular - excreting

(polyphagia) enhances the problem by further elevating the blood glucose.

Ketoacidosis.   When insulin is absent, glucose is unavailable for cellular metabolism and the body chooses alternate sources of energy, principally fat. Consequently, fats break down into fatty acids, and glycerol in fat cells and liver is converted to ketone bodies (β-hydroxybutyric acid, acetoacetic acid, acetone). The ketone bodies can be used as an alternative source of fuel for glucose, but they are used in the cells at a limited rate. Any excess is eliminated in the urine *(ketonuria)* or the lungs (acetone breath). The ketone bodies in the blood *(ketonemia)* are strong acids that lower serum pH, producing *ketoacidosis.* The respiratory system attempts to eliminate the excess carbon dioxide by increased depth and rate—*Kussmaul respirations,* the hyperventilation characteristic of metabolic acidosis.

With cellular death, potassium is released from the cell into the interstitial spaces and then into the bloodstream. It is then excreted by the kidney, where the loss is accelerated by osmotic diuresis. The total body potassium is then decreased, even though the serum potassium level may be elevated as a result of the decreased fluid volume in which it circulates. Alteration in serum and tissue potassium can make cardiac arrest a potential problem.

If these conditions are not reversed by insulin therapy in combination with correction of the fluid deficiency and electrolyte imbalance, progressive deterioration occurs, with dehydration, electrolyte imbalance, acidosis, coma, and death. Diabetic ketoacidosis should be diagnosed promptly and therapy instituted.

Long-Term Complications.   Long-term complications of diabetes involve the small, as well as larger, blood vessels. The principal microvascular complications are *nephropathy* and *retinopathy.* The process appears to be one of *glycosylation,* wherein proteins from the blood become deposited in the basement membrane of small vessels (e.g., glomeruli, retina), where they become trapped by "sticky" glucose compounds (glycosyl radicals). The buildup of these substances over time causes narrowing of the vessels with subsequent interference with microcirculation to the affected areas. With poor control, vascular changes appear as early as 2½ to 3 years after diagnosis; with good control changes have been postponed for 20 or more years.

Neuropathy appears to be an identical process, but glycosylation occurs on the sheath of nerves, interrupting neurotransmission of stimuli. Macrovascular disease develops after 25 years of diabetes and creates the predominant complications in patients with NIDDM. Intensive insulin therapy appears to delay the onset and slow the progression of clinically important retinopathy including vision loss, nephropathy, and neuropathy, by 35% to more than 70% (Nathan, 1993).

Mild Diabetes.   Although most childhood diabetes is recognized during the rapid initial deterioration in carbohydrate metabolism, other cases with more benign disease are being identified with increasing frequency. A few are detected accidentally by urinalysis before overt symptoms are observed. Maturity-onset diabetes of youth (MODY) is sometimes seen in an obese teenager. This type, like NIDDM, can often be controlled with diet restriction. Diabetes is a great imitator; influenza, gastroenteritis, and appendicitis are the conditions most often diagnosed.

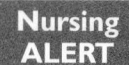 **Nursing ALERT**   Recurrent urinary tract and vaginal infections, especially with *Candida albicans,* are often an early sign of IDDM, especially in adolescents.

Diagnostic Evaluation

Three groups of children who should be considered as possibly diabetic are (1) those who have glycosuria, polyuria, and a history of weight loss or failure to gain despite a hearty appetite; (2) those with transient or persistent glycosuria; and (3) those who display manifestations of metabolic acidosis, with or without stupor or coma. Clinical manifestations of IDDM are outlined in the accompanying box.

Diagnosis is based on *serum glucose levels.* A fasting blood glucose level of >140 mg/dl or a random blood glucose level of ≥200 mg/dl accompanied by classic signs of IDDM is almost certain to be caused by diabetes. Postprandial blood glucose determinations and the traditional oral glucose tolerance tests are not usually necessary for establishing a diagnosis. Serum insulin levels may be normal or moderately elevated at the onset of diabetes; delayed insulin response to glucose indicates the presence of prediabetes.

Ketoacidosis must be differentiated from other causes of acidosis or coma, including hypoglycemia, uremia, gastroenteritis with metabolic acidosis, salicylate intoxication, encephalitis, and other intracranial conditions. *Diabetic ketoacidosis (DKA)* is determined by the presence of hyperglycemia (blood glucose measurement of ≥300 mg/dl), ketonemia (strongly positive), acidosis (pH of <7.30 and bicarbonate of <15 mEq/L), glycosuria, and ketonuria. Tests used to determine glycosuria and ketonuria are the glucose oxidase tapes (Tes-Tape and Clinistix) or Clinitest tablets.

Therapeutic Management

The management of the child with IDDM consists of a multidisciplinary approach involving the family, the child (when appropriate), and professionals, including a pediatric endocrinologist, diabetes nurse educator, and nutritionist as well as an exercise physiologist. Often psychologic support from a mental health professional is also needed. Communication among the team members is essential and extends to other individuals in the child's life, such as teachers, the school nurse, school guidance counselor, and coach.

CLINICAL MANIFESTATIONS OF INSULIN-DEPENDENT DIABETES MELLITUS

Polyphagia	Headache
Polyuria	Frequent infections
Polydipsia	Hyperglycemia:
Weight loss	Elevated blood glucose levels
Child may start bed-wetting	
Irritability and "not himself" or "herself"	Glucosuria
Shortened attention span	Diabetic ketosis:
Lowered frustration tolerance	Ketones as well as glucose in urine
Appears overly tired	No noticeable dehydration
Dry skin	Diabetic ketoacidosis:
Blurred vision	Dehydration
Sores that are slow to heal	Electrolyte imbalance
Flushed skin	Acidosis

Bei Kedrus

The definitive treatment is replacement of insulin. However, insulin needs are affected by nutritional intake, activity, emotions, and other life events, such as illnesses and puberty. Medical and nutritional guidance are primary, but management also includes continuing diabetes education, family guidance, and emotional support.

Insulin Therapy.   Insulin is available in highly purified beef, pork, or beef-pork preparations and in human insulin manufactured by biosynthesis. Most clinicians suggest human insulin as the treatment of choice. It is available in rapid-, intermediate-, and long-acting preparations, and all are packaged in the strength of 100 units/ml. (Other dosages are available for situations where extraordinarily large or small dosages are required.)

The precise dose of insulin needed cannot be predicted. Therefore a regimen of total dosage and the percentage of regular- to intermediate-acting insulin is determined for each child. The amount of insulin is based on capillary blood glucose levels, which the child or family member tests by means of a drop of blood on a chemically treated test strip with the aid of a color chart or a glucose monitor.

Daily insulin is administered subcutaneously by twice-daily injections, by multiple-dose injections, or by means of a portable pump. Diabetes can be controlled satisfactorily in most children with a *twice-daily insulin* regimen consisting of a combination of *rapid-acting (regular)* and *intermediate-acting (NPH or Lente)* insulin given in the same syringe before breakfast and before the evening meal. The amount of insulin is determined by measurements of the blood glucose level after the peak effect of the insulin has occurred. For example, the amount of regular insulin at breakfast is determined by the previous late-morning blood glucose measurement. Regular insulin is best given at least 30 minutes before meals to allow sufficient time for absorption. Some children require more frequent administration of insulin. This includes children with difficult-to-control diabetes and children during the adolescent growth spurt. A *multiple daily injection (MDI)* program has been shown to reduce microvascular complications in young, healthy, patients who have IDDM (Diabetes Control, 1993; Reasner, 1994).

The *insulin pump* is designed to deliver fixed amounts of regular insulin continuously, thereby more closely imitating the release of the hormone by the islet cells. The system consists of a syringe to hold the insulin, a plunger, and a mechanism to drive the plunger. The insulin flows from the syringe through a catheter to a needle inserted into subcutaneous tissue (the abdomen or thigh), and the lightweight device is worn on a belt or a shoulder holster. The needle and catheter are changed every 48 hours by the child or parent, using aseptic technique, and taped in place.

Although the pump provides more even insulin release, it has disadvantages. It cannot be removed for more than 1 hour, which may limit some activities, such as bathing and swimming, although some water-safe models are now available; reactions to the needle are common; and, like any other mechanical device, it is subject to malfunction. However, the pumps are equipped with alarms that signal problems that may arise, such as run-down batteries, blocked needle or tubing, or a malfunction that allows uncontrollable insulin delivery.

Researchers are experimenting with *intranasal insulin administration.* Specially prepared insulin combined with bile salts can be administered by means of an aerosol pump. The insulin is able to cross the nasal mucosa to increase serum levels. The duration of action is not long enough to be a total replacement for injections but may be of value as insulin supplementation at mealtime.

Islet cell or whole pancreas transplantation may offer hope to patients in the future. Viable insulin-producing cells have been injected into the portal vein, where they take root in the liver and eventually produce up to two thirds of the needed insulin. The major use of transplants has been in persons who have serious complications, particularly those whose deteriorating kidneys have required renal transplants and who are receiving immunosuppression therapy. However, islet cell and pancreatic transplants tend not to be sustainable over time despite continuation of therapy. The use of nonhuman islets encapsulated in immunoprotective, semipermeable membranes may have a future in the treatment of IDDM (Brouhard and Rogers, 1993).

Monitoring. *Home blood glucose monitoring (HBGM)* has improved diabetes management and is used successfully by children from the onset of their diabetes. By testing their own blood, children are able to change their insulin regimen to maintain their glucose level in the euglycemic (normal) range of 80 to 120 mg/dl. Diabetes management depends to a great extent on HBGM.

Laboratory measurement of *glycosylated hemoglobin (hemoglobin A_{1c})* levels reflects the average blood glucose levels during the previous 3 months and is of value in assessing glucose control in any person with diabetes. As red blood cells circulate in the bloodstream, glucose molecules gradually attach to the hemoglobin A molecules and remain there for the lifetime of the red blood cell, approximately 120 days.

Urine testing for glucose is no longer used for diabetic management; there is poor correlation between simultaneous glycosuria and blood glucose concentrations. However, urine testing can be carried out to detect evidence of ketonuria.

Nursing ALERT	It is recommended that urine be tested for ketones during an illness and whenever blood glucose is 250 mg/dl or higher when measured twice in a span of 4 to 6 hours.

Nutrition.   Essentially the nutritional needs of children with diabetes are no different from those of unaffected children, except for deletion of concentrated sugars. Children with diabetes require no special foods or supplements. They need sufficient calories to balance daily expenditure for energy and to satisfy the requirement for growth and development.

Normally insulin is secreted in response to food intake. However, insulin injected subcutaneously, has a relatively predictable time of onset, peak effect, duration of action, and absorption rate, depending on the type of insulin used. Consequently the timing of food consumption is regulated to correspond to the time and action of the insulin prescribed. Meals and snacks must be eaten at the same times each day, and the total number of calories and proportions of basic nutrients must be consistent from day to day. The distribution of calories is determined to fit the activity pattern of each child. Alterations in food intake are made so that food, insulin, and exercise are balanced. Extra food is needed for extra activity.

The food intake is based on a balanced diet that incorporates six basic food groups: milk, meat, vegetables, fat, fruit, and bread. The family may follow the exchange system approved by the American Diabetes Association (ADA) or the point system, based on 75 kcal equaling 1 point. The exchange system indicates the amount (portion size) of each food by volume or weight and is prescribed in terms of the number of exchanges from each food group that constitutes each meal and snack. This ensures day-to-day consistency in total calories, protein, fat, and carbohydrate while allowing a choice from a wide variety of foods. Fiber is important in dietary planning because of its influence on digestion, absorption, and metabolism of many nutrients; it diminishes the rise in the blood glucose level after meals.

Exercise. Exercise is encouraged and never restricted unless indicated by other health conditions, because it lowers blood glucose levels. It is included as part of diabetic management and is planned around the child's interests and capabilities. However, in most instances children's activities are unplanned, and the resulting decrease in the blood glucose level can be compensated for by providing extra snacks before (and, if prolonged, during) the activity. Besides providing a feeling of well-being, regular exercise aids in the body's use of food and often decreases insulin requirements.

Hypoglycemia. Even a child with well-controlled diabetes may often experience mild symptoms of hypoglycemia, but if the signs and symptoms are recognized early (see Table 29-2) and relieved promptly by appropriate therapy, the child's activity should not be interrupted for more than a few minutes.

> **Nursing ALERT**
>
> Children on split-mixed insulin dosage schedules tend to experience hypoglycemic episodes at 11:30 AM and 2:30 AM as peaking of insulin occurs.

The most common causes of hypoglycemia, *insulin reaction,* are bursts of physical activity without additional food, or delayed, omitted, or incompletely consumed meals. Reglycosolation of muscles may occur over the ensuing 24 hours. Therefore particular vigilance related to hypoglycemia may be necessary during the night after vigorous exertion.

In the majority of cases simple concentrated sugar, such as honey, that can be held in the mouth for a short time will elevate the blood glucose level and alleviate the symptoms. The simpler the carbohydrate, the more rapidly it will be absorbed. For a mild reaction milk is a good food to use in children. It supplies them with lactose or milk sugar, as well as providing a more prolonged action from the protein and fat (aids in decreased absorption). All children with diabetes should carry with them a source of glucose, such as glucose tablets, Insta-glucose, Life Savers, or sugar cubes. The rapid-releasing sugar is followed by a complex carbohydrate and protein, such as a slice of bread or a cracker spread with peanut butter.

TABLE 29-2. Comparison of manifestations of hypoglycemia and hyperglycemia

VARIABLE	HYPOGLYCEMIA	HYPERGLYCEMIA
Onset	Rapid (minutes)	Gradual (days)
Mood	Labile, irritable, nervous, weepy	Lethargic
Mental status	Difficulty concentrating, speaking, focusing, coordinating	Dulled sensorium
		Confused
Inward feeling	Shaky feeling, hunger	Thirst
	Headache	Weakness
	Dizziness	Nausea/vomiting
		Abdominal pain
Skin	Pallor	Flushed
	Sweating	Signs of dehydration
Mucous membranes	Normal	Dry, crusty
Respirations	Shallow	Deep, rapid (Kussmaul)
Pulse	Tachycardia	Less rapid, weak
Breath odor	Normal	Fruity, acetone
Neurologic	Tremors	Diminished reflexes
	Late: hyperflexia, dilated pupils, convulsion	Paresthesia
Ominous signs	Shock, coma	Acidosis, coma
Blood:		
Glucose	Low: below 60 mg/dl	High: 250 mg/dl or more
Ketones	Negative	High/large
Osmolarity	Normal	High
pH	Normal	Low (7.25 or less)
Hematocrit	Normal	High
HCO$_3$	Normal	Less than 20 mEq/L
Urine:		
Output	Normal	Polyuria (early) to oliguria (late)
Sugar	Negative	High
Ketones	Negative/trace	High

Glucagon is sometimes prescribed for home treatment of hypoglycemia. It is available in a premixed syringe and is administered intramuscularly or subcutaneously. It functions by releasing stored glycogen from the liver and requires about 15 to 20 minutes to elevate the blood glucose level. Once the child is responsive, the lost glycogen stores are replaced by small amounts of sugar-containing fluid administered frequently until the child feels comfortable about trying solid foods.

> **Nursing ALERT** Vomiting may occur after administration of glucagon; therefore precautions against aspiration must be taken, (e.g., placing the child on the side), because the child will be unconscious.

The *somogyi effect* should be recognized as a separate response from hypoglycemia. This phenomenon occurs when the blood glucose level decreases to the point where stress hormones (epinephrine, growth hormone, and corticosteroids) are released, causing a rebound hyperglycemia. Treatment consists of increasing the amount of food eaten and/or decreasing the insulin.

Illness Management. Illness alters diabetes management, and maintaining control is usually related to the seriousness of the illness. As the illness runs its course, the goal of diabetic management is to maintain some euglycemia while recognizing and treating urinary ketones. Some hyperglycemia and ketonuria are expected in most illnesses, even with diminished food intake, and indicate the need for increased insulin. Insulin should never be omitted during an illness, although dosage requirements may increase, decrease, or remain unchanged, depending on the severity of the illness and the child's appetite. Insulin dosage based on a sliding scale according to ABGM should be implemented using regular insulin only and used in place of, not in addition to, prescribed insulin.

Management of Diabetic Ketoacidosis. DKA, the most complete state of insulin deficiency, is a life-threatening situation. The child is admitted to an intensive care facility for management, which consists of rapid assessment, adequate insulin to reduce the elevated blood glucose level, fluids to overcome dehydration, and electrolyte replacement (especially potassium). The preferred method for administering insulin to the child with ketoacidosis is a continuous infusion of low-dose regular insulin.

> **Nursing ALERT** Since insulin can chemically bind to plastic tubing and in-line filters, thereby reducing the amount of the medication reaching the bloodstream, an insulin mixture is run through the tubing to saturate the insulin binding sites before the infusion is begun.

Current trends suggest cautious fluid management to reduce risk of cerebral edema. The fluid deficit is replaced evenly over 24 to 48 hours. Serum potassium levels may be normal on admission, but rapid return of potassium to cells following initiation of fluid and insulin can seriously deplete serum levels, with the attendant risk of cardiac arrhythmias. A cardiac monitor is employed as a guide to therapy and to determine changes that might indicate alterations in potassium concentration.

> **Nursing ALERT** Potassium must never be given until the serum potassium is known to be normal or low and voiding is observed. All IV fluids should include 20 to 40 mg/L of potassium. Never give potassium as a rapid IV bolus, or cardiac arrest may result.

When the critical period is over, the task of regulating insulin dosage to diet and activity is begun. Children should be actively involved in their own care and are given responsibility according to their ability and guidance of the nurse.

❖ Assessment

Daily monitoring of blood glucose levels, periodic urine analysis for ketones, and observation for signs of hypoglycemia, hyperglycemia, or other complications is part of the daily life of the child with diabetes and the family. Diabetes should be suspected in any child who exhibits the manifestations outlined in the box on p. 1051, and the child should be referred for further assessment and appropriate testing.

The signs and symptoms of hypoglycemia are caused by both increased adrenergic activity and impaired brain function, and it is often difficult to distinguish between hyperglycemia and a hypoglycemic reaction (Table 29-2). Since the symptoms are similar and usually begin with changes in behavior, the simplest way to differentiate between the two is to test the blood glucose level (low in hypoglycemia; elevated in hyperglycemia).

The nurse should also be alert to evidence of complications, although these are usually not manifested until adulthood. Assessment of skin for evidence of breakdown is important in order that appropriate care can be implemented to facilitate healing and prevent infection. Because illnesses, such as respiratory infections or gastrointestinal upsets, complicate diabetes management, they should be detected early.

Education is the cornerstone of diabetes management and the major responsibility in diabetes nursing care. Whether teaching is conducted on an outpatient basis or in a preparatory, in-depth manner on an inpatient basis, the ability of the individuals involved to learn must be accurately assessed. This includes assessment of the educational background and emotional stability of the individual(s) involved and the use of appropriate measurement tools, such as a pretest or an objective assessment of the learner's educational level and literacy.

❖ Nursing Diagnoses

A number of nursing diagnoses are prominent in the nursing management of IDDM, and others specific to individual cases become evident. The most common are outlined in the Nursing Care Plan on pp. 1061-1063.

❖ Planning

The goals of care for the child with IDDM and family are as follows:

1. Child and family will be educated about the disease, assessment techniques, and therapy.
2. Child will experience a minimum of complications of diabetes.

3. Child will develop a positive self-image.
4. Child and family will receive adequate support.

❖ Implementation

Once the child with diabetes is diagnosed and insulin therapy initiated, the major nursing responsibility is the education of the family and reinforcement of information. The parents must supervise and manage the child's therapeutic program, but the child should assume responsibility for self-management as soon as he or she is capable. Children can learn to collect their own blood for glucose testing at a relatively young age (4 to 5 years), and most are able to check their blood glucose level and administer insulin at about 9 years of age. In situations in which the parents are inconsistent and/or unreliable, the child is taught self-care at an earlier age.

The first 3 or 4 days after diagnosis is not an optimum time for learning, therefore the family should be given only essential or survival information first and intense information later. A child learns best when sessions are kept short, no more than 15 to 20 minutes. The parents do best in periods of 45 to 60 minutes and, often, longer if they are inquisitive. Education should involve all the senses, and although visual aids are valuable tools, participation is the most effective method for learning. For example, to teach blood testing, the technique is explained; the procedure is demonstrated; the learner is allowed to perform the procedure, followed by a review of the material by visual aids; and the learning is validated by some testing method that includes feedback. Varying the presentation with a number of audiovisual materials, including videotapes, slide-tape programs, and books, stimulates the senses and helps the individual to learn.

Several organizations are prepared to assist with education and dissemination of knowledge about diabetes. The **American Diabetes Association, Inc.,**[*] **Canadian Diabetes Association,**[†] **Juvenile Diabetes Foundation International,**[‡] **Juvenile Diabetes Foundation—Canada,**[§] and **American Association of Diabetes Educators**[‖] are valuable resources for a wide variety of educational materials. The **National Diabetes Information Clearinghouse**[¶] publishes a number of comprehensive annotated bibliographies, including *Educational Materials for and about Young People with Diabetes*, a compilation of resource materials for children, siblings, parents, teachers, and health professionals, and *Sports and Exercise for People with Diabetes*.

Self-management, the ultimate goal for the child with diabetes, is more likely to occur when the child understands the disease and the care it requires. Properly educated, any family should be able to follow a program of regulated control satisfactorily. The following information will allow the family to manage the daily aspects of care.

Identification. One of the first issues to raise with parents is the need for the child to wear a Medic-alert bracelet

for identification. This essential and immediate information can save the child's life.

Nature of Diabetes. The better the parents understand the pathophysiology of diabetes and the function and action of insulin and glucagon in relation to caloric intake and exercise, the better their understanding of the disease and its effect on the child. Parents need answers to a number of questions (voiced or unvoiced), because those answers will provide them with an increased feeling of security in coping with the disease.

Meal Planning. Normal nutrition is a major aspect of the family education program. Diet instruction is usually conducted by the nutritionist, with reinforcement and guidance from the nurse (Fig. 29-3). Learning about foods within specific food groups helps in making choices. Weights and measures of foods, used as eye-training devices in defining food volumes, should be practiced repeatedly, with gradual conversion to estimating foods. Members of the family are also guided in reading labels for the nutritional value of foods and food contents. Meals and snacks are modified according to the child and the present food menu, preserving cultural patterns and preferences as much as possible.

Lists of popular fast-food items and items served at the major fast-food chains can be obtained from the American Diabetes Association (ADA) to help guide food selections. Children are advised to use sugar substitutes with moderation in items such as soft drinks. "Sugar-free" chewing gum and candies made with sorbitol are not usually recommended for children with diabetes. Sorbitol is metabolized to fruc-

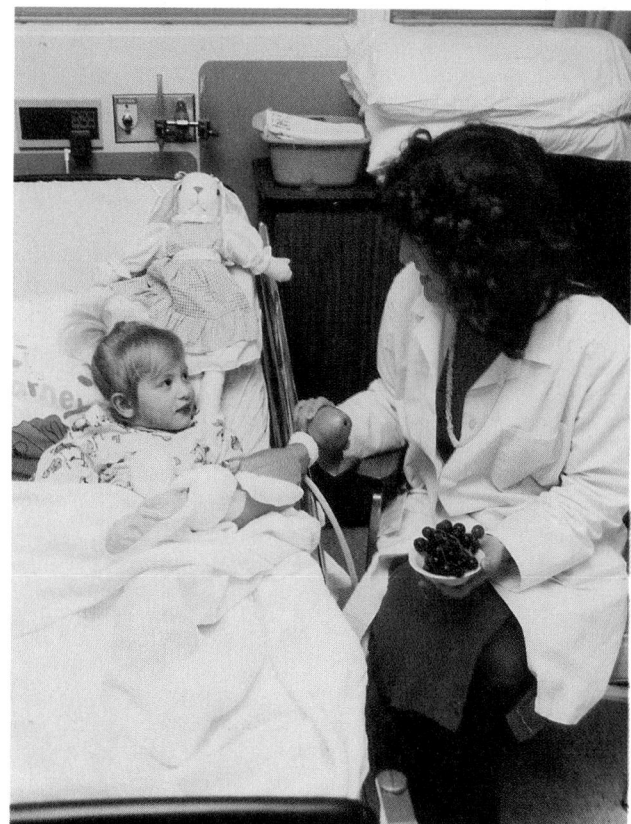

FIG. 29-3. Nutritionist instructs child, using food to explain food exchanges.

---

*1660 Duke St., Alexandria, VA 22314; (800) 232-3472.

†15 Toronto St., Suite 800, Toronto, Ontario, Canada M5C 2E3, (416) 363-3373.

‡432 Park Ave., S., New York, NY 10016; (800) 223-1138.

§89 Granton Dr., Richmond Hill, Ontario, Canada L4B 2N5; (800) 668-0274.

‖500 N. Michigan Ave., Chicago, IL 60611; (800) 338-3633.

¶Box NDIC, 9000 Rockville Pike, Bethesda, MD 20892.

tose and then to glucose, and large amounts of sorbitol can cause an osmotic diarrhea. Dietetic foods that contain sorbitol are more expensive than regular foods, and the caloric content of the food is the same or even greater.

Insulin. Families need to understand the treatment method and the insulin prescribed, including the effective duration, onset, and peak action. They also need to know the characteristics of the various types of insulins, the proper mixing and dilution of insulins, and how to substitute another type when their usual brand is not available (insulin is a nonprescription drug). Insulin need not be refrigerated but should be maintained at a temperature above freezing and below 29.4° C (85° F). An extra supply can be kept in the refrigerator. Freezing renders insulin inactive.

Injection Procedure. Learning to give the insulin injections is a source of anxiety for the family and the child. It is helpful for the learner to know that this important aspect of care will become as routine as brushing the teeth. First, the basic injection technique is taught, using an orange or similar item and normal saline for practice.* To gain the confidence of the child, the nurse demonstrates the technique by giving a skillful injection to the parent, who then returns the demonstration by giving the nurse an injection. With practice family members soon are able to give the insulin injection to the child. Both parents should participate, and as little time as possible should elapse between instruction and the actual injection, especially with parents and the teenage learner.

---

*Home care instructions on subcutaneous injection are available in Wong DL: *Wong and Whaley's Clinical manual of pediatric nursing,* ed 4, St Louis, 1996, Mosby.

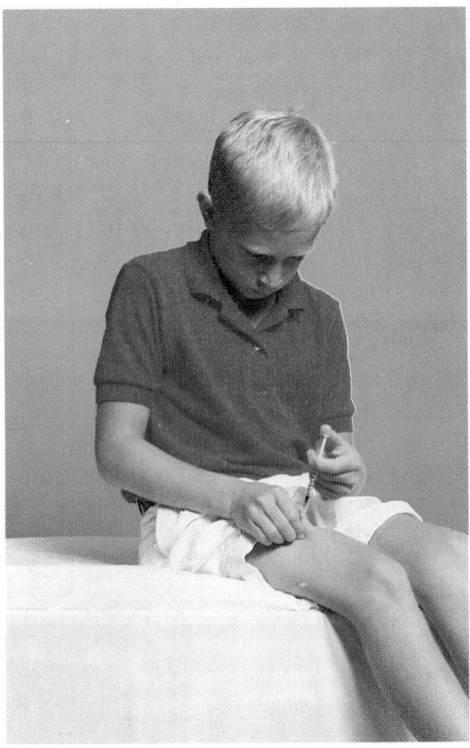

FIG. 29-4. School-age children are able to administer their own insulin.

Insulin can be injected into any area in which there is skin over muscle with fatty tissue in between (Fig. 29-4). The drug is injected at a 90-degree angle; if the child is especially thin or debilitated a 45-degree angle can be used. Newly diagnosed children may have lost adipose tissue, and care should be exercised not to inject into the muscle or blood vessel. Usually the smaller the child, the thinner the skin. The pinch technique is the most effective method for obtaining skin tightness to allow easy entrance of the needle into subcutaneous tissues in children. The site selected will sometimes depend on whether the child or parent administers the insulin. The upper arms, thighs, hips, and abdomen are usual injection sites for insulin. The child can reach the thighs, abdomen, and part of the hip and arm easily but may require help to inject other sites. For example, a parent can pinch a loose fold of skin on the arm while the child injects the insulin.

Injections are rotated to various areas of the body to enhance absorption, since insulin absorption is slowed by the fat pads that develop in overused areas of injection. The parents and child are helped to work out a rotation pattern, which involves giving about four to six injections in one area (each injection about 1 inch, or the diameter of the insulin vial, from the previous injection) and then moving to another area. In this way injection sites for an entire month can be planned in advance on a simple chart or illustration, such as an outline of a body or a teddy bear. It is a good idea for the parents each to give one or two injections a week in the areas that are difficult to reach in order to keep in practice.

It is important to remember that the absorption rate varies in different parts of the body (Table 29-3). Methodically using one anatomic area and then moving to another minimizes variation in absorption rates. Injecting *small* doses of insulin also minimizes changes in plasma glucose levels. Absorption is also altered by vigorous exercise, which enhances absorption from exercised muscles. Therefore it is recommended that excess exercise be avoided during the time the insulin is expected to peak or that other sites be used.

Teaching includes the proper way to equalize pressure in the bottle by injecting an amount of air equal to the amount of solution withdrawn and how to remove air bubbles from the syringe. When insulin dosages are small, an air bubble in the syringe can displace a significant amount of medication. Since the introduction of the 5/10 ml and 3/10 ml syringes, the risk of incorrect dosage has diminished. However, insulin injections of less than 2 units of U100 have an unacceptably large error. Diluted insulin should be used if the prescribed dose is less than 2 units (Casella and others, 1993). Aspiration for blood before injecting the insulin is not routinely done.

Insulin syringes should be compared for accuracy, comfort, and strength. The family and/or child should be able to choose both "their" insulin and "their" syringe from a variety of samples. Use of the same type of syringe (even during hospitalization) is recommended to prevent errors in dosage caused by varying amounts of dead space among syringes.

When the child's dosage requires the injection of both short- and intermediate-acting insulin at the same time, most families prefer to mix the two and use a single injection. However, there are some problems associated with this accepted practice, and the family should understand what happens

TABLE 29-3. Onset and duration of action related to injection site

| | SITE OF INJECTION | | | |
	ABDOMEN	ARM	LEG	BUTTOCK
Rate	Very fast	Fast	Slow	Very slow
Duration	Very short	Short	Long	Very long

From Albisser AM, Sperlich M: Adjusting insulins, *Diabetes Educator* 18(3):211-218, 1992.

when insulins are mixed. Longer-acting insulins contain ingredients that bind to insulin, allowing for gradual release after injection. Some brands contain extra binding compounds that can bind with regular insulin, converting it to the long-acting type and altering the effect on blood glucose. The degree of alteration depends on the type of longer-acting insulin, the ratio of short- to long-acting insulin, and how long the mixture is allowed to stand before injection. The mixture should be injected less than 5 minutes after mixing (before the zinc content of the long-acting insulin affects the action time of the regular or short-acting insulin) or longer than 15 minutes after mixing (to allow the insulins to resume long-acting and short-acting properties).

To obtain the maximum benefit from mixing insulins, the recommended practice is to

1. inject the measured amount of air (equivalent to the dosage) into the longer-acting insulin
2. inject the measured amount of air into the regular insulin and, without removing the needle
3. withdraw the regular insulin
4. insert the needle (already containing the regular insulin) into the longer-acting insulin and withdraw the desired amount

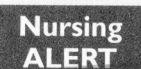

Nursing ALERT When mixing types of insulin, always withdraw regular insulin first, then the longer-acting insulin next to avoid contaminating the regular or short-acting insulin with longer-acting insulin.

It has become acceptable practice to reuse disposable needles and syringes for up to 7 days. Bacteria counts are unaffected, and there is a considerable cost saving. If this method is approved, it is important to stress the importance of vigorous handwashing before handling any equipment, as well as capping the syringe immediately after use and storing it in the refrigerator to decrease the growth of organisms. Nurses should also teach proper disposal of equipment after use in the home. Although it is not standard practice in the hospital, at-home use of a needle clipper is recommended to safely remove and house the used needle. In addition, the syringe plunger can be broken before disposal. An excellent means for syringe disposal is use of an opaque, puncture-resistant container, such as an empty coffee can, bleach bottle, or milk carton which is labeled "bio-hazardous waste" and is discarded with similar material only, not with household refuse.

Other devices are available for insulin injection and may offer advantages to some children. Children who do not wish to give themselves injections can be taught to use a syringe-loaded injector (*Injectease*). With the device, puncture is always automatic. Adolescents respond well to a self-contained and compact device resembling a fountain pen (e.g., *NovoPen*), which eliminates conventional vials and syringes. Preloaded pens may also cause less pain, because the needle is not blunted by piercing the rubber top of the insulin vial (Chantelau and others, 1991).

Some children are considered candidates for continuous subcutaneous insulin infusion with a portable insulin pump. The child and the parents are taught to operate the device, including the mechanics of the pump, battery changes, and alarm systems. They learn how to load the syringe, insert the catheter, adjust the insulin flow for routine needs and for illnesses, and connect and disconnect the catheter. Nurses who work where the pumps are part of the therapeutic regimen should become familiar with the operation of the specific device being used and the protocol of the regimen.

Glucose Monitoring. Nurses should also be prepared to teach and supervise blood glucose monitoring. Blood for testing can be obtained by two different methods: manually or with a spring-loaded puncturing device. The automatic puncture device is recommended because its precise puncture depth produces better blood flow and less pain. However, the child and family should learn to use both methods in the event of mechanical failure. Several lancet devices are available from which to choose, and each provides a means for obtaining enough blood for testing (Fig. 29-5).

Nursing ALERT Caution children not to allow anyone else to use their lancet because of risk of contracting hepatitis B virus or human immunodeficiency virus (HIV).

Repeated finger punctures can be painful, but most children become accustomed to the procedure (see Atraumatic care box on p. 1058). However, persistent signs of redness and soreness at the puncture site should be investigated. It may be evidence of poor technique or poor skin healing relative to poor control.

The least expensive testing method uses a reagent strip to which blood is applied. After blotting, the color change is compared with a color scale for an estimation of the blood glucose level. The strips can be cut in half (although this is not recommended by all professionals) to obtain two readings per strip. This method might be ideal for use at school, where expensive equipment can be lost or broken.

Many types of glucose monitors are available for home use. The family should be shown features of several meters, in-

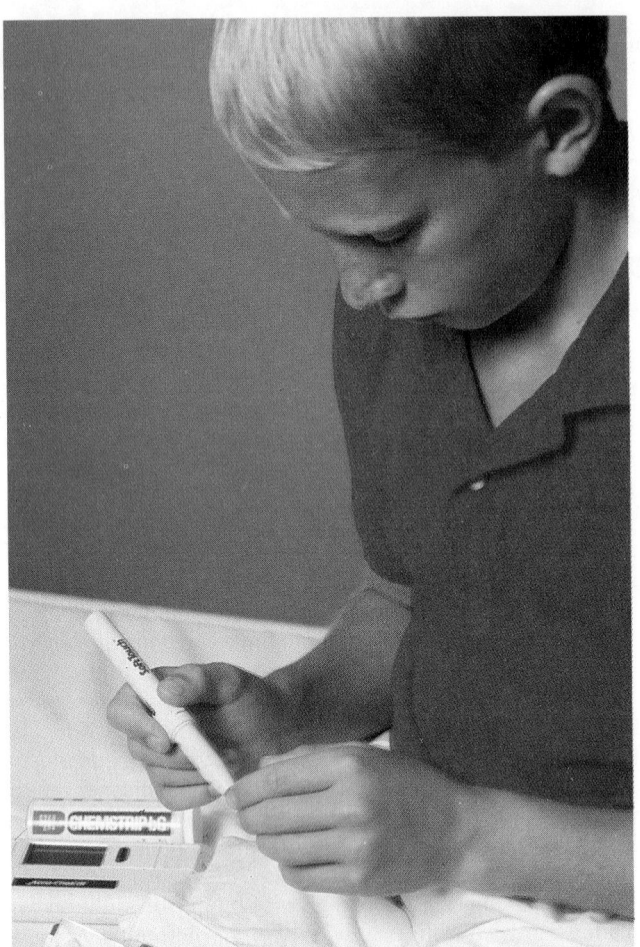

FIG. 29-5. Child using automatic puncture or "finger stick" device to obtain blood sample. Blood glucose monitor and reagent strips are nearby.

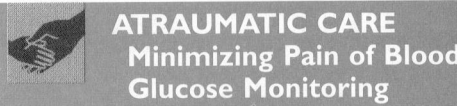

ATRAUMATIC CARE
Minimizing Pain of Blood Glucose Monitoring

To enhance blood flow to the finger, hold it under warm water for a few seconds before the puncture.

When obtaining blood samples, use the ring finger or thumb (blood flows more easily to these areas), and puncture the finger just to the side of the finger pad (more blood vessels and fewer nerve endings).

To prevent a deep puncture, press the platform of the lancet device lightly against the skin and avoid steadying the finger against a hard surface.

Use preloaded insulin devices, (e.g., NovoPen)

Use glucose monitors that require very small blood samples to avoid repunctures, (e.g., Glucometer Elite)

Apply EMLA to puncture site, especially when child is newly diagnosed and skin is still very sensitive (see Pain management, Chapter 21).

cluding advantages and disadvantages, and allowed to choose equipment that best meets their needs. One important consideration is the amount of blood needed. Choosing devices that require small amounts may prevent repunctures.

Urine Testing. Urine testing is easily taught and should include all methods, not just the test to be used for the particular child. Testing for ketones is recommended during times of illness or when glucose readings are high. Since moisture will cause changes to take place in both glucose and ketone strips, families are instructed to discard strips that are discolored, that have been open for a specified time, or after an expiration date. Test strips are available for testing both glucose and ketones.

Hyperglycemia and Hypoglycemia. Severe hyperglycemia is most often caused by illness, growth, or emotional upset. With careful glucose monitoring, any elevation can be managed by adjustment of insulin or food intake. The family should understand how to adjust food, activity, and insulin at the time of illness or when the child is treated for an illness with a medication known to raise the blood glucose level, such as cough syrup or steroids. The hyperglycemia is managed by increasing insulin soon after the increased glucose is noted.

Hypoglycemia is caused by imbalances of food intake, insulin, and activity. Ideally, hypoglycemia should be prevented, and parents need to be prepared to prevent, recognize, and treat the problem. They should be familiar with the signs of hypoglycemia and instructed in treatment, including care of the child with seizures (see Chapter 28). Hypoglycemia can be managed effectively as outlined in Emergency Treatment: Hypoglycemia on p. 1059.

Exercise. Exercise should be planned (as may be necessary for the sedentary teenager) or observed (as in most active children). If the child is more active at one time of the day than at another, food and/or insulin can be altered to meet the activity pattern of the individual. Food should be increased in the summer, when children tend to be more active. Decreased activity on return to school may require a decrease in food intake. The child who is active in team sports will need additional food intake on the days of activity in the form of a snack about ½ hour before the anticipated activity. Races or other competition may call for a slightly higher food intake than practice times.

Food will usually need to be repeated for prolonged activity periods, often as frequently as every 45 minutes to 1 hour. Families should be informed that if increased food is not tolerated, decreased insulin is the next course of action. If the blood glucose level is elevated (240 mg/dl or higher) before planned exercise, the activity should be postponed until the blood glucose is controlled.

Record Keeping. Recording information about food, insulin, blood glucose measurements, and ketonuria is useful to the practitioner, as well as to the family. Insulin reactions are noted, including the time, severity, treatment, and response to treatment. Dietary variations are noted so that an increased blood glucose level can be analyzed in relation to insulin dose, food intake, and activity level.

Self-Management. Self-management is the key to close control. Being able to make changes at the time they are needed rather than waiting until the next contact with health professionals is important for self-management and gives the individual and family the feeling that they have control over the disease. As children grow and assume more and more responsibility for self-management, they develop confidence in their ability to manage their disease and in themselves as persons. Self-management techniques to be mastered are the testing of blood and urine and adjustment of insulin and diet with alterations in day-to-day activities and unusual occurrences.

Hygiene. All aspects of personal hygiene are emphasized for the child with diabetes. The child should be cautioned against wearing shoes without socks, wearing sandals, or walking barefoot. The correct method of nail and extremity care instituted for each particular child (with the guidance of a podiatrist) can begin health practices that last a lifetime. Eyes should be checked once a year, unless the child wears glasses, and then as directed by the ophthalmologist. Regular dental care is emphasized, and cuts and scratches should be treated with plain soap and water unless otherwise indicated.

Acute Care. Children with diabetes may be admitted to the hospital at the time of their initial diagnosis, during illness or surgery, or during episodes of DKA—especially in the small number who exhibit a degree of metabolic lability or who have repeated episodes of DKA. Most children with diabetes are able to keep the disease under control with periodic assessment and adjustment of insulin, diet, and activity as needed under health supervision.

The child with DKA requires intensive nursing care. On admission to the hospital, usually an intensive care unit, an intravenous infusion is started immediately to hydrate the child and to administer insulin, usually as a continuous infusion (see medical management, p. 1054). The blood glucose level is monitored at regular intervals, and the insulin administered as ordered.

Sodium, potassium, and bicarbonate levels are monitored and replaced as indicated. Since potassium and sodium reenter the cells rapidly after administration of insulin, depletion of these electrolytes can be a serious consequence. The child is attached to a cardiac monitor for continual assessment of cardiac status, especially when potassium levels are markedly altered.

Careful and accurate records are maintained, including vital signs, blood pressure, intravenous fluids, electrolytes, insulin, blood glucose level, and intake and output. A urine collection device or retention catheter is used to obtain the urine measurements, which include volume, specific gravity, and glucose and ketone values. The volume relative to the glucose content is important, since 5% glucose in a 300 ml sample is a significantly greater amount than a similar reading from a 75 ml sample. A diabetic flow sheet maintained at the bedside provides an ongoing record of the vital signs, urine and blood tests, amount of insulin given, and intake and output of the patient. The level of consciousness is assessed and recorded at frequent intervals. The comatose child generally regains consciousness fairly soon after initiation of therapy but is managed as is any unconscious child during that time.

Family Support. In any educational program the psychologic needs of the child are just as important as the physical needs. Adjustment to a chronic illness is difficult and follows the grief process (see Chapter 18). A noticeable adjustment cycle occurs during the week-long education course. First, there is interest and perhaps some anger and doubt, fol-

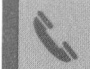

EMERGENCY TREATMENT
Hypoglycemia

Mild Reaction: Adrenergic Symptoms
Give child 10 to 15 g simple, high carbohydrate (preferably liquid, e.g., 3 to 6 oz milk).
Follow with starch-protein snack.

Moderate Reaction: Neuroglycopenic Symptoms
Give child 10 to 15 g simple carbohydrate as above.
Repeat in 10 to 15 minutes if symptoms persist.
Follow with larger starch-protein snack.
Watch child closely.

Severe Reaction: Unresponsive, Unconscious, and/or Seizures
Administer glucagon as prescribed.
Watch child closely for seizures and vomiting (glucagon may take up to 15 minutes to have an effect).
Follow with planned meal or snack when child is able to eat, or add a snack of 10% of daily calories.

Nocturnal Reaction
Give child 10 to 15 g simple carbohydrate.
Follow with snack of 10% of daily calories.

lowed by denial and accompanied by the overwhelming feeling of "Why me?" There are doubts regarding the ability to absorb so much essential information. Then there are the acceptance and synthesis of material, as the learners realize that they are able to state and demonstrate their understanding of the material.

Children in the years before adolescence tend to accept their condition most easily. However, challenges exist, such as providing regular feedings to the sick infant or to the negative toddler. With toddlers and preschoolers insulin injections and glucose testing may be difficult at first. However, they usually accept the procedures when the parents use a matter-of-fact approach without calling attention to a "hurt" and treat the procedure like any other routine part of a child's life. Following the injection, time with some special and positive attention such as reading, talking, or other pleasant activity is one way to convert children who initially refuse injections to those who accept them.

School-age children can understand the basic concepts related to their disease and its treatment. They are able to test blood glucose and urine, recognize food groups, give injections, keep records, and distinguish between feelings of fear, excitement, and hypoglycemia. They understand how to recognize, prevent, and treat hypoglycemia. However, they still need considerable parental involvement.

Adolescents appear to have the most difficulty in adjusting. Adolescence is a time when there is much stress toward being "perfect" and being like peers and, no matter what others say, having diabetes is being different. Some youngsters are more upset about not being able to have a candy bar than about injections, diet, and other aspects of management. If children can accept the difference as a part of life, in other words, that each person is different in some way, then with adequate family support they should be able to adjust well. (See Family Focus box and Critical Thinking Exercise on p. 1060.)

As a nurse caring for adolescents with IDDM I am constantly aware of the wide range of adolescent behaviors that affect the course of this disease. Education of the child and the parents can often make the difference between a disease in control of the teen and a teen in control of the disease.

I have cared for many adolescent females who have episodes of hyperglycemia at the time of menstruation that can result in DKA. I have found that education regarding sick-day protocol with sliding-scale regular insulin instituted at the first sign of hyperglycemia, which may occur 1 to 2 days before onset of menses, can keep the adolescent girl out of the ICU and in control of her diabetes.

Eating disorders, such as bulimia or anorexia nervosa, in the teenager with IDDM pose a serious health hazard. Also, insulin manipulation or omission has been identified as a weight loss method used by some female adolescents (Rodin, Craven, and Daneman, 1989). Nurses working with these adolescents, especially females, must be aware of the hazards and openly discuss the risks with the young person. A referral for specialized intervention may be needed.

Another group of adolescents with diabetes who are at risk are those who drink alcohol. I have found that confusion about the effects of alcohol on blood glucose is common. Teens may believe that alcohol will increase blood glucose levels, when in fact the opposite occurs. Ingestion of alcohol inhibits the release of glycogen from the liver, therefore resulting in hypoglycemia. Teens with diabetes who drink alcohol may become hypoglycemic, but be treated as if they were inebriated (drunk). Behaviors may be similar such as shakiness, combativeness, slurred speech, and loss of consciousness.

Education regarding the effects of alcohol is important and must be included in a teaching plan. If teens insist on drinking alcohol they can be cautioned to use sweetened mixers or eat snacks when consuming alcoholic beverages.

Episodes of hyper- or hypoglycemia may become a serious issue for adolescents who are leaving home for the first time. One teenager confided that her mother always recognized her combative, antisocial behavior as impending hypoglycemia and treated her with the appropriate intervention. The teen feared that a college roommate might be offended by the behavior and leave her alone with impending hypoglycemia.

One young man realized he could not live alone when he "took a nap because of feeling tired" and woke up 4 days later in the hospital. Fortunately, his family realized he was in a coma and summoned emergency medical service. The fatigue signaled the beginning of a viral infection, which led to a blood glucose of 410 mg/dl. Nurses need to address these fears openly and facilitate ways in which the teen can enlist the aid of significant peers who may be available during hyper- or hypoglycemic episodes.

Susan Zekauskas, RN, MSN, PNP

CRITICAL THINKING EXERCISE
Insulin Dependent Diabetes Mellitus (IDDM)

Rebecca, 15 years old, has a 3-year history of IDDM, and has been admitted to the pediatric intensive care unit for treatment of diabetic ketoacidosis (DKA). This is her fifth admission for DKA in one year. Rebecca's parents are divorced and she has four younger siblings. Rebecca's mother has maintained two jobs for the past 5 years and frequently leaves Rebecca in charge of the household. In anticipation of her discharge, you plan a teaching program for Rebecca and her mother. Areas of diabetes management that must be stressed are the need for careful management of her diet, an exercise program, the need for conscientious self-testing of blood glucose with appropriate administration of daily insulin, the use of sliding scale insulin therapy as prescribed, urine ketone testing when blood glucose levels are high, and methods to handle emotional stressors. Of the following issues that might be influencing the recurrent episodes of DKA, which one should you address first?

1. The responsibility Rebecca feels for the care of her four younger siblings
2. Fluctuation of blood glucose levels around the time of menses with inadequate insulin coverage
3. Stress related to the absence of Rebecca's mother and the loss of the close relationship Rebecca shared with her father
4. Adolescent issues, such as seeking independence, feeling different because of IDDM, and alcohol use

The correct answer is two. The nurse should concentrate first on those situations directly related to hyperglycemia. Adolescent females with diabetes tend to have frequent fluctuation of blood glucose levels, especially increased blood glucose immediately before, during, or after their menses. Emotional stress related to increased responsibilities, personal loss from divorce, and normal developmental tasks of adolescence can also precipitate a stress response and elevate blood glucose levels. The nurse should address these issues as time for teaching permits or make a referral for special support services.

stand how to prevent problems and how to handle problems calmly if they occur. (See Compliance, Chapter 22.)

NURSING TIP Ongoing motivation to adhere to a regimen is difficult. An older child and parent (or another caregiver) may enjoy negotiating a day off when the responsibility for testing and recording blood glucose is delegated from the child to the caregiver (or vice-versa).

For all families, daily compliance with numerous procedures and structured living schedules is difficult. Maintaining good blood glucose control requires ongoing motivation. Nurses can encourage families to adhere to treatment regimens and life-style adjustments by emphasizing the benefits of preventing complications, such as hypoglycemia. However, complications can have a favorable impact. Once parents experience the child's having a severe insulin reaction with a seizure or the adolescent has one in a public place, the desire to maintain better control is reinforced. They must under-

Parents develop guilt feelings when they have a child with any chronic disease, especially one with a hereditary component. They cope with these feelings in a number of ways. For example, they may be either overprotective or neglectful. Parents may blame themselves for the disease, consciously or subconsciously. Nevertheless, they must come to realize, through education and counseling, that there was nothing they could have done to prevent the disease and that it was not their fault, since environmental, as well as hereditary, factors may be involved in the development of the disease.

NURSING CARE PLAN
The Child with Diabetes Mellitus

<table>
<tr><td>

Hospital Care

NURSING DIAGNOSIS: High risk for injury related to insulin deficiency

PATIENT GOAL 1: Will exhibit normal blood glucose levels

- **NURSING INTERVENTIONS/*RATIONALES***

Obtain blood glucose level *to determine most appropriate dose of insulin*
*Administer insulin as prescribed *to maintain normal blood glucose level*
Understand the action of insulin
    Understand the differences in composition, time of onset, and duration of action for the various insulin preparations *to ensure accurate insulin administration*
Employ insulin techniques when preparing and administering insulin
    Subcutaneous injection; depth according to thickness of subcutaneous tissue
    Rotation of sites *to enhance absorption of insulin*

- **EXPECTED OUTCOME**

Child demonstrates normal blood glucose levels

NURSING DIAGNOSIS: High risk for injury related to hypoglycemia

PATIENT GOAL 1: Will exhibit no evidence of hypoglycemia

- **NURSING INTERVENTIONS/*RATIONALES***

Recognize signs of hypoglycemia early
    Be particularly alert at times when blood glucose levels are lowest (11:00 AM and 2:30 AM) (e.g., bursts of physical activity without additional food, or delayed, omitted, or incompletely consumed meal or snack)
    Test blood glucose
Offer 10 to 15 g of readily absorbed carbohydrates, such as orange juice, hard candy, or milk, *to elevate blood glucose level and alleviate symptoms of hypoglycemia*
Follow with complex carbohydrate and protein, such as bread or cracker spread with peanut butter or cheese *to maintain blood glucose level*
*Administer glucagon to unconscious child *to elevate blood glucose level;* position child *to minimize risk of aspiration, since vomiting may occur*

- **EXPECTED OUTCOMES**

Child ingests an appropriate carbohydrate
Child displays no evidence of hypoglycemia

</td><td>

Preparation for Home Care

NURSING DIAGNOSIS: Knowledge deficit (diabetes management) related to care of a child with newly diagnosed diabetes mellitus

PATIENT/FAMILY GOAL 1: Will accept teaching provided

- **NURSING INTERVENTIONS/*RATIONALES***

Select methods, vocabulary, and content appropriate to the level of the learner *to maximize learning*
Allow 3 or 4 days for family and child to begin to adjust to the initial impact of the diagnosis
Select an environment conducive to learning
Allow ample time for the education process
Restrict length of teaching sessions *because this is how people learn best*
    Child—15-20 minutes
    Parents—45-60 minutes
Involve all senses and employ a variety of teaching strategies, especially participation *because it is usually the most effective method for learning*
Provide pamphlets or other supplementary materials *for future referral*

- **EXPECTED OUTCOME**

Child and/or family display attitudes conducive to learning

PATIENT/FAMILY GOAL 2: Will demonstrate understanding of disease and its therapy

- **NURSING INTERVENTIONS/*RATIONALES***

Provide information regarding the pathophysiology of diabetes and the function and actions of insulin and glucagon in relation to caloric intake and exercise
Answer questions and clarify misconceptions *to ensure optimum learning*
Explain function and expected effects of procedures and tests, *since these are a necessary part of diabetes management*

- **EXPECTED OUTCOME**

Child and/or family demonstrate an understanding of the disease and its therapy (specify indicators)

PATIENT/FAMILY GOAL 3: Will demonstrate understanding of diet planning

- **NURSING INTERVENTIONS/*RATIONALES***

Enlist the services of a dietitian *to teach diet planning*
Emphasize the relationship between normal nutritional needs and the disease *to encourage a sense of normalcy*
Become familiar with family's culture and food preferences *so that these are included in meal planning*
Teach or reinforce learners' understanding of the basic food groups and the diet plan prescribed (e.g., exchange diet)
Help child and family estimate food weights by volume, *since this is more practical than weighing food*
Suggest low-carbohydrate snack items

</td></tr>
</table>

*Dependent nursing action.

Continued.

Nursing Care Plan
The Child with Diabetes Mellitus—cont'd

Guide family in assessing the labels of food products for carbohydrate content, *since concentrated sugars are avoided in the diet*

Teach or reinforce an understanding of the concept of exchanges, *since exchanges ensure day-to-day consistency in total intake while allowing a choice of foods*

Relate constant carbohydrate equivalents to familiar foods

Retain cultural patterns and family preferences as much as possible, *so that child and family are more likely to adhere to diet requirements*

- **EXPECTED OUTCOME**

Child and/or family demonstrate an understanding of diet planning and food selection (specify indicators)

PATIENT/FAMILY GOAL 4: Will demonstrate knowledge of and ability to administer insulin

- **NURSING INTERVENTIONS/*RATIONALES***

Teach child and family the characteristics of the insulins prescribed for child, *since there are several insulin preparations* (Fig. 29-6).

Teach proper mixing of insulins and acceptable substitutions *when the family brand is unavailable*

Teach injection procedure
   Impress on learners that the procedure will be a routine part of child's life *in order to decrease anxiety and increase cooperation*
   Involve caregivers and child, if old enough, *so that more than one person learns procedure*
   Teach basic techniques using an orange or similar item *so that learner can gain confidence before injecting a person*
   Use demonstration and return demonstration techniques on another before injecting child *because this is usually less stressful*

Help families and child work out a set rotational pattern *because this is important for maximum absorption of insulin*

Teach proper care of insulin and equipment

Teach management of continuous infusion pump (if used)

- **EXPECTED OUTCOMES**

Child and/or family demonstrate an understanding of insulin, its various forms, and action (specify indicators)

Child and/or family demonstrate injection technique correctly

Child and/or family develop a rotation plan

Child and/or family demonstrate correct use of pump and care of injection site

PATIENT/FAMILY GOAL 5: Will demonstrate ability to test blood glucose level

- **NURSING INTERVENTIONS/*RATIONALES***

Teach family and child, if old enough:
   Blood glucose monitoring and/or use of equipment selected for use
   Interpretation of results *so that they learn how to adjust insulin based on blood glucose level*
   Care and maintenance of equipment

- **EXPECTED OUTCOME**

Child and/or family demonstrate correct use of the glucose monitoring equipment

PATIENT/FAMILY GOAL 6: Will demonstrate ability to test urine

- **NURSING INTERVENTIONS/*RATIONALES***

Teach family and child, if old enough:
   Urine ketone testing and interpretation of results
   Proper care of test strips

- **EXPECTED OUTCOME**

Child and/or family demonstrate urine testing and interpretation

PATIENT/FAMILY GOAL 7: Will demonstrate understanding of proper hygiene

- **NURSING INTERVENTIONS/*RATIONALES***

Emphasize the importance of personal hygiene *so that child establishes health practices that last a lifetime*

Encourage regular dental care and yearly ophthalmologic examinations, *since these are important for child's general health*

Teach proper care of cuts and scratches *to minimize risk of infection*

Teach proper foot care, *since this will become a high priority during adulthood*

- **EXPECTED OUTCOME**

Child and family demonstrate an understanding of the importance of proper hygiene

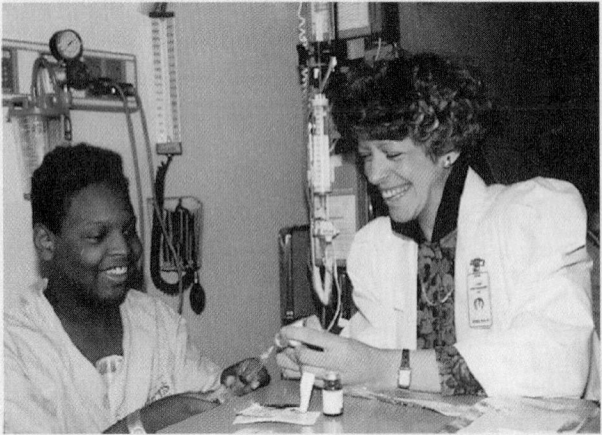

FIG. 29-6. Children learn best when they are active participants in the teaching process. (Courtesy of St. Louis Children's Hospital.)

NURSING CARE PLAN
The Child with Diabetes Mellitus—cont'd

PATIENT/FAMILY GOAL 8: Will demonstrate understanding of importance of exercise regimen

• **NURSING INTERVENTIONS/RATIONALES**

Arrange for occupational therapy program that includes physical activity, *since this is an important part of diabetic management*

Work with child, family, and others (e.g., coaches) to help plan a home exercise program

Reiterate practitioner's instructions regarding adjustment of food and/or insulin to meet child's activity pattern; reinforce with examples *so that child and family are adequately prepared*

• **EXPECTED OUTCOME**

Child and family help child outline and carry out a regular exercise program

PATIENT/FAMILY GOAL 9: Will demonstrate understanding and management of hyperglycemia and hypoglycemia

• **NURSING INTERVENTIONS/RATIONALES**

Instruct learners in how to recognize signs of hyperglycemia and hypoglycemia (especially hypoglycemia) *to prevent delay in treatment*

Explain the relationship of insulin needs to illness, activity, and intense emotion (either positive or negative)

Teach how to adjust food, activity, and insulin at times of illness and during other situations that alter blood glucose levels

Suggest carrying source of carbohydrate, such as sugar cubes or hard candy, in pocket or handbag *so that it is readily available to treat hypoglycemia*

Instruct parents and child in how to treat hypoglycemia with food, simple sugars, or glucagon

• **EXPECTED OUTCOME**

Child and family demonstrate an understanding of the signs and management of a hypoglycemic reaction (specify)

PATIENT GOAL 10: Will wear medical identification

• **NURSING INTERVENTIONS/RATIONALES**

Encourage acquisition of a means of identification, such as an identification bracelet, that explains child's condition *in case of emergency*

Explain to child why identification is important *so that child is more likely to comply*

• **EXPECTED OUTCOME**

Family acquires and child wears identification bracelet

PATIENT/FAMILY GOAL 11: Will keep proper records of insulin administration and testing procedures

• **NURSING INTERVENTIONS/RATIONALES**

Help child and family to design a form for keeping records of the following *because this information is useful to both practitioner and family in managing diabetes:*
Insulin administered
Blood and urine tests
Food intake
Marked variation in exercise
Illness

• **EXPECTED OUTCOME**

Family and child keep an accurate record of insulin administration, glucose testing, etc.

PATIENT GOAL 12: Will engage in self-management

• **NURSING INTERVENTIONS/RATIONALES**

Encourage honesty in recording, such as eating a forbidden candy bar, *so that recording is accurate and useful*

Encourage independence in applying the concepts learned in teaching sessions *since diabetes management is a life-long endeavor*

Instruct when to seek assistance from medical personnel *to prevent delay in treatment*

• **EXPECTED OUTCOME**

Child takes responsibility for management of disease commensurate with age and capabilities

> **NURSING DIAGNOSIS:** Altered family processes related to situational crisis (child with a chronic disorder)

See Nursing Care Plan: The Child with Chronic Illness or Disability, Chapter 18

Problems in the parental response provide a challenge for the nurse to assist through counseling or, if the problems are severe enough, to refer the parents to appropriate resources designed to help them alter their behavior. Times should be set aside during the child's health visit or afterward to meet the needs of the parents. Parents should also be included in special sessions to keep them abreast of the child's management, to help them continue to participate in the child's care, and to provide them with an opportunity to express their own feelings concerning their own or their child's adjustment to the disease. The amount of information that they offer at this time can give clues to their level of support of the child and help assist in decisions concerning the therapeutic management of the child.

Camps for children with diabetes and other special groups are very useful. In the special camp these children learn that they are not alone. As a result, most children become more independent and resourceful outside the camp setting. Camp time also provides parents a respite from the child's daily regimen. Information about such camps and organizations can be obtained from the American Diabetes Association. A free list of accredited camps specifically for children and teens with diabetes is also available.*

---

*Camp Directory, 1660 Duke St., Alexandria, VA 22314; (800) 232-3472.

❖ Evaluation

The effectiveness of nursing interventions is determined by continual reassessment and evaluation of care based on the following observational guidelines and expected outcomes:

1. Interview family to determine their understanding of the disease; have child and family demonstrate and discuss the needed assessment and therapeutic techniques.
2. Interview family regarding their understanding of tight control; analyze and evaluate management records.
3. Discuss child's disease with him or her.
4. Interview family and child regarding their feelings and concerns about the disease.

Expected outcomes:
See Nursing Care Plan, pp. 1061-1063.

KEY POINTS

- The endocrine system has three components: the cell, which sends a chemical message via a hormone; target cells, which receive the message; and the environment through which the chemical is transported from the site of synthesis to the sites of cellular action.
- Pituitary dysfunction is manifested primarily by growth disturbance.
- The main physiologic action of thyroid hormone is to regulate the basal metabolic rate and control the processes of growth and tissue differentiation.
- Disorders of thyroid function include hypothyroidism, autoimmune thyroiditis, goiter, and hyperthyroidism.
- Therapy for hyperthyroidism is directed at retarding the rate of hormone secretion and may include drug therapy, thyroidectomy, or radioiodine therapy.
- Classic forms of hypoparathyroidism in childhood are idiopathic—deficient production of PTH—and pseudohypoparathyroidism—increased PTH production with end-organ unresponsiveness to PTH.
- The adrenal cortex secretes three important groups of hormones: glucocorticoids, mineralocorticoids, and sex steroids.

- Disorders of adrenal function include acute adrenocortical insufficiency, chronic adrenocortical insufficiency, Cushing syndrome, congenital adrenogenital hyperplasia, and hyperaldosteronism.
- Four categories of Cushing syndrome are pituitary, adrenal, ectopic, and iatrogenic.
- Management of congenital adrenogenital hyperplasia includes assignment of a sex according to genotype, administration of cortisone, and, possibly, reconstructive surgery.
- Diabetes mellitus is categorized as insulin-dependent diabetes, non-insulin-dependent diabetes, and maturity-onset diabetes of youth.
- The focus of insulin-dependent diabetes management is insulin replacement, diet, and exercise.
- Education of families includes explanation of diabetes, meal planning, administering insulin injection, monitoring, general hygienic practices, promoting exercise, record keeping, and observing for complications.

REFERENCES

Albisser AM, Sperlich M: Adjusting insulins, *Diabetes Educator* 18(3):211-218, 1992.

Brouhard B, Rogers G: Pancreatic and islet replacement therapy for insulin-dependent diabetes mellitus, *Clin Pediatr* 32(5):258-263, 1993.

Casella S and others: Accuracy and precision of low-dose insulin administration, *Pediatrics* 91(6):1155-1157, 1993.

Chantelau E and others: What makes insulin injections painful? *Br Med J* 303(6793):26-27, 1991.

Diabetes Control and Complications Trial Research Group: The effect of intensive treatment of diabetes on the development and progression of long-term complications in insulin-dependent diabetes mellitus, *N Engl J Med* 329(14):977-986, 1993.

DiGeorge AM: The endocrine system. In Behrman RE, Vaughan VC III: *Textbook of pediatrics*, ed 14, Philadelphia, 1992, WB Saunders.

Drash AL: Insulin-dependent diabetes mellitus in children and adolescents: genetics and etiology, *Curr Opin Pediatr* 1:61-73, 1989.

Gildea J: High and dry—low and wet: the key to DI and SIADH, *Pediatr Nurs* 19(5):478-481, 1993.

Hancock SL, Cox RS, McDougall R: Thyroid diseases after treatment of Hodgkin's disease, *N Engl J Med* 325(9):599-605, 1991.

Moore KC and others: Clinical diagnoses of children with extremely short stature and their response to growth hormone, *J Pediatr* 122(5):687-692, 1992.

Reasner II C: Clinical implications of the DCCT trial, *Contemp Intern Med* 6(2):5-8, 1994.

Rodin G, Craven J, Daneman D: Eating disorders and insulin manipulation in adolescent females with insulin-dependent diabetes mellitus, *Psychosom Med* 51:244-266, 1989.

Ruble JA: Congenital adrenal hyperplasia. In Jackson PL, Vessey JA: *Primary care of the child with a chronic condition*, ed 2, St Louis, 1996, Mosby.

Stabler B: Psychosocial outcomes of short stature, *Pediatr Rounds* 2(1):5-7, 1993.

Tallstedt L and others: Occurrence of ophthalmopathy after treatment for Graves hyperthyroidism, *N Engl J Med* 326(26):1733-1738, 1992.

Winters WE, Chihara T, Schatz D: The genetics of autoimmune diabetes, *Am J Dis Child* 147(12):1282-1290, 1993.

Zekauskas S and others: Human growth hormone and Creutzfeldt-Jakob disease, *J Okla State Med Assoc* 83(9):446-449, 1990.

BIBLIOGRAPHY

Pituitary Dysfunction

Connaughty MS: Accelerated growth in children, *J Pediatr Health Care* 6(5):316-324, 1992.

Giordano BP: The impact of genetic syndromes on children's growth, *J Pediatr Health Care* 6(5):309-315, 1992.

Henry JJ: Routine growth monitoring and assessment of growth disorders, *J Pediatr Health Care* 6(5, pt 2):291-301, 1992.

Jackson PL, Ott MJ: Precocious puberty: the role of the school nurse, *Sch Nurse* 6(1):16-18, 1990.

Kaplowitz P, Webb J: Diagnostic evaluation of short children with height 3 SD or more below the mean, *Clin Pediatr* 33(19):530-35, 1994.

Reiser PA: Educational psychologic, and social aspects of short stature, *J Pediatr Health Care* 6(5):325-332, 1992.

Schwartz ID, Root AW: Puberty in girls: early, incomplete, or precocious? *Contemp Pediatr* 7(1):147-156, 1990.

Disorders of Thyroid Function/Disorders of the Parathyroid Gland/Adrenal Dysfunction

Bertagna X: New causes of Cushing's syndrome, *N Engl J Med* 327(14):1024-1025, 1992.

Burrow GN, Fisher DA, Larsen PR: Maternal and fetal thyroid function, *New Engl J Med* 331(16):1072-78, 1994.

Darland NW: Congenital adrenocortical hyperplasia: supportive nursing interventions, *J Pediatr Nurs* 1(2):117-123, 1986.

Farnklyn JA: The management of hyperthyroidism, *New Engl J Med* 330(24):1731-38, 1994.

Mack R: Thyroid medication—don't overdose on conformity, *Contemp Pediatr* 10(3):105-114, 1993.

Magiakou MA and others: Cushing's syndrome in children and adolescents, *New Engl J Med* 331(10):629-36, 1994.

Page J: The newborn with ambiguous genitalia *Neonat Net* 13(5):15-21, 1994.

Diabetes Mellitus

Bailie MD: Heading off the complications of diabetes, *Contemp Pediatr* 6(1):87-102, 1989.

Balik B, Haig B, Moynihan PM: Diabetes and the school-aged child, *MCN* 11:324-330, 1986.

Chase HP and others: Cyclosporine A for the treatment of new-onset insulin-dependent diabetes mellitus, *Pediatrics* 85:241-245, 1990.

Chase HP and others: Diabetic ketoacidosis in children and the role of outpatient management, *Pediatr Rev* 11(10):297-304, 1990.

Chase HP and others: Prediction of the course of pre-type I diabetes, *J Pediatr* 118(6):838-841, 1991.

Clark LM, Plotnick LP: Insulin pumps in children with diabetes, *J Pediatr Health Care* 4:3-10, 1990.

Dashiff CJ: Parents' perceptions of diabetes in adolescent daughters and its impact on the family, *J Pediatr Nurs* 8(6):361-369, 1993.

Faro B: Students with diabetes: implications of the diabetes control and complications trial for the school setting, *J School Nurs* 11(1):16-21, 1995.

Gallo AM: Family management style in juvenile diabetes: a case illustration, *J Pediatr Nurs* 5:23-32, 1990.

Grey M, Boland EA: Diabetes mellitus (type 1). In Jackson PL, Vessey JA, editors: *Primary care of the child with a chronic condition,* ed 2, St Louis, 1996, Mosby.

Grey M and others: Initial adaptation in children with newly diagnosed diabetes and healthy children, *Pediatr Nurs* 21(1):17-22, 1994.

Hanna KM, Jacobs PM, Guthrie D: Exploring the concept of health among adolescents with diabetes using photography, *J Pediatr Nurs* 10(5):321-327, 1995.

Henry L, Johnson A, Villarosa L: *The black health library guide to diabetes*, New York, 1993, Henry Holt.

Kittler MS, Sucher D: Diet counseling in a multicultural society, *Diabetes Educator* 16(2):127-131, 1990.

Lipman TH and others: A developmental approach to diabetes in children: birth through preschool, *MCN* 14:255-259, 1989.

Lipman TH and others: A developmental approach to diabetes in children: school age—adolescence, *MCN* 14:330-332, 1989.

Lockwood DN, Trand MJ, Mather HM: Is injecting air into insulin bottles necessary? *Br Med J* 297:1315-1316, 1988.

Martin R and others: The infant with diabetes mellitus: a case study, *Pediatr Nurs* 20(1):27-34, 1994.

McNabb WL and others: Increasing children's responsibility for diabetes self-care: in control study, *Diabetes Educator* 20(2):121-124, 1994.

Miller-Johnson S and others: Parent-child relationships and the management of insulin-dependent diabetes mellitus, *J Consult Clin Psychol* 62:603-610, 1994.

Rodrigue JR and others: Parenting satisfaction and efficacy among caregivers of children with diabetes, *Child Health Care* 23:181-191, 1994.

Savinetti-Rose B: Developmental issues in managing children with diabetes, *Pediatr Nurs* 20(1):11-15, 1994.

Snyder AL, Clarke WL: The diabetes control and complications trial: new challenges for the school nurse, *J School Nurs* 11(1):22-25, 1995.

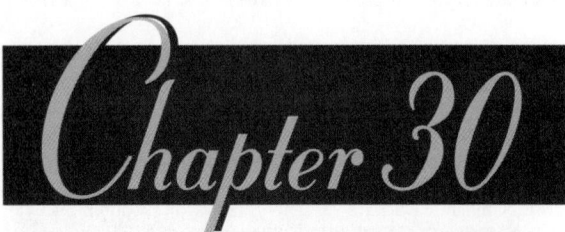

THE CHILD WITH
INTEGUMENTARY DYSFUNCTION

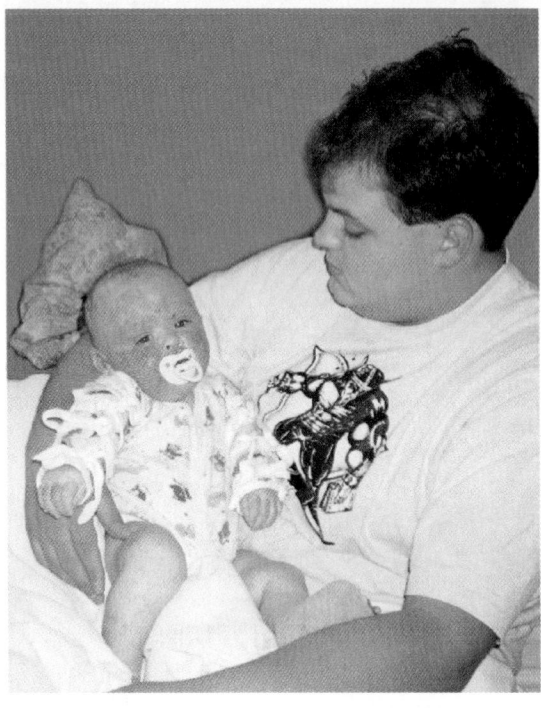

" *In spite of his dermatitis, he is still a happy, developing, and playful baby.* "

Mother of Matthew, age 6½ months, severe atopic dermatitis

RELATED TOPICS

INTEGUMENTARY DYSFUNCTION

SKIN LESIONS

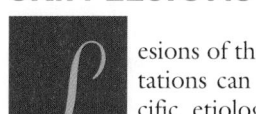

esions of the skin or disorders with skin manifestations can be a result of a wide variety of specific etiologic factors. In general, skin lesions originate from (1) contact with injurious agents, such as infective organisms, toxic chemicals, and physical trauma; (2) hereditary factors; or (3) a systemic disease of which the lesions are a cutaneous manifestation (e.g., measles, lupus erythematosus, nutritional deficiency diseases) or some external factor that produces a reaction in the skin (e.g., allergens). In the case of external factors, the damage is caused by the body's response to the agent rather than by the agent itself. Such responses are highly individualized. An agent that may be harmless to one individual may be damaging to another, and a single agent may produce various types of responses in different individuals.

Among other factors involved in the etiology of skin manifestations is the age of the child. For example, infants are subject to "birthmark" malformations and atopic dermatitis that appear early in life; the school-age child is susceptible to ringworm of the scalp; and acne is a characteristic skin disorder of puberty. Contact dermatitis, such as poison ivy, is seen only where the noxious agent is a feature of the area. Similarly, reactions to insect bites are associated with life cycle and seasonal activities. Although less common in children, tension and anxiety may produce, modify, or prolong many skin conditions.

Skin of Younger Children

The major skin layers arise from different embryologic origins. Early in the embryonic period, a single layer of epithelium forms from the ectoderm, while simultaneously the corium develops from the mesenchyme. In the infant and small child the epidermis is still loosely bound to the dermis. This poor adherence causes the layers to separate readily during an inflammatory process to form blisters. This is especially true in preterm infants, who have an even greater propensity to blister formation and separation during careless handling (such as removal of adhesive tape). The skin is thinner than in older children, and the cells of all strata are more compressed.

Krena Hunter White, MS, MA, RN, revised this chapter.

Several characteristics influence skin responses in infants and young children. Their skin is far more susceptible to superficial bacterial infection. They are more likely to have associated systemic symptoms with some infections and are more apt to react to a primary irritant than to a sensitizing allergen. Infants and young children are more frequently affected by chronic atopic dermatitis (eczema). The infant's skin is much more prone to develop a toxic erythema as a result of skin eruptions or drug reactions and is subject to maceration, infection, and the moisture retention associated with diaper rash.

Pathophysiology of Dermatitis

Over half of dermatologic problems are various forms of dermatitis. This implies a sequence of inflammatory changes in the skin that are grossly and microscopically similar but diverse in course and causation. Acute responses produce intercellular and intracellular edema, the formation of intradermal vesicles, and an initial minimum infiltration of inflammatory cells into the epidermis. In the dermis there is edema, vascular dilation, and early perivascular cellular infiltration. The location and manner of these reactions produce the lesions characteristic of each disorder. The changes are reversible, and the skin ordinarily recovers without blemish and completely intact unless complicating factors such as ulceration from the primary irritant, scratching, and infection are introduced or underlying vascular disease develops. In chronic conditions permanent effects are seen that vary according to the disorder, the general condition of the affected individual, and available therapy.

Diagnostic Evaluation

Although the history and subjective symptoms are explored first, objective findings are often noted simultaneously. One of the more advantageous aspects of skin lesions is that often the diagnosis is readily established after simple, careful inspection.

History and Subjective Symptoms. Many cutaneous lesions are associated with local symptoms, the most common of which is itching *(pruritus)* that varies in kind and intensity. Pain or tenderness often accompanies some skin lesions, and other sensations may be described as burning, prickling, stinging, or crawling. Alterations in local feeling or sensation include absence of sensation *(anesthesia)*, excessive sensitiveness *(hyperesthesia)*, diminished sensation *(hypesthesia* or *hypoesthesia)*, or abnormal sensation, such as burning or prickling *(paresthesia)*. These symptoms may remain localized or may migrate, may be constant or intermittent, and may be aggravated by a specific activity or circumstance, such as exposure to sunlight.

It is also important to determine whether the child has had an allergic condition such as asthma or hay fever or has had previous skin disease. Atopic dermatitis, often associated with allergies, frequently begins in infancy. It should be determined when the lesion or symptom first became apparent, as well as whether it is related to ingestion of a food or other substance, including any medication the child might be taking. It should be kept in mind that the condition may be related to an activity such as contact with plants, insects, or chemicals.

Objective Findings. Much can be determined by the distribution, size, morphology, and arrangement of the lesions. Extrinsic causes usually result from physical, chemical, or allergic irritants or from an infectious agent such as bacteria, fungi, viruses, or animal parasites. Skin manifestations can be produced by such intrinsic causes as a specific infection (such as measles or chickenpox), drug sensitization, or other allergic phenomena. Other diagnostic tools are subjective symptoms, the history, and medical and laboratory studies.

Lesion. According to the nature of the pathologic process, lesions assume more or less distinct characteristics. Names that have been applied to these lesions are important for descriptive purposes in the processes of record keeping and communication. Nurses should also become familiar with the more common terms used to describe skin lesions seen in dermatologic conditions:

Erythema—a reddened area caused by increased amounts of oxygenated blood in the dermal vasculature

Ecchymoses (bruises)—localized red or purple discolorations caused by extravasation of blood into dermis and subcutaneous tissues

Petechiae—pinpoint, tiny, and, sharp circumscribed spots in the superficial layers of the epidermis

Primary lesions—skin changes produced by some causative factor; common primary lesions in pediatric skin disorders are macules, papules, and vesicles (Fig 30-1)

Secondary lesions—changes that result from alteration in the primary lesions, such as those caused by rubbing, scratching, medication, or involution and healing (Fig. 30-2)

Distribution pattern—the pattern in which lesions are distributed over the body, whether local or generalized, and specific areas associated with the lesions

Configuration and arrangement—the size, shape, and arrangement of a lesion or groups of lesions (e.g., *discrete, clustered, diffuse,* or *confluent*).

Laboratory Studies. When it is suspected that a skin problem might be related to a systemic disease, such as one of the collagen diseases or immunodeficiency disease, studies are needed to rule out these possibilities. Diagnostic modalities include microscopic examination, cultures, skin scrapings

Macule—flat; nonpalpable; circumscribed; less than 1 cm in diameter; brown, red, purple, white, or tan in color
Examples: Freckles; flat moles; rubella; rubeola

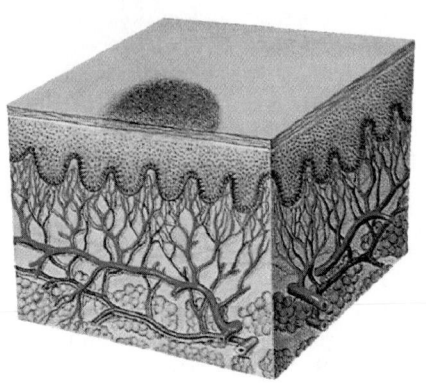

Plaque—elevated; flat topped; firm; rough; superficial papule greater than 1 cm in diameter; may be coalesced papules
Examples: Psoriasis; seborrheic and actinic keratoses

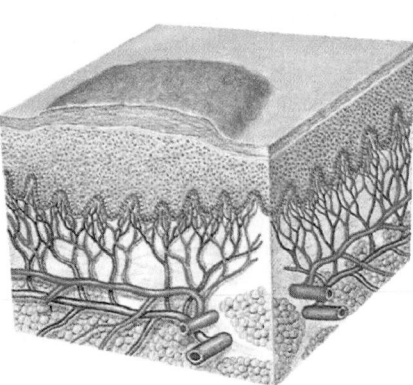

Patch—flat; nonpalpable; irregular in shape; macule that is greater than 1 cm in diameter
Examples: Vitiligo; port-wine marks

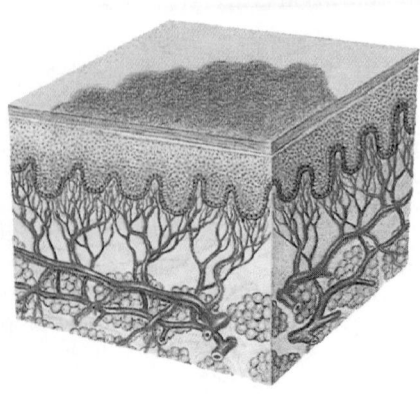

Wheal—elevated, irregular-shaped area of cutaneous edema; solid, transient, changing, variable diameter; pale pink with lighter center
Examples: Urticaria; insect bites

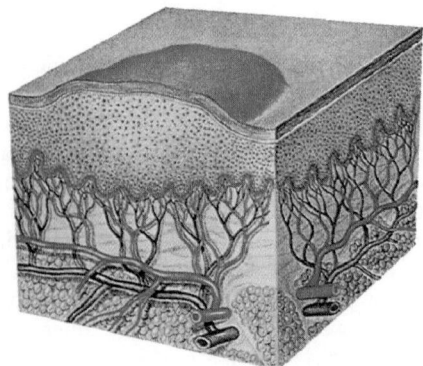

FIG. 30-1. Primary skin lesions. (From Seidel HM and others: *Mosby's guide to physical examination,* ed 3, St Louis, 1995, Mosby.)

Papule—elevated; palpable; firm; circumscribed; less than 1 cm in diameter; brown, red, pink, tan, or bluish red in color
Examples: Warts; drug-related eruptions; pigmented nevi

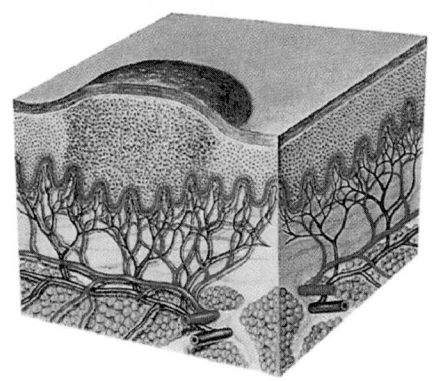

Nodule—elevated; firm; circumscribed; palpable; deeper in dermis than papule; 1 to 2 cm in diameter
Examples: Erythema nodosum; lipomas

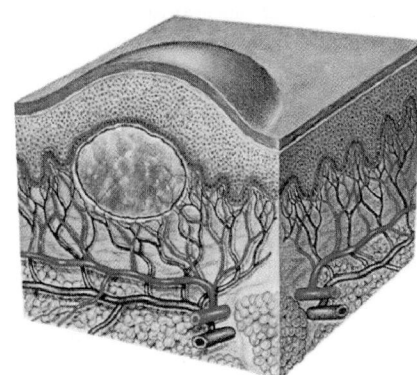

Vesicle—elevated; circumscribed; superficial; filled with serous fluid; less than 1 cm in diameter
Examples: Blister; varicella

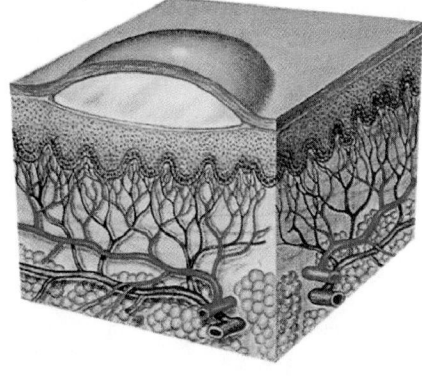

Pustule—elevated; superficial; similar to vesicle but filled with purulent fluid
Examples: Impetigo; acne; variola

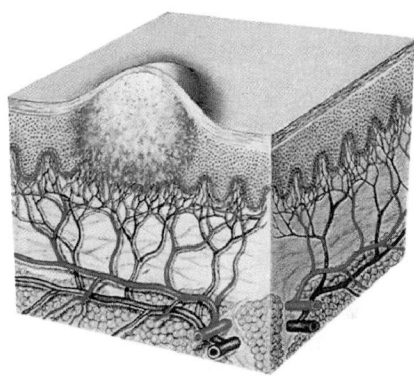

Bulla—vesicle greater than 1 cm in diameter
Examples: Blister; pemphigus vulgaris

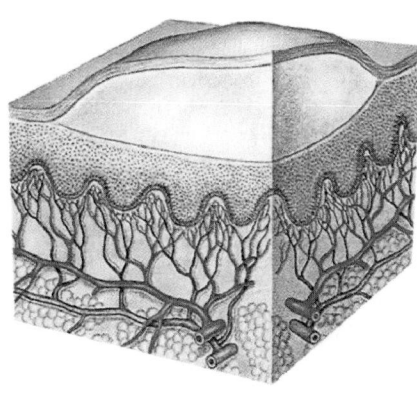

Cyst—elevated; circumscribed; palpable; encapsulated; filled with liquid or semisolid material
Example: Sebaceous cyst

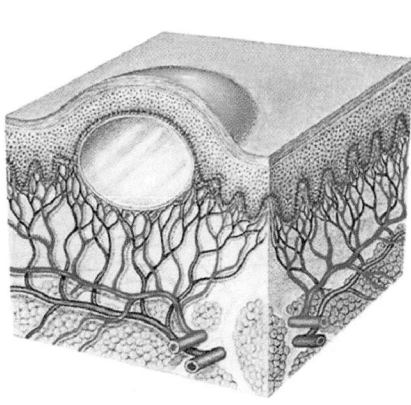

FIG. 30-1, cont'd. Primary skin lesions.

or biopsy, cytodiagnosis, patch testing, and Wood light examination. Allergic skin testing and various other laboratory tests (blood count, sedimentation rate) are used when indicated.

WOUNDS

Wounds are structural or physiologic disruptions of the integument that call for normal or abnormal tissue repair responses. All wounds can be classified as acute or chronic. *Acute wounds* are those that heal uneventfully within the usual time frame. *Chronic wounds* are those that do not heal in the expected time frame or are associated with many complications. In children most wounds are acute and can be prevented from becoming chronic wounds through appropriate nursing care. Wounds are classified in the same manner as burns: partial-thickness, full-thickness, and complex wounds that include muscle and/or bone.

Epidermal Injuries

Abrasions are the most common epidermal wounds of childhood, usually in the form of a skinned knee or elbow. In most injuries the margins of the abraded area are superficial, involving only the outer layers of epidermis, although the central portion may extend into the dermis. Initially the defect is filled by a blood clot and necrotic debris, which subsequently dehydrate to form a scab. Epithelial tissue is composed of *labile cells*, which are constantly destroyed and re-

placed throughout life. Injury to these tissues results in *regeneration* (i.e., rapid replacement by similar cells).

The epithelial wound heals by migration and proliferation of epithelial cells from the wound margin and from cells surviving in transected skin appendages. This response begins within 24 to 48 hours after the wound is incurred. Cell migration ceases when migrating cells make contact with epithelial cells migrating from all other sites. Fixed basal cells adjacent to the wound edge and in skin appendages begin to divide rapidly to replace the migrated cells. As resurfacing is accomplished, the migrated cells begin to divide and thicken the new epithelial layer.

Epithelial cells advance over the wound surface by "flowing." The first cell advances, anchors, and then moves no more. Instead, a cell from behind advances over it, anchors, and subsequently is overridden by other cells that advance over both the primary cells—similar to a leapfrog movement. Epithelial cells move most rapidly in moist environments, and the rate of epithelization depends on a variety of elements, particularly the amount of oxygen supplied to the wound (Hunt, 1990).

Injury to Deeper Tissues

Tissues composed of *permanent cells,* such as muscle and nerve cells, are unable to regenerate. Therefore these tissues repair themselves by substituting fibrous connective tissue for the injured tissue. This fibrous tissue, or *scar,* serves as a patch

FIG. 30-2. Secondary skin lesions. (From Seidel HM and others: *Mosby's guide to physical examination,* ed 3, St Louis, 1995, Mosby.)

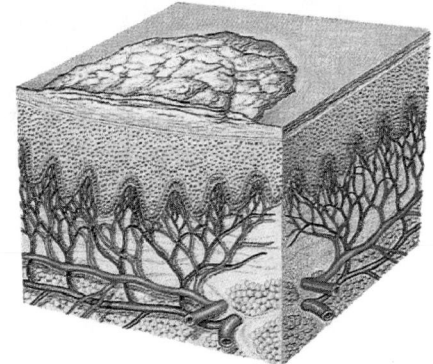

Scale—heaped-up keratinized cells; flaky exfoliation; irregular; thick or thin; dry or oily; varied size; silver, white, or tan in color
Examples: Psoriasis; exfoliative dermatitis

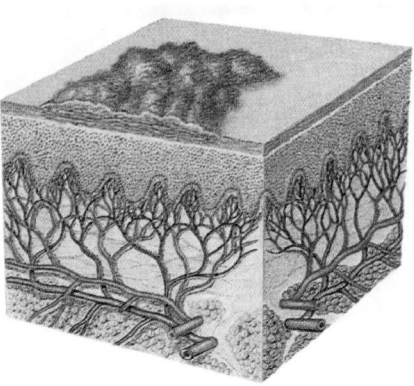

Crust—dried serum, blood, or purulent exudate; slightly elevated; size varies; brown, red, black, tan, or straw in color
Examples: Scab on abrasion; eczema

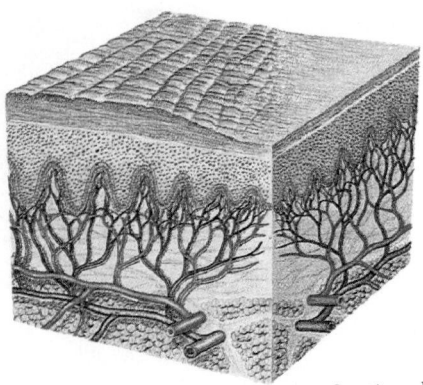

Lichenification—rough, thickened epidermis; accentuated skin markings caused by rubbing or irritation; often involves flexor aspect of extremity
Example: Chronic dermatitis

Continued.

Scar—thin to thick fibrous tissue replacing injured dermis; irregular; pink, red, or white in color; may be atrophic or hypertrophic
Example: Healed wound or surgical incision

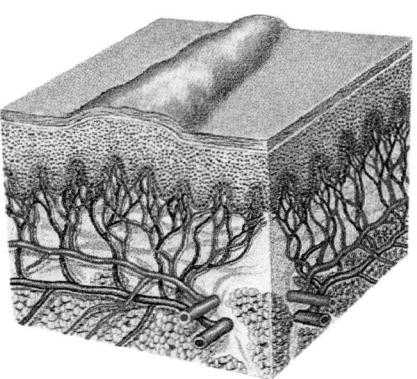

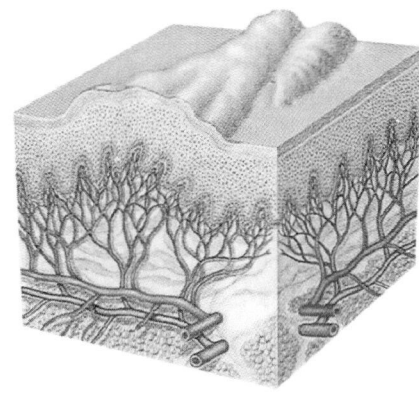

Keloid—irregularly shaped, elevated, progressively enlarging scar; grows beyond boundaries of wound; caused by excessive collagen formation during healing
Example: Keloid from ear piercing or burn scar

Excoriation—loss of epidermis; linear or hollowed-out crusted area; dermis exposed
Examples: Abrasion; scratch

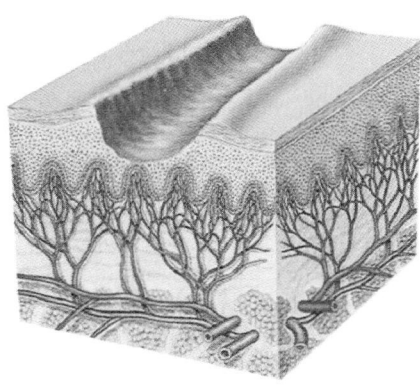

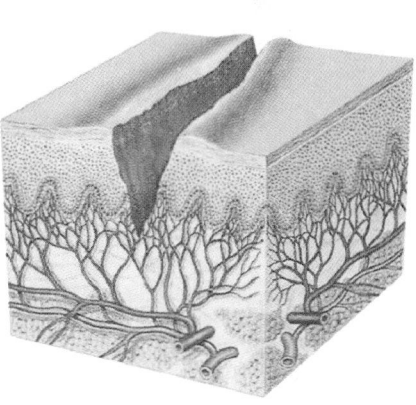

Fissure—linear crack or break from epidermis to dermis; small; deep; red
Examples: Athlete's foot: cheilosis

Erosion—loss of all or part of epidermis; depressed; moist; glistening; follows rupture of vesicle or bulla; larger than fissure
Examples: Varicella; variola following rupture

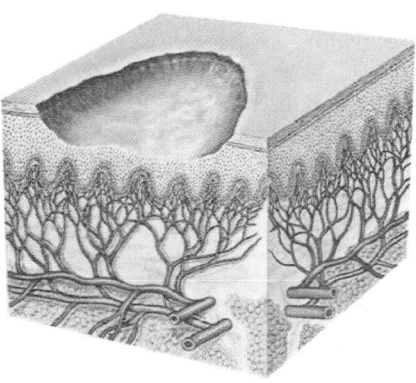

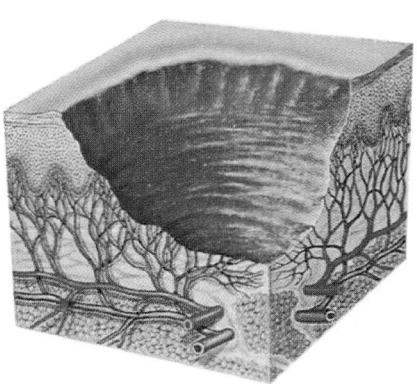

Ulcer—loss of epidermis and dermis; concave; varies in size; exudative; red or reddish blue
Examples: Decubiti; stasis ulcers

FIG. 30-2, cont'd. Secondary skin lesions.

TABLE 30-1. Factors that delay wound healing

FACTOR	EFFECT ON HEALING
Dry wound environment	Allows epithelial cells to dry out and die; impairs migration of epithelial cells across wound surface
Nutritional deficiencies	
Vitamin C	Inhibits formation of collagen fibers and capillary development
Protein	Reduces supply of amino acids for tissue repair
Zinc	Impairs epithelialization
Impaired circulation	Reduces supply of nutrients to wound area
	Inhibits inflammatory response and removal of debris from wound area
Stress (pain, poor sleep)	Releases catecholamines that cause vasoconstriction
Antiseptics	
Hydrogen peroxide	Toxic to fibroblasts; can cause subcutaneous gas formation (mimics gas-forming infection)
Povidone-iodine	Toxic to white and red blood cells and fibroblasts
Chlorhexidine	Toxic to white blood cells
Corticosteroids	Impair phagocytosis
	Inhibit fibroblast proliferation
	Depress formation of granulation tissue
	Inhibit wound contraction
Foreign bodies	Inhibit wound closure
	Increase inflammatory response
Infection	Increases inflammatory response
	Increases tissue destruction
Mechanical friction	Damages or destroys granulation tissue
Fluid accumulation	Accumulation in area inhibits tissues from approximating
Radiation	Inhibits fibroblastic activity and capillary formation
	May cause tissue necrosis
Diseases	
Diabetes mellitus	Inhibits collagen synthesis
	Impairs circulation and capillary growth
	Hyperglycemia impairs phagocytosis
Anemia	Reduces oxygen supply to tissues

to preserve or restore the continuity of the tissue. Wounds involving permanent cells include surgical incisions, lacerations, ulcers, evulsions, and full-thickness burns. Injured cells of glandular organs and bones, composed of *stable* cells, multiply less vigorously and heal more slowly.

Process of Wound Healing

The nonspecific repair mechanism of wound healing with scar formation involves the processes of inflammation, fibroplasia, contraction, and scar maturation. The initial response at the site of injury is *inflammation,* a vascular and cellular response, which prepares the tissues for the subsequent repair process. There is a transient constriction of transected blood vessels, lasting 5 to 10 minutes, followed by active vasodilation of all local small vessels and increased blood flow to the area. This is accompanied by increased permeability of small venules, allowing plasma to leak into surrounding tissues *(edema).* A blood clot is formed along wound edges, forming a framework for future growth of capillaries *(angiogenesis)* and epithelial cells.

At the same time, vessel walls become lined with leukocytes, primarily neutrophils, which pass through the walls and concentrate at the injured site, where they ingest bacteria and debris *(phagocytosis).* The presence of neutrophils is superseded by macrophages, which continue phagocytosis, and also by growth factors needed for skin repair and angiogenesis. Fibroblasts attracted to the area from blood vessels deposit fibrin throughout the clot. Adjacent capillaries begin to form buds that stretch across the supporting fibrin threads, and epithelial cells secrete a fibrolytic enzyme that allows their advancement across the wound. This initial phase of wound healing takes place during the first 3 to 5 days following injury.

Fibroplasia (granulation or *proliferation),* the second phase of healing, lasts from 5 days to 4 weeks. Fibroblasts, immature connective tissue cells, migrate to the healing site and begin to secrete collagen into the meshwork spaces. Granulation tissue is highly vascular, "beefy" red, and shiny connective tissue that organizes and restructures, forming thicker, stronger fibers arranged in orderly layers. A thin layer of epithelial tissue is regenerated over the surface of the wound, and leukocytes gradually disappear from the area.

During *contraction* and *maturation,* the third and fourth phases of wound healing, collagen continues to be deposited and organized into layers, compressing the new blood vessels and gradually ceasing blood flow across the wound. Fibroblasts disappear as the wound becomes stronger. Fibroblast movement causes contraction of the healing area, helping to bring wound edges closer together. A mature scar is then formed. The maturation process may continue for years, and the extent to which the scar remodels and matures varies among individuals.

Children heal aggressively with abundant scar tissue, especially during growth spurts. The highly elastic quality of children's skin pulls on wounds, which defend against the pull by aggressive scarring. Consequently, the child's skin heals with more scar tissue than the less elastic skin of the adult.

Factors That Influence Healing

During the last two decades understanding of wound healing has revolutionized the interventions used to promote healing. Emphasis has shifted from interventions directed at maintaining a dry environment that promoted eschar formation to those that promote a moist, crust-free environment that enhances the migration of epithelial cells across the wound and facilitates resurfacing.

 An acute full-thickness wound kept in a moist environment usually reepithelializes in 12 to 15 days, whereas the same wound when kept open to the air heals in approximately 25 to 30 days (Alvarez, Rozint, and Meehan, 1990).

In addition to knowing what promotes healing, numerous factors have been identified that delay healing (Table 30-1). Many traditional practices, such as the use of antiseptics (hydrogen peroxide and povidone-iodine [Betadine] solutions), thought to prevent infection, actually have a cytotoxic effect on healthy cells and minimal effect on controlling infections. In general, wounds in children heal more rapidly than those in older persons because of children's increased metabolism and good circulation.

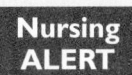 Do not put anything in a wound that you would not put in the eye. The safest solution is normal saline.

GENERAL THERAPEUTIC MANAGEMENT

The human body tends to heal; therefore treatment is directed toward eliminating or ameliorating influences that interfere with normal healing processes. Some disorders may demand aggressive therapy, but by and large the major aim of any treatment is to prevent further damage, eliminate the cause, prevent complications, and provide relief from discomfort while tissues undergo healing. Factors that contribute to the dermatitis and prolong the course of the disease must be eliminated when possible. The most common offenders in pediatrics are environmental factors (such as soaps, bubble baths, shampoos, rough or tight clothing, wet diapers, blankets, and toys) and the natural elements (such as dirt, sand, heat, cold, moisture, and wind). Dermatitis can also be aggravated by home remedies and medications.

Dressings

Dressings are frequently applied to skin lesions and are universally used for wound management. Dressings serve several useful functions: (1) provide a moist healing environment, (2) protect the wound from infection and trauma, (3) provide compression in the event of anticipated bleeding or swelling, (4) apply medication, (5) absorb drainage, (6) debride necrotic tissue, (7) reduce pain, and (8) control odor. To provide a moist environment, open wounds are covered with an occlusive ointment or dressing (Table 30-2). No one dressing meets the needs of all types of wounds. The traditional gauze dressing should not be used on open wounds because it allows the wound surface to dry, does little to prevent bacterial invasion, and adheres to the dried scab so that removal disturbs the newly regenerating epithelial cells.

Topical Therapy

A variety of agents and methods are available for treatment of dermatologic problems. In selecting a therapeutic program

the practitioner considers (1) a choice of active ingredient, (2) a proper vehicle or base, (3) the cosmetic effect, (4) the cost, and (5) instructions for its use. In addition, several basic concepts are kept in mind. Overtreatment is avoided. For example, when the dermatitis is acute, the applications should be mild and bland to avoid further irritation. Broken or inflamed skin, especially in children, is more absorbent than intact skin, and chemicals that are nonirritating to intact skin may be quite irritating to inflamed skin.

Topical applications may be applied to treat the disorder, reduce the itching associated with many diseases, decrease external stimuli, or apply external heat or cold. The emollient action of soaks, baths, and lotions provides a soothing film over the skin surface that reduces external stimuli. Ordinarily lukewarm, tepid, or cool applications offer the greatest relief.

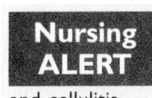 Application of heat tends to aggravate most conditions, and its use is usually reserved for reducing specific inflammatory processes, such as folliculitis and cellulitis.

Topical Corticosteroid Therapy. The glucocorticoids are the therapeutic agents used most widely for skin disorders. Their local antiinflammatory effects are merely palliative so that the medication must be applied until the disease state undergoes a remission or the causative agent is eliminated. Corticosteroids are applied directly to the affected area, and, because they are essentially nonsensitizing and have only minor side effects, they can be applied over prolonged periods with continuing effectiveness. As with the use of any steroids, their use in large amounts may mask signs of infection, and symptoms may be exacerbated following termination of the drug. Families are cautioned that the medication cannot be used for all skin disorders. The concentrations available without prescription are not adequate for some stubborn conditions (e.g., psoriasis) and may cause worsening of inflammation caused by fungus or bacteria. It has also been found that users apply too much topical hydrocortisone; therefore they should be counseled that it is both effective and economical to apply only a thin film and massage it into the skin.

Other Topical Therapies. Other topical treatments include chemical cautery (especially useful for warts), cryosurgery, electrodesiccation (chiefly used for warts, granulomas, and nevi), ultraviolet therapy (primarily used in psoriasis and acne), laser therapy (especially for birthmarks), and special acne therapies such as dermabrasion and chemical peels.

Systemic Therapy

Therapeutic agents are often used as an adjunct to topical therapy in dermatologic disorders, and those most frequently used therapeutically are the corticosteroids and the antibiotics. The corticosteroid hormones with their capacity to inhibit inflammatory and allergic reactions are valuable in the treatment of severe skin disorders. Dosage is carefully adjusted and gradually tapered to the minimum that is effective and tolerated. In infants and children, dosage is larger than is usually calculated from body-weight ratios. However, prolonged use may temporarily suppress growth.

TABLE 30-2. Properties of commonly used occlusive dressings

EXAMPLES	INDICATIONS	ADVANTAGES	DISADVANTAGES	CONSIDERATIONS
Polyurethane Films Op-Site, Tegaderm, Bioclusive, Blister-film, Ensure-it, Ac-cuderm, Uniflex, Opraflex	Protection of partial-thickness red wounds Cover dressing for hydrophilic preparations and hydrogels	Transparent; good adhesion; waterproof; reduces pain; minimizes friction forces to wound; timesaving; easy to store	Adhesive injury to intact and new skin; nonabsorbent; some products difficult to apply; variable barrier function; can promote wound infection	Protect wound margins; avoid in wounds with infection, copious drainage, or tracts; change only if dressing leaks
Hydrocolloids DuoDerm, J&J, Ulcer Dr., Comfeel, Restore, Intact, Intrasite, Tegasorb	Protection of superficial and small, deep red wounds Autolytic debridement of small, noninfected yellow wounds*	Absorbent; nonadhesive to healing tissue; good barrier; waterproof; reduces pain; easy to apply; time saving; easy to store	Nontransparent; may soften and lose shape with heat or friction; odor and brown drainage on removal (melted dressing material)	Frequency of changes will depend on amount of exudate (change as needed for leakage); avoid in wounds with infection
Hydrogel Sheets Vigilon, Geliperm, Elastogel, Cutinova	Protection of superficial and moderately deep red wounds Autolytic debridement of small, noninfected yellow or black wounds* Delivery system for topical antimicrobial creams (increases penetration)	Absorbent; nonadhesive; reduces pain; compatible with topicals; good conformity; easy to store	Poor barrier; semitransparent; requires cover dressing to secure; can promote growth of *Pseudomonas* and yeast; expensive	Avoid in infected wounds; change every 8 hr or as needed for leakage

Slightly modified from Cuzzell JZ: Choosing a wound dressing: a systematic approach, *AACN Clin Issues Crit Care Nurs* 1(3):566-577, 1990.
*NOTE: Users should read package inserts for any contraindications to the use of these products. Some dressings, such as Duoderm CGF, have recently been approved for application to infected wounds, provided that the wound is cultured and treated for the infection. However, Duoderm CGF should not be used on third-degree burns.

Antibiotics, which interfere with the growth of microorganisms, are used in severe or widespread skin infections. However, because they tend to produce a hypersensitivity in the patient, they are used with caution. Antifungal agents are the only means for treating systemic fungal infections.

NURSING CARE OF THE CHILD WITH A SKIN DISORDER

❖ Assessment

To help establish a diagnosis, it is important for nurses to accurately describe any deviation in the character of the skin, using both inspection and palpation. The color, shape, and distribution of the lesions or wounds are noted. The individual lesions are described according to the accepted terminology and may involve more than one type, such as a maculopapular rash. Wounds are assessed for depth of tissue damage, evidence of healing, and signs of infection.

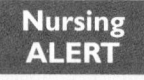 **Nursing ALERT**

Signs of wound infection are:
Increased erythema, especially beyond wound margin
Edema
Purulent exudate
Pain
Increased temperature

To confirm or amplify the findings made by inspection, the skin is gently palpated to detect characteristics such as temperature, moisture, texture, elasticity, and the presence of edema. It should be indicated whether the findings are restricted to the area of the lesion(s) or are generalized.

The child's subjective symptoms provide additional information. Older children are able to describe the condition as painful, itching, or tingling or in other descriptive terms. However, much can be determined by observing the younger child's behavior and the parents' account of these reactions.

Does the child scratch? Is the child restless or irritable? Does the child favor or avoid using a part? A careful history may provide clues. Has the child had access to chemicals or been in the woods or around a woodpile? Has the child eaten a new food? Is the child taking medication? Has the child any known allergy? Do any playmates have a similar lesion? A doubtful diagnosis is frequently confirmed on the basis of history.

❖ Nursing Diagnoses

Nursing diagnoses are determined following an assessment of the child and the skin lesions. The major diagnoses identified for the child with a skin disorder are outlined in the Nursing Care Plan on pp. 1077-1078.

❖ Planning

The goals for the child with a skin condition and the family are as follows:

1. Child will exhibit signs of wound healing.
2. Child will not experience secondary damage to the lesion, such as from infection.
3. Child will demonstrate acceptable level of comfort, especially if pain or itching exist.
4. Child and family will receive appropriate education and support.

❖ Implementation

Therapeutic programs are usually designed to provide general measures such as rest, protection, and relief of discomfort and specific treatments such as a definitive medication or physical technique. Since only a few skin diseases are contagious, it is usually not necessary to isolate the affected child unless there is a danger of acquiring a secondary infection (e.g., the child receiving large doses of corticosteroids or other immunosuppressant drugs or the child with an immunologic deficiency disorder). If the skin manifestation is caused by a viral exanthem, such as measles or chickenpox, the child is prevented from exposing other susceptible children.

Wound Care

Small wounds to the skin are managed by the parents at home. The parents are instructed to wash their hands and then wash the wound gently with mild soap and water for several minutes, followed by thorough rinsing. Open wounds are covered with a dressing, such as a commercial adhesive bandage, although larger wounds may benefit from the use of occlusive dressings (see Table 30-2). If occlusive dressings are applied, instruct the parents on their correct application and removal. For example, hydrocolloid dressings adhere best if a wide margin is left around the wound and the dressing is pressed against intact skin until it adheres.* The edges of the dressing can be secured to the skin with waterproof tape. They are removed if leakage occurs or after a specific time interval, usually 7 days. Dressings are removed carefully to protect intact skin from damage and the epithelial surface of the wound.

NURSING TIP To remove transparent or hydrocolloid dressings, raise one edge of the dressing and pull *parallel* to

---

*Information on the use of the hydrocolloid dressing Duoderm is available from ConvaTec Professional Services, (800) 422-8811.

the skin to loosen the adhesive. The longer the dressings are left on, the easier they are to remove.

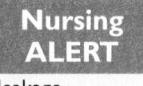 **Nursing ALERT** Advise parents that the yellow gel forming under hydrocolloid dressings may look like pus and has a distinct odor (somewhat fruity) but is normal leakage.

Lacerations present a special challenge. The injured child and family are usually very distressed by the bleeding and are in variable degrees of shock; parental guilt usually accompanies the injury. Because scalp lacerations bleed so profusely, they are especially frightening. The initial nursing intervention is to apply pressure to the area and attempt to calm the child before further examination. Unless there is bleeding from a severed artery, the wound can be cleansed with a forced jet of sterile tepid water or saline (via syringe) and examined for extent, depth, and presence of foreign material such as dirt, glass, or fabric fragments.

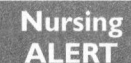 **Nursing ALERT** Hydrogen peroxide and povidone-iodine are contraindicated for cleaning fresh open wounds. Hydrogen peroxide can cause formation of subcutaneous gas when applied under pressure.

The location of the wound also dictates assessment. For example, wounds over bony areas may contain bone chips, and clear fluid seeping from severe head wounds may indicate cerebrospinal fluid. A pressure dressing is applied for transfer to medical care; the child in a medical facility is prepared for suturing. (See Atraumatic Care box.)

Puncture wounds that do not require a tetanus booster are soaked in hot water and soap for several minutes. Causing the wound to rebleed may be helpful. An adhesive bandage can be applied if desired. Puncture wounds of the head, chest, or abdomen or those that could still contain a portion of the puncturing object must be evaluated.

Parents are cautioned against opening blisters or kissing a wound "to make it better." The wound can easily become contaminated from germs in the human mouth. If scabs form, they are allowed to slough off without assistance; pick-

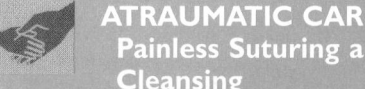
ATRAUMATIC CARE
Painless Suturing and Wound Cleansing

The topical application of lidocaine, adrenaline, and tetracaine (LAT); bupivacaine and norepinephrine; tetracaine, adrenaline, and cocaine (TAC); or AC (without tetracaine) gel to wounds, especially on the head, scalp, and face, provides anesthesia in 10 to 15 minutes (Smith and others, 1996). If further anesthesia is required or if the topical preparations are not available, using *buffered* lidocaine reduces the stinging and burning of the injection (see Pain Management, Chapter 21). The use of a noninvasive tissue adhesive (Histoacryl blue) provides a faster and less painful method of facial laceration repair (Osmond, Klassen, and Quinn, 1995).

ing or early removal may cause scarring. Parents are advised to seek medical help if there is evidence of infection.

Relief of Symptoms

Most of the therapeutic regimens for skin lesions are directed toward relief of pruritus, the most common subjective complaint. Cooling the affected area and increasing the skin pH with measures such as cool baths or compresses to reduce external stimuli to the area and alkaline applications (e.g., baking soda baths) to increase skin pH help to prevent scratching. Clothing and bed linen should be soft and lightweight to decrease the irritation from friction and stimulation.

During any type of treatment, both affected and unaffected skin is protected from damage and secondary infection. Preventing scratching is of primary importance. Older children will usually cooperate, although they may need to be reminded to stop scratching or rubbing; but in smaller and uncooperative children the use of techniques and devices such as mittens, (especially during sleep), or special coverings is required. Keeping fingernails short, well-trimmed, and clean helps reduce the chance of secondary infection.

Antipruritic medications, such as diphenhydramine (Benadryl) or hydroxyzine (Atarax), may be prescribed for severe itching, especially if it disturbs the child's rest. Pain and discomfort are usually managed with nonpharmacologic measures and mild analgesia; severe pain may require more potent medication. Occlusive dressings over wounds reduce pain. For suturing wounds a topical anesthetic or intradermal buffered lidocaine can be used. (See Pain Management, Chapter 21.)

Topical Therapy

Therapy usually involves some type of topical treatment, and the mode of application depends on the nature and location of the lesion being treated. It is especially important to wash the hands before and after application of topical therapies. The skin is assessed before the treatment or application of medication and reassessed after the treatment is completed. Any observed changes are noted and described.

Wet compresses or *dressings* cool the skin by evaporation, relieve itching and inflammation, and cleanse the area by loosening and removing crusts and debris. Any of a variety of ingredients, such as plain water or Burow solution (available without a prescription), can be applied on Kerlix gauze, plain gauze, or (preferably) soft cotton cloths such as freshly laundered handkerchiefs or strips from diaper, sheeting, or pillowcase material.

Dressings immersed in the desired solution are wrung out slightly and applied to the affected area wet but not dripping. They are applied flat and smooth and in such a way that motion is not totally restricted—fingers are wrapped separately, and arms and legs are wrapped so that elbows and knees can bend. Dressings are kept in place by Kerlix or other cotton wrap, tubular stockinette, mittens, and socks (two pairs—one to hold the dressings in place, the other to take up movement) but are left uncovered. When evaporation begins to dry them, the dressings are removed, rewet in the solution, and reapplied to the area using aseptic technique. The solution is not poured or syringed directly over the dressings. As fluid evaporates, the solution becomes increasingly concentrated and thus stronger, which may be damaging to sensitive lesions.

Fresh solution at room temperature is applied at 2-, 3-, or 4-hour intervals and is allowed to remain on the lesion from 30 minutes to 1½ hours. Wet dressings are seldom continued after about 48 hours. The child must be guarded against chilling during treatment, and no more than 20% of the body should be covered at one time to avoid the risk of hypothermia. After treatment, the skin is dried thoroughly by patting with a towel. Application of lotion or other medication may be ordered at this time.

When children are uncooperative in the use of wet dressings, *soaks* are often used for removal of crusts and for their mild astringent action, with the same solution as for wet compresses. Gaining young children's cooperation for hand or foot soaks is difficult unless the procedure is made attractive to them through play.

NURSING TIPS
Older infants and toddlers delight in playing with brightly colored objects or poker chips scattered over the bottom of the receptacle, and preschoolers can be challenged to hold a floating item beneath the water's surface. These activities require supervision; infants and small children will often place items in their mouths, and children can easily lose control with water play.
Washing dishes, cars, dolls, or doll clothes will occupy many children for quite some time.

The older child is able to cooperate but may need something to do during the procedure such as listening to music or to a story, or watching television.

NURSING TIP A single extremity (a foot or a hand) can be easily soaked by placing the solution and the extremity in a plastic sealable bag. The closure is then zipped snugly around the limb.

Baths are especially useful in the treatment of widespread dermatitis by evenly distributing the soothing antipruritic and antiinflammatory effects of the solution, usually oatmeal or mineral oil preparations. The solution is added to a tub of lukewarm water. The temperature of the bath is tepid, and the treatment usually lasts 15 to 30 minutes. Therapeutic baths are always more interesting when the child is accompanied by toy boats or other items for water play.

Topical applications are applied to skin lesions to ease discomfort, prevent further injury, and facilitate healing. Most preparations are placed directly on the skin and left uncovered; others may be applied under an occlusive dressing. A thin application of the ointment or cream is covered with plastic film and anchored with adhesive or covered with a commercial transparent dressing. Occlusive dressings promote moisture retention and nonevaporation of the preparation, which increases the penetration of the medication. Regardless of the type of preparation used, parents need detailed information on how to apply it and how long the preparation should remain on the skin or under an occlusive dressing.

NURSING TIP Apply topical applications systematically with the contour of the body surface (not simply up and down). Children love to be "painted." Therefore lotion applications can be fun when an ordinary paintbrush is used.

NURSING DIAGNOSIS: Impaired skin integrity related to environmental agents, somatic factors, immunologic deficit

---

PATIENT GOAL 1: Will exhibit signs of skin healing

• **NURSING INTERVENTIONS/*RATIONALES***

Carry out therapeutic regimens as prescribed or support and assist parents in carrying out treatment plan *to promote skin healing*

Provide moist environment (dressing or ointment) *for optimum wound healing*

*Administer topical treatments and applications

*Administer systemic medications, if ordered

Prevent secondary infection and autoinoculation, *since these delay healing*

Reduce external stimuli that aggravate condition, *causing delay in healing*

Encourage rest *to support body's natural defenses*

Encourage well-balanced diet *to support body's natural defenses*

Administer skin care and general hygiene measures *to promote skin healing*

• **EXPECTED OUTCOME**

Affected area exhibits signs of healing

NURSING DIAGNOSIS: High risk for impaired skin integrity related to mechanical trauma, body secretions, increased susceptibility to infection

---

PATIENT GOAL 1: Will maintain skin integrity

• **NURSING INTERVENTIONS/*RATIONALES***

Keep intact skin clean and dry; cleanse skin at least once daily *to minimize risk of infection*

Inspect total skin area frequently for evidence of irritation or breakdown *so that appropriate therapy can be initiated*

Protect skinfolds and surfaces that rub together *to prevent mechanical trauma to skin*

Keep clothing and linen clean and dry *to prevent excoriation and infection of skin*

Apply protective lotion to anal and perineal areas, knees, elbows, ankles, and chin, *since excoriation is most likely to occur in these areas*

Carry out good perineal care under urine collection device when applicable *to prevent impaired skin integrity*

Remove adhesives and occlusive dressings carefully *to prevent skin trauma*

• **EXPECTED OUTCOME**

Skin remains clean, dry, and free of irritation

PATIENT GOAL 2: Will exhibit no evidence of secondary infection

• **NURSING INTERVENTIONS/*RATIONALES***

Maintain careful handwashing before handling affected child *to prevent infection*

---
*Dependent nursing action.

Wear surgical gloves when handling or dressing affected parts if indicated by nature of lesion *to prevent contamination of lesion(s)*

Teach child and family hygienic care and medical asepsis *to prevent secondary infection*

Devise methods to prevent secondary infection of lesion in small or uncooperative children

Keep nails short and clean *to minimize trauma and secondary infection*

Apply mittens or elbow restraints *to prevent child from reaching skin lesion(s)*

Dress in one-piece outfit with long sleeves and legs *to keep lesion(s) covered and out of child's reach*

Observe skin lesions for signs of infection (increased erythema, edema, purulent exudate, pain, increased temperature) *so that appropriate therapy can be initiated*

• **EXPECTED OUTCOMES**

Skin lesions remain confined to primary sites

Skin lesions exhibit no signs of secondary infection

PATIENT GOAL 3: Will maintain integrity of healthy skin

• **NURSING INTERVENTIONS/*RATIONALES***

Teach and impress on child importance of keeping hands away from lesion(s) *to prevent spreading lesion(s) and secondary infection*

Help child determine ways of preventing autoinoculation *to increase compliance*

Devise means for keeping small or uncooperative children from spreading infection to other areas

Keep healthy skin dry *to prevent maceration*

• **EXPECTED OUTCOMES**

Healthy skin remains clean and intact

Skin lesions remain confined to primary sites

NURSING DIAGNOSIS: High risk for infection related to presence of infective organisms

---

PATIENT GOAL 1: Will not spread infection to self or others

• **NURSING INTERVENTIONS/*RATIONALES***

Implement universal precautions *to prevent spread of infection*

Isolate affected child from susceptible individuals if indicated *to prevent spread of infection*

Maintain careful handwashing after caring for child *to remove infective organisms*

Avoid unnecessary close contact with affected child during infective stage of disease

Use correct technique for disposal of dressings, solutions, and other fomites in contact with lesion(s) *to safely dispose of infective organisms*

Teach and reinforce positive habits of hygienic care *to decrease risk of infection*

• **EXPECTED OUTCOMES**

Infection remains confined to primary site

Child and family comply with preventive measures

Continued.

NURSING DIAGNOSIS: High risk for impaired skin integrity related to allergenic factors

PATIENT GOAL 1: Will experience no occurrence or recurrence of skin lesion(s)

- **NURSING INTERVENTIONS/*RATIONALES***

Avoid or reduce contact with agents or circumstances known to precipitate skin reaction *to prevent occurrence or recurrence of lesion(s)*

Teach child to recognize agents or circumstances that produce reaction *to prevent occurrence or recurrence of lesion(s)*

- **EXPECTED OUTCOME**

Child avoids precipitating agents

NURSING DIAGNOSIS: Pain related to skin lesions, pruritus

PATIENT GOAL 1: Will exhibit optimum comfort level

- **NURSING INTERVENTIONS/*RATIONALES***

Avoid or reduce external stimuli that aggravate discomfort, such as clothing and bed linen

Implement other appropriate nonpharmacologic pain reduction techniques (see Chapter 21)

*Apply soothing treatments and topical applications as ordered *to relieve pain or pruritus*

*Administer medications *to relieve discomfort and/or restlessness and irritability*

Advocate for child regarding appropriate anesthesia for wound suturing *to prevent unnecessary pain and emotional trauma*

- **EXPECTED OUTCOME**

Child remains calm and exhibits no evidence of discomfort or pruritus

NURSING DIAGNOSIS: Body image disturbance related to perception of appearance

PATIENT GOAL 1: Will demonstrate positive self-image

- **NURSING INTERVENTIONS/*RATIONALES***

Encourage child to express feelings about personal appearance and perceived reactions of others *to facilitate coping*

Discuss with child improvement in skin condition *to instill hope*

- **EXPECTED OUTCOME**

Child verbalizes feelings and concerns

PATIENT GOAL 2: Will receive tactile contact

- **NURSING INTERVENTIONS/*RATIONALES***

Hold child; remember that there is no substitute for the stimulation and comfort of human contact

*Dependent nursing action.

Touch and caress unaffected area *to provide tactile contact without risk of spreading infection*

- **EXPECTED OUTCOMES**

Child exhibits signs of comfort

Child responds positively to tactile stimulation

PATIENT GOAL 3: Will receive adequate support

- **NURSING INTERVENTIONS/*RATIONALES***

Teach self-care where appropriate *to encourage sense of adequacy*

Involve child in planning treatment schedules *to give child some control*

Support and encourage child in efforts to deal with multiple problems that may be associated with disorder, including discomfort, rejection, discouragement, and feelings of self-revulsion *to facilitate coping*

Encourage child to maintain usual activities *so that child experiences normalcy in situation*

Help child improve appearance (e.g., attractive clothing) *to promote positive self-image*

- **EXPECTED OUTCOMES**

Child collaborates in determining means for improving appearance

Child maintains customary activities and relationships

Child participates in own care and treatment

NURSING DIAGNOSIS: Altered family processes related to having a child with a severe skin condition (e.g., eczema, psoriasis, ichthyosis)

PATIENT (FAMILY) GOAL 1: Will receive adequate support

- **NURSING INTERVENTIONS/*RATIONALES***

Teach family skills needed *to carry out therapeutic program*

Provide written instructions *to increase compliance*

Inform family of expected and unexpected results of therapy and a course of action to follow

Help devise special techniques to carry out therapy *to increase compliance and cooperation*

Be aware of overprotectiveness and restrictiveness, *to prevent stifling child's emotional growth*

Allow and encourage family members, particularly the one who cares for the child most of the time, to express negative feelings, such as anger, frustration, and perhaps guilt, *to facilitate coping*

Stress that negative feelings are normal, acceptable, and expected but that they must have an outlet if family members are to remain healthy

Encourage family in efforts to carry out plan of care *to provide support*

Provide assistance when appropriate

Refer to agencies and services that assist with social, financial, and medical problems *to provide ongoing support*

- **EXPECTED OUTCOME**

Family demonstrates necessary skills (specify)

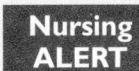

Nursing ALERT Provide written instructions and demonstrate to parents the correct amount of topical medication to apply (e.g., size of a pea; thin film to cover). If more than one preparation is applied, mark the containers 1 and 2 for parents to remember the correct order. Stress that more is not necessarily better with some medications, such as steroids.

Home Care and Family Support

Dermatologic conditions always involve the family. Since few situations require hospitalization and children who are hospitalized will complete a therapy program at home, the family must carry out the treatment plan; therefore their cooperation is essential. Regimens that are simple to accomplish in the hospital or office may be frustrating and baffling at home. The family often needs assistance in adapting equipment available in the home to the therapy.

It is important that the child and family be given as detailed explanations as possible about both the expected and unexpected results of treatment, including any ill effects that might occur. If unexplained reactions do develop, the family is directed to discontinue treatment and report the reactions to the appropriate person(s). The use of over-the-counter medicines is discouraged unless they have first been discussed with the attending practitioner and received approval.

Since the skin is the most visible portion of the body, defects in its surface that alter its appearance are sometimes a source of distress to the child and of revulsion and rejection by others. Parents of other children may fear that their children will "catch" the disorder. Occasionally the affected child's own family members will reduce their interaction with him or her, especially close physical contact, or otherwise demonstrate a distaste for the condition, which the child may interpret as rejection. This is seldom a difficulty with dermatitis of short duration, but chronic conditions can create problems in development of a positive self-concept (see Family Focus.)

FAMILY FOCUS
Skin Lesions and Self-Esteem in the School-Aged Child

When I was 8 years old a lot of small oval tannish-brown spots developed, especially around my neck and waist. The dermatologist said it was a rare condition and it should disappear by the time I was eleven or twelve. They actually disappeared when I was ten. Because the spots were kind of unusual, the dermatologist invited me to attend a dermatology meeting where people with strange skin problems were placed in private clinic rooms and doctors came in and looked at each person's skin. They were all nice, but I felt a little like an animal in the zoo. The thing I mostly remember about the spots was that I always tried to keep them covered. People stared and kids made fun of me. The spots didn't hurt or itch, but I always knew they were there. I would not wear a two-piece swimsuit, even though my friends wore them. My mom and I tried to think of anything that might have caused the spots, but I never knew why they developed on me. I remember thinking it wasn't fair that it happened to me. I learned that many times, people cannot prevent the bad things that happen to them.

Marissa White, age 16
Tulsa, OK

❖ Evaluation

The effectiveness of nursing interventions is determined by continual reassessment and evaluation of care based on the following observational guidelines and expected outcomes:

1. Observe if reasonable care is used in performing nursing activities, and observe lesions and child's reactions to therapies.
2. Observe signs of wound healing.
3. Use assessment techniques to identify relief of discomfort as described in Chapter 21.
4. Reassess skin lesions; observe and interview child and family regarding compliance with therapy.

Expected outcomes:
See Nursing Care Plan, pp. 1077-1078.

INFECTIONS OF THE SKIN

BACTERIAL INFECTIONS

Normally, the skin harbors a variety of bacterial flora, including the major pathogenic varieties of staphylococci and streptococci. The degree of their pathogenicity depends on the invasiveness and toxigenicity of the specific organism, the integrity of the skin, the barrier of the host, and the immune and cellular defenses of the host. Children with immunodeficiency, such as infants, children with congenital immune deficiency disorders, children in a debilitated condition, those on immunosuppressive therapy, and those with a generalized malignancy such as leukemia or lymphoma, are at risk for developing bacterial infections.

Because of the characteristic "walling-off" process of the inflammatory reaction (abscess formation), staphylococci are more difficult to attack, and the local infected area is associated with an increase in numbers of bacteria all over the skin surface that serve as a source of continuing infection. Staphylococcal infections occur most often in children in the younger age-groups, and the incidence decreases with advancing age. All these factors emphasize the importance of careful handwashing and cleanliness when caring for infected children and their lesions to prevent spread of the infection and as an essential prophylactic measure when caring for infants and small children. Common bacterial skin disorders are outlined in Table 30-3.

Nursing Considerations

The major nursing functions related to bacterial skin infections are to prevent the spread of infection and to prevent complications. Handwashing is mandatory before and after contact with an affected child. Handwashing is also emphasized to both the child and the family, and the child should be provided with towels separate from those of other family members. Impetigo contagiosa is easily spread by self-inoculation; therefore the child must be cautioned against touching the involved area. This is difficult to accomplish; distraction or reminders are useful but are not helpful when the child is alone, such as at bedtime.

Children and parents are often tempted to squeeze follicular lesions. They must be warned that squeezing will not hasten the resolution of the infection and that there is a risk of making the lesion worse or spreading the infection. No attempt should be made to puncture the surface of the pustule

TABLE 30-3. Bacterial infections

DISORDER/ ORGANISM	MANIFESTATIONS	MANAGEMENT	COMMENTS
Impetigo Contagiosa (Fig. 30-3)— *Staphylococcus*	Begins as a reddish macule Becomes vesicular Ruptures easily, leaving superficial, moist erosion Tends to spread peripherally in sharply marginated irregular outlines Exudate dries to form heavy, honey-colored crusts Pruritus common Systemic effects: minimal or asymptomatic	Careful removal of undermined skin, crusts, and debris by softening with 1:20 Burow solution compresses Topical application of bactericidal ointment Systemic administration of oral or parenteral antibiotics (penicillin) in severe or extensive lesions	Tends to heal without scarring unless secondary infection Autoinoculable and contagious Very common in toddler, preschooler
Pyoderma— *Staphylococcus, Streptococcus*	Deeper extension of infection into dermis Tissue reaction more severe Systemic effects: fever, lymphangitis	Soap and water cleansing Wet compresses Bathing with antibacterial soap as prescribed	Autoinoculable and contagious May heal with or without scarring
Folliculitis (pimple), furuncle (boil), carbuncle (multiple boils)—*Staphylococcus aureus*	Folliculitis: infection of hair follicle Furuncle: larger lesion with more redness and swelling at a single follicle Carbuncle: more extensive lesion with widespread inflammation and "pointing" at several follicular orifices Systemic effects: malaise, if severe	Skin cleanliness Local warm, moist compresses Topical application of antibiotic agents Systemic antibiotics in severe cases Incision and drainage of severe lesions, followed by wound irrigations with antibiotics or suitable drain implantation	Autoinoculable and contagious Furuncle and carbuncle tend to heal with scar formation A lesion should *never* be squeezed
Cellulitis—*Streptococcus, Staphylococcus, Haemophilus influenzae* (Fig. 30-4)	Inflammation of skin and subcutaneous tissues with intense redness, swelling, and firm infiltration Lymphangitis "streaking" frequently seen Involvement of regional lymph nodes common May progress to abscess formation Systemic effects: fever, malaise	Oral or parenteral antibiotics Rest and immobilization of both affected area and child Hot moist compresses to area	Hospitalization may be necessary for child with systemic symptoms Otitis media may be associated with facial cellulitis
Staphylococcal Scalded Skin Syndrome— *S. aureus*	Macular erythema with "sandpaper" texture of involved skin Epidermis becomes wrinkled (in 2 days or less) and large bullae appear	Systemic administration of antibiotics Gentle cleansing with saline, Burow solution, or 0.25% silver nitrate compresses	Infant subject to fluid loss, impaired body temperature regulation, and secondary infection, such as pneumonia, cellulitis, and septicemia Heals without scarring

with a needle or sharp instrument. A child with a sty may waken with the eyelids of the affected eye sealed shut with exudate. The child or the parents are instructed to gently wipe the lid with clear warm water and a clean washcloth until the exudate has been removed.

The child with limited cellulitis of an extremity is usually managed at home on a regimen of oral antibiotics and warm compresses. The parents are taught the procedures and instructed in administration of the medication. Children with more extensive cellulitis, especially around a joint with lymphadenitis or on the face, are usually admitted to the hospital for parenteral antibiotics. Nurses are responsible for administering the medication, applying compresses, and maintaining the intravenous infusion.

VIRAL INFECTIONS

Viruses are intracellular parasites that produce their effect by using the intracellular substances of the host cells. Composed

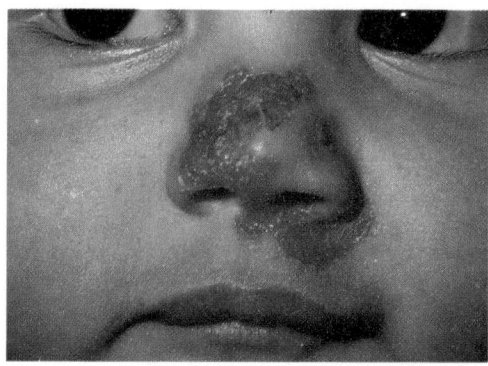

FIG. 30-3. Impetigo contagiosa. (From Weston WL, Lane AT: *Color textbook of pediatric dermatology,* St Louis, 1991, Mosby.)

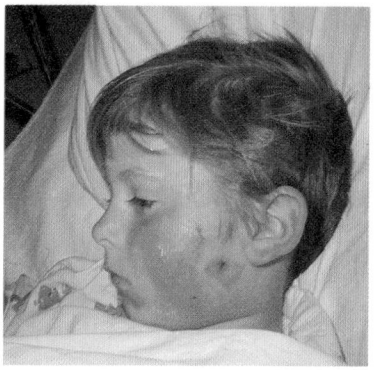

FIG. 30-4. Cellulitis of cheek from puncture wound. (From Weston WL, Lane AT: *Color textbook of pediatric dermatology,* St Louis, 1991, Mosby.)

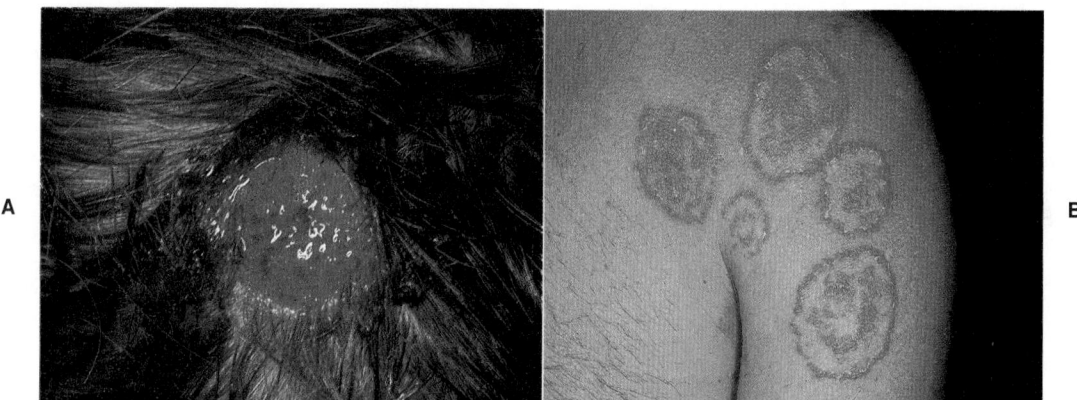

FIG. 30-5. A, Tinea capitis. **B,** Tinea corporis. Both infections are caused by *Microsporum canis,* the "kitten" or "puppy" fungus. (From Habif TP: *Clinical dermatology: a color guide to diagnosis and therapy,* ed 2, St Louis, 1990, Mosby.)

of only a DNA or RNA core enclosed in an antigenic protein shell, viruses are unable to provide for their own metabolic needs or to reproduce themselves. After a virus penetrates a cell of the host organism, it sheds the outer shell and disappears within the cell, where the nucleic acid core stimulates the host cell to form more virus material from its intracellular substance. In a viral infection the epidermal cells react with inflammation and vesiculation (as in herpes simplex) or by proliferating to form growths (warts).

Most of the communicable diseases of childhood are associated with rashes, and each rash is characteristic. The type of lesion and the configuration of the viral exanthems of rubeola, rubella, and chickenpox are described in Table 15-1. Other common viral disorders of the skin are outlined in Table 30-4.

DERMATOPHYTOSES (FUNGAL INFECTIONS)

The dermatophytoses (ringworm) are infections caused by a group of closely related filamentous fungi that invade primarily the stratum corneum, hair, and nails. These are superficial infections that live on, not in, the skin. They are confined to the dead keratin layers and are unable to survive in the deeper layers. Since the keratin is being desquamated constantly, the fungus must multiply at a rate that equals the rate of keratin production to maintain itself; otherwise the infection would be shed with the discarded skin cells. Common dermatophytoses are outlined in Table 30-5.

Dermatophytoses are designated by the Latin word *tinea,* with further designation related to the area of the body where they are found (e.g., tinea capitis [ringworm of the scalp]). Dermatophyte infections are most often transmitted from one person to another or from infected animals to humans. Diagnosis is made from microscopic examination of scrapings taken from the advancing periphery of the lesion, which almost always produces scale.

Nursing Considerations

When teaching families regarding the care of children with ringworm, the nurse should emphasize good health and hygiene. Because of the infectious nature of the disease, several basic hygienic measures are particularly pertinent. Affected children are not to exchange with other children any grooming items, headgear, scarves, or other articles of apparel that have been in proximity to the infected area. Affected children

TABLE 30-4. Viral infections

DISEASE	MANIFESTATIONS	MANAGEMENT	COMMENTS
Verruca (Warts) Cause: human papillomavirus (various types)	Small, benign tumors Usually well-circumscribed, gray or brown, elevated firm papules with a roughened, finely papillomatous texture Occur anywhere, but usually appear on exposed areas such as fingers, hands, face, and soles May be single or multiple Asymptomatic	Not uniformly successful Local destructive therapy, individualized according to location, type, and number—surgical removal, electrocautery, curettage, cryotherapy (liquid nitrogen), caustic solutions (lactic acid and salicylic acid in flexible collodion, retinoic acid, salicylic acid plasters), x-ray treatment	Common in children Tend to disappear spontaneously Course unpredictable Most destructive techniques tend to leave scars Autoinoculable Repeated irritation will cause to enlarge
Verruca plantaris (plantar wart)	Located on plantar surface of feet and, because of pressure, are practically flat; may be surrounded by a collar of hyperkeratosis	Apply caustic solution to wart, wear foam insole with hole cut to relieve pressure on wart; soak 20 min after 2-3 days; repeat until wart comes out	Destructive techniques tend to leave scars, which may cause problems with walking
Herpes Simplex Virus Type I (cold sore, fever blister) Type II (genital)	Grouped, burning, and itching vesicles on inflammatory base, usually on or near mucocutaneous junctions (lips, nose, genitals, buttocks) Vesicles dry, forming a crust, followed by exfoliation and spontaneous healing in 8-10 days May be accompanied by regional lymphadenopathy	Avoidance of secondary infection Burow solution compresses during weeping stages Topical therapy has proved to have effect on recurrences Oral antiviral (Acyclovir) for initial infection or to reduce severity in recurrence	Heal without scarring unless secondary infection Aggravated by corticosteroids Positive psychologic effect from treatment May be fatal in children with depressed immunity
Varicella Zoster Virus (Herpes Zoster; Shingles)	Caused by same virus that causes varicella (chickenpox) Virus has affinity for posterior root ganglia, posterior horn of spinal cord, and skin; crops of vesicles usually confined to dermatome following along course of affected nerve Usually preceded by neuralgic pain, hyperesthesias, or itching May be accompanied by constitutional symptoms	Symptomatic Analgesics for pain Mild sedation sometimes helpful Local moist compresses Drying lotions may be helpful Ophthalmic variety: systemic corticotropin (ACTH) and/or corticosteroids Acyclovir	Pain in children usually minimal Postherpetic pain does not occur in children Chickenpox may follow exposure; isolate affected child from other children in a hospital or school May occur in children with depressed immunity; can be fatal
Molluscum Contagiosum Cause: pox virus	Flesh-colored papules with a central caseous plug (umbilicated) Usually asymptomatic	Cases in well children resolve spontaneously in about 18 months Treatment reserved for troublesome cases Curettage or cryotherapy	Common in school-age children Spread by skin-to-skin contact, including autoinoculation and fomite-to-skin contact

TABLE 30-5. Dermatophytoses (fungal infections)

DISEASE/ORGANISM	MANIFESTATIONS	MANAGEMENT	COMMENTS
Tinea Capitis— *Trichophyton tonsurans, Microsporum audouini, Microsporum canis* (Fig. 30-5, *A* on p. 1081)	Lesions in scalp but may extend to hairline or neck Characteristic configuration of scaly, circumscribed patches and/or patchy, scaling areas of alopecia Generally asymptomatic, but severe, deep inflammatory reaction may occur that manifests as boggy, encrusted lesions (kerions) Pruritic Microscopic examination of scales is diagnostic	Oral griseofulvin Oral ketoconazole for difficult cases Selenium sulfide shampoos Topical antifungal agents (e.g., clotrimazole, haloprogin, miconazole)	Person-to-person transmission Animal-to-person transmission Rarely, permanent loss of hair *M. audouini* transmitted from one human being to another directly or from personal items; *M. canis* usually contracted from household pets, esp. cats Atopic individuals more susceptible
Tinea Corporis— *Trichophyton rubrum, Trichophyton mentagrophytes, M. canis, Epidermophyton* (see Fig. 30-5, *B* on p. 1081)	Generally round or oval, erythematous scaling patch that spreads peripherally and clears centrally; may involve nails (tinea unguium) Diagnosis: direct microscopic examination of scales Usually unilateral	Oral griseofulvin Local application of antifungal preparation such as tolnaftate, haloprogin, miconazole, clotrimazole; apply 1 inch beyond periphery of lesion; continual application 1 to 2 weeks after no sign of lesion	Usually of animal origin from infected pets Majority of infections in children caused by *M. canis* and *M. audouini*
Tinea Cruris ("jock itch")—*Epidermophyton floccosum, T. rubrum, T. mentagrophytes*	Skin response similar to tinea corporis Localized to medial proximal aspect of thigh and crural fold; may involve scrotum in males Pruritic Diagnosis: same as for tinea corporis	Local application of tolnaftate liquid Wet compresses or sitz baths may be soothing	Rare in preadolescent children Health education regarding personal hygiene

Tinea Pedis ("athlete's foot")—*T. rubrum, Trichophyton interdigitale, E. floccosum*	On intertriginous areas between toes or on plantar surface of feet
	Lesions vary:
	  Maceration and fissuring between toes
	  Patches with pinhead-sized vesicles on plantar surface
	  Pruritic
	  Diagnosis: direct microscopic examination of scrapings
		Oral griseofulvin
		Local applications of tolnaftate liquid and antifungal powder containing tolnaftate
		Acute infections: compresses or soaks followed by application of glucocorticoid cream
		Elimination of conditions of heat and perspiration by clean, light socks and well-ventilated shoes; avoidance of occlusive shoes
			Most frequent in adolescents and adults; rare in children, but occurrence increases with wearing of plastic shoes
			Transmission to other individuals rare despite general opinion to contrary
			Ointments not successful

Candidiasis (moniliasis)—*Candida albicans*	Grows in chronically moist areas Inflamed areas with white exudate, peeling, and easy bleeding Pruritic Diagnosis: characteristic appearance	Amphotericin B, nystatin ointment, or other antifungal preparations to affected areas	Common form of diaper dermatitis (see Fig. 30-11) Oral form common in infants (see Chapter 9) May be disseminated in immunosuppressed children

TABLE 30-6. Systemic mycoses

DISORDER/ ORGANISM	SKIN MANIFESTATIONS	SYSTEMIC MANIFESTATIONS	TREATMENT	COMMENTS
North American blastomycosis— *Blastomyces dermatitidis*	Chronic granulomatous lesions and microabscesses in any part of body Initial lesion is a papule; undergoes ulceration and peripheral spread	Pulmonary symptoms, such as cough, chest pain, weakness, and weight loss May have skeletal involvement, with bone destruction and formation of cutaneous abscesses	Intravenous administration of amphotericin B	Usual portal of entry is lungs Source of infection unknown Noninfectious Pulmonary infections may be mild and self-limiting and require no treatment Progressive disease often fatal
Cryptococcosis— *Cryptococcus neoformans (Torula histolytica)*	Usually on face; acneiform, firm, nodular, painless eruption	Central nervous system (CNS) manifestations; headache, dizziness, stiff neck, and signs of increased intracranial pressure Low-grade fever, mild cough, lung infiltration	Intravenous amphotericin B; may be administered intrathecally for CNS involvement 5-Flurocytosine for meningitis Excision and drainage of local lesions	Acquired by inhalation of dust but may enter through skin Prognosis serious Noninfectious Increased incidence in persons receiving corticosteroids with lymphoreticular malignancies, or type II diabetes
Histoplasmosis— *Histoplasma capsulatum*	Not distinctive or uniform but most appear as punched-out or granulomatous ulcers	General systemic symptoms may include pallor, diarrhea, vomiting, irregular spiking temperature, hepatosplenomegaly, and pulmonary symptoms Any tissue of body may be involved with related symptoms	Intravenous amphotericin B for severe cases Oral ketoconazole	Organism cultured from soil, especially where contaminated with fowl droppings Fungus enters through skin or mucous membranes of mouth and respiratory tract Endemic in Mississippi and Ohio River valleys Disseminated diseases most common in infants and children
Coccidioidomycosis (valley fever)— *Coccidioides immitis*	Erythema nodosum Erythema multiforme Erythematous maculopapular rash	Primary lung disease usually asymptomatic May be sign of acute febrile illness Disseminated disease is very serious	Intravenous amphotericin B Intravenous miconazole (synthetic imidazole) Intraventricular miconazole plus oral ketoconazole for CNS involvement Surgical resection of persistent pulmonary cavities	Inhalation of aerospores from soil Endemic in southwestern United States Usually resolves spontaneously Increased incidence in dark-skinned races (Filipino, black, Mexican, Asian)

are provided with their own towels and directed to wear protective caps at night to avoid transmitting the fungus to bedding, especially if they sleep with another person. Since the infection can be acquired by animal-to-human transmission, all household pets should be examined for the presence of the disorder. Other sources of infection are seats with headrests, such as theater seats or seats in public transportation.

Treatment with the drug griseofulvin frequently lasts for weeks or months, and, because subjective symptoms subside, children or parents may be tempted to decrease or discontinue the drug. The nurse should impress on members of the family the importance of maintaining the prescribed dosage schedule. They are also instructed regarding the possibility of side effects from the drug such as headache, gastrointestinal upset, fatigue, insomnia, and photosensitivity. For children who take the drug over many months, periodic testing is required to monitor leukopenia and assess liver and renal function.

SYSTEMIC MYCOTIC (FUNGAL) INFECTIONS

Mycotic (systemic or deep fungal) infections have the capacity to invade the viscera as well as the skin. The best known of these infections are primarily lung diseases, which are usually acquired by inhalation of fungal spores. These fungi produce a variable spectrum of disease, and some are quite common in certain geographic areas. They are not transmitted from person to person but appear to reside in the soil, from which their spores are airborne. The cutaneous lesions caused by deep fungal infections are granulomatous and appear as ulcers, plaques, nodules, fungating masses, and abscesses. The course of deep fungal diseases is chronic with slow progression that favors sensitization (Table 30-6).

SKIN DISORDERS RELATED TO CHEMICAL OR PHYSICAL CONTACTS

CONTACT DERMATITIS

Contact dermatitis is an inflammatory reaction of the skin to chemical substances, natural or synthetic, that evoke a hypersensitivity response or to those agents that cause direct irritation. The initial reaction occurs in an exposed region, most commonly the face and neck, backs of the hands, forearms, male genitalia, and lower legs. There is characteristically a sharp delineation between inflamed and normal skin early in the reaction that ranges from a faint, transient erythema to massive bullae on an erythematous swollen base. Itching is a constant symptom.

The cause may be a primary irritant or a sensitizing agent. A *primary irritant* is one that irritates any skin. A *sensitizing agent* produces an irritation on those who have met the irritant or something chemically related to it, have undergone an immunologic change, and have become sensitized. Prior exposure is not necessarily a factor in the reaction. A sensitizer irritates in relatively low concentrations only persons who are allergic to it. Sometimes with repeated exposure and

reactions the skin loses its capacity to return to normal, or secondary factors become predominant to produce a chronic inflammatory process.

The major goal in treatment is to prevent further exposure of the skin to the offending substance. Provided there is no further irritation, the normal recuperative powers of the skin will produce satisfactory results without treatment. The most frequent offenders are plant and animal irritants, the prototype of which is poison ivy (see below).

The most common contact dermatitis in infants occurs on the convex surfaces of the diaper area (see Diaper Dermatitis, p. 1093). Other agents that frequently produce dermatologic responses from contact are animal irritants such as wool, feathers, and furs; vegetable irritants such as oleoresins, oils, and turpentine; and chemicals of all kinds, including synthetic fabrics (e.g., shoe components), dyes, metals, cosmetics, perfumes, and soaps (including bubble baths). The list is endless.

Nursing Considerations

Nurses frequently detect evidence of contact dermatitis during routine physical assessments. Skin manifestations in specific areas suggest limited contact, such as around the eyes (mascara), areas of the body covered by clothing but not protected by undergarments (wool), or areas of the body not covered by clothing (ultraviolet injury). Generalized involvement is more likely to be caused by bubble bath or soap. Often nurses are able to determine the offending agent and counsel families regarding management. However, if the lesions persist, are extensive, or show evidence of infection, medical evaluation is indicated.

POISON IVY, OAK, AND SUMAC

The prototype of plant offenders is poison ivy (also poison oak and sumac) (Fig. 30-6). Contact with the dry or succulent portions of the plant produces localized, streaked or spotty, oozing and painful impetiginous lesions. The offending substance in these plants is an oil, *urushiol*, that is extremely potent. Sensitivity to urushiol is not inborn but is developed after one or two exposures and may change over a lifetime. All parts of the plants contain the oil, so dried leaves and stems contain the irritant. Even smoke from burning brush piles can produce a reaction.

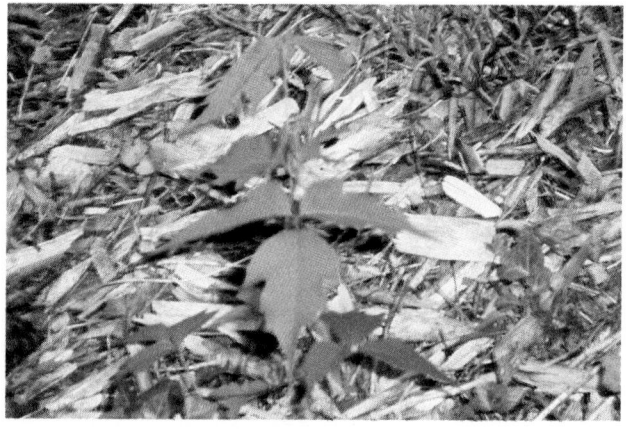

FIG. 30-6. Poison ivy.

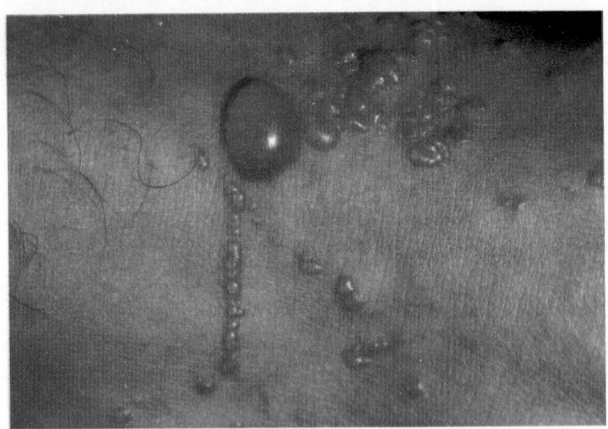

FIG. 30-7. Poison ivy; note "streaked" blisters surrounding one large blister. (From Habif TP: *Clinical dermatology: a color guide to diagnosis and therapy,* ed 2, St Louis, 1990, Mosby.)

Animals do not seem to be affected by the oil; however, dogs or other animals that have run or played in the plants may carry the sap on their fur, and animals who eat the plants can transfer the oil in saliva. Shoes, tools, and toys can transfer the oil. Golf balls that have been in the rough also are sources of contact.

Urushiol takes effect as soon as it touches the skin. It penetrates through the epidermis and bonds with the dermal layer, where it initiates an immune response. The full-blown reaction is evident after about 2 days, with redness, swelling, and itching at the site of contact. Several days later, streaked or spotty blisters oozing serum from damaged cells produce the characteristic impetiginous lesions (Fig. 30-7). The lesions dry and heal spontaneously, and itching stops by 10 to 14 days.

Therapeutic Management

Treatment of the lesions includes calamine lotion, soothing Burow solution compresses, and/or Aveeno baths to relieve discomfort. Topical corticosteroid gel is very effective for prevention or relief of inflammation, especially when applied before blisters form. Oral corticosteroids may be needed for severe reactions, and a sedative such as diphenhydramine (Benadryl) may be ordered.

Nursing Considerations

When it is known that the child has made contact with the plant, the area is immediately flushed (preferably within 15 minutes) with *cold* running water to neutralize the urushiol not yet bonded to the skin. If there is a stream nearby, an effective method is to have the child enter the water (clothes and all) and allow the water to rinse the oil from both skin and clothing. Harsh soap is contraindicated because it removes protective skin oils and dilutes the urushiol, allowing it to spread; also, hard scrubbing irritates the skin. All clothing that has come in contact with the plant is removed with care and thoroughly laundered in hot water and detergent. Every effort is made to prevent the child from scratching the lesions. Although the lesions do not spread by contact with the blister serum or from scratching, they can become secondarily infected.

Prevention. Prevention is best accomplished by avoidance of contact and removal of the plant from the environment when feasible. All children, especially those known to be sensitive, should be taught to recognize the plant. Information regarding means for destroying plants can be obtained from the U.S. Department of Agriculture or Forestry Service. An example of a cream that helps protect exposed skin from poison oak and ivy is Stokogard.*

DRUG REACTIONS

Adverse reactions to drugs are seen more often in the skin than in any other organ, although any organ of the body can be affected. The reaction may be a result of toxicity related to drug concentration, individual intolerance to the average dosage of the drug, or an allergic or idiosyncratic response. The manifestations may be associated with side effects or secondary effects of a drug, either of which are unrelated to its primary pharmacologic actions.

Although any drug is capable of producing almost any form of reaction in the susceptible individual, some have a tendency to produce a particular reaction consistently, and some are more likely than others to produce an untoward effect. Many are allergenic responses following a prior administration of the drug, even a topical application. Other factors influence a drug response in a particular individual. For example, the incidence increases with the number and amount of drugs being given, and intravenous drugs are more likely to cause a reaction than are oral drugs.

Manifestations of drug reactions may be delayed or immediate. Rashes are the most common manifestation of adverse drug reactions in children. However, individual drug reactions may vary from a single lesion to extensive, generalized epidermal necrosis, such as occurs in Stevens-Johnson syndrome (see Table 30-9). Cutaneous manifestations can resemble almost any skin disease and can be seen in almost any degree of severity. With few exceptions, the distribution of a drug eruption is widespread, since it results from a circulating agent, appears as an inflammatory response with itching, is sudden in onset, and may be associated with constitutional symptoms such as fever, malaise, gastrointestinal upsets, anemia, or liver and kidney damage.

 Seven days are usually required for a child to develop sensitivity to a drug that has never been administered previously. With prior sensitivity the manifestations appear almost immediately.

In most cases treatment for simple cutaneous reactions consists of discontinuing the drug. Sometimes a decision is made to continue the drug (such as an antibiotic in an infant or small child) until the cause of the rash is clearly indicated. In urticarial-type eruptions antihistamines may be ordered, and for widespread and severe lesions corticosteroids are beneficial. Severe anaphylactic reactions are a medical emergency (see Anaphylaxis, Chapter 25).

Nursing Considerations

The most effective means of management is prevention. Parents always remember a severe reaction. A careful history will elicit evidence of a previous drug reaction. The history should

---

*Distributed in the USA by: Stockhausen, Inc., Greensboro, NC 27406; (800) 334-0242.

include the name of the drug, nature of the reaction, drug dose, and how soon after administration the reaction occurred (see Chapter 6).

Nurses who suspect that a rash is caused by a medication should withhold any further dose and report the eruption to the practitioner. Frequent offenders in drug reactions are penicillin and sulfonamides, and nurses must be alert to this possibility. However, even commonplace drugs, including aspirin, barbiturates, chemical agents in a number of foods, flavoring agents, and preservatives, are capable of producing an undesired response. Persons who have severe reactions should wear an identification bracelet or chain in case of emergency or inadvertent administration of the offending drug.

FOREIGN BODIES

Small wooden splinters can be removed by parents with a needle and tweezers that have been sterilized with alcohol or a flame. The area around the sliver is washed with soap and water before removal is attempted. The sliver is exposed with the needle, then grasped firmly by the tweezers and pulled out. Suggestions for removing cactus spines are listed below. Some foreign bodies, such as a fishhook, a piece of glass or other difficult-to-see object, or a deeply embedded object, such as a needle in a foot or near a joint, may need medical evaluation.

NURSING TIPS
Cactus prickles or spines are readily removed by one of several methods:
- Apply a thin layer of household glue and cover with gauze. When glue dries, peel off gauze (Martinez and others, 1987).
- Apply commercial hair removal wax or body sugar (Aplon*), let dry, and remove (Hennes, 1988).
- Place cellophane tape, sticky side down, over the spines and lift off (Cooper, 1988).

SKIN DISORDERS RELATED TO INSECT AND ANIMAL CONTACTS

SCABIES

Scabies is an endemic infestation produced by the scabies mite, *Sarcoptes scabiei*. The lesions are created as the impregnated female burrows into the stratum corneum of the epidermis (never into living tissue) to bury her eggs. The inflammatory response and itching occur after the host becomes sensitized to the mite, approximately 30 to 60 days following initial contact. After this time, anywhere the mite has traveled will begin to itch and develop the characteristic eruption (see box above). Consequently, mites will not necessarily be located at all sites of eruption. The picture is often confusing in infants, who often develop an eczematous eruption; therefore the observer must look for discrete papules, burrows, or vesicles.

Nursing Considerations
The treatment of scabies is the application of a scabicide, such as 1% lindane (Kwell, Scavene) in a vanishing cream base.

*Distributed by Corsa, Ltd., Conshohocker, PA 19428.

CLINICAL MANIFESTATIONS OF SCABIES

Lesion
Children—minute grayish-brown, threadlike (mite burrows), pruritic
    Black dot at end of burrow (mite)
Infants—eczematous eruption, pruritic

Distribution
Generally in intertriginous areas—interdigital, axillary-cubital, popliteal, inguinal
Children over 2 years of age—primarily hands and wrists
Children younger than 2 years—primarily feet and ankles

However, crotamiton (Eurax) or permethrin 5% cream (Elimite) is often used to avoid the risk of neurotoxicity from lindane (Taplin and others, 1990). Nurses instructing families in use of the scabicide should emphasize the importance of following the directions accurately. Lindane is applied to cool, dry skin—not following a hot bath—and left on for the recommended time, usually 4 hours for infants and 6 hours for older children and adults. Permethrin is applied for 8 to 14 hours. One liberal application is sufficient, but all persons in the family (including baby-sitters and others who have close contact with the child) should be treated. Families need to know that although the mite will be killed, the rash and the itch will not be eliminated until the stratum corneum is replaced, which takes approximately 2 to 3 weeks. Soothing ointments or lotions can be applied for itching. Antibiotics may be given for secondary infection.

PEDICULOSIS CAPITIS

Pediculosis capitis (head lice, or "cooties") is an infestation of the scalp by *Pediculus humanus capitis*, a very common parasite, especially in school-age children. The adult louse lives only about 48 hours when away from a human host, and the life span of the average female is 1 month. The female lays eggs at the junction of a hair shaft and close to the skin, because they need a warm environment. The *nits*, or eggs, hatch in approximately 7 to 10 days; the egg is thus about 4 mm, or ¼ inch, from the scalp (but may be farther) at the time of hatching.

Diagnostic Evaluation

Diagnosis is made by observation of the white eggs (nits) firmly attached to the base of the hair shafts (see box on p. 1088). Because of their brief life span and mobility, adult lice are more difficult to locate. Nits must be differentiated from dandruff, lint, hair spray, and other items of similar size and shape. Scratch marks and/or inflammatory papules, caused by secondary infection, may also be found on the scalp in the vulnerable areas.

Therapeutic Management

Treatment consists of the application of pediculocides and manual removal of nit cases. A number of effective products are available. Permethrin 1% creme rinse (Nix) kills both lice and nits after one application. This product and preparations of pyrethrin with piperonyl butoxide (RID or A-200 pyri-

---

CLINICAL MANIFESTATIONS OF PEDICULOSIS

Pruritus (caused by crawling insect and insect saliva on skin)
Nits observable on hair shaft (see Fig. 30-8)

Distribution
Occipital area
Behind ears
Nape of neck
Eyebrows and eyelashes (occasionally) (caused by pubic lice)

FAMILY HOME CARE
Preventing the Spread and Recurrence of Pediculosis

Machine wash all washable clothing, towels, and bed linens in hot water and dry in a hot dryer for at least 20 minutes. Dry clean nonwashable items.
Thoroughly vacuum carpets, car seats, pillows, stuffed animals, rugs, mattresses, and upholstered furniture.
Seal nonwashable items in plastic bags for 14 days if unable to dry clean or vacuum.
Soak combs, brushes, and hair accessories in lice-killing products for 1 hour or in boiling water for 10 minutes.

From Clore ER: Dispelling the common myths about pediculosis, *J Pediatr Health Care* 3:28-33, 1989.

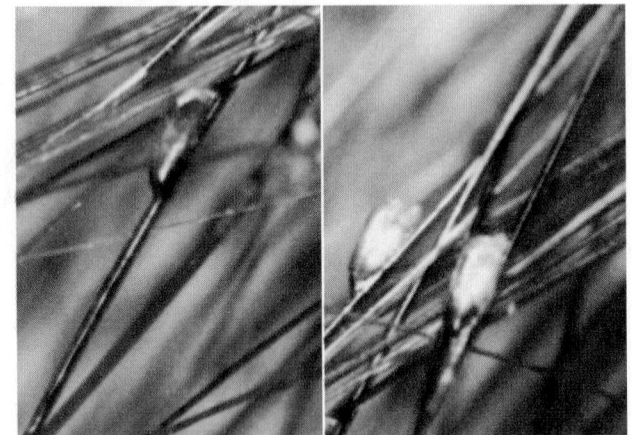

A   **B**

FIG. 30-8. A, Empty nit case. **B,** Viable nits. (From *The contemporary approach to the control of head lice in schools and communities*, Pittsburgh, 1991, SmithKline Beecham.)

nate) can be obtained without a prescription and are more effective and safer than lindane. In fact in a study comparing these pediculicides and other products, as well as their nit-removal combs, Nix (and its comb) was found to be the most effective product (Clore and Longyear, 1993).

Nursing Considerations

Nurses should be aware of several things to successfully manage or assist parents in coping with pediculosis. It should be emphasized that *anyone* can get pediculosis; it has no respect for age, socioeconomic level, or cleanliness. The louse does not jump or fly, but it can be transmitted from one person to another on personal items. Therefore children are cautioned against sharing combs, hats, caps, scarves, coats, and other items used on or near the hair. Children who share lockers are more likely to contract an infestation, and slumber parties place children at risk. Lice are not carried or transmitted by pets.

Nurses or parents should carefully inspect the head of a child who scratches the head more than usual for bite marks, redness, and nits. The hair is systematically spread with two flat-sided sticks or tongue depressors, and the scalp observed for any movement that indicates a louse. Nurses should wear gloves when examining the hair. Lice are small and grayish-tan, have no wings, and are visible to the naked eye. The nits, or eggs, appear as tiny whitish oval specks adhering to the hair shaft about ¼ inch from the scalp. The adherent nature of the nits distinguishes them from dandruff, which falls off readily. *Empty nit cases,* indicating hatched lice, are translucent rather than white and are located more than ¼ inch from the scalp (Fig. 30-8).

If evidence of infestation is found, it is important to perform the treatment according to the directions described on the label of the pediculicide. Parents are advised to read the directions carefully before beginning treatment. Instructions on the labels indicate that dead lice and remaining nits are removed with an extra-fine-tooth comb. Most preparations include a comb to dislodge the firmly adhered nits. A commercial product of formic acid solution (Step 2 or Clear) may be used to loosen attached nits for removal. However, if the comb is ineffective in removing the nit cases, they must be removed with tweezers or between the fingernails.

The child is made as comfortable as possible during the application process, because the pediculicide must remain on the scalp and hair for several minutes. If eye irritation occurs, the eyes must be flushed well with tepid water.

NURSING TIP Playing "beauty parlor" during the shampoo is a useful strategy. The child lies supine, with the head over a sink or basin, and covers the eyes with a dry towel or washcloth. This prevents medication, which can cause chemical conjunctivitis, from splashing into the eyes.

Live lice survive for up to 48 hours away from the host, but nits are shed into the environment and are capable of hatching in 7 to 10 days. Therefore measures must be taken to prevent further infestation (see Family Home Care box). Spraying with insecticide is not recommended because of the danger to children and animals. Families should also be advised that the pediculicide is relatively expensive, especially when several members of the household require treatment.

The psychologic effects of lice infestations can be highly stressful to children. They are influenced by the reactions of others, including their parents, and may be made to feel ashamed or guilty. Parents are strongly cautioned against cutting a child's hair or, worse, shaving a child's head. Lice infest short hair as readily as long hair, and these actions only compound the child's distress and serve as a continual reminder to peers, who are always ready to taunt another with something out of the ordinary.

TABLE 30-7. Skin lesions caused by arthropods

MECHANISM/CHARACTERISTICS	MANIFESTATIONS	MANAGEMENT

Insect Bites—Flies, Gnats, Mosquitoes, Fleas
Mechanism:
  Foreign protein in insects' saliva introduced when skin penetrated for a blood-sucking meal
Distribution:
  Almost everywhere—fleas, mosquitoes, ants
  Suburbs and rural areas—bees
  Urban areas—hornets, wasps, yellow jackets
	Hypersensitivity reaction
	  Papular urticaria
	  Firm papules; may be capped by vesicles or excoriated
	Little or no reaction in nonsensitized person
		Treatment:
		  Use antipruritic agents and baths
		  Administer antihistamines
		  Prevent secondary infection
		Prevention:
		  Avoid contact
		  Remove focus, such as treating furniture, mattresses, carpets, and pets, where insects may live
		  Apply insect repellent when exposure is anticipated

Chiggers—Harvest Mite
Mechanism:
  Creeps into skin pores and hair follicles to feed
Manifestations:
  Erythematous papules
  Intense itching
	Same as insect bites
	Favor warm areas of body, especially intertriginous areas and areas covered with clothing
		Avoid contact, especially in areas of tall grass and underbrush
		Apply insect repellant when exposure is anticipated
		May require systemic steroids for extensive bites

Hymenopteran Stings—Bees, Wasps, Hornets, Yellow Jackets, Fire Ants
Mechanism:
  Injection of venom through stinging apparatus
  Venom contains histamine, allergenic proteins, and often a spreading factor, hyaluronidase
Severe reactions caused by hypersensitivity and/or multiple stings
	Local reaction: small red area, wheal, itching, and heat
	Systemic reactions: may be mild to severe, including generalized edema, pain, nausea and vomiting, confusion, respiratory embarrassment, and shock
		Treatment:
		  Carefully scrape off stinger if present
		  Cleanse with soap and water
		  Apply cool compresses
		  Apply common household product, e.g., lemon juice, paste made with aspirin, baking soda, or Adolph's Meat Tenderizer
		  Administer antihistamines
		  Severe reactions: administer epinephrine, corticosteroids; treat for shock
		Prevention:
		  Teach child to wear shoes, to avoid wearing bright clothing, flowery prints, shiny jewelry, or perfumed grooming products (cologne, scented hairspray) that might attract the insect, and to avoid places where the insect may be contacted
		Hypersensitive children should wear identifying tag to indicate allergy and therapy needed; family should keep emergency medication and be taught its administration

Black Widow Spider
Mechanism:
  Venom injected through a clawlike appendage; has neurotoxic action
Characteristics:
  Spider is shiny black, with a body about 1.25 cm (0.5 inches) long and a red or orange hourglass-shaped marking on underside
  Avoids light and bites in self-defense
	Mild sting at time of bite
	Area becomes swollen, painful, and erythematous
	Dizziness, weakness, and abdominal pain
	May produce delirium, paralysis, convulsions, and (if large amount of venom absorbed) death
		Treatment:
		  Cleanse wound with antiseptic
		  Apply cool compresses
		  Administer antivenin
		  Administer muscle relaxant, such as calcium gluconate; analgesics and/or sedatives; hydrocortisone or diazepam IV
		Prevention:
		  Teach children to avoid places that harbor the spider (e.g., woodpiles)

Continued.

TABLE 30-7. Skin lesions caused by arthropods—cont'd

MECHANISM/CHARACTERISTICS	MANIFESTATIONS	MANAGEMENT
Brown Recluse Spider Mechanism: 　Venom injected via fangs 　Venom contains powerful necrotoxin Characteristics: 　Spider is slender, long-legged, with body length of 1 to 2 cm; color is fawn to dark brown and recognized by fiddle-shaped mark on head 　Shy; bites only when annoyed or surprised 　Prefers dark areas where seldom disturbed	Mild sting at time of bite Transient erythema followed by bleb or blister; mild to severe pain in 2-8 hours; purple, star-shaped area in 3-4 days; necrotic ulceration in 7-14 days (Fig. 30-9) Systemic reactions may include fever, malaise, restlessness, nausea and vomiting, and joint pain Generalized petechial eruption Wounds heal with scar formation	Treatment: 　Apply cool compresses locally 　Administer antibiotics, corticosteroids 　Relieve pain 　Wound may require skin graft Prevention: 　Teach children to avoid possible nesting sites
Scorpions Mechanism: 　Sting by means of a hooked caudal stinger that discharges venom 　Venom of more venomous species contains hemolysins, endotheliolysins, and neurotoxins Characteristics: 　Usual habitat is southwestern United States	Intense local pain, erythema, numbness, burning, restlessness, vomiting Ascending motor paralysis with convulsions, weakness, rapid pulse, excessive salivation, thirst, dysuria, pulmonary edema, coma, and death Some species produce only local tissue reaction with swelling at puncture site (distinctive) Symptoms subside in a few hours Deaths occur among children under 4 years of age, usually in first 24 hours	Treatment: 　Delay absorption of venom by keeping child quiet; place involved area in dependent position 　Administer antivenin 　Relieve pain 　Admit to PICU for surveillance Prevention: 　Teach children to avoid possible nesting sites
Ticks Mechanism: 　In process of sucking blood, head and mouth parts are buried in skin Characteristics: 　Feed on blood of mammals 　Significant in humans because of pathologic organism carried 　May be vectors of various infectious diseases, such as Rocky Mountain spotted fever, Q fever, tularemia, relapsing fever, Lyme disease, tick paralysis 　Must attach and feed 1-2 hours to transmit disease 　Usual habitat is very wooded area	Tick usually attached to skin, head embedded Produce firm, discrete, intensely pruritic nodules at site of attachment May cause urticaria or persistent localized edema	Treatment: 　Grasp tick with tweezers (forceps) as close as possible to point of attachment 　Pull straight up with steady, even pressure; if bare hands, use a tissue to touch tick during removal; wash hands thoroughly with soap and water 　Remove any remaining part (e.g., head) with sterile needle 　Cleanse wounds with soap and disinfectant Prevention: 　Teach children to avoid areas where prevalent 　Inspect skin (especially scalp) after being in wooded areas

Prevention. The increasing incidence of pediculosis in schoolchildren has become a serious concern for school nurses, parents, and community health agencies. School nurses usually coordinate school-community prevention control programs for pediculosis. The *National Pediculosis Association** offers education and advocates a "no nits" policy for treated children's reentry to school.

ARTHROPOD BITES AND STINGS

Bites and stings account for a significant incidence of mild to moderate discomfort, and most are managed by simple symptomatic measures, such as compresses, calamine lotion, and prevention of secondary infection.

Arthropods include insects and arachnids, such as mites, ticks, spiders, and scorpions. Major offending creatures, their manifestations, and management are outlined in Table 30-7.

When an insect stings, its stinger often remains imbedded in the skin. For example, bees have barbed stingers that penetrate the skin, and any pressure on the venom sac at the tip of the barb pushes more venom into the skin. Children who have become sensitized to hymenopteran bites may demonstrate a severe systemic response that can be life-threatening. One sting can produce generalized urticaria, respiratory difficulty (from laryngeal edema), hypotension, and death

*P.O. Box 149, Newton, MA 02161; (617) 449-6487 or (800) 446-4NPA.

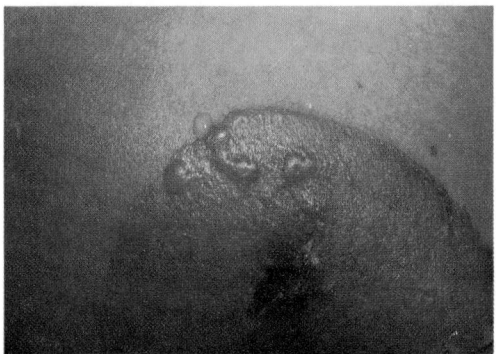

FIG. 30-9. Brown recluse spider bite; note central necrosis surrounded by purplish area and blisters. (From Weston WL, Lane AT: *Color textbook of pediatric dermatology,* St Louis, 1991, Mosby.)

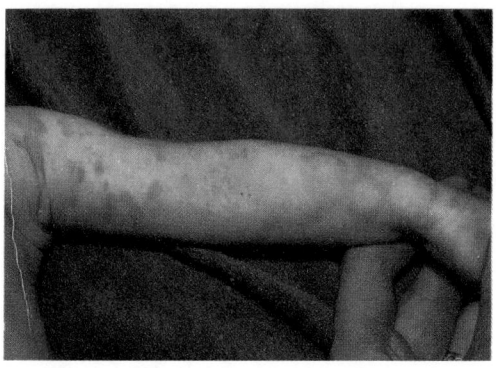

FIG. 30-10. Lyme disease. Note annular red rings in erythema chronicum migrans. (From Weston WL, Lane AT: *Color textbook of pediatric dermatology,* St Louis, 1991, Mosby.)

within 1 hour. Intramuscular administration of epinephrine provides immediate relief and must be available for emergency use.

For hypersensitive children a kit must be available that contains epinephrine and a hypodermic syringe; they also should wear a medical identification device. Families are reminded to check the expiration date on the kit and to replace an outdated one. They should determine if a nurse is available at the school and the school policy regarding administration of drugs. If a school nurse is not present, someone at the school should be designated to inject the epinephrine in case of an emergency.

Most arthropods in the United States are relatively harmless, including tarantulas. Although all spiders produce venom that is injected via fangs, some species are unable to pierce the skin; others produce a venom that is insufficiently toxic to be harmful. Only scorpions and two species of spiders—the brown recluse and the black widow—inject venom deadly enough to require immediate attention. Children bitten by these arachnids must receive medical attention as soon as possible.

INFECTIONS TRANSMITTED BY ARTHROPODS

The organisms responsible for a number of disorders are transmitted to human beings via arthropods (Table 30-8). Rickettsiae are intracellular parasites, similar in size to bacteria, that inhabit the alimentary tract of a wide range of natural hosts. Mammals become infected only through the bites of infected lice, fleas, ticks, and mites, all of which serve as both infectors and reservoirs. Rickettsial diseases are more common in temperate and tropical climates and in areas where humans live in association with arthropods. Infection in humans is incidental (except epidemic typhus) and not necessary for the survival of the rickettsial species. However, once the organism invades a human, it causes a disease that varies in intensity from a benign, self-limiting illness to a fulminating and frequently fatal one.

Lyme disease is a relatively recently recognized disorder caused by a spirochete transmitted by ticks. The disease may first be seen in any of three stages: (1) the tick bite at the time of inoculation: followed in 3 to 32 days by the development of *erythema chronicum migrans (ECM)* at the site of the bite (Fig. 30-10); (2) the most serious stage of the disease: systemic involvement of neurologic, cardiac, and musculoskeletal systems that appears several weeks after the cutaneous phase is completed; and (3) musculoskeletal pains involving the tendons, bursae, muscles and synovia may develop. Arthritis may occur; late neurologic problems may include deafness and chronic encephalopathy.

ANIMAL BITES

Contrary to accepted belief, children are bitten more often by animals belonging to the family or to neighbors than by stray animals. More than half the victims of dog bites are less than 4 years of age. Boys are bitten more often than girls. Most dog or cat injuries are to the upper extremities. However, small children are more likely to be bitten or scratched on the head, face, and neck because they tend to put their heads near the animal's head and to flail their arms rather than protecting their heads. The injuries vary from small puncture wounds to complete evulsion of tissue and can be associated with significant crush injury.

Therapeutic Management

General wound care consists of rinsing the wound with large amounts of saline or Ringer's lactate under pressure (syringe) and washing the surrounding skin with mild soap. A clean pressure dressing is applied, and the extremity elevated if the wound is bleeding. Medical evaluation is advised, since there is danger of tetanus and rabies, although dogs in most urban areas are required to be immunized against rabies. Bites from wild animals, such as squirrels, bats, and raccoons, are potentially dangerous.

Prophylactic antibiotics are indicated for puncture wounds and wounds in areas that may prove to be cosmetically or functionally impaired if infected. Extensive lacerations are debrided and loosely sutured. Tetanus toxoid is administered according to standard guidelines (see Immunizations, Chapter 10), and rabies protocol is followed (see Rabies, Chapter 28). Cat bites become infected more easily than dog bites but no more so than lacerations from other causes. Injuries to

TABLE 30-8. Disorders transmitted by arthropods

DISORDER/ ORGANISM/HOST	MANIFESTATIONS	MANAGEMENT	COMMENTS
Rocky Mountain Spotted Fever— *R. rickettsii* Arthropod: tick Transmission: tick Mammal source: wild rodents; dogs	Gradual onset: fever, malaise, anorexia, myalgia Abrupt onset: rapid temperature elevation, chills, vomiting, myalgia, severe headache Maculopapular or petechial rash primarily on extremities (ankles and wrists) but may spread to other areas, characteristically to palms and soles	Control: protection from tick bite by proper wearing apparel, tick repellent Treatment: Tetracycline or chloramphenicol Vigorous supportive therapy	Usually self-limited in children Onset in children may resemble any infectious disease Severe disease rare in children Children and dogs should be inspected regularly if they play in wooded areas See Table 30-7 for management of ticks
Epidemic Typhus— *R. prowazekii* Arthropod: body louse Transmission: infected feces into broken skin Mammal source: humans	Abrupt onset of chills, fever, diffuse myalgia, headache, malaise Maculopapular rash becomes petechial 4 to 7 days later spreading from trunk outward	Control: immediate destruction of vectors Treatment: Tetracycline or chloramphenicol Supportive	Patient should be isolated until deloused See discussion on p. 1087 for management of pediculosis Excreta from infected lice also in dust—disinfect patient's clothing, bedding, and possessions and wash in hot water
Endemic Typhus— *R. typhi* Arthropod: rat fleas or body lice Transmission: flea bite; inhaling or ingesting flea excreta Mammal source: rats	Headache, arthralgia, backache followed by fever; may last 9-14 days Maculopapular rash after 1-8 days of fever; begins in trunk and spreads to periphery; rarely involves face, palms, soles	Control; eliminate rat reservoir, insect vectors, or both Treatment: Tetracycline or chloramphenicol Supportive	Fairly common in United States Shorter duration than epidemic typhus Mild, seldom fatal illness Difficult to distinguish from epidemic typhus
Rickettsialpox—*R. akari* Arthropod: mouse mite Transmission: mite Mammal source: house mouse	Maculopapular rash following primary lesion; eschar at site of bite, fever, chills, headache	Control: eradication of rodent reservoir and mite vector Treatment: Tetracycline or chloramphenicol Supportive	Self-limited nonfatal disease Endemic in New York City Found in many cities in United States
Lyme Disease— spirochete *Borrelia burgdorferi* Arthropod: tick Transmission: tick bite Mammal source: rodents, deer	Stage 1: tick bite Stage 2: erythema chronicum migrans; papule at bite site progresses to large circumferential ring with a raised edematous doughnutlike border (see Fig. 30-10) Stage 3: systemic involvement—cardiac, neurologic, musculoskeletal	Control: protection from tick bite by proper wearing apparel, tick repellent Treatment: Tetracycline or penicillin Supportive	Regional distribution: Northeast (Massachusetts, Connecticut, Rhode Island, New York, New Jersey, Pennsylvania to Maryland); Midwest (Wisconsin, Minnesota); West (California, Oregon), but becoming more widespread

poorly vascularized areas such as the hands are more likely to become infected than those in more vascularized areas such as the face; puncture wounds are more apt to become infected than lacerations.

Nursing Considerations

The most important aspect related to animal bites is prevention. Children should understand animal behavior and develop a respect for animals. Parents should monitor their children's behavior with a dog and instruct them not to tease or surprise a dog, invade its territory, interfere with its feeding, or sleeping, take its toy, or interact with a sick or injured dog or a dog with pups (Riegger and Guntzelman, 1990). Parents who are contemplating getting a pet, especially a dog, for themselves or their children should receive some advice about the dog that is least likely to be a danger to their children. A categorization of dogs related to their potential interaction with children can be found in the publication *The Right Dog for You*.*

HUMAN BITES

Children often acquire lacerations from the teeth of other humans in rough play, during fights, or as victims of child abuse. Many preschool children bite others out of frustration or anger. Because human dental plaque and gingiva harbor pathogenic organisms, all human bites should receive attention.

If the laceration is less than ¼ inch in length, the wound can be treated at home. The wound is washed thoroughly with soap and water, and a pressure dressing is applied to stop bleeding. Ice applications minimize discomfort and swelling. Increased pain or redness at the wound site is an indication that the child should receive medical attention for antibiotic therapy. Tetanus toxoid is needed if the child is insufficiently immunized. Larger wounds should receive medical attention.

CAT SCRATCH DISEASE (CSD)

CSD is described as a subacute regional adenitis that follows the scratch or bite of an animal, especially a cat (99% of cases). The disease is usually a benign, self-limiting illness that resolves spontaneously in about 2 to 4 months. The diagnosis is made on the basis of three of the following: (1) contact (usually a kitten) and regional inoculation lesion, (2) lymphadenopathy, (3) a positive CSD skin test, and (4) biopsy of lymph node with histopathology compatible with CSD (Margileth and Hadfield, 1990). The disease may persist for several months before gradual resolution. In some children, especially those who are immunocompromised, the adenitis may progress to suppuration and serious complications. Treatment is primarily supportive.

MISCELLANEOUS SKIN DISORDERS

A number of skin lesions are caused by extrinsic or intrinsic factors. Some of these are listed in Table 30-9. There are a number of congenital skin disorders, usually inherited as an autosomal-dominant trait. *Ichthyoses* are a heterogenous group of disorders characterized by scaling that create a challenging problem in treatment. These disorders are not discussed in detail because of their wide variability.

SKIN DISORDERS ASSOCIATED WITH SPECIFIC AGE-GROUPS

Several common and important dermatologic conditions are confined primarily to children in specific age-groups. These conditions include atopic, seborrheic, and diaper dermatitis and the acne of adolescence. The treatment modalities include those previously described. However, there are some special needs and therapies involved with these disorders.

DIAPER DERMATITIS

Diaper dermatitis, one of the most common dermatoses in infants, is one of several acute inflammatory skin disorders caused either directly or indirectly by the wearing of diapers. The peak age of occurrence is 9 to 12 months of age, and the incidence is generally reported as greater in bottle-fed infants than in breast-fed infants.

Pathophysiology and Clinical Manifestations

Diaper dermatitis is caused by prolonged and repetitive contact with an irritant, principally urine, feces, soaps, detergents, ointments, and friction. Although the obvious irritant in the majority of incidences is urine and feces, the specific components that contribute to irritation include a combination of factors.

Prolonged contact of the skin with diaper wetness affects several skin properties. It produces higher friction, greater abrasion damage, increased transepidermal permeability, and increased microbial counts. Therefore healthy skin becomes less resistant to potential irritants.

Although ammonia was once thought to cause diaper rash because of the association between the strong odor on diapers and dermatitis, ammonia alone is not sufficient. The important function of urine is related to an increase in pH from the breakdown of urea in the presence of fecal urease. The increased pH promotes the activity of fecal enzymes, principally proteases and lipases, which act as irritants. Fecal enzymes also increase the permeability of skin to bile salts, another potential irritant in feces.

The eruption of diaper dermatitis can be manifested primarily on convex surfaces or in the folds, and the lesions can represent a variety of types and configurations. Eruptions involving the skin in most intimate contact with the diaper (e.g., the convex surfaces of buttocks, inner thighs, mons pubis, and scrotum) but sparing the folds are likely to be caused by chemical irritants, especially from urine and feces (Fig. 30-11). Other causes are detergents or soaps from inadequately rinsed cloth diapers or the fragrance added to some diapers or disposable wipes. Perianal involvement is usually the result of chemical irritation from feces, especially diarrheal stools. *Candida albicans* infection produces perianal inflammation with satellite lesions (Fig. 30-12).

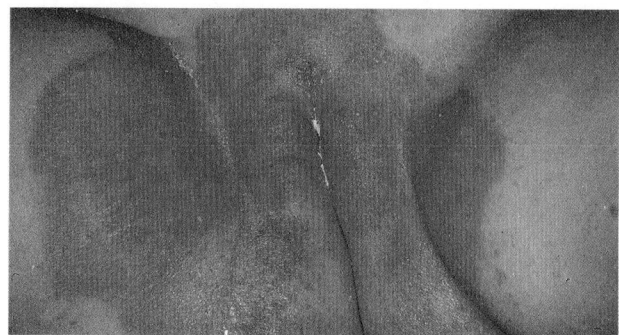

FIG. 30-11. Irritant diaper dermatitis. Note sharply demarcated edges. (From Habif TP: *Clinical dermatology: a color guide to diagnosis and therapy,* ed 2, St Louis, 1990, Mosby.)

TABLE 30-9. Miscellaneous skin disorders

DISEASE/CAUSATIVE AGENT	LOCAL MANIFESTATIONS	MANAGEMENT	COMMENTS
Urticaria—usually allergic response to drugs or infection	Development of wheals Vary in size and configuration and tend to appear quickly, spread irregularly, and fade within a few hours May be constant or intermittent, sparse or profuse, small or large, discrete or confluent May be acute, chronic, or recurrent in acute attacks	Local soothing and antipruritic applications Antihistamines Epinephrine or ephedrine Cortisone or corticotropin (ACTH) in severe cases Severe upper respiratory involvement may require tracheostomy	Known etiology agents should be avoided May be accompanied by malaise, fever, lymphadenopathy Severe cases may involve mucous membranes, internal organs, and joints Obstruction to air passages constitutes medical emergency (see Chapter 25)
Intertrigo—mechanical trauma and aggravating factors of excessive heat, moisture, and sweat retention	Red, inflamed, moist, partially denuded, marginated areas, the shape of which is determined by location Appears where opposing skin surfaces rub together, such as intergluteal folds, groin, neck, and axilla Excessive moisture and obesity are often factors	Affected areas kept clean and dry Skin folds kept separated with a generous supply of nonmedicated powder Expose to air and light Remove excess clothing	A form of diaper irritation Prevent recurrence by keeping susceptible areas clean and dry Frequently associated with overheating from too much clothing
Psoriasis—unknown; hereditary predisposition; may be triggered by stress	Round, thick, dry, reddish patches covered with coarse, silvery scales over trunk and extremities; first lesions commonly appear in scalp; facial lesions more common in children than adults Affected cells proliferate at a much more rapid rate than normal cells	Exposure to sunlight, ultraviolet light Topical corticosteroids Tar derivates Trihydroxyanthracine Keratolytic agents (salicylic acid) Psoralin—ultraviolet A (PUVA)* Emollients may provide relief	Uncommon in children under age 6 years Persons are otherwise healthy individuals Coal tar and psoralin act synergistically with ultraviolet light Keratolytic agents enhance absorption of corticosteroids Humidifiers may help in winter
Alopecia Alopecia areata	Sudden onset of asymptomatic, noninflammatory, round, bald patches in hairy parts of body	Psychologic support Inducement of allergic contact dermatitis to stimulate growth of hair Minoxidil (peripheral vasodilator)	Family history in 10%-26% of cases Some concern regarding drug therapy safety Refer to support groups†
Traumatic alopecia	Traction alopecia around scalp margins from tight hair styles (e.g., braids, pony tails, corn rows)	Counseling regarding hair styling, use of hair cosmetics, hot combs, rollers	More prevalent in black children and adolescents Prolonged traction can produce fibrosis of hair root and permanent loss
Trichotillomania	Compulsive hair pulling	Determine and treat cause	Chronic hair pulling may require psychologic therapy
Tinea capitis	See Table 30-5	See Table 30-5	See Table 30-5

*Still considered investigational.
†*National Alopecia Areata Foundation,* 710 C St, Suite 11, San Rafael, CA 94901; (415) 456-4644.

TABLE 30-9. Miscellaneous skin disorders—cont'd

DISEASE/CAUSATIVE AGENT	LOCAL MANIFESTATIONS	MANAGEMENT	COMMENTS
Erythema Multiforme (Stevens-Johnson Syndrome)—unknown; associated with ingestion of some drugs; often follows upper respiratory infection	Erythematous papular rash Lesions enlarge by peripheral expansion; develop central vesicle Involves most skin surfaces except scalp May extend to mucous membranes, especially oral, ocular, and urethral	Symptomatic and supportive Maintain adequate fluid intake (oral or IV), calorie, and protein Cutaneous hygiene Appropriate treatment of complications Diligent monitoring of urine volume and specific gravity, hemoglobin and hematocrit, serum electrolyte levels, total body weight	Rash often preceded by fever and malaise Complications include renal failure and severe eye disease Respiratory involvement in a number of cases Self-limiting, but recovery may extend for weeks; skin lesions subside without scarring; mucous membrane lesions may persist for months Recurrence rate 20%; mortality as high as 10%
Neurofibromatosis—inherited disorder	Café-au-lait spots, pigmented nevi, axillary freckling Slow-growing cutaneous and subcutaneous neurofibromas	Symptomatic treatment of associated manifestations, e.g., speech defects, seizures, skeletal defects (scoliosis, kyphosis), learning disabilities Surgical removal of troublesome tumors	Autosomal-dominant inheritance pattern High mutation rate Refer to support groups*

National Neurofibromatosis Foundation, Inc. 95 Pine St., 16th Floor, New York, NY 10005; (800) 323-7938, (212) 460-8980.

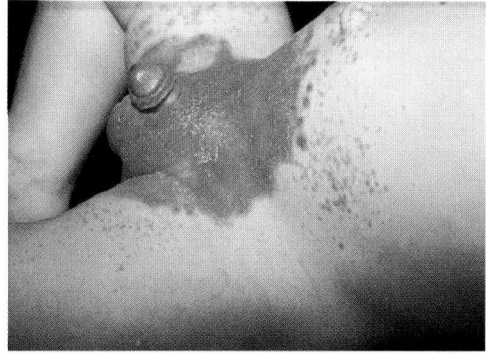

FIG. 30-12. Candidiasis of diaper area. Note beefy-red central erythema with satellite pustules. (From Weston WL, Lane AT: *Color textbook of pediatric dermatology*, St Louis, 1991, Mosby.)

Nursing Considerations

Nursing interventions are aimed at altering the three factors considered to produce dermatitis—wetness, pH, and fecal irritants. The most significant factor amenable to intervention is the moist environment created in the diaper area. Changing the diaper as soon as it becomes wet eliminates a large part of the problem, and removing the diaper to expose healthy skin to air facilitates drying.

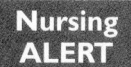 **Nursing ALERT** A heat lamp, hairdryer, or source of oxygen should not be used on very reddened or denuded skin because these interventions dry the skin and retard healing. Instead, occlusive ointments are applied to provide a moist healing environment.

Diaper construction has a significant impact on the incidence and severity of diaper dermatitis. Superabsorbent disposable paper diapers have been shown to reduce diaper dermatitis. They contain an absorbent gelling material. The gel binds water tightly to decrease skin wetness, maintains pH control by providing a buffering capacity, and decreases skin irritation by preventing mixing of urine and feces in the diaper (Wong and others, 1992).

Guidelines for controlling diaper rash are presented in the Family Home Care box on p. 1096.* A common misconception about using cornstarch on skin is that it promotes the growth of *Candida albicans*. A study comparing cornstarch and talc found that neither product supports growth of the fungi under conditions normally found in the diaper area. Cornstarch is also more effective in reducing friction and tends to cake less than talc when the skin is wet (Leyden, 1984). On

---

*Pamphlets describing the development and treatment of diaper rash are *Diaper Rash* from the American Academy of Pediatrics, 141 Northwest Point Blvd., P.O. Box 927, Elk Grove Village, IL 60007, (800) 433-9016; and *An Information Guide for Parents About Diaper Rash* from NAPNAP Diaper Rash Brochure, 718 Main St., Cincinnati, OH 45202-2137.

Keep skin dry
  Use superabsorbent disposable diapers to reduce skin wetness.
  If using cloth diapers, use only overwraps that allow air to circulate; avoid rubber pants.
  Change diapers as soon as soiled, especially with stool, whenever possible, preferably once during the night.
  Expose healthy or only slightly irritated skin to air, not heat, to dry completely.
Apply ointment, such as zinc oxide or petrolatum, to protect skin, especially if skin is very red or has moist, open areas.
  When soiled, wipe off top layer of ointment and reapply.
  To completely remove ointment, especially zinc oxide, use mineral oil; do not wash vigorously.
Avoid overwashing the skin, especially with perfumed soaps or commercial wipes that may be irritating.
  May use a moisturizer such as Derma-Life Skin Care Formula,* or nonsoap cleanser, such as cold cream or Cetaphil, to wipe urine from skin.
  Gently wipe stool from skin using water and mild soap, such as Dove.

NOTE: Powder helps keep the skin dry, but talc is very dangerous if breathed into the lungs. Plain cornstarch or cornstarch-based powder is safer. When using any powder product, shake it first into your hand, then apply it to the diaper area. Store the container away from the infant's reach; keep container closed when not in use.
*Available from Derma-Life Corp., P.O. Box 90638, Albuquerque, NM 87199; (800)658-9341.

the basis of these properties and its safety in terms of inhalation injury, cornstarch is the preferred product.

ATOPIC DERMATITIS (AD) (ECZEMA)

Eczema or eczematous inflammation of the skin refers to a descriptive category of dermatologic diseases and not to a specific etiology. AD is a type of pruritic eczema that usually begins during infancy and is associated with allergy with a hereditary tendency *(atopy)*. AD presents in three forms based on the age of the child and the distribution of lesions:

1. **Infantile (infantile eczema)**—usually begins at 2 to 6 months of age and generally undergoes spontaneous remission by 3 years of age.
2. **Childhood**—may follow the infantile form; it occurs at 2 to 3 years of age, and 90% of the children will manifest the disease by the age 5 years.
3. **Preadolescent and adolescent**—begins at about 12 years of age and may continue into the early adult years or indefinitely.

The diagnosis of AD is based on a combination of history and morphologic findings (see box). Children with the disease have a lower threshold for cutaneous itching, and many authorities believe the dermatologic manifestations appear subsequent to scratching of the intense pruritus. For example, infants will rub their faces against bed linen, and crawling (a form of scratching) results in irritation of knees and elbows. Lesions will disappear if the scratching is stopped.

The majority of children with infantile AD have a family history of eczema, asthma, or allergic rhinitis, which strongly supports a genetic predisposition. The cause is unknown but appears to be related to abnormal function of the skin, in-

---

CLINICAL MANIFESTATIONS OF ATOPIC DERMATITIS

Distribution of Lesions
Infantile form—generalized, especially cheeks, scalp, trunk, and extensor surfaces of extremities (Fig. 30-13)
Childhood form—flexural areas (antecubital and popliteal fossae, neck), wrists, ankles, and feet
Preadolescent and adolescent form—face, sides of neck, hands, feet, face, and antecubital and popliteal fossae (to a lesser extent)

Appearance of Lesions
Infantile form
  Erythema
  Vesicles
  Papules
  Weeping
  Oozing
  Crusting
  Scaling
  Often symmetric
Childhood form
  Symmetric involvement
  Clusters of small erythematous or flesh-colored papules or minimally scaling patches
  Dry and may be hyperpigmented
  Lichenification (thickened skin with accentuation of creases)
  Keratosis pilaris (follicular hyperkeratosis) common
Adolescent/adult form
  Same as childhood manifestations
  Dry, thick lesions (lichenified plaques) common
  Confluent papules

Other Physical Manifestations
Intense itching
Unaffected skin dry and rough
Black children likely to exhibit more papular and/or follicular lesions than white children
May exhibit one or more of the following:
  Lymphadenopathy, especially near affected sites
  Increased palmar creases (many cases)
  Atopic pleats (extra line or groove of lower eyelid)
  Prone to cold hands
  Pityriasis alba (small, poorly defined areas of hypopigmentation)
  Facial pallor (especially around nose, mouth, and ears)
  Bluish discoloration beneath eyes ("allergic shiners")
  Increased susceptibility to unusual cutaneous infections (especially viral)

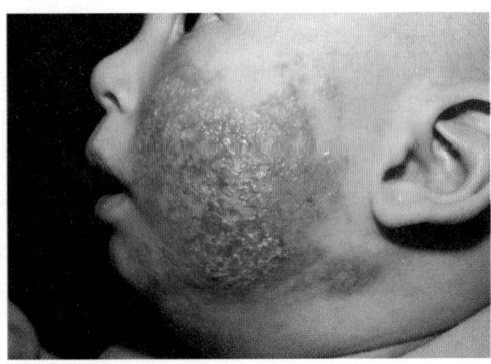

FIG. 30-13. Infantile atopic dermatitis with oozing and crusting of lesions. (From Weston WL, Lane AT: *Color textbook of pediatric dermatology,* St Louis, 1991, Mosby.)

GUIDELINES
Preventing Atopy in Children

Identify Children at Risk
Family history of allergy
Increased IgE in cord blood and postnatal serum

Prenatal Precautions (Last Trimester)
Avoid any known food allergens
Avoid milk and other dairy products, peanuts, and eggs
Minimize ingestion of other hyperallergenic foods

Postnatal Precautions
Breast milk or casein/whey hydrolysate formula (e.g., Nutramigen, Pregestimil, Alimentum) exclusively for at least 6 months
No solid food for 6 months
No cow's milk or soy formula for 12 months
No egg, fish, corn, citrus, peanuts, nuts, or chocolate for 12 months
One new food added at 5-day intervals to identify possible reaction

Environmental Control
Limited exposure to dust, molds, animals, and cigarette smoke

Data from Johnstone D: Strategy for intervention of food allergy in infants, *Int Pediatr* 4(4):319-325, 1989; and Zeiger R and others: Effectiveness of dietary manipulation in the prevention of food allergy in infants, part 2, *J Allergy Clin Immunol* 78(1, pt 2):224-238, 1986.

NURSING DIAGNOSES: THE CHILD WITH ATOPIC DERMATITIS

Impaired skin integrity related to eczematous lesions
High risk for infection related to risk of secondary infection of primary lesions
Altered family processes related to child's discomfort and lengthy therapy

---

cluding alterations in sweating, peripheral vascular function, and heat tolerance. The symptoms are better in humid climates and worse in fall and winter, when homes are heated and environmental humidity is lower. The disorder can be controlled but not cured.

Therapeutic Management

The major goals of management are to (1) relieve pruritus, (2) hydrate the skin, (3) reduce inflammation, and (4) prevent or control secondary infection. Most of the general measures for managing AD serve to reduce pruritus as well as other aspects of the disease. General management includes avoiding exposure to skin irritants, avoiding overheating, improving skin hydration, and administration of medications such as antihistamines, topical steroids, and (sometimes) mild sedatives as indicated.

Differing philosophies regarding cleansing and hydrating the skin of the child with AD generally embrace two methods—the wet and the dry methods. In the *dry method* baths are infrequent, and skin is cleansed with a nonlipid, hydrophilic agent such as Cetaphil. The *wet method* consists of frequent baths (up to four times per day) followed immediately by the application of a lubricant (while the skin is still damp) to trap moisture in the skin. No soap or a very mild, nonperfumed soap (such as Dove, Lowila, or Neutrogena) is used. Some advocate oil or oilated oatmeal baths with light drying so that a protective, oily film remains on the skin. Showers are acceptable as long as a moisturizer is applied within 3 minutes to prevent drying and damaging the skin (Hanifin, 1991).

Enhancing skin hydration can be accomplished by application of preparations that occlude the skin to prevent evaporation and retain moisture in the upper skin layers and/or by replacement of natural moisturizing substances in the skin. A variety of emollients containing petrolatum or lanolin have occlusive properties and are prescribed according to the degree of occlusion desired. For the majority of patients lotions applied twice or three times daily maintain satisfactory hydration. The frequency may be increased if greater hydration is required. Creams or ointments provide more occlusion, and those that contain urea or lactic acid improve the binding of water in the skin and prevent evaporation of moisture.

Sometimes colloid baths, such as the addition of 2 cups of cornstarch to a tub of warm water, provide temporary relief of itching and may help the child sleep if given before bedtime. Cool wet compresses are soothing to the skin and provide antiseptic protection.

Moderate or severe pruritus is usually relieved by administration of oral antihistamine drugs (hydroxyzine [Atarax] or diphenhydramine [Benadryl]); the amount is tailored to the individual child. Since pruritus increases at night, a mild sedative may be needed.

Occasional flare-ups require the use of topical steroids to diminish inflammation. Low-, moderate-, or high-potency topical corticosteroids are prescribed, depending on the degree of involvement, the area of the body to be treated, the age of the child, and the type of vehicle to be used (e.g., cream, lotion, ointment). Secondary infection is managed with appropriate antibiotic therapy. The prevention of AD by limiting the fetus' and child's exposure to allergens is controversial. However, the precautions in the Guidelines box may be recommended.

Prognosis.   The majority of affected children (90%) "outgrow" AD by adolescence. Some continue to have chronic AD in adulthood.

Nursing Considerations

❖ Assessment

Assessment of the child with AD includes a family history for evidence of atopy, a history of previous involvement, and any environmental or dietary factors associated with the present and previous exacerbations. The skin lesions are examined for type, distribution, and evidence of secondary infection. The parents are interviewed regarding the child's behavior, especially in relation to the child's scratching, irritability, and sleeping patterns. The interview should also include exploration of the family's feelings and methods of coping with the situation.

❖ Nursing Diagnoses

A number of nursing diagnoses identified for the child with AD are outlined in the accompanying box. Others will be apparent in individual cases.

❖ **Planning**

The objectives for nursing care of the child with AD and family are as follows:

1. Child will experience no or minimal pruritus.
2. Child will receive appropriate treatment for skin hydration.
3. Child will experience no complications.
4. Child and family will receive adequate support.

❖ **Implementation**

The child with AD presents a nursing challenge. Controlling the intense pruritus is imperative if the disorder is to be successfully managed, since scratching leads to the formation of new lesions and may cause secondary infection. In addition to the medical regimen, other measures can be taken to prevent or minimize the scratching. Fingernails and toenails are cut short, kept clean, and filed frequently to prevent sharp edges. Gloves or cotton stockings may have to be placed over the hands and pinned to shirtsleeves. To prevent any contact with the skin, elbow restraints are sometimes necessary. One-piece outfits with long sleeves and long pants also decrease direct contact with the skin. Whether gloves or restraints are used, the child needs time to be free from such restrictions. An excellent time to remove any protective devices is during the bath or after receiving sedative or antipruritic medication.

> **Nursing ALERT**
> Do not remove elbow restraints during sleep because of the likelihood that the child will scratch while asleep.

Conditions that increase itching are eliminated when possible. Woolen clothes or blankets, rough fabrics, and furry stuffed animals should be removed. Since heat and humidity cause perspiration, which intensifies the itching, proper dress for climatic conditions is essential. Pruritus is often precipitated by exposure to the irritant effects of certain components of common products such as soaps, detergents, fabric softeners, perfumes, and powders. Most children experience less itching when soft cotton fabrics are worn next to the skin. During cold months, synthetic fabrics (not wool) should be used for overcoats, hats, gloves, and snowsuits.

Clothes and sheets are laundered in a mild detergent and rinsed thoroughly in clear water (without fabric softeners and antistatic chemicals). Putting the clothes through a second complete wash cycle without using detergent reduces the amount of residue remaining in the fabric.

Preventing infection is usually secondary to preventing scratching. Personal hygiene is accomplished as described previously. Baths are given as prescribed, the water kept tepid, and soaps (except as indicated) and bubble baths are avoided, as well as the use of oils or powders. Skinfolds and diaper areas need frequent cleansing with plain water.

A room humidifier or vaporizer may benefit children with extremely dry skin.

> **Nursing ALERT**
> If the child is being treated with frequent baths for hydration, it is imperative that the emollient preparation be applied immediately following bathing (while the skin is still slightly moist) to prevent drying.

Soaks and compresses are applied and medications for pruritus or infection are administered as directed. The family is given explicit instructions on the preparation and use of soaks, special baths, and topical medications, including the order of application if more than one is prescribed. If children have difficulty remaining still for a 10- or 15-minute soak, bath, or dressing application, these can be carried out at naptime or when the child is engrossed in television, a story, or playing with tub toys.

Since adequate rest is also important for these children, who are usually fretful and irritable, planning meals, baths, medications, and treatments during awake periods is paramount. Sleepy, tired children are normally cranky, and such behavior only intensifies the urge to scratch. During periods of irritability, these children tend to have a poor appetite, which is worsened by restriction of their usual foods.

Diet modification is another source of frustration to parents. When a hypoallergenic diet is prescribed, parents need help in understanding the reason for the diet and guidelines for following it. Since hypoallergenic diets take time before visible effects are apparent, parents need reassurance that results may not be seen immediately.

Family Support. Parents can be assured that the lesions will not produce scarring (unless secondarily infected) and that the disease is not contagious. However, the child will be subject to repeated exacerbations and remissions.

During periods of acute exacerbation the emotional stress can become intense for the family. They need time to discuss negative feelings and to be reassured that these feelings are normal and acceptable. During acute phases, relieving as much anxiety as possible in both parents and child has a beneficial emotional and physical effect, since stress tends to aggravate the severity of the condition.

❖ **Evaluation**

The effectiveness of nursing interventions is determined by continual reassessment and evaluation of care based on the following observational guidelines and expected outcomes:

1. Observe child's behavior, clothing, and activities.
2. Examine skin for evidence of dryness.
3. Examine skin lesions for evidence of secondary infection.
4. Interview aspects of family and encourage dialogue regarding the child and aspects of care.

Expected outcomes:

1. Child does not scratch and rests or plays quietly.
2. Skin appears well hydrated.
3. There is no evidence of secondary infection.
4. Family members comply with the therapeutic regimen, freely discuss their feelings and concerns, and appear to be coping with the inconveniences imposed by the disorder (specify).

See also Nursing Care Plan: The Child with Atopic Dermatitis (Eczema).*

SEBORRHEIC DERMATITIS

Seborrheic dermatitis is a chronic, recurrent, inflammatory reaction of the skin. It occurs most commonly on the scalp (cradle cap) but may involve the eyelids (blepharitis), exter-

*In Wong DL: *Wong and Whaley's Clinical manual of pediatric nursing,* ed 4, St Louis, 1996, Mosby.

nal ear canal (otitis externa), nasolabial folds, and inguinal region. The cause is unknown, although it is more common in early infancy, when sebum production is increased. The lesions are characteristically thick, adherent, yellowish, scaly, oily patches that may or may not be mildly pruritic. Unlike atopic dermatitis, seborrheic dermatitis is not associated with a positive family history for allergy and is very common in infants shortly after birth and after puberty. Diagnosis is made primarily by the appearance and location of the crusts or scales.

Nursing Considerations

Cradle cap may be prevented with adequate scalp hygiene. Not infrequently, parents omit shampooing the infant's hair for fear of damaging the "soft spots," or fontanels. It is important to discuss how to shampoo the infant's hair and to emphasize that the fontanel is like skin anywhere else on the body—it does not puncture or tear with mild pressure.

When seborrheic lesions are present, the treatment is mainly directed at removing the crusts. Parents are taught the appropriate procedure to clean the scalp, which may require a demonstration. Shampooing should be done daily with a mild soap or commercial baby shampoo; medicated shampoos are not necessary but an antiseborrheic shampoo containing sulfur and salicylic acid may be used (Hurwitz, 1993). Shampoo is applied to the scalp and allowed to penetrate and soften the crusts, and then the scalp is thoroughly rinsed. Using a fine-tooth comb or a soft facial brush after shampooing helps remove the loosened crusts from the strands of hair.

ACNE

There is one skin disorder that although not limited to the adolescent age-group, appears predominantly at this time— *acne vulgaris.* Acne is an almost universal occurrence during these years and involves anatomic, physiologic, biochemical, genetic, immunologic, and psychologic factors of significant import.

It is estimated that about 85% of the population will have had acne by the end of the teenage years. Although the disorder can appear before this time, the peak incidence is in late adolescence, at about age 16 to 17 in girls and 17 to 18 years in boys. It is more common in males than in females. The degree to which an individual is affected may range from nothing more than a few isolated comedones to a severe inflammatory reaction. Although the disease is self-limited and not life-threatening, its significance to the adolescent is great, and it is a mistake to underestimate the impact it can have on young persons.

The etiology of acne is still unclear, although a number of factors appear to be related to its development. Its distribution in families and a high degree of concordance in identical twins suggest that hereditary factors predispose to susceptibility to acne. Androgens are implicated, and the disorder seems to be aggravated by emotional stress, a hot, humid environment, and the premenstrual period in females. There is no positive evidence that any specific foods are factors, except perhaps on an individual basis.

Pathophysiology

Acne is a disease that involves the *pilosebaceous follicles* (the hair follicle and sebaceous gland complex) of the face, neck,

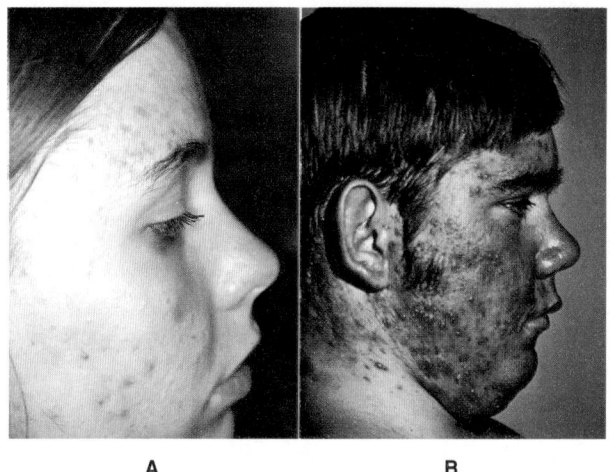

FIG. 30-14. Acne vulgaris. **A,** Comedones with a few inflammatory pustules. **B,** Papulopustular acne. (From Weston WL, Lane AT: *Color textbook of pediatric dermatology,* St Louis, 1991, Mosby.)

shoulders, back, and upper chest—the so-called flush areas of the skin. There are two basic types of lesions seen in acne (Fig. 30-14):

1. *Noninflamed lesions,* called *comedones,* consisting of compact masses of keratin, lipids, fatty acids, and bacteria that dilate the follicular duct, which may be plugged, *closed comedones,* or whiteheads, with no visible opening) or *open comedones,* or blackheads, with visible dilated openings that are discolored as fatty acids are oxidized by air
2. *Inflamed lesions,* which result when the follicular wall ruptures to produce papules, pustules, nodules, and cysts; responsible for the destructiveness and propensity for scarring

A normally harmless bacterium, *Propionibacterium acnes (P. acnes),* is present in larger amounts in persons with acne. Polymorphonuclear leukocytes enter the sebaceous follicle to ingest the bacteria. Hydrolytic enzymes and free fatty acids are released as a byproduct. These fatty acids are the major tissue irritants in the sebum and initiate the inflammatory response.

Adolescents' concern about their appearance tempts them to pick, finger, squeeze, and otherwise manipulate the lesions; this plays an important role in the perpetuation of acne and possible secondary infection. In addition to the precipitating factors mentioned previously, the application of creams and oils, including some suntanning and sunscreen preparations, and some heavy make-up bases that add to the plugging of the follicles may aggravate acne.

Therapeutic Management

There is little evidence that treatment shortens the duration of the entire course of the disease. However, treatment can bolster self-esteem and prevent unnecessary scarring. No single therapeutic agent is effective in the management of acne, except in a few mild cases. It is usually more effective to use a combination of therapies. The treatment most commonly consists of measures directed toward improving the general health of the person, removing comedones, preventing their formation, controlling excessive sebaceous gland activity, controlling infection, and preventing scar formation.

General Measures. Improvement of the adolescent's overall health status is part of the general management. Adequate rest, moderate exercise, a well-balanced diet, reduction of emotional stress, and elimination of any foci of infection are all part of general health promotion. There is no convincing evidence to implicate any single dietary item or combination of foods in the exacerbation of acne. Occasionally a youngster will demonstrate an aggravation of symptoms after each ingestion of a given food. In such instances the food is eliminated for a period of time to assess its influence on the condition.

Medication. There is a wide range of types and combinations of topical agents for the treatment of acne, with selection depending on the type and severity of the lesions. *Tretinoin (retinoic acid, Retin-A)* is the only drug that effectively interrupts the abnormal follicular keratinization that produces microcomedones, precursors of visible comedones. It takes at least 2 to 3 months for significant improvement to be apparent. *Topical* tretinoin is not associated with increased risk of birth defects. Topical *benzoyl peroxide* kills *P. acnes* organisms. The most effective therapy involves the use of benzoyl peroxide, tretinoin, or a combination of these.

Both agents can cause redness and peeling early in their use; therefore the treatment usually begins with graded increases in concentration and/or frequency of application according to the patient's tolerance. Because of these effects, adolescents may be tempted to discontinue their use. The two drugs should not be applied together because the benzoyl peroxide may oxidize the retinoic acid and render it impotent.

NURSING TIP The adolescent can be advised that side effects may be minimized by delaying application of medication until the skin is completely dry (20 to 30 minutes after cleansing).

Systemic antibiotic therapy may be needed for some patients who do not respond to topical therapy. *Isotretinoin, 13-cis retinoic acid (Accutane),* a very potent and effective oral agent, is reserved for severe cystic acne. Since the drug is teratogenic and therefore unsuitable for pregnant women, practitioners must follow strict guidelines when prescribing the drug for female patients. Before treatment, identify whether or not the teen is sexually active. The drug should be given only if he or she uses an effective form of contraception during treatment and has received oral and written warning of the reproductive hazards of the drug (American Academy of Pediatrics, 1992).

Cleansing. Gentle cleansing with a mild cleanser once or twice daily is usually sufficient. Antibacterial soaps are ineffective and may be too drying in combination with topical acne medications. For some adolescents hygiene of the hair and scalp appears to be related to the clinical activity of the acne. In these persons acne of the forehead can be improved by brushing the hair away from the forehead and shampooing more frequently.

Prognosis. Acne will resolve spontaneously over a variable amount of time, depending on the individual.

Nursing Considerations

Because acne is so common and its appearance may seem so mild, the health care provider may underestimate the relative importance of this phenomenon to the adolescent. The nurse should assess the individual adolescent's level of distress, current management, and perceived success of any regimen before initiating a referral. If adolescents do not perceive the acne to be a problem, they will not be motivated to follow the daily routine necessary to treat the acne.

Teenagers need a supportive, caring individual to help them maintain the persistence required to deal with the disorder over such an extended period of time. The adolescent needs education regarding the disease process and instruction in the prescribed therapy. Instruction should be definite and as specific as practical for each individual youngster. A written instruction sheet that describes the etiology and therapeutic regimen is often helpful, and parents should be cautioned against nagging. Adolescents should assume responsibility for following through on the instructions. They are cautioned against damaging the skin through too vigorous scrubbing. Several points are emphasized as particularly important: using only those preparations prescribed for their particular needs; carrying out associated directions, such as hairstyling and shampooing and not leaving cosmetics on the face overnight. Teenagers are subject to the influence of commercial advertising from a variety of media. Washing with a mild, nonabrasive cleanser, such as Dove (unscented), is adequate for cleansing. Most cosmetics do not cause acne, and contrary to once-popular belief, it does not make a difference

---

CRITICAL THINKING EXERCISE
Acne

Kim, who is 16 years old, recently started "breaking out." During her visit to the dermatologist, she was diagnosed as having a mild form of acne and was told to cleanse her face twice a day and apply Retin-A and benzoyl peroxide daily. Which instructions describe the correct skin care schedule?

1. Use a mild facial scrub in the morning and apply the Retin-A; at night use an astringent to remove makeup and apply benzoyl peroxide.
2. Wash the face with soap in the morning and at night; wait 30 minutes after the night cleansing to apply Retin-A, followed by benzoyl peroxide.
3. Wash the face with soap in the morning and apply benzoyl peroxide; wash the face before bedtime and apply Retin-A.
4. Wash the face with soap in the morning and apply benzoyl peroxide; wash the face in the evening and apply Retin-A about 30 minutes later.

The correct answer is four. The most important aspects of the skin care regimen are to apply the topical preparation at different times of the day, because they are less effective when applied close together. Also, the face should be completely dry before applying Retin-A to reduce skin irritation. Although either preparation can be used first, it is preferable to suggest applying Retin-A at night, when the teenager has time to wait after cleansing the skin. Facial scrubs and astringents are not used, because they increase skin dryness.

if a cosmetic is oil-free or not (Bikowski, 1992). Cosmetics that do not cause acne are labeled *noncomedogenic.*

Certain acne preparations, such as retinoic acid and tetracycline, can cause photosensitivity. Adolescents should be advised to apply the medication at night and use a sunscreen with a sun protective factor (SPF) of at least 15 in the daytime. Other measures that minimize sun exposure, such as wearing a tightly woven, wide-brimmed hat or sun visor, are encouraged. Teenagers should be advised not to expect any visible improvement for 4 to 6 weeks after initiation of therapy. Acne may appear to worsen initially. Medications often cause erythema, peeling, itching, burning, and drying when first applied. The use of comedone extractors to remove blackheads is not recommended because this procedure can cause increased scarring. Females taking oral contraceptive pills and oral antibiotics should be instructed to use an additional form of contraception.

During conversations with teenagers the nurse can dispel the common myths often associated with acne and allow youngsters to discuss any feelings related to the disorder, such as self-consciousness or anxieties regarding relationships with others. Sometimes the nurse also can help teenagers explore job or other after-school interests. The acne lesions need not become an excuse to avoid social contacts and activities. (See Critical Thinking Exercise.)

THERMAL INJURY

BURNS

Minor burn injuries are experienced by everyone in day-to-day living and are relatively commonplace in nursing practice. Extensive burns, on the other hand, are relatively uncommon; however, they account for some of the most difficult nursing problems encountered in the pediatric age-group. Serious burn injury accounts for a very large number of children who must undergo prolonged, painful, and restrictive hospitalization. The following discussion of burns focuses on the burn wound; burn prevention is discussed in Chapters 10, 12, 15, and 16.

 When burns are characterized by patients' age and type of injury, the following pattern arises (Adams, Hunt, and Purdue, 1991): (1) toddlers sustain hot water scalds most frequently, and older children are most likely to have received flame-related burns; (2) 10% of all pediatric admissions can be attributed to child abuse; and (3) the most frequent mode of injury is by submersion in hot water.

Burns are caused by thermal, chemical, electrical, or, rarely, radioactive agents. Thermal injuries are the most common, followed by chemical and electrical, respectively.

The extent of tissue destruction is determined by considering the intensity of the heat source, duration of contact or exposure, conductivity of the tissue involved, and the rate at which the heat energy is dissipated by the skin. A brief exposure to high-intensity heat from a flame can produce burn injuries similar to those induced by long exposure to less intense heat in hot water.

Chemical burns can be serious injuries, but with effective emergency treatment the extent of the injury can be minimized. Chemical agents continue to cauterize the tissues until treated.

Electrical burns can be deceptive because although cutaneous injury may be minimal, most of the damage can lie beneath the skin in the tissues of muscle and bone that cannot be seen and initially may be hard to diagnose. Electrical burns are often full-thickness burns involving the muscle and bone (fourth-degree burns). Extremities can become mummified with black, charred eschar present.

Characteristics of Burn Injury

The physiologic responses, therapy, prognosis, and disposition of the injured child are all directly related to the *amount of tissue destroyed;* therefore the severity of the burn injury is assessed on the basis of the percentage of surface burned and the depth of the burn. Also important in determining the seriousness of the injury are the location of the wounds, the age of the child, the causative agent, the presence of respiratory involvement, the general health of the child, and the presence of any associated injury or condition.

Extent of Injury. The extent of a burn is expressed as a percentage of *total body surface area (TBSA).* This is most accurately estimated by using specially designed age-related charts (Fig. 30-15). It is generally more efficient to use any of a variety of charts designed to assign body proportions to children of different ages.

Depth of Injury. A thermal injury is a three-dimensional wound and therefore is also assessed in relation to depth of injury. Traditionally the terms first-, second-, and third-degree have been used to describe the depth of tissue injury. However, with the current emphasis on wound healing, these are gradually being replaced by more descriptive terms based on the extent of destruction to the epithelializing elements of the skin (Fig. 30-16).

Superficial (first-degree) burns are usually of minor significance. There is frequently a latent period followed by erythema. Tissue damage is minimal, protective functions remain intact, and systemic effects are rare. Pain is the predominant symptom, and the burn will heal without scarring in 5 to 10 days.

Partial thickness (second-degree) injuries involve the epidermis and varying degrees of the dermis. These wounds are painful, moist, red, and blistered. *Superficial partial thickness burns* involve the epidermis and part of the dermis. Dermal elements are left intact, and the wound should heal in approximately 14 days with variable amounts of scarring (Fig. 30-17). *Deep dermal burns,* although classified as second-degree or partial-thickness burns, in many respects resemble full-thickness injuries (Fig. 30-18). The difference is that sweat glands and hair follicles are left intact. Although these wounds can heal spontaneously in about 30 days with variable amounts of scarring, they can convert into a full-thickness burn if they become infected.

Full-thickness (third-degree) burns are serious injuries in which all layers of the skin, epidermis and dermis, are destroyed, and the underlying subcutaneous tissue is affected (see Fig. 30-18). Burns extending into the fascia, muscle, and bone are sometimes referred to as *fourth-degree burns* (Fig. 30-19). A full-thickness burn requires surgical excision of burn eschar and grafting to obtain a permanent coverage for the wound. Less scarring occurs with a full-thickness burn

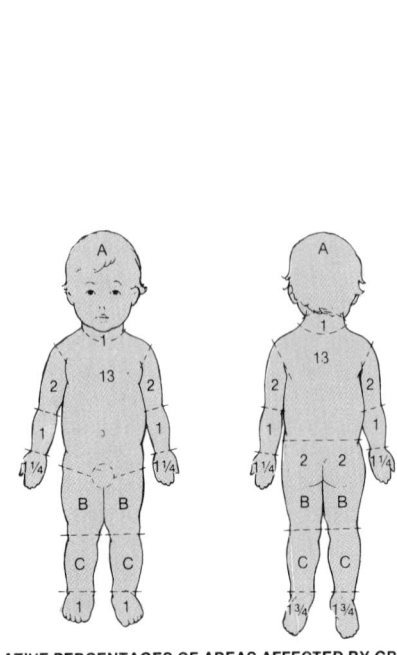
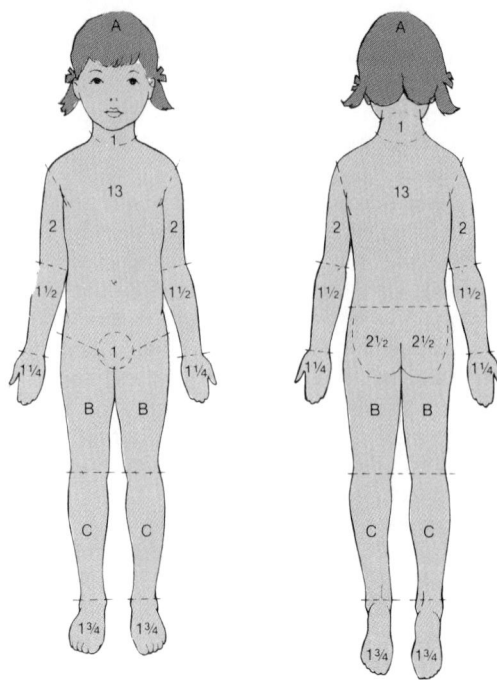

RELATIVE PERCENTAGES OF AREAS AFFECTED BY GROWTH			
AREA	BIRTH	AGE 1 YR	AGE 5 YR
A = ½ of head	9½	8½	6½
B = ½ of one thigh	2¾	3¼	4
C = ½ of one leg	2½	2½	2¾

A

RELATIVE PERCENTAGES OF AREAS AFFECTED BY GROWTH			
AREA	AGE 10 YR	AGE 15 YR	ADULT
A = ½ of head	5½	4½	3½
B = ½ of one thigh	4½	4½	4¾
C = ½ of one leg	3	3¼	3½

B

FIG. 30-15. Estimation of distribution of burns in children. **A,** Children from birth to age 5 years. **B,** Older children.

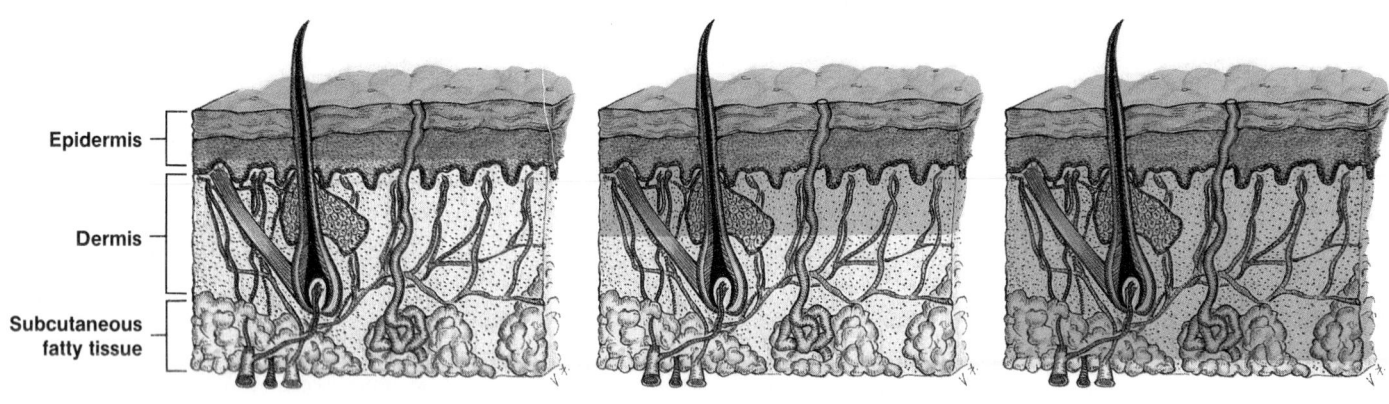

Epidermis

Dermis

Subcutaneous fatty tissue

	Superficial (first degree)	**Partial-thickness (second degree)**	**Full-thickness (third degree)**
Type of burn	Sunburn; low-intensity flash; brief scald	Scalds; flash flame	Fire; contact with hot objects
Appearance	Dry surface; red; blanches on pressure and refills	Blistered; moist; mottled pink or red, reddened; blanches on pressure and refills	Tough, leathery; brown, tan, black, or red; does not blanch on pressure; dull, dry
Sensation	Painful	Very painful	Variable pain, often severe

FIG. 30-16. Classification of burn depth. Blue screen indicates depth of burn. (Modified from Potter PA, Perry AG: *Basic nursing: theory and practice,* ed 2, St Louis, 1991, Mosby.)

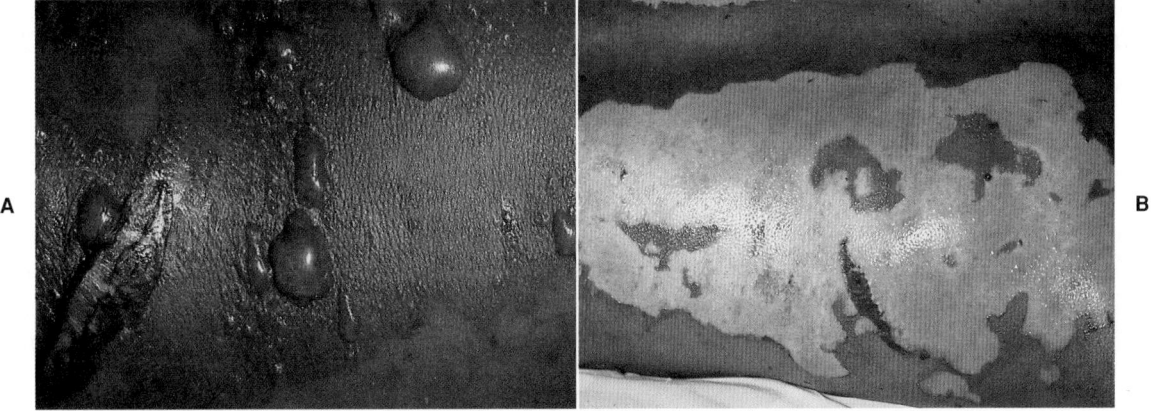

FIG. 30-17. Superficial partial-thickness burns on black child. **A,** Blisters intact. **B,** Blisters removed. (Courtesy of Hillcrest Medical Center, Tulsa, OK.)

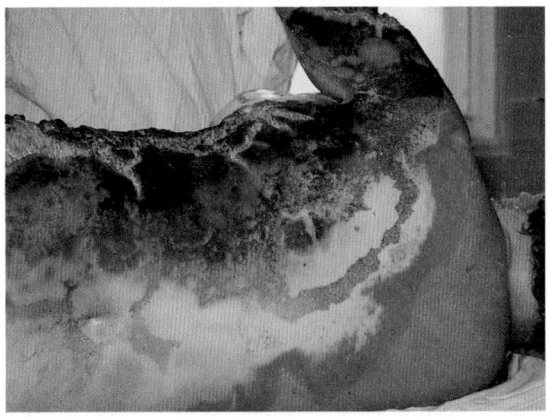

FIG. 30-18. *From bottom to top:* Deep partial-thickness burn *(red area);* full-thickness burn *(white area);* full-thickness burn with eschar *(brown area).* (Courtesy Hillcrest Medical Center, Tulsa, OK.)

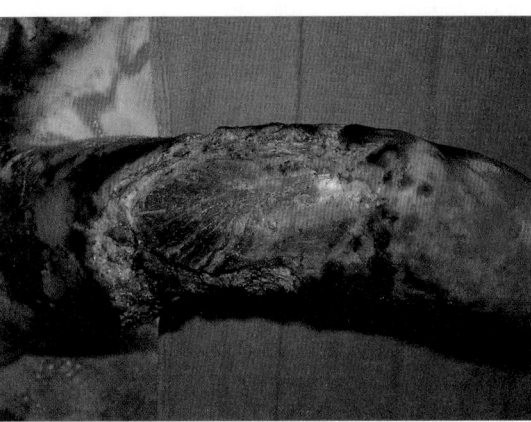

FIG. 30-19. Full-thickness burn with muscle and fascia involved. (Courtesy Hillcrest Medical Center, Tulsa, OK.)

that has had surgical excision of the eschar and grafting than in a deep partial-thickness burn allowed to heal spontaneously.

Theoretically, with a full-thickness burn the nerve endings have been destroyed, and no pain should be associated with this type injury. However, most full-thickness burns occur with superficial and partial-thickness burns in which nerve endings are intact and exposed. Also, excised eschar and donor sites cause exposed nerve fibers. Finally, as peripheral fibers regenerate, painful sensation returns. Consequently, children often experience severe pain that is related to the size and depth of the burn (Atchison and others, 1991). Even when nerve endings are destroyed, children may develop phantom skin pain.

Severity of Injury. Burns are also assessed on the basis of their severity, which is useful in determining the disposition and management of the patient. Burned patients can usually be distinguished as (1) those with a major burn in-

jury, who require the services and equipment of a special burn unit, (2) those with moderate burns, who may be treated in any hospital unit, and (3) those with minor burns, who are able to be treated on an outpatient basis. (See grading system for burn severity in Table 30-10). Because infants' skin is so thin, it is likely to sustain deeper injuries. Children younger than 2 years of age, especially 6 months or younger, have a significantly higher mortality rate than older children with burns of similar magnitude. Acute or chronic illnesses or superimposed injuries also complicate burn care and response to treatment.

Other Factors. Regardless of the amount of tissue destroyed, if inhalation injury is suspected there is risk of airway obstruction. There are two classifications of airway injury: upper airway and lower airway. A patient can have upper airway injury, lower airway injury, or both. Facial edema may endanger the upper airway.

Lower airway injury to the lungs is not the result of direct thermal injury, because the upper airway has the capa-

TABLE 30-10. Severity grading system adopted by the American Burn Association			
	MINOR*	MODERATE	MAJOR
Partial-thickness burns	<10% of TBSA	10%-20% of TBSA	>20% of TBSA
Full-thickness burns			All
Treatment	Usually outpatient; may require 1-2 day admission	Admission to hospital, preferably one with expertise in burn care	Admission to a burn center

From Vaccaro P, Trofino RB: Care of the patient with minor to moderate burns. In Trofino RB, editor: *Nursing care of the burn-injured patient,* Philadelphia, 1991, FA Davis.
*Minor burns exclude any burn involving the face, hands, feet, perineum, or crossing joints; electrical burns; any injury complicated by the presence of inhalation injury or concomitant trauma; children with psychosocial factors impacting the injury.

bility of cooling the heated air before it reaches the lung. Steam is the exception to this rule. Damage to the lung may also be caused by a bronchoscopy.

Pathophysiology

Thermal injuries produce both local and systemic effects that are directly related to the extent of tissue destruction. In superficial burns the tissue damage is minimal. In partial-thickness burns there is considerable edema and more severe capillary damage. With a major burn greater than 30% of TBSA, there is a systemic response involving an increase in capillary permeability, allowing plasma proteins, fluids, and electrolytes to be lost. Maximum edema formation in a small wound occurs about 8 to 12 hours after injury. After a larger injury, hypovolemia, associated with this phenomenon, will slow the rate of edema formation, with maximum effect at 18 to 24 hours.

Another systemic response is anemia, caused by direct heat destruction of red blood cells, hemolysis of injured red cells, and trapping of red cells in the microvascular thrombi of damaged cells. A long-term decrease in the number of red blood cells may result in diminished red blood cell life span. Initially there is an increased blood flow to the heart, brain, and kidneys, with decreased blood flow to the gastrointestinal tract. There is an increase in metabolism to maintain body heat, providing for the increased energy needs of the body.

Complications. Thermally injured children are subject to a number of serious complications, both from the wound and from systemic alterations resulting from the injury. The immediate threat to life is related to airway compromise and profound shock. A less apparent respiratory injury is inhalation of carbon monoxide. Carbon monoxide has a greater affinity for hemoglobin than does oxygen, thereby depriving peripheral tissues and oxygen-dependent organs (such as the heart and brain) of the oxygen needed for survival. Treatment for either of these two problems is 100% oxygen, which reverses the situation rapidly. The child must also be observed for signs of local and generalized sepsis complications.

Pulmonary problems persist as a major cause of fatality in children with either thermal burns or injuries/complications in the respiratory tract. A full range of respiratory insufficiency can occur, including inhalation injuries, aspiration in unconscious patients, bacterial pneumonia, pulmonary ed-

ema, pulmonary embolus, and posttraumatic pulmonary insufficiency. The most common causative factor in respiratory failure in the pediatric age-group is bacterial pneumonia, which requires prolonged intubation and sometimes necessitates a tracheostomy. Because tracheostomies increase the incidence of serious complications, including pneumonia, they are only performed in extreme cases.

Sepsis is the most critical problem in treatment of burns, and it is an ever-present threat after the shock phase. Initially burns are relatively pathogen free, unless the wound is contaminated with potentially infectious material, such as dirt or polluted water. However, dead tissue and exudate provide a fertile field for bacterial growth. Early colonization of the wound surface by a preponderance of gram-positive organisms (primarily staphylococci) changes on about the third postburn day to predominantly gram-negative organisms, particularly *Pseudomonas aeruginosa.* By the fifth postburn day the bacterial invasion is well under way beneath the surface of the wound. Early surgical excision of eschar along with placement of autograft has reduced the incidence of sepsis today.

Superficial mucosal erosion, *Curling ulcers,* that cause recurrent or intermittent gastrointestinal bleeding can be a major complication of burns. Prophylactic administration of antacids, histamine H_2-antagonists, or sucralfate, as well as the early initiation of enteral support, usually prevents the development of serious bleeding.

Therapeutic Management: Emergency Care

The first priority is to stop the burning process (see Emergency Treatment box). The child should then be transported immediately to the nearest medical facility for definitive treatment and evaluation for transfer to a burn center. The child and the family will be extremely frightened and anxious; sensitivity to their emotional state will provide reassurance during the transport process.

Stop the Burning Process. The chief aim of rescue in flame burns is to smother the fire, not fan it. Children tend to panic and run, which only serves to spread the flames and make assistance more difficult. The injured child should be placed in a horizontal position and rolled in a blanket, rug, or similar article, with care taken not to cover the head and face because of the danger of the inhalation of toxic fumes. If nothing is available, the victim should lie down and roll over slowly to extinguish the flames. Remaining in the vertical position may cause the hair to ignite or the inhalation of flames, heat, or smoke.

Major burns with large amounts of denuded skin should not be cooled. Heat is rapidly lost from burned areas, and additional cooling leads to a drop in core body temperature and potential circulatory collapse. Wet dressings also promote vasoconstriction because of cooling, resulting in impaired circulation to the burned area and increased tissue damage. Chemical burns present special circumstances and require continuous flushing with large amounts of water during transport to a medical facility. The use of neutralizing agents on the skin is contraindicated, since a chemical reaction is initiated and further injury may result. If the chemical is in powder form, the addition of water may spread the caustic agent. The powder should be brushed off if possible.

Burned clothing is removed to prevent further damage from smoldering fabric and hot beads of melted synthetic materials. Any jewelry is also removed to eliminate the transfer of heat from the metal and the constriction resulting from edema formation. This also provides better access to the wound and precludes more painful removal later on.

Assess the Victim's Condition. As soon as the flames are extinguished, the condition of the victim is assessed. Airway, breathing, and circulation are the priority concerns. Cardiopulmonary and cerebral emergencies are always a consideration following trauma. Cardiopulmonary complications may result from exposure to electric current, inhalation of toxic fumes and smoke, hypovolemia, and shock. Emergency measures are instituted as appropriate.

Cover the Burn. The burn wound should be covered with a clean cloth to prevent contamination and decrease pain by eliminating air contact. The child with extensive burns is covered to prevent hypothermia. No attempt should be made to treat the burn. Application of topical ointments, oils, or other home remedies is contraindicated.

Transport the Child to Medical Aid. The child with an extensive burn is not given anything by mouth to avoid aspiration in the presence of paralytic ileus and upper airway edema and to prevent water intoxication. The child is transported to the nearest medical facility. If this cannot be accomplished within a relatively short period of time, intravenous access should be established if possible with a large-bore catheter. Oxygen is administered if available at 100%. A report of the initial assessment and any interventions implemented is given to the medical facility assuming responsibility for the care of the child.

Provide Reassurance. Providing reassurance and psychologic support to both the family and the child helps immeasurably during postinjury crisis. Reducing anxiety helps to conserve energy needed to cope with the physiologic and emotional stress of a traumatic injury.

Therapeutic Management: Minor Burns

Treatment of burns classified as minor can usually be managed adequately on an outpatient basis when it is determined that the parent can be relied on to carry out instructions for care and observation. Patients with less than optimal circum-

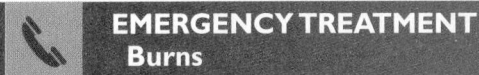

EMERGENCY TREATMENT
Burns

Minor Burns
Stop the burning process:
  Apply cool water to the burn or hold the burned area under cool running water.
Do not disturb any blisters that form.
Do not apply anything to the wound.
Cover with a clean cloth if risk of damage or contamination.
Remove burned clothing and jewelry.

Major Burns
Stop the burning process:
  Flame burns—smother the fire.
  Place victim in the horizontal position.
  Roll victim in a blanket or similar object; avoid covering the head.
Assess for an adequate airway and breathing.
If not breathing, begin mouth-to-mouth resuscitation.
Remove burned clothing and jewelry.
Cover wound with a clean cloth.
Transport to medical aid.
Begin IV and oxygen therapy as prescribed.

stances may require close follow-up to ensure compliance with the treatment program.

The wound is cleansed with a mild soap and tepid water. Debridement of the wound includes removal of any embedded debris, chemicals, and devitalized tissue. Removal of intact blisters remains controversial. Some argue that blisters provide a barrier against infection; others maintain that blister fluid is an effective medium for the growth of microorganisms (Peate, 1992). Most practitioners favor covering the wound with an antimicrobial ointment to reduce the risk of infection and to provide some form of pain relief. The dressing consists of a fine-mesh gauze placed over the ointment and a light wrap of gauze dressing that avoids interference with movement. This helps to keep the wound clean and protect it from trauma. The caregiver is instructed to wash the wound twice a day, reapply the dressing, and return the child to the office or clinic as directed for wound observation.

Other practitioners prefer an occlusive dressing, such as a hydrocolloid, which is placed over the wound after cleansing. The dressing is changed once leakage occurs or at regular intervals, usually every 7 days. This method provides a moist healing environment and eliminates the discomfort associated with frequent dressing changes but impairs visualization of the wound surface.

If there is a high probability of infection or other complications or if there is doubt about the ability to carry out instructions, the parents may be directed to return daily for dressing changes and inspection, or a nurse may be assigned to make a home visit for that purpose. Frequent removal of the dressing is an effective mode of debridement. Soaking the dressing in tepid water before removal will help loosen the dressing and debris and reduce discomfort. Burns of the face are usually treated by exposure. The wound is washed and debrided in the same manner, and a thin film of antimicrobial ointment is applied twice a day.

A tetanus history is obtained on admission. When there is

no history of immunization or more than 5 years have passed since the last immunization, tetanus prophylaxis is administered. Administration of antibiotics for minor burns is controversial. A mild analgesic, such as acetaminophen, is usually sufficient to relieve discomfort; the antipyretic effect of the drug also alleviates the sensation of heat.

Prognosis.   Most minor burns heal without difficulty, but if the wound margin becomes erythematous, gross purulence is noted, or the child develops evidence of systemic reaction, such as fever or tachycardia, hospitalization is indicated. The child should also be evaluated for functional impairment, and the caregiver should be instructed in the exercise and ambulation program. Following wound healing, an evaluation of scar maturation and range of motion will indicate any need for further therapy.

Therapeutic Management: Major Burns

Establishment of an Adequate Airway.   The first priority of care is airway maintenance. If there is evidence of respiratory involvement, 100% oxygen is administered; and blood gases, including carbon monoxide, are quickly determined. If the child exhibits air hunger or otherwise appears in critical condition, an endotracheal tube is inserted to maintain the airway. Since early edema subsides within 24 to 48 hours and many have been managed successfully for longer periods of time without significant damage with nasotracheal intubation, tracheostomy is rarely used because of the increased risk of complications.

Frequently, placing the child in a tent or under an oxygen hood with a high flow of oxygen and maximum humidity is sufficient to reduce reflex bronchospasm produced by trauma to the bronchial mucosa. When the child has a facial burn, the bed is elevated 80 to 90 degrees to reduce swelling and the risk of upper airway obstruction.

Fluid Replacement Therapy.   The objectives of fluid therapy are to (1) compensate for water and sodium lost to traumatized areas and interstitial spaces, (2) replenish sodium deficits, (3) restore plasma volume, (4) obtain adequate perfusion, (5) correct acidosis, and (6) improve renal function.

Fluid replacement is required during the first 24 hours because of fluid shifts that are occurring. There are many formulas used to calculate these needs, and the one adopted depends on practitioner preference. Crystalloid solutions are used during this initial phase of therapy. Adequacy of fluid resuscitation is determined by several parameters, such as vital signs (especially heart rate), urine output volume, adequacy of capillary filling, and state of sensorium.

After the initial 24-hour period, theoretically there is a capillary seal, and capillary permeability is restored. Colloid solutions such as albumin, plasmalyte, or fresh frozen plasma are useful in maintaining plasma volume.

Oral fluids are usually withheld in the early resuscitative phase but may be administered in 24 to 48 hours. Fluid balance may continue to be a problem throughout the course of treatment, especially during the periods in which there may be considerable evaporative loss from the wound.

Nutrition.   The enhanced metabolic requirements and catabolism in severe burns make nutritional needs of paramount importance and often difficult to provide. The diet must provide sufficient calories to meet the increased metabolic needs and protein to avoid protein breakdown.

Many burn patients are able to eat; a high-protein, high-calorie diet is encouraged as soon as possible after resolution of paralytic ileus. However, many of these children have poor appetites and are unable to meet energy requirements solely by oral feeding. Most children with burns in excess of 25% of the TBSA require supplementation with tube feeding. Absence of bowel sounds does not preclude enteral nutrition. Since the small bowel maintains motility and absorptive capabilities, the placement of a small-bore feeding tube into the duodenum allows for the safe delivery of enteral nutrition during periods of paralytic ileus associated with trauma, sepsis, and anesthesia (Jenkins, Gottschlich, and Warden, 1994). Protection from aspiration is achieved by means of a nasogastric tube to decompress the stomach.

If nutritional requirements cannot be met entirely by the enteral route, parenteral hyperalimentation can be used to supplement intake. However, enteral nutrition is preferred because it eliminates the risk of catheter-related sepsis, maintains intestinal integrity and function, and allows more efficient utilization of nutrients, especially protein.

To facilitate growth and proliferation of epithelial cells, administration of vitamins A and C is begun early in the postburn period. Zinc is also supplemented because of its important role in wound healing and epithelialization.

Medication.   Controversy also exists regarding the use of antibiotics during the first few days after injury. Antibiotics are not generally given prophylactically but are administered to treat specific infections. When a patient has elevated temperature, it is appropriate to obtain blood, sputum, and urine cultures to isolate the source of the infection. Otitis media must not be overlooked as a source of fever. When the source and particular organism are identified, appropriate antibiotics can be administered.

Some form of sedation and analgesia is required in the care of burned children. Morphine sulfate is the drug of choice for severe burn injuries. Morphine has extensive distribution, although it is eliminated rapidly; continuous infusion or frequent administration is needed for pain management in burns. Morphine is administered intravenously and titrated to individual need. The unstable circulatory status and edema formation preclude intramuscular or subcutaneous administration. The addition of scheduled methadone to intermittent morphine administration for painful procedures has proved effective in managing burn pain in some children. Nonopioid/opioid combinations, such as acetaminophen with codeine, are often effective for less severe injuries.

The use of short-acting anesthetic agents, such as ketamine, propofol, and nitrous oxide, has proved beneficial in eliminating procedural pain. Ketamine is a dissociative anesthetic agent that can be administered either orally, intravenously, or intramuscularly. Unconsciousness following intravenous administration occurs within 30 seconds and lasts approximately 10 minutes (Groeneveld and Inkson, 1992). Pharyngeal reflexes remain intact, thus ensuring a patent airway. Propofol (Deprivan) is an intravenous sedative hypnotic agent that produces sedation in less than 1 minute and lasts only a few minutes (Fig. 30-20).

Nitronox is a useful short-term analgesic mixture of gases on a fixed ratio of 50% nitrous oxide and 50% oxygen. Initiation of action is approximately 1 minute with peak effect reached in 3 to 5 minutes. Nitronox is useful to alleviate anxi-

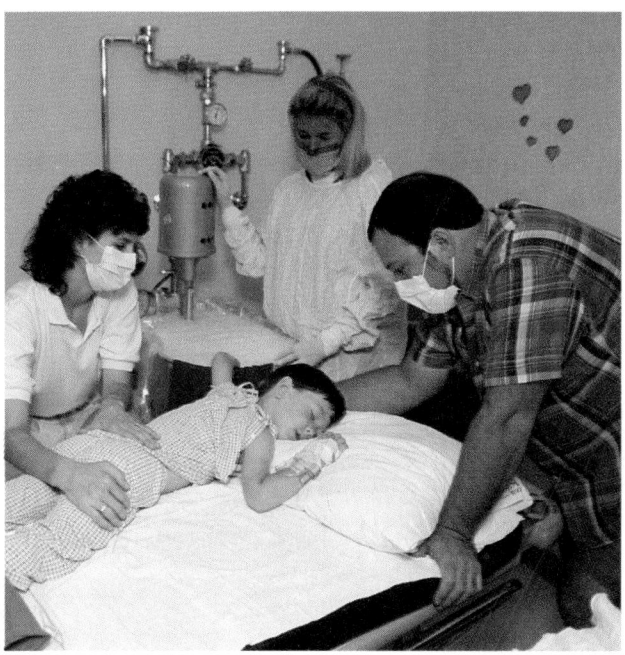

FIG. 30-20. Pain control during burn care. Child is well sedated with oral ketamine and midazolam.

ety and raise the threshold of pain during procedures. The child must be able to follow instructions to hold the face mask and may self-administer the Nitronox with assistance (Selbst, 1993). For any conscious or unconscious sedation, the child is monitored continuously during the procedure (see Preoperative Care, Chapter 22, and Chapter 21 for a discussion of pain assessment and management).

Care of Burn Wounds. After the initial period of shock and the restoration of fluid balance, the primary concern is the burn wound. The objectives of wound management include the prevention of infection, removal of devitalized tissue, and closure of the wound. The application of dressings and topical antimicrobial therapy reduce pain by minimizing the exposure to air.

Primary Excision. In children with large, full-thickness burn wounds, excision is performed as soon as the patient is hemodynamically stable after initial resuscitation. Since the burn wound is precipitating the exaggerated physiologic response, many associated complications do not resolve until the eschar is excised and the wound is closed (Finkelstein and others, 1992). Early excision of deep partial-thickness and full-thickness burns has reduced the incidence of infection and the threat of sepsis.

Debridement. Hydrotherapy is employed to cleanse the wound and involves soaking in a tub or showering once or twice a day for no more than 20 minutes. Hydrotherapy helps to cleanse not only the wound but the entire body and also aids in maintenance of range of motion.

TABLE 30-11. Comparison of common topical preparations

ADVANTAGES	DISADVANTAGES
Silver Nitrate 0.5% (AgNO₃)	
Greatly reduces evaporative losses; does not interfere with wound healing; bacteriostatic action against major burn flora, including *Pseudomonas* and *Staphylococcus;* inexpensive	Does not penetrate eschar; ineffective on established burn wound infections; little effect on *Klebsiella* and *Aerobacter* groups; stains skin, clothing, linens; makes assessment of the wound difficult because of staining; hypotonicity pulls electrolytes from the wound, depleting sodium, potassium, chloride, and magnesium; stings on application
Silver Sulfadiazine 1% (Silvadene) (AgSD)	
Little pain on application; bactericidal by altering DNA and cell metabolism; effective against gram-positive and gram-negative bacteria; easy to apply; nontoxic	Transient neutropenia; does not penetrate eschar; forms proteinaceous gel on wound surface that is painful to remove; occasional rashes and pruritus; decreases granulocyte formation
Mafenide Acetate 10% (Sulfamylon)	
Penetrates eschar and diffuses rapidly into burn wound and underlying tissues; effective in deep flame, electrical, and infected wounds; biostatic against many gram-positive and gram-negative organisms, including *Pseudomonas* and *Clostridium*	Difficult and painful to remove cream; pain on application; metabolic acidosis, hypercapnia, and carbonic anhydrase inhibition; inhibits wound healing; hypersensitivity in some patients
Povidone-Iodine (Betadine Ointment)	
Microbicidal against gram-positive, gram-negative organisms, yeast, fungi, and viruses; ease of application	Painful on application; elevation of protein-bound iodine may result in metabolic acidosis; stains clothes, linens, and the wound, making evaluation difficult; allergic reaction to iodine
Bacitracin	
Bactericidal and bacteriostatic against gram-positive organisms; low toxicity; painless application; ease of application	Limited activity against gram-negative organisms; allergic reaction in sensitive individuals

Partial-thickness wounds require debridement of devitalized tissue to promote healing. Debridement is very painful and requires some type of analgesia before the procedure. The water acts to loosen and remove sloughing tissue, exudate, and topical medications. Mesh gauze serves to entrap the exudative slough and is readily removed during hydrotherapy. Any loose tissue is carefully trimmed away before the wound is redressed.

Topical Antimicrobial Agents. Methods used for managing the burn wound are the following:

Exposure—Wounds are left open to air; crust forms on partial-thickness wounds, and eschar forms on full-thickness burns.

Open—Topical antimicrobial agent is applied directly to the wound surface, and the wound is left uncovered.

Modified—Antimicrobial is applied directly or impregnated into thin gauze and applied to the wound; gauze or net secures the area

Occlusive—Antimicrobial is impregnated in gauze or applied directly to the wound; multiple layers of bulky gauze are placed over the primary layer and secured with gauze or net.

All meet the objective of preparation for permanent wound coverage and all employ some type of topical agent.

Topical agents do not eliminate organisms from the wound but can effectively inhibit bacterial growth. To be effective, a topical application must be nontoxic, capable of diffusing through eschar, harmless to viable tissue, inexpensive, and easy to apply. It should not encourage the development of resistant strains of bacteria and should produce minimum electrolyte derangement. A comparison of commonly used agents is summarized in Table 30-11.

Biologic Skin Coverings. Temporary closure of the burn wound by the use of material other than the patient's own skin has become commonplace. Biologic dressings are used during the acute phase of therapy to cover the wound surface, protect the wound from bacterial contamination, reduce fluid and protein loss, increase the rate of epithelialization, reduce pain, and facilitate movement of joints to retain range of motion.

Allograft (homograft) skin is obtained from human cadavers that are screened for communicable diseases. Homograft is particularly useful in the coverage of surgically excised deep partial-thickness and full-thickness wounds in extensive burns when available donor sites are limited. Severe immunosuppression occurs in massively burned children, and the allograft becomes adherent. The homograft can remain in place until suitable donor sites become available. Typically, rejection is seen approximately 14 days after application. The use of homograft is limited by the availability of tissue banks and a supply of suitable donors.

Xenograft from a variety of species, most notably pigs, is commercially available. Split-thickness pigskin adheres less than allografts and replaced daily or every 2 to 3 days. They are particularly effective in children with partial-thickness scald burns of the hands and face, since they allow relatively pain-free movement, which reduces contracture formation and has the added benefit of improving appetite and morale.

When applied early to a superficial partial-thickness injury, biologic dressings create an environment at the wound surface that is conducive to epithelial growth and faster wound healing. Biologic dressings must be applied to clean wounds. If the dressing covers areas of heavy microbial contamination,

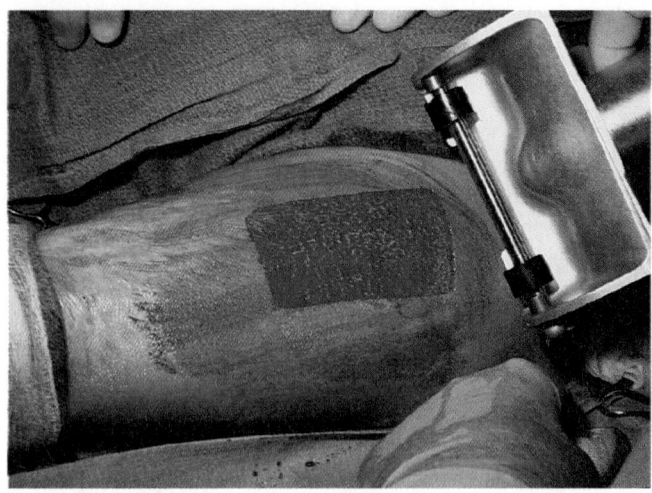

FIG. 30-21. Removal of split-thickness skin graft with a dermatome.

 ATRAUMATIC CARE
Skin Grafting

The removal of skin with a dermatome is a very painful procedure. The child should be given conscious or unconscious sedation in combination with the use of the topical anesthetic, EMLA, placed on the donor site 2 hours before the procedure.

infection occurs beneath the dressing. In the case of partial-thickness burns, such infection may convert the wound to a full-thickness injury.

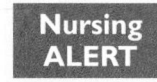 **Nursing ALERT** Observe the wound daily for any sign of an infectious process, such as purulence, erythema, or cellulitis around the wound edges or temperature elevation.

Synthetic skin coverings are available for the management of partial-thickness burn wounds. Ideally the dressing should provide many of the properties of human skin: adherence, elasticity, durability, and hemostasis. Synthetic skin substitutes are readily available, have an indefinite shelf life, and are relatively inexpensive.

Synthetic dressings are composed of a variety of materials and can be used very successfully in the management of superficial partial-thickness burns and donor sites. Examples include adherent elastic films, hydroactive materials, or colloidal suspensions that are usually permeable to air, vapor, and fluids. Another product that consists of a nylon fabric bonded to a silicone rubber membrane is used by many burn centers. Calcium alginate is gaining popularity for the treatment of donor sites with both patients and staff because of its significant reduction in discomfort. As with biologic dressings, it is important that the wound be free of debris before the dressing is applied.

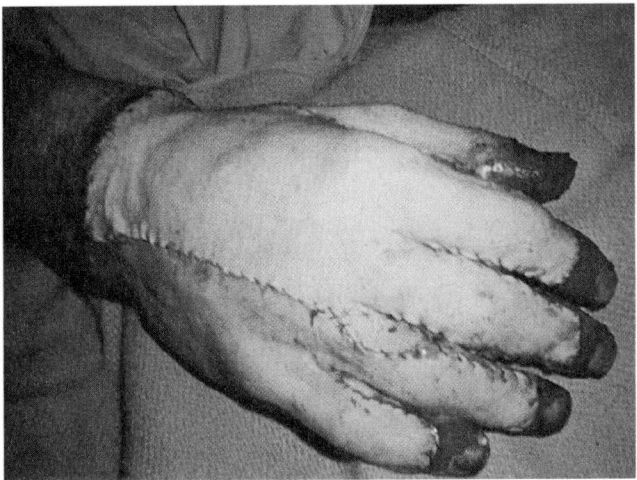

FIG. 30-22. Sheet graft.

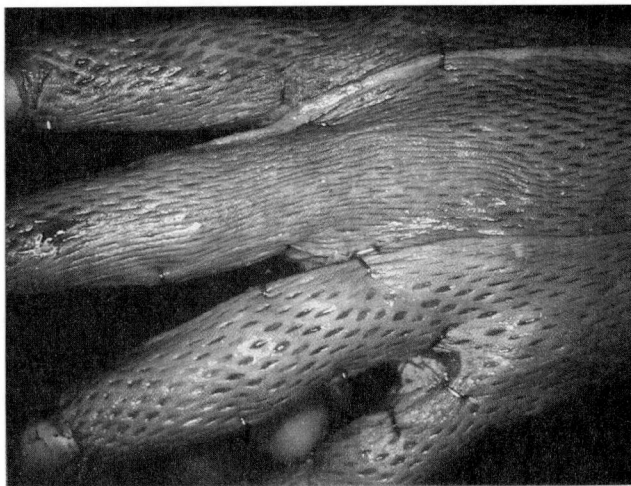

FIG. 30-23. Mesh graft.

Permanent Skin Coverings. Permanent coverage of deep partial-thickness and full-thickness burns is usually accomplished with a split-thickness skin graft. This graft consists of the epidermis and a portion of the dermis removed from an intact area of skin by a special instrument, the *dermatome* (Fig. 30-21) (see Atraumatic Care box on p. 1108).

With extensive burns it is often difficult to find enough viable skin to cover the wounds; therefore, available donor sites are used to the best advantage by special techniques. The various types of split-thickness skin grafts are:

Sheet graft—A sheet of skin, removed from the donor site, is placed intact over the recipient site and sutured in place; used in areas where cosmetic results are most visible (Fig. 30-22).

Mesh graft—A sheet of skin is removed from the donor site and passed through a mesher, which produces tiny slits in the skin that allow the skin to cover 1½ to 9 times the area of the sheet graft; results in a less desirable cosmetic and functional outcome (Fig. 30-23).

The donor site is dressed with synthetic wound coverings or fine-mesh gauze until the dressing separates at 10 to 14 days when the wound is healed. Dressings are not changed on donor sites to avoid damage to newly healed, delicate epithelium. Healed donor sites are available for reharvesting in patients with extensive burns and limited undamaged skin, but the quality of skin is decreased when multiple grafts are taken.

Cultured Epithelium. When burns are extensive and donor sites for split-thickness skin grafting are limited, it is possible to culture cells from a full-thickness skin biopsy and produce coherent sheets that can be applied to clean, excised full-thickness wounds. Some children have been successfully treated with this autologous cultured epithelium (Boyce and others, 1993). Long-term followup studies are currently being conducted to determine pathologic changes and functional properties. Epithelial cell culture grafts offer the possibility of an unlimited source of autografts in patients with extensive burns.

Prognosis. Children differ from adults in their responses to thermal injury, and the mortality rates in young children are significantly higher than those in older children and adults. Mortality is greatest for children younger than 48 months of age (Erickson and others, 1991). Many children who do survive have long-term functional and cosmetic impairments.

Nursing Considerations

❖ Assessment

Initial assessment of the burned child includes the wound assessment described on p. 1101, as well as a comprehensive assessment of the child's general condition and behavior. The child with severe and/or extensive burns requires constant observation and assessment, with special attention to signs of complications. Each major phase of care has areas of greatest threat: fluid and electrolyte disturbances (especially shock) in the acute phase, infection in the management phase, and healing and functional disturbances from scar formation in the rehabilitative phase. Respiratory, cardiac, and renal complications may appear early in the postburn period.

> **Nursing ALERT**
>
> Disorientation in the burned patient is one of the first signs of overwhelming sepsis. A spiking fever and diminished bowel sounds accompanied by paralytic ileus are noted and progressively increase over 48 to 72 hours, after which the temperature falls to subnormal limits. At this time the wound deteriorates, the white blood cell count is depressed, and septic shock becomes manifest.

❖ Nursing Diagnoses

Nursing diagnoses identified for the child with severe or extensive burns are included in the Nursing Care Plan on pp. 1114-1116. Additional diagnoses may be ascertained for individual children.

❖ Planning

The goals for the child with a burn injury and the family are as follows:

1. Child will experience reduction of pain.
2. Child will exhibit evidence of wound healing.

3. Child will receive adequate nutrition and will achieve reduction in metabolic losses.
4. Child will not experience acute complications during management phase.
5. Child will not experience long-term complications during rehabilitative phase.
6. Child and family will receive emotional support.

❖ Implementation

Prevent Acute Complications. The primary emphasis during the initial phases of burn care is on prevention of burn shock. Checking vital signs, monitoring the intravenous infusion, and measuring urine output are ongoing nursing activities in the hours immediately after injury. The intravenous infusion is started immediately by intracatheter or cutdown and is regulated according to urine output and specific gravity, laboratory data, and objective signs of adequate hydration. Urine volume, measured at least every hour, should be 1-2 ml/kg/hr.

> **Nursing ALERT**
> Monitor the child's urine for the presence of pigmented myoglobin, a by-product of muscle breakdown, to prevent kidney damage. Testing can be done at the bedside using a reagent strip (Hemastix).

Dextrosticks should be used at least every 4 hours for the first 24 to 48 hours to monitor the blood glucose level. Careful monitoring of the child's serum sodium levels and accurate intake and output records are indicated. A complication associated with hyponatremia is the possibility of seizures.

Children with major burns should initially have nothing by mouth. Placement of a nasogastric tube to a low wall suction is indicated to prevent paralytic ileus during the first 24 hours.

Edema formation in a burned extremity with full-thickness burns must be observed closely for signs of circulatory impairment (i.e., loss of sensation, deep throbbing pain, and loss of pulse—late sign).

> **Nursing ALERT**
> Evaluate the extremity and check the pulse every hour. If unable to palpate, use Doppler to ascertain loss of circulation and pulse. If the pulse is lost, escharotomy may be necessary to relieve the edema causing pressure on blood vessels, to restore adequate circulation.

The burn wound is treated according to the protocol of the specific burn facility. Extensive wounds may require the use of special beds and other equipment, such as CircOelectric beds, flotation beds, alternating pressure mattresses, and many other devices, depending on the extent and location of the wound.

The course of treatment is often long and emotionally laden for the child, the family, and the nursing staff. The severe pain of the wound and the therapies, the anxiety generated by these experiences, and the conscious and unconscious interpretations of traumatic events contribute to the psychologic reactions frequently observed in burned children. Much of the difficulty encountered in managing burned children is related to these factors. Soon after hospitalization many burned children become irritable, depressed, hostile, and aggressive toward the members of the health team. In their helplessness, children often resort to angry outbursts against anything and anybody.

Relieve Pain. The burn pain is overwhelming, engulfing, and irrepressible. Consequently, the pain causes anxiety and a feeling of profound helplessness in the child and can produce reactions of confusion, fear, and panic. Compounding the pain is the child's interpretation of it and of the procedures; this is closely related to the developmental level of the child. Many burned children believe their pain is punishment for past misdeeds and therefore deserved. There are often feelings of anger, guilt, and depression and, as in all illness, regressive behavior. When children appear to accept their pain and show little or no aggressive behavior, psychologic consultation is usually in order.

It is always difficult to deal with a child in pain, and to inflict pain on a helpless child is contrary to the empathic nature of nursing. Adequate management of pain is essential to reduce the discomfort of the burn and the necessary therapeutic procedures. Management of pain consists of (1) choosing the correct analgesic, (2) using a sufficient dosage, and (3) observing appropriate timing. For example, to relieve pain adequately, the *onset* of action of the drug must be considered so that the peak effect occurs when the treatment is performed. An oral analgesic administered shortly before the procedure will exert its effect *after* the procedure is completed. Management of pain follows the principles described in Chapter 21.

NURSING TIP To relieve pain effectively during burn treatments, administer IV narcotics immediately before the procedure but oral nonnarcotics 1 hour before the procedure.

Facilitate Wound Healing. The nurse has the major responsibility for cleansing, debriding, and applying topical medication and dressings to the burn wound. Because dressing removal is a painful procedure, children should receive adequate analgesia before the scheduled tubbing. It should be administered so that the peak effect of the drug coincides with the procedure. Both nurses and children must recognize it for exactly what it is—a dreadful but absolutely necessary procedure.

Research has demonstrated that children are more cooperative and demonstrate less anxiety and depression when they are allowed to be active participants in their care (Kavanagh and others, 1991). Predictability and controllability are promoted during dressing changes. Predictability is increased by providing cues (nurses wearing specific clothing for dressing changes), focusing the patient on the procedure, and providing children with information about physical sensations they are likely to experience (e.g., pulling, stinging, pressure) before they experience them. Controllability is enhanced by providing the children with as many choices as possible during the burn care and encouraging active participation. These strategies are unlike the traditional approaches of distraction and passivity. "Learned helplessness" is most intense when the outcomes are unpleasant and the situation is perceived to be unchangeable (see box).

Outer dressings (if any) are removed before the child is placed in the shower, but adherent dressings are more easily removed after soaking with the water. Loose or easily detached tissue is also removed during hydrotherapy, and children are encouraged to move about as much as possible to exercise muscles and reduce contracture formation. They need to be encouraged and to be made aware of every little bit of healing as evidence that they are getting better. Merely saying that they are better is insufficient as they gaze at unsightly wounds. In dressing the wound, it is important that all areas be clean, that medication be amply applied, and that no two burned surfaces touch each other, such as fingers or toes, or the ears touching the head; for example, a 4 × 4 inch gauze pad can be placed between fingers and toes.

Application of the medication can be a painful experience also, especially when mafenide acetate (Sulfamylon) cream is the agent used. This is used on electrical and fourth-degree burns because of its ability to penetrate eschar, but it can cause metabolic acidosis. Both the nurse and the child must understand that a painful sensation often described as "burning" may have special significance for burned children. They must be reassured that the medication is not inflicting further injury and that the sensation is only a transient discomfort.

When occlusive dressings are applied, elastic (Ace) bandages are worn over dressings to prevent epithelial breakdown, edema, stimulate circulation, and make mobility easier. This is especially important when the child is ambulatory.

Provide Nutrition. After the initial phase of care, children are usually allowed oral feedings (unless paralytic ileus persists). Because children frequently lack an appetite, a great deal of encouragement, help, and patience is required on the part of the nursing staff. Consultation with the parents and the dietitian is arranged to determine the best way to provide needed nutrients in foods the child will be more likely to eat. Children who are old enough to participate should be included in the planning.

Nourishing snacks (high-protein milkshakes and enriched supplements such as Pedi-Ensure) are provided between regularly scheduled mealtimes, and if children eat better at a time other than a scheduled mealtime, that is the time to feed them. Most important, meals should not be scheduled immediately after a dressing change. Most children are too physically exhausted and too emotionally upset to eat at this time. If they will not eat, a 72-hour calorie count is taken to determine if tube feeding is necessary, and every effort should be made to encourage oral intake. (See Chapter 22 for suggestions for feeding the sick child.)

Prevent Long-Term Complications. The chief dangers in this phase of burn care are wound infection, generalized sepsis, and bacterial pneumonia. Most burn patients are treated in a protected environment. Children are placed in burn units or private rooms in general units. Staff typically change into "scrub" clothing, and visitors change into gowns, wash their hands, and wear gloves before entering the child's room. In some burn centers wearing masks and caps is an additional requirement.

The value of strict isolation in preventing infection in the burn wound is controversial. Studies have found that less strict isolation procedures, such as handwashing and wearing gloves, caps, masks, and nonpermeable aprons when providing direct patient contact or when in contact with body secretions, were actually more effective than strict isolation procedures. The use of a simplified isolation protocol can effectively reduce the nosocomial transmission of organisms, increase the compliance with isolation technique, and decrease cost (Lee and others, 1990).

It is important to make accurate ongoing assessments. Wound cultures are obtained at least three times a week, and a blood culture is indicated in any child with a rectal temperature of 39.5° C (103° F) or higher. Urine and sputum cultures may be helpful in isolating the source(s) of infection.

> **Nursing ALERT** Signs and symptoms of sepsis are (1) disorientation, (2) tachypnea, (3) temperature above 39.5° C (103° F), (4) hypothermia, and (5) distention of the abdomen or development of intestinal ileus.

To reduce metabolic expenditure as much as possible, the ambient temperature of the environment is maintained between 28° and 33° C (82.4° to 91.4° F) to avoid both overheating and underheating. An overhead warming unit may be provided to maintain body heat. Heat is often provided by means of a heat cradle over the child, but if used, the heat source should be situated well away from the child's body. Other methods include using electric heaters, which should be situated 4 to 5 feet away to avoid overheating, and maintaining the room temperature sufficiently elevated to reduce evaporative loss.

Antacids are usually administered prophylactically to prevent or minimize the effect of Curling (stress) ulcer, a frequent complication of severe burns, but nurses must be alert for any signs of bleeding.

Because the child is reluctant to move and doing so causes pain or discomfort, stiffness and joint contracture develop easily. In an effort to prevent this complication, the child is encouraged to move whenever feasible, and active physiotherapy is included as an essential aspect of burn care. When the child is resting or sleeping, contracture is prevented by proper splinting. Frog-legging, where the hips rotate outward and the knees are bent, can be prevented by placing a roll on either side of the legs to promote proper positioning. Children have a natural tendency to be active, and they will usually move spontaneously unless the pain is severe.

Care for Skin Graft. Effort in the care of children with skin grafts is directed toward facilitating a "take." Trauma, infection, and bleeding must be avoided for a successful transplantation to occur. When the grafted area is left exposed, the child must be immobilized to prevent the graft from becoming dislodged. Flat surfaces usually pose few problems, but grafts over irregular or mobile areas may require special techniques, such as splints or bulky surgical dressings.

The grafted areas have sutures to anchor the graft over the excised area. These are removed about 5 to 7 days after surgery. When the surgical dressings are removed, on approximately the fourth day after surgery, a dressing of fine mesh gauze impregnated with a topical antibiotic ointment (e.g., neomycin) is placed over the new graft and wrapped with Kling to help secure it in place. After the graft is completely healed, it may be left exposed (Fig. 30-24). The child may resume activities after the surgical dressings are removed, with the exception of grafts on the legs, which require bed rest for 7 to 10 days.

Wound contraction and scar tissue formation are normal parts of wound healing. Scar tissue is metabolically active tissue that continually rearranges itself; as a result, disabling contractures, deformity, and disfigurement are ever-present possibilities. Physical therapy, splints, and other methods are used to minimize these long-term effects. Pressure splints and elastic bandages or elasticized (Jobst) garments help reduce scar hypertrophy and may be worn for months to 2 years after hospitalization (Fig. 30-25).

Scar tissue has some properties that are significant, particularly for growing children. Intense itching occurs in healing burn wounds and scar tissue (especially on the legs and arms, but not the face). It is usually treated with administration of hydroxyzine (Atarax) or diphenhydramine (Benadryl) and frequent application of a moisturizer such as Eucerin cream, cocoa butter, or Nivea. Because scar tissue has no sweat glands, children with extensive scarring may have difficulty during hot weather or when they develop a fever. Parents need to be informed of this characteristic so that they can be prepared to find alternative cooling methods when indicated.

Severely burned children must return to the hospital periodically for additional skin grafts and scar revisions, especially to release contractures over joint spaces and for cosmetic considerations. Achievement of optimum results frequently requires years. In the meantime, burn scars are unsightly, and although improvements can be made, hope should not be extended to the parents and child for complete cosmetic and functional repair.

Support Child and Family. A critical component of burn care is support for the child and family. Throughout the acute phase of care, the child's emotional needs must not be overlooked. Children are frightened, uncomfortable, and often confused. They are isolated from familiar persons and surroundings, and the often overwhelming physical needs at this time are the primary focus of the staff and parents. Children need reassurance that they are all right and that they will get better.

The child is encouraged to participate in as many aspects of care as possible. With illness, children always regress to the

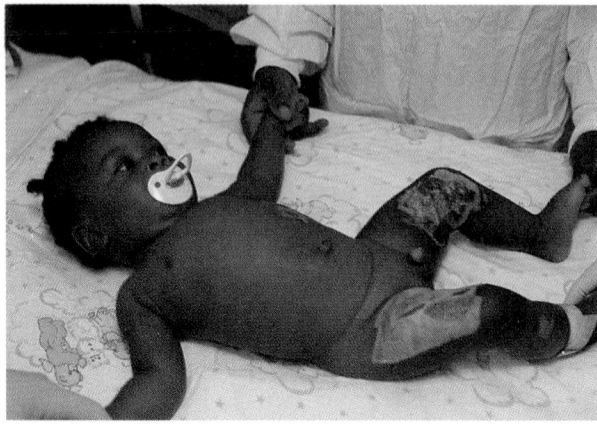

FIG. 30-24. Appearance of donor (right leg) and graft (left leg) sites 9 days after grafting. Dark areas on graft site are engrafted skin.

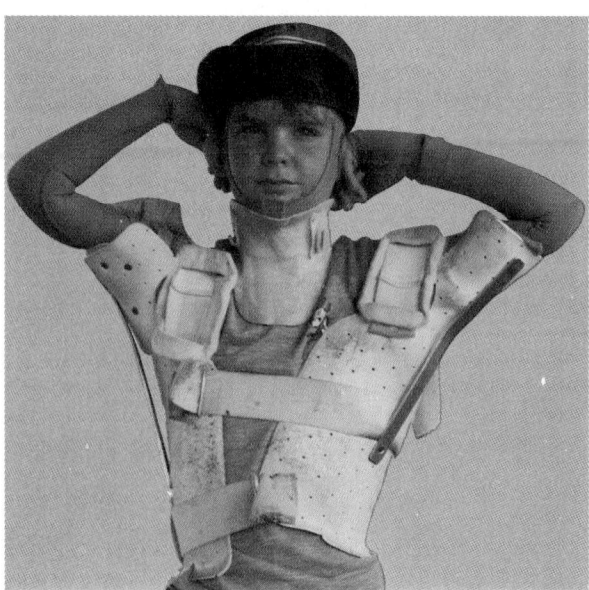

FIG. 30-25. Child in elasticized garment (Jobst) and "airplane" splints.

developmental level that allows them to deal with the stress. As their condition permits, children can be expected to do things that they were capable of doing for themselves before they were burned, such as oral hygiene, face washing, feeding themselves, and playing. Allowing children to make choices and to help make decisions about the time of their care and recreational activities makes them feel a part of the team and provides them with a measure of control. Children will probably require assistance; however, as they see themselves contributing to their care, they gain confidence and self-esteem.

The psychologic pain and sequelae of severe burn trauma are as intense as the physical trauma. Each burned child goes through a tremendous amount of pain, often continuous for varying periods, and is often separated from the family for extended periods. In addition, there is a continual barrage of painful therapeutic and diagnostic procedures that are inflicted by others. They wonder why this has happened to *them*—what they have done that they should be punished so. Past experiences cannot serve them in this crisis. They do not understand the "ugliness" and disfigurement they see as their body.

The impact of such severe injury taxes the capabilities of children at all ages, but young children who suffer acutely from separation anxiety and adolescents who are developing an identity are probably most affected psychologically. Toddlers cannot begin to comprehend why the parents whom they love and who have protected them from hurt can leave them in such a dreadful place and allow others to inflict such painful indignities on them.

Adolescents in the process of achieving independence from their parents and seeking to find out who they are in the world find themselves in a dependent position with a damaged body. Being different from others at a time when conformity and being like one's peers are so important is difficult to accept. These children need understanding adults to help them deal with the struggles concerning resentment and other feelings generated by such a catastrophe.

Members of the family, as well as the child, feel the impact of severe burn injury. They are concerned about the child's survival, recovery, and future appearance. Nurses are in the most opportune position to assist parents in coping with the stresses of the child's illness and their feelings of guilt and helplessness. The parents need to be informed of the child's progress and helped in their efforts to cope with their feelings while providing support to the child (Fig. 30-26). The nurse is the person who can help them understand that it is not selfish to look after themselves and their own needs so that they can better meet the needs of the child. For parents whose response to the illness is too severe or whose response to stress is manifested in destructive behavior, professional help may be needed. Additional information on burn care and prevention can be obtained from the **American Burn Association.***

The **Alisa Ann Ruch California Burn Foundation†** provides assistance to burn victims and burn centers, supports research to improve burn care and treatment, and promotes

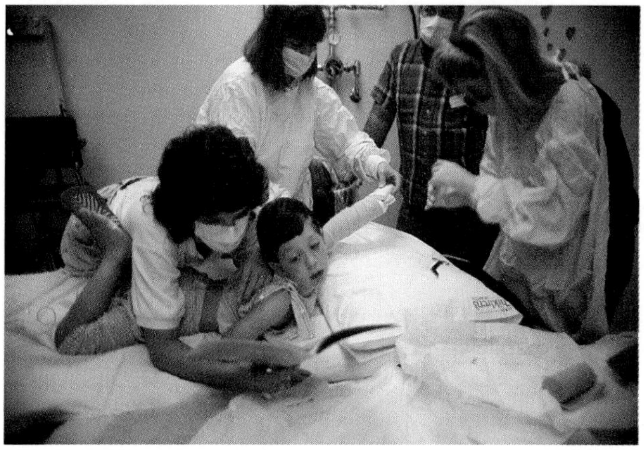

FIG. 30-26. Parents play a critical role in helping their child cope with the burn injury. Here a parent uses distraction by reading her child a book during burn care.

public education in fire and burn prevention. The **Shriners Burns Institutes** are staffed to treat patients with acute burns and patients needing plastic or reconstructive surgery as a result of healed burns, with severe scarring resulting in contractures or interference in proper limb mobility, or with scarring and deformity of the face. Applications can be obtained through the Shrine Temple, Shrine Club, or Shriners Hospitals or by contacting the **International Shrine Headquarters.***

Prepare for Discharge and Home Care. In most burn centers the nurse participates as part of an interdisciplinary discharge team that includes physicians, social workers, physical and occupational therapists, and child development specialists who plan with the patient and family for dismissal. The family's willingness to assume responsibility and their capability to administer care effectively are assessed. Home, school, and other environmental settings are explored; financial concerns and available community resources are discussed; and a specific plan of care for the child with an anticipated follow-up program is developed.

Because the family and/or other caregivers play a vital role in the successful reintroduction of burned children into the social and educational system, health education by the nurse is essential. The parents should observe wound care and at least two to five dressing changes until they feel comfortable in performing the procedure. It is recommended that the parents actually perform at least one dressing change before discharge so that the nurse can determine their knowledge and ability in accomplishing the task successfully. The parents must also be able to explain signs and symptoms of infection to the nurse.

Arrangements with the family for discharge medications and supplies for dressing changes are provided. If the parents are unable to perform wound care and dressing changes, it is important to ensure that the prescribed care will be maintained. This may be accomplished by designating caregivers other than the parents to perform the procedures or by requiring daily visits to a clinic.

---

*New York-Cornell Medical Center, 525 E. 68th St., Room L-706, New York, NY 10021; (800) 548-BURN.
†20944 Sherman Way, Suite 115, Canoga Park, CA 91303; (818) 883-7700.

---

*2900 Rocky Point Dr., Tampa, FL 33607; (800) 237-5055 (in Florida [800] 282-9161).

NURSING CARE PLAN

The Child with Burns: Management and Rehabilitative Stages

NURSING DIAGNOSIS: Impaired skin integrity related to thermal injury

PATIENT GOAL 1: Will exhibit evidence of wound healing

• **NURSING INTERVENTIONS/*RATIONALES***

Shave hair to a 2-inch margin from the wound and area immediately surrounding the burn *to remove a reservoir for infection*

Thoroughly cleanse the wound and surrounding skin *to decrease the risk of infection;* debride devitalized tissue *to promote healing*

Keep child from scratching and picking at the wound
Provide distraction appropriate to child's age
Older child: explain reasons to encourage cooperation
Young child: supervise activity as needed

Maintain care in handling the wound *to avoid damaging epithelializing and granulating tissues*

Offer high-calorie, high-protein meals and snacks *to meet augmented protein and calorie requirements caused by increased metabolism and catabolism*

Prevent infection, which can delay healing and convert partial-thickness wounds to full-thickness wounds

Administer supplementary vitamins and minerals—vitamins A, B, C, iron, and zinc—*to facilitate wound healing and epithelialization*

Pad burned ears *to prevent tissue necrosis caused by minimal blood flow to cartilage*

Monitor for signs/symptoms of wound infection *to ensure prompt recognition and treatment*

Wrap fingers and toes separately *to avoid tissue adherence from prolonged contact*

• **EXPECTED OUTCOME**

Wounds heal without evidence of damage or inflammation

PATIENT GOAL 2: Will maintain integrity of skin graft

• **NURSING INTERVENTIONS/*RATIONALES***

Position for minimal mechanical disturbance of graft site
Restrain if necessary *to prevent graft from being dislodged*
Maintain splints or dressings *if needed for protection of the graft*
Observe grafts for evidence of hematoma/fluid accumulation; aspirate or express fluids *to ensure contact of the graft with the base*

• **EXPECTED OUTCOME**

Skin graft remains intact

NURSING DIAGNOSIS: Pain related to skin trauma, therapies

PATIENT GOAL 1: Will experience reduction of pain to a level acceptable to the child

• **NURSING INTERVENTIONS/*RATIONALES***

Assess need for medication (see Pain Assessment, Chapter 21)
Recognize that burn pain is often overwhelming, engulfing, and irrepressible
Position in extension to minimize pain resulting from exercising to regain extension
Implement passive and active exercising *to minimize contracture formation*
Reduce irritation to prevent increased pain
Touch/stroke unburned areas *to provide physical contact and comfort*
Employ appropriate nonpharmacologic pain-reduction techniques (see Pain Management, Chapter 21)
Promote control and predictability during painful procedures (see box on p. 1111)
Anticipate the need for pain medication and administer before the onset of severe pain and at regular intervals *to prevent recurrence* (see Pain Management, Chapter 21)

• **EXPECTED OUTCOME**

Child exhibits reduction of pain to level acceptable to child

---

NURSING DIAGNOSIS: High risk for infection related to denuded skin, presence of pathogenic organisms, and altered immune response

PATIENT GOAL 1: Will exhibit no evidence of wound infection

• **NURSING INTERVENTIONS/*RATIONALES***

Implement and maintain infection control precautions according to unit policy
Maintain careful handwashing by members of staff and visitors *to minimize exposure to infectious agents*
Wear clean or sterile gown, cap, mask, and gloves when handling wound area *to minimize exposure to infectious agents*
Debride eschar, crust, and blisters *to eliminate the reservoir for organisms*
Avoid patient contact with persons who have upper respiratory or skin infection
Cover the wound and/or patient according to the protocol of the unit *to provide a barrier to organisms*
Administer good oral hygiene
*Apply prescribed topical antimicrobial preparation and dressings to the wound *to control bacterial proliferation*
Obtain baseline and serial wound cultures *to ascertain any increase or changes in wound flora*
Monitor closely for signs of sepsis and infection (disorientation, tachypnea, temperature above 39.5° C [103° F], hypothermia, distention of the abdomen or intestinal ileus, change in wound appearance)

---

*Dependent nursing action.

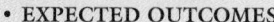

- **EXPECTED OUTCOMES**

Possible sources of infection are eliminated
Wound displays minimal or no evidence of infection

> **NURSING DIAGNOSIS:** Altered nutrition: less than body requirements related to increased catabolism and metabolism, loss of appetite

PATIENT GOAL 1: Will receive optimum nourishment

- **NURSING INTERVENTIONS/*RATIONALES***

Encourage oral feeding (see Feeding the Sick Child, Chapter 22)
Provide high-calorie, high-protein meals and snacks *to avoid protein breakdown and meet augmented calorie requirements*
Provide foods child likes, *to stimulate appetite*
Allow self-help *to encourage cooperation*
Provide meals when child is most likely to eat well
Provide attractive meals and surroundings *to encourage eating*
Provide companionship at meals *to create a more homelike environment*
Use "contract" with older children *to encourage compliance*
Administer supplemental enteral feedings as prescribed *to meet calculated needs*
Obtain weekly weight *to monitor nutritional status*
Record accurate intake and output *to evaluate sufficiency of intake*
Monitor for diarrhea/constipation and institute prompt treatment *to avoid feeding intolerance*

- **EXPECTED OUTCOME**

Child consumes a sufficient amount of nutrients (specify) and maintains preburn weight

> **NURSING DIAGNOSIS:** Impaired physical mobility (specify level) related to pain, impaired joint movement, scar formation

PATIENT GOAL 1: Will achieve optimum physical functioning

- **NURSING INTERVENTIONS/*RATIONALES***

Carry out range-of-motion exercises *to maintain optimum joint and muscle function*
Encourage mobility if child is able to move extremities
Ambulate as soon as feasible
Splint involved joints in extension at night and during rest periods *to minimize contracture formation*
Encourage and promote self-help activities *to increase mobility*
Administer analgesia before painful activity (e.g., physical therapy) *so that child is more likely to cooperate and be mobile*
Encourage participation in activities of daily living and play activities *to incorporate exercise into enjoyable events*

Use lotion and massage on healed areas before exercise *to soften tissues and promote relaxation*

PATIENT GOAL 2: Will exhibit minimal scarring

- **NURSING INTERVENTIONS/*RATIONALES***

Position in a functional attitude for minimal deformity and optimum functioning
Apply splints as ordered and designed *to minimize contracture*
Wrap healing tissue with elastic bandage or dress in elastic garments as ordered *to help reduce scar hypertrophy by compressing collagen and decreasing vascularity*
Carry out physical therapy *to minimize deformity related to scar contracture formation*
Provide treatment for pruritus *to minimize scratching and irritation of newly healed tissue*

- **EXPECTED OUTCOME**

Wound heals with minimal scar formation; joints remain flexible and functional

> **NURSING DIAGNOSIS:** Body image disturbance related to perception of appearance and mobility

PATIENT GOAL 1: Will receive adequate emotional support

- **NURSING INTERVENTIONS/*RATIONALES***

Convey positive attitude toward child *to demonstrate acceptance and so that child expects to get better*
Encourage parents to participate in care *to prevent the stress of separation and prepare for reintegration into the community*
Encourage as much independence as condition allows *to give child a sense of control*
Arrange for continued schooling *to encourage optimum development and sense of normalcy*
Promote peer contact where possible *to decrease isolation*
Be honest with child and family *to create a trusting nurse-client relationship*
Encourage activities appropriate to age and capabilities *to promote normalcy and increase self-esteem*
Prepare peers for child's appearance *to encourage acceptance and support*
Provide opportunities for child and family to discuss the impact of the change in appearance and life-style *to increase coping*
Support behaviors suggesting adaptation *to build on strengths*

- **EXPECTED OUTCOMES**

Child accepts efforts of family and caregivers
Child engages in activities with others according to age and capabilities

Continued.

NURSING CARE PLAN
The Child with Burns: Management and Rehabilitative Stages—cont'd

PATIENT GOAL 2: Will demonstrate improved body image

• NURSING INTERVENTIONS/*RATIONALES*

Explore feelings concerning physical appearance *to facilitate coping with body image changes*

Discuss feelings about returning to home, family, school, and friends *to build coping mechanisms*

Provide reinforcement of positive aspects of appearance and capabilities *to recognize and build on strengths*

Point out evidence of healing *to encourage a sense of hope*

Discuss aids that camouflage disfigurement *to facilitate coping*
Wigs
Clothing (e.g., turtleneck sweaters)
Makeup

Provide recreational and diversional activities *to promote a sense of normalcy*

Promote constructive thinking in child *to encourage positive coping*

Help child devise a plan to address and cope with the reactions of others *to increase the sense of control*

• EXPECTED OUTCOMES

Child discusses feelings and concerns regarding appearance and the perceived reactions of others

Child verbalizes positive suggestions for adjusting to appearance and community/peer response

PATIENT GOAL 3: Will engage in self-care activities

• NURSING INTERVENTIONS/*RATIONALES*

Assist with self-care activities as needed

Encourage self-care according to capabilities

Begin early in hospitalization to discuss "going home" *so that child expects to get better*

Accept regressive behavior where appropriate *because this is how child is coping with stress*

Help child develop independence and self-help capabilities *to increase self-esteem*

• EXPECTED OUTCOMES

Child verbalizes and otherwise demonstrates interest in going home

Child engages in self-help activities

> **NURSING DIAGNOSIS:** Altered family processes related to situational crisis (child with a serious injury)

PATIENT GOAL 1: Will be prepared for discharge and home care

• NURSING INTERVENTIONS/*RATIONALES*

Teach wound care to caregiver *to achieve proficiency and increase confidence*

Discuss diet, rest, and activity *to assist in planning for a home care regimen*

Explore attitudes toward child's reentry into the family *to facilitate coping and identify a possible need for intervention*

Explore family's concept regarding child's capabilities and the possible restrictions and freedom they will allow *to assist them in planning realistically for an altered life-style*

Help family set realistic goals for themselves, the child, and other family members *to clarify and validate the plan of home care*

Help family acquire needed equipment and supplies *to reduce anxiety*

• EXPECTED OUTCOMES

Family demonstrates an understanding of child's needs and the impact child's condition will have on them

Family sets realistic goals for selves, child, and others

PATIENT/FAMILY GOAL 2: Will participate in follow-up care

• NURSING INTERVENTIONS/*RATIONALES*

Coordinate team management of child and family for ongoing care *to provide continuity*

Arrange for return visits

Assess the needs of the family *to determine appropriate plan of care*

Arrange for referral agencies based on needs assessment

Collaborate with school nurse *to help with child's reintegration into school and the world of peers*

Visit the school, if possible, to prepare teacher and peers *to encourage acceptance of child*

• EXPECTED OUTCOMES

Family maintains contact with health providers

Child attends school regularly and interacts with age-mates

See also:
Nursing Care Plan: The Child in the Hospital, Chapter 21
Nursing Care Plan: The Family of the Ill or Hospitalized Child, Chapter 21

Some burn centers have a back-to-school reentry program for school-age burn patients to assist the child in returning to a classroom of peers. The program provides information about burn wound care, scarring, and rehabilitation therapy to help the child's classmates understand what the child has experienced and what the child must anticipate. It is hoped that sharing the child's experiences will help the other students appreciate the obstacles the child must overcome to return to normal childhood activities. The intent of the reentry program is to gain peer support for the burned child and allow peers to empathize with and understand the needs of the burned child.

❖ Evaluation

The effectiveness of nursing interventions is determined by continual reassessment and evaluation of care based on the following observational guidelines and expected outcomes:

1. Observe child's behavior during all aspects of care; listen to verbal cues; use a pain assessment record to evaluate the effectiveness of analgesia.
2. Observe the burn wound and child's general condition.
3. Observe child's eating behavior and the amount of food consumed; weigh daily or as indicated.
4. Inspect the burn wound for signs of infection; take vital signs; observe for evidence of gastric bleeding, respiratory complications, weight loss, hemoglobin level, and neurologic signs.
5. Observe for evidence of healing and scar formation; assess effectiveness of physical therapy and appliances (splints, pressure garments).
6. Observe child's and family's behaviors; interview child and family regarding their feelings and concerns.

Expected outcomes:
See Nursing Care Plan, pp. 1114-1116.

SUNBURN

Sunburn is a very common skin injury caused by overexposure to ultraviolet light waves. The sun emits a continuous spectrum of visible and nonvisible light rays that range in length from very short to very long. The shorter, higher-frequency waves are more damaging than longer wavelengths, but much of the light is filtered out as it travels through the atmosphere. Of the light that does filter through, *ultraviolet A (UVA) waves* are the longest and cause only minimum burning, but they potentiate *ultraviolet B (UVB)* effects and play a significant role in photosensitive and photoallergic reactions and premature aging. UVB waves are shorter and responsible for tanning, burning, and most of the harmful effects attributed to sunlight, especially skin cancer.

Numerous factors influence the amount of UVB exposure. Maximum exposure occurs at midday (10 AM to 3 PM), when the distance from the sun to a given spot on the earth is shortest. There is more exposure at higher altitudes, less when the sky is hazy (although the amount of ultraviolet radiation that does penetrate is easily underestimated); window glass effectively screens out UVB but not UVA rays. Fresh snow and water reflect ultraviolet rays, especially when the sun is directly overhead; some rays are reflected by sand.

Nursing Considerations

Protection from sunburn is the major goal of medical and nursing management, and the harmful effects of the sun on the delicate skin of infants and children is receiving increased attention. To protect skin exposed to the sun for extended periods, skin should be covered with clothing, and FDA-approved sun protective agents should be applied.

Two types of products are available for sun protection: *topical sunscreens,* which partially absorb ultraviolet light, and *sun blockers,* which block out ultraviolet rays by reflecting sunlight. The most frequently recommended sun blockers are zinc oxide and titanium dioxide ointments. Sunscreens are products containing a *sun protection factor (SPF)* based on evaluation of effectiveness against ultraviolet rays. The SPF is indicated by a number, such as 15, which indicates that if individuals normally burn in 10 minutes without a sunscreen, use of a sunscreen with SPF 15 allows them to remain in the sun 15 × 10 or 150 minutes (2½ hours) before burning to the same degree. The most effective sunscreens against UVB are *p-aminobenzoic acid (PABA)* and *PABA-esters.*

Claims such as "broad-spectrum" or "UVA-UVB sunblock" are usually unsubstantiated. One product that affords protection against UVA is *Parsol 1789,* found in Photoplex and UVA Guard.

Sunscreens are applied evenly to all exposed areas, with special attention to skinfolds and areas that might become exposed as clothing shifts. Parents are directed to read labels of sunscreen products carefully for the SPF and follow the manufacturer's directions for application.

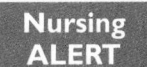 **Nursing ALERT** Sunscreens are not recommended for infants under 6 months of age. Infants should be kept out of the sun or physically shaded from it. Dry fabric with a tight weave, such as cotton, and in darker colors offers good protection (Stanford and others, 1995).

Sunburn is usually an epidermal burn, although severe sunburn can be a partial-thickness burn with blister formation. Treatment involves stopping the burning process, decreasing the inflammatory response, and rehydrating the skin. Local application of cool tap water soaks, or immersion in a tepid water bath for 20 minutes or until the skin is cool limits tissue destruction and relieves the discomfort. Moisturizing lotion is then applied. Partial-thickness burns are treated the same as those from any heat source (see earlier discussion on burns).

COLD INJURY

Cold injuries are most commonly seen in very cold regions. The nature of the heat-regulating mechanisms of the body are such that the inner portion of the body, or core, produces heat and the periphery, or outer area, conserves or dissipates heat. When the body attempts to conserve heat, the outer tissues are subjected to low temperatures, and local trauma may result.

Chilblain, redness and swelling of the skin, occurs when extremities, usually the hands, are exposed intermittently to temperatures of −1.1° to 15.5° C (30° to 60° F). The response may vary but is characterized by intense vasodilation that increases the temperature of involved tissues above that of unaffected tissue and produces edematous, reddish-blue patches that itch and burn. As warming takes place, the sensations become more intense, but ordinarily subside in a few days.

Frostbite results from sufficient exposure that heat loss to local tissues allows ice crystals to form in tissues, resulting in variable degrees of loss of tissue and function. The frostbitten part appears white or blanched, feels solid, and is without sensation. Rapid rewarming produces a flush (sometimes deep purple) and a return of sensation, which is extremely painful. In 24 to 48 hours after rewarming, large blisters appear, which begin to reabsorb within 5 to 10 days, followed by the formation of a hard black eschar. Superficial injury often heals without incident. Rewarming is accomplished by immersing the part in well-agitated water at 100° to 108° F. Discomfort is managed with analgesics and sedatives. Care of blistered skin is similar to that described for burns. It is seldom possible to estimate the extent of tissue loss until new skin layers are revealed after the eschar layer separates.

KEY POINTS

- Therapeutic management of skin disorders includes a variety of methods and agents to cool, soothe, and reduce the irritating effects of external stimuli.
- A moist environment promotes healing of wounds.
- Skin infections can be caused by bacteria, viruses, or fungi.
- Some diseases manifested in the skin are transmitted by arthropod vectors, especially ticks.
- The most common skin infestations of childhood—scabies and pediculosis capitis—can affect children of any age and from any social class.
- Contact dermatitis may involve a primary irritant or a sensitizing agent.
- Adverse reactions to drugs are manifested more often in the skin than in any other body organ.
- The most common skin disorders of infancy are diaper dermatitis, seborrheic dermatitis, and atopic dermatitis.
- Acne, a disorder affecting a large proportion of adolescents, is related to maturation of pilosebaceous follicles and increased androgen secretion.
- Noninflammatory acne is predominantly an obstructive disease characterized by open and closed comedones; lesions of inflammatory acne consist of papules, pustules, nodules, and cysts.
- Burns are caused by thermal, chemical, electric, or radioactive agents.
- Burns are assessed on the extent, depth, and severity of the wound.
- Essentials of emergency care of burn injury include stopping the burning process, covering the burn, transporting the injured child to medical aid, and providing reassurance to the child and family.
- Management of minor burns consists of facilitating wound healing, relieving discomfort, and preventing complications.
- Management of major burns consists of facilitating wound healing, relieving discomfort, replacing destroyed skin, preventing and/or treating complications, and providing rehabilitation.
- Sunscreen is recommended for use when the skin is exposed to the damaging effects of the sun's rays.
- Thermal injuries to the skin can result from exposure to extreme cold.

REFERENCES

Adams LE, Hunt JL, Purdue GF: Tap water scald burns: awareness is not the problem, *J Burn Care Rehabil* 12(1):91-95, 1991.

Alvarez O, Rozint J, Meehan M: Principles of moist wound healing: indications for chronic wounds. In Krasner D, editor: *Chronic wound care: a clinical source book for health care professionals,* King of Prussia, PA, 1990, Health Management.

American Academy of Pediatrics, Committee on Drugs: Retinoid therapy for severe dermatological disorders, *Pediatrics* 90:119-120, 1992.

Atchison NE and others: Pain during burn dressing change in children: relationship to burn area, depth and analgesic regimens, *Pain* 47:41-45, 1991.

Bikowski J: Effectively treating acne vulgaris, *Phys Sports Med* 20:100-107, 1992.

Boyce ST and others: Skin anatomy and antigen expression after burn wound closure with composite grafts of cultures, skin cells and biopolymers, *Plast Reconstr Surg* 91:632-641, 1993.

Clore ER, Longyear LA: A comparative study of seven pediculides and their packaged nit removal combs, *J Pediatr Health Care* 7(2):55-60, 1993.

Cooper LI: Removing cactus spines *Am J Dis Child* 142:1140, 1988 (letter).

Erickson EJ and others: Differences in mortality from thermal injury between pediatric and adult patients, *J Pediatr Surg* 26(7):821-825, 1991.

Finkelstein JL and others: Pediatric burns: an overview, *Pediatr Clin North Am* 39:1145-1163, 1992.

Groeneveld A, Inkson T: Ketamine: a solution to procedural pain in burned children, *Can Nurse* 88(8):28-31, 1992.

Hanifin JM: Atopic dermatitis in infants and children, *Pediatr Clin North Am* 38(4):763-790, 1991.

Hunt TK: Basic principles of wound healing, *J Trauma* 30 (12, suppl):S122-S128, 1990.

Hurwitz S: Skin lesions in the first year of life, *Contemp Pediatr* 10(1):110-128, 1993.

Jenkins M, Gottschlich M, Warden G: Enteral support during operative procedures, *J Burn Care Rehabil* 15:199-205, 1994.

Kavanagh CK and others: Learned helplessness and the pediatric burn patient: dressing change behavior and serum cortisol and β-endorphin. In Barness LA, editor: *Advances in pediatrics,* vol 38, St Louis, 1991, Mosby.

Lee JJ and others: Infection control in a burn center, *J Burn Care Rehabil* 11(6):575-580, 1990.

Leyden JJ: Cornstarch, Candida albicans, and diaper rash, *Pediatr Dermatol* 1(4):322-325, 1984.

Margileth A, Hadfield T: A new look at old cat-scratch, *Contemp Pediatr* 7(12):25-48, 1990.

Martinez TT and others: Removal of cactus spines from the skin, *Am J Dis Child* 141:1291-1292, 1987.

Osmond MH, Klassen TP, Quinn JV: Economic comparison of a tissue adhesive and suturing in the repair of pediatric facial lacerations, *J Pediatr* 126(6):892-895, 1995.

Peate WF: Outpatient management of burns, *Am Fam Physician* 45:1321-1330, 1992.

Riegger M, Guntzelman J: Prevention and amelioration of stress and consequences of interaction between children and dogs, *JAMA* 196(11):1781-1785, 1990.

Selbst SM: Pain management in the emergency department. In Schechter N, Berde C, Yaster M: *Pain in infants, children, and adolescents,* Baltimore, 1993, Williams & Wilkins.

Smith GA and others: Comparison of topical anesthetics without cocaine to tetracaine-adrenaline-cocaine and lidocaine infiltration during repair of lacerations: bupivacaine-norepinephrine is an effective new topical anesthetic agent, *Pediatrics* 97(3):301-307, 1996.

Stanford DG and others: Sun protection by a summer weight garment: the effects of washing and wearing, *Med J Aust* 162(8):422-425, 1995.

Taplin D and others: Comparison of crotamiton 10% cream (Eurax) and permethrin 5% cream (Elimite) for the treatment of scabies in children, *Pediatr Dermatol* 7(1):67-73, 1990.

Wong DL and others: Diapering choices: a critical review of the issues, *Pediatr Nurs* 18(1):41-54, 1992.

BIBLIOGRAPHY

Skin Disorders: General

Bolton L, Rijswijk LV: Wound dressings: meeting clinical and biological needs, *Dermatol Nurs* 3(1):146-161, 1991.

Carney M: A suture nurse program in a pediatric emergency department, *J Emerg Nurs* 20:517-520, 1994.

Ching D, Mell D: Use of adhesive dressings in skin care: DuoDerm Extra Thin, *J Pediatr Health Care* 4(3):155-156, 1990.

Cuzzell JZ, Stotts NA: Trial and error yields to knowledge, *Am J Nurs* 90(10):53-63, 1990.

Engebo DA: Safe and effective use of tetracaine, adrenaline, and cocaine (TAC) solution anesthetic for anesthetizing of lacerations, *J Emerg Nurs* 16:100-101, 1990.

Ernst AA and others: Lidocaine adrenaline tetracaine gel versus tetracaine adrenaline cocaine gel for topical anesthesia in linear scalp and facial lacerations in children aged 5 to 17 years, *Pediatrics* 95(2):255-258, 1995.

Hagelgans NA: Pediatric skin care issues for the home care nurse, *Pediatr Nurs* 19(5):499-507, 1993.

Hurwitz S: *Clinical pediatric dermatology: a textbook of skin disorders of childhood and adolescence,* ed 2, Philadelphia, 1993, WB Saunders.

Schilling CG and others: Tetracaine, epinephrine (adrenalin), and cocaine (TAC) versus lidocaine, epinephrine, and tetracaine (LET) for anesthesia of lacerations in children, *Ann Emerg Med* 25:203-208, 1995.

Smith DP, Kemper JY: Skin therapy. In Smith DP and others, editors: *Comprehensive child and family nursing skills,* St Louis, 1991, Mosby.

Wysocki A: Skin structure. In Bryant RA, editor: *Acute and chronic wounds: nursing management,* St Louis, 1992, Mosby.

Wounds

Bryant RA, editor: *Acute and chronic wounds: nursing management,* St Louis, 1992, Mosby–Year Book.

Cuzzell JZ, Stotts NA: Wound care: trial and error yields to knowledge, *Am J Nurs* 90(10):53-63, 1990.

Garvin G: Wound healing in pediatrics, *Nurs Clin North Am* 25(1):181-192, 1990.

Harding KG: Wound care: putting theory into clinical practice, *Wounds* 2(1):21-32, 1990.

Norris S, Provo B, Stotts N: Physiology of wound healing and risk factors that impede the healing process, *AACN Clin Issues Crit Care Nurs* 1(3):545-552, 1990.

Oberg MS, Lindsey D: Do not put hydrogen peroxide or povidone-iodine into wounds! *Am J Dis Child* 141(1):27-28, 1987.

O'Hanlon-Nichols T: Commonly asked questions about wound healing, *Am J Nurs* 95(4):22-24, 1995.

Ratner MH: A short course in wound care for children, *Contemp Pediatr* 8(8):22-38, 1991.

Rodeheaver G and others: Wound healing and wound management: focus on debridement, *Adv Wound Care* 7(1):22-39, 1994.

Infections/Infestations

Brady M: Common viral skin problems of childhood: warts and molluscum, *J Pediatr Health Care* 2:208-210, 1988.

Brimhall CL, Esterly NB: Uninvited guests: skin infestations of childhood, *Contemp Pediatr* 7(1):18-57, 1990.

Brozena SJ: Scabies: update on diagnosis and treatment, *J Sch Nurs* 8(4):15-19, 1992.

Halpern JS: Recognition and treatment of pediculosis (head lice) in the emergency department, *J Emerg Nurs* 20(2):130-133, 1994.

Krugman S and others: *Infectious diseases of children,* ed 9, St Louis, 1992, Mosby.

Molinaro F: Treatment of pediculosis and scabies, *Pediatr Nurs* 18(6):600-602, 1992.

Rasmussen JE: Cutaneous fungus infections in children, *Pediatr Rev* 13(4):152-156, 1992.

Rasmussen JE: Impetigo: changing bacteria, changing therapies, *Contemp Pediatr* 9(2):14-22, 1992.

Sokoloff F: Identification and management of pediculosis, *Nurs Pract* 19(8):62-64, 1994.

Walker DH, Dumler JS: Emerging and reemerging rickettsial diseases, *New Engl J Med* 331(24):1651-1652, 1994.

Age-Related Skin Disorders

Berg R: Etiology and pathophysiology of diaper dermatitis, *Adv Dermatol* 3:75-98, 1988.

Casimir GJA and others: Atopic dermatitis: role of food and house dust mite allergens, *Pediatrics* 92(2):252-256, 1993.

Castiglia PT: Acne, *J Pediatr Health Care* 3:259-261, 1989.

Farrington E: Diaper dermatitis, *Pediatr Nurs* 18(1):81-82, 1992.

Garvin G: Skin care considerations in the neonate for the ET nurse, *J Enterostom Ther* 17(6):225-230, 1990.

Holaday B and others: Diaper type and fecal contamination in child day care, *J Pediatr Health Care* 9(2):67-74, 1995.

Holaday B and others: Fecal contamination in child day care centers: cloth vs paper, *Am J Public Health* 85(1):30-33, 1995.

Hurwitz S: Acne treatment for the '90s, *Contemp Pediatr* 12(8):19-32, 1995.

Jick SS and others: First trimester topical tretinoin and congenital disorders, *Lancet* 341:1181-1182, 1993.

Kubiak M and others: Comparison of stool containment in cloth and single-use diapers using a simulated infant feces, *Pediatrics* 91(3):632-636, 1993.

Lane A, Rehder P, Helm K: Evaluations of diapers containing absorbent gelling material with conventional disposable diapers in newborn infants, *Am J Dis Child* 144(3):315-318, 1990.

Novick NL: Diaper rashes, *Pharmacol Times* 57(5):41-47, 1991.

Novotny J: Adolescents, acne, and the side-effects of Accutane, *Pediatr Nurs* 15:247-248, 1989.

Pairaudeau P and others: Inhalation of baby powder: an unappreciated hazard, *Br Med J* 302:1200-1201, 1991.

Rothman KF, Lucky AW: Acne vulgaris, *Adv Dermatol* 8:347-374, 1993.

White KH: Diapering and skin care. In Smith DP and others, editors: *Comprehensive child and family nursing skills*, St Louis, 1991, Mosby.

Bites, Stings, and Other Animal-Related Disorders

Adamski DB: Assessment and treatment of allergic response to stinging insects, *J Emerg Nurs* 16:77-80, 1990.

Agre F, Schwartz R: The value of early treatment of deer tick bites for the prevention of Lyme disease, *Am J Dis Child* 147:945-947, 1993.

Carithers H, Margileth A: Cat-scratch disease: acute encephalopathy and other neurologic manifestations, *Am J Dis Child* 145(1):98-101, 1991.

Clore ER: Dispelling the common myths about pediculosis, *J Pediatr Health Care* 3:28-33, 1989.

Clore ER: Head-lice screening, *Sch Health Watch* 5(2):2, 1994.

Collipp PJ: Cat-scratch disease: therapy with trimethoprim-sulfamethoxazole, *Am J Dis Child* 146(4):397-399, 1992.

Distinguishing Lyme disease from its look-alikes, *Emerg Med* 24(11):28-50, 1992.

Guin JD, Kligman AM, Maibach HI: Managing the poison-plant rashes, *Patient Care* 26(8):63-66, 70-72, 1992.

Hibel JA, Clore ER: Prevention and primary care treatment of stings from imported fire ants, *Nurse Practitioner* 17(6):65-71, 1992.

Koehler JE: Progress in cat scratch disease, *JAMA* 271:531, 1994.

Protecting yourself from poison ivy, oak, and sumac, *Patient Care* 26(8):77-78, 1992.

Shewell PC, Nancarrow JD: Dogs that bite, *Br Med J* 303(6816):1512-1513, 1991.

Slota M, O'Connor K: Recognizing and treating cat scratch disease with encephalopathy in children, *Crit Care Nurse* 12(6):39-42, 1992.

Sofer S, Shahak E, Gueron M: Scorpion envenomation and antivenom therapy, *J Pediatr* 124:973-978, 1994.

Stafford CT, Moffitt JE, Yates AB: Insect sting anaphylaxis referral is imperative, *Emerg Med* 24(11):230-231, 1992.

Walker DH: Rocky Mountain spotted fever: a seasonal alert, *Clin Infect Dis* 20(5):1111-1117, 1995.

Miscellaneous Skin Disorders

Ansell BM, Falcini F, Woo P: Scleroderma in childhood, *Clin Dermatol* 12:299-307, 1994.

Castiglia PT: Alopecia, *J Pediatr Health Care* 5(1):44-46, 1991.

Hofman KJ and others: Neurofibromatosis type 1: the cognitive phenotype, *J Pediatr* 124(4):S1-S8, 1994.

Kaminester LH: The many guises of psoriasis, *J Emerg Med* 25(7):27-41, 1993.

Korf BR: Diagnostic outcome in children with multiple café au lait spots, *Pediatrics* 90(6):924-927, 1992.

Mackreth B: Poison ivy, don't rub it the wrong way, *Patient Care* 16(8):21-25, 1991.

Nigro JF, Esterly NB: Psoriasis—chronic but controllable, *Contemp Pediatr* 10(10):114-128, 1993.

New retinoid gel studied for psoriasis, *Dermatol Nurs* 7(1):65, 1995.

Phillips T, Dover J: Recent advances in dermatology, *N Engl J Med* 326(3):167-178, 1992.

Rasmussen JE: Erythema multiforme, Stevens-Johnson syndrome, and toxic epidermal necrolysis, *Dermatol Nurs* 7(1):37-43, 1995.

Thermal Injuries

Adler R: Burns are different: the child psychiatrist on the pediatric burns ward, *J Burn Care Rehabil* 13(1):28-32, 1992.

Bargoil SC, Erdman LK: Safe tan, an oxymoron, *Cancer Nurs* 16(2):139-144, 1993.

Carr DB, Osgood PF, Szyfelbein SK: Treatment of pain in acutely burned children. In Schechter N, Berde C, Yaster M: *Pain in infants, children, and adolescents*, Baltimore, 1993, Williams & Wilkins.

Faldmo L, Kravitz M: Management of acute burns and burn shock resuscitation, *AACN Clin Issues* 4:351-366, 1993.

Gottschlich MM, Alexander JW, Bower RH: Enteral nutrition in patients with burns or trauma. In Rombeau JL, Caldwell MD, editors: *Enteral and tube feeding*, Philadelphia, 1990, WB Saunders.

Harrell D, Hoelker L, Maley MS: Community burn prevention, *Proc Am Burn Assoc* 26:66, 1994.

Helvig E: Pediatric burn injuries, *AACN Clin Issues* 4:433-442, 1993.

Hendricks L and others: Subanesthetic ketamine for painful nonoperative procedures in pediatric burn patients, *Proc Am Burn Assoc* 23:52, 1991.

Hermans M, Hermans R: Burns: Duoderm, an alternative dressing for smaller burns, *Burns* 12(3):214-219, 1986.

Herndon DN, Rutan RL, Rutan TC: Management of the pediatric patient with burns, *J Burn Care Rehabil* 14:3-8, 1993.

Holaday M, Blakeney P: A comparison of psychologic functioning in children and adolescents with severe burns on the Rorschach and the child behavior checklist, *J Burn Care Rehabil* 15(5):412-415, 1994.

Housinger TA, Hills J, Warden GD: Management of pediatric facial burns, *J Burn Care Rehabil* 15(5):408-411, 1994.

Housinger TA, Wondrely L, Warden GD: The use of Biobrane for pediatric donor sites, *J Burn Care Rehabil* 14:26-28, 1993.

Jessee PO: Perception of body image in children with burns, five years after burn injury, *J Burn Care Rehabil* 13(1):33-38, 1992.

Kinner MA, Daly WL: Skin transplantation, *Crit Care Nurs Clin North Am* 4:173-178, 1992.

Maley M: Scald in the kitchen, *Information Exchange* 9:1-5, 1993.

Martinez S: Ambulatory management of burns in children, *J Pediatr Health Care* 6(1):32-37, 1992.

Munster AM: *Severe burns: a family guide to medical and emotional recovery*, Baltimore, 1993, Johns Hopkins University Press.

Osgood PF, Szyfelbein SK: Management of burn pain in children, *Pediatr Clin North Am* 36:1001-1013, 1989.

Patterson DR: Practical applications of psychological techniques in controlling burn pain, *J Burn Care Rehabil* 13(1):13-18, 1992.

Rieg LS, Jenkins M: Burn injuries in children, *Crit Care Clin North Am* 3:457-470, 1991.

Rumsfield J: Sunscreen: what you and your patients should know, *Dermatol Nurs* 2(3):139-147, 1990.

Sheridan RL and others: Midazolam infusion in pediatric patients with burns who are undergoing mechanical ventilation, *J Burn Care Rehabil* 15(6):515-518, 1994.

Sullivan SA: How severe is this frostbite? *Am J Nurs* 93(2):59-64, 1993.

Taking the bite out of frostbite, *Emerg Med* 24(2):121-138, 1992.

Truhan AP: Sun protection in childhood, *Clin Pediatr* 30(7):412-421, 1991.

U.S. Consumer Product Safety Commission: Child-resistant lighter standard moves forward, *News from CPSS*, Release no. 92-123, July 29, 1992.

Vitale M, Fields-Blanche C, Luterman A: Severe itching in the patient with burns, *J Burn Care Rehabil* 12(4):330-333, 1991.

Walter P: Burn wound management, *AACN Clin Issues* 4:378-387, 1993.

Warden GD: Burn shock resuscitation, *World J Surg* 16:16-23, 1992.

Yarbrough DR: Improving survival in the burned patient, *J S C Med Assoc* 86(6):347-349, 1990.

Zingg BM: Managing burns in children: an intraoperative nursing care plan, *AORN J* 54:568-575, 1991.

Chapter 31

THE CHILD WITH MUSCULOSKELETAL OR ARTICULAR DYSFUNCTION

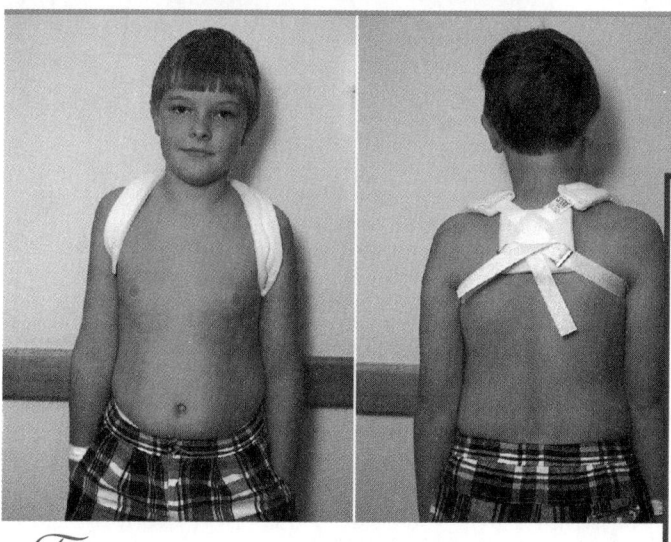

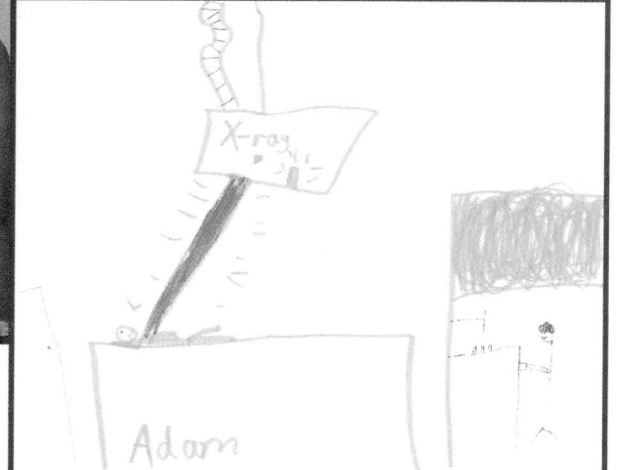

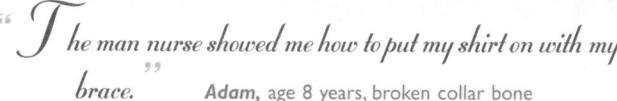

"The man nurse showed me how to put my shirt on with my brace." **Adam,** age 8 years, broken collar bone

RELATED TOPICS

THE IMMOBILIZED CHILD

IMMOBILIZATION

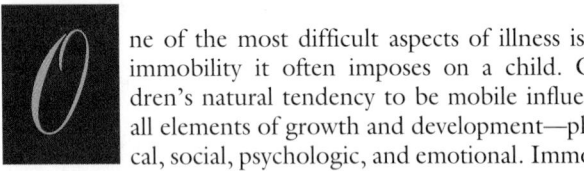 ne of the most difficult aspects of illness is the immobility it often imposes on a child. Children's natural tendency to be mobile influences all elements of growth and development—physical, social, psychologic, and emotional. Immobility restricts expression and causes anxiety and frustration. For these reasons children are immobilized only when necessary and for the shortest time possible.

Physiologic Effects of Immobilization

Functional and metabolic responses to restricted movement can be noted in most of the body systems, all of which have a direct influence on the child's growth and development, because homeostatic mechanisms thrive on normal use and need feedback to maintain dynamic equilibrium. Most of the pathologic changes that take place during immobilization arise from decreased muscle strength and mass, decreased metabolism, and bone demineralization, which are closely interrelated. Some results of immobilization are primary and produce a direct effect; others seem to be more indirect, or secondary and affect more than one body system.

The major effects of immobilization are outlined briefly in Table 31-1. They are related directly or indirectly to decreased muscle activity, which produces numerous primary changes in both muscular and bone structures with secondary alterations in the cardiovascular, respiratory, metabolic, and renal systems. The major consequences are the following:

1. Significant loss of muscle strength, endurance, and muscle mass (atrophy)
2. Bone demineralization leading to osteoporosis
3. Loss of joint mobility and contractures

The larger the portion of the body immobilized and the longer the immobilization, the greater the hazards of immobility.

Psychologic Effects of Immobilization

Throughout childhood, physical activity is an integral part of daily life and is essential for physical growth and development. The activity helps children deal with a variety of feelings and impulses and provides a mechanism by which they can exert control over inner tensions. Children respond to anxiety with increased activity. Removal of this power deprives them of necessary input and a natural outlet for their feelings and fantasies.

When children are immobilized by disease or as part of a treatment regimen, they experience diminished environmental stimuli with a loss of tactile input and an altered perception of themselves and their environment. Sudden or gradual immobilization narrows the amount and variety of environmental stimuli children receive by means of all of their senses: touch, sight, hearing, taste, smell, and proprioception—a feeling of where they are in their environment. This sensory deprivation frequently leads to feelings of isolation and boredom, and of being forgotten, especially by peers (see Family Focus box on p. 1124).

Physical interference with the activity of infants and young children gives them a feeling of helplessness. Even speech and language skills require sensorimotor activity and experience. Children who are restrained by casts, splints, or straps during the first 3 years of life may have more difficulty with language than children whose activities are unrestricted.

For the toddler, exploration and imitative behaviors are essential to developing a sense of autonomy; the preschooler's expression of initiative is evidenced by the need for vigorous physical activity; the school-age child's development is strongly influenced by physical achievement and competition; and the adolescent relies on mobility to achieve independence. The quest for mastery at every stage of development is related to mobility.

The monotony of immobilization can lead to sluggish intellectual and psychomotor responses, decreased communication skills, increased fantasizing, and even hallucinations and disorientation. Children are likely to become depressed over loss of ability to function or the marked changes in body image. They may seek the attention of others by reverting to earlier developmental behaviors, such as wanting to be fed, bed-wetting, and baby talk.

Shona Swenson Lenss, BSN, RN, revised this chapter.

TABLE 31-1. Summary of physical effects of immobilization*

PRIMARY EFFECTS	SECONDARY EFFECTS	PRIMARY EFFECTS	SECONDARY EFFECTS
Muscular System		**Cardiovascular System—cont'd**	
Decreased muscle strength, tone, and endurance	Decreased venous return and decreased cardiac output	Altered distribution of blood volume	Decreased cardiac workload Decreased exercise tolerance
	Decreased metabolism and need for oxygen	Venous stasis	Pulmonary emboli and/or thrombi
	Decreased exercise tolerance	Dependent edema	Tissue breakdown and susceptibility to infection
	Bone demineralization		
Disuse atrophy and loss of muscle mass	Catabolism Loss of strength	**Respiratory System**	
Loss of joint mobility	Contractures, ankylosis of joints	Decreased need for oxygen	Altered oxygen—carbon dioxide exchange and metabolism
Weak back muscles	Secondary spinal deformities	Decreased chest expansion and diminished vital capacity	Diminished oxygen intake Dyspnea and inadequate arterial oxygen saturation; acidosis
Weak abdominal muscles	Impaired respiration		
Skeletal System		Poor abdominal tone and distention	Interference with diaphragmatic excursion
Bone demineralization—osteoporosis, hypercalcemia	Negative calcium balance Pathologic fractures Calcium deposits Extraosseous bone formation, especially at hip, knee, elbow, and shoulder Renal calculi	Mechanical or biochemical secretion retention	Hypostatic pneumonia Bacterial and viral pneumonia Atelectasis
		Loss of respiratory muscle strength	Poor cough Upper respiratory infection
Negative calcium balance	Life-threatening electrolyte imbalance	**Gastrointestinal System**	
Metabolism		Distention caused by poor abdominal muscle tone	Interference with respiratory movements
Decreased metabolic rate	Slowing of all systems Decreased food intake	No specific primary effect	Difficulty in feeding in prone position; gravitation effect on feces through ascending colon, or weakened smooth muscle tone may cause constipation Anorexia
Negative nitrogen balance	Decline in nutritional state Impaired healing		
Hypercalcemia	Electrolyte imbalance		
Decreased production of stress hormones	Decreased physical and emotional coping capacity	**Urinary System**	
		Alteration of gravitational force	Difficulty in voiding in prone position
Cardiovascular System		Impaired ureteral peristalsis	Urinary retention in calyces and bladder Infection Renal calculi
Decreased efficiency of orthostatic neurovascular reflexes	Inability to adapt readily to upright position Pooling of blood in extremities in upright posture	**Integumentary System**	
Diminished vasopressor mechanism	Orthostatic hypotension with syncope—hypotension, decreased cerebral blood flow, tachycardia	No specific primary effect	Decreased circulation and pressure leading to tissue injury and decreased healing capacity Difficulty with personal hygiene

*Not all problems will apply in every situation.

FAMILY FOCUS
Immobilization and Self-Esteem

Immobilization, as with any illness or disorder that is debilitating in some way, may restrict children from participating in age-appropriate activities. These children may be labeled as "different," and over time, this may result in a child feeling unaccepted. In young children, acceptance from their peers is an important component in the formulation of their self-esteem. The assessment of self-esteem in young children is a critical attribute to their well-being. It is important to educate children about their illness and encourage them to engage in activities. Children who have a strong sense of self-worth and confidence are able to initiate activities and explore their environment. They approach tasks and relationships with the expectation that they will be well received and successful.

Also, limbs in casts or traction transmit less than normal sensory data. Children who have limited ability to feel others touching them not only experience less tactile stimuli in a physical sense but are also deprived of warm, loving feelings that arise from being touched. The loss of feeling derived from touch can further add to their sense of being isolated and unwanted.

Children may react to immobility by active protest, anger, and aggressive behavior, or they may become quiet, passive, and submissive. Children should be allowed to discharge their anger, but it should be within the limits of safety to their self-esteem and not damaging to the integrity of others. For example, providing an object to attack rather than a person or a valued possession is safe and therapeutic. When children are unable to express anger, aggression is often displayed inappropriately through regressive behavior and outbursts of crying or temper tantrums.

Effect on Families

Brief periods of immobilization have few effects on the family; however, catastrophic illness or disability may severely tax their resources.

The family's needs often must be met by the services of a multidisciplinary team, and nurses play a key role in anticipating the services they will need and in coordinating conferences to plan care. In preparation for discharge, home visits are advisable, and home management is frequently planned weeks in advance of the actual discharge, including special considerations for cultural, economic, physical, and psychologic needs. A child with a severe disability is very dependent, and caregivers need rest periods to revitalize themselves. Individual and group counseling is beneficial for preproblem-solving situations and provides an emotional support system. Parent groups are also helpful and often allow nonthreatening social contact. The families of children with permanent disabilities need long-term resources, since some of the most difficult problems arise as they try to sustain high-quality care for many years (see Chapter 20).

Nursing Considerations

❖ Assessment

Assessment of the child who is immobilized as a result of an injury or a degenerative disease includes not only the injured part such as a fracture or damaged joint, but also the functioning of other systems that may be affected secondarily—the circulatory, renal, respiratory, muscular, and gastrointestinal systems. In long-term immobilization there may also be neurologic impairment and metabolic changes in electrolytes (especially calcium), nitrogen balance, and general metabolic rate.

Nursing assessment includes psychosocial data, as well as physical manifestations, since long-term immobilization has a profound effect on the child and family. Nursing approaches are evaluated frequently and continued, discontinued, or modified to meet the changing problems and goals.

❖ Nursing Diagnoses

Nursing diagnoses for the immobilized child are outlined in the Nursing Care Plan on p. 1125. Others will be identified in specific cases.

❖ Planning

The general goals of care for the immobilized child and family include the following:

1. Child will experience no physical injury.
2. Child will experience no psychologic complications.
3. Child will engage in appropriate diversional activities.
4. Child and family will receive adequate support.

❖ Implementation

Frequent position changes help to prevent dependent edema and fluid movement and to stimulate circulation, respiratory function, gastrointestinal motility, and neurologic sensations. The use of antiembolism stockings or Ace wraps may minimize or prevent dependent edema and fluid shifts to third spaces. Metabolism is increased by activity within the limitations of the disability and capabilities of the child. High-protein, high-calorie foods are encouraged for correction of negative nitrogen balance, which may be difficult to correct by diet, especially if there is loss of appetite. Stimulating the appetite with small servings of attractively arranged, preferred foods may be sufficient. Sometimes supplementary nasogastric feedings, gastrostomy feedings, or total parenteral nutrition may be needed.*

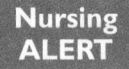 Lying in a prone position during feeding increases the risk of aspiration. Therefore suction is kept nearby.

Adequate hydration promotes bowel and kidney function and helps prevent complications in these systems. It is also a primary measure for managing hypercalcemia, in addition to restricting high-calcium foods.

Children are encouraged to be as active as their condition and restrictive devices allow. This poses few problems for children, whose innate ingenuity and natural inclination toward mobility provide them with the impetus for physical activity. They need the opportunity, the materials or objects to stimulate activity, and the encouragement and participation of oth-

---

*Home care instructions on giving nasogastric tube feedings and gastrostomy tube feedings are available in Wong DL: *Wong and Whaley's Clinical manual of pediatric nursing,* ed 4, St Louis, 1996, Mosby.

NURSING CARE PLAN
The Child Who Is Immobilized

NURSING DIAGNOSIS: Impaired physical mobility related to mechanical restrictions, physical disability (specify level)

PATIENT GOAL 1: Will have opportunity for mobilization

- **NURSING INTERVENTIONS/RATIONALES**

Transport child by gurney, stroller, wagon, bed, wheelchair, or other conveyance from confines of room *to provide for mobilization despite restrictions.*

Change position of bed in room *to alter monotony of immobilization.*

Change position in bed when possible *to decrease feelings of being immobilized.*

- **EXPECTED OUTCOMES**

Child moves from confines of room or within room.

Child's position is changed when possible.

PATIENT GOAL 2: Will maintain optimum autonomy

- **NURSING INTERVENTIONS/RATIONALES**

Provide mobilizing devices (orthoses, crutches, wheelchair).

Assist with acquisition of specialized equipment *to encourage independence.*

Instruct in use of equipment *to ensure safety.*

Encourage activities that require mobilization.

Allow as much freedom of movement as possible and encourage normal activities *to maintain a sense of autonomy.*

Encourage child to participate in own care as much as possible *to encourage sense of autonomy and independence.*

Allow child to make choices (e.g., daily routine, food, clothes) *to encourage sense of autonomy despite limitations.*

- **EXPECTED OUTCOMES**

Child moves about without assistance.

Child engages in activities appropriate to limitations and developmental level.

NURSING DIAGNOSIS: High risk for impaired skin integrity related to immobility, therapeutic appliances

PATIENT GOAL 1: Will maintain skin integrity

- **NURSING INTERVENTIONS/RATIONALES**

Place child on pressure-reducing surface *to prevent tissue breakdown and pressure necrosis.*

Change position frequently, unless contraindicated, *to prevent dependent edema and stimulate circulation.*

Protect pressure points (e.g., trochanter, sacrum, ankle, shoulder, occiput) with proper positioning and cushioning (i.e., pillow between legs) *to prevent decreased bloodflow to area.*

Inspect skin surfaces regularly for signs of irritation, redness, evidence of pressure.

Eliminate mechanical factors causing pressure, friction, or irritation (e.g., keep linen and clothing free of wrinkles).

Maintain meticulous skin cleanliness.

Gently massage with or without lubricating substance *to stimulate circulation.*

- **EXPECTED OUTCOME**

Skin remains clean and intact with no evidence of irritation.

NURSING DIAGNOSIS: High risk for injury related to impaired mobility

PATIENT GOAL 1: Will experience no physical injury

- **NURSING INTERVENTIONS/RATIONALES**

Teach correct use of mobilizing devices and/or apparatus *to ensure safety.*

Assist with moving and/or ambulating as needed *to ensure safety.*

Remove hazards from environment (specify).

Modify environment as needed (specify).

Keep call button within reach.

Keep siderails up at all times *to prevent falls.*

Help child to use bathroom or commode if possible.

Implement safety measures appropriate to child's developmental age (specify).

- **EXPECTED OUTCOME**

Child remains free of injury.

NURSING DIAGNOSIS: Diversional activity deficit related to impaired mobility, musculoskeletal impairment, confinement to hospital or home

PATIENT GOAL 1: Will engage in diversional activity

- **NURSING INTERVENTIONS/RATIONALES AND EXPECTED OUTCOMES**

See Nursing Care Plan: The Child in the Hospital, Chapter 21.

NURSING DIAGNOSIS: Altered family processes related to a child with disability, illness

PATIENT (FAMILY) GOAL 1: Will receive adequate support

- **NURSING INTERVENTIONS/RATIONALES AND EXPECTED OUTCOMES**

See Nursing Care Plan: The Family of the Ill or Hospitalized Child, Chapter 21.

ers. Those who are unable to move need passive exercise and movement.

Whenever possible, transporting the child by stretcher, stroller, or wagon outside the confines of the room increase environmental stimuli and provide social contact with others. While hospitalized, children benefit from frequent visitors, clocks and calendars, and a program of diversional therapy, all of which help them to function in a more normal way. As soon as possible, they should wear "street clothes" and resume school and preinjury hobbies. The use of play (see Chapter 21) and any activity that is tolerated (e.g., turning in bed or changing the position of a bed in the room) help to alter the monotony of immobilization and decrease tension and frustration.

Using dolls to illustrate and explain the restraining method is a valuable tool for small children. Placing a cast, tubing, or other restraining equipment on the doll offers the child a nonthreatening opportunity to express, through the doll, feelings concerning the restrictions and feelings toward the nurse and other health providers. It also provides a means for anticipatory teaching and explanation of needed restraining devices.

One of the most useful interventions to help children cope with immobility is participation in their own care. Self-care to the maximum extent is usually well received by children. They can help plan their daily routine, select their diet (when possible), and choose the clothes they are to wear, including innovative adornment, such as a baseball cap, brightly colored stockings, or other items of apparel that express each child's autonomy and individuality. They are encouraged to do as much for themselves as they are able in order to keep muscles active and their interest alive. If feasible, they should be placed where they can benefit from the company of other children who are immobilized, which assures them that they are not singled out for this treatment.

It is important for children to understand behavioral limitations or rules, and their questions should be answered. For example, they need to know the reasons for medical, nursing, occupational, and physical therapy and to know that schedules are necessary. In some areas they have a choice; in others they do not. They may or may not be permitted to sleep late, but they can choose their own clothing. Most of children's activity of daily living is play; therefore therapies that incorporate this concept are more apt to gain their cooperation.

Visits from significant persons, such as family members and friends, offer occasions for emotional support and also provide opportunities for learning how to care for the child. Some privacy is needed, particularly by the teenager, and most long-term health care facilities recognize that rooms shared by two to four children, rather than large wards, are better environments for habilitation or rehabilitation. Selecting roommates according to age and companionship gives each child the chance to test out thoughts and feelings safely with others. If a traumatic incident caused the child's disability, guilt feelings may be displayed overtly or masked behind regressive or aggressive behavior. The feeling that "I must have been bad for this to happen" is common, and honest feedback stating, "It just happened—it was an accident," needs to be repeated many times.

For a child with greatly restricted movement (e.g., the quadriplegic child or the child with a large bilateral hip spica cast), nursing care is a challenge. These situations require long-term care either in the hospital or at home, but wherever the care occurs, consistent planning and coordination of activities with professionals and significant others are vital nursing functions.

Family Support and Home Care.   The needs of a child with severe disabilities can be very complex, and family members require time to assimilate the teachings and demonstrations needed to understand the child's situation and care. Even the child who is confined on a short-term basis can be a challenge for the family, which is usually unprepared for the problems imposed by the child's special needs. Home modification is usually needed for facilitating care, especially when it involves traction, large casts, or extended confinement. Suitable child care may be needed for times when all family members work.

Just as in the hospital, the child at home is encouraged to be as independent as possible and to follow a schedule that approximates his or her normal life-style as nearly as possible, such as continuing school lessons, regular bedtime, and suitable recreational activities.

❖ Evaluation

The effectiveness of nursing interventions is determined by continual reassessment and evaluation of care based on the following observational guidelines and expected outcomes:

1. Observe vital signs, neurologic signs, and respiratory, gastrointestinal, and renal functioning; inspect skin; observe effects of correct functioning of equipment and appliances (restraints, traction, cast, braces).
2. Observe child's behavior; engage in dialogue to elicit feelings, concerns, and interests.
3. Observe child's activities and interests.
4. Interview child and family regarding their feelings and concerns; observe family interaction at home, if possible.

Expected outcomes:
See Nursing Care Plan, p. 1125.

TRAUMATIC INJURY

SOFT TISSUE INJURY

Injuries to the muscles, ligaments, and tendons are common in children (Fig. 31-1). In young children, soft tissue injury usually results from mishaps during play. In older children and adolescents, participation in sports is the more common cause.

Contusions

A contusion is damage to the soft tissue, subcutaneous structures, and muscle. The tearing of these tissues and small blood vessels and the inflammatory response lead to hemorrhage, edema, and associated pain when the child attempts to move the injured part. The escape of blood into the tissues is observed as *ecchymosis*, a black-and-blue discoloration. Immediate treatment consists of cold application, as in the treatment of sprains described below. Return to participation is allowed when the strength and range of motion of the affected extremity are equal to those of the opposite extremity.

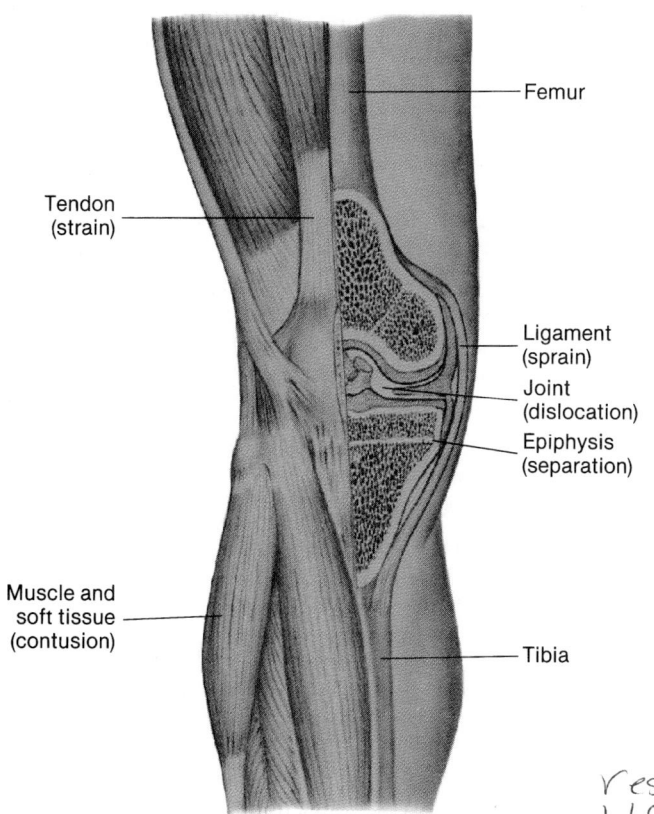

Tendon
(strain)

Femur

Ligament
(sprain)

Joint
(dislocation)

Epiphysis
(separation)

Muscle and
soft tissue
(contusion)

Tibia

FIG. 31-1. Sites of injuries to bones, joints, and soft tissues.

Related to contusions are crush injuries that occur in children when they slam their fingers (in doors, folding chairs, or equipment) or hit their fingers (as when hammering a nail). A severe crush injury involves the bone, with swelling and bleeding beneath the nail (subungual) and sometimes laceration of the pulp of the distal phalanx. The subungual hematoma can be released by drilling holes at the proximal end of the nail. The time-honored method of applying a heated paper clip or needle to melt or puncture a small hole in the nail is highly effective and causes few problems. However, any procedure should be performed with aseptic technique. If the bone is fractured, any communication with the skin essentially renders it an open fracture.

Dislocations *Back in joint – reduce*

Long bones are held in approximation to one another at the joint by ligaments. A dislocation occurs when the force of stress on the ligament is so great as to displace the normal position of the opposing bone ends or the bone end to its socket. The predominant symptom is pain that increases with attempted passive or active movement of the extremity. In dislocations there may be an obvious deformity and inability to move the joint. Temporary restriction of the joint, with a sling or bandage that secures the arm to the chest in a shoulder dislocation, provides sufficient comfort and immobilization until the child can receive medical help.

Simple dislocations should be reduced as soon as possible with the child under conscious sedation and often local anesthesia. Also, the use of anesthetics, such as nitrous oxide, parenteral or oral ketamine, or intravenous propofol, can be

used to produce partial or complete analgesia (Bostrom, McCormick, and Hooke, 1993; Tobias and others, 1992; Wattenmaker, Kasser, and McGravey, 1990). An unreduced dislocation will be complicated by increased swelling, making reduction difficult and increasing the risk of neurovascular problems. Reduction is accomplished by simple traction and slight flexion, followed by immobilization in a splint for 10 to 16 days or up to 3 weeks or more for healing of torn ligaments.

Sprains

A sprain occurs when trauma to a joint is so severe that a ligament is partially or completely torn or stretched by the force created as a joint is twisted or wrenched, often accompanied by damage to associated blood vessels, muscles, tendons, and nerves.

The presence of joint laxity is the most valid indicator of the severity of a sprain. In a severe injury the child complains of the joint "feeling loose" or as if "something is coming apart" and may describe hearing a "snap," "pop," or "tearing." Pain is seldom the principal subjective symptom. There is a rapid onset with swelling, often diffuse, accompanied by immediate disability and appreciable reluctance to use the injured joint.

Strains *long-term repetitive* *pulling + twisting motion*

rest ice comp elevate

A strain is a microscopic tear to the musculotendinous unit and has features in common with sprains. The area is painful to touch and swollen. Most strains are incurred over time rather than suddenly, and the rapidity of the appearance provides clues regarding severity. In general, the more rapidly the strain occurs, the more severe the injury. When the strain involves the muscular portion, there is more bleeding, often palpable soon after injury and before edema obscures the hematoma. *very swollen* *more painful than sprain*

Therapeutic Management

The first 6 to 12 hours is the most critical period for virtually all soft tissue injuries. Basic principles of managing sprains and other soft tissue injuries are summarized in the acronyms ***RICE*** or ***ICES:***

R—rest	**I**—ice
I—ice *20-30min intervals*	**C**—compression
C—compression	**E**—elevation
E—elevation	**S**—support

Soft tissue injuries should be iced immediately. This is best accomplished with crushed ice wrapped in a towel or encased in a screw-top ice bag or resealable storage bag. A wet elastic wrap, which transfers cold better than dry wrap, is applied to provide compression and to keep the ice pack in place. Ice has a rapid cooling effect on tissues that reduces the pain threshold. However, ice should never be applied for more than 30 minutes at a time.

NURSING TIP A plastic bag of frozen vegetables, such as peas, serves as a convenient ice pack for soft tissue injuries. It is clean, watertight, and easily molded to the injured part. When available, snow placed in a plastic bag works well also.

Elevating the extremity uses gravity to facilitate venous return and reduce edema formation in the damaged area. The

small children
subluxation of radial head – elbow

point of injury should be kept several inches above the level of the heart for therapy to be effective. Several pillows can be used effectively for elevation. Allowing the extremity to be dependent causes excessive fluid accumulation in the area of injury, delaying healing and causing painful swelling.

Torn ligaments, especially those in the knee, are usually treated by immobilization with a cast for 3 to 4 weeks or strapping of the joint with adhesive or Elastoplast bandage. Passive leg exercises, gradually increased to active ones, are begun as soon as sufficient healing has taken place. Parents and children are cautioned against using any form of liniment or other heat-producing preparation before examination. If the injury requires casting or splinting, the heat generated in the enclosed space can cause extreme discomfort and may even cause tissue damage.

FRACTURES _reduce line it up_

Bones fracture when the resistance of bone against the stress being exerted yields to the stress force. Fractures are a common injury at any age but are more likely to occur in children and older adults. Because of the characteristics of the child's skeleton, the pattern of fractures, problems of diagnosis, and methods of treatment differ in the child and the adult.

Fracture injuries in children are a result of traumatic incidents at home, at school, in a motor vehicle, or in association with recreational activities. Children's everyday activities include vigorous play that predisposes them to injury—climbing, falling down, running into immovable objects, and receiving blows to any part of their bodies.

Aside from automobile accidents, true injuries that cause fractures rarely occur in infancy; therefore bone injury in children of that age-group warrants further investigation. In any small child radiographic evidence of fractures at various stages of healing are, with few exceptions, the result of physical abuse. Fractures in school-age children are often the result of bicycle-automobile or skateboard injuries. Adolescents are vulnerable to multiple and severe trauma, because they are mobile on bikes and motorcycles and are active in sports.

Speed and congested surroundings often intensify the impact. Young children and teenagers usually do not calculate risks as they learn to manipulate their environment and achieve developmental goals. Therefore injuries are a part of most childhood experience.

Types of Fractures

A fractured bone consists of fragments—the fragment closer to the midline, or the proximal fragment, and the fragment farther from the midline, or the distal fragment. When fracture fragments are separated, the fracture is **complete;** when fragments remain attached, the fracture is **incomplete.** The fracture line can be any of the following:

Transverse—crosswise, at right angles to the long axis of the bone
Oblique—slanting but straight, between a horizontal and a perpendicular direction
Spiral—slanting and circular, twisting around the bone shaft

The twisting of an extremity while the bone is breaking results in a spiral break. If the fracture does not produce a break in the skin, it is a **simple,** or **closed, fracture. Open,** or **compound, fractures** are those with an open wound through which the bone is or has protruded. If the bone fragments cause damage to other organs or tissues (such as the lung or bladder), the injury is said to be a **complicated fracture.** When small fragments of bone are broken from the fractured shaft and lie in the surrounding tissue, the injury is a **comminuted fracture.** This type of fracture is rare in children. The types of fractures seen most often in children are described in the accompanying box and in Fig. 31-2.

TYPES OF FRACTURES IN CHILDREN

Bends—occurs when the bone is bent but not broken. A child's flexible bone can be bent 45 degrees or more before breaking. However, if bent, the bone will straighten slowly, but not completely, to produce some deformity but without the angulation seen when the bone breaks. Bends occur most commonly in the ulna and fibula, often in association with fractures of the radius and tibia.
Buckle, or torus, fracture—produced by compression of the porous bone; appears as a raised or bulging projection at the fracture site. These fractures occur in the most porous portion of the bone near the metaphysis (the portion of the bone shaft adjacent to the epiphysis) and are more common in young children.
Green-stick fracture—occurs when a bone is angulated beyond the limits of bending. The compressed side bends, and the tension side fails, causing an incomplete fracture similar to the break observed when a green stick is broken.
Complete fracture—divides the bone fragments. These fragments often remain attached by a periosteal hinge, which can aid or hinder reduction.

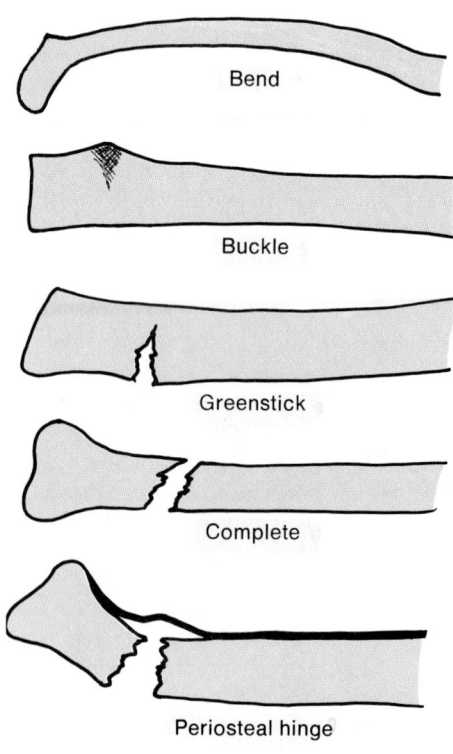

FIG. 31-2. Types of fractures in children.

femur humerus radius

Nursing ALERT	A spiral fracture in children may indicate child abuse. Further assessment and immediate involvement of interdisciplinary team members, such as a social worker, is necessary.

pulling + turning

Immediately after a fracture occurs, the muscles contract and physiologically splint the injured area. This phenomenon accounts for the muscle tightness observed over a fracture site and the deformity that is produced as the muscles pull the bone ends out of alignment. This muscle response must be overcome by traction or complete muscle relaxation (i.e., anesthesia) in order to realign the distal bone fragment to the proximal bone fragment.

Bone Healing and Remodeling

Bone healing is characteristically rapid in children because of the thickened periosteum and generous blood supply. When there is a break in the continuity of bone, the osteoblasts are stimulated to maximum activity. New bone cells are formed in immense numbers almost immediately after the injury and, in time, are evidenced by a bulging growth of new bone tissue between the fractured bone fragments. This is followed by deposition of calcium salts to form a *callus.*

Fractures heal in less time in children than in adults. The approximate healing times for a femoral shaft are as follows:

- Neonatal period—2 to 3 weeks
- Early childhood—4 weeks
- Later childhood—6 to 8 weeks
- Adolescence—8 to 12 weeks

Diagnostic Evaluation

A history is often lacking in childhood injuries. Infants are unable to communicate, and older children seldom volunteer information (even under direct questioning) when the injury occurred during forbidden activities. Unless they are witnesses to the injury, parents may misinterpret what the child is trying to say. In cases of child abuse, parents may give false information to protect themselves.

The child exhibits the same manifestations seen in adults (see box). However, often a fracture is remarkably stable because of intact periosteum. The child may even be able to use an affected arm or walk on a fractured leg.

Nursing ALERT	A fracture should be strongly suspected in a small child who refuses to walk or move an upper extremity.

CLINICAL MANIFESTATIONS OF A FRACTURE

Signs of injury
  Generalized swelling
  Pain or tenderness
  Diminished functional use of affected part
May be
  Bruising
  Severe muscular rigidity
  Crepitus (grating sensation at fracture site)

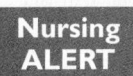

EMERGENCY TREATMENT
Fracture

Assess extent of injury—5 "Ps":
  Pain and point of tenderness
  Pulse—distal to the fracture site
  Pallor
  Paresthesia—sensation distal to the fracture site
  Paralysis—movement distal to the fracture site
Determine the mechanism of injury.
Move injured part as little as possible.
  Cover open wounds with sterile or clean dressing.
Immobilize the limb, including joints above and below the fracture site; do not attempt to reduce fracture or push protruding bone under the skin.
  Soft splint (pillow or folded towel)
  Rigid splint (rolled newspaper or magazine)
  Uninjured leg can serve as splint for leg fracture if no splint available
Reassess neurovascular status.
Apply traction if circulatory compromise is present.
Elevate the injured limb if possible.
Apply cold to the injured area.
Call Emergency Medical Service or transport to medical facility.

cast above + below the joint wher fx is

Radiographic examination is the most useful diagnostic tool for assessing skeletal trauma. The calcium deposits in bone make the entire structure radiopaque. Radiographic films are taken after fracture reduction and, in some cases, may be taken during the healing process to determine satisfactory progress.

Therapeutic Management

The majority of children's fractures heal well, and nonunion is rare. Most fractures are readily reduced by simple traction and immobilization until healing takes place. However, the position of the bone fragments in relation to one another influences the rapidity of healing and the residual deformity. Healing is prompt and complete with end-to-end apposition, but a gap between fragments delays (or prevents) healing. The goals of fracture management are the following:

1. To regain alignment and length of the bony fragments (reduction)
2. To retain alignment and length (immobilization)
3. To restore function to the injured parts

In children the bone fragments are usually realigned and immobilized by traction or by closed manipulation and casting until adequate callus is formed. Weight bearing on lower extremity fractures and active movement for the purpose of regaining function can begin after the fracture site is stable. The child's natural tendency to be active is usually sufficient to restore normal mobility, and physical therapy is rarely needed. In most cases children's fractures can be managed by closed reduction and plaster immobilization, which is most often provided on an outpatient basis with reevaluation in 7 to 10 days.

Children are most frequently hospitalized for fractures of the femur and the supracondylar area of the distal humerus. If simple reductions cannot be achieved or if a neurovascular problem is detected after injury, observation in a hospital is indicated. Severe contusions with profound swelling cannot be treated with a cast, which would act as a tourniquet on the extremity. A badly malaligned fracture requires traction for a period of time before a cast is applied.

The major methods for immobilizing a fracture, casting and traction, are described in the following section in relation to the nursing care involved.

Nursing Considerations

Nurses are frequently the persons who make the initial assessment of a child with a suspected fracture (see Emergency Treatment box). The child and parents are frightened and upset, the child is in pain, and since most fractures are obvious, the parents and (frequently) the child are already convinced of the diagnosis. Therefore, if the child is alert and there is no evidence of hemorrhage, the initial nursing interventions are directed toward calming and reassuring the child and parents so that a more extensive assessment can be more easily accomplished.

While remaining calm and speaking in a quiet voice, the nurse can ask the parents and older child to describe what happened and how they feel about it. Since the child usually arrives with the limb supported in some manner, this time does not delay or endanger the treatment. Initially it is best not to touch the child but to ask him or her to point to the painful area and to wiggle the fingers or toes. By this time the child usually feels relatively safe and will allow someone to gently touch the area just enough to feel the pulse and test for sensation. A child's anxiety is greatly influenced by previous experiences with injury and with health personnel. However, he or she needs to be told what will happen and what to do to help. The affected limb need not be palpated, and it should not be moved unless properly splinted. If the child is at home or if the practitioner is not present to examine the child, some type of splint is applied carefully for transport to the medical facility.

THE CHILD IN A CAST

The completeness of the fracture, the type of bone involved, and the amount of weight bearing influence how much of the extremity must be included in the cast to immobilize the fracture site completely. In most cases the joints above and below the fracture are immobilized to eliminate the possibility of movement that might cause displacement at the fracture site. Four major categories of casts are used for fractures: *upper extremity* to immobilize the wrist and/or elbow, *lower extremity* to immobilize the ankle and/or knee, *spinal* and *cervical* for immobilization of the spine, and *spica casts* to immobilize the hip and knee.

The Cast

When a cast is to be applied, the nurse often must set up the cast materials and hold the extremity in alignment. In most instances only the cast material is required; however, special cast tables that hold the child's body are used for applying large hip spica casts. If possible, children should be allowed to play with a doll that has a cast so that they understand what will be done.

Before the cast is applied, the extremities are checked for any abrasions, cuts, or other alterations in the skin surface and for the presence of rings or other items that might cause

constriction from swelling; such objects are removed. Identification bands are placed on a noninjured extremity if hospitalization is anticipated.

Casts are constructed from gauze strips and bandages impregnated with plaster of Paris or, more commonly, from synthetic lighter-weight and water-resistant materials (e.g., fiberglass and polyurethane resin). With plaster of Paris, a heat-producing chemical reaction occurs between the plaster and water as the plaster becomes a crystalline gypsum; the drying process takes 10 to 72 hours, depending on the size of the cast. Synthetic materials dry in 5 to 30 minutes, depending on the type of cast.

 Synthetic casts have special advantages for children. They come in different colors and with designs (e.g., cartoons and stripes). They are lightweight, durable, easy to clean, and water resistant. With a special Gore-Tex liner, the cast can be immersed in water. One drawback—their rough surface is harder to autograph!

A tube of stockinette is stretched over the area to be casted, and bony prominences are padded with soft cotton sheeting. Dry rolls of casting material are immersed in a pail of water. The wet rolls are put on in a bandage fashion and molded to the extremity. During application of the cast the underlying stockinette is pulled over the raw edges of the cast and secured with a layer of wet plaster ½ to 1 inch below the rim to form a smooth, padded edge to protect the skin.

If the operator does not form such a protective edge with stockinette, the raw edges of the cast can be protected by a "petaled" edge. Small pieces approximately 2 to 3 inches long are cut from 1- or 1½-inch-wide adhesive tape. The edges are rounded with scissors, and these "petals" are placed over the edge of the cast, with each petal slightly overlapping the previous petal to form a smooth, neat edge. It is easier to apply the petal to the underside of the cast first and then bring the unadhered edge to the front, pressing firmly so that the edges remain securely attached. Adhesive bandages can be used instead of the tape petals for quicker preparation and a slightly padded cast edge.

Nursing Considerations

The complete evaporation of the water from a hip spica cast can take 24 to 48 hours when older types of plaster materials are used. Drying occurs within minutes with new quick-drying substances. The cast must remain uncovered to allow it to dry from the inside out. Turning the child in a plaster cast at least every 2 hours will help to dry a body cast evenly and prevent complications related to immobility. A regular fan or cool-air hairdryer to circulate air may be helpful when the humidity is high.

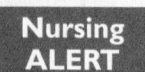 Heated fans or dryers are not used, since they cause the cast to dry on the outside and remain wet beneath or cause burns from heat conduction by way of the cast to the underlying tissue.

A wet cast should be supported by a pillow that is covered with plastic and handled by the palms of the hands to prevent indenting the cast, which can create pressure areas. A dry plaster of Paris cast produces a hollow sound when it is tapped with the finger. If "hot spots" are felt on the cast surface (usually indicating infection beneath the area), this should be reported so that a window can be made in the cast to observe the site.

During the first few hours after a cast is applied, the chief concern is that the extremity may continue to swell to the extent that the cast becomes a tourniquet, shutting off circulation and producing neurovascular complications. To reduce the likelihood of this potential problem, the body part can be elevated, thereby increasing venous return. If edema is excessive, casts are bivalved (i.e., cut to make anterior and posterior halves that are held together with an elastic bandage). The cast and the involved extremity are observed frequently for neurovascular integrity and any signs of compromise.

 Nursing ALERT   Observations such as pain, swelling, discoloration (pallor or cyanosis) of the exposed portions, lack of pulsation and warmth, or the inability to move the exposed part(s) are reported immediately.

When casting an extremity that has sustained an open fracture, a window is often left over the wound area to allow for observation and for dressing of the wound. A surgical reduction is usually casted as for a closed fracture. For the first few hours after surgery, there may be substantial bleeding that will soak through the cast. Periodically the circumscribed blood-stained area should be outlined with a ball-point pen or pencil, and the time indicated to provide a guide for assessing the amount of bleeding.

Usually the child is discharged to home care after a cast is applied in the emergency room or clinic. Parents need instructions on drying and caring for the cast and checking for signs and symptoms that indicate the cast is too tight (see Family Home Care box). They should also be told to take the child to the health professional for attention if the cast becomes too loose, since a loose cast no longer serves its purpose. A cast is a badge of honor for the child and serves as visible evidence of an otherwise invisible injury.

Cast Removal.   Cutting the cast to remove it or to relieve tightness is frequently a frightening experience for children. They fear the sound of the cast cutter and are terrified that their flesh, as well as the cast, will be cut. Since it works by vibration, a cast cutter cuts only the hard surface of the cast. This can be demonstrated on the nurse or person removing the cast. The oscillating blade vibrates very rapidly back and forth and will not cut when placed lightly on the skin. Children have described it as producing a "tickly" sensation. The vibration also generates heat that may be felt by the child. Both these feelings should be explained.

Preparation for the procedure will help reduce anxiety, especially if a trusting relationship has been established between the child and the nurse. Many young children come to regard the cast as part of themselves, which intensifies their fear of removal (Fig. 31-3). Using the analogy of having fingernails or hair cut sometimes helps reduce their anxiety. They need continual reassurance that all is going well and that their behavior is accepted.

Nurses can help families adapt the child's home environment to meet the temporary encumbrance of a cast. Home care creates problems of various magnitude, especially for children in large casts (e.g., a hip spica). Commonplace situations become problematic, (e.g., returning the child home

FAMILY HOME CARE
Cast Care

Keep the casted extremity elevated on pillows or similar support for the first day, or as directed by the health professional.

Avoid indenting the cast while still wet to avoid creating pressure points.

Observe the extremities (fingers or toes) for any evidence of swelling or discoloration (darker or lighter than a comparable extremity) and contact the health professional if noted.

Check movement and sensation of the visible extremities frequently.

Follow health professional's orders regarding any restriction of activities.

Restrict strenuous activities for the first few days.
  Engage in quiet activities but encourage use of muscles.
  Move the joints above and below the cast on the affected extremity.

Encourage frequent rest for a few days, keeping the injured extremity elevated while resting.

Avoid allowing the affected limb to hang down for any length of time.
  Keep an injured upper extremity elevated (e.g., in a sling) while upright.
  Elevate a lower limb when sitting and avoid standing for too long.

Do not allow the child to put anything inside the cast.
  Keep small items that might be placed inside the cast away from small children

Keep a clear path for ambulation.
  Remove toys, hazardous floor rugs, pets, or other items over which the child might stumble.

Use crutches appropriately if lower limb fracture.
  The crutches should fit properly, have a soft rubber tip to prevent slipping, and be well padded at the axilla.

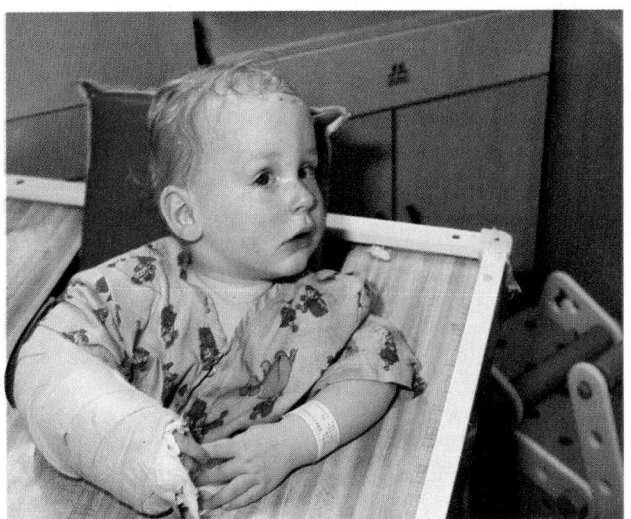

FIG. 31-3. Young children come to regard a cast as part of their body. They usually adapt well but may fear its removal. (Courtesy St. Louis Children's Hospital.)

safely and comfortably). Standard seat belts and car seats are not readily adapted for use by children in casts (see p. 1141 and Fig. 31-15). Sitting can be impossible in a spica cast, and leg casts require extra space.

Children in spica casts usually find the prone position easier for self-feeding from a small table placed next to the dining table. The use of a conventional toilet is almost impossible. Small bedpans or other containers offer alternatives for elimination. The nurse may suggest waterproofing methods, by devising plastic wraps, for elimination and showers. Baths are possible only if the plaster cast is kept out of the water and covered to prevent it from becoming wet from splashes. Synthetic casts can be immersed in water if a special type of cast liner is used.

After the cast is removed, the skin surface will be caked with desquamated skin and sebaceous secretions. Simple soaking in a bathtub is usually sufficient for their removal, but a period of several days may be required to eliminate the accumulation completely. Application of olive oil or lotion may provide comfort. The parents and child should be instructed not to pull or forcibly remove this material with vigorous scrubbing, because it may cause excoriation and bleeding.*

See also Nursing Care Plans: The Child with a Fracture†.

THE CHILD IN TRACTION

Bone fragments that cannot be aligned initially by simple traction and stabilization with a cast require the extended pulling force supplied by continuous traction. Traction may be used for other purposes also:

- To provide rest for an extremity
- To help prevent or improve contracture deformity
- To correct a deformity
- To treat a dislocation
- To allow preoperative or postoperative positioning and alignment
- To provide immobilization of specific areas of the body
- To reduce muscle spasms (rare in children)

In most of these cases the traction is often applied at night and intermittently during the day. Muscle relaxants may be administered for muscle spasms.

Purposes of Traction

The three essential components of traction management are traction, countertraction, and friction (Fig. 31-4). To reduce or realign a fracture site, *traction* (forward force) is produced by attaching weight to the distal bone fragment; body weight provides *countertraction* (backward force); and the patient's contact with the bed constitutes the *frictional* force. These forces are used to align the distal and proximal bone fragments by adjusting the line of pull upward or downward and adducting or abducting the extremity.

To attain equilibrium, the amount of forward force is adjusted by adding weight to or subtracting weight from the traction, and/or countertraction can be increased by elevating the foot of the bed to create a greater gravitational

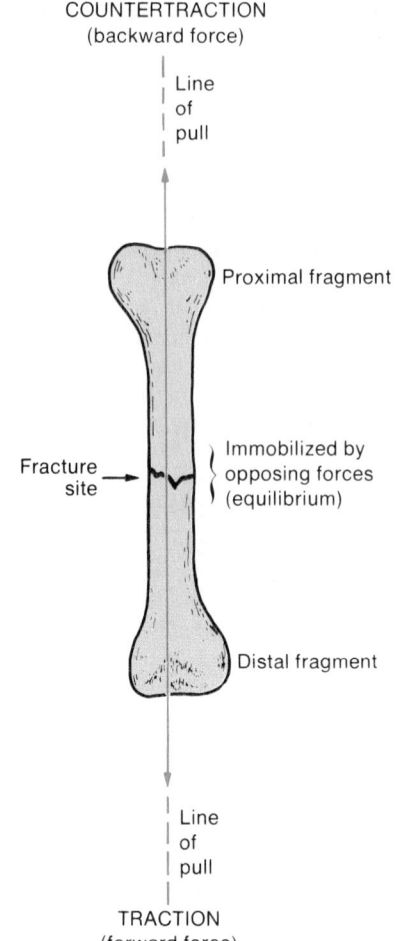

FIG. 31-4. Application of traction for maintaining equilibrium.

pull to the backward force. A bed board placed under the mattress of heavy children prevents sagging, which might otherwise change the direction of the forces applied to the fracture.

The three primary purposes of traction for reduction of fractures are the following:

- To fatigue the involved muscle and reduce muscle spasm so that bones can be realigned
- To position the distal and proximal bone ends in desired realignment to promote satisfactory bone healing
- To immobilize the fracture site until realignment has been achieved and sufficient healing has taken place to permit casting or splinting

The *all-or-none law,* characteristic of muscle contractibility, influences the complete relaxation. When muscle is stretched, muscle spasm ceases and permits the realignment of the bone ends. The continuous maintenance of traction is important during this phase because releasing the traction allows the normal contracting ability of the muscle to again cause a malpositioning of the bone ends.

The realignment of the fragments is a gradual process that is achieved more rapidly in infants, who have limited muscle tone, than in muscular teenagers. The desired line of pull and callus formation are checked periodically by radiographic examination. The traction pull to some degree immobilizes the fracture site; however, adjunctive immobilizing devices such as splints or casts are sometimes used with skeletal traction. In injuries in which there is severe soft tissue swelling or vascular and nerve damage, it is customary to use traction until these complications have been resolved and it is safe to apply a cast. Immobilization with traction will be maintained until the bone ends are in satisfactory realignment, after which a less confining type of immobilization, usually a cast, will be applied.

Types of Traction (General)

The pull needed for traction can be applied to the distal bone fragment in several ways (see box). *Manual traction* is used in uncomplicated arm or leg fractures in which there is little overriding of the bones and minimal muscle pull to overcome. Manual traction is used to realign bone fragments for immediate cast application. *Skin traction* is applied when there is minimal displacement and little muscle spasticity, but it is contraindicated when there is associated skin damage. Skin traction has specific limits of weight that it can pull without causing tissue breakdown. *Skeletal traction* is used when significant traction pull must be applied to achieve realignment and immobilization. By inserting a pin or wire into the bone, the stress is placed on the bone and not on the surrounding tissue.

The type of traction applied is determined primarily by the age of the child, the condition of the soft tissues, and the type and degree of displacement of the fracture. Fractures most commonly treated by application of traction are those involving the humerus, femur, and vertebrae. The major types of traction for specific fractures are discussed in the following sections.

Upper Extremity Traction

Treatment of fractures of the humerus by traction is accomplished by (1) overhead suspension, in which the arm, bent at the elbow, is suspended vertically by skin or skeletal attachment and traction is applied to the distal end of the humerus, or (2) Dunlop traction. With *Dunlop traction* (Fig. 31-5), the arm is suspended horizontally, using either skin or skeletal attachment. A skeletal wire placed in the upper arm to allow additional weight may be applied in certain instances, such as a supracondylar fracture. When skin traction is used, straps are placed on the lower and upper arm with the arm flexed to accomplish pull in two directions: one along the lon-

---

TYPES OF TRACTION

Manual traction—applied to the body part by the hand placed distally to the fracture site. Nurses frequently provide manual traction during cast application.

Skin traction—applied directly to the skin surface and indirectly to the skeletal structures. The pulling mechanism is attached to the skin with adhesive material or an elastic bandage. Both types are applied over soft, foam-backed traction straps to distribute the traction pull.

Skeletal traction—applied directly to the skeletal structure by a pin, wire, or tongs inserted into or through the diameter of the bone distal to the fracture.

---

gitudinal direction of the upper arm and one to maintain vertical alignment of the lower arm.

Fractures of the humerus, which usually result from a fall with the arm in extension, frequently involve the supracondylar portion. These fractures especially place the patient at risk for nerve damage and angulation deformities; therefore they must be reduced carefully, sometimes with the patient under anesthesia. Because of the danger of complications, children with closed reduction of supracondylar fractures are often hospitalized for observation. In severely malaligned fractures, closed reduction with the patient under anesthesia is followed by application of skeletal traction for 2 to 3 weeks, after which a long arm cast is applied for an additional 2 to 3 weeks.

Lower Extremity Traction

The severity of the fracturing force and the ability of the muscles to hold the fracture out of alignment will determine the degree of bone fragment displacement. A fracture in the middle third of the shaft results in significant overriding but minimal displacement. In a fracture in the lower one third of the shaft, the pull of the gastrocnemius muscle causes the distal fragment to become downwardly displaced.

Fractures of the femur can often be reduced with immediate application of a hip spica cast in young children. When traction is required, several types may be used, based on the initial assessment.

Bryant traction is a type of running traction in which the pull is only in one direction. Skin traction is applied to the legs, which are flexed at a 90° angle at the hips. The child's

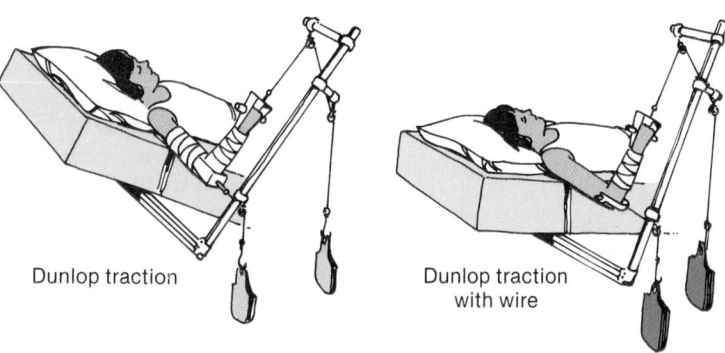

Dunlop traction

Dunlop traction with wire

FIG. 31-5. Dunlop traction.

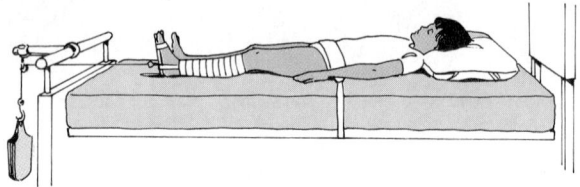

FIG. 31-6. Buck extension traction.

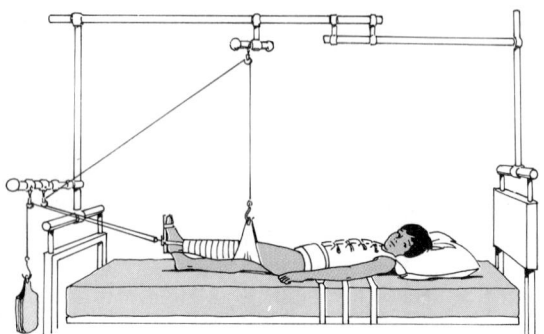

FIG. 31-7. Russell traction.

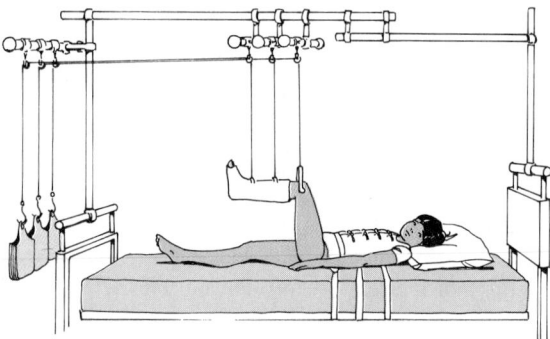

FIG. 31-8. Ninety-degree—ninety-degree traction.

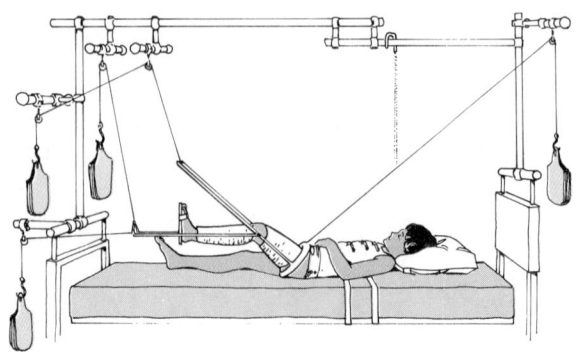

FIG. 31-9. Balance suspension with Thomas ring splint and Pearson attachment.

trunk (buttocks are raised slightly off the bed) provides countertraction.

Nursing ALERT Bryant traction is not recommended because of the gravitational vascular draining of the elevated extremities, the possible tourniquet effect of the bandages, and the effect of the traction, which can trigger vasospasms and avascular necrosis.

Buck extension (Fig. 31-6) is a type of skin traction with the legs in an extended position. Except for fracture cases, turning from side to side with care is permitted, to maintain the involved leg alignment. Buck extension is used primarily for short-term immobilization, preoperatively with dislocated hips, for correcting contractures, or for bone deformities such as Legg-Calvé-Perthes disease.

Russell traction (Fig. 31-7) uses skin traction on the lower leg and a padded sling under the knee. Two lines of pull, one along the longitudinal line of the lower leg and one perpendicular to the leg, are produced. This combination of pulls allows realignment of the lower extremity and immobilizes the hip and knee in a flexed position. The hip flexion must be kept at the prescribed angle to prevent fracture malalignment, since there is no direct support under the fracture and the skin traction may slip. Special nursing measures include carefully checking the position of the traction so that the amount of desired hip flexion is maintained and damage to the common peroneal nerve under the knee does not produce footdrop. *Split-Russell traction,* in which the lines of pull are modified, is a variation of classic Russell traction.

Ninety-degree—ninety-degree traction is the most common skeletal traction (Fig. 31-8). The lower leg is put in a boot cast and a skeletal Steinmann pin or Kirschner wire is placed in the distal fragment of the femur. From a nursing standpoint, this traction easily facilitates position changes, toileting, and prevention of traction complications.

Balance suspension traction (Fig. 31-9) may be used with or without skin or skeletal traction. Unless used with another traction, the balanced suspension merely suspends the leg in a desired flexed position to relax the hip and hamstring muscles and does not exert any traction directly on a body part. A *Thomas splint* extends from the groin to midair above the foot, and a *Pearson attachment* supports the lower leg. Towels or pieces of felt covered with stockinette are clipped or pinned to the splints for leg support. When the child is lifted off the bed, the traction lifts with the child without loss of alignment. This traction requires very careful checking of splints and ropes to make certain that no slippage or fraying has occurred. The traction is of great value in an older and heavier child when it is essential to lift the patient for care.

Cervical Traction

The cervical area is a vulnerable site for flexion or extension injuries to muscle, vertebrae, and/or the spinal cord. Cervical muscle trauma without other complications is treated with a cervical soft or hard collar to relieve the weight of the head from the fracture site. Intermittent cervical skin traction might be used with a child halter and weight to decrease muscle spasms (Fig. 31-10).

Cervical traction is usually accomplished by the insertion of *Crutchfield* or *Barton tongs* through burr holes in the

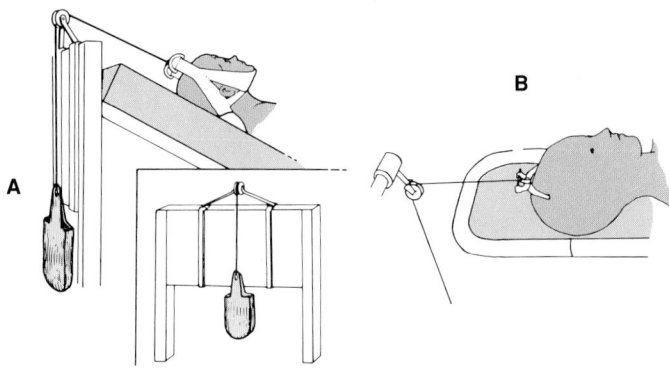

FIG. 31-10. Cervical traction. **A,** With chin strap. **B,** With Crutchfield tongs. (Figs 31-5 to 31-10 redrawn from Hilt NE, Schmitt EW: *Pediatric orthopedic nursing,* St Louis, 1975, Mosby.)

skull and weights attached to the hyperextended head. As the neck muscles fatigue with constant traction pull, the vertebral bodies gradually separate so that the cord is no longer pinched between the vertebrae. Immobilization until fracture healing can occur is an essential goal of cervical traction. If the injury has been limited to a vertebral fracture without neurologic deficit, a halo cast can be applied to permit earlier ambulation.

Nursing Considerations

Generally the child in traction is hospitalized under the direct care of nurses who develop individualized nursing care plans based on an understanding of correct traction management. Evaluating the therapeutic effects and possible negative consequences is essential to good patient care. Many of the nursing problems associated with a child in traction are related to immobility. However, it is important that nurses understand the basic principles of traction and their role in its maintenance.

Skeletal traction is never released by the nurse, except under certain circumstances, such as in the child with Legg-Calvé-Perthes disease or scoliosis. The nurse may remove nonadhesive skin traction. In these cases intermittent traction is periodically released and reapplied as ordered. When skin traction must be constantly maintained, such as in fractures, nurses may occasionally remove and reapply the elastic bandage if this is approved by the practitioner, provided that *someone manually maintains the traction during the rewrapping process.* It is not uncommon for a child to have several types of traction at one time, and each traction must be assessed separately to avoid problems.

NURSING TIP A small hand mirror facilitates visualization of inaccessible skin areas.

When the child is first placed in traction, an increase in discomfort is common as a result of the traction pull fatiguing the muscle. It has been determined that orthopedic conditions are associated with a higher-than-average number of painful events and a higher percentage of bodily symptoms than other common conditions (Wong and Baker, 1988). An-

algesics, including opioids, and muscle relaxants help during this phase of care and should be administered liberally.

Children are given an explanation at their level of understanding about what is happening and why they must remain in the device. Children are reassured of the presence of someone who will aid them in adjusting to the traction and coping with the problems of immobilization.

The specific nursing responsibilities for the patient in traction are outlined in the Guidelines box on p. 1136.

DISTRACTION

Unlike traction, which helps bones realign and fuse properly, distraction is the process of separating opposing bone to encourage regeneration of new bone in the created space. Distraction can also be used when limbs are of unequal lengths and new bone is needed to elongate the shorter limb.

Ilizarov External Fixator (IEF)

The IEF uses a system of wires, rings, and telescoping rods that permits limb lengthening to occur by manual distraction. In addition to lengthening bones, the device can be used to correct angular or rotational defects or to immobilize fractures. The device is attached surgically by securing a series of external full or half rings to the bone with wires. External telescoping rods connect the rings to each other. Manual distraction is accomplished by manipulating the rods to increase the distance between the rings. A percutaneous ostomy is performed when the device is applied to create a "false" growth plate. A special osteotomy or corticotomy involves cutting only the cortex of the bone while preserving its blood supply, bone marrow, endosteum, and periosteum. Capillary blood flow to the transected area is essential for proper bone growth. Cut bone ends typically grow at a rate of 1 cm/month. The IEF can result in up to a 15-cm gain in length (Carlino, 1991).

Nursing Considerations

Success of the IEF depends on the child's and family's cooperation; therefore, before surgery they must be fully informed of the appearance of the device, how it accomplishes bone growth, alterations in activities, and home and follow-up care. Children are involved in learning to adjust the device to accomplish distraction. Children who participate actively in their care report less discomfort. Since the device is external, the child and family need to be prepared for the reactions of others and assisted in camouflaging the device with appropriate apparel, such as wide-legged pants that close with self-adhering fasteners around the device (Fig. 31-11). Partial weight bearing is allowed, and the child needs to learn to walk with crutches. Alterations in activity include modifications at school and in physical education. Full weight bearing is not allowed until the distraction is completed and bone consolidation has occurred. Follow-up care is essential to maintaining appropriate distraction until the desired leg length is achieved. The device is removed surgically after the bone has consolidated, and the child may need to use crutches or have a cast for about 1 month following removal.

AMPUTATION

A child may be born with the congenital absence of a body part, have a traumatic loss of an extremity, or need a surgical

GUIDELINES
Traction Care

Understand Therapy
Understand purpose of traction
Understand function of traction in each specific situation

Maintain Traction
Check desired line of pull and relationship of distal fragment to proximal fragment
  Check whether fragment is being directed upward, adducted, or abducted
Check function of each component
  Position of bandages, frames, splints
  Ropes: in center tract of pulley, taut, no fraying, knots tied securely
  Pulleys:
    In original position on attachment bar; have not slid from original site
    Wheels freely movable
  Weights:
    Correct amount of weight
    Hanging freely
    In safe location
Check bed position—head or foot elevated as directed for desired amount of pull and countertraction
Do not remove skeletal traction or adhesive traction straps on skin traction

Maintain Alignment
Observe for correct body alignment with emphasis on alignment of shoulder, hip, and leg
Check after child has moved
Apply restraints when indicated
Maintain correct angles at joints

Skin Traction
Replace nonadhesive straps and/or elastic bandage on skin traction *when permitted* and/or absolutely necessary, but make certain that traction on limb is maintained by someone during procedure
Assess bandages to ascertain if they are correctly applied (diagonal or spiral), not too loose or too tight, which could cause slippage and malalignment of traction

Skeletal Traction
Check pin sites frequently for signs of bleeding, inflammation, or infection
Cleanse and dress pin sites as ordered
Apply topical antiseptic or antibiotic daily as ordered
Cover ends of pins with protective cord or padding to prevent child's being scratched by pin
Note pull of traction on pin; pull should be even
Check pin screws to be certain that screws are tight in metal clamp that attaches traction apparatus to pin

Prevent Skin Breakdown
Provide sheepskin, waffle mattress, or alternating-pressure mattress underneath hips and back
Make total body skin checks for redness or breakdown, especially over areas that receive greatest pressure (see Nursing Tip)
Wash and dry skin at least daily
Stimulate circulation with gentle massage over pressure areas
Change position at least every 2 hours to relieve pressure

Prevent Complications
Check pulse in affected area and compare with pulse in contralateral site
Assess circular dressings for excessive tightness
Assess restraining devices
  Make certain that they are not too loose or too tight
  Remove periodically and check for pressure areas
Encourage deep breathing frequently with maximum inspiratory chest expansion
Note any neurovascular changes, such as:
  Color in skin and nail beds
  Alterations in sensation, increased pain
  Alterations in motor ability
Take immediate action to correct problem or report to practitioner if neurovascular changes are found
Record findings of neurovascular changes
Carry out passive, active, or active-with-resistance exercises of uninvolved joints
Note if any tightness, weakness, or contractures are developing in uninvolved joints and muscles
Take measures to correct or prevent further development of weakness, such as applying foot plate to prevent footdrop

---

amputation for a pathologic condition such as osteogenic sarcoma. With today's surgical technology and the quick thinking of bystanders who save a traumatically amputated body part, some children have had fingers and arms sewn back on with variable degrees of functional use regained. A severed part should be wrapped lightly in a clean cloth or gauze saturated with normal saline and sealed in a watertight plastic bag. One should avoid using ice, which might come in contact with the tissue and make implantation impossible. The bag should be labeled with the child's name, the date, and the time and taken to the hospital with the child.

Surgical amputation or the surgical repair of a permanently severed limb focuses on constructing an adequately nourished stump. A smooth, healthy, padded stump, free of nerve endings, is important in prosthesis fitting and subsequent ambulation. In some situations in which there is no vascular or neurologic deficit, a cast is applied to the stump immediately af-

ter the procedure, and a pylon, metal extension, and artificial foot are attached so that the patient can walk on the temporary prosthesis within a few hours.

Nursing Considerations

Stump shaping is done postoperatively with special elastic bandaging using a figure-eight bandage, which applies pressure in a cone-shaped fashion. This technique decreases stump edema, controls hemorrhage, and aids in developing desired contours so that the child will bear weight on the posterior aspect of the skin flap rather than on the end of the stump. Stump elevation may be used during the first 24 hours, but after this time the extremity should not be left in this position, because contractures in the proximal joint will develop and seriously hamper ambulation. Monitoring proper body alignment will further decrease the risk of flexion contractures.

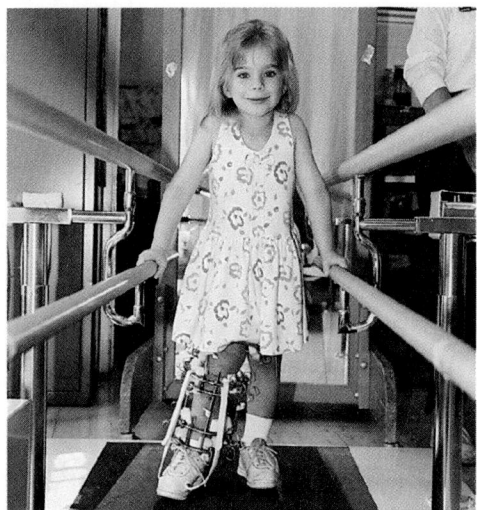

FIG. 31-11. Children with the Ilizarov external fixator must cope with the visible nature of the device.

For older children and adolescents, arm exercises and bed pushups, as well as parallel bars, which are used in prosthesis-training programs, help build up the arm muscles necessary for walking with crutches. Full range-of-motion exercises of joints above the amputation must be performed several times daily, using active and isotonic exercises. Young children are spontaneously active and require little encouragement.

Depending on the age of the child, children or their parents will need to learn stump hygiene, including careful soap and water washing every day and checking for skin irritation, breakdown, or infection. A tube of stockinette or powder is used to slide the prosthesis on more easily. Skin must be checked carefully every time the prosthesis is removed, and prosthesis tolerance time must be adjusted to prevent skin breakdown.

For children who have had an amputation, *phantom limb sensation* is an expected experience because the nerve-brain connections are still present. Gradually these sensations fade. Preoperative discussion of this phenomenon will aid a child in understanding these "unusual feelings" and not hiding the experiences from others. Limb pain, especially pain that in-

creases with ambulation, should be evaluated for the possibility of a neuroma at the free nerve endings in the stump (see also p. 1152).

CONGENITAL DEFECTS

There are numerous skeletal defects that can be diagnosed at or shortly after birth. The alert nurse is frequently the person who detects the defect and refers the family for correction of the condition. The deviation is often difficult to detect without careful inspection. Therefore it is imperative that nurses become acquainted with signs of these defects and understand the principles of therapy in order to direct others in the care and management of these children.

DEVELOPMENTAL DYSPLASIA OF THE HIP (DDH)

The broad term *developmental dysplasia of the hip* describes a group of disorders related to abnormal development of the hip. A change in terminology from congenital hip dysplasia (CHD) and congenital dislocation of the hip (CHD) to DDH more properly reflects a variety of hip abnormalities in which there is a shallow acetabulum, subluxation, or dislocation. DDH has an incidence of 1 to 2 cases per 1000 live births in the United States. It occurs more commonly in females at a ratio of 6:1 (Bennett and MacEwen, 1989). One fifth of the cases involve both hips, and when only one hip is involved, the left hip is affected three times more often than the right.

Pathophysiology
Three degrees of DDH can be identified (Fig. 31-12):

Acetabular dysplasia (or preluxation)—the mildest form, in which there is neither subluxation nor dislocation. The dysplasia reflects an apparent delay in acetabular development evidenced by osseous hypoplasia of the acetabular roof that is oblique and shallow, although the cartilaginous roof is comparatively intact. The femoral head remains in the acetabulum.

Subluxation—accounts for the largest percentage of congenital hip dysplasias. Subluxation implies incomplete dislocation of the hip and is sometimes regarded as an intermediate state in the devel-

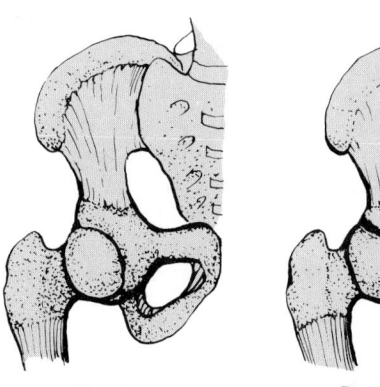
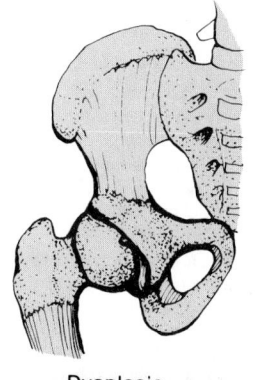
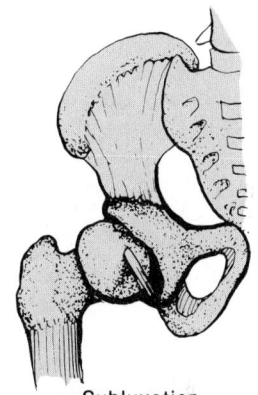
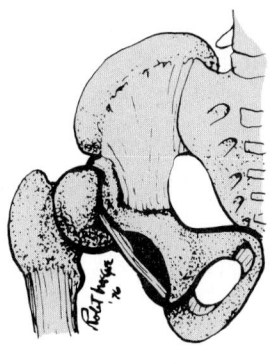

Normal   Dysplasia   Subluxation   Dislocation

FIG. 31-12. Configuration and relationship of structures in congenital hip deformities.

[handwritten: complete dislocation—cant move leg back in.]

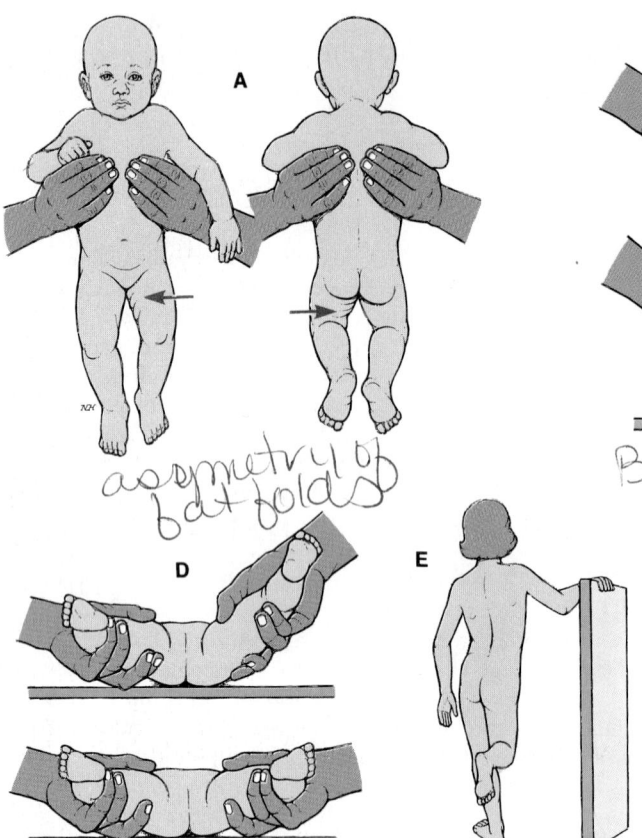

[handwritten: assymetry of fat folds]

[handwritten: Allis sign] *[handwritten: beet flat on btable notevent clunk if it dislocate]*

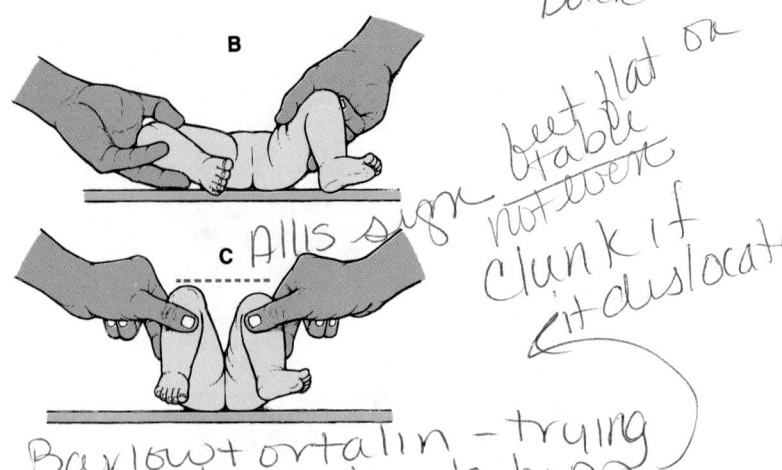

[handwritten: Barlow + ortalin —trying to dislocate hips]

FIG. 31-13. Signs of developmental dysplasia of hip. **A,** Assymetry of gluteal and thigh folds. **B,** Limited hip abduction, as seen in flexion. **C,** Apparent shortening of femur, as indicated by level of knees in flexion. **D,** Ortolani click (if infant is under 4 weeks of age). **E,** Positive Trendelenburg sign or gain (if child is weight bearing).

opment from primary dysplasia to complete dislocation. The femoral head remains in contact with the acetabulum, but a stretched capsule and ligamentum teres cause the head of the femur to be partially displaced. Pressure on the cartilaginous roof inhibits ossification and produces a flattening of the socket.

Dislocation—in which the femoral head loses contact with the acetabulum and is displaced posteriorly and superiorly over the fibrocartilaginous rim. The ligamentum teres is elongated and taut.

Prenatal factors that influence development of hip abnormalities are maternal hormone secretion and mechanical factors of intrauterine posture. The maternal hormone secretion, principally of estrogen, that produces laxity of the maternal pelvis toward the end of gestation affects the fetal joints as well. Reliable evidence indicates an association between a higher incidence of developmental hip deformities with breech presentations and cesarean section (often necessitated by abnormal intrauterine position). Legs in frank breech position (i.e., with the hips acutely flexed and knees extended) is an important factor. Other prenatal factors that contribute to hip dysplasia include twinning and large infant size. (See also Cultural Awareness box.)

Diagnostic Evaluation

[handwritten: #1 law suit in nursery missing hip duplasa]

The diagnosis of DDH should be made in the newborn period if possible, since treatment initiated before 2 months of age is most successful (see box). In the newborn period dysplasia usually appears as hip joint laxity rather than as outright dislocation (Fig. 31-13). Subluxation and the tendency to dislocate can be demonstrated by the Ortolani or Barlow tests (Fig. 31-13, *B*, *C*, and *D*). There are cases in which

---

🌐 CULTURAL AWARENESS
Developmental Dysplasia of the Hip

A striking relationship exists between the development of the dislocation and methods of handling infants. Among the cultures with the highest incidence of dislocation, newly born infants are tightly wrapped in blankets or other swaddling material or are strapped to cradle boards. In cultures such as the Far East, where mothers traditionally carry infants on their backs or hips in the widely abducted straddle position, the disorder is virtually unknown.

CLINICAL MANIFESTATIONS OF DEVELOPMENTAL DYSPLASIA OF THE HIP

Infant
Shortening of limb on affected side (Galleazzi sign, Allis sign)
Restricted abduction of hip on affected side
Unequal gluteal folds (infant prone)
Positive Ortolani test *[handwritten:]downward pressure*
Positive Barlow test *[handwritten: trying to dislocate hip]*

Older Infant and Child
Affected leg shorter than the other
Telescoping or piston mobility of joint
   Head of femur can be felt to move up and down in buttock
     when extended thigh is pushed first toward child's head
     and then pulled distally
Trendelenburg sign
   When child stands first on one foot and then on the other
     (holding onto a chair, rail, or someone's hands) bearing
     weight on affected hip, pelvis tilts downward on normal
     side instead of upward, as it would with normal stability
Greater trochanter is prominent and appears above a line from
   anterior superior iliac spine to tuberosity of ischium
Marked lordosis (bilateral dislocations)
Waddling gait (bilateral dislocations)

dislocation is not diagnosed by these standard tests, and the disorder may not be apparent at birth. Therefore it is recommended that hip examination be included as part of health supervision until the child begins to walk and the gait is obviously normal.

In older infants and children radiographic examination is useful in confirming the diagnosis. An upward slope in the roof of the acetabulum (the acetabular angle) greater than 40 degrees with upward and outward displacement of the femoral head is a frequent finding in older children. Radiographic examination in early infancy is not reliable, because the bones are largely cartilaginous and difficult to visualize. However, the cartilaginous head can be visualized directly with real-time high-resolution ultrasonography.

Therapeutic Management

Treatment is begun as soon as the condition is recognized, since early intervention is more favorable to the restoration of normal bony architecture and function. The longer treatment is delayed, the more severe the deformity, the more difficult the treatment, and the less favorable the prognosis. The treatment varies with the age of the child and the extent of the dysplasia.

Newborn to Age 6 Months. The hip joint is maintained by splinting with the proximal femur centered in the acetabulum in an attitude of flexion. Of the numerous devices available, the *Pavlik harness* is the most widely used, and with time, motion, and gravity the hip works into a more abducted, reduced position (Fig. 31-14). The harness is worn continuously until the hip is clinically and radiographically stable, usually in about 3 to 6 months.

When adduction contracture is present, other devices (such as skin traction) are used to slowly and gently stretch the hip to full abduction, after which wide abduction is maintained until stability is attained. When there is difficulty in maintaining stable reduction, a hip spica cast is applied and changed periodically to accommodate the child's growth. After 3 to 6 months, sufficient stability is acquired to allow transfer to a removable protective abduction brace. The duration of treatment depends on development of the acetabulum but is usually accomplished within the first year.

Ages 6 to 18 Months. In this age-group the dislocation is not recognized until the child begins to stand and walk, when attendant shortening of the limb and contractures of hip adductor and flexor muscles become apparent. Gradual reduction by traction is followed by cast immobilization, which is maintained until radiographic examination confirms a stable joint. Often soft tissue may obstruct and complicate reduction and subsequent joint development. In this case open reduction is performed to remove the obstruction; followed by postoperative spica cast immobilization, and later replacement with an abduction splint.

Older Child. Correction of the hip deformity in older children is inherently more difficult than in the preceding age-groups, since secondary adaptive changes complicate the condition. Operative reduction, which may involve preoperative traction, tenotomy of contracted muscles, and any one of several innominate osteotomy procedures designed to construct an acetabular roof, is usually required. After the cast is removed and before weight bearing is permitted, range-of-motion exercises help restore movement. Next, rehabilitative

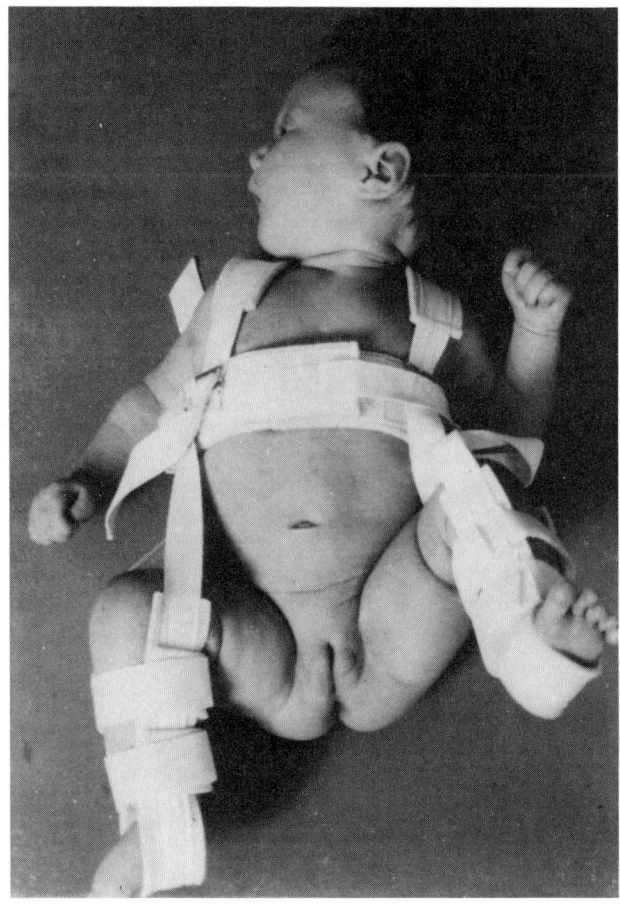

FIG. 31-14. Child in Pavlik harness.

Keep hips abducted

CRITICAL THINKING EXERCISE
The Diagnosis of DDH

During Kiasha's four-week well-child visit, her mother comments on a skin fold on the left inner thigh. History includes a normal pregnancy. A cesarean section was necessary due to breech presentation at 42 weeks' gestation. Given the facts, what intervention should you take, if any?

1. Reassure the mother that her infant has normal vital signs and weight gain and appears very healthy.
2. Explain to the mother that it is adipose tissue, which accumulates rapidly during the first 6 months.
3. Discuss concerns of the presented "skin fold" with the physician for further examination.
4. Order blood tests.

The correct answer is three. Clinical manifestations of developmental dysplasia of the hip in an infant include unequal gluteal folds, shortening of limb on affected side, restricted abduction of hip on affected side, positive Ortolani test, and positive Barlow test.

The first intervention is not correct, because a thorough assessment should be completed first. The second response is true; however, the key finding is the gluteal fold on the left inner thigh. In general, serum results are not necessary for diagnostic measures. Radiographic examination may be helpful, but it is not always reliable in infants.

measures are instituted. Successful reduction and reconstruction become increasingly difficult after the age of 4 years and are usually impossible or inadvisable in children over 6 years of age because of severe shortening and contracture of muscles and deformity of the femoral and acetabular structures.

Nursing Considerations

❖ Assessment

Nurses are in a unique position to detect DDH in the newborn. During the infant assessment process and routine nurturing activities the hips and extremities are inspected for any deviations from normal. Usually only nurses specially trained in the technique are permitted to perform Ortolani and Barlow tests, but any nurse can be alert to other signs of DDH. These observations are reported to the attending practitioner, and the ambulatory child who displays a limp or an unusual gait should be referred for evaluation. This may indicate an orthopedic or neurologic problem. Nonambulatory children with cerebral palsy should also be assessed for evidence of dislocation (see Critical Thinking Exercise on p. 1139).

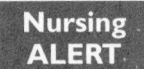 **Nursing ALERT** Observations during routine care, such as diapering, provide an excellent opportunity to observe the infant for limited movement and a wide perineum, which is an indication to assess for leg shortening, unequal gluteal folds, and limited abduction.

❖ Nursing Diagnoses

Nursing diagnoses identified for the child with congenital hip dysplasia are listed in the accompanying box. Other diagnoses will be apparent in specific situations.

❖ Planning

The goals of care for the child in a mechanical device for correction of DDH are as follows:

1. Child will maintain correct position of hip in acetabulum.
2. Child will experience no complications related to wearing corrective device.
3. Family will adapt routine nurturing activities to accommodate corrective device.

❖ Implementation

The major nursing problems in the care of an infant or child in a cast or other device are related to maintenance of the device and adaptation of nurturing activities to meet the needs of the infant or child. Generally, treatment and follow-up care of these children are carried out in a clinic, practitioner's office, or outpatient unit. Hospitalization may be necessary for cast application or brace fitting but seldom exceeds 24 to 48 hours. Longer hospitalization is required for open reduction.

The primary nursing goal is teaching parents to apply and maintain the reduction device. The Pavlik harness allows for easy handling of the infant and usually produces less apprehension in the parent than heavy braces and casts. It is important that parents understand the correct use of the appliance, which may or may not allow for its removal during bathing. When the infant has a harness that is not removed, a sponge bath is recommended, and the skin beneath the harness is assessed daily for irritation. Powders and lotions are not used, because they tend to cake or "ball" underneath straps or clothing.

To prevent skin irritation from the straps, long socks and a shirt are worn under the device. Extensions on the shirt that snap at the crotch help keep the shirt in place (Speers and Speers, 1992). Unbuckling or removal of the harness is determined individually on the basis of the family's level of understanding and the degree of deformity in the hip. In general, parents should not adjust the harness without supervision. The child should be examined by the practitioner before any adjustment is attempted to make certain the hips are in correct placement before the harness is resecured.

Casts and orthotics devices ("braces") offer more challenging nursing problems, since they cannot be removed for routine care, although sometimes a brace may be removed for bathing. Care of an infant or small child with a cast requires nursing innovation to reduce irritation and to maintain cleanliness of both the child and the cast, particularly in the diaper area. (See p. 1130 for care of the child in a cast.)

Parents are taught the proper care of the cast (or orthotic device) and are helped to devise means for maintaining cleanliness. A superabsorbent disposable diaper (newborn size) is tucked beneath the entire perineal opening of the cast. A larger (toddler size) diaper can be applied and fastened over the small diaper and cast.

For tightly fitting casts, transparent film dressings can be cut into strips as for petaling (see p. 1130), and one edge applied to the cast edge and the other directly to the perineum; this forms a continuous, waterproof bridge between the perineum and the cast to prevent leakage. An additional advantage to the use of this transparent dressing is that it keeps both the skin and the cast dry while allowing for observation of skin beneath the dressing.

Older infants and small children may stuff bits of food, small toys, or other items under the cast; parents should be alerted to this possibility so that suitable preventive measures can be initiated.

Feeding the infant in a hip spica cast offers problems of positioning. Very young infants can be fed in the supine position with the head elevated, and with the infant's hips and legs supported on a pillow at the side, the parent can cuddle the infant in his or her arms during feeding. A somewhat similar position can be used for breast-feeding (i.e., with the infant supported on pillows or held in a "football" hold facing the mother with the legs behind her). An alternate position is to hold the infant upright on the caregiver's lap with the legs of the infant astride the adult's leg.

NURSING DIAGNOSES: THE CHILD WITH DEVELOPMENTAL DYSPLASIA OF THE HIP

Impaired physical mobility related to correction device
High risk for impaired skin integrity related to presence of correction device
Altered family processes related to care of a child in a corrective device

Infants who are able to sit up can be fed while sitting at a feeding table or in a modified high chair. Parents may be able to fashion a tilt board with a padded seat or an adjustable chair. The table or chair provides an excellent place for the child to play in an upright position. The child's car seat is also a vital consideration. Modifications can be made on several standard, government-approved car seats.* A specially designed car restraint for a young child in a spica cast is shown in Fig. 31-15.

It is important for nurses, parents, and other caregivers to understand that children in corrective devices need to be involved in all the activities of any child in the same age-group. Toys are chosen that can be used in a prone position on the floor or in the seats devised for feeding and other activities. Confinement in a cast or appliance should not exclude children from family (or unit) activities. They can be held astride the lap for comfort and transported to areas of activity. The child may be allowed to walk in a cast or orthotic device. An adapted wheelchair, stroller, or scooter can offer mobility to the older infant or child.

❖ Evaluation

The effectiveness of nursing interventions is determined by continual reassessment and evaluation of care based on the following observational guidelines and expected outcomes:

1. Inspect corrective device regularly.
2. Inspect child's skin and circulation regularly.
3. Observe family's behavior with child and interview them regarding identified problems and solutions.

Expected outcomes:

1. Hip remains in desired position; corrective device is positioned properly.
2. Skin remains free of irritation; circulation is unimpaired.
3. Family adjusts nurturing activities to accommodate corrective device.

CONGENITAL CLUBFOOT

The general term *clubfoot* is used to describe a common deformity in which the foot is twisted out of its normal shape or position. Any foot deformity involving the ankle is called *talipes,* derived from *talus,* meaning ankle, and *pes,* meaning foot. Deformities of the foot and ankle are described according to the position of the ankle and foot. The more common positions involve the following variations:

Talipes varus—an inversion or a bending inward
Talipes valgus—an eversion or bending outward
Talipes equinus—plantar flexion in which the toes are lower than the heel
Talipes calcaneus—dorsiflexion, in which the toes are higher than the heel

Most clubfeet are a combination of these positions, and the most frequently occurring type of clubfoot (approximately 95%) is the composite deformity *talipes equinovarus (TEV),* in which the foot is pointed downward and inward in varying degrees of severity (Fig. 31-16). Unilateral club-

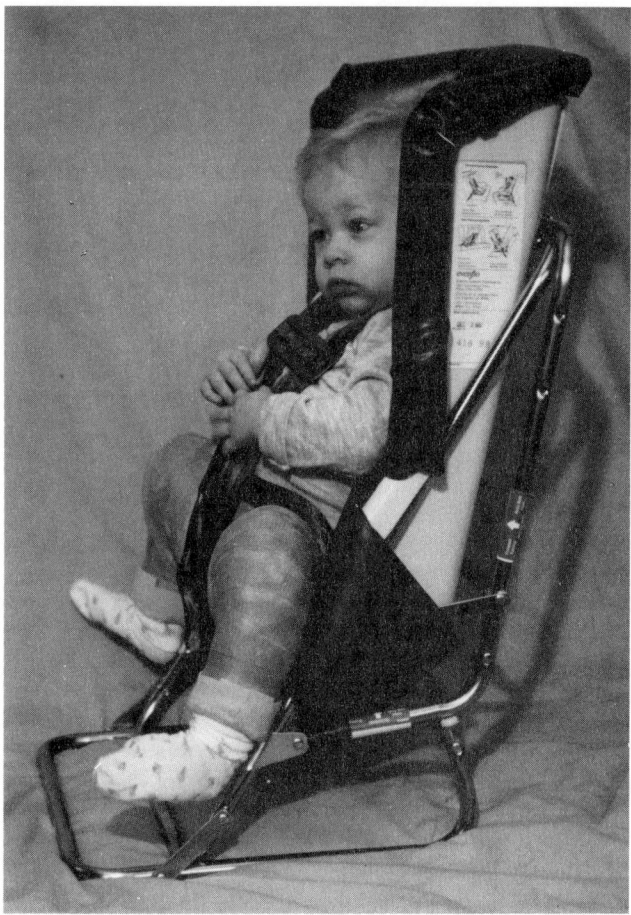

FIG. 31-15. Child in specially designed car restraint (Spelcast).

foot is somewhat more common than bilateral clubfoot and may occur as an isolated defect or in association with other disorders or syndromes, such as chromosomal aberrations, arthrogryposis (a generalized immobility of the joints), cerebral palsy, or spina bifida.

The frequency of clubfoot in the general population is 1:700 to 1:1000 live births, with boys affected twice as often as girls. There is a 35% concordance in monozygotic twins, as opposed to a 3% concordance in dizygotic twins, which indicates a hereditary component.

Pathophysiology

The precise cause of clubfoot is unknown. Some authorities attribute the defect to abnormal positioning and restricted movement in utero, although the evidence is not conclusive. Other experts implicate arrested or abnormal embryonic development. Arrested development during this early stage tends to result in a rigid deformity, whereas mechanical pressures from intrauterine positioning are likely causes of more flexible deformities.

Diagnostic Evaluation

The deformity is readily apparent and easily detected prenatally through ultrasonography or at birth. However, it must be differentiated from some positional deformities that can be passively corrected or overcorrected. The true clubfoot is

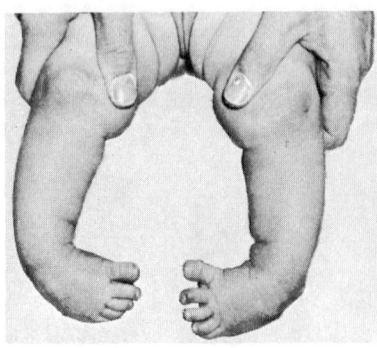

FIG. 31-16. Bilateral congenital talipes equinovarus (congenital clubfoot) in 2-month-old infant. (From Brashear HR Jr, Raney RB: *Handbook of orthopaedic surgery,* ed 10, St Louis, 1986, Mosby.)

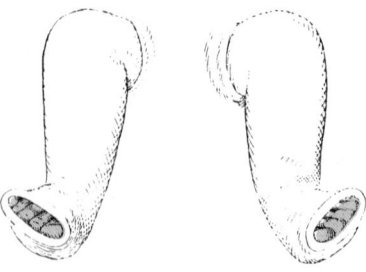

FIG. 31-17. Feet casted for correction of bilateral congenital talipes equinovarus. (From Brashear HR Jr, Raney RB: *Handbook of orthopaedic surgery,* ed 10, St Louis, 1986, Mosby.)

fixed. Paralytic changes in the lower extremity of children with neuromuscular involvement often produce equinovarus deformity.

slow serial casting to stretch ligaments into place

Therapeutic Management

Treatment is begun as soon as the deformity is recognized and involves three stages: (1) correction of the deformity, (2) maintenance of the correction until normal muscle balance is regained, and (3) follow-up observation to avert possible recurrence of the deformity. Some feet respond to treatment readily; some respond only to prolonged, vigorous, and sustained efforts; and the improvement in others remains disappointing even with maximum effort on the part of all concerned.

Correction of TEV is most reliably accomplished by manipulation and the application of a series of casts begun immediately or shortly after birth and continued until marked overcorrection is reached (Fig. 31-17). Successive casts allow for gradual stretching of tight structures on the medial side of the foot and gradual contraction of lax structures on the lateral side. Manipulation and casting are repeated frequently (every few days for 1 to 2 weeks, then at 1- to 2-week intervals) to accommodate the rapid growth of early infancy. The extremity or extremities are casted until the desired result is achieved.

Nursing Considerations

Nursing care of the child with nonsurgical correction of clubfoot is the same as for any child who has a cast (p. 1130). Because the child will spend considerable time in a corrective device, nursing care plans include both long-term and short-term goals. Conscientious observation of the skin and circulation is particularly important in young infants because of their normally rapid growth rate. Since treatment and follow-up care are handled in the orthopedist's office, clinic, or outpatient department, parent education and support are important in nursing care of these children.

Parents need to understand the overall treatment program, the importance of regular cast changes, and the role they play in the long-term effectiveness of the therapy. Reinforcing and clarifying the orthopedist's explanations and instructions; teaching parents about care of the cast or appliance (including vigilant observation for potential problems), and encour-

aging parents to facilitate normal development within the limitations imposed by the deformity or therapy are all part of nursing responsibilities.

METATARSUS ADDUCTUS (VARUS)

Metatarsus adductus, or metatarsus varus, is probably the most common congenital foot deformity. In most instances it is a result of abnormal intrauterine positioning and is usually detected at birth. The deformity is characterized by medial adduction of the toes and forefoot, frequently in association with inversion, and by convexity of the lateral border of the foot. Unlike TEV, with which it is often confused, the angulation occurs at the tarsometatarsal joint, while the heel and ankle remain in a neutral position. This deformity often causes a pigeon-toed gait in the child.

Management depends on the rigidity of the deformity. Correction can usually be accomplished by gentle manipulation and passive stretching of the foot, which the parent is taught to perform. Repeated and consistent stretching is continued for the first 6 weeks, after which the treatment is based on the flexibility of the foot. Those feet that do not respond to the manipulation require orthopedic therapy. If the child is able to actively overcorrect the deformity voluntarily on stimulation, continued stretching is generally sufficient. If the foot cannot be actively or passively overcorrected, the feet are stretched and manipulated and held with casts and/or orthoses.

Nursing Considerations

The nursing role primarily involves identifying the defect, so that early therapy and instruction of the parents can be initiated. The nurse teaches the parents how to hold the heel firmly and to stretch only the forefoot; otherwise, undue force on the heel may produce a valgus deformity. If casting is needed, the nurse instructs the parents in cast care and observation (see p. 1131).

SKELETAL LIMB DEFICIENCY

Congenital limb deficiencies, or reduction malformations, are manifested by a variety of degrees of loss of functional capacity. They are characterized by underdevelopment of skeletal elements of the extremities. The range of malformation can extend from minor defects of the digits to serious abnormalities, such as *amelia,* absence of an entire extremity, or *meromelia,* partial absence of an extremity, which includes *phocomelia* (seal limbs), an interposed deficiency of long bones

casting not always successful
1/2 still need surgery

with relatively good development of hands and feet attached at or near the shoulder or the hips.

In rare instances prenatal destruction of limbs has been reported, but most reduction deformities are primary defects of development (agenesis, aplasia). Therefore, congenital amputations in the literal sense are not amputations, since nonexistent limbs cannot be amputated.

Pathophysiology

Limb deficiencies can be attributed to both heredity and environment and can originate at any stage of limb development. Formation of limbs may be suppressed at the time of limb bud formation, or there may be interference in later stages of differentiation and growth. Heredity appears to play a prominent role, and prenatal environmental insults have been implicated in a number of cases, such as the well-publicized thalidomide tragedy of the 1950s and early 1960s, which demonstrated a clear relationship between the time of exposure of the pregnant woman to the antiemetic drug and the presence and type of limb deformity in the newborn.

Therapeutic Management

Children with congenital limb deficiencies should be fitted with prosthetic devices whenever possible, and the devices should be applied at the earliest possible stage of development in an attempt to match the motor readiness of the infant. This favors natural progression of prosthetic use. For example, a young infant with an upper extremity deficiency is fitted with a simple passive device, such as a mitten prosthesis, to encourage limb exploration, sitting (with the extremities needed for support), and bilateral hand activities.

Lower limb prostheses are applied when the infant is ready to pull to a standing position. In preparation for prosthetic devices, surgical modification is often necessary to ensure the most favorable use of the device, since severe deformity can interfere with its effective use. Phocomelic digits are preserved for controlling switches of externally powered appliances in upper extremities. Digits (in both upper and lower extremities) provide the child with surfaces for tactile exploration and stimulation. Prostheses are replaced to accommodate growth and increasing capabilities of the child.

Nursing Considerations

Prosthetic application training and habilitation are most successfully carried out in a center that specializes in meeting the special needs of these children, especially very young children and those with multiple amputations. It involves a team of health professionals and the parents, who must encourage the child in making age-commensurate adjustments to the environment. Although these children need assistance, excessive overprotection may produce overdependency, with later maladjustment to school and other situations.

OSTEOGENESIS IMPERFECTA (OI)

OI refers to a group of heterogenous inherited disorders of connective tissue characterized by connective tissue and bone defects. The inheritance pattern is autosomal-dominant in the majority of cases, although the most severe form demonstrates autosomal-recessive inheritance (see Appendix B).

Persons with OI appear to have abnormal precollagen that prevents the formation of collagen, the major component of connective tissue. At present OI is believed to consist of four different variations (see box). Type II, the most severe form of OI, is characterized by multiple intrauterine or perinatal fractures, severe deformity, and, often, early death. The brittle bones easily fracture from the slightest trauma.

The diseases of later onset run a milder course. The tendency to fracture appears later (at variable ages) and disappears after puberty. During childhood the shafts of long bones are slender, with reduced cortical thickness resulting from defective periosteal bone formation. In addition to the features already described, the child with OI has thin skin, hyperextensibility of ligaments, a tendency toward recurrent epistaxis, excess diaphoresis, a tendency to bruise easily, and mild hyperpyrexia. The disease shows variable expressivity; that is, the number and extent of pathologic features appear in any individual range, from severe to minimal involvement. The incidence of fractures decreases at puberty, when the body's production of hormones helps strengthen bones.

Therapeutic Management

The treatment is primarily supportive. Several drugs have been tried but appear to be of limited benefit. Lightweight braces and splints help support limbs, prevent fractures, and aid in ambulation. Physical therapy helps prevent disuse osteoporosis and strengthens muscles, which in turn improves bone density. Exercises are usually simple ones against light resistance or water exercises with swimming. Patients with milder disease are encouraged to participate in appropriate sports.

Surgery is sometimes used to help treat the manifestations of the disease. Surgical techniques are used to correct deformities that interfere with bracing, standing, or walking. For the child with recurrent fractures, inserting an intermedullary rod provides stability to bones. Unfortunately, the rods

CLASSIFICATION OF OSTEOGENESIS IMPERFECTA

Type		Characteristics
I*		Mild bone fragility; blue sclerae; normal teeth; presenile deafness (age 20-30 years); autosomal-dominant inheritance
	B	Same as A except dentinogenesis imperfecta instead of normal teeth
	C	Same as B; no bone fragility
II		Lethal; stillborn or die in early infancy; severe bone fragility, multiple fractures at birth; 10% of OI cases; autosomal-recessive inheritance
III		Severe bone fragility leads to severe progressive deformities; normal sclerae; marked growth failure; most autosomal-recessive; few autosomal-dominant
IV	A	Mild to moderate bone fragility; normal sclerae; short stature; variable deformity; autosomal-dominant
	B	Same as A except dentinogenesis imperfecta instead of normal teeth; approximately 6% of OI cases

*Two thirds of cases are type I.

must be replaced as the child grows; otherwise fractures may occur through the unprotected portion of the bone.

Nursing Considerations

Infants and children with this disorder require careful handling to prevent fractures. They must be supported when they are being turned, positioned, moved, and fondled. Even changing a diaper may cause a fracture in severely affected infants. These children should never be held by the ankles when being diapered but should be gently lifted by the buttocks.

Both parents and the affected child need education regarding the child's limitations and guidelines in planning suitable activities that promote optimum development, as well as protect the child from harm. Realistic occupational planning and genetic counseling are part of the long-term goals of care. Educational materials and information can be obtained from the *Osteogenesis Imperfecta Foundation, Inc,** which also has a network that can put a family in contact with other families with a similar problem.

ACQUIRED DEFECTS

LEGG-CALVÉ-PERTHES DISEASE

Legg-Calvé-Perthes disease, sometimes called *coxa plana* or *osteochondritis deformans juvenilis,* is a self-limited disorder in which there is aseptic necrosis of the femoral head. The disease affects children 3 to 12 years of age, but most cases occur in males between ages 4 and 8 years as an isolated event. In approximately 10% to 15% of cases the involvement is bilateral; most of the affected children have a skeletal age significantly below their chronologic age. The male/female ratio is 4:1 or 5:1; white children are affected 10 times more frequently than black children.

Pathophysiology

The cause of the disease is unknown, but there is a disturbance of circulation to the femoral capital epiphysis that produces an ischemic aseptic necrosis of the femoral head. Dur-

*5005 W. Laurel St., Tampa, FL 33607-3836; (813) 282-1161.

ing middle childhood, circulation to the femoral epiphysis is more tenuous than at other ages and can become obstructed by trauma, inflammation, coagulation defects, and a variety of other causes. The pathologic events seem to take place in four stages (see box). The entire process may encompass as little as 18 months or continue for several years. The reformed femoral head may be severely altered or appear entirely normal.

Diagnostic Evaluation

The diagnosis is suspected from clinical manifestations (see box) and established by radiographic examination.

Therapeutic Management

Since deformity occurs early in the disease process, the aim of treatment is to keep the head of the femur contained in the acetabulum, which serves as a mold to preserve the spherical shape of the head and to maintain a full range of motion. The initial therapy is rest, which helps reduce inflammation and restore motion. Active motion is encouraged. In some cases traction is applied to stretch tight adductor muscles.

Containment can be accomplished by non-weightbearing devices, such as an abduction brace, leg casts, or a leather harness sling that prevents weight bearing on the affected limb; by various weight-bearing appliances, such as abduction-ambulation braces or casts, after a period of bed rest and traction; and by surgical reconstructive and containment procedures. Conservative therapy must be continued for 2 to 4 years, although braces constructed from lightweight materials allow the child to maintain a nearly normal activity level. Surgical correction returns the child to normal activities within 3 to 4 months.

The disease is self-limited, but the ultimate outcome of therapy depends on early and efficient treatment and the age of onset of the disorder. Younger children, whose epiphyses are more cartilaginous, have the brightest prognosis for complete recovery. The later the diagnosis is made, the more damage has occurred before treatment is implemented. In most cases, with good patient compliance the prognosis is excellent.

Nursing Considerations

Nurses are often the first health professionals to identify affected children and to refer them for medical evaluation. They are also persons on whom the child and the family can rely

---

STAGES OF LEGG-CALVÉ-PERTHES DISEASE

Stage I: Aseptic necrosis or infarction of the femoral capital epiphysis with degenerative changes producing flattening of the upper surface of the femoral head—the *avascular stage*

Stage II: Capital bone absorption and revascularization with fragmentation (vascular resorption of the epiphysis) that gives a mottled appearance on radiographs—the *fragmentation,* or *revascularization, stage*

Stage III: New bone formation, which is represented on radiographs as calcification and ossification or increased density in the areas of radiolucency; this filling-in process appears to take place from the periphery of the head centrally—the *reparative stage*

Stage IV: Gradual reformation of the head of the femur without radiolucency and, it is hoped, to a spherical form—the *regenerative stage*

CLINICAL MANIFESTATIONS OF LEGG-CALVÉ-PERTHES DISEASE

Insidious onset
Intermittent appearance of limp on affected side
Pain
  Soreness or aching
  In hip, along entire length of thigh, or in vicinity of knee
  Most evident on rising or at end of a long day
  Usually accompanied by joint dysfunction and limited range of motion
Stiffness
Point tenderness over hip capsule
External hip rotation (late sign)

CLINICAL MANIFESTATIONS OF SLIPPED FEMORAL CAPITAL EPIPHYSIS

Obese or tall, lanky youngster
Limp on affected side
Pain in hip
   Continuous or intermittent
    Frequently referred to groin, anteromedial aspect of thigh, or knee
Restricted internal rotation on adduction with external rotation deformity
Loss of abduction and internal rotation as severity increases

docrine abnormalities such as hypothyroidism, renal osteodystrophy, and growth hormone therapy.

The pathologic processes as seen in radiographs involve first a rarefaction of bone on the lower femoral side of the epiphysis with widening of the growth plate. After trauma or slight injury the femoral portion of the epiphysis slides upward but remains attached by the thick, continuous periosteum. As slipping increases, the epiphyseal displacement becomes posterior and inferior. The slipping produces deformity of the femoral head and stretches the blood vessels to the epiphysis.

Diagnostic Evaluation

The disorder is suspected when an adolescent or preadolescent youngster displays clinical signs or complains of pain (see box). The diagnosis is confirmed by radiographic examination.

Therapeutic Management *surgical stabilization*

The treatment varies with the degree of displacement but involves surgical stabilization and correction of deformity. In mild cases simple pin fixation is sufficient. More extensive displacement requires skeletal traction followed by pin fixation or osteotomy. The prognosis depends on the degree of deformity and the occurrence of complications, such as avascular necrosis and cartilaginous necrosis. As in other disorders, early diagnosis and implementation of therapy increase the likelihood of a satisfactory cure. *severe—put in traction fir...*

Nursing Considerations

Nursing care is the same as that for a child in a cast or a child in traction, as discussed earlier in this chapter.

KYPHOSIS AND LORDOSIS

Kyphosis is an abnormally increased convex angulation in the curvature of the thoracic spine (Fig. 31-18, *B*). It can occur secondary to disease processes such as tuberculosis, chronic arthritis, osteodystrophy, or compression fractures of the thoracic spine. The most common form of kyphosis is "postural." Children, especially during the time when skeletal growth outpaces growth of muscle, are prone to exaggeration of a tendency toward kyphosis. They assume abnormal sitting and standing positions. This is particularly common in self-conscious adolescent girls who assume a round-shouldered slouching posture in an attempt to hide their developing breasts.

Postural kyphosis is almost always accompanied by a com-

to help them understand and adjust to the therapeutic measures. Since most of the child's care is conducted on an outpatient basis, the major emphasis of nursing care is teaching the family the care and management of the corrective appliance selected for therapy. The family needs to learn the purpose, function, application, and care of the corrective device and the importance of compliance in order to achieve the desired outcome.

One of the most difficult aspects associated with the disorder is coping with a normally active child who feels well but must remain relatively inactive. Suitable activities must be devised to meet the needs of the child in the process of developing a sense of initiative or industry. Activities that meet the creative urges are well received. This is also an opportune time to encourage the child to begin a hobby, such as collections, model building, or crafts (see Family Focus box).

SLIPPED FEMORAL CAPITAL EPIPHYSIS *no infectious process*

Slipped femoral capital epiphysis, or *coxa vara,* refers to the spontaneous displacement of the proximal femoral epiphysis in a posterior and inferior direction. It develops most frequently shortly before or during accelerated growth and the onset of puberty (children between the ages of 10 and 16 years—median age, 13 for boys, 11 for girls) and is most frequently observed in obese children. Bilateral involvement has been reported as 16% to 40%.

Pathophysiology *Backwards + down*

The cause of coxa vara is unknown, but it occurs most often in "overlarge" youngsters or very tall, thin, rapidly growing children. There has been some evidence to implicate hormonal factors, such as decreased growth hormone and increased sex hormone. It has also been associated with en-

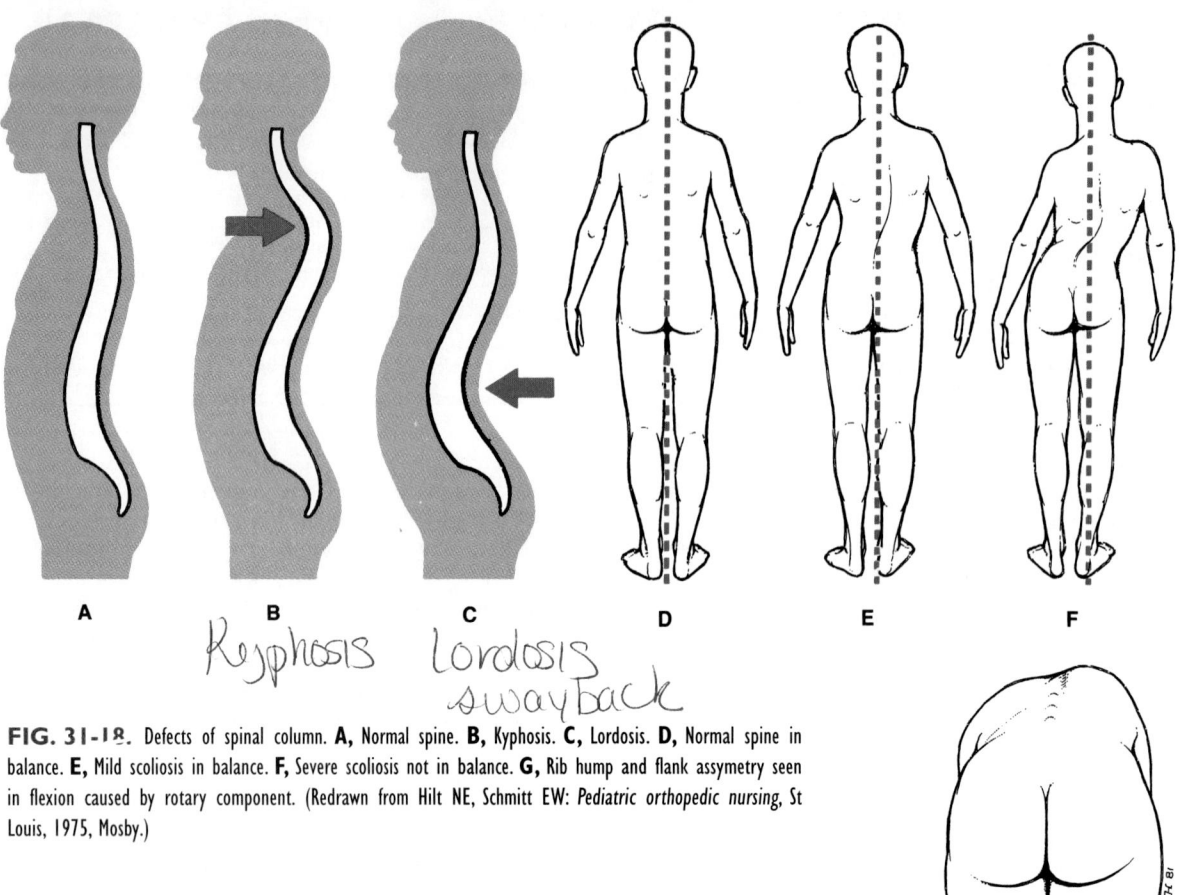

Kyphosis   Lordosis
              swayback

FIG. 31-18. Defects of spinal column. **A,** Normal spine. **B,** Kyphosis. **C,** Lordosis. **D,** Normal spine in balance. **E,** Mild scoliosis in balance. **F,** Severe scoliosis not in balance. **G,** Rib hump and flank assymetry seen in flexion caused by rotary component. (Redrawn from Hilt NE, Schmitt EW: *Pediatric orthopedic nursing,* St Louis, 1975, Mosby.)

pensatory postural lordosis, an abnormally exaggerated concave lumbar curvature. Treatment consists of postural exercises to strengthen shoulder and abdominal muscles and bracing for more marked deformity. Unfortunately, treatment is difficult; the normal rebellious tendencies of the adolescent, together with continual parental nagging to "stand up straight," often interfere with compliance to a therapeutic regimen. The best approach is to emphasize the cosmetic value of corrective therapy and to place the responsibility on the adolescent for carrying out an exercise program at home with regular visits to and assessments by a therapist. Most adolescents respond well to selected sports as a supplement to regular exercise. Boys prefer weight lifting (preferably performed from a prone or supine position on a bench) and track sports. Girls respond well to dancing classes (ballet or modern dancing). Swimming is excellent and has the added advantages of exercising all muscles, eliminating gravity, and teaching breath control.

Lordosis is an accentuation of the cervical or lumbar curvature beyond physiologic limits (Fig. 31-18, *C*). It may be a secondary complication of a disease process, a result of trauma, or idiopathic. It is often seen in association with flexion contractures of the hip, obesity, congenital dislocated hip, and slipped femoral capital epiphysis. During the pubertal growth spurt lordosis of varying degrees is observed in teenagers, especially girls. In obese children the weight of the abdominal fat alters the center of gravity, causing a compensatory lordosis. Unlike kyphosis, severe lordosis is usually accompanied by pain.

Treatment involves management of the predisposing cause when possible, such as weight loss and correction of deformities. Postural exercises and/or support garments are helpful in relieving symptoms in some cases; however, these do not usually effect a permanent cure.

SCOLIOSIS

Scoliosis, the most common spinal deformity, is a lateral curvature of the spine usually associated with a rotary deformity that eventually causes cosmetic and physiologic alterations in the spine, chest, and pelvis. It can be congenital, or it can develop during infancy or childhood, but it is most common during the growth spurt of early adolescence.

Etiology

Scoliosis can be caused by a number of conditions and may occur alone or in association with other diseases, particularly neuromuscular conditions. In most cases, however, there is no apparent cause, and it is called *idiopathic scoliosis.* There is evidence that it may be genetic and transmitted as an autosomal-dominant trait with incomplete penetrance, or it may be multifactorial.

Diagnostic Evaluation

Diagnosis is made by observation and radiographic examination. Discomfort is rarely present, and there are few outward signs until the deformity is well established. Early detection and treatment are essential to successful management (see also Spine, Chapter 7). The undressed child viewed from the posterior side often reveals primary curvature and a compensatory curvature that places the head in alignment with the gluteal fold (Fig. 31-18, *E*). In uncompensated scoliosis the head and hips are not in alignment (Fig. 31-18, *F*). In advanced cases with rotary deformity, rib hump and flank asymmetry are observed when the child bends from the waist unsupported by the arms (Fig. 31-18, *G*). Radiographs taken in the standing position establish the degree of curvature.

 Not all spinal curvatures are scoliosis. A curve of less than 10 degrees is considered a postural variation. Curves of under 20 degrees are mild and, if nonprogressive, do not require treatment.

Therapeutic Management

A thorough examination, history, and assessment of the child are carried out to evaluate the status of the deformity, factors contributing to the defect, and factors that may influence the outcome of therapy. Treatment is best undertaken in a center in which a team is available that specializes in management of scoliosis. Current management involves straightening and realignment of the vertebrae by either external (bracing) or internal (surgical) fixation techniques. Bracing is not curative but may slow the progression of the deformity until the spine has reached skeletal maturity.

Bracing and Exercise. Exercises alone are rarely of value with scoliosis. However, supplemental exercises are employed daily in and out of the brace to prevent atrophy of spinal and abdominal muscles. Nonoperative treatment by application of a properly constructed and well-fitted external bracing device and close supervision are successful in halting the progression of most curvatures. The two most commonly used types of braces are (1) the **Boston brace**, or underarm orthosis, customized from prefabricated plastic shells, with corrective forces for each patient, using lateral pads and decreasing lumbar lordosis, and (2) the **Milwaukee brace**, an individually adapted plastic and metal brace that includes a neck ring and can be used for curves with an apex of higher than T8 (Fig. 31-19).

The type of brace and wearing schedule (usually between 16 and 23 hours a day) is based on the nature of the curve, the age of the child, and any underlying condition associated with the curve. The underarm brace is usually more cosmetically acceptable to the child, since it is easily hidden under loose-fitting clothing.

Electrical Stimulation. Mild to moderate curvatures may be treated with electrical stimulation. An electrical stimulator generates an electrical pulse that is transmitted to muscles on the convex side of the curvature. This causes the muscles to contract at regular and frequent intervals, possibly straightening the spine. The device is worn at night, allowing unrestricted activity during the waking hours. Not all authorities believe that this therapy is effective.

Surgical Correction. Surgical intervention may be required for correction. With few exceptions the techniques consist of spinal realignment and straightening by way of external or internal fixation and instrumentation combined with bony fusion (arthrodesis) of the realigned spine. The age of

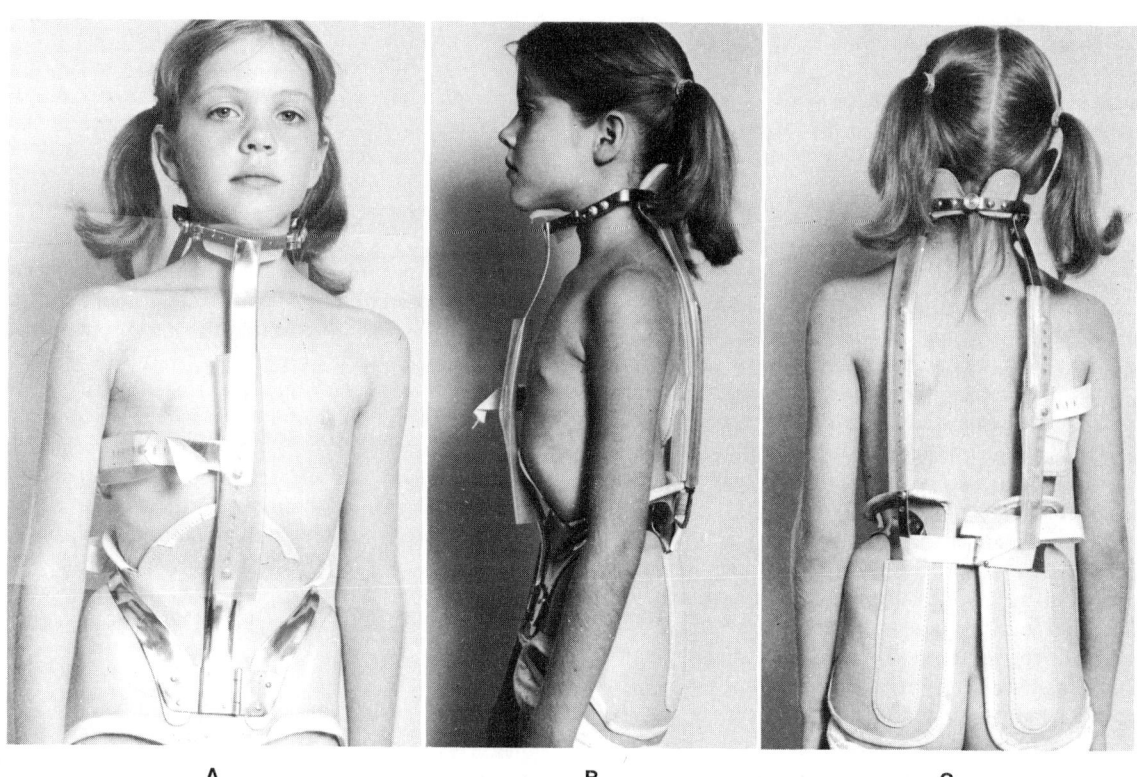

FIG. 31-19. Milwaukee brace. **A,** Front view. **B,** Side view. **C,** Rear view. (From Blount WP, Mueller KH, *Praxis* 8:139-149, 1972.)

the child and location of the curvature influence the decision for surgery, and any curve that does not respond to more conservative measures requires surgical correction.

For the most severe scoliotic curvatures, traction is often needed for a time before spinal fusion to provide partial correction and more flexibility. Methods incorporating either continuous or intermittent traction are used. One type consists of a leather head halter and pelvic girdle attached to a system of ropes and pulleys that can be manipulated by the patient. More rigid deformities are best managed by skeletal traction techniques.

When surgical intervention is elected, a variety of spinal fusion techniques may be used. Depending on the surgical procedure, casting or a removable brace may be used for a period of 6 months to a year to produce satisfactory results. The surgical techniques for internal vertebral fixation include the following:

Harrington instrumentation—implantation of metal rods by way of clips to hold the vertebrae and bone fragments for permanent fusion; postoperatively the child is logrolled to prevent spinal motion. A molded plastic jacket is used to provide external stabilization of the spine while the child resumes activities

Luque segmental spinal instrumentation—a flexible L-shaped metal rod fixed by wires to the bases of the spinous processes; patient can walk within a few days, and no postoperative immobilization is necessary

Dwyer instrumentation—a titanium cable through cannulated screws transfixed to each vertebra; child is cared for in bed following surgery

Zielke procedure—combination of Harrington and Dwyer procedures; requires an anterior approach

Cotrel-Dubousset (CD) procedure—a form of bilateral segmental fixation that uses two knurled rods and multiple hooks that provide secure attachment to the spine so that casting or bracing is not needed

Texas Scottish Rite Hospital (TSRH) System—use of bilateral rods, hooks, and cross-link plates; if needed, system allows for easier surgical revision than CD instrumentation

Nursing Considerations

Treatment for scoliosis extends over a significant portion of the affected child's period of growth. In adolescents this period is the one in which their identity, physical and psychologic, is formed. For some youngsters much of this time is spent in the hospital setting, immobilized in complex, unattractive appliances. For those treated on an outpatient basis, it means a modified life-style and being "different" from their peers, even though they are usually able to engage in many activities enjoyed by other youngsters.

When a child first faces the prospect of a prolonged period in a brace, cast, or other device, the therapy program and the nature of the device must be explained thoroughly to both the child and the parents so that they will have an understanding of the anticipated results, how the appliance corrects the defect, the freedoms and constraints imposed by the device, and what they can do to help achieve the desired goal. The management involves the skills and services of a team of specialists, including the orthopedist, physical therapist, orthotist (a specialist in fitting orthopedic braces), nurse, social worker, and sometimes a pulmonary specialist.

It is difficult for a child to be restricted at any phase of development, but the teenager needs continual positive rein-

forcement, encouragement, and as much independence as can be safely assumed during this time. Guidance and assistance regarding anticipated problems, such as selection of clothing and participation in social activities, are appreciated by adolescents. Socialization with peers is encouraged, and every effort is expended to help the adolescent feel attractive and worthwhile.

Preoperative Care. The child hospitalized for surgical management requires preparation for the procedures involved, which are puzzling and often frightening to the very young patient. The child needs to know what is going to happen and deserves a full explanation of why the procedure is necessary and the potential outcome of the surgery.

Postoperative Care. Following surgery patients are monitored in an intensive care unit and logrolled when changing position to prevent damage to the fusion and instrumentation. Skin care is very important, and pressure-relieving mattresses or beds may be needed to prevent pressure wounds (see Maintaining Healthy Skin, Chapter 22).

In addition to the usual postoperative assessments—of wound, circulation, and vital signs—the neurologic status of the patient's extremities requires special attention. There is usually some degree of paralytic ileus following the procedure; therefore nursing includes care of the nasogastric intubation and assessment for returning bowel function. Urinary retention is common and often requires insertion of an indwelling catheter. Because of the extensive blood loss during the surgical procedure and renal hypoperfusion, observation of urine output is especially important.

The child usually has considerable pain for the first few days following surgery and requires frequent administration of pain medication, preferably the use of opioids administered on a regular schedule administered intravenously or epidurally. For children able to understand the concept, patient-controlled analgesia (PCA) is a recommended alternative (see Pain Assessment; Pain Management, Chapter 21).

All patients are started on physiotherapy as soon as they are able, beginning with range-of-motion exercises and many of the activities of daily living. Self-care, such as washing and eating, is always encouraged. Some simple physical therapy may be begun during this acute stage. Throughout the hospitalization diversional activities and contact with family and friends are important parts of nursing care and planning.

The family is encouraged to become involved with the patient's care to facilitate the transition from hospital to home management. Family members learn to apply and care for the brace or learn cast care. An organization that provides education and services to both families and professionals is the **National Scoliosis Foundation, Inc.*** The **Scoliosis Research Society,†** an organization of physicians and scientists, has published an excellent book, *Scoliosis: A Handbook for Patients.*

See also Nursing Care Plan: The Child with Structural Scoliosis.‡

---

*5 Cabot Place, Stoughton, MA 02072; (617)341-6333.
†6300 River Rd., Rosemont, IL 60018; (847) 698-1627. The book can be purchased by sending $1.00 to the organization.
‡In Wong DL: *Wong and Whaley's Clinical manual of pediatric nursing*, ed 4, St Louis, 1996, Mosby.

INFECTIONS OF BONES AND JOINTS

OSTEOMYELITIS

Osteomyelitis is an infectious process of bone that can occur at any age but that occurs most frequently between 5 and 14 years of age. It is twice as common in boys as in girls.

Pathophysiology

Osteomyelitis can be acquired from exogenous or hematogenous sources. *Exogenous osteomyelitis* is acquired by invasion of the bone by direct extension from the outside as a result of a penetrating wound, open fracture, contamination during surgery, or secondary extension from an overlying abscess or burn. *Hematogenous osteomyelitis* occurs from spread of organisms from preexisting infectious foci, including furuncles, skin abrasions, impetigo, upper respiratory tract infections, acute otitis media, tonsillitis, abscessed teeth, pyelonephritis, or infected burns.

Any organism can cause osteomyelitis, and there is some relationship between the age of the child and the type of organism responsible. In older children staphylococci are the most common organisms, approximately 80% of which are *Staphylococcus aureus;* in younger children other organisms predominate, especially *Haemophilus influenzae.* In children with sickle cell anemia, *Salmonella* organisms are frequently the responsible agents. Other factors that predispose to development of osteomyelitis are poor physical condition, inadequate nutrition, and surroundings that are not hygienic.

Infective emboli from the focus of infection travel to the small end arteries in the bone metaphysis, where they set up an infectious process that leads to local bone destruction and abscess formation.

Diagnostic Evaluation

The signs and symptoms of *acute hematogenous osteomyelitis* begin abruptly and build up to a maximum intensity during the first few days of the disease, usually less than 1 week (see box). Symptoms often resemble those observed in other disorders involving bones (e.g., leukemia, arthritis). There is marked leukocytosis and an elevated erythrocyte sedimentation rate. Blood culture is usually positive during the early stage, and radiographic findings are often negative or show only soft tissue swelling for 10 to 14 days. After this time the radiographic findings reveal new bone formation. Tomography may reveal bone changes at an early stage. (See Critical Thinking Exercise.)

Most cases involve the femur or tibia and to a lesser extent the humerus and hip. In infants the diagnosis is more difficult because of a lack of systemic symptoms, and the disease may involve multiple bones or joints because of the difficulty in confining an infectious process in children in this age-group.

In *subacute hematogenous osteomyelitis,* symptoms have been present for a longer period of time, and the child sometimes has been treated with antibiotics, often for another infection, which modifies the clinical symptoms. In some instances the infection may produce a walled-off abscess rather than a spreading infection.

Therapeutic Management

As soon as blood cultures have been drawn, prompt and vigorous intravenous antibiotic therapy is initiated. The choice of antibiotic is influenced by age, and the dosage determined is sufficient to ensure high blood and tissue levels. The appropriate antibiotic is usually continued for at least 3 to 4 weeks, but the length of therapy is determined by the duration of symptoms, the initial response to treatment, and the sensitivity of the organism in the specific case. Because of prolonged high-dose therapy, it is important to monitor hematologic, renal, hepatic, and other organ systems that might be adversely affected by the drugs (e.g., ototoxic).

Antibiotic therapy is accompanied by local treatment. The child is placed on complete bed rest. Immobilization of the affected extremity, which may require a splint or bivalved cast, is continued throughout therapy to limit the spread of infection and, when it is a complication of a fracture, to maintain alignment of bone fragments.

Opinions differ regarding surgical intervention, but many advocate sequestrectomy (removal of dead bone) and surgical drainage to prevent abscess formation. When surgical

Culture before antibiotics

CLINICAL MANIFESTATIONS OF ACUTE OSTEOMYELITIS

General Manifestations
History of trauma to affected bone (frequent)
Child appears very ill
Irritability
Restlessness
Elevated temperature
Rapid pulse
Dehydration

Local Manifestations
Tenderness
Increased warmth
Diffuse swelling over involved bone
Involved extremity painful, especially on movement
Involved extremity held in semiflexion
Surrounding muscles tense and resist passive movement

CRITICAL THINKING EXERCISE

Acute Osteomyelitis

Luis, a 12-year-old male, is in the emergency room with a 102° F temperature and a heart rate of 94. He is restless and complains of right leg pain. Laboratory results show an elevated erythrocyte sedimentation rate and leukocytosis. History includes a recent automobile accident that resulted in hospitalization. During the hospital stay he had acquired a nosocomial *Staphylococcus aureus* infection. What findings would you expect from a thorough assessment?

1. Localized warmth, tenderness, and diffuse swelling above his right knee
2. Ability to extend right leg to full flexion
3. Slight pain with ambulation
4. All of the above

The correct answer is one, which indicates the clinical manifestations of acute osteomyelitis. Other signs would include inability to fully extend the leg and significant pain with ambulation.

drainage is carried out, polyethylene tubes are placed in the wound—one tube instills an antibiotic solution directly into the infected area by gravity, and the other, connected to a suction apparatus, provides drainage.

Nursing Considerations

During the acute phase of illness any movement of the affected limb will cause discomfort; therefore the child is positioned comfortably with the affected limb supported. Moving and turning are carried out carefully and gently to minimize pain. Pain medication is administered to provide comfort. Vital signs are taken and recorded frequently, and measures are implemented to reduce a significant temperature elevation.

Antibiotic therapy requires careful observation and monitoring of the intravenous equipment and site. Since more than one antibiotic is usually administered, the compatibility of the drugs is determined, and care is taken to avoid mixing noncompatible drugs. For long-term antibiotic therapy, an intermittent infusion device or peripherally inserted central catheter (PICC) is used (see Venous Access Devices, Chapter 22). Antibiotic therapy is often continued at home.

The child with an open wound may be placed on contact isolation. The wound is managed as prescribed. Antibiotic solution administered directly into the wound is most efficiently accomplished with a regular intravenous infusion setup that is prepared and regulated in the same manner as any other. The drainage tubes are connected to low Gomco or wall suction for continuous removal. Intake and output are measured and recorded, and the character of the wound drainage is noted. The amount and character of drainage on the wound dressing are also noted.

Casts are sometimes used for immobilization, and, if so, routine cast care is carried out. The extremity is examined for sensation, circulation, and pain, and the area over the inflammation is usually left open for observation. The affected area, casted or uncasted, is assessed for color, swelling, heat, and tenderness.

The child usually has a poor appetite at first. Nourishment in the form of high-calorie liquids, such as fruit juices, gelatin, and juice bars, is encouraged until the child begins to feel better. The appetite returns as the acute symptoms subside. During convalescence adequate nutrition must be maintained to aid healing and formation of new bone.

When the acute stage subsides, the child begins to feel better, the appetite improves, and the child becomes interested in the surroundings and relationships, and may move about in bed. However, weight bearing on the affected limb is not permitted until healing is well under way in order to avoid pathologic fractures. Diversional and constructive activities become important nursing interventions. The child is usually confined to bed for some time after the acute phase but may be allowed to move about in a wheelchair when isolation and bed rest are no longer necessary. As the infection subsides, physical therapy is instituted to ensure restoration of optimum function.

SEPTIC (SUPPURATIVE, PYOGENIC, PURULENT) ARTHRITIS

Infection of the joints, like infection of bone, usually develops through hematogenous dissemination from another fo-

---

> **CLINICAL MANIFESTATIONS OF SEPTIC ARTHRITIS**
>
> History of a traumatic injury to the affected joint (often)
> Fever
> Involved joint is:
>   Warm and tender
>   Erythematous
>   Swollen
>   Painful on even gentle pressure
> Superficial involved joints are exquisitely painful
> Deep-seated involved joints show little superficial evidence

cus; occasionally it results from direct extension of a soft tissue infection. Joint infections occur predominantly in males, especially in the adolescent age-group. In infancy, however, the incidence in boys and girls is more nearly equal. Any joint may be involved, but the hip, knee, shoulder, and other large joints are more commonly affected. Usually only one joint is involved.

Diagnostic Evaluation

The signs and symptoms of suppurative arthritis, unlike those of osteomyelitis, are usually characteristic (see box). Fever, leukocytosis, and an increased erythrocyte sedimentation rate are present but may not be demonstrated in affected infants. The most common pathogens are *Staphylococcus aureus*, group A streptococci, and *Haemophilus influenzae*. Diagnosis is made from blood culture, joint fluid aspirate, and radiographs.

Therapeutic Management

Treatment consists of open surgical drainage of hip and shoulder joint disease and repeated needle aspirations of the joint space in other joints. The goals are (1) to cleanse the joint to avoid destruction of articular cartilage, (2) to decompress the joint to avoid interference with the blood supply to the epiphysis, (3) to eradicate the infection with adequate antibiotic therapy, and (4) to prevent secondary bone infection and hematogenous spread. Therapy is similar to that for osteomyelitis: intravenous antibiotic therapy, relief of pain, immobilization of the joint, and prohibition of weight bearing until healing is complete.

Nursing Considerations

Nursing care is the same as that for osteomyelitis.

TUBERCULOSIS

Tubercular infection of the bones is acquired by hematogenous dissemination from a primary tubercular focus. The most common sites in infants and small children are the carpals and phalanges and the corresponding bones of the feet. One or several bones may be involved, with spindle-shaped swelling and tenderness as soft tissues are affected. The process, relatively painless, persists with intermittent symptoms for several months and may leave a permanent deformity. The affected areas are immobilized with a splint or cast.

Tuberculosis of the Spine (Tuberculous Spondylitis)

In older children the infection attacks the body of one or more vertebrae, destroying the bone, and spreads to all the

---

CLINICAL MANIFESTATIONS OF TUBERCULOSIS OF THE BONE

Spinal Manifestations

Insidious onset

Irritability

Child complains of persistent or intermittent pain over areas innervated by spinal nerves that arise adjacent to affected vertebrae

Muscle splinting and pain when there is increased pressure applied to head

Child assumes position that best eases weight on diseased vertebrae, such as avoiding bending, walking stiffly and carefully on toes, and resting on abdomen or across a chair or a lap

Hip Manifestations

Limp that occurs intermittently

Limp occurs most often on arising in the morning or after exercise

Pain

Thigh gradually becomes fixed and adducted with internal rotation

May be swelling around hip

CLINICAL MANIFESTATIONS OF BONE TUMORS

Pain localized at affected site
  May be severe or dull
  Often relieved by position of flexion
  Frequently brought to attention when child:
    Limps
    Curtails own physical activity
    Is unable to hold heavy objects

---

articular tissues, producing a kyphotic deformity. The lower thoracic spine is most frequently affected (see box for manifestations).

Treatment consists of immobilization until there is no evidence of active infection, followed by spinal fusion. Antimicrobial therapy and drainage of tubercular abscess are standard therapies. The reparative process is slow, but in most instances recovery takes place with little or no deformity.

Tuberculosis of the Hip

The hip is the joint most often affected by tuberculosis, but the process usually begins in the epiphysis of the femoral head and then erupts into the joint capsule. There is progressive destruction of the femoral head with accompanying symptoms (see box). There may be abscess formation.

Treatment involves bed rest, traction to reduce muscle spasm, and appropriate drug therapy. Hip fusion may be necessary in severe cases.

BONE AND SOFT TISSUE TUMORS*

GENERAL CONCEPTS: BONE TUMORS

Neoplastic disease can arise from any tissues involved in bone growth. In children the two types that account for 85% of all primary malignant bone tumors are osteogenic sarcoma (osteosarcoma) and Ewing sarcoma.

The peak ages during childhood are 15 to 19 years. The sexes are affected equally until puberty, at which time the ratio approaches 2:1 in favor of males. This propensity for males, with a peak incidence during adolescence, is thought to be related to the accelerated growth rate of osseous tissue. These two bone tumors have several characteristics in

common, which are discussed, and then specific information about each tumor is detailed.

Diagnostic Evaluation

A primary objective in diagnosis of bone neoplasm is to rule out causes such as trauma or infection. A history and careful questioning regarding pain help determine the duration and rate of tumor growth (see box above). Physical assessment focuses on the functional status of the affected area, signs of inflammation, size of the mass, involvement of regional lymph nodes, and any systemic indication of generalized malignancy.

Definitive diagnosis is based on radiologic studies (particularly computerized tomography), radioisotope bone scans, and/or surgical bone biopsy to identify the histologic type. Radiologic findings are characteristic for each type of tumor: a "sunburst" appearance produced by needlelike bone projections in osteogenic sarcoma and an "onionskin" appearance caused by layers of new bone in Ewing sarcoma. In both types of bone tumors, soft tissue infiltration may be apparent.

At present there is no reliable biochemical test for bone cancers, although elevated alkaline phosphatase levels may occur in osteoid tumors. Several tests may be performed to rule out metastatic disease from other neoplasms; lung tomography is especially important, since pulmonary metastasis is the most common complication of primary bone tumors. Bone marrow aspiration is helpful in diagnosing Ewing sarcoma in the rare event the child has bone marrow metastasis.

OSTEOGENIC SARCOMA

Osteogenic sarcoma is the most frequently encountered malignant bone cancer in children, with a peak incidence between 10 and 25 years of age (Link and Eilber, 1993). Most primary tumor sites are in the metaphysis of long bones (wider part of the shaft, next to epiphyseal growth plate), especially in the lower extremities. More than half occur in the femur, particularly the distal portion, with the rest involving the humerus, tibia, pelvis, jaw, and phalanges.

Therapeutic Management

Optimum treatment of osteosarcoma is controversial. The traditional approach has consisted of radical surgical resection or amputation of the affected area. Depending on the tumor site, surgery consists of amputation of the affected extremity at least 7.5 cm (3 inches) above the proximal tumor margin or above the joint proximal to the involved bone (Link and Eilber, 1993). With tumors of the distal femur, preservation of the hip joint may be possible. Other procedures include

---

*Marilyn Hockenberry-Eaton, PhD, RN,C, PNP, and Nancy E. Kline, MS, RN, CPNP, revised this section.

an above-the-knee amputation for tumors of the tibia or fibula, a hemipelvectomy for tumors of the innominate (hip) bone, and a forequarter amputation (removal of arm, scapula, and portion of the clavicle on the affected side) for tumors of the upper humerus. For selected patients, *limb salvage procedures* are performed; this involves primary tumor resection with prosthetic replacement of the involved bone. For example, with a tumor in the distal femur, a total femur and joint replacement is performed.

Antineoplastic drugs, such as high-dose methotrexate, adriamycin, bleomycin, actinomycin D, cyclophosphamide, ifosfamide, and cisplatin, may be administered in combination or singly both before and after either type of surgery.

Prognosis. With surgery, such as amputation to resect the primary tumor or thoracotomy for pulmonary metastasis, combined with chemotherapy, survival statistics are improving. Survival rates depend on the treatment and are influenced by other factors, such as the site of the primary tumor and the presence or absence of metastatic disease at diagnosis. However, approximately 50% of children with osteogenic sarcoma can expect long-term survival, and various cancer centers are reporting higher percentages (Jaffe, 1991).

Nursing Considerations

Nursing care depends on the type of surgical approach, and in either instance preparation of the child and family is crucial. Obviously, the family may have more difficulty adjusting to an amputation than a limb salvage procedure. Straightforward honesty is essential to gain the cooperation and trust of the child. The diagnosis of cancer should not be disguised with falsehoods such as "infection." To accept the need for radical surgery, the child must be aware of the lack of alternatives for treatment. Although the task of informing the child is the responsibility of the physician, the nurse should be present for the discussion or be aware of exactly what is said to the child. The child should be told a few days before surgery, so that he or she has time to think about the diagnosis and consequent treatment and to ask questions.

Sometimes children have many questions about the prosthesis, limitations on physical ability, and prognosis in terms of cure. At other times they react with silence or with a calm manner that masks their concern and fear. Either response is part of the grieving process that accompanies a loss and must be accepted. Children should not be overwhelmed with information. A supportive approach is to answer their questions without offering additional information and to show a willingness to talk, with such expressions as, "Anytime you would like to talk or ask questions about the surgery, tell me." The nurse should not push the topic unless the child initiates the discussion. Silence does not always mean nonacceptance.

The child is also informed of the need for chemotherapy. Again, caution must be exercised in offering too much information at one time. It is wise to discuss hair loss with emphasis on positive aspects, such as wearing a wig or baseball cap. Since bone tumors affect adolescents and young adults, it is not unusual for them to become angry over all the radical body alterations.

If an amputation is performed, the child may be fitted with a temporary prosthesis immediately after surgery, which permits early functioning and fosters psychologic adjustment. If

this is not done, the child requires stump care, which is the same as for any amputee. A permanent prosthesis is usually fitted within 6 to 8 weeks. During hospitalization the child begins physical therapy to become proficient in the use and care of the device.

Phantom limb pain may develop following amputation. This symptom is characterized by pain, tingling, itching, burning, and/or cramping in the area of the amputated leg. The child and family need to know that the sensations are real, not imagined. Amitriptyline (Elavil) has been used successfully in children to decrease the pain (Rogers, 1989). However, several pharmacologic and nonpharmacologic interventions, such as transcutaneous electrical nerve stimulation (TENS), may need to be tried to successfully treat phantom limb pain (Rounseville, 1992).

Discharge planning must begin early during the postoperative period. Every effort is made to promote normality and gradual resumption of realistic preamputation activities.* Role playing in anticipation of such experiences is very beneficial in preparing the child for the inevitable confrontation by others. Environmental barriers, such as stairs, are assessed in terms of the accessibility of the school and/or home, especially since the child may need to use crutches or a wheelchair before complete healing and prosthetic competency are achieved.

The family and child need a great deal of support in adjusting not only to a life-threatening diagnosis but also to alteration in body image and function. Since loss of a limb requires a grieving process, those caring for the child need to recognize that anger and depression are normal, necessary reactions. Often parents view the anger as a direct affront to them for allowing the amputation, or they view the depression as rejection. These are not personal attacks but the child's attempts to cope with the loss.

See also Nursing Care Plan: The Child with Cancer (Chapter 26) and Nursing Care Plan: The Child with a Bone Tumor.†

EWING SARCOMA

Ewing sarcoma arises in the marrow spaces of the bone rather than from osseous tissue. The principal sites of origin are shafts of long bones (femur, tibia, fibula, humerus, ulna), trunk bones (vertebra, scapula, ribs, pelvis), and skull (Pizzo and Poplack, 1993). The disease occurs almost exclusively in individuals under age 30, with most occurrences in individuals between 4 and 25 years of age.

Therapeutic Management

Surgical amputation is not routinely recommended but may be considered when the results of radiotherapy render the extremity useless or deformed (such as from retarded growth in young children) or the tumor appears resectable. The treat-

---

*Information about special programs for children with amputations, such as "Sunshine Skiers," is available from the **Candlelighters Childhood Cancer Foundation,** 1901 Pennsylvania Ave., N.W., Suite 1001, Washington, DC 20006. Information about prostheses can be obtained from the **National Amputation Foundation, Inc.,** 3840 Church St., Malverne, NY 11565; (516) 887-3600. In Canada: **War Amputations of Canada,** 2827 Riverside Dr., Ottawa, Ontario K1V 0C4; (613) 731-3821.

†In Wong DL: *Wong and Whaley's: Clinical manual of pediatric nursing,* ed 4, St Louis, 1996, Mosby.

ment of choice is intensive irradiation of the involved bone combined with chemotherapy. A widely used drug regimen includes vincristine, actinomycin D, cyclophosphamide, or ifosphamide, VP-16, and adriamycin.

Prognosis. The prognosis is best for children who do not have metastasis at the time of diagnosis. Children with massive tumors or lung and bone marrow metastasis have a much poorer prognosis. Children with distal lesions have the best chance for cure.

Nursing Considerations

The psychologic adjustment to Ewing sarcoma is typically less traumatic than to osteogenic sarcoma because of the preservation of the affected limb. Many families accept the diagnosis with a sense of relief in knowing that this type of bone cancer does not necessitate amputation, and initially they may not be aware of the deleterious effects on the irradiated site, especially severely affected growth, function, and appearance. Consequently, they need preparation for the various diagnostic tests, including bone marrow aspiration and surgical biopsy, and adequate explanation of the treatment regimen.

High-dose radiotherapy often causes a skin reaction of dry or moist desquamation followed by hyperpigmentation. The nurse advises the child to wear loose-fitting clothes over the irradiated area to minimize additional skin irritation. Because of increased sensitivity, the area is protected from sunlight and sudden changes in temperature, such as avoiding use of heating pads or ice packs. The child is encouraged to use the extremity as tolerated. Occasionally an active exercise program may be planned by the physical therapist to preserve maximum function.

The child needs the same considerations as any other patient with cancer in adjusting to the effects of chemotherapy, such as hair loss, severe nausea and vomiting, peripheral neuropathy, and possibly cardiotoxicity. Every effort should be made to outline a treatment plan that allows the child maximum resumption of a normal lifestyle and activities.

See also Nursing Care Plan: The Child with Cancer (Chapter 26).

RHABDOMYOSARCOMA

Soft tissue sarcomas are malignant neoplasms that originate from undifferentiated mesenchymal cells in muscles, tendons, bursae, and fascia or from such cells in fibrous, connective, lymphatic, or vascular tissue. They are the fourth most common type of solid tumor in children. These disorders derive their name from the specific tissue(s) of origin, such as *myosarcoma (myo—muscle)*. *Rhabdomyosarcoma (rhabdo—striated)* is the most common soft tissue sarcoma in children. Because striated (skeletal) muscle is found almost anywhere in the body, these tumors occur in many sites, the most common of which are the head and neck, especially the orbit. The disease occurs most commonly in children younger than 5 years of age.

Diagnostic Evaluation

The initial signs and symptoms are related to the site of the tumor and compression of adjacent organs (see box). Some tumor locations, particularly the orbit, produce symptoms early in the course of the illness and contribute to rapid diagnosis and improved prognosis. Other tumors, such as those of the retroperitoneal area, produce no symptoms until they are large, invasive, and widely metastasized. Unfortunately, many of the signs and symptoms attributable to rhabdomyosarcoma are vague and frequently suggest a common childhood illness, such as "earache" or "runny nose." In some instances a primary tumor site is never identified.

Diagnosis begins with a careful examination of the head and neck area, particularly palpation of a nontender, firm, hard mass. The nasopharynx and oropharynx are inspected for any evidence of a visible mass. Radiographic studies are performed to isolate a tumor site, accompanied by chest radiographic examinations, lung tomograms, bone surveys, and bone marrow aspiration to rule out metastasis. A lumbar puncture is indicated for head and neck tumors. An excisional biopsy is performed to confirm the histologic type.

Therapeutic Management

Since this tumor is highly malignant, with metastasis frequently occurring at the time of diagnosis, aggressive multimodal therapy is recommended. Complete removal of the primary tumor is advocated whenever possible. However, biopsy is required only in certain tumor locations, such as those of the orbit when followed by radiation and chemotherapy.

CLINICAL MANIFESTATIONS OF RHABDOMYOSARCOMA ACCORDING TO TUMOR SITE

Orbit
Rapidly developing unilateral proptosis
Ecchymosis of conjunctiva
Loss of extraocular movements (strabismus)

Nasopharynx
Stuffy nose (earliest sign)
Nasal obstruction—dysphagia, nasal voice (obstruction of posterior nasal conchae), serous otitis media (obstruction of eustachian tube)
Pain (sore throat and ear)
Epistaxis
Palpable neck nodes
Visible mass in oropharynx (late sign)

Paranasal Sinuses
Nasal obstruction
Local pain
Discharge
Sinusitis
Swelling

Middle Ear
Signs of chronic serous otitis media
Pain
Sanguinopurulent drainage
Facial nerve palsy

Retroperitoneal Area
Usually a "silent" tumor
Abdominal mass
Pain
Signs of intestinal or genitourinary obstruction

Perineum
Visible superficial mass
Bowel or bladder dysfunction (from tumor compression)

This avoids the devastating effects of enucleation, amputation, or pelvic exenteration.

High-dose irradiation to the primary tumor is recommended for most tumors. Radiation usually begins after several chemotherapy courses have been given to shrink the tumor. Drugs that are cytotoxic for rhabdomyosarcoma are *vincristine, actinomycin D,* and *cyclophosphamide* (collectively known as *VAC*), with or without adriamycin. Other drugs also may be used for more extensive disease.

Prognosis. With current treatment protocols survival rates for children with tumors detected at all clinical stages have increased considerably. Data suggest that children who remain disease free for 2 years are probably cured; however, if relapse occurs, the prognosis for long-term survival is extremely poor (Raney and others, 1993).

Nursing Considerations

The nursing responsibilities are similar to those for other types of cancer, especially the solid tumors when surgery is used. Specific objectives include (1) careful assessment for signs of the tumor, especially during well-child examinations; (2) preparation of the child and family for the multiple diagnostic tests; and (3) supportive care during each stage of multimodal therapy. The reader is urged to review Nursing Considerations under Leukemias in Chapter 26 for physical care of the child, and Chapter 18 for emotional support of the family in the event of a poor prognosis.

DISORDERS OF JOINTS

JUVENILE RHEUMATOID ARTHRITIS (JRA)

Clinically and pathologically, JRA is an inflammatory disease with an unknown cause. There are two peak ages of onset: between 2 and 5 years of age and between 9 and 12 years of age. Females are affected somewhat more frequently than males. In many instances the disease remains undiagnosed for years.

JRA is not a single disease, but a heterogeneous group of diseases. Three major types can be identified. *Systemic-onset disease* is associated with daily temperature spikes (usually in the afternoon) for at least 2 weeks, with or without a maculopapular rash. It accounts for about 30% of all cases. The *polyarticular onset* involves five or more joints and is seen in 25% of cases. The *pauciarticular onset* involves four or fewer joints and is the most common type, accounting for 45% of all cases.

Pathophysiology

The rheumatic process is characterized by a chronic inflammation of the synovium with joint effusion and eventual erosion, destruction, and fibrosis of the articular cartilage. Adhesions between joint surfaces and ankylosis of joints occur if the process persists long enough.

Whether a single joint or multiple joints are involved, the general manifestations (see box) result from edema, joint effusion, and synovial thickening. The limited motion, early in the disease, is the result of muscle spasm and joint inflamma-

---

CLINICAL MANIFESTATIONS OF JUVENILE RHEUMATOID ARTHRITIS

Involved joints:
  Stiffness
  Swelling
  Tenderness
  Painful to touch or relatively painless
  Warm to touch (seldom red)
  Loss of motion
  Characteristic morning stiffness or "gelling" on arising in the morning or after inactivity

---

tion; later it is caused by ankylosis or soft tissue contracture. Infections, injuries, or operations often precipitate a flare-up of the arthritis; therefore it is necessary to recognize and treat infections promptly.

Growth may be retarded during periods of active disease, usually with growth spurts during remissions. In severe longstanding cases growth is significantly retarded. Corticosteroid therapy can be a contributing factor.

Diagnostic Evaluation

There are no definitive serologic tests for JRA. The diagnosis is based on criteria established by the American Rheumatism Association (Emery and Miller, 1993). The erythrocyte sedimentation rate may or may not be elevated, depending on the degree of inflammation present. Leukocytosis is generally present in the early stages of classic systemic disease. The latex fixation test, the most common test used to detect the presence of rheumatoid factor (RF) in adults, is negative in 90% of juvenile cases. RFs are found in some children, usually those with disease of later onset. Antinuclear antibodies (ANAs) are found in some types of JRA, especially early-onset pauciarticular disease.

Radiographic findings are variable, but the earliest manifestations are widening joint spaces followed by gradual evidence of fusion and articular destruction.

Therapeutic Management

There is no specific cure for JRA. The major goals of therapy are to preserve joint function, prevent physical deformities, and relieve symptoms without iatrogenic harm. The child is treated at home under the supervision of the health team, and intermittent treatment by qualified professionals is administered. Hospitalization may be needed during severe exacerbations or when intercurrent illness warrants. *Iridiocyclitis,* also known as *uveitis* (inflammation of the iris and ciliary body) is a serious disorder unique to JRA that requires the attention of an ophthalmologist.

Drugs. Several drugs, given alone or in combination, are effective in suppressing the inflammatory process and relieving pain:

Nonsteroidal antiinflammatory drugs (NSAIDs)—(e.g., aspirin, tolmetin sodium, ibuprofen, and naproxen) daily dose usually divided into two or four doses

Slower-acting antirheumatic drugs (SAARDS)—(gold, D-penicillamine, and hydroxychloroquine) may be added to the regimen when one or two NSAIDs have been ineffective

Cytotoxic drugs—(e.g., cyclophosphamide, azathioprine, chlorambucil, and methotrexate) reserved for patients with severe debilitating disease and those who have responded poorly to NSAIDs and SAARDs (White and Ansell, 1992)

Corticosteroids—potent antiinflammatory agents are used for life-threatening disease, incapacitating systemic disease (unresponsive to other antiinflammatory therapy), and iridocyclitis; administered in the lowest effective dose, on alternate days (rather than daily), and for the shortest period possible; undesirable chronic side effects

Physical Management.   Programs of physical management are individualized for each child and designed to reach the ultimate goal—preserving function and/or preventing deformity. Physical therapy is directed toward specific joints, focusing on strengthening muscles, mobilizing restricted joint motion, and preventing or correcting deformities. Occupational therapy assumes responsibility for generalized mobility and performance of activities of daily living.

General treatment or maintenance programs varies; physiotherapists may be involved several times weekly to monthly in management of a home program, or their visits may be limited to infrequent review of the home program for compliance, effectiveness, and need. Normal activities of daily living and the child's natural tendency to be active are usually sufficient to maintain muscle strength and joint mobility.

Exercising in a pool is excellent therapy, since it allows freedom of movement with support and minimum gravitational pull. When joints are inflamed, heavy resistance aggravates the pain; at such times simple isometric or tensing exercises that do not involve joint movement are generally tolerated and should be encouraged. Range-of-motion exercises are an important aspect of therapy and are continued after evidence of disease has disappeared in order to detect any signs of recurrence.

Most practitioners recommend splinting and positioning during rest to help minimize pain and prevent or reduce flexion deformity. Joints most frequently splinted are the knees, wrists, and hands. Positioning during rest is also important. The child rests on a firm mattress with no pillow or a very low one and has no support under the knee. Loss of extension in the knee, hip, and wrist causes special problems and requires vigilance to detect the earliest signs of involvement and vigorous attention to prevent deformity with specialized passive stretching, positioning, and resting splints.

Prognosis.   The course of JRA is highly variable. Thirty percent to 40% of patients have active disease 10 years after the diagnosis, have substantial disability as adults, and require long-term drug therapy. The prognosis is best for children with pauciarticular JRA and worst for children with chronic, polyarticular disease, especially those positive for RF (Wallace and Levinson, 1991).

NURSING DIAGNOSES: THE CHILD WITH JUVENILE RHEUMATOID ARTHRITIS

Chronic pain related to joint inflammation
Impaired physical mobility related to joint discomfort and stiffness
Bathing/hygiene, dressing/grooming, feeding, or toileting self-care deficit related to impaired joint mobility
Altered family processes related to a situational crisis (child with a chronic illness)

Nursing Considerations

❖ Assessment

Nursing the child with JRA involves assessment of the child's general health, the status of involved joints, and the child's emotional response to all ramifications of the disease—discomfort, physical restrictions, therapies, and self-concept.

❖ Nursing Diagnoses

Nursing diagnoses and management identified for the child with JRA are outlined in the accompanying box. Others will be apparent in individual cases.

❖ Planning

Goals for the child with JRA and family include the following:

1. Child will experience reduction of pain to level acceptable to child.
2. Child will remain healthy.
3. Child will exhibit signs of adequate joint function.
4. Child will perform activities of daily living.
5. Child and family will receive adequate support.

❖ Implementation

The effects of the disease are manifested in every aspect of the child's life—in physical activities, social experiences, and personality development. Much of the children's adjustment to the stresses and demands of the disease and the level of functioning they achieve are directly related to the reaction and support they receive from their family and the health professionals concerned with their care and management.

Relieve Pain.   The pain of JRA is related to several aspects of the disease—disease severity, functional status, individual pain threshold, family variables, and psychologic adjustment. Although complete pain relief would be highly desirable, it is probably unrealistic. The aim is to provide as much relief as possible with antiinflammatory medication and other therapies to help children tolerate the pain and cope as effectively as possible (Lovell and Walco, 1989). At present, opioid administration is not a routine therapy for the chronic pain. Nonpharmacologic modalities have proved effective in modifying pain perception (see Pain Management, Chapter 21) and activities that aggravate pain.

Promote General Health.   The general health of children and their siblings must be considered and is frequently overlooked as parents and health personnel concentrate on the disease. A well-balanced diet and assessment of nutritional status are integral parts of health supervision. The discomfort and increased need for rest may create problems of weight control. Excess weight causes additional strain on inflamed joints, especially those of the lower extremities. Excessive fatigue and overexertion should be avoided by regular periods of rest, especially during acute flare-ups of arthritis. Symptoms may exacerbate during a viral illness.

Posture and body mechanics are important for children with JRA, both when they are at rest and when they are active. They must have a firm mattress to maintain good alignment of spine, hips, and knees and no pillow or a very thin one. Children who are confined to bed either at home or in the hospital may require supports or splints to maintain positioning. Waterbeds or an electric blanket (or electric sheet) placed under the bottom sheet provides comforting warmth.

Lying in the prone position is encouraged to straighten hips and knees, which they can do during rest periods or while watching television. The family is instructed in the principles and purposes of splints so that they can use them judiciously.

Children are encouraged to attend school, even on days when there may be some pain or discomfort. The aid of the school nurse is enlisted so that a child is permitted to take the prescribed medication at school and to arrange for rest in the nurse's office during the day. Split days or half days may help a child remain involved in school. Permitting the child to come to school late allows time to gain joint movement and reduces the time at school to avoid exhaustion. It is important that the child attend school to learn skills and engage in social interaction, especially if the JRA continues to limit physical skills. Arranging for two sets of textbooks eliminates the need to carry heavy or numerous books to and from school, thus reducing discomfort and difficulty ambulating.

Facilitate Compliance. The child and family are involved in the therapeutic plan. They need to know the purpose and correct use of any splints and appliances and the medication regimen. The family is instructed regarding administration of medications, as well as the value of a regular schedule of administration to maintain a satisfactory drug level in the body. They need to know that aspirin, as well as most NSAIDs, should not be given on an empty stomach and to be alert for signs of aspirin toxicity, which include hyperventilation as a sign of acidosis, bleeding from decreased clotting capacity, tinnitus (ringing in the ears) as a sign of cranial nerve VIII involvement, and undue drowsiness that may indicate central nervous system depression. If evidence of drug toxicity is noted, the family is instructed to stop the medication and notify the health professional.

Encourage Heat and Exercise. Heat has been shown to be beneficial to children with arthritis. Moist heat is best for relieving pain and stiffness, and the most efficient and practical method is in the bathtub. The temperature and duration of the bath are specified by the therapist but usually do not exceed 10 minutes at 37.8° C (100° F). Sometimes a daily whirlpool bath, paraffin bath, or hot packs may be used as needed for temporary relief of acute swelling and pain. Hot packs are easily applied using a bath towel wrung out after being immersed in hot water or heated in a microwave oven, applied to the area, and covered with plastic for 20 minutes. Commercial pads that warm in only a few minutes in the microwave are also available. Painful hands or feet can be immersed in a pan of water for 10 minutes two or three times daily in addition to tub baths.

Pool therapy is the easiest method for exercising a large number of joints. Swimming activities strengthen muscles and maintain mobility in larger joints. Children in urban areas have access to a therapy pool, although transportation may be a problem for some families. Very small children who are frightened of the water can carry out their exercises in the bathtub. Small children love to splash, kick, and throw things in the water.

Activities of daily living provide satisfactory exercise for older children to maintain maximum mobility with minimum pain. These children are encouraged in their efforts and patiently allowed to dress and groom themselves, to assume daily tasks, and to care for their belongings. It is often difficult for stiff fingers to manipulate buttons, comb or brush hair, and turn faucets, but parents and other caregivers should not offer assistance to them. In addition, children should learn and understand why others do not help them. Many helpful devices, such as self-adhering fasteners, tongs for manipulating difficult items, and grab bars installed in bathrooms for safety, can be used to facilitate tasks. A raised toilet seat often makes the difference between dependent and independent toileting, since weak quadriceps muscles and sore knees inhibit the ability to raise the body from a low sitting position.

A child's natural affinity for play offers many opportunities for incorporating therapeutic exercises. Throwing or kicking a ball, hanging from monkey bars, and riding a tricycle (with seat raised to achieve maximum leg extension) are excellent moving and stretching exercises for a very young child whose daily living activities are physically limited.

An effective approach to beginning the day's activities is to awaken children early to give them the medication and then to allow them to sleep for an hour. On arising, children take a hot bath (or shower) and perform a simple ritual of limbering-up exercises, after which they commence the activities of the day, such as going to school. Exercise, heat, and rest are spaced throughout the remainder of the day according to individual needs and schedules. Parents are instructed in exercises that meet the needs of the child.

NURSING TIP Another method of supplying warmth before the child arises is to plug an electric blanket into an appliance timer. Set the blanket to medium or high and adjust the timer to turn on the blanket 1 hour before the child awakens (McIlvain-Simpson and Singsen, 1991).

The **Arthritis Foundation*** and the **American Juvenile Arthritis Foundation*** provide services for both parents and professionals, and nurses should refer families to these agencies as an added resource.

Support Child and Family. Rheumatoid arthritis affects every aspect of the child's daily life. The physical pain and limitations interfere with performance of normal tasks and provision of self-care. There may be school difficulties related to transportation to and from school, stairs, and loss of time as a result of exacerbations and hospitalization. Physical limitations interfere with participation in many activities, both curricular and extracurricular, which limits peer contacts and interaction and increases social isolation. Changes in personality usually accompany JRA, as they do in any child with a chronic illness. They may be temporary, such as demanding, irritable behavior, or they may be manifested in more permanent ways, such as passive hostility, uncommunicativeness, and manipulativeness. Efforts should be made to break through the child's defenses and to identify his or her anxieties, concerns, and conflicts in order to intervene early to prevent the development of permanent personality problems.

Most of the reactions, problems, and concerns of families of a child with JRA are those of any family of a chronically ill and/or disabled child. The problems and needs of these fami-

---

*1314 Spring St., N.W., Atlanta, GA 30309; (404) 872-7100 or (800) 283-7800. In Canada: the **Arthritis Society,** 250 Bloor St., E., Suite 401, Toronto, Ontario, Canada M4W 3P2; (416) 967-5679.

lies are discussed in Chapter 18, and the reader is directed to this chapter for guidance in planning care.

❖ Evaluation

The effectiveness of nursing interventions is determined by continual reassessment and evaluation of care based on the following observational guidelines and expected outcomes:

1. Observe child's behavior and use pain assessment techniques.
2. Conduct routine assessment of child's general health.
3. Observe child during planned and unplanned activities, assess mobility of joints, and observe the use of prescribed appliances.
4. Observe child's ability to perform activities of daily living.
5. Observe and interview child and family regarding feelings and concerns.

Expected outcomes:

1. Child is able to move with minimum or no discomfort.
2. Child attains and maintains optimum health status (specify).
3. Child engages in activities suitable to interests, capabilities, and developmental level; joints are mobile, flexible, and free of deformity.
4. Child is involved in self-care activities to maximum capabilities.
5. Child and family demonstrate an understanding of the child's disease and therapies; they verbalize their feelings and concerns.

See also Nursing Care Plan: The Child with Juvenile Rheumatoid Arthritis.*

SYSTEMIC LUPUS ERYTHEMATOSUS (SLE)

SLE, or lupus erythematosus (LE), is a chronic inflammatory disease of the collagen or supporting tissues of the body. It characteristically follows an unpredictable course of remis-

---

*In Wong DL: *Wong and Whaley's Clinical manual of pediatric nursing,* ed 4, St Louis, 1996, Mosby.

---

sions and exacerbations. Because connective tissue is found practically everywhere, almost any organ or structure can be affected.

SLE in childhood consists of two basic types: a transient neonatal disease apparently related to maternal pathology and a group of chronic diseases (usually having their onset after infancy) that correspond to the diseases seen in adults. The major portion of the discussion is limited to SLE in childhood.

The cause of SLE is not known, although it is believed that some inciting event, such as stress, infection, extreme fatigue, or exposure to various chemicals, drugs, or excessive sunburn triggers a reaction that alters the body's immune response to its own tissues. The disease shows a tendency to occur within families.

Diagnostic Evaluation

Because SLE can affect almost any tissue, the clinical manifestations are variable (see box), and the diagnosis is established by demonstration of any 4 of 11 diagnostic criteria (see box). However, rapid involvement of vital organs, primarily the kidneys, can herald an accelerated course with minimum or absent involvement of other sites.

Therapeutic Management

The objectives of medical treatment are (1) to reverse the autoimmune and inflammatory processes and (2) to prevent exacerbations and complications. Therapy involves the use of specific and supportive medications and regulation of activity and diet. The principal drugs used to control inflammation are corticosteroids administered in doses sufficient to suppress symptoms, then tapered to the lowest suppressive dose. Other drugs include the immunosuppressive agents; antimalarial preparations, which are useful against dermatologic, arthritic, and renal symptoms of the disease; and nonsteroidal antiinflammatory agents, which relieve muscle and joint pains and reduce tissue inflammation. Drugs used to control various complications include antiepileptics, antihypertensives, and antibiotics.

The goal of restricted activity is to prevent a recurrence of the disease. An effective schedule must provide for gradual resumption of pre–lupus erythematosus activity and maximum rest periods, usually 8 to 10 hours of sleep a night and one or two rest times during the day. The most frequently prescribed diet modification, if needed, is moderate- or low-

---

CLINICAL MANIFESTATIONS OF SYSTEMIC LUPUS ERYTHEMATOSUS RELATED TO TISSUES INVOLVED

Cutaneous lesions—erythematous blush or scaly erythematous patches over bridge of nose and extending to each cheek symmetrically ("butterfly rash"); may extend to scalp, neck, chest, and extremities; sometimes pruritic; resemble severe sunburn or hives or may become bullous

Musculoskeletal system—generalized weakness, usually accompanied by arthritis, myalgia, joint swelling, and stiffness; usually not severe enough to cause deformity; pain may cause temporary disability

Central nervous system—varies from forgetfulness, excitability, and headache to seizures and frank psychosis; seizures may be early sign; any cranial nerves can be affected; paralysis (spinal cord involvement)

Heart and lungs—serous linings may be inflamed; pleurisy (lungs), pericarditis (heart); usually reversible with rest

Kidneys—glomerulus is usual site of destruction; proteinuria; kidney failure

Blood—anemia from decreased erythrocytes is common; amenorrhea secondary to anemia; platelets and plasma proteins may be affected

Lymphoid system—spleen and cervical, axillary, and inguinal lymph nodes are enlarged (sometimes); LE hepatitis may develop

Gastrointestinal tract—nausea, vomiting, diarrhea, and abdominal pain are possible

---

CRITERIA FOR DIAGNOSIS OF SYSTEMIC LUPUS ERYTHEMATOSUS

Butterfly rash
Discoid rash
Photosensitivity
Oral ulcers
Arthritis
Serositis
Renal disorder
Neurologic disorder(s) (psychosis, coma, seizures, paresis)
Hematologic disorder(s) (anemia, thrombocytopenia, leukopenia)
Immunologic disorder(s) (anti-DNA, LE prep, anti-SM, STS)
Antinuclear antibody (ANA)

salt intake. Low-protein diets may be necessary to prevent elevated nitrogen levels. Weight reduction, if indicated, may help preserve maximum joint function and conserve energy.

Nursing Considerations

The principal nursing goal is to help the child and family adjust to the limitations and treatments of the disease and to prevent exacerbations and complications. Since older female adolescents are the most likely group to be affected, the nurse must be aware of their special needs, such as body image changes, present and future vocational activities, and social relationships. (See Chapter 18 for a discussion on adjusting to a chronic illness.)

Family members need an understanding of the disease process to gain an appreciation of the need for regular, uninterrupted drug administration, moderate activity, and any diet modifications that may be imposed. Usually, diagnostic tests are performed during hospitalization, which allows the nurse an opportunity to help the child and parents learn about the disease. Several organizations have been formed to help children and families learn about and adjust to the disease. These groups include the **American Lupus Society,*** the **Lupus Foundation of America Inc.,*** and the **Arthritis Foundation** (see p. 1156).†

In teaching the child with SLE and the family, the nurse stresses the importance of adequate rest and the need to adhere to the medication schedule. Individuals who are sensitive to the sun must avoid exposure. It is important to emphasize that sun filtered through clouds or reflected from snow, water, or white surfaces (such as cement) can cause a severe reaction. Although clothes can protect most areas of the body, sunblocking or sunscreening agents with a high sun protection factor (SPF) are needed on exposed areas such as the face (see Sunburn, Chapter 30). A large-brimmed hat helps in partially shading the face.

Affected persons are advised to maintain regular medical supervision and to seek additional attention during periods of stress, illness, or before elective surgical procedures, such as dental extraction, because the body may require larger amounts of a drug. People with SLE should carry medical identification emphasizing their dependence on steroids.

---

*P.O. Box 9610, Marina Del Rey, CA 90215; (310) 390-6888.

*4 Research Place, Suite 180, Rockville, MD 20850; (301) 670-9292 or (800) 558-0121.
†A recommended booklet available from the foundation is *Meeting the Challenge: A Young Person's Guide to Living with Lupus.*

KEY POINTS

- Immobility has a profound effect on all aspects of growth and development.
- The major physical consequences of immobilization are loss of muscle strength, endurance, and muscle mass; bone demineralization; loss of joint mobility; and contractures.
- Features of children's fractures not observed in the adult include presence of growth plate, thicker and stronger periosteum, bone porosity, more rapid healing, and less joint stiffness.
- The goals of fracture management are to regain alignment and length of bony fragments, retain alignment and length, and restore function to injured parts.
- The method of fracture reduction is determined by the age of the child, degree of displacement, amount of overriding, amount of edema, condition of the skin and soft tissues, sensation, and circulation distal to the fracture.
- The primary purposes of traction are to fatigue involved muscles and reduce muscle spasm, position bone ends in desired realignment, and immobilize the fracture site until realignment has been achieved to permit casting or splinting.
- The development of developmental dysplasia of the hip appears to be related to intrauterine, genetic, and cultural factors.
- Treatment of clubfoot consists of manipulation and casting to correct the deformity, maintenance of the correction, and prevention of possible recurrence of the deformity.
- Acquired hip deformities are managed with non-weight-bearing devices (coxa plana) or surgical stabilization (coxa vara).
- Observation for scoliosis is an important part of a routine physical assessment.
- Scoliosis is managed by bracing and exercise, or surgical correction.
- Bone infections are managed with vigorous antibiotic therapy, immobilization of the affected part, and (sometimes) surgical drainage.
- Osteosarcoma is a neoplasm of bone-forming tissues; Ewing sarcoma is a neoplasm that arises from bone marrow spaces.
- Rhabdomyosarcoma may occur almost anywhere in the body, but the most common sites are the head and neck.
- Nursing care of the child with juvenile arthritis consists of promoting general health, relieving discomfort, preventing deformity, and preserving function.
- Lupus erythematosus is a chronic autoimmune disorder that affects the collagen tissues of the body.

REFERENCES

Bennett JT, MacEwen GD: Congenital dislocation of the hip, *Clin Orthop* 247:15-21, 1989.

Bostrom B, McCormick P, Hooke C: Painless procedures with propofol, *J Pediatr Oncol Nurs* 10(2):64-65, 1993.

Carlino HY: The child with an Ilizarov external fixator, *Pediatr Nurs* 17(4):355-358, 1991.

Emery HM, Miller ML: *Ambulatory pediatric care*, ed. 2, Philadelphia, 1993, JB Lippincott.

Jaffe N: Osteosarcoma, *Pediatr Rev* 12(11):333-343, 1991.

Link MP and Eilber F: Osteosarcoma. In Pizzo PA, Poplack DG: *Principles and practice of pediatric oncology*, ed 2, Philadelphia, 1993, JB Lippincott.

Lovell DJ, Walco GA: Pain associated with juvenile rheumatoid arthritis, *Pediatr Clin North Am* 36:1015-1027, 1989.

McIlvain-Simpson G, Singsen B: Decreasing morning stiffness, *Small Talk* 3(6):8, 1991.

Pizzo PA, Poplack DG: *Principles and practice of pediatric oncology*, ed 2, Philadelphia, 1993, JB Lippincott.

Raney RB and others: Rhabdomysarcoma and the undifferentiated sarcomas. In Pizzo PA, Poplack DG: *Principles and practice of pediatric oncology*, ed 2, Philadelphia, 1993, JB Lippincott.

Rogers AG: Use of amitriptyline (Elavil) for phantom limb pain in younger children, *J Pain Symptom Manage* 4(2):96, 1989.

Rounseville C: Phantom limb pain: the ghost that haunts the amputee, *Orthop Nurs* 11(2):67-71, 1992.

Speers AT, Speers M: Care of the infant in a Pavlik harness, *Pediatr Nurs* 18(3):229-232, 252, 1992.

Tobias JD and others: Oral ketamine premedication to alleviate the distress of invasive procedures in pediatric oncology patients, *Pediatrics* 90(4):537-541, 1992.

Wallace CA, Levinson JE: Juvenile rheumatoid arthritis: outcome and treatment for the 1990s, *Rheum Dis Clin North Am* 17:891-905, 1991.

Wattenmaker I, Kasser JR, McGravey A: Self administered nitrous oxide for fracture reduction in children in an emergency room setting, *J Orthop Trauma* 4(1):35-38, 1990.

White PH, Ansell BM: Methotrexate for juvenile rheumatoid arthritis, *N Engl J Med* 326(16):1077-1078, 1992.

Wong D, Baker C: Pain in children: comparison of assessment scales, *Pediatr Nurs* 14(1):9-17, 1988.

BIBLIOGRAPHY

Immobilization

Brady M, Grey M: Growing pains: a myth or a reality, *J Pediatr Health Care* 3:219-220, 1989.

Bubulka GM, Cipolla F: Preparing for pediatric emergencies, *J Emerg Nurs* 17(4):236-240, 1991.

Mehmert PA, Delaney CW: Validating impaired physical mobility, *Nurs Diagn* 2(4):143-154, 1991.

National Association of Orthopaedic Nurses: Cues for orthopaedic patient care: common concerns, *Orthop Nurs* 10(5):73-74, 1991.

Olson EV: The hazards of immobility, *Am J Nurs* 90:43-52, 1990.

Quellet LL, Rush KL: A synthesis of selected literature on mobility: a basis for studying impaired mobility, *Nurs Diagn* 3(2):72-80, 1992.

Sills EM: What's causing the back pain? *Contemp Pediatr* 5(11):85-96, 1988.

Szer IS: Are those limb pains "growing" pains? *Contemp Pediatr* 6(3):143-148, 1989.

Traumatic Injury

Alexander R and others: Serial abuse in children who are shaken, *Am J Dis Child* 144:58-60, 1990.

Campbell LS, Campbell JD: Musculoskeletal trauma in children, *Crit Care Nurs Clin North Am* 3(3):445-456, 1991.

Davis JM, Kuppermann N, Fleisher G: Serious sports injuries requiring hospitalization seen in a pediatric emergency department, *Am J Dis Child* 147(9):1001-1004, 1993.

DuRant RH and others: Findings from the preparticipation athletic examination and athletic injuries, *Am J Dis Child* 146:85-91, 1992.

Dyment PG: How to make the sports physical exciting, *Contemp Pediatr* (10):93-106, 1991.

Feller NG, Stroup K, Christian L: Helping staff nurses become mini-specialists, *Am J Nurs* 89:991-992, 1989.

Hansell MJ: Fractures and the healing process, *Orthop Nurs* 7(1):43-49, 1988.

Hergenroeder AC: Acute shoulder, knee, and ankle injuries, Part 1: diagnosis and management, *Adolescent Health Update* 8(2):1-8, 1996.

Hergenroeder AC: Acute shoulder, knee, and ankle injuries, Part 2: Rehabilitation, *Adolescent Health Update* 8(3):1-8, 1996.

Kelly JP and others: Concussion in sports, *JAMA* 266(20):2867-2869, 1991.

Leyendecker M and others: Rescuing a multiple trauma victim, *Nursing 89* 19(10):54-61, 1989.

Mansfield MJ, Emans SJ: Growth in female gymnasts: should training decrease during puberty? *J Pediatr* 122(2):237-240, 1993.

Newman DML, Fawcett J: Caring for a young child in a body cast: impact on the care giver, *Orthop Nurs* 14(1):41-46, 1995.

Nypaver M, Treloar D: Neutral cervical spine positioning in children, *Ann Emerg Med* 23(2):208-211, 1994.

Reed JL, Keegan MJ: Fat embolism syndrome: a complication of trauma, *Crit Care Nurse* 13(3):33-37, 1993.

Sonzogni JJ, Gross M: Hip and pelvic injuries in the young: fractures and special disorders, part 2, *Emerg Med* 25(8):18-20+, 1993.

Varela CD, Lorfing KC, Schmidt TL: Intravenous sedation for the closed reduction of fractures in children, *J Bone Joint Surg* 77(3):340-345, 1995.

Congenital Defects

Bender LH: Osteogenesis imperfecta, *Orthop Nurs* 10(4):23-32, 1991.

Cmiel PA, Cavanaugh CE: Digital replantation in children, *Am J Nurs* 89:1158-1161, 1989.

McGrath PA, Hillier LM: Phantom limb sensations in adolescents: a case study to illustrate the utility of sensation and pain logs in pediatric clinical practice, *J Pain Symptom Manage* 7:46-53, 1992.

Rounseville C: Phantom limb pain: the ghost that haunts the amputee, *Orthop Nurs* 11(2):67-71, 1992.

Varni JW and others: Family functioning, temperament, and psychologic adaptation in children with congenital or acquired limb deficiencies, *Pediatrics* 84:323-330, 1989.

Williamson VC: Amputation of the lower extremity: an overview, *Orthop Nurs* 11(2):55-65, 1992.

Orthopedic Infections

Bender LH: Osteogenesis imperfecta, *Orthop Nurs* 10(4):23-32, 1991.

Dunst RM: Legg-Calvé-Perthes disease, *Orthop Nurs* 9(2):18-27, 35-6, 1990.

Ekeberg DRE: Promoting a positive attitude in pediatric patients undergoing limb lengthening, *Orthop Nurs* 13(1):41-49, 1994.

Faden H, Grossi M: Acute osteomyelitis in children, *Am J Dis Child* 145(1):65-69, 1991.

Hart K: Using the Ilizarov external fixator in bone transport, *Orthop Nurs* 13(1):35-40, 1994.

Jacobs NM: Pneumococcal osteomyelitis and arthritis in children, *Am J Dis Child* 145(1):70-74, 1991.

Kerrick RC, French C: Torticollis: a head and neck immobilizer, *Am J Occup Ther* 47(1):79-80, 1993.

Ledwith CA, Fleisher GR: Slipped capital femoral epiphysis without hip pain leads to missed diagnosis, *Pediatrics* 89(4):660-662, 1992.

Nance DK, Mardjetko SM: Technical aspects and nursing considerations of limb lengthening, *Orthop Nurs* 13(1):21-33, 1994.

Scoliosis

Brosnan H: Nursing management of the adolescent with idiopathic scoliosis, *Nurs Clin North Am* 26(1):17-31, 1991.

Bunnel WP: Outcome of spinal screening, *Spine* 18(12):1572-1580, 1993.

Cassella M, Hall JE: Current treatment approaches in the nonoperative and operative management of adolescent idiopathic scoliosis, *Phys Ther* 71(12):897-909, 1991.

Cotton LA: Unit rod segmental spinal instrumentation for the treatment of neuromuscular scoliosis, *Orthop Nurs* 10(5):17-23, 1991.

Jacobs-Zacny JM, Horn MJ: Nursing care of adolescents having posterior spinal fusion with Cotrel-Dubousset instrumentation, *Orthop Nurs* 7(1):17-21, 1988.

Johnson JB, Killman-Young J: Adolescence, anxiety, and adaptation: preparing for posterior spine fusion with instrumentation, *J Pediatr Nurs* 3:348-349, 1988.

Murrel GAC and others: An assessment of the reliability of the scoliometer, *Spine* 18(6):709-712, 1993.

National Association of School Nurses Position Paper: Postural screening, *NASN Newsletter* (2):10, 1995.

Rauen KK, Ho M: Children's use of patient-controlled analgesia after spine surgery, *Pediatr Nurs* 15:589-593, 1989.

Richardson A, Taylor M, Murphree B: TSRH instrumentation: evolution of a new system, *Orthop Nurs* 9(6):15-21, 1990.

Scoloveno MA, Yarcheski A, Mahon NE: Scoliosis treatment effects on selected variables among adolescents, *West J Nurs Res* 12(5):616-619, 1990.

Voznak L: My life with scoliosis, *Orthop Nurs* 7(1):22-26, 1988.

Willers U and others: Long-term results of Harrington instrumentation in idiopathic scoliosis, *Spine* 18(6):713-717, 1993.

Bone and Soft Tissue Tumors

Bohm P, Wirth CJ, Jansson V: Limb-preserving operations in the treatment of malignant bone tumors, *Arch Orthop Trauma Surg* 108:218-224, 1989.

Bonilla JA, Healy GB: Management of malignant head and neck tumors in children, *Pediatr Clin North Am* 36(6):1443-1450, 1989.

Hockenberry MJ, Lane B: Limb salvage procedures in children with osteosarcoma, *Cancer Nurs* 11(1):2-8, 1988.

Loughlin KR and others: Genitourinary rhabdomyosarcoma in children, *Cancer* 63:1600-1606, 1989.

Maurer HM, Ragab AH: Rhabdomyosarcoma. In Fernbach DJ, Vietti TJ, editors: *Clinical pediatric oncology,* ed 4, St Louis, 1991, Mosby.

Rofary C, Flament F, Donaldson SS: An attempt to use a common staging system in rhabdomyosarcoma: a report of an international workshop initiated by the International Society of Pediatric Oncology, *Med Pediatr Oncol* 17:210-215, 1989.

Shochat S: Update on solid tumor management in children, *Pediatr Surg* 72(6):1417-1427, 1992.

Juvenile Rheumatoid Arthritis

Arnett FC: Revised criteria for the classification on rheumatoid arthritis, *Orthop Nurs* 9(2):58-64, 1990.

Fantini F: Future trends in pediatric rheumatology, *J Rheumatol Suppl* 37:49-53, 1992.

Hughes RB, D'Ambrosia K: Nursing management of a child with juvenile rheumatoid arthritis, *Orthop Nurs* 12(5):17-22, 1993.

Lavigne JV and others: Evaluation of a psychological treatment package for treating pain in juvenile rheumatoid arthritis, *Arthritis Care Res* 5(2):101-110, 1992.

McIlvain-Simpson G: Juvenile rheumatoid arthritis. In Jackson PL, Vessey JA, editors: *Primary care of the child with a chronic condition,* ed 2, St Louis, 1996, Mosby.

Page GG: Chronic pain and the child with juvenile rheumatoid arthritis, *J Pediatr Health Care* 5(1):18-23, 1991.

Quirk ME, Young MH: The impact of JRA on children, adolescents, and their families: current research and implications for future studies, *Arthritis Care Res* 3(1):36-43, 1990.

Rose CD: Pharmacological management of juvenile rheumatoid arthritis, *Drugs* 43(6):849-863, 1992.

Sipos DA: M.P. implants for rheumatoid arthritis of the hand, *Orthop Nurs* 12(5):7-14, 1993.

Southwood TR and others: Unconventional remedies used for patients with juvenile arthritis, *Pediatrics* 85:150-154, 1990.

Swann M: The surgery of juvenile chronic arthritis: an overview, *Clin Orthop* (259):70-75, 1990.

Systemic Lupus Erythematosus

Feutren G and others: Effects of cyclosporine in severe systemic lupus erythematosus, *J Pediatr* 111:1063-1068, 1987.

Fuller C, Hartley B: Systemic lupus erythematosus in adolescents, *J Pediatr Nurs* 6(4):251-257, 1991.

Lee LA, Weston WL: Lupus erythematosus in childhood, *Dermatol Clin* 4:151-160, 1986.

Lehman TJA and others: Systemic lupus erythematosus in the first year of life, *Pediatrics* 83:235-239, 1989.

McCurdy DK and others: Lupus nephritis: prognostic factors in children, *Pediatrics* 89(2):240-246, 1992.

Olson NY, Lindsley CB: Neonatal lupus syndrome, *Am J Dis Child* 141:908-910, 1987.

Ramirez-Seijas F, Cepero-Akselrad A: Systemic lupus erythematosus in children, *Int Pediatr* 8(3):334-343, 1993.

Venables PJW: Diagnosis and treatment of systemic lupus erythematosus, *Br Med J* 307:663-666, 1993.

Chapter 32

THE CHILD WITH NEUROMUSCULAR OR MUSCULAR DYSFUNCTION

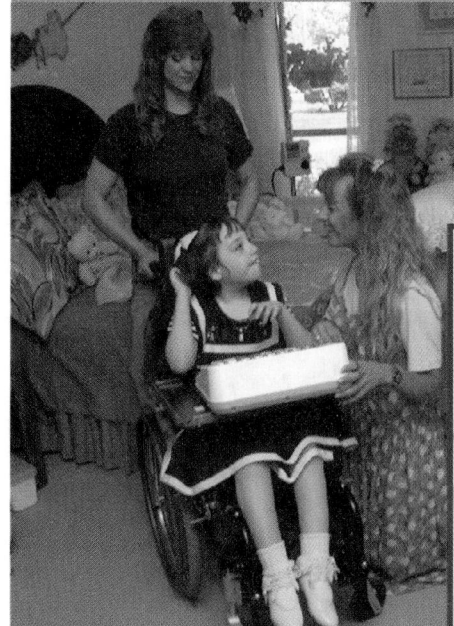

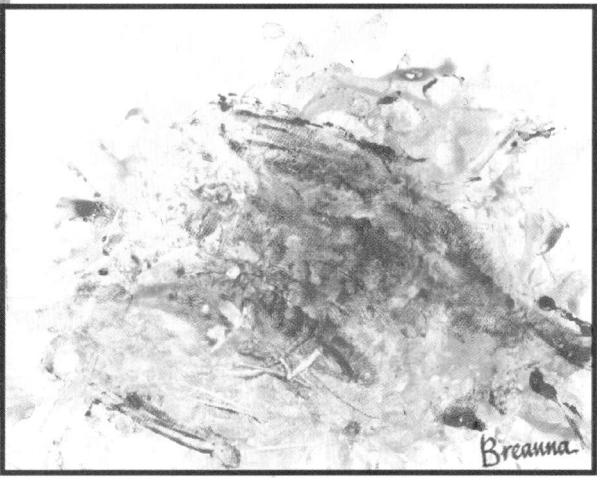

One of the hardest things was adjusting and accepting Breanna's health and the feeling of helplessness to her and her mother — being unable to solve their problems and only offer support and love.

Helen, grandmother of Breanna, age 7½ years, Rett syndrome

Breanna

RELATED TOPICS

LEARNING OBJECTIVES

On completion of this chapter the reader will be able to:

- Discuss the nursing role in helping parents cope with a child with cerebral palsy
- Formulate a nursing care plan for the preoperative and
- postoperative care of a child with myelomeningocele
- Outline a plan of care for a child with Duchenne muscular dystrophy
- Discuss the prevention and treatment of tetanus
- Identify the causes of botulism in infants and children
- List three causes of spinal cord injury in children

1161

CONGENITAL NEUROMUSCULAR OR MUSCULAR DISORDERS

CEREBRAL PALSY (CP)

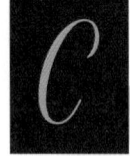

CP is a nonspecific term applied to disorders characterized by impaired movement and posture and early onset. It is nonprogressive and may be accompanied by perceptual problems, language deficits, and intellectual impairment. The etiology, clinical features, and course are variable and are characterized by abnormal muscle tone and coordination as the primary disturbances. CP is the most common permanent physical disability of childhood, and the incidence is reported as 1.9 to 2.3 in every 1000 live births.

A variety of prenatal, perinatal, and postnatal factors contribute to the etiology of CP singly or multifactorially. Although the prevalent hypothesis has been that CP results from perinatal problems, especially birth asphyxia, it is now known that CP results more often from existing *prenatal* brain abnormalities. Premature delivery continues to be the single most important determinant of CP; however, in approximately 24% of the cases, no cause is determined.

Pathophysiology

It is difficult to establish a precise location of neurologic lesions based on etiology or clinical signs because no characteristic pathologic picture exists. Some patients have gross malformations of the brain; others may have evidence of vascular occlusion, atrophy, loss of neurons, and degeneration. *Anoxia* plays the most significant role in the pathologic state of brain damage, which occurs frequently secondary to other causative mechanisms.

David Wilson, MS, RNC, revised this chapter.

CLINICAL CLASSIFICATION OF CEREBRAL PALSY

Spastic—May involve one or both sides
  Hypertonicity with poor control of posture, balance, and co-ordinated motion
  Impairment of fine and gross motor skills
  Active attempts at motion increase abnormal postures and overflow of movement to other parts of the body
Dyskinetic—Abnormal involuntary movement
  Athetosis, characterized by slow, wormlike, writhing movements that usually involve the extremities, trunk, neck, facial muscles, and tongue
  Involvement of the pharyngeal, laryngeal, and oral muscles causes drooling and dysarthria (imperfect speech articulation)
  Involuntary movements may take on choreoid (involuntary, irregular, jerking movements) and dystonic (disordered muscle tone) manifestations that increase in intensity with emotional stress and around adolescence
Ataxic
  Wide-based gait
  Rapid repetitive movements performed poorly
  Disintegration of movements of the upper extremities when the child reaches for objects
Mixed type—Combination of spasticity and athetosis

CP has been classified in several ways, but the most useful classification is based on the nature and distribution of neuromuscular dysfunction (see box).

Diagnostic Evaluation

The neurologic examination and history are the primary modalities for diagnosis of CP. A thorough knowledge of normal variations of motor development is required for detecting abnormal progress, and a careful history is elicited to detect possible etiologic factors. The alert observer may be suspicious when a child demonstrates some of the manifestations outlined in the box. The child's spontaneous movements and behavior are observed, including posture, attitude, and muscle size, function, and tone. Persistence of primitive reflexes may be of value, and two of these aid in the diagnoses:

CLINICAL MANIFESTATIONS OF CEREBRAL PALSY

Delayed Gross Motor Development
A universal manifestation
Delay in all motor accomplishments
Increases as growth advances

Abnormal Motor Performance
Very early preferential unilateral hand use
Abnormal and asymmetric crawl
Standing or walking on toes
Uncoordinated or involuntary movements
Poor sucking
Feeding difficulties
Persistent tongue thrust

Alterations of Muscle Tone
Increased or decreased resistance to passive movements
Opisthotonic postures (exaggerated arching of back)
Feels stiff on handling or dressing
Difficulty in diapering
Rigid and unbending at the hip and knee joints when pulled to sitting position (an early sign)

Abnormal Postures
Maintains hips higher than trunk in prone position with legs and arms flexed or drawn under the body
Scissoring and extension of legs, with the feet plantar flexed in supine position
Persistent infantile resting and sleeping posture:
  Arms abducted at shoulders
  Elbows flexed
  Hands fisted

Reflex Abnormalities
Persistence of primitive infantile reflexes:
  Obligatory tonic neck reflex at any age
  Nonpersistence beyond 6 months of age
Persistence or hyperactivity of the Moro, plantar, and palmar grasp reflexes
Hyperreflexia, ankle clonus, and stretch reflexes elicited in many muscle groups on fast passive movements

Associated Disabilities*
Subnormal learning and reasoning (mental retardation in about two thirds of individuals)
Seizures
Impaired behavioral and interpersonal relationships
Sensory impairment (vision, hearing)

---

*May or may not be present.

the asymmetric tonic neck reflex and the crossed extensor reflex.

Supplemental diagnostic tests may be employed, such as electroencephalography, tomography, screening for metabolic defects, and serum electrolyte values. The possibility that the manifestations are those of slowly progressive degenerative disease or early-onset, slowly growing brain tumors must be ruled out.

Therapeutic Management

The goals of therapy for children with CP are early recognition and promotion of an optimum developmental course to enable affected children to attain their potential within the limits of their brain dysfunction. The disorder is permanent, and therapy is chiefly symptomatic and preventive.

The broad aims of therapy are (1) to establish locomotion, communication, and self-help; (2) to gain optimum appearance and integration of motor functions; (3) to correct associated defects as effectively as possible; (4) to provide educational opportunities adapted to the individual child's needs and capabilities; and (5) to promote socialization experiences with other affected and unaffected children. Each child is evaluated and managed on an individual basis. The plan of therapy may involve a variety of settings, facilities, and specially trained persons, including the parents.

Ankle-foot orthoses (AFOs, braces) are worn by many of these children and are used to help prevent or reduce deformity, increase the energy efficiency of gait, and control alignment. Other mobilization devices include wheeled scooter boards that allow children to propel themselves while on the abdomen, wheeled go-carts that provide sitting balance and serve as early "wheelchair" experience for young children, and special devices that leave the upper extremities free (Figs. 32-1 and 32-2).

> **Nursing ALERT** The use of infant walkers is discouraged. They pose a risk of injury to normal children and are especially hazardous for children with CP. Also, jumping seats, such as those that hang in doorways, should not be used.

Orthopedic surgery may be required to correct contracture or spastic deformities, to provide stability for an uncontrollable joint, and to provide balanced muscle power. This includes tendon-lengthening procedures (especially heel-cord lengthening), release of spastic wrist flexor muscles, and correction of hip and adductor muscle spasticity or contracture to improve locomotion. *Selective dorsal rhizotomy* has provided marked improvement in some children with CP. However, achieving the benefits from the surgery requires intensive physical therapy and family commitment (Brucker, 1990). Because the procedure results in flaccid muscles, the child must be retaught to sit, stand, and walk.

Surgical intervention is usually reserved for the child who does not respond to the more conservative measures, but it is also indicated for the child whose spasticity causes progressive deformities. Surgery is primarily used to improve function rather than for cosmetic purposes and is followed by physical therapy. Neurosurgical procedures are used only in selected patients.

Drugs that decrease spasticity have little usefulness in improving function in CP. Antianxiety agents have been used to some extent to relieve excessive motion and tension, particularly in the athetoid child. Skeletal muscle relaxants, such as dantrolene (Dantrium), baclofen, and methocarbamol

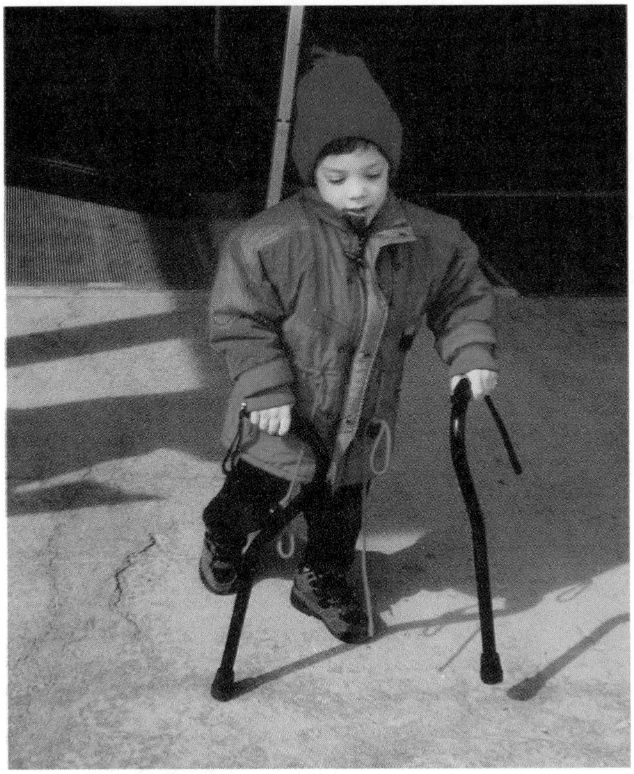

FIG. 32-1. Mobilization device for child.

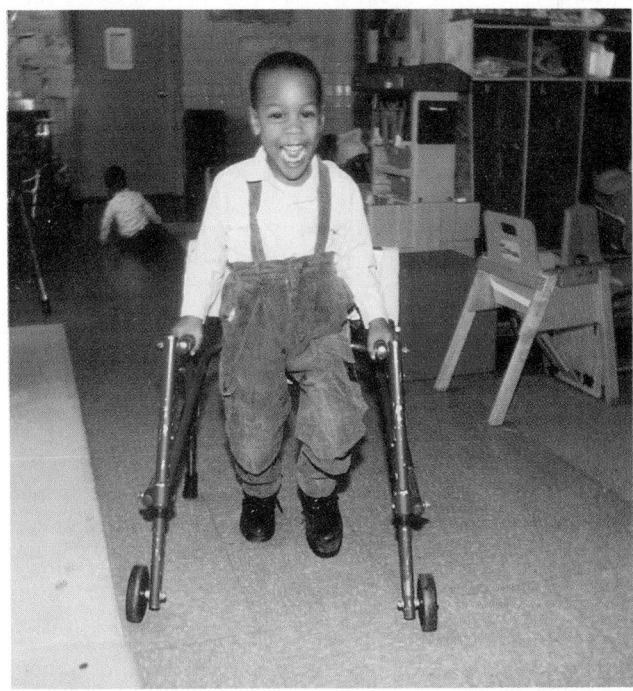

FIG. 32-2. Child ambulating with use of assistive device.

(Robaxin) may be used on a short-term basis for older children and adolescents. Diazepam (Valium) is used frequently but should be restricted to older children and adolescents. A local nerve block to motor points of a muscle with a neurolytic agent such as phenol solution reduces spasticity temporarily. Botulinum toxin (Botox) is also being used to paralyze a specific muscle.

Antiepileptic medications, especially phenobarbital and phenytoin, are prescribed routinely for children who have seizures, and hyperactive, dyskinetic children perform better when given dextroamphetamine or other drugs used for the child with attention deficit–hyperactivity disorder. Care of visual and auditory deficits requires the attention of appropriate specialists, and speech therapy involves the services of a speech therapist. Dental care is especially important. Regular visits to the dentist and prophylaxis, including brushing, fluoride, and flossing, should be instituted as soon as the teeth erupt. This is especially important for children given phenytoin, who often develop gum hyperplasia.

A wide variety of technical aids are available to improve the functioning of children with CP. These include electromechanical toys that employ the concept of biofeedback and operate from a head unit. The toy is manipulated only when the head and trunk are in correct alignment. Eye-hand coordination can also be enhanced by appropriately designed toys and games. Microcomputers combined with voice synthesizers aid children with speech difficulties to "speak." These and others print messages onto screen monitors and paper. These devices have made it apparent that some children have been erroneously considered to be mentally retarded.

Many other electronic devices allow independent functioning. Sensors can be activated and deactivated by using a head-stick, tongue, or other voluntary muscle movement over which the child has control. The application of this technology makes it possible for persons with CP to function eventually in their own residences and can be extended into the workplace (see Fig. 19-3).

Physical therapy is one of the most frequently used conservative treatment modalities. It requires the specialized skills of a qualified therapist with an extensive repertoire of exercise methods who can design a program to stimulate each child to achieve his or her functional goals.

An active therapy program involves the family, the physical therapist, and often other members of the health team, especially the nurse. The major approach employs traditional types of therapeutic exercises that consist of stretching, passive, active, and resisted movements applied to specific muscle groups or joints to maintain or increase range of motion, strength, or endurance.

Prognosis. Survival rates of children with moderate disability from CP are about the same as for unaffected children for the first 20 years of life. Children with severe disability have a probability of about 50% for surviving 20 or more years (Hutton, Cooke, and Pharaoh, 1994).

Nursing Considerations

❖ Assessment

Early recognition of CP is often a result of alert observation by the nurse. Detection begins at birth, and the nurse should be especially observant for signs in an infant who has a his-

---

WARNING SIGNS OF CEREBRAL PALSY

Physical Signs
Poor head control after 3 months of age
Stiff or rigid arms or legs
Pushing away or arching back
Floppy or limp body posture
Cannot sit up without support by 8 months
Uses only one side of the body, or only the arms to crawl

Behavioral Signs
Extreme irritability or crying
Failure to smile by 3 months
Feeding difficulties
   Persistent gagging or choking when fed
   After 6 months of age, tongue pushes soft food out of the mouth

Data from Pathways Awareness Foundation: *Parents . . . if you see any of these warning signs . . . don't delay,* Chicago, 1991, The Foundation.

---

tory that includes any of the prenatal or perinatal conditions that predispose to brain damage. Unusual manifestations in a newborn can be signs of a variety of conditions, but an infant who displays poor feeding, rigidity, tenseness, or hypotonia merits closer scrutiny. A history of these unexplained signs is cause for repeated assessment. The disorder is not readily identifiable in the early months of life; often evidence is not apparent until the child begins to walk. Delayed attainment of developmental milestones is one of the most valuable clues to recognizing CP; therefore slow development in a child offers one of the earliest indications of neurologic impairment (see box).

❖ Nursing Diagnoses

Based on a thorough assessment, several nursing diagnoses identified for the child with CP are primarily related to self-help and to facilitating mobility (see Nursing Care Plan, pp. 1167-1168). Other diagnoses may apply in specific cases.

❖ Planning

The goals of nursing care for the child with CP and the family are as follows:

1. Child will acquire mobility within personal capabilities.
2. Child will acquire communication skills or use appropriate assistive devices.
3. Child will engage in self-help activities.
4. Child will receive appropriate education.
5. Child will develop a positive self-image.
6. Family will receive appropriate education and support in their efforts to meet the child's needs.
7. Child will receive appropriate care if hospitalized.

❖ Implementation

Since children are being treated at an earlier age, parents are participating earlier in treatment programs for their disabled child. They are taught the proper handling and home care of young children with CP and need carefully programmed steps so that their change of role from parent to therapist can be melded into the already-established relationship. Nurses reinforce the therapeutic plan and assist the family in devising and modifying equipment and activities to continue the therapy program in the home.

Therapeutic interventions are those that are most appropriate for the specific problem and that best suit the needs of the individual child at any given time. Passive range-of-motion exercises, stretching, and elongation exercises are valuable at any age, even at early ages when the child is unable to cooperate. They are of particular value for postural abnormalities around various joints.

Training in manual skills and activities of daily living proceeds along developmental lines and according to the child's functional level. Sitting, balancing, crawling, and walking are encouraged at appropriate ages, accompanied by stimulation of protective extension and equilibrium reactions. Hand activities are begun early to improve motor function and provide the child with sensory experiences and information about the environment. As the child progresses from simple feeding and self-care activities, training is extended to include other tasks, such as cooking or typing, that are within the child's developmental and functional capabilities. It should be remembered that a child should not be expected to learn a task until he or she is at the developmental stage at which it would normally be accomplished.

Incorporating play into the therapeutic program often requires great ingenuity and inventiveness from those involved in the child's care. Objects and toys are chosen to provide needed sensory input, using a variety of shapes, forms, and textures. Nurses can help parents integrate therapy into play activities in natural ways.

The child may need considerable help (and patience) in learning to feed, dress, and care for personal hygiene needs. Children should be fed in the normal eating position. When they have difficulty with sucking and swallowing, it is a temptation to hold them in a semireclining posture to make use of gravity flow. This method does not promote active swallowing, however, and the neck hyperextension may even interfere with swallowing. A more flexed sitting position with arms brought forward to decrease the tendency toward back and neck extension is more natural during bottle- or spoon-feeding and encourages active swallowing.

Because jaw control is compromised, more normal control can be achieved if the feeder provides stability of the oral mechanism from the side or front of the face. When directed from the front, the middle finger of the nonfeeding hand is placed posterior to the body portion of the chin, the thumb is placed below the bottom lip, and the index finger is placed parallel to the child's mandible (Fig. 32-3). Manual jaw control from the side assists with head control, correction of neck and trunk hyperextension, and jaw stabilization. The middle finger of the nonfeeding hand is placed posterior to the bony portion of the chin, the index finger is placed on the chin below the lower lip, and the thumb is placed obliquely across the cheek to provide lateral jaw stability (Fig. 32-4).

Speech training under the supervision of a speech therapist is begun early, before the child learns poor habits of communication. Parents and others can help by following the directions of the speech therapist and by talking to the child slowly and using pictures or handling objects about which the adult is speaking. Feeding techniques such as forcing the child to use the lips and tongue in eating help to facilitate speech (e.g., placing food at the side of the tongue, first one side then the other; making the child use the lips to take food from a spoon rather than placing it directly on the tongue; and avoiding using the teeth to remove the food from the utensil). If severe dysarthria prevents articulate speech and the child has reasonable intelligence, nonverbal communication, such as sign language, is taught.

As in all aspects of care, educational requirements are determined by the child's needs and potential. Children with mild to moderate involvement are generally able to participate, for varying amounts of time, in regular classes. Resource rooms are available in most schools to provide more individualized attention to a child's particular needs. Integration of these children into regular classrooms should be the initial goal. For those who are unable to benefit from formal education, a training program may be appropriate. At adolescence, prevocational and vocational counseling and guidance are arranged. At any phase or in any setting, education is geared toward the child's assets.

Recreational outlets and after-school activities should be

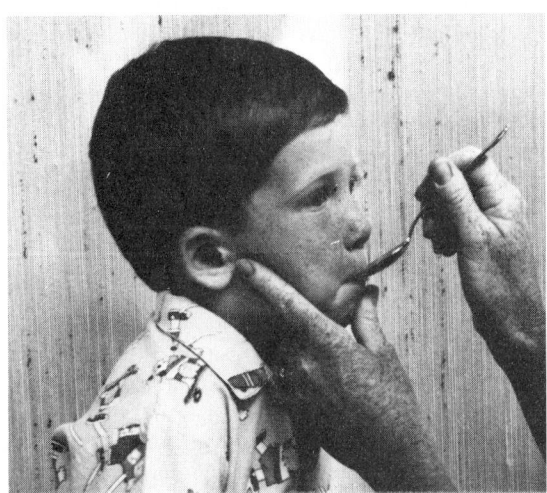

FIG. 32-3. Manual jaw control provided anteriorly.

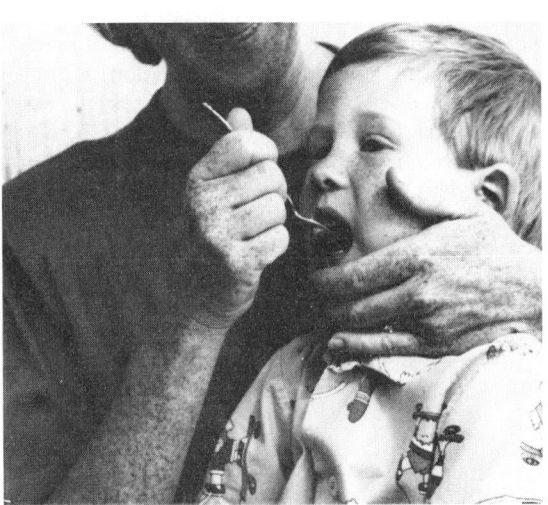

FIG. 32-4. Manual jaw control provided posteriorly.

considered for the child who is unable to participate in the regular athletic programs and other peer activities. Some children can compete in athletic and artistic endeavors, and many games and pasttimes are suited to their capabilities. Competitive sports are also becoming increasingly available to children with disabilities and offer an added dimension to physical activities. Information on training programs and competition on local, state, regional, and national levels can be obtained from the **National Association of Sports for Cerebral Palsy.***

Recreational activities serve to stimulate children's interest and curiosity, help them adjust to their disability, improve their functional abilities, and build self-esteem. Any accomplishment that helps children approach a "normal" way of life enhances their self-concept.

Support Family. Probably the nursing interventions most valuable to the family are support and help in coping with the emotional aspects of the disorder, many of which are discussed in relation to the child with a disability (see Chapter 18). Initially the parents need supportive counseling directed toward understanding the implications of the diagnosis and all the feelings that it engenders. Later they need clarification regarding what they can expect from the child and from health professionals. Having a child with CP implies numerous problems of daily management and changes in family life.

The nurse needs to support the parents in their frustration, their problem solving, their concerns, their approaches to helping the child, and their lack of gratification, as well as the positive approaches they use. All these aspects must be explored and discussed. Parents, as well as other members of the family, require much support and counseling. Siblings of a child with a disability are affected and may respond to the presence of the child with overt or less evident behavioral problems. The family needs a relationship with nurses who can provide continued contact, support, and encouragement through the long process of habilitation.

Parents can also find help and solace from parent groups, with whom they can share problems and concerns and from whom they can derive comfort and practical information. Parent support groups are most helpful through sharing experiences and accomplishments. For example, parents can understand from others what it is like to have a child with CP, which is generally not possible from professionals (see Family Focus box). The national organization, **United Cerebral Palsy Associations,**† has branches in most communities. The address of the nearest branch can be obtained from a local telephone directory, local agency directory, or a local health department or by writing to the national headquarters. The association provides a variety of services for children and families. A number of excellent books also are available to serve as guides for parents and nurses who work with the child with CP.

Support Hospitalized Child. CP is not a disorder that requires hospitalization; therefore, when children with CP are hospitalized, they are usually admitted for another rea-

---

*710 Penn Plaza, Suite 804, New York, NY 10001; (800) USA-1UCP. In Canada: **Ontario Federation of Cerebral Palsy,** 1021 Lawrency Ave., W., Suite 303, Toronto, Ontario, M6A 1C8, Canada; (416) 787-4595.
†See previous footnote.

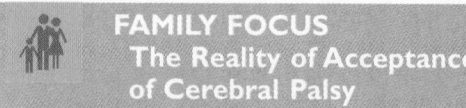

FAMILY FOCUS
The Reality of Acceptance of Cerebral Palsy

Acceptance is rarely achieved in the length of time implied in the literature.

In the first place, what is it? To me, it is the end of comparing my son with every other child I see. I focus on *his* gains, not society's expectations.

It is also being able to laugh periodically *at* his "clumsiness." It is "gallows humor" as he achieves adulthood; jokes about CP can be funny now.

The bitterness is gone; I am now happy for people who have children without CP.

I no longer feel sorry for my son, but rather for the people who cannot see him for the great person he is; the CP does *not* come first.

He is now a young man of 25 years and I am learning to accept his independence.

It is a "never-ending story."

Elaine A. Dunham, RN
Shriner's Hospital
Springfield, MA

son or for corrective surgery. Consequently, many nurses are not accustomed to handling these children. Nurses who have never been associated with a child with CP may react in a variety of ways, including fear, revulsion, or overwhelming pity. The basic concept to keep in mind when caring for these children is that they are, first of all, children, who happen to be afflicted with a disorder that limits their capacities in performing some activities of daily living and, for some, in communicating with others.

Children with CP should be approached and treated the same as any child in the hospital. The nurse's actions should convey acceptance, affection, and friendliness and promote a feeling of trust and dependability in the child. This is especially true with older children who have normal intelligence but who may have communication problems. Speech impairment is common in children with CP. All too frequently, nurses tend to "talk down" to these children and do things for them that they are perfectly capable of doing for themselves, although not as adeptly. This is especially humiliating to teenagers, who value their independence and self-esteem.

To facilitate the care and management of these children, the therapy program should be continued, insofar as their condition allows, during the time they are hospitalized. This should be incorporated into the nursing care plan and every effort expended to make certain that the ground that has been so laboriously gained is not lost. Encouraging the parent to room-in and actively participate in the child's care facilitates a continuation of the home therapy program and helps the child adjust to an unfamiliar environment. However, it is equally important to remember that a hospitalization may be the first time a parent can defer care to a nurse and not be the primary caregiver. This respite may be crucial to the parent's well-being.

NURSING DIAGNOSIS: Impaired physical mobility related to neuromuscular impairment

PATIENT GOAL 1: Will acquire locomotion within capabilities

- **NURSING INTERVENTIONS/RATIONALES**

Encourage sitting, crawling, and walking at appropriate ages

Carry out therapies that strengthen and improve control *to facilitate optimum development*

Assist child in using reciprocal leg motion when learning to walk

Provide incentives to locomote (e.g., place toy out of child's reach)

Ensure adequate rest before attempting locomotion activities *to encourage success*

Incorporate play that encourages desired behavior, *since this encourages cooperation*

Employ aids such as parallel bars and crutches *to facilitate locomotion*

Prepare child and family for surgical procedures if indicated

- **EXPECTED OUTCOME**

Child acquires locomotion within capabilities (specify)

PATIENT GOAL 2: Will experience no or minimal deformity

- **NURSING INTERVENTIONS/RATIONALES**

Apply and correctly use orthoses *for maximum benefit*

Carry out and teach family to perform stretching exercises *to prevent deformities*

Employ appropriate range-of-motion exercises *to facilitate muscle development and flexibility of joints*

Perform preoperative and postoperative care for child who requires corrective surgery

- **EXPECTED OUTCOME**

Alignment and flexibility are maintained within child's limits

NURSING DIAGNOSIS: Bathing/hygiene, dressing/grooming, feeding, toileting self-care deficits related to physical disability

PATIENT GOAL 1: Will engage in self-help activities of daily living

- **NURSING INTERVENTIONS/RATIONALES**

Encourage child to assist with care as age and capabilities permit *to facilitate optimum development*

Select toys and activities that allow maximum participation by child and that improve motor function and sensory input *so that child is more able to care for self*

Avoid undue persistence *because child may be unable or not ready to accomplish a goal*

Encourage activities that require both unimanual and bi-manual activities *to encourage optimum development*

Assist with jaw control during feeding *to facilitate eating*

Encourage use of adapted utensils, foods, and clothing *to facilitate self-help* (e.g., large-bowled spoon with padded handle; finger foods and foods that adhere to, rather than slip from, utensil; clothing that opens from front with self-adhering closings rather than buttons)

Assist parents in toilet training child, *since methods may need to be individualized according to child's abilities*

- **EXPECTED OUTCOME**

Child engages in self-help activities commensurate with capabilities

NURSING DIAGNOSIS: High risk for injury related to physical disability, neuromuscular impairment, perceptual and cognitive impairment

PATIENT GOAL 1: Will experience no physical injury

- **NURSING INTERVENTIONS/RATIONALES**

Provide safe physical environment
    Padded furniture *for protection*
    Siderails on bed *to prevent falls*
    Sturdy furniture that does not slip *to prevent falls*
    Avoid scatter rugs and polished floors *to prevent falls*

Select toys appropriate to age and physical limitations *to prevent injuries*

Encourage sufficient rest *because fatigue can increase risk of injuries*

Use restraints when child is in chair or vehicle

Provide child who is prone to falls with protective helmet and enforce its use *to prevent head injuries*

Institute seizure precautions for susceptible child

*Administer antiepileptic drugs as prescribed *to prevent seizures*

- **EXPECTED OUTCOMES**

Family provides a safe environment for child (specify)
Child is free of injury

NURSING DIAGNOSIS: Impaired verbal communication

PATIENT GOAL 1: Will engage in communication process within limits of impairment

- **NURSING INTERVENTIONS/RATIONALES**

Enlist the services of a speech therapist early *before child learns poor habits of communication*

Talk to child slowly *to give child time to understand speech*

Use articles and pictures *to reinforce speech and encourage understanding*

Employ feeding techniques *that help facilitate speech*, such as using lips, teeth, and various tongue movements

Teach and use nonverbal communication methods (e.g., sign language) for child with severe dysarthria

Help family acquire electronic equipment *to facilitate nonverbal communication* (e.g., typewriter, microcomputer with voice synthesizer)

---

*Dependent nursing action.

Continued.

NURSING CARE PLAN
The Child with Cerebral Palsy—cont'd

- **EXPECTED OUTCOME**

Child is able to communicate needs to caregivers (specify desired communication and means of accomplishment)

NURSING DIAGNOSIS: Fatigue related to increased energy expenditure

PATIENT GOAL 1: Will receive optimum nutrition

- **NURSING INTERVENTIONS/*RATIONALES***

Provide extra calories *to meet energy demands of increased muscle activity*
Monitor weight gain *to evaluate adequacy of nutritional intake*
Provide vitamin, mineral, and/or protein supplements if eating habits are poor
Devise aids and techniques to facilitate feeding *so that child receives adequate nourishment*

- **EXPECTED OUTCOMES**

Child eats a balanced diet
Weight remains within acceptable limits (specify)

PATIENT GOAL 2: Will receive optimum rest

- **NURSING INTERVENTIONS/*RATIONALES***

Maintain a well-regulated schedule that allows for adequate rest and sleep periods *to prevent fatigue*
Be alert for evidence of fatigue, which tends to aggravate symptoms

- **EXPECTED OUTCOME**

Child is sufficiently rested

PATIENT GOAL 3: Will maintain good general health

- **NURSING INTERVENTIONS/*RATIONALES***

Ensure regular routine health maintenance *to promote general health*
    Physical assessment
    Dental care
    Immunizations

- **EXPECTED OUTCOMES**

Child receives regular health assessments (specify schedule)
Child receives appropriate immunizations (specify) and dental care (specify)

NURSING DIAGNOSIS: Body image disturbance related to perception of disability

PATIENT GOAL 1: Will demonstrate positive body image

- **NURSING INTERVENTIONS/*RATIONALES***

Demonstrate acceptance of child through own behavior, *since children are sensitive to affective attitude of the professional*
Capitalize on child's assets and provide compensation for liabilities *to encourage positive self-image*
Praise child for accomplishments and "near" accomplishments, such as partial completion of a task
Plan activities and goals *with* the child that provide opportunities for success *to encourage cooperation and positive self-image*
Encourage grooming and age-appropriate dress *to promote acceptance by others and positive body image*
See Nursing diagnosis: Body image disturbance, in Nursing Care Plan: The Child with Chronic Illness or Disability, Chapter 18

- **EXPECTED OUTCOME**

Child exhibits behaviors that indicate positive body image (specify)

NURSING DIAGNOSIS: Altered family processes related to a child with a lifelong disability

PATIENT (FAMILY) GOAL 1: Will receive adequate support

- **NURSING INTERVENTIONS/*RATIONALES***

See Nursing diagnosis: Altered family processes, in Nursing Care Plan: The Child with Chronic Illness or Disability, Chapter 18
Refer to special support group(s) and agencies *for ongoing support*

- **EXPECTED OUTCOME**

Family contacts special support group
See also:
    Nursing Care Plan: The Child with Chronic Illness or Disability, Chapter 18
    Nursing Care Plan: The Child with Mental Retardation, Chapter 19
    Nursing Care Plan: The Child with Hearing Impairment, Chapter 19

❖ Evaluation

The effectiveness of nursing interventions is determined by continual reassessment and evaluation of care based on the following observational guidelines and expected outcomes:

1. Observe child's movements and use of mobilization devices.
2. Observe child's speech and ability to use communication devices.
3. Observe child's activities, especially those related to self-care.
4. Interview family regarding child's activities and school attendance.
5. Observe child's interactions with others and choice of activities; interview child regarding feelings and concerns.
6. Interview family regarding their feelings and concerns and observe family members' interaction with the child.
7. Observe child's behavior and responses during hospitalization.

Expected outcomes:
See Nursing Care Plan, pp. 1167-1168.

SPINA BIFIDA
(MYELOMENINGOCELE)*

Abnormalities that are derived from the embryonic neural tube *(neural tube defects [NTDs])* constitute the largest group of congenital anomalies that is consistent with multifactorial inheritance. Normally the spinal cord and cauda equina are encased in a protective sheath of bone and meninges (Fig. 32-5, *A*). Failure of neural tube closure produces defects of varying degrees (see box). They may involve the entire length of the neural tube or may be restricted to a small area.

In the United States, rates of NTDs have declined from 1.3 per 1000 births in 1970 to 0.6 per 1000 births in 1989. A partial explanation is the increased use of prenatal diagnostic techniques and termination of pregnancies.

Myelodysplasia refers broadly to any malformation of the spinal canal and cord. Midline defects involving failure of the osseous (bony) spine to close are called *spina bifida (SB),* the most common defect of the central nervous system. SB is categorized into two types: spina bifida occulta and spina bifida cystica.

Spina bifida occulta refers to a defect that is not visible externally. It occurs most frequently in the lumbosacral area (L5 and S1) (Fig. 32-5, *B*). SB occulta may not be apparent unless there are associated cutaneous manifestations or neuromuscular disturbances.

Spina bifida cystica refers to a visible defect with an external saclike protrusion. The two major forms of SB cystica are *meningocele,* which encases meninges and spinal fluid, but no neural elements (Fig. 32-5, *C*); and *myelomeningocele* (or *meningomyelocele*), which contains meninges, spinal fluid, and nerves (Fig. 32-5, *D*). Meningocele is not associated with neurologic deficit, which occurs in varying, often serious, degrees in myelomeningocele. Clinically the term *spina bifida* is used to refer to myelomeningocele.

---

*Jeanne O'Connor Egan, MSN, RN, and David Wilson, MS, RNC, revised this section.

SIGNIFICANT NEURAL TUBE DEFECTS

Cranioschisis—A skull defect through which various tissues protrude
Exancephaly—Brain is totally exposed or extruded through an associated skull defect; fetus usually aborted
Anencephaly—If fetus with exancephaly survives, the brain degenerates to a spongiform mass with no bony covering; incompatible with life usually beyond a few days
Encephalocele—Herniation of brain and meninges through a defect in the skull producing a fluid-filled sac
Rachischisis or **spina bifida**—Fissure in the spinal column that leaves the meninges and spinal cord exposed
Meningocele—Hernial protrusion of a saclike cyst of meninges filled with spinal fluid (Fig. 32-5, *C*)
Myelomeningocele (meningomyelocele)—Hernial protrusion of a saclike cyst containing meninges, spinal fluid, and a portion of the spinal cord with its nerves (Fig. 32-5, *D*)

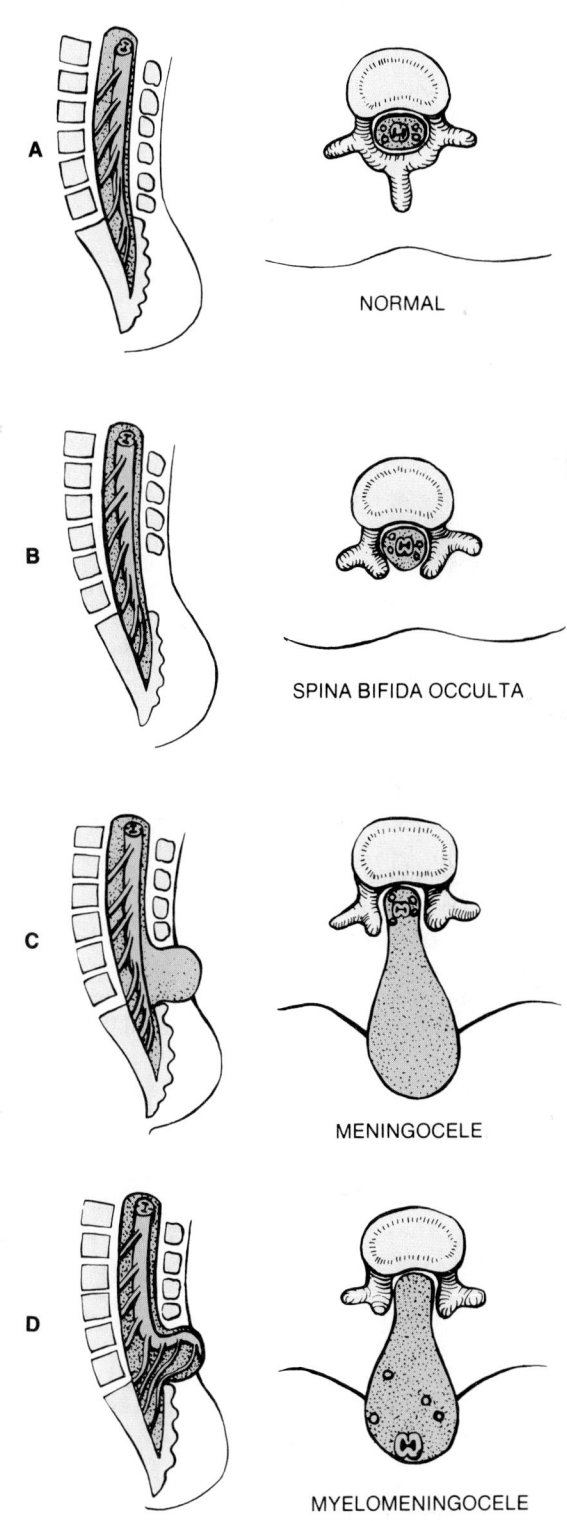

A NORMAL

B SPINA BIFIDA OCCULTA

C MENINGOCELE

D MYELOMENINGOCELE

FIG. 32-5. Midline defects of osseous spine with varying degrees of neural herniations.

The cause of NTDs is unknown. However, studies have shown that women at high risk for having a child with an NTD because they had previously delivered an infant or fetus with SB, anencephaly, or encephalocele, significantly reduced the recurrence rate by taking supplements of the ***B vitamin folic acid*** (4 mg) before conception. The American Academy of Pediatrics (1993) recommends daily intake of folic acid for all women of childbearing age. The daily dose of 0.4 mg is the recommended dietary allowance (RDA). Folic acid taken before conception and during early pregnancy can reduce the risk of NTDs, such as SB, by at least 50% (Knowledge, 1995).*

>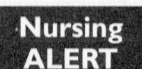
> **Nursing ALERT**   Educate childbearing adolescent females about the need for folic acid to prevent neural tube birth defects. The daily dose of 0.4 mg is most easily obtained from a multivitamin supplement. For women needing a daily dose of 4 mg, special supplements are necessary.

Pathophysiology   *heart +61*

Most authorities believe that the primary defect in NTDs is a failure of neural tube closure during early development of the embryo. However, evidence indicates that the defects are a result of splitting of the already-closed neural tube as a result of an abnormal increase in cerebrospinal fluid pressure during the first trimester. The degree of neurologic dysfunction is directly related to the anatomic level of the defect and thus the nerves involved. Most myelomeningoceles involve the lumbar or lumbosacral area, and hydrocephalus is a frequently associated anomaly (90% of patients).

Diagnostic Evaluation

The diagnosis of SB is made on the basis of clinical manifestations (see box) and examination of the meningeal sac. Diagnostic measures used to evaluate the brain and spinal cord include magnetic resonance imaging (MRI), ultrasound, computed tomography (CT), and myelography.

Laboratory examinations are used primarily to determine causative organisms for the major complications of myelomeningocele—meningitis and urinary tract infections. Infants with urinary tract incontinence may require urinalysis, culture, and evaluation of blood urea nitrogen (BUN) and creatinine clearance.

Prenatal Detection.   It is possible to determine the presence of some major open NTDs prenatally. Ultrasound scanning of the uterus and elevated concentrations of alpha-fetoprotein (AFP), a fetal-specific gamma-1 globulin, in amniotic fluid may indicate the presence of anencephaly or myelomeningocele. The optimum time for performing these diagnostic tests is between 16 and 18 weeks of gestation, before AFP concentrations normally diminish and in sufficient time to permit a therapeutic abortion. It is recommended that such diagnostic procedures be considered for all mothers who have borne an affected child, and testing is offered to all pregnant women. In addition, elective prelabor cesarean birth may result in less motor dysfunction.

---

*As of this writing, the U.S. Food and Drug Administration (FDA) has required that folic acid be added to most enriched breads, flours, rice, grits, and other grain products. However, the supplementation may only be 10% of the RDA.

> ### CLINICAL MANIFESTATIONS OF SPINA BIFIDA
>
> **Spina Bifida Cystica**
> Sensory disturbances usually parallel motor dysfunction
>   Below second lumbar vertebra:
>   Flaccid, are flexic partial paralysis of lower extremities
>   Varying degrees of sensory deficit
>   Overflow incontinence with constant dribbling of urine
>   Lack of bowel control
>   Rectal prolapse (sometimes)
>   Below third sacral vertebra:
>   No motor impairment
>   May be saddle anesthesia with bladder and anal sphincter paralysis
> Joint deformities (sometimes produced in utero):
>   Talipes valgus or varus contractures
>   Kyphosis
>   Lumbosacral scoliosis
>   Hip dislocations
>
> **Spina Bifida Occulta**
> Frequently no observable manifestations
> May be associated with one or more cutaneous manifestations:
>   Skin depression or dimple
>   Port-wine angiomatous nevi
>   Dark tufts of hair
>   Soft, subcutaneous lipomas
> May be neuromuscular disturbances:
>   Progressive disturbance of gait with foot weakness
>   Bowel and bladder sphincter disturbances

Therapeutic Management

Management of the child who has a myelomeningocele requires a multidisciplinary approach involving the specialties of neurology, neurosurgery, pediatrics, urology, orthopedics, rehabilitation, and physical therapy, as well as intensive nursing care in a variety of specialty areas. The collaborative efforts of these specialists are focused on (1) the myelomeningocele and the problems associated with the defect—hydrocephalus, paralysis, orthopedic deformities, and genitourinary abnormalities; (2) possible acquired problems that may or may not be associated, such as meningitis, hypoxia, and hemorrhage; and (3) other abnormalities, such as cardiac or gastrointestinal malformations.

Infancy.   Initial care of the newborn involves prevention of infection; neurologic assessment, including observation for associated anomalies; and dealing with the impact of the anomaly on the family. Although meningoceles are repaired early, especially if there is danger of rupture of the sac, the philosophy regarding skin closure of myelomeningocele varies. Most authorities believe that early closure, within the first 24 to 72 hours, offers the most favorable outcome. Early closure, preferably in the first 12 to 18 hours, not only prevents local infection and trauma to the exposed tissues, but also avoids stretching of other nerve roots, which may occur as the meningeal sac expands during the first hours after birth, thus preventing further motor impairment.

Other experts contend that surgical repair is best delayed until after further assessment of neurologic function, intellectual potential, and extent of complications. This delay increases the infant's ability to tolerate the surgical procedure, allows for better epithelialization of the sac (thus reducing the risk of infection), and permits easier mobilization of skin for closure.

A variety of neurosurgical and plastic surgical procedures can be used for skin closure without disturbing the neural elements or removing any portion of the sac (e.g., Fig. 32-6, *B*). The objective is satisfactory skin coverage of the lesion and meticulous closure. Wide excision of the large membranous covering may damage functioning neural tissue.

Associated problems are assessed and managed by appropriate surgical and supportive measures. Shunt procedures provide relief from imminent or progressive hydrocephalus (see Chapter 28). Meningitis, urinary tract infection, and pneumonia are treated with vigorous antibiotic therapy and supportive measures.

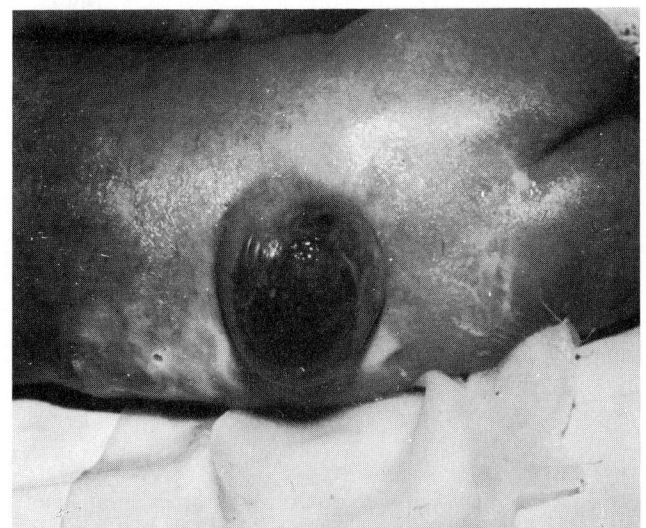

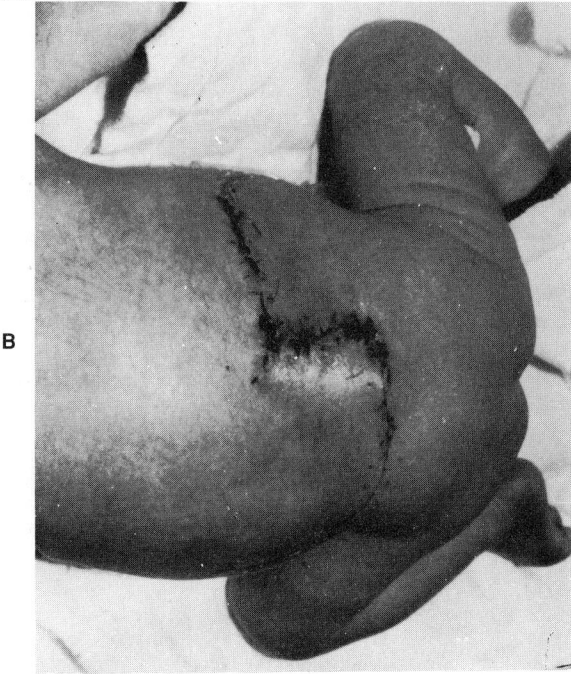

FIG. 32-6. A, Myelomeningocele before surgery. **B,** Same patient after surgery. (Courtesy MC Gleason, MD, San Diego. From Ingalls AJ, Salerno MC: *Maternal and child health nursing,* ed 7, St Louis, 1991, Mosby.)

Orthopedic Considerations. According to most orthopedists, musculoskeletal problems that will affect later locomotion should be evaluated early, and treatment, where indicated, should be instituted without delay. Neurologic assessment will determine the neurosegmental level of the lesion, recognition of spasticity and progressive paralysis, potential for deformity, and functional expectations. Orthopedic management includes prevention of joint contractures, correction of the deformity, prevention of skin breakdown, and obtaining the best possible locomotor function. The status of the neurologic deficit remains the most important factor in determining the child's ultimate functional abilities.

A variety of devices are available to provide mobility to children with spinal cord lesions, including lightweight braces, special "walking" devices, and custom-built wheelchairs (see also Chapter 19). Corrective procedures, when indicated, are best initiated at an early age so that the child will not lag significantly behind age-mates in developmental progress. Where there is little hope for lower extremity functioning, surgery is seldom recommended.

Management of Genitourinary Function. Myelomeningocele is one of the most common causes of *neuropathic (neurogenic) bladder dysfunction* among children. In infants the goal of treatment is to preserve renal function. In older children the goal is to achieve urinary continence (Fernandes and others, 1994). Urinary incontinence, a chronic, often debilitating problem, typically arises from the dysfunctional bladder. In addition, neuropathic bladder dysfunction may predispose the child to *urinary system distress* (infection, ureterohydronephrosis, and vesicoureteral reflux). The characteristics of bladder dysfunction in children vary according to the level of the lesion and the influence of bony growth and development on the spine. Therefore urodynamic testing during infancy and early childhood is important because bladder function changes. The presence of hydrocephalus has the potential to affect bladder function, although spinal influences are predominant.

Treatment of renal problems includes (1) regular urologic care with prompt and vigorous treatment of infections; (2) some type of regular emptying of the bladder, such as clean intermittent catheterization (CIC) taught to and performed by parents and self-catheterization taught to children; (3) medications to improve bladder storage and continence, such as oxybutynin chloride (Ditropan), propantheline (Pro-Banthine), and ephedrine; and (4) surgical procedures such as *vesicostomy* (stoma created on the abdominal wall for urinary drainage) and *augmentation enterocytoplasty* (increases bladder capacity and reduces high bladder pressures).

Infrequently, children with myelodysplasia may develop severe dysfunction of the bladder that compromises renal function or produces debilitating urinary incontinence that is intractable to other means. *Urinary diversion,* typically using a continent neobladder constructed from bowel or stomach, may be required. Whenever feasible, the neobladder is constructed in a way that allows continence, and CIC is used to regularly evacuate urine.

Bowel Control. Some degree of fecal continence can usually be achieved in most children with myelomeningocele with diet modification, regular toilet habits, and prevention of constipation and impaction. It is frequently a lengthy process. Fiber supplements, laxatives, suppositories, and/or enemas aid in producing regular evacuation.

Latex Allergy. Latex allergy has been identified as a serious health hazard in children with SB. These children are at high risk for developing latex allergy because of repeated exposure to latex products during surgery and from numerous bladder catheterizations. Allergic reactions range from urticaria, wheezing, watery eyes, and rashes to anaphylactic shock. More severe reactions tend to occur when latex comes in contact with mucous membranes, wet skin, and the bloodstream and in individuals with atopic disorders. The incidence of latex allergy in children with SB ranges from an estimated 18% to 60%.

The most important goals are prevention of latex allergy and identification of children with a known hypersensitivity (see Guidelines box). Allergy testing with the latex extract may be performed with the skin prick test; however, skin testing can cause an allergic reaction. The *radioallergosorbent test (RAST)* is the most specific test for immunoglobulin E antibody. Children who are allergic to latex must avoid all latex products and may be given antihistamines and steroids (dexamethasone) before and after surgery to reduce the possibility of a serious reaction.

Prognosis. The early prognosis for the child with myelomeningocele depends on the neurologic deficit present at birth, including motor ability and bladder innervation and the presence of associated cerebral anomalies. Early surgical repair of the spinal defect, antibiotic therapy to reduce the incidence of meningitis and ventriculitis, prevention of urinary system dysfunction, and correction of hydrocephalus have significantly increased the survival rate. Based on current medical knowledge and ethical considerations, aggressive management is favored for the child with meningomyelocele.

With the widespread use of folate supplementation during the childbearing years, the incidence of SB should decrease dramatically. Whether folic acid will lessen the se-

verity of the defect in infants born with SB despite supplementation is unknown.

❖ Assessment

At birth an examination is performed to assess the intactness of the membranous cyst. During transport to the nursery, every effort is made to prevent trauma to this protective covering. In addition to the routine assessment of the newborn (see Chapter 8), the infant is assessed for level of neurologic involvement. Movement of extremities or skin response, especially an anal reflex, that might provide clues to the degree of motor or sensory impairment is noted. It is important to observe the infant's behavior in conjunction with the stimulus, since limb movements can be induced in response to spinal cord reflex activity that has no connection with the higher centers. Observation of urine output, especially if a diaper remains dry, may indicate urinary retention. The head circumference is measured daily (see Chapter 7), and the fontanels are examined for signs of tension or bulging.

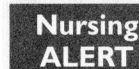

| **Nursing ALERT** | Avoid measuring rectal temperatures in infants with SB. Since bowel sphincter function is frequently affected, the thermometer can cause irritation and rectal prolapse. |

❖ Nursing Diagnoses

Nursing diagnoses identified for the infant with myelomeningocele (SB) are listed in the box. Others will be evident in specific cases and with the child's advancing years.

❖ Planning

The goals for the infant with myelomeningocele and the family include the following:

1. Infant will not experience damage to the myelomeningocele sac.
2. Infant will not experience complications.
3. Family will receive support and education.

❖ Implementation

Care of the Myelomeningocele Sac. The infant is usually placed in an incubator or warmer so that temperature can be maintained without clothing or covers that might irritate the delicate lesion. When an overhead warmer is used, the dressings over the defect require more frequent moistening because of the dehydrating effect of the radiant heat.

Before surgical closure the myelomeningocele is prevented from drying by the application of a sterile, moist, nonadher-

---

NURSING DIAGNOSES: THE INFANT WITH MYELOMENINGOCELE

High risk for infection related to nonepithelialized meningeal sac

High risk for neurologic trauma related to spinal defect

High risk for impaired skin integrity related to unprotected meningeal sac; bowel and bladder dysfunction

Altered family processes related to birth of a child with a congenital defect

High risk for impaired parent-infant attachment related to birth of a child with a chronic congenital defect

ent dressing over the defect. The moistening solution is usually sterile normal saline. Dressings are changed frequently (every 2 to 4 hours), and the sac is closely inspected for leaks, abrasions, irritation, or any signs of infection. The sac must be carefully cleansed if it becomes soiled or contaminated. Sometimes the sac ruptures during delivery or transport, and any opening in the sac greatly increases the risk of infection to the central nervous system.

> **Nursing ALERT**
>
> Observe for early signs of infection, such as elevated temperature (axillary), irritability, lethargy, and nuchal rigidity, and for signs of increased intracranial pressure (ICP), which might indicate developing hydrocephalus.

NURSING TIP To prevent stool contamination of the SB defect preoperatively, obtain a surgical drape (e.g., Steri Drape*). Cut a portion of the drape to fit the infant's sacrum using nonlatex tape to secure the plastic drape to the sacrum. The rest of the drape is placed loosely over the dressing covering the defect, thus preventing exposure to stool.

One of the most difficult, important, and challenging aspects in the early care of the infant with myelomeningocele is positioning. Before surgery the infant is kept in the prone position to minimize tension on the sac and the risk of trauma. The prone position allows for optimum positioning of the legs, especially in cases of associated hip dysplasia. The infant is placed flat with the hips only slightly flexed to reduce tension on the defect. The legs are maintained in abduction with a pad between the knees to counteract hip subluxation, and a small roll is placed under the ankles to maintain a neutral foot position. A variety of aids, including diaper rolls, pads, small sandbags, or specially designed frames and appliances, can be used to maintain the desired position.

Prevent Complications. The prone position affects other aspects of the infant's care. For example, in this position the infant is more difficult to keep clean, pressure areas are a constant threat, and feeding becomes a problem. The infant's head is turned to one side for feeding. Fortunately, most defects are repaired early, and the infant can be held for feeding as soon as the surgical site is sufficiently healed to permit handling.

Diapering the infant is contraindicated until the defect has been repaired and healing is well advanced or epithelialization has taken place. The padding beneath the diaper area is changed as needed to keep the skin dry and free of irritation. When urinary retention is detected, CIC is employed.* Since the bowel sphincter is frequently affected, there is continual passage of stool, often misinterpreted as diarrhea, which is a constant irritant to the skin and a source of infection to the spinal lesion.

Areas of sensory and motor impairment are subject to skin breakdown and therefore require meticulous care. Placing the infant on a soft foam or fleece pad reduces pressure on the knees and ankles. Periodic cleansing, application of lotion, and gentle massage aid circulation.

Gentle range-of-motion exercises are sometimes carried out to prevent contractures, and stretching of contractures is performed when indicated. However, these exercises may be restricted to the foot, ankle, and knee joint. Where the hip joints are unstable, stretching against tight hip flexors or adductor muscles, which act much like bowstrings, may aggravate a tendency toward subluxation. A physical therapist is usually consulted.

Some infants with unrepaired myelomeningocele are unable to be held in the arms and cuddled as unaffected infants are, so their need for tactile stimulation is met by caressing, stroking, and other comfort measures. To facilitate handling and to reduce parental anxiety, the infant can recline on a pillow placed in the parent's lap. Black-and-white drawings or geometric shapes can be placed within the infant's view, and other stimulation usually provided for infants is appropriate. All infants respond to pleasant sounds.

Provide Postoperative Care. Postoperative care of the infant with myelomeningocele involves the same basic care as that of any postsurgical infant: monitoring vital signs, monitoring intake and output, nourishment, observation for signs of infection, and pain management as needed. Wound management is carried out under direction of the surgeon and includes close observation for signs of leakage of cerebrospinal fluid. General care is continued as preoperatively.

The prone position is maintained after surgical closure, although many neurosurgeons allow a side-lying or partial side-lying position unless it aggravates a coexisting hip dysplasia or permits undesirable hip flexion. This offers an opportunity for position changes, which reduces the risk of pressure sores and facilitates feeding. If permitted, the infant can be held upright against the body, with care taken to avoid pressure on the operative site. Once the effects of anesthesia have subsided and the infant is alert, feedings may be resumed unless there are other anomalies or associated complications.

Since children who have SB are prone to develop an allergy to latex, reducing exposure to latex, from birth on, is hoped to decrease the chance of allergy development. Latex, a natural product derived from the rubber tree, is used in combination with other chemicals to provide elasticity, strength, and durability to many products.

Avoiding latex products is the most important intervention. The establishment of a nonlatex environment is being accomplished in many health care facilities where patients (and health care workers) are at high risk.

> **Nursing ALERT**
>
> Ask *all* patients about allergic reactions to latex, not only those at risk, during the health interview with the parent and/or child. Be sure this is a routine part of all preoperative histories.

Support Family and Educate About Home Care. As soon as the parents are able to cope with the infant's condition, they are encouraged to become involved in care. They need to learn how to continue at home the care that has been initiated in the hospital—positioning, feeding, skin care, and range-of-motion exercises when appropriate. They are taught CIC technique when prescribed.* They need to know the

---

*3M, St. Paul, MN.

*Home care instructions on performing clean intermittent self-catheterization (CIC) are available in Wong DL: *Wong and Whaley's Clinical manual of pediatric nursing*, ed 4, St Louis, 1996, Mosby.

signs of complications and how to obtain assistance when needed. When the defect has not been repaired, they are taught to care for the lesion.

The long-range planning with and support of the parents and child begin in the hospital and extend throughout childhood and even beyond. Long-term care of these children is of uncertain length. Nurses assume an important role as a central member of the health team. As a coordinator, the nurse reviews information with the family, takes responsibility for family teaching, and acts as a liaison between inpatient and outpatient services. The child may need numerous hospitalizations over the years, and each one will be a source of stress, to which the younger child is especially vulnerable. (See Chapter 18 for a discussion of care of the child with a disability.)

Habilitation involves not only solving problems of self-help and locomotion, but also solving the most distressing problem of incontinence, which threatens the child's social acceptability. Assistance with preparing the child and the school regarding the special needs of the child helps provide a better initial adjustment to this broader social experience. The **Spina Bifida Association of America*** is organized to provide services and support for families of children with spinal lesions.

❖ Evaluation

The effectiveness of nursing interventions is determined by continual reassessment and evaluation of care based on the following observational guidelines and expected outcomes:

1. Inspect spinal defect, take appropriate measurements (weight, vital signs, head circumference), observe child's general health status, and check completed care against the preoperative checklist.
2. Take vital signs, inspect operative site (or preoperative lesion), inspect skin (especially dependent areas), measure head circumference, and assess range of motion of lower extremities.
3. Observe parent-infant interactions and behavior of family members, and interview family members regarding their feelings and concerns.

Expected outcomes:

1. Child is physically prepared for surgical repair of the defect.
2. Child exhibits no evidence of infection (skin, meningeal, or renal), deformities of extremities, or pressure necrosis; signs of complications (e.g., hydrocephalus, hip dysplasia) are detected early and appropriate interventions initiated.
3. Family members discuss their feelings and concerns and participate in infant's care; family makes contact with appropriate community agencies and facilities.

See also Nursing Care Plan: The Infant with Myelomeningocele.†

PROGRESSIVE INFANTILE SPINAL MUSCULAR ATROPHY (WERDNIG-HOFFMANN DISEASE)

Progressive infantile spinal muscular atrophy (Werdnig-Hoffmann disease) is a disorder characterized by progressive

---

*4590 McArthur, N.W., Washington, DC 20007; (202) 944-3285 or (800) 621-3141.
†In Wong DL: *Wong and Whaley's Clinical manual of pediatric nursing,* ed 4, St Louis, 1996, Mosby.

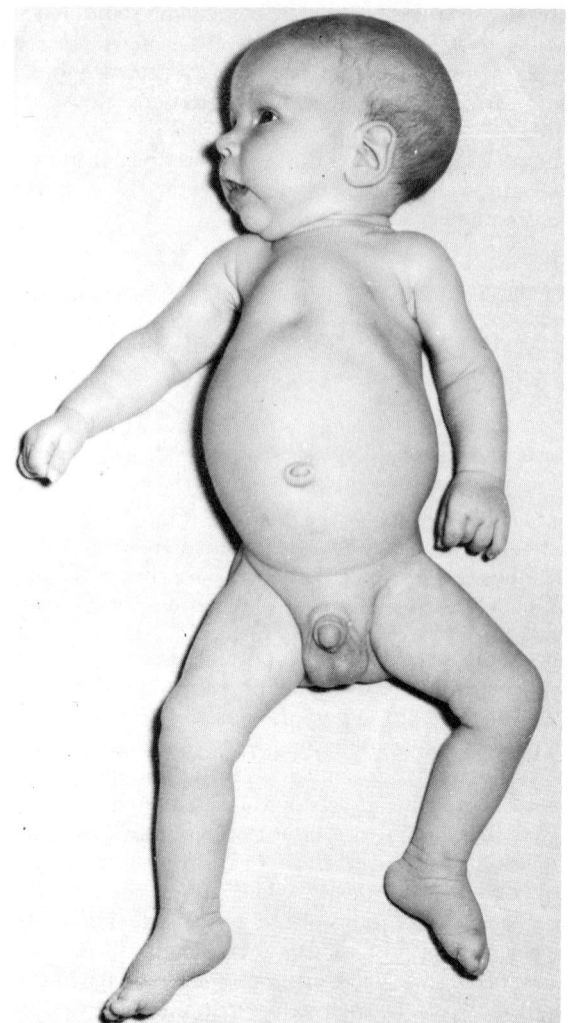

FIG. 32-7. Child with group I Werdnig-Hoffmann disease lying in typical posture of abduction of legs at hips and flexion of knees. Arms are flexed slightly with little movement at shoulders. Movements of fingers and toes are present. Pectus excavatum deformity of chest is common and is a result of unopposed diaphragmatic breathing. (From Swaiman KF, Wright FS: *The practice of pediatric neurology,* ed 2, St Louis, 1982, Mosby.)

weakness and wasting of skeletal muscles caused by degeneration of anterior horn cells. It is inherited as an autosomal-recessive trait and is the most common paralytic form of the "floppy infant syndrome." The site of the pathologic condition is the anterior horn cells of the spinal cord and the motor nuclei of the brainstem, but the primary effect is atrophy of skeletal muscles (Fig. 32-7).

Therapeutic Management

The diagnosis is suspected on the basis of clinical manifestations (see box). It is established by electromyography demonstrating a denervation pattern and is confirmed by muscle biopsy. Treatment is symptomatic and preventive, primarily preventing infection and treating orthopedic problems, the most serious of which is scoliosis. Many children benefit from powered chairs, lifts, special mattresses, and accessible environmental controls. Vigorous antibiotic therapy and pulmo-

CLINICAL MANIFESTATIONS OF WERDNIG-HOFFMANN DISEASE

Group 1
Disease acquired in utero or during first 2 months of life
Inactivity is most prominent feature
Infant lies in the frog position with legs externally rotated, abducted, and flexed at hips (Fig. 32-7)
Weakness
Limited movements of shoulder and arm muscles
Active movement is usually limited to fingers and toes
Diaphragmatic breathing with sternal retractions
Weak cry and cough
Secretions tend to pool in pharynx
Alert facies
Normal sensation and intellect
Affected infants do not progress to sit alone, roll over, or walk
Early death (usually by 3 years of age) from respiratory failure or infection

Group 2
Disease manifested between 2 and 12 months of age
Early—weakness confined to arms and legs
Later—weakness becomes generalized
Legs usually involved to greater extent than arms
Prominent pectus excavatum
Movements absent during complete relaxation or sleep
Some infants able to sit if placed in position
Life span varies from 7 months to 7 years

Group 3
Onset of symptoms in second year of life
Normal head control and can sit unassisted by 6 to 8 months of age
Thigh and hip muscles weak
In those who manage to walk:
  Lumbar lordosis
  Waddling gait
  Genu recurvatum
  Protuberant abdomen
  Ambulation becomes increasingly difficult
  Confined to a wheelchair by second decade of life
Deep tendon reflexes may be present early but disappear

---

nary physical therapy are implemented during upper respiratory infections.

Prognosis. Prognosis varies according to age of onset or group as described in the box. However, recent observations suggest that the classification is not valid. Individuals with group 1 manifestations had a life span of 4 months to 31 years. Also, some affected persons did not demonstrate progressive loss of strength and function (Russman and others, 1992).

Nursing Considerations
The infant or small child with extensive paralysis requires frequent change of position to prevent physical injury and complications, especially pneumonia. The pharynx requires suctioning to remove secretions, and feeding must be carried out slowly and carefully to prevent aspiration. Since these children are intellectually normal, verbal, tactile, and auditory stimulation are important aspects of care. Supporting them so that they can see the activities around them and transporting them in appropriate conveyances (i.e., carriage, wagon, wheelchair) for a change of environment provide stimulation and a broader scope of contacts.

Children who are able to sit require proper support and attention to alignment to prevent deformities and other complications. Children who survive beyond infancy will need attention to educational needs and opportunities for social interaction with other children. The parents of a child who is chronically or potentially fatally ill require much support and encouragement (see Chapter 18). The parents of a child with a genetically transmitted disorder also need to be encouraged to seek genetic counseling.

JUVENILE SPINAL MUSCULAR ATROPHY (KUGELBERG-WELANDER DISEASE)

Juvenile spinal muscular atrophy (Kugelberg-Welander disease, juvenile proximal hereditary muscular atrophy) is also the result of anterior horn cell and motor nerve degeneration. The disease is characterized by a pattern of muscular weakness similar to that of infantile spinal muscular atrophy. Several modes of inheritance have been reported for the disease: autosomal-recessive, autosomal-dominant, and X-linked recessive.

The onset occurs from less than 1 year of age into adulthood, with symptoms resembling group 3 infantile spinal muscular atrophy; proximal muscle weakness (especially of the lower limbs) and muscular atrophy are the predominant features. The disease runs a slowly progressive course. Some children lose the ability to walk 8 to 9 years after the onset of symptoms, but many can still walk after 30 years or more. Many affected persons have a normal life expectancy.

Therapeutic Management and Nursing Considerations
The management is primarily symptomatic and supportive and is related to maintaining mobility as long as possible, preventing complications, and providing support to the child and family.

MUSCULAR DYSTROPHIES (MDs)
MDs constitute the largest and most important single group of muscle diseases of childhood. They all have a genetic origin in which there is gradual degeneration of muscle fibers, and they are characterized by progressive weakness and wasting of symmetric groups of skeletal muscles, with increasing disability and deformity. In all forms of MD there is insidious loss of strength, but each type differs in regard to muscle groups affected (Fig. 32-8), age of onset, rate of progression, and inheritance patterns. The most common form, *Duchenne muscular dystrophy,* is considered separately in the next section.

Facioscapulohumeral (Landouzy-Déjérine) muscular dystrophy is inherited as an autosomal-dominant disorder with onset in early adolescence. It is characterized by difficulty in raising the arms over the head, lack of facial mobility, and a forward slope of the shoulders. The progression is slow.

Limb-girdle muscular dystrophy is an autosomal-recessive disease of later childhood or adolescence with variable but usually slow progression; it is characterized by weakness of proximal muscles of the pelvic and shoulder girdles.

Treatment of the MDs consists mainly of supportive measures, including physical therapy, orthopedic procedures to

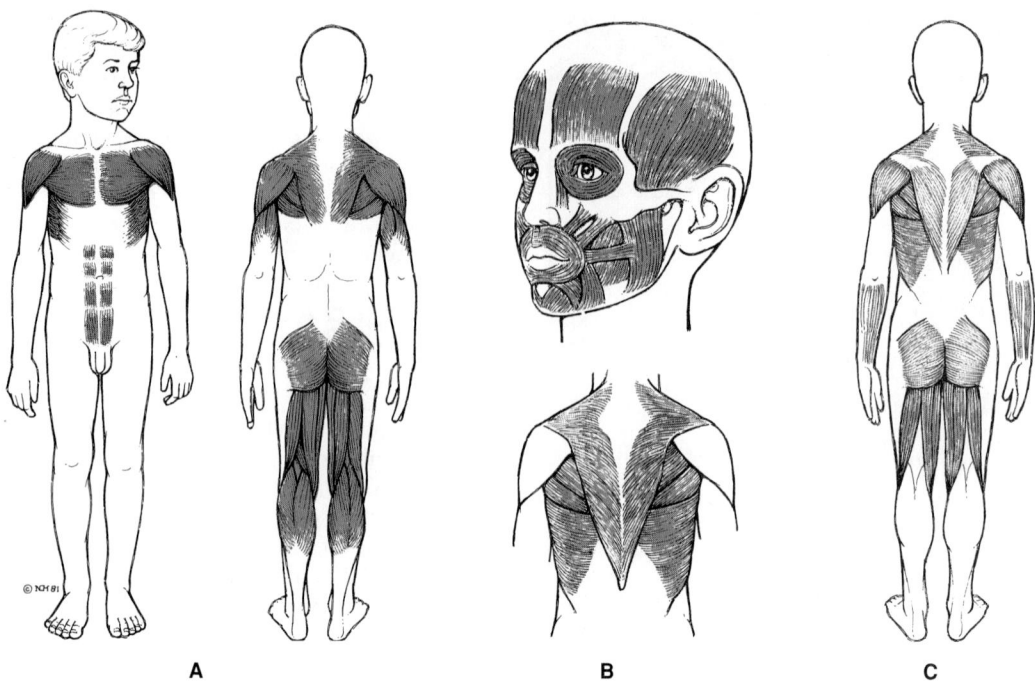

FIG. 32-8. Initial muscle groups involved in muscular dystrophies. **A,** Pseudohypertrophic. **B,** Facioscapulohumeral. **C,** Limb-girdle.

minimize deformity, and assistance for the affected child in meeting the demands of daily living.

PSEUDOHYPERTROPHIC (DUCHENNE) MUSCULAR DYSTROPHY (DMD)

DMD is the most severe and the most common muscular dystrophy of childhood. An X-linked inheritance pattern is identified in most patients; about one third of all cases represent fresh mutations. As in all X-linked disorders, males are affected almost exclusively. The incidence is approximately 1:3500 male births (Multicenter Study Group, 1992). The box describes the characteristics of DMD.

Evidence of muscle weakness usually appears during the third year, although there may have been a history of delay in motor development, particularly walking. Difficulties in running, riding a bicycle, and climbing stairs are usually the first symptoms noted. Later, abnormal gait on a level surface becomes apparent. In the early years, rapid developmental gains may mask the progression of the disease. Questioning the parents may reveal that the child has difficulty in rising

from a sitting or supine position. Occasionally the parents notice enlarged calves.

The term *pseudohypertrophy* is derived from muscular enlargement caused by fatty infiltration. Profound muscular atrophy occurs in later stages, and as the disease progresses, contractures and deformities involving large and small joints are common complications. Ambulation usually becomes impossible by 12 years of age. Facial, oropharyngeal, and respiratory muscles are spared until the terminal stages of the disease. Ultimately the disease process involves the diaphragm and auxiliary muscles of respiration, and cardiomegaly is common. The cause of death is usually respiratory tract infection or cardiac failure.

Diagnostic Evaluation

The disease is suspected on the basis of clinical manifestations (see box) and confirmed by serum enzyme measurement, muscle biopsy, and electromyography (EMG). The serum creatine phosphokinase, aldolase, and serum glutamic-oxaloacetic transaminase (SGOT) (more recent term, aspartate aminotransferase, AST) levels are extremely high in the first 2 years of life before the onset of clinical weakness. They diminish with muscle deterioration but do not reach normal levels until severe muscle wasting and incapacitation have occurred. Muscle biopsy reveals degeneration of muscle fibers, with fibrosis and fatty tissue replacement. EMG readings show a decrease in amplitude and duration of motor unit potentials.

Therapeutic Management

No effective treatment exists for childhood MD. Increased muscle bulk and muscle power have been reported after a course of corticosteroids; however, this therapy requires further evaluation before it becomes routine management. Maintaining function in unaffected muscles for as long as pos-

---

CHARACTERISTICS OF DUCHENNE MUSCULAR DYSTROPHY

Early onset, usually between 3 and 5 years of age
Progressive muscular weakness, wasting, and contractures
Calf muscle hypertrophy in most patients
Loss of independent ambulation by 9 to 11 years of age
Slowly progressive, generalized weakness during teenage years
Relentless progression until death from respiratory or cardiac failure

---

CLINICAL MANIFESTATIONS OF DUCHENNE MUSCULAR DYSTROPHY

Waddling gait
Lordosis
Frequent falls
Gower sign (child turns onto side or abdomen, flexes knees to assume a kneeling position, then with knees extended gradually pushes torso to an upright position by "walking" the hands up the legs)
Enlarged muscles (especially thighs and upper arms)
Feel unusually firm or woody on palpation
Later stages: profound muscular atrophy
Mental deficiency (common)
Mild (about 20 IQ points below normal)
Frank mental deficit present in 25% of patients
Complications:
Contracture deformities of hips, knees, and ankles
Disuse atrophy
Obesity

---

sible is the primary goal. It has been found that children who remain as active as possible are able to avoid wheelchair confinement for a longer time. Early recourse to a wheelchair accelerates deconditioning and promotes the development of lower extremity contractures. Maintenance of function often includes range-of-motion exercises, surgery to release contracture deformities, bracing, and performance of activities of daily living. Genetic counseling is recommended for parents, female siblings, and maternal aunts and their female offspring.

Nursing Considerations

The major emphasis of nursing care is to assist the child and family cope with the progressive, incapacitating, and fatal nature of the disease; to help design a program that will afford a greater degree of independence and reduce the predictable and preventable disabilities associated with the disorder; and to help the child and family deal constructively with the limitations the disease imposes on their daily lives.

Working closely with other team members, nurses assist the family in developing the child's self-help skills to give the child the satisfaction of being as independent as possible for as long as possible. This requires continual evaluation of the child's capabilities, which are often difficult to assess. It is not always possible to know when children seek parental assistance because they want a little extra attention, when parents are being overprotective, or when the muscles are overtired. Fortunately, most children with MD instinctively recognize this need to become as independent as possible and strive to do so.

Practical difficulties faced by families are physical limitations of housing and mobility. Parents also need assistance in buying and modifying clothing for their child. It is difficult to find clothing and footwear to wear comfortably in a wheelchair, to fit over contracted limbs, and to fit hypertrophied muscles. The parent's social activities are also restricted, and the family's activities must be continually modified to the needs of the affected child.

When the child becomes increasingly helpless, the family may consider a skilled nursing facility or respite care to provide the care needed. Nurses can assist with decision making and support the family in the decision.

No matter how successful the program or how well the family adapts to the disorder, superimposed on the physical and emotional problems associated with a child with a long-term disability is the constant presence of the ultimate outcome of the disease. All the manifestations seen in the child with a chronic fatal illness are encountered in these families (see Chapter 18). The guilt feelings of the mother may be particularly pronounced in this disorder because of the mother-to-son transmission of the defective gene.

Nurses are especially valuable health professionals as they come to know the family and the family's problems. Nurses can be alert to the problems and needs of the families and make necessary referrals when supplementary services are indicated. The **Muscular Dystrophy Association of America, Inc.*** has branches in most communities to provide assistance to families in which there is a member with muscular dystrophy.

ACQUIRED NEUROMUSCULAR DISORDERS

GUILLAIN-BARRÉ SYNDROME (GBS) (INFECTIOUS POLYNEURITIS)

GBS, also known as infectious polyneuritis, is an uncommon acute demyelinating polyneuropathy with a progressive, usually ascending flaccid paralysis. Children are less often affected than adults, with children between ages 4 and 10 years having higher susceptibility. Both sexes are affected with equal frequency.

Pathophysiology

GBS is an immune-mediated disease often associated with a number of viral or bacterial infections or the administration of vaccines. It has been associated with infectious mononucleosis, measles, mumps, *Borrelia burgdorferi* (Lyme disease), *Helicobacter pylori,* and *Mycoplasma* and *Pneumocystis* infections. Pathologic changes in spinal and cranial nerves consist of inflammation and edema with rapid, segmented demyelination and compression of nerve roots within the dural sheath. Nerve conduction is impaired, producing ascending partial or complete paralysis of muscles innervated by the involved nerves.

Diagnostic Evaluation

Diagnosis of GBS is based on the paralytic manifestations (see box on p. 1178) and/or EMG findings. Cerebrospinal fluid analysis reveals an increased protein concentration, but other laboratory studies are noncontributory. The symmetric nature of the paralysis helps differentiate this disorder from spinal paralytic poliomyelitis, which usually affects sporadic muscles.

Therapeutic Management

Treatment of GBS is symptomatic. In some reports, corticosteroid therapy has been of benefit in the early stages. Respi-

---

*10 E. 40th St., Room 4105, New York, NY 10019; (212) 679-6215 or (212) 689-9040. In Canada: **Muscular Dystrophy Association of Canada,** 150 Eglinton Ave, E., Suite 400, Toronto, Ontario M4P 1E8; (416) 488-0030.

ratory and pharyngeal involvement requires assisted ventilation, frequently with tracheostomy. Plasma exchange (plasmapheresis) may be beneficial both in shortening the length of illness and in lessening the long-term disability; intravenous immunoglobulin is also advocated (Vajsar and others, 1994).

Course and Prognosis. Better outcomes are associated with younger age, no requirement for respiratory assistance, slower progression of disease, normal peripheral nerve function on EMG, and treatment by plasmapheresis.

Almost all deaths are caused by respiratory failure; therefore early diagnosis and access to respiratory support are especially important. Muscle function begins to return 2 days to 2 weeks after the onset of symptoms, and recovery is complete in most patients. The rate of recovery is usually related to the degree of involvement, which may extend from a few weeks to months. The greater the degree of paralysis, the longer is the recovery phase.

Nursing Considerations

Nursing care is essentially supportive and is the same as that required for quadriplegia from any cause. The emphasis of care is on close observation to assess the extent of paralysis and on prevention of complications.

During the acute phase of GBS the child's condition should be carefully observed for possible difficulty in swallowing and respiratory involvement. The child's cardiorespiratory function is monitored, and a ventilator, suction apparatus, tracheostomy tray, and vasoconstrictor drugs are kept available at the bedside. Vital signs and level of consciousness are monitored frequently. For the child who develops respiratory dysfunction, the care is the same as that for any child with respiratory distress requiring mechanical ventilation.

Throughout the recovery phase, special emphasis is placed on prevention of complications, including proper postural alignment, frequent change of position, and passive range-

of-motion exercises. Children with oral and pharyngeal involvement are usually fed via a nasogastric tube to ensure adequate feeding. Bowel and bladder care is needed to avoid constipation and urine retention. Sensory impairment makes the child susceptible to burns and trophic ulcers.

Physical therapy is limited to passive range-of-motion exercises during the evolving phase of the disease. Later, as the disease stabilizes and recovery begins, an active physical therapy program is implemented to prevent contracture deformities and facilitate muscle recovery. This may include active exercise, gait training, and bracing.

Throughout the course of the illness, support of the child and parents is paramount. The usual rapidity of the paralysis and the long period of recovery greatly tax the emotional reserves of all family members. The parents and child benefit from repeated reassurance that recovery is occurring and from realistic information regarding the possibility of permanent disability. In the event of a residual disability, the family needs assistance in accepting and adjusting to the loss of function (see Chapter 18). The **Guillain-Barré Syndrome Support Group*** is a nonprofit organization devoted to support, education, and research. It provides support to families from recovered persons, publishes informational literature and a newsletter, and maintains a list of practitioners experienced with the disease.

TETANUS

Tetanus, or *lockjaw,* is an acute, preventable, and often fatal disease caused by an exotoxin produced by the anaerobic spore-forming, gram-positive bacillus *Clostridium tetani.* The disorder is characterized by painful muscular rigidity primarily involving the masseter and neck muscles. There are four requirements for the development of tetanus: (1) presence of tetanus spores or vegetative forms of the bacillus, (2) injury to the tissues, (3) wound conditions that encourage multiplication of the organism, and (4) a susceptible host.

Tetanus spores are found in soil, dust, and the intestinal tracts of humans and animals, especially herbivorous animals. The organisms are more prevalent in rural areas but are readily carried to urban areas by the wind. The organisms are not invasive but enter the body by way of wounds, particularly a puncture wound, burn, or crushed area. They may enter through a very minor, unnoticed break in the skin, such as a thorn or needle prick, bee sting, or scratch. In the newborn, infection may occur through the umbilical cord, usually in situations in which infants are delivered in severely contaminated surroundings. The disease has the greatest incidence in months when persons are more involved in outdoor activities. Substance abusers are especially susceptible from poor injection technique and the use of street heroin, which is often mixed with quinine, a protoplasmic poison that favors the growth of the organism.

Pathophysiology

When conditions are favorable, the organisms proliferate and elaborate a potent exotoxin that affects the central nervous system to produce the clinical manifestations of the disease. The ideal conditions for growth of the organisms are devitalized tissues without access to air, such as wounds that have not been washed or kept clean and those that have crusted

---
*P.O. Box 262, Wynnewood PA 19096.

over, trapping pus beneath. The exotoxin appears to reach the central nervous system by way of either the neuron axons or the vascular system. The toxin becomes fixed on nerve cells of the anterior horn of the spinal cord and the brainstem. The toxin acts at the myoneural junction to produce muscular stiffness and lower the threshold for reflex excitability.

Several forms of the disease exist, but the generalized form is the most common and most dangerous. The incubation period for tetanus varies from 3 days to 3 weeks but generally averages 8 days. The traditional belief that the more extensive the injury, the shorter the incubation period and the more severe the symptoms, has not been confirmed in the United States.

The manner of onset varies, but the initial symptoms are usually a progressive stiffness and tenderness of the muscles in the neck and jaw. Eventually all voluntary muscles are affected (see box). As the child recovers from the disease, the paroxysms become less frequent and gradually subside. Survival beyond 4 days usually indicates recovery, but complete recovery may require weeks.

The mortality rate is about 30%, but the disease is almost invariably fatal in the newborn. The incubation period is short, with the appearance of symptoms 3 to 10 days after exposure. The first symptom is difficulty sucking, which progresses to total inability to suck, excessive crying, irritability, and nuchal rigidity.

Therapeutic Management

Preventive measures are based on the immune status of the affected child and the nature of the injury. Specific prophylactic therapy after trauma is administration of either *tetanus toxoid* or *tetanus antitoxin* (see Immunizations, Chapter 10).

The unprotected or inadequately immunized child who sustains a "tetanus-prone" wound (such as, but not limited to, wounds contaminated with dirt, feces, soil, and saliva; puncture wounds; avulsions; and wounds resulting from missiles, crushing, burns, and frostbite) should receive *tetanus immune globulin (TIG)*. Concurrent administration of both TIG and tetanus toxoid at separate sites is recommended both to provide protection and to initiate the active immune process. Completion of active immunization is carried out according to the usual pattern.

The affected child is best treated in an intensive care facility where close and constant observation and equipment for monitoring and respiratory support are readily available. A quiet environment is preferred to reduce external stimuli. Neonates are placed in an open warmer unit or incubator to maintain a constant environmental temperature.

General supportive care, including maintenance of adequate fluid and electrolyte balance and caloric intake, is indicated. Indwelling oral or nasogastric feedings are used whenever possible, but severe laryngospasm may necessitate intravenous parenteral nutrition or gastrostomy feeding. Recurrent laryngospasm or excessive accumulation of secretions may require endotracheal intubation.

TIG therapy to neutralize toxins is the most specific therapy for tetanus. Antibiotics are administered to control the proliferation of the vegetative forms of the organism at the site of infection. Local care of the wound by surgical débridement and cleansing helps reduce the numbers of proliferating organisms at the site of injury. The cleansing should be repeated several times during the first 48 hours, and deep, infected lacerations are usually exposed and debrided.

Sedatives or muscle relaxants are administered to help reduce muscle spasm and prevent convulsions. The most widely used is diazepam (Valium), but phenobarbital, chloral hydrate, the phenothiazines, and paraldehyde may be employed. Patients with severe tetanus and those who do not respond to other sedatives require the administration of a neuromuscular blocking agent, usually pancuronium bromide (Pavulon) or vecuronium. Because of their paralytic effect on respiratory muscles, use of these drugs requires mechanical ventilation with endotracheal intubation or tracheostomy and constant attendance by trained personnel until muscle spasms are controlled. Endotracheal tube insertion or tracheostomy is often indicated and should be performed before severe respiratory distress develops. Administration of corticosteroids has met with success in some instances.

Nursing Considerations

In caring for the child with tetanus, every effort is made to control or eliminate stimulation from sound, light, and touch. Although a darkened room is ideal, sufficient light is essential in order that the child can be carefully observed; light appears to be less irritating than vibratory or auditory stimuli. The infant or child is handled as little as possible, and extra effort is expended to avoid any sudden and/or loud noise.

Medications are administered as prescribed, and vital signs are observed and recorded at frequent intervals. The location and extent of muscle spasms and assessment of their severity

---

CLINICAL MANIFESTATIONS OF TETANUS

Initial Symptoms

Progressive stiffness and tenderness of muscles in neck and jaw
Characteristic difficulty in opening the mouth (trismus)
Risus sardonicus (sardonic smile) caused by facial muscle spasm

Progressive Involvement

Opisthotonos
Boardlike rigidity of abdominal and limb muscles
Difficulty swallowing
High sensitivity to external stimuli (slight noise, gentle touch, or bright light):
  Trigger paroxysmal muscular contractions that last seconds to minutes
  Contractions recur with increased frequency until almost continuous
Laryngospasm and tetany of respiratory muscles:
  Accumulated secretions
  Respiratory arrest
  Atelectasis
  Pneumonia

Other Aspects

Mentation unaffected; patient alert
Pain and distress are reflected in:
  Rapid pulse
  Sweating
  Anxious expression
Fever usually absent or only mild

are important nursing observations. Respiratory status is carefully evaluated for any signs of distress, and appropriate emergency equipment is kept available at all times. Muscle relaxants and sedatives that may be prescribed can also cause respiratory depression; therefore the child must be assessed for excessive central nervous system depression. Oxygen saturation is monitored, and when needed, blood gases are obtained frequently to evaluate respiratory status. Attention to hydration and nutrition may involve monitoring an intravenous infusion, monitoring nasogastric or gastrostomy feedings, and suctioning oropharyngeal secretions when indicated.

If a potent muscle relaxant such as pancuronium bromide is used, the total paralysis makes oral communication impossible. Therefore all the child's needs must be anticipated and procedures carefully explained beforehand. As the dose of medication is decreased, the child regains movement of the eyelids and facial muscles, which gives the child some opportunity to express emotions and indicate choices through a signal system, for example, blinking the lids to indicate "yes" or "no."

Since their mental status is clear, children with tetanus are aware of what is happening to them and are often in a state of terror. They should not be left alone, and all efforts should be made to reduce anxiety, which can contribute to muscular spasms. A calm and reassuring manner and sympathetic understanding can assist immeasurably in helping a child through this crisis situation. Parents are encouraged to stay with the child to offer security and support.

BOTULISM

Botulism is a serious food poisoning that results from ingestion of the preformed toxin produced by the anaerobic bacillus *Clostridium botulinum*. The most common source of the toxin is improperly sterilized home-canned foods. Central nervous system symptoms appear abruptly about 12 to 36 hours after ingestion of contaminated food and may or may not have been preceded by acute digestive disturbance (see box).

CLINICAL MANIFESTATIONS OF BOTULISM

General Signs
Weakness
Dizziness
Headache
Difficulty talking and speaking
Diplopia
Vomiting
Progressive, life-threatening respiratory paralysis

Infant Botulism
Constipation (a common symptom)
Generalized weakness
Decrease in spontaneous movements
Diminished or absent deep tendon reflexes
Loss of head control
Difficulty feeding
Weak cry
Reduced gag reflex
Progressive respiratory paralysis

Treatment consists of intravenous administration of botulism antitoxin and general supportive measures, primarily respiratory and nutritional. Toxins vary in protein-binding capacity. Some have a relatively short half-life and do not bind to tissues firmly; therefore therapy is continued until paralysis abates. Other toxins appear to bind irreversibly to nerve endings and are therefore not amenable to neutralization. Respiratory support is often needed and should be available at the bedside, ready for use if indicated.

Infant Botulism

Infant botulism, unlike the disease in older persons, is caused by ingestion of spores or vegetative cells of *C. botulinum* and the subsequent release of the toxin from organisms colonizing the gastrointestinal tract. There appears to be no common food or drug source of the organisms; however, the *C. botulinum* organisms have been found in honey and light or dark corn syrup fed to affected infants (American Academy of Pediatrics, 1994).

There is wide variation in the severity of the disease, from mild constipation to progressive sequential loss of neurologic function and respiratory failure (see box). The affected infant is usually well before the onset of symptoms. Constipation is a common presenting symptom, and almost all infants exhibit generalized weakness and a decrease in spontaneous movements. Deep tendon reflexes are usually diminished or absent; cranial nerve deficits are common, as evidenced by loss of head control, difficulty in feeding, weak cry, and reduced gag reflex. The most frequently recognized form of the disease is consistent with the hypotonic infant. Botulism toxin exerts its effect by inhibiting the release of acetylcholine at the myoneural junction, thereby impairing motor activity of muscles innervated by affected nerves.

Diagnosis is made on the basis of the history, physical examination, and laboratory detection of the organism in the patient or the implicated food. Treatment consists of supportive measures, primarily respiratory and nutritional. Botulism antitoxin, used in adults and older children, is not administered to infants. Evidence indicates that infants recover without it and that its therapeutic efficacy is lacking.

The prognosis is generally good if the patient is adequately supported, although recovery may be very slow, requiring weeks to months following severe illness. An infant who is recovering from botulism must avoid contact with other infants for about 3 months or until excretion of organisms has ceased.

Nursing Considerations

Nursing responsibilities include observing for and reporting signs of muscle impairment and providing intensive nursing care when the infant is hospitalized (see Nursing Care of the High-Risk Newborn and Family, Chapter 9). Parental support and reassurance are important. Most infants recover when the disorder is recognized and therapy is implemented. Parents should be aware that during recovery, patients tire easily when muscular action is sustained. This has important implications for timing the resumption of feedings, because of the risk of aspiration. Parents should also be advised that normal bowel action may not return for several weeks; therefore a stool softener can be beneficial. Cathartics and enemas are not advised.

Home supervision of the outpatient and education regarding possible modes of infection (e.g., use of honey or corn syrup as a formula sweetener) are nursing responsibilities. Since the prime sources of botulism toxin are inadequately cooked or improperly canned food, families are advised about the danger of home-canned foods, especially vegetables, fruits, fish, and condiments. Boiling water is not always adequate, particularly in high altitudes where water boils at a lower temperature, which does not destroy the organisms.

SPINAL CORD INJURIES

Spinal cord injuries with major neurologic involvement are not a common cause of physical disability in childhood. However, a sufficient number of children with these injuries are admitted to major medical centers, and because of the increased survival rate as a result of improved management, nurses are more likely to become involved with such children.

Mechanisms of Injury

In motor vehicle accidents (MVAs), most spinal cord injuries in children are a result of indirect trauma caused by sudden hyperflexion or hyperextension of the neck, often combined with a rotational force. Trauma to the spinal cord without evidence of vertebral fracture or dislocation is particularly likely to occur in an MVA when proper restraints are not used. An unrestrained child becomes a projectile during sudden deceleration and is subject to injury from contact with a variety of objects inside and outside the vehicle. Individuals who use only a lap seat belt restraint are at greater risk of spinal cord injury than those who use a combination lap and shoulder restraint.

Falling from heights occurs less often in children than in adults, but vertebral compression from blows to the head or buttocks can occur in water sports (diving and surfing), falls from horses, or other athletic activities. Birth injuries may occur in breech deliveries from traction force on the spinal cord during delivery of the head and shoulders. An increasing number of teenagers receive spinal cord injuries when they are shot or stabbed in the back.

The injury sustained can affect any of the spinal nerves, and the higher the injury, the more extensive the damage. The child can be left with complete or partial paralysis of the lower extremities *(paraplegia)* or with damage at a higher level and without functional use of any of the four extremities *(quadriplegia).* A high cervical cord injury that affects the phrenic nerve paralyzes the diaphragm and leaves the child dependent on a ventilator.

A mild but equally frightening form of cord trauma is *spinal cord compression,* a temporary neural dysfunction without visible damage to the cord. Complete quadraplegia can result but initially may not be differentiated from serious cord injury.

Therapeutic Management

The management of the child with spinal cord injury is complex and controversial. Initial care begins at the scene of the accident; therefore education and training of rescue personnel in stabilization and transfer techniques to prevent or reduce the severity of injury are critically important. In any situation in which spinal cord injury is suspected or a possibility, the child should be calmed, reassured, and told not to move; no one should be allowed to move the child unless they are able to stabilize the head and trunk correctly to avoid twisting or bending the spine. If conscious, the child is placed supine on a rigid surface to prevent sagging. Infants and small children are removed in their car seats; no attempt should be made to take them out of the seat. Because of the complexity and relative infrequency of these injuries, it is usually recommended that these persons be transferred to a spinal injury center for care by specially trained personnel.

Nursing Considerations

The nursing care of the paraplegic or quadriplegic child is complex and challenging. As a member of the acute care and rehabilitation teams, the nurse is involved in all aspects of care. Ideally, initial care takes place in a special intensive care unit with personnel trained to handle spinal cord injuries. Nursing management is concerned primarily with prevention of complications and maintenance of function.

Once the acute period is over, the lesion is usually static and nonprogressive, regardless of whether the paralysis is secondary to trauma, a congenital defect, infection, a treated tumor, or surgery. The nurse is a member of a team of specialists, including physicians from a number of specialty areas, physical and occupational therapists, psychologists, social workers, teachers, and vocational counselors. Each team member has a unique contribution to make, and mutual agreement for specific areas of responsibility and evaluation of progress are determined during regularly scheduled team conferences.

To meet the needs of these children, the reader is referred to the extensive discussion in Wong (1995) or to texts devoted to children with spinal cord injuries.

KEY POINTS

- Clinical manifestations of cerebral palsy include delayed gross motor development, abnormal motor performance, alterations of muscle tone, abnormal postures, reflex abnormalities, and associated disabilities such as mental retardation, seizures, attention deficit disorder, and sensory impairment.

- Therapy for cerebral palsy takes into account the nature of the physical disability, defects associated with the disorder, and interpersonal and social influences encountered by the affected child.
- Care of the infant and child with myelomeningocele is directed toward protecting the meningeal sac, pre-

venting infection and skin breakdown, and observing for signs of complications.

- Werdnig-Hoffmann disease is characterized by progressive weakness and wasting of skeletal muscles caused by degeneration of anterior horn cells of the spinal cord.
- Muscular dystrophies are the greatest and most important cause of muscular dysfunction of childhood.
- Major complications of Duchenne muscular dystrophy include joint contractures, disuse atrophy, infections, obesity, and cardiopulmonary problems.
- Nursing care of the child with Guillain-Barré syn-

drome consists of monitoring vital signs, ensuring alignment and positioning, providing physical therapy, and providing support to the child and family.
- Tetanus occurs when tetanus spores or vegetative bacilli enter a wound and multiply in a susceptible host.
- Infant botulism results from the release of toxins from *Clostridium botulinum* colonizing the gastrointestinal tract.
- Therapeutic management of spinal cord injury is directed toward preventing further neuronal damage, avoiding complications, and maintaining vital functions.

REFERENCES

American Academy of Pediatrics: *Report of the Committee on Infectious Diseases,* ed 23, Elk Grove Village, IL, 1994, The Academy.

American Academy of Pediatrics, Committee on Genetics: Folic acid for the prevention of neural tube defects, *Pediatrics* 92(3):493-494, 1993.

Brucker JM: Selective dorsal rhizotomy: neurosurgical treatment of cerebral palsy, *J Pediatr Nurs* 5:105-114, 1990.

Fernandes ET and others: Neurogenic bladder dysfunction in children: review of pathophysiology and current management, *J Pediatr* 124(1):1-7, 1994.

Hutton JL, Cooke T, Pharaoh P: Life expectancy in children with cerebral palsy, *Br Med J* 309(6952):431-435, 1994.

Knowledge and use of folic acid by women of childbearing age—United States, 1995, *MMWR* 44(38):716-718, 1995.

Multicenter Study Group: Diagnosis of Duchenne and Becker muscular dystrophies by polymerase chain reaction, *JAMA* 267(19):2609-2615, 1992.

Russman BS and others: Spinal muscular atrophy: new thoughts on the pathogenesis and classification schema, *J Child Neurol* 7(4):347-353, 1992.

Vajsar J and others: Plasmapheresis vs intravenous immunoglobulin treatment in childhood Guillain-Barré syndrome, *Arch Pediatr Adolesc Med* 148(11):1210-1211, 1994.

Wong D: Whaley and Wong's *Nursing Care of Infants and Children,* ed 5, St Louis, 1995, Mosby.

BIBLIOGRAPHY

Cerebral Palsy/Spina Bifida

Appleton PL, Minchom PE, Ellis NC: The self-concept of young people with spina bifida, *Dev Med Child Neurol* 36(3):198-215, 1994.

Blasco PA: Primitive reflexes: their contribution to the early detection of cerebral palsy, *Clin Pediatr* 33(7):388-397, 1994.

Dormans JP: Orthopedic management of children with cerebral palsy, *Pediatr Clin North Am* 40(3):645-657, 1993.

Eicher PS, Batshaw ML: Cerebral palsy, *Pediatr Clin North Am* 40(3):537-551, 1993.

Farley JA, Dunleavy MJ: Myelodysplasia. In Jackson PL, Vessey JA: *Primary care of the child with a chronic illness,* ed 2, St Louis, 1996, Mosby.

Hobdell EF: Perceptual accuracy and gender-related differences in parents of children with myelomeningocele, *J Neurosci Nurs* 27(4):240-244, 1995.

Knutson LM, Clark DE: Orthotic devices for ambulation in children with cerebral palsy and myelomeningocele, *Phys Ther* 71(12):947-960, 1991.

Kuban KC, Leviton A: Medical progress: cerebral palsy, *N Engl J Med* 330(3):188-195, 1994.

Morrow JD: Temperament of the infant with myelomeningocele, *J Pediatr Nurs* 10(2):99-104, 1995.

Nehring WM, Steele S: Cerebral palsy. In Jackson PL, Vessey JA: *Primary care of the child with a chronic condition,* ed 2, St Louis, 1996, Mosby.

Park TS, Owen JH: Surgical management of spastic diplegia in cerebral palsy, *N Engl J Med* 326(11):745-749, 1992.

Peacock WJ, Staudt LA: Management of spasticity in cerebral palsy, *Int Pediatr* 7(2):181-184, 1992.

Peterson PM and others: Spina bifida: the transition into adulthood begins in infancy, *Rehabil Nurs* 19(4):229-238, 1994.

Polivka BJ, Nickel JT, Wilkins III Jr: Cerebral palsy: evaluation of a model of risk, *Res Nurs Health* 16(2):113-122, 1993.

Romanczuk AN, Brown JP: Folic acid will reduce risk of neural tube defects, *MCN Am J Matern Child Nurs* 19(6):331-334, 1994.

Sackett CK: Spina bifida, *Urol Nurs* 13(2):58-61, 1993.

Segal ES, Deatrick JA, Hagelgans NA: The determinants of successful self-catheterization programs in children with myelomeningoceles, *J Pediatr Nurs* 10(2):82-88, 1995.

Sprague JB: Surgical management of cerebral palsy, *Orthop Nurs* 11(4):11-19, 1992.

Turnbull JD: Early intervention for children with or at risk of cerebral palsy, *Am J Dis Child* 147(1):54-59, 1993.

Walker MJ: Selective dorsal rhizotomy, reducing spasticity in patients with cerebral palsy, *AORN J* 54(4):759-761, 1991.

Zickler CF, Dodge NN: Office management of the young child with cerebral palsy and difficulty in growing, *J Pediatr Health Care* 8(3):111-120, 1994.

Neuromuscular Dysfunction

Bechler-Karsch A, Berro E: Infant botulism, *MCN Am J Matern Child Nurs* 19(5):275-280, 1994.

Hardy EM, Rittenberry K: Myasthenia gravis: an overview, *Orthopaed Nurs* 13(6):37-42, 1994.

Iannaccone ST and others: Prospective study of spinal muscular atrophy before age 6 years: DCN/SMA Group, *Pediatr Neurol* 9(3):187-193, 1993.

Jansen PW, Perkins RM, Ashwal S: Guillain-Barré syndrome in childhood: natural course and efficacy of plasma pheresis, *Pediatr Neurol* 9(1):16-20, 1993.

Khan MA: Corticosteroid therapy in Duchenne muscular dystrophy, *J Neurol Sci* 120(1):8-14, 1993.

McGhee B, Jarjour IT: Single-dose intravenous immune globulin for treatment of Guillain-Barré syndrome, *Am J Hosp Pharm* 51(1):97-99, 1994.

Mygrant BI and others: Infant botulism, *Heart Lung* 23(2):164-168, 1994.

Pentland B, Donald SM: Pain in the Guillain-Barré syndrome: a clinical review, *Pain* 59(2):159-164, 1994.

Rantala H and others: Epidemiology of Guillain-Barré syndrome in children: relationship of oral polio vaccine administration to occurrence, *J Pediatr* 124(2):220-223, 1994.

Vallee L and others: Intravenous immune globulin is also an efficient therapy of acute Guillain-Barré syndrome in affected children, *Neuropediatrics* 24(4):235-236, 1993.

Wise EJ: Preventing complications in infant botulism, *DCCN* 14(2):86-91, 1995.

Spinal Cord Injury

Ditunno JF, Formal CS: Current concepts: chronic spinal cord injury, *N Engl J Med* 330(8):550-556, 1994.

Joy C: Pediatric spinal cord injury, *Crit Care Nurs Clin North Am* 2(3):415-419, 1990.

Lang SM, Bernardo LM: SCIWORA syndrome: nursing assessment . . . spinal cord injury without radiographic abnormality, *Dimens Crit Care Nurs* 12(5):247-254, 1993.

Mulcahey MJ and others: Outcomes of tendon transfer surgery and occupational therapy in a child with tetraplegia, *Am J Occup Ther* 49(7):607-617, 1995.

Rathbone D and others: Spinal cord concussion in pediatric athletes, *J Pediatr Orthop* 12:616-620, 1992.

Wineman NM, Durand EJ, Steiner R: A comparative analysis of coping behaviors in persons with multiple sclerosis or a spinal cord injury, *Res Nurs Health* 17(3):185-194, 1994.

Yoshimura O and others: Spinal cord injury in a child: a long term follow-up study. Case report, *Paraplegia* 33(6):362-363, 1995.

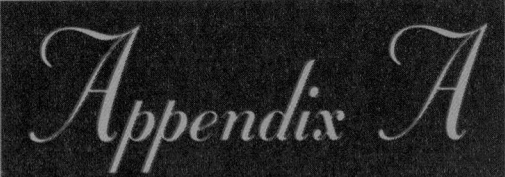

Family APGAR questionnaire

PART I

The following questions have been designed to help us better understand you and your family. You should feel free to ask questions about any item in the questionnaire.

The space for comments should be used when you wish to give additional information or if you wish to discuss the way the question is applied to your family. Please try to answer all questions.

Family is defined as the individual(s) with whom you usually live. If you live alone, your "family" consists of persons with whom you now have the strongest emotional ties.*

For each question, check only one box

	Almost always	Some of the time	Hardly ever
I am satisfied that I can turn to my family for help when something is troubling me. Comments: _____	☐	☐	☐
I am satisfied with the way my family talks over things with me and shares problems with me. Comments: _____	☐	☐	☐
I am satisfied that my family accepts and supports my wishes to take on new activities or directions. Comments: _____	☐	☐	☐
I am satisfied with the way my family expresses affection and responds to my emotions, such as anger, sorrow, and love. Comments: _____	☐	☐	☐
I am satisfied with the way my family and I share time together. Comments:	☐	☐	☐

A

*According to which member of the family is being interviewed the interviewer may substitute for the word "family" either spouse, significant other, parents, or children.

FIG. A-1. Family APGAR questionnaire; may be photocopied for clinical use. **A,** Part I. (Modified from Smilkstein G: The Family APGAR: a proposal for a family function test and its use by physicians, *J Fam Pract* 6(6):1231-1239, 1978.)

Family APGAR questionnaire

PART II

Who lives in your home?* List by relationship (e.g., spouse, significant other,†child, or friend).

Please check below the column that best describes how you now get along with each member of the family listed.

Relationship	Age	Sex	Well	Fairly	Poorly
_____	—	—	☐	☐	☐
_____	—	—	☐	☐	☐
_____	—	—	☐	☐	☐
_____	—	—	☐	☐	☐
_____	—	—	☐	☐	☐
_____	—	—	☐	☐	☐

If you don't live with your own family, please list below the individuals to whom you turn for help most frequently. List by relationship, (e.g., family member, friend, associate at work, or neighbor).

Please check below the column that best describes how you now get along with each person listed.

Relationship	Age	Sex	Well	Fairly	Poorly
_____	—	—	☐	☐	☐
_____	—	—	☐	☐	☐
_____	—	—	☐	☐	☐
_____	—	—	☐	☐	☐
_____	—	—	☐	☐	☐

*If you have established your own family, consider home to be the place where you live with your spouse, children, or significant other; otherwise, consider home as your place of origin, e.g., the place where your parents or those who raise you live.
†"Significant other" is the partner you live with in a physically and emotionally nurturing relationship, but to whom you are not married.

B

FIG. A-1, cont'd. B, Part II.

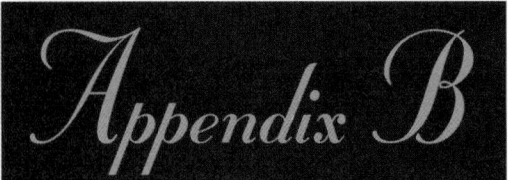

Patterns of Inheritance

GLOSSARY

congenital The condition is present at birth. The disorder may be brought about by genetic causes, nongenetic causes, or a combination of these.

familial A disorder that "runs in families" or is present in more members of a family than would be expected by chance.

genetic The disorder is caused by a single harmful gene, by several genes, or by a deviation in chromosome number or structure. It may or may not be apparent at birth.

genotype The genetic constitution that determines the physical and chemical characteristics of an individual.

heterozygous Having dissimilar genes at a given position (locus) on a pair of chromosomes.

homozygous Having the same genes at a given position (locus) on a pair of chromosomes.

inherited (heritable, hereditary) Synonymous with genetic, although in the past often used to describe a disorder that appeared in parent and offspring over several generations.

mutation Structural or chemical alteration in genetic material that, when changed, remains changed and is transmitted to future generations. Mutations usually occur naturally *(spontaneous)*, or can be *induced* by a variety of external agents, or *mutagens*, including temperature, certain chemicals, and radiation.

phenotype The physical or chemical characteristics of an individual, produced by the interaction of the environment with the genotype.

MODIFICATIONS OF BASIC INHERITANCE PATTERNS

heterogeneity The same or similar manifestations that result from (1) different mutant genes at the same location on a chromosome or (2) mutant genes at different locations on a chromosome (such as the hemophilias, which produce defects in coagulation, and the muscular dystrophies, which produce muscular weakness), but that exhibit different inheritance patterns.

linkage Some genes are located too close together on a chromosome, so they segregate and migrate together during cell division; therefore, the characteristics they produce always appear together in the phenotype.

penetrance The regularity with which an inherited trait is manifested in the person who carries the gene. When a gene produces its effect on the phenotype each time it is present in the genotype, it is said to be *fully penetrant* or to exhibit *complete penetrance*. For example, achondroplasia (a form of dwarfism) is always evident whenever the gene is present. If a trait is not recognized in a person who carries the responsible gene, it is said to be *nonpenetrant* in that individual. This phenomenon accounts for what appears to be skipped generations.

pleiotropy The multiple, different, and seemingly unrelated effects associated with a particular disorder; the varied clinical features that constitute a syndrome. For example, Marfan syndrome, a disorder of the elastic fibers of connective tissue, may be manifested in an individual by any or all of the symptoms associated with it—aortic aneurysm, dislocation of the optic lens, or any of a number of skeletal deformities.

variable expressivity The degree of severity of, or the variability in, the manifestations seen in persons of a particular genotype. For instance, polydactyly can be expressed as any number of extra digits, or the extra digits may be fingers in one generation and toes in another. The severity of a disorder may be so mild as to be almost undetected or so severe that the affected individual is totally incapacitated.

Autosomal Dominant Inheritance

Characteristics of a condition caused by a dominant gene on an autosome include the following (Fig. B-1):

1. Males and females are affected with equal frequency.
2. Affected individuals have an affected parent (unless the condition is caused by a fresh mutation).
3. Half the children of a heterozygous affected parent will possess the defective gene, although it may be nonpenetrant.
4. Unaffected children of affected parents will have unaffected children (unless the gene is nonpenetrant).

		Affected parent	
	Gametes	A	a
Normal parent	a	A a Affected	a a Normal
	a	A a Affected	a a Normal

FIG. B-1. Possible offspring of mating between normal parent, aa, and parent with an autosomal-dominant trait, Aa.

Autosomal Recessive Inheritance

Characteristics of a condition caused by a recessive gene on an autosome include the following (Fig. B-2):

1. Males and females are affected with equal frequency.
2. Affected individuals have unaffected parents who are heterozygous for the trait.
3. There is a one in four chance that any child of two unaffected heterozygous parents will be affected.
4. Two affected parents will have affected children exclusively.
5. Affected individuals married to unaffected individuals will have normal children, all of whom will be carriers.
6. There is usually no evidence of the trait in previous generations—a negative family history.

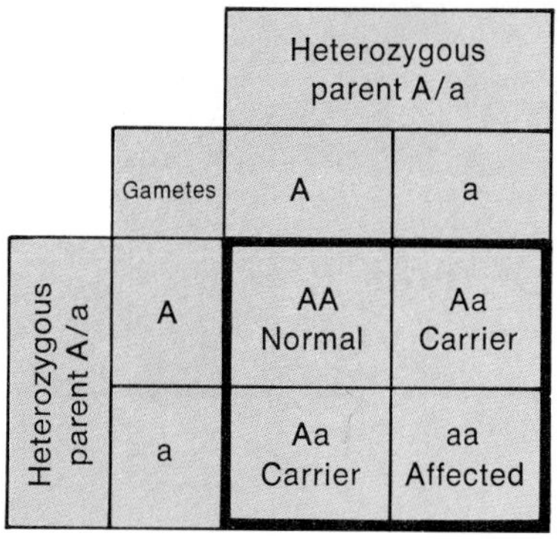

FIG. B-2. Possible offspring of mating between two parents with a recessive gene, a, on an autosome.

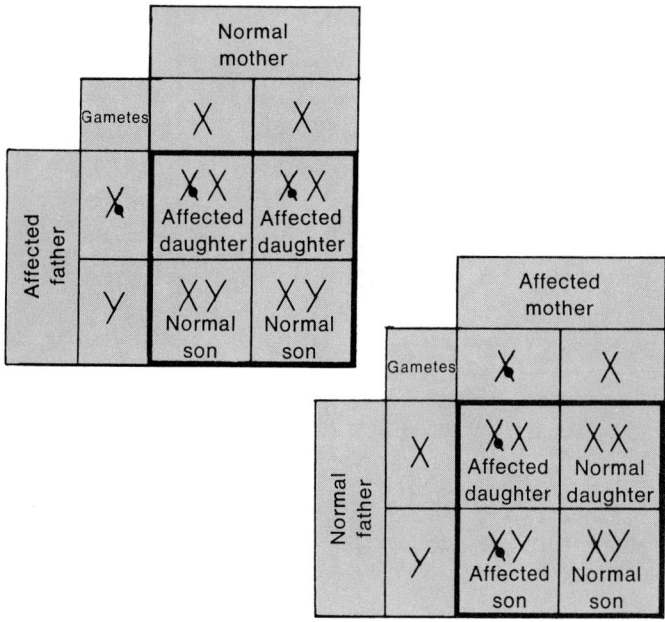

FIG. B-3. Sex differences in offspring ratios in X-linked dominant inheritance. ● = Dominant allele on X chromosome.

X-Linked Dominant Inheritance

Characteristics of a condition caused by a dominant gene on an X chromosome include the following (Fig. B-3):

1. Affected individuals have an affected parent.
2. All the daughters but none of the sons of an affected male will be affected.
3. Half the sons and half the daughters of an affected female will be affected.
4. Normal children of an affected parent will have normal offspring.
5. There are no carriers.
6. The inheritance pattern shows a positive family history.

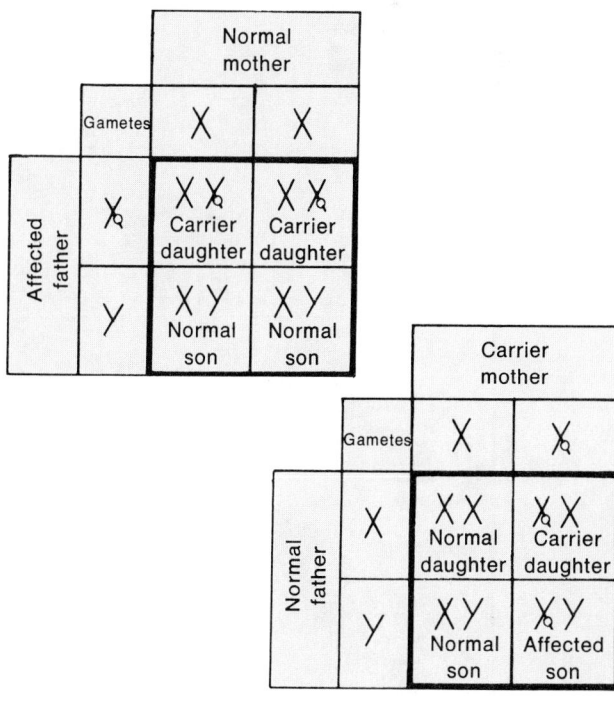

FIG. B-4. Differences in offspring ratios in X-linked recessive inheritance. ○ = Recessive allele on X chromosome.

X-Linked Recessive Inheritance

Characteristics of a disorder caused by a recessive gene on the X chromosome include the following (Fig. B-4):

1. Affected individuals are principally males.
2. Affected individuals have unaffected parents (except in the rare possibility that the father is affected and the mother is a carrier).
3. Half of the female siblings of an affected male will be carriers of the trait.
4. Unaffected male siblings of an affected male cannot transmit the disorder.
5. Sons of an affected male are unaffected.
6. Daughters of an affected male are carriers.
7. The unaffected male children of a carrier female do not transmit the disorder.

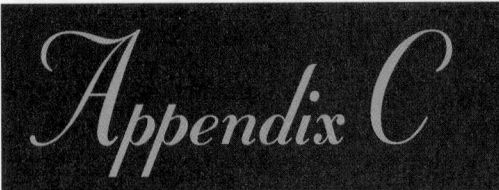

Developmental/Sensory Assessment

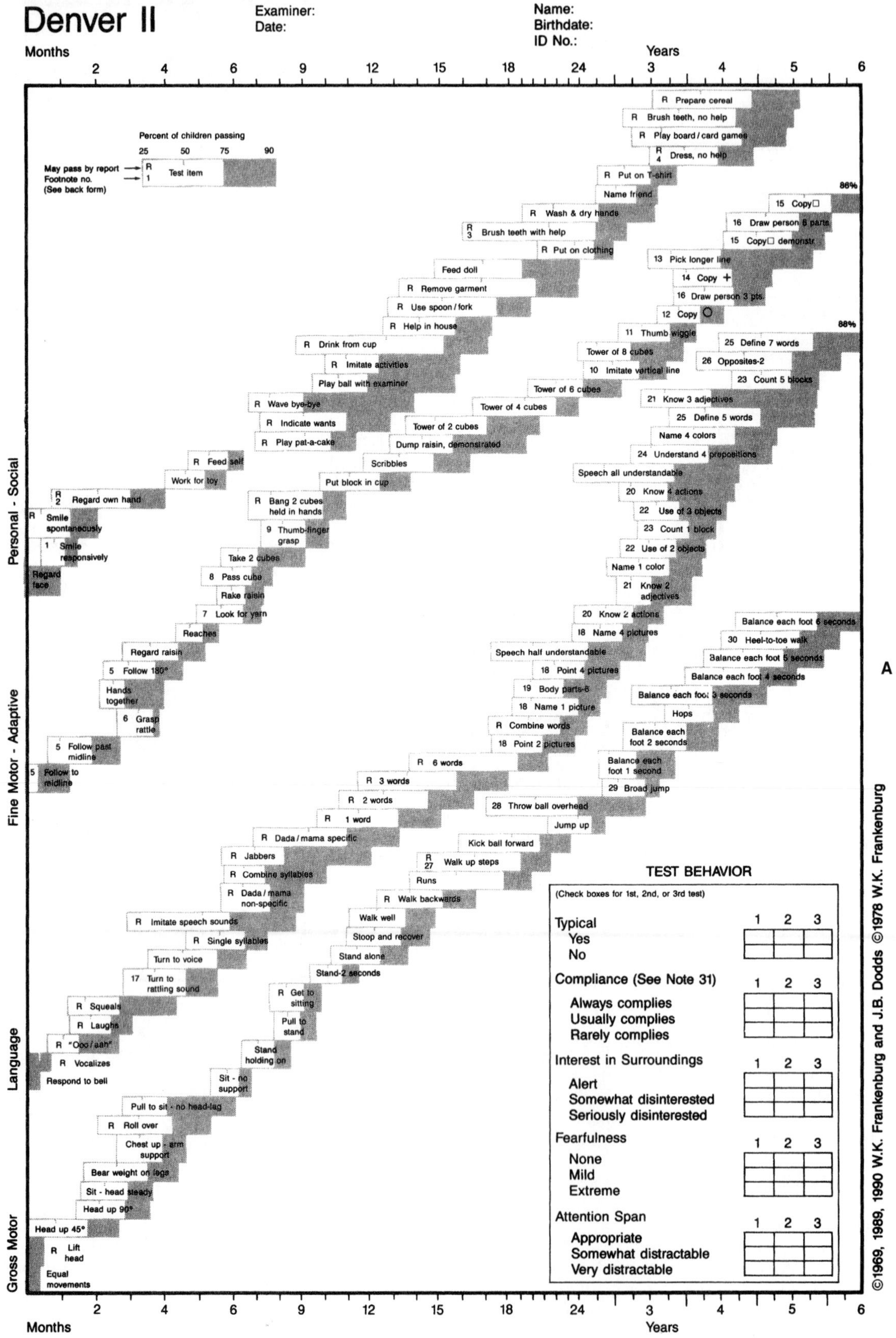

Denver II

Examiner:
Date:

Name:
Birthdate:
ID No.:

Months 2 · 4 · 6 · 9 · 12 · 15 · 18 · 24 | Years 3 · 4 · 5 · 6

Percent of children passing
25 50 75 90

May pass by report →
Footnote no. →
(See back form)

R — Test item
1

Personal - Social
- Equal movements
- Regard face
- Smile responsively
- Smile spontaneously
- R Regard own hand
- Work for toy
- R Feed self
- R Wave bye-bye
- R Indicate wants
- R Play pat-a-cake
- R Drink from cup
- R Imitate activities
- Play ball with examiner
- Feed doll
- R Remove garment
- R Use spoon / fork
- R Help in house
- R Wash & dry hands
- R Brush teeth with help
- R Put on clothing
- R Put on T-shirt
- Name friend
- R Prepare cereal
- R Brush teeth, no help
- R Play board / card games
- R Dress, no help

Fine Motor - Adaptive
- Follow to midline
- Follow past midline
- Hands together
- Follow 180°
- Regard raisin
- Reaches
- Look for yarn
- Rake raisin
- Pass cube
- Take 2 cubes
- 6 Grasp rattle
- 9 Thumb-finger grasp
- R Bang 2 cubes held in hands
- Put block in cup
- Scribbles
- Dump raisin, demonstrated
- Tower of 2 cubes
- Tower of 4 cubes
- Tower of 6 cubes
- Imitate vertical line
- Tower of 8 cubes
- Thumb wiggle
- 12 Copy ○
- 16 Draw person 3 pts.
- 14 Copy +
- 13 Pick longer line
- 15 Copy ○ demonstr.
- 16 Draw person 6 parts
- 15 Copy □

Language
- Respond to bell
- R Vocalizes
- R "Ooo / aah"
- R Laughs
- R Squeals
- 17 Turn to rattling sound
- Turn to voice
- R Single syllables
- R Imitate speech sounds
- R Dada / mama non-specific
- R Combine syllables
- R Jabbers
- R Dada / mama specific
- R 1 word
- R 2 words
- R 3 words
- R 6 words
- R Combine words
- 18 Point 2 pictures
- 18 Name 1 picture
- 19 Body parts-6
- 18 Point 4 pictures
- Speech half understandable
- 18 Name 4 pictures
- 20 Know 2 actions
- 21 Know 2 adjectives
- Name 1 color
- 22 Use of 2 objects
- 23 Count 1 block
- 22 Use of 3 objects
- 20 Know 4 actions
- Speech all understandable
- 24 Understand 4 prepositions
- Name 4 colors
- 25 Define 5 words
- 21 Know 3 adjectives
- 23 Count 5 blocks
- 26 Opposites-2
- 25 Define 7 words

Gross Motor
- Lift head
- Head up 45°
- Head up 90°
- Sit - head steady
- Bear weight on legs
- Chest up - arm support
- R Roll over
- Pull to sit - no head lag
- Stand holding on
- Pull to stand
- R Get to sitting
- Stand-2 seconds
- Stand alone
- Stoop and recover
- Walk well
- Walk backwards
- R Dada / mama non-specific
- Runs
- R 27 Walk up steps
- Kick ball forward
- Jump up
- 28 Throw ball overhead
- 29 Broad jump
- Balance each foot 1 second
- Balance each foot 2 seconds
- Hops
- Balance each foot 3 seconds
- Balance each foot 4 seconds
- Balance each foot 5 seconds
- 30 Heel-to-toe walk
- Balance each foot 6 seconds

86%

88%

TEST BEHAVIOR
(Check boxes for 1st, 2nd, or 3rd test)

	1	2	3
Typical			
Yes			
No			

Compliance (See Note 31)	1	2	3
Always complies			
Usually complies			
Rarely complies			

Interest in Surroundings	1	2	3
Alert			
Somewhat disinterested			
Seriously disinterested			

Fearfulness	1	2	3
None			
Mild			
Extreme			

Attention Span	1	2	3
Appropriate			
Somewhat distractable			
Very distractable			

A

FIG. C-1. A, Denver II. (From Frankenburg WK, Dodds JB, 1990.)

DIRECTIONS FOR ADMINISTRATION

1. Try to get child to smile by smiling, talking or waving. Do not touch him/her.
2. Child must stare at hand several seconds.
3. Parent may help guide toothbrush and put toothpaste on brush.
4. Child does not have to be able to tie shoes or button/zip in the back.
5. Move yarn slowly in an arc from one side to the other, about 8" above child's face.
6. Pass if child grasps rattle when it is touched to the backs or tips of fingers.
7. Pass if child tries to see where yarn went. Yarn should be dropped quickly from sight from tester's hand without arm movement.
8. Child must transfer cube from hand to hand without help of body, mouth, or table.
9. Pass if child picks up raisin with any part of thumb and finger.
10. Line can vary only 30 degrees or less from tester's line.
11. Make a fist with thumb pointing upward and wiggle only the thumb. Pass if child imitates and does not move any fingers other than the thumb.

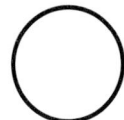   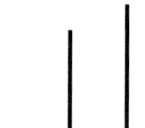   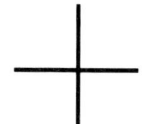   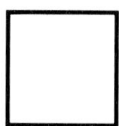

12. Pass any enclosed form. Fail continuous round motions.
13. Which line is longer? (Not bigger.) Turn paper upside down and repeat. (pass 3 of 3 or 5 of 6)
14. Pass any lines crossing near midpoint.
15. Have child copy first. If failed, demonstrate.

When giving items 12, 14, and 15, do not name the forms. Do not demonstrate 12 and 14.

16. When scoring, each pair (2 arms, 2 legs, etc.) counts as one part.
17. Place one cube in cup and shake gently near child's ear, but out of sight. Repeat for other ear.
18. Point to picture and have child name it. (No credit is given for sounds only.)
   If less than 4 pictures are named correctly, have child point to picture as each is named by tester.

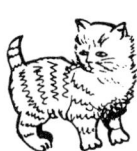   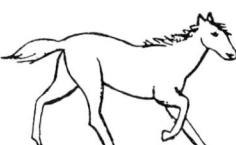   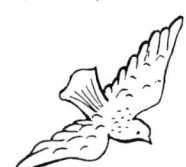   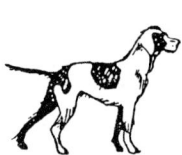   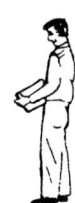

19. Using doll, tell child: Show me the nose, eyes, ears, mouth, hands, feet, tummy, hair. Pass 6 of 8.
20. Using pictures, ask child: Which one flies?... says meow?... talks?... barks?... gallops? Pass 2 of 5, 4 of 5.
21. Ask child: What do you do when you are cold?... tired?... hungry? Pass 2 of 3, 3 of 3.
22. Ask child: What do you do with a cup? What is a chair used for? What is a pencil used for?
   Action words must be included in answers.
23. Pass if child correctly places <u>and</u> says how many blocks are on paper. (1, 5).
24. Tell child: Put block **on** table; **under** table; **in front of** me, **behind** me. Pass 4 of 4.
   (Do not help child by pointing, moving head or eyes.)
25. Ask child: What is a ball?... lake?... desk?... house?... banana?... curtain?... fence?... ceiling? Pass if defined in terms of use, shape, what it is made of, or general category (such as banana is fruit, not just yellow). Pass 5 of 8, 7 of 8.
26. Ask child: If a horse is big, a mouse is __? If fire is hot, ice is __? If the sun shines during the day, the moon shines during the __? Pass 2 of 3.
27. Child may use wall or rail only, not person. May not crawl.
28. Child must throw ball overhand 3 feet to within arm's reach of tester.
29. Child must perform standing broad jump over width of test sheet (8 1/2 inches).
30. Tell child to walk forward, ∞∞∞➤ heel within 1 inch of toe. Tester may demonstrate.
   Child must walk 4 consecutive steps.
31. In the second year, half of normal children are non-compliant.

OBSERVATIONS:

FIG. C-1, cont'd. **B,** Directions for administration of numbered items on Denver II. (From Frankenburg WK, Dodds JB, 1990.)

```
┌─────────────────────────────────────────────────┐
│        DENVER ARTICULATION SCREENING EXAM        │   Name:
│        for children 2½ to 6 years of age         │
│                                                   │   Hosp. No.:
│   Instructions:  Have child repeat each word after│
│   you.  Circle the underlined sounds that he pro- │   Address:_____
│   nounces correctly.  Total correct sounds is the │
│   Raw Score.  Use charts on reverse side to score │           _____
│   results.                                        │
└─────────────────────────────────────────────────┘
```

Date: _____   Child's age: _____   Examiner: _____   Raw score: ____
Percentile: _____   Intelligibility: _____   Result: _____

1. table   6. zipper   11. sock   16. wagon   21. leaf
2. shirt   7. grapes   12. vacuum   17. gum   22. carrot
3. door   8. flag   13. yarn   18. house
4. trunk   9. thumb   14. mother   19. pencil
5. jumping   10. toothbrush 15. twinkle   20. fish

Intelligibility: (circle one)
        1. Easy to understand   3. Not understandable
        2. Understandable ½ the time   4. Can't evaluate

Comments:

Date: _____   Child's age: _____   Examiner: _____   Raw score: ____
Percentile: _____   Intelligibility: _____   Result: _____

1. table   6. zipper   11. sock   16. wagon   21. leaf
2. shirt   7. grapes   12. vacuum   17. gum   22. carrot
3. door   8. flag   13. yarn   18. house
4. trunk   9. thumb   14. mother   19. pencil
5. jumping   10. toothbrush 15. twinkle   20. fish

Intelligibility: (circle one)
        1. Easy to understand   3. Not understandable
        2. Understandable ½ the time   4. Can't evaluate

Comments:

A

Date: _____   Child's age: _____   Examiner: _____   Raw score ____
Percentile: _____   Intelligibility: _____   Result: _____

1. table   6. zipper   11. sock   16. wagon   21. leaf
2. shirt   7. grapes   12. vacuum   17. gum   22. carrot
3. door   8. flag   13. yarn   18. house
4. trunk   9. thumb   14. mother   19. pencil
5. jumping   10. toothbrush 15. twinkle   20. fish

Intelligibility: (circle one)
        1. Easy to understand   3. Not understandable
        2. Understandable ½ the time   4. Can't evaluate

FIG. C-2. A, Denver Articulation Screening examination for children 2½ to 6 years of age. (Modified from Drumwright AF, University of Colorado Medical Center, 1971.)

To score DASE words: Note raw score for child's performance. Match raw score line (extreme left of chart) with column representing child's age (to the closest previous age group). Where raw score line and age column meet number in that square denotes percentile rank of child's performance when compared to other children that age. Percentiles above heavy line are ABNORMAL percentiles, below heavy line are NORMAL.

PERCENTILE RANK

Raw Score	2.5 yr.	3.0	3.5	4.0	4.5	5.0	5.5	6 years
2	1							
3	2							
4	5							
5	9							
6	16							
7	23							
8	31	2						
9	37	4	1					
10	42	6	2					
11	48	7	4					
12	54	9	6	1	1			
13	58	12	9	2	3	1	1	
14	62	17	11	5	4	2	2	
15	68	23	15	9	5	3	2	
16	75	31	19	12	5	4	3	
17	79	38	25	15	6	6	4	
18	83	46	31	19	8	7	4	
19	86	51	38	24	10	9	5	1
20	89	58	45	30	12	11	7	3
21	92	65	52	36	15	15	9	4
22	94	72	58	43	18	19	12	5
23	96	77	63	50	22	24	15	7
24	97	82	70	58	29	29	20	15
25	99	87	78	66	36	34	26	17
26	99	91	84	75	46	43	34	24
27		94	89	82	57	54	44	34
28		96	94	88	70	68	59	47
29		98	98	94	84	84	77	68
30		100	100	100	100	100	100	100

B

To score intelligibility:

	NORMAL	ABNORMAL
2½ years	Understandable ½ the time, or, "easy"	Not understandable
3 years and older	Easy to understand	Understandable ½ time Not understandable

Test result: 1. NORMAL on Dase and Intelligibility = NORMAL

2. ABNORMAL on Dase and/or Intelligibility = ABNORMAL

*If abnormal on initial screening, rescreen within 2 weeks.
If abnormal again, child should be referred for complete speech evaluation.

FIG. C-2, cont'd. B, Percentile rank. (From Drumwright AF, University of Colorado Medical Center, 1971.)

DENVER EYE SCREENING TEST

Name:
Hospital No.:
Ward:
Address:

Vision Tests

Vision Tests	1st Screening: Date: Right Eye Normal	Abnormal	Untestable	Left Eye Normal	Abnormal	Untestable	Rescreening: Date: Right Eye Normal	Abnormal	Untestable	Left Eye Normal	Abnormal	Untestable
1. "E" (3 years and above—3 to 5 trials)	3P	3F	U	3P	3F	U	3P	3F	U	3P	3F	U
2. Picture card (2 1/2 – 2 11/12 yrs.—3 to 5 trials)	3P	3F	U	3P	3F	U	3P	3F	U	3P	3F	U
3. Fixation (6 months – 2 5/12 years)	P	F	U	P	F	U	P	F	U	P	F	U
4. Squinting		yes			yes			yes			yes	

Tests for Non-Straight Eyes

Tests for Non-Straight Eyes	1st Screening Normal	Abnormal	Untestable	Rescreening Normal	Abnormal	Untestable
1. Do your child's eyes turn in or out, or are they ever not straight?	NO	YES	U	NO	YES	U
2. Cover Test	P	F	U	P	F	U
3. Pupillary Light Reflex	P	F	U	P	F	U

Total Test Rating (Both Eyes)

Normal (passed vision test plus no squint, plus passed 2/3 tests for non-straight eyes) .... Normal .... Normal

Abnormal (abnormal on any vision test, squinting or 2 of 3 procedures for non-straight eyes) .... Abnormal .... Abnormal

Untestable (untestable on any vision test or untestable on 2/3 tests for non-straight eyes) .... Untestable .... Untestable

Future Rescreening Appointment for Total Test Rating (Abnormal or Untestable) .... Date: .... Date:

FIG. C-3. Denver Eye Screening Test. (From Frankenburg WK, Dobbs JB, University of Colorado Medical Center, 1969.)

SNELLEN SCREENING*
Preparation

1. Hang the Snellen chart on a light-colored wall so that the 20- to 30-foot lines are at eye level when children 6 to 12 years old are tested in the standing position.
2. Secure the chart to the wall with double-stick tape on the back side of all four corners. If the chart must be reversed for use of the letter or E chart, secure it at the top and bottom with tacks. Make sure that the chart does not swing when in place.
3. The illumination intensity on the chart should be 10 to 30 foot candles, without any glare from windows or light fixtures. The illumination should be checked with a light meter.
4. Mark an exact 20-foot distance from the chart. Mark the floor with a piece of tape or "footprints" positioned so that the heels touch the 20-foot line.

Procedure

1. Place child at the 20-foot mark, with the heel edging the line if child is standing or with the back of the chair placed at the marker if child is seated.
2. If the E chart is used, accustom child to identifying which direction the "legs of the E" are pointing. Use a demonstration E card for this purpose.
3. Teach child to use the occluder to cover one eye. Instruct child to keep both eyes open during the test. Provide a clean cover card for each child and then discard after use.
4. If child wears glasses, test only with glasses on.
5. Test both eyes together, then right eye, then left eye.

*Modified from recommendations of the National Society to Prevent Blindness: *Guide to testing distance visual acuity.* Schaumburg, IL, 1988, The Society.

6. Begin with the 40- or 30-foot line and proceed with test to include the 20-foot line.
7. With child suspected of low vision, begin with the 200-foot line, and proceed until child can no longer correctly read three out of four or four out of six symbols on a line.
8. Use covers on the Snellen chart to expose only one symbol or one line at a time. When screening kindergarten or older children, expose one line but may use a pointer to point to one symbol at a time.

Recording and Referral

1. Record the last line the child read correctly (three out of four or four out of six symbols).
2. Record visual acuity as a fraction. The numerator represents the distance from the chart, and the denominator represents the last line read correctly. For example, 20/30 means that the child read the 30-foot line at a 20-foot distance.
3. Observe the child's eyes during testing and record any evidence of squinting, head tilting, thrusting the head forward, excessive blinking, tearing, or redness.
4. Only make referrals after a second screening has been made on children who are potential candidates for referral.
5. The following children should be referred for a complete eye examination:
   a. Three-year-old children with vision in either eye of 20/50 or less (inability to correctly identify one more than half the symbols on the 40-foot line) *or* a two-line difference in visual acuity between the eyes in the passing range (e.g., 20/20 in one eye and 20/40 in the other)
   b. All other ages and grades with vision in either eye of 20/40 or less (inability to correctly identify one more than half the symbols on the 30-foot line)
   c. All children who consistently show any of the signs of possible visual disturbances, regardless of visual acuity

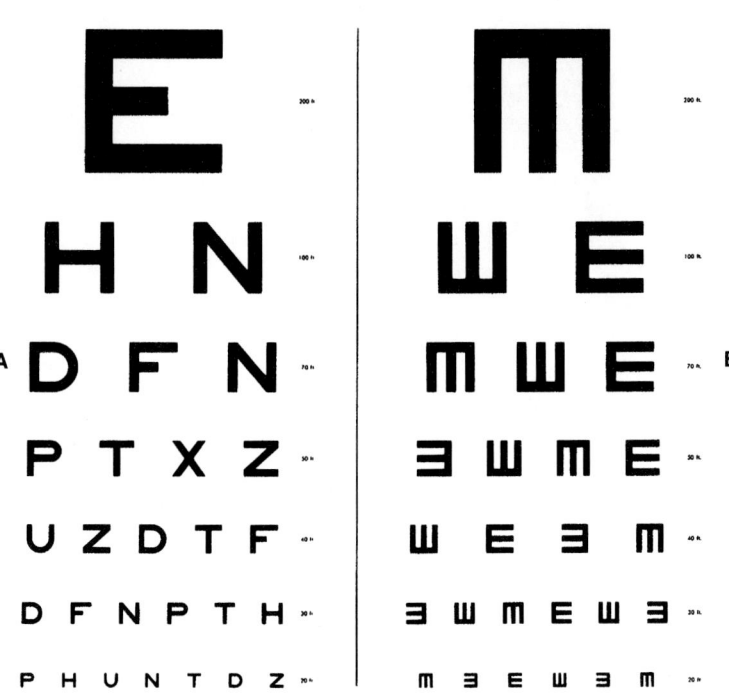

FIG. C-4. Snellen chart. **A,** Letter (alphabet) chart. **B,** Symbol E chart. (From National Society to Prevent Blindness, Schaumburg, IL.)

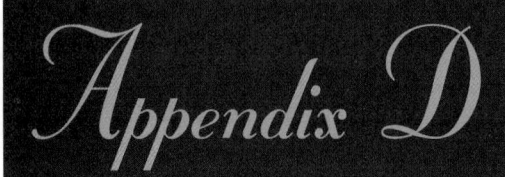

Appendix D Growth Measurements

HEIGHT AND WEIGHT MEASUREMENTS FOR BOYS

	HEIGHT BY PERCENTILES						WEIGHT BY PERCENTILES					
	5		50		95		5		50		95	
AGE*	cm	inches	cm	inches	cm	inches	kg	lb	kg	lb	kg	lb
Birth	46.4	18¼	50.5	20	54.4	21½	2.54	5½	3.27	7¼	4.15	9¼
3 months	56.7	22¼	61.1	24	65.4	25¾	4.43	9¾	5.98	13¼	7.37	16¼
6 months	63.4	25	67.8	26¾	72.3	28½	6.20	13¾	7.85	17¼	9.46	20¾
9 months	68.0	26¾	72.3	28½	77.1	30¼	7.52	16½	9.18	20¼	10.93	24
1	71.7	28¼	76.1	30	81.2	32	8.43	18½	10.15	22½	11.99	26½
1½	77.5	30½	82.4	32½	88.1	34¾	9.59	21¼	11.47	25¼	13.44	29½
2†	82.5	32½	86.8	34¼	94.4	37¼	10.49	23¼	12.34	27¼	15.50	34¼
2½†	85.4	33½	90.4	35½	97.8	38½	11.27	24¾	13.52	29¾	16.61	36½
3	89.0	35	94.9	37¼	102.0	40¼	12.05	26½	14.62	32¼	17.77	39¼
3½	92.5	36½	99.1	39	106.1	41¾	12.84	28¼	15.68	34½	18.98	41¾
4	95.8	37¾	102.9	40½	109.9	43¼	13.64	30	16.69	36¾	20.27	44¾
4½	98.9	39	106.6	42	113.5	44¾	14.45	31¾	17.69	39	21.63	47¾
5	102.0	40¼	109.9	43¼	117.0	46	15.27	33¾	18.67	41¼	23.09	51
6	107.7	42½	116.1	45¾	123.5	48½	16.93	37¼	20.69	45½	26.34	58
7	113.0	44½	121.7	48	129.7	51	18.64	41	22.85	50¼	30.12	66½
8	118.1	46½	127.0	50	135.7	53½	20.40	45	25.30	55¾	34.51	76
9	122.9	48½	132.2	52	141.8	55¾	22.25	49	28.13	62	39.58	87¼
10	127.7	50¼	137.5	54¼	148.1	58¼	24.33	53¾	31.44	69¼	45.27	99¾
11	132.6	52¼	143.3	56½	154.9	61	26.80	59	35.30	77¾	51.47	113½
12	137.6	54¼	149.7	59	162.3	64	29.85	65¾	39.78	87¾	58.09	128
13	142.9	56¼	156.5	61½	169.8	66¾	33.64	74¼	44.95	99	65.02	143¼
14	148.8	58½	163.1	64¼	176.7	69½	38.22	84¼	50.77	112	72.13	159
15	155.2	61	169.0	66½	181.9	71½	43.11	95	56.71	125	79.12	174½
16	161.1	63½	173.5	68¼	185.4	73	47.74	105¼	62.10	137	85.62	188¾
17	164.9	65	176.2	69¼	187.3	73¾	51.50	113½	66.31	146¼	91.31	201¼
18	165.7	65¼	176.8	69½	187.6	73¾	53.97	119	68.88	151¾	95.76	211

Modified from National Center for Health Statistics (NCHS), Health Resources Administration, Department of Health, Education and Welfare, Hyattsville, MD. Conversion of metric data to approximate inches and pounds by Ross Laboratories, 1977.
*Years unless otherwise indicated
†Height data include some recumbent length measurements, which make values slightly higher than if all measurements had been of stature (standing height).

HEIGHT AND WEIGHT MEASUREMENTS FOR GIRLS

AGE*	HEIGHT BY PERCENTILES						WEIGHT BY PERCENTILES					
	5		50		95		5		50		95	
	cm	inches	cm	inches	cm	inches	kg	lb	kg	lb	kg	lb
Birth	45.4	17¾	49.9	19¾	52.9	20¾	2.36	5¼	3.23	7	3.81	8½
3 months	55.4	21¾	59.5	23½	63.4	25	4.18	9¼	5.4	12	6.74	14¾
6 months	61.8	24¼	65.9	26	70.2	27¾	5.79	12¾	7.21	16	8.73	19¼
9 months	66.1	26	70.4	27¾	75.0	29½	7.0	15½	8.56	18¾	10.17	22½
1	69.8	27½	74.3	29¼	79.1	31¼	7.84	17¼	9.53	21	11.24	24¾
1½	76.0	30	80.9	31¾	86.1	34	8.92	19¾	10.82	23¾	12.76	28¼
2†	81.6	32¼	86.8	34¼	93.6	36¾	9.95	22	11.8	26	14.15	31¼
2½†	84.6	33¼	90.0	35½	96.6	38	10.8	23¾	13.03	28¾	15.76	34¾
3	88.3	34¾	94.1	37	100.6	39½	11.61	25½	14.1	31	17.22	38
3½	91.7	36	97.9	38½	104.5	41¼	12.37	27¼	15.07	33¼	18.59	41
4	95.0	37½	101.6	40	108.3	42¾	13.11	29	15.96	35¼	19.91	44
4½	98.1	38½	105.0	41¼	112.0	44	13.83	30½	16.81	37	21.24	46¾
5	101.1	39¾	108.4	42¾	115.6	45½	14.55	32	17.66	39	22.62	49¾
6	106.6	42	114.6	45	122.7	48¼	16.05	35½	19.52	43	25.75	56¾
7	111.8	44	120.6	47½	129.5	51	17.71	39	21.84	48¼	29.68	65½
8	116.9	46	126.4	49¾	136.2	53½	19.62	43¼	24.84	54¾	34.71	76½
9	122.1	48	132.2	52	142.9	56¼	21.82	48	28.46	62¾	40.64	89½
10	127.5	50¼	138.3	54½	149.5	58¾	24.36	53¾	32.55	71¾	47.17	104
11	133.5	52½	144.8	57	156.2	61½	27.24	60	36.95	81½	54.0	119
12	139.8	55	151.5	59¾	162.7	64	30.52	67¼	41.53	91½	60.81	134
13	145.2	57¼	157.1	61¾	168.1	66¼	34.14	75¼	46.1	101¾	67.3	148¼
14	148.7	58½	160.4	63¼	171.3	67½	37.76	83¼	50.28	110¾	73.08	161
15	150.5	59¼	161.8	63¾	172.8	68	40.99	90¼	53.68	118¼	77.78	171½
16	151.6	59¾	162.4	64	173.3	68¼	43.41	95¾	55.89	123¼	80.99	178½
17	152.7	60	163.1	64¼	173.5	68¼	44.74	98¾	56.69	125	82.46	181¾
18	153.6	60½	163.7	64½	173.6	68¼	45.26	99¾	56.62	124¾	82.47	181¾

Modified from National Center for Health Statistics, Health Resources Administration, Department of Health, Education and Welfare, Hyattsville, MD, 1977. Conversion of metric data to approximate inches and pounds by Ross Laboratories.
*Years unless otherwise indicated.
†Height data include some recumbent length measurements, which make values slightly higher than if all measurements had been of stature.

GROWTH STANDARDS OF HEALTHY CHINESE CHILDREN

AGE (MONTHS OR YEARS)	WEIGHT (kg)		HEIGHT (cm)		HEAD CIRCUMFERENCE	
	BOYS	GIRLS	BOYS	GIRLS	BOYS	GIRLS
Birth	3.27	3.17	50.6	50.0	34.3	33.7
1 month	4.97	4.64	56.5	55.5	38.1	37.3
2 months	5.95	5.49	59.6	58.4	39.7	38.7
3 months	6.73	6.23	62.3	60.9	41.0	40.0
4 months	7.32	6.69	64.4	62.9	42.0	41.0
5 months	7.70	7.19	65.9	64.5	42.9	41.9
6 months	8.22	7.62	68.1	66.7	43.9	42.8
8 months	8.71	8.14	70.6	69.0	44.9	43.7
10 months	9.14	8.57	72.9	71.4	45.7	44.5
12 months	9.56	9.04	75.6	74.1	46.3	45.2
15 months	10.15	9.54	78.3	76.9	46.8	45.6
18 months	10.67	10.08	80.7	79.4	47.3	46.2
21 months	11.18	10.56	83.0	81.7	47.8	46.7
24 months	11.95	11.37	86.5	85.3	48.2	47.1
2.5 years	12.84	12.28	90.4	89.3	48.8	47.7
3 years	13.63	13.16	93.8	92.8	49.1	48.1
3.5 years	14.45	14.00	97.2	96.3	49.4	48.5
4 years	15.26	14.89	100.8	100.1	49.7	48.9
4.5 years	16.07	15.63	103.9	103.1	50.0	49.1
5 years	16.88	16.46	107.2	106.5	50.2	49.4
5.5 years	17.65	17.18	110.1	109.2	50.5	49.6
6 years	19.25	18.67	114.7	113.9	50.8	50.0
7 years	21.01	20.35	120.6	119.3	51.1	50.2
8 years	23.08	22.43	125.3	124.6	51.4	50.6
9 years	25.33	24.57	130.6	129.5	51.7	50.9
10 years	27.15	27.05	134.4	134.8	51.9	51.3
11 years	30.13	30.51	139.2	140.6	52.3	51.7
12 years	33.05	34.74	144.2	146.6	52.7	52.3
13 years	36.90	38.52	149.8	150.7	53.0	52.8

Data from Bejing Children's Hospital, 1987, China.

HEAD CIRCUMFERENCE CHARTS

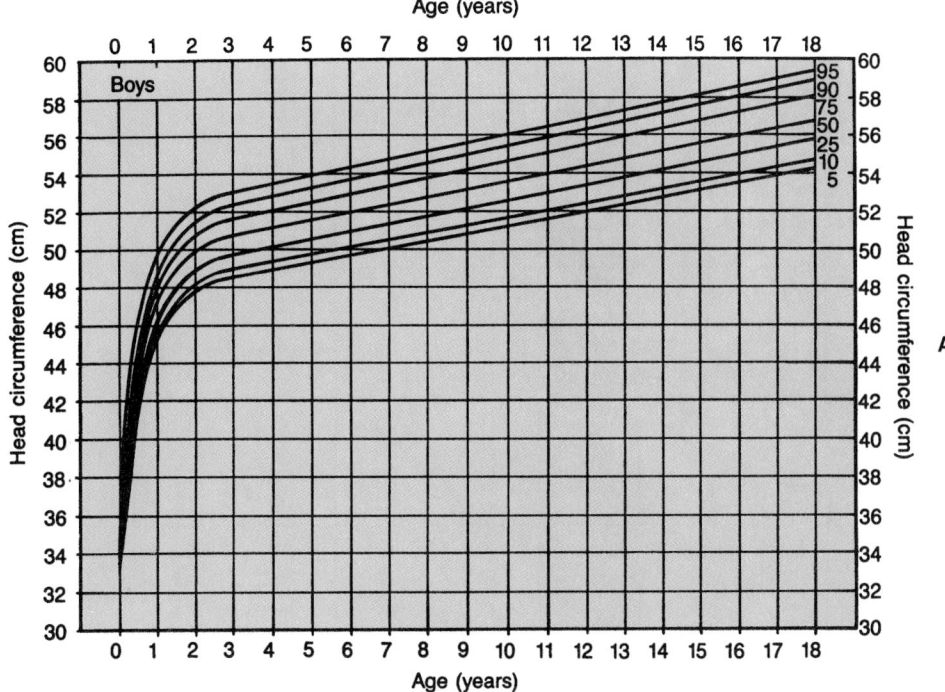

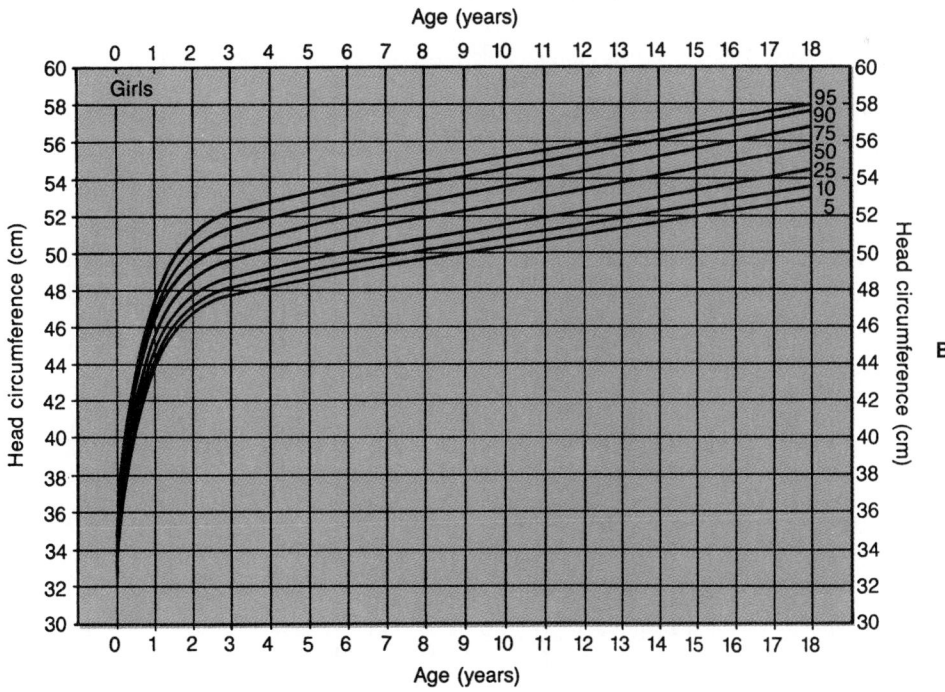

FIG. D-I. Selected percentiles for smoothed head circumference values of children from birth to 18 years. **A,** Boys. **B,** Girls. (From Roche AF and others: Head circumference reference data: birth to 18 years, Pediatrics 79(5):706-712, 1987.)

PERCENTILES FOR TRICEPS SKINFOLD

AGE-GROUP (YEARS)	TRICEPS SKINFOLD PERCENTILES (mm)									
	MALES					FEMALES				
	5	25	50	75	95	5	25	50	75	95
1-1.9	6	8	10	12	16	6	8	10	12	16
2-2.9	6	8	10	12	15	6	9	10	12	16
3-3.9	6	8	10	11	15	7	9	11	12	15
4-4.9	6	8	9	11	14	7	8	10	12	16
5-5.9	6	8	9	11	15	6	8	10	12	18
6-6.9	5	7	8	10	16	6	8	10	12	16
7-7.9	5	7	9	12	17	6	9	11	13	18
8-8.9	5	7	8	10	16	6	9	12	15	24
9-9.9	6	7	10	13	18	8	10	13	16	22
10-10.9	6	8	10	14	21	7	10	12	17	27
11-11.9	6	8	11	16	24	7	10	13	18	28
12-12.9	6	8	11	14	28	8	11	14	18	27
13-13.9	5	7	10	14	26	8	12	15	21	30
14-14.9	4	7	9	14	24	9	13	16	21	28
15-15.9	4	6	8	11	24	8	12	17	21	32
16-16.9	4	6	8	12	22	10	15	18	22	31
17-17.9	5	6	8	12	19	10	13	19	24	37
18-18.9	4	6	9	13	24	10	15	18	22	30
19-24.9	4	7	10	15	22	10	14	18	24	34

From Frisancho A: New norms of upper limb fat and muscle areas for assessment of nutritional status, *Am J Clin Nutr* 34:2540-2545, 1981.

PERCENTILES OF UPPER ARM CIRCUMFERENCE

AGE-GROUP (YEARS)	ARM CIRCUMFERENCE PERCENTILES (mm)									
	MALES					FEMALES				
	5	25	50	75	95	5	25	50	75	95
1-1.9	142	150	159	170	183	138	148	156	164	177
2-2.9	141	153	162	170	185	142	152	160	167	184
3-3.9	150	160	167	175	190	143	158	167	175	189
4-4.9	149	162	171	180	192	149	160	169	177	191
5-5.9	153	167	175	185	204	153	165	175	185	211
6-6.9	155	167	179	188	228	156	170	176	187	211
7-7.9	162	177	187	201	230	164	174	183	199	231
8-8.9	162	177	190	202	245	168	183	195	214	261
9-9.9	175	187	200	217	257	178	194	211	224	260
10-10.9	181	196	210	231	274	174	193	210	228	265
11-11.9	186	202	223	244	280	185	208	224	248	303
12-12.9	193	214	232	254	303	194	216	237	256	294
13-13.9	194	228	247	263	301	202	223	243	271	338
14-14.9	220	237	253	283	322	214	237	252	272	322
15-15.9	222	244	264	284	320	208	239	254	279	322
16-16.9	244	262	278	303	343	218	241	258	283	334
17-17.9	246	267	285	308	347	220	241	264	295	350
18-18.9	245	276	297	321	379	222	241	258	281	325
19-24.9	262	288	308	331	372	221	247	265	290	345

From Frisancho A: New norms of upper limb fat and muscle areas for assessment of nutritional status, *Am J Clin Nutr* 34:2540-2545, 1981.

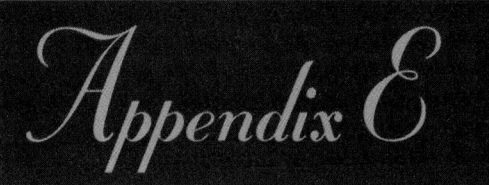

Common Laboratory Tests*

TEST/SPECIMEN	AGE/SEX/REFERENCE	CONVENTIONAL UNITS	INTERNATIONAL UNITS (SI)
		NORMAL RANGES	
Acetaminophen			
Serum or plasma	Therap. conc.	10-30 µg/ml	66-200 µmol/L
	Toxic Conc.	>200 µg/ml	>1300 µmol/L
Ammonia nitrogen			
Plasma or serum	Newborn	90-150 µg/dl	64-107 µmol/L
	0-2 wk	79-129 µg/dl	56-92 µmol/L
	>1 mo	29-70 µg/dl	21-50 µmol/L
	Thereafter	15-45 µg/dl	11-32 µmol/L
Urine, 24 hr		500-1200 mg/d	36-86 mmol/d
Antistreptolysin O titer (ASO)			
Serum	2-4 yr	<160 Todd units	
	School-age children	170-330 Todd units	
Base excess			
Whole blood	Newborn	(−10)-(−2) mEq/L	(−10)-(−2) mmol/L
	Infant	(−7)-(−1) mEq/L	(−7)-(−1) mmol/L
	Child	(−4)-(+2) mEq/L	(−4)-(+2) mmol/L
	Thereafter	(−3)-(+3) mEq/L	(−3)-(+3) mmol/L
Bicarbonate (HCO_3)			
Serum	Arterial	21-28 mEq/L	21-28 mmol/L
	Venous	22-29 mEq/L	22-29 mmol/L

		Premature (mg/dl)	Full term (mg/dl)	Premature (µmol/L)	Full term (µmol/L)
Bilirubin, total					
Serum	Cord	<2.0	<2.0	<34	<34
	0.1 d	8.0	<6.0	<137	<103
	1-2 d	12.0	<8.0	<205	<137
	2-5 d	16.0	<12.0	<274	<205
	Thereafter	2.0	0.2-1.0	<34	3.4-17.1

TEST/SPECIMEN	AGE/SEX/REFERENCE	CONVENTIONAL UNITS	INTERNATIONAL UNITS (SI)
Bilirubin, direct (conjugated)			
Serum		0.0-0.2 mg/dl	0-3.4 µmol/L
Bleeding time			
Blood from skin puncture			
Ivy	Normal	2-7 min	2-7 min
	Borderline	7-11 min	7-11 min
Simplate (G-D)		2.75-8 min	2.75-8 min
Blood volume			
Whole blood	Male	52-83 ml/kg	0.052-0.083 L/kg
	Female	50-75 ml/kg	0.050-0.075 L/kg

Modified from Behrman RE and others, editors: *Nelson textbook of pediatrics,* ed 14, Philadelphia, 1992, WB Saunders.
*For a description of abbreviations see p. 1209.

Continued.

COMMON LABORATORY TESTS—cont'd

TEST/SPECIMEN	AGE/SEX/REFERENCE	CONVENTIONAL UNITS	INTERNATIONAL UNITS (SI)
		NORMAL RANGES	
C-reactive protein (CRP)			
Serum	Cord	52-1330 ng/ml	52-1330 µg/L
	Adult	67-1800 ng/ml	67-1800 µg/L
Calcium, ionized			
Serum, plasma, or whole blood	Cord	50-60 mg/dl	1.25-1.50 mmol/L
	Newborn, 3-24 hr	4.3-5.1 mg/dl	1.07-1.27 mmol/L
	24-48 hr	4.0-4.7 mg/dl	1.00-1.17 mmol/L
	Thereafter	4.8-4.92 mg/dl or 2.24-2.46 mEq/L	1.12-1.23 mmol/L
Calcium, total			
Serum	Cord	9.0-11.5 mg/dl	2.25-2.88 mmol/L
	Newborn, 3-24 hr	9.0-10.6 mg/dl	2.3-2.65 mmol/L
	24-48 hr	7.0-12.0 mg/dl	1.75-3.0 mmol/L
	4-7 d	9.0-10.9 mg/dl	2.25-2.73 mmol/L
	Child	8.8-10.8 mg/dl	2.2-2.70 mmol/L
	Thereafter	8.4-10.2 mg/dl	2.1-2.55 mmol/L
Carbon dioxide, partial pressure (Pco_2)			
Whole blood, arterial	Newborn	27-40 mm Hg	3.6-5.3 kPa
	Infant	27-41 mm Hg	3.6-5.5 kPa
	Thereafter: Male	35-48 mm Hg	4.7-6.4 kPa
	Female	32-45 mm Hg	4.3-6.0 kPa
Carbon dioxide, total (tCO_2)			
Serum or plasma	Cord	14-22 mEq/L	14-22 mmol/L
	Premature (1 wk)	14-27 mEq/L	14-27 mmol/L
	Newborn	13-22 mEq/L	13-22 mmol/L
	Infant, child	20-28 mEq/L	20-28 mmol/L
	Thereafter	23-30 mEq/L	23-30 mmol/L
Cerebrospinal fluid (CSF)			
Pressure		70-180 mm water	70-180 mm water
Volume	Child	60-100 ml	0.06-0.10 L
	Adult	100-160 ml	0.1-0.16 L
Chloride			
Serum or plasma	Cord	96-104 mEq/L	96-104 mmol/L
	Newborn	97-110 mEq/L	97-110 mmol/L
	Thereafter	98-106 mEq/L	98-106 mmol/L
Sweat	Normal (homozygote)	<40 mEq/L	<40 mmol/L
	Marginal (e.g., asthma, Addison disease, malnutrition)	45-60 mEq/L	45-60 mmol/L
	Cystic fibrosis	>60 mmol/L	>60 mmol/L
Cholesterol, total			
Serum or plasma*	Acceptable	<170 mg/dl	<4.4 mmol/L
	Borderline	170-199 mg/dl	4.4-5.1 mmol/L
	High	≥200 mg/dl	≥5.2 mmol/L
Clotting time (Lee-White)			
Whole blood		5-8 min (glass tubes)	5-8 min
		5-15 min (room temp)	5-15 min
		30 min (silicone tube)	30 min

*From National Cholesterol Education Program: Report of the expert panel on blood cholesterol levels in children and adolescents, *Pediatrics* 89 (3, pt 2):527, 1992.

TEST/SPECIMEN	AGE/SEX/REFERENCE	CONVENTIONAL UNITS	INTERNATIONAL UNITS (SI)
		NORMAL RANGES	
Creatine kinase (CK, CPK)			
Serum	Cord blood	70-380 U/L	70-380 U/L
	5-8 hr	214-1175 U/L	214-1175 U/L
	24-33 hr	130-1200 U/L	130-1200 U/L
	72-100 hr	87-725 U/L	87-725 U/L
	Adult	5-130 U/L	5-130 U/L
Creatinine			
Serum	Cord	0.6-1.2 mg/dl	53-106 μmol/L
	Newborn	0.3-1.0 mg/dl	27-88 μmol/L
	Infant	0.2-0.4 mg/dl	18-35 μmol/L
	Child	0.3-0.7 mg/dl	27-62 μmol/L
	Adolescent	0.5-1.0 mg/dl	44-88 μmol/L
	Adult: Male	0.6-1.2 mg/dl	53-106 μmol/L
	Female	0.5-1.1 mg/dl	44-97 μmol/L
Urine, 24 hr	Premature	8.1-15.0 mg/kg/24 hr	72-133 μmol/kg/24 hr
	Full term	10.4-19.7 mg/kg/24 hr	92-174 μmol/kg/24 hr
	1.5-7 yr	10-15 mg/kg/24 hr	88-133 μmol/kg/24 hr
	7-15 yr	5.2-41 mg/kg/24 hr	46-362 μmol/kg/24 hr
Creatinine clearance (endogenous)			
Serum or plasma and urine	Newborn	40-65 ml/min/1.73 m^2	
	<40 yr: Male	97-137 ml/min/1.73 m^2	
	Female	88-128 ml/min/1.73 m^2	
Digoxin			
Serum, plasma; collect at least 12 hr after dose	Therap. conc.		
	CHF	0.8-1.5 ng/ml	1.0-1.9 nmol/L
	Arrhythmias	1.5-2.0 ng/ml	1.9-2.6 nmol/L
	Toxic conc		
	Child	>2.5 ng/ml	>3.2 nmol/L
	Adult	>3.0 ng/ml	>3.8 nmol/L
Eosinophil count			
Whole blood, capillary blood		50-350 cells/mm^3 (μl)	50-350 × 10^6 cells/L
Erythrocyte (RBC) count			
Whole blood	Cord	3.9-5.5 million/mm^3	3.9-5.5 × 10^{12} cells/L
	1-3 d	4.0-6.6 million/mm^3	4.0-6.6 × 10^{12} cells/L
	1 wk	3.9-6.3 million/mm^3	3.9-6.3 × 10^{12} cells/L
	2 wk	3.6-6.2 million/mm^3	3.6-6.2 × 10^{12} cells/L
	1 mo	3.0-5.4 million/mm^3	3.0-5.4 × 10^{12} cells/L
	2 mo	2.7-4.9 million/mm^3	2.7-4.5 × 10^{12} cells/L
	3-6 mo	3.1-4.5 million/mm^3	3.1-4.5 × 10^{12} cells/L
	0.5-2 yr	3.7-5.3 million/mm^3	3.7-5.3 × 10^{12} cells/L
	2-6 yr	3.9-5.3 million/mm^3	3.9-5.3 × 10^{12} cells/L
	6-12 yr	4.0-5.2 million/mm^3	4.0-5.2 × 10^{12} cells/L
	12-18 yr: Male	4.5-5.3 million/mm^3	4.5-5.3 × 10^{12} cells/L
	Female	4.1-5.1 million/mm^3	4.1-5.1 × 10^{12} cells/L
Erythrocyte sedimentation rate (ESR)			
Whole blood			
Westergren (modified)	Child	0-10 mm/hr	0-10 mm/hr
	<50 yr: Male	0-15 mm/hr	0-15 mm/hr
	Female	0-20 mm/hr	0-20 mm/hr
Wintrobe	Child	0-13 mm/hr	0-13 mm/hr
	Adult: Male	0-9 mm/hr	0-9 mm/hr
	Female	0-20 mm/hr	0-20 mm/hr

Continued.

COMMON LABORATORY TESTS—cont'd

TEST/SPECIMEN	AGE/SEX/REFERENCE	CONVENTIONAL UNITS	INTERNATIONAL UNITS (SI)
		NORMAL RANGES	
Fibrinogen			
Plasma	Newborn	125-300 mg/dl	1.25-3.00 g/L
	Thereafter	200-400 mg/dl	2.00-4.00 g/L
Galactose			
Serum	Newborn	0-20 mg/dl	0-1.11 mmol/L
	Thereafter	<5 mg/dl	<0.03 mmol/L
Urine	Newborn	≤60 mg/dl	≤3.33 mmol/L
	Thereafter	<14 mg/dl	<0.08 mmol/d
Glucose			
Serum	Cord	45-96 mg/dl	2.5-5.3 mmol/L
	Newborn, 1 d	40-60 mg/dl	2.2-3.3 mmol/L
	Newborn, >1 d	50-90 mg/dl	2.8-5.0 mmol/L
	Child	60-100 mg/dl	3.3-5.5 mmol/L
	Thereafter	70-105 mg/dl	3.9-5.8 mmol/L
Whole blood	Adult	65-95 mg/dl	3.6-5.3 mmol/L
CSF	Adult	40-70 mg/dl	2.2-3.9 mmol/L
Urine (quantitative)		<0.5 g/d	<2.8 mmol/d
(Qualitative)		Negative	Negative

Glucose tolerance test (GTT), oral
Serum

Dosages		Normal	Diabetic	Normal	Diabetic
Adult: 75 g	Fasting	70-105 mg/dl	>115 mg/dl	3.9-5.8 mmol/L	>6.4 mmol/L
Child: 1.75 g/kg of ideal	60 min	120-170 mg/dl	≥200 mg/dl	6.7-9.4 mmol/L	≥11 mmol/L
weight up to maximum of	90 min	100-140 mg/dl	≥200 mg/dl	5.6-7.8 mmol/L	≥11 mmol/L
75 g	120 min	70-120 mg/dl	≥140 mg/dl	3.9-6.7 mmol/L	≥7.8 mmol/L

TEST/SPECIMEN	AGE/SEX/REFERENCE	CONVENTIONAL UNITS	INTERNATIONAL UNITS (SI)
Growth hormone (hGH, somatotropin)			
Plasma	Cord	10-50 ng/ml	10-50 µg/L
Fasting, at rest	Newborn	10-40 ng/ml	10-40 µg/L
	Child	<5 ng/ml	<5 µg/L
	Adult: Male	<5 ng/ml	<5 µg/L
	Female	<8 ng/ml	<8 µg/L
Hematocrit (HCT, Hct)			
Whole blood	1 d (cap)	48%-69%	0.48-0.69 vol. fraction
	2 d	48%-75%	0.48-0.75 vol. fraction
	3 d	44%-72%	0.44-0.72 vol. fraction
	2 mo	28%-42%	0.28-0.42 vol. fraction
	6-12 yr	35%-45%	0.35-0.45 vol. fraction
	12-18 yr: Male	37%-49%	0.37-0.49 vol. fraction
	Female	36%-46%	0.36-0.46 vol. fraction
Hemoglobin (Hb)			
Whole blood	1-3 d (cap)	14.5-22.5 g/dl	2.25-3.49 mmol/L
	2 mo	9.0-14.0 g/dl	1.40-2.17 mmol/L
	6-12 yr	11.5-15.5 g/dl	1.78-2.40 mmol/L
	12-18 yr: Male	13.0-16.0 g/dl	2.02-2.48 mmol/L
	Female	12.0-16.0 g/dl	1.86-2.48 mmol/L
Hemoglobin A			
Whole blood		>95% of total	0.95 fraction of Hb

TEST/SPECIMEN	AGE/SEX/REFERENCE	CONVENTIONAL UNITS	INTERNATIONAL UNITS (SI)
		NORMAL RANGES	
Hemoglobin F			
Whole blood	1 d	63%-92% HbF	0.62-0.92 mass fraction HbF
	5 d	65%-88% HbF	0.65-0.88 mass fraction HbF
	3 wk	55%-85% HbF	0.55-0.85 mass fraction HbF
	6-9 wk	31%-75% HbF	0.31-0.75 mass fraction HbF
	3-4 mo	<2%-59% HbF	<0.02-0.59 mass fraction HbF
	6 mo	<2%-9% HbF	<0.02-0.09 mass fraction HbF
	Adult	<2.0% HbF	<0.02 mass fraction HbF
Immunoglobulin A (IgA)			
Serum	Cord blood	1.4-3.6 mg/dl	14-36 mg/L
	1-3 mo	1.3-53 mg/dl	13-530 mg/L
	4-6 mo	4.4-84 mg/dl	44-840 mg/L
	7 mo-1 yr	11-106 mg/dl	110-1060 mg/L
	2-5 yr	14-159 mg/dl	140-1590 mg/L
	6-10 yr	33-236 mg/dl	330-2360 mg/L
	Adult	70-312 mg/dl	700-3130 mg/L
Immunoglobulin D (IgD)			
Serum	Newborn	None detected	None detected
	Thereafter	0-8 mg/dl	0-80 mg/L
Immunoglobulin E (IgE)			
Serum	M	0-230 IU/ml	0-230 kIU/L
	F	0-170 IU/ml	0-170 kIU/L
Immunoglobulin G (IgG)			
Serum	Cord blood	636-1606 mg/dl	6.36-16.06 g/L
	1 mo	251-906 mg/dl	2.51-9.06 g/L
	2-4 mo	176-601 mg/dl	1.76-6.01 g/L
	5-12 mo	172-1069 mg/dl	1.72-10.69 g/L
	1-5 yr	345-1236 mg/dl	3.45-12.36 g/L
	6-10 yr	608-1572 mg/dl	6.08-15.72 g/L
	Adult	639-1349 mg/dl	6.39-13.49 g/L
Immunoglobulin M (IgM)			
Serum	Cord blood	6.3-25 mg/dl	63-250 mg/L
	1 mo-4 mo	17-105 mg/dl	170-1050 mg/L
	5 mo-9 mo	33-126 mg/dl	330-1260 mg/L
	10 mo-1 yr	41-173 mg/dl	410-1730 mg/L
	2-8 yr	43-207 mg/dl	430-2070 mg/L
	9-10 yr	52-242 mg/dl	520-2420 mg/L
	Adult	56-352 mg/dl	560-3520 mg/L
Iron			
Serum	Newborn	100-250 μg/dl	17.90-44.75 μmol/L
	Infant	40-100 μg/dl	7.16-1790 μmol/L
	Child	50-120 μg/dl	8.95-21.48 μmol/L
	Thereafter: Male	50-160 μg/dl	8.95-28.64 μmol/L
	Female	40-150 μg/dl	7.16-26.85 μmol/L
	Intoxicated child	280-2550 μg/dl	50.12-456.5 μmol/L
	Fatally poisoned child	>1800 μg/dl	>322.2 μmol/L
Iron-binding capacity, total (TIBC)			
Serum	Infant	100-400 μg/dl	17.90-71.60 μmol/L
	Thereafter	250-400 μg/dl	44.75-71.60 μmol/L

Continued.

COMMON LABORATORY TESTS—cont'd

TEST/SPECIMEN	AGE/SEX/REFERENCE	CONVENTIONAL UNITS		INTERNATIONAL UNITS (SI)
		NORMAL RANGES		
Lead				
Whole blood	Child	<10 μg/dl		<0.48 μmol/L
Urine, 24 hr		<80 μg/L		<0.39 μmol/L
Leukocyte count (WBC count)		× 1000 cells/mm³ (μl)		× 10⁹ cells/L
Whole blood	Birth	9.0-30.0		9.0-30.0
	24 hr	9.4-34.0		9.4-34.0
	1 mo	5.0-19.5		5.0-19.5
	1-3 yr	6.0-17.5		6.0-17.5
	4-7 yr	5.5-15.5		5.5-15.5
	8-13 yr	4.5-13.5		4.5-13.5
	Adult	4.5-11.0		4.5-11.0
		× 1000 cells/mm³ (μl)		× 10⁶ cells/L
CSF	Premature	0-25 mononuclear		0-25
		0-100 polymorphonuclear		0-100
		0-1000 RBC		0-1000
	Newborn	0-20 mononuclear		0-20
		0-70 polymorphonuclear		0-70
		0-800 RBC		0-800
	Neonate	0-5 mononuclear		0-5
		0-25 polymorphonuclear		0-25
		0-50 RBC		0-50
	Thereafter	0-5 mononuclear		0-5
Leukocyte differential count				
Whole blood	Myelocytes	0%	0 cells/mm³ (μl)	Number fraction 0
	Neutrophils—"bands"	3%-5%	150-400 cells/mm³ (μl)	Number fraction 0.03-0.05
	Neutrophils—"segs"	54%-62%	3000-5800 cells/mm³ (μl)	Number fraction 0.54-0.62
	Lymphocytes	25%-33%	1500-3000 cells/mm³ (μl)	Number fraction 0.25-0.33
	Monocytes	3%-7%	285-500 cells/mm³ (μl)	Number fraction 0.03-0.07
	Eosinophils	1%-3%	50-250 cells/mm³ (μl)	Number fraction 0.01-0.03
	Basophils	0%-0.75%	15-50 cells/mm³ (μl)	Number fraction 0-0.0075
Mean corpuscular hemoglobin (MCH)				
Whole blood	Birth	31-37 pg/cell		0.48-0.57 fmol/L
	1-3 d (cap)	31-37 pg/cell		0.48-0.57 fmol/L
	1 wk-1 mo	28-40 pg/cell		0.43-0.62 fmol/L
	2 mo	26-34 pg/cell		0.40-0.53 fmol/L
	3-6 mo	25-35 pg/cell		0.39-0.54 fmol/L
	0.5-2 yr	23-31 pg/cell		0.36-0.48 fmol/L
	2-6 yr	24-30 pg/cell		0.37-0.47 fmol/L
	6-12 yr	25-33 pg/cell		0.39-0.51 fmol/L
	12-18 yr	25-35 pg/cell		0.39-0.54 fmol/L
	18-49 yr	26-34 pg/cell		0.40-0.53 fmol/L

TEST/SPECIMEN	AGE/SEX/REFERENCE	CONVENTIONAL UNITS	INTERNATIONAL UNITS (SI)
		NORMAL RANGES	
Mean corpuscular hemoglobin concentration (MCHC)			
Whole blood	Birth	30%-36% Hb/cell or g Hb/dl RBC	4.65-5.58 mmol or Hb/L RBC
	1-3 d (cap)	29%-37% Hb/cell or g Hb/dl RBC	4.50-5.74 mmol or Hb/L RBC
	1-2 wk	28%-38% Hb/cell or g Hb/dl RBC	4.34-5.89 mmol or Hb/L RBC
	1-2 mo	29%-37% Hb/cell or g Hb/dl RBC	4.50-5.74 mmol or Hb/L RBC
	3 mo-2 yr	30%-36% Hb/cell or g Hb/dl RBC	4.65-5.58 mmol or Hb/L RBC
	2-18 yr	31%-37% Hb/cell or g Hb/dl RBC	4.81-5.74 mmol or Hb/L RBC
	>18 yr	31%-37% Hb/cell or g Hb/dl RBC	4.81-5.74 mmol or Hb/L RBC
Mean corpuscular volume (MCV)			
Whole blood	1-3 d (cap)	95-121 μm^3	95-121 fl
	0.5-2 yr	70-86 μm^3	70-86 fl
	6-12 yr	77-95 μm^3	77-95 fl
	12-18 yr: Male	78-98 μm^3	78-98 fl
	Female	78-102 μm^3	78-102 fl
Osmolality			
Serum	Child, adult:	275-295 mOsmol/kg H_2O	
Urine, random		50-1400 mOsmol/kg H_2O, depending on fluid intake; after 12 hr fluid restriction: >850 mOsmol/kg H_2O	
Urine, 24 hr		≃300-900 mOsmol/kg H_2O	
Oxygen, partial pressure (Po_2)			
Whole blood, arterial	Birth	8-24 mm Hg	1.1-3.2 kPa
	5-10 min	33-75 mm Hg	4.4-10.0 kPa
	30 min	31-85 mm Hg	4.1-11.3 kPa
	>1 hr	55-80 mm Hg	7.3-10.6 kPa
	1 d	54-95 mm Hg	7.2-12.6 kPa
	Thereafter (decreased with age)	83-108 mm Hg	11-14.4 kPa
Oxygen saturation (Sao_2)			
Whole blood, arterial	Newborn	85%-90%	Fraction saturated 0.85-0.90
	Thereafter	95%-99%	Fraction saturated 0.95-0.99
Partial thromboplastin time (PTT)			
Whole blood (Na citrate)			
Nonactivated		60-85 s (Platelin)	60-85 s
Activated		25-35 s (differs with method)	25-35 s
pH			H^+ concentration:
Whole blood, arterial	Premature (48 hr)	7.35-7.50	31-44 nmol/L
	Birth, full term	7.11-7.36	43-77 nmol/L
	5-10 min	7.09-7.30	50-81 nmol/L
	30 min	7.21-7.38	41-61 nmol/L
	>1 hr	7.26-7.49	32-54 nmol/L
	1 d	7.29-7.45	35-51 nmol/L
	Thereafter	7.35-7.45	35-44 nmol/L
	Must be corrected for body temperature		

Continued.

COMMON LABORATORY TESTS—cont'd

TEST/SPECIMEN	AGE/SEX/REFERENCE	CONVENTIONAL UNITS	INTERNATIONAL UNITS (SI)
		NORMAL RANGES	
Urine, random	Newborn/neonate	5-7	0.1-10 μmol/L
	Thereafter (average ≃6)	4.5-8	0.01-32 μmol/L (average ≃1.0 μmol/L)
Stool		7.0-7.5	31-100 nmol/L
Phenylalanine			
Serum	Premature	2.0-7.5 mg/dl	120-450 μmol/L
	Newborn	1.2-3.4 mg/dl	70-210 μmol/L
	Thereafter	0.8-1.8 mg/dl	50-110 μmol/L
Urine, 24 hr	10 d-2 wk	1-2 mg/d	6-12 μmol/d
	3-12 yr	4-18 mg/d	24-110 μmol/d
	Thereafter	trace-17 mg/d	trace-103 μmol/d
Plasma volume			
Plasma	Male	25-43 ml/kg	0.025-0.043 L/kg
	Female	28-45 ml/kg	0.028-0.045 L/kg
Platelet count (thrombocyte count)			
Whole blood (EDTA)	Newborn	$84\text{-}478 \times 10^3/mm^3$ (μl)	$84\text{-}478 \times 10^9/L$
	(After 1 wk, same as adult)		
	Adult	$150\text{-}400 \times 10^3/mm^3$ (μl)	$150\text{-}400 \times 10^9/L$
Potassium*			
Serum	Newborn	3.0-6.0 mEq/L	3.0-6.0 mmol/L
	Thereafter	3.5-5.0 mEq/L	3.5-5.0 mmol/L
Plasma (heparin)		3.4-4.5 mEq/L	3.4-4.5 mmol/L
Urine, 24 hr		2.5-125 mEq/d varies with diet	2.5-125 mmol/L
Protein			
Serum, total	Premature	4.3-7.6 g/dl	43-76 g/L
	Newborn	4.6-7.4 g/dl	46-74 g/L
	1-7 yr	6.1-7.9 g/dl	61-79 g/L
	8-12 yr	6.4-8.1 g/dl	64-81 g/L
	13-19 yr	6.6-8.2 g/dl	66-82 g/L
Total			
Urine, 24 hr		1-14 mg/dl	10-140 mg/L
		50-80 mg/d (at rest)	50-80 mg/d
		<250 mg/d after intense exercise	<250 mg/d after exercise
Total			
CSF		Lumbar: 8-32 mg/dl	80-320 mg/L
Prothrombin time (PT)			
One-stage (Quick)			
Whole blood (Na citrate)	In general	11-15 s (varies with type of thromboplastin)	11-15 s
	Newborn	Prolonged by 2-3 sec	Prolonged by 2-3 sec
Two-stage modified (Ware and Seegers)			
Whole blood (Na citrate)		18-22 sec	18-22 sec
RBC count, see erythrocyte count			
Red blood cell volume			
Whole blood	Male	20-36 ml/kg	0.020-0.036 L/kg
	Female	19-31 ml/kg	0.019-0.031 L/kg

*Potassium ranges are from Johns Hopkins Hospital: *The Harriet Lane handbook,* ed 12, St Louis, 1991, Mosby, p 383.

TEST/SPECIMEN	AGE/SEX/REFERENCE	CONVENTIONAL UNITS	INTERNATIONAL UNITS (SI)
		NORMAL RANGES	
Reticulocyte count			
Whole blood	Adults	0.5%-1.5% of erythrocytes or 25,000-75,000/mm³ (µl)	0.005-0.015 (number fraction) 25,000-75,000 × 10⁶/L
Capillary	1 d	0.4%-6.0%	0.004-0.060 (number fraction)
	7 d	<0.1%-1.3%	<0.001-0.013 (number fraction)
	1-4 wk	<0.1%-1.2%	<0.001-0.012 (number fraction)
	5-6 wk	<0.1%-2.4%	<0.001-0.024 (number fraction)
	7-8 wk	0.1%-2.9%	0.001-0.029 (number fraction)
	9-10 wk	<0.1%-2.6%	<0.001-0.026 (number fraction)
	11-12 wk	0.1%-1.3%	0.001-0.013 (number fraction)
Salicylates			
Serum, plasma	Therap. conc.	15-30 mg/dl	1.1-2.2 mmol/L
	Toxic conc.	>30 mg/dl	>2.2 mmol/L
Sedimentation rate: see erythrocyte sedimentation rate			
Sodium			
Serum or plasma	Newborn	136-146 mEq/L	134-146 mmol/L
	Infant	139-146 mEq/L	139-146 mmol/L
	Child	138-145 mEq/L	138-145 mmol/L
	Thereafter	136-146 mEq/L	136-146 mmol/L
Urine, 24 hr		40-220 mEq/L (diet dependent)	40-220 mmol/L
Sweat	Normal	<40 mEq/L	<40 mmol/L
	Indeterminate	45-60 mEq/L	45-60 mmol/L
	Cystic fibrosis	>60 mEq/L	>60 mmol/L
Specific gravity			
Urine, random	Adult	1.002-1.030	1.002-1.030
	After 12 hr fluid restriction	>1.025	>1.025
Urine, 24 hr		1.015-1.025	
Theophylline			
Serum, plasma	Therap. conc.		
	Bronchodilator	10-20 µg/ml	56-110 µmol/L
	Premature apnea	6-10 µg/ml	28-56 µmol/L
	Toxic conc.	>20	>166 µmol/L
Thrombin time			
Whole blood (Na citrate)		Control time ± 2 sec when control is 9-13 sec	Control time ± 2 sec when control is 9-13 sec
Thyroxine, total (T₃)			
Serum	Cord	8-13 µg/dl	103-168 nmol/L
	Newborn	11.5-24 (lower in low-birth-weight infants)	148-310 nmol/L
	Neonate	9-18 µg/dl	116-232 nmol/L
	Infant	7-15 µg/dl	90-194 nmol/L
	1-5 yr	7.3-15 µg/dl	94-194 nmol/L
	5-10 yr	6.4-13.3 µg/dl	83-172 nmol/L
	Thereafter	5-12 µg/dl	65-155 nmol/L
	Newborn screen (filter paper)	6.2-22 µg/dl	80-284 nmol/L

Continued.

COMMON LABORATORY TESTS—cont'd

TEST/SPECIMEN	AGE/SEX/REFERENCE	CONVENTIONAL UNITS		INTERNATIONAL UNITS (SI)	
		NORMAL RANGES			
Tourniquet test (capillary fragility)		<5-10 petechiae in 2.5 cm circle on forearm (halfway between systolic and diastolic); pressure for 5 min; 0-8 petechiae in 6 cm circle (50 torr for 15 min); 10-20 petechiae in 5 cm circle (80 mm Hg)		<5-10 petechiae in 2.5 cm circle on forearm (halfway between systolic and diastolic); pressure for 5 min; 0-8 petechiae in 6 cm circle (50 torr for 15 min); 10-20 petechiae in 5 cm circle (80 mm Hg)	
Triglycerides (TG) Serum, after ≥12 hr fast		mg/dl		g/L	
		M	F	M	F
	Cord blood	10-98	10-98	0.10-0.98	0.10-0.98
	0-5 yr	30-86	32-99	0.30-0.86	0.32-0.99
	6-11 yr	31-108	35-114	0.31-1.08	0.35-1.14
	12-15 yr	36-138	41-138	0.36-1.38	0.41-1.38
	16-19 yr	40-163	40-128	0.40-1.63	0.40-1.28
Triiodothyronine, free Serum	Cord	20-240 pg/dl		0.3-3.7 pmol/L	
	1-3 d	200-610 pg/dl		3.1-9.4 pmol/L	
	6 wk	240-560 pg/dl		3.7-8.6 pmol/L	
	Adults (20-50 yr)	230-660 pg/dl		3.5-10.0 pmol/L	
Triiodothyronine, total (T_3-RIA) Serum	Cord	30-70 ng/dl		0.46-1.08 nmol/L	
	Newborn	72-260 ng/dl		1.16-4.00 nmol/L	
	1-5 yr	100-260 ng/dl		1.54-4.00 nmol/L	
	5-10 yr	90-240 ng/dl		1.39-3.70 nmol/L	
	10-15 yr	80-210 ng/dl		1.23-3.23 nmol/L	
	Thereafter	115-190 ng/dl		1.77-2.93 nmol/L	
Urea nitrogen Serum or plasma	Cord	21-40 mg/dl		7.5-14.3 mmol urea/L	
	Premature (1 wk)	3-25 mg/dl		1.1-9 mmol urea/L	
	Newborn	3-12 mg/dl		1.1-4.3 mmol urea/L	
	Infant/child	5-18 mg/dl		1.8-6.4 mmol urea/L	
	Thereafter	7-18 mg/dl		2.5-6.4 mmol urea/L	
Urine volume Urine, 24 hr	Newborn	50-300 ml/d		0.050-0.300 L/d	
	Infant	350-550 ml/d		0.350-0.500 L/d	
	Child	500-1000 ml/d		0.500-1.000 L/d	
	Adolescent	700-1400 ml/d		0.700-1.400 L/d	
	Thereafter: Male	800-1800 ml/d		0.800-1.800 L/d	
	Female	600-1600 ml/d (varies with intake and other factors)		0.600-1.600 L/d	
WBC, see leukocyte					

ABBREVIATIONS USED IN LABORATORY TESTS

Abbreviation	Term
cap	capillary
CHF	congestive heart failure
conc.	concentration
CSF	cerebrospinal fluid
d	day; diem
EDTA	ethylenediaminetetraacetate
g	gram
m	meter
hr	hour
L, l	liter
mEq	milliequivalent
min	minute
mm	millimeter
mm^3	cubic millimeter
mo	month
mol	mole
mOsmol	milliosmole
s	second
SI	International system of units
Therap.	therapeutic
U	International unit of enzyme activity
vol	volume
wk	week
yr	year
>	greater than
≥	greater than or equal to
<	less than
≤	less than or equal to
±	plus/minus
≃	approximately equal to

PREFIXES DENOTING DECIMAL FACTORS

Prefix	Symbol	Amount
deci	d	one tenth (10^{-1})
centi	c	one hundredth (10^{-2})
milli	m	one thousandth (10^{-3})
micro	μ	one millionth (10^{-6})
nano	n	one billionth (10^{-9})
pico	p	one trillionth (10^{-12})
femto	f	one quadrillionth (10^{-15})

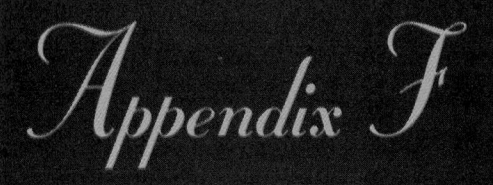

Recommended Daily Dietary Allowances

CATEGORY	AGE (YEARS) OR CONDITION	WEIGHT[b] (kg)	WEIGHT[b] (lb)	HEIGHT[b] (cm)	HEIGHT[b] (in)	PROTEIN (g)	FAT-SOLUBLE VITAMINS VITAMIN A (μ RE)[c]	VITAMIN D (μg)[d]	VITAMIN E (mg/α-TE)[e]	VITAMIN K (μg)
Infants	0.0-0.5	6	13	60	24	13	375	7.5	3	5
	0.5-1.0	9	20	71	28	14	375	10	4	10
Children	1-3	13	29	90	35	16	400	10	6	15
	4-6	20	44	112	44	24	500	10	7	20
	7-10	28	62	132	52	28	700	10	7	30
Males	11-14	45	99	157	62	45	1000	10	10	45
	15-18	66	145	176	69	59	1000	10	10	65
	19-24	72	160	177	70	58	1000	10	10	70
	25-50	79	174	176	70	63	1000	5	10	80
	51+	77	170	173	68	63	1000	5	10	80
Females	11-14	46	101	157	62	46	800	10	8	45
	15-18	55	120	163	64	44	800	10	8	55
	19-24	58	128	164	65	46	800	10	8	60
	25-50	63	138	163	64	50	800	5	8	65
	51+	65	143	160	63	50	800	5	8	65
Pregnant						60	800	10	10	65
Lactating	1st 6 months					65	1300	10	12	65
	2nd 6 months					62	1200	10	11	65

From Food and Nutrition Board, National Research Council: *Recommended dietary allowances,* ed 10, Washington, DC, 1989, National Academy of Sciences.

[a]The allowances, expressed as average daily intakes over time, are intended to provide for individual variations among most normal persons as they live in the United States under usual environmental stresses. Diets should be based on a variety of common foods in order to provide other nutrients for which human requirements have been less well defined.

[b]Weights and heights of reference adults are actual medians for the U.S. population of the designated age, as reported by National Health and Nutrition Examination Survey (NHANES) II. The median weights and heights of those under 19 years of age were taken from Hamill PV and others: Physical growth: National Center for Health Statistics percentiles, *Am J Clin Nutr* 32:607-629, 1979. The use of these figures does not imply that the height-to-weight ratios are ideal.

[c]Retinol equivalent. 1 retinol equivalent = 1 μg retinol or 6 μ β-carotene.

[d]As cholecalciferol. 10μg cholecalciferol = 400 IU vitamin D.

[e]α-Tocopherol equivalents. 1 mg d-α-tocopherol = 1 α-TE.

[f]1 NE (niacin equivalent) is equal to 1 mg of niacin or 60 mg of dietary tryptophan.

WATER-SOLUBLE VITAMINS							MINERALS						
VITA-MIN C (mg)	THIAMIN (mg)	RIBO-FLAVIN (mg)	NIACIN (mg NE)[f]	VITA-MIN B^6 (mg)	FOLATE (μg)	VITA-MIN B$_{12}$ (μg)	CALCIUM (mg)	PHOS-PHORUS (mg)	MAGNE-SIUM (mg)	IRON (mg)	ZINC (mg)	IODINE (μg)	SELE-NIUM (μg)
30	0.3	0.4	5	0.3	25	0.3	400	300	40	6	5	40	10
35	0.4	0.5	6	0.6	35	0.5	600	500	60	10	5	50	15
40	0.7	0.8	9	1.0	50	0.7	800	800	80	10	10	70	20
45	0.9	1.1	12	1.1	75	1.0	800	800	120	10	10	90	20
45	1.0	1.2	13	1.4	100	1.4	800	800	170	10	10	120	30
50	1.3	1.5	17	1.7	150	2.0	1200	1200	270	12	15	150	40
60	1.5	1.8	20	2.0	200	2.0	1200	1200	400	12	15	150	50
60	1.5	1.7	19	2.0	200	2.0	1200	1200	350	10	15	150	70
60	1.5	1.7	19	2.0	200	2.0	800	800	350	10	15	150	70
60	1.2	1.4	15	2.0	200	2.0	800	800	350	10	15	150	70
50	1.1	1.3	15	1.4	150	2.0	1200	1200	280	15	12	150	45
60	1.1	1.3	15	1.5	180	2.0	1200	1200	300	15	12	150	50
60	1.1	1.3	15	1.6	180	2.0	1200	1200	280	15	12	150	55
60	1.1	1.3	15	1.6	180	2.0	800	800	280	15	12	150	55
60	1.0	1.2	13	1.6	180	2.0	800	800	280	10	12	150	55
70	1.5	1.6	17	2.2	400	2.2	1200	1200	320	30	15	175	65
95	1.6	1.8	20	2.1	280	2.6	1200	1200	355	15	19	200	75
90	1.6	1.7	20	2.1	260	2.6	1200	1200	340	15	16	200	75

Estimated safe and adequate daily dietary intakes of selected vitamins and minerals[a]

CATEGORY	AGE (YEARS)	VITAMINS	
		BIOTIN (μg)	PANTOTHENIC ACID (mg)
Infants	0-0.5	10	2
	0.5-1	15	3
Children and adolescents	1-3	20	3
	4-6	25	3-4
	7-10	30	4-5
	11+	30-100	4-7
Adults		30-100	4-7

From Food and Nutrition Board, National Research Council: *Recommended dietary allowances,* ed 10, Washington, DC, 1989, National Academy of Sciences.
[a]Because there is less information on which to base allowances, these figures are not given in the main table of RDAs and are provided here in the form of ranges of recommended intakes.
[b]Since the toxic levels for many trace elements may be only several times usual intakes, the upper levels for the trace elements given in this table should not be habitually exceeded.

Estimated sodium, chloride, and potassium minimum requirements of healthy persons[a]

AGE	WEIGHT (kg)[a]	SODIUM (mg)[a,b]	CHLORIDE (mg)[a,b]	POTASSIUM (mg)[c]
Months				
0-5	4.5	120	180	500
6-11	8.9	200	300	700
Years				
1	11.0	225	350	1000
2-5	16.0	300	500	1400
6-9	25.0	400	600	1600
10-18	50.0	500	750	2000
>18[d]	70.0	500	750	2000

From Food and Nutrition Board, National Research Council: *Recommended dietary allowances,* ed 10, Washington, DC, 1989, National Academy of Sciences.
[a]No allowance has been included for large, prolonged losses from the skin through sweat.
[b]There is no evidence that higher intakes confer any health benefit.
[c]Desirable intakes of potassium may considerably exceed these values (~3500 mg for adults).
[d]No allowance included for growth. Values for those younger than 18 years of age assume a growth rate at the 50th percentile reported by the National Center for Health Statistics and averaged for males and females.

TRACE ELEMENTS[b]

COPPER (mg)	MANGANESE (mg)	FLUORIDE (mg)	CHROMIUM (µG)	MOLYBDENUM (µg)
0.4-0.6	0.3-0.6	0.1-0.5	10-40	15-30
0.6-0.7	0.6-1.0	0.2-1.0	20-60	20-40
0.7-1.0	1.0-1.5	0.5-1.5	20-80	25-50
1.0-1.5	1.5-2.0	1.0-2.5	30-120	30-75
1.0-2.0	2.0-3.0	1.5-2.5	50-200	50-150
1.5-2.5	2.0-5.0	1.5-2.5	50-200	75-250
1.5-3.0	2.0-5.0	1.5-4.0	50-200	75-250

Median heights and weights and recommended energy intake

CATEGORY	AGE (YEAR) OR CONDITION	WEIGHT (kg)	WEIGHT (lb)	HEIGHT (cm)	HEIGHT (in)	REE[a] (kcal/day)	AVERAGE ENERGY ALLOWANCE (kcal)[b] MULTIPLES OF REE	AVERAGE ENERGY ALLOWANCE (kcal)[b] PER kg	AVERAGE ENERGY ALLOWANCE (kcal)[b] PER DAY[c]
Infants	0.0-0.5	6	13	60	24	320		108	650
	0.5-1.0	9	20	71	28	500		98	850
Children	1-3	13	29	90	35	740		102	1300
	4-6	20	44	112	44	950		90	1800
	7-10	28	62	132	52	1130		70	2000
Males	11-14	45	99	157	62	1440	1.70	55	2500
	15-18	66	145	176	69	1760	1.67	45	3000
	19-24	72	160	177	70	1780	1.67	40	2900
	25-50	79	174	176	70	1800	1.60	37	2900
	51+	77	170	173	68	1530	1.50	30	2300
Females	11-14	46	101	157	62	1310	1.67	47	2200
	15-18	55	120	163	64	1370	1.60	40	2200
	19-24	58	128	164	65	1350	1.60	38	2200
	25-50	63	138	163	64	1380	1.55	36	2200
	51+	65	143	160	63	1280	1.50	30	1900
Pregnant	1st trimester								+0
	2nd trimester								+300
	3rd trimester								+300
Lactating	1st 6 months								+500
	2nd 6 months								+500

From Food and Nutrition Board, National Research Council: *Recommended dietary allowances,* ed 10, Washington, DC, 1989, National Academy of Sciences.

[a]Resting energy expenditure.

[b]In the range of light to moderate activity, the coefficient of variation is ±20%.

[c]Figure is rounded.

The data in this table have been assembled from the observed median heights and weights of children together with desirable weights for adults for the mean heights of men (70 inches) and women (64 inches) between the ages of 18 and 34 years as surveyed in the United States population (HEW/NCHS data). The energy allowances for the young adults are for men and women doing light work. The allowances for the two older age-groups represent mean energy needs over these age spans, allowing for a 2% decrease in basal (resting) metabolic rate per decade and a reduction in activity of 200 kcal/day for men and women between 51 and 75 years of age, 500 kcal for men over 75, and 400 kcal for women over 75. The customary range of daily energy output is shown for adults in parentheses and is based on a variation in energy needs of ±400 kcal at any one age, emphasizing the wide range of energy intakes appropriate for any group of people. Energy allowances for children through age 18 are based on medium energy intakes of children these ages followed in longitudinal growth studies. The values in parentheses are 10th and 90th percentiles of energy intake, to indicate the range of energy consumption among children of these ages.

Appendix G   NANDA–Approved Nursing Diagnoses*

Activity intolerance
Activity intolerance, risk for
Adaptive capacity, decreased: intracranial
Adjustment, impaired
Airway clearance, ineffective
Anxiety
Aspiration, risk for
Body image disturbance
Body temperature, altered, risk for
Bowel incontinence
Breastfeeding, effective
Breastfeeding, ineffective
Breastfeeding, interrupted
Breathing pattern, ineffective
Cardiac output, decreased
Caregiver role strain
Caregiver role strain, risk for
Communication, impaired verbal
Community coping, potential for enhanced
Community coping, ineffective
Confusion, acute
Confusion, chronic
Constipation
Constipation, colonic
Constipation, perceived
Coping, defensive
Coping, family: potential for growth
Coping, ineffective family: compromised
Coping, ineffective family: disabling
Coping, ineffective individual
Decisional conflict (specify)
Denial, ineffective
Diarrhea
Disuse syndrome, risk for
Diversional activity deficit
Dysreflexia
Energy field disturbance
Environmental interpretation syndrome:
  impaired
Family processes, altered: alcoholism
Family processes, altered
Fatigue
Fear
Fluid volume deficit
Fluid volume deficit, risk for
Fluid volume excess
Gas exchange, impaired

Grieving, anticipatory
Grieving, dysfunctional
Growth and development, altered
Health maintenance, altered
Health-seeking behaviors (specify)
Home maintenance management, impaired
Hopelessness
Hyperthermia
Hypothermia
Incontinence, functional
Incontinence, reflex
Incontinence, stress
Incontinence, total
Incontinence, urge
Infant behavior, disorganized
Infant behavior, disorganized: risk for
Infant behavior, organized: potential for
  enhanced
Infant feeding pattern, ineffective
Infection, risk for
Injury, perioperative positioning: risk for
Injury, risk for
Knowledge deficit (specify)
Loneliness, risk for
Management of therapeutic regimen, commu-
  nity: ineffective
Management of therapeutic regimen, families:
  ineffective
Management of therapeutic regimen, individu-
  als: effective
Management of therapeutic regimen, individu-
  als: ineffective
Memory, impaired
Mobility, impaired physical
Noncompliance (specify)
Nutrition, altered: less than body require-
  ments
Nutrition, altered: more than body require-
  ments
Nutrition, altered: risk for more than body
  requirements
Oral mucous membrane, altered
Pain
Pain, chronic
Parent/Infant/Child attachment altered,
  risk for
Parental role conflict
Parenting, altered
Parenting, altered, risk for

Peripheral neurovascular dysfunction, risk for
Personal identity disturbance
Poisoning, risk for
Post-trauma response
Powerlessness
Protection, altered
Rape-trauma syndrome
Rape-trauma syndrome: compound reaction
Rape-trauma syndrome: silent reaction
Relocation stress syndrome
Role performance, altered
Self-care deficit, bathing/hygiene
Self-care deficit, dressing/grooming
Self-care deficit, feeding
Self-care deficit, toileting
Self-esteem disturbance
Self-esteem, chronic low
Self-esteem, situational low
Self-mutilation, risk for
Sensory/perceptual alterations (specify) (visual,
  auditory, kinesthetic, gustatory, tactile,
  olfactory)
Sexual dysfunction
Sexuality patterns, altered
Skin integrity, impaired
Skin integrity, impaired, risk for
Sleep pattern disturbance
Social interaction, impaired
Social isolation
Spiritual distress (distress of the human
  spirit)
Spiritual well-being, potential for enhanced
Suffocation, risk for
Swallowing, impaired
Thermoregulation, ineffective
Thought processes, altered
Tissue integrity, impaired
Tissue perfusion, altered (specify type) (renal,
  cerebral, cardiopulmonary, gastrointestinal,
  peripheral)
Tissue perfusion: coronary, decreased
Trauma, risk for
Unilateral neglect
Urinary elimination, altered
Urinary retention
Ventilation, inability to sustain spontaneous
Ventilatory weaning process, dysfunctional
Violence, risk for: self-directed or directed at
  others

*Includes those approved in 1992.

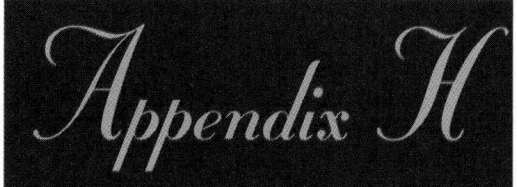

Which Face Shows How Much Hurt You Have Now?

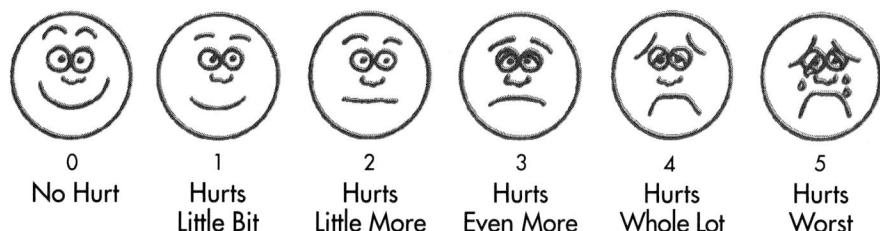

0	1	2	3	4	5
No Hurt	Hurts Little Bit	Hurts Little More	Hurts Even More	Hurts Whole Lot	Hurts Worst

Explain to the person that each face is for a person who feels happy because he has no pain (hurt) or sad because he has some or a lot of pain. **Face 0** is very happy because he doesn't hurt at all. **Face 1** hurts just a little bit. **Face 2** hurts a little more. **Face 3** hurts even more. **Face 4** hurts a whole lot. **Face 5** hurts as much as you can imagine, although you don't have to be crying to feel this bad. Ask the person to choose the face that best describes how he is feeling.

Rating scale is recommended for persons age 3 years and older.

*The *brief word instructions* under each face can also be used. Point to each face using the words to describe the pain intensity. Ask the child to choose face that best describes own pain and record the appropriate number. *Note:* In a study of 148 children ages 4 to 5 years, there were no differences in pain scores when children used the original or brief word instructions. (In Wong D, Baker C: Reference manual for the Wong-Baker FACES Pain Rating Scale, Duarte, CA, 1996, City of Hope Mayday Pain Resource Center.)

Spanish

Expliquele a la persona que cada cara representa una persona que se siente feliz porque no tiene dolor o triste porque siente un poco o mucho dolor. **Cara 0** se siente muy feliz porque no tiene dolor. **Cara 1** tiene un poco de dolor. **Cara 2** tiene un poquito más de dolor. **Cara 3** tiene más dolor. **Cara 4** tiene mucho dolor. **Cara 5** tiene el dolor más fuerte que usted pueda imaginar, aunque usted no tiene que estar llorando para sentirse asi de mal. Pidale a la persona que escoja la cara que mejor describe su proprio dolor.

Esta escala se puede usar con personas de tres años de edad o más.

French

Expliquez à la personne que chaque visage représent un personne qui est heureux parce qu'elle n'a pas point du mal ou triste parce qu'il a un peu ou beaucoup du mal. **Visage 0** est trés heureux parce qu'elle n'a pas point du mal. **Visage 1** a un petit peu de mal. **Visage 2** a plus du mal. **Visage 3** a encore plus du mal. **Visage 4** a beaucoup du mal. **Visage 5** a autant mal que vous pouvez imaginer, bien que ces mauvais sentiments ne finissent pas nécessairement a vous faire pleurer. Demandez à la personne de choisir le visage qui convient le mieux avec ses sentiments.

Ces evaluations sont recommendés pour des personnes de trois ans et davantage.

Wong-Baker FACES Pain Rating Scale: Available at no charge from The Purdue Frederick Company, 100 Connecticut Ave., Norwalk, CT 06850-3590; (203) 853-0123, ext. 7378. Spanish and Portuguese translations by Ellen Johnsen; French translation by Irene Sherman Liguori and Robert Marino; Italian translation by Madeline Mitchko and Ida DiPietropaolo; Romanian translation by Florin Nicolae; Vietnamese translation by Yen B. Isle; Chinese translation by Hung-Shen Lin; Japanese translation from *After the announcement of cancer*, Tokyo, 1993, Iwanami Shoten, Pub.

Italian

Spiegare a la persona che ogni facien è per una persona che si sente felice perchè non tiene dolore oppure triste perchè ha poco o molto dolore. **Faccia O** è molto felice perchè non tiene dolor. **Faccia 1** tiene poco dolore. **Faccia 2** tiene un po più di dolore. **Faccia 3** tiene più dolore. **Faccia 4** tiene molto dolore. **Faccia 5** tiene molto dolore che non puoi immaginare però non devi piangere per tenere dolore. Domandi ala persona di scegliere quale faccia meglio descrive come si sente.

Grado scale è raccomandata a la persona di tre anni in sù.

Portuguese

Explique a pessoa que cada face representa uma pessoa que está feliz porque não têm dor, ou triste por ter um pouco ou muita dor. **Face 0** está muito feliz porque não têm nenhuma dor. **Face 1** tem apenas um pouco de dor. **Face 2** têm um pouco mais de dor. **Face 3** têm ainda mais dor. **Face 4** têm muita dor. **Face 5** têm uma dor máxima, apesar de que nem sempre provoca o choro. Peça a pessoa que escolhe a face que melhor descreve como ele se sente.

Esta escala é aplicável a pessoas de tres anos de idade ou mais.

Romanian

Explică persoanei că fiecare faţă este specifică diferitelor stări fizice; o persoană este ferioita pentru că nu are nici o durere ori tristă pentru că suferă puţin sau mai mult. **Faţa 0** este foarte ferioită pentru că nu are absolut nici o durere. **Faţa 1** are un pic de durere. **Faţa 2** are ceva mai mult. **Faţa 3** suferă şi mai mult. **Faţa 4** suferă foarte mult. **Faţa 5** este greu de imaginat cât de mult suferă, căci nu trebuie neapărat să plângi, oricat de tare te-ar durea. Intreabă persoana să indice figura care-i desorie cel mai bine starea fizică.

Acest **grad de durere** este racomandat pentru persoanele de la 3 ani în sus.

Vietnamese

Xin cắt nghĩa cho mỗi người, từng khuôn mặt của một người cảm thấy vui vẽ tại vì không có sự đau đớn hoặc, buồn vì có chút ít hay rất nhiều sự đau đớn.

Cái **mặt** với **số 0** thì rất là vui tại vì mặt ấy không có sự đau đớn. **Mặt số 1** chỉ đau một chút thôi. **Mặt số 2** hơi đau hơn một chút nữa. **Mặt số 3** đau hơn chút nữa. **Mặt số 4** đau thật nhiều. **Mặt số 5** đau không thể tưởng tượng, mặc dù người ta không cần phải khóc mới cảm thấy được sự buồn khổ như thế.

Bạn hỏi từng người tự chọn khuôn mặt nào diễn tả được sự đau đớn của chính mình.

Japanese

3歳以上の患者に望ましい。それぞれの顔は、患者の痛み (pain, hurt) がないのでご機嫌な感じ、または、ある程度の痛み・沢山の痛みがあるので悲しい感じを表現していることを説明して下さい。0＝痛みがまったくないから、とても幸せな顔をしている、1＝ほんの少し痛い、2＝もう少し痛い、3＝もっと痛い、4＝とっても痛い、5＝痛くて涙を流す必要はないけれども、これ以上の痛みは考えられないほど痛い。今、どのように感じているか最もよく表わしている顔を選ぶよう、患者に求めて下さい。

Chinese

解釋給人聽用每張臉譜來代表著一個人的感覺是因爲沒有疼痛〔傷痛〕而感快樂或是因爲些許疼痛或者是許多疼痛而感傷心。第零張臉是很快樂的因爲他一點也不覺得疼痛。第一張臉只痛一丁點兒。第二張臉又痛多了一些。第三張臉痛得更多了。第四張臉是非常痛了。第五張臉是爲人們所能想像到的劇痛既使感到這樣難過，卻不一定哭出來。請這人選擇出最能代表他現在感覺的一張臉譜。此量表適用於三歲以上的人。

Index

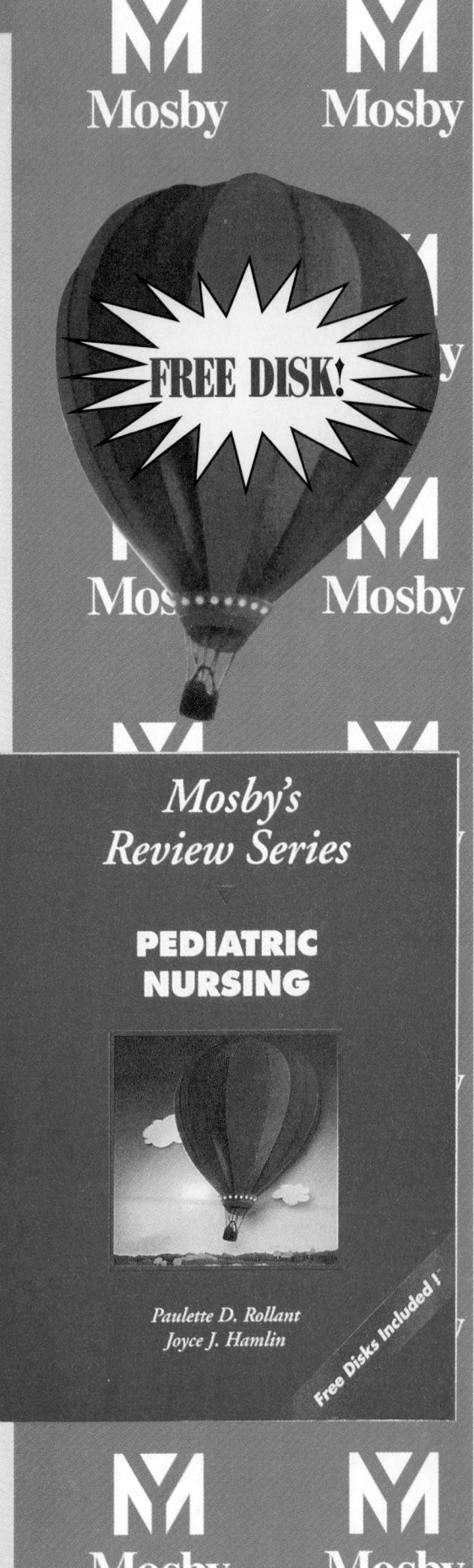

NORMAL HEART RATES FOR INFANTS AND CHILDREN

Age	Rate (beats/min)		
	Resting (awake)	Resting (sleeping)	Exercise (fever)
Newborn	100-180	80-160	Up to 220
1 week to 3 months	100-220	80-200	Up to 220
3 months to 2 years	80-150	70-120	Up to 200
2 years to 10 years	70-110	60-90	Up to 200
10 years to adult	55-90	50-90	Up to 200

From Gillette PC: Dysrhythmias. In Adams FH, Emmanouilides GC, Riemenschneider TA, editors: *Moss' heart disease in infants, children, and adolescents,* ed 4, Baltimore, 1989, Williams & Wilkins.

NORMAL RESPIRATORY RATES FOR CHILDREN

Age	Rate (breaths/min)
Newborn	35
1 to 11 months	30
2 years	25
4 years	23
6 years	21
8 years	20
10 years	19
12 years	19
14 years	18
16 years	17
18 years	16-18

NORMAL BLOOD PRESSURE READINGS FOR CHILDREN
BOYS

Age	Systolic blood pressure percentile					Age	Diastolic blood pressure* percentile				
	5th	10th	50th	90th	95th		5th	10th	50th	90th	95th
1 day	54	58	73	87	92	1 day	38	42	55	68	72
3 days	55	59	74	89	93	3 days	38	42	55	68	71
7 days	57	62	76	91	95	7 days	37	41	54	67	71
1 mo	67	71	86	101	105	1 mo	35	39	52	64	68
2 mo	72	76	91	106	110	2 mo	33	37	50	63	66
3 mo	72	76	91	106	110	3 mo	33	37	50	63	66
4 mo	72	76	91	106	110	4 mo	34	37	50	63	67
5 mo	72	76	91	105	110	5 mo	35	39	52	65	68
6 mo	72	76	90	105	109	6 mo	36	40	53	66	70
7 mo	71	76	90	105	109	7 mo	37	41	54	67	71
8 mo	71	75	90	105	109	8 mo	38	42	55	68	72
9 mo	71	75	90	105	109	9 mo	39	43	55	68	72
10 mo	71	75	90	105	109	10 mo	39	43	56	69	73
11 mo	71	76	90	105	109	11 mo	39	43	56	69	73
1 yr	71	76	90	105	109	1 yr	39	43	56	69	73
2 yr	72	76	91	106	110	2 yr	39	43	56	68	72
3 yr	73	77	92	107	111	3 yr	39	42	55	68	72
4 yr	74	79	93	108	112	4 yr	39	43	56	69	72
5 yr	76	80	95	109	113	5 yr	40	43	56	69	73
6 yr	77	81	96	111	115	6 yr	41	44	57	70	74
7 yr	78	83	97	112	116	7 yr	42	45	58	71	75
8 yr	80	84	99	114	118	8 yr	43	47	60	73	76
9 yr	82	86	101	115	120	9 yr	44	48	61	74	78
10 yr	84	88	102	117	121	10 yr	45	49	62	75	79
11 yr	86	90	105	119	123	11 yr	47	50	63	76	80
12 yr	88	92	107	121	126	12 yr	48	51	64	77	81
13 yr	90	94	109	124	128	13 yr	45	49	63	77	81
14 yr	93	97	112	126	131	14 yr	46	50	64	78	82
15 yr	95	99	114	129	133	15 yr	47	51	65	79	83
16 yr	98	102	117	131	136	16 yr	49	53	67	81	85
17 yr	100	104	119	134	138	17 yr	51	55	69	83	87
18 yr	102	106	121	136	140	18 yr	52	56	70	84	88

Reprinted with permission from the Second Task Force on Blood Pressure Control in Children, National Heart, Lung and Blood Institute, Bethesda, MD. Tabular data prepared by Dr. B. Rosner, 1987.
*K4 was used for ages less than 13; K5 was used for ages 13 and over.